HEMATOLOGY-ONCOLOGY THERAPY

SECOND EDITION

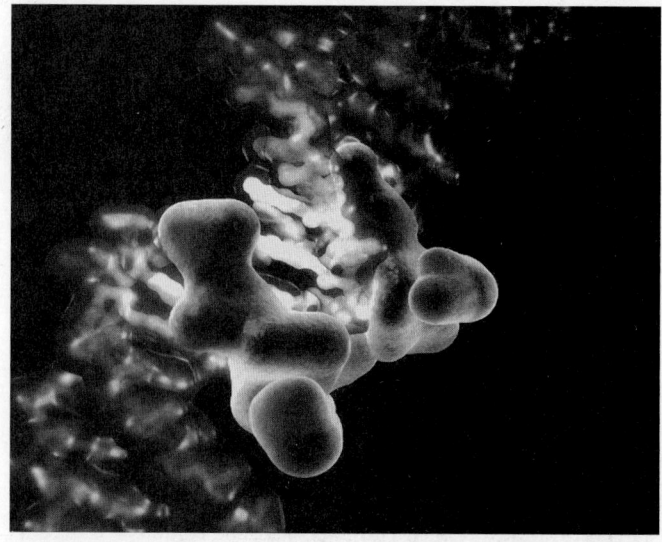

MICHAEL M. BOYIADZIS, MD, MHSc
Associate Professor of Medicine
Division of Hematology-Oncology
Department of Medicine
University of Pittsburgh School of Medicine
University of Pittsburgh Cancer Institute
Pittsburgh, Pennsylvania

JAMES N. FRAME, MD, FACP
Clinical Professor of Medicine
Robert C. Byrd Health Sciences Center
West Virginia University School of Medicine
Medical Director, David Lee Cancer Center
Charleston Area Medical Center Health Systems
Charleston, West Virginia

DAVID R. KOHLER, PharmD
Oncology Clinical Pharmacy Specialist
Bethesda, Maryland

TITO FOJO, MD, PhD
Senior Investigator
Medical Oncology
Center for Cancer Research
National Cancer Institute
National Institutes of Health
Bethesda, Maryland

McGraw Hill Education Medical

New York   Chicago   San Francisco   Athens   London   Madrid
Mexico City   Milan   New Delhi   Singapore   Sydney   Toronto

Hematology-Oncology Therapy, Second Edition

1 2 3 4 5 6 7 8 9 0   QVS/QVS   18 17 16 15 14 13

ISBN 978-0-07-163789-3
MHID 0-07-163789-3

Notice

Medicine is an ever-changing science. As new research and clinical experience broaden our knowledge, changes in treatment and drug therapy are required. The authors and the publisher of this work have checked with sources believed to be reliable in their efforts to provide information that is complete and generally in accord with the standards accepted at the time of publication. However, in view of the possibility of human error or changes in medical sciences, neither the authors nor the publisher nor any other party who has been involved in the preparation or publication of this work warrants that the information contained herein is in every respect accurate or complete, and they disclaim all responsibility for any errors or omissions or for the results obtained from use of the information contained in this work. Readers are encourage to confirm the information contained herein with other sources. For example and in particular, readers are advised to check product information sheet included in the package of each drug they plan to administer to be certain that the information contained in this work is accurate and that changes have not been made in the recommended dose or in the contraindications for administration. This recommendation is of particular importance in connection with new or infrequently used drugs.

This book was set in Centaur MT by Thomson Digital.
The editors were Jim Shanahan and Harriet Lebowitz.
The production supervisor was Richard Ruzycka.
The book designer was Eve Siegel.
Project management was provided by Ritu Joon, Thomson Digital.
Cover Designer: Anthony Landi
Image Credit: © XVIVO LLC / Phototake
The cover illustration is a gene bound by a molecule of estrogen in the nucleus of an estrogen-sensitive breast cancer cell.
Quad Graphics/Versailles was printer and binder.

Library of Congress Cataloging-in-Publication Data

Hematology-oncology therapy / [edited by] Michael M. Boyiadzis, James N. Frame, David R. Kohler, Tito Fojo.—Second edition.
    p. ; cm.
Includes index.
Preceded by Hematology-oncology therapy / Michael M. Boyiadzis . . . [et al.]. c2007.
ISBN 978-0-07-163789-3 (softcover)—ISBN 0-07-163789-3 (softcover)
I. Boyiadzis, Michael M., editor. II. Frame, James N., editor. III. Kohler, David R., editor. IV. Fojo, Antonio Tito, 1952- editor.
[DNLM: 1. Neoplasms—therapy. 2. Drug Therapy, Combination—methods. 3. Hematologic Diseases. QZ 266]
RC270.8
616.99'406—dc23
                                                        2014014802

To the patients our profession has the privilege to serve, and to our colleagues whose compassionate care and research efforts continue to extend the spectrum of hope.

Contents

Authors

Nadine Abi-Jaoudeh, MD
Physician, Assistant Professor
Radiology & Imaging Sciences
National Institutes of Health
Bethesda, Maryland
Hepatocellular Carcinoma

Ivan Aksentijevich, MD
Virginia Cancer Specialists
Specialist in Medical Oncology and Hematology
Alexandria, Virginia
Leukemia, Acute Lymphoblastic (ADULT); Leukemia, Acute Myeloid

Carmen Joseph Allegra, MD
Professor and Chief Hematology and Oncology
Department of Medicine
University of Florida Health
Gainesville, Florida
Colorectal Cancer

Kenneth C. Anderson, MD
Professor of Medicine, Department of Medicine,
Harvard Medical School
Physician, Oncology, Brigham and Women's Hospital
Medical Director, Kraft Family Blood Center,
Dana-Farber Cancer Institute
Boston, Massachusetts
Multiple Myeloma

Andrea Apolo, MD
Head, Bladder Cancer Section
Genitourinary Malignancies Branch
Center for Cancer Research, National Cancer Institute
National Institutes of Health
Bethesda, Maryland
Bladder Cancer

Dean Bajorin, MD
Member and Professor of Medicine
Genitourinary Oncology Service
Memorial Sloan-Kettering Cancer Center
New York, New York
Bladder Cancer

John R. Bartholomew, MD, FACC, MSVM
Professor of Medicine and
Section Head of Vascular Medicine
Cardiovascular Medicine and Hematology
Cleveland Clinic
Cleveland, Ohio
Heparin-Induced Thrombocytopenia

James C. Barton, MD
Medical Director, Southern Iron Disorders Center
Clinical Professor of Medicine
University of Alabama at Birmingham
Birmingham, Alabama
Hemochromatosis

Susan Bates, MD
Senior Investigator
Head, Molecular Therapeutics Section
Medical Oncology
National Cancer Institute, National Institutes of Health
Bethesda, Maryland
Renal Cell Cancer

Kenneth A. Bauer, MD
Professor of Medicine, Harvard Medical School
Director, Thrombosis Clinical Research,
Beth Israel Deaconess Medical Center
Boston, Massachusetts
The Hypercoagulable State

Ann Berger, MSN, MD
Chief, Pain and Palliative Care Service
National Institutes of Health Clinical Center
Bethesda, Maryland
Cancer Pain: Assessment and Management

Giada Bianchi, MD
Department of Medical Oncology
Dana Farber Cancer Institute
Harvard Medical School
Boston, Massachusetts
Multiple Myeloma

Michael R. Bishop, MD
Professor of Medicine
Director, Hematopoietic Stem Cell Transplantation Program
The University of Chicago Medicine
Chicago, Illinois
Complications and Follow-Up After Hematopoietic Cell Transplantation

Jean-Yves Blay, MD
Professor of Medicine in Medical Oncology
Head of the Medical Oncology Department
Centre Leon Berard of the Université Claude Bernard
Scientific Director, Canceropole Lyon Rhône Alpes
Lyon, France
Sarcomas

George J. Bosl, MD
Chair, Department of Medicine, and
Member, Memorial Sloan Kettering Cancer Center
Professor of Medicine, Weill Cornell Medical College
Testicular Cancer

Leslie Boyd, MD
Assistant Professor of Gynecology
Perlmutter Cancer Center
NYU Langone Medical Center
New York, New York
Vaginal Cancer

Michael M. Boyiadzis, MD, MHSc
Associate Professor of Medicine
Division of Hematology-Oncology
Department of Medicine
University of Pittsburgh School of Medicine
University of Pittsburgh Cancer Institute
Pittsburgh, Pennsylvania
*Leukemia, Acute Lymphoblastic (ADULT); Leukemia, Acute Myeloid;
Complications and Follow-Up After Hematopoietic Cell Transplantation;
Aplastic Anemia; Myelodysplastic Syndromes*

Kathleen A. Calzone, PhD, RN, APNG, FAAN
Senior Nurse Specialist, Research
National Cancer Institute
Center for Cancer Research, Genetics Branch
Bethesda, Maryland
Cancer Screening; Genetics of Common Inherited Cancer Syndromes

Carla Casulo, MD
Assistant Professor of Medicine
University of Rochester Medical Center at Strong Memorial Hospital
Rochester, New York
Lymphoma, Non-Hodgkin

Julia Lee Close, MD
Assistant Professor, University of Florida
Section Chief, Hematology/Oncology,
Gainesville VA Medical Center
Gainesville, Florida
Colorectal Cancer

Jennifer Cuellar-Rodriguez, MD
Staff Clinician
Laboratory of Clinical Infectious Diseases
National Institute of Allergy and Infectious Diseases
Bethesda, Maryland
Fever and Neutropenia

William L. Dahut, MD
Principal Investigator
Medical Oncology
Genitourinary Malignancies Branch
Center for Cancer Research
National Cancer Institute, National Institutes of Health
Bethesda, Maryland
Prostate Cancer

Nancy E. Davidson, MD
Director, University of Pittsburgh Cancer Institute
UPMC Cancer Center
Associate Vice Chancellor for Cancer Research
Professor of Medicine, University of Pittsburgh
Pittsburgh, Pennsylvania
Breast Cancer

Michael W.N. Deininger, MD, PhD
Chief, Division of Hematology and Hematologic Malignancies
M.M. Wintrobe Professor of Medicine
University of Utah
Huntsman Cancer Institute
Salt Lake City, Utah
Leukemia, Chronic Myelogenous

Bruce J. Dezube, MD
Associate Professor of Medicine
Beth Israel Deaconess Medical Center
Harvard Medical School
Boston, Massachusetts
HIV-Related Malignancies

Volker Diehl, MD
Emeritus Professor of Medicine, Hematology, Oncology
University of Cologne
Germany
Lymphoma, Hodgkin

Brian J. Druker, MD
Director, Oregon Health & Science University Knight Cancer Institute
JELD-WEN Chair of Leukemia Research
Investigator, Howard Hughes Medical Institute
Portland, Oregon
Leukemia, Chronic Myelogenous

Dennis A. Eichenauer, MD
First Department of Internal Medicine and German
Hodgkin Study Group
University Hospital Cologne
Cologne, Germany
Lymphoma, Hodgkin

Sara Ekeblad, MD, PhD
Uppsala University Hospital
Stockholm, Sweden
Pancreatic Endocrine Tumors

Jennifer Eng-Wong, MD, MPH
Assistant Medical Director
Genentech
South San Francisco, California
Cancer Screening

Jonas W. Feilchenfeldt, MD
Attending Physician
FMH Internal Medicine and Medical Oncology
Department of Medical Oncology
Hôpital du Valais
Sion, Switzerland
Gastric Cancer

Darren R. Feldman, MD
Assistant Member, Department of Medicine
Memorial Sloan Kettering Cancer Center, and
Assistant Professor in Medicine, Weill Cornell Medical College
New York, New York
Testicular Cancer

Enriqueta Felip, MD, PhD
Department of Medical Oncology
Vall d'Hebron University Hospital
Barcelona, Spain
Lung Cancer

Howard Fine, MD
Director, Division of Hematology and Oncology
Director, NYU Brain Tumor Center
Deputy Director, NYU Cancer Institute
Director, Bellevue Hospital Cancer Center
The New York University (NYU) Langone Medical Center
NYU Cancer Institute
New York, New York
Brain Cancer

Richard Fisher, MD
President and CEO
Fox Chase Cancer Center - Temple Health
Senior Associate Dean
Temple University School of Medicine
Philadelphia, Pennsylvania
Lymphoma, Non-Hodgkin

Tito Fojo, MD, PhD
Senior Investigator
Medical Oncology
Center for Cancer Research
National Cancer Institute
National Institutes of Health
Bethesda, Maryland
Adrenocortical Cancer; Pheochromocytoma; Sarcomas; Guidelines for Chemotherapy Dosage Adjustment; Oncologic Emergencies

Kenneth Foon, MD
Vice President, Global Medical Affairs, Lymphoma and CLL
Medical Affairs
Celgene Corporation
Summit, New Jersey
Leukemia, Chronic Lymphocytic

James N. Frame, MD, FACP
Clinical Professor of Medicine
Robert C. Byrd Health Sciences Center
West Virginia University School of Medicine
Medical Director, David Lee Cancer Center
Charleston Area Medical Center Health Systems
Charleston, West Virginia
Indications for Growth Factors in Hematology-Oncology; Indications for Bone-Modifying Agents in Hematology-Oncology; Heparin-Induced Thrombocytopenia; Autoimmune Hemolytic Anemia; Sickle Cell Disease: Acute Complications

Jonathan W. Friedberg, MD, MMSc
Director, James P. Wilmot Cancer Center
Samuel Durand Professor of Medicine and Oncology
University of Rochester
Rochester, New York
Lymphoma, Non-Hodgkin

Michael Fuchs, MD
Head of the Trial Coordination Center German Hodgkin Study Group
Department of Internal Medicine
University Hospital of Cologne
Cologne, Germany
Lymphoma, Hodgkin

Naseema Gangat, MD
Assistant Professor of Medicine
Division of Hematology
Mayo Clinic
Rochester, Minnesota
Myeloproliferative Neoplasms

Juan C. Gea-Banacloche, MD
Chief, Infectious Diseases Consultation Service
Experimental Transplantation and Immunology Branch
National Cancer Institute, National Institute of Health
Bethesda, Maryland
Fever and Neutropenia; Complications and Follow-Up After Hematopoietic Cell Transplantation

James N. George, MD
George Lynn Cross Professor
Departments of Medicine, Biostatistics & Epidemiology
University of Oklahoma Health Sciences Center
Oklahoma City, Oklahoma
Thrombotic Thrombocytopenic Purpura/Hemolytic Uremic Syndrome; Idiopathic Thrombocytopenic Purpura

Irene M. Ghobrial, MD
Associate Professor of Medicine
Dana-Farber Cancer Institute
Harvard Medical School
Boston, Massachusetts
Multiple Myeloma

Giuseppe Giaccone, MD, PhD
Associate Director for Clinical Research
Georgetown Lombardi Comprehensive Cancer Center
Director of Clinical Research, MedStar Georgetown Health Cancer Network's Washington Region
Georgetown University Medical Center
Washington, DC
Thymic Malignancies

Amanda L. Gillespie-Twardy, MD
University of Pittsburgh School of Medicine
Pittsburgh, Pennsylvania
Melanoma

Eli Glatstein, MD
Professor, Department of Radiation Oncology
University of Pennsylvania
Philadelphia, Pennsylvania
Radiation Complications

Ann Gramza, MD
Staff Clinician
Center for Cancer Research
National Cancer Institute, NIH
Bethesda, Maryland
Thyroid Cancer

F. Anthony Greco, MD
Clinical Researcher and Director
Sarah Cannon Research Institute
Nashville, Tennessee
Carcinoma of Unknown Primary

Tim Greten, MD, PhD
Senior Investigator
Gastrointestinal Malignancy Section
Center for Cancer Research
National Cancer Institute
Bethesda, Maryland
Biliary: Gallbladder Cancer and Cholangiocarcinoma; Hepatocellular Carcinoma

Thomas E. Hughes, PharmD, BCOP
Oncology Clinical Pharmacy Specialist
Pharmacy Department
National Institutes of Health Clinical Center
Bethesda, Maryland
Prophylaxis and Treatment of Chemotherapy-Induced Nausea and Vomiting

Jimmy Hwang, MD
Chief, GI Medical Oncology
Levine Cancer Institute
Carolinas Healthcare System
Charlotte, North Carolina
Esophageal Cancer

Rachel C. Jankowitz, MD
Assistant Professor of Medicine
University of Pittsburgh Cancer Institute
UPMC Magee Women's Cancer Program
Pittsburgh, Pennsylvania
Breast Cancer

Irfan Jawed, MD
Medical Oncologist/Pain Medicine/Hospice & Palliative Care
Lawrence Memorial Hospital Oncology Center
Lawrence, Kansas
Anal Cancer

Steven J. Jubelilirer, MD
Clinical Professor of Medicine
West Virginia University-Charleston
Division Director, CAMC Hemophilia Treatment Center
Charleston Area Medical Center
Charleston, West Virginia
Hemophilia

Judith Karp, MD
Professor of Oncology and Medicine
John Hopkins University School of Medicine
Baltimore, Maryland
Leukemia, Acute Lymphoblastic (ADULT); Leukemia, Acute Myeloid

Lyndon Kim, MD
Division of Neuro-Oncology
Department of Neurological Surgery
Department of Medical Oncology
Thomas Jefferson University Hospital
Philadelphia, Pennsylvania
Brain Cancer

John M. Kirkwood, MD
Usher Professor of Medicine, Dermatology and Translational Science
Co-Director, Melanoma and Skin Cancer Program
University of Pittsburgh Cancer Institute
Pittsburgh, Pennsylvania
Melanoma

Joseph E. Kiss, MD
Associate Professor of Medicine
Department of Medicine
Division of Hematology/Oncology
Medical Director, Hemapheresis and Blood Services
University of Pittsburgh
Pittsburgh, Pennsylvania
Transfusion Therapy

David R. Kohler, PharmD
Oncology Clinical Pharmacy Specialist
Bethesda, Maryland
*Drug Preparation and Administration;
Antineoplastic Drugs: Preventing and Managing Extravasation*

Kiarash Kojouri, MD, MPH
Skagit Valley Hospital Regional Cancer Care Center
Seattle Cancer Care Alliance
Hematologist-Oncologist
Skagit Valley Hospital Regional Cancer Care Clinic
Mount Vernon, Washington
*Thrombotic Thrombocytopenic Purpura/Hemolytic Uremic Syndrome;
Idiopathic Thrombocytopenic Purpura*

Patricia Kropf, MD
Assistant Professor of Medicine
Fox Chase Cancer Center
Temple Health
Philadelphia, Pennsylvania
Leukemia, Chronic Lymphocytic

Peter F. Lebowitz, MD, PhD
Global Head of Oncology Research and Development
Janssen, Pharmaceutical Companies of Johnson & Johnson
Spring House, Pennsylvania
Adrenocortical Cancer

John R. Lurain, MD
Marcia Stenn Professor of Gynecologic Oncology
Gynecologic Oncology Fellowship Program Director
Northwestern University, Feinberg School of Medicine
Chicago, Illinois
Gestational Trophoblastic Neoplasia

Pier M. Mannucci, MD
Professor
Scientific Direction
IRCCS Ca' Granda Maggiore Policlinico Hospital Foundation
Milano, Italy
von Willebrand Disease

Maurie Markman, MD
Senior Vice President for Clinical Affairs
Cancer Treatment Centers of America
Clinical Professor of Medicine
Drexel University of College of Medicine
Philadelphia, Pennsylvania
Endometrial Cancer

John Marshall, MD
Director, The Ruesch Center for the Cure of GI Cancers
Chief, Hematology and Oncology
Lombardi Comprehensive Cancer Center
Georgetown University Medical Center
Washington, DC
Anal Cancer; Esophageal Cancer

Pamela W. McDevitt, PharmD, BCOP
Oncology Clinical Pharmacy Specialist
David Lee Cancer Center
Charleston, West Virginia
*Guidelines for Chemotherapy Dosage Adjustment;
Indications for Growth Factors in Hematology-Oncology*

Franco Muggia, MD
Professor of Medicine (Oncology)
Perlmutter Cancer Center
NYU Langone Medical Center
New York, New York
Vaginal Cancer

Ashok Nambiar, MD
Health Science Associate Clinical Professor
Department of Laboratory Medicine
Director, Transfusion Medicine
Director, Moffitt-Long & Mt. Zion Hospital Tissue Banks
UCSF Medical Center
University of California, San Francisco
San Francisco, California
Transfusion Therapy

Naomi P. O'Grady, MD
Medical Director, Procedures, Vascular Access,
and Conscious Sedation Services
Department of Critical Care Medicine
National Institutes of Health
Bethesda, Maryland
Catheter-Related Bloodstream Infections: Management and Prevention

Karel Pacak, MD, PhD, DSc
Senior Investigator
Chief, Section on Medical Neuroendocrinology
Eunice Kennedy Shriver NICHD, National Institutes of Health
Bethesda, Maryland
Pheochromocytoma

Mauricio Burotto Pichun, MD
Medical Oncology
Center for Cancer Research
National Cancer Institute, National Institutes of Health
Bethesda, Maryland
Oncologic Emergencies

Sheila Prindiville, MD, MPH
Director, Coordinating Center for Clinical Trials
National Cancer Institute
Bethesda, Maryland
Cancer Screening; Genetics of Common Inherited Cancer Syndromes

Margaret Ragni, MD, MPH
Professor of Medicine and Clinical Translational Science
Department of Medicine
Division of Hematology-Oncology
University of Pittsburgh
Director, Hemophilia Center of Western Pennsylvania
Pittsburgh, Pennsylvania
Hemophilia

Arun Rajan, MD
Staff Clinician
Center for Cancer Research
National Cancer Institute, National Institutes of Health
Bethesda, Maryland
Thymic Malignancies

Ramesh K. Ramanathan, MD, PhD, Sc
Virginia G. Piper Cancer Center - Clinical Trials
Scottsdale Health Care
Scottsdale, Arizona
Clinical Professor of Medicine, Translational Genomics Research
Institute and College of Medicine
University of Arizona
Phoenix, Arizona
Pancreatic Cancer

Eddie Reed, MD
Clinical Director
National Institute on Minority Health and Health Disparities
National Institutes of Health
Bethesda, Maryland
Ovarian Cancer

Ramesh Rengan, MD, PhD
Associate Professor
Associate Member, Fred Hutchinson Cancer Research Center
Medical Director, SCCA Proton Therapy
Department of Radiation Oncology
University of Washington
Radiation Complications

Olivier Rixe, MD, PhD
Professor of Medicine
Director, Experimental Therapeutics Program
Leader, Neuro-Oncology Program
Georgia Regents University Cancer Center
Augusta, Georgia
Renal Cell Cancer

Aldo Roccaro, MD, PhD
Dana Farber Cancer Institute
Harvard Medical School
Boston, Massachusetts
Multiple Myeloma

Griffin P. Rodgers, MD, MACP
Chief, Molecular and Clinical Hematology Branch
National Heart, Lung and Blood Institute
Director, National Institute of Diabetes,
Digestive and Kidney Diseases
National Institutes of Health
Bethesda, Maryland
Sickle Cell Disease: Acute Complications

Peter G. Rose, MD
Section Head Gynecologic Oncology
Cleveland Clinic Foundation
Tenured Professor of Surgery, Oncology and Reproductive Biology
Case Western Reserve University
Cleveland, Ohio
Cervical Cancer

Rafael Rosell, MD
Director, Cancer Biology and Precision Medicine Program
Catalan Institute of Oncology,
Hospital Germans Trias i Pujol, Badalona
Pangaea Biotech, Quirón-Dexeus University Hospital
Barcelona, Spain
Lung Cancer

Julia Schaefer-Cutillo, MD
Medical Oncologist
Hudson Valley Hematology Oncology
Poughkeepsie, New York
Lymphoma, Non-Hodgkin

Werner Scheithauer, MD
Professor
Department of Internal Medicine I
Division of Oncology
Vienna University Medical School, Vienna University Hospital
Vienna, Austria
Biliary: Gallbladder Cancer and Cholangiocarcinoma

Lee S. Schwartzberg, MD, FACP
Chief, Division of Hematology Oncology
Professor of Medicine
The University of Tennessee Health Science Center
Memphis, Tennessee
Indications for Growth Factors in Hematology-Oncology

Avni Shah, MD
Medical Oncologist
Genitourinary Malignancies Branch
Center for Cancer Research
National Cancer Institute, National Institutes of Health
Bethesda, Maryland
Prostate Cancer

Manish A. Shah, MD
Associate Professor of Medicine
Director, Gastrointestinal Oncology
Weill Cornell Medical College of Cornell University
New York-Presbyterian
New York, New York
Gastric Cancer

Reem Abozena Shalabi, PharmD, BCOP
Clinical Pharmacy Specialist
Blood and Marrow Transplantation
National Institutes of Health
Bethesda, Maryland
Indications for Bone-Modifying Agents in Hematology-Oncology

Britt Skogseid, MD, PhD
Professor of Endocrine Tumorbiology
Department of Endocrine Oncology
Uppsala University Hospital
Uppsala, Sweden
Pancreatic Endocrine Tumors

Roy E. Smith, MD, MS
Professor of Medicine
Division of Hematology/Oncology
University of Pittsburgh Cancer Institute
Pittsburgh, Pennsylvania
Venous Catheter-Related Thrombosis

Pol Specenier, MD, PhD
Antwerp University Hospital
Edegem, Belgium
Head and Neck Cancers

David R. Spigel, MD
Director, Lung Cancer Research Program
Sarah Cannon Research Institute
Nashville, Tennessee
Carcinoma of Unknown Primary

Diana C. Stripp, MD
Assistant Professor
Department of Radiation Oncology
University of Pennsylvania
Hospital of University of Pennsylvania
Philadelphia, Pennsylvania
Radiation Complications

Martin S. Tallman, MD
Chief of the Leukemia Service
Department of Medicine
Memorial Sloan Kettering Cancer Center
Professor of Medicine
Weill Cornell Medical College
New York, New York
Leukemia, Hairy Cell

Ahmad A. Tarhini, MD, PhD
Associate Professor of Medicine, Clinical and Translational Science
Department of Medicine
Division of Hematology/Oncology
University of Pittsburgh
Pittsburgh, Pennsylvania
Melanoma

Ayalew Tefferi, MD
Professor of Medicine
Division of Hematology
Mayo Clinic
Rochester, Minnesota
Myeloproliferative Neoplasms

Arafat Tfayli, MD
Associate Professor of Clinical Medicine
NK Basile Cancer Institute
American University of Beirut Medical Center
Beirut, Lebanon
Thrombotic Thrombocytopenic Purpura/Hemolytic Uremic Syndrome;
Idiopathic Thrombocytopenic Purpura

Anish Thomas, MD
Thoracic and Gastrointestinal Oncology Branch
National Cancer Institute, National Institutes of Health
Bethesda, Maryland
Mesothelioma

Susanna Ulahannan, MD
Center for Cancer Research
National Cancer Institute, National Institutes of Health
Bethesda, Maryland
Biliary: Gallbladder Cancer and Cholangiocarcinoma

Verna Vanderpuye, MD
Radiotherapy Consultant
National Centre of Radiotherapy and Nuclear Medicine
Korle Bu Teaching Hospital
Accra, Ghana
Mesothelioma

JB Vermorken, MD, PhD
Emeritus Professor of Oncology
Department of Medical Oncology
Antwerp University Hospital
Antwerp, Belgium
Head and Neck Cancers

Daniel D. Von Hoff, MD, FACP
Physician in Chief, Distinguished Professor
Translational Genomics Research Institute
Professor of Medicine, Mayo Clinic
Chief Scientific Officer, Scottsdale Healthcare
Medical Director of Research and Scientific Medical Officer,
US Oncology Research
Senior Investigator
Clinical Professor of Medicine
Translational Genomics Research Institute
University of Arizona Cancer Center
Phoenix, Arizona
Pancreatic Cancer

Nicholas J. Vogelzang, MD
Medical Oncologist
U.S. Oncology
Comprehensive Cancer Centers of Nevada
Las Vegas, Nevada
Mesothelioma

Charles F. von Gunten, MD, PhD
Vice President, Medical Affairs
Hospice and Palliative Medicine for OhioHealth
Columbus, Ohio
Hospice Care and End-of-Life Issues

David E. Weissman, MD
Director of the Palliative Care Center
Professor of Medicine
Division of Hematology and Oncology
Medical College of Wisconsin
Milwaukee, Wisconsin
Hospice Care and End-of-Life Issues

Sam Wells, MD
Center for Cancer Research
National Cancer Institute, National Institutes of Health
Bethesda, Maryland
Thyroid Cancer

Brigitte Widemann, MD
Senior Investigator
Pediatric Oncology Branch
Center for Cancer research
National Cancer Institute, National Institutes of Health
Bethesda, Maryland
Sarcomas

Neal S. Young, MD
Chief, Hematology Branch
National Heart, Lung, and Blood Institute,
National Institutes of Health
Bethesda, Maryland
Aplastic Anemia; Myelodysplastic Syndromes

Wenhui Zhu, MD, PhD
Seidman Cancer Center
Southwest General Hospital
Middleburg Heights, Ohio
Prostate Cancer

Jeffrey I. Zwicker, MD
Assistant Professor of Medicine
Division of Hematology-Oncology
Beth Israel Deaconess Medical Center, Harvard Medical School
Boston, Massachusetts
The Hypercoagulable State

Preface

The practical need for a readily accessible, up-to-date, comprehensive therapy resource, supported by referenced literature, was the original inspiration of the first edition of *Hematology-Oncology Therapy*. The book received considerable acclaim and filled a void in the medical literature as a practical guide and reference for practicing oncologists and hematologists. The rapid and numerous advances in the field of hematology-oncology are reflected in the updated information of this second edition. Over 500 treatment regimens are presented in a concise and uniform format that includes oncologic disorders, non-neoplastic hematologic disorders, and supportive care.

The three sections of *Hematology-Oncology Therapy* are:

I.   Oncology
II. Supportive Care, Drug Preparation, Complications, and Screening
III. Selected Hematologic Diseases.

Section I provides detailed information about the administration, supportive care, toxicity, dose modification, monitoring, and efficacy of commonly used and recently approved chemotherapeutic regimens, drugs, and biological agents. Each chapter is focused on a specific cancer, and contains information about epidemiology, pathology, work-up, and staging, as well as survival data. In addition, each chapter has a new feature, Expert Opinion, in which experts in the field provide treatment recommendations and guidance on the use of the included regimens.

Section II consists of topics commonly encountered in clinical hematology-oncology practice. Section III provides an authoritative guide to therapy for principal diseases in consultative hematology.

Hematology-Oncology Therapy integrates extensive information that is critical to both office- and hospital-based clinical practice of hematology and oncology. This comprehensive approach makes the book invaluable to all practitioners involved in the care of patients with cancer or hematologic diseases and complements other excellent book references in hematology-oncology.

We wish to express our appreciation to the many contributors to this book, whose expert knowledge in their fields makes *Hematology-Oncology Therapy* a unique addition to the medical literature. They helped us compile the extensive and detailed therapy information contained in this book, which is a testament to the efforts of so many to improve the treatment of patients with oncologic and hematologic diseases. We also wish to thank our editors at McGraw-Hill for their continued support, patience, and faith in our vision and concept for this book. Their professional support has earned our praise and debt of gratitude. Finally, we would like to thank those with whom we work and those we love for their support during the writing and editing of the second edition.

Michael M. Boyiadzis, MD, MHSc
James N. Frame, MD, FACP
David R. Kohler, PharmD
Tito Fojo, MD, PhD

SECTION I. Oncology

(Continued on following page)

(Continued on following page)

1. Adrenocortical Cancer

Peter F. Lebowitz, MD, PhD and Tito Fojo, MD, PhD

Epidemiology

Incidence: 0.5 to 2.0 cases per one million population
Deaths: 0.2% of cancer deaths
Median age: Bimodal median, at age 4 years and ages 40–50 years
Male to female ratio: 1:1.3

Cohn K et al. Surgery 1986;100:1170–1177
Wooten MD, King DK. Cancer 1993;72:3145–3155

Stage at Presentation
Stage I: 3%
Stage II: 29%
Stage III: 19%
Stage IV: 49%

Pathology

1. Unlike renal cell carcinoma, adrenocortical cancer stains positive for vimentin
2. >20 mitoses per HPF—median survival 14 months

    ≤20 mitoses per HPF—median survival 58 months
3. Tumor necrosis—poor prognosis
4. Vascular invasion—poor prognosis
5. Capsular invasion—poor prognosis

Weiss LM et al. Am J Surg Pathol 1989;13:202–206

Survival After Complete Resection

5-Year Actuarial Survival	
Stages I–II	54%
Stage III	24%
1-Year survival	
Stage IV	9%

Icard P et al. Surgery 1992;112:972–980; discussion 979–980
Icard P et al. World J Surg 1992;16:753–758

Work-up

1. CT scan of chest, abdomen, and pelvis to determine extent of disease
2. MRI of abdomen may help to identify and follow liver metastases
3. If IVC is compressed, consider IVC contrast study, ultrasound, or MRI to assess disease involvement before surgical exploration, although apparent extent of involvement should not deter exploration
4. Serum and 24-hour urinary cortisol; 24-hour urinary 17-ketosteroid
5. Additional studies can be performed to determine the functional status of the tumor including: serum estradiol, estrone, testosterone, dehydroepiandrosterone sulfate (S-DHAS), 17-OH-progesterone, and androstenedione

Staging

Stage I	<5-cm tumor confined to adrenal
Stage II	>5-cm tumor confined to adrenal
Stage III	Positive lymph nodes or local invasion with tumor outside adrenal in fat or adjacent organs
Stage IV	Distant metastasis

Macfarlane DA. Ann R Coll Surg Engl 1958;23:155–186
Sullivan M et al. J Urol 1978;120:660–665

Expert Opinion

1. *Primary therapy:* Primary therapy is complete surgical resection

2. *Surgery and Radio Frequency Ablation (RFA) as therapies for recurrences:* When possible, local recurrences should be addressed surgically. Some advocate surgical resection of metastatic disease, and although it may improve survival, firm evidence is lacking. Radio frequency ablation may be used as an alternative if the recurrence is deemed amenable to ablation and has an expendable margin. Just as incomplete resections should not be embarked on, neither should incomplete ablations be performed

3. *Management of excess hormone production:* Excess hormone production should not be ignored. Manage severe hypercortisolism aggressively. Because chemotherapy is usually ineffective, treatment of hormonal excess should not be delayed in expectation that chemotherapy will reduce the tumor burden and improve symptoms. Instead, use steroidogenesis inhibitors either singly or in combination. **Mitotane** is the cornerstone of any strategy and should be started as soon as a diagnosis has been made. Use mitotane at the highest tolerable dose. However, because a therapeutic mitotane level and steady state will not be reached for several months, other agents must be initiated concurrently. In patients with LFT results not more than 3 times normal range, begin therapy with **ketoconazole**, mindful of the potential for a pharmacokinetic interaction with other drugs. If LFTs are elevated, if an aggressive ketoconazole dose escalation is unsuccessful in controlling symptoms, or if toxicity develops, use **metyrapone***, either alone or in combination with ketoconazole. Cortisol levels must be monitored frequently to adjust steroidogenesis inhibitor drug doses and to avoid adrenal insufficiency, which occurs infrequently in patients with cortisol-producing tumors. Should adrenal insufficiency occur, hydrocortisone and mineralocorticoid replacement should be instituted as indicated below
   - *Mitotane:* Refer to section describing mitotane as a regimen for ACC
   - *Ketoconazole:* In patients with ACC and frank Cushing syndrome, treatment can start with 200 mg/dose given 3 or 4 times per day. The dose can then be increased by 400 mg/day every few days to a maximum single doses of 1200–1600 mg administered 3 or 4 doses per day (ie, total daily doses = 3600–6400 mg) while monitoring liver function. Because ketoconazole requires stomach acidity for absorption, proton pump inhibitors should be avoided, and achlorhydria should be suspected in elderly individuals who do not respond to therapy
   - *Metyrapone*:* Metyrapone is begun at a low dose of 500–1000 mg (250–500 mg 2–4 times daily) and is escalated every few days to the maximum daily dose. The dose needed to inhibit cortisol production ranges from 500–6000 mg/day, although little is gained with total daily doses greater than 2000 mg

4. *Chemotherapy for unresectable, advanced, and recurrent disease:* Chemotherapy is recommended for patients with metastatic disease, although evidence of survival benefit is not and will never be available. EDP (etoposide + doxorubicin + cisplatin) plus mitotane or streptozocin plus mitotane should be used as first-line therapy. "Novel targeted therapies" that may seem attractive have not been proved and should not be substituted for these chemotherapies that have known activity in ACC

5. *Adjuvant mitotane:* A recent analysis of 177 patients with ACC compared the outcome in 47 patients treated with adjuvant mitotane therapy with 130 patients who received no additional therapy (Terzolo et al., 2007). Surprisingly, when used at "more tolerable" daily doses of 2000–3000 mg, the authors reported that mitotane demonstrated significant benefit in the adjuvant setting. However, the results of this retrospective nonrandomized study must be viewed cautiously. Because the advantage was confined to time to recurrence and not to overall survival, the value of adjuvant mitotane is diminished. Furthermore, the short follow-up period of patients treated with mitotane leaves the conclusions in doubt. The lack of convincing evidence and the difficulty of administering mitotane has often guided a recommendation that "adjuvant" mitotane therapy should be used only in cases where a tumor cannot be fully removed surgically or in patients with a high likelihood of recurrence; that is, large tumors with extensive necrosis, capsular, lymphatic, or venous invasion, a high mitotic or Ki67 labeling index, and small or questionable surgical margins. Until further data are available, this continues to be the most reasonable approach

6. *Long-term mitotane monotherapy:* Administer mitotane long-term only to patients who tolerate it well and experience a therapeutic response or those who are at high-risk for recurrence. The optimal duration of therapy is not known: a recommendation of "indefinite" is most conservative. *Prolonged therapy is often made possible by the fact that after months of therapy body stores are finally saturated, and the dose needed to maintain serum levels is then markedly reduced.* In this case the tolerability improves markedly. However, suboptimal therapy (judged by serum mitotane levels) that is limited by side effects should not be continued; in this setting there is little chance of benefit in the face of continued toxicity. Although suboptimal therapy cannot be accurately defined, blood levels of 10–14 mg/L are often cited as optimal based on two small studies, but lower levels are likely of some value; a clinical observation also noted in the recent retrospective analysis of adjuvant mitotane (Terzolo et al., 2007)

*At present, metyrapone is not available in pharmacies. To obtain metyrapone (Metopirone), a pharmacist or physician must call Novartis Pharmaceuticals Corporation at 1-800-988-7768

Ng L, Libertino JM. J Urol 2003;169:5–11
Terzolo M et al. N Engl J Med 2007;356:2372–2380
Vassilopoulou-Sellin R, Shultz PN. Cancer 2001;92:1113–1121
Veytsman I et al. J Clin Oncol 2009;27:4619–4629
Wajchenberg BL et al. Cancer 2000;88:711–736

REGIMEN

MITOTANE (*o,p'*-DDD)

Luton J-P et al. N Engl J Med 1990;322:1195–1201

Mitotane 2000–20,000 mg/day; administer orally as a single dose or in 2–4 divided doses

Glucocorticoid replacement is necessary in all patients:
Hydrocortisone 15–20 mg; administer orally every morning, *plus:*
Hydrocortisone 7.5–10 mg; administer orally every afternoon around 4 PM
Mineralocorticoid replacement is also recommended:
Fludrocortisone acetate 100–200 mcg/day; administer orally every morning, *or:*
Fludrocortisone acetate 100 mcg/day; administer orally every morning and every evening

Supportive Care
Antiemetic prophylaxis
Emetogenic potential: **MINIMAL**
See Chapter 39 for antiemetic recommendations

Hematopoietic growth factor (CSF) prophylaxis
Primary prophylaxis is NOT indicated
See Chapter 43 for more information

Antimicrobial prophylaxis
Risk of fever and neutropenia is LOW
  Antimicrobial primary prophylaxis to be considered:
  • Antibacterial—not indicated
  • Antifungal—not indicated
  • Antiviral—not indicated unless patient previously had an episode of HSV
See Chapter 47 for more information

Mitotane is available in the United States for oral administration in tablets that contain 500 mg mitotane. Lysodren (mitotane tablets). Bristol-Myers Squibb Company, Princeton, NJ

Patient Population Studied

A study of 59 patients with adrenocortical carcinoma treated with mitotane at different times in relation to surgery

Efficacy (N = 37)

Overall response rate	22%
Stable disease >12 months	5%
Clinical benefit rate	27%

Complete responses have been reported in other studies but are rare

Toxicity

Adverse Event	% Patients	No. of Patients
Anorexia/nausea	93	
Vomiting	82	
Diarrhea	68	28
Skin rash	32	
Confusion/sleepiness	100	
Ataxia	39	
Depression	33	
Dysarthria	28	18
Tremor	22	
Visual disturbance	17	
Leukopenia	17	

Van Slooten H et al. Eur J Cancer Clin Oncol 1984;20:47–53

Treatment Modifications

Adverse Event	Dose Modification
General Guidelines: First step with most side effects, especially if they occur as mitotane dose is advanced: (1) stop mitotane; (2) wait up to 7 days for symptoms to resolve; (3) restart mitotane at lower dose (500–1000 mg/day less than previous dose) or at previously tolerated dose; (4) increase dose in 500-mg/day increments at 1-week intervals	
Anorexia Nausea/vomiting	Administer mitotane in divided doses, and/or most of dose before bedtime. Crush tablets and dissolve in vehicle. Use antiemetics as needed. Reassess adrenal replacement
Diarrhea	Administer as divided doses. Use loperamide or diphenoxylate/ atropine
Altered mental status	Stop therapy. Follow general guidelines. Obtain imaging study only if symptoms persist after 1 week off therapy
Skin rash	If not severe, continue mitotane and treat rash with local measures and antipruritics

Therapy Monitoring

1. Check mitotane level at least every 4 weeks initially. Patients receiving long-term mitotane therapy can have monitoring reduced to every 2–3 months
2. Adrenal function can be monitored by measuring ACTH, but this alone is not reliable and should be interpreted together with clinical assessment
3. *Response assessment:* Initially every 6–8 weeks. Patients receiving long-term mitotane therapy can have monitoring reduced to every 3–6 months

Notes

1. Begin mitotane administration at a low dosage, usually no more than 2000 mg/day

2. Increase dose in increments of 500 mg to a maximum of 1000 mg/day, usually at intervals of not less than 1 week

3. Do not increase mitotane if a patient is experiencing side effects; follow General Guidelines in the Treatment Modifications section. Although mitotane is considered to have low to no emetogenic potential, it often produces low-grade nausea that is difficult to tolerate because it occurs every day. In some patients, chronic administration of antiemetics is required. See Chapter 39

4. The optimal dosage is not known; however, mitotane levels should be monitored with a goal of attaining a level of 14–20 mcg/mL. Levels greater than 20 mcg/mL are usually associated with intolerable side effects

5. A dosage of 4000–6000 mg/day usually results in a therapeutic level of mitotane in most patients after 6–10 weeks; however, some patients tolerate or require doses as high as 10,000–12,000 mg/day

6. Therapeutic levels can be achieved more quickly by administering higher doses and by increasing doses more aggressively, but this strategy usually fails because of side effects that result

7. With long-term administration of mitotane, the dosage required to maintain a therapeutic level may be substantially less, even as low as 500–1000 mg/day

8. Chronic administration results in adrenal insufficiency requiring steroid replacement therapy, as recommended in Regimen. Some physicians prefer to begin replacement therapy at the time mitotane therapy is started; others wait until there is evidence of incipient adrenal insufficiency, usually 6–8 weeks after the start of therapy. Replacement therapy is recommended with twice-daily hydrocortisone and with once- or twice-daily fludrocortisone replacement. Measuring ACTH levels to monitor the adequacy of replacement therapy is of limited value, because normal ACTH levels are difficult if not impossible to achieve. Patients should be instructed to obtain and wear identification that warns health care providers about possible adrenal insufficiency

9. Even without effecting a reduction in tumor size, mitotane may reduce circulating hormone levels, so that mitotane therapy can be continued solely to control the signs and symptoms of hormonal excess. Furthermore, if, after a period of mitotane administration, there is evidence of disease progression, discontinuing mitotane will result in a recurrence of the signs and symptoms of hormonal excess. The latter may appear gradually as mitotane is slowly cleared, but may eventually be worse than before mitotane therapy because of interval growth of the tumor. In these patients, consider continuing mitotane or begin an alternate drug to control hormonal excess

Haak HR et al. Br J Cancer 1994;69:947–951
Hoffman DL, Mattox VR. Med Clin North Am 1972;56:999–1012
Van Slooten H et al. Eur J Cancer Clin Oncol 1984;20:47–53

REGIMEN

CISPLATIN + MITOTANE

Bukowski RM et al. J Clin Oncol 1993;11:161–165

Hydration: ≥2000 mL 0.9% Sodium Chloride injection (0.9% NS), at ≥100 mL/hour before and after cisplatin administration. Also encourage increased oral fluid intake. Monitor and replace magnesium/electrolytes as needed

Cisplatin 75–100 mg/m²; administer intravenously in 50–250 mL of 0.9% NS over 30 minutes on day 1 every 3 weeks (total dosage per cycle = 75–100 mg/m²)
Mitotane* 4000 mg/day; administer orally, continually

Glucocorticoid replacement is necessary in all patients:
Hydrocortisone 15–20 mg; administer orally every morning, *plus*
Hydrocortisone 7.5–10 mg; administer orally every evening, continually
Mineralocorticoid replacement is also recommended
Fludrocortisone acetate 100–200 mcg/day; administer orally every morning, *or*
Fludrocortisone acetate 100 mcg/day; administer orally every morning and every evening, continually

Supportive Care
Antiemetic prophylaxis
Emetogenic potential on day 1: **HIGH**. *Potential for delayed symptoms*
Emetogenic potential on days with mitotane alone: **MINIMAL**
See Chapter 39 for antiemetic recommendations

Hematopoietic growth factor (CSF) prophylaxis
Primary prophylaxis is NOT indicated
See Chapter 43 for more information

Antimicrobial prophylaxis
Risk of fever and neutropenia is LOW
   Antimicrobial primary prophylaxis to be considered:
   • Antibacterial—not indicated
   • Antifungal—not indicated
   • Antiviral—not indicated unless patient previously had an episode of HSV
See Chapter 47 for more information

*Mitotane therapy may be better tolerated if started at a dose of 2000 mg/day, increasing by 500–1000 mg/day at 1-week intervals. The total daily mitotane dosage can be taken in 2–4 divided doses or as a single daily dose, which often is best tolerated at bedtime

Mitotane is available in the United States for oral administration in tablets that contain 500 mg mitotane Lysodren (mitotane tablets). Bristol-Myers Squibb Company, Princeton, NJ

Treatment Modifications

Adverse Event	Dose Modification
CrCl 30–50 mL/min (0.5–0.83 mL/s)	Hold cisplatin until CrCl ≥50 mL/min (≥0.83 mL/s), then reduce dose to 75 mg/m² if previous dose was 100 mg/m² or 60 mg/m² if previous dose was 75 mg/m²
CrCl <30 mL/min (<0.5 mL/s)	Discontinue cisplatin
Unacceptable GI or neuromuscular side effects from mitotane	Reduce mitotane to 2000 mg/day
Unacceptable side effects from mitotane at 2000 mg/day	Reduce mitotane to 1000 mg/day
Unacceptable side effects from mitotane at 1000 mg/day	Discontinue mitotane

CrCl, creatinine clearance

Patient Population Studied

A trial of 42 patients with metastatic or residual adrenocortical carcinoma because complete resection was not possible. Prior therapy with mitotane was allowed

Efficacy (N = 37)

Complete response	2.7%
Partial response	27%
Median response duration	7.9 months
Median time to response	76 days

Toxicity (N = 36)

Adverse Event	% G1/2	% G3/4
Hematologic		
Anemia	8	8
Leukopenia	36	6
Thrombocytopenia	—	3
Nonhematologic		
Nausea/vomiting	75	22
Diarrhea	11	—
Mucositis	6	—
Increased bilirubin	6	—
Renal	17	8
Peripheral neuropathy	3	6
Myalgias	17	6

N = 36, but reported as percent of 37 eligible patients

Therapy Monitoring

1. CBC with leukocyte differential count, serum creatinine and electrolytes, serum magnesium, and LFTs on day 1

2. *Response assessment:* Repeat imaging studies every 2 cycles; 24-hour urine cortisol and 17-ketosteroids with each cycle, if abnormal at baseline

3. Mitotane level at least every 4 weeks initially. A level of 14–20 mcg/mL is desirable

4. Adrenal function can be monitored by measuring ACTH, but this alone is not reliable and should be interpreted together with clinical assessment

ADVANCED OR METASTATIC ADRENAL CANCER REGIMEN

ETOPOSIDE + DOXORUBICIN + CISPLATIN + MITOTANE (EDP-M)

Fassnacht M et al. N Engl J Med 2012;366:2189–2197

Mitotane 500–5000 mg/day; administer orally, continually

- If possible, mitotane is started a minimum of 1 week before cytotoxic treatment is initiated. The ultimate goal is to attain mitotane concentrations in blood of 14–20 mcg/mL over time, as tolerated, trying not to exceed these values as side effects worsen with higher values. Note that side effects may preclude this range from being attained
- Initiate treatment with doses of 1000–1500 mg per day at bedtime to minimize sedative effects during waking hours, and escalate doses as tolerated
- Large daily doses may be divided in ≥2 doses

Doxorubicin 40 mg/m²; administer by intravenous injection over 3–5 minutes on day 1, every 4 weeks (total dosage/cycle = 40 mg/m²)

Prehydration for cisplatin: ≥500 mL 0.9% sodium chloride injection (0.9% NS) per day; administer intravenously at ≥100 mL/hour for 2 consecutive days, starting before cisplatin on days 3 and 4

Cisplatin 40 mg/m² per day; administer intravenously in 50–500 mL of 0.9% NS over 30–60 minutes for 2 doses on 2 consecutive days, days 3 and 4, every 4 weeks (total dosage/cycle = 80 mg/m²)

Posthydration for cisplatin: ≥500 mL 0.9% NS per day; administer intravenously at ≥100 mL/ hour for 2 consecutive days, after cisplatin on days 3 and 4. Encourage increased oral fluid intake. Monitor and replace magnesium and electrolytes as needed

± Mannitol diuresis: May be given to patients who have received adequate hydration

Mannitol 12.5–25 g may be administered by intravenous injection before or during cisplatin administration, *or*

Mannitol 10–40 g; administer intravenously over 1–4 hours before or during cisplatin administration, or may be prepared as an admixture with cisplatin

Note: Diuresis with mannitol requires maintaining hydration with intravenously administered fluid during and for hours after mannitol administration

Etoposide 100 mg/m² per dose; administer intravenously diluted to a concentration within the range 0.2–0.4 mg/mL in 5% dextrose injection or 0.9% NS over at least 60 minutes for 3 consecutive days, on days 2, 3, and 4, every 4 weeks (total dosage/cycle = 300 mg/m²)

Glucocorticoid replacement is necessary in all patients taking mitotane
Hydrocortisone 15–20 mg orally every morning, *plus:*
Hydrocortisone 7.5–10 mg orally every evening
Mineralocorticoid replacement is also recommended:
Fludrocortisone acetate 100–200 mcg/day orally every morning, *or:*
Fludrocortisone acetate 100 mcg/day orally every morning and every evening

Supportive Care
Antiemetic prophylaxis
Emetogenic potential on day 1: **MODERATE**
Emetogenic potential on day 2: **LOW**
Emetogenic potential on days 3 and 4: **HIGH.** *Potential for delayed symptoms*
See Chapter 39 for antiemetic recommendations

Hematopoietic growth factor (CSF) prophylaxis
Primary prophylaxis is NOT indicated
See Chapter 43 for more information

Antimicrobial prophylaxis
Risk of fever and neutropenia is LOW
Antimicrobial primary prophylaxis to be considered:
- Antibacterial—not indicated
- Antifungal—not indicated
- Antiviral—not indicated unless patient previously had an episode of HSV

See Chapter 47 for more information

Patient Population Studied

Patients with histologically confirmed adrenocortical carcinoma not amenable to radical surgical resection who had not received any previous treatment with cytotoxic drugs, except mitotane, and had an Eastern Cooperative Oncology Group (ECOG) performance status of 0, 1, or 2. One hundred fifty-one patients received etoposide + doxorubicin + cisplatin + mitotane

Age (y)	
Median	51.9
Range	19.0–76.2
Sex—Number (%)	
Male	60 (39.7)
Female	91 (60.3)
Tumor stage—Number (%)	
III	0
IV	151 (100.0)
Endocrine symptoms—Number (%)	
Cushing syndrome ± other symptoms	60 (39.7)
Conn syndrome only	2 (1.3)
Virilization only	6 (4.0)
Feminization only	3 (2.0)
No symptoms	70 (46.4)
Missing data	10 (6.6)
ECOG performance status score—Number (%)	
0	73 (48.3)
1	64 (42.4)
2	13 (8.6)
4	1 (0.7)
Time since primary diagnosis—Months	
Median	7.3
Range	0–183.7
Number of affected sites*	
Median	3
Range	1–7

*The following sites were calculated as separate sites of adrenocortical carcinoma: adrenal gland (including local recurrence), liver, lung, bone, peritoneum, retroperitoneum, pleura, mediastinum, central nervous system, soft tissue, spleen, and ovary

Treatment Modifications

Adverse Event	Dose Modification
Day 1 WBC <1000/mm^3 *or* platelet count <100,000/mm^3 *or* G >2 nonhematologic toxicity	Delay chemotherapy until WBC ≥1000/mm^3 and platelet count ≥100,000/mm^3, or nonhematologic toxicity G ≤1 for a maximum delay of 2 weeks
>2-week delay in reaching WBC >1000/mm^3 *or* platelet count >100,000/mm^3 *or* for resolution of non-hematologic toxicity to G ≤1	Discontinue therapy
G4 ANC or G ≥3 platelet counts	Reduce dosages of all drugs by 25% except mitotane
Creatinine clearance <50 to 60 mL/min	Hold cisplatin until creatinine clearance >50–60 mL/min

Efficacy

Efficacy in the Intention-to-Treat Population
Randomized Comparison versus Streptozocin + Mitotane*

Variable	EDP-M (N = 151)[†]	Sz-M (N = 153)[†]	P-Value
Type of response—no. (%)			
Complete response	2 (1.3)	1 (0.7)	
Disease-free by time of surgery[‡]	4 (2.6)	2 (1.3)	
Partial response	29 (19.2)	11 (7.2)	
Stable disease[§]	53 (35.1)	34 (22.2)	
Progressive disease	43 (28.5)	88 (57.5)	
Did not receive treatment	3 (2.0)	4 (2.6)	
Not evaluable for response	17 (11.3)	13 (8.5)	
Objective response[ϵ]			
Number of patients	35	14	
% (95% CI)	23.2 (16.7–30.7)	9.2 (5.1–14.9)	<0.001
Disease control**			
Number of patients	88	48	
% (95% CI)	58.3 (50.0–66.2)	31.4 (24.1–39.4)	<0.001
	EDP-M (N = 151)[†]	Sz-M (N = 153)[†]	HR [95%CI]; P-Value
Progression-free survival	5.0 months	2.1 months	0.55 [0.42–0.68]; <0.001
Overall survival[††]	14.8 months	12.0 months	0.79 [0.61–1.02]; 0.07

*Responses according to Response Evaluation Criteria in Solid Tumors (RECIST)
[†]EDP + M = etoposide + doxorubicin + cisplatin + mitotane; Sz + M = streptozocin + mitotane
[‡]Surgery performed >PR to study treatment; not included in PR category
[§]Stable disease was defined as no disease progression for at least ≥8 weeks and no objective response to treatment. Confirmatory scans were not required for this determination, according to the study protocol
[ϵ]Objective response = CR + PR
**Disease control + CR + PR + SD
[††]Patients classified according to first-line therapy, but they were allowed to receive the alternate therapy in second line

Toxicity

Event	Number of Patients (%)
Any serious adverse event	86 (58.1)
Adrenal insufficiency	5 (3.4)
Bone marrow toxicity	17 (11.5)
Cardiovascular or thromboembolic event	10 (6.8)
Fatigue or general health deterioration	8 (5.4)
Gastrointestinal disorder	6 (4.1)
Impaired liver function	0
Impaired renal function	1 (0.7)
Infection	10 (6.8)
Neurologic toxicity	5 (3.4)
Respiratory disorder	9 (6.1)
Other	15 (10.1)

Therapy Monitoring

1. CBC with leukocyte differential count, serum creatinine and electrolytes, serum magnesium, and LFTs on day 1 of each cycle
2. *Response assessment:* Repeat imaging studies every 2 cycles; 24-hour urine 17-ketosteroids and cortisol with each cycle if abnormal at baseline
3. Mitotane level at least every 4 weeks initially. A level of 14–20 mcg/mL is desirable but may not be attained
4. Adrenal function can be monitored by measuring ACTH, but this alone is not reliable and should be interpreted together with clinical assessment

REGIMEN

DOXORUBICIN

Decker RA et al. Surgery 1991;110:1006–1013

Doxorubicin 60 mg/m^2; administer by intravenous injection over 3–5 minutes on day 1, every 3 weeks to a maximum cumulative lifetime dosage of 500 mg/m^2 (total dosage per cycle = 60 mg/m^2)

Supportive Care
Antiemetic prophylaxis
Emetogenic potential: **HIGH**
See Chapter 39 for antiemetic recommendations

Hematopoietic growth factor (CSF) prophylaxis
Primary prophylaxis may be indicated
See Chapter 43 for more information

Antimicrobial prophylaxis
Risk of fever and neutropenia is LOW
   Antimicrobial primary prophylaxis to be considered:
   • Antibacterial—not indicated
   • Antifungal—not indicated
   • Antiviral—not indicated unless patient previously had an episode of HSV
See Chapter 47 for more information

Patient Population Studied

A study of 31 patients with unresectable adrenocortical carcinoma with ECOG PS 0–3. Fifteen of the 31 patients had been treated with mitotane immediately before doxorubicin

Efficacy (N = 31)

	Response Rate	No. of Patients
Initial treatment with chemotherapy (doxorubicin); no prior mitotane	19%	16
Tumor did not respond, or progressed when treated with mitotane	0%	15

Toxicity (N = 31)

	% Mild/ Moderate	% Severe
Hematologic		
Any hematologic	48	19
Nonhematologic		
Nausea/vomiting	45	3
Diarrhea	19	3
Skin/mucosa	16	0
Neurologic	13	0
Hepatic	6	0

Bear HD et al. J Clin Oncol 2003;21:4165–4174

Therapy Monitoring

1. CBC with leukocyte differential count, serum creatinine, electrolytes, and LFTs on day 1

2. *Response assessment:* Repeat imaging studies every 2 cycles; 24-hour urine cortisol and 17-hydroxycorticosteroids with each cycle if abnormal at baseline

Treatment Modifications

Adverse Event	Dose Modification
Day 1 ANC <1500/mm^3, platelet count <75,000/mm^3	Delay chemotherapy until ANC >1500/mm^3 and platelet counts >75,000/mm^3 for a maximum delay of 2 weeks. Use filgrastim or pegfilgrastim in subsequent cycles if delay for low ANC
Febrile neutropenia	Filgrastim or pegfilgrastim in subsequent cycles
Febrile neutropenia on filgrastim or pegfilgrastim	Reduce doxorubicin dosage by 25%
G ≥3 Nonhematologic toxicity	Hold therapy until resolution to G1. Reduce doxorubicin dosage by 25% if recovery occurs in <2 weeks

Bear HD et al. J Clin Oncol 2003;21:4165–4174

Notes

The recommended limit for total cumulative lifetime doxorubicin dosage of 450–500 mg/m^2 may be exceeded, provided that adequate cardiac monitoring is conducted before every or every other chemotherapy cycle

ADVANCED OR METASTATIC ADRENAL CANCER REGIMEN
STREPTOZOCIN + MITOTANE (Sz-M)

Fassnacht M et al. N Engl J Med 2012;366:2189–2197

Mitotane 500–5000 mg/day; administer orally, continually

- If possible, mitotane is started a minimum of 1 week before cytotoxic treatment is initiated. The ultimate goal is to attain mitotane concentrations in blood of 14–20 mcg/mL over time, as tolerated, trying not to exceed these values as side effects worsen with higher values. Note that side effects may preclude this range from being attained
- Initiate treatment with doses of 1000–1500 mg/day at bedtime to minimize sedative effects during waking hours, and escalate doses as tolerated
- Large daily doses may be divided in ≥2 doses

Hydration for streptozocin (all cycles): 1000 mL 0.9% sodium chloride injection (0.9% NS) per day; administer intravenously with 500 mL given before streptozocin and 500 mL given after streptozocin

First cycle: **Streptozocin** 1000 mg/day; administer intravenously in 50–500 mL of 0.9% NS or 5% dextrose injection (D5W) over 30–60 minutes for 5 doses on 5 consecutive days, days 1–5, every 3 weeks (total dose/cycle = 5000 mg)

Second and subsequent cycles: **Streptozocin** 2000 mg; administer intravenously in 50–500 mL of 0.9% NS or D5W over 30–60 minutes on day 1, every 3 weeks (total dose/cycle = 2000 mg)

Glucocorticoid replacement is necessary in all patients taking mitotane
Hydrocortisone 15–20 mg orally every morning, *plus*:
Hydrocortisone 7.5–10 mg orally every evening
Mineralocorticoid replacement is also recommended:
Fludrocortisone acetate 100–200 mcg/day orally every morning, *or*:
Fludrocortisone acetate 100 mcg/day orally every morning and every evening

Supportive Care
Antiemetic prophylaxis
*Emetogenic potential is **HIGH** each day streptozocin is administered. Potential for delayed symptoms*
See Chapter 39 for antiemetic recommendations

Hematopoietic growth factor (CSF) prophylaxis
Primary prophylaxis is NOT indicated
See Chapter 43 for more information

Antimicrobial prophylaxis
Risk of fever and neutropenia is LOW
Antimicrobial primary prophylaxis to be considered:
- Antibacterial—not indicated
- Antifungal—not indicated
- Antiviral—not indicated unless patient previously had an episode of HSV

See Chapter 47 for more information

Patient Population Studied
Patients with histologically confirmed adrenocortical carcinoma not amenable to radical surgical resection who had not received any previous treatment with cytotoxic drugs, except mitotane, and had an Eastern Cooperative Oncology Group (ECOG) performance status of 0, 1, or 2. One-hundred fifty-three patients received streptozocin + mitotane

Age (y)	
Median	50.0
Range	18.8–72.8

Sex—Number (%)	
Male	61 (39.9)
Female	92 (60.1)

Tumor stage—Number (%)	
III	1 (0.7)
IV	152 (99.3)

Endocrine symptoms—Number (%)	
Cushing syndrome ± other symptoms	64 (41.8)
Conn syndrome only	3 (2.0)
Virilization only	7 (4.6)
Feminization only	2 (1.3)
No symptoms	68 (44.4)
Missing data	9 (5.9)

ECOG performance status score—Number (%)	
0	72 (47.1)
1	60 (39.2)
2	21 (13.7)
4	0

Time since primary diagnosis—Months	
Median	4.5
Range	0–111.6

Number of affected sites*	
Median	3
Range	1–8

*The following sites were calculated as separate sites of adrenocortical carcinoma: adrenal gland (including local recurrence), liver, lung, bone, peritoneum, retroperitoneum, pleura, mediastinum, central nervous system, soft tissue, spleen, and ovary

Treatment Modifications

Adverse Event	Dose Modification
Day 1 WBC <1000/mm³ *or* platelet count <100,000/mm³ *or* G >2 nonhematologic toxicity	Delay chemotherapy until WBC ≥1000/mm³ and platelet count ≥100,000/mm³, or nonhematologic toxicity G ≤1 for a maximum delay of 2 weeks
>2-week delay in reaching WBC, >1000/mm³ *or* platelet count >100,000/mm³, or for resolution of nonhematologic toxicity to G ≤1	Discontinue therapy
G4 ANC *or* G ≥3 platelet counts	Reduce streptozocin dose by 25%
Creatinine clearance <50–60 mL/min	Hold streptozocin until creatinine clearance >50–60 mL/min

Efficacy

Efficacy in the Intention-to-Treat Population
Randomized Comparison vs. Etoposide + Doxorubicin + Cisplatin + Mitotane*

Variable	EDP-M (N = 151)[†]	Sz-M (N = 153)[†]	P-Value
Type of response—no. (%)			
Complete response	2 (1.3)	1 (0.7)	
Disease-free by time of surgery[‡]	4 (2.6)	2 (1.3)	
Partial response	29 (19.2)	11 (7.2)	
Stable disease[§]	53 (35.1)	34 (22.2)	
Progressive disease	43 (28.5)	88 (57.5)	
Did not receive treatment	3 (2.0)	4 (2.6)	
Not evaluable for response	17 (11.3)	13 (8.5)	
Objective response[ϵ]			
Number of patients	35	14	
% (95% CI)	23.2 (16.7–30.7)	9.2 (5.1–14.9)	<0.001
Disease control**			
Number of patients	88	48	
% (95% CI)	58.3 (50.0–66.2)	31.4 (24.1–39.4)	<0.001
	EDP-M (N = 151)[†]	Sz-M (N = 153)[†]	HR [95% CI]; P-Value
Progression-free Survival	5.0 months	2.1 months	0.55 [0.42–0.68]; <0.001
Overall Survival[††]	14.8 months	12.0 months	0.79 [0.61–1.02]; 0.07

*Responses according to Response Evaluation Criteria in Solid Tumors (RECIST)
[†]EDP + M = etoposide + doxorubicin + cisplatin + mitotane; Sz + M = streptozocin + mitotane
[‡]Surgery performed >PR to study treatment; not included in PR category
[§]Stable disease was defined as no disease progression for at least 8 weeks and no objective response to treatment.
Confirmatory scans were not required for this determination, according to the study protocol
[ϵ]Objective response = CR + PR
**Disease control + CR + PR + SD
[††]Patients classified according to first-line therapy, but they were allowed to receive the alternate therapy in second line

Toxicity

Event	Number of Patients (%)
Any serious adverse event	62 (41.6)
Adrenal insufficiency	1 (0.7)
Bone marrow toxicity	3 (2.0)
Cardiovascular or thromboembolic event	0
Fatigue or general health deterioration	7 (4.7)
Gastrointestinal disorder	12 (8.1)
Impaired liver function	7 (4.7)
Impaired renal function	6 (4.0)
Infection	4 (2.7)
Neurologic toxicity	4 (2.7)
Respiratory disorder	5 (3.4)
Other	13 (8.7)

Therapy Monitoring

1. CBC with leukocyte differential count, serum creatinine, electrolytes, and LFTs on day 1; obtain creatinine clearance on day 1 if an elevation in serum creatinine is observed

2. Twenty-four–hour urine for protein on day 1

3. *Response assessment:* Repeat imaging studies every 2 cycles; 24-hour urine 17-ketosteroids and cortisol with each cycle if abnormal at baseline

4. Mitotane level at least every 4 weeks initially. A level of 14–20 mcg/mL is desirable, but may not be attained

5. Adrenal function can be monitored by measuring ACTH, but this alone is not reliable and should be interpreted together with clinical assessment

2. Anal Cancer

Irfan Jawed, MD and John Marshall, MD

Epidemiology

Incidence: 7,210 (male: 2,660; female: 4,550. Estimated new cases for 2014 in the United States)
1.5 per 100,000 male per year, 1.9 per 100,000 female
Deaths: Estimated 950 in 2014 (male: 370; female: 580)
Median age at diagnosis: 60 years
Male to female ratio: Slight female predominance

Stage at Presentation
Stages I/II: 50%
Stage III: 29–40%
Stage IV: 10–13%

Daling JR et al. J Natl Cancer Inst 2000;92:1500–1510
Fred Hutchinson Cancer Research Center, Changing Trends in Sexual Behavior May Explain Rising Incidence of
Anal Cancer Among American Men and Women. Fred Hutchinson Cancer Research Center (fhcrc.org). 2004-07-06. Retrieved 2010-04
Frisch M et al. Gynecol Oncol 2009;114:395–398
Maggard MA et al. Dis Colon Rectum 2003;46:1517–1523; discussion 1523–1524; author reply 1524
Ryan DP et al. Int J Cancer 2010;127:675–684
Ryan DP et al. N Engl J Med 2000;342:792–800
Siegel R et al. CA Cancer J Clin 2014;64:9–29
Surveillance, Epidemiology and End Results (SEER) Program, available from http://seer.cancer.gov (accessed in 2013)
Uronis HE and Bendell JC. Oncologist 2007;12:524–534

Work-up

All stages
1. Sigmoidoscopy with biopsy
2. CT scan of abdomen and pelvis, or MRI
3. Chest x-ray or chest CT
4. Consider HIV testing
5. Consider PET-CT scan
6. Gynecologic exam for women, including screening for cervical cancer

Positive inguinal lymph node on imaging
1. Fine-needle aspiration or biopsy of node

Pathology

By convention, anal cancer should now refer only to *squamous cell cancers* arising in the anus. Earlier surgical series often did not make this distinction. *Adenocarcinomas* occurring in the anal canal should be treated according to the same principles applied to rectal adenocarcinoma. Similarly, melanomas and sarcomas should be treated according to the same principles applied to those tumor types at other sites

The distal anal canal is lined by squamous epithelium, and tumors arising in this portion are often keratinizing. Around the dentate line, the mucosa transitions from squamous mucosa to the nonsquamous rectal mucosa. Tumors arising in this transitional zone are often nonkeratinizing and previously were referred to as basaloid or cloacogenic

Clark MA et al. Lancet Oncol 2004;5:149–157
Ryan DP et al. N Engl J Med 2000;342:792–800

Five-Year Survival (After Chemoradiation)

Stages I/II: 80%
Stage III: 60%
Stage IV: 30.5%

Howlader N et al., eds. SEER Cancer Statistics Review, 1975–2008. Bethesda, MD: National Cancer Institute, http://seer.cancer.gov/csr/1975_2008/, based on November 2010 SEER data submission, posted to the SEER website, 2011

Poor Prognostic Factors
1. Nodal involvement
2. Skin ulceration
3. Male gender
4. Tumor >5 cm

Bartelink F et al. J Clin Oncol 1997;15:2040–2049
Comments: Highlights of Gastrointestinal Cancer Research 1999;3:539–552
Gunderson LL et al. Proc Am Soc Clin Oncol 2011;29:257s [abstract 4005]
UKCCR (UK Co-ordinating Committee on Cancer Research). Lancet 1996;348:1049–1054

Staging

Primary Tumor (T)

TX	Primary tumor cannot be assessed
T0	No evidence of primary tumor
Tis	Carcinoma *in situ* (Bowen disease, High-grade Squamous Intraepithelial Lesion (HSIL), Anal Intraepithelial Neoplasia II–III (AIN II–III)
T1	Tumor 2 cm or less in greatest dimension
T2	Tumor more than 2 cm but not more than 5 cm in greatest dimension
T3	Tumor more than 5 cm in greatest dimension
T4	Tumor of any size invades adjacent organ(s), eg, vagina, urethra, bladder*

*Direct invasion of the rectal wall, perirectal skin, subcutaneous tissue, or the sphincter muscle(s) is not classified as T4

Regional Lymph Nodes (N)

NX	Regional lymph nodes cannot be assessed
N0	No regional lymph node metastasis
N1	Metastasis in perirectal lymph node(s)
N2	Metastasis in unilateral internal iliac and/or inguinal lymph node(s)
N3	Metastasis in perirectal and inguinal lymph nodes and/or bilateral internal iliac and/or inguinal lymph nodes

Distant Metastasis (M)

M0	No distant metastasis (no pathologic M0; use clinical M to complete stage group)
M1	Distant metastasis

Group	T	N	M
0	Tis	N0	M0
I	T1	N0	M0
II	T2	N0	M0
	T3	N0	M0
IIIA	T1	N1	M0
	T2	N1	M0
	T3	N1	M0
	T4	N0	M0
IIIB	T4	N1	M0
	Any T	N2	M0
	Any T	N3	M0
IV	Any T	Any N	M1

Edge SB, Byrd DR, Compton CC, Fritz AG, Greene FL, Trotti A, eds. *AJCC Cancer Staging Manual.* 7th ed. New York, NY: Springer; 2010

Expert Opinion

Locoregional disease *(squamous cell cancers)*

Anal canal cancer

- Concurrent chemoradiation is the recommended primary treatment for patients with anal canal cancer that has not metastasized, with fluorouracil 1000 mg/m² per day by continuous intravenous infusion over 24 hours for 4 consecutive days on days 1–4, *plus* mitomycin 10 mg/m² by slow intravenous injection on day 1, every 28 days for 2 cycles (see Regimens below)
- Long-term update of U.S. GI intergroup RTOG 98-11 phase III trial for anal carcinoma: disease-free and overall survival with RT + fluorouracil + mitomycin versus RT + fluorouracil + cisplatin

Long-term Update of U.S. GI Intergroup RTOG 98-11

Gunderson LL et al. Proc Am Soc Clin Oncol 2011;29:257s [abstract 4005]

	# Patients	DFS TF	DFS %, 5-Years	OS TF	OS %, 5-Years	CFS TF	CFS %, 5-Years	LRF TF	LRF %, 5-Years	DM TF	DM %, 5-Years	CF TF	CF %, 5-Years
RT + fluorouracil + mitomycin	325	117	67.7	80	78.2	101	71.8	67	20.0	45	13.1	38	11.9
RT + fluorouracil + cisplatin	324	156	57.6	108	70.5	126	64.9	86	26.5	60	17.8	55	17
p Value			0.0044		0.021		0.053		0.089		0.12		0.075

CF, colostomy failure; CFS, colostomy-free survival; DFS, Disease-free survival; DM, distant metastases; LRF, locoregional failure; OS, overall survival; RT, radiation therapy; TF, total failures

- Locoregional failure rate is 10–30%. If locally persistent or progressive disease is present, consider abdominoperineal resection (APR). If positive lymph nodes are found, perform groin dissection with RT (if RT was not previously administered) or without RT

Anal margin cancer

- A well-differentiated anal margin lesion characterized as T1, N0, can be treated with margin negative excision alone with close follow-up
- For T2–T4 or any N, the recommended treatment is chemoradiation: fluorouracil 1000 mg/m² per day by continuous intravenous infusion over 24 hours for 4 consecutive days on days 1–4, *plus* mitomycin 10 mg/m² intravenously on day 1, every 28 days for 2 cycles (see Regimens below)

Metastatic anal cancer *(squamous cell cancers)*

Metastatic disease should be treated with cisplatin-based chemotherapy or enrollment in a clinical trial

Faivre C et al. Bull Cancer 1999;86:861–865

(continued)

Expert Opinion (continued)

Fluorouracil 1000 mg/m² per day administer by continuous intravenous infusion over 24 hours for 5 consecutive days on days 1–5, every 4 weeks, *plus*
Cisplatin 100 mg/m² administer intravenously over 30–60 minutes on day 2, every 4 weeks
- The regimen of choice
- Should be repeated until there is evidence of disease progression or toxicity requires cessation of treatment
Note: If the above regimen fails, no other regimen has been shown to be effective

Supportive Care/Alternate Treatments
- Radiotherapy might be delivered with less toxicity by means of 3D conformal radiotherapy or IMRT followed by conventional radiotherapy as shown in RTOG 0529 trial (2-year outcomes of RTOG 0529: a phase II evaluation of dose-painted IMRT in combination with fluorouracil and mitomycin for the reduction of acute morbidity in carcinoma of the anal canal). However, IMRT is not recommended in obese patients with nonreproducible external skin contours or patients with a major component of tumor outside the anal canal

Two-Year Outcomes of RTOG 0529

Kachnic LA et al. J Clin Oncol 2011;29(Suppl 4) [abstract 368]

End Point	0529 (N = 52)		9811 (N = 325)	
	Events	2-Year % (95% CI)	Events	2-Year % (95% CI)
LRF	10	20 (9, 31)	67	19 (14, 23)
CF	4	8 (0.4, 15)	38	11 (8, 14)
OS	7	88 (75, 94)	80	91 (87, 94)
DFS	12	77 (62, 86)	117	76 (70, 80)
CFS	7	86 (73, 93)	101	83 (79, 87)

CF, colostomy failures; CFS, colostomy-free survival; DFS, disease-free survival; LRF, Locoregional failure; OS, overall survival

- Capecitabine has been assessed in a phase II trial as a replacement for fluorouracil, but, to date, there is insufficient evidence to recommend substitution (Glynne-Jones R et al. Int J Radiat Oncol Biol Phys 2008;72:119–126)
- Tolerance to treatment can be maximized with antibiotics, antifungals, antiemetics, analgesia, skin care, advice regarding nutrition, and psychological support

Prevention of Anal Cancer
The U.S. Food and Drug Administration in 2010 approved recombinant human papillomavirus quadrivalent vaccine (Gardasil) for use in females and males ages 9 through 26 years for indications, including the prevention of anal intraepithelial neoplasia and associated precancerous lesions caused by human papillomavirus (HPV) types 6, 11, 16, and 18

Management of HIV Positive Patients
HIV-positive patients are generally treated similarly to those without HIV infection, however dosage may need to be adjusted (or treat without mitomycin) specifically if CD4 count is <200 cells/mm³ or patients with a history of HIV-related complications as outcomes appear to be comparable but treatment-related toxicity may be worse

Post-treatment surveillance
There are no prospective trials to guide the post-treatment surveillance strategy for patients treated for anal cancer
- For patients who have a complete remission at 8–12 weeks from initial chemoradiotherapy, guidelines from the NCCN suggest the following every three to six months for five years:
  - Digital rectal examination
  - Anoscopy
  - Inguinal node palpation
  - If initially T3-4 disease or inguinal node-positive, or for those with persistent disease at the initial post-treatment biopsy who regress on serial examinations, consider imaging of the chest/abdomen and pelvis annually for three years
- For patients who have persistent disease at 8–12 weeks on DRE, it is recommended to re-evaluate in four weeks, and, if regression is observed on serial exams, continue to observe and re-evaluate in 3 months. If progressive disease is documented, perform a biopsy and restage
- For patients who undergo APR for biopsy-proven progressive or recurrent disease, perform inguinal node palpation every three to six months for five years, and annual radiographic imaging of the chest/abdomen/pelvis for three years

Allal AS et al. Effectiveness of surgical salvage therapy for patients with locally uncontrolled anal carcinoma after sphincter-conserving treatment. Cancer 1999;86:405–409
Faivre C et al. 5-fluorouracile and cisplatin combination chemotherapy for metastatic squamous-cell anal cancer. Bull Cancer 1999;86:861–865
Glynne-Jones R et al. EXTRA—a multicenter phase II study of chemoradiation using a 5 day per week oral regimen of capecitabine and intravenous mitomycin C in anal cancer. Int J Radiat Oncol Biol Phys 2008;72:119–126
Gunderson LL et al. Long-term update of U.S. GI intergroup RTOG 98-11 phase III trial for anal carcinoma: disease-free and overall survival with RT + fluorouracil-mitomycin versus RT + fluorouracil-cisplatin [abstract 4005]. J Clin Oncol 2011;29:257s
Kachnic LA et al. Two-year outcomes of RTOG 0529: a phase II evaluation of dose-painted IMRT in combination with 5-fluorouracil and mitomycin-C for the reduction of acute morbidity in carcinoma of the anal canal. J Clin Oncol 2011;29(Suppl 4) (2011 Gastrointestinal Cancers Symposium, American Society of Clinical Oncology; abstract 368)
Kreuter A et al. Anal carcinoma in human immunodeficiency virus-positive men: results of a prospective study from Germany. Br J Dermatol 2010;162:1269–1277
Schiller DE et al. Outcomes of salvage surgery for squamous cell carcinoma of the anal canal. Ann Surg Oncol 2007;14:2780–2789

REGIMEN

MITOMYCIN + FLUOROURACIL + RADIATION THERAPY (RTOG 8704/ECOG 1289 AND RTOG-0529)

Flam M et al. J Clin Oncol 1996;14:2527–2539
Kachnic LA et al. J Clin Oncol 2011;29(Suppl 4) (American Society of Clinical Oncology 2011 Gastrointestinal Cancers Symposium, abstract 368)

Mitomycin 10 mg/m^2 single dose (maximum dose = 20 mg); administer by intravenous injection over 3–5 minutes on day 1 every 4 weeks for 2 cycles (days 1 and 29 of radiation) (total dosage/cycle = 10 mg/m^2, but *not* greater than 20 mg)

Fluorouracil 1000 mg/m^2 per day (maximum daily dose = 2000 mg); administer by continuous intravenous infusion over 24 hours for 4 consecutive days, on days 1–4 every 4 weeks for 2 cycles (days 1–4 and 29–32 of radiation therapy) (total dosage/cycle = 4000 mg/m^2, but *not* greater than 8000 mg)

External beam radiation therapy 1.8 Gy/fraction; administer daily 5 days/week for 5 weeks (total dose to pelvis/complete course = 45 Gy in 5 weeks)
For patients with T3, T4, or N+ lesions or T2 lesions with residual disease after 45 Gy, current RTOG protocol recommends an additional 10–14 Gy to a reduced field

Alternate RT regimen: dose-painted (DP) IMRT
DP-IMRT prescribed as follows:
- T2N0: 42-Gy elective nodal and 50.4-Gy anal tumor planning target volumes (PTVs), 28 fractions
- T3-4N0-3: 45-Gy elective nodal, 50.4-Gy ≤3 cm, and 54-Gy >3 cm metastatic nodal and 54-Gy anal tumor PTVs, 30 fractions

Note: IMRT is not recommended in obese patients with nonreproducible external skin contours, or patients with a major component of tumor outside the anal canal

Supportive Care
Antiemetic prophylaxis
Emetogenic potential is **LOW**
See Chapter 39 for antiemetic recommendations

Hematopoietic growth factor (CSF) prophylaxis
Primary prophylaxis is NOT indicated
See Chapter 43 for more information

Antimicrobial prophylaxis
Risk of fever and neutropenia is LOW
  Antimicrobial primary prophylaxis to be considered:
  - Antibacterial—not indicated
  - Antifungal—not indicated
  - Antiviral—not indicated, unless patient previously had an episode of HSV
See Chapter 47 for more information

Diarrhea management
Latent or delayed onset diarrhea:
  Loperamide 4 mg orally initially after the first loose or liquid stool, *then*
  Loperamide 2 mg orally every 2 hours during waking hours, *plus*
  Loperamide 4 mg orally every 4 hours during hours of sleep
  - Continue for at least 12 hours after diarrhea resolves
  - Recurrent diarrhea after a 12-hour diarrhea free interval is treated as a new episode
  - Rehydrate orally with fluids and electrolytes during a diarrheal episode
  - If a patient develops blood or mucus in stool, dehydration, or hemodynamic instability, or if diarrhea persists >48 hours despite loperamide, stop loperamide and hospitalize the patient for IV hydration

  Alternatively, a trial of **Diphenoxylate hydrochloride** 2.5 mg **with Atropine sulfate** 0.025 mg (eg, Lomotil®)
  - Initial adult dose is two tablets four times daily until control has been achieved, after which the dose may be reduced to meet individual requirements. Control may often be maintained with as little as two tablets daily

(continued)

Treatment Modifications

Adverse Event	Dose Modification
G3/4 Diarrhea or stomatitis	Reduce fluorouracil dosage 50% during second cycle
G3 Radiation dermatitis	
G4 Radiation dermatitis	Do not give second cycle of chemotherapy
ANC <500/mm^3 or platelets <50,000/mm^3	Reduce fluorouracil and mitomycin dosages 50%
G3/4 Hematologic or nonhematologic events	Suspend chemoradiation until recovers to G ≤2

Based on RTOG protocol 98-11

Toxicity (N = 146)

	% G4/5
Acute (≤90 days after starting treatment)	25
Hematologic	18
Nonhematologic (diarrhea, skin, mucositis)	7
Late (>90 days after starting treatment)	5
Any grade 4 adverse event	23
Toxic death rate*	2.8

*All treatment-related deaths occurred in a setting of neutropenia and sepsis
NCI Common Toxicity Criteria, version 2.0

Efficacy (N = 129–146)

Positive biopsy after induction	8%
5-Year locoregional failure	36%
5-Year colostomy rate	22%
5-Year colostomy-free survival	64%
5-Year disease-free survival	67%
5-Year overall survival	67%

Flam M et al. Classic Papers and Current Comments: Highlights of Gastrointestinal Cancer Research 1999;3:539–552

(*continued*)

- Clinical improvement of acute diarrhea is usually observed within 48 hours. If improvement of chronic diarrhea after treatment with a maximum daily dose of 8 tablets is not observed within 10 days, control is unlikely with further administration

Persistent diarrhea:

Octreotide 100–150 mcg subcutaneously 3 times daily. Maximum total daily dose is 1500 mcg

Antibiotic therapy during latent or delayed onset diarrhea:

A fluoroquinolone (eg, **Ciprofloxacin** 500 mg orally every 12 hours) if absolute neutrophil count <500/mm³ with or without accompanying fever in association with diarrhea

- Antibiotics should also be administered if patient is hospitalized with prolonged diarrhea and should be continued until diarrhea resolves

*Rothenberg ML et al. J Clin Oncol 2001;19:3801–3807
Wadler S et al. J Clin Oncol 1998;16:3169–3178
Abigerges D et al. J Natl Cancer Inst 1994;86:446–449

Oral care

Prophylaxis and treatment for mucositis/stomatitis

General advice:

- Encourage patients to maintain intake of non-alcoholic fluids
- Evaluate patients for oral pain and provide analgesic medications
- Consider histamine (H$_2$-subtype) receptor antagonists (eg, ranitidine, famotidine), or a proton pump inhibitor for epigastric pain
- *Lactobacillus* sp.-containing probiotics may be beneficial in preventing diarrhea

Patients with intact oral mucosa:

- Clean the mouth, tongue, and gums by brushing after every meal and at bedtime with an ultra-soft toothbrush with fluoride toothpaste
- Floss teeth gently every day unless contraindicated. If gums bleed and hurt, avoid bleeding or sore areas, but floss other teeth
- Patients may use saline or commercial bland, non-alcoholic rinses
  - Do not use mouthwashes that contain alcohols

If mucositis or stomatitis is present:

- Keep the mouth moist utilizing water, ice chips, sugarless gum, sugar-free hard candies, or a saliva substitute
- Rinse mouth several times a day to remove debris
  - Use a solution of ¼ teaspoon (1.25 g) each of baking soda and table salt (sodium chloride) in one quart (~950 mL) of warm water. Follow with a plain water rinse
  - Do not use mouthwashes that contain alcohols
- Foam-tipped swabs (eg, Toothettes®) are useful in moisturizing oral mucosa, but ineffective for cleansing teeth and removing plaque
- Advise patients who develop mucositis to:
  - Choose foods that are easy to chew and swallow
  - Take small bites of food, chew slowly, and sip liquids with meals
  - Encourage soft, moist foods such as cooked cereals, mashed potatoes, and scrambled eggs
  - For trouble swallowing, soften food with gravies, sauces, broths, yogurt, or other bland liquids
  - Avoid sharp, crunchy foods; hot, spicy or highly acidic foods (eg, citrus fruits and juices); sugary foods; toothpicks; tobacco products; alcoholic drinks

Patient Population Studied

A study of 146 patients with localized (nonmetastatic) squamous cell cancer of the anal canal

Therapy Monitoring

1. *Every week:* CBC with differential
2. *Response assessment:* PE 6 weeks after completion of chemoradiotherapy. If there is regression of tumor on exam, then 12 weeks after completion of therapy repeat PE, perform sigmoidoscopy and obtain CT scan. If there is a residual mass or thickening, a biopsy should be performed. If there is residual disease at 12 weeks or if there is progression of disease on exam, consider salvage abdominoperineal resection

Notes

Severely immunocompromised patients or HIV-positive patients with low CD4 counts should be treated with caution. Consider omitting and/or reducing the dose of chemotherapy

REGIMEN

FLUOROURACIL + CISPLATIN + EXTERNAL BEAM RADIATION THERAPY

Doci R et al. J Clin Oncol 1996;14:3121–3125

Fluorouracil 750 mg/m² per day; administer by continuous intravenous infusion in 500–1000 mL 0.9% sodium chloride injection (0.9% NS) or 5% dextrose injection (D5W) over 24 hours for 4 consecutive days, on days 1–4, every 21 days for 2 cycles (total dosage/cycle = 3000 mg/m²)
(Days 1–4 and 21–24 of radiation therapy)
Hydration before cisplatin ≥1000 mL 0.9% NS; administer intravenously over a minimum of 2–4 hours
Cisplatin 100 mg/m²; administer intravenously in 50–250 mL 0.9% NS over 60 minutes, on day 1 every 21 days for 2 cycles (total dosage/cycle = 100 mg/m²)
(Days 1 and 21 of radiation therapy)
Hydration after cisplatin ≥1000 mL 0.9% NS; administer intravenously over a minimum of 2–4 hours. Encourage patients to supplement their usual oral hydration with extra non–alcohol-containing fluids for at least 24 hours after receiving cisplatin
External beam radiation therapy 1.8 Gy/fraction; administer daily 5 days/week up to 54–58 Gy

Supportive Care
Antiemetic prophylaxis
Emetogenic potential on days with cisplatin, fluorouracil, and RT is **HIGH**. *Potential for delayed symptoms*
Emetogenic potential on days with fluorouracil and RT is **LOW**
See Chapter 39 for antiemetic recommendations

Hematopoietic growth factor (CSF) prophylaxis
Primary prophylaxis is NOT indicated
See Chapter 43 for more information

Antimicrobial prophylaxis
Risk of fever and neutropenia is LOW
Antimicrobial primary prophylaxis to be considered:
- Antibacterial—not indicated
- Antifungal—not indicated
- Antiviral—not indicated unless patient previously had an episode of HSV

See Chapter 47 for more information

Diarrhea management
Latent or delayed onset diarrhea*:
Loperamide 4 mg orally initially after the first loose or liquid stool, *then*
Loperamide 2 mg orally every 2 hours during waking hours, *plus*
Loperamide 4 mg orally every 4 hours during hours of sleep
- Continue for at least 12 hours after diarrhea resolves
- Recurrent diarrhea after a 12-hour diarrhea-free interval is treated as a new episode
- Rehydrate orally with fluids and electrolytes during a diarrheal episode
- If a patient develops blood or mucus in stool, dehydration, or hemodynamic instability, or if diarrhea persists >48 hours despite loperamide, stop loperamide and hospitalize the patient for IV hydration

Alternatively, a trial of **Diphenoxylate hydrochloride** 2.5 mg **with Atropine sulfate** 0.025 mg (eg, Lomotil®)
- Initial adult dose is two tablets four times daily until control has been achieved, after which the dose may be reduced to meet individual requirements. Control may often be maintained with as little as two tablets daily
- Clinical improvement of acute diarrhea is usually observed within 48 hours. If improvement of chronic diarrhea after treatment with a maximum daily dose of 8 tablets is not observed within 10 days, control is unlikely with further administration

(continued)

Patient Population Studied
A study of 35 patients with previously untreated basaloid (n = 5) or squamous cell carcinoma (n = 30) of the anus. In all patients, the cancer was located in the anal canal; in 28, the tumor extended to adjacent sites. Nine patients had nodal metastases; no patient had distant metastases

Efficacy (N = 35)

Complete response	94%
Partial response*	6%
Local recurrence	6%
At median follow-up of 37 months	
No evidence of disease	94%
Colostomy free	86%

Normal anal function preserved in 30 of 35 patients
*Two partial responses in 2 of 5 (40%) patients with T3 tumors

Toxicity* (N = 35)

	% G1	% G2	% G3
Hematologic (leukopenia)	40	31	—
Vomiting	40	33	10
Dermatitis, proctitis, diarrhea	8.5	88.5	3
Cardiac	—	3†	—

*Acute toxicities. Chronic toxicities not reported.
No grade 4 toxicities reported
†Transient at end of first cycle; resolved
WHO criteria

(*continued*)

Persistent diarrhea:
   Octreotide 100–150 mcg subcutaneously 3 times daily. Maximum total daily dose is 1500 mcg

Antibiotic therapy during latent or delayed onset diarrhea:
   A fluoroquinolone (eg, **Ciprofloxacin** 500 mg orally every 12 hours) if absolute neutrophil count <500/mm³ with or without accompanying fever in association with diarrhea
   • Antibiotics should also be administered if patient is hospitalized with prolonged diarrhea and should be continued until diarrhea resolves

*Rothenberg ML et al. J Clin Oncol 2001;19:3801–3807
Abigerges D et al. J Natl Cancer Inst 1994;86:446–449
Wadler S et al. J Clin Oncol 1998;16:3169–3178

Oral care

Prophylaxis and treatment for mucositis/stomatitis
General advice:
• Encourage patients to maintain intake of non-alcoholic fluids
• Evaluate patients for oral pain and provide analgesic medications
• Consider histamine (H₂-subtype) receptor antagonists (eg, ranitidine, famotidine), or a proton pump inhibitor for epigastric pain
• *Lactobacillus* sp.-containing probiotics may be beneficial in preventing diarrhea

Patients with intact oral mucosa:
• Clean the mouth, tongue, and gums by brushing after every meal and at bedtime with an ultra-soft toothbrush with fluoride toothpaste
• Floss teeth gently every day unless contraindicated. If gums bleed and hurt, avoid bleeding or sore areas, but floss other teeth
• Patients may use saline or commercial bland, non-alcoholic rinses
   ▪ Do not use mouthwashes that contain alcohols

If mucositis or stomatitis is present:
• Keep the mouth moist utilizing water, ice chips, sugarless gum, sugar-free hard candies, or a saliva substitute
• Rinse mouth several times a day to remove debris
   ▪ Use a solution of ¼ teaspoon (1.25 g) each of baking soda and table salt (sodium chloride) in one quart (~950 mL) of warm water. Follow with a plain water rinse
   ▪ Do not use mouthwashes that contain alcohols
• Foam-tipped swabs (eg, Toothettes®) are useful in moisturizing oral mucosa, but ineffective for cleansing teeth and removing plaque
• Advise patients who develop mucositis to:
   ▪ Choose foods that are easy to chew and swallow
   ▪ Take small bites of food, chew slowly, and sip liquids with meals
   ▪ Encourage soft, moist foods such as cooked cereals, mashed potatoes, and scrambled eggs
   ▪ For trouble swallowing, soften food with gravies, sauces, broths, yogurt, or other bland liquids
   ▪ Avoid sharp, crunchy foods; hot, spicy or highly acidic foods (eg, citrus fruits and juices); sugary foods; toothpicks; tobacco products; alcoholic drinks

Note: The RTOG has amended the above regimen as follows:
Two cycles of chemotherapy are given before external beam radiation therapy commences; that is, radiation therapy begins coincident with the start of chemotherapy cycle 3
The chemotherapy regimen used has been modified as follows:
Fluorouracil 1000 mg/m² per day; administer by continuous intravenous infusion in 500–1000 mL 0.9% NS or D5W over 24 hours for 4 consecutive days on days 1–4, every 28 days for 4 cycles (total dosage/cycle = 4000 mg/m²)
Cisplatin 75 mg/m²; administer intravenously in 250 mL 0.9% NS over 60 minutes on day 1 every 28 days for 4 cycles on days 1, 29, 57, and 85 (total dosage/cycle = 75 mg/m²)

Treatment Modifications

Adverse Event	Dose Modification
ANC <500/mm³ or platelets <50,000/mm³	Decrease fluorouracil and cisplatin dosages by 50%
G3/4 diarrhea or stomatitis	Decrease fluorouracil dosage by 50%
G3 radiation dermatitis	
G4 radiation dermatitis	Hold radiation until dermatitis resolves to G ≤2, and do not administer additional fluorouracil
Creatinine 1.5–2.0 mg/dL (133–177 μmol/L)	Decrease cisplatin dosage by 50%
Creatinine >2.0 mg/dL (>177 μmol/L)	Hold cisplatin

Recommended by RTOG 98-11

Therapy Monitoring

1. *Before each cycle:* CBC with differential, BUN, creatinine, magnesium, and electrolytes
2. *Response assessment:* PE 4–6 weeks after completion of chemoradiotherapy. Perform a biopsy only in the absence of a response to therapy. If there has been a response to therapy, reevaluate at 12 weeks with PE, sigmoidoscopy, and CT scan. If residual tumor is suspected, biopsy the affected area. If residual disease is documented at 12 weeks or if there is progression of disease on exam, consider salvage abdominoperineal resection

ADVANCED DISEASE REGIMEN

CISPLATIN + FLUOROURACIL BY CONTINUOUS INTRAVENOUS INFUSION

Faivre C et al. Bull Cancer 1999;86:861–865

Hydration before, during, and after cisplatin administration ± mannitol:

- *Pre-cisplatin hydration* with ≥1000 mL 0.9% sodium chloride injection (0.9% NS); administer intravenously with potassium and magnesium supplementation as needed based on pretreatment values

- *Mannitol diuresis:* May be given to patients who have received adequate hydration. A dose of **mannitol** 12.5–25 g may be administered by intravenous injection or a short infusion before or during cisplatin administration, or prepared as an admixture with cisplatin. Continued intravenous hydration is essential

- *Continued mannitol diuresis:* In an inpatient or day-hospital setting, one may administer additional mannitol in the form of an intravenous infusion: **mannitol** 10–40 g administer intravenously over 1–4 hours. This can be done either during or immediately after cisplatin, but requires maintenance of adequate intravenously administered fluids during and for hours after mannitol administration

- Post-cisplatin hydration with ≥1000 mL 0.9% NS; administer intravenously with potassium and magnesium supplementation as needed based on measured values. Encourage patients to supplement their usual oral hydration with extra non–alcohol-containing fluids for at least 24 hours after receiving cisplatin

Cisplatin 100 mg/m²; administer intravenously in 100–500 mL 0.9% NS over 30–60 minutes on day 2, every 4 weeks (total dosage/cycle = 100 mg/m²)

Fluorouracil 1000 mg/m² per day; administer by continuous intravenous infusion in 50–1000 mL 0.9% NS or 5% dextrose injection over 24 hours for 5 consecutive days, on days 1–5, every 4 weeks (total dosage/cycle = 5000 mg/m²)

Notes:
- Ten patients received further local treatment
- Carboplatin used instead of cisplatin in the event of renal toxicity

Supportive Care

Antiemetic prophylaxis
*Emetogenic potential on days with cisplatin is **HIGH**. Potential for delayed symptoms*
*Emetogenic potential on days with fluorouracil alone is **LOW***
See Chapter 39 for antiemetic recommendations

Hematopoietic growth factor (CSF) prophylaxis
Primary prophylaxis is NOT indicated
See Chapter 43 for more information

Antimicrobial prophylaxis
Risk of fever and neutropenia is LOW
  Antimicrobial primary prophylaxis to be considered:
  - Antibacterial—not indicated
  - Antifungal—not indicated
  - Antiviral—not indicated unless patient previously had an episode of HSV

See Chapter 47 for more information

Diarrhea management
Latent or delayed onset diarrhea:
  Loperamide 4 mg orally initially after the first loose or liquid stool, *then*
  Loperamide 2 mg orally every 2 hours during waking hours, *plus*
  Loperamide 4 mg orally every 4 hours during hours of sleep
  - Continue for at least 12 hours after diarrhea resolves
  - Recurrent diarrhea after a 12-hour diarrhea-free interval is treated as a new episode
  - Rehydrate orally with fluids and electrolytes during a diarrheal episode
  - If a patient develops blood or mucus in stool, dehydration, or hemodynamic instability, or if diarrhea persists >48 hours despite loperamide, stop loperamide and hospitalize the patient for IV hydration

(continued)

Treatment Modifications

Adverse Event	Dose Modification
G3/4 hematologic	Reduce fluorouracil and cisplatin dosages by 20%
Hand-foot syndrome (palmar-plantar erythrodysesthesia)	Interrupt fluorouracil therapy until symptoms resolve. Then, reduce fluorouracil dosage by 20%, or discontinue fluorouracil
Mucositis	Interrupt fluorouracil therapy until symptoms resolve. Then, reduce fluorouracil dosage by 20%
Diarrhea	
Reduction in creatinine clearance* to ≤60% of on study value	Delay therapy for 1 week. If creatinine clearance does not recover to pretreatment values, consider reducing cisplatin dose or replace cisplatin with carboplatin
Creatinine clearance* 40–60 mL/min (0.66–1 mL/s)	Consider reducing cisplatin dose, so that dose in milligrams equals the creatinine clearance* value expressed in mL/min[†]. Alternatively, replace cisplatin with carboplatin
Creatinine clearance* <40 mL/min (<0.66 mL/s)	Hold cisplatin
Clinically significant ototoxicity	Discontinue cisplatin
Clinically significant sensory loss	Discontinue cisplatin

*Creatinine clearance is used as a measure of glomerular filtration rate
[†]This also applies to patients with creatinine clearance of 40–60 mL/min before commencing treatment

Patient Population Studied

Study of 19 patients (3 males, 16 females), median age 58 years, WHO performance status: G0-1 in 68% and G2 in 32%. Metastasis were synchronous in 6 patients and metachronous in 13 patients. Metastatic sites included liver (10/19 patients), lymph nodes (11/19 patients: paraaortic 5, iliac 4, and inguinal 2) and pulmonary (3/11 patients). In 9 of 19 patients lymph node metastases were isolated; in 7 of 19 patients liver metastases were isolated

(continued)

Alternatively, a trial of **Diphenoxylate hydrochloride** 2.5 mg **with Atropine sulfate** 0.025 mg (eg, Lomotil®)
- Initial adult dose is two tablets four times daily until control has been achieved, after which the dose may be reduced to meet individual requirements. Control may often be maintained with as little as two tablets daily
- Clinical improvement of acute diarrhea is usually observed within 48 hours. If improvement of chronic diarrhea after treatment with a maximum daily dose of 8 tablets is not observed within 10 days, control is unlikely with further administration

Persistent diarrhea:
Octreotide 100–150 mcg subcutaneously 3 times daily. Maximum total daily dose is 1500 mcg

Antibiotic therapy during latent or delayed onset diarrhea:
A fluoroquinolone (eg, **Ciprofloxacin** 500 mg orally every 12 hours) if absolute neutrophil count <500/mm^3 with or without accompanying fever in association with diarrhea
- Antibiotics should also be administered if patient is hospitalized with prolonged diarrhea and should be continued until diarrhea resolves

*Rothenberg ML et al. J Clin Oncol 2001;19:3801–3807
Abigerges D et al. J Natl Cancer Inst 1994;86:446–449
Wadler S et al. J Clin Oncol 1998;16:3169–3178

Oral care
Prophylaxis and treatment for mucositis/stomatitis
General advice:
- Encourage patients to maintain intake of non-alcoholic fluids
- Evaluate patients for oral pain and provide analgesic medications
- Consider histamine (H$_2$-subtype) receptor antagonists (eg, ranitidine, famotidine), or a proton pump inhibitor for epigastric pain
- *Lactobacillus* sp.-containing probiotics may be beneficial in preventing diarrhea

Patients with intact oral mucosa:
- Clean the mouth, tongue, and gums by brushing after every meal and at bedtime with an ultra-soft toothbrush with fluoride toothpaste
- Floss teeth gently every day unless contraindicated. If gums bleed and hurt, avoid bleeding or sore areas, but floss other teeth
- Patients may use saline or commercial bland, non-alcoholic rinses
  - Do not use mouthwashes that contain alcohols

If mucositis or stomatitis is present:
- Keep the mouth moist utilizing water, ice chips, sugarless gum, sugar-free hard candies, or a saliva substitute
- Rinse mouth several times a day to remove debris
  - Use a solution of ¼ teaspoon (1.25 g) each of baking soda and table salt (sodium chloride) in one quart (~950 mL) of warm water. Follow with a plain water rinse
  - Do not use mouthwashes that contain alcohols
- Foam-tipped swabs (eg, Toothettes®) are useful in moisturizing oral mucosa, but ineffective for cleansing teeth and removing plaque
- Advise patients who develop mucositis to:
  - Choose foods that are easy to chew and swallow
  - Take small bites of food, chew slowly, and sip liquids with meals
  - Encourage soft, moist foods such as cooked cereals, mashed potatoes, and scrambled eggs
  - For trouble swallowing, soften food with gravies, sauces, broths, yogurt, or other bland liquids
  - Avoid sharp, crunchy foods; hot, spicy or highly acidic foods (eg, citrus fruits and juices); sugary foods; toothpicks; tobacco products; alcoholic drinks

Toxicity, N = 19*

Hematologic	
G3/4 thrombocytopenia	24%
G3/4 neutropenia	13%
Febrile neutropenia	0
Nonhematologic	
G3/4 nausea/vomiting	30%
G3/4 diarrhea	0
G3/4 mucositis	0
Neurotoxicity	0
Ototoxicity	0
G1–2 nephrotoxicity	11.1%
Mean fluorouracil dose intensity during cycles 1 and 2	92.5%
Mean cisplatin dose intensity during cycles 1 and 2	95%

*WHO criteria

Efficacy (N = 18)*

Overall response rate	66%
Complete response	5.5%
Partial response	61.1%
Stable disease	22.2%
Progressive disease	11.1%
Median number of cycles (range)	4 (2–7)
1-Year survival	62.2%
5-Year survival	32.2%
Overall survival	34.5 months

*WHO criteria
Note: Three patients who were alive at 4, 5, and 7 years, respectively, had received additional local treatment (1 patient received chemotherapy after hepatic resection and 2 patients were treated after response to the FUP regimen with surgery or radiotherapy)

Treatment Monitoring

1. CBC with diff, electrolytes (including sodium, potassium, magnesium), and serum creatinine and LFTs before each cycle
2. Assessment evaluation: every 8 weeks

3. Biliary: Gallbladder Cancer and Cholangiocarcinoma

Tim Greten, MD, PhD, Susanna Ulahannan, MD, and Werner Scheithauer, MD

Epidemiology

Gallbladder Cancer & Other Biliary

Incidence: 10,650 (male: 4,960; female: 5,690. Estimated new cases for 2014 in the United States)

Deaths: Estimated 3,630 in 2014 (male: 1,610; female: 2,020)

Median age, cholangiocarcinoma: 65 years

Gallbladder: 7th decade

Gallbladder cancer: Women are two to six times more likely to develop gallbladder cancer than men

Cholangiocarcinoma: Slighlty more common in men

Siegel R et al. CA Cancer J Clin 2014;64:9–29

Work-up

1. Early diagnosis of gallbladder or cholangiocellular carcinoma is nearly impossible or can only be realized in exceptional cases

2. In a patient with specific clinical symptoms or ultrasound suspicion of biliary tract cancer, a spiral CT and chest x-ray should be performed

3. Medically fit, nonjaundiced patients whose disease appears *potentially resectable* may proceed directly to surgical exploration without needle biopsy to avoid tumor spread. Consider a laparoscopic evaluation before open surgery owing to the common occurrence of otherwise nonvisible metastatic spread to the peritoneum

4. If the potential to perform a resection remains *uncertain* and for those with jaundice, a more precise assessment of tumor extent and lymph node involvement should be obtained with MRCP ± MRA, which may help to rule out vascular invasion and anomalous anatomic findings for surgical planning

5. If it is obvious that a resection will *not* be possible or if distant metastases are present, fine-needle biopsy for tissue confirmation should be obtained

6. In *nonresectable jaundiced* patients, depending on the location of the biliary obstruction, a percutaneous transhepatic cholangiography (PTC) or an endoscopic retrograde cholangiography (ERC) should be considered to guide placement of a stent

Fong Y et al. Cancer of the liver and biliary tree. In: Principles and Practice of Oncology, 6th ed. Baltimore, MD: Lippincott Williams & Wilkins 2001:1162–1203

Pathology

1. Gallbladder cancer		(60%)
2. Cholangiocarcinoma		(40%)
Intrahepatic		10%
Perihilar (Klatskin tumor)		40–60%
Distal		20–30%
Multifocal		<10%

Histopathology

1. Adenocarcinoma	80–90%
Papillary, nodular, tubular, medullary	
2. Pleomorphic giant cell carcinoma	>10%
3. Squamous cell carcinoma	5%
4. Mucoid carcinoma	<1%
5. Anaplastic carcinoma	<1%
6. Cystadenocarcinoma	<1%
7. Clear cell carcinoma	<1%
8. Other rare forms	<1%

Lazcano-Ponce EC et al. CA Cancer J Clin 2001;51:349–364
Nakeeb A et al. Ann Surg 1996;224:463–475

Five-Year Survival (Cholangiocarcinoma and Gallbladder Cancer)*

Stage IA	85–100%
Stage IB	30–40% to 70–90%
Stage II	10–60%
Stage III	10–40%
Stage IV	0%

*Statistics for gallbladder cancer not certain because few cases reported in the literature

Staging

Gallbladder Cancer

Primary Tumor (T)	
TX	Primary tumor cannot be assessed
T0	No evidence of primary tumor
Tis	Carcinoma *in situ*
T1	Tumor invades lamina propria or muscular layer
T1a	Tumor invades lamina propria
T1b	Tumor invades muscular layer
T2	Tumor invades perimuscular connective tissue; no extension beyond serosa or into liver
T3	Tumor perforates the serosa (visceral peritoneum) and/or directly invades the liver and/or one other adjacent organ or structure, such as the stomach, duodenum, colon, pancreas, omentum, or extrahepatic bile ducts
T4	Tumor invades main portal vein or hepatic artery or invades 2 or more extrahepatic organs or structures

Regional Lymph Nodes (N)	
NX	Regional lymph nodes cannot be assessed
N0	No regional lymph node metastasis
N1	Metastases to nodes along the cystic duct, common bile duct, hepatic artery, and/or portal vein
N2	Metastases to periaortic, pericaval, superior mesentery artery, and/or celiac artery lymph nodes

Distant Metastasis (M)

M0	No distant metastasis		
M1	Distant metastasis		

Group	T	N	M
0	Tis	N0	M0
I	T1	N0	M0
II	T2	N0	M0
IIIA	T3	N0	M0
IIIB	T1-3	N1	M0
IVA	T4	N0-1	M0
IVB	Any T	N 2	M0
	Any T	Any N	M1

Intrahepatic Bile Duct Staging

Primary Tumor (T)	
TX	Primary tumor cannot be assessed
T0	No evidence of primary tumor
Tis	Carcinoma *in situ* (intraductal tumor)
T1	Solitary tumor without vascular invasion
T2a	Solitary tumor with vascular invasion
T2b	Multiple tumors, with or without vascular invasion
T3	Tumor perforating the visceral peritoneum or involving the local extra hepatic structures by direct invasion
T4	Tumor with periductal invasion

Regional Lymph Nodes (N)	
NX	Regional lymph nodes cannot be assessed
N0	No regional lymph node metastasis
N1	Regional lymph node metastasis present

Distant Metastasis (M)

M0	No distant metastasis		
M1	Distant metastasis		

Group	T	N	M
0	Tis	N0	M0
I	T1	N0	M0
II	T2	N0	M0
III	T3	N0	M0
IVA	T4	N0	M0
IVB	Any T	N1	M0
	Any T	Any N	M1

(continued)

Staging (continued)

Perihilar Bile Ducts Staging

Primary Tumor (T)	
TX	Primary tumor cannot be assessed
T0	No evidence of primary tumor
Tis	Carcinoma *in situ*
T1	Tumor confined to the bile duct, with extension up to the muscle layer or fibrous tissue
T2a	Tumor invades beyond the wall of the bile duct to surrounding adipose tissue
T2b	Tumor invades adjacent hepatic parenchyma
T3	Tumor invades unilateral branches of the portal vein or hepatic artery
T4	Tumor invades main portal vein or its branches bilaterally; or the common hepatic artery; or the second-order biliary radicals bilaterally; or unilateral second-order biliary radicals with contralateral portal vein or hepatic artery involvement

Regional Lymph Nodes (N)	
NX	Regional lymph nodes cannot be assessed
N0	No regional lymph node metastasis
N1	Regional lymph node metastasis (including nodes along the cystic duct, common bile duct, hepatic artery, and portal vein)
N2	Metastasis to periaortic, pericaval, superior mesentery artery, and/or celiac artery lymph nodes

Distant Metastasis (M)	
M0	No distant metastasis
M1	Distant metastasis

Distal Bile Duct Staging

Primary Tumor (T)	
TX	Primary tumor cannot be assessed
T0	No evidence of primary tumor
Tis	Carcinoma *in situ*
T1	Tumor confined to the bile duct histologically
T2	Tumor invades beyond the wall of the bile duct
T3	Tumor invades the gallbladder, pancreas, duodenum or other adjacent organs without involvement of the celiac axis, or the superior mesenteric artery
T4	Tumor involves the celiac axis, or the superior mesenteric artery

Regional Lymph Nodes (N)	
NX	Regional lymph nodes cannot be assessed
N0	No regional lymph node metastasis
N1	Regional lymph node metastasis

Distant Metastasis (M)			
M0	No distant metastasis		
M1	Distant metastasis		
Group	T	N	M
0	Tis	N0	M0
IA	T1	N0	M0
IB	T2	N0	M0
IIA	T3	N0	M0
IIB	T1	N1	M0
IIB	T2	N1	M0
IIB	T3	N1	M0
III	T4	Any N	M0
IV	Any T	Any N	M1

Edge SB, Byrd DR, Compton CC, Fritz AG, Greene FL, Trotti A, editors. AJCC Cancer Staging Manual. 7th ed. New York: Springer; 2010

Expert Opinion

Biliary tract malignancies include carcinoma of the gallbladder as well as of the intrahepatic, perihilar, and distal bile ducts. Complete surgical resection remains the only curative modality for gallbladder cancer (cholecystectomy, en bloc hepatic resection, and lymphadenectomy with or without bile duct excision). Postoperative therapy for patients who undergo an operative resection might be considered with adjuvant chemotherapy and/or fluoropyrimidine-based radiochemotherapy, in selected cases. Patients with unresectable tumor without obvious metastatic disease and without jaundice may benefit from a regimen of fluorouracil- or capecitabine-based chemotherapy $\pm$ radiation. Metastatic disease is typically treated with systemic chemotherapy. Interventional procedures including brachytherapy and photodynamic therapy represent a therapeutic option for selected patients. However, overall survival of such patients remains poor (Razumilava and Gores, 2013)

Less than 20% of all patients have disease that is deemed resectable, and even after having undergone potential curative resection, recurrence rates are high. Thus for the majority of patients, systemic chemotherapy is the mainstay of treatment. The problem concerning chemotherapy is the fact that most studies conducted in the past have been single-center, nonrandomized, phase II studies with relatively small patient numbers (Hezel and Zhu, 2008). Heterogeneous inclusion criteria, inherent difficulties in measuring tumor response, and the lack of studies having applied RECIST (Response Evaluation Criteria in Solid Tumors) methodology for confirmation of treatment effects further contribute to our limited knowledge how to best treat patients with advanced tumors (Eckel and Schmid, 2007)

In the absence of validated data from prospective randomized studies, patients with biliary cancer were usually treated with gemcitabine or fluoropyrimidines $\pm$ platinum compounds. This, however, changed with the publication of the results from the ABC-01 trial that evaluated patients with locally advanced or metastatic cholangiocarcinoma, gallbladder cancer, or ampullary cancer (Valle et al, 2010). After a median follow-up of 8.2 months, the median overall survival was 11.7 months in the cisplatin plus gemcitabine group and 8.1 months in the gemcitabine group (HR, 0.64; 95% CI, 0.52 to 0.80; $P < 0.001$). The median progression-free survival was 8 months in the cisplatin plus gemcitabine group and 5 months in the gemcitabine-only group ($P < 0.001$). Adverse events were similar in both groups, with the exception of neutropenia—higher in the cisplatin plus gemcitabine group—although the number of neutropenia-associated infections was similar in the 2 groups. Consequently, a cisplatin + gemcitabine regimen has become the standard of care on this indication

Novel agents, such as epidermal growth factor receptor blockers, MEK inhibitors and angiogenesis inhibitors, may hold promise for improving the therapeutic results obtained with conventional chemotherapy alone, but clinical study results are pending (Sasaki et al, 2013)

Intrahepatic cholangiocarcinoma
Patients who have undergone a tumor resection with or without ablation with negative margins may be followed up with observation, because there is no definitive adjuvant regimen to improve their overall survival. For individuals whose disease is resectable but who are left with positive margins after resection: (a) consider additional resection, (b) ablative therapy, or (c) combined radiation with or without chemotherapy using either fluorouracil- or capecitabine-based regimens or gemcitabine (Horgan et al, 2012). For patients with unresectable disease, therapeutic options include, depending on tumor location, extent of disease, and performance status: (a) chemotherapy with cisplatin plus gemcitabine or a fluorouracil- or capecitabine-based regimen, (b) combined radiochemotherapy, or (c) best supportive care

Extrahepatic cholangiocarcinoma
Patients with positive margins after resection should be considered candidates for either cisplatin plus gemcitabine or fluorouracil- or capecitabine-based chemotherapy with radiation (external beam therapy or brachytherapy) (Valero et al, 2012). The addition of adjuvant therapy in patients after potential curative surgical resection remains a subject of clinical investigation. Patients whose disease is deemed unresectable at the time of surgery should undergo biliary drainage if required, ideally nonsurgically; that is, by using a stent. Photodynamic therapy has demonstrated to be even more effective than stenting alone (Ortner et al, 2003). Given their overall poor prognosis, further options for patients with unresectable disease, include: (a) chemotherapy with cisplatin plus gemcitabine, (b) a clinical trial, (c) chemoradiation (fluorouracil- or capecitabine-based chemotherapy/RT), and (d) best supportive care

Eckel F et al. Br J Cancer 2007;96:896–902
Hezel AF et al. Oncologist 2008;13:415–423
Horgan AM et al. J Clin Oncol 2012; 30:1934–1940
Ortner ME et al. Gastroenterology 2003;125:1355–1363
Razumilava N, Gores GJ. Clin Gastroenterol Hepatol 2013;11:13–21
Sasaki T et al. Korean J Intern Med 2013;28:515–524
Valero V et al. Expert Rev Gastroenterol Hepatol 2012;6:481–495
Valle J et al. N Engl J Med 2010;362:1273–1281

(continued)

Expert Opinion (continued)

First-Line Chemotherapy in Advanced Biliary Cancer
Phase III and Randomized Phase II Trials

Regimen	#	%RR	PFS/TTP*		OS*		References
Phase III							
GEM + CDDP	204	26.1[†]	8.0	P<0.001	11.7	HR = 0.64 (95% CI, 0.52–0.80) P<0.001	Valle
GEM	206	15.5[†]	5.0		8.1		
GEM + oxaliplatin	26	30.8[‡]	8.5	P<0.001	9.5	P = 0.039	Sharma
5-FU + folinic acid	28	14.3[‡]	3.5		4.6		
BSC	27	0	2.8		4.5		
Randomized Phase II							
GEM + CDDP	41	19.5	5.8	HR = 0.66 (95% CI, 0.41–1.05) P = 0.077	11.2	HR = 0.69 (95% CI, 0.42–1.13) P = 0.139	Okusaka
GEM	42	11.9	3.7		7.7		
GEM + S-1	30	20.0	5.6	95% CI 2.0–10.5	8.9	95% CI 5.8–11.9	Sasaki
GEM	32	9.4	4.3	95% CI 1.9–5.7	9.2	95% CI 5.2–14.6	
GEM + S-1	51	36.4	7.1	HR = 0.437 (95% CI, 0.286–0.669) P<0.0001	12.5	HR = 0.859 (95% CI, 0.543–1.360) P = 0.52	Morizane
S-1	50	17.4	4.2		9.0		
GEM + CDDP	49	19.6	5.7	HR = 0.85 (95% CI 0.52–1.36) P = 0.488	10.1	HR = 0.72 (95% CI 0.45–1.17) P = 0.187	Kang
S-1 + CDDP	47	23.8	5.4		9.9		

#, number of patients enrolled; %RR, percent response rate; BSC, best supportive care; CDDP, cisplatin; 5FU, Fluorouracil; GEM, gemcitabine; S-1, an oral anticancer drug, consisting of the fluorouracil prodrug tegafur and 2 biochemical modulators, 5-chloro-2,4-dihydroxypyridine (CDHP) and potassium oxonate (Oxo)
*Median values in months
[†]Not significant
[‡]p<0.001

Kang et al. Acta Oncol 2012;51:860–866
Morizane et al. Cancer Sci 2013;104:1211–1216
Okusaka et al. Br J Cancer 2010;103(4):469–474
Sasaki et al. Cancer Chemother Pharmacol 2013;71:973–979
Sharma et al. J Clin Oncol 2010;28:4581–4586
Valle J et al. N Engl J Med 2010;362:1273–1281

ADVANCED DISEASE REGIMEN
CISPLATIN + GEMCITABINE

Valle J et al. N Engl J Med 2010;362:1273–1281

Note: Biliary obstruction per se is not considered to be disease progression in the absence of radiologically confirmed disease progression, and treatment can be recommenced after initial or further biliary stenting and normalization of liver function

Hydration before cisplatin: ≥1000 mL 0.9% sodium chloride injection (0.9% NS); administer by intravenous infusion over ≥1 hour

Cisplatin 25 mg/m² per dose; administer intravenously in 50–1000 mL 0.9% NS over 1 hour for 2 doses on days 1 and 8, every 3 weeks for 4 cycles (total dosage/cycle = 50 mg/m²), *followed by:*

Hydration after cisplatin: ≥1000 mL 0.9% NS; administer by intravenous infusion over ≥1 hour

Gemcitabine 1000 mg/m² per dose; administer intravenously in 50–250 mL 0.9% NS over 30 minutes for 2 doses on days 1 and 8, every 3 weeks, for 4 cycles (total dosage/cycle = 2000 mg/m²)
• Gemcitabine may be administered concurrently with hydration after cisplatin administration is completed

Note: In the absence of disease progression at 12 weeks, treatment with the same regimen may continue for an additional 12 weeks

Supportive Care
Antiemetic prophylaxis
Emetogenic potential is **HIGH**
See Chapter 39 for antiemetic recommendations

Hematopoietic growth factor (CSF) prophylaxis
Primary prophylaxis is NOT indicated
See Chapter 43 for more information

Antimicrobial prophylaxis
Risk of fever and neutropenia is LOW
   Antimicrobial primary prophylaxis to be considered:
    • Antibacterial—not indicated
    • Antifungal—not indicated
    • Antiviral—not indicated, unless patient previously had an episode of HSV
See Chapter 47 for more information

Treatment Modifications

Adverse Event	Dose Modification
Cisplatin	
Any G ≥3 adverse event Hematologic toxicity, abnormal renal function, nausea, vomiting, edema, or tinnitus	Decrease cisplatin dosage by 25%
Reduction in creatinine clearance* to ≤60% of onstudy value	Delay therapy 1 week. If creatinine clearance does not recover to pretreatment values, then consider reducing cisplatin dose
Creatinine clearance* 40–60 mL/min (0.66–1 mL/s)	Consider reducing cisplatin so that dose in milligrams equals the creatinine clearance* value in mL/min (mL/s × 1/0.0166)†
Creatinine clearance* <40 mL/min (<0.66 mL/s)	Hold cisplatin
Clinically significant ototoxicity	Discontinue cisplatin
Persistent (>14 days) peripheral neuropathy without functional impairment	Decrease cisplatin dosage by 50%
Clinically significant sensory loss— persistent (>14 days) peripheral neuropathy with functional impairment	Discontinue cisplatin
Day 1 WBC count <2000/mm³ or platelet count <100,000/mm³	Delay cisplatin and gemcitabine for 1 week or until myelosuppression resolves
Recurrent treatment delay because of myelosuppression	Delay cisplatin for 1 week, or until myelosuppression resolves, then decrease cisplatin and gemcitabine dosages by 25% during subsequent treatments
Sepsis during an episode of neutropenia	

*Creatinine clearance is used as a measure of glomerular filtration rate
†This also applies to patients with creatinine clearance (GFR) of 40–60 mL/min at the outset of treatment

Patient Population Studied

Patients with a diagnosis of nonresectable, recurrent, or metastatic biliary tract carcinoma (intrahepatic or extrahepatic cholangiocarcinoma, gallbladder cancer, or ampullary carcinoma); an Eastern Cooperative Oncology Group performance status of 0, 1, or 2; and an estimated life expectancy of more than 3 months. Other eligibility criteria included a total bilirubin level ≤1.5 times the upper limit of the normal range; liver-enzyme levels that were ≤5 times the upper limit of the normal range; renal function with levels of serum urea and serum creatinine that were <1.5 times the upper limit of the normal range; and an estimated glomerular filtration rate ≥45 mL/minute (≥0.75 mL/s)

Efficacy (N = 161)*

	All Patients (N = 161)	Gallbladder Tumors[†] (N = 61)	Bile Duct and Ampullary Tumors[†] (N = 100)
Complete response	0.6%	0	1%
Partial response	25.5%	37.7%	18%
Stable disease[‡]	55.3%	47.5%	60%
Progressive disease	18.6%	14.8%	21%
Median progression-free survival	8.0 months	—	—
Median overall survival	11.7 months	—	—

*RECIST (Response Evaluation Criteria in Solid Tumors) (Therasse P et al. J Natl Cancer Inst 2000;92:205–216)
[†]No differences in RR between gallbladder and cholangiocarcinoma subgroups
[‡]Not defined

Toxicity (N = 198)

	% G3/4
Hematologic	
Decreased WBC	15.7
Decreased platelet counts	8.6
Decreased hemoglobin concentration	7.6
Decreased ANC	25.3
Any hematologic toxic effect	32.3
Liver Function	
Increased alanine amino transferase level	9.6
Other abnormal liver function	13.1
Any abnormal liver function	16.7
Nonhematologic	
Alopecia	1
Anorexia	3
Fatigue	18.7
Nausea	4
Vomiting	5.1
Impaired renal function	1.5
Infection	
Without neutropenia	6.1
With neutropenia	10.1
Biliary sepsis	4.0
Any type	18.2
Deep vein thrombosis	2.0
Thromboembolic event	3.5
Other	54.5
Any G3/4 toxic effect	70.7

NCI Common Terminology Criteria for Adverse Events v3.0

Therapy Monitoring

1. *Between days 8 and 10:* CBC with differential
2. *Before each cycle:* Electrolytes, renal function, LFTs
3. *Response assessment:* Every 2–3 cycles

ADVANCED DISEASE REGIMEN
GEMCITABINE + OXALIPLATIN (GEMOX)

André T et al. Ann Oncol 2004;15:1339–1343

Gemcitabine 1000 mg/m²; administer by intravenous infusion in 250 mL 0.9% sodium chloride injection at an infusion rate of 10 mg/m² per minute (over 100 minutes) on day 1, every 2 weeks (total dosage every 2 weeks = 1000 mg/m²)

Oxaliplatin 100 mg/m²; administer by intravenous infusion in 250–500 mL of 5% dextrose injection over 2 hours on day 2, every 2 weeks (total dosage every 2 weeks = 100 mg/m²)

Supportive Care
Antiemetic prophylaxis
Emetogenic potential with gemcitabine (day 1) is **LOW**
Emetogenic potential with oxaliplatin (day 2) is **MODERATE**
See Chapter 39 for antiemetic recommendations

Hematopoietic growth factor (CSF) prophylaxis
Primary prophylaxis is NOT indicated
See Chapter 43 for more information

Antimicrobial prophylaxis
Risk of fever and neutropenia is LOW
  Antimicrobial primary prophylaxis to be considered:
  • Antibacterial—not indicated
  • Antifungal—not indicated
  • Antiviral—not indicated unless patient previously had an episode of HSV
See Chapter 47 for more information

Treatment Modifications

Adverse Event	Dose Modification
Nadir WBC <1000/mm³, ANC <500/mm³, or platelets <50,000/mm³	Decrease gemcitabine and oxaliplatin dosages by 25% in subsequent cycles
G ≥3 nonhematologic adverse event during the previous treatment cycle	
WBC <3000/mm³ or platelets <75,000/mm³ on day of treatment	Delay chemotherapy for up to 2 weeks
Treatment delay >2 weeks for recovery from hematologic adverse events	Discontinue treatment

Therapy Monitoring

1. *Every week:* CBCs with differential
2. *Before each cycle:* Complete biochemical profile
3. *Response assessment:* Every 2 months

Patient Population Studied

A study of 33 patients with advanced biliary tract carcinoma

Efficacy (N = 31)*

Overall response rate	35.5%
Stable disease	26%
Progressive disease	38.5%
Median progression-free survival	5.7 months
Overall survival	14.3 months

*André T et al. Ann Oncol 2004;15:1339–1343

Complete Response	7.7%
Partial Response	23%
Stable Disease	38%
Progressive Disease	31%
Median Overall Survival	9.5 months
Median Progression-free Survival	8.5 months

Sharma et al. J Clin Oncol 2010;28:4581–4586

Toxicity (N = 56)

G3 Neutropenia	12.5%
G3 Thrombocytopenia	9%
Peripheral sensory neuropathy	7.1%
G2 Alopecia	5.3%
G3 Nausea/vomiting	3.5%
G3 Diarrhea	—

NCI, CTC, National Cancer Institute (USA) Common Toxicity Criteria, version 2.0. At: http://ctep.cancer.gov/protocolDevelopment/electronic_applications/ctc.htm [accessed December 7, 2013]

ADVANCED DISEASE REGIMEN

GEMCITABINE + CAPECITABINE

Koeberle D et al. J Clin Oncol 2008;26:3702–3708

Gemcitabine 1000 mg/m^2 per dose; administer intravenously in 50–250 mL 0.9% Sodium Chloride Injection over 30 minutes for 2 doses on days 1 and 8, every 3 weeks (total dosage/cycle = 2000 mg/m^2)

Capecitabine 650 mg/m^2 per dose; administer orally twice daily (approximately every 12 hours) for 14 consecutive days (28 doses), days 1–14, every 3 weeks (total dosage/cycle = 18,200 mg/m^2)

Supportive Care
Antiemetic prophylaxis
Emetogenic potential is LOW
See Chapter 39 for antiemetic recommendations

Hematopoietic growth factor (CSF) prophylaxis
Primary prophylaxis is NOT indicated
See Chapter 43 for more information

Antimicrobial prophylaxis
Risk of fever and neutropenia is LOW
  Antimicrobial primary prophylaxis to be considered:
  • Antibacterial—not indicated
  • Antifungal—not indicated
  • Antiviral—not indicated, unless patient previously had an episode of HSV
See Chapter 47 for more information

Treatment Modifications

Adverse Event	Dose Modification
Nadir WBC <1000/mm^3, ANC <500/mm^3, or Platelets <50,000/mm^3	Delay chemotherapy for up to 3 weeks until adverse events are G ≤1, then reduce gemcitabine dosage by 25%
Any G3 nonhematologic toxicity during a previous cycle	Delay chemotherapy for up to 3 weeks until adverse events are G ≤1, then decrease gemcitabine and capecitabine dosages by 25%
Any G4 nonhematologic toxicity during a previous cycle	Delay chemotherapy for up to 3 weeks until adverse events are G ≤1, then decrease gemcitabine and capecitabine dosages by 50%

Patient Population Studied

A study of 44 chemotherapy-naïve patients with unresectable, locally advanced or metastatic biliary tract cancer. Patients were required to be symptomatic and have at least 1 of the following characteristics at baseline: Karnofsky performance score between 60 and 80, average analgesic consumption of ≥10 mg of morphine equivalents per day, and average pain intensity score of ≥20 mm out of a maximum of 100 mm based on a linear analog self-assessment (LASA ≥2/10) scale. No prior chemotherapy for advanced disease was allowed

Efficacy (N = 44)

Complete response	1 (2%)
Partial responses	10 (23%)
Stable disease*	24 (55%)
Progression/nonassessable	9 (20%)
Median time to progression	7.2 months
Median overall survival	13.2 months

*Stable disease lasting for ≥8 weeks
RECIST Criteria (Response Evaluation Criteria in Solid Tumors) (Therasse P et al. J Natl Cancer Inst 2000;92:205–216)

Toxicity (N = 44)

	% G1/2	% G3/4
Hematologic		
Anemia	91	2
Leukocytopenia	71	11
Thrombocytopenia	63	7
Nonhematologic		
Nausea	50	5
Vomiting	32	2
Diarrhea	21	2
Stomatitis	9	0
Anorexia	52	7
Fatigue	62	11
Hand-foot syndrome	11	0

NCI, CTC, National Cancer Institute (USA) Common Toxicity Criteria, version 2.0. At: http://ctep.cancer.gov/protocolDevelopment/electronic_applications/ctc.htm [accessed December 7, 2013]

Therapy Monitoring

1. *Between days 8 and 10:* CBC with differential
2. *Before each cycle:* Electrolytes, renal function, LFTs
3. *Response assessment:* Every 3 cycles

ADVANCED DISEASE REGIMEN

CAPECITABINE + OXALIPLATIN

Nehls O et al. Br J Cancer 2008;98:309–315

Capecitabine 1000 mg/m^2 per dose; administer orally twice daily (approximately every 12 hours) for 14 consecutive days (28 doses) on days 1–14, every 3 weeks (total dosage/cycle = 28,000 mg/m^2)

Oxaliplatin 130 mg/m^2; administer intravenously in 250–500 mL 5% dextrose injection over 2 hours on day 1, every 3 weeks (total dosage/cycle = 130 mg/m^2)

Supportive Care

Antiemetic prophylaxis
Emetogenic potential for oxaliplatin is **MODERATE**
Emetogenic potential on days with capecitabine alone is **LOW**
See Chapter 39 for antiemetic recommendations

Hematopoietic growth factor (CSF) prophylaxis
Primary prophylaxis is NOT indicated
See Chapter 43 for more information

Antimicrobial prophylaxis
Risk of fever and neutropenia is LOW
    Antimicrobial primary prophylaxis to be considered:
- Antibacterial—not indicated
- Antifungal—not indicated
- Antiviral—not indicated, unless patient previously had an episode of HSV

See Chapter 47 for more information

Treatment Modifications

Adverse Event	Dose Modification
Capecitabine	
Any G ≥2 adverse event except alopecia	Interrupt/delay capecitabine until adverse event improves to G ≤1, and decrease capecitabine dosage by 25% during subsequent cycles
Second occurrence of G ≥2 adverse event	Interrupt/delay capecitabine until adverse event improves to G ≤1 and decrease capecitabine dosage by 50% during subsequent cycles
Third occurrence of G ≥2 adverse event	Discontinue capecitabine use permanently
Oxaliplatin	
Any G ≥3 adverse event	Decrease oxaliplatin dosage by 25%
Persistent (>14 days) peripheral neuropathy without functional impairment	Decrease oxaliplatin dosage by 50%
Persistent (>14 days) peripheral neuropathy with functional impairment	Discontinue oxaliplatin use permanently

Patient Population Studied

A study of 65 chemotherapy-naïve patients with advanced biliary tract cancer (adenocarcinomas of the gallbladder [GBC] or the intrahepatic [ICC] or extrahepatic [ECC] biliary tract) not amenable to curative surgical treatment strategies, ECOG performance status ≤2. Patients were stratified prospectively between 2 groups based on location of the primary, that is, gallbladder cancer or extrahepatic cholangiocarcinoma versus intrahepatic cholangiocarcinoma

Efficacy*

	GBC/ECC (N = 47)	ICC (N = 18)
Complete response	2 (4%)	0
Partial response	11 (23%)	0
Stable disease†	23 (49%)	6 (33%)
Progression	11 (23%)	12 (67%)
Median time to progression	6.5 months	2.2 months
Median overall survival	12.8 months	5.2 months

*WHO Criteria
†Stable disease was defined as a reduction <50% for an unspecified duration or an increase <25% of measurable lesions according to the previous method, with the absence of any new lesions

Toxicity (N = 65)

	% G2	% G3	% G4
Hematologic			
Anemia	18	0	0
Neutropenia	14	0	2
Thrombocytopenia	20	9	2
Nonhematologic			
Nausea/vomiting	29	6	0
Diarrhea	18	5	2
Stomatitis	2	0	0
Hand-foot syndrome	9	5	NA
Infection	15	0	3
Thromboembolic event	0	0	2
Peripheral neuropathy	35	15	2

NCI, CTC, National Cancer Institute (USA) Common Toxicity Criteria, version 2.0. At: http://ctep.cancer.gov/protocolDevelopment/electronic_applications/ctc.htm [accessed December 7, 2013]

Therapy Monitoring

1. *Between days 8 and 10:* CBC with differential
2. *Before each cycle:* Electrolytes, renal function, LFTs
3. *Response assessment:* Every 2–3 cycles

REGIMEN

GEMCITABINE

Penz M et al. Ann Oncol 2001;12:183–186

Gemcitabine 2200 mg/m²; administer by intravenous infusion in 250 mL 0.9% sodium chloride injection over 30 minutes on day 1, every 2 weeks for 6 months (total dosage per 2-week cycle = 2200 mg/m²)

Supportive Care
Antiemetic prophylaxis
Emetogenic potential is LOW
See Chapter 39 for antiemetic recommendations

Hematopoietic growth factor (CSF) prophylaxis
Primary prophylaxis is NOT indicated
See Chapter 43 for more information

Antimicrobial prophylaxis
Risk of fever and neutropenia is LOW
   Antimicrobial primary prophylaxis to be considered:
   • Antibacterial—not indicated
   • Antifungal—not indicated
   • Antiviral—not indicated, unless patient previously had an episode of HSV
See Chapter 47 for more information

Patient Population Studied

A study of 32 chemotherapy-naïve patients with locally advanced or metastatic biliary tract cancer

Efficacy (N = 32)

Overall response rate	21.9%
Stable disease	43.7%
Progressive disease	34.4%
Median progression-free survival	5.6 months
Median overall survival	11.5 months

WHO criteria

Toxicity (N = 32)

	% G1	% G2	% G3
Hematologic			
Neutropenia	19	22	6
Thrombocytopenia	12	3	6
Anemia	31	25	3
Nonhematologic			
Nausea/vomiting	22	22	—
Diarrhea	3	9	—
Constipation	6	3	—
Stomatitis	6	3	—
Fatigue	22	9	—
Alopecia	6	12	—
Fever	9	12	—
Cutaneous	6	3	—
Serum transaminases	12	9	—

No grade 4 toxicities
WHO criteria

Treatment Modifications

Adverse Event	Dose Modification
Nadir WBC <1000/mm³, ANC <500/mm³, or platelets <50,000/mm³	Reduce gemcitabine dosage by 25% in subsequent cycles
G ≥3 nonhematologic adverse event during the previous treatment cycle	
WBC <3000/mm³ or platelets <75,000/mm³ on day of treatment	Delay chemotherapy for up to 2 weeks
Treatment delay >2 weeks for recovery from hematologic adverse event	Discontinue treatment

Therapy Monitoring

1. *Every week:* CBCs with differential LFTs
2. *Before each cycle:* Complete biochemical profile
3. *Response assessment:* Every 2 months

REGIMEN

MITOMYCIN + CAPECITABINE

Kornek GV et al. Ann Oncol 2004;15:478–483

Mitomycin 8 mg/m^2; administer by intravenous injection over 2–3 minutes on day 1, every 4 weeks (total dosage/cycle = 8 mg/m^2)

Capecitabine 1000 mg/m^2 per dose; administer orally twice daily (approximately every 12 hours) for 14 consecutive days (28 doses) on days 1–14, every 4 weeks (total dosage/cycle = 28,000 mg/m^2)

(Capecitabine is taken with water within 30 minutes after food ingestion)

Supportive Care

Antiemetic prophylaxis
*Emetogenic potential with capecitabine with or without mitomycin is **LOW***
See Chapter 39 for antiemetic recommendations

Hematopoietic growth factor (CSF) prophylaxis
Primary prophylaxis is NOT indicated
See Chapter 43 for more information

Antimicrobial prophylaxis
Risk of fever and neutropenia is LOW
 Antimicrobial primary prophylaxis to be considered:
 • Antibacterial—not indicated
 • Antifungal—not indicated
 • Antiviral—not indicated, unless patient previously had an episode of HSV
See Chapter 47 for more information

Treatment Modifications

Adverse Event	Dose Modification
Nadir WBC <1000/mm^3, ANC <500/mm^3, or platelets <50,000/mm^3	Delay chemotherapy for up to 2 weeks until adverse events are G ≤1, then decrease subsequent mitomycin and capecitabine dosages by 25%
Any G ≥3 nonhematologic adverse events during the previous treatment cycle	
Duration of treatment delay >2 weeks for recovery from adverse events	Discontinue treatment

Therapy Monitoring

1. *Weekly:* CBC with differential
2. *Before each cycle:* Biochemical profile
3. *Response assessment:* Every 2 cycles

Patient Population Studied

A study of 26 chemotherapy-naïve patients with advanced biliary tract cancer

Efficacy (N = 26)

Partial responses	30.8%
Stable disease	34.6%
Progressive disease	34.6%
Median progression-free survival	5.35 months
Median overall survival	9.25 months

WHO Criteria

Toxicity (N = 24)

	% G1/2	% G3
Hematologic		
Neutropenia	N/A	17
Thrombocytopenia	48	17
Nonhematologic		
Nausea/vomiting	42	—
Fatigue	42	—
Diarrhea	28	—
Hand-foot syndrome	17	—
Alopecia	12	—
Increased liver function results*	54	—

Fever without documented infection: 8%

*Possibly a result of progressive disease because >80% of patients had liver involvement
WHO criteria

4. Bladder Cancer

Andrea Apolo, MD and Dean Bajorin, MD

Epidemiology

Incidence: 74,690 (male: 56,390; female: 18,300 Estimated new cases for 2014 in the United States)
20.7 per 100,000 male and female per year (36.6 per 100,000 men, 8.9 per 100,000 women)

Deaths: Estimated 15,580 in 2014 (male: 11,170; female: 4,410)

Median age: Seventh decade

Male to female ratio: 3:1

Stage at Presentation:

Stage I:	70%
Stages II/III:	25%
Stage IV:	5%

Siegel R et al. CA Cancer J Clin 2014;64:9–29
Surveillance, Epidemiology and End Results (SEER) Program, available from http://seer.cancer.gov (accessed in 2013)

Work-up

Stage I	H&P, cystoscopy, exam under anesthesia, transurethral resection of the bladder tumor (TURBT), and cytology. Consider CT or MRI of the abdomen and pelvis prior to TURBT if sessile or high grade. Consider upper tract imaging with either CT urogram, retrograde pyelogram, or intravenous pyelogram (IVP). Transurethral biopsy of prostate if clinically indicated
Stages II/III	H&P, cystoscopy, exam under anesthesia, TURBT, and cytology. CT or MRI of the abdomen and pelvis prior to TURBT. CT of chest. Consider upper tract imaging with either CT urogram, retrograde pyelogram, or IVP. Bone scan if alkaline phosphatase is elevated or symptoms. Transurethral biopsy of prostate if clinically indicated
Stage IV	H&P, cystoscopy, exam under anesthesia, TURBT, and cytology. CT or MRI of the abdomen and pelvis prior to TURBT. CT of chest. Upper tract imaging with either CT urogram, retrograde pyelogram, or IVP. Bone scan if alkaline phosphatase is elevated or symptoms

Pathology

Transitional cell carcinoma	90–95%
Squamous cell carcinoma	5%
Adenocarcinoma	2%
Small cell carcinoma	1%

Histopathologic evaluation should include a description of cell type(s), whether or not there are areas of differing differentiation and the extent of differentiation, whether the tumor is a micropapillary or nested variant, grade (low [G1] vs. high [G2, G3]), presence or absence of lymphatic invasion, the depth of invasion, and whether or not there is muscle in the specimen. Pathologic grade is important in the management of noninvasive tumors

McDougal WS et al. Cancer of the bladder, ureter, and renal pelvis. In: Devita VT, Lawrence TS, Rosenberg SA, eds. Cancer: Principles and Practice of Oncology. Philadelphia: Lippincott Williams and Wilkins, 2008

Expert Opinion

1. MVAC is the historic standard of care for systemic therapy of patients with metastatic bladder cancer based on high response rates and cure in a subset of patients. A phase III trial demonstrated that the 2-drug doublet of gemcitabine and cisplatin (GC) and MVAC are similar in response and survival but that GC has a better toxicity profile. A phase III trial compared dose dense or high dose (DD) MVAC (plus granulocyte-colony stimulating factor (G-CSF) on 2 week cycles) to standard MVAC (on a 4-week cycle) [1–2]. Although there was no significant difference in median survival, DD MVAC was superior in response rate, 5-year survival rates and progression fee survival. DD- M-VAC is another first-line chemotherapy option for metastatic bladder cancer

   After completion of therapy, imaging with CT or MRI of the abdomen and pelvis, chest x-ray or CT of the chest, urine cytology (if applicable), creatinine and electrolytes recommended at 3–6 month intervals for 2 years and then as clinically indicated

(continued)

Staging

Primary Tumors of the Bladder (T)

TX	Primary tumor cannot be assessed
T0	No evidence of primary tumor
Ta	Noninvasive papillary carcinoma
Tis	Carcinoma in situ (ie, flat tumor)
T1	Tumor invades subepithelial connective tissue
T2	Tumor invades muscularis propria
pT2a	Tumor invades superficial muscularis propria (inner half)
pT2b	Tumor invades deep muscularis propria (outer half)
T3	Tumor invades perivesical tissue
pT3a	Microscopically
pT3b	Macroscopically (extravesical mass)
T4	Tumor invades any of the following: prostatic stroma, seminal vesicles, uterus, vagina, pelvic wall, abdominal wall
T4a	Tumor invades the prostatic stroma, uterus, vagina
T4b	Tumor invades the pelvic wall, abdominal wall

Regional Lymph Nodes for Urothelial Tumors (N)

NX	Regional lymph nodes cannot be assessed
N0	No lymph node metastasis
N1	Single regional lymph node metastasis in the true pelvis (hypogastric, obturator, external iliac, or presacral node)
N2	Multiple regional lymph node metastases in the true pelvis (hypogastric, obturator, external iliac, or presacral node)
N3	Lymph node metastasis to the common iliac lymph nodes

Distant Metastasis for Urothelial Tumors (M)

M0	No distant metastasis
M1	Distant metastasis

Anatomic Stage

Stage 0a	Ta	N0	M0
Stage 0is	Tis	N0	M0
Stage I	T1	N0	M0
Stage II	T2a	N0	M0
	T2b	N0	M0
Stage III	T3a	N0	M0
	T3b	N0	M0
	T4a	N0	M0
Stage IV	T4b	N0	M0
	Any T	N1–3	M0
	Any T	any	M1

Edge SB, Byrd DR, Compton CC, Fritz AG, Greene FL, Trotti A, editors. AJCC Cancer Staging Manual. 7th ed. New York: Springer; 2010

Five-Year Survival*

Stage 0	98.4%
Stage I	87.7%
Stage II	62.6%
Stage III	45.5%
Stage IV	14.8%

*Lynch CF et al. Chapter 23. Cancer of the urinary bladder. In: Ries LAG, Young JL, Keel GE, Eisner MP, Lin YD, Horner M-J, eds. SEER Survival Monograph: Cancer Survival Among Adults: U.S. SEER Program, 1988–2001, Patient and Tumor Characteristics. Bethesda, MD, National Cancer Institute, SEER Program, NIH Pub. No. 07-6215, 2007

Expert Opinion (continued)

2. Because MVAC includes doxorubicin, the regimen should be avoided in patients with preexisting cardiac disease unless cleared by a cardiologist familiar with doxorubicin-induced cardiac toxicity

3. Patients with marginal renal function (60–70 mL/min) may benefit from administering cisplatin divided over 2 days rather than over 1 day

4. Patients with inadequate renal function for cisplatin (creatinine clearance <60 mL/min [<1 mL/s]) and stage IV disease should be treated with carboplatin-based therapy. Gemcitabine and carboplatin is a regimen well-studied in randomized studies and is considered a standard of care based on a higher response rate and less toxicity than carboplatin, vinblastine, and methotrexate

5. Encourage neoadjuvant cisplatin-based chemotherapy (either DD MVAC or GC) in patients with muscle-invasive bladder cancer who have a good performance status and adequate renal function. Adjuvant chemotherapy is a consideration for patients at high risk of relapse after cystectomy if neoadjuvant chemotherapy was not administered

   After cystectomy, imaging with CT or MRI of the abdomen and pelvis, urine cytology, creatinine, and electrolytes recommended at 3–6 month intervals for 2 years and then as clinically indicated

6. Patients with metastatic bladder cancer, as well as those with organ-confined, muscle-invasive bladder cancer, should be considered for clinical trials

REGIMEN

METHOTREXATE + VINBLASTINE + DOXORUBICIN + CISPLATIN (MVAC)

von der Maase H et al. J Clin Oncol 2000;17:3068–3077
von der Maase H et al. J Clin Oncol 2005;21:4602–4608

Methotrexate 30 mg/m² per dose; administer by intravenous injection over 15–60 seconds for 3 doses on days 1, 15, and 22, every 28 days for a maximum of 6 cycles (total dosage/cycle = 90 mg/m²)

Vinblastine 3 mg/m² per dose; administer by intravenous injection over 1–2 minutes for 3 doses on days 2, 15, and 22, every 28 days for a maximum of 6 cycles (total dosage/cycle = 9 mg/m²)

Doxorubicin 30 mg/m²; administer by intravenous injection over 3–5 minutes on day 2, every 28 days for a maximum of 6 cycles (total dosage/cycle = 30 mg/m²)

Hydration before and after cisplatin administration: Administer intravenously ≥1000 mL 0.9% sodium chloride injection (0.9% NS) over at least 2 hours, both before and after cisplatin administration. Also encourage patients to increase oral intake of non-alcoholic fluids. Monitor serum electrolytes and replace as needed (potassium, magnesium, sodium)

Cisplatin 70 mg/m²; administer intravenously in 100–1000 mL 0.9% NS over 1 to 8 hours on day 2, every 28 days for a maximum of 6 cycles (total dosage/cycle = 70 mg/m²)

Supportive Care: Antiemetic prophylaxis
Emetogenic potential on days 1, 15, and 22: **LOW**
Emetogenic potential on day 2: **HIGH**. *Potential for delayed symptoms*
See Chapter 39 for antiemetic recommendations

Hematopoietic growth factor (CSF) prophylaxis
Primary prophylaxis may be indicated between doses of myelosuppressive chemotherapy
See Chapter 43 for more information

Antimicrobial prophylaxis
Risk of fever and neutropenia is LOW
Antimicrobial primary prophylaxis to be considered:
• Antibacterial—not indicated
• Antifungal—not indicated
• Antiviral—not indicated unless patient previously had an episode of HSV
See Chapter 47 for more information

Oral care: Encourage patients to maintain intake of non-alcoholic fluids
If mucositis or stomatitis is present:
• Rinse mouth several times a day with ¼ teaspoon (1.25 g) each of baking soda and table salt in one quart of warm water. Follow with a plain water rinse
• Do not use mouthwashes that contain alcohols

Patient Population Studied

Study of 202 patients with locally advanced or metastatic transitional cell urothelial cancer without prior systemic chemotherapy or immunotherapy. Prior local intravesical therapy, immunotherapy, or RT were allowed. Karnofsky Performance Status ≥70; and measured creatinine clearance ≥60 mL/min (≥1 mL/s)

Efficacy (N = 196)

Complete response	11.9%
Partial response	33.8%
Median overall survival	14.8 months
Median time to treatment failure	4.6 months
Median time to disease progression	7.4 months
Median duration of response	9.6 months

Therapy Monitoring

1. *Prior to each cycle:* CBC with differential count, serum electrolytes, BUN, creatinine, and LFTs
2. *Days 15 and 22:* CBC with differential count
3. *Response evaluation every 2–3 cycles:* CT or MRI of chest, abdomen or pelvis, or chest x-ray for lung lesions every 2–3 cycles. (von der Maase H et al. J Clin Oncol 2000;17:3068–3077)
4. *Follow-up after completion of therapy:* Imaging with CT or MRI of the abdomen and pelvis, chest x-ray or CT of the chest, urine cytology (if applicable), creatinine and electrolytes recommended at 3–6 months intervals for 2 years, and then as clinically indicated

Toxicity (N = 202)
(WHO Criteria)

Toxicity	% G3	% G4
Hematologic Toxicities		
Anemia	15.5	2.1
Thrombocytopenia	7.7	12.9
Neutropenia	17.1	65.2
Nonhematologic Toxicities		
Mucositis	17.7	4.2
Nausea	19.2	1.6
Alopecia	54.2	1.0
Infection	9.9	5.2
Diarrhea	7.8	0.5
Pulmonary	2.6	3.1
Hematuria	2.3	0
Constipation	2.6	0.5
Hemorrhage	2.1	0
State of consciousness	3.1	0.5
Fever	3.1	0

Treatment Modifications

Adverse Events	Treatment Modifications
Day 1 if WBC <3000/mm³, or platelet counts <100,000/mm³	Delay chemotherapy for 1 week
Day 15 or 22 if WBC ≤2900/mm³ or platelet count ≤74,000/mm³	Hold dose of methotrexate and vinblastine
G3/4 mucositis*	Reduce methotrexate dosage by 33% (all remaining doses and into next cycle)
Severe neurotoxicity	Reduce vinblastine dosage by 33%
Clinical evidence of CHF	Discontinue doxorubicin

*Leucovorin may be given 24 hours after methotrexate for patients who experienced G3/4 mucositis after previously administered doses

Notes

1. Give 6 cycles unless document disease progression
2. Avoid this regimen in patients with preexisting cardiac disease without guidance from a cardiologist familiar with effects of doxorubicin

BLADDER CANCER REGIMEN

GEMCITABINE + CISPLATIN (GC)

von der Maase H et al. J Clin Oncol 2000;17:3068–3077

Gemcitabine 1000 mg/m² per dose; administer intravenously in 50–250 mL 0.9% sodium chloride injection (0.9% NS) over 30–60 minutes for 3 doses on days 1, 8, and 15, every 28 days for a maximum of 6 cycles, (total dosage/cycle = 3000 mg/m²)

Hydration before and after cisplatin administration: ≥500 mL 0.9% NS intravenously over a minimum of 1 hour both before and after cisplatin. Encourage increased oral fluid intake
Cisplatin 70 mg/m²; administer intravenously in 100–250 mL 0.9% NS over 1 hour on day 2, every 28 days for a maximum of 6 cycles (total dosage/cycle = 70 mg/m²)

Supportive Care
Antiemetic prophylaxis
Emetogenic potential on days 1, 8, and 15: **LOW**
Emetogenic potential on day 2 is: **HIGH**. *Potential for delayed symptoms*
See Chapter 39 for antiemetic recommendations

Hematopoietic growth factor (CSF) prophylaxis
Primary prophylaxis may be indicated between doses of myelosuppressive chemotherapy
See Chapter 43 for more information

Antimicrobial prophylaxis
Risk of fever and neutropenia is LOW
  Antimicrobial primary prophylaxis to be considered:
  • Antibacterial—not indicated
  • Antifungal—not indicated
  • Antiviral—not indicated unless patient previously had an episode of HSV
See Chapter 47 for more information

Patient Population Studied

Study of 203 patients with locally advanced or metastatic transitional cell urothelial cancer without prior systemic chemotherapy or immunotherapy. Prior local intravesical therapy, immunotherapy, or RT were allowed. Karnofsky performance status ≥70; and measured creatinine clearance ≥60 mL/minute (≥1 mL/s)

Efficacy (N = 200)

Complete response	12.2%
Partial response	37.2%
Median overall survival	13.8 months
Median time to disease progression	5.4 months
Median time to treatment failure	7.8 months
Median duration of response	9.6 months

Treatment Modifications

Adverse Events	Treatment Modifications
Day 1 WBC count <3000/mm³ or platelet count <100,000/mm³	Hold chemotherapy until WBC count is >3000/mm³ and platelet count >100,000/mm³
Days 8 or 15 WBC count ≤1990/mm³ or platelet count ≤49,000/mm³	Omit gemcitabine on that day*
Treatment delay >4 weeks	Discontinue treatment

*Missed chemotherapy doses are not given. If gemcitabine is omitted on day 15, the cycle duration may be shortened to 21 days

Therapy Monitoring

1. *Prior to each cycle for 6 cycles:* CBC with differential count, serum electrolytes, BUN, and creatinine
2. *On all treatment days:* CBC with differential count
3. *Response evaluation every 2–3 cycles:* CT or MRI of chest, abdomen or pelvis, or chest x-ray for lung lesions every 2–3 cycles. (von der Maase H et al. J Clin Oncol 2000;17:3068–3077)
4. *Follow-up after completion of therapy:* Imaging with CT or MRI of the abdomen and pelvis, chest x-ray or CT of the chest, urine cytology (if applicable), creatinine and electrolytes recommended at 3–6 month intervals for 2 years, and then as clinically indicated

Notes

1. Give 6 cycles unless disease progression can be documented

Toxicity (N = 203)
(WHO Criteria)

Toxicity	% G3	% G4
Hematologic Toxicities		
Anemia	23.5	3.5
Thrombocytopenia	28.5	28.5
Neutropenia	41.2	29.9
Nonhematologic Toxicities		
Mucositis	1.0	0
Nausea	22	0
Alopecia	10.5	0
Infection	2.0	0.5
Diarrhea	3.0	0
Pulmonary	2.5	0.5
Hematuria	4.5	0
Constipation	1.5	0
Hemorrhage	2.0	0
State of consciousness	0.5	0
Fever	0	0

REGIMEN

GEMCITABINE + CARBOPLATIN

De Santis M et al. J Clin Oncol 2009;27:5634–5639
De Santis M et al. J Clin Oncol 2012;30(2):191–199

Gemcitabine 1000 mg/m² per dose; administer intravenously 50–250 mL 0.9% sodium chloride injection over 30 minutes for 2 doses on days 1 and 8, every 21 days × 6 cycles (total dosage/cycle = 2000 mg/m²)
Carboplatin* (calculated dose) AUC = 4.5 mg/mL · min administer intravenously in 50–150 mL 5% dextrose injection over 60 minutes after gemcitabine on day 1, every 21 days × 6 cycles (total dose/cycle calculated to produce an AUC = 4.5 mg/mL · min)

*Carboplatin dose is based on Calvert et al.'s formula to achieve a target area under the plasma concentration versus time curve (AUC) (AUC units = mg/mL · min)

$$\text{Total carboplatin Dose (mg)} = (\text{target AUC}) \times (\text{GFR} + 25)$$

In practice, creatinine clearance (Clcr) is used in place of glomerular filtration rate (GFR). Clcr can be calculated from the equation of Cockcroft and Gault:

$$\text{For males, Clcr} = \frac{(140 \pm \text{age [years]}) \times \text{body weight [kg]}}{72 \times (\text{Serum creatinine [mg/dL]})}$$

$$\text{For females, Clcr} = \frac{(140 - \text{age [years]}) \times \text{body weight [kg]}}{72 \times (\text{Serum creatinine [mg/dL]})} \times 0.85$$

Note: A carboplatin dose calculated with an IDMS-measured serum creatinine result using the Calvert formula could exceed an expected exposure (AUC) and result in increased drug-related toxicity. The FDA recommends capping an estimated GFR at 125 mL/min for any targeted AUC value. [online] May 23, 2013. Available from: http://www.fda.gov/AboutFDA/CentersOffices/OfficeofMedicalProductsandTobacco/CDER/ucm228974.htm [accessed February 26, 2014]

Calvert AH et al. J Clin Oncol 1989;7:1748–1756
Cockcroft DW, Gault MH. Nephron 1976;16:31–41
Jodrell DI et al. J Clin Oncol 1992;10:520–528
Sorensen BT et al. Cancer Chemother Pharmacol 1991;28:397–401

Supportive Care
Antiemetic prophylaxis—first regimen
Emetogenic potential on day 1: **HIGH**. *Potential for delayed symptoms*
Emetogenic potential on days 8: **LOW**
See Chapter 39 for antiemetic recommendations

Hematopoietic growth factor (CSF) prophylaxis
Primary prophylaxis is NOT indicated
See Chapter 43 for more information

Antimicrobial prophylaxis
Risk of fever and neutropenia is LOW
Antimicrobial primary prophylaxis to be considered:
• Antibacterial—not indicated
• Antifungal—not indicated
• Antiviral—not indicated, unless patient previously had an episode of HSV
See Chapter 47 for more information

Patient Population Studied

Study of 88 patients with either transitional cell tumors of the urothelial tract that are unresectable and measurable, or those with metastatic (N+ or M+) tumors. Patients "unfit" for cisplatin met any of the following criteria: (a) ECOG performance status of 2; (b) GFR <60 mL/min but >30 mL/min and normal cardiovascular and hepatic function

Efficacy (N = 88)

Complete response	3.4%
Partial response	34%
Median overall survival	Too early

Serious Adverse Toxicity (N = 119)

Death	2.3%
G3 Mucositis	1.1%
G4 Thrombocytopenia plus bleeding	3.4%
Neutropenia and fever	5.7%
Grades 3/4 renal toxicity	3.4%

Data above are from the phase II portion of a randomized phases II/III study. More definitive data will be available with completion of accrual and maturation of the phase III part of the trial

Treatment Modifications

Adverse Events	Treatment Modifications
Day 1 ANC <1500/mm³, platelets <100,000/mm³, or mucositis present	Hold treatment until ANC >1500/mm³, platelets >100,000/mm³, and mucositis resolves
Day 8 ANC 500–1000/mm³ or platelets 50,000–99,000/mm³	Reduce gemcitabine dosage by 50% on day of treatment
G4 neutropenia and fever, G4 thrombocytopenia >3 days, or thrombocytopenia and active bleeding	Reduce doses of both drugs by 25%

Therapy Monitoring

1. *Day 1:* CBC with differential count, serum electrolytes, BUN, and creatinine
2. *Day 8:* CBC with differential count
3. *Treatment evaluation after C3 and C6:* CT (or MRI) scan of the initial evaluable/measurable sites
4. *Duration of treatment:* Treat for 6 cycles unless progression documented
5. *Follow-up after completion of therapy:* Imaging with CT or MRI of the abdomen and pelvis, chest x-ray or CT of the chest, urine cytology (if applicable), creatinine, and electrolytes recommended at 3–6 month intervals for 2 years, and then as clinically indicated

Notes

1. Give platelet transfusions if platelet <20,000/mm³
2. Treat for 6 cycles unless progression documented

REGIMEN

NEOADJUVANT METHOTREXATE + VINBLASTINE + DOXORUBICIN + CISPLATIN (MVAC) BEFORE RADICAL CYSTECTOMY

Grossman HB et al. N Engl J Med 2003;349:859–866. Erratum in: N Engl J Med 2003;349:1880

Methotrexate 30 mg/m² per dose; administer by intravenous injection over 15–60 seconds on days 1, 15, and 22, every 28 days for 3 cycles (total dosage/cycle = 90 mg/m²)

Vinblastine 3 mg/m² per dose; administer by intravenous injection over 1–2 minutes on days 2, 15, and 22, every 28 days for 3 cycles (total dosage/cycle = 9 mg/m²)

Doxorubicin 30 mg/m²; administer by intravenous injection over 3–5 minutes on day 2, every 28 days for 3 cycles (total dosage/cycle = 30 mg/m²)

Hydration before and after cisplatin administration: Administer intravenously ≥1000 mL 0.9% sodium chloride injection (0.9% NS), at ≥100 mL/hour before and after cisplatin administration. Also encourage patients to increase oral intake of non-alcoholic fluids. Monitor serum electrolytes and replace as needed (potassium, magnesium, sodium)

Cisplatin 70 mg/m²; administer intravenously in 100–250 mL 0.9% NS over 70 minutes on day 2 every 28 days for 3 cycles (total dosage/cycle = 70 mg/m²)

Supportive Care
Antiemetic prophylaxis
Emetogenic potential on days 1, 15, and 22: **LOW**
Emetogenic potential on day 2: **HIGH**. *Potential for delayed symptoms*
See Chapter 39 for antiemetic recommendations

Hematopoietic growth factor (CSF) prophylaxis
Primary prophylaxis may be indicated between doses of myelosuppressive chemotherapy
See Chapter 43 for more information

Antimicrobial prophylaxis
Risk of fever and neutropenia is LOW
Antimicrobial primary prophylaxis to be considered:
- Antibacterial—not indicated
- Antifungal—not indicated
- Antiviral—not indicated unless patient previously had an episode of HSV

See Chapter 47 for more information

Oral care
Encourage patients to maintain intake of non-alcoholic fluids
If mucositis or stomatitis is present:
- Rinse mouth several times a day with ¼ teaspoon (1.25 g) each of baking soda and table salt in one quart of warm water. Follow with a plain water rinse
- Do not use mouthwashes that contain alcohols

Treatment Modifications

Adverse Events	Treatment Modifications
On day 1 if WBC count <3000/mm³ or platelet count <100,000/mm³	Delay chemotherapy for 1 week
On day 15 or 22: WBC count ≤2900/mm³ or platelet count ≤74,000/mm³	Hold dose of methotrexate and vinblastine
Severe mucositis (G3 or G4)*	Reduce methotrexate dosage by 33% (for all doses and into next cycle)
Severe neurotoxicity	Reduce vinblastine dosage by 33%
Clinical evidence of congestive heart failure	Discontinue doxorubicin

*Leucovorin may be started 24 hours after methotrexate infusion

Toxicity (N = 150*)

Adverse Event	% G3†	% G4‡
Hematologic Toxicities		
Granulocytopenia	23	33
Thrombocytopenia	5	0
Anemia	6	1
Nonhematologic Toxicities		
Nausea or vomiting	6	0
Stomatitis	10	0
Diarrhea or constipation	4	0
Renal effects	1	0
Neuropathy	2	0
Fatigue, lethargy, and malaise	3	0
All Toxicities		
Maximal grade of any adverse effect	35	37

*Patients who received any methotrexate, vinblastine, doxorubicin, and cisplatin
†Grade 3 described as adverse events of moderate severity
‡Grade 4 described as severe adverse events

Therapy Monitoring

1. *Prior to each cycle:* CBC with differential count, serum electrolytes, BUN, creatinine, and LFTs
2. *Weekly:* CBC with differential
3. *Response evaluation:* None needed during neoadjuvant therapy
4. *Follow-up after cystectomy:* Imaging with CT or MRI of the abdomen and pelvis, chest x-ray, urine cytology, creatinine, and electrolytes recommended at 3–6 month intervals for 2 years, and then as clinically indicated

Efficacy (N = 153)
(Intention-to-Treat Analysis)

Median survival	77 months
5-Year survival	57%

Patient Population Studied

Study of 153 patients with muscle-invasive bladder tumors without nodal or metastatic disease eligible for radical cystectomy. No previous pelvic radiation; adequate renal, hepatic, hematologic function; ECOGG performance status ≤1

REGIMEN

NEOADJUVANT GEMCITABINE + CISPLATIN (GC)

Dash A et al. Cancer 2008;113:2471–2477

Gemcitabine 1000 mg/m² per dose; administer intravenously in 50–250 mL 0.9% sodium chloride injection (0.9% NS) over 30–60 minutes for 2 doses on days 1 and 8, every 21 days for 4 cycles (total dosage/cycle = 2000 mg/m²)

Hydration before and after cisplatin administration: Administer ≥500 mL 0.9% NS intravenously over a minimum of 1 hour both before and after cisplatin. Encourage patients to increase oral intake of non-alcoholic fluids. Monitor serum electrolytes and replace as needed (potassium, magnesium, sodium)

Cisplatin 70 mg/m² single dose; administer intravenously in 100–250 mL 0.9% NS over 60 minutes on day 1, every 21 days for 4 cycles (total dosage/cycle = 70 mg/m²)*

or

Cisplatin 35 mg/m² per dose; administer intravenously in 100–250 mL 0.9% NS over 60 minutes for 2 doses, after gemcitabine on days 1 and 8, every 21 days for 4 cycles (total dosage/cycle = 70 mg/m²)[†]

*Soto Parra H et al. Ann Oncol 2002;13:1080–1086
[†]Hussain SA et al. Br J Cancer 2004;91:844–849

Supportive Care
Antiemetic prophylaxis
Emetogenic potential on days with cisplatin and gemcitabine: **HIGH**. *Potential for delayed symptoms*
Emetogenic potential on days with gemcitabine alone: **LOW**
See Chapter 39 for antiemetic recommendations

Hematopoietic growth factor (CSF) prophylaxis
Primary prophylaxis is NOT indicated
See Chapter 43 for more information

Antimicrobial prophylaxis
Risk of fever and neutropenia is LOW
Antimicrobial primary prophylaxis to be considered:
- Antibacterial—not indicated
- Antifungal—not indicated
- Antiviral—not indicated, unless patient previously had an episode of HSV

See Chapter 47 for more information

Efficacy (Response at Cystectomy, N = 52)

Cisplatin dose intensity achieved	90%
Gemcitabine dose intensity achieved	90%
Pathologic complete response	26%
<pT2 disease	36%
Median overall survival	Not reached
Median duration of response	9.6 months

Patient Population Studied

Study of 52 patients with locally advanced transitional cell urothelial cancer defined as muscle invasive (T2-T4a) without evidence of adenopathy (N0) and without prior systemic chemotherapy. Prior local intravesical therapy and/or immunotherapy were allowed. Karnofsky performance status ≥70; and measured creatinine clearance ≥60 mL/min (≥1 mL/s)

Notes

1. Administer 4 cycles followed by CT scan and cystectomy
2. This study randomized patients with multiple malignancies and not just urothelial cancer to 3-week (days 1 and 8) or 4-week (days 1, 8, 15) GC

Treatment Modifications

Adverse Events	Treatment Modifications
Day 1 WBC count <3000/mm³, or platelet count <100,000/mm³	Hold chemotherapy until WBC count >3000/mm³ and platelet count >100,000/mm³
Day 8 WBC count ≤1000/mm³, or platelet count ≤100,000/mm³	Hold chemotherapy and reduce following doses of gemcitabine by 10%
Febrile neutropenia or G4 thrombocytopenia	Reduce following gemcitabine doses by 10%

Missed chemotherapy doses are not given

Toxicity with 21-Day GC (N = 53)

Toxicity	% G3	% G4
Hematologic Toxicities		
Anemia	9.4	0
Thrombocytopenia	3.7	1.8
Neutropenia	16.9	5.6
Nonhematologic Toxicities		
Mucositis	1.8	1.8
Nausea	5.6	0
Alopecia	0	0
Infection	1.8	0
Fatigue	3.0	0
Cardiac	1.8	0
Fever	0	0

Soto Parra H et al. Ann Oncol 2002;13:1080–1086

Therapy Monitoring

1. *Prior to each dose of cisplatin:* CBC with differential count, serum electrolytes, BUN, and creatinine
2. *On all treatment days:* CBC with differential count
3. *Response evaluation after 4 cycles:* CT scan
4. *Follow-up after cystectomy:* Imaging with CT or MRI of the abdomen and pelvis, chest x-ray, urine cytology, creatinine, and electrolytes recommended at 3–6 month intervals for 2 years, and then as clinically indicated

ADVANCED TRANSITIONAL CELL CARCINOMA (TCC) REGIMEN

HIGH-DOSE (INTENSITY) OR DOSE-DENSE METHOTREXATE, VINBLASTINE, ADRIAMYCIN, AND CISPLATIN (HD-MVAC OR DD-MVAC)

Plimack et al. J Clin Oncol 2012;30, suppl; abstr 4526
Sternberg CN et al. J Clin Oncol 2001;19:2638–2646
Sternberg CN et al. Eur J Cancer 2006;42:50–54

Methotrexate 30 mg/m^2; administer by intravenous injection over ≤1 minute *or* intravenously in 10–100 mL 0.9% sodium chloride injection (0.9% NS) or 5% dextrose injection (D5W) over 10–30 minutes on day 1, every 14 days (total dosage/14-day cycle = 30 mg/m^2)
Hydration before cisplatin: 1000 mL 0.9% NS; administer intravenously over a minimum of 1 hour before commencing cisplatin administration
Vinblastine 3 mg/m^2; administer by intravenous injection over 1–2 minutes on day 2, every 14 days (total dosage/14-day cycle = 3 mg/m^2)
Doxorubicin 30 mg/m^2; administer by intravenous injection over 3–5 minutes on day 2, every 14 days (total dosage/14-day cycle = 30 mg/m^2)
Cisplatin 70 mg/m^2; administer intravenously in 50–500 mL 0.9 NS over 30–60 minutes on day 2, every 14 days (total dosage/14-day cycle = 70 mg/m^2)
Hydration after cisplatin: 1000 mL 0.9% NS; administer intravenously over a minimum of 2 hours. Monitor and replace magnesium and other electrolytes as needed. Encourage patients to increase their intake of non-alcoholic fluids
OR
2000 mL 0.45% NS; administer intravenously over a minimum of 2 hours
± *Mannitol diuresis:* May be given to patients who have received adequate hydration
Mannitol 37.5 grams; administer intravenously over 1–4 hours before or during cisplatin administration, or may be prepared as an admixture with cisplatin
Note: Diuresis with mannitol requires maintaining hydration with intravenously administered fluid during and for hours after mannitol administration

Filgrastim 240 mcg/m^2 per dose; administer subcutaneously, daily for 7 consecutive days, on days 4–10, every 14 days
• Calculated doses may be rounded by ±10% to use the most economical combination of commercially available products
• Filgrastim is discontinued when patients achieve a post-nadir ANC = 30,000/mm^3
• The duration of filgrastim use may be extended to a total of 14 consecutive days if neutrophil recovery is inadequate after a 7-day course

Supportive Care
Antiemetic prophylaxis
Emetogenic potential on Day 1 is **MINIMAL**
Emetogenic potential on Day 2 is **HIGH**. *Potential for delayed symptoms*
See Chapter 39 for antiemetic recommendations

Hematopoietic growth factor (CSF) prophylaxis
Primary prophylaxis with granulocyte-colony stimulating factor is an integral part of the treatment regimen

Antimicrobial prophylaxis
Risk of fever and neutropenia is LOW
Antimicrobial primary prophylaxis to be considered:
• Antibacterial—not indicated
• Antifungal—not indicated
• Antiviral—not indicated, unless patient previously had an episode of HSV
See Chapter 47 for more information

Oral care
Encourage patients to maintain intake of non-alcoholic fluids
If mucositis or stomatitis is present:
• Rinse mouth several times a day with ¼ teaspoon (1.25 g) each of baking soda and table salt in one quart of warm water. Follow with a plain water rinse
• Do not use mouthwashes that contain alcohols

Dose Modifications

Adverse Event	Treatment Modification
G3/4 hematologic toxicity	Extend the duration of filgrastim treatment as needed, up to a total of 14 consecutive days
ANC >30,000/mm^3	Discontinue filgrastim
G3/4 mucositis	Reduce methotrexate dosage by 33%
G3/4 neurotoxicity	Reduce vinblastine dosage by 33%
Clinical evidence of congestive heart failure	Discontinue doxorubicin

Patient Population Studied

263 patients with metastatic or advanced transitional-cell carcinoma (TCC) were randomly assigned to HD-MVAC (2-week cycles) or MVAC (4-week cycles). Eligibility criteria included the presence of TCC of the urinary tract (bladder, ureter, urethra, or renal pelvis) and bi-dimensionally measurable metastatic or locally advanced disease, no prior systemic cytotoxic or biologic treatment, and a World Health Organization (WHO) performance status of 0, 1, or 2; the median WHO performance status was 1. Sixty to 65% of patients were considered at low risk, 30–35% intermediate risk, and 5% high risk; 15–20% had had prior radiotherapy, and 73–75% had prior surgery. Sites of origin included bladder (82–88%), the renal pelvis (8–12%), and other sites (ureter, urethra, or prostatic ducts). Visceral metastases were present in 28–36%. The majority of patients had abdominal masses (pelvic, extranodal, or retroperitoneal masses) and more than one disease site

Toxicity (WHO Grade)

Toxicity	Grade	MVAC (n = 129) #Patients	%	HD-MVAC (n = 134) #Patients	%	P (trend)
WBC		2	2	4	3	
	0	8	6	46	34	
	1	11	8	29	21	<0.001
	2	28	22	28	21	
	3	59	46	16	12	
	4	21	16	11	8	
Platelets		2	2	4	3	
	0	80	62	48	43	
	1	10	8	22	16	0.033
	2	15	12	22	16	
	3	14	11	14	11	
	4	8	6	14	11	
Mucositis		7	5	10	8	
	0	31	24	43	32	
	1	43	33	44	33	0.034
	2	26	20	24	18	
	3	18	14	12	9	
	4	4	3	1	1	
Creatinine		2	2	5	4	
	0	113	88	118	88	
	1	7	5	4	3	0.815
	2	3	2	2	2	
	3	4	3	5	4	
Nausea and/or vomiting		4	3	7	5	
	0	9	7	3	2	
	1	27	21	20	15	0.025
	2	52	40	55	41	
	3	32	25	42	31	
	4	5	4	7	5	
Neurotoxicity		7	5	10	8	
	0	70	54	63	47	
	1	38	30	44	33	0.170
	2	12	9	10	8	
	3	2	2	5	4	
	4	0	0	2	2	
Alopecia		7	5	9	7	
	0	11	9	16	12	
	1	13	10	19	14	0.180
	2	36	28	33	25	
	3	62	48	57	43	
	4	0	0	0	0	

Efficacy

Response Rates

	M-VAC (n = 129)	HD-M-VAC (n = 134)	P-Value
Number evaluable	113 (88%)	114 (85%)	
CR + PR	65 (58%)	83 (72%)	0.016 (2-sided)
CR	12 (11%)	28 (25%)	0.006 (2-sided)
PR	53 (47%)	55 (48%)	

Endpoint	Time/Percent (95% CI)	Time/Percent (95% CI)	P-Value HR (95% CI)
Progression-free survival	8.1 months (7.0–9.9)	9.5 months (7.6–12.2)	P = 0.017 HR = 0.73 (0.56–0.95)
Overall survival	14.9 months	15.1 months	P = 0.042 HR 0.76 (0.58–0.99)
2-year survival rate	26.2% (18.4–34%)	36.7% (28.3–45%)	
5-year survival	13.5% (7.4–19.6%)	21.8% (14.5–29.2%)	P = 0.042
7.3-year survival rate*	13.2%	24.6%	
Cancer death	76%	64.9%	

*Median follow-up

MUSCLE-INVASIVE BLADDER CANCER REGIMEN

NEOADJUVANT CISPLATIN, METHOTREXATE, AND VINBLASTINE

International Collaboration of Trialists. Lancet 1999;354:533–540
International Collaboration of Trialists. J Clin Oncol 2011;29:2171–2177

Methotrexate 30 mg/m^2 per dose; administer by intravenous injection over ≤1 minute *or* intravenously in 10–100 mL 0.9% sodium chloride Injection (0.9% NS) or 5% dextrose injection (D5W) over 5–30 minutes for 2 doses on days 1 and 8, every 21 days for 3 cycles (total dosage/cycle = 60 mg/m^2)

Vinblastine 4 mg/m^2 per dose; administer by intravenous injection over 1–2 minutes for 2 doses on days 1 and 8, every 21 days for 3 cycles (total dosage/cycle = 8 mg/m^2)

Hydration before cisplatin: 1000 mL 0.9% NS; administer intravenously over a minimum of 1 hour on day 2 before commencing cisplatin administration

Cisplatin 100 mg/m^2; administer intravenously in 50–500 mL 0.9 NS over 30–60 minutes on day 2, every 21 days for 3 cycles (total dosage/cycle = 100 mg/m^2)

Hydration after cisplatin: 1000 mL 0.9% NS; administer intravenously over a minimum of 2 hours. Monitor and replace magnesium and other electrolytes as needed. Encourage patients to increase their intake of non-alcoholic fluids

Leucovorin calcium 15 mg; administer orally or intravenously every 6 hours commencing 24 hours after methotrexate was administered for 4 doses on day 2 and 4 doses on day 9 (total dose/cycle = 120 mg)

• *Alternatively,* **Levoleucovorin calcium** 7.5 mg may be given orally or intravenously every 6 hours commencing 24 hours after methotrexate was administered for 4 doses starting on day 2 and 4 doses starting on day 9 (total dose/cycle = 60 mg)

Supportive Care

Antiemetic prophylaxis
Emetogenic potential on Days 1, 8, and 9 is **MINIMAL**
Emetogenic potential on Day 2 is **HIGH**. *Potential for delayed symptoms*
See Chapter 39 for antiemetic recommendations

Hematopoietic growth factor (CSF) prophylaxis
Primary prophylaxis may be indicated
See Chapter 43 for more information

Antimicrobial prophylaxis
Risk of fever and neutropenia is LOW
  Antimicrobial primary prophylaxis to be considered:
  • Antibacterial—not indicated
  • Antifungal—not indicated
  • Antiviral—not indicated, unless patient previously had an episode of HSV
See Chapter 47 for more information

Diarrhea management
Latent or delayed-onset diarrhea*:
  Loperamide 4 mg; administer orally initially after the first loose or liquid stool, *then*
  Loperamide 2 mg every 2 hours while awake; every 4 hours during sleep
  Alternatively, a trial of **Diphenoxylate hydrochloride** 2.5 mg with **Atropine sulfate** 0.025 mg (eg, Lomotil®) two tablets four times daily until control is achieved.
Persistent diarrhea:
  Octreotide acetate (solution) 100–150 mcg; administer subcutaneously 3 times daily.
Antibiotic therapy during latent or delayed-onset diarrhea:
  A fluoroquinolone (eg, **Ciprofloxacin** 500 mg orally every 12 hours) if absolute neutrophil count <500/mm^3

*Abigerges D, et al. J Natl Cancer Inst 1994;86:446–449
Rothenberg ML, et al. J Clin Oncol 2001;19:3801–3807
Wadler S, et al. J Clin Oncol 1998;16:3169–3178

Dose Modifications

Adverse Event	Treatment Modification
G3/4 mucositis	Reduce methotrexate dosage by 33%
G3/4 neurotoxicity	Reduce vinblastine dosage by 33%
Creatinine clearance <50 mL/min (<0.83 mL/s)	Hold cisplatin until creatinine clearance >50 mL/min (>0.83 mL/s)

Patient Population Studied

Patients with T2 G3, T3, T4a, N0-NX, or M0 transitional-cell carcinoma of the bladder undergoing curative cystectomy or full-dose external-beam radiotherapy were randomly assigned three cycles of neoadjuvant chemotherapy (cisplatin, methotrexate, and vinblastine, with folinic acid rescue (n = 491) or no chemotherapy (n = 485). Thirty-four, 58, and 8% of patients had T2, T3, and T4a disease, respectively. Eighty-eight percent of patients had grade 3 disease, and 65% had N0. The median age was 64 years; 88% of patients were male; and 43%, 50%, and 7% of patients chose as local radical treatment radiotherapy, cystectomy, and a combination of radiotherapy and cystectomy, respectively

Toxicity

Chemotherapy-related mortality	1%
Nausea and vomiting	Common despite antiemetics
WHO G3/4 leucopenia	16%
WHO G3/4 thrombocytopenia	6.5%
Fever and neutropenia	10%
G1/2 nephrotoxicity requiring dose reduction/delay	26%
Postoperative wound infections	8% (20/249)
Wound dehiscence	2.4% (6/249)
Urinary or fecal fistulae	2% (5/249)
Dysuria (worse or severe)	31% (53/171)
G3/4 diarrhea	12.7% (23/181)

Efficacy					
Endpoint	Time	No CMV	CMV	HR 95% CI	P-Value
Overall survival	3 y	50%	56%	0.84 0.72–0.99	0.037
	5 y	43%	49%		
	10 y	30%	36%		
Metastases-free survival	3 y	44%	53%	0.77 0.66–0.90	0.001
	5 y	38%	47%		
	10 y	23%	33%		
Locoregional disease-free survival	3 y	41%	46%	0.87 0.75–1.01	0.067
	5 y	34%	39%		
	10 y	22%	27%		
Disease-free survival	3 y	38%	45%	0.82 0.70–0.95	0.008
	5 y	32%	39%		
	10 y	20%	27%		
Locoregional control	3 y	55%	56%	0.96 0.80–1.15	0.632
	5 y	50%	51%		
	10 y	39%	40%		

5. Brain Cancer

Lyndon Kim, MD and Howard Fine, MD

Epidemiology

Incidence: 23,380 (male: 12,820; female: 10,560. Estimated new cases for 2014 in the United States)
7.7 per 100,000 men 5.4 per 100,000 women
Deaths: Estimated 14,320 in 2014 (male: 8,090; female: 6,230)
Median age at diagnosis: 57 years
Male to female ratio: Slight male predominance in the incidence of malignant brain tumors

Siegel R et al. CA Cancer J Clin 2014;64:9–29
Surveillance, Epidemiology and End Results (SEER) Program, available from http://seer.cancer.gov (accessed in 2013)

Work-up

1. Neuroimaging study (MRI of the brain preferred over CT)

No other staging work-up is required except:

2. *Primary CNS lymphoma:* MRI of spine, lumbar puncture, and ophthalmologic examination
3. *PNET/medulloblastoma:* MRI of spine and lumbar puncture when safe to do so

Pathology

I. **Neuroepithelial Tumors**
   A. Glial tumors
      1. Astrocytic tumors (45–50%)
         - Glioblastoma multiforme (GBM grade IV): 50%
         - Anaplastic astrocytoma (AA grade III): 30%
         - Diffuse astrocytoma (grade II): 20%
         - Gliosarcoma (grade IV): <5% of GBM
         - Pilocytic astrocytoma (grade I): <1%
      2. Oligodendrogliomas/ oligoastrocytomas (5–10%)
         - Oligodendroglioma (O grade II)
         - Anaplastic oligodendroglioma (AO grade III)
         - Oligoastrocytoma (OA grade II)
         - Anaplastic oligoastrocytoma (AOA grade III)
      3. Ependymal tumors (5%)
         - Myxopapillary ependymoma (grade I)
         - Ependymoma (grade II)
         - Anaplastic ependymoma (grade III)
         - Subependymoma
   B. Neuronal and mixed glial-neuronal tumors (<1%)
      - Central neurocytoma
      - Dysembryoplastic neuroepithelial tumor
      - Desmoplastic infantile astrocytoma/ganglioma
      - Ganglioma
      - Paraganglioma
   C. Nonglial tumors
      1. Embryonal tumors (<5%)
         - Primitive neuroectodermal tumors (PNET)
         - Medulloblastoma
         - Ependymoblastoma
      2. Choroid plexus tumors (<1%)
         - Choroid plexus papilloma
      3. Pineal tumors (<1%)
         - Pineoblastoma
         - Pineocytoma

II. **Meningeal Tumors (15–28%)**
   - Benign meningioma (grade I): >90%
   - Atypical meningioma (grade II): 6%
   - Anaplastic meningioma (grade III): 2%
   - Hemangiopericytoma

III. **Germ Cell Tumors (<1%)**

IV. **Nerve Sheath Tumors (4–8%)**
   - Schwannoma

V. **Primary CNS Lymphoma (PCNSL) (1–5%)**

VI. **Metastatic Tumors**

Adesina AM et al. Histopathology of primary tumors of the central nervous system. In: Prados M, ed. Brain Cancer: American Cancer Society Atlas of Clinical Oncology. Hamilton, Ontario, Canada: BC Decker Inc.; 2002:16–47
Greenberg H et al. Brain Tumors. Oxford University Press, 1999:1–26
WHO Classification of Tumors. IARC Press, 2000:6–7

Staging

(TNM staging does not apply to most brain tumors because they rarely metastasize. Ependymal tumors such as medulloblastoma are exceptions to this rule)

WHO Designation*	WHO Grade*					St. Anne–Mayo Grade†
	Grade	Nuclear Atypia	Mitosis	Endothelial Proliferation	Necrosis	
Pilocytic astrocytoma	I	—	—	—	—	Astrocytoma grade 1 (no criteria present)
Diffuse astrocytoma	II	+	Usually —	—	—	Astrocytoma grade 2 (1 criterion present)
Anaplastic astrocytoma	III	+	+	±	—	Astrocytoma grade 3 (2 criteria present)
Glioblastoma	IV	+	+, Active	Usually +	Usually +	Astrocytoma grade 4 (3 or 4 criteria present)

*The current 2000 WHO grading system stratifies previous low-grade astrocytomas (WHO grades I and II) into different subtypes. WHO grade I pilocytic astrocytoma is characteristically well circumscribed, cystic, and localized. WHO grade II diffuse astrocytoma, like WHO grades III and IV, is characteristically infiltrative and progressive
†In the St. Anne–Mayo grading system, the grades are based on the total number of criteria present. The criteria are similar to those in the WHO system: nuclear atypia, mitosis, endothelial proliferation, and necrosis

Daumas-Duport et al. Cancer 1988;62:2152–2165
Kleihues P et al. Histological Typing Tumours of the Central Nervous System. 2nd ed. WHO. Berlin: Springer-Verlag, 1993
WHO Classification of Tumors. Lyons, France: IARC Press, 2000:6–7

Prognosis

Median Survival*

Grade I	>10 years
Grade II	5–8 years
Grade III	3–5 years
Grade IV	0.9–1 year

*Because oligodendrogliomas and oligoastrocytomas are uniquely sensitive to both chemotherapy and radiation therapy with better overall survival and prognosis, every effort should be made to look for oligodendroglial cell components and provide proper treatment options based on the pathology

Burger PC et al. Cancer 1985;56:1106–1111
Piepmeier J et al. Neurosurgery 1987;67:177–181

Expert Opinion

Grade I Astrocytoma (Pilocytic Astrocytoma)

Pilocytic astrocytoma is a rare tumor commonly seen in the pediatric or young adult population. The tumor is well circumscribed and MRI findings reveal a homogenously enhancing lesion with an associated macrocyst commonly seen in the cerebellum, brainstem, and optic pathways

1. **Observation following surgery:** Most patients can be cured with surgery alone. Following surgery, patients can be simply observed. The role of radiation therapy for incomplete resection remains undetermined

Grade II Astrocytomas (Diffuse Astrocytoma)

Diffuse astrocytoma patients can be seen in the young adult population. Although considered as a low grade, the prognosis is still not optimal with overall survival of 5–8 years. MRI usually reveals nonenhancing lesion that could be best seen on T2 or FLAIR images

1. **Observation:** Patients with the following good prognostic factors can be closely monitored with serial scans:

- Young age (<40 years)
- Asymptomatic
- Good performance score (KPS >70)
- Near or complete resection
- Small nonenhancing lesion
- Low Ki-67 or MIB-1 proliferative index
- Presence of IDH1 or IDH2 mutation

Note: About a third of patients who have nonenhancing lesions may ultimately prove on biopsy to have anaplastic tumors. Thus, close surveillance (particularly early on until the natural course of the diseases becomes apparent) is recommended for all patients with diffuse astrocytomas for whom a watch-and-wait strategy is employed

(continued)

Expert Opinion (*continued*)

2. Treatment: General indications for treatment include:

- Older patient (>40 years)
- Symptomatic
- Large or inoperable lesion
- Enhancement on imaging studies
- High Ki-67 or MIB-1 proliferative index
- Lack of IDH1 or IDH2 mutation

    a. Radiation therapy: Radiation therapy was considered as the standard treatment until the randomized phase III RTOG 9802 trial revealed a significantly longer survival for radiation therapy plus PCV chemotherapy over radiation therapy alone for high-risk low-grade gliomas. Radiation therapy can be still considered for those who could not tolerate chemoradiation therapy or chemotherapy. Delayed radiation-mediated neurotoxicity remains a concern, although prospective studies suggest it occurs less commonly than was once feared. Factors that increase the chance of clinically significant delayed radiation-induced neurotoxicity include:

- Large radiation fields
- Large fraction dose and total dose
- Older age
- Underlying neurodegenerative disease
- Radiation of temporal and frontal lobes

    For patients considered at significant risk of radiation-induced neurotoxicity, treatment with temozolomide alone is a consideration, although the data suggest that the period of tumor control is generally relatively short

    b. Chemotherapy: Chemotherapy with deferred radiation therapy can be considered especially for those patients with large inoperable tumors or whose tumor has mutated IDH1 and IDH2 unable to tolerate radiation therapy or chemoradiation therapy. Recently, temozolomide, an oral agent, has shown efficacy in unirradiated low-grade gliomas. It causes no delayed neurotoxicity and can be considered as a treatment option for low-grade gliomas requiring treatment to defer radiation therapy. At a median follow-up of 45.5 months and after the tumors of 246/477 patients had progressed, there was no statistical difference in the primary end point, progression-free survival (PFS). Overall toxicity was mild. Grade 3 hematologic toxicity was observed in 9% of the temozolomide-treated patients [temozolomide chemotherapy versus radiotherapy in molecularly characterized (1p loss) low-grade glioma: a randomized phase III intergroup study by the EORTC/NCIC-CTG/TROG/MRC-CTU (EORTC 22033-26033), Baumert et al. Abstract 2007, ASCO 2013 Annual Meeting]

    c. Chemoradiation therapy: Radiation followed by PCV chemotherapy is now considered as the standard of care for patients with high-risk low grade gliomas (astrocytomas, oligoastrocytomas, oligodendrogliomas, and neurofibromatosis). Recent long-term follow-up result of the phase III RTOG 9802* clinical trial revealed a significant survival benefit for patients who were randomized to radiation followed by PCV chemotherapy over radiation therapy alone. Median survival time was 13.3 years and 7.8 years, respectively. Additional molecular and genetic studies are ongoing to further identify patients who would most likely benefit from chemotherapy. Patients who are felt to be appropriate candidates for radiation therapy or chemotherapy should be considered for chemoradiation therapy

*A Phase II Study of Observation in Favorable Low-Grade Glioma and A Phase III Study of Radiation with or without PCV Chemotherapy in Unfavorable Low-Grade Glioma. NCI Press Release February 03, 2014

Grade III Astrocytoma (Anaplastic Astrocytoma)

Anaplastic astrocytoma is an aggressive tumor that has overall survival of 3–5 years. MRI often reveals heterogeneous enhancement that is usually intermixed with nonenhancing tumor, although as many as half of all anaplastic astrocytomas may be largely nonenhancing. Mitosis, endothelial proliferation, and atypia can be seen

1. Treatment:

    a. Radiation therapy: Radiation therapy remains as standard of care

    b. Chemotherapy: The standard of care for anaplastic gliomas had been surgery followed by radiotherapy. The role of chemotherapy for anaplastic astrocytomas remains unclear. In patients with newly diagnosed anaplastic gliomas (anaplastic oligodendroglioma, oligoastrocytoma, and astrocytoma), the NOA-04 phase III trial compared the efficacy and safety of radiotherapy followed by chemotherapy at progression with the reverse sequence. The results showed comparable results with either initial radiotherapy or initial chemotherapy (Wick et al, 2009). [Median TTF hazard ratio HR = 1.2; 95% CI, 0.8–1.8, PFS HR = 1.0; 95% CI, 0.7–1.3, and overall survival HR = 1.2; 95% CI, 0.8–1.9] were similar for radiotherapy and procarbazine, lomustine, and vincristine (PCV)/temozolomide. A more recent phase III study of anaplastic gliomas (NOA-08) randomly assigned patients to receive either chemotherapy (PCV or temozolomide) versus radiation therapy as initial treatment. This study showed no difference in time to treatment failure, progression free survival, or overall survival [median overall survival 8.6 months (95% CI 7.3–10.2) in the temozolomide group and 9.6 months (8.2–10.8) in the radiotherapy group HR 1.09, 95% CI 0.84–1.42, noninferiority = 0.033], leading the authors to concluded temozolomide alone is noninferior to radiotherapy alone in the treatment of elderly patients with malignant astrocytoma (Wick et al, 2012)

    c. Chemoradiation Therapy: The use of concurrent and postirradiation temozolomide therapy, an approach employed in newly diagnosed glioblastoma (grade IV astrocytoma) also has become widely accepted for the treatment of other types of malignant gliomas

Wick W et al. J Clin Oncol 2009;27:5874–5880
Wick W et al. Lancet Oncol 2012;13:707–715

(*continued*)

Expert Opinion (continued)

Grade IV Astrocytomas (Glioblastomas)

Glioblastomas are the most common malignant tumors of the elderly population. The tumor grows rapidly and causes significant morbidity and mortality with overall survival of 14–18 months. Imaging studies usually reveal a heterogeneously enhancing lesion or lesions with a significant amount of surrounding edema. Increased number of mitosis, endothelial proliferation, atypia, and necrosis are commonly seen

1. Treatment:

Chemoradiation therapy:

Initial therapy:

- For patients age 18–70 years, combined radiation therapy with low-dose daily temozolomide followed by monthly temozolomide is the standard of care (Stupp et al, 2005)
- Combined radiation therapy with low-dose daily temozolomide followed by monthly temozolomide can be also considered for patients who are older than 70 years with a good performance status
- Alternatively, for patients 70 years or older with a poor performance status, temozolomide or radiation therapy alone can be an option. A 2- or 3-week course of hypofractionated radiation therapy could be an option for patients with poor performance status
- Radiation therapy followed by one of the nitrosoureas (carmustine [BCNU] or lomustine [CCNU]) is an option for those who could not receive temozolomide

Recurrent disease:

- Bevacizumab is the treatment of choice for patients for whom it is not medically or neurologically contraindicated (Kreisl et al, 2009)
- *Retreatment with a continuous low-dose (metronomic) temozolomide dosing schedule is an option especially for patients who have never been treated with bevacizumab and responded well to their original temozolomide with the last treatment greater than 6 months and whose tumor has a methylated MGMT status (see Table below)*
- Other molecular targeted drugs such as erlotinib can be considered for malignant gliomas expressing EGFR or EGFRviii
- Second-line chemotherapeutic agents such as BCNU, CCNU, or carboplatin are also options
- Participation in a well-designed clinical trial is highly recommended

Kreisl TN et al. J Clin Oncol 2009;27:740–745
Stupp R et al. N Engl J Med 2005;352:987–996

Phase II Trials of Continuous Low-dose Temozolomide for Patients with Recurrent Malignant Glioma

Reference	N	TMZ Daily Dose, Schedule	ORR (%)	PFS6 (%)	Median OS (months)
Khan	27	75 mg/m², 42/70 days	14	27	8
Brandes	33	75 mg/m², 21/28 days	9	30	10
Wick	64	150 mg/m², 7/14 days	15	44	9
Perry	33	*Early progression on adjuvant TMZ, 50 mg/m², 28/28 days*	3	27	NA
	27	*Progression on extended TMZ, 50 mg/m², 28/28 days*	0	7	NA
	28	*Rechallenge, 50 mg/m², 28/28 days*	11	36	NA
Kong	38	40–50 m², 28/28 days	5	32	13
Abacioglu	16	100 mg/m², 21/28 days	7	25	7
Verhoeff	15	50 mg/m², 28/28 days + bevacizumab 10 mg/kg q21d	NA	7	4
Desjardins	32	50 mg/m², 28/28 days + bevacizumab 10 mg/kg q14d	28	19	6
Omuro	37	All patients, 50 mg/m², 28/28 days	11	19	7
		Bevacizumab failures, 50 mg/m², 28/28 days	0	11	4
		Bevacizumab naïve, 50 mg/m², 28/28 days	20	26	13

NA, not available; ORR, objective response rate (complete + partial responses); PFS6, progression-free at 6 months; TMZ, temozolomide

Abacioglu U et al. J Neurooncol 2011;103:585–593
Brandes AA et al. Br J Cancer 2006;95:1155–1160
Desjardins A et al. Cancer 2011;118:1302–1312
Khan RB et al. Neuro Oncol 2002;4:39–43
Kong DS et al. Neuro Oncol 2010;12:289–296
Omuro A et al. Neuro Oncol 2013;15:242–250
Perry JR et al. J Clin Oncol 2010;28:2051–2057
Verhoeff JJ et al. Ann Oncol 2010;21:1723–1727
Wick A et al. J Clin Oncol 2007;25:3357–3361

(continued)

Expert Opinion (continued)

Oligodendroglioma (WHO grade II)

Oligodendrogliomas are rare tumors that can respond extremely well to radiation and chemotherapy. They appear as fried egg, round cells under the microscope and imaging studies that show calcifications can help establish the diagnosis. Co-deletion of 1p and 19q usually confers a good prognosis

1. **Observation:** Patients with the following good prognostic factors can be closely monitored with serial scans:

   - Young age (<40 years)
   - Asymptomatic
   - Good performance score (KPS >70)
   - Small non-enhancing lesion
   - Nearly or completely resected tumor
   - Low Ki-67 or MIB-1 proliferative index
   - Co-deletion of 1p and 19q
   - Presence of IDH1 or IDH2 mutation

2. **Treatment:**

   General indications for treatment include: Older patient (>40 years)

   - Symptomatic
   - Poor performance score (<70)
   - Large or inoperable, enhancing tumor
   - High Ki-67 or MIB-1 proliferative index
   - Lack of IDH1 or IDH2 mutation
   - Intact 1p and 19q status

   a. **Chemotherapy:** If the tumor cannot be completely resected, radiation therapy or chemotherapy can be considered as oligodendrogliomas can respond to either treatment extremely well. However, because oligodendrogliomas with 1p, 19q co-deletion can be exquisitely sensitive to chemotherapy, temozolomide or PCV can be offered as alternative treatments, especially for young patients with good prognostic features, in order to avoid the potential for delayed neurotoxicity

   b. **Radiation therapy:** Radiation therapy is usually reserved for patients with poor prognostic features, who are unable to tolerate chemotherapy or for chemotherapy resistant and progressive disease

   c. **Combined chemotherapy and radiation therapy:** Recent RTOG 9802* phase III trial for high-risk low-grade gliomas (astrocytomas, oligodendrogliomas, oligoastrocytomas, and neurofibromatosis) reveled a significant long-term survival benefit for patients who were randomized to radiation followed by PCV chemotherapy over radiation therapy alone. Median survival time was 13.3 years for radiation plus PCV arm and 7.8 years for radiation alone arm. Based on these findings, this combination therapy is now considered as the standard treatment for high-risk low-grade gliomas especially when oligodendrogliomas are well known to be extremely sensitive to radiation therapy and chemotherapy. Additional molecular and genetic studies are ongoing to further identify patients who would most likely benefit from chemotherapy. Patients who are felt to be appropriate candidates for radiation therapy or chemotherapy should be considered for chemoradiation therapy

*A Phase II Study of Observation in Favorable Low-Grade Glioma and A Phase III Study of Radiation with or without PCV Chemotherapy in Unfavorable Low-Grade Glioma. NCI Press Release. February 03, 2014

Anaplastic Oligodendroglioma (WHO grade III)

Anaplastic oligodendrogliomas, like grade II oligodendrogliomas, can be extremely sensitive to radiation and chemotherapy. Co-deletion of 1p and 19q confers a good prognosis

1. **Treatment:** Combined chemotherapy with PCV and pre- or postradiation therapy is standard of treatment. Radiation therapy alone and chemotherapy alone are no longer considered as standard of care and they are reserved for patients who could not tolerate combination therapy

   a. **Combined chemotherapy and radiation therapy:** Two recent long-term follow-up results from the phase III randomized trials for newly diagnosed anaplastic oligodendrogliomas revealed a significant survival benefit for combination PCV chemotherapy and radiation therapy over radiation therapy alone (van den Bent et al, 2012; Cairncross et al, 2012). These trials also validated the role of 1p, 19q as a predictive biomarker for survival. Therefore, PCV chemotherapy given either pre- or postradiation therapy is now considered as the standard of treatment. However, because PCV chemotherapy compared to temozolomide carries a greater toxicity with a less-favorable dosing schedule and administration, many still debate accepting PCV chemotherapy as standard of care. The role of concurrent radiation and postradiation chemotherapy with temozolomide, the treatment standard for glioblastomas, is now commonly adopted for the treatment of other malignant gliomas like anaplastic oligodendrogliomas

Cairncross JG et al. 2012 ASCO Annual Meeting. Abstract 2008b
van den Bent MJ et al. J Clin Oncol 2006;24:2715–2722
van den Bent MJ et al. J Clin Oncol 2012;43:2229

(continued)

Expert Opinion (continued)

Medulloblastoma and Primitive Neuroectodermal Tumors

These tumors usually occur in children and young adults. They are aggressive in nature and have a high propensity to spread through the cerebrospinal fluid resulting in distant metastasis within the central nervous system. A thorough staging work up, including a careful examination of the cerebrospinal fluid and spine, are required. Medulloblastoma usually arises in the posterior fossa causing hydrocephalus and associated obstructive symptoms, including headaches, nausea, vomiting, and gait difficulties requiring urgent ventriculoperitoneal shunt placement to relieve the intracranial pressure

1. Treatment:

   a. **Radiation Therapy:** Craniospinal radiation therapy is the standard of care

   b. **Chemotherapy:** Chemotherapy is usually provided after the completion of radiation therapy. When chemotherapy is considered, craniospinal radiation dose can be reduced to minimize the toxicity (Packer et al, 2006). For recurrent disease, stereotactic radiation therapy, chemotherapy or high dose chemotherapy with stem cell rescue can be considered

Packer et al. J Clin Oncol 2006;24:4202–4208

Primary Central Nervous System Lymphomas

Primary central nervous system lymphomas are rare non-Hodgkin lymphomas arising within the central nervous system without systemic involvement. They occur mostly in the elderly population and in patients who are immunocompromised. The most common type is diffuse large B-cell lymphoma and they invariably express CD20. MRI findings usually reveal homogenously enhancing lesion(s) involving periventricle or splenium (butterfly lesion). If a primary central system lymphoma is suspected, a stereotactic biopsy is sufficient to establish the diagnosis as this tumor can be successfully treated with radiation and methotrexate containing chemotherapy with high cure rates. However, in the presence of significant mass effect, partial or total resection can be considered. As an initial work up, a thorough examination of eyes and cerebrospinal fluid are required because of the propensity to involve these sites. If a primary central nervous system lymphoma is suspected, the administration of steroids is discouraged as steroids can be oncolytic and could cause a decrease in the size of the tumor making the diagnosis difficult. Steroids are usually administered after a biopsy or surgery

1. Treatment:

   a. **Chemotherapy:** High-dose methotrexate ($3.5–8$ g/m²) given alone or as part of multiagent regimen remains as the standard therapy (Batchelor et al, 2003). Even at high dose as a single agent the treatment is well tolerated and causes minimal side effects. The complete response and survival rates are found to be comparable or better than radiation therapy. Delayed neurotoxicity commonly seen in long-term survivors of whole-brain radiation therapy is less frequent. Because of high central nervous system penetration of the drug, patients with ocular, cerebrospinal fluid or leptomeningeal involvement can be safely treated with high-dose methotrexate alone without concurrent radiation or intraocular or intrathecal chemotherapy. CD20-directed rituximab in combination with high-dose methotrexate is also commonly used (Chamberlain and Johnston, 2010). Patients who receive high-dose methotrexate alone can be treated with rituximab as maintenance therapy following high-dose methotrexate. For recurrence, retreatment with high-dose methotrexate with and without rituximab, (Chamberlain and Johnston, 2010) topotecan, (Voloschin et al, 2008) high-dose cytarabine or temozolomide can be considered. If chemotherapy is not considered as a good option because of the patient's high comorbidities, renal failure, or inability to tolerate chemotherapy, radiation therapy could be an alternative option

   Recent long-term follow-up results of a phase II high-dose methotrexate-based multiagent chemotherapy followed by consolidation, reduced-dose radiation therapy, and high-dose cytarabine for newly diagnosed primary central nervous system lymphoma patients revealed a high rate of response and overall survival with favorable cognitive outcomes compared to historical controls treated with whole-brain radiation therapy alone (Morris et al, 2013). A randomized phase III Radiation Therapy Oncology Group trial based on an earlier phase II regimen with or without reduced-dose whole-brain radiation therapy is currently underway

   In newly diagnosed primary central nervous system lymphoma patients who responded to a chemotherapy trial, a phase II study of a methotrexate-based chemotherapy regimen followed by high-dose chemotherapy with autologous stem cell transplantation and reduced-dose whole-brain radiation therapy revealed an encouraging high response rate and survival results that warrants further investigation in a larger phase III trial (Colombat et al, 2006)

   b. **Radiation therapy:** Radiation therapy was a standard of care in the past, but because of high treatment failure and high incidence of delayed neurotoxicity commonly seen in long-term survivors, this approach is no longer considered as first-line therapy. However, radiation therapy is still considered for patients who have poor performance status and/or are unable to tolerate chemotherapy or for recurrent disease

Batchelor TJ Clin Oncol 2003;21:1044–1049
Chamberlain and Johnston. Neuro Oncol 2010;2:736–744
Colombat P et al. Bone Marrow Transplant 2006;38:417–420
Morris PG et al. J Clin Oncol 2013;31:3971–3979
Voloschin AD et al. J Neurooncol 2008;86:211–215

(continued)

Expert Opinion (*continued*)

Meningiomas

Meningiomas are rare brain tumors arising from the meninges. They usually affect the elderly population and have a slight female preponderance. Calcifications and bone involvement can be seen on CT scan. MRI scan usually reveals a dural-based homogenously enhancing lesion that has a typical tail sign

Treatment options include observation of asymptomatic patients and surgery for those who have symptoms

Benign Meningiomas (Grade I):

1. **Observation:** Grade I meningiomas are slow growing benign tumors that have an excellent prognosis with overall survival greater than 10 years. They can be simply followed without any therapeutic intervention

2. **Treatment:**

    a. Surgery: If the tumor grows and or a patient becomes symptomatic, surgery may be indicated

Atypical Meningiomas (Grade II):

1. **Observation:** For most atypical meningioma (grade II) patients, close observation following surgery is usually sufficient if the patient is asymptomatic and the pathology showed a low Ki-67 or MIB-1 proliferation index

2. **Treatment:**

    a. Radiation therapy: Radiation can be considered if the patient is symptomatic and or the pathology showed a high Ki-67 or MIB-1 proliferation index

Malignant meningiomas (Grade III):

Malignant meningiomas (grade III) are a rapidly growing tumor that carries a poor prognosis with overall survival less than 2–3 years. MRI scan typically reveals a significant vasogenic edema

1. **Treatment:**

    a. Surgery followed by radiation therapy: For recurrent tumors, surgery, additional radiation therapy, or stereotactic radiation therapy can be considered. Immunomodulating agents, such as α-interferon (Chamberlain and Glantz, 2008) and somatostatin analogs for somatostatin receptor-positive tumors (positive octreotide scan) (Chamberlain et al, 2007) have shown some modest responses that can be durable. Chemotherapeutic agents, such as hydroxyurea (Chamberlain, 2012) and platinum compounds, also have shown some modest benefits. Bevacizumab, as a single agent or in combination with chemotherapy (Lou et al, 2012), can be safely administered and it appears to have encouraging antitumor effects. Further trials to investigate the efficacy and side effects are warranted

Chamberlain M. J Neurooncol 2012;107:315–321
Chamberlain M, Glantz MJ. Cancer 2008;113:2146–2151
Lou E et al. J Neurooncol 2012;109:63–70

Targeted Therapy for Recurrent High-grade Meningioma (Adapted from Chamberlain MC and Johnston SK, 2011)

Inhibitor [Reference]	Target	Number of Patients	Radiographic RR (%)	Progression-free Survival	
				Median	6-months
Bevacizumab [Nayak, 2011]	VEGF	6	0	4.0 months	NS
Sunitinib [Kaley, 2010]	VEGFR	30	0	5.1 months	36%
Vatalanib [Grimm, 2010]	VEGFR	21	5.8	3.65 months	37.5%
Imatinib [Wen, 2006 and Wen, 2009]	PDGFR	10	0	2.0 months	29.4%
Erlotinib [Norden, 2010]	EGFR	25	0	2.0 months	25%
Pasireotide [Hammond, 2011]	SST	17	0	4.0 months	12%
Sandostatin LAR [Chamberlain, 2007]	SST	8	25	3.0 months	25%

EGFR, epidermal growth factor receptor; NS, not stated; PDGFR, platelet-derived growth factor receptor; RR, response rate; SST, somatostatin receptor; VEGF, vascular endothelial growth factor; VEGFR, vascular endothelial growth factor receptor

Chamberlain MC et al. Neurology 2007;69:969–973
Chamberlain MC, Johnston SK. J Neurooncol 2011;104:765–771
Grimm SA et al. J Clin Oncol 2010;29(15S):151s (Abstract #2046)
Hammond S et al. J Clin Oncol 2011;29(15S):150s (Abstract #2040)
Kaley TJ et al. Neuro Oncol 2010;12(s4):iv75–iv76
Nayak L et al. Neurology 2011;76:A96 (Abstract P02.011)
Norden AD et al. J Neurooncol 2010;96:211–217
Wen PY et al. Neuro Oncol 2009;11:853–860
Wen PY et al. Clin Cancer Res 2006;12:4899–4907

REGIMEN

TEMOZOLOMIDE

Bower M et al. Cancer Chemother Pharmacol 1997;40:484–488

Cycle 1:
Temozolomide 150 mg/m^2 per day; administer orally for 5 consecutive days, on days 1–5 of a 4-week cycle (total dosage/cycle = 750 mg/m^2)

Cycle 2 and subsequent cycles:
Temozolomide 200 mg/m^2 per day; administer orally for 5 consecutive days, on days 1–5, every 4 weeks (total dosage/cycle = 1000 mg/m^2)

Supportive Care
Antiemetic prophylaxis
Emetogenic potential: ***MODERATE***
See Chapter 39 for antiemetic recommendations

Hematopoietic growth factor (CSF) prophylaxis
Primary prophylaxis is NOT indicated
See Chapter 43 for more information

Antimicrobial prophylaxis
Risk of fever and neutropenia is LOW
  Antimicrobial primary prophylaxis to be considered:
  • Antibacterial—not indicated
  • Antifungal—not indicated
  • Antiviral—not indicated unless patient previously had an episode of HSV
See Chapter 47 for more information

Treatment Modifications

Adverse Event	Dose Modification
G ≤1 myelosuppression in cycle 1	Escalate temozolomide dosage to 200 mg/m^2 per day, days 1–5
WBC <3000/mm^3 or platelets <100,000/mm^3 on day 1 of any cycle	Delay retreatment for 1 week
After a 1-week delay, if WBC <2000/mm^3 or platelets <75,000/mm^3	Reduce temozolomide dosage by 25%
After a 1-week delay, if WBC <1000/mm^3 or platelets <25,000/mm^3	Reduce temozolomide dosage by 50%

Efficacy (N = 103)

Objective response	11%
Stable disease	47%
Median survival	5.8 months
Progression-free survival at 6 months	22%

The study included 18 patients not evaluable for response

NOA-04 Randomized Phase III Trial of Sequential Radiochemotherapy of Anaplastic Glioma with Procarbazine, Lomustine, and Vincristine (PCV) or Temozolomide (TMZ)

Wick W et al. J Clin Oncol 2009;27:5874–5880

TTF, PFS, and OS	Radiotherapy (n = 139)		PCV or TMZ (n = 135)	
	Median	95% CI	Median	95% CI
TTF, months	42.7+		43.8	37.4–NR
Anaplastic astrocytoma	32.0	23.3–NR	29.4	19.0–NR
Anaplastic oligoastrocytoma	54+		54+	
Anaplastic oligodendroglioma	54+		54+	
Treatment failure at 48 months, %	55.5	46.3–64.6	46.4	36.7–56.2
PFS, months	30.6	16.3–42.8	31.9	21.1–37.3
Anaplastic astrocytoma	10.8	8.9–28.3	18.2	12.1–24.2
Anaplastic oligoastrocytoma Anaplastic oligodendroglioma	52.1	36.5–NR	52.7	33.9–NR
OS, months	72.1		82.6	
OS at 48 months, %	72.6	63.8–81.4	64.6	54.6–74.7

NR, not reached; OS, overall survival; PFS, progression-free survival; TTF, time to treatment failure

Temozolomide Chemotherapy Alone Versus Radiotherapy Alone for Malignant Astrocytoma in the Elderly: The NOA-08 Randomized, Phase III Trial*

Wick W et al. Lancet Oncol 2012;13:707–715

Entire Temozolomide Group[†]	
Overall survival at 6 months	66.7% (95% CI 60.0–73.0)
Overall survival at 1 year	34.4% (95% CI 27.6–41.4)
Median overall survival	8.6 months (95% CI 7.3–10.2)
Event-free survival at 6 months	30.1% (95% CI 23.6–36.6)
Event-free survival at 1 year	12.0% (95% CI 7.9–17.1)
Median event-free survival	3.3 months (95% CI 3.2–4.1)
Patients with Methylated MGMT Promoter	
Median overall survival	NR (95% CI 10.1–NR)[‡]
Median event-free survival	8.4 months (95% CI 5.5–11.7)[§]

95% CI, 95% confidence interval; MGMT, O$_6$-methylguanine-DNA-methyltransferase; NR, not reached
*Designed as a noninferiority trial
[†]Values are for ITT (intent-to-treat) population. The noninferiority of temozolomide for overall survival and event-free survival were also confirmed in the per-protocol population
[‡]Compared with 7 months (95% CI 5.7–8.7) for patients with an unmethylated tumor MGMT promoter
[§]Compared with 3.3 months (95% CI 3.0–3.5) for patients with an unmethylated tumor MGMT promoter

Toxicity (N = 101)

	% CTC Grade				
	None	G1	G2	G3	G4
Hematologic					
Neutropenia	82	6	8	1	4
Thrombocytopenia	53	29	6	6	7
Anemia	64	32	4	0	1
Lymphopenia	12	10	20	43	16
Nonhematologic					
Nausea	40	18	21	22	0
Vomiting	41	8	27	24	1
Constipation	59	13	17	12	0
Mucositis	76	14	8	3	0
Increased ALT	53	36	9	3	0
Increased ALP	75	26	0	0	0
Increased bilirubin	95	0	5	0	1

	None	Mild	Moderate	Severe
Lethargy*	49	5	14	33
Anorexia*	64	17	10	10

*No CTC grading available. National Cancer Institute (USA) Common Toxicity Criteria (CTC) and Common Terminology Criteria for Adverse Events (CTCAE), all versions. At: http://ctep.cancer.gov/protocolDevelopment/electronic_applications/ctc.htm [accessed December 7, 2013]

NOA-04 Randomized Phase III Trial of Sequential Radiochemotherapy of Anaplastic Glioma (Anaplastic Oligodendroglioma, Oligoastrocytoma, Astrocytoma) with Procarbazine, Lomustine, and Vincristine (PCV) or Temozolomide (TMZ)

Wick W et al. J Clin Oncol 2009;27:5874–5880

Toxicity in the First and Recurrence Treatments

Grade 2/3 Adverse Event According to CTCAE	TMZ (N = 108)
Allergic reaction	1 (0.9%)
Alopecia/local skin reaction	0
Cephalgia	1 (0.9%)
Diarrhea	3 (2.8%)
Hematologic (grades 3 to 4)	6 (5.6%)
Herpes zoster infection	2 (1.8%)
Infection (grades 2 to 4)	2 (1.8%)
Obstipation	2 (1.8%)
Polyneuropathy	0
Pneumonia	2 (1.8%)
Pneumonitis	0
Tumor bleed, thromboembolic events	3 (2.8%)
Transaminase elevation	2 (1.8%)

CTCAE, National Cancer Institute (USA) Common Terminology Criteria for Adverse Events

(*continued*)

Patient Population Studied

A multicenter phase II trial of 103 patients with progressive or recurrent supratentorial high-grade gliomas

Toxicity (N = 101) *(continued)*

NOA-04 Randomized Phase III Trial of Sequential Radiochemotherapy of Anaplastic Glioma (Anaplastic Oligodendroglioma, Oligoastrocytoma, Astrocytoma) with Procarbazine, Lomustine, and Vincristine (PCV) or Temozolomide (TMZ)

Wick W et al. Lancet Oncol 2012;13:707–715

(N = 195)

	Numbers of Grades 2–4 Adverse Events*		
	Grade 2	Grade 3	Grade 4
Hematologic Toxic Effects			
Neutropenia	56	12	4
Lymphocytopenia	60	44	2
Thrombocytopenia	36	12	2
Nonhematologic Toxic Effects			
Liver enzyme elevation	42	26	4
Infection	54	26	9
Thromboembolic event	16	18	6
Asthenia/fatigue	37	21	3
Nausea/vomiting	32	6	0
Weight loss/inappetence	8	2	0
Neurologic symptoms	73	27	9
Seizures	14	15	2
Cutaneous (dermatitis, allergic rash, alopecia)	15	1	0

*Note: N = 195 refers to number of patients. However, number of events are total events and if the grade of an adverse event had returned to 1, subsequent events of grades 2 to 4 were counted as new events, so that a patient could have more than 1 event

Therapy Monitoring

1. *Weekly:* CBC with differential
2. *Every 4 weeks:* Serum electrolytes, mineral panel, and LFTs

REGIMEN

TEMOZOLOMIDE WITH RADIATION THERAPY

Stupp R et al. J Clin Oncol 2002;20:1375–1382
Stupp R et al. N Engl J Med 2005;352:987–996

Temozolomide with radiation therapy:
Temozolomide 75 mg/m² per day; administer orally, continually, 7 days/week for 6–7 weeks in a fasting state 1 hour before radiation therapy (RT), and in the morning in a fasting state on days without RT (total dosage/6- to 7-week cycle = 3150–3675 mg/m²)
Radiation therapy once daily at 2 Gy/fraction for 5 days/week for a total of 60 Gy

Adjuvant temozolomide starting 4 weeks after completing RT:
Temozolomide 200 mg/m² per day; administer orally for 5 consecutive days, on days 1–5 every 28 days for up to 6 cycles (total dosage/cycle = 1000 mg/m²)

Supportive Care
Antiemetic prophylaxis
Emetogenic potential: *MODERATE*
See Chapter 39 for antiemetic recommendations

Hematopoietic growth factor (CSF) prophylaxis
Primary prophylaxis is NOT indicated
See Chapter 43 for more information

Antimicrobial prophylaxis
Risk of fever and neutropenia is LOW
Antimicrobial primary prophylaxis to be considered:
- Antibacterial—not indicated
- Antifungal—not indicated
- Antiviral—not indicated unless patient previously had an episode of HSV

See Chapter 47 for more information

Treatment Modifications

Adverse Event	Dose Modification
WBC <3000/mm³ or platelets <100,000/mm³ on day 1 of any cycle	Delay retreatment for 1 week
After a 1-week delay, if WBC <2000/mm³ or platelets <75,000/mm³	Reduce temozolomide dosage by 25%
After a 1-week delay, if WBC <1000/mm³ or platelets <25,000/mm³	Reduce temozolomide dosage by 50%

Adapted from Stupp R et al. J Clin Oncol 2002;20:1375–1382, in which dose modifications were not specified

Patient Population Studied

A multicenter phase III trial of 573 patients with newly diagnosed GBM in which 287 patients received temozolomide with RT

Efficacy (N = 287)

Median Survival	14.6 months
1-Year survival	61.1%
2-Year survival	26.5%

Therapy Monitoring

1. *Weekly:* CBC with differential
2. *Every 4 weeks:* Serum electrolytes, chemistry panel, and LFTs

Toxicity (N = 287)
Temozolomide with Radiation Therapy (N = 287)

Toxicity	% CTC Grade	
	G2	G3/G4
Hematologic Toxicity		
Leucopenia	N/A	2
Neutropenia	N/A	4
Thrombocytopenia	N/A	3
Anemia	N/A	<1
Any	N/A	7
Nonhematologic Toxicity		
Fatigue	26	7
Other constitutional symptoms	7	2
Rash/other dermatologic	9	1
Infection	1	3
Vision	14	1
Nausea/vomiting	13	<1

Adjuvant Temozolomide After RT (N = 287)

Toxicity	% CTC Grade	
	G2	G3/4
Hematologic Toxicity		
Leukopenia	N/A	5
Neutropenia	N/A	4
Thrombocytopenia	N/A	11
Anemia	N/A	1
Any	N/A	14
Nonhematologic Toxicity		
Fatigue	25	6
Other constitutional symptoms	4	2
Rash/other dermatologic	5	2
Infection	2	5
Vision	10	<1
Nausea/vomiting	18	1

CTC, National Cancer Institute (USA) Common Toxicity Criteria, version 2.0. At: http://ctep.cancer.gov/protocolDevelopment/electronic_applications/ctc.htm [accessed December 7, 2013]

REGIMEN
CARMUSTINE (BCNU)

Levin VA et al. Cancer Treat Rep 1976;60:719–724
Walker MD et al. J Neurosurg 1978;49:333–343

Carmustine 80 mg/m^2 per dose; administer intravenously in 100–250 mL 5% dextrose injection (D5W) over at least 60 minutes for 3 consecutive days, on days 1–3, every 6–8 weeks (total dosage/cycle = 240 mg/m^2)

or

Carmustine 200 mg/m^2; administer intravenously in 100–500 mL D5W over at least 60 minutes, given on day 1, every 6–8 weeks (total dosage/cycle = 200 mg/m^2)
Note: Both schedules are comparable. However, there is no good rationale for the 3-day treatment schedule

Supportive Care
Antiemetic prophylaxis
Emetogenic potential: **MODERATE** *(3-day regimen)* **to HIGH** *(1-day regimen)*
See Chapter 39 for antiemetic recommendations

Hematopoietic growth factor (CSF) prophylaxis
Primary prophylaxis is NOT indicated
See Chapter 43 for more information

Antimicrobial prophylaxis
Risk of fever and neutropenia is LOW
  Antimicrobial primary prophylaxis to be considered:
  • Antibacterial—not indicated
  • Antifungal—not indicated
  • Antiviral—not indicated unless patient previously had an episode of HSV
See Chapter 47 for more information

Patient Population Studied

A phase III randomized study of supportive care alone in 303 patients with newly diagnosed malignant gliomas versus BCNU and/or radiation therapy

Walker MD et al. J Neurosurg 1978;49:333–343

Efficacy (N = 222)

Therapy	Median Survival
Best conventional care only	14 weeks
Carmustine only	18.5 weeks
Radiation therapy only	36 weeks
Radiation therapy + carmustine	34.5 weeks

Note: The addition of carmustine to radiation therapy failed to alter median survival significantly. However, there was a significantly greater surviving percentage of patients at the end of 18 months among those who received combination therapy

Walker MD et al. J Neurosurg 1978;49:333–343

Toxicity (N = 51 for BCNU Group)

	% Patients
Thrombocytopenia: Platelets <100,000/mm^3	54
Platelets <50,000/mm^3	30
Leukopenia: WBC <4000/mm^3	61
WBC <2000/mm^3	18
Anemia	Occasional; no profound anemia encountered
Nausea	Occasional
Vomiting	Occasional
Elevated LFTs	Occasional

Therapy Monitoring

1. *Weekly:* CBC with differential
2. *A minimum of every 6 weeks:* LFTs, BUN, creatinine
3. *Every 2–3 cycles:* Pulmonary function test

Treatment Modifications

Adverse Event	Dose Modification
Nadir prior cycle: WBC 2000–3000/mm^3 or platelets 25,000–75,000/mm^3	Delay treatment until WBC ≥3000/mm^3 and platelets ≥100,000/mm^3, then resume treatment with carmustine dosage reduced by 10–25%
Nadir prior cycle: WBC <2000/mm^3 or platelets <25,000/mm^3	Delay treatment until WBC ≥3000/mm^3 and platelets ≥100,000/mm^3, then resume treatment with carmustine dosage reduced by 25–50%
Cumulative carmustine dosage >1400 mg/m^2 or worsening forced vital capacity (FVC) or carbon monoxide diffusing capacity (DL$_{co}$)	Discontinue carmustine

Note: Usually no more than 5–6 cycles (total cumulative dose of 1000–1200 mg/m^2) of carmustine is recommended. Patients receiving >1400 mg/m^2 cumulative carmustine dosage have a higher risk of developing pulmonary toxicity. Patients with a baseline FVC or DL$_{co}$ <70% are particularly at risk. BiCNU® (carmustine for injection); product label, May 2011. Ben Venue Laboratories, Inc., Bedford, OH

Notes

Two meta-analyses showed a survival benefit for patients treated with nitrosoureas after radiation

Fine HA et al. Cancer 1993;71:2585–2597
Stewart LA et al. Lancet 2002;359:1011–1018

REGIMEN

LOMUSTINE (CCNU)

Batchelor TT, J Clin Oncol 31:3212–3218

Lomustine 110 mg/m^2; administer orally as a single dose on day 1, every 6–8 weeks for a total of 6 cycles (total dosage/cycle = 110 mg/m^2)

Supportive Care
Antiemetic prophylaxis
Emetogenic potential on day 1 is **MODERATE–HIGH**
See Chapter 39 for antiemetic recommendations

Hematopoietic growth factor (CSF) prophylaxis
Primary prophylaxis is NOT indicated
See Chapter 43 for more information

Antimicrobial prophylaxis
Risk of fever and neutropenia is LOW
  Antimicrobial primary prophylaxis to be considered:
  • Antibacterial—not indicated
  • Antifungal—not indicated
  • Antiviral—not indicated unless patient previously had an episode of HSV
See Chapter 47 for more information

Treatment Modifications

Adverse Event	Dose Modification
WBC nadir during the prior cycle 2000–3000/mm^3, or platelets 25,000–75,000/mm^3	Reduce lomustine dosage by 10–25%
WBC nadir during the prior cycle <2000/mm^3, or platelets <25,000/mm^3	Reduce lomustine and dosage by 25–50%
Cumulative lomustine dosage >1100 mg/m^2, or worsening forced vital capacity (FVC) or carbon monoxide diffusing capacity (DLco)*	Discontinue lomustine

*Note: Usually no more than a total of 6–7 cycles of lomustine (660–770 mg/m^2) is recommended. Patients receiving cumulative lomustine dosages >1100 mg/m^2 are at increased risk for developing pulmonary toxicity. Patients with baseline FVC or DLco<70% are particularly at risk
(CCNSB™ (lomustine) Capsules; May 2013 product label. Next Source Biotechnolgy, LLC, Miami, FL)

Patient Population Studied

Patients with recurrent glioblastoma, prior treatment with a temozolomide-containing chemotherapy regimen, prior treatment with radiation, Karnofsky performance status (KPS) ≥70, Mini-Mental Status Examination score ≥15, and who had not received any prior anti-VEGF therapy or cranial radiation within 3 months before study entry

Toxicity

Grades 3/4 Adverse Events	Placebo + Lomustine (n = 64)	
	Number	%
Any AE, ≥ grade 3	39	60.9
Thrombocytopenia	14	22
Neutropenia	2	3.1
Fatigue	6	9.4
Leukopenia	3	4.7
Platelet count decreased	1	1.6
Anemia	0	
Hypertension	0	
ALT increased	0	
GGT increased	2	3.1
WBC decreased	3	4.7
Diarrhea	1	1.6
Pulmonary embolism	4	6.3
Lymphopenia	5	7.8
Convulsion	3	4.7
Intracranial hemorrhage	2	3.1

AE, adverse event; GGT, γ-glutamyltransferase

Efficacy

Best Overall Response	Lomustine + Placebo (n = 56)	
	Number	%
Overall response rate	5	8.9
Complete response (CR)	0	—
Partial response (PR)	5	8.9
Stable disease	23	41.1
Unconfirmed CR	0	—
Unconfirmed PR	2	3.6
PD	16	28.6
Nonevaluable	5	8.9

Median reduction in contrast-enhanced tumor area	+14% increase
APF6 proportions	25%
Corticosteroid usage	+5%

Median progression-free survival	82 days (first quartile = 42 days, third quartile = 168 days)
Median overall survival	9.8 months

REGIMEN

CARBOPLATIN

Yung WK et al. J Clin Oncol 1991;9:860–864

Carboplatin 400 mg/m^2; administer intravenously over 30 minutes to 2 hours in 250 mL 5% dextrose injection (D5W) or 0.9% sodium chloride injection (0.9% NS) on day 1, every 4 weeks (total dosage/cycle = 400 mg/m^2)

or

Carboplatin (calculated dose) AUC = 5–7 mg/mL • min; administer intravenously over 30 minutes to 2 hours in a volume of D5W or 0.9% NS sufficient to produce a concentration ≥0.5 mg/mL, on day 1, every 4 weeks (total dosage/cycle calculated to produce an AUC = 5–7 mg/mL • min)

Supportive Care
Antiemetic prophylaxis
Emetogenic potential is **MODERATE–HIGH**. *Potential for delayed symptoms*
See Chapter 39 for antiemetic recommendations

Hematopoietic growth factor (CSF) prophylaxis
Primary prophylaxis is NOT indicated
See Chapter 43 for more information

Antimicrobial prophylaxis
Risk of fever and neutropenia is LOW
  Antimicrobial primary prophylaxis to be considered:
  • Antibacterial—not indicated
  • Antifungal—not indicated
  • Antiviral—not indicated unless patient previously had an episode of HSV
See Chapter 47 for more information

Carboplatin dose is based on a formula described by Calvert et al. to achieve a target area under the plasma concentration versus time curve (AUC)

$$\text{Total carboplatin dose (mg)} = (\text{Target AUC}) \times (\text{GFR} + 25)$$

In practice, creatinine clearance (Clcr) is used in place of glomerular filtration rate (GFR). Clcr can be calculated from the equation of Cockcroft and Gault, thus:

$$\text{For males, Clcr} = \frac{(140 - \text{age [years]}) \times \text{body weight [kg]}}{72 \times (\text{serum creatinine [mg/dL]})}$$

$$\text{For females, Clcr} = \frac{(140 - \text{age [years]}) \times \text{body weight [kg]}}{72 \times (\text{serum creatinine [mg/dL]})} \times 0.85$$

Calvert AH et al. J Clin Oncol 1989;7:1748–1756
Cockcroft DW, Gault MH. Nephron 1976;16:31–41
Jodrell DI et al. J Clin Oncol 1992;10:520–528
Sorensen BT et al. Cancer Chemother Pharmacol 1991;28:397–401

Note: On October 8, 2010, the FDA identified a potential safety issue with carboplatin dosing based on recent changes in the measurement of serum creatinine. By the end of 2010, all clinical laboratories in the United States will use the standardized Isotope Dilution Mass Spectrometry (IDMS) method to measure serum creatinine, which could result in an overestimation of the GFR in some patients with normal renal function. A carboplatin dose calculated with an IDMS-measured serum creatinine result using the Calvert formula could exceed an expected exposure (AUC) and result in increased drug-related toxicity
Provided actual GFR measurements are made to assess renal function, carboplatin can be safely dosed according to the Calvert formula described in product labeling
If GFR (or creatinine clearance) is estimated based on serum creatinine measurements by the IDMS method, the FDA recommended for patients with normal renal function capping an estimated GFR at 125 mL/min for any targeted AUC value. No greater estimated GFR values should be used
U.S. FDA. Carboplatin dosing. [online] October 8, 2010. Available from: http://www.fda.gov/AboutFDA/CentersOffices/OfficeofMedicalProductsandTobacco/CDER/ucm228974.htm [accessed February 26, 2014]

Patient Population Studied

A study of 30 patients with recurrent malignant gliomas

Treatment Modifications

Adverse Event	Dose Modification
Day 1 WBC <3000/mm^3 or platelets <50,000/mm^3	Delay treatment until WBC ≥3000/mm^3 and platelets ≥100,000/mm^3
ANC nadir <500/mm^3 or platelets <50,000/mm^3	Reduce carboplatin dosage by 25%
Cycle 1 ANC nadir ≥1500/mm^3 and platelet nadir ≥100,000/mm^3	Increase carboplatin dosage by 12.5%

Toxicity (N = 29)

Nonhematologic Toxicity

Toxicity	Percent Cycles with Toxicity		
	Mild	Moderate	Severe
Nausea/vomiting	8	24	2.4
Malaise	18		—

Hematologic Toxicity at 400 mg/m^2

Toxicity	Percent of Patients
Neutropenia (ANC <500/mm^3)	7
Thrombocytopenia* <50,000/mm^3	7

*Although the incidence of thrombocytopenia in this study was low, significant thrombocytopenia often follows carboplatin treatment

Efficacy (N = 29)

Partial response (PR)	7%
Minor response (MR)	7%
Stable disease (S)	34%
Median time to progression (PR/MR/S)	26 weeks
Median survival time (PR/MR/S)	50 weeks

Therapy Monitoring

1. *Weekly:* CBC with differential
2. *Every 28 days:* LFTs. BUN, serum creatinine, serum calcium, magnesium, and uric acid
3. *Every other cycle:* Urine for creatinine clearance
4. *When clinically indicated:* Audiogram

Notes

Adjust the dose based on hematologic toxicity and/or urine creatinine clearance

REGIMEN

PROCARBAZINE, LOMUSTINE (CCNU), VINCRISTINE (PCV)

Levin VA et al. Cancer Treat Rep 1980;64:237–241

Special instructions:
Because procarbazine is a weak monoamine oxidase inhibitor, one should restrict tyramine-containing foods in patients receiving procarbazine

Anon. Med Lett Drugs Ther 1989;31:11–12
DaPrada M et al. J Neural Transm 1988;26:31–56
McCabe BJ. J Am Diet Assoc 1986 86:1059–1064

Lomustine (CCNU) 110 mg/m^2; administer orally as a single dose on day 1, every 6–8 weeks (total dosage/cycle = 110 mg/m^2)
Procarbazine 60 mg/m^2 per day; administer orally for 14 consecutive days on days 8–21, every 6–8 weeks (total dosage/cycle = 840 mg/m^2)
Vincristine 1.4 mg/m^2 per dose (maximum single dose = 2 mg); administer by intravenous injection over 1–2 minutes for 2 doses, on days 8 and 29, every 6–8 weeks (total dosage/cycle = 2.8 mg/m^2, but *not* >4 mg/cycle)

Supportive Care
Antiemetic prophylaxis
Emetogenic potential on day 1 and days 8–21 is **MODERATE–HIGH**
Emetogenic potential on day 29 is **MINIMAL**
See Chapter 39 for antiemetic recommendations

Hematopoietic growth factor (CSF) prophylaxis
Primary prophylaxis is NOT indicated
See Chapter 43 for more information

Antimicrobial prophylaxis
Risk of fever and neutropenia is LOW
  Antimicrobial primary prophylaxis to be considered:
  • Antibacterial—not indicated
  • Antifungal—not indicated
  • Antiviral—not indicated unless patient previously had an episode of HSV
See Chapter 47 for more information

Treatment Modifications

Adverse Event	Dose Modification
Nadir prior cycle: WBC 2000–3000/mm^3 or platelets 25,000–75,000/mm^3	Reduce lomustine and procarbazine dosages by 10–25%
Nadir prior cycle: WBC <2000/mm^3 or platelets <25,000/mm^3	Reduce lomustine and procarbazine dosages by 25–50%
Severe neurotoxicity, eg, painful paresthesia or peripheral weakness	Discontinue vincristine
Cumulative lomustine dosage >1100 mg/m^2 or worsening forced vital capacity (FVC) or carbon monoxide diffusing capacity (DL$_{co}$)*	Discontinue lomustine

*Note: Usually no more than a total of 6–7 cycles (660–770 mg/m^2) of lomustine is recommended. Patients receiving >1100 mg/m^2 cumulative lomustine dosage have a higher risk of developing pulmonary toxicity. Patients with a baseline FVC or DLco <70% are particularly at risk

(CCNSB™ (lomustine) Capsules; May 2013 product label. NextSource Biotechnolgy, LLC, Miami, FL)

Efficacy (N = 46)

Objective response (OR)	26%
Stable disease (SD)	35%
Median time to progression (OR + SD)	26 weeks
Progression-free survival at 12 months	30%

NOA-04 Randomized Phase III Trial of Sequential Radiochemotherapy of Anaplastic Glioma with Procarbazine, Lomustine, and Vincristine (PCV) or Temozolomide (TMZ)

Wick W et al. J Clin Oncol 2009;27:5874–5880

TTF, PFS, and OS	Radiotherapy (n = 139)		PCV or TMZ (n = 135)	
	Median	95% CI	Median	95% CI
TTF, months	42.7+		43.8	37.4–NR
Anaplastic astrocytoma	32.0	23.3–NR	29.4	19.0–NR
Anaplastic oligoastrocytoma	54+		54+	
Anaplastic oligodendroglioma	54+		54+	
Treatment failure at 48 months, %	55.5	46.3–64.6	46.4	36.7–56.2
PFS, months	30.6	16.3–42.8	31.9	21.1–37.3
Anaplastic astrocytoma	10.8	8.9–28.3	18.2	12.1–24.2
Anaplastic oligoastrocytoma Anaplastic oligodendroglioma	52.1	36.5–NR	52.7	33.9–NR
OS, months	72.1		82.6	
OS at 48 months, %	72.6	63.8–81.4	64.6	54.6–74.7

OS, overall survival; PFS, progression-free survival; TTF, time to treatment failure

Toxicity (N = 72)

	%G1	%G2	%G3	%G4
Hematologic				
Leukopenia	14	43	15	8
Thrombocytopenia	13	17	15	11
Nonhematologic				
Nausea/vomiting	21	15	11	0
Neuropathy	15	15	8	0

Occasionally a rash is observed

Northern California Oncology Group Criteria
Levin VA et al. J Neurosurg 1985;63:218–223. Toxicity data obtained from a similar study

NOA-04 Randomized Phase III Trial of Sequential Radiochemotherapy of Anaplastic Glioma (Anaplastic Oligodendroglioma, Oligoastrocytoma, Astrocytoma) with Procarbazine, Lomustine, and Vincristine (PCV) or Temozolomide (TMZ)

Wick W et al. J Clin Oncol 2009;27:5874–5880

Toxicity in the First and Recurrence Treatments

Grades 2/3 Adverse Event According to CTCAE	PCV (N = 100)
Allergic reaction	13 (13%)
Alopecia/local skin reaction	0
Cephalgia	0
Diarrhea	0
Hematologic (grades 3 to 4)	22 (22%)
Herpes zoster infection	4 (4%)
Infection (grades 2 to 4)	4 (4%)
Obstipation	0
Polyneuropathy	16 (16%)
Pneumonia	3 (3%)
Pneumonitis	1 (1%)
Tumor bleed, thromboembolic events	3 (3%)
Transaminase elevation	23 (23%)

CTCAE, National Cancer Institute (USA) Common Terminology Criteria for Adverse Events, all versions.
At: http://ctep.cancer.gov/protocolDevelopment/electronic_applications/ctc.htm [accessed December 7, 2013]

Patient Population Studied

A phase II study of 46 patients with recurrent malignant brain tumor

Therapy Monitoring

1. *Weekly:* CBC with differential
2. *Before each treatment:* LFTs
3. *Every 3–4 cycles:* Pulmonary function test

Notes

This regimen has been particularly effective for the treatment of high risk low grade gliomas following radiation therapy, anaplastic oligodendrogliomas and oligoastrocytomas

Cairncross JG et al. Ann Neurol 1988;23:360–364
Kim L et al. J Neurosurg 1996;85:602–607

REGIMEN

ADJUVANT PROCARBAZINE, LOMUSTINE (CCNU), AND VINCRISTINE (PCV)
NEWLY DIAGNOSED ANAPLASTIC OLIGODENDROGLIOMA

van den Bent MJ et al. J Clin Oncol 2013;31:344–350
van den Bent MJ et al. J Clin Oncol 2006;24:2715–2722

Special instructions:
Because procarbazine is a weak monoamine oxidase inhibitor, clinicians should guide patients who receive the drug in limiting their dietary intake of tyramine-containing foods and beverages

Anon. Med Lett Drugs Ther 1989;31:11–12
DaPrada M et al. J Neural Transm Suppl 1988;26:31–56
McCabe BJ. J Am Diet Assoc 1986;86:1059–1064

PCV chemotherapy started within 4 weeks after the end of RT
Lomustine 110 mg/m^2; administer orally as a single dose on day 1, every 6 weeks for a total of 6 cycles (total dosage/cycle = 110 mg/m^2)
Procarbazine 60 mg/m^2 per day; administer orally for 14 consecutive days on days 8–21, every 6 weeks for a total of 6 cycles (total dosage/cycle = 840 mg/m^2)
Vincristine 1.4 mg/m^2; administer per dose (maximum single dose = 2 mg); administer by intravenous injection over 1–2 minutes for 2 doses, on days 8 and 29, every 6 weeks for a total of 6 cycles (total dosage/cycle = 2.8 mg/m^2; maximum dose/cycle = 4 mg)
Radiotherapy within 6 weeks after surgery. 45 Gy is administered to the planning target volume-1 (PTV-1) in twenty-five 1.8-Gy fractions, 5 days/week over 5 weeks. Thereafter, a boost of 14.4 Gy (up to a cumulative dose of 59.4 Gy) is delivered to the PTV-2 in 8 fractions of 1.8 Gy, 1 fraction per day, 5 fractions per week. PTV-2 is to include the nonenhancing tumor area and/or the enhancing area as visible on the postoperative CT scan with contrast with a 1.5-cm margin; in case of a nonenhancing tumor on CT scan, a postoperative MRI scan with and without gadolinium is recommended to further define the tumor volume

Supportive Care
Antiemetic prophylaxis
Emetogenic potential on day 1 and days 8–21 is **MODERATE–HIGH**
Emetogenic potential on day 29 is **MINIMAL**
See Chapter 39 for antiemetic recommendations

Hematopoietic growth factor (CSF) prophylaxis
Primary prophylaxis is NOT indicated
See Chapter 43 for more information

Antimicrobial prophylaxis
Risk of fever and neutropenia is LOW
 Antimicrobial primary prophylaxis to be considered:
 • Antibacterial—not indicated
 • Antifungal—not indicated
 • Antiviral—not indicated unless patient previously had an episode of HSV
See Chapter 47 for more information

Note: Treatment at the time of progression was left to the discretion of local investigators, but the study protocol strongly advised treating physicians to consider (PCV) chemotherapy, especially for patients in the RT-only arm

Treatment Modifications

Adverse Event	Dose Modification
WBC nadir during the prior cycle 2000–3000/mm^3, or platelets 25,000–75,000/mm^3	Reduce lomustine and procarbazine dosages by 10–25%
WBC nadir during the prior cycle <2000/mm^3, or platelets <25,000/mm^3	Reduce lomustine and procarbazine dosages by 25–50%
Severe neurotoxicity; eg, painful paresthesia or peripheral weakness	Discontinue vincristine
Cumulative lomustine dosage >1100 mg/m^2, or worsening forced vital capacity (FVC) or carbon monoxide diffusing capacity (DL$_{co}$)*	Discontinue lomustine

*Note: Usually no more than a total of 6–7 cycles of lomustine (660–770 mg/m^2) is recommended. Patients receiving cumulative lomustine dosages >1100 mg/m^2 are at increased risk for developing pulmonary toxicity. Patients with baseline FVC or DL$_{co}$ <70% are particularly at risk

Patient Population Studied

Patient Characteristic	Radiotherapy Plus PCV (N = 185)	Radiotherapy Only (N = 183)
	Number of Patients (Percent)	
Age, years: median (range)	48.6 (18.6–68.7)	49.8 (19.2–68.7)
Sex: Male/Female	102/83	110/73
WHO performance status: 0/1/2	155 (84)/30 (16)	153/30/84/16
Previous resection for low-grade tumor: Yes/No	27 (15)/156 (84)	25 (14)/157 (86)
Enhancement of the tumor: Yes/No	144 (78)/33 (18)	140 (77)/29 (16)
Tumor localization: Frontal/Elsewhere	89 (48)/96 (52)	84 (47)/98 (53)
MMSE score: 27–30/<27	116 (63)/46 (25)	14 (62)/53 (29)
Extent of resection* Biopsy Partial resection Total resection	27 (15) 100 (54) 58 (31)	25 (14) 83 (45) 75 (41)
Pathology Oligodendroglioma Oligoastrocytoma Missing	139 (75) 44 (24) 2 (1)	126 (69) 56 (31) 1 (1)
1p/19q determined 1p/19q loss 1p loss 19q loss No loss	155 42 (27) 24 (15) 18 (12) 71 (46)	156 36 (23) 24 (15) 20 (13) 76 (49)

MMSE, Mini-Mental State Examination; PCV, procarbazine, lomustine, and vincristine
*The extent of resection as assessed by the neurosurgeon

Toxicity

- Most patients who discontinued PCV prematurely did so for (usually asymptomatic) hematologic toxicity or for tumor progression
- A quality-of-life analysis that was part of this study has shown that patients in the RT/PCV arm complained more frequently of nausea/vomiting, loss of appetite, and drowsiness during and shortly after PCV chemotherapy
- However, no long-term effects of PCV chemotherapy on quality of life were identified

G3/4 Toxicity in the Patients Who Started PCV Chemotherapy (N = 161)

Toxicity	Grade 3	Grade 4
	Number of Patients (Percent)	
WBC count	43 (27)	5 (3)
Neutrophils	39 (24)	13 (8)
Platelets	23 (14)	11 (7)
Hemoglobin	10 (6)	1 (1)
Any hematologic toxicity	51 (32)	23 (14)
Nausea	9 (6)	—
Vomiting	10 (6)	—
Polyneuropathy	3 (2)	—
Allergic skin reactions	2 (1)	—

PCV, procarbazine, lomustine, and vincristine

Efficacy*

Median and 5-Year Overall Survival and Progression-Free Survival According to Assigned Treatment in the Various Subgroups

	Overall Survival				Progression-free Survival			
	Median	95% CI	% 5-y	95% CI	Median	95% CI	% 5-y	95% CI
Intent-to-treat Population (N_{RT} = 183; $N_{RT/PCV}$ = 185)								
RT	30.6	21.5–44.5	37.0	30.0–44.0	13.2	9.2–17.9	22	16.0–27.9
RT/PCV	42.3	28.7–62.0	43.4	36.2–50.5	24.3	17.4–40.7	37.5	30.5–44.4
1p/19q Status								
Deleted 1p/19q (N = 80)								
RT	111.8	75.7–134.3	73.0	55.6–84.4	49.9	27.8–101.8	46.0	29.6–60.9
RT/PCV	NR		76.2	60.3–86.4	156.8	68.1–NR	71.4	55.2–82.7
	HR, 0.56 (95% CI, 0.31–1.03); P = 0.0594				HR, 0.42 (95% CI, 0.24 to 0.74); P = 0.002			
Nondeleted 1p/19q (N = 236)								
RT	21.1	17.6–28.7	25.1	17.7–33.0	8.7	7.1–11.7	13.5	8.1–20.3
RT/PCV	25.0	18.0–36.8	31.6	23.3–40.2	14.8	9.9–21.1	25.4	17.8–33.7
	HR, 0.83 (95% CI, 0.62–1.10); P = 0.185				HR, 0.73 (95% CI, 0.56–0.97); P = 0.026			
IDH Status								
Mutated (N = 81)								
RT	64.8	36.9–111.8	52.8	35.5–67.4	36.0	17.2–58.6	33.3	18.8–48.6
RT/PCV	NR		68.2	52.3–79.8	71.2	47.1–NR	59.1	43.2–71.9
Wild type (N = 97)								
RT	14.7	11.9–19.1	16.0	7.5–27.4	6.8	5.4–8.6	4.0	0.74–12.1
RT/PCV	19.0	14.6–30.2	21.3	11.0–33.8	10.0	7.8–18.2	17.0	8.0–29.0
MGMT Promoter								
Methylated (N = 136)								
RT	43.3	21.9–66.2	41.9	29.6–53.8	15.2	8.7–34.5	21.0	11.9–31.8
RT/PCV	70.9	42.0–136.8	54.8	42.7–65.4	55.6	20.4–73.6	48.0	36.2–58.8
Unmethylated (N = 47)								
RT	15.6	11.4–19.1	8.3	1.4–23.3	7.1	4.4–8.7	4.2	0.3–17.6
RT/PCV	16.3	9.1–30.3	17.4	5.4–35.0	9.8	4.6–15.4	17.4	5.4–35.0
Confirmed Anaplastic Oligodendroglial Histology at Central Review (N_{RT} = 126; $N_{RT/PCV}$ = 131)								
RT	28.7	19.3–41.7	33.0	25.0–41.3	10.4	8.4–16.9	17.9	11.8–25.1
RT/PCV	35.0	24.2–56.2	41.5	33.0–49.8	19.1	15.2–40.0	35.4	27.3–43.6
	HR, 0.73 (95% CI, 0.55–0.96)							

CI, confidence interval; IDH, isocitrate dehydrogenase; MGMT, O_6-methylguanine-DNA methyltransferase; NR, not reached; PCV, procarbazine, lomustine, and vincristine; RT, radiotherapy

*The increase in OS was achieved despite the fact that the median number of PCV cycles was 3, with only 30% of patients completing the intended 6 cycles; most patients that discontinued PCV prematurely did so for (usually asymptomatic) hematologic toxicity or for tumor progression

Therapy Monitoring

1. *Weekly:* CBC with differential
2. *Before each treatment:* LFTs
3. *Every 3–4 cycles:* Pulmonary function tests

REGIMEN

HIGH-DOSE TAMOXIFEN

Couldwell WT et al. Clin Cancer Res 1996;2:619–622

Initial dose and schedule:
Tamoxifen 20 mg/dose; administer orally, twice daily for 4 days (total dose/4 days = 160 mg)

If tolerated advance dose as follows:
Increase the tamoxifen dose every week in increments of 20 mg/dose (40 mg/day) to achieve after 1 month the target doses indicated below

Target dose for females:
Tamoxifen 80 mg/dose; administer orally, twice daily, continually (total dose/30 days = 4800 mg)

Target dose for males:
Tamoxifen 100 mg/dose; administer orally, twice daily, continually (total dose/30 days = 6000 mg)

Supportive Care
Antiemetic prophylaxis
Emetogenic potential: **MINIMAL**
See Chapter 39 for antiemetic recommendations

Hematopoietic growth factor (CSF) prophylaxis
Primary prophylaxis is NOT indicated
See Chapter 43 for more information

Antimicrobial prophylaxis
Risk of fever and neutropenia is LOW
   Antimicrobial primary prophylaxis to be considered:
   • Antibacterial—not indicated
   • Antifungal—not indicated
   • Antiviral—not indicated, unless patient previously had an episode of HSV
See Chapter 47 for more information

Treatment Modifications

Adverse Event	Dose Modification
Deep venous thrombosis	Discontinue tamoxifen
Nausea/vomiting	Hold tamoxifen. Restart previously tolerated dose when symptoms resolve to G ≤1
G3 fatigue	Hold tamoxifen. Restart previously tolerated dose when symptoms resolve to G ≤1

Therapy Monitoring

1. *Weekly:* CBC with differential
2. *Weekly while escalating dose:* LFTs, BUN, and serum creatinine
3. *Every 2 months when not escalating dose:* LFTs, BUN, and serum creatinine

Patient Population Studied

A phase II study of 32 patients with recurrent malignant gliomas

Efficacy (N = 32)

Clinical and radiographic responses	25%
Stable disease	19%
Median survival	10.1 months

Toxicity (N = 32)

	% Patients
Deep vein thrombosis	6
Nausea	3
Hot flashes	3
Fatigue	6

REGIMEN

ERLOTINIB (TARCEVA)

Prados MD et al. Neuro Oncol 2006;8:67–78
Raizer JJ et al. Proc Am Soc Clin Oncol 2004;22:107s (abstract #1502)
Yung A et al. Proc Am Soc Clin Oncol 2004;22:120s (abstract #1555)

Patients receiving non–enzyme-inducing antiepileptic drugs (NEIAED)
Erlotinib 200 mg per day; administer orally, continually, every day of a 4-week cycle
(total dosage/cycle = 5600 mg)

Patients receiving enzyme-inducing antiepileptic drugs (EIAED)
Erlotinib 500 mg per day; administer orally, continually, every day of a 4-week cycle
(total dosage/cycle = 14,000 mg)

Supportive Care
Antiemetic prophylaxis
Emetogenic potential: **MINIMAL**
See Chapter 39 for antiemetic recommendations

Hematopoietic growth factor (CSF) prophylaxis
Primary prophylaxis is NOT indicated
See Chapter 43 for more information

Antimicrobial prophylaxis
Risk of fever and neutropenia is LOW
Antimicrobial primary prophylaxis to be considered:
• Antibacterial—not indicated
• Antifungal—not indicated
• Antiviral—not indicated unless patient previously had an episode of HSV
See Chapter 47 for more information

Diarrhea management
Latent or delayed onset diarrhea*:
Loperamide 4 mg orally initially after the first loose or liquid stool, *then*
Loperamide 2 mg orally every 2 hours during waking hours, *plus*
Loperamide 4 mg orally every 4 hours during hours of sleep

• Continue for at least 12 hours after diarrhea resolves
• Recurrent diarrhea after a 12-hour diarrhea free interval is treated as a new episode
• Rehydrate orally with fluids and electrolytes during a diarrheal episode
• If a patient develops blood or mucus in stool, dehydration, or hemodynamic instability, or if diarrhea persists >48 hours despite loperamide, stop loperamide and hospitalize the patient for IV hydration
Alternatively, a trial of Diphenoxylate hydrochloride 2.5 mg with Atropine sulfate 0.025 mg (eg, Lomotil®)
• Initial adult dose is two tablets four times daily until control has been achieved, after which the dose may be reduced to meet individual requirements. Control may often be maintained with as little as two tablets daily
• Clinical improvement of acute diarrhea is usually observed within 48 hours. If improvement of chronic diarrhea after treatment with a maximum daily dose of 8 tablets is not observed within 10 days, control is unlikely with further administration
Persistent diarrhea:
Octreotide 100–150 mcg subcutaneously 3 times daily. Maximum total daily dose is 1500 mcg
Antibiotic therapy during latent or delayed onset diarrhea:
A fluoroquinolone (eg, **Ciprofloxacin** 500 mg orally every 12 hours) if absolute neutrophil count <500/mm³ with or without accompanying fever in association with diarrhea
• Antibiotics should also be administered if patient is hospitalized with prolonged diarrhea and should be continued until diarrhea resolves

*Rothenberg ML et al. J Clin Oncol 2001;19:3801–3807
Abigerges D et al. J Natl Cancer Inst 1994;86:446–449
Wadler S et al. J Clin Oncol 1998;16:3169–3178

Treatment Modifications

Adverse Event	Dose Modification
Pulmonary symptoms (dyspnea, cough, fever)	Hold erlotinib
Interstitial lung disease	Discontinue erlotinib
G1/2 diarrhea	Administer loperamide, 2 mg orally several times a day; if symptoms do not improve, hold erlotinib until symptoms resolve and then reduce dose
G2+/3/4 diarrhea	Reduce dose, *or* hold erlotinib until symptoms resolve and then reduce dose
G1/2 rash, skin reaction	Hold erlotinib. Administer supportive care. If symptoms resolve, restart the same dose
G2+/3/4 rash, skin reaction	Hold erlotinib. Administer supportive care. If symptoms resolve, restart at a reduced dose

Patient Population Studied

• A phase I study of 83 patients with stable or progressive malignant primary glioma (Prados et al.)
• A phase II study of 48 patients with glioblastoma in first relapse
• A phase II study of 45 patients with recurrent malignant gliomas not on EIAED

Yung A et al. Proc Am Soc Clin Oncol 2004;22:120s (abstract #1555)

Toxicity* (N = 83)

	% All Grades	% G1	% G2	% G3	% G4
Rash	84	34	37	13	0
Fatigue	67	20	41	5	0
Diarrhea	64	43	17	4	0
White blood cell count	40	24	13	2	0
Headache	35	27	7	1	0
Liver dysfunction	32	25	5	1	0
Constipation	29	17	12	0	0
Nausea/vomiting	26	11	12	2	0
Dry mouth	24	24	0	0	0
Platelet count	16	4	0	5	7
Pruritus	12	7	5	0	0
Infection	11	1	8	0	1[†]
Kidney dysfunction	10	7	1	1	0

*Includes all patients on erlotinib alone or combined with temozolomide)
[†]Grade 5; thought to be temozolomide-associated myelosuppression with infection

Prados MD et al. Neuro Oncol 2006;8:67–78

Toxicity (N = 22)

		No EIAED		+ EIAED	
Adverse Event	% of All Patients	% Erlotinib Alone	% Erlotinib + Temozolomide	% Erlotinib Alone	% Erlotinib + Temozolomide
Rash	50	18	18	9	14
Thrombocytopenia	10	9	14	0	23
Fatigue	18	9	9	0	0
Diarrhea	14	4.5	0	9	0
Neutropenia	9	0	0	0	9
Headache	4.5	0	4.5	0	0
Liver dysfunction	4.5	0	0	0	4.5
Nausea/vomiting	9	4.5	4.5	0	0
Infections	4.5	4.5	0	0	0
Kidney dysfunction	4.5	0	0	0	4.5

Prados MD et al. Neuro Oncol 2006;8:67–78

Efficacy (N = 57)

Partial response	14%
PFS >6 months	10.5% (including 4/6 with PR)

Prados MD et al. Neuro Oncol 2006;8:67–78

Efficacy (N = 48)

Complete response	2%
Partial response	2%
Stable disease	21%

Yung A et al. Proc Am Soc Clin Oncol 2004;22:120s (abstract #1555)

Efficacy (N = 45)

Glioblastoma Multiforme (GBM)— 30 Patients	
Stable disease	13%
Median progression-free survival	12 weeks
Anaplastic Glioma—15 Patients	
Partial response	7%
Stable disease	13%
Median progression-free survival	8.6 weeks

Raizer JJ et al. Proc Am Soc Clin Oncol 2004;22: 107s (abstract #1502)

Therapy Monitoring

1. *Weekly:* CBC with differential
2. *Every 4 weeks:* Serum electrolytes, mineral panel, and LFTs

Notes

This regimen might be useful particularly for patients whose tumor expresses EGFR or EGFRviii, which are commonly found in GBM

REGIMEN

BEVACIZUMAB (AVASTIN) ± IRINOTECAN

Kreisl T et al. J Clin Oncol 2009;27:740–745

Initial therapy:
Bevacizumab 10 mg/kg per dose; administer intravenously in 100 mL 0.9% sodium chloride injection, USP (0.9% NS) every 14 days on a 28-day cycle (total dosage/cycle = 20 mg/kg)
• First dose is administered over 90 minutes
• Second dose may be administered over 60 minutes, if the first dose was well tolerated
• Third and subsequent doses may be administered over 30 minutes, if doses administered over 60 minutes were well tolerated

Therapy after documented tumor progression:
Bevacizumab 10 mg/kg per dose; administer intravenously in 100 mL 0.9% NS every 14 days on a 28-day cycle (total dosage/cycle = 20 mg/kg), *plus*
Irinotecan
  Patients receiving non–enzyme-inducing antiepileptic drugs (NEIAED)
    125 mg/m²; administer intravenously over 90 minutes in 250 mL 0.9% NS or 5% dextrose injection, USP (D5W), every 14 days on a 28-day cycle (total dosage per cycle = 250 mg/m²)
  Patients receiving enzyme-inducing antiepileptic drugs (EIAED)
    340 mg/m²; administer intravenously over 90 minutes in 250 mL 0.9% NS or D5W every 14 days on a 28-day cycle (total dosage per cycle = 680 mg/m²)

Supportive Care
Antiemetic prophylaxis
Emetogenic potential with bevacizumab alone is **MINIMAL**
Emetogenic potential with bevacizumab + irinotecan is **MODERATE**
See Chapter 39 for antiemetic recommendations

Hematopoietic growth factor (CSF) prophylaxis
Primary prophylaxis is NOT indicated
See Chapter 43 for more information

Antimicrobial prophylaxis
Risk of fever and neutropenia is LOW
  Antimicrobial primary prophylaxis to be considered:
  • Antibacterial—not indicated
  • Antifungal—not indicated
  • Antiviral—not indicated, unless patient previously had an episode of HSV
See Chapter 47 for more information

Acute cholinergic syndrome
Atropine sulfate 0.25–1 mg administer subcutaneously or intravenously if abdominal cramping or diarrhea develop during or within 1 hour after irinotecan administration
• If symptoms are severe, add as primary prophylaxis at least 30 min before irinotecan during subsequent cycles
• For irinotecan, acute cholinergic syndrome may be characterized by: abdominal cramping, diarrhea, diaphoresis, hypotension, flushing, bradycardia, rhinitis, increased salivation, meiosis, and lacrimation

Diarrhea management
Latent or delayed onset diarrhea*:
  Loperamide 4 mg orally initially after the first loose or liquid stool, *then*
  Loperamide 2 mg orally every 2 hours during waking hours, *plus*
  Loperamide 4 mg orally every 4 hours during hours of sleep
  • Continue for at least 12 hours after diarrhea resolves
  • Recurrent diarrhea after a 12-hour diarrhea free interval is treated as a new episode
  • Rehydrate orally with fluids and electrolytes during a diarrheal episode
  • If a patient develops blood or mucus in stool, dehydration, or hemodynamic instability, or if diarrhea persists >48 hours despite loperamide, stop loperamide and hospitalize the patient for IV hydration

(continued)

Toxicity (N = 48)

Toxicity	% G1	% G2	% G3	% G4
Thrombo-embolic events			4.2	8.4
Hypertension		8.4	4.2	
Hypophos-phatemia		4.2	6.3	
Thrombo-cytopenia		4.2	2.1	
Hepatic dysfunction			2.1	
Proteinuria	2.1			
Bowel perforation			2.1	

Patient Population Studied

A phase II study of 48 patients with recurrent glioblastoma

Efficacy (N = 48)

Partial response	71%
6-Month survival rate	57%
6-Month progression-free survival	29%
Median overall survival	31 weeks
Median progression-free survival	16 weeks

Note: Of 19 patients treated with bevacizumab plus irinotecan at progression, there were no objective radiographic responses

Therapy Monitoring

1. *Every 2 weeks:* CBC with differential, urinalysis for urine protein: creatinine ratio, BP check
2. *Every 4 weeks:* CBC with differential, serum electrolytes, mineral panel, and LFTs

(*continued*)

Alternatively, a trial of **Diphenoxylate hydrochloride** 2.5 mg **with Atropine sulfate** 0.025 mg (eg, Lomotil®)
- Initial adult dose is two tablets four times daily until control has been achieved, after which the dose may be reduced to meet individual requirements. Control may often be maintained with as little as two tablets daily
- Clinical improvement of acute diarrhea is usually observed within 48 hours. If improvement of chronic diarrhea after treatment with a maximum daily dose of 8 tablets is not observed within 10 days, control is unlikely with further administration

Persistent diarrhea:
Octreotide 100–150 mcg subcutaneously 3 times daily. Maximum total daily dose is 1500 mcg

Antibiotic therapy during latent or delayed onset diarrhea:
A fluoroquinolone (eg, **Ciprofloxacin** 500 mg orally every 12 hours) if absolute neutrophil count <500/mm^3 with or without accompanying fever in association with diarrhea
- Antibiotics should also be administered if patient is hospitalized with prolonged diarrhea and should be continued until diarrhea resolves

*Rothenberg ML et al. J Clin Oncol 2001;19:3801–3807; Abigerges D et al. J Natl Cancer Inst 1994;86:446–449; Wadler S et al. J Clin Oncol 1998;16:3169–3178

Treatment Modifications: Bevacizumab-Related Adverse Events

Note: There are no recommended dose reductions for the use of bevacizumab. Consequently, bevacizumab use is either temporarily interrupted or discontinued

Adverse Event	Toxicity Grade	Dose Modification/Action to Be Taken
Allergic reactions or Acute infusional reactions/ cytokine release syndrome	G1–3	Premedications should be given before the next dose, and infusion time may not be shortened for subsequent infusions For patients with G3 reactions, bevacizumab infusion should be stopped and not restarted on the same day. At a physician's discretion, bevacizumab may be permanently discontinued or reinstituted with premedications and at a rate designed to complete administration over 90 ± 15 minutes. If bevacizumab is reinstituted, the patient should be closely monitored for a duration comparable to or longer than the duration of the previous reactions
	G4	Discontinue bevacizumab
Arterial thrombosis • Cardiac ischemia/infarction • CNS ischemia (TIA, CVA) • Any peripheral or visceral arterial ischemia/thrombosis	G2 (if new or worsened after starting bevacizumab therapy)	Discontinue bevacizumab
	G3/4	Discontinue bevacizumab
Venous thrombosis	G3 or asymptomatic G4	• Hold bevacizumab treatment. If the planned duration of full-dose anticoagulation is <2 weeks, bevacizumab should be withheld until the full-dose anticoagulation period is over. Prophylaxis against pulmonary emboli can be accomplished through placement of an IVC filter • If the planned duration of full-dose anticoagulation is >2 weeks, permanently discontinue bevacizumab • If thromboemboli worsen/recur upon resumption of therapy, discontinue bevacizumab
	G4 (symptomatic)	Discontinue bevacizumab
Hypertension (Treat with antihypertensive medications as needed. The goal of BP control should be consistent with general medical practice)	If BP is controlled medically	Continue bevacizumab
	Persistent or symptomatic HTN	Hold bevacizumab. If treatment is delayed for >4 weeks because of uncontrolled hypertension, discontinue bevacizumab
	G4	Discontinue bevacizumab
Proteinuria (Proteinuria should be monitored by urine analysis for urine protein:creatinine [UPC] ratio prior to every dose of bevacizumab)	UPC ratio <3.5	Continue bevacizumab
	UPC ratio ≥3.5	Hold bevacizumab until UPC recovers to <3.5. If therapy is held for >2 months because of proteinuria, discontinue bevacizumab
	G4 or nephrotic syndrome	Discontinue bevacizumab
Wound dehiscence requiring medical or surgical intervention		Discontinue bevacizumab
GI perforation, GI leak or fistula		Discontinue bevacizumab

REGIMEN

HIGH-DOSE METHOTREXATE FOR PRIMARY CNS LYMPHOMA

Batchelor T et al. J Clin Oncol 2003;21:1044–1049

Induction phase:
Methotrexate every 14 days until complete response (CR) or a maximum of 8 cycles are delivered

Consolidation phase:
For patients achieving a CR during induction, give 2 cycles of methotrexate every 14 days, then give:

Maintenance phase:
Eleven cycles of methotrexate every 28 days

Hydration before, during, and after methotrexate:
Before methotrexate administration:
5% Dextrose injection (D5W) or 5% dextrose/0.45% sodium chloride injection (D5W/0.45% NS) with 50–100 mEq sodium bicarbonate injection/L; administer intravenously at 100–150 mL/hour
- Adjust infusion rate to achieve and maintain a urine output ≥100 mL/hour for ≥4 hours before starting methotrexate
- Adjust sodium bicarbonate to produce a urine pH within the range ≥7.0 to ≤8.0 before starting methotrexate

During methotrexate administration:
No additional hydration (see below)

After methotrexate administration:
D5W or D5W/0.45% NS with 50–100 mEq sodium bicarbonate injection/L; administer intravenously at 100–150 mL/hour until serum methotrexate concentration <0.1 μmol/L
- Adjust infusion rate to maintain urine output ≥100 mL/hour
- Adjust sodium bicarbonate to maintain urine pH ≥7.0 to ≤8.0

Methotrexate 8000 mg/m^2 in 500–1000 mL D5W with 50–100 mEq sodium bicarbonate per dose; administer intravenously over 4 hours (total dosage every 14 days [induction and consolidation cycles] and every 28 days [maintenance cycles] = 8000 mg/m^2)
(Add sodium bicarbonate in amounts sufficient to produce a bicarbonate concentration equivalent to fluid used for the same volume of hydration fluid given over a 4-hour period)
Leucovorin calcium 25 mg per dose; administer intravenously every 6 hours for 4 doses, starting 24 hours after methotrexate administration began
Six hour after the last dose of intravenously administered leucovorin, start oral leucovorin or continue with intravenous leucovorin calcium every 6 hours if patient is nauseated or vomiting otherwise:
Leucovorin calcium 25 mg per dose; administer orally or intravenously every 6 hours until serum methotrexate concentration <0.1 μmol/L

Supportive Care
Antiemetic prophylaxis
Emetogenic potential is **MODERATE**
See Chapter 39 for antiemetic recommendations

Hematopoietic growth factor (CSF) prophylaxis
Primary prophylaxis is NOT indicated
See Chapter 43 for more information

Antimicrobial prophylaxis
Risk of fever and neutropenia is LOW
  Antimicrobial primary prophylaxis to be considered:
  - Antibacterial—not indicated
  - Antifungal—not indicated
  - Antiviral—not indicated, unless patient previously had an episode of HSV
See Chapter 47 for more information

Patient Population Studied

A multicenter phase II trial of 25 patients with newly diagnosed non–AIDS-related primary CNS lymphoma (PCNSL). Previous radiation therapy was not allowed

Efficacy (N = 24)

Complete response*	50%
Partial response	21%
Stable disease	4.2%
Median progression-free survival	12.8 months
Median overall survival	>22.8 months

*Median number of cycles to CR = 6

Treatment Modifications

Methotrexate dosage is based on a measured creatinine clearance before treatment commences. For any creatinine clearance <100 mL/min, methotrexate dosage is calculated by multiplying the planned dosage (8000 mg/m^2) by the ratio between the measured creatinine clearance (Clcr) and 100

Example:
For a measured Clcr = 75 mL/min:

$$\frac{75}{100} = 0.75 \text{ (ie, 75\%)}$$

Thus, the adjusted methotrexate dosage is:

$$8000 \text{ mg/m}^2 \times 0.75 = 6000 \text{ mg/m}^2$$

Toxicity

(N = 25 Patients; N = 287 Cycles)

Toxicity	% Patients
G ≥3/4 toxicity	48
No G3/4 toxicity	52
Leukoencephalopathy	—

Batchelor T et al. J Clin Oncol 2003;21:1044–1049

(N = 31 Patients; N = 375 Cycles)*

Toxicity	% Cycles
Leukopenia (<2000 WBC/mm³)	1
Nonoliguric acute renal failure	1
G3 mucositis	2
Leukoencephalopathy	—
Acute cerebral dysfunction	—
Delayed methotrexate clearance[†]	13

Guha-Thakurta N et al. J Neurooncol 1999;43:259–268

*Treatment:
1. Methotrexate 8000 mg/m² for ≥3 induction cycles
2. Methotrexate 3500–8000 mg/m²/cycle until CR
3. Methotrexate 3500 mg/m²/month for 3 months
4. Methotrexate 3500 mg/m²/3 months indefinitely

Median: 10 cycles/patient (range: 3–30 cycles)

[†]Risk factors for delayed methotrexate clearance:
1. Cycle intervals <10 days
2. Concurrent SIADH or diabetes insipidus
3. Acute renal failure
4. "Third-space" fluid compartments (eg, effusions)

Therapy Monitoring

Before each treatment cycle:
1. CBC with differential
2. Serum electrolytes
3. LFTs
4. 24-hour urine collection for creatinine clearance

During hospitalization:
1. Check urine output and pH frequently
2. Daily CBC with differential and serum electrolytes
3. Monitor daily methotrexate levels starting the day after methotrexate administration begins and continue until serum methotrexate concentrations are <0.1 μmol/L. In patients with renal impairment or pleural effusion, continue leucovorin and check serum methotrexate concentrations daily until methotrexate is undetectable

Notes

1. The regimen is for the treatment of primary central nervous system lymphoma for which radiation therapy has been deferred
2. In patients with renal impairment or an effusion, consider empirically continuing leucovorin calcium administration until serum methotrexate concentrations become undetectable

CNS LYMPHOMA REGIMEN

RITUXIMAB, METHOTREXATE, PROCARBAZINE, AND VINCRISTINE FOLLOWED BY CONSOLIDATION, REDUCED-DOSE WHOLE-BRAIN RADIOTHERAPY, AND CYTARABINE (R-MPV → RT + C) NEWLY DIAGNOSED PRIMARY CNS LYMPHOMA

Morris PG et al. J Clin Oncol 2013;31:3971–3979
Shah GD et al. J Clin Oncol 2007;25:4730–4735

Induction Chemotherapy: Five 14-Day Cycles

Premedication for rituximab:
Acetaminophen 650–1000 mg orally, *plus*
Diphenhydramine 25–50 mg orally or intravenously, 30–60 minutes before starting rituximab
Rituximab 500 mg/m²; administer intravenously in 0.9% sodium chloride injection (0.9% NS) or 5% dextrose injection (D5W), USP, diluted to a concentration within the range 1–4 mg/mL on day 1, every 2 weeks, for 5–7 cycles (total dosage/cycle = 500 mg/m²)

Notes on rituximab administration:
- Administer initially at a rate of 50 mg/h. If hypersensitivity or infusion reactions do not occur during the first 30 minutes, increase the rate by 50 mg/h every 30 minutes as tolerated to a maximum rate of 400 mg/h
- During subsequent treatments, if previous rituximab administration was well tolerated, start at 100 mg/hour and increase by 100 mg/hour every 30 minutes as tolerated to a maximum rate of 400 mg/hour
- Interrupt rituximab administration for fever, chills, edema, congestion of the head and neck mucosa, hypertension, and other serious adverse events. Resume rituximab administration after adverse events abate

Methotrexate 3500 mg/m²; administer intravenously over 2 hours on day 2, every 2 weeks, for 5–7 cycles (total dosage/cycle *not* including intrathecal therapy = 3500 mg/m²)
Note: For logistical practicality and efficiency, parenteral admixtures containing methotrexate may include a portion or all of the fluid and sodium bicarbonate needed to meet hydration and urinary alkalinization requirements during methotrexate administration

Hydration before, during, and after methotrexate:
Administer 1500–3000 mL/m² per day. Use a solution containing a total amount of sodium not greater than 0.9% sodium chloride injection (ie, ≤154 mEq/1000 mL), by intravenous infusion during methotrexate administration and for at least 24 hours afterward

- Commence fluid administration 2–12 hours before starting methotrexate, depending upon a patient's fluid status
- Urine output should be at least 100 mL/h before starting methotrexate infusion
- Maintain hydration at a rate that maintains urine output of at least 100 mL/h until the serum methotrexate concentration is <0.05 µmol/L
- Adverse effects attributable to methotrexate are related to systemic methotrexate concentrations *and* the duration for which concentrations are maintained

Sodium bicarbonate 50–150 mEq/1000 mL is added to parenteral hydration solutions to maintain urine pH ≥7.0 to ≤8.0

Base Solution Sodium Content	Sodium Bicarbonate Additive	Total Sodium Content
0.45% Sodium Chloride Injection (0.45% NS)		
77 mEq/L	50–75 mEq	125–152 mEq/L
0.2% Sodium Chloride Injection (0.2% NS)		
34 mEq/L	100–125 mEq	134–159 mEq/L
5% Dextrose Injection (D5W)		
0	125–150 mEq	125–150 mEq/L
D5W/0.45% NS		
77 mEq/L	50–75 mEq	125–152 mEq/L
D5W/0.2% NS		
34 mEq/L	100–125 mEq	134–159 mEq/L

(continued)

Treatment Modifications

Adverse Event	Dose Modification
WBC nadir during the previous cycle 2000–3000/mm³, or platelets 25,000–75,000/mm³	Reduce procarbazine dosage by 10–25%
WBC nadir during the previous cycle <2000/mm³, or platelets <25,000/mm³	Reduce procarbazine dosage by 25–50%
Severe neurotoxicity; eg, painful paresthesia or peripheral weakness	Discontinue vincristine
Leucovorin doses	See leucovorin guidelines

Patient Population Studied

Clinical Characteristics (N = 30)

Characteristic	
Age (years), median/range	57 (30–76)
Sex, Male/Female	17/13
Karnofsky performance score, median/range	70 (50–90)
Positive CSF	6
Ocular involvement	3

(*continued*)

Leucovorin calcium 25 mg/m²; administer intravenously in 25–250 mL 0.9% NS or D5W over 15–30 minutes every 6 hours starting 24 hours after methotrexate administration began, for at least 72 hours (≥12 doses) or until serum methotrexate concentrations are ≤0.05 μmol/L or undetectable, every 2 weeks, for 5–7 cycles

Leucovorin Rescue Guidelines

Clinical Situation	Serum Methotrexate Concentration*	Leucovorin Dosage, Schedule, and Duration
Normal Methotrexate Elimination	• ≤10 μmol/L at 24 hours, *or* • ≤1 μmol/L at 48 hours, *or* • ≤0.2 μmol/L at 72 hours	• Give leucovorin calcium 25 mg/m² intravenously every 6 hours until serum methotrexate concentrations are <0.1 μmol/L (<1 × 10⁻⁷ mol/L or <100 nmol/L), then give leucovorin calcium 25 mg orally every 6 hours for 8 doses
Delayed/Late Methotrexate Elimination	• ≥10 μmol/L at 24 hours, *or* • ≥1 μmol/L at 48 hours, *or* • ≥0.1 μmol/L at 72 hours, *or* • ≥0.05 μmol/L at 96 hours *or* • ≥100% increase in serum creatinine concentration at 24 hours after methotrexate administration	• Give leucovorin calcium 100 mg/m² intravenously every 3 hours • When serum methotrexate concentration results are <0.1 μmol/L the leucovorin dosage may be decreased to 10 mg/m² intravenously given every 3 hours until the serum methotrexate concentration is <0.05 μmol/L or undetectable

*After methotrexate administration began
Methotrexate concentration conversions: 1 μmol/L = 10⁻⁶ mol/L = 1000 nmol/L

Vincristine 1.4 mg/m² (maximum dose = 2.8 mg); administer by intravenous injection over 1–2 minutes on day 2, every 2 weeks, for 5–7 cycles (total dosage/cycle = 1.4 mg/m²; maximum dose/cycle = 2.8 mg)

Procarbazine 100 mg/m² per day; administer orally for 7 consecutive days on days 1 through 7, *only* during odd-numbered cycles (cycles 1, 3, 5 ± 7; ie, every 4 weeks) for 3 or 4 cycles (total dosage/cycle = 700 mg/m²)

For patients with cerebrospinal fluid cytologically positive for lymphoma:
Preservative-free methotrexate 12 mg; administer intrathecally via intraventricular catheter or reservoir (eg, Ommaya) once per cycle between days 5 and 8, every 2 weeks, for 5–7 cycles

Supportive Care
Antiemetic prophylaxis
Emetogenic potential on day 1 is **MINIMAL**
Emetogenic potential on day 2 during odd-numbered cycles (with procarbazine) is **MODERATE–HIGH**
Emetogenic potential on day 2 during even-numbered cycles (without procarbazine) is **MODERATE**
See Chapter 39 for antiemetic recommendations

Hematopoietic growth factor (CSF) prophylaxis
Primary prophylaxis is indicated with:
  Filgrastim (G-CSF) 5 mcg/kg per day, by subcutaneous injection
• Begin use during odd-numbered cycles on day 8 (24 hours after the last dose of procarbazine)
• Begin use during even-numbered cycles 24 hours after serum methotrexate concentrations are <0.01 μmol/L(<1 × 10⁻⁸ mol/L, <10 nmol/L, or undetectable)
• Discontinue daily filgrastim use at least 24 hours before resuming myelosuppressive treatment
See Chapter 43 for more information

(*continued*)

Efficacy

Response Rate to R-MPV (n = 27)

Time Point	Complete Response Number (Percent)	Partial Response Number (Percent)	Overall Response Number (Percent)
After ≥5 cycles	12 (44%)	13 (59%)	25 (93%)
After all cycles	21 (78%)	4 (15%)	25 (93%)

R-MPV, rituximab, methotrexate, procarbazine, and vincristine

Efficacy*

Reduced-dose Whole-brain Radiotherapy (rdWBRT) (N = 31)

Median PFS†	7.7 years	
Median OS†	Not reached	
Median PFS <60 years†	Not reached	*P* = 0.02
Median PFS ≥60 years†	4.4 years	
Median OS <60 years†	Not reached	*P* = 0.17
Median OS ≥60 years†	Not reached	
1-year PFS	84% (95% CI, 71–97%)	
2-year PFS	77% (95% CI, 63–92%)	
3-year PFS	71% (95% CI, 55–87%)	
1-year OS	94% (95% CI, 85–100%)	
2-year OS	90% (95% CI, 80–100%)	
3-year OS	87% (95% CI, 75–99%)	
5-year OS	80% (95% CI, 66–94%)	
1-year PFS patients <60 years	94% (95% CI, 82–100%)	
2-year PFS patients <60 years	94% (95% CI, 82–100%)	
3-year PFS patients <60 years	88% (95% CI, 71–100%)	
1-year PFS patients ≥60 years	73% (95% CI, 51–96%)	
2-year PFS patients ≥60 years	60% (95% CI, 35–85%)	
3-year PFS patients ≥60 years	53% (95% CI, 28–79%)	

(*continued*)

(continued)

Antimicrobial prophylaxis

Risk of fever and neutropenia is INTERMEDIATE

Antimicrobial primary prophylaxis to be considered:

- Antibacterial—consider a fluoroquinolone or no prophylaxis; *Pneumocystis jirovecii* prophylaxis is recommended (eg, cotrimoxazole)
- Antifungal—recommended; consider use during periods of neutropenia
- Antiviral—antiherpes antivirals (eg, acyclovir, famciclovir, valacyclovir)

See Chapter 47 for more information

Infusion reactions associated with rituximab

Fevers, chills, and rigors

1. Interrupt rituximab administration for severe symptoms, and give:
   - **Acetaminophen** 650 mg; administer orally for fever. For persistent or recurrent symptoms, repeat administration every 4–6 hours as needed during rituximab administration
   - **Diphenhydramine** 25–50 mg; administer orally or by intravenous injection for pruritus, hypotension, or angioedema. For persistent or recurrent symptoms, repeat administration every 4–6 hours as needed during rituximab administration
   - **Meperidine** 12.5–25 mg; administer by intravenous injection every 10–20 minutes as needed for shaking chills (generally, cumulative doses >100 mg are not needed; use repeated doses with caution in persons with moderate or more severely impaired renal function)
2. If rituximab administration was interrupted, resume infusion at a slower rate than the maximum rate previously attempted. Rate escalation may be reattempted at smaller incremental steps with close monitoring. Do not exceed the maximum recommended rate of 400 mg/hour

Dyspnea or wheezing without allergic findings (urticaria, or tongue or laryngeal edema)

1. Interrupt rituximab administration immediately
2. Give **hydrocortisone** 100 mg; administer by intravenous injection (or an alternative steroid with equivalent glucocorticoid potency)
3. Give a **histamine (H$_2$) receptor antagonist** (ranitidine 50 mg, cimetidine 300 mg, or famotidine 20 mg); administer intravenously over 15–30 minutes
4. After symptoms resolve, resume rituximab administration at 25 mg/hour with close monitoring. Do not increase the administration rate

CONSOLIDATION AFTER RADIOTHERAPY: TWO 28-DAY CYCLES

Cytarabine 3000 mg/m² per day (maximum daily dose = 6000 mg); administer intravenously in 25–500 mL 0.9% NS or D5W over 3 hours for 2 days (2 doses), on days 1 and 2, every 28 days (total dosage/cycle = 6000 mg/m²; maximum dose/cycle = 12,000 mg)

Supportive Care

Antiemetic prophylaxis

Emetogenic potential is MODERATE

See Chapter 39 for antiemetic recommendations

Hematopoietic growth factor (CSF) prophylaxis

Primary prophylaxis is indicated with one of the following:

Filgrastim (G-CSF) 5 mcg/kg per day; administer by subcutaneous injection, *or*

Pegfilgrastim (pegylated filgrastim) 6 mg/0.6 mL; administer by subcutaneous injection for 1 dose

- Begin use from 24–72 hours after cytarabine is completed
- Continue daily filgrastim use until ANC ≥10,000/mm³ on two measurements separated temporally by ≥12 hours
- Discontinue daily filgrastim use at least 24 hours before administering myelosuppressive treatment. Do not administer pegfilgrastim within 14 days before resuming myelosuppressive treatment

See Chapter 43 for more information

(continued)

Efficacy* (continued)

Entire Cohort (N = 52)

Median PFS‡	3.3 years	
Median OS‡	6.6 years	
Median PFS <60 years‡	7.7 years	*P* = 0.09
Median PFS ≥60 years‡	1.4 years	
Median OS <60 years‡	Not reached	*P* = 0.14
Median OS ≥60 years‡	5.5 years	
1-year PFS	65% (95% CI, 52–78%)	
2-year PFS	57% (95% CI, 44–71%)	
3-year PFS	51% (95% CI, 38–65%)	
1-year OS	85% (95% CI, 75–94%)	
2-year OS	81% (95% CI, 70–91%)	
3-year OS	77% (95% CI, 65–88%)	
5-year OS	70% (95% CI, 57–83%)	
1-year PFS patients <60 years	68% (95% CI, 50–86%)	
2-year PFS patients <60 years	64% (95% CI, 45–83%)	
3-year PFS patients <60 years	64% (95% CI, 45–83%)	
1-year PFS patients ≥60 years	63% (95% CI, 45–81%)	
2-year PFS patients ≥60 years	47% (95% CI, 28–66%)	
3-year PFS patients ≥60 years	38% (95% CI, 19–57%)	

*The favorable regimen performance in patients expected to have a poor prognosis (elderly and low KPS) abrogated the predictive value of the Memorial Sloan Kettering Cancer Center RPA class, and no differences were seen in PFS or OS according to methotrexate pharmacokinetic parameters
†Median follow-up of 5.9 years for survivors
‡Median follow-up of 5.6 years for survivors

(continued)

Antimicrobial prophylaxis
Risk of fever and neutropenia is INTERMEDIATE
   Antimicrobial primary prophylaxis to be considered:
   • Antibacterial—consider a fluoroquinolone or no prophylaxis; *Pneumocystis jirovecii* prophylaxis is recommended (eg, cotrimoxazole)
   • Antifungal—recommended; consider use during periods of neutropenia
   • Antiviral—antiherpes antivirals (eg, acyclovir, famciclovir, valacyclovir)
See Chapter 47 for more information

Keratitis prophylaxis
Steroid ophthalmic drops (prednisolone 1% or dexamethasone 0.1%) by intraocular instillation daily until 24 hours after high-dose cytarabine is completed

Patients with CSF evidence of malignancy received 12 mg of intra-Ommaya methotrexate between cycles

Response Assessment After Five Induction Chemotherapy Cycles*

Assessment	Plan
Complete Response (CR)	Reduced-dose whole-brain radiotherapy (rdWBRT) (23.40 Gy in 1.8-Gy fractions × 13 fractions) 3–5 weeks after chemotherapy completion. Opposed lateral radiation fields were used to include the whole brain down to the level of C2 (so-called German helmet shape) and excluded the anterior two-thirds of the orbit
Partial Response (PR)	Two additional cycles of R-MPV, and, if a CR was achieved, rdWBRT was given as previously described. Otherwise, a standard dose of WBRT (45 Gy in 25 fractions) was offered
Stable or progressive disease	Standard WBRT. Patients with ocular involvement were irradiated without orbital shielding to the full dose of 23.40 Gy (patients in CR) or to a dose of 36 Gy (patients with less than a CR)

*Response was assessed using International PCNSL Collaborative Group criteria, based on imaging, corticosteroid use, and CSF cytology and slit-lamp examination in case of CSF or ocular involvement

Therapy Monitoring

1. *Weekly:* CBC with differential
2. *Before each treatment:* serum creatinine and liver function tests
3. *Every 3–4 cycles:* pulmonary function test

Toxicity (N = 52)*

Acute renal failure	3%
Septic shock	2%
Fatal febrile neutropenia >2 cycles	2%
G4/5 neutropenia[†]	13%
G3 anemia	10%
G3 thrombocytopenia	27%
G3 lymphopenia	40%
G3 neutropenia	20%

*Median number of R-MPV (rituximab, methotrexate, procarbazine, and vincristine) cycles received was 5 (range: 0–7)
[†]Includes 2 of the first 5 treated patients; the protocol was the amended to require prophylactic filgrastim

Toxicity

Exploratory Neuropsychological and Imaging Correlates (N = 12 treated with rdWBRT)

• At baseline: Cognitive impairment present in several domains
• After induction chemotherapy: significant improvement in executive (P <0.01) and verbal memory (P <0.05)
• During follow-up: no evidence of significant cognitive decline except for motor speed (P <0.05)
• During follow-up: no evidence of depressed mood, and self-reported quality of life remained stable during the follow-up period
• *At baseline:* 5/12 patients had G ≥2 white matter disease
• *After induction chemotherapy:* 1/12 patients had G ≥2 white matter disease
• *At 4-year evaluation:* 5/12 patients had G2 and 2/12 patients had G3 white matter disease
• *During follow-up:* no patient developed Fazekas scores of 4 or 5

REGIMEN

HIGH-DOSE METHOTREXATE AND RITUXIMAB WITH DEFERRED RADIOTHERAPY
NEWLY DIAGNOSED PRIMARY B-CELL CNS LYMPHOMA

Chamberlain MC, Johnson SK. Neuro Oncol 2010;12:736–744

INDUCTION (≥4 BI-WEEKLY CYCLES)

Methotrexate; administer intravenously over 6 hours on day 1, every 2 weeks

Methotrexate Dosage

Estimated or measured creatinine clearance	≥60 mL/minute (≥1 mL/s)	<60 mL/minute (<1 mL/s)
Methotrexate	8000 mg/m² (total dosage/2-week cycle = 8000 mg/m²)	4000 mg/m² (total dosage/2-week cycle = 4000 mg/m²)

Notes: For logistical practicality and efficiency, parenteral admixtures containing methotrexate may include a portion or all of the fluid and sodium bicarbonate needed to meet hydration and urinary alkalinization requirements during methotrexate administration

Hydration before, during, and after methotrexate:
Administer intravenously 1500–3000 mL/m² per day. Administer a solution containing a total amount of sodium not greater than 0.9% sodium chloride injection (ie, 154 mEq/1000 mL) by intravenous infusion during methotrexate administration and for at least 24 hours afterward

- Commence fluid administration 2–12 hours before starting methotrexate, depending upon a patient's fluid status
- Urine output should be at least 100 mL/hour before starting methotrexate infusion
- Urine pH should be ≥7.0 but ≤8.0 before, during, and after methotrexate administration
- Maintain hydration at a rate that maintains urine output of at least 100 mL/hours until the serum methotrexate concentration is <0.1 μmol/L
- Adverse effects attributable to methotrexate are related to systemic methotrexate concentrations *and* the duration for which concentrations are maintained

Sodium bicarbonate 50–150 mEq/1000 mL is added to parenteral hydration solutions to maintain urine pH ≥7.0 to ≤8.0

Base Solution Sodium Content	Sodium Bicarbonate Additive	Total Sodium Content
0.45% Sodium chloride injection (0.45% NS)		
77 mEq/L	50–75 mEq	125–152 mEq/L
0.2% Sodium chloride injection (0.2% NS)		
34 mEq/L	100–125 mEq	134–159 mEq/L
5% Dextrose injection (D5W)		
0	125–150 mEq	125–150 mEq/L
D5W/0.45% NS		
77 mEq/L	50–75 mEq	125–152 mEq/L
D5W/0.2% NS		
34 mEq/L	100–125 mEq	134–159 mEq/L

Leucovorin calcium 10 mg/m²; administer intravenously in 25–250 mL 0.9% NS or D5W over 15–30 minutes every 6 hours starting 24 hours after methotrexate administration begins, and continue until serum methotrexate concentrations are ≤0.1 μmol/L, every 2 weeks for a minimum of 4 cycles. When serum methotrexate concentrations are ≤0.1 μmol/L, discontinue intravenous hydration and leucovorin, *then:*

- Give **leucovorin** calcium 25 mg; administer orally every 6 hours for 2 days (8 doses), *and*
- Continue hydration orally with >1500 mL/m² (>50 fluid ounces/m²) for 3 days after intravenous hydration is discontinued

(continued)

Treatment Modifications

Adverse Event	Treatment Modification
G ≥3 hematologic toxicity on day 1 of a cycle or G >1 nonhematologic toxicity on day 1 of a cycle	Withhold treatment until all hematologic toxicity has resolved to G ≤2 and all nonhematologic toxicity has resolved to G ≤1
G ≥4 toxicity ascribed to methotrexate	Reduce the methotrexate dosage by 50%
G ≥3 toxicity ascribed to methotrexate after the dosage has been reduced by 50%	Discontinue methotrexate

Patient Population Studied

Patient Characteristics
N = 40

Forty patients (25 men; 15 women), ages 18–93 years (median: 61.5 years), with newly diagnosed B-cell primary central nervous system lymphoma (PCNSL). Histopathology was determined by stereotactic biopsy in 29 patients, resective surgery in 9 patients, cerebrospinal fluid (CSF) flow cytometry in 1, and vitrectomy in 1 patient

Variables	Number of Patients (Percent)
Age, Median (range)	61.5 y (18–93 y)
≥50 y/≥70 y	33 (82.5)/17 (42.5)
Sex, Male/Female	25 (62.5)/15 (37.5)
Location of tumor	
Frontal	18 (45)
Temporal	3 (7.5)
Parietal	9 (22.5)
Corpus callosum	9 (22.5)
Deep gray nuclei	5 (12.5)
Occipital	2 (5)
Cerebellum	3 (7.5)
Brainstem	1 (2.5)
Subarachnoid/ventricular	2 (5)
Multilobar	12 (30)

(continued)

(*continued*)

Rituximab 375 mg/m²; administer intravenously in 0.9% NS or D5W diluted to a concentration within the range 1–4 mg/mL between days 7 and 10 every 2 weeks for a minimum of 4 cycles; ie, within a 2-week cycle, during the week when methotrexate is not given (total dosage/2-week cycle = 375 mg/m²)

Notes on rituximab administration:
- Administer initially at a rate of 50 mg/hour. If hypersensitivity or infusion reactions do not occur during the first 30 minutes, increase the rate by 50 mg/hour every 30 minutes as tolerated to a maximum rate of 400 mg/hour
- During subsequent treatments, if previous rituximab administration was well tolerated, start at 100 mg/hour and increase the rate by 100 mg/hour every 30 minutes as tolerated to a maximum rate of 400 mg/hour
- Interrupt rituximab administration for fever, chills, edema, congestion of the head and neck mucosa, hypertension, and other serious adverse events. Resume rituximab administration after adverse events abate

MAINTENANCE (4-WEEK CYCLES)
Methotrexate; administer intravenously over 6 hours on day 1, every 4 weeks

Methotrexate Dosage

Estimated or measured creatinine clearance	≥60 mL/minute (≥1 mL/s)	<60 mL/minute (<1 mL/s)
Methotrexate	8000 mg/m² (Total dosage/4-week cycle = 8000 mg/m²)	4000 mg/m² (Total dosage/4-week cycle = 4000 mg/m²)

Notes: For logistical practicality and efficiency, parenteral admixtures containing methotrexate may include a portion or all of the fluid and sodium bicarbonate needed to meet hydration and urinary alkalinization requirements during methotrexate administration

Hydration before, during, and after methotrexate:
Administer intravenously 1500–3000 mL/m² per day. Administer a solution containing a total amount of sodium not greater than 0.9% sodium chloride injection (ie, 154 mEq/1000 mL) by intravenous infusion during methotrexate administration and for at least 24 hours afterward

- Commence fluid administration 2–12 hours before starting methotrexate, depending upon a patient's fluid status
- Urine output should be at least 100 mL/hour before starting methotrexate infusion
- Urine pH should be ≥7.0 but ≤8.0 before, during, and after methotrexate administration
- Maintain hydration at a rate that maintains urine output of at least 100 mL/hour until the serum methotrexate concentration is <0.1 μmol/L
- Adverse effects attributable to methotrexate are related to systemic methotrexate concentrations *and* the duration for which concentrations are maintained

Sodium bicarbonate 50–150 mEq/1000 mL is added to parenteral hydration solutions to maintain urine pH ≥7.0 to ≤8.0

Base Solution Sodium Content	Sodium Bicarbonate Additive	Total Sodium Content
0.45% Sodium Chloride Injection (0.45% NS)		
77 mEq/L	50–75 mEq	125–152 mEq/L
0.2% Sodium Chloride Injection (0.2% NS)		
34 mEq/L	100–125 mEq	134–159 mEq/L
5% Dextrose Injection (D5W)		
0	125–150 mEq	125–150 mEq/L
D5W/0.45% NS		
77 mEq/L	50–75 mEq	125–152 mEq/L
D5W/0.2% NS		
34 mEq/L	100–125 mEq	134–159 mEq/L

(*continued*)

Patient Population Studied
(*continued*)

Extent of initial surgery	
Subtotal resection	9 (22.5)
Biopsy	29 (72.5)
Vitrectomy	1 (2.5)
Response to up-front chemotherapy	
Complete response	24 (60)
Partial response	8 (20)
Progressive disease	8 (20)
Progression-free survival to up-front chemotherapy	
Median (range)	21 mo (2–78 mo)
Salvage therapy at recurrence	
Temozolomide	9 (22.5)
Procarbazine, Lomustine (CCNU), Vincristine	5 (12.5)
Methotrexate	1 (2.5)
Whole brain irradiation	8 (20)
Response to salvage therapy	
Complete response	2 (9)
Partial response	12 (67)
Progressive disease	4 (22)
Progression-free survival to salvage therapy	
Median (range)	6 mo (1 − 38+ mo)
Overall survival	
Median (range)	29 mo (6 − 80+ mo)
Alive and disease free	20 (50)
≤50 y of age	7/9 (78)
>50 y of age	8/31 (26)
>60 y of age	0/20 (0)

(continued)

Leucovorin calcium 10 mg/m^2; administer intravenously in 25–250 mL 0.9% NS or D5W over 15–30 minutes every 6 hours starting 24 hours after methotrexate administration begins, and continue until serum methotrexate concentrations are ≤0.1 μmol/L, every 4 weeks

- When serum methotrexate concentrations are ≤0.1 μmol/L, discontinue intravenous hydration and leucovorin, *then:*
  - Give **leucovorin calcium** 25 mg; administer orally every 6 hours for 2 days (8 doses), *and*
  - Continue hydration orally with >1500 mL/m^2 (>50 fluid ounces/m^2) for 3 days after intravenous hydration is discontinued

Leucovorin Rescue Guidelines

Clinical Situation	Serum Methotrexate Concentration*	Leucovorin Dosage, Schedule, and Duration
Normal methotrexate elimination	• ≤10 μmol/L at 24 hours, *or* • ≤1 μmol/L at 48 hours, *or* • ≤0.2 μmol/L at 72 hours	• Give leucovorin calcium 10 mg/m^2 intravenously every 6 hours until serum methotrexate concentrations are <0.1 μmol/L (<1 × 10^{-7} mol/L, or <100 nmol/L), then give leucovorin calcium 25 mg orally every 6 hours for 8 doses
Delayed/late methotrexate elimination	• ≥10 μmol/L at 24 hours, *or* • ≥1 μmol/L at 48 hours, *or* • ≥0.1 μmol/L at 72 hours, *or* • ≥0.05 μmol/L at 96 hours, *or* • ≥100% increase in serum creatinine concentration at 24 hours after methotrexate administration	• Give leucovorin calcium 100 mg/m^2 intravenously every 3 hours • When serum methotrexate concentration results are <0.1 μmol/L the leucovorin dosage may be decreased to 10 mg/m^2 intravenously given every 3 hours until the serum methotrexate concentration is <0.05 μmol/L or undetectable

*After methotrexate administration is begun
Methotrexate concentration conversions: 1 μmol/L = 10^{-6} mol/L = 1000 nmol/L

Toxicity

Toxicity	G2	G3	G4	G5	Total
Anemia	1	2	0	0	3
Fatigue	6	1	0	0	7
Hepatic	2	1	0	0	3
Hyperglycemia	6	2	0	0	8
Neutropenia without fever	1	4	0	0	5
Nausea	2	0	0	0	2
Renal	13	4	2	0	19
Thrombophlebitis	0	2	0	0	2
Totals	31	16	2	0	49

Treatment Monitoring

1. CBC with differential every week
2. Serum creatinine and liver function tests at the beginning of each cycle
3. Serum creatinine levels and serum methotrexate concentrations at 24 hours, 48 hours, and 72 hours after administration of methotrexate began, continuing at least until a serum methotrexate concentration ≤0.1 μmol/L is achieved

Efficacy (N = 40)

Following induction with 4–6 cycles of methotrexate/rituximab (N = 40)	
Complete radiographic response	24 (60%)
Partial radiographic response	8 (20%)*
Progressive disease	8 (20%)
Following maintenance methotrexate (N = 40)	
Progression during maintenance	4 (10%)
At conclusion of induction and maintenance methotrexate (N = 28)†	
Complete radiographic response	27/28
Partial radiographic response	1/28
Median OS	33.5 months (11−80 months)
Median PFS	21.0 months (95% CI, 13.8−28.2)
Entire cohort (N = 40)	
Median overall survival, entire cohort	29.0 months (95% CI, 19.7−38.3)
Probability of disease-free survival, <50 years	86% (6/7)
Probability of disease-free survival, 50–59 years	33% (4/12)
Probability of disease-free survival, 60–69 years	25% (1/4)
Probability of disease-free survival, >70 years	0 (0/17)

*Six of the 8 patients (75%) with a PR to induction methotrexate/rituximab converted to a complete response with maintenance methotrexate
†6–8 months of total therapy

RECURRENT MENINGIOMA
LONG-ACTING OCTREOTIDE ACETATE

Chamberlain MC et al. Neurology 2007;69:969–973

Long-acting octreotide acetate 30 mg; administer by intramuscular injection (intragluteally) every 4 weeks (total dose/cycle = 30 mg)

Note: If after 2 cycles of therapy a patient has achieved stable disease or a better response and has tolerated a 30-mg dose, the dose of long-acting octreotide acetate may be increased to 40 mg every 4 weeks for the third and subsequent cycles of therapy (total dose/cycle = 40 mg)
Note: For patients not previously treated with subcutaneously-administered octreotide acetate, it is recommended to start with the administration of subcutaneous octreotide at a dosage of 0.1 mg 3 times daily for a short period (approximately 2 weeks) to assess the response and systemic tolerability of octreotide before initiating the treatment with long-acting octreotide acetate
Note: Limited published data indicate somatostatin analogs might decrease the metabolic clearance of compounds known to be metabolized by cytochrome P450. Use with caution drugs mainly metabolized by CYP3A4 and which have a low therapeutic index (eg, quinidine, terfenadine)

Supportive Care
Antiemetic prophylaxis
Emetogenic potential is **MINIMAL**
See Chapter 39 for antiemetic recommendations

Hematopoietic growth factor (CSF) prophylaxis
Primary prophylaxis is NOT indicated
See Chapter 43 for more information

Antimicrobial prophylaxis
Risk of fever and neutropenia is LOW
Antimicrobial primary prophylaxis to be considered:
- Antibacterial—*Pneumocystis jirovecii* prophylaxis is recommended (eg, cotrimoxazole)
- Antifungal—not indicated
- Antiviral—not indicated unless patient previously had an episode of HSV

See Chapter 47 for more information

Treatment Modifications

Adverse Event	Treatment Modification
Asymptomatic gallstones	Continue long-acting octreotide acetate depending on reassessment of the benefit-to-risk ratio. Either way, no action is required except to continue monitoring with increased frequency if treatment with long-acting octreotide acetate is continued
Symptomatic gallstones	Long-acting octreotide acetate may be either stopped or continued, depending on reassessment of the benefit-to-risk ratio. Either way, the gallstones should be treated like any other symptomatic gallstones

Efficacy

Partial response	4/16
Stable disease	5/16
Progressive disease	7/16
6-Month progression-free survival	44% (7/16)
Median duration of response	5.0 months (range: 2–20+ months)
Median overall survival	7.5 months (range: 3–20+ months)

Treatment/Therapy Monitoring

1. Ultrasound examination of the gallbladder prior to commencing octreotide treatment and at approximately 6-month intervals throughout treatment
2. Monitor vitamin B_{12} levels in patients who have a history of vitamin B_{12} deprivation

Toxicity
Adverse Drug Reactions Reported in Clinical Studies

Gastrointestinal Disorders	
Very common	Diarrhea, abdominal pain, nausea, constipation, flatulence
Common	Dyspepsia, vomiting, abdominal bloating, steatorrhea, loose stools, discoloration of feces

Nervous System Disorders	
Very common	Headache
Common	Dizziness

Endocrine Disorders	
Common	Hypothyroidism, thyroid dysfunction (eg, decreased TSH, decreased total T_4, and decreased free T_4)

Hepatobiliary Disorders	
Very common	Cholelithiasis
Common	Cholecystitis, biliary sludge, hyperbilirubinemia

Metabolism and Nutrition Disorders*	
Very common	Hyperglycemia
Common	Hypoglycemia, impaired glucose tolerance, anorexia
Uncommon	Dehydration

General Disorders and Administration Site Reactions	
Very common	Localized pain at injection site

Laboratory Investigations	
Common	Elevated transaminase levels
Uncommon	Depressed vitamin B_{12} levels and abnormal Schilling tests

Skin and Subcutaneous Tissue Disorders	
Common	Pruritus, rash, alopecia

Respiratory Disorders	
Common	Dyspnea

Cardiac Disorders	
Common	Bradycardia
Uncommon	Tachycardia

Very common: ≥1/10; Common: ≥1/100, <1/10; Uncommon: ≥1/1000, <1/100
*Note: Because of its inhibitory action on growth hormone, glucagon, and insulin release, long-acting somatostatin may affect glucose regulation. Postprandial glucose tolerance may be impaired. In some instances, a state of persistent hyperglycemia may be induced as a result of chronic administration

Patient Characteristics and Individual Efficacy

Age/Gender	PATH	LOC	SUR	RT, Gy	SUR	EBRT	SRT	CHEMORx	KPS	#Cy	RESP	OS
M/62	I/Yes	LF LFP RCS	No	No	No	No	15	Celebrex (SD)	90	11	PR/12*	12*
M/83	III/Yes	LF LT Falx SS	STR	No	No	No	No	No	80	15	PR/15*	15*
F/41	I/No	CS LSW	STR	54	X2	No	18	TAM 30 (SD) HU 4.5 (PD)	90	8	PR/8	20+
M/67	III/No	BF	GTR	55	X2	No	No	No	60	8	SD/8*	8*
F/65	III/No	LTP	STR	58.4	X2	No	12.9	TMZ + erlotinib2 (PD)	70	2	PD/2	10
F/68	II/No	RSW	STR	58.4	X1	No	No	αIFN 12 (SD)	90	6	PR/6	11+
F/26	III/Yes	RT RF Spine CSF	GTR	59.4	X4	No	12	HU 2 (PD) TMZ 2 (PD)	60	2	PD/2	3
F/45	I/No	RSB RSF CbPA	STR	No	No	No	18	No	80	5	SD/5*	5*
F/52	I/No	LS LCS	No	No	No	No	No	HU 3 (PD)	90	6	SD/20	20+
F/87	II/Yes	RF	STR	No	X1	61	No	No	70	3	PD/3	4
F/51	I/No	LF	GTR	54	No	No	No	HU 3 (PD)	80	3	PD/3	8+†
M/61	I/No	RF RP	GTR	No	X2	54	18	HU 3 (PD)	60	3	PD/3	7+†
F/51	III/No	RF	STR	54	X1	No	18	Thal 13 (SD) HU 3 (PD)	50	6	PD/3	7+†
F/84	II/No	RCS	Bx	No	No	No	No	HU 3 (PD)	80	5	SD/5*	5*
FX/74	I/No	LSW	GTR	No	No	54	No	HU 3 (PD)	80	3	PD/3	4
M/72	I/No	LCS	Bx	54	No	No	No	HU 6 (PD)	70	6	PR/6	7+

Column descriptions (in left-to-right order): Age/Gender (in years); PATH, histology, WHO grade/multifocal; LOC, tumor location; SUR, surgery; RT, radiotherapy; Gy, Gray; EBRT, external beam radiotherapy; SRT, stereotactic radiotherapy; CHEMORx, chemotherapy, number of cycles* (best response); KPS, Karnofsky performance status; #Cy, number of cycles (cycle defined as 4 weeks); RESP, response assessment/duration in months; OS, overall survival
LOC (tumor location) (in order listed): LF, left frontal; LFP, left frontoparietal; RCS, right cavernous sinus; LT, left temporal; SS, sphenoid sinus; CS, cavernous sinus; LSW, left sphenoid wing; BF, bifrontal; LTP, left temporoparietal; RSW, right sphenoid wing; RT, right temporal; RF, right frontal, RSB, right skull; base; CbA, cerebellopontine angle; LS, left sphenoid; LCS, left cavernous sinus
Other (alphabetically): αIFN, interferonalfa; Bx, biopsy; CR, complete response; GTR, gross total resection; HU, hydroxyurea; NE, nonevaluable; PD, progressive disease; PR, partial response; SD, stable disease; STR, subtotal resection; TAM, tamoxifen; Thal, thalidomide; TMZ, temozolomide
*Alive on octreotide acetate
†Alive

RECURRENT MENINGIOMA

INTERFERON ALFA

Chamberlain MC, Glantz MJ. Cancer 2008;113:2146–2151

Interferon alfa-2b 10 million Units/m²; administer subcutaneously every-other-day for 4 weeks (total dose/week [4 doses] = 40 million Units/m²)

Supportive Care
Antiemetic prophylaxis
Emetogenic potential is **MODERATE**
See Chapter 39 for antiemetic recommendations

Hematopoietic growth factor (CSF) prophylaxis
Primary prophylaxis is NOT indicated
See Chapter 43 for more information

Antimicrobial prophylaxis
Risk of fever and neutropenia is LOW
   Antimicrobial primary prophylaxis to be considered:
- Antibacterial—*Pneumocystis jirovecii* prophylaxis is recommended (eg, cotrimoxazole)
- Antifungal—not indicated
- Antiviral—not indicated unless patient previously had an episode of HSV

See Chapter 47 for more information

Toxicity

Toxicity	G2	G3	G4	G5	All Grades
Alopecia	1				1
Anemia	8	3			11
Constipation	3	1			4
Diarrhea	3				3
Fatigue	17	4	2		23
Granulocytopenia	2	1			3
Infection, neutropenia	1				1
Leukopenia	6	3			9
Nausea	4				4
Thrombocytopenia	2				2
Thrombophlebitis	2				2
Vomiting	2				2
Totals	51	12	2	0	65

Treatment Modifications

Adverse Event	Treatment Modification
G3/4 hematologic toxicity on day 1 of a cycle	Withhold interferon alfa-2b until all hematologic toxicity is G ≤2, then resume at 50% of the previous dose
G2/3/4 nonhematologic toxicity on day 1 of a cycle	Withhold interferon alfa-2b until all nonhematologic toxicity is G ≤1, then resume at 50% of the previous dose if toxicity was G3/4
G3/4 hematologic or nonhematologic toxicity after dosage reduced to 50%	Discontinue therapy
ALT/AST >5× to 10× the upper limit of normal range	Withhold interferon alfa-2b until adverse reactions abate, then resume at 50% of the previous dose

Efficacy

Intention to Treat
(N = 35)

Median OS	8 months (range: 3–28 months; 95% confidence interval, 5.6–10.4 months)
PFS at 6 months	54%
PFS at 12 months	31%
Median time to tumor progression	7 months (range: 2–24 months; 95% confidence interval, 4.9–9.1 months)

Treatment Monitoring

1. CBC with differential, serum electrolytes, BUN, creatinine, and liver function tests initially 3 times per week, then every week, and, eventually, monthly
2. Serum TSH level at start of treatment and at 3 and 6 months

Patient Characteristics and Individual Efficacy

| Age/ Gender | PATH | Tumor Location | Adjuvant Rx | | Therapy at Disease Recurrence | | | | | | |
| | | | | | SUR | RTGy | | CHEMORx | Interferon-α Therapy | | |
			SUR	RTGy		EBRT	SRT		#Cy	RESP	OS
65/M	1/+	LF/LP/LCS	STR	54	No	No	15	HU2 (PD)	14	SD/14	18
84/M	1/+	LF/LT/Falx	STR	54	STR	No	14	HU4 (PD)	16	SD/16	19
49/F	1/−	RCS/RSW	STR	54	STR×2	No	12	HU6 (SD)	8	SD/12	14
68/F	1/−	LF	GTR	No	STR	54	No	HU3 (PD)	9	SD/12	15
58/F	1/−	LP	STR	54	STR	No	15	HU9 (SD)	6	SD/8	10
70/F	1/−	LSW	STR	50.4	STR	No	15	HU6 (SD)	12	SD/14	16
36/F	1/+	LT/LF	STR	54	STR×3	No	14	HU2 (PD)	8	SD/9	12
55/F	1/−	LSB/CbPA	STR	55	No	No	14	HU6 (SD)	6	SD/8	10
59/F	1/−	RSS/RCS	Bx	54	No	No	12	HU3 (PD)	6	SD/20	24
88/F	1/−	LF	GTR	No	STR	54	14	HU6 (PD)	12	SD/14	16
54/F	1/−	RF	GTR	No	GTR	54	15	HU3 (PD)	6	SD/7	8
66/M	1/−	LF/LP	STR	55	STR	No	16	HU3 (PD)	3	PD/3	5
57/F	1/−	RT	GTR	No	STR	54	15	HU3 (PD)	6	SD/7	8
80/F	1/−	LCS	Bx	54	No	No	12	HU3 (PD)	18	SD/24	28
54/M	1/+	LF/RP	STR	54	STR×2	No	15	TMZ 2 (PD)	6	SD/6	8
87/F	1/−	LF	STR	54	No	No	No	HU 3 (PD)	12	SD/14	17
58/F	1/−	RF	STR	54	STR	No	No	TMZ 2 (PD)	4	SD/4	4
69/M	1/−	LT	GTR	No	GTR	54	No	TMZ 4 (SD)	4	SD/4	4
66/F	1/−	RF	STR	54	No	No	No	TMZ 4 (SD)	4	SD/4	4
53/F	1/−	LP	Bx	54	No	No	18	TMZ 2 (PD)	4	SD/4	4
54/F	1/−	RF	STR	54	No	No	18	TMZ 4 (SD)	4	PD/4	4
66/F	1/−	Lten	STR	54	STR	No	No	TMZ 4 (SD)	2	PD/2	3
67/F	1/−	LCS	Bx	54	No	No	18	TMZ 4 (PD)	2	PD/2	3
59/F	1/−	LF	GTR	No	STR	54	No	CPT 1 (SD)	4	SD/4	4
61/F	1/−	LP	STR	54	No	No	18	CPT 2 (SD)	3	PD/3	4
54/F	1/−	LP	Bx	54	No	No	14	CPT 1 (SD)	3	PD/3	4
55/F	1/−	LF	STR	54	No	No	18	CPT 2 (SD)	3	PD/3	4
66/F	1/−	Lten	STR	54	STR	No	No	CPT 2 (SD)	3	PD/3	4
47/F	1/−	LF	GTR	No	GTR	54	No	CPT 1 (SD)	3	PD/3	4
61/F	1/−	LF	STR	54	No	No	No	HU 3 (PD) SS 3 (PD)	6	SD/8	9
61/M	1/−	RFP	GTR	No	GTR×2	54	18	HU 3 (PD) SS 3 (PD)	6	SD/7	8
61/F	1/−	LCS	STR	50.4	STR	No	20	Bev +Cel*	3	SD/3	6
42/F	1/+	RF/RP	STR	50.4	No	No	No	HU 6 (PD)	4	SD/4	4†
70/F	1/−	LF	GTR	No	No	54	No	HU 4 (SD)	20	SD/20	21†
68/F	1/−	RSW	STR	58.4	STR	No	No	None	12	SD/18	23†

Column descriptions (in left-to-right order): Age/Gender (age in years); PATH, WHO grade/multifocal; SUR, surgery; RT, radiotherapy; Gy, gray; EBRT, external beam radiotherapy; SRT, stereotactic radiotherapy; CHEMORx, chemotherapy, number cycles* (best response); #Cy, number of cycles; RESP, response assessment/duration in months; OS, overall survival
Tumor location (in order listed): LF, left frontal; LP, left parietal; LCS, left cavernous sinus; LT, left temporal; RCS, right cavernous sinus; RSW , right sphenoid wing; LSW, left sphenoid wing; LSB, left skull base; CbPA, cerebellopontine angle; RSS, right sphenoid sinus; RCS, cavernous sinus; RF, right frontal; LP, left parietal; RT, right temporal; RP, right parietal; RF, right frontal; Lten, left tentorium; RFP, right frontoparietal; RSW, right sphenoid wing
Other (alphabetically): Bx, biopsy; GTR, gross total resection; HU, hydroxyurea; PD, progressive disease; SD, stable disease; SS, long-acting octreotide acetate (Sandostatin LAR); STR, subtotal resection; TMZ, temozolomide
*Bevacizumab plus celecoxib
†Alive

RECURRENT MENINGIOMA

HIGH-GRADE MENINGIOMA REFRACTORY TO RECURRENT SURGERY AND RADIATION HYDROXYUREA

Chamberlain MC. J Neurooncol 2012;107:315–321

Hydroxyurea 1000 mg/m^2 per day; administer orally, continually for 28 consecutive days, every 4 weeks (total dosage/cycle = 28,000 mg/m^2)

Supportive Care
Antiemetic prophylaxis
*Emetogenic potential is **MINIMAL–LOW***
See Chapter 39 for antiemetic recommendations

Hematopoietic growth factor (CSF) prophylaxis
Primary prophylaxis is NOT indicated
See Chapter 43 for more information

Antimicrobial prophylaxis
Risk of fever and neutropenia is LOW
   Antimicrobial primary prophylaxis to be considered:
   • Antibacterial—*Pneumocystis jirovecii* prophylaxis is recommended (eg, cotrimoxazole)
   • Antifungal—not indicated
   • Antiviral—not indicated unless patient previously had an episode of HSV
See Chapter 47 for more information

Efficacy

Hydroxyurea for Recurrent Meningioma
(Adapted from Chamberlain and Johnston)

Sources	Grades 2/3*	Prior RT	Response (%)	Median TTP†	G ≥3 Toxicity (%)
Newton 2000 Newton 2004	17 (4)	7	SD (88)	20 months	25 (15)
Mason 2002	20 (4)	8	SD (60)	30 months	15
Rosenthal 2002	15 (10)	1	SD (73)	10 months	27 (20)
Hahn 2005	21 (17)	21 (concurrent)	SD (52)	14 months	53 (0)
Loven2004	12 (4)	6	SD (8)	13 months	33 (25)

*Number with grades 2/3 on pathology review
†TTP, time to progression

Chamberlain MC, Johnston SK. J Neurooncol 2011;104:765–771
Hahn BM et al. J Neurooncol 2005;74:157–165
Loven D et al. J Neurooncol 2004;67:221–226
Mason WP et al. J Neurosurg 2002;97:341–346
Newton HB et al. Br J Neurosurg 2004;18:495–499
Newton HB et al. J Neurooncol 2000;49:165–170
Rosenthal MA et al. J Clin Neurosci 2002;9:156–158

Treatment Modifications

Adverse Event	Dose Modification
WBC count <2500/mm^3, or platelet count <100,000/mm^3	Withhold therapy until WBC count is >2500/mm^3, and platelet count is >100,000/mm^3
Severe anemia	Continue hydroxyurea
Severe gastric distress, such as nausea, vomiting, and anorexia	Withhold therapy until symptoms improve

Toxicity
(N = 35)

Toxicity	Grade 2	Grade 3	Total
Anemia	4	1	5
Constipation	6	0	6
Fatigue	10	2	12
Infection, without neutropenia	2	0	2
Lymphopenia	5	0	5
Nausea	2	0	2
Neutropenia	3	0	3
Thrombophlebitis	2	0	2
Totals	34	3	37

Treatment Monitoring

1. Complete blood counts and neurologic examination on day 1 of each 28-day cycle
2. Every 8 weeks and following 2 cycles of hydroxyurea, reevaluate with contrast cranial MR

Patient Characteristics and Individual Efficacy

Age/ Gender	Tumor Location	Initial Therapy			Salvage Therapy			Hydroxyurea Therapy		
		SUR	RT	SRS	SUR	RT	SRSGy	#Cy	RESP	PFS
86/F	LF	GTR	60	No	No	No	15	0.5	PD	0.5
75/M	RF	STR	59.4	No	STR	No	14	0.5	PD	0.5
70/F	RCS, RSW	STR	54	No	STR	No	12	0.5	PD	0.5
68/F	LF	GTR	60	No	STR	No	14	1	PD	1
56/F	RP	GTR	60	No	STR	No	15	1	PD	1
73/F	RSW	STR	60	No	No	No	15	1	PD	1
42/M	RT, RF	STR	60	No	STR x2	No	14	1	PD	1
61/F	LtenCbPA	GTR	60	No	STR x1	No	14	1	PD	1
58/F	RSW	STR	60	No	No	No	15	1	PD	1
80/F	RF	GTR	60	No	STR	No	14	1.5	PD	1.5
52/M	LF	GTR	59.4	No	GTR	No	15	1.5	PD	1.5
66/F	RF, RP	STR	60	No	STR	No	16	1.5	PD	1.5
67/F	LT	GTR	60	No	STR	No	15	1.5	PD	1.5
68/M	RCS	Bx	60	No	No	No	12	2	PD	2
51/M	RF, RP	STR	59.4	No	STR x2	No	15	2	PD	2
78/F	RF	GTR	60	No	No	No	12	2	PD	2
63/F	LF	GTR	60	No	STR	No	14	2	PD	2
69/F	RT	GTR	59.4	No	GTR	No	15	2	PD	2
66/F	LF, RF	STR	60	No	No	No	14	2	PD	2
50/M	RP	Bx	59.4	No	No	No	18	2	PD	2
40/F	LF	GTR	60	No	No	No	18	2.5	SD	2.5
63/F	Rten	GTR	59.4	No	STR	No	14	2.5	SD	2.5
62/F	RCS	Bx	60	No	No	No	18	3	SD	3
48/F	RF	GTR	60	No	STR	No	14	3	SD	3
63/M	RP	STR	59.4	No	No	No	18	3	SD	3
60/F	LF, LP	Bx	60	No	No	No	14	3.5	SD	3.5
76/F	LF, RF	STR	59.4	No	No	No	12	3.5	SD	3.5
64/F	Rten	GTR	59.4	No	STR	No	14	4	SD	4
79/F	RF	GTR	60	No	STR	No	15	4	SD	4
70/F	RF	GTR	59.4	No	GTR	No	15	4.5	SD	4.5
34/M	RF, RP	GTR	60	No	GTR	No	14	4.5	SD	4.5
38/F	RCS	Bx	59.4	No	No	No	15	5	SD	5
82/F	RT,falx, RSW	STR	60	No	STR	No	14	5	SD	5
62/F	LCS, LSW	STR	59.4	No	No	No	14	6	SD	6
47/F	LF, RF	STR	No	No	STR	No	12	7	SD	7

Column descriptions (in left-to-right order): Age/Gender (age in years); SUR, surgery; RT, radiotherapy; Gy, gray; SRT, stereotactic radiotherapy; CHEMORx, chemotherapy, number cycles* (best response); #Cy, number of cycles; RESP, response assessment/duration in months; PFS, progression-free survival (in months)

Tumor location (in order listed): LF, left frontal; RF, right frontal; RCS, cavernous sinus; RSW, right sphenoid wing; RP, right parietal; RT, right temporal; Lten, left tentorium; CbPA, cerebellopontine angle; LT, left temporal; RCS, right cavernous sinus; Rten, right tentorium; LP, left parietal; LCS, left cavernous sinus; LSW, left sphenoid wing

Other (alphabetically): Bx, biopsy; GTR, gross total resection; PD, progressive disease; SD, stable disease; STR, subtotal resection

6. Breast Cancer

Rachel C. Jankowitz, MD and Nancy E. Davidson, MD

Epidemiology

Incidence: 235,030 (male: 2,360; female: 232,670. Estimated new cases for 2014 in the United States)
123.8 per 100,000 females per year
Deaths: Estimated 40,430 in 2014 (male: 430; female: 40,000)
Median age: 61 years
Male to female ratio: 1:160

Stage at Presentation
Stage I: 49%
Stage II: 39%
Stage III: 7%
Stage IV: 5%

Siegel R et al. CA Cancer J Clin 2014;64:9–29
Surveillance, Epidemiology and End Results (SEER) Program, available from http://seer.cancer.gov (accessed in 2013)

Pathology

Invasive Carcinoma

1. Ductal: 49–75%
2. Lobular: 5–16%
3. Medullary: 3–9%
4. Mucinous: 1–2%
5. Tubular: 1–3%

Ductal Carcinoma In Situ

1. Comedo
2. Cribriform
3. Micropapillary
4. Papillary
5. Solid

Harris JR et al. Disease of the Breast, 4th ed.
Philadelphia: Lippincott Williams & Wilkins, 2010

Work-up

In situ:

1. History and physical
2. Bilateral diagnostic mammogram
3. Pathology review with ER status
4. Genetic counseling if patient is high risk for hereditary breast cancer

Stages I & II:

1. History and physical
2. CBC with platelets
3. LFTs and alkaline phosphatase
4. Diagnostic bilateral mammogram
5. Pathology review with ER/PR/HER-2 status
6. Genetic counseling if the patient is at high risk for hereditary breast cancer

Stage III:

1. History and physical
2. CBC with platelets
3. LFTs and alkaline phosphatase
4. Diagnostic bilateral mammogram
5. Pathology review with ER/PR/HER-2 status
6. Consider bone scan, abdominal ± pelvis CT or US or MRI, and chest imaging
7. Genetic counseling if the patient is at high risk for hereditary breast cancer

Stage IV:

1. History and physical
2. CBC with platelets
3. LFTs and alkaline phosphatase
4. Diagnostic bilateral mammogram
5. Pathology review with ER/PR/HER-2 status
6. Chest imaging
7. Bone scan, X-rays of symptomatic bones and long or weight-bearing bones and bones abnormal on bone scan
8. Consider abdominal ± pelvis CT or MRI
9. Biopsy at first recurrence with pathology review
10. Genetic counseling if the patient is at high risk for hereditary breast cancer

Staging

Primary Tumor (T)

TX	Primary tumor cannot be assessed
T0	No evidence of primary tumor
Tis	Carcinoma in situ
Tis (DCIS)	Ductal carcinoma in situ
Tis (LCIS)	Lobular carcinoma in situ
Tis (Paget)	Paget disease of the nipple is NOT associated with invasive carcinoma and/or carcinoma in situ (DCIS and/or LCIS) in the underlying breast parenchyma. Carcinomas in the breast parenchyma associated with Paget's disease are categorized based on the size and characteristics of the parenchymal disease, although the presence of Paget disease should still be noted
T1	Tumor ≤20 mm in greatest dimension
T1mi	Tumor ≤1 mm in greatest dimension
T1a	Tumor >1 mm but ≤5 mm in greatest dimension
T1b	Tumor >5 mm but ≤10 mm in greatest dimension
T1c	Tumor >10 mm but ≤20 mm in greatest dimension
T2	Tumor >20 mm but ≤50 mm in greatest dimension
T3	Tumor >50 mm in greatest dimension
T4	Tumor of any size with direct extension to the chest wall and/or to the skin (ulceration or skin nodules)*
T4a	Extension to the chest wall, not including only pectoralis muscle adherence/invasion
T4b	Ulceration and/or ipsilateral satellite nodules and/or edema (including peau d'orange) of the skin which do not meet the criteria for inflammatory carcinoma
T4c	Both T4a and T4b
T4d	Inflammatory carcinoma†

*Invasion of the dermis alone does not qualify as T4
†Inflammatory carcinoma is restricted to cases with typical skin changes involving a third or more of the skin of the breast. Although the histologic presence of invasive carcinoma invading dermal lymphatics is supportive of the diagnosis, it is not required, nor is dermal lymphatic invasion without typical clinical findings sufficient for a diagnosis of inflammatory breast cancer

Distant Metastasis (M)

M0	No clinical or radiographic evidence of distant metastases (no pathologic M0; use clinical M to complete stage group)
cM0(i+)	No clinical or radiographic evidence of distant metastases, but deposits of molecularly or microscopically detected tumor cells in circulating blood, bone marrow or other nonregional nodal tissue that are no larger than 0.2 mm in a patient without symptoms or signs of metastases
M1	Distant detectable metastases as determined by classic clinical and radiographic means and/or histologically proven larger than 0.2 mm

Regional Lymph Nodes (N)

NX	Regional lymph nodes cannot be assessed (eg, previously removed)
pNX*	Regional lymph nodes cannot be assessed (eg, previously removed, or not removed for pathologic study)
N0	No regional lymph node metastases
pN0	No regional lymph node metastasis identified histologically
pN0(i-)	No regional lymph node metastases histologically, negative IHC
pN0(i+)	Malignant cells in regional lymph node(s) no greater than 0.2 mm (detected by H&E or IHC including ITC)
pN0(mol-)	No regional lymph node metastases histologically, negative molecular findings (RT-PCR)
pN0(mol+)	Positive molecular findings (RT-PCR), but no regional lymph node metastases detected by histology or IHC
N1	Metastases to movable ipsilateral level I, level II axillary lymph node(s)
pN1	Micrometastases; or metastases in 1–3 axillary lymph nodes; and/or in internal mammary nodes with metastases detected by sentinel lymph node biopsy but not clinically detected†
pN1mi	Micrometastases (greater than 0.2 mm and/or more than 200 cells, but none greater than 2.0 mm)
pN1a	Metastases in 1–3 axillary lymph nodes, at least 1 metastasis greater than 2.0 mm
pN1b	Metastases in internal mammary nodes with micrometastases or macrometastases detected by sentinel lymph node biopsy but not clinically detected†
pN1c	Metastases in 1–3 axillary lymph nodes and in internal mammary lymph nodes with micrometastases or macrometastases detected by sentinel lymph node biopsy but not clinically detected†
N2	Metastases in ipsilateral level I, level II axillary lymph nodes that are clinically fixed or matted; or in clinically detected* ipsilateral internal mammary nodes in the *absence* of clinically evident axillary lymph node metastases
pN2	Metastases in 4–9 axillary lymph nodes; or in clinically detected‡ internal mammary lymph nodes in the *absence* of axillary lymph node metastases
N2a	Metastases in ipsilateral axillary lymph nodes fixed to one another (matted) or to other structures
pN2a	Metastases in 4–9 axillary lymph nodes (at least 1 tumor deposit greater than 2.0 mm)
N2b	Metastases only in clinically detected‡ ipsilateral internal mammary nodes and in the *absence* of clinically evident axillary lymph node metastases

(continued)

Staging (continued)

Staging

0	Tis	N0	M0
IA	T1*	N0	M0
IB	T0	N1mi	M0
	T1*	N1mi	M0
IIA	T0	N1†	M0
	T1*	N1†	M0
	T2	N0	M0
IIB	T2	N1	M0
	T3	N0	M0
IIIA	T0	N2	M0
	T1*	N2	M0
	T2	N2	M0
	T3	N1	M0
	T3	N2	M0
IIIB	T4	N0	M0
	T4	N1	M0
	T4	N2	M0
Stage IIIC	Any T	N3	M0
Stage IV	Any T	Any N	M1

*T1 includes T1mi
†T0 and T1 tumors with nodal micrometastases only are excluded from Stage IIA and are classified Stage IB

Edge SB, Byrd DR, Compton CC, Fritz AG, Greene FL, Trotti A, editors. AJCC Cancer Staging Manual. 7th ed. New York: Springer; 2010

Adjusted Survival

	5-Year	8-Year
In situ	98%	97%
Stage I	96%	92%
Stage II	82%	72%
Stage III	53%	41%
Stage IV	17%	9%

SEER data (1977–1983) from Seidman et al. CA Cancer J Clin 1987;37(5):258–290

Regional Lymph Nodes (N) (continued)

pN2b	Metastases in clinically detected‡ internal mammary lymph nodes in the absence of axillary lymph node metastases
N3	Metastases in ipsilateral infraclavicular (level III axillary) lymph node(s) with or without level I, level II axillary lymph node involvement; or in clinically detected* ipsilateral internal mammary lymph node(s) with clinically evident level I, level II axillary lymph node metastases; or metastases in ipsilateral supraclavicular lymph node(s) with or without axillary or internal mammary lymph node involvement
pN3	Metastases in 10 or more axillary lymph nodes; or in infraclavicular (level III axillary) lymph nodes; or in clinically detected‡ ipsilateral internal mammary lymph nodes in the *presence* of 1 or more positive level I, level II axillary lymph nodes; or in more than 3 axillary lymph nodes and in internal mammary lymph nodes with micrometastases or macrometastases detected by sentinel lymph node biopsy but not clinically detected†; or in ipsilateral supraclavicular lymph nodes
N3a	Metastases in ipsilateral infraclavicular lymph node(s)
pN3a	Metastases in 10 or more axillary lymph nodes (at least 1 tumor deposit greater than 2.0 mm); or metastases to the infraclavicular (level III axillary lymph) nodes
N3b	Metastases in ipsilateral internal mammary lymph node(s) and axillary lymph node(s)
pN3b	Metastases in clinically detected‡ ipsilateral internal mammary lymph nodes in the *presence* of 1 or more positive axillary lymph nodes; or in more than 3 axillary lymph nodes and in internal mammary lymph nodes with micrometastases or macrometastases detected by sentinel lymph node biopsy but not clinically detected†
N3c	Metastases in ipsilateral supraclavicular lymph node(s)
pN3c	Metastases in ipsilateral supraclavicular lymph nodes

*Classification is based on axillary lymph node dissection with or without sentinel lymph node biopsy. Classification based solely on sentinel lymph node biopsy without subsequent axillary lymph node dissection is designated (sn) for "sentinel node," for example, pN0(sn)
†*Not clinically detected* is defined as not detected by imaging studies (excluding lymphoscintigraphy) or not detected by clinical examination
‡*Clinically detected* is defined as detected by imaging studies (excluding lymphoscintigraphy) or by clinical examination and having characteristics highly suspicious for malignancy or a presumed pathologic macrometastasis based on fine-needle aspiration biopsy with cytologic examination. Confirmation of clinically detected metastatic disease by fine-needle aspiration without excision biopsy is designated with an (f) suffix, for example, cN3a(f). Excisional biopsy of a lymph node or biopsy of a sentinel node, in the absence of assignment of a pT, is classified as a clinical N, for example, cN1. Information regarding the confirmation of the nodal status will be designated in site-specific factors as clinical, fine-needle aspiration, core biopsy, or sentinel lymph node biopsy. Pathologic classification (pN) is used for excision or sentinel lymph node biopsy only in conjunction with a pathologic T assignment
Note: Isolated tumor cell clusters (ITC) are defined as small clusters of cells not greater than 0.2 mm, or single tumor cells, or a cluster of fewer than 200 cells in a single histologic cross-section. ITCs may be detected by routine histology or by immunohistochemical (IHC) methods. Nodes containing only ITCs are excluded from the total positive node count for purposes of N classification but should be included in the total number of nodes evaluated

Expert Opinion

DCIS
- Local treatment consists of lumpectomy plus radiation versus mastectomy
- Tamoxifen is used to lower the likelihood of in-breast recurrence and/or contralateral DCIS and invasive breast cancer

Early Stage Breast Cancer
- Local treatment is lumpectomy plus radiation versus mastectomy
- Decisions regarding adjuvant therapy must be individualized, but general guidelines are outlined below
- Molecular assays such as the 21-gene recurrence score can be incorporated into decision making regarding chemotherapy treatment for patients with node-negative ER-positive disease
- In patients with ER-positive and/or PR-positive disease, adjuvant hormonal therapy should be used
- If ovarian suppression is given, it should be given with tamoxifen, not an aromatase inhibitor (AI)
- In women who are pre-/perimenopausal at diagnosis, tamoxifen with or without ovarian suppression/ablation should be used for 5 years. After 5 years, if a patient still is premenopausal, an additional 5 years of tamoxifen should be considered. If after 5 years, the patient is postmenopausal, consider an additional 5 years of tamoxifen or 5 years of an AI
- In women who are postmenopausal at diagnosis, an AI should be used in one of the following adjuvant dosing strategies based on assessment of risk and patient preference:
  - **Upfront** (AI for 5 years),
  - **Sequential** (tamoxifen for 2–3 years followed by an AI to complete 5 years of therapy *or* an AI for 2–3 years followed by tamoxifen to complete 5 years of therapy),
  - **Extended** (tamoxifen for 5 years followed by an AI for 5 years)
- At this time, there is no evidence to support continuing AI therapy beyond 5 years until trials in progress mature

Locally Advanced Breast Cancer
- Neoadjuvant chemotherapy incorporating an anthracycline and a taxane allows for higher rates of breast conservation than adjuvant chemotherapy
- Neoadjuvant endocrine therapy may be considered for hormone receptor-positive postmenopausal patients

Metastatic Disease
Chemotherapy: In general, single chemotherapy agents (monotherapy) may be used sequentially. If a rapid clinical response is needed, combination chemotherapy regimens may be used
Hormonal therapy: For patients with ER-positive and/or PR-positive disease without visceral involvement or with low-volume disease, hormonal therapy is preferred. For postmenopausal women there is a survival benefit with aromatase inhibitor vs. other endocrine therapies. For premenopausal women, ovarian suppression/ablation should be used with an AI if a patient has previously received tamoxifen
HER2-positive disease (IHC 3+ or FISH+): Trastuzumab and pertuzumab should be used in combination with a taxane for patients with ER- and PR-negative disease, and for patients with ER-positive and/or PR-positive disease whose tumors are refractory to endocrine therapies
Bone Disease Present: Add denosumab, zoledronic acid, or pamidronate disodium

Gradishar WJ. Ann Oncol 2013;24:2492–2500
Jankowitz RC et al. Breast 2013;22(Suppl 2):S165–S170
Jelovac D, Emens LA. Oncology (Williston Park) 2013;27:166–175

SYSTEMIC ADJUVANT TREATMENT GUIDELINES

Less-Favorable Histologies: Ductal, Lobular, Mixed, and Metaplastic

1. **Hormone receptor-positive–HER2-negative**
   pT1, pT2, or pT3 and pN0 or pN1mi:

   Tumor ≤0.5 cm or microinvasive:
   - N0: consider adjuvant endocrine therapy
   - N1mi: Adjuvant endocrine therapy ± adjuvant chemotherapy

   Tumor >0.5 cm (consider 21-gene RT-PCR assay):
   - Assay not done: adjuvant endocrine therapy ± adjuvant chemotherapy
   - Low recurrence score (<18): adjuvant endocrine therapy
   - Intermediate recurrence score (18–30): adjuvant endocrine therapy ± adjuvant chemotherapy
   - High recurrence score (≥31): adjuvant endocrine therapy + adjuvant chemotherapy

   Node positive:
   - Adjuvant endocrine therapy + adjuvant chemotherapy

2. **Hormone receptor-positive–HER2-positive**
   pT1, pT2, or pT3 and pN0 or pN1mi:

   Tumor ≤0.5 cm or micro-invasive:
   - N0: consider adjuvant endocrine therapy
   - N1mi: adjuvant endocrine therapy ± adjuvant chemotherapy + trastuzumab

   Tumor 0.6–1.0 cm:
   - Adjuvant endocrine therapy ± adjuvant chemotherapy and trastuzumab

   Tumor >1.0 cm:
   - Adjuvant endocrine therapy + adjuvant chemotherapy + trastuzumab

   Node positive:
   - Adjuvant endocrine therapy + adjuvant chemotherapy + trastuzumab

3. **Hormone receptor-negative–HER2-positive**
   pT1, pT2, or pT3 and pN0 or pN1mi:

   Tumor ≤0.5 cm or micro-invasive:
   - N0: no adjuvant therapy
   - N1mi: consider adjuvant chemotherapy + trastuzumab

   Tumor 0.6–1.0 cm:
   - Consider adjuvant chemotherapy + trastuzumab

   Tumor >1.0 cm:
   - Adjuvant chemotherapy + trastuzumab

   Node positive:
   - Adjuvant chemotherapy + trastuzumab

4. **Hormone receptor-negative–HER2-negative:**
   pT1, pT2, or pT3 and pN0 or pN1mi:

   Tumor ≤0.5 cm or microinvasive:
   - N0: no adjuvant therapy
   - N1mi: Consider adjuvant chemotherapy

   Tumor 0.6–1.0 cm:
   - Consider adjuvant chemotherapy

   Tumor >1.0 cm:
   - Adjuvant chemotherapy

   Node positive:
   - Adjuvant chemotherapy

Favorable Histologies: Tubular, Colloid

1. **ER-positive and/or PR-positive**
   pT1, pT2, or pT3 and pN0 or pN1mi:

   Tumor <1.0 cm:
   - No adjuvant therapy

   Tumor 1.0–2.9 cm:
   - Consider adjuvant endocrine therapy

   Tumor ≥3.0 cm:
   - Adjuvant endocrine therapy

   Node positive:
   - Adjuvant endocrine therapy ± adjuvant chemotherapy

2. **ER-negative and PR-negative:**
   Repeat ER and PR status; if truly negative, treat as usual breast cancer histology

PREFERRED *ADJUVANT CHEMOTHERAPY REGIMENS*

Non-Trastuzumab Regimens
1. TAC (docetaxel/doxorubicin/cyclophosphamide)
2. Dose-dense AC (doxorubicin and cyclophosphamide) followed by paclitaxel every 2 weeks
3. AC (doxorubicin/cyclophosphamide) followed by weekly paclitaxel
4. TC (docetaxel and cyclophosphamide)
5. AC (doxorubicin/cyclophosphamide)

Other Adjuvant Regimens
1. FEC (fluorouracil/epirubicin/cyclophosphamide)
2. CMF (cyclophosphamide/methotrexate/fluorouracil)
3. AC (doxorubicin/cyclophosphamide) followed by docetaxel every 3 weeks
4. FEC followed by docetaxel
5. FEC followed by weekly paclitaxel

Trastuzumab-Containing Regimens
Preferred adjuvant trastuzumab-containing regimens:
Pertuzumab should be administered to patients receiving neoadjuvant therapy with ≥T2 or ≥N1, HER2-positive, early-stage breast cancer
1. TCH (docetaxel/carboplatin/trastuzumab)
2. AC (doxorubicin/cyclophosphamide) followed by a taxane + concurrent trastuzumab

Other adjuvant trastuzumab-containing regimens:
1. Docetaxel + trastuzumab followed by FEC (fluorouracil/epirubicin/cyclophosphamide)
2. AC (doxorubicin/cyclophosphamide) followed by docetaxel with trastuzumab

PREFERRED CHEMOTHERAPY FOR *METASTATIC BREAST CANCER (MBC)*

Single Agents
Anthracyclines:
1. Doxorubicin
2. Epirubicin
3. Doxorubicin HCl liposomal injection

Taxanes:
1. Paclitaxel (preferred agent with bevacizumab)
2. Docetaxel
3. Paclitaxel protein bound particles for injectable suspension (albumin-bound)

Antimetabolites:
1. Capecitabine
2. Gemcitabine

Other microtubule inhibitors:
1. Vinorelbine
2. Eribulin

Other Single Agents
1. Cyclophosphamide
2. Mitoxantrone
3. Cisplatin
4. Etoposide (oral)
5. Ixabepilone

Preferred Chemotherapy Combinations
1. FEC (fluorouracil/epirubicin/cyclophosphamide)
2. AC (doxorubicin/cyclophosphamide)
3. CMF (cyclophosphamide /methotrexate/fluorouracil)
4. Docetaxel/capecitabine
5. GT (gemcitabine/paclitaxel)

Other Combinations
1. Ixabepilone + capecitabine

Preferred First-line Agents for HER2-Positive Disease
1. Pertuzumab + trastuzumab + docetaxel
2. Pertuzumab + trastuzumab + paclitaxel

Other First-line Agents for HER2-Positive Disease
Trastuzumab alone or in combination with:
1. Paclitaxel + carboplatin
2. Paclitaxel
3. Docetaxel
4. Vinorelbine
5. Capecitabine

Preferred Agents for Trastuzumab-Exposed HER2-Positive Disease
1. ado-Trastuzumab emtansine (TDM-1)

Other Agents for Trastuzumab-exposed HER2-Positive Disease
1. Lapatinib + capecitabine
2. Trastuzumab + capecitabine
3. Trastuzumab + lapatinib

ADJUVANT, METASTATIC REGIMEN

DOCETAXEL + DOXORUBICIN + CYCLOPHOSPHAMIDE (TAC)

Nabholtz JM et al. J Clin Oncol 2001;19:314–321 [Treatment for metastatic disease]
Nabholtz J-M et al. Proc Am Soc Clin Oncol 2002;21:36a [Abstract 141; adjuvant treatment]

Premedication:
Dexamethasone 8 mg/dose; administer orally twice daily for 3 days, starting on the day before docetaxel administration (total dose/cycle = 48 mg)
Hydration with 1000 mL 0.9% sodium chloride injection (0.9% NS); administer intravenously 500 mL before starting cyclophosphamide and 500 mL after completing cyclophosphamide

Doxorubicin HCl 50 mg/m^2; administer by intravenous injection over 3–5 minutes on day 1, every 3 weeks for 6 cycles (total dosage/cycle = 50 mg/m^2), *followed by:*
Cyclophosphamide 500 mg/m^2; administer intravenously in 100–500 mL 0.9% NS or 5% dextrose injection (D5W), over 15–60 minutes on day 1, every 3 weeks for 6 cycles (total dosage/cycle = 500 mg/m^2), *followed by:*
Docetaxel 75 mg/m^2; administer intravenously in a volume of 0.9% NS or D5W sufficient to produce a docetaxel concentration within the range 0.3–0.74 mg/mL over 60 minutes on day 1, every 3 weeks for 6 cycles (total dosage/cycle = 75 mg/m^2)

Supportive Care
Antiemetic prophylaxis
Emetogenic potential is **HIGH**. *Potential for delayed symptoms*
See Chapter 39 for antiemetic recommendations

Hematopoietic growth factor (CSF) prophylaxis
Primary prophylaxis is indicated with one of the following:
 Filgrastim (G-CSF) 5 mcg/kg per day, by subcutaneous injection, *or*
 Pegfilgrastim (pegylated filgrastim) 6 mg/0.6 mL, by subcutaneous injection for 1 dose
 • Begin use from 24–72 hours after myelosuppressive chemotherapy is completed
 • Continue daily filgrastim until ANC ≥5000/mm^3
See Chapter 43 for more information

Antimicrobial prophylaxis
Risk of fever and neutropenia is LOW
 Antimicrobial primary prophylaxis to be considered:
 • Antibacterial—not indicated
 • Antifungal—not indicated
 • Antiviral—not indicated, unless patient previously had an episode of HSV
See Chapter 47 for more information

Steroid-associated gastritis
Add a **proton pump inhibitor** during steroid use to prevent gastritis and duodenitis

Patient Population Studied

Nabholtz JM et al. J Clin Oncol 2001;19:314–321 [Treatment for metastatic disease]
Nabholtz J-M et al. Proc Am Soc Clin Oncol 2002;21:36a [Abstract 141]

Study of 745 patients with node-positive primary breast cancer treated with adjuvant TAC and 54 patients with metastatic breast cancer and no prior chemotherapy for metastatic disease. All patients were anthracycline-naïve

Efficacy

Nabholtz J-M et al. 2002

	TAC (N = 745)	FAC (N = 746)
Disease-free survival*	82%	74%
Overall survival	TAC demonstrated a reduction in risk of 25% compared with FAC	

*Median follow-up was 33 months

Toxicity (N = 745)

Nabholtz J-M et al. 2002

Toxicity	Percent
Febrile neutropenia	24%
G3/4 infection	2.8%
G3/4 asthenia	11%
G3/4 stomatitis	7%
CHF	1.2%

Therapy Monitoring

Before each cycle: CBC with differential and platelet count, LFTs, and serum electrolytes

Treatment Modifications

Adverse Events	Treatment Modifications
Febrile neutropenia or documented infection after treatment	Reduce docetaxel dosage to 60 mg/m^2 during subsequent cycles
G3 or G4 nausea, vomiting, or diarrhea despite appropriate prophylaxis	Reduce doxorubicin dosage to 40 mg/m^2 during subsequent cycles
First episode of G3 or G4 stomatitis	Reduce doxorubicin dosage to 40 mg/m^2 during subsequent cycles
Second episode of G3 or G4 stomatitis	Reduce docetaxel dosage to 60 mg/m^2 during subsequent cycles
G3 or G4 neuropathy	Discontinue treatment
Other severe adverse events	Hold treatment until toxicity resolves to G ≤1, then resume at decreased dosages appropriate for the toxicity

Note: Dosages reduced for adverse events are not re-escalated

ADJUVANT REGIMEN

DOSE-DENSE DOXORUBICIN + CYCLOPHOSPHAMIDE, THEN PACLITAXEL EVERY 2 WEEKS (ddAC → P)

Citron ML et al. J Clin Oncol 2003;21:1431–1439

Note: Doxorubicin and cyclophosphamide (ddAC) are given in combination, followed sequentially by paclitaxel (P). Both ddAC and P are given for 4 complete cycles

Hydration with 1000 mL 0.9% sodium chloride injection (0.9% NS); administer intravenously 500 mL before starting cyclophosphamide and 500 mL after completing cyclophosphamide

Doxorubicin HCl 60 mg/m^2; administer by intravenous injection over 3–5 minutes on day 1, every 14 days for 4 cycles (total dosage/cycle = 60 mg/m^2)

Cyclophosphamide 600 mg/m^2; administer intravenously in 100–500 mL 0.9% NS or 5% dextrose injection (D5W) over 15–60 minutes on day 1, every 14 days for 4 cycles (total dosage/cycle = 600 mg/m^2)

Filgrastim 5 mcg/kg per day; administer subcutaneously for 7 consecutive days on days 3–9, every 14 days for 4 cycles
• Calculated doses may be rounded by ±10% to use the most economical combination of commercially available products
  (containing 300 mcg or 480 mcg)

After 4 cycles, doxorubicin + cyclophosphamide are followed by:

Premedication:

Dexamethasone 10 mg/dose; administer orally for 2 doses 12 hours and 6 hours before paclitaxel (total dose/cycle = 20 mg), *or*

Dexamethasone 20 mg; administer intravenously over 10–15 minutes, 30–60 minutes before paclitaxel (total dose/cycle = 20 mg)

Note: Dexamethasone doses may be gradually decreased in the absence of hypersensitivity reactions during repeated paclitaxel treatments

Diphenhydramine 50 mg; administer by intravenous injection 30–60 minutes before paclitaxel

Cimetidine 300 mg (or Ranitidine 50 mg, Famotidine 20 mg, or an equivalent histamine receptor [H$_2$]-subtype antagonist); administer intravenously over 15–30 minutes, 30–60 minutes before paclitaxel

Paclitaxel 175 mg/m^2; administer intravenously in a volume of 0.9% NS or D5W sufficient to produce a concentration within the range 0.3–1.2 mg/mL over 3 hours, on day 1, every 14 days for 4 cycles (total dosage/cycle = 175 mg/m^2)

Filgrastim 5 mcg/kg per day; administer subcutaneously for 7 consecutive days on days 3–9, every 14 days for 4 cycles
• Calculated doses may be rounded by ±10% to use the most economical combination of commercially available products
  (containing 300 mcg or 480 mcg)

Supportive Care with Doxorubicin + Cyclophosphamide (AC) Chemotherapy

Antiemetic prophylaxis

*Emetogenic potential is **HIGH**. Potential for delayed symptoms*

See Chapter 39 for antiemetic recommendations

Hematopoietic growth factor (CSF) prophylaxis

Primary prophylaxis, is indicated as described in the regimens

See Chapter 43 for more information

Antimicrobial prophylaxis

Risk of fever and neutropenia is LOW

  Antimicrobial primary prophylaxis to be considered:

  • Antibacterial—not indicated

  • Antifungal—not indicated

  • Antiviral—not indicated, unless patient previously had an episode of HSV

See Chapter 47 for more information

Supportive Care with Paclitaxel (P) Chemotherapy

Antiemetic prophylaxis

Emetogenic potential is LOW

See Chapter 39 for antiemetic recommendations

Hematopoietic growth factor (CSF) prophylaxis

Primary prophylaxis, is indicated as described in the regimens

See Chapter 43 for more information

Antimicrobial prophylaxis

Risk of fever and neutropenia is LOW

  Antimicrobial primary prophylaxis to be considered:

  • Antibacterial—not indicated

  • Antifungal—not indicated

  • Antiviral—not indicated, unless patient previously had an episode of HSV

See Chapter 47 for more information

Treatment Modifications

Adverse Events	Treatment Modifications
ANC <1000/mm^3, or platelets <100,000/mm^3 at start of cycle	Delay treatment until ANC ≥1000/mm^3 and platelets ≥100,000/mm^3. If a treatment delay is >3 weeks, consider decreasing implicated drug dosage by 25%
G3/4 nonhematologic toxicity	If adjustment indicated, decrease implicated drug dosage by 25%
G3/4 neuropathy	Discontinue paclitaxel

Patient Population Studied

Women with node-positive operable breast cancer. Chemotherapy was given adjuvantly after recovery from surgery. A total of 2005 females were randomly assigned to receive one of the following regimens: (1) Sequential A × 4 → P × 4 → C × 4 with doses every 3 weeks; (2) sequential A × 4 → P × 4 → C × 4 every 2 weeks with filgrastim; (3) concurrent AC × 4 → P × 4 every 3 weeks, or (4) concurrent AC × 4 → P × 4 every 2 weeks with filgrastim

Toxicity

Toxicity	AC → P (N = 495)	A → P → C (N = 493)
	G3/4	G3/4
Hematologic Toxicity		
Leukopenia	6%	<1%
Neutropenia	9%	3%
Thrombocytopenia	<1%	0
Anemia	<1%	<1%
RBC transfusions	13% of cycles	1% of cycles
Nonhematologic Toxicity		
Nausea	8%	7%
Vomiting	6%	4%
Diarrhea	1%	3%
Stomatitis	3%	1%
Cardiac function	<1%	1%
Phlebitis/thrombosis	1%	1%
Sensory	4%	4%
Myalgias/arthralgias	5%	5%
Infection	3%	4%

Efficacy

		Survival*	
		Disease-Free	Overall
Dose-dense regimens (every 2 weeks)	N = 988	82%	92%
Standard 3-week-interval regimens	N = 985	75%	90%

*Median follow-up of 36 months; no difference between sequential and concurrent arms in efficacy

Therapy Monitoring

Before each cycle: CBC with differential and platelet count, LFTs, and serum electrolytes

ADJUVANT REGIMEN

DOXORUBICIN + CYCLOPHOSPHAMIDE, THEN WEEKLY PACLITAXEL (AC → P)

Perez EA et al. J Clin Oncol 2001;19:4216–4223
Seidman AD et al. J Clin Oncol 1998;16:3353–3361
Sparano JA. N Engl J Med 2008;258:1663–1671

Hydration with 1000 mL 0.9% sodium chloride injection (0.9% NS); administer intravenously 500 mL before starting cyclophosphamide and 500 mL after completing cyclophosphamide

Doxorubicin HCl 60 mg/m^2; administer by intravenous injection over 3–5 minutes on day 1 every 21 days for 4 cycles (total dosage/cycle = 60 mg/m^2)

Cyclophosphamide 600 mg/m^2; administer intravenously in 100–500 mL 0.9% NS or 5% dextrose injection (D5W) over 30–60 minutes on day 1, every 21 days for 4 cycles (total dosage/cycle = 600 mg/m^2), *followed after 4 cycles by:*

Premedication:
Dexamethasone 10 mg/dose; administer orally for 2 doses at 12 hours and 6 hours before paclitaxel (total dose/cycle = 20 mg), *or*
Dexamethasone 20 mg; administer intravenously over 10–15 minutes, 30–60 minutes before starting paclitaxel (total dose/cycle = 20 mg)
Diphenhydramine 50 mg; administer intravenously 30 minutes prior to starting paclitaxel
Cimetidine 300 mg (or ranitidine 50 mg, or famotidine 20 mg, or an equivalent histamine receptor [H$_2$]-subtype antagonist); administer intravenously over 15–30 minutes, 30–60 minutes before starting paclitaxel

Paclitaxel 80 mg/m^2 per dose; administer intravenously in a volume of 0.9% NS or D5W sufficient to produce a concentration within the range 0.3–1.2 mg/mL over 60 minutes, weekly for 12 consecutive weeks (total dosage/21-day cycle = 240 mg/m^2)

Supportive Care with Doxorubicin + Cyclophosphamide (AC) Chemotherapy
Antiemetic prophylaxis
Emetogenic potential is **HIGH**. *Potential for delayed symptoms*
See Chapter 39 for antiemetic recommendations

Hematopoietic growth factor (CSF) prophylaxis
Primary prophylaxis may be indicated
See Chapter 43 for more information

Antimicrobial prophylaxis
Risk of fever and neutropenia is LOW
   Antimicrobial primary prophylaxis to be considered:
   • Antibacterial—not indicated
   • Antifungal—not indicated
   • Antiviral—not indicated, unless patient previously had an episode of HSV
See Chapter 47 for more information

Supportive Care with Paclitaxel (P) Chemotherapy
Antiemetic prophylaxis
Emetogenic potential is **LOW**
See Chapter 39 for antiemetic recommendations

Hematopoietic growth factor (CSF) prophylaxis
Primary prophylaxis is NOT indicated
See Chapter 43 for more information

Antimicrobial prophylaxis
Risk of fever and neutropenia is LOW
   Antimicrobial primary prophylaxis to be considered:
   • Antibacterial—not indicated
   • Antifungal—not indicated
   • Antiviral—not indicated, unless patient previously had an episode of HSV
See Chapter 47 for more information

Treatment Modifications: AC

Bear HD et al. J Clin Oncol 2003;21:4165–4174
Citron ML et al. J Clin Oncol 2003;21:1431–1439

Adverse Events	Treatment Modifications
Absolute neutrophil count (ANC) <1500/mm³ or platelets <100,000/mm³ at start of cycle*	Delay treatment until ANC ≥1500/mm³ and platelets ≥100,000/mm³. Give filgrastim after chemotherapy during subsequent cycles
First episode of febrile neutropenia	Give filgrastim after chemotherapy during subsequent cycles†
Second episode of febrile neutropenia	During subsequent cycles, consider prophylaxis with ciprofloxacin‡
Third episode of febrile neutropenia	Decrease both doxorubicin and cyclophosphamide dosages by 25%

*Although an ANC of 1500/mm³ is often identified as a minimum acceptable ANC to safely proceed with treatment, recent data shows that an ANC ≥1000/mm³ is acceptable if filgrastim is given after chemotherapy
†Filgrastim 5 mcg/kg per day; administer subcutaneously starting at least 24 hours after completing chemotherapy until ANC >5000/mm³
‡Ciprofloxacin 500 mg orally twice daily for 7 consecutive days starting on day 5

Treatment Modifications: Paclitaxel

Adverse Events	Treatment Modifications
ANC ≤800/mm³ or platelets ≤50,000/mm³	Hold treatment until ANC >800/mm³ and platelets >50,000/mm³, then resume with weekly paclitaxel dosage reduced by 10 mg/m²
G2 motor or sensory neuropathies	Reduce weekly paclitaxel dosage by 10 mg/m² without interrupting planned treatment
Other nonhematologic adverse events G2 or G3	Hold treatment until adverse events resolve to G ≤1, then resume with weekly paclitaxel dosage reduced by 10 mg/m²
Patients who cannot tolerate paclitaxel at 60 mg/m² per week	Discontinue treatment
Treatment delay >2 weeks	Decrease weekly paclitaxel dosage by 10 mg/m² or consider discontinuing treatment

Patient Population Studied

Sparano JA. N Engl J Med 2008;258:1663–1671

Study of 4950 patients with operable, hormone receptor positive adenocarcinoma of the breast with either (a) histologically involved lymph nodes (tumor stage T1, T2, or T3 and nodal stage N1 or N2) or (b) "high-risk, axillary node-negative disease" (T2 or T3, N0) without distant metastases. Of the study patients, 88% were node-positive and 19% HER2neu+. All patients received 4 cycles of intravenous doxorubicin and cyclophosphamide at 3-week intervals and were assigned to intravenous paclitaxel or docetaxel given at 3-week intervals for 4 cycles or at 1-week intervals for 12 cycles. The primary end point was disease-free survival

Efficacy (N = 4950)

Sparano JA. N Engl J Med 2008;258:1663–1671

	Number of Patients	5-Year DFS (%)	Hazard Ratio for DFS*	5-Year OS (%)	Hazard Ratio for OS*
Paclitaxel every 3 weeks	1253	76.9	1	86.5	1
Weekly Paclitaxel	1231	81.5	1.27, p = 0.006	89.7	1.32, p = 0.01
Docetaxel every 3 weeks	1236	81.2	1.23, p = 0.020	87.3	1.13, p = 0.25
Weekly docetaxel	1230	77.6	1.09, p = 0.290	86.2	1.02, p = 0.80

DFS, Disease-free survival; OS, overall survival
*Hazard ratio >1 favors the group receiving that therapy

Toxicity of Paclitaxel and Docetaxel

Sparano JA. N Engl J Med 2008;258:1663–1671

Toxicity*	Paclitaxel Every 3 Weeks	Weekly Paclitaxel	Docetaxel Every 3 Weeks	Weekly Docetaxel
	Percent			
Neutropenia[†]	4	2	46	3
Febrile neutropenia[†]	<1	1	16	1
Infection	3	3	13	4
Stomatitis	<1	0	5	2
Fatigue	2	3	9	11
Myalgia	7	2	6	1
Arthralgia	6	2	6	1
Lacrimation	<1	0	<1	5
G3/4 neuropathy	5	8	4	6
G2/3/4 neuropathy	20	27	16	16

*Tabulation of G3/4 toxic effects and G2/3/4 neuropathies resulting from the taxane component of therapy that occurred in at least 5% of all treated patients
[†]Information on only G4 neutropenia (ANC <500/mm³) was collected

Therapy Monitoring

1. *Weekly:* CBC with differential and platelet count
2. *Monthly:* LFTs and serum electrolytes

ADJUVANT REGIMEN

DOCETAXEL + CYCLOPHOSPHAMIDE (TC) EVERY 3 WEEKS × 4 CYCLES

Jones S et al. J Clin Oncol 2006;24:5381–5387
Jones S et al. J Clin Oncol 2009;27:1177–1183

Hydration with 1000 mL 0.9% sodium chloride injection (0.9% NS); administer intravenously 500 mL before starting cyclophosphamide and 500 mL after completing cyclophosphamide

Premedication:
Dexamethasone 8 mg/dose; administer orally every 12 hours for 3 days starting on the day before docetaxel administration (total dose/cycle = 48 mg)
Docetaxel 75 mg/m²; administer intravenously in a volume of 0.9% NS or 5% dextrose injection (D5W) sufficient to produce a docetaxel concentration within the range 0.3–0.74 mg/mL over 30–60 minutes on day 1 every 21 days for 4 cycles (total dosage/cycle = 75 mg/m²)
Cyclophosphamide 600 mg/m²; administer intravenously in 100–500 mL 0.9% NS or D5W over 30–60 minutes on day 1 every 21 days for 4 cycles (total dosage/cycle = 600 mg/m²)

Supportive Care
Antiemetic prophylaxis
Emetogenic potential is **MODERATE**
See Chapter 39 for antiemetic recommendations

Hematopoietic growth factor (CSF) prophylaxis
Primary prophylaxis is NOT indicated
See Chapter 43 for more information

Antimicrobial prophylaxis
Risk of fever and neutropenia is LOW
  Antimicrobial primary prophylaxis to be considered:
  • Antibacterial—not indicated
  • Antifungal—not indicated
  • Antiviral—not indicated, unless patient previously had an episode of HSV
See Chapter 47 for more information

Steroid-associated gastritis
Add a **proton pump inhibitor** during steroid use to prevent gastritis and duodenitis

Treatment Modifications

Patients were taken off treatment if administration of any study drug was delayed more than 2 weeks as a result of drug-related toxicities. *No dose reductions were permitted.* No prophylactic growth factors were used and the use of oral prophylactic antibiotics was at the discretion of the treating physician

Patient Population Studied

Phase III randomized prospective clinical trial comparing 4 cycles of doxorubicin + cyclophosphamide (AC) with 4 cycles of docetaxel + cyclophosphamide (TC) as adjuvant chemotherapy in 1016 women with operable stages I to III invasive breast cancer. Eligible patients had a Karnofsky performance status of ≥80% and no evidence of metastatic disease. Before treatment, a complete surgical excision of the primary tumor (lumpectomy and axillary dissection or modified radical mastectomy) was performed. Neoadjuvant chemotherapy was *not* permitted. Eligible primary tumor size was ≥1.0 cm and <7.0 cm. Patients were randomly assigned to 4 cycles of either standard-dose AC (60 and 600 mg/m², respectively) or TC (75 and 600 mg/m², respectively) administered on day 1 of each 21-day cycle for 4 cycles as adjuvant treatment after complete surgical excision of the primary tumor. Chemotherapy was administered before radiation therapy (XRT) when XRT was indicated (breast conservation or postoperative XRT for patient with 4 or more involved axillary lymph nodes). On completion of 4 cycles of chemotherapy (±XRT), tamoxifen was administered to all patients with hormone receptor-positive breast cancer for 5 years. The majority (71%) of patients had breast cancer that was estrogen receptor (ER)-positive and/or progesterone receptor (PR)-positive. The number of patients with node-negative disease was balanced between groups (47% TC and 49% AC); 12% of TC and 9% of AC patients had ≥4 positive nodes

Efficacy

	7-Year DFS		7-Year OS	
TC × 4 (N = 506)	81%	HR = 0.74 [95% CI, 0.56–0.98] P = 0.033	87%	HR = 0.69 [95% CI, 0.50–0.97] P = 0.032
AC × 4 (N = 510)	75%		82%	

Unplanned, exploratory analyses of disease-free survival hazard ratios (HR) and CI

	Hazard Ratio	95% Confidence Interval (CI)
HER2− (TC = 55; AC = 69)	0.56	0.30–1.05
HER2+ (TC = 28; AC = 18)	0.73	0.32–1.70
ER− and PR− (TC = 136; AC = 158)	0.70	0.44–1.10
ER+ or PR+ (TC = 368; AC = 351)	0.79	0.56–1.13
Age ≥65 (TC = 78; AC = 82)	0.70	0.40–1.24
Age <65 (TC = 428; AC = 428)	0.76	0.55–1.04

AC, doxorubicin + cyclophosphamide; DFS, Disease-free survival; ER, estrogen receptor; OS, overall survival; PR, progesterone receptor; TC, docetaxel + cyclophosphamide

Toxicity*

Frequency of Most Common Adverse Events (All Grades)*

	TC Patients (N = 506)				AC Patients (N = 510)			
	Grade (%)				Grade (%)			
	1	2	3	4	1	2	3	4
Hematologic								
Anemia	3	2	<1	<1	4	2	1	<1
Neutropenia	<1	1	10	51	1	2	12	43
Thrombocytopenia	<1	<1	0	<1	<1	<1	1	0
Nonhematologic								
Asthenia	43	32	3	<1	41	31	4	<1
Edema	27	7	<1	0	17	3	<1	<1
Fever	14	5	3	2	11	4	2	<1
Infection	8	4	7	<1	7	5	8	<1
Myalgia	22	10	1	<1	11	5	<1	<1
Nausea	38	13	2	<1	43	32	7	<1
Phlebitis	8	3	<1	0	1	1	0	0
Stomatitis	23	10	<1	<1	29	15	1	1
Vomiting	9	5	<1	<1	21	16	5	<1

AC, doxorubicin and cyclophosphamide; TC, Docetaxel and cyclophosphamide
*NCI-Common Toxicity Criteria v1. Treatment-related toxicities were reported using Coding Symbols for a Thesaurus of Adverse Reaction Terms (COSTART) and summarized by highest grade per patient

Therapy Monitoring

1. *Baseline:* LFTs, serum chemistry, CBC with differential and platelet count
2. *Follow-up:* CBC with differential and platelet count at start of each cycle

ADJUVANT, NEOADJUVANT METASTATIC REGIMEN

DOXORUBICIN + CYCLOPHOSPHAMIDE (AC)

Fisher B et al. J Clin Oncol 1997;15:1858–1869

Hydration with 1000 mL 0.9% sodium chloride injection (0.9% NS); administer intravenously 500 mL before starting cyclophosphamide and 500 mL after completing cyclophosphamide

Doxorubicin HCl 60 mg/m²; administer by intravenous injection over 3–5 minutes on day 1, every 21 days for 4 cycles (total dosage/cycle = 60 mg/m²)
Cyclophosphamide 600 mg/m²; administer intravenously in 100–500 mL 0.9% NS or 5% dextrose injection over 15–60 minutes on day 1, every 21 days for 4 cycles (total dosage/cycle = 600 mg/m²)

Supportive Care
Antiemetic prophylaxis
Emetogenic potential is **HIGH**. *Potential for delayed symptoms*
See Chapter 39 for antiemetic recommendations

Hematopoietic growth factor (CSF) prophylaxis
Primary prophylaxis may be indicated
See Chapter 43 for more information

Antimicrobial prophylaxis
Risk of fever and neutropenia is LOW
  Antimicrobial primary prophylaxis to be considered:
  • Antibacterial—not indicated
  • Antifungal—not indicated
  • Antiviral—not indicated, unless patient previously had an episode of HSV
See Chapter 47 for more information

Toxicity*

Toxicity	G3	G4
Neutropenia	4.8%	1.6%
Infection	2.4%	0.3%
Sepsis	NR	3.3%
Nausea	8.5%	NR
Vomiting	12.4%	1.2%
Stomatitis	1.3%	0
Other Toxicities		
Alopecia (pronounced)		91%
CHF responsive to therapy		0.1%
AML		0.1%
Myelodysplastic syndrome		0.1%

*NCI Common Toxicity Criteria; Fisher B et al. J Clin Oncol 1997;15:1858–1869

Therapy Monitoring

Before each cycle: CBC with differential and platelet counts, LFTs, serum electrolytes, BUN, and creatinine

Treatment Modifications

Bear HD et al. J Clin Oncol 2003;21:4165–4174
Citron ML et al. J Clin Oncol 2003;21:1431–1439

Adverse Events	Treatment Modifications
Absolute neutrophil count (ANC) <1500/mm³ or platelets <100,000/mm³ at start of cycle*	Delay treatment until ANC ≥1500/mm³ and platelets ≥100,000/mm³. Give filgrastim after chemotherapy during subsequent cycles
First episode of febrile neutropenia	Give filgrastim after chemotherapy during subsequent cycles†
Second episode of febrile neutropenia	During subsequent cycles, consider prophylaxis with ciprofloxacin‡
Third episode of febrile neutropenia	Decrease both doxorubicin and cyclophosphamide dosages by 25%

*Although an ANC of 1500/mm³ is often identified as a minimum acceptable ANC to safely proceed with treatment, recent data shows that an ANC ≥1000/mm³ is acceptable if filgrastim is given after chemotherapy
†Filgrastim 5 mcg/kg per day; administer subcutaneously starting at least 24 hours after completing chemotherapy until ANC ≥5000/mm³
‡Ciprofloxacin 500 mg orally twice daily for 7 consecutive days starting on day 5

Patient Population Studied

Fisher B et al. J Clin Oncol 1997;15:1858–1869

Study of 764 patients with node-positive primary breast cancer who were treated with AC for adjuvant therapy. This regimen has also been studied in the neoadjuvant and metastatic settings

Efficacy

Jones S et al. J Clin Oncol 2009;27:1177–1183

	7-Year DFS		7-Year OS	
TC × 4 (N = 506)	81%	HR = 0.74 [95% CI, 0.56–0.98] *P* = 0.033	87%	HR = 0.69 [95% CI, 0.50–0.97] *P* = 0.032
AC × 4 (N = 510)	75%		82%	

Unplanned, exploratory analyses of disease-free survival hazard ratios (HR) and CI

	Hazard Ratio	95% Confidence Interval (CI)
HER2− (TC = 55; AC = 69)	0.56	0.30–1.05
HER2+ (TC = 28; AC = 18)	0.73	0.32–1.70
ER− and PR− (TC = 136; AC = 158)	0.70	0.44–1.10
ER+ or PR+ (TC = 368; AC = 351)	0.79	0.56–1.13
Age ≥65 (TC = 78; AC = 82)	0.70	0.40–1.24
Age <65 (TC = 428; AC = 428)	0.76	0.55–1.04

AC, doxorubicin + cyclophosphamide; DFS, Disease-free survival; ER, estrogen receptor; OS, overall survival; PR, progesterone receptor; TC, docetaxel + cyclophosphamide

ADJUVANT, METASTATIC REGIMEN
CYCLOPHOSPHAMIDE + EPIRUBICIN + FLUOROURACIL
(FEC 100)

Bonneterre et al. J Clin Oncol 2004;22:3070–3079
French Adjuvant Study Group. J Clin Oncol 2001;19:602–611

Fluorouracil 500 mg/m²; administer by intravenous injection over 1–3 minutes on day 1, every 21 days for 6 cycles (total dosage/cycle = 500 mg/m²)
Epirubicin HCl 100 mg/m²; administer by intravenous injection over 3–5 minutes on day 1, every 21 days for 6 cycles (total dosage/cycle = 100 mg/m²)

Hydration with 1000 mL 0.9% sodium chloride injection (0.9% NS); administer intravenously 500 mL before starting cyclophosphamide and 500 mL after completing cyclophosphamide
Cyclophosphamide 500 mg/m²; administer intravenously in 100–500 mL 0.9% NS or 5% dextrose injection over 15–60 minutes on day 1, every 21 days for 6 cycles (total dosage/cycle = 500 mg/m²)

Supportive Care
Antiemetic prophylaxis
Emetogenic potential is **HIGH**. *Potential for delayed symptoms*
See Chapter 39 for antiemetic recommendations

Hematopoietic growth factor (CSF) prophylaxis
Primary prophylaxis is indicated with one of the following:
   Filgrastim (G-CSF) 5 mcg/kg per day by subcutaneous injection, *or*
   Pegfilgrastim (pegylated filgrastim) 6 mg/0.6 mL by subcutaneous injection for 1 dose
   • Begin use from 24–72 hours after myelosuppressive chemotherapy is completed
   • Continue daily filgrastim until ANC ≥5000/mm³
See Chapter 43 for more information

Antimicrobial prophylaxis
Risk of fever and neutropenia is LOW
   Antimicrobial primary prophylaxis to be considered:
   • Antibacterial—not indicated
   • Antifungal—not indicated
   • Antiviral—not indicated, unless patient previously had an episode of HSV
See Chapter 47 for more information

Patient Population Studied

Premenopausal and postmenopausal women with histologically proven axillary lymph node involvement (at least 5 axillary nodes resected) with more than 3 positive nodes or between 1 and 3 positive nodes with Scarff-Bloom-Richardson (SBR) grade ≥2 and hormone receptor negativity (both estrogen and progesterone) were enrolled. Postmenopausal status was defined as an amenorrhea for at least 1 year. Main eligibility criteria included a World Health Organization (WHO) performance status ≤2, no cardiac dysfunction (baseline left ventricular ejection fraction [LVEF] ≥50%). Patients were randomized after surgery to receive either fluorouracil 500 mg/m², epirubicin 50 mg/m², and cyclophosphamide 500 mg/m² every 21 days for 6 cycles (FEC 50), or the same regimen except with epirubicin dose of 100 mg/m² (FEC 100). Treatment was begun within 42 days of surgery

Treatment Modifications

Adverse Events	Treatment Modifications
ANC <1500/mm³, or platelets <100,000/mm³ at start of cycle	Delay treatment until ANC ≥1500/mm³ and platelets ≥100,000/mm³
Hematologic recovery >3 weeks	Discontinue treatment
First episode of febrile neutropenia	During subsequent cycles, consider prophylaxis with ciprofloxacin*
Second episode of febrile neutropenia	Decrease chemotherapy doses by 20% (epirubicin by 20 mg/m², fluorouracil and cyclophosphamide by 100 mg/m²) and administer ciprofloxacin*
First episode of G4 documented infection	Add ciprofloxacin prophylaxis during subsequent cycles*
Second episode of G4 documented infection	Decrease chemotherapy doses by 20% (epirubicin by 20 mg/m², fluorouracil and cyclophosphamide by 100 mg/m²) and administer ciprofloxacin*
Third episode of G4 documented infection	Discontinue chemotherapy
Serum total bilirubin levels 2 to 3 mg/dL (34.2 to 51.3 mmol/L)	Reduce epirubicin dose by 50%
Serum bilirubin levels ≥3 mg/dL (≥51.3 mmol/L)	Discontinue treatment

*Ciprofloxacin 500 mg orally twice daily for 7 consecutive days starting on day 5

Efficacy

5-Year DFS and OS Rates

Group	5-Year DFS			5-Year OS		
	FEC 50	FEC 100		FEC 50	FEC 100	
All patients	54.8%	66.3%	P = 0.03	65.3%	77.4%	P = 0.007
1–3 Nodes	77.6%	71.0%	P = 0.42	83.8%	78.2%	P = 0.63
>3 Nodes	49.6%	65.3%	P = 0.005	60.9%	77.2%	P = 0.001

DFS, Disease-free survival; FEC 50, fluorouracil + cyclophosphamide + epirubicin 50 mg/m²; FEC 100, fluorouracil + cyclophosphamide + epirubicin 100 mg/m²; OS, overall survival

Toxicity

Toxicity	FEC 50 (N = 278)		FEC 100 (N = 268)		
	G1/2	G3/4	G1/2	G3/4	P Value
Hematologic Toxicity					
Neutropenia	43.5%	11.1%	30.1%	25.2%	0.001
Anemia	11.1%	0	41.6%	0.8%	0.001
Nonhematologic Toxicity					
Nausea/vomiting	61.6%	23.3%	58%	34.7%	0.008
Stomatitis	7.8%	0	24.1%	3.8%	0.001
Infection	15.9%	0	17.2%	3.4%	0.003
Cardiac, all	6/278		4/268		
Cardiac, acute	1/278 (MI)		1/268 (↓LVEF)		
Cardiac, delayed	5/278		3/268		

After more than 8 years of follow-up, the cardiac toxicity observed after adjuvant treatment with FEC 100 consists of 2 cases of well-controlled congestive heart failure and 18 cases of asymptomatic left ventricular dysfunction. In the majority of women with primary breast cancer, the benefits of treatment with FEC 100 in terms of disease-free and overall survival outweigh the risks, and cardiac risk factors should be carefully evaluated in patient selection

Therapy Monitoring

1. *Weekly:* CBC with differential and platelet count
2. *Before each cycle:* CBC with differential and platelet count, LFTs, and serum electrolytes

ADJUVANT, METASTATIC REGIMEN
CYCLOPHOSPHAMIDE + METHOTREXATE + FLUOROURACIL
(CMF; ORAL)

Amadori D et al. J Clin Oncol 2000;18:3125–3134

Cyclophosphamide 100 mg/m² per day; administer orally for 14 consecutive days on days 1–14, every 4 weeks for 6 cycles, (total dosage/cycle = 1400 mg/m²)
Note: Encourage patients to supplement their usual oral hydration with (extra) non–alcohol-containing fluids, 1000–2000 mL/day, to take cyclophosphamide doses at the beginning of a waking cycle, and to void urine frequently while taking cyclophosphamide
Methotrexate 40 mg/m² per dose; administer by intravenous injection over ≤1 minute for 2 doses on days 1 and 8, every 4 weeks for 6 cycles (total dosage/cycle = 80 mg/m²)
Fluorouracil 600 mg/m² per dose; administer by intravenous injection over 1–3 minutes for 2 doses on days 1 and 8, every 4 weeks for 6 cycles (total dosage/cycle = 1200 mg/m²)

Supportive Care
Antiemetic prophylaxis
Emetogenic potential on Days 1–14 is **LOW–MODERATE**
See Chapter 39 for antiemetic recommendations

Hematopoietic growth factor (CSF) prophylaxis
Primary prophylaxis is NOT indicated
See Chapter 43 for more information

Antimicrobial prophylaxis
Risk of fever and neutropenia is LOW
  Antimicrobial primary prophylaxis to be considered:
  • Antibacterial—not indicated
  • Antifungal—not indicated
  • Antiviral—not indicated, unless patient previously had an episode of HSV
See Chapter 47 for more information

Treatment Modifications

Adverse Events	Treatment Modifications
WBC <3500/mm³ or platelets <100,000/mm³ on first day of a cycle	Delay treatment for a maximum of 2 weeks until WBC >3500/mm³ and platelets >100,000/mm³. Continue at full dosages if counts recover within 2 weeks
If after 2 weeks WBC <3500/mm³ or platelets <100,000/mm³ reduce all drugs' dosages as follows:	
WBC 3000–3499/mm³, or platelets 75,000–99,999/mm³	Reduce dosages by 25%
WBC 2500–2999/mm³ and platelets ≥75,000/mm³	Reduce dosages by 50%
WBC <2500/mm³, or platelets <75,000/mm³	Hold treatment
ANC <1500/mm³, or platelets <100,000/mm³ at start of cycle	Delay treatment until ANC ≥1500/mm³ and platelets ≥100,000/mm³. Give filgrastim* in subsequent cycles
Hematologic recovery >3 weeks	Discontinue treatment
First episode of febrile neutropenia	Give filgrastim* during subsequent cycles
Second episode of febrile neutropenia	During subsequent cycles, consider prophylaxis with ciprofloxacin†
Third episode of febrile neutropenia	Decrease chemotherapy doses by 20% and administer filgrastim* + ciprofloxacin†
First episode of G4 documented infection	Add filgrastim* and ciprofloxacin† prophylaxis during subsequent cycles
Second episode of G4 documented infection	Decrease chemotherapy doses by 20% and administer filgrastim* + ciprofloxacin†
Third episode of G4 documented infection	Discontinue chemotherapy
G3 stomatitis	Reduce methotrexate and fluorouracil dosage by 50% during subsequent cycles
G4 non-hematologic toxicity	Discontinue chemotherapy

*Filgrastim 5 mcg/kg per day; administer subcutaneously for 8 consecutive days (days 3–10)
†Ciprofloxacin 500 mg orally twice daily for 7 consecutive days starting on day 5

Patient Population Studied

Amadori D et al. J Clin Oncol 2000;18:3125–3134

Study of 281 women with node-negative resectable breast cancer. CMF was given as adjuvant therapy within 6 weeks of surgery. All patients had rapidly proliferating tumors as determined by thymidine-labeling index

Toxicity

Boccardo F et al. J Clin Oncol 2000;18:2718–2727
Bonnadonna G et al. N Engl J Med 1976;294:405–410

Toxicity (N = 207)	% of Patients
Leukocytes = 2500–3900/mm³	67%
Leukocytes <2500/mm³	4%
Platelets = 75,000–129,000/mm³	57%
Platelets <75,000/mm³	14%
Oral mucositis	18%
Conjunctivitis	25%
Hair loss	55%
Cystitis	28%
Amenorrhea	54%
Febrile neutropenia	3%

Efficacy

Early Breast Cancer Trialists' Collaborative Group. Lancet 1998;352:930–942

Absolute Risk Reduction with Adjuvant Chemotherapy (Primarily CMF)

	5-year	
	Recurrence	Mortality
Node+, Age <50 years	15.4%	12.4%
Node+, Age >50 years	5.4%	2.3%
Node−, Age <50 years	10.4%	5.7%
Node−, Age >50 years	5.7%	6.4%

Note: Anthracycline-containing regimens may be superior to CMF with additional absolute risk reductions of 3.2% for recurrence and 2.7% for mortality

Therapy Monitoring

Before each cycle: CBC with differential and platelet counts

ADJUVANT, NEOADJUVANT REGIMEN
DOXORUBICIN + CYCLOPHOSPHAMIDE THEN DOCETAXEL EVERY 3 WEEKS (AC → T)

Bear HD et al. J Clin Oncol 2003;21:4165–4174

AC (Doxorubicin + Cyclophosphamide) × 4 cycles
Hydration with 0.9% sodium chloride injection (0.9% NS); administer intravenously 500 mL before and 500 mL after cyclophosphamide

Doxorubicin HCl 60 mg/m^2; administer by intravenous injection over 3–5 minutes on day 1, every 21 days for 4 cycles (total dosage/cycle = 60 mg/m^2)
Cyclophosphamide 600 mg/m^2; administer intravenously in 100–500 mL 0.9% NS or 5% dextrose injection (D5W), over 15–60 minutes on day 1, every 21 days for 4 cycles (total dosage/cycle = 600 mg/m^2), *followed after 4 cycles by:*

T (Docetaxel) × 4 cycles
Premedication:
Dexamethasone 8 mg/dose; administer orally twice daily for 3 days, starting on the day before docetaxel administration (total dose/cycle = 48 mg)

Docetaxel 100 mg/m^2; administer intravenously in a volume of 0.9% NS or D5W sufficient to produce a docetaxel concentration within the range 0.3–0.74 mg/mL over 60 minutes on day 1, every 21 days for 4 cycles (total dosage/cycle = 100 mg/m^2)

Supportive Care for Doxorubicin + Cyclophosphamide (AC) Chemotherapy
Antiemetic prophylaxis
Emetogenic potential is **HIGH**. *Potential for delayed symptoms*
See Chapter 39 for antiemetic recommendations

Hematopoietic growth factor (CSF) prophylaxis
Primary prophylaxis may be indicated
See Chapter 43 for more information

Antimicrobial prophylaxis
Risk of fever and neutropenia is LOW
   Antimicrobial primary prophylaxis to be considered:
   • Antibacterial—not indicated
   • Antifungal—not indicated
   • Antiviral—not indicated, unless patient previously had an episode of HSV
See Chapter 47 for more information

Supportive Care for Docetaxel (T) Chemotherapy
Antiemetic prophylaxis
Emetogenic potential is **LOW**
See Chapter 39 for antiemetic recommendations

Hematopoietic growth factor (CSF) prophylaxis
Primary prophylaxis is indicated with one of the following:
   Filgrastim (G-CSF) 5 mcg/kg per day, by subcutaneous injection, *or*
   Pegfilgrastim (pegylated filgrastim) 6 mg/0.6 mL, by subcutaneous injection for 1 dose
   • Begin use from 24–72 hours after myelosuppressive chemotherapy is completed
See Chapter 43 for more information

Antimicrobial prophylaxis
Risk of fever and neutropenia is LOW
   Antimicrobial primary prophylaxis to be considered:
   • Antibacterial—not indicated
   • Antifungal—not indicated
   • Antiviral—not indicated, unless patient previously had an episode of HSV
See Chapter 47 for more information

Steroid-associated gastritis
Add a **proton pump inhibitor** during steroid use to prevent gastritis and duodenitis

Patient Population Studied
Study of 1584 women with primary breast cancer with tumor size >1 cm *or* lymph nodes with clinical evidence of malignant disease. Regimen was given as neoadjuvant therapy in this study, but is also often given as adjuvant therapy in node-positive disease. The regimen is 1 of 3 arms in NSABP B-30

Efficacy (N = 752/1534)

Neoadjuvant Therapy	AC → T (N = 752)	AC (N = 1534)
Overall response	91%	85%
CR (pathologic)	26%	13%

Toxicity (for Docetaxel) (N = 1584)
NCI Common Toxicity Criteria (CTC)

Toxicity	G3	G4
Neutropenia	2%	<0.5%
Febrile neutropenia	NA	21%
Infection	0.7%	6%
Nausea/vomiting	0.5%	0.4%
Stomatitis	2.2%	0.4%
Diarrhea	NR	0.6%
Thrombosis	NR	0.7%
Allergy	NR	0.3%
Neuropathy	2.3%	0.1%

Therapy Monitoring
Before each cycle: CBC with differential and platelet count, LFTs, and serum electrolyte

Treatment Modifications

Doxorubicin and Cyclophosphamide

Adverse Events	Treatment Modifications
ANC <1500/mm³, or platelets <100,000/mm³ at start of cycle*	Delay treatment until ANC ≥1500/mm³ and platelets ≥100,000/mm³. Administer filgrastim[†] during subsequent cycles*
First episode of febrile neutropenia	Give filgrastim during subsequent cycles
Second episode of febrile neutropenia	Consider ciprofloxacin[‡] prophylaxis in subsequent cycles
Third episode of febrile neutropenia	Decrease both doxorubicin and cyclophosphamide dosages by 25% and administer ciprofloxacin[‡]
First episode of G4 documented infection	Add filgrastim[†] and ciprofloxacin[‡] prophylaxis during subsequent cycles
Second episode of G4 documented infection	Decrease both doxorubicin and cyclophosphamide dosages by 25%. Administer filgrastim[†] and ciprofloxacin[‡] during subsequent cycles
Third episode of G4 documented infection	Discontinue chemotherapy

Docetaxel

Adverse Events	Treatment Modifications
ANC <1500/mm³ on day of planned treatment*	Delay treatment until ANC ≥1500/mm³; administer filgrastim[†] during subsequent cycles*
First episode of febrile neutropenia	Reduce docetaxel dosage to 75 mg/m² during subsequent cycles
Second episode of febrile neutropenia	Continue docetaxel 75 mg/m² and give filgrastim[†] during subsequent cycles
Third episode of febrile neutropenia	Add ciprofloxacin[‡]
First episode of G4 documented infection	Reduce docetaxel dosage to 75 mg/m² during subsequent cycles
Second episode of G4 documented infection	Continue docetaxel at 75 mg/m² per dose and give filgrastim[†] and ciprofloxacin[‡] during subsequent cycles
Third episode of G4 documented infection	Discontinue docetaxel

*Although an ANC of 1500/mm³ is often identified as a minimum acceptable ANC to safely proceed with treatment, recent data shows that an ANC ≥1000/mm³ is acceptable if filgrastim is given after chemotherapy
[†]Filgrastim 5 mcg/kg per day; administer subcutaneously starting at least 24 hours after completing chemotherapy until ANC ≥5000/mm³
[‡]Ciprofloxacin 500 mg orally twice/day for 7 days starting on day 5

ADJUVANT REGIMEN
CYCLOPHOSPHAMIDE + EPIRUBICIN + FLUOROURACIL
(FEC) × 3 CYCLES → DOCETAXEL × 3 CYCLES

Roché HJ. Clin Oncol 2006;24:5664–5671

FEC (Cyclophosphamide + Epirubicin + Fluorouracil) × 3 cycles
Hydration before and after cyclophosphamide with 0.9% sodium chloride injection (0.9% NS); administer intravenously 500 mL before starting cyclophosphamide and 500 mL after completing cyclophosphamide

Fluorouracil 500 mg/m^2; administer by intravenous injection over 1–3 minutes on day 1, every 21 days for 3 cycles (total dosage/cycle = 500 mg/m^2)
Epirubicin HCl 100 mg/m^2; administer by intravenous injection over 3–5 minutes on day 1, every 21 days for 3 cycles (total dosage/cycle = 100 mg/m^2)
Cyclophosphamide 500 mg/m^2; administer intravenously in 100–500 mL 0.9% NS or 5% dextrose injection (D5W) over 30–60 minutes on day 1, every 21 days for 3 cycles (total dosage/cycle = 500 mg/m^2)

Supportive Care
Antiemetic prophylaxis
Emetogenic potential is **HIGH**. *Potential for delayed symptoms*
See Chapter 39 for antiemetic recommendations

Hematopoietic growth factor (CSF) prophylaxis
Primary prophylaxis may be indicated
See Chapter 43 for more information

Antimicrobial prophylaxis
Risk of fever and neutropenia is LOW
 Antimicrobial primary prophylaxis to be considered:
 • Antibacterial—not indicated
 • Antifungal—not indicated
 • Antiviral—not indicated, unless patient previously had an episode of HSV
See Chapter 47 for more information

Docetaxel × 3 cycles
Premedication:
Dexamethasone 8 mg/dose; administer orally twice daily for 3 days, starting on the day before docetaxel administration (total dose/cycle = 48 mg)
Docetaxel 100 mg/m^2; administer intravenously in a volume of 0.9% NS or D5W sufficient to produce a final docetaxel concentration of 0.3–0.74 mg/mL over 30–60 minutes on day 1, every 21 days for 3 cycles (total dosage/cycle = 100 mg/m^2)

Supportive Care
Antiemetic prophylaxis
Emetogenic potential is **LOW**
See Chapter 39 for antiemetic recommendations

Hematopoietic growth factor (CSF) prophylaxis
Primary prophylaxis is indicated with one of the following:
 Filgrastim (G-CSF) 5 mcg/kg per day, by subcutaneous injection, *or*
 Sargramostim (GM-CSF) 250 mcg/m^2 per day, by subcutaneous injection
 • Begin use from 24–72 h after myelosuppressive chemotherapy is completed
See Chapter 43 for more information

Antimicrobial prophylaxis
Risk of fever and neutropenia is LOW
 Antimicrobial primary prophylaxis to be considered:
 • Antibacterial—not indicated
 • Antifungal—not indicated
 • Antiviral—not indicated, unless patient previously had an episode of HSV
See Chapter 47 for more information

Treatment Modifications

Adverse Events	Treatment Modifications
WBC <3500/mm^3 or platelets <100,000/mm^3 on first day of a cycle	Delay treatment for a maximum of 2 weeks until WBC >3500/mm^3 and platelets >100,000/mm^3. Continue at full dosages if counts recover within 2 weeks
If after 2 weeks WBC <3500/mm^3 or platelets <100,000/mm^3, reduce all drugs' dosages as follows:	
WBC 3000–3499/mm^3, or platelets 75,000–99,999/mm^3	Reduce dosages by 25%
WBC 2500–2999/mm^3 and platelets ≥75,000/mm^3	Reduce dosages by 50%
WBC <2500/mm^3, or platelets <75,000/mm^3	Hold treatment
ANC <1500/mm^3, or platelets <100,000/mm^3 at start of cycle	Delay treatment until ANC ≥1500/mm^3 and platelets ≥100,000/mm^3. Give filgrastim* in subsequent cycles
Hematologic recovery >3 weeks	Discontinue treatment
Second episode of febrile neutropenia	During subsequent cycles, consider prophylaxis with ciprofloxacin†
Third episode of febrile neutropenia	Decrease chemotherapy doses by 20% (epirubicin by 20 mg/m², fluorouracil and cyclophosphamide by 100 mg/m², and docetaxel by 20 mg/m²) and administer filgrastim* + ciprofloxacin†
First episode of G4 documented infection	During subsequent cycles, consider prophylaxis with ciprofloxacin†
Second episode of G4 documented infection	Decrease chemotherapy doses by 20% (epirubicin by 20 mg/m², fluorouracil and cyclophosphamide by 100 mg/m², and docetaxel by 20 mg/m²) and administer filgrastim* + ciprofloxacin†
Third episode of G4 documented infection	Discontinue chemotherapy
Serum bilirubin levels 2–3 mg/dL (34.1–51.3 mmol/L)	Reduce epirubicin dose by 50%
Bilirubin levels ≥3 mg/dL (≥51.3 mmol/L)	Discontinue treatment
G3 stomatitis	Reduce epirubicin and fluorouracil dosage by 50% during subsequent cycles
G4 nonhematologic toxicity	Discontinue chemotherapy
G2 motor or sensory neuropathies	Reduce docetaxel dosage by 20–50 mg/m²
G3/4 motor or sensory neuropathies	Discontinue docetaxel

*Filgrastim 5 mcg/kg per day; administer subcutaneously starting at least 24 hours after completing chemotherapy until ANC ≥5000/mm^3
†Ciprofloxacin 500 mg; administer orally twice daily for 7 days starting on day 5

Patient Population Studied

Study of 1999 patients with operable node-positive breast cancer who were randomly assigned to receive fluorouracil 500 mg/m², epirubicin 100 mg/m², and cyclophosphamide 500 mg/m² (FEC) intravenously on day 1 every 21 days for 6 cycles or the same regimen of FEC for 3 cycles followed by docetaxel 100 mg/m² intravenously on day 1 every 21 days for 3 cycles

Efficacy

Analysis of Events in the ITT Population

	FEC (N = 996)		FEC-D (N = 1003)				
	No of Pts	%	No of Pts	%	HR	95%CI	p*
First event[†]	264	26.5	218	21.7	0.80	0.67–0.96	0.012
Relapse of breast cancer	235	23.6	190	18.9	0.78	0.64–0.94	0.010
Local only	40	4	28	2.8			
Regional (± local)	15	1.5	12	1.2			
Distant (± local or regional)	180	18.1	150	14.9			
Contralateral breast cancer	23	2.3	21	2.1	0.80	0.47–1.37	0.43
Any death	135	13.5	100	10.0	0.73	0.56–0.94	0.017
Of breast cancer	123	12.3	89	8.9			

FEC, fluorouracil, epirubicin, and cyclophosphamide; FEC-D, fluorouracil, epirubicin, and cyclophosphamide followed by docetaxel; HR, hazard ratio; ITT, Intention-to-treat
*Log-rank test adjusted for nodal involvement and age
[†]First event defined according to the disease-free survival criteria (ie, local relapse, regional relapse, distant relapse, contralateral breast cancer, death of any cause)

Cox Regression Model Analysis for Disease-Free Survival (DFS) in the Intention-to-Treat (ITT) Population

	HR	95% CI	p-Value
FEC	1	—	—
FEC-D	0.82	0.69 to 0.99	0.034

DFS and OS by Kaplan-Meier Method

	FEC	FEC-D	p-Value
5-Year DFS	73.2%	78.4%	0.012
5-Year OS	86.7%	90.7%	0.017

Toxicity*

Event	Percent of Patients		
	FEC (N = 995)	FEC-D (N = 1001)	P
G3/4 Hematologic			
Neutropenia on day 21	33.6	28.1	0.008
Neutropenia on day 21, cycles 4–6	20.2	10.9	<0.001
Febrile neutropenia	8.4	11.2	0.03
Febrile neutropenia, cycles 4–6	3.7	7.4	0.005
GCSF	27	22.2	0.01
GCSF, cycles 5 and 6	24.8	9.5	<0.001
Infection	1.6	1.6	0.99
Anemia	1.4	0.7	0.12
Thrombocytopenia	0.3	0.4	0.71
Nonhematologic			
G3/4 Nausea-vomiting	20.5	11.2	<0.001
G3/4 Nausea-vomiting, cycles 4–6	11	1.6	<0.001
G3/4 Stomatitis	4.0	5.9	0.054
G3/4 Stomatitis, cycles 4–6	2.3	4.0	0.030
Alopecia grade 3	83.9	82.6	0.40
Edema moderate or severe, cycles 4–6	0.3	4.8	<0.001
Nail disorder moderate or severe, cycles 4–6	1.0	10.3	<0.001
Any cardiac event reported as SAE[†]	1.3	0.4	0.030

*Toxicity graded according to WHO criteria and serious adverse events (SAEs) defined according to International Conference on Harmonization (ICH) guidelines
[†]Although rare overall, there were fewer cardiac events after FEC-D (P = 0.03), attributable mainly to the lower anthracycline cumulative dose

Therapy Monitoring

1. *Before each cycle:* CBC with differential and platelet count, serum total bilirubin
2. *Before each cycle with docetaxel:* Neurologic examination

ADJUVANT REGIMEN

CYCLOPHOSPHAMIDE + EPIRUBICIN + FLUOROURACIL (FEC) × 4 CYCLES → WEEKLY PACLITAXEL × 8 CYCLES

Martin et al. J Natl Cancer Inst 2008;100:805–814

FEC × 4 cycles

Hydration with 0.9% sodium chloride injection (0.9% NS); administer intravenously 500 mL before starting cyclophosphamide and 500 mL after completing cyclophosphamide

Fluorouracil 600 mg/m^2; administer by intravenous injection over 1–3 minutes on day 1, every 21 days for 4 cycles (total dosage/cycle = 600 mg/m^2)

Epirubicin HCl 90 mg/m^2; administer by intravenous injection over 3–5 minutes on day 1, every 21 days for 4 cycles (total dosage/cycle = 90 mg/m^2)

Cyclophosphamide 600 mg/m^2; administer intravenously in 100–500 mL 0.9% NS or 5% dextrose injection (D5W) over 30–60 minutes on day 1, every 21 days for 4 cycles (total dosage/cycle = 600 mg/m^2)

Supportive Care

Antiemetic prophylaxis
Emetogenic potential is **HIGH**. *Potential for delayed symptoms*
See Chapter 39 for antiemetic recommendations

Hematopoietic growth factor (CSF) prophylaxis
Primary prophylaxis may be indicated
See Chapter 43 for more information

Antimicrobial prophylaxis
Risk of fever and neutropenia is LOW
  Antimicrobial primary prophylaxis to be considered:
  • Antibacterial—not indicated
  • Antifungal—not indicated
  • Antiviral—not indicated, unless patient previously had an episode of HSV
See Chapter 47 for more information

Paclitaxel, weekly × 8 weeks

Follows 3 weeks after completing 4 cycles of FEC

Premedication:
Dexamethasone 10 mg/dose; administer orally or intravenously for 2 doses at 12 hours and 6 hours before paclitaxel, *or*
Dexamethasone 20 mg; administer intravenously 30–60 minutes before paclitaxel (total dose/cycle = 20 mg)
Note: Dexamethasone doses may be gradually decreased in the absence of hypersensitivity reactions during repeated paclitaxel treatments
Diphenhydramine 50 mg; administer by intravenous injection 30–60 minutes before paclitaxel
Cimetidine 300 mg (or ranitidine 50 mg, or famotidine 20 mg, or an equivalent histamine receptor [H$_2$]-subtype antagonist); administer intravenously over 15–30 minutes, 30–60 minutes before starting paclitaxel administration

Paclitaxel 100 mg/m^2; administer intravenously in a volume of 0.9% NS or D5W sufficient to produce a concentration within the range 0.3–1.2 mg/mL over 60 minutes, once weekly for 8 weeks (total dosage/week = 100 mg/m^2)

Supportive Care

Antiemetic prophylaxis
Emetogenic potential is **LOW**
See Chapter 39 for antiemetic recommendations

Hematopoietic growth factor (CSF) prophylaxis
Primary prophylaxis may be indicated
See Chapter 43 for more information

Antimicrobial prophylaxis
Risk of fever and neutropenia is LOW
  Antimicrobial primary prophylaxis to be considered:
  • Antibacterial—not indicated
  • Antifungal—not indicated
  • Antiviral—not indicated, unless patient previously had an episode of HSV
See Chapter 47 for more information

(continued)

(*continued*)

Notes:

On completion of chemotherapy, tamoxifen (20 mg daily; administer orally for 5 years) was mandatory for all patients whose tumors were positive for estrogen receptor, progesterone receptor, or both (according to institutional guidelines). Subsequently an amendment to the study protocol allowed the use of aromatase inhibitors in postmenopausal women

1. Radiotherapy was mandatory after breast-conserving surgery, and was administered after mastectomy according to the guidelines of each participating institution, mostly to women with tumors >5 cm or with ≥4 affected lymph nodes

2. Prophylaxis with filgrastim (granulocyte colony-stimulating factor) was not routine. However, secondary prophylaxis with filgrastim was mandatory among patients who had at least 1 episode of febrile neutropenia or an infection

Treatment Modifications–FEC

Adverse Events	Treatment Modifications
WBC <3500/mm³ or platelets <100,000/mm³ on first day of a cycle	Delay treatment for a maximum of 2 weeks until WBC >3500/mm³ and platelets >100,000/mm³. Continue at full dosages if counts recover within 2 weeks
If after 2 weeks WBC <3500/mm³ or platelets <100,000/mm³ reduce all drugs' dosages as follows:	
WBC 3000–3499/mm³, or platelets 75,000–99,999/mm³	Reduce dosages by 25%
WBC 2500–2999/mm³ and platelets ≥75,000/mm³	Reduce dosages by 50%
WBC <2500/mm³, or platelets <75,000/mm³	Hold treatment
ANC <1500/mm³, or platelets <100,000/mm³ at start of cycle	Delay treatment until ANC ≥1500/mm³ and platelets ≥100,000/mm³. Give filgrastim* in subsequent cycles
Hematologic recovery >3 weeks	Discontinue treatment
First episode of febrile neutropenia	Give filgrastim* during subsequent cycles
Second episode of febrile neutropenia	During subsequent cycles, consider prophylaxis with ciprofloxacin†
Third episode of febrile neutropenia	Decrease chemotherapy doses by 20% (epirubicin by 20 mg/m², fluorouracil and cyclophosphamide by 100 mg/m²) and administer filgrastim* + ciprofloxacin†
First episode of G4 documented infection	Add filgrastim* and ciprofloxacin† prophylaxis during subsequent cycles
Second episode of G4 documented infection	Decrease chemotherapy doses by 20% (epirubicin by 20 mg/m², fluorouracil and cyclophosphamide by 100 mg/m²) and administer filgrastim* + ciprofloxacin†
Third episode of G4 documented infection	Discontinue chemotherapy
Serum bilirubin levels 2 to 3 mg/dL (34.1 to 51.3 mmol/L)	Reduce epirubicin dose by 50%
Bilirubin levels ≥3 mg/dL (≥51.3 mmol/L)	Discontinue treatment
G3 stomatitis	Reduce epirubicin and fluorouracil dosage by 50% during subsequent cycles
Any other G3 nonhematologic toxicity	Reduce the dosage of all drugs 25%
G4 nonhematologic toxicity	Discontinue chemotherapy

Treatment Modifications–Paclitaxel

Adverse Events	Treatment Modifications
ANC ≤800/mm³ or platelets ≤50,000/mm³	Hold treatment until ANC >800/mm³ and platelets >50,000/mm³, then resume with weekly paclitaxel dosage reduced by 10 mg/m²
G2 motor or sensory neuropathies	Reduce weekly paclitaxel dosage by 10 mg/m² without interrupting planned treatment
Other nonhematologic adverse events G2 or G3	Hold treatment until adverse events resolve to G ≤1, then resume with weekly paclitaxel dosage reduced by 10 mg/m²
Patients who cannot tolerate paclitaxel at 60 mg/m² per week	Discontinue treatment
Treatment delay >2 weeks	Decrease weekly paclitaxel dosage by 10 mg/m² or consider discontinuing treatment

*Filgrastim 5 mcg/kg per day; administer subcutaneously starting at least 24 hours after completing chemotherapy until ANC ≥5000/mm³
†Ciprofloxacin 500 mg administer orally twice daily for 7 days starting on day 5

Patient Population Studied

Study of 1246 women who had undergone primary curative surgery (ie, mastectomy, tumorectomy, or lumpectomy) with axillary lymph node dissection (in which at least 6 lymph nodes were isolated) for operable unilateral carcinoma of the breast (stage T1–T3) and were found to have node-positive breast cancer. All patients had at least 1 axillary lymph node that was positive for cancer on histologic examination. The margins of resected specimens had to be histologically free of invasive carcinoma and ductal carcinoma in situ. A complete staging work-up was carried out within 16 weeks before registration in the study. Criteria for exclusion included advanced disease (ie, stage T4, N2 or N3, or M1) and motor or sensory neuropathy of NCI Common Toxicity Criteria G2 or more

Efficacy

Analysis of Events in the ITT Population

	FEC (N = 632)		FEC-P (N = 614)	
	No of Pts	%	No of Pts	%
No event	439	69.5	468	76.2
An event	193	30.5	146	23.8
Relapse of breast cancer	174	27.6	113	18.4
Local only, regional only or both	30	4.8	11	1.8
Distant	141	22.3	101	16.4
Local and second primary	1	0.2	0	0
Second primary cancer	16	2.5	23	3.7
Contralateral breast cancer	4	0.6	7	1.1

FEC, Fluorouracil, epirubicin, and cyclophosphamide; FEC-P, FEC + paclitaxel

DFS, RFS, and OS by Kaplan-Meier Method

	FEC	FEC-P	p-Value	HR	CI
Unadjusted 5-year DFS	72.1%	78.5%	0.006	0.74	0.60–0.92
Adjusted 5-year DFS*			0.006	0/77	0.62–0.95
5-Year distant RFS	78.1%	83.8%	0.006	0.70	0.54–0.90
5-Year OS	87.1%	89.9%	0.109	0.78	0.57–1.06

CI, confidence interval; DFS, Disease-free survival; FEC, fluorouracil, epirubicin, and cyclophosphamide; FEC-P, FEC + paclitaxel; HR, hazard ratio; RFS, relapse-free survival; OS, overall survival
*Adjusted for lymph node status, age, tumor size, histology, hormone receptor status, and hormonal therapy

Toxicity*

Toxicity	FEC	FEC-P
G3/4 neutropenia	25.5%	19.1%
G3/4 febrile neutropenia	9.5%	5.1%
G3/4 fatigue	2.4%	4.2%
G3/4 nausea	5.9%	5.4%
G3/4 vomiting	9.9%	7.3%
G3/4 stomatitis	4.9%	3.1%
Amenorrhea	58%	65%
G2 alopecia	>90%	>90%
G2 neuropathy	N/A	22.2%
G3 neuropathy	N/A	3.7%
G2 arthralgia/myalgia	N/A	20.6%
G3 arthralgia/myalgia	N/A	2.8%
G2 LV dysfunction	7.2%	7.8%

*Comparison of treatment arms as follows:
FEC, Six 21-day cycles of fluorouracil 600 mg/m², epirubicin 90 mg/m², and cyclophosphamide 600 mg/m²
FEC-P, Four 21-day cycles of the same FEC schedule and, after 3 weeks of no treatment, eight 1-week courses of paclitaxel 100 mg/m²

Therapy Monitoring

1. *Before each cycle:* CBC with differential and platelet count, serum total bilirubin
2. *Before each treatment with paclitaxel:* Neurologic examination

ADJUVANT, NEOADJUVANT REGIMEN
DOCETAXEL + CARBOPLATIN + TRASTUZUMAB (TCH)

Slamon S et al. N Engl J Med 2011;365:1273–1283
(Third Interim Analysis Phase III Randomized Trial Comparing Doxorubicin and Cyclophosphamide Followed by Docetaxel [AC → T] with Doxorubicin and Cyclophosphamide Followed by Docetaxel and Trastuzumab [AC → TH] with Docetaxel, Carboplatin and Trastuzumab [TCH] in Her2neu Positive Early Breast Cancer Patients: BCIRG 006 Study)

TCH regimen
Premedication:
Dexamethasone 8 mg/dose; administer orally twice daily for 3 days, starting on the day before docetaxel administration (total dose/cycle = 48 mg)

Docetaxel 75 mg/m²; administer intravenously in a volume of 0.9% sodium chloride injection (0.9% NS) or 5% dextrose injection (D5W) sufficient to produce a final docetaxel concentration of 0.3–0.74 mg/mL over 30–60 minutes on day 1, every 3 weeks for 6 cycles (total dosage/cycle = 75 mg/m²)
Carboplatin target AUC = 6 mg/mL · min; administer intravenously in 250 mL D5W or 0.9% NS over 30–60 minutes on day 1, every 3 weeks for 6 cycles (total dose/cycle calculated to achieve a target AUC = 6 mg/mL · min), *concurrently with:*
Trastuzumab every 21 days for 6 cycles:
   Loading Dose: **Trastuzumab** 8 mg/kg; administer intravenously in 250 mL 0.9% NS over 90 minutes as a loading dose on day 1, cycle 1 only (total dosage during the first cycle = 8 mg/kg), *followed 3 weeks later by:*
   Maintenance Doses: **Trastuzumab** 6 mg/kg; administer intravenously in 250 mL 0.9% NS over 30 minutes on day 1, every 3 weeks for 5 cycles (total dosage/cycle = 6 mg/kg)

Three weeks after completing combination (TCH) chemotherapy:
Trastuzumab 6 mg/kg; administer intravenously in 250 mL 0.9% NS over 30 minutes every 3 weeks for 11 doses (total dosage/3-week cycle = 6 mg/kg)

Supportive Care
Antiemetic prophylaxis
Emetogenic potential on days with TCH combination chemotherapy is **HIGH**. *Potential for delayed symptoms*
Emetogenic potential on days with trastuzumab alone is **LOW**
See Chapter 39 for antiemetic recommendations

Hematopoietic growth factor (CSF) prophylaxis
Primary prophylaxis may be indicated
See Chapter 43 for more information

Antimicrobial prophylaxis
Risk of fever and neutropenia is LOW
   Antimicrobial primary prophylaxis to be considered:
   • Antibacterial—not indicated
   • Antifungal—not indicated
   • Antiviral—not indicated, unless patient previously had an episode of HSV
See Chapter 47 for more information

(continued)

Treatment Modifications

Adverse Events	Treatment Modifications
WBC <3500/mm³, or absolute neutrophil count (ANC) <1500/mm³, or platelets <100,000/mm³ on first day of a cycle	Delay treatment for a maximum of 2 weeks until WBC >3500/mm³, ANC >1500/mm³, and platelets >100,000/mm³. Continue at full dosages if counts recover within 2 weeks. Give filgrastim* in subsequent cycles
If after 2 weeks WBC <3500/mm³, ANC <1500/mm³, or platelets <100,000/mm³, reduce all drugs' dosages as follows:	
WBC 3000–3499/mm³, ANC 1000–1500/mm³, or platelets 75,000–99,999/mm³	Reduce dosages by 20%
WBC 2500–2999/mm³, ANC 500–1000/mm³, or platelets ≥ 75,000/mm³	Reduce dosages by 50%
WBC <2500/mm³, ANC <500/mm³, or platelets <75,000/mm³	Hold treatment
Hematologic recovery >3 weeks	Discontinue treatment
First episode of febrile neutropenia or documented infection after treatment	Filgrastim* prophylaxis administered during subsequent cycles
Second episode of febrile neutropenia or documented infection after treatment	Reduce docetaxel dosage to 60 mg/m² during subsequent cycles, administer filgrastim* and consider prophylaxis with ciprofloxacin†
Third episode of febrile neutropenia or documented infection after treatment	Discontinue chemotherapy
G3/4 stomatitis	Reduce docetaxel dosage to 60 mg/m² during subsequent cycles
G3/4 neuropathy	Discontinue treatment

(continued)

(continued)

Trastuzumab infusion reactions:

- A symptom complex most commonly consisting of chills and/or fever may occur in as many as 40% of patients during the first infusion of trastuzumab. These symptoms occur infrequently with subsequent trastuzumab infusions. Other signs and/or symptoms may include nausea, vomiting, pain (in some cases at tumor sites), rigors, headache, dizziness, dyspnea, hypotension, rash, and asthenia. Although the symptoms are usually mild to moderate in severity, infrequently, trastuzumab may need to be discontinued

- When such a symptom complex is observed it can be treated with or without reduction in the rate of trastuzumab infusion, and:

  - **Acetaminophen** 650 mg; administer orally

  - **Diphenhydramine** 25–50 mg; administer orally or by intravenous injection, and

  - **Meperidine** 12.5–25 mg; administer by intravenous injection every 10 minutes if needed for shaking chills (generally, cumulative doses >50 mg are not needed; use with caution in persons with moderate or more severely impaired renal function)

  - With or without reduction in the rate of trastuzumab infusion

Treatment plan notes:

- LVEF assessment (MUGA or echocardiography) every 3 months in patients receiving trastuzumab

- One year of trastuzumab therapy = 51 weeks or 17 total doses (6 doses [cycles] with docetaxel and carboplatin and 11 doses [cycles] of single agent trastuzumab)

Carboplatin dose

Carboplatin dose is based on a formula described by Calvert et al. to achieve a target area under the plasma concentration versus time curve (AUC)

$$\text{Total Carboplatin Dose (mg)} = (\text{target AUC})(\text{GFR} + 25)$$

In practice, creatinine clearance (Clcr) is used in place of glomerular filtration rate (GFR). Clcr can be estimated from the equation of Cockcroft and Gault, thus:

$$\text{For males, Clcr} = \frac{(140 - \text{age[years]}) \times (\text{body weight [kg]})}{72 \times (\text{serum creatinine [mg/dL]})}$$

$$\text{For females, Clcr} = \frac{(140 - \text{age[years]}) \times (\text{body weight [kg]})}{72 \times (\text{serum creatinine [mg/dL]})} \times 0.85$$

Calvert AH et al. J Clin Oncol 1989;7:1748–1756
Cockcroft DW, Gault MH. Nephron 1976;16:31–41
Jodrell DI et al. J Clin Oncol 1992;10:520–528
Sorensen BT et al. Cancer Chemother Pharmacol 1991;28:397–401

Note: On October 8, 2010, the U.S. Food and Drug Administration (FDA) identified a potential safety issue with carboplatin dosing based on recent changes in the measurement of serum creatinine. By the end of 2010, all clinical laboratories in the United States will use the standardized isotope dilution mass spectrometry (IDMS) method to measure serum creatinine, which could result in an overestimation of the GFR in some patients with normal renal function. A carboplatin dose calculated with an IDMS-measured serum creatinine result using the Calvert formula could exceed an expected exposure (AUC) and result in increased drug-related toxicity. Provided actual GFR measurements are made to assess renal function, carboplatin can be safely dosed according to the Calvert formula described in product labeling. If GFR (or creatinine clearance) is estimated based on serum creatinine measurements by the IDMS method, the FDA recommended for patients with normal renal function capping an estimated GFR at 125 mL/min for any targeted AUC value. No greater estimated GFR values should be used U.S. Food and Drug Administration. Carboplatin dosing. May 23, 2013. Available from: http://www.fda.gov/AboutFDA/CentersOffices/OfficeofMedicalProductsandTobacco/CDER/ucm228974.htm [accessed February 26, 2014]

Treatment Modifications
(continued)

Adverse Events	Treatment Modifications
Other severe adverse events	Hold treatment until toxicity resolves to G ≤1, then resume at decreased dosages appropriate for the toxicity
Asymptomatic decreases in ejection fraction	Monitor patient closely for evidence of clinical deterioration
Clinically significant congestive heart failure	Discontinue trastuzumab

*Filgrastim 5 mcg/kg per day; administer subcutaneously starting at least 24 hours after completing chemotherapy until ANC ≥5000/mm³
†Ciprofloxacin 500 mg; administer orally twice daily for 7 days starting on day 5
Note: Dosages reduced for adverse events are not re-escalated

Patient Population Studied

Study of 3222 women with HER2+ by FISH, T1–3, N0/N1, M0 breast cancer (AC → T: 1073; AC→TH: 1074; TCH: 1075). Stratified by nodes and hormonal receptor status

Therapy Monitoring

1. *Before each cycle:* CBC with differential and platelet count, LFTs, serum electrolytes, BUN, and creatinine
2. *Assessment of ejection fraction:* Every 3 months or as clinically indicated
3. *Hearing test:* At baseline and as needed

Note

In the neoadjuvant setting, consider adding Pertuzumab to TCH chemotherapy
Give pertuzumab every 21 days for 6 cycles:
Loading dose: **Pertuzumab** 840 mg; administer intravenously in 250 mL of 0.9% NS over 90 minutes on day 1 after trastuzumab, cycle 1 only (total dose during the first cycle = 840 mg), *followed 3 weeks later by:*
Maintenance doses: **Pertuzumab** 420 mg; administer intravenously in 250 mL of 0.9% NS over 30–60 minutes on day 1 after trastuzumab, every 3 weeks for 5 cycles (total dose/cycle = 420 mg)

Schneeweiss A et al. Ann Oncol 2013;24:2278–2284

Efficacy

Third Planned Efficacy Analysis: 65 Months Follow Up*

	AC → T	AC → TH	AC → TH vs. AC → T		TCH	TCH vs. AC → T		AC → TH vs. TCH
			HR	p-Value		HR	p-Value	p-Value
All Patients								
	N = 1073	N = 1074			N = 1075			
DFS	75%	84%	0.64	<0.001	81%	0.75	0.04	0.21
OS	87%	92%	0.63	<0.001	91%	0.77	0.038	0.14
Patients with Negative Lymph Nodes								
	N = 309	N = 310			N = 309			
DFS	85%	93%	0.47	0.003	90%	0.64	0.057	—
OS	93%	97%	0.38	0.02	96%	0.56	0.11	—
Patients with Positive Lymph Nodes								
	N = 764	N = 764			N = 766			
DFS	71%	80%	0.68	0.0003	78%	0.78	0.013	—
Patients with ≥4 Positive Lymph Nodes								
	N = 350	N = 350			N = 352			
DFS	61%	73%	0.66	0.002	72%	0.66	0.002	—

AC → T, doxorubicin (Adriamycin) + cyclophosphamide followed by docetaxel; AC → TH, doxorubicin + cyclophosphamide followed by docetaxel plus trastuzumab (Herceptin) then trastuzumab alone; DFS, disease-free survival; OS, overall survival; TCH, docetaxel plus carboplatin plus concurrent trastuzumab then trastuzumab alone
*DFS and OS values are at 65 months

Toxicity						
	AC → T N = 1050		AC → TH N = 1068		TCH N = 1056	
	% All G	% G3/4	% All G	% G3/4	% All G	% G3/4
Nonhematologic Toxicity						
Neuropathy, sensory	48.6		49.7		36.1*	
Neuropathy, motor	5.2		6.3		4.2*	
Nail changes	49.3		43.6		28.7*	
Myalgia	52.8	5.2	55.5	5.2	38.6*	1.8*
Renal failure	0		0		0.1	
G3/4 creatinine	0.6		0.3		0.1	
Arthralgia		3.2		3.3		1.4*
Fatigue		7		7.2		7.2
Hand-foot syndrome		1.9		1.4		0*
Stomatitis		3.5		2.9		1.4*
Diarrhea		3.0		5.6		5.4
Nausea		5.9		5.7		4.8
Vomiting		6.1		6.7		3.5*
Irregular menses		27		24.3		26.5
Hematologic Toxicity						
Neutropenia		63.5		71.6		66.2*
Leucopenia		51.9		60.4		48.4*
Neutropenic infection		9.3		10.9		9.6
Febrile neutropenia		11.5		12.1		11.2
Anemia		2.4		3.1*		5.8
Thrombocytopenia		1.6		2.1*		6.1
Acute leukemia	0.6		0.1		0.1	
Cardiac Toxicity						
G3/4 LV dysfunction (CHF)[†]	7/1050		21/1068		4/1056	
>10% Relative LVEF decline[‡]	11%		19%		9%	

AC → T, doxorubicin (Adriamycin) + cyclophosphamide followed by docetaxel; AC→TH, doxorubicin + cyclophosphamide followed by docetaxel plus trastuzumab (Herceptin) then trastuzumab alone; CHF, congestive heart failure; LV, left ventricular; LVEF, left ventricular ejection fraction; TCH, docetaxel plus carboplatin plus concurrent trastuzumab then trastuzumab alone
*Less statistically significantly events than the comparator groups
[†]AC → T vs. AC → TH: p = 0.0121; AC → TH vs. TCH: p <0.001; AC → T vs. TCH: p = 0.3852
[‡]AC → T vs. AC → TH: p <0.001; AC → TH vs. TCH: p <0.001; AC → T vs. TCH: p = 0.19

ADJUVANT, NEOADJUVANT REGIMEN
DOXORUBICIN + CYCLOPHOSPHAMIDE, THEN PACLITAXEL + TRASTUZUMAB, THEN TRASTUZUMAB ALONE
(AC × 4 → TH × 12 WEEKS → H × 40 WEEKS)

Romond EH et al. N Engl J Med 2005;353:1673–1684
Seidman AD et al. J Clin Oncol 2001;19:2587–2595

AC (doxorubicin + cyclophosphamide) regimen
Hydration with 0.9% sodium chloride injection (0.9% NS); administer intravenously 500 mL before starting cyclophosphamide and 500 mL after completing cyclophosphamide administration

Doxorubicin HCl 60 mg/m^2; administer by intravenous injection over 3–5 minutes on day 1, every 21 days for 4 cycles (total dosage/cycle = 60 mg/m^2)
Cyclophosphamide 600 mg/m^2; administer intravenously in 100–500 mL 0.9% NS or 5% dextrose injection (D5W) over 15–60 minutes on day 1, every 21 days for 4 cycles (total dosage/cycle = 600 mg/m^2)

Supportive Care
Antiemetic prophylaxis
Emetogenic potential is **HIGH**. *Potential for delayed symptoms*
See Chapter 39 for antiemetic recommendations

Hematopoietic growth factor (CSF) prophylaxis
Primary prophylaxis is NOT indicated
See Chapter 43 for more information

Antimicrobial prophylaxis
Risk of fever and neutropenia is LOW
   Antimicrobial primary prophylaxis to be considered:
   • Antibacterial—not indicated
   • Antifungal—not indicated
   • Antiviral—not indicated, unless patient previously had an episode of HSV
See Chapter 47 for more information

Weekly TH (paclitaxel + trastuzumab) regimen

Schedule for first week of paclitaxel + trastuzumab
Trastuzumab 4 mg/kg (loading dose); administer intravenously in 250 mL 0.9% NS over at least 90 minutes, 1 day before the first dose of paclitaxel is administered (total trastuzumab dosage during the first treatment week = 4 mg/kg), *followed 1 day later by:*

Premedication for paclitaxel:
Dexamethasone 10 mg; administer intravenously 30–60 minutes before paclitaxel (total dose/cycle = 10 mg)
Note: Dexamethasone doses may be gradually reduced in 2- to 4-mg increments if a patient has no hypersensitivity reactions during repeated paclitaxel treatments
Diphenhydramine 50 mg; administer intravenously 30–60 minutes before paclitaxel
Cimetidine 300 mg (or ranitidine 50 mg, or famotidine 20 mg, or an equivalent histamine receptor [H$_2$]-subtype antagonist); administer intravenously over 15 to 30 minutes, 30 to 60 minutes before starting paclitaxel administration

Paclitaxel 80 mg/m^2; administer intravenously in a volume of 0.9% NS or D5W sufficient to produce a concentration within the range 0.3–1.2 mg/mL over 60 minutes (total dosage = 80 mg/m^2)

Paclitaxel + trastuzumab during the second and subsequent weeks
Premedication for paclitaxel:
Dexamethasone 10 mg; administer intravenously 30–60 minutes before paclitaxel
Note: If a patient does not experience any manifestations of hypersensitivity or an allergic reaction after 8 paclitaxel infusions, the **dexamethasone** dose may be reduced as follows:
• Weeks 9 and 10:   **Dexamethasone** 8 mg IV
• Weeks 11 and 12:   **Dexamethasone** 6 mg IV
• Weeks 13 and beyond: **Dexamethasone** 4 mg IV
Diphenhydramine 50 mg; administer by intravenous injection 30–60 minutes before paclitaxel
Cimetidine 300 mg (or ranitidine 50 mg, or famotidine 20 mg, or an equivalent histamine receptor [H$_2$]-subtype antagonist); administer intravenously over 15–30 minutes, 30–60 minutes before starting paclitaxel administration

(continued)

(continued)

Paclitaxel 80 mg/m² per week; administer intravenously in a volume of 0.9% NS or D5W sufficient to produce a concentration within the range 0.3–1.2 mg/mL over 60 minutes, weekly, for 11 weeks (total dosage/week = 80 mg/m²), *followed immediately afterward by:*
Trastuzumab 2 mg/kg per week; administer intravenously in 250 mL 0.9% NS over 30 minutes, weekly, for 11 weeks
(total trastuzumab dosage/week during the second and later weeks = 2 mg/kg)
Note: The duration of trastuzumab administration may be decreased from an initial infusion duration of 90 to 30 minutes if administration over longer durations is well tolerated

Supportive Care
Antiemetic prophylaxis
Emetogenic potential is **LOW**
See Chapter 39 for antiemetic recommendations

Hematopoietic growth factor (CSF) prophylaxis
Primary prophylaxis is NOT indicated
See Chapter 43 for more information

Antimicrobial prophylaxis
Risk of fever and neutropenia is LOW
   Antimicrobial primary prophylaxis to be considered:
   • Antibacterial—not indicated
   • Antifungal—not indicated
   • Antiviral—not indicated, unless patient previously had an episode of HSV
See Chapter 47 for more information

Weekly H (*trastuzumab*) regimen
Trastuzumab 2 mg/kg per week; administer intravenously in 250 mL 0.9% NS over 30 minutes, weekly, for 40 weeks
(total trastuzumab dosage/week = 2 mg/kg)

Supportive Care
Antiemetic prophylaxis
Emetogenic potential is **MINIMAL**
See Chapter 39 for antiemetic recommendations

Hematopoietic growth factor (CSF) prophylaxis
Primary prophylaxis is NOT indicated
See Chapter 43 for more information

Antimicrobial prophylaxis
Risk of fever and neutropenia is LOW
   Antimicrobial primary prophylaxis to be considered:
   • Antibacterial—not indicated
   • Antifungal—not indicated
   • Antiviral—not indicated, unless patient previously had an episode of HSV
See Chapter 47 for more information

Trastuzumab infusion reactions
• A symptom complex most commonly consisting of chills and/or fever may occur in as many as 40% of patients during the first infusion of trastuzumab. These symptoms occur infrequently with subsequent trastuzumab infusions. Other signs and/or symptoms may include nausea, vomiting, pain (in some cases at tumor sites), rigors, headache, dizziness, dyspnea, hypotension, rash, and asthenia. Although the symptoms are usually mild to moderate in severity, infrequently, trastuzumab may need to be discontinued
• When such a symptom complex is observed it can be treated with or without reduction in the rate of trastuzumab infusion, and:
   ▪ **Acetaminophen** 650 mg; administer orally
   ▪ **Diphenhydramine** 25–50 mg; administer orally or by intravenous injection, and
   ▪ **Meperidine** 12.5–25 mg; administer by intravenous injection every 10 minutes if needed for shaking chills (generally, cumulative doses >50 mg are not needed; use with caution in persons with moderate or more severely impaired renal function)
   ▪ With or without reduction in the rate of trastuzumab infusion

Treatment Plan Notes:
• LVEF assessment (MUGA or echocardiography) every 3 months in patients receiving trastuzumab

Treatment Modifications: Cyclophosphamide + Doxorubicin

Adverse Events	Treatment Modifications
Absolute neutrophil count (ANC) <1500/mm³, or WBC <3500/mm³, or platelets <100,000/mm³ at start of cycle*	Delay treatment for a maximum of 2 weeks until ANC ≥1500/mm³, WBC ≥3500/mm³, and platelets ≥100,000/mm³. Continue at full dosages if counts recover within 2 weeks. Give filgrastim† after chemotherapy during subsequent cycles
If after 2 weeks ANC <1500/mm³, or WBC <3500/mm³, or platelets <100,000/mm³, reduce all drug dosages as follows:	
ANC 1000–1500/mm³, WBC 3000–3499/mm³, or platelets 75,000–99,999/mm³	Reduce cyclophosphamide and doxorubicin dosages by 20%
ANC 500–1000/mm³, WBC 2500–2999/mm³, and platelets ≥75,000/mm³	Reduce cyclophosphamide and doxorubicin dosages by 50%
ANC <500/mm³, WBC <2500/mm³, or platelets <75,000/mm³	Hold treatment
First episode of febrile neutropenia	Give filgrastim† after chemotherapy during subsequent cycles
Second episode of febrile neutropenia	During subsequent cycles, consider prophylaxis with ciprofloxacin‡
Third episode of febrile neutropenia	Decrease both doxorubicin and cyclophosphamide dosages by 25%

*Although an ANC of 1500/mm³ is often identified as a minimum acceptable ANC to safely proceed with treatment, recent data shows that an ANC ≥1000/mm³ is acceptable if filgrastim is given after chemotherapy
†Filgrastim 5 mcg/kg per day; administer subcutaneously starting at least 24 hours after completing chemotherapy until ANC ≥5000/mm³
‡Ciprofloxacin 500 mg; administer orally twice daily for 7 days starting on day 5

Treatment Modifications: Paclitaxel

Adverse Events	Adverse Events
ANC ≤800/mm³, platelets ≤50,000/mm³, or documented infection	Hold treatment until ANC >1000/mm³, platelets >100,000/mm³, and/or infection resolved, then resume with weekly paclitaxel dosage reduced by 10 mg/m²
G2 motor or sensory neuropathies	Reduce weekly paclitaxel dosage by 10 mg/m² without interrupting planned treatment
G2 nonhematologic adverse events (other than sensory or motor neuropathies)	Hold treatment until adverse events resolve to G ≤1, then resume with weekly paclitaxel dosage reduced by 10 mg/m²
G3 nonhematologic adverse events (other than sensory or motor neuropathies)	Hold treatment until adverse events resolve to G ≤1, then resume with weekly paclitaxel dosage reduced by 20 mg/m²
Patients who cannot tolerate paclitaxel at 60 mg/m² per week	Discontinue treatment
Treatment delay >2 weeks	Decrease weekly paclitaxel dosage by 10 mg/m² or consider discontinuing treatment

Patient Population Studied

Romond EH et al. J Clin Oncol 2005;16:1673–1684: Report of two trials that treated 1672 women with a regimen of AC followed by paclitaxel with trastuzumab, followed by trastuzumab alone [AC → P + H → H]. Two studies were combined in one analysis: (a) National Surgical Adjuvant Breast and Bowel Project trial B-31 and (b) North Central Cancer Treatment Group trial N9831. Both trials enrolled women with a pathologic diagnosis of adenocarcinoma of the breast with immunohistochemical staining for HER2 protein of 3+ intensity or amplification of the *HER2* gene on fluorescence in situ hybridization. Initially, required patients to have histologically proven, node-positive disease; subsequently, N9831 was amended to include patients with high-risk node-negative disease (defined as a tumor that was more than 2 cm in diameter and positive for estrogen receptors or progesterone receptors or as a tumor that was more than 1 cm in diameter and negative for both estrogen receptors and progesterone receptors). Other requirements included a left ventricular ejection fraction (LVEF) that met or exceeded the lower limit of normal. Complete resection of the primary tumor and axillary-node dissection were required (negative sentinel-node biopsy was allowed in trial N9831). Patients were ineligible if they had one of several cardiac risk factors

Note

In the neoadjuvant setting, consider adding pertuzumab to paclitaxel and trastuzumab Give pertuzumab every 21 days for 4 cycles:
Loading dose: **Pertuzumab** 840 mg; administer intravenously in 250 mL of 0.9% NS over 90 minutes on the same day as trastuzumab, but after completing trastuzumab administration (total dose during the first cycle = 840 mg), *followed 3 weeks later by:*
Maintenance doses: **Pertuzumab** 420 mg; administer intravenously in 250 mL of 0.9% NS over 30–60 minutes after trastuzumab, every 3 weeks for 3 cycles (total dose/3-week cycle = 420 mg)

Schneeweiss A et al. Ann Oncol 2013;24:2278–2284

Efficacy (Combined Analysis of NSABP B-31 and NCCTG N9831)

Romond EH et al. N Eng J Med 2005;353:1673–1684

	AC → PTX N = 1679	AC → P + H → H N = 1672	Hazard Ratio
3-Year DFS	75.4%	87.1%	0.48
4-Year DFS	67.1%	85.3%	
3 Years free of distant recurrence	81.5%	90.4%	0.47
4 Years free of distant recurrence	79.3%	89.7%	
3-Year OS	91.7%	94.3%	0.67
4-Year OS	86.6%	91.4%	
Isolated brain metastases as first event, B-31*	11/872	21/864	
Isolated brain metastases as first event, N9831*	4/807	12/808	
Brain metastases as first/subsequent event, B-31*	35/872	28/864	0.79

AC → PTX, doxorubicin (Adriamycin) + cyclophosphamide followed by paclitaxel; AC → P + H → H, doxorubicin + cyclophosphamide followed by paclitaxel plus trastuzumab (Herceptin) then trastuzumab alone; DFS, disease-free survival; OS, overall survival

*The imbalance in brain metastases as first events can be attributed to earlier failures at other distant sites among patients in the control group

Toxicity

(Romond EH et al. N Eng J Med 2005;353:1673–1684)

	AC → PTX N = 1679	AC → P + H → H N = 1672
NYHA III/IV CHF* or cardiac death at 3 yrs, B-31[†]	0.8%[‡]	4.1%[§]
NYHA III/IV CHF* or cardiac death at 3 yrs, N9831[†]	0	2.9%[¶]
Interstitial pneumonitis, B-31		4/864**
Interstitial pneumonitis, N9831		5/808[††]
Other toxicities	Similar CTC v2 toxicities[‡‡]	

AC → PTX, doxorubicin (Adriamycin) + cyclophosphamide followed by paclitaxel; AC → P + H → H, doxorubicin + cyclophosphamide followed by paclitaxel plus trastuzumab (Herceptin) then trastuzumab alone

*New York Heart Association classes III or IV congestive heart failure

[†]Cumulative incidence in patients who remained free of cardiac symptoms during doxorubicin and cyclophosphamide therapy and who had LVEF values that met requirements for the initiation of trastuzumab therapy

[‡]Four patients had congestive heart failure, and 1 died from cardiac causes

[§]Thirty-one patients had congestive heart failure. (Amongst 27 patients followed ≥6 months after onset of CHF, only 1 reported persistent symptoms of CHF)

[¶]Twenty patients had congestive heart failure; 1 died of cardiomyopathy

**One died

[††]G3+ pneumonitis or pulmonary infiltrates; 1 died

[‡‡]During treatment with paclitaxel alone or with trastuzumab, there was little imbalance between treatment groups in the incidence of any Common Toxicity Criteria version 2.0

Therapy Monitoring

General:
1. *At intervals:* CBC with differential and platelet count, LFTs, serum electrolytes, BUN, and creatinine
2. *Assessment of ejection fraction:* Every 3 months or as clinically indicated

For doxorubicin + cyclophosphamide:
1. *Each cycle:* CBC with differential and platelet count, serum electrolytes, LFTs

For weekly paclitaxel
1. *Every week:* CBC with differential and platelet count
2. *Every 3 to 4 weeks:* LFTs, serum electrolytes, calcium, and magnesium

For trastuzumab cycles:
Assessment of ejection fraction: Every 3 months or as clinically indicated

Notes:
- In NSABP B31 and NCCTG N9831, cardiac ejection fraction assessed before entry, after completion of doxorubicin/cyclophosphamide, and 6, 9, and 18 months after initiation of trastuzumab
- Initiation of trastuzumab required cardiac ejection fraction to be in the normal range with no more than a 16-percentage point decrease from baseline
- At 6 and 9 months assessment, if the cardiac ejection fraction had declined by ≥16% from initial or was 10–15% below the normal range, trastuzumab was held for 4 weeks and reassessed. Trastuzumab could be restarted if the cardiac ejection fraction recovered

ADJUVANT REGIMEN

DOCETAXEL + TRASTUZUMAB FOLLOWED BY CYCLOPHOSPHAMIDE + EPIRUBICIN + FLUOROURACIL (FEC)

Joensuu H et al. N Engl J Med 2006;354:809–820
Joensuu H et al. J Clin Oncol 2009;27:5685–5692

Docetaxel + Trastuzumab: weeks 1 through 9
Trastuzumab 4 mg/kg (loading dose); administer intravenously in 250 mL 0.9% sodium chloride injection (0.9% NS) over at least 90 minutes, 1 day before the first dose of docetaxel is administered (total trastuzumab dosage during the first treatment week = 4 mg/kg), *followed during subsequent weeks by:*
Trastuzumab 2 mg/kg per week; administer intravenously in 250 mL 0.9% NS over 30 minutes, weekly, continually for 8 weeks (total trastuzumab dosage/week during the second to ninth weeks = 2 mg/kg)
Notes:
Trastuzumab administration preceded docetaxel administration on days when both drugs were administered
Trastuzumab administration duration may be decreased from 90 to 30 minutes if administration over longer durations is well tolerated

Premedication:
Dexamethasone 8 mg/dose; administer orally twice daily for 3 days, starting on the day before docetaxel administration (total dose/cycle = 48 mg)

Docetaxel 80 mg/m² or 100 mg/m²; administer by intravenous infusion in a volume of 0.9% NS or 5% dextrose injection (D5W) sufficient to produce a final docetaxel concentration of 0.3–0.74 mg/mL over 60 minutes on day 1, every 21 days for 3 cycles (total dosage/cycle = 80 mg/m² or 100 mg/m²)
Note:
An independent study monitoring committee recommended the docetaxel dosage be reduced because of a high incidence of febrile neutropenia following treatment. Therefore, 41% of patients received docetaxel 100 mg/m² and 59% received docetaxel 80 mg/m² as the starting dose

Supportive Care
Antiemetic prophylaxis
Emetogenic potential is **LOW**
See Chapter 39 for antiemetic recommendations

Hematopoietic growth factor (CSF) prophylaxis
Primary prophylaxis may be indicated
See Chapter 43 for more information

Antimicrobial prophylaxis
Risk of fever and neutropenia is LOW–INTERMEDIATE
(risk varies directly with docetaxel dosage)
  Antimicrobial primary prophylaxis to be considered:
  • Antibacterial—consider a fluoroquinolone or no prophylaxis
  • Antifungal—not indicated
  • Antiviral—not indicated, unless patient previously had an episode of HSV
See Chapter 47 for more information

Trastuzumab infusion reactions
• A symptom complex most commonly consisting of chills and/or fever may occur in as many as 40% of patients during the first infusion of trastuzumab. These symptoms occur infrequently with subsequent trastuzumab infusions. Other signs and/or symptoms may include nausea, vomiting, pain (in some cases at tumor sites), rigors, headache, dizziness, dyspnea, hypotension, rash, and asthenia. Although the symptoms are usually mild to moderate in severity, infrequently, trastuzumab may need to be discontinued
• When such a symptom complex is observed it can be treated with or without reduction in the rate of trastuzumab infusion, and:
  ▪ **Acetaminophen** 650 mg; administer orally
  ▪ **Diphenhydramine** 25–50 mg; administer orally or by intravenous injection, and

(continued)

Treatment Modifications

Adverse Events	Treatment Modifications
WBC <3500/mm³ or platelets <100,000/mm³ on the first day of a cycle	Delay treatment for a maximum of 2 weeks until WBC >3500/mm³ and platelets >100,000/mm³. Continue at full dosages if counts recover within 2 weeks
If after 2 weeks WBC <3500/mm³ or platelets <100,000/mm³, reduce all drug dosages as follows:	
WBC 3000–3499/mm³, or platelets 75,000–99,999/mm³	Reduce dosages by 20%
WBC 2500–2999/mm³ and platelets ≥75,000/mm³	Reduce dosages by 50%
WBC <2500/mm³, or platelets <75,000/mm³	Hold treatment
ANC <1500/mm³, or platelets <100,000/mm³ at start of cycle	Delay treatment until ANC ≥1500/mm³ and platelets ≥100,000/mm³. Give filgrastim* in subsequent cycles
Hematologic recovery >3 weeks	Discontinue treatment
First episode of febrile neutropenia or documented infection after treatment	Filgrastim* prophylaxis administered during subsequent cycles
Second episode of febrile neutropenia or documented infection after treatment	Reduce docetaxel dosage to 60 mg/m² during subsequent cycles; administer filgrastim* and consider prophylaxis with ciprofloxacin†
Third episode of febrile neutropenia or documented infection after treatment	Discontinue chemotherapy

(continued)

(continued)

- Meperidine 12.5–25 mg; administer by intravenous injection every 10 minutes if needed for shaking chills (generally, cumulative doses >50 mg are not needed; use with caution in persons with moderate or more severely impaired renal function)
- With or without reduction in the rate of trastuzumab infusion

Treatment Plan Notes:
- LVEF assessment (MUGA or echocardiography) every 3 months in patients receiving trastuzumab

FEC (Cyclophosphamide + Epirubicin + Fluorouracil): weeks 10 through 18
Hydration with 0.9% sodium chloride injection (0.9% NS); administer intravenously 500 mL before starting cyclophosphamide and 500 mL after completing cyclophosphamide administration

Fluorouracil 600 mg/m^2; administer by intravenous injection over 1–3 minutes on day 1, every 21 days for 3 cycles (total dosage/cycle = 600 mg/m^2)
Epirubicin HCl 60 mg/m^2; administer by intravenous injection over 3–5 minutes on day 1, every 21 days for 3 cycles (total dosage/cycle = 60 mg/m^2)
Cyclophosphamide 600 mg/m^2; administer intravenously in 100–500 mL 0.9% NS or D5W over 30–60 minutes on day 1, every 21 days for 3 cycles (total dosage/cycle = 600 mg/m^2)

Supportive Care
Antiemetic prophylaxis
Emetogenic potential is **HIGH***. Potential for delayed symptoms*
See Chapter 39 for antiemetic recommendations

Hematopoietic growth factor (CSF) prophylaxis
Primary prophylaxis is NOT indicated

Antimicrobial prophylaxis
Risk of fever and neutropenia is LOW
Antimicrobial primary prophylaxis to be considered:
- Antibacterial—not indicated
- Antifungal—not indicated
- Antiviral—not indicated, unless patient previously had an episode of HSV
See Chapter 47 for more information

Efficacy

	Patient Number	Recurrence				Deaths
		Distant	Local or Regional	Contralateral Breast Cancer	Any	
All Study Participants						
Docetaxel/FEC	502	12.2	3.2	1.6	13.3	7.8
Vinorelbine/FEC	507	18.7	5.3	2.6	21.5	10.8
Patients with HER2-Positive Cancers						
Docetaxel/FEC/ trastuzumab	54	5.6	3.7	1.9	9.3	7.4
Docetaxel/FEC	58	25.9	10.3	1.7	25.9	17.2
Vinorelbine/FEC/ trastuzumab	61	27.9	8.2	4.9	36.1	13.1
Vinorelbine/FEC	58	25.9	6.9	0	27.6	19.0

Joensuu H et al. J Clin Oncol 2009;27:5685–5692

Treatment Modifications
(continued)

Adverse Events	Treatment Modifications
G3/4 stomatitis	Reduce docetaxel dosage to 60 mg/m^2 during subsequent cycles. Reduce epirubicin and fluorouracil dosage by 50% during subsequent cycles
G3/4 neuropathy	Discontinue treatment
Serum bilirubin levels 2 to 3 mg/dL (34.2 to 51.3 mmol/L)	Reduce epirubicin dosage by 50%
Bilirubin levels ≥3 mg/dL (≥51.3 mmol/L)	Discontinue treatment
Any other G3 nonhematologic toxicity	Hold treatment until toxicity resolves to G ≤1, then resume treatment with dosages of all drugs reduced by 25%
G4 nonhematologic toxicity	Discontinue chemotherapy
Asymptomatic decreases in ejection fraction	Monitor patient closely for evidence of clinical deterioration
Clinically significant congestive heart failure	Discontinue trastuzumab

*Filgrastim 5 mcg/kg per day; administer subcutaneously starting at least 24 hours after completing chemotherapy until ANC ≥5000/mm^3
†Ciprofloxacin 500 mg; administer orally twice daily for 7 days starting on day 5
Note: Dosages reduced for adverse events are not re-escalated

Patient Population Studied

Joensuu H et al. N Engl J Med 2006;354:809–820

Study of 1010 women with axillary node-positive or high-risk node-negative breast cancer were randomly assigned to receive 3 cycles of docetaxel or vinorelbine, followed in both groups by 3 cycles of fluorouracil, epirubicin, and cyclophosphamide (FEC). Women with HER2-positive cancer (n = 232) were further assigned to either receive or not receive trastuzumab for 9 weeks with docetaxel or vinorelbine. The median follow-up time was 62 months after random assignment

Toxicity

Adverse Event	Docetaxel No Trastuzumab (N = 447)		Docetaxel + Trastuzumab (N = 54)	
	% G1/2	% G3/4	% G1/2	% G3/4
Anemia	66	0.5	63	0
Neutropenia	1.6	98.5	0	100
Thrombocytopenia	3.7	0	0	0
Neutropenic fever	0	23	0	29.6
Infection/no neutropenia	39.2	5	43.1	5.9
Vomiting	10.2	0.5	11.8	0
Stomatitis	71.1	2.7	66	4
Alopecia	98	N/A	100	N/A
Nail problems	55.9	N/A	47.9	N/A
Skin rash	55.6	0.9	60	0
Phlebitis	8.9	0	6	0
Allergic reaction	11.7	2	13.5	5.8
Neuropathy, motor	30.5	1.4	27.5	0
Neuropathy, sensory	49.5	0.2	57.4	0
Edema	61.6	1.6	62	0
Fatigue	83	8.2	76	8
Any adverse effect	100	10	100	100

Joensuu H et al. N Engl J Med 2006;354:809–820

FEC Toxicity (N = 632)*

Toxicity	Percent of Patients
G3/4 neutropenia	25.5%
G3/4 febrile neutropenia	9.5%
G3/4 fatigue	2.4%
G3/4 nausea	5.9%
G3/4 vomiting	9.9%
G3/4 stomatitis	4.9%
Amenorrhea	58%
G2 alopecia	>90%
G2 neuropathy	N/A
G3 neuropathy	N/A
G2 arthralgia/myalgia	N/A
G3 arthralgia/myalgia	N/A
G2 LV dysfunction	7.2%

*FEC = Six 21-day cycles of fluorouracil 600 mg/m², epirubicin 90 mg/m², and cyclophosphamide 600 mg/m²

Martin et al. J Natl Cancer Inst 2008;100:805–814

Therapy Monitoring

General:

1. *Before each cycle:* CBC with differential and platelet count, LFTs, serum electrolytes, BUN, and creatinine
2. *Assessment of ejection fraction:* Every 3 months or as clinically indicated

Note:

Before initiation of trastuzumab, cardiac ejection fraction should be documented to be in the normal range

Toxicity: Left Ventricular Ejection Fraction (LVEF) During Follow-up Among Study Participants Who Had Breast Cancer with *HER2/neu* Amplification

Treatment Group	Before Chemotherapy	Last Cycle of Chemotherapy	12 Months > Chemotherapy	36 Months > Chemotherapy
Docetaxel Plus FEC (N = 58)				
Median LVEF (%)	67	64	64	64
Range LVEF (%)	53–83	48–78	45–79	52–76
No. of patients	56	51	49	24
Docetaxel Plus FEC and trastuzumab (N = 54)				
Median LVEF (%)	66	65	66	69
Range LVEF (%)	49–82	51–78	51–83	49–77
No. of patients	50	48	48	30

Joensuu H et al. N Engl J Med 2006;354:809–820

FEC Toxicity*,† (N = 995)

Event	Percent (%) of Patients
Neutropenia on day 21	33.6
Neutropenia on day 21, cycles 4–6	20.2
Febrile neutropenia	8.4
Febrile neutropenia, cycles 4–6	3.7
GCSF	27
GCSF, cycles 5 and 6	24.8
Infection	1.6
Anemia	1.4
Thrombocytopenia	0.3
G3/4 nausea-vomiting	20.5
G3/4 nausea-vomiting, cycles 4–6	11
G3/4 stomatitis	4.0
G3/4 stomatitis, cycles 4–6	2.3
Alopecia grade 3	83.9
Edema moderate or severe, cycles 4–6	0.3
Nail disorder moderate or severe, cycles 4–6	1.0
Any cardiac event reported as SAE	1.3

*FEC = Three 21-day cycles of fluorouracil 500 mg/m², epirubicin 100 mg/m², and cyclophosphamide 500 mg/m²; GCSF, granulocyte-colony stimulating factor
†Toxicity graded according to WHO criteria and serious adverse events (SAEs) defined according to International Conference on Harmonization (ICH) guidelines

Roche H. J Clin Oncol 2006;24:5664–5671

ADJUVANT, NEOADJUVANT REGIMEN

DOXORUBICIN + CYCLOPHOSPHAMIDE (AC) FOLLOWED BY DOCETAXEL WITH TRASTUZUMAB (TH) (AC → TH)

Slamon D et al. N Engl J Med 2011;365:1273–1283
Slamon D. Abstract 62. SABCS 2009
(Third Interim Analysis Phase III Randomized Trial Comparing Doxorubicin and Cyclophosphamide Followed by Docetaxel [AC → T] with Doxorubicin and Cyclophosphamide Followed by Docetaxel and Trastuzumab [AC → TH] with Docetaxel, Carboplatin and Trastuzumab [TCH] in Her2neu Positive Early Breast Cancer Patients: BCIRG 006 Study)

Hydration with 0.9% sodium chloride injection (0.9% NS); administer 500 mL before starting cyclophosphamide and 500 mL after completing cyclophosphamide administration

Doxorubicin HCl 60 mg/m²; administer by intravenous injection over 3–5 minutes on day 1, every 21 days for 4 cycles (total dosage/cycle = 60 mg/m²)
Cyclophosphamide 600 mg/m²; administer intravenously in 100–500 mL 0.9% NS or 5% dextrose injection (D5W) over 15–60 minutes on day 1, every 21 days for 4 cycles (total dosage/cycle = 600 mg/m²)

Supportive Care
Antiemetic prophylaxis
Emetogenic potential is **HIGH**. Potential for delayed symptoms
See Chapter 39 for antiemetic recommendations

Hematopoietic growth factor (CSF) prophylaxis
Primary prophylaxis is NOT indicated
See Chapter 43 for more information

Antimicrobial prophylaxis
Risk of fever and neutropenia is LOW
  Antimicrobial primary prophylaxis to be considered:
  • Antibacterial—not indicated
  • Antifungal—not indicated
  • Antiviral—not indicated, unless patient previously had an episode of HSV
See Chapter 47 for more information

Followed by:
Trastuzumab every 21 days for 4 cycles,
Loading Dose: **Trastuzumab** 4 mg/kg; administer intravenously in 250 mL 0.9% NS over 90 minutes on day 1 only during the first cycle, *then*
Maintenance Dose: **Trastuzumab** 2 mg/kg per dose; administer intravenously in 250 mL 0.9% NS over 30 minutes, once weekly on days 8 and 15 during cycle 1, and days 1, 8, and 15 during cycles 2–4 (total dosage during the first cycle = 8 mg/kg; total dosage during cycles 2–4 = 6 mg/kg)

Premedication:
Dexamethasone 8 mg/dose; administer orally twice daily for 3 days, starting on the day before docetaxel administration (total dose/cycle = 48 mg)

Docetaxel 100 mg/m²; administer intravenously in a volume of 0.9% NS or D5W sufficient to produce a final docetaxel concentration within the range of 0.3–0.74 mg/mL over 60 minutes on day 1 after trastuzumab, every 21 days for 4 cycles (total dosage/cycle = 100 mg/m²)

Supportive Care
Antiemetic prophylaxis
Emetogenic potential is **LOW**
See Chapter 39 for antiemetic recommendations

Hematopoietic growth factor (CSF) prophylaxis
Primary prophylaxis may be indicated
See Chapter 43 for more information

Antimicrobial prophylaxis
Risk of fever and neutropenia is INTERMEDIATE
  Antimicrobial primary prophylaxis to be considered:
  • Antibacterial—consider a fluoroquinolone or no prophylaxis
  • Antifungal—not indicated
  • Antiviral—not indicated, unless patient previously had an episode of HSV
See Chapter 47 for more information

(continued)

Treatment Modifications

Adverse Events	Treatment Modifications
WBC <3500/mm³, or absolute neutrophil count (ANC) <1500/mm³, or platelets <100,000/mm³ on first day of a cycle	Delay treatment for a maximum of 2 weeks until WBC >3500/mm³, ANC >1500/mm³, and platelets >100,000/mm³. Continue at full dosages if counts recover within 2 weeks. Give filgrastim* in subsequent cycles
If after 2 weeks, WBC <3500/mm³, ANC <500/mm³, or platelets <100,000/mm³, reduce all drug dosages as follows:	
WBC 3000–3499/mm³, ANC 1000–1500/mm³, or platelets 75,000–99,999/mm³	Reduce dosages by 20%
WBC 2500–2999/mm³, ANC 500–1000/mm³, or platelets ≥75,000/mm³	Reduce dosages by 50%
WBC <2500/mm³, ANC <500/mm³, or platelets <75,000/mm³	Hold treatment
Hematologic recovery >3 weeks	Discontinue treatment
First episode of febrile neutropenia or documented infection after treatment	Filgrastim* prophylaxis administered during subsequent cycles
Second episode of febrile neutropenia or documented infection after treatment	Reduce docetaxel dosage to 60 mg/m² *or* doxorubicin and cyclophosphamide dosages by 25% during subsequent cycles; administer filgrastim* and consider prophylaxis with ciprofloxacin†
Third episode of febrile neutropenia or documented infection after treatment	Discontinue chemotherapy

(continued)

(continued)

Four cycles of trastuzumab and docetaxel are followed by:
Trastuzumab 6 mg/kg; administer intravenously in 250 mL 0.9% NS over 30 minutes on day 1, every 21 days for 9 months to complete 1 year of trastuzumab

Supportive Care
Antiemetic prophylaxis
Emetogenic potential is **LOW**
See Chapter 39 for antiemetic recommendations

Hematopoietic growth factor (CSF) prophylaxis
Primary prophylaxis is NOT indicated
See Chapter 43 for more information

Antimicrobial prophylaxis
Risk of fever and neutropenia is LOW
   Antimicrobial primary prophylaxis to be considered:
- Antibacterial—not indicated
- Antifungal—not indicated
- Antiviral—not indicated, unless patient previously had an episode of HSV
See Chapter 47 for more information

Trastuzumab infusion reactions
- A symptom complex most commonly consisting of chills and/or fever may occur in as many as 40% of patients during the first infusion of trastuzumab. These symptoms occur infrequently with subsequent trastuzumab infusions. Other signs and/or symptoms may include nausea, vomiting, pain (in some cases at tumor sites), rigors, headache, dizziness, dyspnea, hypotension, rash, and asthenia. Although the symptoms are usually mild to moderate in severity, infrequently, trastuzumab may need to be discontinued
- When such a symptom complex is observed it can be treated with or without reduction in the rate of trastuzumab infusion, and:
  - **Acetaminophen** 650 mg; administer orally
  - **Diphenhydramine** 25–50 mg; administer orally or by intravenous injection, and
  - **Meperidine** 12.5–25 mg; administer by intravenous injection every 10 minutes if needed for shaking chills (generally, cumulative doses >50 mg are not needed; use with caution in persons with moderate or more severely impaired renal function)
  - With or without reduction in the rate of trastuzumab infusion

Treatment Plan Notes:
- LVEF assessment (MUGA or echocardiography) every 3 months in patients receiving trastuzumab

Note
In the neoadjuvant setting, consider adding pertuzumab with docetaxel and trastuzumab chemotherapy
Give Pertuzumab every 21 days for 4 cycles:
   Loading dose: **Pertuzumab** 840 mg; administer intravenously in 250 mL of 0.9% NS over 90 minutes on day 1 after trastuzumab, cycle 1 only (total dose during the first cycle = 840 mg), *followed 3 weeks later by:*
   Maintenance doses: **Pertuzumab** 420 mg; administer intravenously in 250 mL of 0.9% NS over 30–60 minutes on day 1 after trastuzumab, every 3 weeks for 3 cycles (total dose/cycle = 420 mg)

Schneeweiss A et al. Ann Oncol 2013;24:2278–2284

Treatment Modifications
(continued)

Adverse Events	Treatment Modifications
G3/4 stomatitis	Reduce docetaxel dosage to 60 mg/m² or doxorubicin dosage by 25% during subsequent cycles
G3/4 neuropathy	Discontinue treatment
Other severe adverse events	Hold treatment until toxicity resolves to G ≤1, then resume at decreased dosages appropriate for the toxicity
Asymptomatic decreases in ejection fraction	Monitor patient closely for evidence of clinical deterioration
Clinically significant congestive heart failure	Discontinue trastuzumab

*Filgrastim 5 mcg/kg per day; administer subcutaneously starting at least 24 hours after completing chemotherapy until ANC ≥5000/mm³
†Ciprofloxacin 500 mg; administer orally twice daily for 7 days starting on day 5
Note: Dosages reduced for adverse events are not re-escalated

Patient Population Studied
Study of 3222 women with HER2+ by FISH, T1–3, N0/N1, M0 breast cancer (AC → T: 1073; AC → TH: 1074; TCH: 1075). Stratified by nodes and hormonal receptor status

Therapy Monitoring
1. *Before each cycle:* CBC with differential and platelet count, LFTs, serum electrolytes, BUN, and creatinine
2. *Assessment of ejection fraction:* Every 3 months or as clinically indicated
3. *Hearing test:* At baseline and as needed

Efficacy

Third Planned Efficacy Analysis: 65 Months Follow Up*

	AC → T	AC → TH	AC → TH vs. AC → T		TCH	TCH vs. AC → T		AC → TH vs. TCH
			HR	p-Value		HR	p-Value	p-Value
All Patients								
	N = 1073	N = 1074			N = 1075			
DFS	75%	84%	0.64	<0.001	81%	0.75	0.04	0.21
OS	87%	92%	0.63	<0.001	91%	0.77	0.038	0.14
Patients with Negative Lymph Nodes								
	N = 309	N = 310			N = 309			
DFS	85%	93%	0.47	0.003	90%	0.64	0.057	—
OS	93%	97%	0.38	0.02	96%	0.56	0.11	—
Patients with Positive Lymph Nodes								
	N = 764	N = 764			N = 766			
DFS	71%	80%	0.68	0.0003	78%	0.78	0.013	—
Patients with ≥4 Positive Lymph Nodes								
	N = 350	N = 350			N = 352			
DFS	61%	73%	0.66	0.002	72%	0.66	0.002	—

AC → T, doxorubicin (Adriamycin) + cyclophosphamide followed by docetaxel; AC → TH, doxorubicin + cyclophosphamide followed by docetaxel plus trastuzumab (Herceptin) then trastuzumab alone; DFS, disease-free survival; OS, overall survival; TCH, docetaxel plus carboplatin plus concurrent trastuzumab, then trastuzumab alone
*DFS and OS values are at 65 months

Toxicity

	AC → T N = 1050		AC → TH N = 1068		TCH N = 1056	
	% All G	%G3/4	% All G	% G3/4	% All G	% G3/4
Nonhematologic Toxicity						
Neuropathy, sensory	48.6		49.7		36.1*	
Neuropathy, motor	5.2		6.3		4.2*	
Nail changes	49.3		43.6		28.7*	
Myalgia	52.8	5.2	55.5	5.2	38.6*	1.8*
Renal failure	0		0		0.1	
G3/4 creatinine	0.6		0.3		0.1	
Arthralgia		3.2		3.3		1.4*
Fatigue		7		7.2		7.2
Hand-foot syndrome		1.9		1.4		0*
Stomatitis		3.5		2.9		1.4*
Diarrhea		3.0		5.6		5.4
Nausea		5.9		5.7		4.8
Vomiting		6.1		6.7		3.5*
Irregular menses		27		24.3		26.5
Hematologic Toxicity						
Neutropenia		63.5		71.6		66.2*
Leucopenia		51.9		60.4		48.4*
Neutropenic infection		9.3		10.9		9.6
Febrile neutropenia		11.5		12.1		11.2
Anemia		2.4		3.1*		5.8
Thrombocytopenia		1.6		2.1*		6.1
Acute leukemia	0.6		0.1		0.1	
Cardiac Toxicity						
G3/4 LV dysfunction (CHF)†	7/1050		21/1068		4/1056	
>10% Relative LVEF decline‡	11%		19%		9%	

AC → T, doxorubicin (Adriamycin) + cyclophosphamide followed by docetaxel; AC → TH, doxorubicin + cyclophosphamide followed by docetaxel plus trastuzumab (Herceptin) then trastuzumab alone; TCH, docetaxel plus carboplatin plus concurrent trastuzumab, then trastuzumab alone; LV, left ventricular; CHF, congestive heart failure; LVEF, left ventricular ejection fraction
*Less statistically significantly events than the comparator groups
†AC → T vs. AC → TH: p = 0.0121; AC → TH vs. TCH: p <0.001; AC → T vs. TCH: p = 0.3852
‡AC → T vs. AC → TH: p <0.001; AC → TH vs. TCH: p <0.001; AC → T vs. TCH: p = 0.19

POSTMENOPAUSAL HORMONE RECEPTOR-POSITIVE ADVANCED BREAST CANCER REGIMEN

EVEROLIMUS + EXEMESTANE

Baselga J et al. N Engl J Med 2012;366:520–529

Everolimus 10 mg/day; administer orally, continually (total dose/week = 70 mg)
Exemestane 25 mg/day; administer orally, continually (total dose/week = 175 mg)
or
Placebo (formulated to match everolimus); administer orally, continually
Exemestane 25 mg/day; administer orally, continually (total dose/week = 175 mg)

Efficacy

	Everolimus and Exemestane (N = 485)	Placebo and Exemestane (N = 239)	P Value	Hazard Ratio
Local Assessment				
Events—no. (%)	202 (42)	157 (66)	<0.001	0.43 (0.35–0.54)
PFS months (95% CI)	6.9 (6.4–8.1)	2.8 (2.8–4.1)		
CR	0.4%	0		
PR	9.1%	0.4%		
SD	70.1%	58.6%		
PD	9.9%	31.4%		
Objective response	9.5%	0.4%	<0.001	
Central Assessment				
Events—no. (%)	114 (24)	104 (44)	<0.001	0.36 (0.27–0.47)
PFS months (95% CI)	10.6	4.1		
CR	0.0	0.0		
PR	7.0	0.4		
SD	74.6	64.4		
PD	5.6	21.8		
Objective response	7.0	0.4	<0.001	

Patient Population Studied

The Breast Cancer Trials of Oral Everolimus-2 (BOLERO-2) was an international, double-blind, phase 3 study in which 724 women with hormone receptor-positive breast cancer refractory to nonsteroidal aromatase inhibitors were randomly assigned to either everolimus + exemestane (485 patients) or exemestane + placebo (239 patients) (2:1 assignment ratio favoring everolimus + exemestane; patients were stratified according to the presence of visceral metastasis and previous sensitivity to endocrine therapy). Median age was 62 y; 56% of patients had visceral involvement, 76% had bone metastases, and 69% had measurable disease. All patients had ER-positive and Her2-negative disease, and had previously received aromatase inhibitor therapy; 68% had prior chemotherapy and 84% had previous sensitivity to endocrine therapy

Toxicity

	Everolimus and Exemestane (N = 482)			Placebo and Exemestane (N = 238)		
	Any Event (%)	G3 (%)	G4 (%)	Any Event (%)	G3 (%)	G4 (%)
Stomatitis	56	8	0	11	1	0
Rash	36	1	0	6	0	0
Fatigue	33	3	<1	26	1	0
Diarrhea	30	2	<1	16	1	0
Nausea	27	<1	<1	27	1	0
Decreased weight	19	1	0	5	0	0
Dyspnea	18	4	0	9	1	<1
Arthralgia	16	1	0	16	0	0
Anemia	16	5	1	4	<1	<1
Epistaxis	15	0	0	1	0	0
Vomiting	14	<1	<1	11	<1	0
Peripheral edema	14	1	0	6	<1	0
AST increase	13	3	<1	6	1	0
Constipation	13	<1	0	11	<1	0
Hyperglycemia	13	4	<1	2	<1	0
Pneumonitis	12	3	0	0	0	0
Thrombocytopenia	12	2	1	<1	0	<1

Treatment Modifications for Everolimus

Adverse Event	Dose Modification
Noninfectious pneumonitis	
Grade 1 (asymptomatic radiologic changes suggestive of pneumonitis)	No dosage adjustment necessary; monitor appropriately
Grade 2 (symptomatic but not interfering with ADL	Consider interrupting treatment, rule out infection, and consider corticosteroids until symptoms improve to G ≤1; reinitiate at a lower dose. Discontinue if recovery does not occur within 4 weeks
Grade 3 (symptomatic, interferes with ADL; oxygen indicated)	Interrupt treatment until symptoms improve to G ≤1; rule out infection and consider corticosteroid treatment; may reinitiate at a lower dose. If G3 toxicity recurs, consider discontinuing
Grade 4 (life-threatening; ventilatory support indicated)	Discontinue treatment; rule out infection; consider corticosteroid treatment

Treatment Modifications for Everolimus (continued)

Adverse Event	Dose Modification
Stomatitis (avoid the use of products containing alcohol, hydrogen peroxide, iodine, or thyme derivatives)	
Grade 1 (minimal symptoms, normal diet)	No dosage adjustment necessary; manage with mouth washes several times a day (see Supportive Care recommendations)
Grade 2 (symptomatic but can eat and swallow modified diet)	Interrupt treatment until symptoms improve to G $\leq$1; reinitiate at same dose; if stomatitis recurs with G2 severity, interrupt treatment until symptoms improve to G $\leq$1 and then reinitiate at a lower dose. Also manage with topical (oral) analgesics (eg, benzocaine, butyl aminobenzoate, tetracaine, menthol, or phenol) $\pm$ topical (oral) corticosteroids (eg, triamcinolone)
Grade 3 (symptomatic and unable to orally aliment or hydrate adequately)	Interrupt treatment until symptoms improve to G $\leq$1; then reinitiate at a lower dose. Also manage with topical (oral) analgesics (eg, benzocaine, butyl aminobenzoate, tetracaine, menthol, or phenol) $\pm$ topical (oral) corticosteroids (eg, triamcinolone)
Grade 4 (life-threatening symptoms)	Discontinue treatment; initiate appropriate medical intervention
Metabolic toxicity (eg, hyperglycemia, dyslipidemia)	
Grade 1	No dosage adjustment necessary; initiate appropriate medical intervention and monitor
Grade 2	No dosage adjustment necessary; manage with appropriate medical intervention and monitor
Grade 3	Temporarily interrupt treatment; reinitiate at a lower dose; manage with appropriate medical intervention and monitor
Grade 4	Discontinue treatment; manage with appropriate medical intervention
Nonhematologic toxicities (excluding pneumonitis, stomatitis, or metabolic toxicity)	
Grade 1	If toxicity is tolerable, no dosage adjustment necessary; initiate appropriate medical intervention and monitor
Grade 2	If toxicity is tolerable, no dosage adjustment necessary; initiate appropriate medical intervention and monitor. If toxicity becomes intolerable, temporarily interrupt treatment until improvement to G $\leq$1 and reinitiate at the same dose; if toxicity recurs at G2, temporarily interrupt treatment until improvement to G $\leq$1 and then reinitiate at a lower dose
Grade 3	Temporarily interrupt treatment until improvement to G $\leq$1; initiate appropriate medical intervention and monitor. May reinitiate at a lower dose; if toxicity recurs at G3, consider discontinuing
Grade 4	Discontinue treatment; initiate appropriate medical intervention
Everolimus dose modifications for organ dysfunction	
Mild hepatic impairment	Everolimus 7.5 mg daily
Moderate hepatic impairment	Everolimus 5 mg daily
Severe hepatic impairment	Maximum dose, Everolimus 2.5 mg daily
Renal Impairment	No adjustment needed

ADL, activities of daily life

Therapy Monitoring

1. *Baseline and Monthly:* CBC with differential and platelet count, and serum electrolytes and LFTs
2. Lipid profile every 6 weeks

METASTATIC REGIMEN

DOXORUBICIN, EVERY 3 WEEKS

Chan S et al. J Clin Oncol 1999;17:2341–2354

Doxorubicin 75 mg/m^2; administer intravenously over 15–20 min on day 1, every 3 weeks for 7 cycles (total dosage/cycle = 75 mg/m^2)

Notes:
- A maximum of 7 cycles was established because of the unacceptable incidence of CHF associated with cumulative doxorubicin dosages >550 mg/m^2. Continuation of treatment is given on a case-by-case basis
- Doxorubicin use is discontinued for either a decrease in LVEF (cardiac ejection fraction) ≥10% (absolute units) or a LVEF decline to <50%

Supportive Care
Antiemetic prophylaxis
Emetogenic potential is **HIGH**. *Potential for delayed emetic symptoms*
See Chapter 39 for antiemetic recommendations

Hematopoietic growth factor (CSF) prophylaxis
Primary prophylaxis may be indicated
See Chapter 43 for more information

Antimicrobial prophylaxis
Risk of fever and neutropenia is LOW
Antimicrobial primary prophylaxis to be considered:
- Antibacterial—not indicated
- Antifungal—not indicated
- Antiviral—not indicated, unless patient previously had an episode of HSV

See Chapter 47 for more information

Treatment Modifications

Adverse Event	Dose Modification
G4 neutropenia	Administer 75% dosage
ANC <1000/mm^3	Delay next cycle until ANC ≥1000/mm^3
Platelet count <100,000/mm^3	Delay next cycle until platelet count ≥100,000/mm^3
G3/4 nonhematologic toxicity	Delay next cycle until nonhematologic toxicities decrease to G ≤1
Bilirubin 1.2–3.0 mg/dL (21–51 μmol/L)	Administer 50% dosage
Bilirubin 3.1–5 mg/dL (53–86 μmol/L)	Administer 25% dosage

Patient Population Studied

Study of 326 patients with MBC randomized to either doxorubicin 75 mg/m^2 or docetaxel 100 mg/m^2 every 3 weeks. All patients had previously received alkylating agent chemotherapy (eg, cyclophosphamide, methotrexate, and fluorouracil [CMF], or its variants) either in the adjuvant setting or for advanced disease. Criteria for exclusion included: more than 1 line of chemotherapy for advanced or metastatic disease; previous treatment with anthracyclines, anthracenes, or a taxane; no alkylating agent in last chemotherapeutic regimen

Efficacy* (N = 147)

WHO Criteria

% Complete response	4.8
% Partial response	28.5

Median time to progression	21 weeks
Median time to treatment failure	18 weeks
Median overall survival	14 months[†]

*All randomized patients. Evaluated by WHO Criteria
[†]26% of patients received taxane-containing therapy

Toxicity (N = 193)

NCI CTCAE

Toxicity	Percent of Patients
Neutropenia, all grades	96.7
G3 neutropenia	11.1
G4 neutropenia	77.8
Febrile neutropenia	12.3
G3/4 infection	4.3
G3/4 anemia	16.1
RBC transfusion	20.9
G4 thrombocytopenia	7.5
>20% LVEF decrease*	31.7
>40% LVEF decrease*	16

*Number of patients assessable for LVEF: 101

Therapy Monitoring

1. CBC with differential and platelet count, and serum LFTs and bilirubin before each treatment. Consider intracycle assessment in early cycles
2. LVEF assessment (MUGA or echocardiography) before starting doxorubicin, after completing 300 mg/m^2, then before every subsequent treatment

METASTATIC REGIMEN

WEEKLY DOXORUBICIN OR EPIRUBICIN

Gasparini G et al. Am J Clin Oncol 1991;14:38–44

Doxorubicin HCl 20 mg/m^2; administer by intravenous injection over 3–5 minutes every week, continually (total dosage/week = 20 mg/m^2)

or

Epirubicin HCl 20 mg/m^2; administer by intravenous injection over 3–5 minutes every week, continually (total dosage/week = 20 mg/m^2)

Notes:
Cumulative doxorubicin and epirubicin dosages >550 mg/m^2 are associated with an unacceptable incidence of CHF. Continuation of treatment is given on a case-by-case basis
Doxorubicin or Epirubicin use is discontinued for either a decrease in LVEF ≥10% (absolute units) or a LVEF (cardiac ejection fraction) decline to <50%

Supportive Care

Antiemetic prophylaxis
Emetogenic potential is **MODERATE**
See Chapter 39 for antiemetic recommendations

Hematopoietic growth factor (CSF) prophylaxis
Primary prophylaxis is NOT indicated
See Chapter 43 for more information

Antimicrobial prophylaxis
Risk of fever and neutropenia is LOW
  Antimicrobial primary prophylaxis to be considered:
  • Antibacterial—not indicated
  • Antifungal—not indicated
  • Antiviral—not indicated, unless patient previously had an episode of HSV
See Chapter 47 for more information

Treatment Modifications

Adverse Events	Treatment Modifications
WBC <3000/mm^3, or platelets <100,000/mm^3	Hold treatment for at least 1 week
LVEF <50%, or symptomatic congestive heart failure	Discontinue therapy

Patient Population Studied

Study of 49 patients with advanced breast cancer whose disease had progressed after or during cyclophosphamide, methotrexate, and fluorouracil (CMF regimen) ± endocrine therapy were randomly assigned to receive weekly treatment with either doxorubicin or epirubicin

Efficacy WHO Criteria

Objective Responses and Durations	Epirubicin (N = 22) Number (%)	Doxorubicin (N = 21) Number (%)
Overall response rate (95% CI)	36% (16–56%)	38% (18–58%)
Complete	0 (–)	1 (5)
Partial	8 (36)	7 (33)
Stable disease	6 (27)	9 (43)
Progressive disease	8 (36)	4 (19)
Median duration of response	4.5 months	7 months
Median duration of complete response	—	14 months
Median duration of partial response	4.5 months (3+ to 10)	7 months (5 to 11)
Median duration of stable disease	4.5 months (2 to 11)	4 months (3 to 7)
Median overall survival	12 months	11 months
ORR (Previous CMF: Major response)	87.5 (7/8)	86% (6/7)
ORR (Previous CMF: Minor/No response)	8% (1/13)	13% (2/15)

Toxicity (WHO Scale)

Hematologic Toxicities

	Number of Patients	
	Epirubicin (N = 22)	Doxorubicin (N = 21)
Leukopenia (WBC nadir)		
% G0 ($\geq$4000/mm^3)	68	38
% G1 (3000–3999/mm^3)	23	29
% G2 (2000–2999/mm^3)	9.1	29
% G3 (1000–1999/mm^3)	0	4.7
% G4 (<1000/mm^3)	0	0
Thrombocytopenia (platelet nadir)		
% G0 (>100,000/mm^3)	91	81
% G1 (75,000–99,999/mm^3)	9.1	14
% G2 (50,000–74,999/mm^3)	0	4.7
% G3 (25,000–49,999/mm^3)	0	0
% G4 (<25,000/mm^3)	0	0
Anemia (Hgb/dL)		
% G0 (>11 g/dL)	91	90
% G1 (9.5–10.9 g/dL)	9.1	9.5
% G2 (8–9.4 g/dL)	0	0
% G3 (6.5–7.9 g/dL)	0	0
% G4 (<6.5 g/dL)	0	0

Nonhematologic Toxicities

	Epirubicin (N = 22)					Doxorubicin (N = 21)				
WHO toxicity grade	0	1	2	3	4	0	1	2	3	4
Gastrointestinal										
Nausea and vomiting	64	23	14	0	0	48	29	19	4.7	0
Stomatitis	68	23	9.1	0	0	57	24	19	0	0
Dermatologic/Vascular										
Alopecia	64	27	4.5	4.5	0	57	29	9.5	4.7	0
Phlebitis	91	4.5	4.5	0	0	21	0	0	0	0
Cardiac										
Acute arrhythmias	91	0	9.1	0	0	86	0	14	0	0
Function*	100	0	0	0	0	95	0	0	0	4.7
Infection	95	0	4.5	0	0	100	0	0	0	0

Treatment delays	1 patient (9%)	7 patients (38%); p = 0.05

*No significant differences were evident; however, the only case that developed symptomatic congestive heart failure was in the doxorubicin arm, after a cumulative dose of 820 mg/m^2 at 11.5 months

Therapy Monitoring

1. *Before each doxorubicin or epirubicin treatment:* CBC with leukocyte differential count and platelet counts, and serum LFTs including total bilirubin

2. *Before starting doxorubicin or epirubicin, after receiving a total cumulative lifetime dosage of 300 mg/m^2, then before every third subsequent treatment:* LVEF assessment (MUGA or echocardiography). Consider more frequent assessment in patients with cardiac disease or previous radiation therapy to fields involving the mediastinum

METASTATIC REGIMEN

DOXORUBICIN HCl LIPOSOME INJECTION (LIPOSOMAL DOXORUBICIN)

O'Brien MER et al. Ann Oncol 2004;15:440–449

Doxorubicin HCl liposome injection 40–50 mg/m^2; administer intravenously in 250 mL (doses ≤90 mg) or 500 mL (doses >90 mg) 5% dextrose injection over 60 minutes on day 1, every 3 weeks (total dosage/cycle = 40–50 mg/m^2)

Note: Liposomal doxorubicin is administered at an initial rate of 1 mg/min to minimize the risk of infusion reactions. If no infusion-related adverse reactions are observed within 15 min after starting administration, the infusion rate may be increased to complete administration over 1 hour

Supportive Care

Antiemetic prophylaxis
Emetogenic potential is LOW
See Chapter 39 for antiemetic recommendations

Hematopoietic growth factor (CSF) prophylaxis
Primary prophylaxis is NOT indicated
See Chapter 43 for more information

Antimicrobial prophylaxis
Risk of fever and neutropenia is LOW
  Antimicrobial primary prophylaxis to be considered:
  • Antibacterial—not indicated
  • Antifungal—not indicated
  • Antiviral—not indicated, unless patient previously had an episode of HSV
See Chapter 47 for more information

Patient Population Studied

Study of 509 women with stages IIIB, IV MBC and normal cardiac function were randomly assigned to receive either liposomal doxorubicin 50 mg/m^2 every 4 weeks, or doxorubicin 60 mg/m^2 every 3 weeks

Efficacy WHO Criteria

	Liposomal Doxorubicin*	Doxorubicin*
Overall response rate (CR + PR)	33%	38%
Stable disease	25%	25%
Progressive disease	18%	11%
Median duration of response	7.3 months	7.1 months
Median overall survival	21 months	22 months

*The HR for PFS was 1.00 (95% CI for HR 0.82–1.22); consistent with noninferiority of liposomal doxorubicin compared with doxorubicin

Treatment Modifications

DOXIL (Doxorubicin HCl Liposome Injection) Product Label, November 2010. Centocor Ortho Biotech Products, L.P.

Adverse Events	Treatment Modifications
Hematologic Adverse Events	
ANC 500–1500/mm^3 or platelets 25,000–75,000/mm^3	Delay treatment until ANC >1500/mm^3 and platelets >75,000/mm^3, then resume treatment at the same dosage and schedule
ANC <500/mm^3 or platelets <25,000/mm^3	Delay treatment until ANC >1500/mm^3 and platelets >75,000/mm^3, then resume treatment with dosage reduced by 25% from the last dose administered, *or* add hematopoietic growth factor
Stomatitis	
G2	Delay treatment until stomatitis resolves to G ≤1
G3/4	Delay treatment until stomatitis resolves to G ≤1, then resume treatment with liposomal doxorubicin dosage decreased by 25%
For delays >2 weeks because of stomatitis	Discontinue treatment
Other G3 adverse events (except nausea, vomiting, or alopecia)	Delay treatment until stomatitis resolves to G1, then resume treatment with liposomal doxorubicin dosage decreased by 25%
Guidelines for Cardiac Toxicity	
LVEF decreases by ≥15% from baseline, or to <45%	Discontinue pegylated liposomal doxorubicin

(continued)

Treatment Modifications (continued)

Adverse Events	Treatment Modifications		
	Guidelines for Palmar-Plantar Erythrodysesthesia		
Grade of Toxicity	4 Weeks > Dose	5 Weeks > Dose	6 Weeks > Dose
G1: Mild erythema, swelling, or desquamation not interfering with daily activities	Redose unless patient has previous G3/4 skin toxicity. If so, delay an additional week	Redose unless patient has previous G3/4 skin toxicity. If so, delay an additional week	Redose at 25% dosage reduction; return to 4-week interval or discontinue therapy
G2: Erythema, desquamation, or swelling interfering with, but not precluding, normal physical activities; small blisters or ulcerations <2 cm in diameter	Delay treatment 1 week	Delay treatment 1 week	Redose at 25% dosage reduction; return to 4-week interval or discontinue therapy
G3: Blistering, ulceration, or swelling interfering with walking or normal daily activities; cannot wear regular clothing	Delay treatment 1 week	Delay treatment 1 week	Discontinue therapy
G4: Diffuse or local process causing infectious complications, or a bedridden state, or hospitalization	Delay treatment 1 week	Delay treatment 1 week	Discontinue therapy

Richardson et al. J Clin Oncol 2006;24:3113–3120

Therapy Monitoring

1. *Before each dose:* CBC with differential and platelet count. Consider intracycle assessment during first few cycles
2. *Every other cycle or every third cycle during therapy:* LFTs, serum electrolytes, cardiac function by ECHO

Toxicity NCI-CTC

	% All Grades	% G3/4
Nonhematologic Toxicities		
PPE	48	17
Nausea	37	3
Mucositis	23	4
Stomatitis	22	5
Alopecia	20	0
Vomiting	19	<1
Fatigue	12	<1
Anorexia	11	1
Asthenia	10	1
Rash	10	2
Abdominal pain	8	1
Constipation	8	<1
Abnormal pigmentation	8	<1
Fever	8	0
Diarrhea	7	1
Erythema	7	<1
Weakness	6	<1
Mouth ulceration	5	<1
Hematologic Toxicities		
Anemia	5	<1
Leukopenia	2	<1
Neutropenia	4	1
Thrombocytopenia	1	0

	Liposomal Doxorubicin N = 254	Doxorubicin N = 255
Cardiotoxicity (yes signs/symptoms of CHF)	0	4% (10/255)
Cardiotoxicity (no signs/symptoms of CHF)	4% (10/254)	15% (38/255)

METASTATIC REGIMEN

WEEKLY PACLITAXEL

Perez EA et al. J Clin Oncol 2001;19:4216–4223

Premedication:

Dexamethasone 10 mg/dose; administer orally for 2 doses 12 hours and 6 hours before paclitaxel (total dose/cycle = 20 mg), *or*

Dexamethasone 20 mg; administer intravenously over 10–15 minutes, 30–60 minutes before paclitaxel (total dose/cycle = 20 mg)

Note: Dexamethasone doses may be gradually decreased in the absence of hypersensitivity reactions during repeated paclitaxel treatments

Diphenhydramine 25–50 mg; administer orally 60 minutes before paclitaxel, *or* administer by intravenous injection 30–60 minutes before paclitaxel

Cimetidine 300 mg (or ranitidine 150 mg, famotidine 20–40 mg, or an equivalent histamine receptor [H_2]-subtype antagonist); administer orally 60 minutes before paclitaxel, *or* cimetidine 300 mg (or ranitidine 50 mg, famotidine 20 mg); administer intravenously over 15–30 minutes, 30–60 minutes before paclitaxel

Paclitaxel 80 mg/m² per dose; administer intravenously in a volume of 0.9% sodium chloride injection or 5% dextrose injection sufficient to produce a concentration within the range 0.3–1.2 mg/mL over 60 minutes, weekly for 4 consecutive weeks, every 4 weeks (total dosage/4-week cycle = 320 mg/m²)

Supportive Care

Antiemetic prophylaxis
Emetogenic potential is **LOW**
See Chapter 39 for antiemetic recommendations

Hematopoietic growth factor (CSF) prophylaxis
Primary prophylaxis is NOT indicated
See Chapter 43 for more information

Antimicrobial prophylaxis
Risk of fever and neutropenia is LOW
Antimicrobial primary prophylaxis to be considered:
- Antibacterial—not indicated
- Antifungal—not indicated
- Antiviral—not indicated, unless patient previously had an episode of HSV

See Chapter 47 for more information

Treatment Modifications

Adverse Events	Treatment Modifications
ANC ≤800/mm³ or platelets ≤50,000/mm³	Hold treatment until ANC >800/mm³ and platelets >50,000/mm³, then resume with weekly paclitaxel dosage reduced by 10 mg/m²
G2 motor or sensory neuropathies	Reduce weekly paclitaxel dosage by 10 mg/m² without interrupting planned treatment
Other nonhematologic adverse events G2 or G3	Hold treatment until adverse events resolve to G ≤1, then resume with weekly paclitaxel dosage reduced by 10 mg/m²
Patients who cannot tolerate paclitaxel at 60 mg/m² per week	Discontinue treatment
Treatment delay >2 weeks	Decrease weekly paclitaxel dosage by 10 mg/m² or consider discontinuing treatment

Patient Population Studied

Study of 212 women with metastatic breast cancer who had previously received up to 2 chemotherapy regimens for metastatic disease. Prior taxane treatment was allowed if the administration interval was every 3 weeks or less frequently

Efficacy (N = 177 Evaluable) as Defined

Overall response	21.5%
Partial response	19.2%
Complete response	2.3%
Stable disease	41.8%
Median overall survival (OS)	12.8 months
Median time to progression (TTP)	4.7 months

Toxicity NCI Common Toxicity Criteria Scale (N = 211)

Toxicity	%G1/2	%G3	%G4
Hematologic Toxicity			
Neutropenia	40	10	5
Thrombocytopenia	25	0.5	0.5
Anemia	83	9	0
Febrile neutropenia	0	1	0
Infection	3	0	0
Nonhematologic Toxicity			
Anaphylaxis	1	0.5	0.5
Neuropathy	59	9	0
Arthralgia/myalgia	23	2	0
Asthenia	44	4	0
Edema	16	0.5	0
Nausea	25	1	0
Vomiting	9	1	0
Diarrhea	22	0.5	0
Stomatitis	19	0.5	0
Alopecia	43	0	0
Nail changes	20	0	0
Rash	18	0.5	0

Therapy Monitoring

1. *Before each dose:* CBC with leukocyte differential count and platelet counts
2. *Every third or every fourth cycle during therapy:* LFTs, serum electrolytes

METASTATIC REGIMEN

PACLITAXEL EVERY 3 WEEKS

Nabholtz J-M et al. J Clin Oncol 1996;14:1858–1867

Premedication:

Dexamethasone 10 mg/dose; administer orally for 2 doses 12 hours and 6 hours before paclitaxel (total dose/cycle = 20 mg), *or*

Dexamethasone 20 mg; administer intravenously over 10–15 minutes, 30–60 minutes before paclitaxel (total dose/cycle = 20 mg)

Note: Dexamethasone doses may be gradually decreased in the absence of hypersensitivity reactions during repeated paclitaxel treatments

Diphenhydramine 25–50 mg; administer orally 60 minutes before paclitaxel, *or* administer by intravenous injection 30–60 minutes before paclitaxel

Cimetidine 300 mg (or ranitidine 150 mg, famotidine 20–40 mg, or an equivalent histamine receptor $[H_2]$-subtype antagonist); administer orally 60 minutes before paclitaxel, *or* cimetidine 300 mg (or ranitidine 50 mg or famotidine 20 mg); administer intravenously over 15–30 minutes, 30–60 minutes before paclitaxel

Paclitaxel 175 mg/m²; administer intravenously in a volume of 0.9% sodium chloride injection or 5% dextrose injection sufficient to produce a concentration within the range 0.3–1.2 mg/mL over 3 hours on day 1, every 3 weeks (total dosage/cycle = 175 mg/m²)

Supportive Care
Antiemetic prophylaxis
Emetogenic potential is **LOW**
See Chapter 39 for antiemetic recommendations

Hematopoietic growth factor (CSF) prophylaxis
Primary prophylaxis is NOT indicated
See Chapter 43 for more information

Antimicrobial prophylaxis
Risk of fever and neutropenia is LOW
Antimicrobial primary prophylaxis to be considered:
• Antibacterial—not indicated
• Antifungal—not indicated
• Antiviral—not indicated, unless patient previously had an episode of HSV
See Chapter 47 for more information

Treatment Modifications

Adverse Events	Treatment Modifications
WHO G3/4 neutropenia for ≥7 days	Decrease paclitaxel dosage by 25%
Platelet counts ≤100,000/mm³ for ≥7 days	
Febrile neutropenia, documented infection, or hemorrhage	
WHO G3 mucositis	
WHO G >2 paresthesias	Discontinue therapy
Symptomatic arrhythmia or heart block >1°	
Other major organ toxicities WHO G >2	
Severe hypersensitivity reaction	

Patient Population Studied

Study of 471 women with measurable metastatic breast cancer who had received 1 prior chemotherapy regimen (as adjuvant therapy or for metastatic disease), or 2 prior regimens (1 adjuvant and 1 for metastatic disease)

Efficacy (N = 471)

WHO Criteria

	Paclitaxel Dosage (mg/m²)	
	175	135
Complete response	5%	2%
Partial response	24%	20%
Stable disease (>4 weeks)	43%	42%
Progressive disease	27%	36%
Median progression-free survival	4.2 months	3.0 months
Median overall survival	11.7 months	10.5 months
Response According to Pretreatment Characteristics		
ECOG performance status 0	35% (33/95)	32% (30/93)
ECOG performance status 1	27% (25/91)	15% (15/100)
ECOG performance status 2	19% (7/37)	18% (6/34)
Disease in soft tissue only	50% (19/38)	31% (10/32)
Disease in bone ± soft tissue	37% (10/27)	22% (6/27)
Visceral ± bone ± soft tissue	23% (36/158)	21% (35/168)
Prior adjuvant therapy only	36% (25/69)	29% (20/68)
Prior metastatic therapy only	26% (23/88)	14% (12/87)
Adjuvant and metastatic therapy	26% (17/66)	26% (19/72)

Toxicity (N = 471)

WHO Toxicity Criteria

Toxicity	Paclitaxel Dosage (mg/m^2)	
	175	135
Hematologic Toxicity		
G3 or G4 leukopenia	34%	24%
G3 or G4 neutropenia	67%	50%
G3/4 neutropenia for ≥7 days	11%	5%
G3 or G4 thrombocytopenia	3%	2%
G3 or G4 anemia	4%	2%
Febrile neutropenia	4%	2%
Infection any grade	23%	15%
Nonhematologic Toxicity		
Severe hypersensitivity*	—	<1%
Bradycardia <50 BPM	3%	4%
G3 or G4 peripheral neuropathy	7%	3%
G3 arthralgia/myalgia	16%	9%
Edema, any grade	13%	16%
G3 or G4 nausea/vomiting	5%	5%
G3 mucositis	3%	<1%

*Includes any of the following: hypotension requiring vasopressors, angioedema, respiratory distress requiring bronchodilators, or generalized urticaria

Therapy Monitoring

Before each cycle: CBC with differential and platelet count. Consider intracycle monitoring during first few cycles

METASTATIC REGIMEN

WEEKLY DOCETAXEL

Burstein HJ et al. J Clin Oncol 2000;18:1212–1219

Premedication:

Dexamethasone 8 mg/dose; administer orally for 3 doses at approximately 12 hours and 1 hour before docetaxel, and 12 hours after docetaxel administration (total dose/week = 24 mg)

Diphenhydramine 50 mg; administer by intravenous injection 30 minutes before docetaxel

Docetaxel 40 mg/m²; administer intravenously in a volume of 0.9% sodium chloride injection or 5% dextrose injection sufficient to produce a final docetaxel concentration within the range 0.3–0.74 mg/mL over 60 minutes, every week for 6 consecutive weeks, every 8 weeks (total dosage/8-week cycle = 240 mg/m²)

Supportive Care

Antiemetic prophylaxis

Emetogenic potential is **LOW**

See Chapter 39 for antiemetic recommendations

Hematopoietic growth factor (CSF) prophylaxis

Primary prophylaxis is NOT indicated

See Chapter 43 for more information

Antimicrobial prophylaxis

Risk of fever and neutropenia is LOW

Antimicrobial primary prophylaxis to be considered:

- Antibacterial—not indicated
- Antifungal—not indicated
- Antiviral—not indicated, unless patient previously had an episode of HSV

See Chapter 47 for more information

Treatment Modifications

Adverse Events	Treatment Modifications
G2 neurotoxicity	Decrease docetaxel dosage by 25%*
Febrile neutropenia	
G4 thrombocytopenia	
Any G3 nonhematologic adverse event	
G4 nonhematologic toxicity	Consider discontinuing treatment
ANC <1000/mm³	Hold treatment until ANC >1000/mm³, platelets >100,000/mm³, bilirubin normalizes, and AST <1.5 × ULN. If delay is >3 weeks, consider discontinuing therapy
Platelets <100,000/mm³	
Bilirubin greater than upper limit of normal (ULN) range	
AST >1.5 ULN	
ANC <1000/mm³ for >2 weeks	Consider adding filgrastim during subsequent cycles
Patients who miss 1–2 weekly treatments in a cycle, but remain eligible for retreatment	Consider retreatment during week 7 of the affected cycle

*Do not re-escalate dose after a dosage decrease

Patient Population Studied

Study of 29 women with metastatic breast cancer with prior treatment of metastatic disease limited to 1 prior chemotherapy regimen. No limitation on prior hormonal therapy

Efficacy (N = 29)

Partial response	41%
Stable disease ≥6 months	17%

Toxicity (N = 29)

NCI Common Toxicity Criteria Scale		
Toxicity	% G1/2	% G3/4
Hematologic Toxicity		
Neutropenia	28	14
Anemia	86	0
Nonhematologic Toxicity		
Nausea/vomiting	34	3
Gastritis	24	3
Diarrhea	24	3
Stomatitis	17	0
Constipation	3	3
Alopecia	66	0
Fatigue	59	14
Excessive lacrimation	52	0
Fluid retention	45	0
Pleural effusion	31	0
Dysgeusia	24	0
Sensory neuropathy	17	3
Motor neuropathy	3	3
Arthralgia	14	0
Dry mouth	14	0
Phlebitis	14	0
Hypersensitivity	3	0

Therapy Monitoring

1. *Weekly, before each docetaxel dose:* CBC with differential and platelet count
2. *Every other week:* Liver function tests

METASTATIC REGIMEN

DOCETAXEL EVERY 3 WEEKS

Chan S et al. J Clin Oncol 1999;17:2341–2354

Premedication:

Dexamethasone 8 mg/dose; administer orally twice daily for 3 days, starting on the day before docetaxel administration (total dose/cycle = 48 mg)

Docetaxel 100 mg/m²; administer intravenously in a volume of 0.9% sodium chloride injection or 5% dextrose injection sufficient to produce a final docetaxel concentration within the range 0.3–0.74 mg/mL over 60 minutes on day 1, every 3 weeks (total dosage/cycle = 100 mg/m²)

Supportive Care

Antiemetic prophylaxis

Emetogenic potential is **LOW**

See Chapter 39 for antiemetic recommendations

Hematopoietic growth factor (CSF) prophylaxis

Primary prophylaxis is NOT indicated

See Chapter 43 for more information

Antimicrobial prophylaxis

Risk of fever and neutropenia is LOW

   Antimicrobial primary prophylaxis to be considered:

   • Antibacterial—not indicated

   • Antifungal—not indicated

   • Antiviral—not indicated, unless patient previously had an episode of HSV

See Chapter 47 for more information

Treatment Modifications

Adverse Events	Treatment Modifications
First episode of hematologic or nonhematologic adverse events G ≥3 other than alopecia and anemia	Reduce docetaxel dosage from 100 mg/m² to 75 mg/m²
Second episode of hematologic or nonhematologic adverse events G3 other than alopecia and anemia	Reduce docetaxel dosage from 75 mg/m² to 55 mg/m²

Patient Population Studied

Study of 159 women with metastatic breast cancer who had previously received chemotherapy containing an alkylating agent in the adjuvant setting or for advanced disease. No prior taxoid treatment. Performance status of at least 60% Karnofsky index

Efficacy (N = 148)

WHO Criteria

	Randomized Patients	Assessable Patients
Overall response	47.8% (95% CI, 40.1–55.5%)	52% (95% CI, 44–60.1%)
Complete response	6.8%	7.4%
Median time to progression	26 weeks	27 weeks
Median time to treatment failure	—	22 weeks
Median overall survival	—	15 months

Toxicity

NCI Common Toxicity Criteria

Toxicity	%G3/4	% Overall
Hematologic Toxicity		
Neutropenia	93.5	97.4
Anemia	4.4	88.6
Thrombocytopenia	1.3	4.4
Febrile neutropenia	—	5.7
Infection	2.5	—
Nonhematologic Toxicity		
Acute		
Nausea	3.1	39.6
Vomiting	3.1	22.6
Stomatitis	5	59.7
Diarrhea	10.7	50.3
Skin toxicity	1.9	37.7
Allergy	2.5	17.6
Chronic		
Alopecia	—	91.2
Asthenia	14.5	59.7
Nail disorder	2.5	44
Neurosensory	5	42.8
Neuromotor	5	18.2
Fluid retention	5	59.7

Therapy Monitoring

1. *Weekly:* CBC with differential and platelet count
2. *Before each docetaxel dose:* CBC with differential and platelet count, LFTs, and serum electrolytes

METASTATIC REGIMEN

ALBUMIN-BOUND PACLITAXEL

Gradishar WJ et al. J Clin Oncol 2009;27:3611–3619

Paclitaxel protein-bound particles for injectable suspension (albumin-bound paclitaxel, *nab*-paclitaxel) 100 mg/m^2 or 150 mg/m^2 per dose*; administer intravenously (undiluted) for 3 doses on days 1, 8, and 15, every 4 weeks (total dosage/cycle may range from 300–450 mg/m^2, depending on the amount of drug given per dose event)

*Initial Dosages in Patients with Hepatic Impairment

ALT (SGOT)		Serum Bilirubin	Initial Dosage (% of Planned Dosage)†
<10 × ULN		> ULN to ≤1.25 × ULN	100%
<10 × ULN	AND	1.26–2 × ULN	75%
<10 × ULN		2.01–5 × ULN	50%
>10 × ULN	OR	>5 × ULN	Withhold *nab*-paclitaxel

ULN, Upper limit of normal range
†Extrapolated from product labeling for Abraxane for injectable suspension (paclitaxel protein-bound particles for injectable suspension) (albumin bound), October 2013; Celgene Corporation, Summit, NJ

Supportive Care
Antiemetic prophylaxis
Emetogenic potential is **LOW**
See Chapter 39 for antiemetic recommendations

Hematopoietic growth factor (CSF) prophylaxis
Primary prophylaxis is NOT indicated
See Chapter 43 for more information

Antimicrobial prophylaxis
Risk of fever and neutropenia is LOW
  Antimicrobial primary prophylaxis to be considered:
   • Antibacterial—not indicated
   • Antifungal—not indicated
   • Antiviral—not indicated, unless patient previously had an episode of HSV
See Chapter 47 for more information

Patient Population Studied

Study of 302 patients with stage IV metastatic breast cancer who had not previously received treatment for metastatic disease who were randomly assigned to 1 of 3 treatment regimens with *nab*-paclitaxel or docetaxel. Prior neoadjuvant or adjuvant chemotherapy was allowed if at least 1 year had elapsed since administration. Forty-three percent of patients had previously received chemotherapy in the adjuvant or neoadjuvant settings, and 10% of patients had grade 1 neuropathy before receiving study therapy

Treatment Modifications

Adverse Event	Treatment Modification
ANC <500/mm^3 for ≥1 week	Withhold *nab*-paclitaxel until symptoms resolve to G ≤1, then resume at a dosage decreased by 25%
Sensory neuropathy G2	Delay *nab*-paclitaxel until symptoms resolve to G ≤1, then resume treatment at the same dosage and schedule
Sensory neuropathy G ≥3	Withhold *nab*-paclitaxel until symptoms resolve to G ≤1, then resume on the same administration schedule with a dosage decreased by 25%. Do not re-escalate *nab*-paclitaxel dosage during subsequent use
Second recurrence of sensory neuropathy G ≥3 after dosage reduction	Withhold *nab*-paclitaxel until symptoms resolve to G ≤1, then resume on the same administration schedule with a dosage decreased by an additional 25% (total 50% dosage reduction). Do not re-escalate *nab*-paclitaxel dosage during subsequent use
Third recurrence of sensory neuropathy G ≥3 after 2 dosage reductions	Discontinue *nab*-paclitaxel
Severe hypersensitivity reaction	Discontinue *nab*-paclitaxel
Hypotension, during the 30-minute infusion (may occur in 5% of patients)	Most often occurs without symptoms and requires neither specific therapy nor treatment discontinuation
Bradycardia, during the 30-minute infusion (may occur in <1% of patients)	Most often occurs without symptoms and require neither specific therapy nor treatment discontinuation

Efficacy
RECIST*

	nab-Paclitaxel		
	300 mg/m² every 3 wks	100 mg/m² weekly*	150 mg/m² weekly†
Overall response rate	37%	45%	49%
Partial response	36%	45%	49%
Complete response	1%	0	0
Stable disease ≥16 weeks	32%	30%	31%
Median progression-free survival	11 months	12.9 months	12.9 months

*RECIST, Response Evaluation Criteria in Solid Tumors (Therasse P et al. J Natl Cancer Inst 2000;92:205–216)
†Weekly regimens are given for 3 consecutive weeks followed by 1 week without retreatment during a 4-week cycle

Toxicity
NCI Common Terminology Criteria for Adverse Events

Toxicity	300 mg/m² every 3 wks	100 mg/m² weekly*	150 mg/m² weekly*
Percent of Patients Experiencing Toxicity			
G1/2 neutropenia	49	55	47
G1/2 sensory neuropathy	56	50	54
G1/2 fatigue	31	34	42
G1/2 arthralgia	31	19	35
Alopecia	47	57	53
G3/4 neutropenia	44	25	44
G3/4 sensory neuropathy	17	8	14
G3/4 fatigue	5	0	3
G3/4 arthralgia	1	0	0

*Weekly regimens are given for 3 consecutive weeks followed by 1 week without retreatment during a 4-week cycle

Therapy Monitoring

1. *Before each dose:* CBC with differential count and platelet count, LFTs, and neurologic exam
2. *Weekly:* CBC with differential and platelet count through cell count nadirs, particularly for a 150-mg/m² for 3-weeks-out-of-4-weeks regimen

METASTATIC REGIMEN

CAPECITABINE

Bajetta E et al. J Clin Oncol 2005;23:2155–2161
Blum JL et al. J Clin Oncol 1999;17:485–493
Blum JL et al. Cancer 2001;92:1759–1768
Reichardt P et al. Ann Oncol 2003;14:1227–1233
Xeloda (capecitabine) Tablets, Film Coated for Oral Use Product Label, December 2013. Genentech USA, Inc., South San Francisco, CA

Capecitabine 1250 mg/m^2 per dose; administer orally twice daily within 30 minutes after a meal for 14 consecutive days (28 doses) on days 1–14, every 3 weeks (total dosage/cycle = 35,000 mg/m^2)

Notes:

• Capecitabine is given for 2 consecutive weeks followed by 1 week without treatment

• Doses are rounded to use combinations of 500-mg and 150-mg tablets that most closely approximate calculated values

• In practice, treatment often is begun with capecitabine 1000 mg/m^2 per dose twice daily for 14 consecutive days on days 1–14, every 3 weeks, because of a high rate of dose reduction with higher dosages (total dosage/cycle = 28,000 mg/m^2)

• Initial capecitabine dosage should be decreased by 25% in patients with moderate renal impairment (baseline creatinine clearance = 30–50 mL/min [0.5–0.83 mL/s]); ie, a dosage reduction from 1250 mg/m^2 per dose, to 950 mg/m^2 per dose, twice daily. Capecitabine use is contraindicated in persons with severe renal impairment (creatinine clearance <30 mL/min [<0.5 mL/s])

• Although food decreases the rate and extent of drug absorption and the time to peak plasma concentration and systemic exposure (AUC) for both capecitabine and fluorouracil, product labeling recommends giving capecitabine within 30 minutes after the end of a meal because established safety and efficacy data are based on administration with food

Supportive Care

Antiemetic prophylaxis
Emetogenic potential is **LOW**
See Chapter 39 for antiemetic recommendations

Hematopoietic growth factor (CSF) prophylaxis
Primary prophylaxis is NOT indicated
See Chapter 43 for more information

Antimicrobial prophylaxis
Risk of fever and neutropenia is LOW
   Antimicrobial primary prophylaxis to be considered:
   • Antibacterial—not indicated

   • Antifungal—not indicated

   • Antiviral—not indicated, unless patient previously had an episode of HSV
See Chapter 47 for more information

Diarrhea management

Latent or delayed onset diarrhea:
   Loperamide 4 mg orally initially after the first loose or liquid stool, *then*
   Loperamide 2 mg orally every 2 hours during waking hours, *plus*
   Loperamide 4 mg orally every 4 hours during hours of sleep
   • Continue for at least 12 hours after diarrhea resolves

   • Recurrent diarrhea after a 12-hour diarrhea-free interval is treated as a new episode

   • Rehydrate orally with fluids and electrolytes during a diarrheal episode

   • If a patient develops blood or mucus in stool, dehydration, or hemodynamic instability, or if diarrhea persists >48 hours despite loperamide, stop loperamide and hospitalize the patient for IV hydration

   Alternatively, a trial of **Diphenoxylate hydrochloride** 2.5 mg **with Atropine sulfate** 0.025 mg (eg, Lomotil)
   • Initial adult dose is 2 tablets 4 times daily until control has been achieved, after which the dose may be reduced to meet individual requirements. Control may often be maintained with as little as 2 tablets daily

   • Clinical improvement of acute diarrhea is usually observed within 48 hours. If improvement of chronic diarrhea after treatment with a maximum daily dose of 8 tablets is not observed within 10 days, control is unlikely with further administration

Hand-foot reaction

For patients who develop a hand-foot reaction, use topical emollients (eg, Aquaphor), topical or orally administered steroids, antihistamine agents (H$_1$-receptor antagonists), or pyridoxine 50–150 mg/day administer orally

Treatment Modifications

Adapted from NCI of Canada CTC

Adverse Event	Dose Modification
First G2 toxicity	Hold capecitabine and resume after adverse events resolve to G ≤1. No change in dosage required
Second G2 toxicity	Hold capecitabine and resume after adverse events resolve to G ≤1. Reduce dosage by 25%
Third G2 toxicity	Hold capecitabine and resume after adverse events resolve to G ≤1. Reduce dosage by 50%
Fourth G2 toxicity	Discontinue capecitabine
First G3 toxicity	Hold capecitabine and resume after adverse events resolve to G ≤1. Reduce dosage by 25%
Second G3 toxicity	Hold capecitabine and resume after adverse events resolve to G ≤1. Reduce dosage by 50%
Third G3 toxicity	Discontinue capecitabine
First G4 toxicity	Hold capecitabine and resume after adverse events resolve to G ≤1. Reduce dosage by 50%
Second G4 toxicity	Discontinue capecitabine
Diarrhea, nausea, and vomiting	Treat symptomatically. Resume previous dosage if toxicity is adequately controlled within 2 days after initiation of treatment. If control takes longer, reduce the capecitabine dosage, or if it occurs despite prophylaxis, reduce the capecitabine dosage 25–50%

Toxicity

Xeloda (capecitabine) Tablets, Film Coated for Oral Use Product Label, December 2013. Genentech USA, Inc., South San Francisco, CA
Incidence of selected adverse reactions possibly or probably related to treatment in ≥5% of patients participating in a single arm trial in stage IV breast cancer (n = 162)
(Adapted from Blum et al. J Clin Oncol 1999;17:485–493)*

Adverse Events	% All Grades	% G3/4
Hematologic Toxicity		
Neutropenia	26	4
Anemia	72	4
Thrombocytopenia	24	4
Lymphopenia	94	59
Nonhematologic Toxicity		
Diarrhea	57	15
Hand-foot syndrome	57	11
Nausea	53	4
Fatigue	41	8
Vomiting	37	4
Dermatitis	37	1

(continued)

Patient Population Studied

Study of 75 patients with metastatic breast cancer who developed disease progression during or after taxane-containing chemotherapy (Blum JL et al. Cancer 2001;92:1759–1768)

Efficacy (N = 75)

Blum JL et al. Cancer 2001;92:1759–1768

WHO Criteria	
Intention-to-treat overall response	26%
Intention-to-treat stable disease >6 weeks	31%
Median time to progressive disease	3.2 months (95% CI, 2.3–4.3)
Median time to treatment failure in all patients	3.2 months (95% CI, 2.2–4.4)
Median duration of response in 17 patients with PR	8.3 months (95% CI, 7–9.9)
Median survival in intention-to-treat population	12.2 months (95% CI, 8.0–15.3)
Median survival in 21 patients with stable disease	12.9 months
Median survival in 17 patients with CR/PR	Not reached

Subgroup Analysis	CR/PR
Paclitaxel pretreated	27%
Paclitaxel failed	33%
Paclitaxel resistant	20%
Docetaxel pretreated	28%
Docetaxel failed	38%
Docetaxel resistant	17%

CR, Complete response; PR, partial response

Toxicity (*continued*)

Adverse Events	% All Grades	% G3/4
Stomatitis	24	7
Anorexia	23	3
Hyperbilirubinemia	22	11
Paresthesia	21	1
Abdominal pain	20	4
Constipation	15	1
Eye irritation	15	—
Pyrexia	12	1
Dyspepsia	8	—
Nail disorder	7	—
Laboratory Abnormalities		
Hyperbilirubinemia	22	11
Increased alkaline phosphatase	—	3.7

*Twice-daily oral capecitabine at 1255 mg/m^2 per dose given for 2 treatment weeks, followed by a 1-week rest period and repeated in 3-week cycles (total daily dose = 2510 mg/m^2)

Therapy Monitoring

1. *Before starting each cycle:* CBC with differential and platelet counts. Consider intracycle monitoring in first few cycles
2. *Every other cycle:* Serum electrolytes, serum creatinine and BUN, and LFTs
3. Frequently monitor anticoagulant response (INR or PT) in patients who use coumarin anticoagulants (eg, warfarin) and capecitabine concomitantly, and adjust anticoagulant dose accordingly, or consider alternative anticoagulant agents

METASTATIC REGIMEN

GEMCITABINE

Blackstein M et al. Oncology 2002;62:2–8
Carmichael J et al. J Clin Oncol 1995;13:2731–2736

Gemcitabine 800–1200 mg/m² per dose; administer by intravenous infusion in 50–250 mL 0.9% sodium chloride injection (0.9% NS) over 30 minutes on days 1, 8, and 15, every 28 days for up to 8 cycles (total dosage/cycle = 2400–3600 mg/m²)

Note: Gemcitabine use in patients with concurrent liver metastases or a preexisting history of hepatitis, alcoholism, or liver cirrhosis, may lead to exacerbation of the underlying hepatic insufficiency

Supportive Care

Antiemetic prophylaxis
Emetogenic potential is LOW
See Chapter 39 for antiemetic recommendations

Hematopoietic growth factor (CSF) prophylaxis
Primary prophylaxis is NOT indicated
See Chapter 43 for more information

Antimicrobial prophylaxis
Risk of fever and neutropenia is LOW
Antimicrobial primary prophylaxis to be considered:
- Antibacterial—not indicated
- Antifungal—not indicated
- Antiviral—not indicated, unless patient previously had an episode of HSV

See Chapter 47 for more information

Treatment Modifications

Adverse Events	Treatment Modifications
ANC 1000–1499/mm³, WBC 1000–1999/mm³, or platelets 50,000–99,999/mm³ on day of treatment	Reduce dosage by 25%
ANC and WBC <1000/mm³ or platelets <50,000/mm³ on day of treatment	Hold treatment until ANC and WBC >1000/mm³, and platelets >50,000/mm³. Resume treatment with gemcitabine dosage reduced by 50%
ANC and WBC <500/mm³, or platelets <25,000/mm³ on day of treatment	Consider discontinuing therapy
WHO G3 nonhematologic adverse events (excluding nausea, vomiting, and alopecia)	Decrease dosage by 50%, or withhold treatment until recovery to G ≤1
WHO G4 nonhematologic adverse events	Hold treatment until resolution to G ≤1 then resume with a 50% dose reduction

Patient Population Studied

Blackstein M et al. Oncology 2002;62:2–8

Study of 39 patients with metastatic breast cancer who had not previously received chemotherapy for metastatic disease

Efficacy (N = 35)

Blackstein M et al. Oncology 2002;62:2–8

WHO Criteria

Overall response rate	37.1% (95% CI, 21.5–55.1)
Complete response rate	5.7%
Partial response rate	31.4%
Median time to progression	5.1 months (95% CI, 3.5–5.8)
Median response duration in 13 responders	8.8 months (95% CI, 5.2–12.7)
Median overall survival	21.1 months (95% CI, 11–26.9)
Estimated 1-year survival	65%

Toxicity (N = 39)

Blackstein M et al. Oncology 2002;62:2–8

WHO Criteria

Toxicity	% G1/2	% G3/4
Hematologic Toxicity		
Anemia	60.6	9.1
Neutropenia*	36.4	30.3
Thrombocytopenia*	25	6.3
Laboratory Abnormalities		
Alkaline phosphatase increase	35.3	0
Alanine aminotransferase increase	58.8	5.9
Bilirubin increase	2.9	2.9
Nonhematologic Toxicity		
Allergic	12.9	0
Cutaneous	30.7	2.6
Diarrhea	23.1	0
Fever	15.4	0
Infection	10.3	2.6
Nausea/vomiting	41.1	10.3
Pulmonary	12.9	5.2
Alopecia	46.2	0

Dose Delivery

Total cycles completed	211
Median cycles/patient	4 (Range: 0–4)
Dosage reductions	102
Dose omissions	69
Dose delays	5
Median dosage intensity	1053 mg/m² per week (Range: 400–1212 mg/m² week)

*Leukopenia was the most common reason for gemcitabine dosage reductions (78.4%) and omissions (58.0%), while thrombocytopenia resulted in 14% and 13% of reductions and omissions, respectively

Therapy Monitoring

Before starting each treatment: CBC with differential and platelet count, LFTs, serum creatinine and BUN, and serum electrolytes. Consider intracycle assessment in first few cycles

METASTATIC REGIMEN

WEEKLY VINORELBINE

Nisticò C et al. Breast Cancer Res Treat 2000;59:223–229
Zelek L et al. Cancer 2001;92:2267–2272

Vinorelbine 25–30 mg/m^2 per dose; administer by intravenous infusion in a volume of 0.9% sodium chloride injection or 5% dextrose injection sufficient to produce a vinorelbine concentration within the range 0.5–2 mg/mL over 20 minutes, every week, continually (total dosage/week = 25–30 mg/m^2)

Supportive Care

Antiemetic prophylaxis
Emetogenic potential is **MINIMAL**
See Chapter 39 for antiemetic recommendations

Hematopoietic growth factor (CSF) prophylaxis
Primary prophylaxis is NOT indicated
See Chapter 43 for more information

Antimicrobial prophylaxis
Risk of fever and neutropenia is LOW
  Antimicrobial primary prophylaxis to be considered:
- Antibacterial—not indicated
- Antifungal—not indicated
- Antiviral—not indicated, unless patient previously had an episode of HSV

See Chapter 47 for more information

Treatment Modifications

Burstein HJ et al. J Clin Oncol 2001;19:2722–2730
Nisticò C et al. Breast Cancer Res Treat 2000;59:223–229

Adverse Event	Treatment Modifications
ANC >1250/mm^3 and platelets >100,000/mm^3 on treatment day	Give starting dose
ANC 750–1250/mm^3 or platelets 50,000–99,000/mm^3 on treatment day	Reduce vinorelbine dosage to 75% of starting dose
ANC <750/mm^3 or platelets <50,000/mm^3	Hold vinorelbine dose until ANC >750/mm^3 and platelets >50,000/mm^3 then resume at dose as determined by ANC and platelets
Treatment delays for neutropenia ≥2 weeks	Add filgrastim
For treatment delays >3 weeks	Consider discontinuing treatment
Total bilirubin 2–3 mg/dL (34.2–51.3 μmol/L)	Give vinorelbine at 12.5 mg/m^2
Total bilirubin >3 mg/dL (>51.3 μmol/L)	Hold vinorelbine
G2 neurologic adverse events	Hold vinorelbine until adverse events resolve to G ≤1, then resume treatment with dosage decreased by 25%
G3 nonhematologic adverse events	Hold vinorelbine dose until adverse events resolve to G ≤1, then resume treatment with dosage decreased by 25%
G4 nonhematologic adverse events	Consider discontinuing treatment

Patient Population Studied

Nisticò C et al. Breast Cancer Res Treat 2000;59:223–229

Study of 40 women with metastatic breast cancer, prior treatment with at least 1 anthracycline-containing regimen in the adjuvant or metastatic setting

Efficacy (N = 40)

Nisticò C et al. Breast Cancer Res Treat 2000;59:223–229

WHO Criteria	
Overall response	52.5% (95% CI, 37–68)
Complete response	12.5%
Partial response	40%
Median duration of response	10 months (Range: 5–21)
Median time to progression	9 months (Range: 1–27)
Estimated overall survival	19 months (Range: 2–54+)

Toxicity (N = 40)

Nisticò C et al. Breast Cancer Res Treat 2000;59:223–229

Toxicity	% G1/2	% G3/4
Hematologic Toxicity		
Neutropenia	57.5	25
Anemia	65	10
Thrombocytopenia	7.5	0
Nonhematologic Toxicity		
Nausea/vomiting	30	0
Mucositis	10	0
Neuropathy	22.5	0
Phlebitis	45	15
Constipation	40	0
Alopecia	42.5	12.5

Asthenia
  Mild
  Moderate
  Severe
	12.5
	47.5
	17.5	

Therapy Monitoring

1. *Before each dose:* CBC with differential count and platelet count
2. *Every other week:* LFTs

METASTATIC REGIMEN

ERIBULIN MESYLATE

Cortes J et al. J Clin Oncol 2010;28:3922–3928
Cortes J et al. Lancet 2011;377:914–923

Eribulin mesylate 1.4 mg/m² per dose*; administer (undiluted) by slow intravenous injection over 2–5 minutes for 2 doses on days 1 and 8, every 21 days (total dosage/cycle = 2.8 mg/m²)

*Dosage Recommendations for Impaired Liver and Renal Function

Condition	Dosage (days 1 and 8; 21-day cycle)
Mild hepatic impairment (Child-Pugh A)	1.1 mg/m² per dose (total dosage/cycle = 2.2 mg/m²)
Moderate hepatic impairment (Child-Pugh B)	0.7 mg/m² per dose (total dosage/cycle = 1.4 mg/m²)
Moderate renal impairment (creatinine clearance: 30–50 mL/min [0.5–0.83 mL/s])	1.1 mg/m² per dose (total dosage/cycle = 2.2 mg/m²)

Supportive Care

Antiemetic prophylaxis
*Emetogenic potential is **LOW***
See Chapter 39 for antiemetic recommendations

Hematopoietic growth factor (CSF) prophylaxis
Primary prophylaxis is *NOT* indicated
See Chapter 43 for more information

Antimicrobial prophylaxis
Risk of fever and neutropenia is LOW
Antimicrobial primary prophylaxis to be considered:
- Antibacterial—not indicated
- Antifungal—not indicated
- Antiviral—not indicated, unless patient previously had an episode of HSV
See Chapter 47 for more information

Treatment Modifications

Eribulin Mesylate Dosage Levels

Dosage Level 1	1.4 mg/m²
Dosage Level −1	1.1 mg/m²
Dosage Level −2	0.7 mg/m²

Adverse Events	Treatment Modifications
ANC <1000/mm³ on cycle days 1 or 8	Hold eribulin mesylate. Administer when ANC >1000/mm³
Platelet count <75,000/mm³ on cycle days 1 or 8	Hold eribulin mesylate. Administer when platelet count >75,000/mm³
Nonhematologic toxicities G ≥3 on cycle days 1 or 8	Hold eribulin mesylate. Administer when toxicities < G2
ANC <1000/mm³ on cycle day 8 resolved by day 15	Give eribulin mesylate at a dosage decreased by 1 dose level but do not administer less than 0.7 mg/m². Initiate a subsequent cycle no sooner than 2 weeks later
Platelet count <75,000/mm³ on cycle day 8 resolved by day 15	
Nonhematologic toxicities G ≥3 on cycle day 8 resolved by day 15	
ANC <1000/mm³ on cycle day 8 and still <1000/mm³ on day 15	Omit day 8 eribulin mesylate dose
Platelet count <75,000/mm³ on cycle day 8 and still <75,000/mm³ on day 15	
Nonhematologic toxicities G ≥3 on cycle day 8 and still G ≥3 on day 15	
ANC <500/mm³ for >7 days	Permanently decrease eribulin mesylate dosage by one dosage level but do not administer less than 0.7 mg/m²
ANC <1000/mm³ with fever or infection	
Platelet count <25,000/mm³	
Platelet count <50,000/mm³ requiring transfusion	
Nonhematologic toxicities G ≥3 lasting >7 days	
Omission or delay of a day 8 dose during the previous cycle for toxicity	

Note: After any dosage decrease, do not re-escalate eribulin mesylate dosages during subsequent treatments

Patient Population Studied

Cortes J et al. Lancet 2011;377:914–923

EMBRACE trial (study E7389-G000-305). A phase 3 open-label, multicenter study that enrolled women with locally recurrent or metastatic breast cancer and randomly allocated them (2:1) to eribulin mesylate or treatment of physician's choice (TPC). Patients were previously treated for locally recurrent or metastatic breast cancer (508 eribulin mesylate vs. 254 TPC). Patients were heavily pretreated (median of 4 previous chemotherapy regimens); 559 (73%) of 762 patients had received capecitabine previously. No TPC patient received supportive care alone; most (238 [96%] of 247) received chemotherapy, which was most often vinorelbine, gemcitabine, or capecitabine. Overall, 16% (123 of 762 patients) had HER2- positive disease, and 19% (144 patients) had triple-negative disease. The most common metastatic sites were bone and liver; 386 (51%) of 762 patients had metastatic disease involving 3 or more organs. Randomization was stratified by geographical region, previous capecitabine treatment, and human epidermal growth factor receptor 2 status. The primary end point was overall survival in the intention-to-treat population

Efficacy (N = 508)

RECIST

	Independent Review	Investigator Review
Median overall survival	13.1 months	
1-Year survival rates	53.9%	
Median duration of treatment	3.9 months (Range: 0.7–16.3)	
Median progression-free survival	3.7 months (95% CI, 3.3–3.9)	3.6 months (95% CI, 3.3–3.7)

Best Overall Tumor Response

	Independent Review	Investigator Review
Complete response	3 (1%)	1 (<1%)
Partial response	54 (12%)	61 (13%)
Stable disease	208 (44%)	219 (47%)
Progressive disease	190 (41%)	176 (38%)
Not evaluable	12 (3%)	11 (2%)
Unknown	1 (<1%)	0
Objective response rate	57 (12%) (95% CI, 9.4–15.5)	62 (13%) (95% CI, 10.3–16.7)

RECIST, Response Evaluation Criteria in Solid Tumors (Therasse P et al. J Natl Cancer Inst 2000;92:205–216)

Therapy Monitoring

1. ECG at baseline (pretreatment on cycle 1, day 1), prior to treatment on day 8, and prior to all eribulin mesylate treatments in patients with CHF or bradyarrhythmias, and in patients concomitantly using drugs known to prolong the QT/QTc interval. Avoid use in patients with congenital long QT syndrome
2. *Before each dose:* CBC with differential and platelet count, serum sodium, potassium, magnesium, creatinine and BUN, and LFTs. Correct electrolyte abnormalities before commencing treatment
3. *Before each cycle:* Neurologic examination

Toxicity (N = 503)*

NCI-CTCAE

	% All Grades	% G3	% G4
Hematologic			
Neutropenia	52	21	24
Leucopenia	23	12	2
Anaemia	19	2	<1
Nonhematologic			
Asthenia/fatigue	54	8	1
Alopecia	45	—	—
Peripheral neuropathy[†]	35	8	<1
Nausea	35	1	0
Constipation	25	1	0
Arthralgia/ myalgia	22	<1	0
Weight loss	21	1	0
Pyrexia	21	<1	0
Anorexia	19	<1	0
Headache	19	<1	0
Diarrhea	18	0	0
Vomiting	18	1	<1
Back pain	16	1	<1
Dyspnea	16	4	0
Cough	14	0	0
Bone pain	12	2	0
Pain in extremity	11	1	0
Mucosal inflammation	9	1	0
Palmar-plantar erythrodysesthesia	1	<1	0

NCI-CTCAE, National Cancer Institute, Common Terminology Criteria for Adverse Events, v.3.0. At: http://ctep.cancer.gov/protocolDevelopment/ electronic_applications/ctc.htm [accessed December 7, 2013]
*Dose interruptions, delays, and reductions were undertaken in 28 (6%), 248 (49%), and 145 (29%) of 503 patients, respectively
†Peripheral neuropathy includes neuropathy peripheral, neuropathy, peripheral motor neuropathy, polyneuropathy, peripheral sensory neuropathy, peripheral sensorimotor neuropathy, demyelinating polyneuropathy, and paraesthesia

METASTATIC REGIMEN

IXABEPILONE

Perez EA et al. J Clin Oncol 2007;25:3407–3414

Premedication:

Diphenhydramine 50 mg or an equivalent histamine receptor [H_1-subtype] antagonist); administer orally 60 minutes before ixabepilone
Ranitidine 150–300 mg (or cimetidine 300 mg, famotidine 20 mg, or an equivalent histamine receptor [H_2-subtype] antagonist); administer orally 60 minutes before ixabepilone

Ixabepilone 40 mg/m²; administer by intravenous infusion in a volume of lactated Ringer injection, or, alternatively, 0.9% sodium chloride injection with sodium bicarbonate (2 mEq/250–500 mL) sufficient to produce an ixabepilone concentration within the range 0.2–0.6 mg/mL over 3 hours on day 1, every 21 days (total dosage/cycle = 40 mg/m²)

Notes:
- Ixabepilone is a substrate for catabolism by cytochrome P450 (CYP) CYP3A subfamily enzymes
- Concomitant use of ixabepilone with strong CYP3A4 inhibitors or inducers should be avoided
- Grapefruit juice may also increase plasma ixabepilone concentrations and should be avoided
- If a strong CYP3A4 INHIBITOR and ixabepilone must be coadministered, a decrease in ixabepilone dosage to 20 mg/m² is predicted to adjust the ixabepilone AUC to the range observed without inhibitors
- If a concomitantly administered strong CYP3A4 inhibitor is discontinued, a period of approximately 1 week should elapse before the ixabepilone dosage is increased to the indicated (unmodified) dosage
- If a strong CYP3A4 INDUCER and ixabepilone must be coadministered (ie, no alternatives are feasible), based on extrapolation from a drug interaction study with rifampin, after a patient has been maintained on a strong CYP3A4 inducer, the dose of ixabepilone may be gradually increased from 40 mg/m² to 60 mg/m², depending on tolerance, which is predicted to adjust the AUC to the range observed without inducers
- Proceed cautiously; there are no clinical data with this dose adjustment in patients receiving strong CYP3A4 inducers
- Patients whose dose is increased >40 mg/m² should be monitored carefully for toxicities. If the strong inducer is discontinued, the ixabepilone dosage should be decreased to the (unmodified) dosage indicated without a strong CYP3A4 inducer

Supportive Care

Antiemetic prophylaxis
Emetogenic potential is **LOW**
See Chapter 39 for antiemetic recommendations

Hematopoietic growth factor (CSF) prophylaxis
Primary prophylaxis is NOT indicated
See Chapter 43 for more information

Antimicrobial prophylaxis
Risk of fever and neutropenia is LOW
  Antimicrobial primary prophylaxis to be considered:
  - Antibacterial—not indicated
  - Antifungal—not indicated
  - Antiviral—not indicated, unless patient previously had an episode of HSV
See Chapter 47 for more information

Patient Population Studied

One-hundred twenty-eight women with metastatic or locally advanced breast cancer resistant to anthracyclines (doxorubicin or epirubicin), taxanes (paclitaxel or docetaxel), and capecitabine were enrolled in a phase II, multicenter, single-arm study designed to evaluate objective response rates to ixabepilone monotherapy administered every 21 days in repeated treatment cycles. Treatment continued for ≤18 cycles or until disease progression or unacceptable toxicity

Treatment Modifications

Ixabepilone Dosage Levels

Dosage level 1	40 mg/m²
Dosage level −1	32 mg/m²
Dosage level −2	25 mg/m²

Adverse Events	Treatment Modifications
On day 1 of repeated cycles, an ANC <1500/mm³	Withhold treatment until ANC >1500/mm³ then administer dosage administered in previous cycle
On day 1 of repeated cycles, a platelet count <100,000/mm³	Withhold treatment until platelet count >100,000/mm³ then administer dosage administered in previous cycle
On day 1 of repeated cycles, nonhematologic toxicities ≥ G2 are present	Withhold treatment until nonhematologic toxicities are G1 or have resolved, then administer dosage administered in previous cycle
Transient G3 arthralgia/myalgia or fatigue	Continue same ixabepilone dosage
ANC <500/mm³ for ≥7 days	Reduce ixabepilone dosage by 1 dosage level
Febrile neutropenia	
Platelet count <25,000/mm³, or platelets <50,000/mm³ with bleeding	
G2 neuropathy lasting ≥7 days	
G3 neuropathy independent of duration	
G3 nonhematologic toxicity other than transient G3 arthralgia/myalgia or fatigue	
ANC still <1500/mm³ 2 weeks after planned start of cycle	Discontinue ixabepilone treatment
Platelet count still <100,000/mm³ 2 weeks after planned start of cycle	
G3 neuropathy lasting ≥7 days or disabling neuropathy	
Any G4 toxicity	
Hypersensitivity reaction to ixabepilone administration despite H₁ and H₂ antagonists	In addition to H₁- and H₂-antihistamines prophylaxis, administer **dexamethasone** 20 mg orally 60 minutes before commencing ixabepilone administration, *or* **Dexamethasone** 20 mg intravenously at least 30 minutes prior to starting ixabepilone administration

Efficacy

RECIST

IRF Best Response (N = 113)*	
Partial response	12%
Stable disease	50%
Progressive disease	32%
Median duration of response	5.7 months (95% CI, 4.4–7.3)
Median time to response	6.1 weeks (range: 5–19)
Stable disease >6 months	13.3%

RECIST, Response Evaluation Criteria in Solid Tumors (Therasse P et al. J Natl Cancer Inst 2000;92:205–216)
*Defined by Response Evaluation Criteria in Solid Tumors and assessed by an Independent Radiology Facility

Toxicity NCI-CTC	% Total	% G2	% G3	% G4
Nonhematologic Toxicities				
Peripheral sensory neuropathy	60	30	13	1
Fatigue/asthenia	50	21	13	1
Myalgia/arthralgia	49	26	8	0
Alopecia	39	39	0	0
Nausea	42	11	2	0
Stomatitis/mucositis	29	7	6	1
Vomiting	29	9	1	0
Diarrhea	22	5	1	0
Musculoskeletal pain	20	9	3	0
Anorexia	19	3	2	0
Constipation	16	6	2	0
Abdominal pain	13	3	2	0
Headache	11	6	0	0
Peripheral motor neuropathy*	10	7	1	0
Dyspnea	9	2	1	0
Nail disorder	9	4	0	0
Pain	8	2	3	0
Palmar plantar erythrodysesthesia (PPE)	8	3	2	0
Fever	8	2	1	0
Dizziness	7	2	0	0
Hypersensitivity	5	2	1	0
Hematologic Toxicities				
Anemia	84	26	6	2
Neutropenia	79	17	31	23
Thrombocytopenia	44	4	6	2

*Peripheral neuropathy
1. Primarily, sensory neuropathy was the most common nonhematologic adverse event: G1/2 neuropathy in 49% of patients, G3/4 in 13% of patients
2. Severe peripheral neuropathy generally was characterized by paresthesias of the hands and feet, and developed after a median of 4 cycles (range: 1–11 cycles)
3. Peripheral neuropathy G ≥3 resolved to baseline or G1 in 13 of 17 patients, with a median time to resolution of 5.4 weeks
4. Median time to resolution of neuropathy G ≥2 was 4 weeks
5. Patients whose ixabepilone dosage was decreased because of neuropathy received a median of 3 additional treatment cycles, among whom 20 of 23 patients did not experience additional worsening or an improvement in their conditions

NCI-CTC, National Cancer Institute (USA) Common Toxicity Criteria. At: http://ctep.cancer.gov/protocolDevelopment/electronic_applications/ctc.htm [accessed December 7, 2013]

Therapy Monitoring

1. *Before each cycle:* Neurologic examination, CBC with differential and platelet count, serum creatinine, BUN, and LFTs. Consider intracycle assessments in first few cycles
2. *During concomitant use with CYP3A4 inhibitors or inducers:* Frequently monitor CBC with differential and platelet count as means to guide ixabepilone dosage adjustments based on altered pharmacodynamic responses

METASTATIC REGIMEN

PACLITAXEL PLUS BEVACIZUMAB

Miller K et al. N Engl J Med 2007;357:2666–2676

Premedication:

Dexamethasone 10 mg/dose; administer orally for 2 doses 12 hours and 6 hours before paclitaxel (total dose/cycle = 20 mg), *or*

Dexamethasone 20 mg; administer intravenously over 10–15 minutes, 30–60 minutes before paclitaxel (total dose/cycle = 20 mg)

Note: Dexamethasone doses may be gradually decreased in the absence of hypersensitivity reactions during repeated paclitaxel treatments

Diphenhydramine 25–50 mg; administer orally 60 minutes before paclitaxel, *or* administer by intravenous injection 30–60 minutes before paclitaxel

Cimetidine 300 mg (or **ranitidine** 150 mg, **famotidine** 20–40 mg, or an equivalent histamine receptor [H_2]-subtype antagonist); administer orally 60 minutes before paclitaxel, *or* **cimetidine** 300 mg (or **ranitidine** 50 mg, **famotidine** 20 mg); administer intravenously over 15–30 minutes, 30–60 minutes before paclitaxel

Paclitaxel 90 mg/m² per dose; administer intravenously in a volume of 0.9% sodium chloride injection (0.9% NS) or 5% dextrose injection sufficient to produce a concentration within the range 0.3–1.2 mg/mL over 60 minutes, for 3 doses on days 1, 8, and 15, every 28 days (total dosage/cycle = 270 mg/m²)

Bevacizumab 10 mg/kg per dose; administer intravenously in 100 mL 0.9% NS every 2 weeks (days 1 and 15) every 28 days (total dosage/cycle = 20 mg/kg)

Note: The initial bevacizumab dose is administered over 90 minutes. If administration is well tolerated, the administration duration may be decreased stepwise during subsequent administrations to 60 minutes, and, finally, to a minimum duration of 30 minutes

Note:

- Bevacizumab therapy is not withheld or discontinued for paclitaxel-related toxic effects. If paclitaxel use is discontinued, patients whose disease has not progressed may continue to receive bevacizumab at the same dosage and schedule previously administered during combination therapy with paclitaxel

- Treat with antihypertensive medication as needed. The goal of BP control should be consistent with general medical practice

Supportive Care

Antiemetic prophylaxis

*Emetogenic potential is **LOW***

See Chapter 39 for antiemetic recommendations

Hematopoietic growth factor (CSF) prophylaxis

Primary prophylaxis is NOT indicated

See Chapter 43 for more information

Antimicrobial prophylaxis

Risk of fever and neutropenia is LOW

Antimicrobial primary prophylaxis to be considered:

- Antibacterial—not indicated

- Antifungal—not indicated

- Antiviral—not indicated, unless patient previously had an episode of HSV

See Chapter 47 for more information

Treatment Modifications

Adverse Event	Treatment Modification
ANC 1000–1499/mm³	Reduce paclitaxel dosage to 65 mg/m² for the next dose given
Platelet count 75,000–99,000/mm³	
AST (SGOT) >5 times, but ≤10 times the upper limit of normal range	
Total bilirubin 1.6–2.5 mg/dL (27.4–42.8 μmol/L)	
Prolonged neutropenia	Permanently reduce paclitaxel dosage to 65 mg/m²
Febrile neutropenia	
Platelet count ≤40,000/mm³ with bleeding	
Any platelet count ≤20,000/mm³	
G3 neuropathy	Withhold paclitaxel until neuropathy improves to G ≤1, then resume paclitaxel at 65 mg/m²
Hypersensitivity reactions G ≥3	Permanently discontinue paclitaxel use*
G ≥3 neuropathy persisting >3 weeks	
Neuropathy recurrent after paclitaxel dosage reduction	
>2+ proteinuria by dipstick	Collect 24-hour urine for protein analysis
24-hour urine protein is <2000 mg	Continue same bevacizumab dosage
24-hour urine protein is ≥2000 mg	Withhold bevacizumab until 24-hour urine protein <2000 mg. Discontinue bevacizumab if 24-hour urine protein does not recover to <2000 mg after 4 weeks of bevacizumab interruption

(continued)

Toxicity*
(N = 365)
NCI-CTC

	% G3	% G4
Hematologic Toxicities		
Neutropenia	0	0
Anemia	0	3
Thrombocytopenia	0	0
Febrile neutropenia	0.5	0.3
Nonhematologic Toxicities		
Allergic reaction	3.0	0.3
Infection	8.8	0.5
Fatigue	8.8	0.3
Nausea	3.3	0
Vomiting	2.7	0
Stomatitis	1.1	0
Anorexia	0.5	0.3
Increased aspartate aminotransferase	1.4	0
Sensory neuropathy	23.0	0.5
Arthralgia	2.7	0.5
Myalgia	1.6	0.5
Hypertension	14.5	0.3
Thrombosis or embolism	1.6	0.5
Cerebrovascular ischemia	0.8	1.1
Left ventricular dysfunction	0.8	0
Hemorrhage	0.5	0
Gastrointestinal perforation	0.5	0
Headache	2.2	0
Proteinuria	2.7	0.8

*Toxic effects are graded according to the National Cancer Institute Common Toxicity Criteria, version 2.0. At: http://ctep.cancer.gov/protocolDevelopment/electronic_applications/ctc.htm [accessed December 7, 2013] The worst grade considered at least possibly related to treatment is given

Therapy Monitoring

- *Before each dose of paclitaxel:* CBC with leukocyte differential count and platelet count, serum creatinine and BUN, and LFTs, and neurologic examination
- *Before each dose of bevacizumab:* Urinalysis for protein excretion (dipstick screening for proteinuria or quantitative analysis)

Treatment Modifications
(continued)

Adverse Event	Treatment Modification
G1 HTN (SBP 120–139 mm Hg or DBP 80–89 mm Hg)	Consider increased BP monitoring; start antihypertensive medication if appropriate
G2 HTN, asymptomatic (SBP 140–159 mm Hg or DBP 90–99 mm Hg)	Begin antihypertensive therapy and continue bevacizumab
G2 HTN, symptomatic (SBP 140–159 mm Hg or DBP 90–99 mm Hg)	Start or adjust antihypertensive medication Hold bevacizumab until symptoms resolve *and* BP <160/90 mm Hg. Resume bevacizumab after BP under control (<160/99 mm Hg)
G3 HTN (SBP ≥160 mm Hg or DBP ≥100 mm Hg)	For refractory hypertension requiring delay of bevacizumab for >4 wk, discontinue bevacizumab
G4 HTN (hypertensive crisis or malignant hypertension)	Permanently discontinue bevacizumab

Patient Population Studied

Study of 722 patients who were randomly assigned to receive initial treatment for metastatic breast cancer with either paclitaxel alone or paclitaxel plus bevacizumab in an open-label study

Efficacy (N = 347)

RECIST

Overall response rate	36.9%
Median progression-free survival	11.8 months
Median overall survival	26.7 months
1-Year survival rate	81.2%

METASTATIC REGIMEN

DOCETAXEL + CAPECITABINE

O'Shaughnessy J et al. J Clin Oncol 2002;12:2812–2823

Premedication:

Dexamethasone 8 mg/dose; administer orally twice daily for 3 days, starting on the day before docetaxel administration (total dose/cycle = 48 mg)

Docetaxel 75 mg/m^2; administer intravenously in a volume of 0.9% sodium chloride injection (0.9% NS) or 5% dextrose injection (D5W) sufficient to produce a final docetaxel concentration within the range 0.3–0.74 mg/mL over 60 minutes on day 1, every 3 weeks for 4 cycles (total dosage/cycle = 75 mg/m^2)

Capecitabine 1250 mg/m^2 per dose; administer orally twice daily with approximately 200 mL water within 30 minutes after a meal for 14 consecutive days on days 1–14 (28 doses), every 3 weeks (total dosage/cycle = 35,000 mg/m^2)

Notes:

• Capecitabine is given for 2 consecutive weeks followed by 1 week without treatment

• Doses are rounded to use combinations of 500-mg and 150-mg tablets that most closely approximate calculated values

• In practice, treatment often is begun with capecitabine 1000 mg/m^2 per dose twice daily for 14 consecutive days on days 1–14, every 3 weeks, because of a high rate of dose reduction with higher dosages (total dosage/cycle = 28,000 mg/m^2)

• Initial capecitabine dosage should be decreased by 25% in patients with moderate renal impairment (baseline creatinine clearance = 30–50 mL/min [0.5–0.83 mL/s]); ie, a dosage reduction from 1250 mg/m^2 per dose to 950 mg/m^2 per dose, twice daily. Capecitabine use is contraindicated in persons with severe renal impairment (creatinine clearance <30 mL/min [<0.5 mL/s])

• Although food decreases the rate and extent of drug absorption and the time to peak plasma concentration and systemic exposure (AUC) for both capecitabine and fluorouracil, product labeling recommends giving capecitabine within 30 minutes after the end of a meal because established safety and efficacy data are based on administration with food

Supportive Care

Antiemetic prophylaxis

Emetogenic potential is **LOW**

See Chapter 39 for antiemetic recommendations

Hematopoietic growth factor (CSF) prophylaxis

Primary prophylaxis is NOT indicated

See Chapter 43 for more information

Antimicrobial prophylaxis

Risk of fever and neutropenia is LOW

Antimicrobial primary prophylaxis to be considered:

• Antibacterial—not indicated

• Antifungal—not indicated

• Antiviral—not indicated, unless patient previously had an episode of HSV

See Chapter 47 for more information

Diarrhea management

Latent or delayed onset diarrhea:

Loperamide 4 mg orally initially after the first loose or liquid stool, *then*

Loperamide 2 mg orally every 2 hours during waking hours, *plus*

Loperamide 4 mg orally every 4 hours during hours of sleep

• Continue for at least 12 hours after diarrhea resolves

• Recurrent diarrhea after a 12-hour diarrhea free interval is treated as a new episode

• Rehydrate orally with fluids and electrolytes during a diarrheal episode

• If a patient develops blood or mucus in stool, dehydration, or hemodynamic instability, or if diarrhea persists >48 hours despite loperamide, stop loperamide and hospitalize the patient for IV hydration

Alternatively, a trial of **Diphenoxylate hydrochloride** 2.5 mg **with Atropine sulfate** 0.025 mg (eg, Lomotil)

• Initial adult dose is 2 tablets 4 times daily until control has been achieved, after which the dose may be reduced to meet individual requirements. Control may often be maintained with as little as 2 tablets daily

• Clinical improvement of acute diarrhea is usually observed within 48 hours. If improvement of chronic diarrhea after treatment with a maximum daily dose of 8 tablets is not observed within 10 days, control is unlikely with further administration

Hand-foot reaction

For patients who develop a hand-foot reaction, use topical emollients (eg, Aquaphor), topical or orally administered steroids, antihistamine agents (H$_1$-receptor antagonists), or pyridoxine 50–150 mg/day; administer orally

Treatment Modifications

NCI of Canada CTC

Adverse Event	Treatment Modification
First G2*	Withhold chemotherapy until adverse events resolve to G ≤1, then resume
Recurrent G2 (second episode)* or Any G3	Withhold chemotherapy for up to 2 weeks • If adverse events resolve to G ≤1 within 2 weeks, resume treatment with docetaxel and capecitabine dosage decreased by 25% • If adverse events do not resolve to G ≤1 within 2 weeks, docetaxel is permanently discontinued, but capecitabine treatment may resume after adverse events resolve to G ≤1 at a dosage decreased by 25%
Recurrent G2 (third episode)* or Recurrent G3 (second episode) or Any G4	Permanently discontinue docetaxel. Withhold capecitabine for up to 2 weeks. If adverse events resolve to G ≤1 within 2 weeks, resume capecitabine treatment at 50% of the previous dosage
Recurrent G2 (fourth episode)* or Recurrent G3 (third episode) or Recurrent G4 (second episode)	Permanently discontinue capecitabine
Patients who continue capecitabine alone without evidence of adverse events G ≥2 during a cycle	Capecitabine dosage may be escalated by 25% greater than the previously administered dose during each subsequent cycle
G3/4 neutropenia	Withhold docetaxel. Resume docetaxel only after ANC ≥1500/mm³; continue capecitabine treatment without interruption
G3/4 neutropenia + any other G2 clinical adverse event	Discontinue capecitabine. Consider hospitalization for management
Neutropenia + fever ≥38°C	
ANC <500/mm³ for >7 days at 75 mg/m² docetaxel	Withhold docetaxel until ANC ≥1500/mm³ and patient is afebrile for ≥48 hours, then resume docetaxel at 55 mg/m²
ANC <500/mm³ for >7 days at 55 mg/m² docetaxel	Permanently discontinue docetaxel

*Except isolated neutropenia

Efficacy (N = 256)

WHO Criteria

Response category	Percent	95% Confidence Interval
Overall response	42%	36–48%
Complete response	5%	2–8%
Stable disease >6 weeks	38%	32–44%
Median time to progression	6.1 months	5.4–6.5 months
12-Month survival	57%	51–63%
Median survival	14.5 months	12.3–16.3 months

Patient Population Studied

Study of 255 patients with metastatic breast cancer with prior anthracycline, no prior docetaxel, and less than 3 prior chemotherapy regimens

Toxicity (N = 251)

NCI of Canada CTC

Toxicity	% G3*	% G4*
Hematologic Toxicity		
Neutropenia[†‡]	5	11
Febrile neutropenia[‡§]	3	13
Nonhematologic Toxicity		
Hand-foot syndrome	24	N/A
Stomatitis	17	0.4
Diarrhea	14	0.4
Nausea	6	—
Fatigue/asthenia	8	0.4
Alopecia	6	—
Laboratory Abnormalities[‡]		
Hyperglycemia	13	1
Hyperbilirubinemia	6.8	2
Elevated ALT/AST	1.6	2.8

*National Cancer Institute of Canada common toxicity criteria scale, except hand-foot syndrome
†Requiring medical intervention; eg, antibiotics, hematopoietic growth factor support. The overall incidence of G3 or G4 adverse events was greatest during the first treatment cycle (38%)
‡Six patients withdrew from further treatment for adverse events, including neutropenia, thrombocytopenia, and increased liver transaminases, each in 1 patient, respectively, and hyperbilirubinemia in 3 patients
§The most common cause of hospitalization was febrile neutropenia (12%)
Dose reductions, treatment interruptions:
• 65% of patients required dose reduction of capecitabine alone (4%), docetaxel alone (10%), or both drugs (51%) for adverse events
• Capecitabine treatment interruption was required in 34% of cycles
• Adverse events, either alone or in combination, most frequently leading to capecitabine treatment interruption, included:
  ▪ Hand-foot syndrome (11.1%)
  ▪ Diarrhea (8.5%)
  ▪ Stomatitis (4.6%)
Note: Deaths classified as probably, possibly, or remotely related to study treatment, during or within 28 days after completing study, occurred in 3 patients (1.2%) in association with enterocolitis, sepsis, and pulmonary edema, each in 1 patient

Therapy Monitoring

Start of each cycle: CBC with leukocyte differential count and platelet counts, LFTs, and serum electrolytes. Consider intracycle assessment in first few cycles

METASTATIC REGIMEN

PACLITAXEL AND GEMCITABINE

Albain KS et al. J Clin Oncol 2008;26:3950–3957

Premedication:

Dexamethasone 10 mg/dose; administer orally for 2 doses 12 hours and 6 hours before paclitaxel (total dose/cycle = 20 mg), *or*

Dexamethasone 20 mg; administer intravenously over 10–15 minutes, 30–60 minutes before paclitaxel (total dose/cycle = 20 mg)

Note:

Dexamethasone doses may be gradually decreased in the absence of hypersensitivity reactions during repeated paclitaxel treatments

Diphenhydramine 25–50 mg administer orally 60 minutes before paclitaxel, *or* administer by intravenous injection 30–60 minutes before paclitaxel

Cimetidine 300 mg (or ranitidine 150 mg, famotidine 20–40 mg, or an equivalent histamine receptor [H_2]-subtype antagonist); administer orally 60 minutes before paclitaxel, *or* cimetidine 300 mg (or ranitidine 50 mg, famotidine 20 mg); administer intravenously over 15–30 minutes, 30–60 minutes before paclitaxel

Paclitaxel 175 mg/m²; administer intravenously in a volume of 0.9% sodium chloride injection (0.9% NS) or 5% dextrose injection sufficient to produce a concentration within the range 0.3–1.2 mg/mL over 3 hours, on day 1 before gemcitabine, every 21 days (total dosage/cycle = 175 mg/m²)

Gemcitabine 1250 mg/m² per dose; administer intravenously in 50–250 mL 0.9% NS over 30–60 minutes for 2 doses on days 1 and 8, every 21 days (total dosage/cycle = 2500 mg/m²)

Supportive Care

Antiemetic prophylaxis

Emetogenic potential is LOW

See Chapter 39 for antiemetic recommendations

Hematopoietic growth factor (CSF) prophylaxis

Primary prophylaxis is NOT indicated

See Chapter 43 for more information

Antimicrobial prophylaxis

Risk of fever and neutropenia is LOW

Antimicrobial primary prophylaxis to be considered:

- Antibacterial—not indicated
- Antifungal—not indicated
- Antiviral—not indicated, unless patient previously had an episode of HSV

See Chapter 47 for more information

Patient Population Studied

Women with locally recurrent or metastatic breast carcinoma after 1 neoadjuvant/adjuvant regimen participated in a multicenter, open-label, phase III trial, in which 266 patients were randomly assigned to receive gemcitabine + paclitaxel and 263 to receive paclitaxel alone. All patients assigned to a treatment arm were analyzed for efficacy on the basis of intention-to-treat, and all who received at least 1 dose of chemotherapy were evaluated for safety

Efficacy (N = 266)

	% Response or Duration	95% CI
Overall response rate	41.4%	35.4–47.3
Complete responses	7.9%	
Partial response	33.5%	

(continued)

Treatment Modifications

Adverse Events	Treatment Modifications
ANC 1000–1499/mm³ or platelets 50,000–99,999/mm³ on days 1 and 8	Proceed with treatment, but decrease gemcitabine dosage by 25%
ANC <1000/mm³ or platelets <50,000/mm³ on day 1	Withhold treatment until ANC is >1000/mm³ and platelets >50,000/mm³, then resume treatment and give filgrastim from day 9 until postnadir ANC >5000/mm³
ANC <500/mm³ on day of treatment, febrile neutropenia during cycle, or ANC <500/mm³ for ≥7 days during cycle	Withhold treatment until ANC is >1000/mm³, then resume treatment with gemcitabine dosage decreased by 25%, and give filgrastim from day 9 until post-nadir ANC >5000/mm³
ANC <500/mm³ on day of treatment (second episode) after decreasing gemcitabine dosage and with filgrastim use	Withhold treatment until ANC is >1000/mm³, then resume treatment with gemcitabine and paclitaxel dosages decreased by 25%, and give filgrastim from day 9 until postnadir ANC >5000/mm³
Platelet count <25,000/mm³ on day of treatment	Withhold treatment until platelet count is >50,000/mm³, then resume treatment with paclitaxel dosage decreased by 25%
G3 nonhematologic adverse events (excluding nausea, vomiting, and alopecia)	Withhold treatment until adverse events recover to G ≤1, then resume treatment with gemcitabine and paclitaxel dosages decreased by 25%
G4 nonhematologic adverse events	Withhold treatment until adverse events recover to G ≤1, then resume treatment with gemcitabine and paclitaxel dosages decreased by 50%
G >2 paresthesias	Discontinue paclitaxel; consider alternative treatment
Symptomatic arrhythmia or heart block >1°	
Other major organ toxicities G >2	
Severe hypersensitivity reaction	

Efficacy (N = 266) *(continued)*

	% Response or Duration	95% CI
Overall response rate, nonvisceral sites only	56.9%	
Overall response rate, visceral sites	35.6%	
Duration of response	9.89 months	8.31–11.73
Median time to progression	6.14 months	5.32–6.70
Progression-free survival	5.9 months	
Median overall survival	18.6 months	

Toxicity (N = 261)

National Cancer Institute Common Toxicity Criteria, version 2.0

	G2 (%)	% G3	% G4
Hematologic Toxicities*			
Neutropenia	13.4	30.3	17.6
Febrile neutropenia	1.1	4.6	0.4
Thrombocytopenia	1.5	5.7	0.4
Anemia	22.2	5	0.8
Nonhematologic Toxicities			
Alopecia	63.6	13.4	3.8
Fatigue[†]	12.3	6.1	0.8
Sensory neuropathy	18.4	5.3	0.4
Motor neuropathy	6.1	2.3	0.4
Myalgia	16.5	4.2	0
Nausea	19.9	1.1	0
Emesis	13.4	1.9	0
Arthralgia	11.5	2.7	0
Diarrhea	8	3.1	0
Stomatitis/pharyngitis	3.8	1.1	0.4
Dyspnea	3.4	1.5[‡]	0.4[‡]
Bone pain	4.2	1.5	0
Laboratory Abnormalities			
Increased ALT	4.2	5	0
Increased AST	6.5	1.5	0

*Treatment delays were most often related to hematologic toxicities
†G3/4 fatigue often not associated with anemia
‡Patients who developed G3/4 dyspnea had active disease in the lungs or pleura

Therapy Monitoring

1. *Start of each cycle:* CBC with leukocyte differential count and platelet count, LFTs, neurologic examination
2. *Before gemcitabine:* CBC with leukocyte differential count and platelet count. Consider intracycle monitoring in early cycles

METASTATIC REGIMEN

IXABEPILONE + CAPECITABINE

Sparano JA et al. J Clin Oncol 2010;28:3256–3263

Premedication:

Diphenhydramine 50 mg or an equivalent histamine receptor [H_1]-subtype antagonist); administer orally 60 minutes before ixabepilone

Ranitidine 150–300 mg (or cimetidine 300 mg, famotidine 20 mg, or an equivalent histamine receptor [H_2]-subtype antagonist); administer orally 60 minutes before ixabepilone

Ixabepilone 40 mg/m^2; administer intravenously in a volume of lactated Ringer injection, or, alternatively, 0.9% sodium chloride injection with sodium bicarbonate (2 mEq/250–500 mL) sufficient to produce an ixabepilone concentration within the range 0.2–0.6 mg/mL over 3 hours on day 1, every 21 days (total dosage/cycle = 40 mg/m^2)

Capecitabine 1000 mg/m^2 per dose; administer orally twice daily with approximately 200 mL water within 30 minutes after a meal for 14 consecutive days on days 1–14 (28 doses), every 3 weeks (total dosage/cycle = 28,000 mg/m^2)

Notes:

• Ixabepilone is a substrate for catabolism by cytochrome P450 (CYP) CYP3A subfamily enzymes

• Concomitant use of ixabepilone with strong CYP3A4 inhibitors or inducers should be avoided

• Grapefruit juice may also increase plasma ixabepilone concentrations and should be avoided

• If a strong CYP3A4 INHIBITOR and ixabepilone must be coadministered, a decrease in ixabepilone dosage to 20 mg/m^2 is predicted to adjust the ixabepilone AUC to the range observed without inhibitors

• If a concomitantly administered strong CYP3A4 inhibitor is discontinued, a period of approximately 1 week should elapse before the ixabepilone dosage is increased to the indicated (unmodified) dosage

• If a strong CYP3A4 INDUCER and ixabepilone must be coadministered (ie, no alternatives are feasible), based on extrapolation from a drug interaction study with rifampin, after a patient has been maintained on a strong CYP3A4 inducer, the dose of ixabepilone may be gradually increased from 40 mg/m^2 to 60 mg/m^2, depending on tolerance, which is predicted to adjust the AUC to the range observed without inducers

  ▪ Proceed cautiously: there are no clinical data with this dose adjustment in patients receiving strong CYP3A4 inducers

  ▪ Patients whose dose is increased >40 mg/m^2 should be monitored carefully for toxicities. If the strong inducer is discontinued, the ixabepilone dosage should be decreased to the (unmodified) dosage indicated without a strong CYP3A4 inducer

• Capecitabine is given for 2 consecutive weeks followed by 1 week without treatment

• Doses are rounded to use combinations of 500-mg and 150-mg tablets that most closely approximate calculated values

• Initial capecitabine dosage should be decreased by 25% in patients with moderate renal impairment (baseline creatinine clearance = 30–50 mL/min [0.5–0.83 mL/s]); ie, a dosage reduction from 1000 mg/m^2 per dose, to 750 mg/m^2 per dose, twice daily. Capecitabine use is contraindicated in persons with severe renal impairment (creatinine clearance <30 mL/min [<0.5 mL/s])

• Although food decreases the rate and extent of drug absorption and the time to peak plasma concentration and systemic exposure (AUC) for both capecitabine and fluorouracil, product labeling recommends giving capecitabine within 30 minutes after the end of a meal because established safety and efficacy data are based on administration with food

Supportive Care

Antiemetic prophylaxis

Emetogenic potential on days with ixabepilone + capecitabine is **LOW–MODERATE**

Emetogenic potential on days with capecitabine alone is **LOW**

See Chapter 39 for antiemetic recommendations

Hematopoietic growth factor (CSF) prophylaxis

Primary prophylaxis is NOT indicated

See Chapter 43 for more information

Antimicrobial prophylaxis

Risk of fever and neutropenia is LOW

  Antimicrobial primary prophylaxis to be considered:

  • Antibacterial—not indicated

  • Antifungal—not indicated

  • Antiviral—not indicated, unless patient previously had an episode of HSV

See Chapter 47 for more information

Diarrhea management

Latent or delayed onset diarrhea:

Loperamide 4 mg orally initially after the first loose or liquid stool, *then*

Loperamide 2 mg orally every 2 hours during waking hours, *plus*

Loperamide 4 mg orally every 4 hours during hours of sleep

• Continue for at least 12 hours after diarrhea resolves

• Recurrent diarrhea after a 12-hour diarrhea free interval is treated as a new episode

(continued)

(*continued*)

- Rehydrate orally with fluids and electrolytes during a diarrheal episode
- If a patient develops blood or mucus in stool, dehydration, or hemodynamic instability, or if diarrhea persists >48 hours despite loperamide, stop loperamide and hospitalize the patient for IV hydration

Alternatively, a trial of **Diphenoxylate hydrochloride** 2.5 mg **with Atropine sulfate** 0.025 mg (eg, Lomotil)

- Initial adult dose is 2 tablets 4 times daily until control has been achieved, after which the dose may be reduced to meet individual requirements. Control may often be maintained with as little as 2 tablets daily
- Clinical improvement of acute diarrhea is usually observed within 48 hours. If improvement of chronic diarrhea after treatment with a maximum daily dose of 8 tablets is not observed within 10 days, control is unlikely with further administration

Hand-foot reaction

For patients who develop a hand-foot reaction, use topical emollients (eg, Aquaphor), topical or orally administered steroids, antihistamine agents (H_1-receptor antagonists), or pyridoxine 50–150 mg/day administer orally

Treatment Modifications

Adverse Events	Treatment Modifications
General Dose Modifications: Ixabepilone and Capecitabine	
On day 1 of repeated cycles ANC <1500/mm³	Withhold treatment until ANC >1500/mm³, then administer dosage administered in previous cycle
On day 1 of repeated cycles platelet count <100,000/mm³	Withhold treatment until platelet count >100,000/mm³, then administer dosage administered in previous cycle
On day 1 of repeated cycles nonhematologic toxicities G ≥2 are present	Withhold treatment until nonhematologic toxicities are G1 or have resolved, then administer dosage administered in previous cycle

Ixabepilone Dose Modifications	
Ixabepilone Dosage Levels	
Dosage level 1	40 mg/m²
Dosage level −1	32 mg/m²
Dosage level −2	25 mg/m²
Transient G3 arthralgia/myalgia or fatigue	Continue same ixabepilone dosage
ANC <500/mm³ for ≥7 days	Reduce ixabepilone dosage by one dosage level
Febrile neutropenia	
Platelet count <25,000/mm³ (G4), or platelets 25,000 to 50,000/mm³ (G3) with bleeding	
G2 neuropathy lasting ≥7 days	
G3 neuropathy independent of duration	
G3 nonhematologic toxicity other than transient G3 arthralgia/myalgia or fatigue	

(*continued*)

Patient Population Studied

Study of 1221 patients with metastatic or locally advanced breast cancer who had prior treatment with anthracyclines and taxanes who were randomly assigned to receive either ixabepilone plus capecitabine (n = 609) or capecitabine alone (n = 612) at 199 sites across 29 countries from November 2003 to August 2006. A total of 1198 patients were treated: 595 with the combination and 603 with capecitabine alone

Treatment Modifications (continued)

Adverse Events	Treatment Modifications
ANC still <1500/mm^3 2 weeks after planned start of cycle	Discontinue ixabepilone treatment
Platelet count still <100,000/mm^3 2 weeks after planned start of cycle	
G3 neuropathy lasting ≥7 days or disabling neuropathy	
Any G4 toxicity	
Hypersensitivity reaction to ixabepilone administration despite H$_1$ and H$_2$ antagonists	In addition to H$_1$- and H$_2$-antihistamines prophylaxis, administer **dexamethasone** 20 mg orally 60 minutes before commencing ixabepilone administration, *or* **Dexamethasone** 20 mg intravenously at least 30 minutes prior to starting ixabepilone administration

Dose Adjustments for Capecitabine

Adverse Event	Dose Modification
First G2 toxicity	Hold capecitabine and resume after adverse events resolve to G ≤1. No change in dosage required
Second G2 toxicity	Hold capecitabine and resume after adverse events resolve to G ≤1. Reduce dosage by 25%
Third G2 toxicity	Hold capecitabine and resume after adverse events resolve to G ≤1. Reduce dosage by 50%
Fourth G2 toxicity	Discontinue capecitabine
First G3 toxicity	Hold capecitabine and resume after adverse events resolve to G ≤1. Reduce dosage by 25%
Second G3 toxicity	Hold capecitabine and resume after adverse events resolve to G ≤1. Reduce dosage by 50%
Third G3 toxicity	Discontinue capecitabine
First G4 toxicity	Hold capecitabine and resume after adverse events resolve to G ≤1. Reduce dosage by 50%
Second G4 toxicity	Discontinue capecitabine
Diarrhea, nausea, and vomiting	Treat symptomatically. Resume previous dosage if toxicity adequately controlled within 2 days after initiation of treatment. If control takes longer, reduce the capecitabine dosage, or if occurs despite prophylaxis, reduce the capecitabine dosage 25 to 50%

Efficacy

RECIST

Efficacy Parameter	Percent or Duration	95% CI
Median overall survival	16.4 months	14.9–17.9 months
Median progression-free survival	6.2 months	5.59–6.77 months
Overall response rate	43.3%	38.7–47.9 months
Complete response	3%	
Partial response	40%	
Progressive disease	12%	
Stable disease	37%	
Month 6 stable disease rate	15%	11.8–18.5%

Toxicity* (N = 595)

NCI-CTCAE

Adverse Event	% G1	% G2	% G3	% G4	% Any Grade
Nonhematologic Abnormality					
Peripheral neuropathy	17	25	24	0.7	66
Peripheral sensory neuropathy†	16	26	22	0.7	65
Peripheral motor neuropathy	3	3	4	0	9
Hand-foot syndrome	21	23	21	NA	64
Nausea	26	20	5	0	51
Diarrhea	22	14	7	0.2	43
Fatigue	16	14	11	0.8	42
Vomiting	18	16	6	0	39
Alopecia	12	29	NA	NA	41
Nail disorder	17	11	4	0	32
Anorexia	17	9	1	0	27
Myalgia	8	10	4	0.2	23
Stomatitis	10	8	2	0	21
Constipation	13	5	0.2	0.2	19
Asthenia	5	8	6	0	19
Arthralgia	6	6	3	0	16
Mucositis	8	4	2	0	13
Hematologic Abnormality					
Leukopenia (N = 591)	10	23	48	15	96
Neutropenia (N = 590)	6	13	34	39	92
Anemia (N = 591)	45	39	4	1	89
Thrombocytopenia (N = 590)	44	8	4	2	59
Febrile neutropenia	0	0.2	5	2	7

*NCI-CTCAE, National Cancer Institute (USA) Common Terminology Criteria for Adverse Events, version 3.0. At: http://ctep.cancer.gov/protocolDevelopment/electronic_applications/ctc.htm [accessed December 7, 2013]
†Included the MedDRA version 9.1 terms of burning sensation, dysesthesia, hyperesthesia, hypoesthesia, neuralgia, neuritis, neuropathy, neuropathy peripheral, neurotoxicity, painful response to normal stimuli, paresthesia, pallanesthesia, peripheral sensory neuropathy, polyneuropathy, and polyneuropathy toxicity

Therapy Monitoring

1. *Before each cycle:* Neurologic examination, CBC with leukocyte differential count and platelet count, serum creatinine, BUN, and LFTs. Consider intracycle assessments in first few cycles

2. *During concomitant use with CYP3A4 inhibitors or inducers:* Frequently monitor CBC with differential and platelet count as means to guide ixabepilone dosage adjustments based on altered pharmacodynamic responses

METASTATIC REGIMEN

TRASTUZUMAB

Esteva FJ et al. J Clin Oncol 2002;20:1800–1808
Leyland-Jones B et al. J Clin Oncol 2003;21:3965–3971
Vogel CL et al. J Clin Oncol 2002;20:719–726

Trastuzumab 4 mg/kg initial (loading) dose; administer intravenously in 250 mL 0.9% sodium chloride injection (0.9% NS), over at least 90 minutes (total initial dosage = 4 mg/kg), *followed at weekly intervals by:*

Trastuzumab 2 mg/kg per dose; administer intravenously in 250 mL 0.9% NS over 30–90 minutes, every week, continually (total dosage/week = 2 mg/kg)

Note: Administration duration may be decreased from 90 to 30 minutes if administration over longer durations is well tolerated

or

Trastuzumab 8 mg/kg initial (loading) dose; administer intravenously in 250 mL 0.9% NS over at least 90 minutes (total initial dosage = 8 mg/kg), *followed 3 weeks later by:*

Trastuzumab 6 mg/kg per dose; administer intravenously in 250 mL 0.9% NS over 30–90 minutes, every 3 weeks, continually (total dosage/3-week cycle = 6 mg/kg)

Note: Administration duration may be decreased from 90 to 30 minutes if administration over longer durations is well tolerated

Supportive Care

Antiemetic prophylaxis
Emetogenic potential is **MINIMAL**
See Chapter 39 for antiemetic recommendations

Hematopoietic growth factor (CSF) prophylaxis
Primary prophylaxis is NOT indicated
See Chapter 43 for more information

Antimicrobial prophylaxis
Risk of fever and neutropenia is LOW
  Antimicrobial primary prophylaxis to be considered:
  • Antibacterial—not indicated
  • Antifungal—not indicated
  • Antiviral—not indicated, unless patient previously had an episode of HSV
See Chapter 47 for more information

Trastuzumab infusion reactions
• A symptom complex most commonly consisting of chills and/or fever may occur in as many as 40% of patients during the first infusion of trastuzumab. These symptoms occur infrequently with subsequent trastuzumab infusions. Other signs and/or symptoms may include nausea, vomiting, pain (in some cases at tumor sites), rigors, headache, dizziness, dyspnea, hypotension, rash, and asthenia. Although the symptoms are usually mild to moderate in severity, infrequently, trastuzumab may need to be discontinued
• When such a symptom complex is observed, it can be treated with or without reduction in the rate of trastuzumab infusion, and:
  ▪ **Acetaminophen** 650 mg; administer orally
  ▪ **Diphenhydramine** 25–50 mg; administer orally or by intravenous injection, and
  ▪ **Meperidine** 12.5–25 mg; administer by intravenous injection every 10 minutes if needed for shaking chills (generally, cumulative doses >50 mg are not needed; use with caution in persons with moderate or more severely impaired renal function)
  ▪ **With or without reduction in the rate of trastuzumab infusion**

Treatment Plan Notes:
• LVEF assessment (MUGA or echocardiography) every 3 months in patients receiving trastuzumab

Patient Population Studied

Vogel CL et al. J Clin Oncol 2002;20:719–726

Study of 84 women with HER2-overexpressing (IHC 3+) metastatic breast cancer with no prior cytotoxic chemotherapy for metastatic disease. Also enrolled were 27 women with HER-2 (IHC 2+) metastatic breast cancer

Treatment Modifications

Adverse Events	Treatment Modifications
Left ventricle ejection fraction <45%, or symptomatic congestive heart failure	Discontinue trastuzumab

Efficacy (N = 84*)

Vogel CL et al. J Clin Oncol 2002;20:719–726

Overall response[†]	35%*
Complete response[†]	8%*
Clinical benefit[‡]	48%*

*Patients with 3+ HER2 overexpression by IHC
[†]>50% of objective responses lasted >12 months
[‡]CR, PR, MR, or stable disease for >6 months

Toxicity

Seidman A et al. J Clin Oncol 2002;20:1215–1221
Vogel CL et al. J Clin Oncol 2002;20:719–726

NCI-CTC

Toxicity	Severity	

Cardiac Toxicity

	Any	NYHA Classes III/IV
Cardiac dysfunction	3–7%	2–4%

Noncardiac Toxicity

	Any	Severe
Pain	59%	8%
Asthenia	53%	7%
Nausea	37%	3%
Fever	36%	2%
Chest pain	25%	3%
Chills	22%	0
Rash	20%	0
Dyspnea	15%	0

Therapy Monitoring

Every 3 to 4 months: Evaluate cardiac ejection fraction

METASTATIC BREAST CANCER

PERTUZUMAB + TRASTUZUMAB + DOCETAXEL

Baselga J et al. N Engl J Med 2012;366:109–119

Trastuzumab 8 mg/kg initial (loading) dose; administer intravenously in 250 mL 0.9% sodium chloride injection (0.9% NS) over at least 90 minutes (total initial dosage = 8 mg/kg), *followed 3 weeks later by:*
Trastuzumab 6 mg/kg per dose; administer intravenously in 250 mL 0.9% NS over 30–90 minutes, every 3 weeks, continually (total dosage/3-week cycle = 6 mg/kg)
Note: Administration duration may be decreased from 90 to 30 minutes if administration over longer durations is well tolerated

Premedication for docetaxel:
Dexamethasone 8 mg/dose; administer orally every 12 hours for 3 days starting on the day before docetaxel administration (total dose/cycle = 48 mg)
Docetaxel 75 mg/m^2; administer intravenously in a volume of 0.9% NS or 5% dextrose injection (D5W) sufficient to produce a docetaxel concentration within the range 0.3–0.74 mg/mL over 60 minutes on day 1, every 3 weeks for at least 6 cycles (total dosage/cycle = 75 mg/m^2)

Pertuzumab 840 mg initial (loading) dose; administer intravenously in 250 mL 0.9% NS over 60 minutes (total initial dose = 840 mg), *followed 3 weeks later by:*
Pertuzumab 420 mg per dose; administer intravenously in 250 mL 0.9% NS over 30–60 minutes, every 3 weeks, continually (total dose/3-week cycle = 420 mg)

Note: Treatment continued until disease progression or the development of adverse effects that could not be effectively managed

Supportive Care
Antiemetic prophylaxis
Emetogenic potential is **LOW**
See Chapter 39 for antiemetic recommendations

Hematopoietic growth factor (CSF) prophylaxis
Primary prophylaxis may be indicated
See Chapter 43 for more information

Antimicrobial prophylaxis
Risk of fever and neutropenia is LOW
Antimicrobial primary prophylaxis to be considered:
- Antibacterial—not indicated
- Antifungal—not indicated
- Antiviral—not indicated unless patient previously had an episode of HSV

See Chapter 47 for more information

Trastuzumab infusion reactions
- A symptom complex most commonly consisting of chills and/or fever may occur in as many as 40% of patients during the first infusion of trastuzumab. These symptoms occur infrequently with subsequent trastuzumab infusions. Other signs and/or symptoms may include nausea, vomiting, pain (in some cases at tumor sites), rigors, headache, dizziness, dyspnea, hypotension, rash, and asthenia. Although the symptoms are usually mild to moderate in severity, infrequently, trastuzumab may need to be discontinued
  - When such a symptom complex is observed it can be treated with or without reduction in the rate of trastuzumab infusion, and:
    - **Acetaminophen** 650 mg orally
    - **Diphenhydramine** 25–50 mg orally or by intravenous injection, and
    - **Meperidine** 12.5–25 mg by intravenous injection every 10 minutes if needed for shaking chills (generally, cumulative doses >50 mg are not needed; use with caution in persons with moderate or more severely impaired renal function)
- Include in treatment plan notes:
  - LVEF assessment (MUGA or echocardiography) every 3 months in patients receiving trastuzumab

Diarrhea management
Latent or delayed onset diarrhea*:
Loperamide 4 mg orally initially after the first loose or liquid stool, *then*
Loperamide 2 mg orally every 2 hours during waking hours, *plus*
Loperamide 4 mg orally every 4 hours during hours of sleep
- Continue for at least 12 hours after diarrhea resolves
- Recurrent diarrhea after a 12-hour diarrhea-free interval is treated as a new episode
- Rehydrate orally with fluids and electrolytes during a diarrheal episode
- If a patient develops blood or mucus in stool, dehydration, or hemodynamic instability, or if diarrhea persists >48 hours despite loperamide, stop loperamide and hospitalize the patient for IV hydration

(continued)

(continued)

Alternatively, a trial of **Diphenoxylate hydrochloride** 2.5 mg **with Atropine sulfate** 0.025 mg (eg, Lomotil)
- Initial adult dose is 2 tablets 4 times daily until control has been achieved, after which the dose may be reduced to meet individual requirements. Control may often be maintained with as little as 2 tablets daily
- Clinical improvement of acute diarrhea is usually observed within 48 hours. If improvement of chronic diarrhea after treatment with a maximum daily dose of 8 tablets is not observed within 10 days, control is unlikely with further administration

*Rothenberg ML et al. J Clin Oncol 2001;19:3801–3807
Wadler S et al. J Clin Oncol 1998;16:3169–3178

Oral care
Prophylaxis and treatment for mucositis/stomatitis
General advice:
- Encourage patients to maintain intake of non-alcoholic fluids
- Evaluate patients for oral pain and provide analgesic medications
- Consider histamine (H_2-subtype) receptor antagonists (eg, ranitidine, famotidine), or a proton pump inhibitor for epigastric pain
- *Lactobacillus* sp.-containing probiotics may be beneficial in preventing diarrhea

Patients with intact oral mucosa:
- Clean the mouth, tongue, and gums by brushing after every meal and at bedtime with an ultrasoft toothbrush with fluoride toothpaste
- Floss teeth gently every day unless contraindicated. If gums bleed and hurt, avoid bleeding or sore areas, but floss other teeth
- Patients may use saline or commercial bland, nonalcoholic rinses
  - Do not use mouthwashes that contain alcohols

If mucositis or stomatitis is present:
- Keep the mouth moist utilizing water, ice chips, sugarless gum, sugar-free hard candies, or a saliva substitute
- Rinse mouth several times a day to remove debris
  - Use a solution of ¼ teaspoon (1.25 g) each of baking soda and table salt (sodium chloride) in 1 quart (~950 mL) of warm water. Follow with a plain water rinse
  - Do not use mouthwashes that contain alcohols
- Foam-tipped swabs (eg, Toothettes) are useful in moisturizing oral mucosa, but ineffective for cleansing teeth and removing plaque
- Advise patients who develop mucositis to:
  - Choose foods that are easy to chew and swallow
  - Take small bites of food, chew slowly, and sip liquids with meals
  - Encourage soft, moist foods such as cooked cereals, mashed potatoes, and scrambled eggs
  - For trouble swallowing, soften food with gravies, sauces, broths, yogurt, or other bland liquids
  - Avoid sharp, crunchy foods; hot, spicy or highly acidic foods (eg, citrus fruits and juices); sugary foods; toothpicks; tobacco products; alcoholic drinks

Patient Population Studied

The Clinical Evaluation of Pertuzumab and Trastuzumab (CLEOPATRA) study was a randomized, double-blind, placebo-controlled, phase 3 trial involving patients with HER2-positive metastatic breast cancer in which the efficacy and safety of pertuzumab versus placebo were evaluated in combination with trastuzumab plus docetaxel as first-line treatment for patients with HER2-positive metastatic breast cancer. It was a randomized, double-blind, placebo-controlled, phase 3 trial involving patients with HER2-positive metastatic breast cancer. Among 808 patients enrolled in the study, 402 were assigned to receive pertuzumab and 406 to receive placebo (control), both in combination with trastuzumab and docetaxel. Eligible patients had locally recurrent, unresectable, or metastatic HER2-positive breast cancer and may have received 1 hormonal treatment for metastatic breast cancer before randomization. Patients may have received adjuvant or neoadjuvant chemotherapy with or without trastuzumab before randomization, with an interval of at least 12 months between completion of the adjuvant or neoadjuvant therapy and the diagnosis of metastatic breast cancer. Median age was 54 y; 78% of patients had visceral involvement, and about 50% of patients had ER-positive and 50% ER-negative disease. Approximately half of the patients had not previously received adjuvant/neoadjuvant chemotherapy, and among them, approximately 10% had received trastuzumab. Patients were stratified according to geographic region (Asia, Europe, North America, or South America) and prior treatment status (prior adjuvant or neoadjuvant chemotherapy vs. no prior treatment)

Efficacy

Overall Response, Independent Review

	Placebo + Trastuzumab + Docetaxel (N = 336)	Pertuzumab + Trastuzumab + Docetaxel (N = 343)
	no. (%)	no. (%)
Objective response	233 (69.3)	275 (80.2)
CR	14 (4.2)	19 (5.5)
PR	219 (65.2)	256 (74.6)
SD	70 (20.8)	50 (14.6)
PD	28 (8.3)	13 (3.8)

Toxicity

Adverse Event	Placebo + Trastuzumab + Docetaxel (N = 397)	Pertuzumab + Trastuzumab + Docetaxel (N = 407)
	no. (%)	
Most Common Events, all grades		
Diarrhea	184 (46.3)	272 (66.8)
Alopecia	240 (60.5)	248 (60.9)
Neutropenia	197 (49.6)	215 (52.8)
Nausea	165 (41.6)	172 (42.3)
Fatigue	146 (36.8)	153 (37.6)
Rash	96 (24.2)	137 (33.7)
Decreased appetite	105 (26.4)	119 (29.2)
Mucosal inflammation	79 (19.9)	113 (27.8)
Asthenia	120 (30.2)	106 (26.0)
Peripheral edema	119 (30.0)	94 (23.1)
Constipation	99 (24.9)	61 (15.0)
Dry skin	17 (4.3)	43 (10.6)
Grade ≥3 Events		
Neutropenia	182 (45.8)	199 (48.9)
Febrile neutropenia	30 (7.6)	56 (13.8)
Leukopenia	58 (14.6)	50 (12.3)
Anemia	14 (3.5)	10 (2.5)
Diarrhea	20 (5.0)	32 (7.9)
Peripheral neuropathy	7 (1.8)	11 (2.7)
Asthenia	6 (1.5)	10 (2.5)
Fatigue	13 (3.3)	9 (2.2)
Left ventricular systolic dysfunction	11 (2.8)	5 (1.2)
Dyspnea	8 (2.0)	4 (1.0)

Treatment Modifications

Adverse Event	Dose Modification
Pertuzumab-related infusion reactions	Slow or interrupt pertuzumab infusion. Consider use of supportive medication to treat symptoms (H_1- and H_2-receptor antagonist antihistamines, steroids) if needed. Reinitiate at a slower rate only when symptoms abate
Serious hypersensitivity	Discontinue immediately. Consider permanent discontinuation of pertuzumab
If trastuzumab is withheld	Pertuzumab also should be withheld
Cardiotoxicity: Left ventricular ejection fraction (LVEF) declines to <40% *or* LVEF between 40 and 45% with ≥10% absolute decrease from pretreatment values	Withhold pertuzumab and trastuzumab for at least 3 weeks. Pertuzumab and trastuzumab treatment may resume if LVEF returns to >45% *or* to 40–45% with <10% absolute decrease below pretreatment values. If after a repeat assessment within ~3 weeks LVEF has not improved (or has declined further), consider discontinuing pertuzumab and trastuzumab unless the benefit of continuing treatment outweighs risks

Dose modifications for organ dysfunction

Hepatic impairment	No adjustment needed
Renal impairment	No adjustment needed

Note: Pertuzumab dose reductions are not recommended

Therapy Monitoring

1. Assess left ventricular ejection fraction at baseline, every 9 weeks during the treatment period, every 6 months in the first year after treatment is discontinued, and annually thereafter for up to 3 years
2. *Day 1 (Every cycle):* CBC with differential and platelet count and serum electrolytes and LFTs

METASTATIC REGIMEN

DOCETAXEL EVERY 3 WEEKS + WEEKLY TRASTUZUMAB

Marty M et al. J Clin Oncol 2005;23:4265–4274

Premedication:

Dexamethasone 8 mg/dose; administer orally twice daily for 3 days, starting on the day before docetaxel administration (total dose/cycle = 48 mg)

Docetaxel 100 mg/m²; administer intravenously in a volume of 0.9% sodium chloride injection (0.9% NS) or 5% dextrose injection sufficient to produce a docetaxel concentration within the range 0.3–0.74 mg/mL over 60 minutes on day 1, every 3 weeks for 6 cycles (total dosage/cycle = 100 mg/m²)

Trastuzumab 4 mg/kg initial (loading) dose; administer intravenously in 250 mL 0.9% NS, over at least 90 minutes (total initial dosage = 4 mg/kg), *followed at weekly intervals by:*

Trastuzumab 2 mg/kg per dose; administer intravenously in 250 mL 0.9% NS over 30–90 minutes, every week, continually until disease progression (total dosage/week = 2 mg/kg)

Notes: Administration duration may be decreased from 90 to 30 minutes if administration over longer durations is well tolerated

Patients who tolerated combination treatment and did not develop disease progression may receive docetaxel for more than 6 cycles

Supportive Care

Antiemetic prophylaxis

Emetogenic potential is **LOW**

See Chapter 39 for antiemetic recommendations

Hematopoietic growth factor (CSF) prophylaxis

Primary prophylaxis is indicated with one of the following:

Filgrastim (G-CSF) 5 mcg/kg per day by subcutaneous injection, *or*

Pegfilgrastim (pegylated filgrastim) 6 mg/0.6 mL by subcutaneous injection for 1 dose

- Begin use from 24–72 hours after myelosuppressive chemotherapy is completed

See Chapter 43 for more information

Antimicrobial prophylaxis

Risk of fever and neutropenia is LOW–INTERMEDIATE

Antimicrobial primary prophylaxis to be considered:

- Antibacterial—consider a fluoroquinolone or no prophylaxis
- Antifungal—not indicated
- Antiviral—not indicated, unless patient previously had an episode of HSV

See Chapter 47 for more information

Trastuzumab infusion reactions

- A symptom complex most commonly consisting of chills and/or fever may occur in as many as 40% of patients during the first infusion of trastuzumab. These symptoms occur infrequently with subsequent trastuzumab infusions. Other signs and/or symptoms may include nausea, vomiting, pain (in some cases at tumor sites), rigors, headache, dizziness, dyspnea, hypotension, rash, and asthenia. Although the symptoms are usually mild to moderate in severity, infrequently, trastuzumab may need to be discontinued

- When such a symptom complex is observed, it can be treated with or without reduction in the rate of trastuzumab infusion, and:

  - **Acetaminophen** 650 mg; administer orally
  - **Diphenhydramine** 25–50 mg; administer orally or by intravenous injection, and
  - **Meperidine** 12.5–25 mg; administer by intravenous injection every 10 minutes if needed for shaking chills (generally, cumulative doses >50 mg are not needed; use with caution in persons with moderate or more severely impaired renal function)

Treatment Plan Notes:

- LVEF assessment (MUGA or echocardiography) every 3 months in patients receiving trastuzumab

Treatment Modifications

Adverse Events	Treatment Modifications
Left ventricle ejection fraction <45%, or symptomatic congestive heart failure	Discontinue trastuzumab
First episode of hematologic or nonhematologic adverse events G ≥3 other than alopecia and anemia	Reduce docetaxel dosage from 100 mg/m² to 75 mg/m²
Second episode of hematologic or nonhematologic adverse events G3 other than alopecia and anemia	Reduce docetaxel dosage from 75 mg/m² to 55 mg/m²

Patient Population Studied

Study of 188 patients with HER2-positive MBC included in an open-label, comparative, randomized, multicenter, multinational trial comparing the efficacy and safety of first-line trastuzumab plus docetaxel *vs.* docetaxel alone

Efficacy (N = 92)

WHO Criteria	
Outcome	Percent or Duration
Overall response rate	61%
Complete response	7%
Partial response	54%
Stable disease	27%
Median duration of response	11.7 months
Median time to progression	11.7 months
Median overall survival*	31.2 months

*Kaplan-Meier estimate

Toxicity (N = 92)

NCI-CTC

Adverse Events	% Total	% G3/4
Nonhematologic Toxicity		
Alopecia	67	10
Asthenia	45	10
Nausea	45	0
Diarrhea	43	5
Peripheral edema	40	1
Paraesthesia	32	0
Vomiting	29	3
Pyrexia	30	1
Constipation	27	2
Myalgia	27	3
Arthralgia	27	4
Rash	24	1
Fatigue	24	3
Mucosal inflammation	23	2
Erythema	23	1
Anorexia	22	2
Headache	21	5
Increased lacrimation	21	1
Epistaxis	20	0
Hematologic Toxicity		
Anemia	—	1
Thrombocytopenia	—	0
Leukopenia	—	20
Neutropenia	—	32
Febrile neutropenia/neutropenic sepsis	—	23

Changes in Left Ventricular Ejection Fraction from Baseline: Worst Value Up to 6 Cycles and Overall

	Worse Up to Cycle 6	Overall
Increase or no change	41	20
Absolute decrease <15%	48	63
Absolute decrease ≥15%	11	17
Absolute value <40%	1	1

NCI-CTC, National Cancer Institute (USA) Common Toxicity Criteria, version 2.0. At: http://ctep.cancer.gov/protocolDevelopment/electronic_applications/ctc.htm [accessed December 7, 2013]

Therapy Monitoring

1. *Every 3 to 4 months:* Evaluate cardiac ejection fraction
2. *Start of each cycle:* CBC with leukocyte differential count and platelet counts, LFTs, and serum electrolytes. Consider intracycle assessment in first few cycles

METASTATIC REGIMEN
WEEKLY DOCETAXEL + TRASTUZUMAB

Esteva FJ et al. J Clin Oncol 2002;20:1800–1808

Initial treatment (first cycle):
Trastuzumab 4 mg/kg (loading dose); administer intravenously in 250 mL 0.9% sodium chloride injection (0.9% NS), over at least 90 minutes 1 day before the first dose of docetaxel is administered (total initial dosage = 4 mg/kg)

Premedication for docetaxel:
Dexamethasone 8 mg/dose; administer orally for 3 doses at approximately 12 hours and 1 hour before docetaxel, and 12 hours after docetaxel administration (total dose during week 1 = 24 mg)
Docetaxel 35 mg/m²; administer intravenously in a volume of 0.9% NS or 5% dextrose injection (D5W), sufficient to produce a final docetaxel concentration within the range 0.3–0.74 mg/mL over 30 minutes, the day after the initial (loading) dose of trastuzumab

Second and subsequent treatments:
Premedication for docetaxel:
Dexamethasone 8 mg/dose; administer orally for 3 doses at approximately 12 hours and 1 hour before docetaxel, and 12 hours after docetaxel administration (total dose during week 1 = 24 mg)
• Initially, dexamethasone is given approximately every 12 hours for 3 doses, starting the evening before docetaxel administration
• If no significant fluid retention or hypersensitivity reactions occur during the first 2 cycles, give dexamethasone 8 mg/dose orally every 12 hours for 2 doses on the day of docetaxel administration, with the first dose given at least 1 hour before docetaxel
• If there is no evidence of fluid retention after a fourth cycle, give a single dose of dexamethasone 8 mg orally just before docetaxel administration

Docetaxel 35 mg/m² per dose; administer intravenously in a volume of 0.9% NS or D5W sufficient to produce a final docetaxel concentration within the range 0.3–0.74 mg/mL over 30 minutes, weekly for 3 consecutive weeks (days 1, 8, and 15), every 4 weeks (total dosage/4-week cycle = 105 mg/m²), *followed by:*
Trastuzumab 2 mg/kg per dose; administer intravenously in 250 mL 0.9% NS over 30–90 minutes, weekly for 3 consecutive weeks (days 1, 8, and 15), every 4 weeks (after an initial 4-mg/kg dose, the total dosage/4-week cycle for the second and subsequent cycles = 6 mg/kg)

Note: Trastuzumab administration duration may be decreased from 90 to 30 minutes if administration over longer durations is well tolerated

Supportive Care
Antiemetic prophylaxis
Emetogenic potential on days with trastuzumab alone is **MINIMAL–LOW**
Emetogenic potential on days with docetaxel is **LOW**
See Chapter 39 for antiemetic recommendations

Hematopoietic growth factor (CSF) prophylaxis
Primary prophylaxis is NOT indicated
See Chapter 43 for more information

Antimicrobial prophylaxis
Risk of fever and neutropenia is LOW
  Antimicrobial primary prophylaxis to be considered:
  • Antibacterial—not indicated
  • Antifungal—not indicated
  • Antiviral—not indicated, unless patient previously had an episode of HSV
See Chapter 47 for more information

Trastuzumab infusion reactions
• A symptom complex most commonly consisting of chills and/or fever may occur in as many as 40% of patients during the first infusion of trastuzumab. These symptoms occur infrequently with subsequent trastuzumab infusions. Other signs and/or symptoms may include nausea, vomiting, pain (in some cases at tumor sites), rigors, headache, dizziness, dyspnea, hypotension, rash, and asthenia. Although the symptoms are usually mild to moderate in severity, infrequently, trastuzumab may need to be discontinued
• When such a symptom complex is observed, it can be treated with or without reduction in the rate of trastuzumab infusion, and:
  ▪ **Acetaminophen** 650 mg; administer orally
  ▪ **Diphenhydramine** 25–50 mg; administer orally or by intravenous injection, and
  ▪ **Meperidine** 12.5–25 mg; administer by intravenous injection every 10 minutes if needed for shaking chills (generally, cumulative doses >50 mg are not needed; use with caution in persons with moderate or more severely impaired renal function)

Treatment Plan Notes:
• LVEF assessment (MUGA or echocardiography) every 3 months in patients receiving trastuzumab

Treatment Modifications

Adverse Events	Treatment Modifications*
ANC <500/mm^3	
Febrile neutropenia	
Platelets <50,000/mm^3	Reduce docetaxel dosage by 5 mg/m^2 per week
G2 nonhematologic adverse events	
G3 nonhematologic adverse events (except fatigue)	Reduce docetaxel dosage by 10 mg/m^2 per week
G3 fatigue	Reduce docetaxel dosage by 5 mg/m^2 per week
Left ventricle ejection fraction <45% or congestive heart failure	Discontinue trastuzumab

*Minimum docetaxel dosage to continue treatment = 20 mg/m^2

Patient Population Studied

Study of 30 women with HER2-overexpressing (FISH+ or IHC 3+) metastatic breast cancer who had not received >3 prior chemotherapy regimens. No limitation on prior hormonal therapy

Therapy Monitoring

1. *Before each docetaxel dose:* CBC with differential and platelet count and LFTs
2. *Every second or third cycle:* Serum electrolytes, calcium, magnesium
3. *Every 3–4 months:* Cardiac ejection fraction

Efficacy (N = 30)

ECOG Criteria	
Overall response	63% (95% CI, 44% to 80%)
Complete response	None
Partial response	63%
Minor response	7%
Stable disease >4 months	20%

Toxicity (N = 30)

NCI of Canada CTC

	G1/2	G3	G4
Hematologic Toxicity			
Neutropenia	49%	16%	10%
Anemia	56%	0	0
Thrombocytopenia	3%	0	0
Febrile neutropenia	0	3%	0
Nonhematologic Toxicity			
Left ventricle dysfunction	26%	3%	0
Diarrhea	60%	6%	0
Alopecia	80%	NR	NR
Fatigue	62%	20%	0
Excessive lacrimation	93%	0	0
Edema	46%	0	0
Pleural effusion	26%	3%	0
Myalgia	60%	NR	NR
Neuropathy	36%	3%	0
Onycholysis	50%	0	0
Hypersensitivity	0	6%	0

NR, Not reported

METASTATIC REGIMEN
TRASTUZUMAB + PACLITAXEL, EVERY 3 WEEKS

Leyland-Jones B et al. J Clin Oncol 2003;21:3965–3971
Slamon DJ et al. N Engl J Med 2001;344:783–792

Initial treatment (first cycle):
Premedication for paclitaxel:
Dexamethasone 20 mg/dose; administer orally for 2 doses at 12 hours and 6 hours before paclitaxel (total dose/cycle = 40 mg)
Diphenhydramine 50 mg; administer by intravenous injection 30–60 minutes before paclitaxel
Cimetidine 300 mg (or **ranitidine** 50 mg, **famotidine** 20 mg, or an equivalent histamine receptor [H_2]-subtype antagonist); administer intravenously in 20–50 mL 0.9% sodium chloride injection (0.9% NS) or 5% dextrose injection (D5W) over 15–30 minutes, 30–60 minutes before paclitaxel
Paclitaxel 175 mg/m²; administer intravenously in a volume of 0.9% NS or D5W sufficient to produce a concentration within the range 0.3–1.2 mg/mL over 3 hours, 24 hours before the first dose of trastuzumab (total dosage = 175 mg/m²)
Trastuzumab 8 mg/kg (loading dose); administer intravenously in 250 mL 0.9% NS over at least 90 minutes, 24 hours after the initial paclitaxel dose (total initial dosage = 8 mg/kg)

Second and subsequent treatments:
Trastuzumab 6 mg/kg per dose; administer intravenously in 250 mL 0.9% NS over 30–90 minutes, on day 1 before paclitaxel, every 3 weeks (total dosage/cycle = 6 mg/kg)
Note: Trastuzumab administration duration may be decreased from 90 to 30 minutes if administration over longer durations is well tolerated
Premedication for paclitaxel:
Dexamethasone 20 mg/dose; administer orally for 2 doses at 12 hours and 6 hours before paclitaxel (total dose/cycle = 40 mg)
Diphenhydramine 50 mg; administer by intravenous injection 30–60 minutes before paclitaxel
Cimetidine 300 mg (or **ranitidine** 50 mg, **famotidine** 20 mg, or an equivalent histamine receptor [H_2]-subtype antagonist); administer intravenously in 20–50 mL 0.9% NS or D5W over 15–30 minutes, 30–60 minutes before paclitaxel
Paclitaxel 175 mg/m²; administer intravenously in a volume of 0.9% NS or D5W sufficient to produce a concentration within the range 0.3–1.2 mg/mL over 3 hours, on day 1 starting 30 minutes after completing trastuzumab administration, every 3 weeks for a total of 6 cycles (total dosage/cycle = 175 mg/m²)

Supportive Care
Antiemetic prophylaxis
Emetogenic potential on days with docetaxel is **LOW**
Emetogenic potential on days with trastuzumab alone is **MINIMAL–LOW**
See Chapter 39 for antiemetic recommendations

Hematopoietic growth factor (CSF) prophylaxis
Primary prophylaxis is NOT indicated
See Chapter 43 for more information

Antimicrobial prophylaxis
Risk of fever and neutropenia is LOW
  Antimicrobial primary prophylaxis to be considered:
  • Antibacterial—not indicated
  • Antifungal—not indicated
  • Antiviral—not indicated, unless patient previously had an episode of HSV
See Chapter 47 for more information

Trastuzumab infusion reactions
• A symptom complex most commonly consisting of chills and/or fever may occur in as many as 40% of patients during the first infusion of trastuzumab. These symptoms occur infrequently with subsequent trastuzumab infusions. Other signs and/or symptoms may include nausea, vomiting, pain (in some cases at tumor sites), rigors, headache, dizziness, dyspnea, hypotension, rash, and asthenia. Although the symptoms are usually mild to moderate in severity, infrequently, trastuzumab may need to be discontinued
• When such a symptom complex is observed, it can be treated with or without reduction in the rate of trastuzumab infusion, and:
  ▪ **Acetaminophen** 650 mg; administer orally
  ▪ **Diphenhydramine** 25–50 mg; administer orally or by intravenous injection, and
  ▪ **Meperidine** 12.5–25 mg; administer by intravenous injection every 10 minutes if needed for shaking chills (generally, cumulative doses >50 mg are not needed; use with caution in persons with moderate or more severely impaired renal function)

Treatment Plan Notes:
• LVEF assessment (MUGA or echocardiography) every 3 months in patients receiving trastuzumab

Treatment Modifications

Nabholtz J-M et al. J Clin Oncol 1996;14:1858–1867

Adverse Events	Treatment Modifications
G3/4 ANC for ≥7 days	Reduce paclitaxel dosage by 25%
Any thrombocytopenia for >7 days	
Febrile neutropenia, documented infection, or hemorrhage	
G3 mucositis	
G3/4 neuropathy	Discontinue paclitaxel
Symptomatic arrhythmia or heart block other than first degree	Discontinue trastuzumab
Left ventricular ejection fraction <45% or NYHA classes III/IV cardiac dysfunction	
Severe hypersensitivity reaction	

Patient Population Studied

Leyland-Jones B et al. J Clin Oncol 2003;21:3965–3971

Study of 92 women with HER2 (IHC 2+, IHC 3+, or FISH+) progressive metastatic breast cancer that had not previously received chemotherapy for metastatic disease

Efficacy (N = 32)

Leyland-Jones B et al. J Clin Oncol 2003;21:3965–3971

WHO Criteria	
Overall response	59%
Complete response	13%
Partial response	47%
Median duration of response	10.5 months

Therapy Monitoring

1. *Every 3 weeks:* CBC with differential and platelet count, LFTs, and serum electrolytes. Consider intracycle assessment in early cycles
2. *Every 3–4 months:* Cardiac ejection fraction

Note

Consider adding pertuzumab in combination with trastuzumab + paclitaxel chemotherapy
Loading dose: **Pertuzumab** 840 mg; administer intravenously in 250 mL of 0.9% NS over 90 minutes after trastuzumab, cycle 1 only (total dose during the first cycle = 840 mg), *followed 3 weeks later by:*
Maintenance doses: **Pertuzumab** 420 mg; administer intravenously in 250 mL of 0.9% NS over 30–60 minutes on day 1 after trastuzumab, every 3 weeks (total dose/cycle = 420 mg)

Datko F et al. Cancer Research 2012;72(24 Suppl 3) [Cancer Therapy & Research Center-American Association of Cancer Research. 35th annual San Antonio Breast Cancer Symposium; poster P5-18–20]

Toxicity (N = 91)

Slamon DJ et al. N Engl J Med 2001;344:783–792

NCI-CTCv2		
Toxicity	% All	% Severe
Hematologic Toxicity		
Leukopenia	24	6
Anemia	14	1
Infection	46	1
Nonhematologic Toxicity		
Any type		
Abdominal pain	34	3
Asthenia	62	8
Back pain	36	8
Chest pain	30	3
Chills	42	1
Fever	47	2
Headache	36	7
Infection	46	1
Pain	60	10
Cardiac dysfunction	13	2*
Digestive Tract		
Anorexia	24	1
Constipation	25	0
Diarrhea	45	1
Nausea	50	3
Stomatitis	10	0
Vomiting	37	9
Musculoskeletal System		
Arthralgia	37	9
Myalgia	38	7
Nervous System		
Paresthesia	47	2
Respiratory system		
Increased coughing	42	0
Dyspnea not related to heart failure	28	1
Pharyngitis	22	0
Skin		
Alopecia	56	26
Rash	38	1

*New York Heart Association classes III or IV

METASTATIC REGIMEN
WEEKLY PACLITAXEL + TRASTUZUMAB

Seidman AD et al. J Clin Oncol 2008;26:1642–1649

Initial treatment (first week)
Trastuzumab 4 mg/kg (loading dose); administer intravenously in 250 mL 0.9% sodium chloride injection (0.9% NS) over at least 90 minutes, 1 day before the first dose of paclitaxel is administered (total dosage during the first treatment week = 4 mg/kg)

Premedication for paclitaxel:
Dexamethasone 10 mg; administer intravenously over 10–15 minutes, 30–60 minutes before paclitaxel
Diphenhydramine 50 mg; administer by intravenous injection 30–60 minutes before paclitaxel
Cimetidine 300 mg (or **ranitidine** 50 mg, **famotidine** 20 mg, or an equivalent histamine receptor [H_2]-subtype antagonist); administer in 20–50 mL 0.9% NS or 5% dextrose injection (D5W) over 15–30 minutes, 30–60 minutes before paclitaxel
Paclitaxel 80–90 mg/m²; administer intravenously in a volume of 0.9% NS or D5W sufficient to produce a concentration within the range 0.3–1.2 mg/mL over 60 minutes (total dosage = 80–90 mg/m²)

Schedule for second and subsequent weeks
Premedication for paclitaxel:
Dexamethasone 10 mg; administer intravenously over 10–15 minutes, 30–60 minutes before paclitaxel
Note: Dexamethasone doses may be gradually reduced in 2- to 4-mg increments if the patient has no hypersensitivity reactions during repeated paclitaxel treatments
Diphenhydramine 50 mg; administer intravenously per push 30–60 minutes before paclitaxel
Cimetidine 300 mg (or **ranitidine** 50 mg, **famotidine** 20 mg, or an equivalent histamine receptor [H_2]-subtype antagonist); administer in 20–50 mL 0.9% NS or D5W over 15–30 minutes, 30–60 minutes before paclitaxel
Paclitaxel 80–90 mg/m² per dose; administer intravenously in a volume of 0.9% NS or D5W sufficient to produce a concentration within the range 0.3–1.2 mg/mL over 60 minutes, every week, continually (total dosage/week = 80–90 mg/m²), *followed by:*
Trastuzumab 2 mg/kg per dose; administer intravenously in 250 mL 0.9% NS over 30–90 minutes, every week, continually (total dosage/week during the second & subsequent weeks = 2 mg/kg)
Note: The duration of trastuzumab administration may be decreased from 90 to 30 minutes if administration over longer durations is well tolerated

Supportive Care
Antiemetic prophylaxis
Emetogenic potential on days with trastuzumab alone is **MINIMAL–LOW**
Emetogenic potential on days with paclitaxel is **LOW**
See Chapter 39 for antiemetic recommendations

Hematopoietic growth factor (CSF) prophylaxis
Primary prophylaxis is NOT indicated
See Chapter 43 for more information

Antimicrobial prophylaxis
Risk of fever and neutropenia is LOW
  Antimicrobial primary prophylaxis to be considered:
- Antibacterial—not indicated
- Antifungal—not indicated
- Antiviral—not indicated, unless patient previously had an episode of HSV

See Chapter 47 for more information

Trastuzumab infusion reactions
- A symptom complex most commonly consisting of chills and/or fever may occur in as many as 40% of patients during the first infusion of trastuzumab. These symptoms occur infrequently with subsequent trastuzumab infusions. Other signs and/or symptoms may include nausea, vomiting, pain (in some cases at tumor sites), rigors, headache, dizziness, dyspnea, hypotension, rash, and asthenia. Although the symptoms are usually mild to moderate in severity, infrequently, trastuzumab may need to be discontinued
- When such a symptom complex is observed, it can be treated with or without reduction in the rate of trastuzumab infusion, and:
  - **Acetaminophen** 650 mg; administer orally
  - **Diphenhydramine** 25–50 mg; administer orally or by intravenous injection, and
  - **Meperidine** 12.5–25 mg; administer by intravenous injection every 10 minutes if needed for shaking chills (generally, cumulative doses >50 mg are not needed; use with caution in persons with moderate or more severely impaired renal function)

Treatment Plan Notes:
- LVEF assessment (MUGA or echocardiography) every 3 months in patients receiving trastuzumab

Treatment Modifications

Adverse Events	Treatment Modifications
ANC <1000/mm³ or platelets <100,000/mm³ on a day of planned treatment	Hold paclitaxel until ANC ≥1000/mm³ and platelets ≥100,000/mm³
If >2 weeks are required for recovery to ANC ≥1000/mm³ and platelets ≥100,000/mm³	Reduce paclitaxel dosage by 20 mg/m²
Platelet nadir count ≤50,000/mm³	
Documented infection	
G2 nonhematologic adverse events	Reduce paclitaxel dosage by 10 mg/m²
G3 nonhematologic adverse events	Hold paclitaxel until toxicity resolves to G ≤2 and reduce paclitaxel dosage by 20 mg/m² during subsequent treatments
Left ventricular ejection fraction <45% or NYHA classes III or IV cardiac dysfunction	Discontinue trastuzumab

Efficacy

Patients	Paclitaxel Dose Frequency	Response (%)	95% CI	OR	95% CI for OR	P Value
All patients (combined)	3-Weekly / Weekly	29 / 42	25–34 / 37–47	1.75	1.28–2.37	0.0004
All patients (limited)	3-Weekly / Weekly	35 / 42	28–41 / 37–47	1.36	0.96–1.23	0.093
HER2-negative (limited)	3-Weekly / Weekly	24 / 42	16–34 / 34–51	2.29	1.27–4.08	0.0063
HER2-negative (limited)	No trastuzumab / Trastuzumab	32 / 39	23–41 / 29–48	1.35	0.78–2.34	0.29
HER2-positive (limited)	3-Weekly / Weekly	59 / 55	46–69 / 45–65	0.99	0.49–1.63	0.71

Toxicity

NCI-CTC

G3 and G4 Hematologic Toxicity by Paclitaxel Dosing (n = 572)

Measure	Treatment Arm	% G3	% G4
WBC	3-Weekly / Weekly	8 / 6	1 / 2
Platelets	3-Weekly / Weekly	2 / 1	0 / 1
Hemoglobin	3-Weekly / Weekly	3 / 5	0 / <1
Granulocytes/bands	3-Weekly / Weekly	10 / 5	5 / 3
Lymphocytes	3-Weekly / Weekly	8 / 15	4 / 4

(continued)

Patient Population Studied

Patients were randomly assigned to paclitaxel 175 mg/m² every 3 weeks or 80 mg/m² weekly. After the first 171 patients, all HER-2–positive patients received trastuzumab; HER-2 non-overexpressers were randomly assigned to receive or not receive trastuzumab, in addition to paclitaxel. A total of 577 patients were treated on 9840 (limited). An additional 158 patients (158 patients from the 175-mg/m² arm of CALGB 9342) were included in analyses, for a total of 735 patients

Therapy Monitoring

1. *Every week:* CBC with differential and platelet count
2. *Every other cycle:* LFTs, serum electrolytes, calcium, and magnesium
3. *Every 3–4 months:* Cardiac ejection fraction

Note

Consider adding pertuzumab in combination with trastuzumab + paclitaxel chemotherapy
Loading dose: **Pertuzumab** 840 mg; administer intravenously in 250 mL of 0.9% NS over 90 minutes after trastuzumab, cycle 1 only (total dose during the first cycle = 840 mg), *followed 3 weeks later by:*
Maintenance Doses: **Pertuzumab** 420 mg; administer intravenously in 250 mL of 0.9% NS over 30–60 minutes on the same day as trastuzumab but after trastuzumab, every 3 weeks (total dose/cycle = 420 mg)

Datko F et al. Cancer Research 2012;72(24 Suppl 3) [Cancer Therapy & Research Center-American Association of Cancer Research. 35th annual San Antonio Breast Cancer Symposium; poster P5-18–20]

Toxicity (continued)

NCI-CTC

G3 and G4 Hematologic Toxicity by Trastuzumab Use (n = 572)

Measure	Trastuzumab	% G3	% G4
WBC	No trastuzumab	8	3
	Trastuzumab	5	<10
Platelets	No trastuzumab	2	<1
	Trastuzumab	0	<1
Hemoglobin	No trastuzumab	5	0
	Trastuzumab	3	<1
Granulocytes/bands	No trastuzumab	7	6
	Trastuzumab	8	2
Lymphocytes	No trastuzumab	15	6
	Trastuzumab	10	2

G3 and G4 Nonhematologic Toxicity by Paclitaxel Dosing Schedule (n = 572)

Toxicity	Treatment	% G3	% G4
Infection	3-Weekly	4	0
	Weekly	5	1
Diarrhea	3-Weekly	3	0
	Weekly	5	0
Dyspnea	3-Weekly	3	1
	Weekly	5	2
Edema	3-Weekly	1	0
	Weekly	5	1
Neurosensory	3-Weekly	12	0
	Weekly	24	<1
Neuromotor	3-Weekly	4	0
	Weekly	9	0
Malaise/fatigue	3-Weekly	5	0
	Weekly	6	<1
Hyperglycemia	3-Weekly	7	1
	Weekly	4	1

NCI, CTC, National Cancer Institute (USA) Common Toxicity Criteria and Common Terminology Criteria for Adverse Events, all versions. At: http://ctep.cancer.gov/protocolDevelopment/electronic_applications/ctc.htm [accessed December 7, 2013]

HER2-POSITIVE ADVANCED BREAST CANCER REGIMEN

ado-TRASTUZUMAB (TRASTUZUMAB EMTANSINE, T-DM1) *OR* LAPATINIB + CAPECITABINE

Verma S et al. N Engl J Med 2012;367:1783–1791

ado-Trastuzumab 3.6 mg/kg; administer intravenously in 250 mL 0.9% sodium chloride injection on day 1, every 21 days (total dosage/cycle = 3.6 mg/kg)

Exposure	Administration Rate	Monitoring
First infusion	Intravenously over 90 minutes	• Patients should be observed closely for infusion-related reactions, especially during the first infusion • Administration should be slowed or interrupted if a patient develops an infusion-related reaction • Permanently discontinue ado-trastuzumab for life-threatening infusion-related reactions
Second and subsequent infusions	• Intravenously over 30 minutes if prior administration were was tolerated • Subsequent doses may be administered at the rate tolerated during the most recently administered treatment	

or

Lapatinib 1250 mg/dose; administer orally, once daily, continually, for 21 consecutive days either at least one hour before or at least one hour after a meal (total dose/21-day cycle = 26,250 mg) *plus*
Capecitabine 1000 mg/m² per dose (maximum planned daily dose = 2000 mg/m²); administer orally within 30 minutes after eating food every 12 hours for 14 consecutive days (28 doses), on days 1–14, every 21 days (total dosage/21-day cycle = 28,000 mg/m²; maximum planned dosage/21-day cycle = 28,000 mg/m²)

Notes:
• Capecitabine is given for 2 consecutive weeks followed by 1 week without treatment
• Doses are rounded to use combinations of 500-mg and 150-mg tablets that most closely approximate calculated values
• In practice, treatment often is begun with capecitabine 1000 mg/m² per dose twice daily for 14 consecutive days on days 1–14, every 3 weeks, because of a high rate of dose reduction with higher dosages (total dosage/cycle = 28,000 mg/m²)
• Initial capecitabine dosage should be decreased by 25% in patients with moderate renal impairment (baseline creatinine clearance = 30–50 mL/min [0.5–0.83 mL/s]); ie, a dosage reduction from 1250 mg/m² per dose to 950 mg/m² per dose, twice daily. Capecitabine use is contraindicated in persons with severe renal impairment (creatinine clearance <30 mL/min [<0.5 mL/s])
• Although food decreases the rate and extent of drug absorption and the time to peak plasma concentration and systemic exposure (AUC) for capecitabine, product labeling recommends giving capecitabine within 30 minutes after the end of a meal because established safety and efficacy data are based on administration with food

Supportive Care (ado-trastuzumab or lapatinib + capecitabine)
Antiemetic prophylaxis
*Emetogenic potential for ado-trastuzumab and for lapatinib + capecitabine is **LOW***
See Chapter 39 for antiemetic recommendations

Hematopoietic growth factor (CSF) prophylaxis
Primary prophylaxis is NOT indicated
See Chapter 43 for more information

Antimicrobial prophylaxis
Risk of fever and neutropenia is LOW
   Antimicrobial primary prophylaxis to be considered:
   • Antibacterial—not indicated
   • Antifungal—not indicated
   • Antiviral—not indicated, unless patient previously had an episode of HSV
See Chapter 47 for more information

Supportive Care (lapatinib + capecitabine only)
Hand-foot reaction (palmar-plantar erythrodysesthesia, PPE)
For patients who develop a hand-foot reaction, use topical emollients (eg, Aquaphor), topical or orally administered steroids, antihistamine agents (H₁-receptor antagonists), or pyridoxine
Pyridoxine may provide relief for discomfort/pain associated with PPE although the mechanism through which this occurs remains unclear
• The suggested pyridoxine starting dose is 50 mg/day, which may be increased to a maximum of 200 mg/day

(continued)

(continued)

Oral care
Prophylaxis and treatment for mucositis/stomatitis
General advice:
- Encourage patients to maintain intake of nonalcoholic fluids
- Evaluate patients for oral pain and provide analgesic medications
- Consider histamine (H_2-subtype) receptor antagonists (eg, ranitidine, famotidine), or a proton pump inhibitor for epigastric pain
- *Lactobacillus* sp.-containing probiotics may be beneficial in preventing diarrhea

Patients with intact oral mucosa:
- Clean the mouth, tongue, and gums by brushing after every meal and at bedtime with an ultrasoft toothbrush with fluoride toothpaste
- Floss teeth gently every day unless contraindicated. If gums bleed and hurt, avoid bleeding or sore areas, but floss other teeth
- Patients may use saline or commercial bland, nonalcoholic rinses
  - Do not use mouthwashes that contain alcohols

If mucositis or stomatitis is present:
- Keep the mouth moist utilizing water, ice chips, sugarless gum, sugar-free hard candies, or a saliva substitute
- Rinse mouth several times a day to remove debris
  - Use a solution of ¼ teaspoon (1.25 g) each of baking soda and table salt (sodium chloride) in 1 quart (~950 mL) of warm water. Follow with a plain water rinse
  - Do not use mouthwashes that contain alcohols
- Foam-tipped swabs (eg, Toothettes) are useful in moisturizing oral mucosa, but ineffective for cleansing teeth and removing plaque
- Advise patients who develop mucositis to:
  - Choose foods that are easy to chew and swallow
  - Take small bites of food, chew slowly, and sip liquids with meals
  - Encourage soft, moist foods such as cooked cereals, mashed potatoes, and scrambled eggs
  - For trouble swallowing, soften food with gravies, sauces, broths, yogurt, or other bland liquids
  - Avoid sharp, crunchy foods; hot, spicy or highly acidic foods (eg, citrus fruits and juices); sugary foods; toothpicks; tobacco products; alcoholic drinks

Efficacy

| | Independent Review | | | |
	Lapatinib Plus Capecitabine (N = 389)	ado-Trastuzumab (N = 397)	Difference	P Value
	no. (%)	no. (%)		
CR or PR	120 (30.8)	173 (43.6)	12.7 (6.0–19.4)	<0.001
CR	2 (0.5)	4 (1.0%)		
PR	118 (30.3)	169 (42.6)		
Duration of CR or PR (months)				
Median	6.5	12.6		
95% CI	5.5–7.2	8.4–20.8		

Patient Population Studied

The EMILIA study, a randomized phase 3 trial, assessed the efficacy and safety of lapatinib plus capecitabine (496 patients) versus ado-trastuzumab (495 patients) in patients with HER2-positive advanced breast cancer previously treated with trastuzumab and a taxane. In both treatment arms, 61% of patients had previously received anthracycline therapy, 41% endocrine therapy, 84% had received trastuzumab, and 39% >1 prior chemotherapy regimen for locally advanced or metastatic disease

Therapy Monitoring

1. *Before each cycle:* CBC with differential and platelet count, serum electrolytes and LFTs
2. *LVEF assessment:* recommended at baseline and repeat serially every 3–4 months for adjuvant treatment, or with the development of cardiac symptoms and/or regimen changes for metastatic treatment

Toxicity

	Lapatinib Plus Capecitabine (N = 488)		ado-Trastuzumab (N = 490)	
	All Grades (%)	G3/4 (%)	All Grades (%)	G3/4 (%)
Diarrhea	389 (79.7)	101 (20.7)	114 (23.3)	8 (1.6)
Palmar-plantar erythrodysesthesia	283 (58.0)	80 (16.4)	6 (1.2)	0
Vomiting	143 (29.3)	22 (4.5)	93 (19.0)	4 (0.8)
Neutropenia	42 (8.6)	21 (4.3)	29 (5.9)	10 (2)
Hypokalemia	42 (8.6)	20 (4.1)	42 (8.6)	11 (2.2)
Fatigue	136 (27.9)	17 (3.5)	172 (35.1)	12 (2.4)
Nausea	218 (44.7)	12 (2.5)	192 (39.2)	4 (0.8)
Mucosal Inflammation	93 (19.1)	11 (2.3)	33 (6.7)	1 (0.2)
Anemia	39 (8.0)	8 (1.6)	51 (10.4)	13 (2.7)
Elevated ALT	43 (8.8)	7 (1.4)	83 (16.9)	14 (2.9)
Elevated AST	46 (9.4)	4 (0.8)	110 (22.4)	21 (4.3)
Thrombocytopenia	12 (2.5)	1 (0.2)	137 (28.0)	63 (12.9)

Treatment Modification for ado-Trastuzumab

ado-Trastuzumab Dose Levels	Dosage
Starting dosage	3.6 mg/kg
First dose reduction	3 mg/kg
Second dose reduction	2.4 mg/kg
Requirement for further dose reduction	Discontinue ado-trastuzumab

Dose delays	If significant related toxicities (other than those described below) have not recovered to G1 or baseline, dose may be delayed for up to 42 days from the last dose. If treatment resumes, it may be at either the same dose level or one dose level lower
Platelet nadir 25,000–50,000/mm^3	Withhold ado-trastuzumab until platelet count recovers to $\geq$75,000/mm^3, then resume treatment at the same dose level
Platelet nadir <25,000/mm^3	Withhold ado-trastuzumab until platelet count recovers to $\geq$75,000/mm^3, then resume treatment with ado-trastuzumab 3 mg/kg every 3 weeks
AST or ALT >2× to $\leq$5× ULN (G2)	Treat at the same ado-trastuzumab dose level
AST or ALT >5× to $\leq$20× ULN (G3)	Withhold ado-trastuzumab until AST and ALT recover to G $\leq$2, then resume ado-trastuzumab with dosage decreased by one dose level
AST or ALT >20× ULN (G4)	Permanently discontinue ado-trastuzumab
Total bilirubin >1.5× to $\leq$3× ULN (G2)	Withhold ado-trastuzumab until total bilirubin recovers to G $\leq$1, then resume ado-trastuzumab at the same dose level
Total bilirubin >3× to $\leq$10× ULN (G3)	Withhold ado-trastuzumab until total bilirubin recovers to G $\leq$1, then resume ado-trastuzumab with dosage decreased by one dose level
Total bilirubin >10× ULN (G4)	Permanently discontinue ado-trastuzumab

(continued)

Treatment Modification for ado-Trastuzumab (*continued*)

ado-Trastuzumab Dose Levels	Dosage
AST or ALT >3× ULN and total bilirubin >2× ULN	Permanently discontinue ado-trastuzumab
Patients diagnosed with nodular regenerative hepatic hyperplasia	Permanently discontinue ado-trastuzumab
Symptomatic CHF (G ≥3 left ventricular systolic dysfunction per NCI CTCAE v3.0)	Discontinue ado-trastuzumab
LVEF <40%	Withhold ado-trastuzumab. Repeat LVEF assessment within 3 weeks. If LVEF <40% is confirmed, discontinue ado-trastuzumab
LVEF 40% to ≤45%, and decrease is ≥10% points from baseline measurement	Withhold ado-trastuzumab. Repeat LVEF assessment within 3 weeks. If LVEF has not recovered to within 10% points from baseline, discontinue ado-trastuzumab
LVEF 40% to ≤45%, and decrease is <10% points from baseline	Continue ado-trastuzumab treatment. Repeat LVEF assessment within 3 weeks
LVEF >45%	Continue treatment with ado-trastuzumab
G3/4 peripheral neuropathy	Withhold ado-trastuzumab until symptoms abate to G ≤2 then resume treatment with ado-trastuzumab
Patients diagnosed with interstitial lung disease or pneumonitis	Permanently discontinue ado-trastuzumab
Life-threatening infusion-related reactions	Permanently discontinue ado-trastuzumab

Notes: ado-trastuzumab dosages should not be re-escalated after a dosage reduction is made

If a planned dose is delayed or missed, it should be administered as soon as possible: Do not wait until the next planned cycle. The schedule of administration should be adjusted to maintain a 3-week interval between doses

Treatment Modifications for Lapatinib

Geyer CE et al. N Engl J Med 2006;355:2733–2743
TYKERB® (lapatinib) tablets, for oral use; product label October 2013. GlaxoSmithKline, Research Triangle Park, NC

Adverse Event	Modification
First occurrence ANC 1000–1500/mm³ or platelet count 50,000–74,999/mm³ (G2 toxicity)	Withhold lapatinib until ANC >1000/mm³ and platelet count is >50,000/mm³, or for up to 14 days. Resume lapatinib at the same dose if toxicity resolves within 14 days, otherwise discontinue lapatinib use
Second occurrence ANC 1000–1500/mm³ or platelet count 50,000–74,999/mm³ (G2 toxicity)	Withhold lapatinib until ANC >1000/mm³ and platelet count is >50,000/mm³, or for up to 14 days. Resume lapatinib with dose decreased to 1000 mg/day if toxicity resolves within 14 days, otherwise discontinue lapatinib use
Any G3/4 toxicities	Withhold lapatinib until adverse events abate to G ≤1 or for up to 14 days. Resume lapatinib with dose decreased to 1000 mg/day if toxicity resolves within 14 days, otherwise discontinue lapatinib use
Recurrent G3/4 toxicities	Permanently discontinue lapatinib
Decreased LVEF G ≥2 per NCI CTCAE v3.0	Permanently discontinue lapatinib
LVEF decreased to less than institutional LLN	Withhold lapatinib for at least 2 weeks. Repeat LVEF assessment, and if LVEF returns to within normal range, resume lapatinib with dosage decreased to 1000 mg/day
Patients with pre-existing severe hepatic impairment (Child-Pugh class C)	Decrease lapatinib dose to 750 mg/day
G ≥3 increase in ALT or AST	Permanently discontinue lapatinib

(*continued*)

Treatment Modifications for Lapatinib (continued)

Adverse Event	Modification
G3 diarrhea, or G1/2 diarrhea with complicating features (moderate to severe abdominal cramping, nausea with significantly decreased oral intake or vomiting [2–5 episodes/24 h], decreased performance status, fever, sepsis, neutropenia, frank bleeding, or dehydration)	Withhold lapatinib until diarrhea decreases to G ≤1. Consider resuming lapatinib treatment at dosage decreased by 20–25% or discontinuing lapatinib
G4 diarrhea	Permanently discontinue lapatinib
Pulmonary symptoms indicative of interstitial lung disease or pneumonitis G ≥3	Permanently discontinue lapatinib
Hypokalemia or hypomagnesemia before starting or during treatment with lapatinib	Correct hypokalemia and hypomagnesemia before starting or continuing lapatinib
Other G2 adverse events	Withhold lapatinib until the adverse condition decreases to G ≤1, then resume lapatinib treatment at dosage decreased by 20–25%
Recurrent G2 and G ≥3 adverse events other than conditions described above	Permanently discontinue lapatinib

ALT, alanine aminotransferase (SGPT); AST, aspartate aminotransferase (SGOT); CHF, congestive heart failure; LLN, lower limit of normal range; LVEF, left ventricular ejection fraction; ULN, upper limit of normal range

NCI, CTCAE, National Cancer Institute (USA) Common Terminology Criteria for Adverse Events, version 3. At: http://ctep.cancer.gov/protocolDevelopment/electronic_applications/ctc.htm [accessed December 7, 2013]

Treatment Modifications for Capecitabine

Adapted from NCI of Canada CTC

Adverse Event	Dose Modification
First G2 toxicity	Hold capecitabine and resume after adverse events resolve to G ≤1. No change in dosage required
Second G2 toxicity	Hold capecitabine and resume after adverse events resolve to G ≤1. Reduce dosage by 25%
Third G2 toxicity	Hold capecitabine and resume after adverse events resolve to G ≤1. Reduce dosage by 50%
Fourth G2 toxicity	Discontinue capecitabine
First G3 toxicity	Hold capecitabine and resume after adverse events resolve to G ≤1. Reduce dosage by 25%
Second G3 toxicity	Hold capecitabine and resume after adverse events resolve to G ≤1. Reduce dosage by 50%
Third G3 toxicity	Discontinue capecitabine
First G4 toxicity	Hold capecitabine and resume after adverse events resolve to G ≤1. Reduce dosage by 50%
Second G4 toxicity	Discontinue capecitabine

Diarrhea, nausea, and vomiting	Treat symptomatically. Resume previous dosage if toxicity is adequately controlled within 2 days after initiation of treatment. If control takes longer, reduce the capecitabine dosage, or if it occurs despite prophylaxis, reduce the capecitabine dosage 25–50%

METASTATIC REGIMEN

WEEKLY VINORELBINE + TRASTUZUMAB

Burstein HJ et al. J Clin Oncol 2001;19:2722–2730
Burstein HJ et al. Cancer 2007;110:965–972
Jahanzeb M et al. Oncologist 2002;7:410–417

Preferred Regimen

First week:

Trastuzumab 4 mg/kg (loading dose); administer intravenously in 250 mL 0.9% sodium chloride injection (0.9% NS) over at least 90 minutes before vinorelbine (total dosage during the first week = 4 mg/kg)

Second and subsequent weeks:

Trastuzumab 2 mg/kg per dose; administer intravenously in 250 mL 0.9% NS over 30–90 minutes before vinorelbine administration, weekly, continually (total dosage during the second and subsequent weeks = 2 mg/kg)

Note: The duration of trastuzumab administration may be decreased from 90 to 30 minutes if administration over longer durations is well tolerated

Every week:

Vinorelbine 25 mg/m^2 per dose; administer by peripheral or central venous access in a volume of 0.9% NS or 5% dextrose injection (D5W) sufficient to produce a concentration within the range 1.5–3 mg/mL over 6–10 minutes after completing trastuzumab administration, weekly, continually (total dosage/week = 25 mg/m^2)

Alternate Regimen

First cycle:

Trastuzumab 4 mg/kg (loading dose); administer intravenously in 250 mL 0.9% NS over at least 90 minutes, on the day before the first dose of vinorelbine is administered

Vinorelbine 30 mg/m^2 per dose; administer by peripheral or central venous access in a volume of 0.9% NS or D5W sufficient to produce a concentration within the range 1.5–3 mg/mL over 6–10 minutes, for 4 doses on days 1, 8, 15, and 22, every 28 days (total dosage/cycle = 120 mg/m^2)

Trastuzumab 2 mg/kg per dose; administer intravenously in 250 mL 0.9% NS over 30–90 minutes for 3 doses on days 8, 15, and 22, before vinorelbine administration, every 28 days (total dosage during the first cycle = 10 mg/kg)

Note: The duration of trastuzumab administration may be decreased from 90 to 30 minutes if administration over longer durations is well tolerated

Second and subsequent cycles

Trastuzumab 2 mg/kg per dose; administer intravenously in 250 mL 0.9% NS over 30–90 minutes for 4 doses on days 1, 8, 15, and 22, before vinorelbine administration, every 28 days (total dosage/cycle = 8 mg/kg)

Note: The duration of trastuzumab administration may be decreased from 90 to 30 minutes if administration over longer durations is well tolerated

Vinorelbine 30 mg/m^2 per dose; administer by peripheral or central venous access in a volume of 0.9% NS or D5W sufficient to produce a concentration within the range 1.5–3 mg/mL over 6–10 minutes for 4 doses on days 1, 8, 15, and 22, every 28 days (total dosage/cycle = 120 mg/m^2)

Supportive Care

Antiemetic prophylaxis

Emetogenic potential on days with trastuzumab alone is **MINIMAL–LOW**

Emetogenic potential on days with vinorelbine is **LOW**

See Chapter 39 for antiemetic recommendations

Hematopoietic growth factor (CSF) prophylaxis

Primary prophylaxis is NOT indicated

See Chapter 43 for more information

Antimicrobial prophylaxis

Risk of fever and neutropenia is LOW

Antimicrobial primary prophylaxis to be considered:

- Antibacterial—not indicated

- Antifungal—not indicated

- Antiviral—not indicated, unless patient previously had an episode of HSV

See Chapter 47 for more information

(continued)

Treatment Modifications

Burstein HJ et al. J Clin Oncol 2001;19:2722–2730
Jahanzeb M et al. Oncologist 2002;7:410–417

Adverse Events	Treatment Modifications
ANC >1250/mm^3 and platelets >100,000/mm^3 on day of treatment	No modification, give 100% doses
G ≥2 neurologic toxicity	Delay vinorelbine dosing 1 week. If neurotoxicity abates to G ≤1, resume vinorelbine with dosage decreased to 15 mg/m^2
ANC 750–1250/mm^3 on day of treatment	Reduce vinorelbine dosage to 15 mg/m^2
Platelets count 50,000–99,000/mm^3 on day of treatment	Reduce vinorelbine dosage to 15 mg/m^2
ANC <750/mm^3 or platelets <50,000/mm^3 on day of treatment	Delay vinorelbine dose until ANC >750/mm^3 and platelets >50,000/mm^3
Treatment delay of ≥2 weeks because of low ANC	Consider adding filgrastim prophylaxis after subsequent treatments
Treatment delay >3–4 weeks because of low ANC	Consider discontinuing treatment
Total bilirubin 2–3 mg/dL (34.2–51.3 μmol/L)	Reduce vinorelbine dosage to 12.5 mg/m^2
Total bilirubin >3 mg/dL (>51.3 μmol/L)	Hold vinorelbine
G3 nonhematologic adverse events	Hold vinorelbine until toxicity resolves to G ≤1
G4 nonhematologic adverse events	Consider discontinuing treatment
Left ventricular ejection fraction <45% or congestive heart failure	Discontinue trastuzumab

(*continued*)

Trastuzumab infusion reactions
- A symptom complex most commonly consisting of chills and/or fever may occur in as many as 40% of patients during the first infusion of trastuzumab. These symptoms occur infrequently with subsequent trastuzumab infusions. Other signs and/or symptoms may include nausea, vomiting, pain (in some cases at tumor sites), rigors, headache, dizziness, dyspnea, hypotension, rash, and asthenia. Although the symptoms are usually mild to moderate in severity, infrequently, trastuzumab may need to be discontinued
- When such a symptom complex is observed, it can be treated with or without reduction in the rate of trastuzumab infusion, and:
  - **Acetaminophen** 650 mg; administer orally
  - **Diphenhydramine** 25–50 mg; administer orally or by intravenous injection, and
  - **Meperidine** 12.5–25 mg; administer by intravenous injection every 10 minutes if needed for shaking chills (generally, cumulative doses >50 mg are not needed; use with caution in persons with moderate or more severely impaired renal function)

Treatment Plan Notes:
- LVEF assessment (MUGA or echocardiography) every 3 months in patients receiving trastuzumab

Patient Population Studied

Burstein HJ et al. Cancer 2007;110:965–972

Study of 81 evaluable women with HER2-overexpressing metastatic breast cancer that had not previously received chemotherapy for advanced disease. Patients were randomized 1:1 to receive either trastuzumab with weekly vinorelbine therapy or weekly taxane therapy (paclitaxel or docetaxel at the investigator's choice). Originally planned for 250 patients, the study was closed because of poor accrual with 81 evaluable patients, including 41 patients who received vinorelbine and 40 patients who received taxane for metastatic disease

Efficacy (N = 40)

Burstein HJ et al. Cancer 2007;110:965–972

RECIST

	Percent or Duration
Overall response rate	51% (95% CI 35–67)
Complete response	12%
Partial response	39%
Stable disease	17%
Progressive disease	0
Unevaluable	31%
Median time to progression	8.5 months
Time to treatment failure	5.8 months

RECIST criteria, v.1.0: Response Evaluation Criteria in Solid Tumors, version 1.0. Therasse P et al. J Natl Cancer Inst 2000;92:205–216

Therapy Monitoring

1. *Weekly:* CBC with differential and platelet count and LFTs
2. *Every 3–4 months:* Cardiac ejection fraction

Toxicity

Burstein HJ et al. Cancer 2007;110:965–972

Toxicity	% G1/2	% G3/4
Hematologic Toxicity		
Neutropenia	17	59
Anemia	58	5
Thrombocytopenia	2	0
Infectious		
Infection with neutropenia	0	0
Infection without neutropenia	2	0
Sepsis	0	2
Nonhematologic Toxicity		
Neurologic/psychiatric		
Neuropathy	44	2
Anxiety	15	0
Ear, nose, throat		
Lachrymation	7	0
Taste alteration	10	0
Cardiac/vascular		
Myocardial infarction	0	2
Heart failure	2	0
Phlebitis	7	0
Dermatologic		
Alopecia	34	0
Rash	12	0
Musculoskeletal		
Arthralgia/arthritis	32	0
Myalgia	20	0
Gastrointestinal		
Constipation	39	2
Diarrhea	29	5
Mucositis	17	0
Nausea	46	5
Vomiting	25	5
General health		
Fatigue	68	12
Fluid retention	10	0
Allergy		
Hypersensitivity reaction	7	2

METASTATIC REGIMEN
CAPECITABINE + TRASTUZUMAB

Bartsch R et al. J Clin Oncol 2007;25:3853–3858

Trastuzumab 8 mg/kg initial (loading) dose; administer intravenously in 250 mL sodium chloride injection (0.9% NS) over at least 90 minutes (total initial dosage = 8 mg/kg), *followed 3 weeks later by:*
Trastuzumab 6 mg/kg per dose; administer intravenously in 250 mL 0.9% NS over 30–90 minutes, every 3 weeks, continually (total dosage/3-week cycle = 6 mg/kg)
Note: Administration duration may be decreased from 90 to 30 minutes if administration over longer durations is well tolerated

Capecitabine 1250 mg/m^2 per dose; administer orally twice daily within 30 minutes after a meal for 14 consecutive days on days 1–14, every 3 weeks (total dosage/cycle = 35,000 mg/m^2)
Notes:
• Capecitabine is given for 2 consecutive weeks followed by 1 week without treatment
• Doses are rounded to use combinations of 500-mg and 150-mg tablets that most closely approximate calculated values
• In practice, treatment often is begun with capecitabine 1000 mg/m^2 per dose twice daily for 14 consecutive days on days 1–14, every 3 weeks, because of a high rate of dose reduction with higher dosages (total dosage/cycle = 28,000 mg/m^2)
• Initial capecitabine dosage should be decreased by 25% in patients with moderate renal impairment (baseline creatinine clearance = 30–50 mL/min [0.5–0.83 mL/s]); ie, a dosage reduction from 1250 mg/m^2 per dose to 950 mg/m^2 per dose, twice daily. Capecitabine use is contraindicated in persons with severe renal impairment (creatinine clearance <30 mL/min [<0.5 mL/s])
• Although food decreases the rate and extent of drug absorption and the time to peak plasma concentration and systemic exposure (AUC) for both capecitabine and fluorouracil, product labeling recommends giving capecitabine within 30 minutes after the end of a meal because established safety and efficacy data are based on administration with food

Supportive Care
Antiemetic prophylaxis
Emetogenic potential on days with capecitabine is **LOW**
Emetogenic potential on days with trastuzumab alone is **MINIMAL–LOW**
See Chapter 39 for antiemetic recommendations

Hematopoietic growth factor (CSF) prophylaxis
Primary prophylaxis is NOT indicated
See Chapter 43 for more information

Antimicrobial prophylaxis
Risk of fever and neutropenia is LOW
  Antimicrobial primary prophylaxis to be considered:
  • Antibacterial—not indicated
  • Antifungal—not indicated
  • Antiviral—not indicated, unless patient previously had an episode of HSV
See Chapter 47 for more information

Diarrhea management
Latent or delayed onset diarrhea:
  Loperamide 4 mg orally initially after the first loose or liquid stool, *then*
  Loperamide 2 mg orally every 2 hours during waking hours, *plus*
  Loperamide 4 mg orally every 4 hours during hours of sleep
  • Continue for at least 12 hours after diarrhea resolves
  • Recurrent diarrhea after a 12-hour diarrhea-free interval is treated as a new episode
  • Rehydrate orally with fluids and electrolytes during a diarrheal episode
  • If a patient develops blood or mucus in stool, dehydration, or hemodynamic instability, or if diarrhea persists >48 hours despite loperamide, stop loperamide and hospitalize the patient for IV hydration

(continued)

Treatment Modifications

Dose Adjustments for Capecitabine

Adverse Event	Dose Modification
First G2 toxicity	Hold capecitabine and resume after adverse events resolve to G ≤1. No change in dosage required
Second G2 toxicity	Hold capecitabine and resume after adverse events resolve to G ≤1. Reduce dosage by 25%
Third G2 toxicity	Hold capecitabine and resume after adverse events resolve to G ≤1. Reduce dosage by 50%
Fourth G2 toxicity	Discontinue capecitabine
First G3 toxicity	Hold capecitabine and resume after adverse events resolve to G ≤1. Reduce dosage by 25%
Second G3 toxicity	Hold capecitabine and resume after adverse events resolve to G ≤1. Reduce dosage by 50%
Third G3 toxicity	Discontinue capecitabine
First G4 toxicity	Hold capecitabine and resume after adverse events resolve to G ≤1. Reduce dosage by 50%
Second G4 toxicity	Discontinue capecitabine
Left ventricular ejection fraction <45% or congestive heart failure	Discontinue trastuzumab

Patient Population Studied

Study of 40 patients with advanced breast cancer. All had prior adjuvant or palliative anthracycline and taxane or vinorelbine treatment; further, a minimum of 1 earlier line of trastuzumab-containing therapy for metastatic disease was obligatory

(*continued*)

Alternatively, a trial of **Diphenoxylate hydrochloride** 2.5 mg **with Atropine sulfate** 0.025 mg (eg, Lomotil)

- Initial adult dose is 2 tablets 4 times daily until control has been achieved, after which the dose may be reduced to meet individual requirements. Control may often be maintained with as little as 2 tablets daily
- Clinical improvement of acute diarrhea is usually observed within 48 hours. If improvement of chronic diarrhea after treatment with a maximum daily dose of 8 tablets is not observed within 10 days, control is unlikely with further administration

Hand-foot reaction

For patients who develop a hand-foot reaction, use topical emollients (eg, Aquaphor), topical or orally administered steroids, antihistamine agents (H_1-receptor antagonists), or pyridoxine 50–150 mg/day; administer orally

Trastuzumab infusion reactions

- A symptom complex most commonly consisting of chills and/or fever may occur in as many as 40% of patients during the first infusion of trastuzumab. These symptoms occur infrequently with subsequent trastuzumab infusions. Other signs and/or symptoms may include nausea, vomiting, pain (in some cases at tumor sites), rigors, headache, dizziness, dyspnea, hypotension, rash, and asthenia. Although the symptoms are usually mild to moderate in severity, infrequently, trastuzumab may need to be discontinued
- When such a symptom complex is observed, it can be treated with or without reduction in the rate of trastuzumab infusion, and:
  - **Acetaminophen** 650 mg; administer orally
  - **Diphenhydramine** 25–50 mg; administer orally or by intravenous injection, and
  - **Meperidine** 12.5–25 mg; administer by intravenous injection every 10 minutes if needed for shaking chills (generally, cumulative doses >50 mg are not needed; use with caution in persons with moderate or more severely impaired renal function)

Treatment Plan Notes:
- LVEF assessment (MUGA or echocardiography) every 3 months in patients receiving trastuzumab

Toxicity

WHO Criteria

Toxicity	% G1	% G2	% G3	% G4
Neutropenia	17.5	15	—	—
Thrombocytopenia	10	—	—	—
Anemia	45	5	—	—
Diarrhea	2.5	20	5	—
Fatigue	—	2.5	—	—
Hand-foot syndrome	10	25	15	—
Nausea/vomiting	5	—	—	—
Stomatitis	2.5	5	—	—

Therapy Monitoring

1. *Days 1 and 10 of the first cycle:* Complete blood count with differential
2. *Day 1 during consecutive cycles:* Blood count with differential if no G3/G4 hematologic toxicity observed

Efficacy

International Union Against Cancer Criteria

	All Patients (N = 40)	Second Line (N = 21)	> Second Line (N = 19)
	Percent or duration		
Overall response rate	20	19	21.1
Complete response	2.5	—	5.3
Partial response	17.5	19	15.8
Stable disease ≥6 months	50	47.6	52.6
Stable disease <6 months	2.5	4.8	—
Progressive disease	27.5	28.6	26.3
Median time to progression	8 months (95% CI: 6.07–9.93)	7 months (95% CI: 2.99–11.01)	8 months 95% CI: 5.94–10.06
Median overall survival	24 months 95% CI: 20.23–27.77		

METASTATIC BREAST CANCER
HORMONAL THERAPY AGENTS

Selective Estrogen Receptor Modulators
Tamoxifen 20 mg daily; administer orally

Selective Estrogen Receptor Downregulator
Fulvestrant 500 mg/treatment; administer by intramuscular injection, 250 mg into each buttock, on days 1, 15, 29, and once monthly thereafter

Aromatase Inhibitors
Anastrozole 1 mg daily; administer orally
Letrozole 2.5 mg daily; administer orally
Exemestane 25 mg daily; administer orally

Progestins
Megestrol Acetate 40 mg 4 times daily; administer orally

LHRH Agonists
Goserelin 3.6 mg implant every 28 days; administer subcutaneously
Goserelin 10.8 mg implant every 3 months; administer subcutaneously

Efficacy

Tamoxifen

Prevention:	50% reduction in breast cancer (invasive and noninvasive) in women at increased risk (5-year risk of 1.66%)
Adjuvant:	50% reduction in recurrence, 28% reduction in mortality
Metastatic:	Response rate 30–70% depending on ER/PR status: ER+/PR+ > ER+/PR− > ER−/PR+

Fulvestrant

Metastatic:	At least equivalent to anastrozole

Anastrozole

Adjuvant:	Superior disease-free survival *vs.* tamoxifen
Metastatic:	Likely superior to tamoxifen

Letrozole

Neoadjuvant:	Superior to tamoxifen
Adjuvant:	Improved DFS when started after 5 years of tamoxifen
Metastatic:	Superior to tamoxifen

Exemestane

Metastatic:	Superior to megestrol acetate

Progestins

Metastatic:	Equivalent to tamoxifen

LHRH Agonists

Adjuvant:	Evidence of efficacy in combination with tamoxifen for premenopausal women
Metastatic:	Evidence of efficacy in combination with tamoxifen for premenopausal women

Baum M et al. Lancet 2002;359:2131–2139
Ellis MJ et al. J Clin Oncol 2001;19:3808–3816
Fisher B et al. J Natl Cancer Inst 1998;90:1371–1388
Goss PE et al. N Engl J Med 2003;349:1793–1802
Kaufmann M et al. J Clin Oncol 2000;18:1399–1411
Klijn JGM et al. J Clin Oncol 2001;19:343–353
Mouridsen H et al. J Clin Oncol 2001;19:2596–2606
Nabholtz JM et al. J Clin Oncol 2000;18:3758–3767
Osborne CK et al. J Clin Oncol 2002;20:3386–3395

Toxicity

Note: Pregnancy is contraindicated with all hormonal therapies

Tamoxifen

	Increase Over Placebo Group
Endometrial cancer	1.39 per 1000 women/year
PE*	0.46 per 1000 women/year
DVT†	0.5 per 1000 women/year
CVA‡	0.53 per 1000 women/year
Cataracts	3.1 per 1000 women/year

	Tamoxifen	Placebo
Hot flashes	45.7%	28.7%
Vaginal discharge	29%	13%

Tamoxifen (ATAC DATA)

Hot flashes	39.7%
Vaginal bleeding	8.2%
Endometrial cancer	0.7%
VTE§	3.5%
Fractures	3.7%
Musculoskeletal	21.3%

Fulvestrant

Toxicities similar to anastrozole without musculoskeletal side effects. Injection-site reaction

Anastrozole (ATAC DATA)

Hot flashes	34.3%
Vaginal bleeding	4.5%
Endometrial cancer	0.1%
VTE§	2.1%
Fractures	5.9%
Musculoskeletal	27.8%

Letrozole

Toxicities similar to anastrozole

Exemestane

Toxicities similar to anastrozole with weight gain

Megestrol

Weight gain/edema
Hyperglycemia
Sedation
Thromboemboli

Goserelin

Hot flashes	70%
Tumor flare	23%
Nausea	11%
Edema	5%

*Pulmonary embolism
†Deep venous thrombosis
‡Cerebrovascular accident
§Venous thromboembolism

Baum M et al. Lancet 2002;359:2131–2139
Fisher B et al. J Natl Cancer Inst 1998;90:1371–1388
Robertson JFR et al. Cancer 2003;98:229–238
Stuart NSA et al. Eur J Cancer 1996;32A:1888–1892

Therapy Monitoring

Tamoxifen
1. LFTs >1 month, then every 3–6 months
2. Serum chemistries and LFTs every 6 months

Fulvestrant
1. Clinic visit at 1 month
2. Serum chemistries and LFTs every 6 months

Anastrozole
1. Clinic visit at 1 month
2. Bone density scan at baseline and every 6–12 months when used as adjuvant therapy
3. Serum chemistries and LFTs every 6 months

Letrozole
1. Clinic visit at 1 month
2. Bone density scan at baseline and every 6–12 months when used as adjuvant therapy
3. Serum chemistries and LFTs every 6 months

Exemestane
1. Clinic visit at 1 month
2. Bone density scan at baseline and every 6–12 months when used as adjuvant therapy
3. Serum chemistries and LFTs every 6 months

Megestrol
1. Clinic visit, serum chemistries, and LFTs at 1 month then every 3–6 months
2. Monitor adrenal function every 3 months
3. *Note:* Consider replacement (or stress dose) steroids with withdrawal or physiologic stress

LHRH Agonists (Goserelin)
1. Clinic visit at 1 month
2. Serum chemistries and LFTs every 6 months

7. Carcinoma of Unknown Primary

David R. Spigel, MD and F. Anthony Greco, MD

Epidemiology

Incidence: Unknown* (Estimated at 30,000–45,000 patients/year)
Median age: Varies by histology (usually sixth decade)
Male to female ratio: M ≅ F

Stage at Presentation
Local/regional: <10%
≥2 sites: >90%

*Due to patient heterogeneity and tumor registry misclassification

Cancer Facts and Figures 2013, the America Cancer Society
Greco FA, Hainsworth JD. In: DeVita VT, Jr, Hellman S, Rosenberg SA, eds. Cancer: Principles & Practice of Oncology, 8th ed. Lippincott; 2008:2363–2388
Hainsworth JD et al. J Clin Oncol 1991;9:1931–1938
Hainsworth JD, Greco FA. N Engl J Med 1993;329:257–263

Pathology

Adenocarcinoma (well differentiated or moderately differentiated)	60%
Poorly differentiated carcinoma/ (± features of adenocarcinoma)	29%
Poorly differentiated malignant neoplasm	5%
Squamous carcinoma	5%
Neuroendocrine carcinoma	1%

Greco FA, Hainsworth JD. In: DeVita VT, Jr, Hellman S, Rosenberg SA, eds. Cancer: Principles & Practice of Oncology, 8th ed. Lippincott; 2008:2363–2388
Hainsworth JD, Greco FA. N Engl J Med 1993;329: 257–263

Work-up

Clinical evaluation
- H&P, including pelvic, breast, and rectal exams
- CBC
- Comprehensive metabolic profile
- Urinalysis
- Occult blood in feces
- Lactate dehydrogenase (LDH)
- Serum human chorionic gonadotropin (HCG)
- Alpha-fetoprotein (AFP)
- Carcinoembryonic antigen (CEA)
- CA 19-9, CA 27–29 (or CA 15-3), CA 125
- Chest/abdominal/pelvic CT

Where appropriate:
- Positron emission tomography (PET)
- Prostate specific antigen (PSA)
- Mammography, bronchoscopy, and panendoscopy (particularly for squamous carcinomas)

Pathologic studies
- Core needle or excisional biopsy preferred over fine-needle aspiration (FNA)/cytology (consider rebiopsy if insufficient material from initial biopsy)
- Immunohistochemistry (IHC) analyses for:
  - PSA in men
  - Estrogen receptor (ER) in women
  - Progesterone receptor (PR) in women
  - HER2/neu overexpression in women
  - CD 117
  - Consider gene signature profiling of tissue of origin

Where appropriate:
- Electron microscopy
- Cytogenetic analysis
- Molecular profiling

Focused Work-up

Presentation	Men	Women
Head and neck or supraclavicular adenopathy	• ENT exam • Chest/abdominal CT • PSA, testicular ultrasound	• ENT exam • Chest/abdominal CT • Mammography, ER/PR • Pathologic evaluation
Axillary adenopathy	• Chest/abdominal CT • PSA	• Chest/abdominal CT • Mammography, ER/PR • (Consider ultrasound or MRI)
Mediastinal involvement	• Chest/abdominal CT • HCG/AFP • PSA	• Chest/abdominal CT • HCG/AFP • Mammography, ER/PR
Chest (effusion and/or nodules) involvement	• Chest/abdominal CT • PSA	• Chest/abdominal/pelvic CT • Mammography, ER/PR • CA 125
Peritoneal involvement	• Chest/abdominal/pelvic CT • PSA	• Chest/abdominal/pelvic CT • Mammography, ER/PR • CA 125
Retroperitoneal mass	• Chest/abdominal/pelvic CT • PSA • HCG/AFP • Testicular ultrasound	• Chest/abdominal/pelvic CT • Mammography, ER/PR • CA 125
Inguinal adenopathy	• Abdominal/pelvic CT • PSA	• Abdominal/pelvic CT • Mammography, ER/PR • CA 125
Hepatic involvement	• Chest/abdominal/pelvic CT • Colonoscopy • AFP • PSA	• Chest/abdominal/pelvic CT • Colonoscopy • AFP • Mammography, ER/PR
Skeletal involvement	• Bone scan • PSA	• Bone scan • Mammography, ER/PR
Brain involvement	• Chest/abdominal CT	• Chest/abdominal CT • Mammography, ER/PR

Greco FA, Hainsworth JD. In: DeVita VT, Jr, Hellman S, Rosenberg SA, eds. Cancer: Principles & Practice of Oncology, 8th ed. Lippincott; 2008:2363–2388

Survival

- 1-Year survival: 35–40%
- 2-Year survival: 15–20%
- 3-Year survival: 10–15%
- 5-Year survival: 10%
- 8-Year survival: < 10%

Survival varies by histology and clinical subsets

Expert Opinion

General: For most patients with CUP who do not fit into a favorable prognostic group and presenting with poor prognostic features and disseminated disease, the prognosis is poor, and resistance to available cytotoxic therapy occurs early. However, survival has improved for a minority of patients with otherwise unfavorable prognostic factors. Empiric regimens were the preferred approach in the past and continue to be acceptable alternatives to offer patients however, emerging data suggest that a more tailored approach to therapy is superior. With the emergence of modern molecular testing to help define CUP subtypes, the focus will shift from empiric combinations to more tailored regimens. Clinical features, immunohistochemical evaluation, and molecular profiling used together are likely to better define CUP subsets. The detailed molecular characterization of these tumors is also likely to suggest appropriate and perhaps more effective targeted therapies. Furthermore, as therapies for known primary cancers improve and become more selective based on biomarkers newer therapeutic approaches should be evaluated in the appropriate CUP subsets as well

Recognizing favorable subsets: Most patients with unknown primary cancer have variable clinical and pathologic presentations making treatment selection somewhat empiric. However, approximately 20% of patients present with recognizable features characteristic of known primary cancers where specific therapies are more established. It is important to recognize these favorable clinical and pathologic subsets when choosing therapy, such as local therapy with curative intent in a patient with isolated neck nodes involved with squamous cell carcinoma or a woman with isolated axillary adenocarcinoma

Empiric therapy: Paclitaxel/carboplatin (± etoposide) and gemcitabine/irinotecan are broad-spectrum regimens that can be used in patients who present without characteristic clinical or pathologic features, particularly in patients with adenocarcinomas. Recently, the combination of oxaliplatin and capecitabine was found to have activity as a salvage treatment for patients with CUP. This regimen should be considered in patients with clinical and pathologic features suggesting a primary site in the gastrointestinal tract

Empiric therapy for unknown primary tumors can also include modern regimens in the appropriate clinical setting. When one's clinical suspicion is NSCLC, despite the absence of a definitive primary site, selecting paclitaxel/carboplatin + bevacizumab or pemetrexed/platinum regimens are appropriate for a patient who is otherwise eligible. Likewise, if the clinical impression is of a primary colorectal malignancy, for example in a patient with hepatic metastases and a negative endoscopic evaluation, choosing infusional fluorouracil and oxaliplatin (FOLFOX) + bevacizumab would be a reasonable option

Tailoring therapy: Advances in imaging (PET/CT) and in our use of immunohistochemistry (TTF-1, CDX2, CK20, CK7, etc.) have helped expand our ability to identify a primary site at diagnosis. However, none of these tests are absolute, and still leave clinicians with some degree of uncertainty when assessing prognosis and selecting treatment. Recently, genomic and proteomic technologies have emerged as additional tools to potentially help identify a tumor's primary origin. These tests analyze which genes are active or inactive in the tumor specimen and compare these genetic signatures with gene profiles from known tumor libraries. Several commercial tests are now available, but still require additional prospective validation. Encouraging preliminary results have been obtained by performing molecular profiling with a reverse transcriptase-polymerase chain reaction (RT-PCR) assay (Cancer Type ID; bioTheranostics, Inc., San Diego, CA). The assay can be performed on formalin-fixed paraffin-embedded biopsy specimens. In a recent blinded study, 15 of the 20 assay predictions (75%) were correct (95% confidence interval, 60–85%), corresponding to the actual latent primary sites identified after the initial diagnosis of CUP. Moreover, in a recent large prospective trial 194 patients with CUP received assay-directed site-specific treatment. The median survival was 12.5 months - and longest in tumor types regarded as clinically more responsive (eg breast, colorectal) when compared with more resistant tumor types (eg biliary, pancreatic). As these diagnostic tests improve, along with our understanding of molecular targets critical to cancer cell growth, we will be better able to select optimal therapies for our patients with unknown primary cancers

Greco FA et al. J Natl Cancer Inst. 2013;105:782–789
Greco FA et al. Oncologist 2010;15:500–506
Hainsworth JD et al. J Clin Oncol 2007;25:1747–1752
Hainsworth JD et al. J Clin Oncol. 2013;31:217–223
Varadhachary GR et al. J Clin Oncol 2008;26:4442–4448

REGIMEN

PACLITAXEL + CARBOPLATIN +/– ETOPOSIDE

Hainsworth JD, Greco FA. J Clin Oncol 1997;15:2385–2393

Premedication against hypersensitivity reactions to paclitaxel:
Dexamethasone 20 mg per dose; administer orally for 2 doses at 12 hours and 4 hours before starting paclitaxel
Diphenhydramine 50 mg; administer by intravenous injection, 30–60 minutes before starting paclitaxel
Cimetidine 300 mg (or equivalent histamine H_2 antagonist); administer intravenously in 25–100 mL 0.9% sodium chloride injection (0.9% NS) or 5% dextrose injection (D5W) over 15–30 minutes, before starting paclitaxel
Dexamethasone 20 mg; administer intravenously over 10–15 minutes, 30 minutes before starting paclitaxel

Paclitaxel 200 mg/m²; administer intravenously diluted in 0.9% NS or D5W to a concentration within the range 0.3 to 1.2 mg/mL, over 1 hour, before starting carboplatin on day 1, every 21 days (total dosage/cycle = 200 mg/m²)

Carboplatin [calculated dose] AUC = 6 mg/mL · min; administer intravenously diluted in 0.9% NS or D5W to a concentration >0.5 mg/mL over 20–30 minutes on day 1, every 21 days (total dosage/cycle calculated to produce an AUC = 6 mg/mL · min)

Etoposide 50 mg per dose; administer orally for 5 doses on days 1, 3, 5, 7, and 9, alternating *with:*
Etoposide 100 mg per dose; administer orally for 5 doses on days 2, 4, 6, 8, and 10 (total dose/cycle = 750 mg)

Supportive Care
Antiemetic prophylaxis
Emetogenic potential on day 1 is **HIGH**. *Potential for delayed symptoms*
Emetogenic potential on days 2 to 10 is **LOW**
See Chapter 39 for antiemetic recommendations

Hematopoietic growth factor (CSF) prophylaxis
Primary prophylaxis is NOT indicated
See Chapter 43 for more information

Antimicrobial prophylaxis
Risk of fever and neutropenia is LOW
  Antimicrobial primary prophylaxis to be considered:
  • Antibacterial—not indicated
  • Antifungal—not indicated
  • Antiviral—not indicated unless patient previously had an episode of HSV
See Chapter 47 for more information

Carboplatin dose is based on a formula described by Calvert et al. to achieve a target area under the plasma concentration versus time curve (AUC)

$$\text{Total carboplatin dose (mg)} = (\text{target AUC}) \times (\text{GFR} + 25)$$

In practice, creatinine clearance (Clcr) is used in place of glomerular filtration rate (GFR). Clcr can be estimated from the equation of Cockcroft and Gault, thus:

$$\text{For males, Clcr} = \frac{(140 - \text{age [years]}) \times (\text{body weight [kg]})}{72 \times (\text{serum creatinine [mg/dL]})}$$

$$\text{For females, Clcr} = \frac{(140 - \text{age [years]}) \times (\text{body weight [kg]})}{72 \times (\text{serum creatinine [mg/dL]})} \times 0.85$$

(continued)

Treatment Modifications

Adverse Event	Dose Modification
Day 21: ANC >1500/mm³ and platelets ≥100,000/mm³	Administer 100% doses
Day 21: ANC <1500/mm³ or platelets <100,000/mm³	Delay treatment 1 week or until ANC >1500/mm³ and platelets >100,000/mm³ Then, retreat at 100% doses
Day 8: ANC ≥1000/mm³ and platelets ≥75,000/mm³	Complete 10 days of etoposide
Day 8: ANC <1000/mm³ *or* platelets <75,000/mm³	Hold days 8, 9, and 10 etoposide doses
Hospitalization for febrile neutropenia	Administer 75% of paclitaxel and carboplatin and give etoposide only on days 1–8 (8 daily doses) during all subsequent cycles
Reversible G3 or G4 nonhematologic toxicity (except for alopecia, nausea, and vomiting)	Decrease the dose of the suspected offending drug(s) by 25% during subsequent cycles

Hematopoietic growth factors may be used as secondary prophylaxis at the discretion of a treating physician, but should not substitute for recommended dose modifications for hematological toxicities

Patient Population Studied

A study of 55 patients with carcinoma of unknown primary site were treated and available for assessment. Responding patients received 4 courses of treatment. The following histologies were included: adenocarcinoma (n = 30); poorly differentiated carcinoma or poorly differentiated adenocarcinoma (n = 21); poorly differentiated neuroendocrine carcinoma (n = 3); and squamous carcinoma (n = 1)

(continued)

Note: On October 8, 2010, the U.S. FDA identified a potential safety issue with carboplatin dosing. By the end of 2010, all clinical laboratories in the United States will use the standardized Isotope Dilution Mass Spectrometry (IDMS) method to measure serum creatinine, which could result in an overestimation of the GFR in some patients with normal renal function. A carboplatin dose calculated from an estimated creatinine clearance based on an IDMS-measured serum creatinine could exceed exposure predicted by the Calvert formula and result in increased drug-related toxicity

Provided actual GFR measurements are made to assess renal function, carboplatin can be safely dosed according to the Calvert formula described in product labeling

If GFR (or Clcr) is estimated using serum creatinine measurements by the IDMS method, the FDA recommended for patients with normal renal function limiting estimated GFR (Clcr) to not more than 125 mL/min for any targeted AUC value

Calvert AH et al. J Clin Oncol 1989;7:1748–1756
Cockcroft DW , Gault MH. Nephron 1976;16:31–41
Jodrell DI et al. J Clin Oncol 1992;10:520–528
Sorensen BT et al. Cancer Chemother Pharmacol 1991;28:397–401
U.S. FDA. Carboplatin dosing. [online] October 8, 2010. Available from http://www.fda.gov/AboutFDA/CentersOffices/OfficeofMedicalProductsandTobacco/CDER/ucm228974.htm [accessed February 26, 2014]

Therapy Monitoring

1. *Weekly:* CBC with differential platelet count
2. *Response evaluation:* After 2 treatment cycles. If objective response or stable disease with symptomatic improvement recorded, administer 2 more cycles for a total of 4 cycles

Notes

1. Responses are similar in adenocarcinoma and poorly differentiated carcinoma
2. This regimen is easier to administer and less toxic than cisplatin-based regimens
3. Toxicity is primarily myelosuppression

Efficacy

Complete response	6%
Partial response	30%
Median actuarial survival	9.1 months
1-Year survival	38%
2-Year survival	19%
3-Year survival	12%
5-Year survival	8%
8-Year survival	6%

Greco FA, Hainsworth JD. In: DeVita VT Jr, Hellman S, Rosenberg SA, eds. Cancer: Principles & Practice of Oncology, 6th ed. Lippincott; 2001:2537–2560

Toxicity (N = 55)

	% G3	% G4
Hematologic		
Leukopenia	56	20
Thrombocytopenia	15	11
Febrile neutropenia	—	13
Nonhematologic		
Nausea/vomiting	7	2
Peripheral neuropathy	7	—
Fatigue	7	—
Arthralgia/myalgia	2	—
Hypersensitivity reaction	—	2

Hainsworth JD, Greco FA. J Clin Oncol 1997;15:2385–2393

REGIMEN

GEMCITABINE + IRINOTECAN

Doss HH et al. Proc Am Soc Clin Oncol 2004;23:354 [Abstract 4167]
Greco FA et al. Proc Am Soc Clin Oncol 2002;21:161a [Abstract 642]
Hainsworth JD et al. Cancer 2005;104:1992–1997

Gemcitabine 1000 mg/m² per dose; administer intravenously in 0.9% sodium chloride injection diluted to a concentration ≥0.1 mg/mL over 30 minutes, for 2 doses on days 1 and 8, every 21 days (total dosage per cycle = 2000 mg/m²)

Irinotecan 100 mg/m² per dose; administer intravenously in 5% dextrose injection diluted to a concentration within the range of 0.12–2.8 mg/mL over 90 minutes, for 2 doses on days 1 and 8, every 21 days (total dosage per cycle = 200 mg/m²)

Supportive Care
Antiemetic prophylaxis
Emetogenic potential is **MODERATE**
See Chapter 39 for antiemetic recommendations

Hematopoietic growth factor (CSF) prophylaxis
Primary prophylaxis is NOT indicated
See Chapter 43 for more information

Antimicrobial prophylaxis
Risk of fever and neutropenia is LOW
Antimicrobial primary prophylaxis to be considered:
- Antibacterial—not indicated
- Antifungal—not indicated
- Antiviral—not indicated unless patient previously had an episode of HSV
See Chapter 47 for more information

Diarrhea management
Latent or delayed onset diarrhea*:
Loperamide 4 mg orally initially after the first loose or liquid stool, *then*
Loperamide 2 mg orally every 2 hours during waking hours, *plus*
Loperamide 4 mg orally every 4 hours during hours of sleep
- Continue for at least 12 hours after diarrhea resolves
- Recurrent diarrhea after a 12-hour diarrhea-free interval is treated as a new episode
- Rehydrate orally with fluids and electrolytes during a diarrheal episode
- If diarrhea persists >48 hours despite loperamide, stop loperamide and hospitalize the patient for IV hydration

Alternatively, a trial of **Diphenoxylate hydrochloride 2.5 mg with Atropine sulfate 0.025 mg** (eg, Lomotil®)
- Initial adult dose is two tablets four times daily until control has been achieved, after which the dose may be reduced to meet individual requirements. Control may often be maintained with as little as two tablets daily
- Clinical improvement of acute diarrhea is usually observed within 48 hours. If improvement of chronic diarrhea after treatment with a maximum daily dose of 8 tablets is not observed within 10 days, control is unlikely with further administration

Persistent diarrhea:
Octreotide 100–150 mcg subcutaneously 3 times daily. Maximum total daily dose is 1500 mcg
Antibiotic therapy during latent or delayed onset diarrhea:
A fluoroquinolone (eg, **Ciprofloxacin** 500 mg orally every 12 hours) if absolute neutrophil count is <500/mm³, with or without accompanying fever in association with diarrhea
- Antibiotics should also be administered if patient is hospitalized with prolonged diarrhea and should be continued until diarrhea resolves

*Rothenberg ML et al. J Clin Oncol 2001;19:3801–3807
Wadler S et al. J Clin Oncol 1998;16:3169–3178
Abigerges D et al. J Natl Cancer Inst 1994;86:446–449

(continued)

Treatment Modifications*

Adverse Event	Dose Modification†
ANC >1500/mm³ *and* platelet count >100,000/mm³	Administer 100% dosage
ANC 1000–1500/mm³ *or* platelet count 75,000–100,000/mm³	Reduce gemcitabine and irinotecan dosages by 25%
ANC <1000/mm³ *or* platelet count <75,000/mm³	Delay treatment 1 week, or until ANC >1000/mm³ *and* platelets >100,000/mm³, then administer both drugs at 75% dosages
G3/4 Diarrhea‡	Hold irinotecan until diarrhea G ≤1; reduce irinotecan dosage to 75% for all subsequent doses
Other reversible G3/4 nonhematologic toxicity	Administer 75% dosage of the offending drug in subsequent courses

*Hematopoietic growth factors may be used as secondary prophylaxis at the discretion of a treating physician, but should not substitute for recommended dose modifications for hematological toxicities
†Parameters for both day 1 and day 8
‡G1/2 diarrhea administer 100% irinotecan dosage

Patient Population Studied

A multicenter community-based trial of 31 patients with previously treated (1 prior regimen) CUP (adenocarcinoma, poorly differentiated carcinoma, poorly differentiated adenocarcinoma, or poorly differentiated neuroendocrine carcinoma) who received gemcitabine + irinotecan every 21 days for 6 cycles

Hainsworth JD et al. Cancer 2005;104:1992–1997

(*continued*)

Acute cholinergic syndrome

Atropine sulfate 0.25–1 mg; administer subcutaneously or intravenously if abdominal cramping or diarrhea develop during or within 1 hour after irinotecan administration

• If symptoms are severe, add as primary prophylaxis at least 30 minutes before irinotecan during subsequent cycles

For irinotecan, acute cholinergic syndrome may be characterized by abdominal cramping, diarrhea, diaphoresis, hypotension, flushing, bradycardia, rhinitis, increased salivation, meiosis, and lacrimation

Therapy Monitoring

1. *Before each cycle:* CBC, serum electrolytes, BUN, creatinine, and LFTs
2. *Response evaluation:* Every 2 cycles

Efficacy (N = 31)

Complete response	2.5%
Partial response	7.5%
Stable disease	41%
Median survival	4.5 months
1-Year survival	25%
2-Year survival	13%

Hainsworth JD et al. Cancer 2005;104:1992–1997

Toxicity (N = 31)

	% G3/4
Hematologic	
Neutropenia	30
Thrombocytopenia	8
Anemia	9
Febrile neutropenia	3
Nonhematologic	
Diarrhea	8
Nausea/vomiting	8
Fatigue	8

REGIMEN

BEVACIZUMAB + ERLOTINIB

Hainsworth JD et al. J Clin Oncol 2007;25:1747–1752

Bevacizumab 10 mg/kg per dose; administer intravenously in 100 mL 0.9% sodium chloride injection for 2 doses on days 1 and 15, every 28 days (total dosage/cycle = 20 mg/kg)

Note: Administration duration for the initial dose is 90 minutes. If administration is well tolerated, the administration duration may be decreased stepwise during subsequent treatments to 60 minutes and, finally, to a minimum duration of 30 minutes

Erlotinib 150 mg/day; administer orally at least 1 hour before or 2 hours after meals, continually (total dose/week = 1050 mg)

Supportive Care
Antiemetic prophylaxis
Emetogenic potential is LOW
See Chapter 39 for antiemetic recommendations

Hematopoietic growth factor (CSF) prophylaxis
Primary prophylaxis is NOT indicated
See Chapter 43 for more information

Antimicrobial prophylaxis
Risk of fever and neutropenia is LOW
   Antimicrobial primary prophylaxis to be considered:
   • Antibacterial—not indicated
   • Antifungal—not indicated
   • Antiviral—not indicated, unless patient previously had an episode of HSV
See Chapter 47 for more information

Diarrhea management
Latent or delayed-onset diarrhea*:
   Loperamide 4 mg orally initially after the first loose or liquid stool, *then*
   Loperamide 2 mg orally every 2 hours during waking hours, *plus*
   Loperamide 4 mg orally every 4 hours during hours of sleep
   • Continue for at least 12 hours after diarrhea resolves
   • Recurrent diarrhea after a 12-hour diarrhea-free interval is treated as a new episode
   • Rehydrate orally with fluids and electrolytes during a diarrheal episode
   • If a patient develops blood or mucus in stool, dehydration, or hemodynamic instability, or if diarrhea persists >48 hours despite loperamide, stop loperamide and hospitalize the patient for IV hydration
   Alternatively, a trial of **Diphenoxylate hydrochloride** 2.5 mg **with Atropine sulfate** 0.025 mg (eg, Lomotil®)
   • Initial adult dose is two tablets four times daily until control has been achieved, after which the dose may be reduced to meet individual requirements. Control may often be maintained with as little as two tablets daily
   • Clinical improvement of acute diarrhea is usually observed within 48 hours. If improvement of chronic diarrhea after treatment with a maximum daily dose of 8 tablets is not observed within 10 days, control is unlikely with further administration

Persistent diarrhea:
   Octreotide 100–150 mcg subcutaneously 3 times daily. Maximum total daily dose is 1500 mcg

Antibiotic therapy during latent or delayed onset diarrhea:
   A fluoroquinolone (eg, **Ciprofloxacin** 500 mg orally every 12 hours) if absolute neutrophil count <500/mm³ with or without accompanying fever in association with diarrhea
   • Antibiotics should also be administered if patient is hospitalized with prolonged diarrhea and should be continued until diarrhea resolves

*Rothenberg ML et al. J Clin Oncol 2001;19:3801–3807
Wadler S et al. J Clin Oncol 1998;16:3169–3178
Abigerges D et al. J Natl Cancer Inst 1994;86:446–449

Treatment Modifications

Adverse Event	Dose Modification
Proteinuria ≥2+ by dipstick examination	Hold bevacizumab and obtain a 24-hour urine
Proteinuria ≥2000 mg/ 24 hours	Hold bevacizumab. Resume after proteinuria decreases to <2000 mg/24 hours
G3/4 bleeding	Hold bevacizumab
Life-threatening hemorrhagic event	Discontinue bevacizumab
G3 hypertension on bevacizumab	Treat using standard antihypertensives
G4 hypertension	Interrupt bevacizumab and begin or advance antihypertensive treatment
G1/2 acneiform skin rash and diarrhea	Treat symptoms. Continue same dose of erlotinib
G3/4 skin toxicity	Stop erlotinib for 1 week or until the toxicity improves to G ≤2 then resume erlotinib at full dose
Recurrent G3/4 skin toxicity	Reduce erlotinib dose to 100 mg daily
G3/4 diarrhea not controlled by using standard schedules of loperamide	Interrupt erlotinib for at least one week or until diarrhea has improved to G ≤2. Erlotinib can then be reinstituted at full dose
Recurrence of G3/4 diarrhea	Interrupt erlotinib for at least one week or until diarrhea has improved to G ≤2. Then, resume erlotinib use with dose decreased to 100 mg daily
Other G3/4 toxicities caused by either of these agents or their combination	The offending agent or agents should be discontinued for 2 weeks or until toxicity has improved to G ≤2. Treatment can be reinstituted at full dose at the discretion of the treating physician

Patient Population Studied

Fifty-one patients with histologically or cytologically confirmed carcinoma of unknown primary site were enrolled in this single cohort, multicenter, phase II trial. Eligible tumor histologies included adenocarcinoma, poorly differentiated adenocarcinoma, and poorly differentiated carcinoma. For study purposes, patients were considered to have carcinoma of unknown primary site if the following diagnostic procedures were unrevealing of a primary site: complete history, physical examination, chemistry profile, CT scans of the chest and abdomen, and directed radiologic work-up of the symptomatic areas. Patients previously treated with either one or two chemotherapy regimens were eligible. In addition, previously untreated patients were eligible if they had advanced liver metastases, predominant bone metastases, or ≥3 visceral sites of metastases (ie, clinical settings in which standard chemotherapy has had relatively little effect). Patients were reevaluated after 8 weeks of treatment; those with objective response or stable disease continued treatment until disease progression

Efficacy*

Complete response	0
Partial response	10%, 95% CI = 3 – 23%
Stable disease	61%
Progressive disease	29%
Median overall survival	7.4 months
1-Year overall survival	33%
Median progression-free survival	3.9 months

*RECIST criteria (Response Evaluation Criteria in Solid Tumors, Therasse P et al. J Natl Cancer Inst 2000;92:205–216)

Therapy Monitoring

1. *Before each dose of bevacizumab:* CBC, serum electrolytes, creatinine, LFTs, and urinalysis
2. *Every month:* History and physical exam
3. After 8 weeks of treatment, evaluate for response by imaging

Toxicity

Toxicity Grade

Toxicity	1/2		3		4	
	No	%	No	%	No	%
Fatigue	21	42	8	16	0	0
Rash	39	78	4	8	1	2
Diarrhea	29	58	4	8	0	0
Nausea/vomiting	22	44	4	8	0	0
Proteinuria	31	62	2	4	1	2
Bleeding	4	8	1	2	0	0
Thrombocytopenia	7	14	1	2	0	0
Pruritus	4	8	1	2	0	0
Stomatitis	14	28	1	2	1	2
Edema	5	10	0	0	0	0
Neutropenia	6	12	0	0	0	0
Hypertension	3	6	0	0	0	0
Hypersensitivity reaction	1	2	0	0	0	0

NCI CTCAE, National Cancer Institute (USA) Common Terminology Criteria for Adverse Events, version 3. At: http://ctep.cancer.gov/protocolDevelopment/electronic_applications/ctc.htm [accessed December 7, 2013]

REFRACTORY OR RECURRENT CARCINOMA OF UNKNOWN PRIMARY REGIMEN
OXALIPLATIN + CAPECITABINE

Hainsworth JD et al. Cancer 2010;116:2448–2454

Oxaliplatin 130 mg/m²; administer intravenously in 250–500 mL 5% dextrose injection over 2 hours on day 1, every 21 days (total dosage/cycle = 130 mg/m²)

Capecitabine 1000 mg/m² per dose; administer orally twice daily (approximately every 12 hours) for 28 doses on days 1–14, every 21 days, (total dose/cycle = 28,000 mg/m²)

Notes:
- Capecitabine is given for 2 consecutive weeks followed by 1 week without treatment
- Doses are rounded to use combinations of 500-mg and 150-mg tablets that most closely approximate calculated values
- Although food decreases the rate and extent of drug absorption and the time to peak plasma concentration and systemic exposure (AUC) for both capecitabine and fluorouracil, product labeling recommends giving capecitabine within 30 minutes after the end of a meal because established safety and efficacy data are based on administration with food

Note: Patients with objective response or stable disease after 2 cycles continued treatment for 6 cycles or until disease progression. Patients who continued to benefit and were tolerating treatment well had the option to receive additional treatment cycles at the discretion of their physician

Note: Leukocyte growth factors are not routinely used during cycle 1, but may be used subsequently as secondary prophylaxis according to standard guidelines

Note: The combination of oxaliplatin and capecitabine has activity as a salvage treatment for patients with CUP. Consider in patients with clinical and pathologic features suggesting a primary site in the gastrointestinal tract

Supportive Care
Antiemetic prophylaxis
Emetogenic potential on day 1 is **MODERATE**
Emetogenic potential on days with capecitabine alone is **LOW**
See Chapter 39 for antiemetic recommendations

Hematopoietic growth factor (CSF) prophylaxis
Primary prophylaxis is NOT indicated
See Chapter 43 for more information

Antimicrobial prophylaxis
Risk of fever and neutropenia is LOW
Antimicrobial primary prophylaxis to be considered:
- Antibacterial—not indicated
- Antifungal—not indicated
- Antiviral—not indicated, unless patient previously had an episode of HSV

See Chapter 47 for more information

Hand-foot reaction (palmar-plantar erythrodysesthesia, PPE)
For patients who develop a hand-foot reaction, use topical emollients (eg, Aquaphor®), topical or orally administered steroids, antihistamine agents (H₁-receptor antagonists), or pyridoxine
Pyridoxine may provide relief for discomfort/pain associated with PPE, although the mechanism through which this occurs remains unclear
- The suggested pyridoxine starting dose is 50 mg/day, which may be increased to a maximum of 200 mg/day

Oral care
Prophylaxis and treatment for mucositis/stomatitis
General advice:
- Encourage patients to maintain intake of non-alcoholic fluids
- Evaluate patients for oral pain and provide analgesic medications
- Consider histamine (H₂-subtype) receptor antagonists (eg, ranitidine, famotidine), or a proton pump inhibitor for epigastric pain
- *Lactobacillus* sp.-containing probiotics may be beneficial in preventing diarrhea

Patients with intact oral mucosa:
- Clean the mouth, tongue, and gums by brushing after every meal and at bedtime with an ultra-soft toothbrush with fluoride toothpaste
- Floss teeth gently every day unless contraindicated. If gums bleed and hurt, avoid bleeding or sore areas, but floss other teeth
- Patients may use saline or commercial bland, non-alcoholic rinses
  - Do not use mouthwashes that contain alcohols

(continued)

(*continued*)

If mucositis or stomatitis is present:
- Keep the mouth moist utilizing water, ice chips, sugarless gum, sugar-free hard candies, or a saliva substitute
- Rinse mouth several times a day to remove debris
  - Use a solution of ¼ teaspoon (1.25 g) each of baking soda and table salt (sodium chloride) in one quart (~950 mL) of warm water. Follow with a plain water rinse
  - Do not use mouthwashes that contain alcohols
- Foam-tipped swabs (eg, Toothettes®) are useful in moisturizing oral mucosa, but ineffective for cleansing teeth and removing plaque
- Advise patients who develop mucositis to:
  - Choose foods that are easy to chew and swallow
  - Take small bites of food, chew slowly, and sip liquids with meals
  - Encourage soft, moist foods such as cooked cereals, mashed potatoes, and scrambled eggs
  - For trouble swallowing, soften food with gravies, sauces, broths, yogurt, or other bland liquids
  - Avoid sharp, crunchy foods; hot, spicy or highly acidic foods (eg, citrus fruits and juices); sugary foods; toothpicks; tobacco products; alcoholic drinks

Hand-foot reaction (palmar-plantar erythrodysesthesia, PPE)
For patients who develop a hand-foot reaction, use topical emollients (eg, Aquaphor®), topical or orally administered steroids, antihistamine agents (H_1-receptor antagonists), or pyridoxine
  Pyridoxine may provide relief for discomfort/pain associated with PPE, although the mechanism through which this occurs remains unclear
- The suggested pyridoxine starting dose is 50 mg/day, which may be increased to a maximum of 200 mg/day
- Patients who develop G1/2 PPE while receiving doxorubicin HCl liposome injection may receive a fixed daily dose of pyridoxine 200 mg. This may allow for treatment to be completed without dosage reduction, treatment delay, or recurrence of PPE

Treatment Modifications

Adverse Event	Dose Modification
ANC <1500/mm³ *or* platelet count <75,000/mm³ on day 1 of a cycle	Delay treatment for 1 week and remeasure blood counts. If, after a 1-week delay, ANC ≥1500/mm³ *and* platelet count ≥75,000/mm³, decrease dosages of both agents by 25% and resume treatment
ANC <1500/mm³ *or* platelet count <75,000/mm³ after a 1-week delay	Delay treatment for 1 additional week and remeasure blood counts. If, after a second 1-week delay, ANC ≥1500/mm³ *and* platelet count ≥75,000/mm³, decrease dosages of both agents by 25% and resume treatment
ANC <1500/mm³ *or* platelet count <75,000/mm³ after a second 1-week delay	Discontinue therapy
Hospitalization for fever and neutropenia	Continue therapy with dosages of both drugs decreased by 25% in subsequent cycles
Neutropenia and fever during a 14-day course of capecitabine	Discontinue capecitabine for remainder of cycle
G2 peripheral neuropathy	Reduce dose of oxaliplatin by 25% during subsequent cycles
G3/4 peripheral neuropathy	Discontinue oxaliplatin; continue single agent capecitabine if patient is benefiting
Laryngopharyngeal dysesthesia during oxaliplatin administration	Increase duration of subsequent oxaliplatin infusions from 2 to 6 hours
G >1 hand-foot syndrome during or after capecitabine	Discontinue remaining capecitabine doses for ongoing cycle Delay starting a subsequent cycle of therapy until the hand-foot syndrome recovers to G ≤1 Give capecitabine during subsequent cycles at dosages decreased by 25%
Hand-foot syndrome G >1 after 2 dose reductions, or requiring delay of >2 weeks for symptoms to resolve	Discontinue capecitabine; continue oxaliplatin in patients benefiting from treatment
Other nonhematologic toxicity G >2	Reduce offending agents dosages by 25% during subsequent courses
Irreversible nonhematologic toxicity, or toxicity that requires treatment delay >2 weeks	Discontinue therapy

Patient Population Studied

Histologically or cytologically confirmed CUP. Eligible tumor histologies included adenocarcinoma, poorly differentiated adenocarcinoma, poorly differentiated carcinoma, squamous carcinoma, and poorly differentiated neuroendocrine carcinoma. Patients were required to have been treated previously with 1 chemotherapy regimen, but could not have previously received oxaliplatin, capecitabine, or fluorouracil. Patients may also have had treatment with 1 immunotherapy or targeted therapy regimen

Previous chemotherapy: Taxane/platinum-based: 30 (63%); bevacizumab/erlotinib: 5 (10%); taxane ± bevacizumab: 3 (6%); irinotecan/gemcitabine: 5 (10%); platinum/etoposide: 2 (4%); others (1 regimen each): 3 (6%)—22 of 31 patients had previously received carboplatin or cisplatin

Best response to previous treatment: Complete: 1 (2%); partial: 11 (23%); stable disease or progression: 33 (69%); unknown: 3 (6%)

Therapy Monitoring

At the beginning of each 21-day cycle, patients seen and examined by physician. Complete blood counts and serum electrolytes, creatinine, LFTs performed Response assessment every 2 cycles

Efficacy* (N = 48)

Complete response	0
Partial response	19%
Stable disease at first evaluation[†]	46%
Remission duration in 9 patients who achieved PR	Median 10 months (range: 2–48 months)
Median progression-free survival	3.7 months
Median overall survival[‡]	9.7 months
1 Year PFS	22%

*RECIST criteria (Response Evaluation Criteria in Solid Tumors, Therasse P et al. J Natl Cancer Inst 2000;92:205–216)
[†]8/22 with SD had SD >3 months, and 4/22 had SD >6 months
[‡]28 patients (58%) subsequently received further treatment for CUP

Note: Patients received a median of 12 weeks (4 cycles) of treatment (range: 3–66 weeks). Fifteen patients completed ≥6 cycles with oxaliplatin + capecitabine

Toxicity (N = 48 patients; 209 Treatment Courses)*

	% G3	% G4
Hematologic		
Neutropenia	3 (6%)	—
Thrombocytopenia	4 (8%)	2 (4%)
Anemia	—	1 (2%)
Febrile neutropenia	—	1 (2%)
Nonhematologic		
Nausea/vomiting	24 (50%)	2 (4%)
Dehydration	9 (19%)	—
Diarrhea	2 (4%)	1 (2%)
Peripheral neuropathy	2 (4%)	—
Mucositis	2 (4%)	—
Treatment-related hospitalizations	13 (27%)	
Treatment-related deaths	—	
Treatment discontinued for toxicity	6 (12.5%)	

*NCI CTCAE, National Cancer Institute (USA) Common Terminology Criteria for Adverse Events, version 3. At: http://ctep.cancer.gov/protocolDevelopment/electronic_applications/ctc.htm [accessed December 7, 2013]

8. Cervical Cancer

Peter G. Rose, MD

Epidemiology

Incidence:	12,360 (Estimated new cases for 2014 in the United States)
	7.9 per 100,000 women per year
Deaths:	Estimated 4020 in 2014
Median age:	49 years

Stage at Presentation

Localized:	55%
Regional:	32%
Distant:	8%
Unstaged:	6%

Siegel R et al. CA Cancer J Clin 2013;63:11–30
Surveillance, Epidemiology and End Results (SEER) Program. Available from: <http://seer.cancer.gov>; Accessed 2013

Work-up

Stage IA/Stage IB1:	• H&P
	• CBC with platelet count, LFTs, BUN, creatinine
	• Cervical biopsy (pathologic review)
	• Cone biopsy as indicated
	• Chest x-ray, intravenous pyelogram, for IB1 CT/MRI ± PET ± lymphangiogram
Stage IB2 or greater:	• Chest x-ray, intravenous pyelogram, or CT/MRI ± PET ± lymphangiogram
	• Consider examination under anesthesia
Stages III/IV:	• Consider cystoscopy/proctoscopy

Pathology

Squamous cell carcinomas • Large cell, keratinizing • Large cell, nonkeratinizing • Small cell (not neuroendocrine) • Verrucous carcinoma	75–80%
Adenocarcinomas • Adenoma malignum • Mucinous • Papillary • Endometrioid • Clear cell • Adenoid cystic	17%
Adenosquamous	6%
Glassy cell carcinoma	Rare
Neuroendocrine small cell carcinoma	Rare

Galic V et al. Gynecol Oncol. 2012;125:287–291
Hunter RD. In: Souhami RL, Tannock I, Hohenberger P, Horiot J-C, eds. Oxford Textbook of Oncology, 2nd ed. New York: Oxford University Press; 2002:1835–1837

Histologic Grade

Gx	Cannot be assessed
G1	Well differentiated
G2	Moderately differentiated
G3	Poorly differentiated
G4	Undifferentiated

Staging

Primary Tumor (T)

TNM Category	FIGO Stage	
TX		Primary tumor cannot be assessed
T0		No evidence of primary tumor
Tis	*	Carcinoma *in situ* (preinvasive carcinoma)
T1	I	Cervical carcinoma confined to uterus (extension to corpus should be disregarded)
T1a[†]	IA	Invasive carcinoma diagnosed only by microscopy. Stromal invasion with a maximum depth of 5.0 mm measured from the base of the epithelium and a horizontal spread of 7.0 mm or less. Vascular space involvement, venous or lymphatic, does not affect classification
T1a1	IA1	Measured stromal invasion 3.0 mm or less in depth and 7.0 mm or less in horizontal spread
T1a2	IA2	Measured stromal invasion more than 3.0 mm and not more than 5.0 mm with a horizontal spread 7.0 mm or less
T1b	IB	Clinically visible lesion confined to the cervix or microscopic lesion greater than T1a/IA2
T1b1	IB1	Clinically visible lesion 4.0 cm or less in greatest dimension
T1b2	IB2	Clinically visible lesion more than 4.0 cm in greatest dimension
T2	II	Cervical carcinoma invades beyond uterus but not to pelvic wall or to lower third of vagina
T2a	IIA	Tumor without parametrial invasion
T2a1	IIA1	Clinically visible lesion 4.0 cm or less in greatest dimension
T2a2	IIA2	Clinically visible lesion more than 4.0 cm in greatest dimension
T2b	IIB	Tumor with parametrial invasion
T3	III	Tumor extends to pelvic wall and/or involves lower third of vagina, and/or causes hydronephrosis or non-functioning kidney
T3a	IIIA	Tumor involves lower third of vagina, no extension to pelvic wall
T3b	IIIB	Tumor extends to pelvic wall and/or causes hydronephrosis or non-functioning kidney
T4	IVA	Tumor invades mucosa of bladder or rectum, and/or extends beyond true pelvis (bullous edema is not sufficient to classify a tumor as T4)

*FIGO staging no longer includes Stage 0 (Tis)
[†]All macroscopically visible lesions—even with superficial invasion—are T1b/IB

Regional Lymph Nodes (N)

TNM Category	FIGO Stage	
NX		Regional lymph nodes cannot be assessed
N0		No regional lymph node metastasis
N1	IIIB	Regional lymph node metastasis

Distant Metastasis (M)

TNM Category	FIGO Stage	
		No distant metastasis (no pathologic M0; use clinical M to complete stage group)
M1	IVB	Distant metastasis (including peritoneal spread, involvement of supraclavicular or mediastinal lymph nodes, lung, liver, or bone)

(continued)

Group	T	N	M
Stage 0*	Tis	N0	M0
Stage I	T1	N0	M0
Stage IA	T1a	N0	M0
Stage IA1	T1a1	N0	M0
Stage IA2	T1a2	N0	M0
Stage IB	T1b	N0	M0
Stage IB1	T1b1	N0	M0
Stage IB2	T1b2	N0	M0
Stage II	T2	N0	M0
Stage IIA	T2a	N0	M0
Stage IIA1	T2a1	N0	M0
Stage IIA1	T2a2	N0	M0
Stage IIB	T2b	N0	M0
Stage III	T3	N0	M0
Stage IIIA	T3a	N0	M0
Stage IIIB	T3b	Any N	M0
	T1-3	N1	M0
Stage IVA	T4 Any	N	M0
Stage IVB	Any T	Any N	M1

*FIGO no longer includes Stage 0 (Tis)

Edge SB, Byrd DR, Compton CC, Fritz AG, Greene FL, Trotti A, editors. AJCC Cancer Staging Manual. 7th ed. New York: Springer; 2010

Overall 5-Year Survival Relative to FIGO* Disease Stage

Stage	% Survival
IA1	94.6
IA2	92.6
IB1	90.4
IB2	79.8
IIA	76
IIB	73.3
IIIA	50.5
IIIB	46.4
IVA	29.6
IVB	22

*International Federation of Gynecology and Obstetrics

Expert Opinion

1. The use of concurrent chemotherapy and radiation has reduced the overall mortality rate by nearly 50%

2. Concurrent chemoradiation should be given to women with high-risk local disease or regionally advanced disease

3. In cervical cancer, survival rates and rates of local control appear to correlate with radiation dose and the time of administration. Better results are achieved with higher radiation doses and shorter periods of administration

4. Chemotherapy agents with single-agent activity include:

   • **Cisplatin:** Considered the most active drug with response rates of 20–30%. At a dosage of 50 mg/m², cisplatin remains the platinum compound of choice in chemotherapy naive patients based on a randomized trial performed by the Japanese GOG despite less toxicity with carboplatin

   • **Paclitaxel:** 17% response rate in GOG trial (McGuire WP et al. J Clin Oncol 1996;14:792–795)

   • **Vinorelbine:** 18% response rate in patients with recurrent/metastatic carcinoma of the cervix (Morris M et al. J Clin Oncol 1998;16:1094–1098; Lacava JA et al. J Clin Oncol 1997;15:604–609); and 45% response rate in patients with previously untreated, locally advanced cervical cancer (Lhommé et al. Eur J Cancer 2000;36:194–199)

   • **Toptecan:** 18.6% response rate in advanced, recurrent, or persistent squamous cell carcinoma of the uterine cervix (Muderspach LI et al. Gynecol Oncol 2001;81:213–215)

   • **Gemcitabine:** 11–18% response rate in patients with advanced disease with symptomatic relief in 69–90% of patients (Goedhals L et al. Proc Am Soc Clin Oncol 1996;15:296 [abstract 819]; Hansen HH. Ann Oncol 1996;7[Suppl 1]:29 [abstract 058])

   • **Irinotecan:** 13.3% response rate in patients with recurrent squamous carcinoma of the cervix (Look KY et al. Gynecol Oncol 1998;70:334–338)

   • **Ifosfamide:** Active in patients who have not received prior chemotherapy with response rates of 16–40% (Coleman RE et al. Cancer Chemother Pharmacol 1986;18:280–283; Meanwell CA et al. Cancer Treat Rep 1986;70:727–730; Sutton GP et al. Am J Obstet 1993;168:805–807)

   • **Nab paclitaxel:** Active in women who have had progressive disease following first-line cytotoxic treatment with a 28.6% response rate (95% CI, 14.6–46.3%). It is also well-tolerated in women who have experienced a paclitaxel-associated hypersensitivity reaction (Fader and Rose, Int J Gynecol Cancer 2009;19:1281–1283; Alberts et al. Gynecol Oncol. 2012;127:451–455)

5. Despite activity, single agents have not had much impact on survival

6. Combination chemotherapy is essential if systemic treatment is to have an impact on survival

7. Platinum combinations yield high response rates, particularly in patients with no prior radiation therapy

8. Two randomized trials have shown improvement in progression-free survival (Long HJ III et al. J Clin Oncol 2005;26:4626–4633; Moore DH et al. J Clin Oncol 2004;22:3113–3119), with 1 trial demonstrating an improvement in survival for combinations (Long HJ III et al. J Clin Oncol 2005;26:4626–4633)

9. The GOG completed a randomized phase III trial of 4 cisplatin (CIS)-containing doublet combinations in stage IVB, recurrent or persistent cervical carcinoma. The study demonstrated that in patients with stage IVB, recurrent or persistent cancer, the combination of paclitaxel 135 mg/m² over 24 hours with cisplatin 50 mg/m² was superior to combinations of vinorelbine 30 mg/m², or gemcitabine 1000 mg/m², or topotecan 0.75 mg/m² with cisplatin 50 mg

10. In view of the fact that most patients currently receive cisplatin-based chemoradiation a subsequent trial GOG 240 compared the combination of paclitaxel with cisplatin versus paclitaxel and topotecan. The study had a secondary randomization to bevacizumab. The trial demonstrated that despite prior platinum exposure during chemoradiation, patients who received the combination of paclitaxel with cisplatin had a higher response rate and a progression-free survival but no improvement in overall survival when compared to patients who received paclitaxel and topotecan. Patients who received bevacizumab had a statistically improved survival by 3.7 months

REGIMEN FOR INITIAL THERAPY

CONCURRENT RADIATION THERAPY + CHEMOTHERAPY/ WEEKLY CISPLATIN

Keys HM et al. N Engl J Med 1999;340:1154–1161
Rose PG et al. N Engl J Med 1999;340:1144–1153

Note: Chemotherapy is given concomitantly with radiation therapy

Cisplatin 40 mg/m^2 per dose (maximum weekly dose 70 mg); administer intravenously in 50–250 mL 0.9% sodium chloride injection (0.9% NS) over 60 minutes weekly for 6 doses during weeks 1–6 (days 1, 8, 15, 22, 29, and 36) starting 4 hours before radiation therapy (total dosage/week = 40 mg/m^2)

Optional hydration with cisplatin: ≥500 mL 0.9% NS; administer intravenously at ≥100 mL/hour before and after cisplatin administration. Also, encourage patients to increase oral intake of non-alcoholic fluids and provide electrolyte replacement as needed (potassium, magnesium, sodium)

Supportive Care
Antiemetic prophylaxis
Emetogenic potential is **HIGH***. Potential for delayed symptoms*
See Chapter 39 for antiemetic recommendations

Hematopoietic growth factor (CSF) prophylaxis
Primary prophylaxis is NOT indicated
See Chapter 43 for more information

Antimicrobial prophylaxis
Risk of fever and neutropenia is LOW
  Antimicrobial primary prophylaxis to be considered:
  • Antibacterial—not indicated
  • Antifungal—not indicated
  • Antiviral—not indicated unless patient previously had an episode of HSV
See Chapter 47 for more information

Treatment Modifications

Adverse Event	Dose Modification
WBC <2000/mm^3	Delay radiation therapy for up to 1 week until WBC >2000/mm^3
Radiation-related gastrointestinal or genitourinary toxicity	Delay radiation therapy for up to 1 week until symptoms resolve
WBC <2500/mm^3 or platelet count <50,000/mm^3	Hold cisplatin until WBC >2500/mm^3 and platelet >50,000/mm^3
G2 neurotoxicity	Reduce cisplatin dosage to 30 mg/m^2 per dose or substitute Carboplatin AUC of 2
≥G3 neurotoxicity	Discontinue cisplatin
Serum creatinine ≥2 mg/dL (≥177 μmol/L)	Reduce cisplatin dosage to 30 mg/m^2 per dose
Serum creatinine ≥2 mg/dL (≥177 μmol/L) despite reduction of cisplatin dosage to 30 mg/m^2	Discontinue cisplatin and substitute Carboplatin dosed to achieve a target AUC of 2 mg/mL · min

Patient Population Studied

Women with untreated invasive squamous cell carcinoma, adenosquamous carcinoma, or adenocarcinoma of the cervix of International Federation of Gynecology and Obstetrics stage IIB (localized disease with parametrial involvement), stage III (extension of tumor to the pelvic wall), or stage IVB (involvement of the bladder and rectal mucosa). Patients with disease outside the pelvis and those with metastases to paraaortic lymph nodes or intraperitoneal disease were not eligible

Therapy Monitoring

Every week: CBC with differential, serum magnesium, BUN, and creatinine

Toxicity (N = 176)

	% G1	% G2	% G3	% G4
Hematologic				
Leukopenia	17	26	21	2
Thrombocytopenia	15	4	2	0
Other hematologic	13	27	10	5
Nonhematologic				
Gastrointestinal	32	28	8	4
Genitourinary	11	6	3	2
Cutaneous	7	6	1	1
Neurologic	6	8	1	0
Pulmonary	0	1	0	0
Cardiovascular	0	0	0	0
Fever	2	4	0	0
Fatigue	5	3	0	0
Pain	2	2	0	0
Weight loss	2	2	1	0
Hypomagnesemia	3	2	2	1
Other*	5	2	1	2

NCI Common Toxicity Criteria (version not specified).
All versions available at: http://ctep.cancer.gov/
protocolDevelopment/electronic_applications/ctc.htm
[accessed December 7, 2013]
*Includes G3 renal abnormalities (serum creatinine
3.1–6 times institutional upper limit of normal),
G3 electrolyte imbalance, G3 dehydration, G3 hepatic
infection, G4 lymphopenia, G4 vaginal necrosis,
G4 edema, and G4 renal abnormalities (serum creatinine
>6 times institutional upper limit of normal)

G1, minimal; G2, mild; G3, moderate; G4, severe
Rose PG et al. N Engl J Med 1999;340:1144–1153

Notes

1. Number of cycles of chemotherapy:

No. of Cycles	% of Patients
0	0.6
1	1.1
2	1.1
3	4
4	10.2
5	33.5
≥6	49.4

2. Radiation therapy (RT) administered:

Percentage of patients who received ≥85% of prescribed RT to both points A and B	90%
Median delay in patients receiving ≥85% of prescribed RT	8 days
Median duration of treatment	9 weeks

3. The rate of local recurrences was significantly lower than the comparison arm with hydroxyurea, whereas the rate of distant recurrences, especially in the lungs, was only slightly less. These results suggest that the principal effect of cisplatin is radiosensitization

Efficacy (N = 176)

	%	P value*
Probability of progression-free survival at 48 months	62	0.001
Probability of survival at 48 months	66.5	0.004
Progression-free survival at 24 months	67[2]	—
Local progression	19[†]	—
Lung metastases	20[†]	—

*Compared with control group (RT + hydroxyurea)
[†]In control group (RT + hydroxyurea), progression-free survival at 24 months = 47%, local progression = 30%, and lung metastases = 10%

Rose PG et al. N Engl J Med 1999;340:1144–1153

REGIMEN FOR INITIAL THERAPY

CONCURRENT RADIATION THERAPY + CHEMOTHERAPY/CISPLATIN + FLUOROURACIL

Morris M et al. N Engl J Med 1999;340:1137–1143
Peters WA III et al. J Clin Oncol 2000;18:1606–1613
Whitney CW et al. J Clin Oncol 1999;17:1339–1348

Notes:
- Chemotherapy is given concomitantly with radiation therapy (begins within 16 hours after the first radiation fraction is administered)
- One cycle is administered at the time of the second intracavitary insertion

Cisplatin 50–75 mg/m² per dose; administer intravenously in 100–500 mL 0.9% sodium chloride injection (0.9% NS) over 4 hours every 3 weeks for 3 cycles. Administration commences within 16 hours after starting radiation therapy (total dosage/3-week cycle = 50–75 mg/m²)

Optional hydration with cisplatin: ≥500 mL 0.9% NS; administer intravenously at ≥100 mL/hour before and after cisplatin administration. Also, encourage patients to increase oral intake of nonalcoholic fluids and provide electrolyte replacement as needed (potassium, magnesium, sodium)

Fluorouracil 1000 mg/m² per day; administer by continuous intravenous infusion in 100–1000 mL 0.9% NS or 5% dextrose injection over 24 hours daily for 4 consecutive days (96-hour infusion) every 3 weeks (starting on days 1, 22, and 43). Administration commences immediately after completing cisplatin infusion (total dosage/cycle = 4000 mg/m²)

Supportive Care
Antiemetic prophylaxis
Emetogenic potential on days with cisplatin is **HIGH**. *Potential for delayed symptoms*
Emetogenic potential on days with fluorouracil + RT is **LOW–MODERATE**
See Chapter 39 for antiemetic recommendations

Hematopoietic growth factor (CSF) prophylaxis
Primary prophylaxis is NOT indicated
See Chapter 43 for more information

Antimicrobial prophylaxis
Risk of fever and neutropenia is LOW
Antimicrobial primary prophylaxis to be considered:
- Antibacterial—not indicated
- Antifungal—not indicated
- Antiviral—not indicated unless patient previously had an episode of HSV

See Chapter 47 for more information

Oral care
Encourage patients to maintain intake of non-alcoholic fluids
If mucositis or stomatitis is present:
- Rinse mouth several times a day with ¼ teaspoon (1.25 g) each of baking soda and table salt in one quart of warm water. Follow with a plain water rinse
- Do not use mouthwashes that contain alcohols

Treatment Modifications

Adverse Event	Dose Modification
WBC <2000/mm³	Delay radiation therapy for up to 1 week until WBC >2000/mm³
Radiation-related gastrointestinal or genitourinary toxicity	Delay radiation therapy for up to 1 week until symptoms resolve
WBC <2500/mm³ or platelet count <50,000/mm³	Hold cisplatin until WBC >2500/mm³ *and* platelet >50,000/mm³
WBC <3000/mm³ or platelet count <100,000/mm³	Hold fluorouracil until WBC >3000/mm³ *and* platelet >100,000/mm³
G3 WBC count	Reduce fluorouracil dosage to 750 mg/m²
G4 WBC count	Reduce fluorouracil dosage to 500 mg/m²
G3 platelet count	Reduce fluorouracil dosage to 750 mg/m²
G4 platelet count	Reduce fluorouracil dosage to 500 mg/m²
G3 stomatitis or diarrhea	Reduce fluorouracil dosage to 750 mg/m²
G4 stomatitis or diarrhea	Reduce fluorouracil dosage to 500 mg/m²
G2 neurotoxicity	Reduce cisplatin dosage to 30 mg/m²
G ≥3 neurotoxicity	Discontinue cisplatin
Serum creatinine ≥2 mg/dL (≥177 μmol/L)	Reduce cisplatin dosage to 30 mg/m²
Serum creatinine ≥2 mg/dL (≥177 μmol/L) despite reduction of cisplatin dosage to 30 mg/m²	Discontinue cisplatin

Efficacy (N = 195)

5-Year survival*	73%	$P = 0.004^\dagger$
5-Year disease-free survival*	67%	$P = 0.001^\dagger$
Rate of distant relapse	14%	$P < 0.001^\dagger$
Rate of locoregional recurrence	19%	$P < 0.001^\dagger$

*Estimated from Kaplan-Meier curves
†P value compared with radiation therapy alone with estimated 5-year survival = 58%; estimated 5-year disease-free survival = 40%; rate of distant relapse = 33%; and rate of locoregional recurrence = 35%

Morris M et al. N Engl J Med 1999;340:1137–1143

Patient Population Studied

Women of all ages with squamous cell carcinoma, adenocarcinoma, or adenosquamous carcinoma of the cervix who had stages IIB through IVA according to the staging system of the International Federation of Gynecology and Obstetrics, or stage IB or IIA with a tumor diameter of at least 5 cm, or biopsy-proven metastases to the pelvic lymph nodes. Women who had disease outside the pelvic area or disease that had spread to paraaortic lymph nodes were excluded

Toxicity (N = 193, 195)

Worst Side Effects Reported During Treatment or Within 60 Days After Completion of Treatment (N = 195)

	% G3	% G4	% G5
Skin abnormalities	2	1	0
Nausea and vomiting	7.2	1.5	0
Bowel/rectal abnormalities	6.2	2.6	0
Bladder abnormalities	1	0	0
Hematologic effects	29.2	8.2	0
Other	4.1	1.5	1
Maximal grade of toxicity	33	11	1
Maximal grade of nonhematologic toxicity	8	2	1

G3, moderate toxicity; G4 severe toxicity; G5, fatal

Worst Side Effects of Treatment Occurring or Persisting More Than 60 Days After Completion of Treatment (N = 193)

	% G3	% G4
Skin or subcutaneous tissue	0.5	0
Small bowel	0.5	2.1
Large bowel or rectum	2.1	6.7
Bladder	2.1	0.5
Uterus	0.5	1
Other	1	0.5
Maximal grade of toxicity	4	8

G3, moderate toxicity; G4, severe toxicity

Morris M et al. N Engl J Med 1999;340:1137–1143
Acute Radiation Morbidity Scoring Criteria
Cooperative Group Common Toxicity Criteria
Late Radiation Morbidity Scoring Scheme of the
Radiation Therapy Oncology Group (RTOG) and the
European Organization for Research and Treatment of
Cancer (EORTC)

Therapy Monitoring

1. *Weekly during treatment:* Clinical assessment, CBC with differential and platelet count, and pelvic examination
2. *Before each cycle of chemotherapy:* CBC with differential and platelet count, serum magnesium, creatinine, urea nitrogen, alanine aminotransferase, alkaline phosphatase, and bilirubin
3. *At time of each intracavitary treatment:* Pelvic examination under anesthesia

Notes

Chemotherapy with cisplatin and fluorouracil is more effective than pelvic and paraaortic radiation alone. However, when compared to weekly cisplatin, the combination of cisplatin and 5-FU was associated with more adverse affects. There were significant differences in symptom scores for well-being, anorexia, fatigue, diarrhea, and stomatitis favoring the weekly cisplatin regimen (Likhacheva A et al. Int J Gynecol Cancer. 2013;23:1520–1527)

REGIMEN FOR INITIAL THERAPY

CONCURRENT RADIATION THERAPY + CHEMOTHERAPY/WEEKLY CARBOPLATIN

Duenas-Gonzalez A et al. Int J Radiat Oncol Biol Phys 2003;56:1361–1365
Higgins RV et al. Gynecol Oncol 2003;89:499–503

Carboplatin (calculated dose) AUC = 2 mg/mL · min*; administer by intravenous infusion in 50–150 mL 5% dextrose injection over 30 minutes on day 1 every 3 weeks (total dosage/cycle calculated to produce an AUC = 2 mg/mL · minute)
*Carboplatin dose is based on a formula described by Calvert et al. to achieve a target area under the plasma concentration versus time curve (AUC)

$$\text{Total Carboplatin Dose (mg)} = (\text{Target AUC}) \times (\text{GFR} + 25)$$

In practice, creatinine clearance (Clcr) is used in place of glomerular filtration rate (GFR). Clcr can be estimated from the equation of Cockcroft and Gault, thus:

$$\text{For males, Clcr} = \frac{(140 - \text{age [years]}) \times (\text{body weight [kg]})}{72 \times (\text{serum creatinine [mg/dL]})}$$

$$\text{For females, Clcr} = \frac{(140 - \text{age [years]}) \times (\text{body weight [kg]})}{72 \times (\text{serum creatinine [mg/dL]})} \times 0.85$$

Calvert AH et al. J Clin Oncol 1989;7:1748–1756
Cockcroft DW, Gault MH. Nephron 1976;16:31–41
Jodrell DI et al. J Clin Oncol 1992;10:520–528
Sorensen BT et al. Cancer Chemother Pharmacol 1991;28:397–401

Note: On October 8, 2010, the U.S. FDA identified a potential safety issue with carboplatin dosing based on recent changes in the measurement of serum creatinine. By the end of 2010, all clinical laboratories in the USA will use the standardized Isotope Dilution Mass Spectrometry (IDMS) method to measure serum creatinine, which could result in an overestimation of the GFR in some patients with normal renal function. A carboplatin dose calculated with an IDMS-measured serum creatinine result using the Calvert formula could exceed an expected exposure (AUC) and result in increased drug-related toxicity
Provided actual GFR measurements are made to assess renal function, carboplatin can be safely dosed according to the Calvert formula described in product labeling
If GFR (or creatinine clearance) is estimated based on serum creatinine measurements by the IDMS method, the FDA recommended for patients with normal renal function capping an estimated GFR at 125 mL/min for any targeted AUC value. No greater estimated GFR values should be used
U.S. FDA. Carboplatin dosing. [online] October 8, 2010. Available from: http://www.fda.gov/AboutFDA/CentersOffices/OfficeofMedicalProductsandTobacco/CDER/ucm228974.htm [accessed February 26, 2014]

Supportive Care
Antiemetic prophylaxis
Emetogenic potential is **MODERATE–HIGH**
See Chapter 39 for antiemetic recommendations

Hematopoietic growth factor (CSF) prophylaxis
Primary prophylaxis is NOT indicated
See Chapter 43 for more information

Antimicrobial prophylaxis
Risk of fever and neutropenia is LOW
  Antimicrobial primary prophylaxis to be considered:
  • Antibacterial—not indicated
  • Antifungal—not indicated
  • Antiviral—not indicated unless patient previously had an episode of HSV
See Chapter 47 for more information

Treatment Modifications

Adverse Event	Dose Modification
ANC <500/mm³ or platelet count <50,000/mm³	Delay therapy for 1 week until ANC >500/mm³ *and* platelet count >50,000/mm³
ANC 500–999/mm³ or platelet count 50,000 to 100,000/mm³	Administer radiation therapy without carboplatin

Note: Do not reduce or escalate the dose of carboplatin

Patient Population Studied

Patients with stages IB-1, IB-2, IIA, IIB, IIIA, IIIB, IVA primary, invasive squamous cell carcinoma or adenocarcinoma, or adenosquamous carcinoma of the uterine cervix, not previously treated, without evidence of paraaortic nodal involvement by radiography or surgical evaluation

Efficacy (N = 31)

Complete response	90%
Disease-free at median follow-up 12 months	74%

Higgins RV et al. Gynecol Oncol 2003;89:499–503

Toxicity (N = 29)

	% G1	% G2	% G3	% G4
Hematologic				
Leukopenia	27.6	34.5	10.3	0
Neutropenia	41.4	20.7	3.4	0
Thrombocytopenia	17.2	3.4	6.9	0
Anemia	37.9	27.6	0	0
Nonhematologic				
Gastrointestinal	48.3	6.9	0	0
Genitourinary	34.5	13.8	0	0
Cutaneous	3.4	3.4	0	0

Higgins RV et al. Gynecol Oncol 2003;89:499–503

Therapy Monitoring

1. *Weekly during treatment:* Clinical assessment, CBC with differential and platelet count, and pelvic examination
2. *Weekly or every other week during treatment:* Serum creatinine, urea nitrogen, alanine aminotransferase, alkaline phosphatase, and bilirubin

Notes

Success rate in administering planned carboplatin treatments was 94%

REGIMEN FOR ADVANCED/ RECURRENT CERVICAL CANCER
CISPLATIN + VINORELBINE

Gebbia V et al. Oncology 2002;63:31–37

Hydration before cisplatin: ≥500 mL 0.9% sodium chloride injection (0.9% NS); administer intravenously at ≥100 mL/hour before and after cisplatin administration. Also, encourage patients to increase oral intake of non-alcoholic fluids and provide electrolyte replacement as needed (potassium, magnesium, sodium)

Mannitol diuresis: May be given to patients who have received adequate hydration. Administer 250 mL of a 15–25% mannitol solution intravenously over 1 hour before starting cisplatin or simultaneously with cisplatin. Continued intravenous hydration is essential with adequate fluid input during and for a minimum of 4 hours after the administration of mannitol

Note: The referenced study recommended 18% mannitol. Although this can be compounded, commercially available (ready-to-use) parenteral products in the United States include 5%, 10%, 15%, and 25% solutions

Cisplatin 80 mg/m^2; administer intravenously in 500 mL 0.9% NS over 60 minutes on day 1, every 21 days (total dosage per cycle = 80 mg/m^2)

Vinorelbine 25 mg/m^2 per dose; administer intravenously in a volume of 0.9% NS or 5% dextrose injection sufficient to produce a solution with a concentration of 1.5–3 mg/mL over 6–10 minutes for 2 doses on days 1 and 8 every 21 days (total dosage/cycle = 50 mg/m^2)

Supportive Care
Antiemetic prophylaxis
Emetogenic potential on day 1 is **HIGH**. *Potential for delayed symptoms*
Emetogenic potential on day 8 is **MINIMAL**
See Chapter 39 for antiemetic recommendations

Hematopoietic growth factor (CSF) prophylaxis
Primary prophylaxis may be indicated
See Chapter 43 for more information

Antimicrobial prophylaxis
Risk of fever and neutropenia is LOW
  Antimicrobial primary prophylaxis to be considered:
  • Antibacterial—not indicated
  • Antifungal—not indicated
  • Antiviral—not indicated unless patient previously had an episode of HSV
See Chapter 47 for more information

Decreased bowel motility
Give a bowel regimen based initially on **stool softeners** to prevent constipation

Oral care
Prophylaxis and treatment for mucositis/stomatitis
  General advice:
  • Encourage patients to maintain intake of non-alcoholic fluids
  • Evaluate patients for oral pain and provide analgesic medications
  • Consider histamine (H$_2$-subtype) receptor antagonists (eg, ranitidine, famotidine), or a proton pump inhibitor for epigastric pain
  • *Lactobacillus* sp.-containing probiotics may be beneficial in preventing diarrhea
  Patients with intact oral mucosa:
  • Clean the mouth, tongue, and gums by brushing after every meal and at bedtime with an ultra-soft toothbrush with fluoride toothpaste
  • Floss teeth gently every day unless contraindicated. If gums bleed and hurt, avoid bleeding or sore areas, but floss other teeth
  • Patients may use saline or commercial bland, non-alcoholic rinses
    ▪ Do not use mouthwashes that contain alcohols

(continued)

Treatment Modifications

Adverse Event	Dose Modification
WBC <4000/mm^3 *or* platelet count <100,000/mm^3	Delay therapy for 1 week until WBC >4000/mm^3 *and* platelet count >100,000/mm^3
G >2 neutropenia on day 8	Omit day 8 vinorelbine, and reduce all subsequent doses by 5 mg/m^2
Day 8 platelet count <50,000/mm^3	Omit vinorelbine dose
G2 neurotoxicity	Reduce cisplatin dosage by 20 mg/m^2 and vinorelbine dosage by 5 mg/m^2
G >2 neurotoxicity	Hold cisplatin and vinorelbine until neurotoxicity G ≤1; then reduce cisplatin dosage by 20 mg/m^2 and vinorelbine dosage by 5 mg/m^2
G1 renal toxicity	Reduce all subsequent cisplatin dosages by 20 mg/m^2
G ≥2 renal toxicity	Hold cisplatin dose until renal toxicity G ≤1; then reduce all subsequent cisplatin dosages by 20 mg/m^2
G4 nonhematologic toxicity	Discontinue therapy

Toxicity (N = 42)

	% G1/2	% G3	% G4
Hematologic			
Neutropenia	26	21	12
Thrombocytopenia	19	—	—
Anemia	12	12	5
Nonhematologic			
Vomiting	52	21	—
Mucositis	14	—	—
Diarrhea	5	—	—
Constipation	38	—	—
Peripheral neuropathy	19	—	—
Alopecia	12	—	—

WHO Toxicity Criteria

(*continued*)

If mucositis or stomatitis is present:
- Keep the mouth moist utilizing water, ice chips, sugarless gum, sugar-free hard candies, or a saliva substitute
- Rinse mouth several times a day to remove debris
  - Use a solution of ¼ teaspoon (1.25 g) each of baking soda and table salt (sodium chloride) in one quart (~950 mL) of warm water. Follow with a plain water rinse
  - Do not use mouthwashes that contain alcohols
- Foam-tipped swabs (eg, Toothettes®) are useful in moisturizing oral mucosa, but ineffective for cleansing teeth and removing plaque
- Advise patients who develop mucositis to:
  - Choose foods that are easy to chew and swallow
  - Take small bites of food, chew slowly, and sip liquids with meals
  - Encourage soft, moist foods such as cooked cereals, mashed potatoes, and scrambled eggs
  - For trouble swallowing, soften food with gravies, sauces, broths, yogurt, or other bland liquids
  - Avoid sharp, crunchy foods; hot, spicy, or highly acidic foods (eg, citrus fruits and juices); sugary foods; toothpicks; tobacco products; alcoholic drinks

Patient Population Studied

A study of women with stage IV de novo or metastatic/recurrent cervical cancer no longer amenable to surgery and/or radiation therapy, with adequate hematopoietic, hepatic, and renal parameters, and a GOG performance status of 0–2

Efficacy (N = 42)

Complete response	12%
Partial response	36%
Median time to progression	5.6 months
Median overall survival	9.1 months

WHO Criteria

Therapy Monitoring

1. *Before each cycle:* PE, CBC with differential, serum electrolytes, magnesium, BUN, and creatinine
2. *Every week:* CBC with differential, serum electrolytes, magnesium, BUN, and creatinine
3. *Response evaluation:* Every 3 cycles

REGIMEN FOR ADVANCED/ RECURRENT CERVICAL CANCER

CISPLATIN + TOPOTECAN

Long HJ III et al. J Clin Oncol 2005;23:4626–4633 (GOG 204)

Topotecan HCl 0.75 mg/m² per day; administer intravenously in 50–250 mL 0.9% sodium chloride injection (0.9% NS) or 5% dextrose injection (D5W) over 30 minutes for 3 consecutive days on days 1–3, every 21 days (total dosage/cycle = 2.25 mg/m²)

Hydration before and after cisplatin: ≥1000 mL 0.45% sodium chloride injection; administer intravenously over a minimum of 2–4 hours. Encourage patients to increase oral intake of nonalcoholic fluids, and provide electrolyte replacement as needed (potassium, magnesium, sodium)

Cisplatin 50 mg/m²; administer intravenously in 50–250 mL 0.9% NS at 1 mg/min on day 1, every 21 days (total dosage/cycle = 50 mg/m²)

Note: Administer cisplatin within 4 hours after completing topotecan administration

Supportive Care

Antiemetic prophylaxis
*Emetogenic potential on day 1 is **HIGH**. Potential for delayed symptoms*
*Emetogenic potential on days 2 and 3 is **LOW***
See Chapter 39 for antiemetic recommendations

Hematopoietic growth factor (CSF) prophylaxis
Primary prophylaxis may be indicated
See Chapter 43 for more information

Antimicrobial prophylaxis
Risk of fever and neutropenia is LOW
  Antimicrobial primary prophylaxis to be considered:
  • Antibacterial—not indicated
  • Antifungal—not indicated
  • Antiviral—not indicated unless patient previously had an episode of HSV
See Chapter 47 for more information

Patient Population Studied

A study of women with advanced (stage IVB), recurrent or persistent carcinoma of the uterine cervix, who were unsuitable candidates for curative treatment with surgery and/or radiation therapy. Histologic types included squamous, adenosquamous, and adenocarcinoma. Prior cisplatin therapy was allowed

Treatment Modifications

Cisplatin Dose Levels	
Initial dosage	50 mg/²
Dose level −1	37.5 mg/m²
Dose level −2	25 mg/m²

Topotecan Dose Levels	
Initial dosage	0.75 mg/m² · d × 3 d
Dose level −1	0.6 mg/m² · d × 3 d
Dose level −2	0.45 mg/m² · d × 3 d

Topotecan Dosage Modifications	
Total Bilirubin (mg/dL)	% Starting Topotecan Dosage
≤2.0 (≤34.2 μmol/L)	100
2.1–3.0 (35.9–51.3 μmol/L)	50
>3.0 (>51.3 μmol/L)	25

Adverse Event	Dose Modification
Day 1 ANC <1500/mm³ or platelet count <100,000/mm³	Hold chemotherapy until ANC ≥1500/mm³ *and* platelet count ≥100,000/mm³
G4 thrombocytopenia	Reduce topotecan dosage 1 level; continue with same cisplatin dosage
G3/4 ANC with fever	
G3/4 ANC with fever despite 1 dose level reduction	Administer filgrastim with all subsequent courses
G2/3/4 nephrotoxicity	Hold cisplatin until serum creatinine ≤1.5 mg/dL (≤133 μmol/L); then resume treatment. If creatinine >1.5 mg/dL >2 weeks beyond scheduled start of next cycle, discontinue cisplatin
G2 peripheral neuropathy or ototoxicity*	Reduce cisplatin dosage by 2 levels
G3/4 peripheral neuropathy or ototoxicity	Hold cisplatin until neuropathy G ≤1; then reduce cisplatin dosage by 2 levels. If G3/4 toxicity persists >2 weeks beyond scheduled start of next cycle, discontinue cisplatin
G4 gastrointestinal toxicity	Continue cisplatin at same dosage
Second event of G4 gastrointestinal toxicity	Reduce cisplatin dosage by 1 level
G2/3 mucositis or diarrhea	Reduce topotecan dosage by 1 level
G4 mucositis or diarrhea	Reduce topotecan dosage by 1–2 levels
Recurrent mucositis or diarrhea despite dosage reduction or persistence of mucositis/diarrhea >2 weeks beyond scheduled start of next cycle	Discontinue topotecan

*G2 ototoxicity consists of tinnitus and symptomatic hearing loss

Toxicity (N = 147)

	% G3	% G4
Hematologic		
Leukopenia	39.4	23.8
Granulocytopenia	24.5	45.6
Thrombocytopenia	24.5	6.8
Anemia	40	6.1
Other hematologic	11.6	2.7
Nonhematologic		
Infection	14.2	3.4
Renal	6.1	6.1
Nausea	12.2	1.4
Emesis	13.6	1.4
Other gastrointestinal	10.9	2.7
Metabolic	8.8	4.8
Neuropathy	0.7	—
Other neurologic	2	0.7
Cardiovascular	4.8	4.1
Pulmonary	2.7	—
Pain	19	2
Constitutional	7.5	—
Hemorrhage	5.4	0.7
Hepatic	3.4	1.4

NCI, CTC, National Cancer Institute (USA) Common Toxicity Criteria, version 2.0. At: http://ctep.cancer.gov/protocolDevelopment/electronic_applications/ctc.htm [accessed December 7, 2013]

Efficacy (N = 147)

Complete response	10%
Partial response	16%
Stable disease	45%
Median progression-free survival	4.6 months
Median survival	9.4 months

Gynecologic Oncology Group Criteria

Therapy Monitoring

1. *Once per week:* CBC with differential
2. *Before the start of a cycle:* CBC with differential, serum calcium, magnesium, potassium, bilirubin, and creatinine

REGIMEN FOR ADVANCED/ RECURRENT CERVICAL CANCER

CISPLATIN + PACLITAXEL

Moore DH et al. J Clin Oncol 2004;22:3113–3119
(GOG 204)

Premedication for paclitaxel:

Dexamethasone 20 mg/dose; administer orally or intravenously for 2 doses at 12 hours and 6 hours before paclitaxel

Note: If patient has no acute toxicities to paclitaxel, the dexamethasone doses at 12 hours and 6 hours before paclitaxel may eventually be omitted

Diphenhydramine 50 mg; administer intravenously 30 minutes before paclitaxel

Cimetidine 300 mg, *or* **ranitidine** 50 mg, *or* **Famotidine** 20 mg; administer intravenously over 5–20 minutes, 30 minutes before paclitaxel

Paclitaxel 135 mg/m^2; administer by continuous intravenous infusion in a volume of 0.9% sodium chloride injection (0.9% NS) or 5% dextrose injection (D5W) sufficient to produce a concentration within the range 0.3–1.2 mg/mL over 24 hours on day 1, every 3 weeks for 6 cycles (total dosage/cycle = 135 mg/m^2)

Hydration before and after cisplatin:

≥1000 mL 0.45% sodium chloride injection; administer intravenously over a minimum of 2–4 hours. Encourage patients to increase oral intake of nonalcoholic fluids, and provide electrolyte replacement as needed (potassium, magnesium, sodium)

Cisplatin 50 mg/m^2; administer intravenously in 50–250 mL 0.9% NS at a rate of 1 mg/min on day 2 after completing paclitaxel administration, every 3 weeks for 6 cycles (total dosage/ cycle = 50 mg/m^2)

Note: Begin cisplatin within 4 hours after completing paclitaxel administration

Supportive Care

Antiemetic prophylaxis

Emetogenic potential during paclitaxel administration is **LOW**

Emetogenic potential on day 2 is **HIGH**. *Potential for delayed symptoms*

See Chapter 39 for antiemetic recommendations

Hematopoietic growth factor (CSF) prophylaxis

Primary prophylaxis may be indicated

See Chapter 43 for more information

Antimicrobial prophylaxis

Risk of fever and neutropenia is LOW

Antimicrobial primary prophylaxis to be considered:

- Antibacterial—not indicated
- Antifungal—not indicated
- Antiviral—not indicated unless patient previously had an episode of HSV

See Chapter 47 for more information

Treatment Modifications

Cisplatin Dose Levels	
Initial dosage	50 mg/m^2
Dose level −1	37.5 mg/m^2
Dose level −2	25 mg/m^2

Paclitaxel Dose Levels	
Initial dosage	135 mg/m^2
Dose level −1	110 mg/m^2
Dose level −2	90 mg/m^2

(continued)

Patient Population Studied

A study of women with advanced (stage IVB), recurrent, or persistent squamous cell carcinoma of the uterine cervix, 24% of whom had received prior chemotherapy and radiation

Efficacy (N = 130)

Complete response	15%
Partial response	21%
Overall response rate (ORR)	36%
ORR, prior chemoradiotherapy (n = 31)	32%
ORR, no prior chemoradiotherapy (n = 99)	37%
Progression-free survival	4.8 months
Progression-free survival, no prior therapy	4.9 months
Median survival	9.7 months
Median survival, no prior therapy	9.9 months

Toxicity (N = 129)

	% G1	% G2	% G3	% G4
Hematologic				
Leukopenia	12.4	22.5	35.7	17
Granulocytopenia	7.8	7.8	20.9	45.7
Thrombocytopenia	30.2	3.1	1.6	2.3
Anemia	10.9	31	22.5	5.4
Nonhematologic				
Nausea/vomiting	29.5	20.9	9.3	0.8
Other gastrointestinal	14	9.3	6.2	0.8
Cardiac	1.6	1.6	1.6	0
Neurologic	19.4	13.2	3.1	0
Fever	1.6	13.2	0	0.8
Dermatologic	2.3	1.6	1.6	0.8
Alopecia	11.6	52.7	0	0
Genitourinary	6.2	10.9	0.8	0
Renal	4.7	7	2.3	0

Treatment Modifications
(continued)

Adverse Event	Dose Modification
Day 1 ANC <1500/mm³ *or* platelet count <100,000/mm³	Hold chemotherapy until ANC ≥1500/mm³ *and* platelet count ≥100,000/mm³
ANC <1500/mm³ *or* platelet count <100,000/mm³ persists ≥2 weeks beyond the scheduled start of cycle	Discontinue therapy
G4 thrombocytopenia	Reduce paclitaxel dosage by 1 level; continue with same cisplatin dosage
G3/4 ANC with fever*	
G3/4 ANC with fever despite paclitaxel dosage reduction by 1 dose level	Administer filgrastim with all subsequent courses
G3/4 ANC with fever despite paclitaxel dose reduction and filgrastim	Reduce paclitaxel dosage by 1 level or 20%; continue with same cisplatin dosage
G2 peripheral neuropathy	Reduce paclitaxel dosage by 2 dose levels
G3/4 peripheral neuropathy	Hold paclitaxel until neuropathy G ≤1; then reduce paclitaxel dosage by 2 dose levels. If G3/4 toxicity persists >2 weeks beyond scheduled start of next cycle, discontinue paclitaxel
G2 hepatic toxicity	Hold paclitaxel until toxicity G ≤1; then reduce paclitaxel dosage by 1 dose level
G3/4 hepatic toxicity	Hold paclitaxel until toxicity G ≤1; then reduce paclitaxel dosage by 1–2 dose levels. If G3/4 toxicity persists >2 weeks beyond scheduled start of cycle, discontinue paclitaxel
G2/3/4 nephrotoxicity	Hold cisplatin until serum creatinine ≤1.5 mg/dL (≤133 μmol/L); then resume treatment
	Discontinue cisplatin if creatinine >1.5 mg/dL (>133 μmol/L) >2 weeks beyond scheduled start of next cycle
G2 peripheral neuropathy or ototoxicity†	Reduce cisplatin dosage by 2 dose levels
G3/4 peripheral neuropathy or ototoxicity	Hold cisplatin until neuropathy G ≤1 then reduce cisplatin dosage by 2 dose levels. If G3/4 toxicity persists >2 weeks beyond scheduled start of next cycle, discontinue cisplatin
G4 gastrointestinal toxicity	Continue cisplatin at same dosage
Second event of G4 gastrointestinal toxicity	Reduce cisplatin dosage by 1 dose level

*Use filgrastim if thought beneficial
†G2 Ototoxicity consists of tinnitus and symptomatic hearing loss

Note: Management of paclitaxel hypersensitivity reaction:
1. Discontinue infusion
2. Wait for symptoms to resolve
3. If symptoms were not life-threatening, repeat premedications (dexamethasone, diphenhydramine, and cimetidine or ranitidine or famotidine) in preparation for restarting infusion
4. Administer 1 mL of the original paclitaxel solution diluted in 100 mL of the same base solution over 1 hour, *then*
5. Administer 5 mL of the original paclitaxel solution diluted in 100 mL of the same base solution over 1 hour, *then*
6. Administer 10 mL of the original paclitaxel solution diluted in 100 mL of the same base solution over 1 hour, *then*
7. Administer the remaining original solution at the original infusion rate

Therapy Monitoring

1. *Every 15 minutes for the first hour of the paclitaxel infusion:* Vital signs including blood pressure, respiratory rate, and temperature
2. *Once per week:* CBC with differential
3. *Before the start of a cycle:* CBC with differential, serum calcium, magnesium, potassium, bilirubin, and creatinine

REGIMEN FOR ADVANCED/ RECURRENT CERVICAL CANCER

CISPLATIN + GEMCITABINE

Burnett AF et al. Gynecol Oncol 2000;76:63–66 (GOG 204)

Gemcitabine 1000–1250 mg/m² per dose; administer intravenously diluted to a concentration ≥0.1 mg/mL in 0.9% sodium chloride injection (0.9% NS) over 30 minutes for 2 doses on days 1 and 8, every 21 days (total dosage/cycle = 2500 mg/m²)

Note: After gemcitabine administration, flush the patient's vascular access device with 75–125 mL of 0.9% NS

Hydration before and after cisplatin: ≥1000 mL 0.45% sodium chloride injection; administer by intravenous infusion over a minimum of 2–4 hours. Encourage patients to increase oral intake of non-alcoholic fluids, and provide electrolyte replacement as needed (potassium, magnesium, sodium)
Cisplatin 50 mg/m²; administer intravenously in 50–250 mL 0.9% NS over 60 minutes on day 1 after completing gemcitabine administration, every 21 days (total dosage/cycle = 50 mg/m²)

Note: Administer cisplatin on day 1 within 4 hours after completing gemcitabine

Supportive Care
Antiemetic prophylaxis
Emetogenic potential on day 1 is **HIGH**. *Potential for delayed symptoms*
Emetogenic potential on day 8 is **LOW**
See Chapter 39 for antiemetic recommendations

Hematopoietic growth factor (CSF) prophylaxis
Primary prophylaxis is NOT indicated
See Chapter 43 for more information

Antimicrobial prophylaxis
Risk of fever and neutropenia is LOW
Antimicrobial primary prophylaxis to be considered:
- Antibacterial—not indicated
- Antifungal—not indicated
- Antiviral—not indicated unless patient previously had an episode of HSV

See Chapter 47 for more information

Patient Population Studied

Phase II trial in patients with advanced, persistent, or recurrent squamous cell carcinoma of the cervix

Treatment Modifications

Cisplatin Dose Levels	
Initial dosage	50 mg/m²
Dose level −1	37.5 mg/m²
Dose level −2	25 mg/m²

Gemcitabine Dose Levels	
Initial dosage	1000 mg/m²
Dose level −1	800 mg/m²
Dose level −2	600 mg/m²

Gemcitabine Dosage Modification	
Total Bilirubin (mg/dL)	% of Starting Gemcitabine Dosage
≤2.0 (≤34.2 µmol/L)	100
2.1–3.0 (35.9–51.3 µmol/L)	50
>3.0 (>51.3 µmol/L)	25

Note: Gemcitabine dose reductions at any time after day 1 of cycle 1 will be continued throughout the rest of the study

Adverse Event	Dose Modification
Day 1 ANC <1500/mm³ or platelet count <100,000/mm³	Hold chemotherapy until ANC ≥1500/mm³ *and* platelet count ≥100,000/mm³
ANC <1500/mm³ or platelet count <100,000/mm³ that persists ≥3 weeks beyond the scheduled start of cycle	Discontinue therapy
>2-Weeks delay until ANC ≥1500/mm³ *and* platelet count ≥100,000/mm³	Reduce gemcitabine by 1 dose level
Day 8 ANC ≥1500/mm³ or platelet count ≥100,000/mm³	Administer day 1 gemcitabine dosage on day 8
Day 8 ANC 1000–1499/mm³ or platelet count 75,000–99,000/mm³	Reduce gemcitabine on day 8 by 1 dose level from day 1 level
Day 8 ANC <1500/mm³ or platelet count <100,000/mm³	Withhold day 8 gemcitabine dose; reduce gemcitabine dosage by 1 dose level in ensuing cycles on day 8
G4 thrombocytopenia	Reduce gemcitabine by 1 dose level; continue with same cisplatin dosage
G3/4 ANC with fever*	Reduce gemcitabine dosage by 1 dose level; continue with same cisplatin dosage
G3/4 ANC with fever despite 1 dose level reduction	Administer filgrastim with all subsequent courses
G3/4 ANC with fever despite gemcitabine dose reduction and filgrastim	Reduce gemcitabine dosage by 1 dose level or 20%; continue with same cisplatin dosage
G1 mucositis or diarrhea	Hold gemcitabine until toxicity resolves; then resume with same dosage
G2/3 mucositis or diarrhea	Hold gemcitabine until toxicity G ≤1; reduce subsequent dosages by 1 dose level

(continued)

Treatment Modifications
(*continued*)

Adverse Event	Dose Modification
Mucositis or diarrhea that is G4 or that persists >2 weeks, or repeated episodes of persistent toxicity G ≥2	Hold gemcitabine until toxicity G ≤1; consider discontinuing gemcitabine
G2/3/4 nephrotoxicity	Hold cisplatin until serum creatinine ≤1.5 mg/dL (≤133 μmol/L) then resume treatment. If creatinine >1.5 mg/dL >2 weeks beyond scheduled start of next cycle, discontinue cisplatin
G2 peripheral neuropathy or ototoxicity†	Reduce cisplatin dosage by 2 dose levels
G3/4 peripheral neuropathy or ototoxicity	Hold cisplatin and gemcitabine until neuropathy G ≤1 then reduce cisplatin dosage by 2 dose levels. If G3/4 toxicity persists >2 weeks beyond scheduled start of next cycle, discontinue cisplatin
G4 gastrointestinal toxicity	Continue cisplatin at same dosage
Second event of G4 gastrointestinal toxicity	Reduce cisplatin dosage by 1 dose level

*Use filgrastim if thought beneficial
†G2 ototoxicity consists of tinnitus and symptomatic hearing loss. If neurotoxicity occurs, it will most likely be cisplatin-related

Efficacy (N = 17)

Complete response	5.9%
Partial response*	35.3%
Median survival patients with response	12 months
Median survival patients without response	7 months

*Six patients; 3 had received prior radiation therapy
GOG Response Criteria

Toxicity (N = 82 cycles)

	% G3	% G4
Hematologic		
Neutropenia	7.3	2.4
Anemia	1.2	1.2
Median leukocyte nadir	3145/mm^3	
Median platelet nadir	174,000/mm^3	
Nonhematologic		
Gastrointestinal	2.4	0

Therapy Monitoring

1. *Once per week:* CBC with differential
2. *Before the start of a cycle:* CBC with differential, serum calcium, magnesium, potassium, bilirubin, and creatinine

REGIMEN FOR ADVANCED/RECURRENT CERVICAL CANCER

CISPLATIN + IRINOTECAN

Chitapanarux I et al. Gynecol Oncol 2003;89:402–407

Irinotecan 60 mg/m^2 per dose; administer intravenously diluted in a volume of 5% dextrose injection (D5W) or 0.9% sodium chloride injection (0.9% NS) sufficient to produce a concentration within the range 0.12–2.8 mg/mL over 90 minutes for 3 doses on days 1, 8, and 15, every 28 days (total dosage/cycle = 180 mg/m^2)

Hydration before and after cisplatin:
≥1000 mL 0.45% sodium chloride injection; administer intravenously over a minimum of 2–4 hours
Note: Encourage patients to increase oral intake of nonalcoholic fluids, and provide electrolyte replacement as needed (potassium, magnesium, sodium)

Cisplatin 60 mg/m^2; administer intravenously in 100–500 mL 0.9% NS over 90 minutes on day 1 after completing irinotecan administration, every 28 days (total dosage per cycle = 60 mg/m^2)

Supportive Care
Antiemetic prophylaxis
Emetogenic potential on day 1 is **HIGH**. *Potential for delayed symptoms*
Emetogenic potential on days 8 and 15 with irinotecan alone is **MODERATE**
See Chapter 39 for antiemetic recommendations

Hematopoietic growth factor (CSF) prophylaxis
Primary prophylaxis is NOT indicated
See Chapter 43 for more information

Antimicrobial prophylaxis
Risk of fever and neutropenia is LOW
Antimicrobial primary prophylaxis to be considered:
- Antibacterial—not indicated
- Antifungal—not indicated
- Antiviral—not indicated unless patient previously had an episode of HSV

See Chapter 47 for more information

Acute cholinergic syndrome
Atropine sulfate 0.25–1 mg administer subcutaneously or intravenously if abdominal cramping or diarrhea develop during or within 1 hour after irinotecan administration
- If symptoms are severe, add as primary prophylaxis at least 30 minutes before irinotecan during subsequent cycles
- For irinotecan, acute cholinergic syndrome may be characterized by abdominal cramping, diarrhea, diaphoresis, hypotension, flushing, bradycardia, rhinitis, increased salivation, meiosis, and lacrimation

Diarrhea management
Latent or delayed onset diarrhea*:
    Loperamide 4 mg orally initially after the first loose or liquid stool, *then*
    Loperamide 2 mg orally every 2 hours during waking hours, *plus*
    Loperamide 4 mg orally every 4 hours during hours of sleep
- Continue for at least 12 hours after diarrhea resolves
- Recurrent diarrhea after a 12-hour diarrhea-free interval is treated as a new episode
- Rehydrate orally with fluids and electrolytes during a diarrheal episode
- If a patient develops blood or mucus in stool, dehydration, or hemodynamic instability, or if diarrhea persists >48 hours despite loperamide, stop loperamide and hospitalize the patient for IV hydration

(continued)

Toxicity (N = 30)

	% G1	% G2	% G3	% G4
Hematologic				
Neutropenia	26.7	26.7	30	—
Anemia	13.3	46.6	16.7	—
Thrombocytopenia	—	—	—	—
Nonhematologic				
Alopecia	50	50	—	—
Acute diarrhea	16.7	3.3	—	—
Late-onset diarrhea	33.3	10	—	—
Nausea/vomiting	30	40	23.3	—
Renal	3.3	20	20	6.7

With respect to nonhematologic toxicity, renal dysfunction was the most significant; 2 patients developed G4 creatinine elevations

NCI, CTC, National Cancer Institute (USA) Common Toxicity Criteria, version 2.0. At: http://ctep.cancer.gov/protocolDevelopment/electronic_applications/ctc.htm [accessed December 7, 2013]

Efficacy (N = 30)

Complete response	6.7%
Partial response	60%
Median survival	16.9 months
Median time to progression	13.4 months

WHO Criteria

Patient Population Studied

Chemotherapy-naïve women with metastatic or recurrent cervical cancer, with measurable disease, adequate hematopoietic, renal, and hepatic function, and with a WHO performance status of 0–2

Therapy Monitoring

1. *Before each cycle:* PE, CBC with differential, serum magnesium, BUN, creatinine, electrolytes, and liver function tests
2. *Weekly:* CBC with differential and serum creatinine
3. *Response evaluation:* After cycles 1 and 2 and every 2 cycles thereafter

(*continued*)

Persistent diarrhea:

    Octreotide 100–150 mcg subcutaneously 3 times daily. Maximum total daily dose is 1500 mcg

Antibiotic therapy during latent or delayed onset diarrhea:

    A fluoroquinolone (eg, **Ciprofloxacin** 500 mg orally every 12 hours) if absolute neutrophil count <500/mm³ with or without accompanying fever in association with diarrhea

    • Antibiotics should also be administered if patient is hospitalized with prolonged diarrhea and should be continued until diarrhea resolves

* Rothenberg ML et al. J Clin Oncol 2001;19:3801–3807

Abigerges D et al. J Natl Cancer Inst 1994;86:446–449

Wadler S et al. J Clin Oncol 1998;16:3169–3178

Treatment Modifications

Adverse Event	Dose Modification
WBC <4000/mm³, platelet count <100,000/mm³, *or* diarrhea	Delay start of cycle by 1 week until WBC >4000/mm³, platelet count >100,000/mm³, *and* no diarrhea
Day 8 or 15 WBC <3000/mm³ *or* platelet count <100,000/mm³	Hold irinotecan
G ≥1 diarrhea	Hold irinotecan
If WBC <1000/mm³, platelet count <50,000/mm³, *or* diarrhea G ≥2 at any time in cycle	Reduce subsequent irinotecan dosage by 50%
Serum creatinine >1.5 × upper limits of normal	Reduce cisplatin dosage to 50 mg/m²

REGIMEN FOR ADVANCED/ RECURRENT CERVICAL CANCER

PACLITAXEL PROTEIN-BOUND PARTICLES FOR INJECTABLE SUSPENSION (ALBUMIN-BOUND) (NAB-PACLITAXEL)

Alberts DS et al. Gynecol Oncol 2012;127:451–455

Paclitaxel protein-bound particles for injectable suspension) (albumin-bound) 125 mg/m^2 per dose (maximum single dose = 250 mg); administer intravenously over 30 minutes for 3 doses, on days 1, 8, and 15, every 28 days (total dosage/cycle = 375 mg/m^2; maximum dose/cycle = 750 mg)

Supportive Care
Antiemetic prophylaxis
Emetogenic potential is LOW
See Chapter 39 for antiemetic recommendations

Hematopoietic growth factor (CSF) prophylaxis
Primary prophylaxis may be indicated
See Chapter 43 for more information

Antimicrobial prophylaxis
Risk of fever and neutropenia is LOW
Antimicrobial primary prophylaxis to be considered:
- Antibacterial—not indicated
- Antifungal—not indicated
- Antiviral—not indicated unless patient previously had an episode of HSV
See Chapter 47 for more information

Treatment Modifications

Adverse Event	Dose Modification
Nab-paclitaxel Dose Levels	
Starting dose	125 mg/m^2
Dosage level (−1)	100 mg/m^2
Dosage level (−2)	80 mg/m^2
Hematologic Toxicities	
On day 1 of a cycle ANC <1500 cells/mm^3 and the platelet count <100,000/mm^3	Withhold therapy until ANC ≥1500 /mm^3 and the platelet count is ≥100,000/mm^3. Delay therapy a maximum of 2 weeks
ANC still <1500 cells/mm^3 and platelet count still <100,000/mm^3 2 weeks after cycle start day	Discontinue therapy
First occurrence of febrile neutropenia or documented G4 neutropenia persisting ≥7 days	Reduce nab-paclitaxel dosage by 1 dose level during subsequent cycles
Recurrent febrile neutropenia or recurrent documented G4 neutropenia persisting ≥7 days after an initial dose reduction	Administer filgrastim
G4 thrombocytopenia	Reduce nab-paclitaxel dosage by 1 dose level during subsequent cycles
Non-hematologic Toxicities	
G ≥2 peripheral neuropathy	Reduce nab-paclitaxel dosage by 1 dose level to 100 mg/m^2 and delay start of subsequent therapy for a maximum of 2 weeks until recovered to G1
G ≥2 nephrotoxicity	Reduce nab-paclitaxel dosage by 1 dose level to 100 mg/m^2 and delay start of subsequent therapy for a maximum of 2 weeks until recovered to G1
G ≥3 elevations in SGOT (AST), SGPT (ALT), alkaline phosphatase, or bilirubin	Reduce nab-paclitaxel dosage by 1 dose level and delay start of subsequent therapy for a maximum of 2 weeks until recovered to G1
Nonhematologic toxicity with adverse effect on organ function G ≥2	Reduce nab-paclitaxel dosage by 1 dose level and delay start of subsequent therapy for a maximum of 2 weeks until recovered to G1 or pretherapy baseline
G3 hypersensitivity reactions	Retreat after administering standard paclitaxel premedication (steroids + histamine [H$_1$- and H$_2$-receptor] antagonists)
Any G3/4 toxicity with nab-paclitaxel 80 mg/m^2 per dose	Discontinue therapy

Patient Population Studied

Characteristics of Evaluable Patients (n = 35)

Characteristic	Number of Cases (%)
Age	
<40 y	6 (17.1)
40–49 y	15 (42.9)
50–59 y	10 (28.6)
60–69 y	3 (8.6)
>70 y	1 (2.9)
Race	
African American	3 (8.6)
American Indian	1 (2.9)
White	30 (85.7)
Unreported	1 (2.9)
Performance status	
0	19 (54.3)
1	10 (28.6)
2	6 (17.1)
Cell type	
Squamous	22 (62.8)
Adenocarcinoma	9 (25.7)
Small cell	1 (2.9)
Endometrioid adenocarcinoma	1 (2.9)
Undifferentiated	1 (2.9)
Adenosquamous	1 (2.9)
Grade	
1	3 (8.6)
2	17 (48.6)
3	14 (40)
Unspecified	1 (2.9)
Prior chemotherapy	
1 regimen	35 (100)
Prior radiation	27 (77.1)
Cycles of treatment	
1	2 (5.7)
2	10 (28.6)
3	2 (5.7)
4	5 (14.3)
5	2 (5.7)
>5	14 (40)

Toxicity (N = 35)

Adverse Event	Number of Patients (Percent of Patients)			
	G1	G2	G3	G4
Leukopenia	10 (28.6%)	12 (34.3%)	3 (8.6%)	0
Thrombocytopenia	4 (11.4%)	0	1 (2.9%)	0
Neutropenia	6 (17.1%)	6 (17.1%)	1 (2.9%)	2 (5.7%)
Anemia	6 (17.1%)	22 (62.9%)	4 (11.4%)	0
Nausea/vomiting	11 (31.4%)	9 (25.7%)	0	0
Other gastrointestinal	10 (28.6%)	10 (28.6%)	2 (5.7%)	0
Genitourinary	1 (2.9%)	0	0	0
Neurotoxicity	11 (31.4%)	8 (22.9%)	1 (2.9%)	0
Pain	9 (25.7%)	4 (11.4%)	2 (5.7%)	0
Pulmonary	1 (2.9%)	2 (5.7%)	2 (5.7%)	0
Cardiovascular	0	1 (2.9%)	0	0
Constitutional (fatigue)	7 (20%)	15 (42.9%)	5 (14.3%)	0
Metabolic	5 (14.3%)	2 (5.7%)	4 (11.4%)	0
Dermatologic	1 (2.9%)	3 (8.6%)	1 (2.9%)	0
Alopecia	3 (8.6%)	15 (42.9%)	—	—
Musculoskeletal	2 (5.7%)	1 (2.9%)	0	0
Auditory	0	1 (2.9%)	0	0
Infection	0	4 (11.4%)	4 (11.4%)	0
SGOT (AST)	1 (2.9%)	0	0	0
Alkaline phosphatase	1 (2.9%)	0	0	0
Lymphatics	2 (5.7%)	2 (5.7%)	0	0

Efficacy (N = 35)

Partial response	10* (28.6%, 95% CI: 14.6%–46.3%)
Median duration of response	6.0 months (range: 1.5–9.2)
Stable disease	15 (42.9%)
Median duration of stable disease	5.8 months (range: 3.7–11.4 months)
Progressive disease	8 (22.9%)
Not evaluable	2 (5.7%)
Median progression-free survival	5.0 months
Median overall survival	9.4 months

*Five of the partial responses were documented in viscera (ie, liver in 2 patients, and 1 each in lung, pancreas, and bladder), whereas the other 5 partial responses occurred in the retroperitoneal nodes (3 patients), mediastinal nodes (1 patient) and intraperitoneal nodes (1 patient)

Treatment Monitoring

1. *Prior to the start of a cycle:* CBC with differential, LFTs, BUN, and creatinine
2. *Response Assessment:* Every 2 cycles

REGIMEN FOR ADVANCED/ RECURRENT/ PERSISTENT CERVICAL CANCER NOT CURABLE WITH STANDARD THERAPIES

PACLITAXEL + TOPOTECAN

Tewari KS et al. Gynecol Oncol SGO Abstract Suppl 2013:S5; SGO #1 (GOG 240)
Tiersten AD et al. Gynecol Oncol 2004;92:635–638

Prophylaxis against hypersensitivity reactions to paclitaxel with:

Dexamethasone 10 mg/dose; orally for 2 doses at 12 hours and 6 hours before paclitaxel, *or*
Dexamethasone 20 mg/dose; intravenously over 10–15 minutes, 30–60 minutes before paclitaxel on day 1 (total dose/cycle = 20 mg)
Diphenhydramine 50 mg, by intravenous injection 30–60 minutes before paclitaxel
Cimetidine 300 mg (or **Ranitidine** 50 mg, **Famotidine** 20 mg, or an equivalent histamine [H_2]-subtype receptor antagonist) administer intravenously over 15–30 minutes, 30–60 minutes before paclitaxel
Paclitaxel 175 mg/m^2; administer intravenously, diluted in a volume of 0.9% Sodium Chloride Injection (0.9% NS) or 5% Dextrose Injection (D5W) sufficient to produce a concentration within the range 0.3–1.2 mg/mL over 3 hours on day 1, every 21 days (total dosage/cycle = 175 mg/m^2), *plus:*
Topotecan 0.75 mg/m^2 per dose; administer intravenously, diluted in 50–250 mL 0.9% NS or D5W over 30 minutes for 3 consecutive days, on days 1–3, every 21 days (total dosage/cycle = 2.25 mg/m^2), *or*
Topotecan 1 mg/m^2 per dose; administer intravenously, diluted in 50–250 mL 0.9% NS or D5W over 30 minutes for 5 consecutive days, on days 1–5, every 21 days (total dosage/cycle = 5 mg/m^2)

Treatment Modifications

Adverse Event	Dose Modification
Day 1 ANC <1000/mm^3 or platelet count <100,000/mm^3	Delay therapy until ANC ≥1000/mm^3 and platelet count is ≥100,000/mm^3. Consider reducing topotecan dosage by 10–20% and paclitaxel dosage to 120–135 mg/m^2 based on dosages previously given. If treatment delay is >2 weeks, consider discontinuing therapy
G ≥2 arthralgias/myalgias	Add dexamethasone as secondary prophylaxis
G3 arthralgia/myalgia despite dexamethasone prophylaxis	Reduce paclitaxel dosage to 135 mg/m^2
G2 neurotoxicity	Reduce paclitaxel dosage to 135 mg/m^2
G3/4 neurotoxicity	Delay therapy until G ≤2, then reduce paclitaxel dosage to 100–120 mg/m^2
G ≥2 AST (SGOT) or ALT (SGPT), or G ≥3 bilirubin	Stop paclitaxel
Moderate hypersensitivity during paclitaxel infusion	Patient may be retreated. Base a decision to retreat on reaction severity and a medically responsible care provider's judgment
Severe hypersensitivity during paclitaxel infusion	Discontinue therapy
Febrile neutropenia	Reduce topotecan and paclitaxel dosages by 25%
Bleeding associated with thrombocytopenia	
Pulmonary symptoms indicative of interstitial lung disease (eg, cough, fever, dyspnea, and/or hypoxia)	Discontinue topotecan and evaluate. If a new diagnosis of interstitial lung disease is confirmed topotecan should be discontinued

Efficacy (N = 13)

Tiersten AD et al. Gynecol Oncol 2004;92: 635–638

	Number (%)
Overall response	7 (54%)
Complete response	1 (8%)
Partial response	6 (46%)
Stable disease	3 (23%)
Progressive disease	3 (23%)

Efficacy*

Tewari KS et al. Gynecol Oncol SGO Abstract Suppl 2013: S5; SGO #1

	Cisplatin + Paclitaxel (N = 229)	Topotecan + Paclitaxel (N = 223)
	15 months	12.5 months
Median OS	HR=1.20 (98.74% CI; 0.82–1.76) P (one-sided) = 0.880	
Overall response rate	38%	27.4%

*Topotecan + paclitaxel was shown to not be neither superior nor inferior to cisplatin + paclitaxel

(continued)

Supportive Care
Antiemetic prophylaxis
Emetogenic potential is LOW
See Chapter 39 for antiemetic recommendations

Hematopoietic growth factor (CSF) prophylaxis
Primary prophylaxis may be indicated
See Chapter 43 for more information

Antimicrobial prophylaxis
Risk of fever and neutropenia is LOW
Antimicrobial primary prophylaxis to be considered:
• Antibacterial—not indicated
• Antifungal—not indicated
• Antiviral—not indicated, unless patient previously had an episode of HSV
See Chapter 47 for more information

Treatment Monitoring

1. Prior to the start of a cycle: CBC with differential, LFTs, BUN, and creatinine
2. Response Assessment: Every 2 cycles

Patient Population Studied

Patient Demographics and Baseline Characteristics (N = 15)*

Tiersten AD et al. Gynecol Oncol 2004;92:635–638

	Number (%)
Age, Median (Range)	52 years (32–68 y)
Histologic type, n (%)	
Squamous cell carcinoma	9 (60%)
Adenocarcinoma	4 (27%)
Adenosquamous	2 (13%)
Prior chemotherapy*	10 (67%)
At time of recurrence*	5 (33%)
Prior radiotherapy	14 (93%)
At time of recurrence	
Pelvic recurrence	6 (40%)
Sites of metastases	
Lung	5 (33%)
Liver	3 (20%)
Pelvis	5 (33%)
Neck	1 (7%)
Psoas muscle	1 (7%)

*Note: Eligible patients could not have received prior taxane or camptothecin therapy or >2 prior chemotherapy regimens

Toxicity

G3/4 Hematologic and Nonhematologic Toxicities
Evaluable for Toxicity = 15 Patients (100%)/(86 Cycles)

Tiersten AD et al. Gynecol Oncol 2004;92:635–638

Adverse Event	Episodes, Number (%)
Hematologic	
Anemia	23 (26.7%)
Leukopenia	16 (18.6%)
Thrombocytopenia	6 (7%)
Febrile neutropenia	6 (7%)
Non-hematologic	
Neurotoxicity	3 (3.5%)
Diarrhea	2 (2.3%)
Pain	2 (2.3%)
Nausea/vomiting	1 (1.2%)
Elevated creatinine	1 (1.2%)
Tolerability	
Treatment delays due to toxicity*	3 (3.5%)
Dose reductions	3 patients (20%)†

*Five patients experienced treatment delays, but only 3 of the 10 cycles that were delayed were related to treatment toxicities (7 were the result of holidays or patient vacation)
†Dose successfully re-escalated in the subsequent cycle for 1 patient (affected drugs not specified)

REGIMEN FOR ADVANCED/ RECURRENT/ PERSISTENT CERVICAL CANCER NOT CURABLE WITH STANDARD THERAPIES

PACLITAXEL + CISPLATIN + BEVACIZUMAB

GOG 240: Tewari KS et al. J Clin Oncol 2013;31:[Abstract 3]

Prophylaxis against hypersensitivity reactions to paclitaxel with:

Dexamethasone 10 mg/dose; orally for 2 doses at 12 hours and 6 hours before paclitaxel, *or*
Dexamethasone 20 mg/dose; intravenously over 10–15 minutes, 30–60 minutes before paclitaxel on day 1 (total dose/cycle = 20 mg)
Diphenhydramine 50 mg, by intravenous injection 30–60 minutes before paclitaxel
Cimetidine 300 mg (or **Ranitidine** 50 mg, **Famotidine** 20 mg, or an equivalent histamine [H_2]-subtype receptor antagonist) intravenously over 15–30 minutes, 30–60 minutes before paclitaxel
Paclitaxel 135–175 mg/m² intravenously, diluted in a volume of 0.9% Sodium Chloride Injection (0.9% NS) or 5% Dextrose Injection (D5W) sufficient to produce a concentration within the range 0.3–1.2 mg/mL over 3 hours on day 1, every 21 days (total dosage/cycle = 135–175 mg/m²)

Hydration before cisplatin: 1000 mL 0.9% NS; intravenously over a minimum of 1 hour before commencing cisplatin administration
Cisplatin 50 mg/m²; intravenously, diluted in 100–500 mL 0.9% NS over 30–90 minutes on day 1, every 21 days (total dosage/cycle = 50 mg/m²)

Hydration after cisplatin: Administer by intravenous infusion ≥1000 mL 0.9% NS over a minimum of 2 hours. Encourage patients to increase oral intake of non-alcoholic fluids, and provide electrolyte replacement as needed (potassium, magnesium, sodium)

Bevacizumab 15 mg/kg; intravenously, diluted in 100 mL 0.9% NS over 30–90 minutes on day 1, every 21 days (total dosage/cycle = 15 mg/kg)

(*continued*)

Treatment Modifications

Dose escalations are not recommended. Dosage reductions are based on toxicity encountered during a previous cycle

Adverse Event	Dose Modification
G≥2 arthralgias/myalgias	Add dexamethasone as secondary prophylaxis
G3 arthralgia/myalgia despite dexamethasone prophylaxis	Reduce paclitaxel dosage to 100–135 mg/m²
G2 neurotoxicity	Reduce paclitaxel dosage to 120–135 mg/m²
G3 neurotoxicity	Reduce paclitaxel dosage to 100–120 mg/m²
G3/4 neurotoxicity	Delay therapy until neurotoxicity abates to G ≤2, then reduce paclitaxel dosage to 100–120 mg/m²
Recurrent G3/4 neurotoxicity at a paclitaxel dosage of 100–120 mg/m²	Delay therapy until neurotoxicity abates to G ≤2, then reduce cisplatin dosage by 25%
G ≥2 AST (SGOT) or G ≥2 ALT (SGPT), or G ≥3 bilirubin	Withhold paclitaxel
Moderate hypersensitivity during paclitaxel infusion	Patient may be retreated. Base a decision to retreat on reaction severity and caregiver's discretion
Severe hypersensitivity during paclitaxel infusion	Discontinue therapy
Day 1 ANC <1500/mm³ or platelet count <100,000/mm³	Delay therapy until ANC ≥1500/mm³ and platelet count is ≥100,000/mm³. If treatment delay is >2 weeks, consider discontinuing therapy
Febrile neutropenia	Reduce cisplatin and paclitaxel dosages by 25%
Bleeding associated with thrombocytopenia	Reduce cisplatin and paclitaxel dosages by 25%
Serum creatinine 1.6–2 mg/dL (141–177 μmol/L)	Reduce cisplatin dosage by 25%
Serum creatinine ≥2 mg/dL (≥177 μmol/L)	Hold cisplatin until serum creatinine is <2.0 mg/dL (<177 μmol/L)
Chest pain or arrhythmia during chemotherapy	Immediately stop chemotherapy and evaluate patient
Symptomatic arrhythmias or AV block ≥ second-degree, or documented ischemic event	Stop treatment
Gastrointestinal perforation	Discontinue bevacizumab permanently
Serious bleeding	Discontinue bevacizumab permanently
Wound dehiscence requiring medical intervention	Discontinue bevacizumab permanently
Nephrotic syndrome	Discontinue bevacizumab permanently
Hypertensive crisis	Discontinue bevacizumab permanently
Moderate to severe proteinuria or severe hypertension not controlled with medical management	Hold bevacizumab pending further evaluation (eg, 24-hour urine protein or work-up and treatment of hypertension)

Note: Bevacizumab use should be suspended at least several weeks before elective surgery and should not be resumed until a surgical incision is fully healed
AVASTIN® (bevacizumab) Solution for intravenous infusion; product label, March 2013. Genentech Inc., South San Francisco, CA

(continued)

Notes about bevacizumab administration: The duration of administration for the initial dose is 90 minutes. If administration is well tolerated, the administration duration may be decreased stepwise during subsequent administrations to 60 minutes and, finally, to a minimum duration of 30 minutes

Supportive Care
Antiemetic prophylaxis
Emetogenic potential on a treatment day with cisplatin is **HIGH**. Potential for delayed emetic symptoms
See Chapter 39 for antiemetic recommendations

Hematopoietic growth factor (CSF) prophylaxis
Primary prophylaxis may be indicated
See Chapter 43 for more information

Antimicrobial prophylaxis
Risk of fever and neutropenia is LOW
Antimicrobial primary prophylaxis to be considered:
- Antibacterial—not indicated
- Antifungal—not indicated
- Antiviral—not indicated, unless patient previously had an episode of HSV

See Chapter 47 for more information

Patient Population Studied

Multicenter study. More than 70% of patients had previously received platinum-based therapy. Patients were randomly assigned to 1 of 4 treatment arms:

Arm I.	Paclitaxel and cisplatin on days 1 *or* 2, every 21 days
Arm II.	Paclitaxel on day 1 plus cisplatin and bevacizumab on days 1 *or* 2, every 21 days
Arm III.	Paclitaxel on day 1, and topotecan on days 1–3, every 21 days
Arm IV.	Paclitaxel and bevacizumab on day 1, and topotecan on days 1–3, every 21 days

Efficacy
(N = 425; Median Follow-up = 20.8 months)

	Cisplatin + Paclitaxel (N = 225)	Cisplatin + Paclitaxel + Bevacizumab (N = 227)
Complete response rate	6.2% (14)	12.3% (28)
Overall response rate	36%	48%
	2-sided p = 0.00807	
Median PFS	5.9 months	8.2 months
	HR = 0.67 (95% CI, 0.54−0.82; 2-sided p = 0.0002)	
Median OS*	13.3 months	17 months
	HR = 0.71 (95% CI, 0.54−0.94; p = 0.0035)	

CI, Confidence interval; HR, hazard ratio; OS, Overall survival; PFS, progression-free survival
*Advantage seen with bevacizumab in:
Patients between the ages of 48–56 years
Patients with recurrent/persistent disease
Patients with squamous histology
Patients with disease in the previously irradiated pelvis

Toxicity

	Cisplatin + Paclitaxel (N = 225)	Cisplatin + Paclitaxel + Bevacizumab (N = 227)
Treatment cycles, median (range)	6 (0–30)	7 (0–36)
Grade 5 adverse events	4 (1.8%)	4 (1.8%)
G ≥2 gastrointestinal, nonfistula	96 (44%)	114 (52%)
G ≥3 gastrointestinal fistula	0	7 (3%)
Gastrointestinal perforation (G ≥3)	0	5 (2%)
Thromboembolism	3 (1%)	18 (8%)
G ≥3 genitourinary fistula	0	6 (2%)
G ≥2 hypertension	4 (2%)	54 (25%)
G ≥3 proteinuria	0	4 (2%)
G ≥4 neutropenia	57 (26%)	78 (35%)
G ≥3 febrile neutropenia	12 (5%)	12 (5%)
G 3-4 bleeding	3 (1%)	12 (5%)
CNS bleeding (any grade)	0	0
G ≥2 pain	62 (28%)	71 (32%)

Treatment Monitoring

1. Prior to the start of a cycle: H&P; CBC with differential; serum LFTs; serum chemistries, including magnesium, potassium, and sodium; serum BUN and creatinine
2. Every week: CBC with differential and platelet count; monitor blood pressure at least weekly or more often as needed
3. Response Assessment: Every 2 cycles

9. Colorectal Cancer

Julia Lee Close, MD and Carmen Joseph Allegra, MD

Epidemiology

Incidence
Colon cancer: 96,830 (male: 48,450; female: 48,380. Estimated new cases for 2014 in the United States)
Rectum cancer: 40,000 (male: 23,380; female: 16,620. Estimated new cases for 2014 in the United States) 52.2 per 100,000 male, 39.3 per 100,000 female for colon and rectum cancer
Deaths: Estimated 50,310 in 2014 for colon and rectum cancer (male: 26,270; female: 24,040)

Median age at diagnosis: 69 years
Male to female ratio: 1.7:1

Siegel R et al. CA Cancer J Clin 2014;64:9–29
Surveillance, Epidemiology and End Results (SEER) Program, available from http://seer.cancer.gov (accessed in 2013)

Stage at presentation:

Stage I:	15%
Stage II:	20–30%
Stage III:	30–40%
Stage IV:	20–25%

Skibber JM et al. Cancer of the colon. In: Devita VT Jr, Hellman S, Rosenberg SA, editors. Cancer: Principles and Practice of Oncology, 6th ed. Philadelphia: Lippincott Williams & Wilkins, 2001:1216–1270

Five-Year Survival

	Colon	Rectal
I	>90%	>90%
II	75–85%	70–85%
IIIA	59%	55%
IIIB	42%	35%
IIIC	27%	24%
IV	<5%	<5%

A large proportion of colorectal cancer patients are potential candidates for adjuvant therapies for stage II or III disease.

AJCC Cancer Staging Manual, 6th ed. New York: Springer-Verlag, 2002:113–123
Greene FL et al. Ann Surg 2002;236:416–421
Greene FL et al. Proc Am Soc Clin Oncol 2003;22:251 [abstract 1007]

Work-up

In situ and Stage I	H&P, carcinoembryonic antigen and (CEA), full colonoscopy, and pathology review
Stage II	H&P, CBC, serum electrolytes, LFTs, serum creatinine, BUN, and CEA. Full colonoscopy, CT scan of thorax and abdomen, and pelvis, pathology review *Rectal lesions:* MRI. Determine whether there is a loss of heterozygosity at chromosome 18q and ascertain the presence of microsatellite instability (MSI). Patient at high risk based on loss of heterozygosity at 18q and MSI status can be recommended for adjuvant treatment
Stage III	As above for stages I–II. If patient has potentially resectable disease, additional studies may be needed before laparotomy to confirm resectability, including spiral CT scan, contrast MRI, PET scan, angiography, and laparoscopy
Stage IV	As above plus KRAS status

de Gramont A et al. Gastrointest Cancer Res 2008,2: S2–S6

Skibber JM et al. Cancer of the colon. In: Devita VT Jr, Hellman S, Rosenberg SA, editors. Cancer: Principles and Practice of Oncology, 6th ed. Philadelphia: Lippincott Williams & Wilkins, 2001:1216–1270

Pathology

World Health Organization Classification

1. Adenocarcinoma (>90%)
2. Mucinous adenocarcinoma
3. Adenosquamous carcinoma
4. Small cell carcinoma
5. Medullary carcinoma
6. Signet ring adenocarcinoma
7. Squamous cell carcinoma
8. Undifferentiated

Skibber JM et al. Cancer of the colon. In: Devita VT Jr, Hellman S, Rosenberg SA, editors. Cancer: Principles and Practice of Oncology, 6th ed. Philadelphia: Lippincott Williams & Wilkins, 2001:1216–1270

Staging

Primary Tumor (T)

TX	Primary tumor cannot be assessed
T0	No evidence of primary tumor
Tis	Carcinoma in situ: intraepithelial or invasion of lamina propria*
T1	Tumor invades submucosa
T2	Tumor invades muscularis propria
T3	Tumor invades through the muscularis propria into pericolorectal tissues
T4a	Tumor penetrates to the surface of the visceral peritoneum†
T4b	Tumor directly invades or is adherent to other organs or structures*,‡

*Tis includes cancer cells confined within the glandular basement membrane (intraepithelial) or mucosal lamina propria (intramucosal) with no extension through the muscularis mucosae into the submucosa.
†Tumor that is adherent to other organs or structures, grossly, is classified cT4b. However, if no tumor is present in the adhesion, microscopically, the classification should be pT1-4a depending on the anatomical depth of wall invasion. The V and L classifications should be used to identify the presence or absence of vascular or lymphatic invasion whereas the PN site-specific factor should be used for perineural invasion.
‡Direct invasion in T4 includes invasion of other organs or other segments of the colorectum as a result of direct extension through the serosa, as confirmed on microscopic examination (for example, invasion of the sigmoid colon by a carcinoma of the cecum) or, for cancers in a retro-peritoneal or subperitoneal location, direct invasion of other organs or structures by virtue of extension beyond the muscularis propria (ie, respectively, a tumor on the posterior wall of the descending colon invading the left kidney or lateral abdominal wall; or a mid or distal rectal cancer with invasion of prostate, seminal vesicles, cervix or vagina).

(continued)

Expert Opinion

Stage II colon cancer:

- Given the relatively low risk for recurrence for most patients with *stage II* colon cancer, the routine use of adjuvant chemotherapy for medically fit patients with stage II colon cancer is not recommended. The QUASAR trial is the only study to have shown a statistical benefit for fluorouracil/leucovorin
- Most experts recommend that adjuvant chemotherapy be considered for patients with *high-risk stage II* disease. Those considered at higher risk for recurrence include patients with:
  - Inadequately sampled nodes (<12)
  - T4 lesions
  - Perforation
  - Poorly differentiated histology, or
  - Lymphatic/vascular invasion
- Deficiency of mismatch repair proteins (MMR) is found in 15–20% of colon cancers. This deficiency has been associated with a low risk of recurrence. Only 1 retrospective study showed no or worse outcomes with fluorouracil, but this has never been validated by other studies. This tumor specific information needs to be considered in advising individual patients relative to adjuvant therapy

Stage III colon cancer:

- Systemic combined chemotherapy is the principal adjuvant therapy for *stage III* colon cancer
- The combinations of oxaliplatin with bolus or infusional fluorouracil/leucovorin
- (FOLFOX 4 or FLOX) have shown improved disease-free survival and overall survival compared with fluorouracil/leucovorin, and have become the standard
- Capecitabine can probably be used in place of bolus or infusional fluorouracil
- FOLFOX 4 or FLOX are associated with ~30% reduction in the risk of disease recurrence, and 22–32% reduction in mortality rate
- Trials testing the benefit of irinotecan, bevacizumab and cetuximab have all been negative in the adjuvant setting

Stage IV colon and rectal cancer:

- The choice of therapy is based on consideration of
  - The type and timing of the prior therapy that has been administered
  - The differing toxicity profiles of the constituent drugs
  - The possibility of resection of metastases
- Approximately 35% of patients have stage IV disease at presentation and 20% to 50% with stage II or III disease progress to stage IV
- Patients can be classified as potentially curable or noncurable
- Up to 60% of patients presenting with liver metastases who underwent a surgical resection were alive at 5 years in a report from Memorial Sloan-Kettering Cancer Center (MSKCC)
- Patients with previously untreated metastatic disease may be treated initially with FOLFOX (or XELOX) or FOLFIRI plus bevacizumab. The median survival approaches 2 years for patients with metastatic colorectal cancer treated initially with multi-agent therapy sets a benchmark
- Unfortunately, patients whose cancers harbor a BRAF mutation have a particularly poor outcome regardless of chemotherapeutic intervention
- Patients with progressive disease who have received fluorouracil–based therapy may be treated with chemotherapy consisting of FOLFIRI, irinotecan or FOLFOX (or XELOX) in addition to continuation of anti-vascular endothelial growth factor (VEGF) therapy or the addition of anti-epidermal growth factor receptor (EGFR) antibody therapy for those patients whose cancers do not contain a mutation in KRAS
- The oral anti-VEGF protein kinase inhibitor, regorafenib, has been shown to have activity in patients with disease that is refractory to the above listed agents

Rectal cancer:

- Preoperative chemoradiotherapy and postoperative chemoradiotherapy yield similar DFS and OS for patients with full thickness muscularis involvement T3), adjacent structure invasion (T4), and/or regional node involvement (N1/N2)
- Preoperative chemoradiotherapy, generally favored as a sphincter-sparing operation, is more likely to be technically feasible when compared to an upfront surgical approach
- Adjuvant chemotherapy is offered to patients who have undergone preoperative chemoradiotherapy
- Adjuvant chemotherapy for stages II and III is firmly established, albeit in the pre-neoadjuvant era. It remains the standard of care in the United States and Europe

Alberts SR et al. JAMA 2012;307:1383–1393
Allegra CJ et al. J Clin Oncol 2013;31:359–364
André T et al. J Clin Oncol 2009;27:3109–3116
Bertagnolli MM et al. J Clin Oncol 2011;29:3153–3162
Cassidy J et al. J Clin Oncol 2008;26:2006–2012
Fong Y et al. Ann Surg 1999;230:309–321
Grothey A et al. Lancet 2013;381:303–312
Haller DG et al. J Clin Oncol 2011;29:1465–1471
Hurwitz H et al. N Engl J Med 2004;350:2335–2342
Quasar Collaborative Group, Gray R et al. Lancet 2007;370:2020–2029
Saltz LB et al. J Clin Oncol 2007;25:3456–3461
Sauer R et al. N Engl J Med 2004;351:1731–1740
Seymour MT et al. Lancet 2007;370:143–152
Van Cutsem E et al. J Clin Oncol 2011;29:2011–2019

Staging (continued)

Regional Lymph Node (N)

NX	Regional lymph nodes cannot be assessed
N0	No regional lymph node metastasis
N1	Metastasis in one to three regional lymph nodes
N1a	Metastasis in one regional lymph node
N1b	Metastasis in two to three regional lymph nodes
N1c	Tumor deposit(s) in the subserosa, mesentery, or nonperitonealized pericolic or perirectal tissues without regional nodal metastasis
N2	Metastasis in four or more regional lymph nodes
N2a	Metastasis in four to six regional lymph nodes
N2b	Metastasis in seven or more regional lymph nodes

Distant Metastasis (M)

M0	No distant metastasis
M1	Distant metastasis
M1a	Metastasis confined to one organ or site (eg, liver, lung, ovary, nonregional node)
M1b	Metastases in more than one organ/site or the peritoneum

Anatomic Stage/Prognostic Groups

Stage	T	N	M	Dukes
0	Tis	N0	M0	—
I	T1	N0	M0	A
	T2	N0	M0	A
IIA	T3	N0	M0	B
IIB	T4a	N0	M0	B
IIC	T4b	N0	M0	B
IIIA	T1-2	N1/N1c	M0	C
	T1	N2a	M0	C
IIIB	T3-T4a	N1/N1c	M0	C
	T2-T3	N2a	M0	C
	T1-T2	N2b	M0	C
IIIC	T4a	N2a	M0	C
	T3-T4a	N2b	M0	C
	T4b	N1-N2	M0	C
IVA	Any T	Any N	M1a	—
IVB	Any T	Any N	M1b	—

Edge SB, Byrd DR, Compton CC, Fritz AG, Greene FL, Trotti A, editors. AJCC Cancer Staging Manual. 7th ed. New York: Springer; 2010

ADJUVANT AND ADVANCED REGIMEN

BOLUS FLUOROURACIL + LEUCOVORIN (ROSWELL PARK REGIMEN)

Petrelli N et al. J Clin Oncol 1989;7:1419–1426
Wolmark N et al. J Clin Oncol 1999;17:3553–3559

Adjuvant therapy:

Leucovorin calcium 500 mg/m^2; administer intravenously in 250 mL 0.9% sodium chloride injection (0.9% NS) over 2 hours once per week for 6 consecutive weeks (weeks 1–6), every 8 weeks (total dosage/cycle = 3000 mg/m^2)

Fluorouracil 500 mg/m^2; administer by intravenous injection over 1–2 minutes, starting 1 hour after leucovorin once per week for 6 consecutive weeks (weeks 1–6), every 8 weeks (total dosage/cycle = 3000 mg/m^2)

Advanced colorectal cancer:

Leucovorin calcium 500 mg/m^2; administer intravenously in 250 mL 0.9% NS over 2 hours once per week for 6 consecutive weeks (weeks 1–6), every 8 weeks (total dosage/cycle = 3000 mg/m^2)

Fluorouracil 600 mg/m^2; administer by intravenous injection over 1–2 minutes, starting 1 hour after leucovorin once per week for 6 consecutive weeks (weeks 1–6), every 8 weeks (total dosage/cycle = 3600 mg/m^2)

Supportive Care

Antiemetic prophylaxis

Emetogenic potential is **LOW**

See Chapter 39 for antiemetic recommendations

Hematopoietic growth factor (CSF) prophylaxis

Primary prophylaxis is NOT indicated

See Chapter 43 for more information

Antimicrobial prophylaxis

Risk of fever and neutropenia is LOW

Antimicrobial primary prophylaxis to be considered:

- Antibacterial—not indicated

- Antifungal—not indicated

- Antiviral—not indicated unless patient previously had an episode of HSV

See Chapter 47 for more information

Diarrhea management

Latent or delayed onset diarrhea*:

Loperamide 4 mg orally initially after the first loose or liquid stool, *then*

Loperamide 2 mg orally every 2 hours during waking hours, *plus*

Loperamide 4 mg orally every 4 hours during hours of sleep

- Continue for at least 12 hours after diarrhea resolves

- Recurrent diarrhea after a 12-hour diarrhea-free interval is treated as a new episode

- Rehydrate orally with fluids and electrolytes during a diarrheal episode

- If diarrhea persists >48 hours despite loperamide, stop loperamide and hospitalize the patient for IV hydration

Persistent diarrhea:

Octreotide 100–150 mcg subcutaneously 3 times daily. Maximum total daily dose is 1500 mcg

Antibiotic therapy during latent or delayed onset diarrhea:

A fluoroquinolone (eg, **Ciprofloxacin** 500 mg orally every 12 hours) if absolute neutrophil count is <500/mm^3 with or without accompanying fever in association with diarrhea

- Antibiotics should also be administered if patient is hospitalized with prolonged diarrhea and should be continued until diarrhea resolves

*Abigerges D et al. J Natl Cancer Inst 1994;86:446–449
Rothenberg ML et al. J Clin Oncol 2001;19:3801–3807
Wadler S et al. J Clin Oncol 1998;16:3169–3178

(continued)

Treatment Modifications

Adverse Event	Dose Modification*
Any G1 toxicity	Maintain dose
Any G2 toxicity	Hold treatment until toxicity resolves to G ≤1. If toxicity occurs after the fourth weekly dose, stop until the next cycle; then resume at same dosage. If diarrhea occurs, reduce fluorouracil to 400 mg/m^2 per dose
Any G3/4 toxicity	Hold treatment until toxicity resolves to G ≤1. If toxicity occurs after the fourth weekly dose, stop until next cycle; then resume with fluorouracil 400 mg/m^2 per dose. If diarrhea occurs, reduce fluorouracil to 350 mg/m^2 per dose
Further toxicity	Reduce fluorouracil to 300 mg/m^2 per dose. If diarrhea occurs, reduce fluorouracil to 250 mg/m^2 dose

*Leucovorin dosage remains constant at 500 mg/m^2 per dose

Adapted from NSABP C-07 protocol
Wolmark et al. Proc Am Soc Clin Oncol 2005;23:246S (abstract 3500)

(continued)

Oral care

Prophylaxis and treatment for mucositis/stomatitis

General advice:

- Encourage patients to maintain intake of non-alcoholic fluids
- Evaluate patients for oral pain and provide analgesic medications
- Consider histamine (H_2-subtype) receptor antagonists (eg, ranitidine, famotidine), or a proton pump inhibitor for epigastric pain
- *Lactobacillus* sp.-containing probiotics may be beneficial in preventing diarrhea

Patients with intact oral mucosa:

- Clean the mouth, tongue, and gums by brushing after every meal and at bedtime with an ultra-soft toothbrush with fluoride toothpaste
- Floss teeth gently every day unless contraindicated. If gums bleed and hurt, avoid bleeding or sore areas, but floss other teeth
- Patients may use saline or commercial bland, non-alcoholic rinses
  - Do not use mouthwashes that contain alcohols

If mucositis or stomatitis is present:

- Keep the mouth moist utilizing water, ice chips, sugarless gum, sugar-free hard candies, or a saliva substitute
- Rinse mouth several times a day to remove debris
  - Use a solution of ¼ teaspoon (1.25 g) each of baking soda and table salt (sodium chloride) in one quart (~950 mL) of warm water. Follow with a plain water rinse
  - Do not use mouthwashes that contain alcohols
- Foam-tipped swabs (eg, Toothettes®) are useful in moisturizing oral mucosa, but ineffective for cleansing teeth and removing plaque
- Advise patients who develop mucositis to:
  - Choose foods that are easy to chew and swallow
  - Take small bites of food, chew slowly, and sip liquids with meals
  - Encourage soft, moist foods such as cooked cereals, mashed potatoes, and scrambled eggs
  - For trouble swallowing, soften food with gravies, sauces, broths, yogurt, or other bland liquids
  - Avoid sharp, crunchy foods; hot, spicy or highly acidic foods (eg, citrus fruits and juices); sugary foods; toothpicks; tobacco products; alcoholic drinks

Patient Population Studied

Patients with stage II (Dukes B) or III (Dukes C) colorectal cancer after potentially curative resection (duration of therapy was 4 cycles). Now, the standard regimen as adjuvant therapy is FOLFOX-4, 6 months For advanced disease this regimen has to be considered for special cases (old patients…)

Wolmark N et al. J Clin Oncol 1999;17:3553–3559

Efficacy (N = 691)

	5-Year DFS	5-Year Overall Survival
All patients	65%	74%
Stage II	75%	84%
Stage III	57%	67%

DFS, disease-free survival

Toxicity (N = 691)

Most Common Toxicities by Grade

Toxicity	% G0	% G1	% G2	% G3	% G4
Overall	4	16	45	26	9
Diarrhea	21	15	37	22	5
Stomatitis	72	18	9	1	<1
Vomiting	66	14	15	3	2
Hematologic					<2
Neurologic					2% ataxia
Death					4 patients

Wolmark N et al. J Clin Oncol 1999;17:3553–3539

Therapy Monitoring

1. *Before each cycle:* H&P, CBC with differential, CEA, serum electrolytes, creatinine, BUN, and LFTs
2. *Every 2–3 months:* CT scans to assess cancer status in patients presenting with advanced colorectal cancer

ADJUVANT AND ADVANCED REGIMEN
BOLUS FLUOROURACIL

Francini G et al. Gastroenterology 1994;106:899–906
Poon MA et al. J Clin Oncol 1989;7:1407–1418
Van Cutsem E et al. J Clin Oncol 2001;19:4097–4106

Leucovorin calcium 20 mg/m² per day; administer by intravenous injection over 30 seconds on 5 consecutive days, given on days 1–5, every 4 weeks, for 6 cycles (total dosage/cycle = 100 mg/m²)
Fluorouracil 425 mg/m² per day; administer by intravenous injection over 1–2 minutes after leucovorin on 5 consecutive days, given on days 1–5, every 4 weeks, for 6 cycles (total dosage/cycle = 2125 mg/m²)

or

Leucovorin calcium 200 mg/m² per day; administer by intravenous injection at a rate <160 mg/minute on 5 consecutive days, given on days 1–5, every 4 weeks, for 6 cycles (total dosage/cycle = 1000 mg/m²)
Fluorouracil 400 mg/m² per day; administer by intravenous injection over 1–2 minutes after leucovorin on 5 consecutive days, given on days 1–5, every 4 weeks, for 6 cycles (total dosage/cycle = 2000 mg/m²)

Supportive Care
Antiemetic prophylaxis
Emetogenic potential is **LOW**
See Chapter 39 for antiemetic recommendations

Hematopoietic growth factor (CSF) prophylaxis
Primary prophylaxis is NOT indicated
See Chapter 43 for more information

Antimicrobial prophylaxis
Risk of fever and neutropenia is LOW
Antimicrobial primary prophylaxis to be considered:
- Antibacterial—not indicated
- Antifungal—not indicated
- Antiviral—not indicated unless patient previously had an episode of HSV

See Chapter 47 for more information

Diarrhea management
Latent or delayed onset diarrhea*:
Loperamide 4 mg orally initially after the first loose or liquid stool, *then*
Loperamide 2 mg orally every 2 hours during waking hours, *plus*
Loperamide 4 mg orally every 4 hours during hours of sleep
- Continue for at least 12 hours after diarrhea resolves
- Recurrent diarrhea after a 12-hour diarrhea-free interval is treated as a new episode
- Rehydrate orally with fluids and electrolytes during a diarrheal episode
- If diarrhea persists >48 hours despite loperamide, stop loperamide and hospitalize the patient for IV hydration

Persistent diarrhea:
Octreotide 100–150 mcg subcutaneously 3 times daily. Maximum total daily dose is 1500 mcg
Antibiotic therapy during latent or delayed onset diarrhea:
A fluoroquinolone (eg, **Ciprofloxacin** 500 mg orally every 12 hours) if absolute neutrophil count <500/mm³ with or without accompanying fever in association with diarrhea
- Antibiotics should also be administered if patient is hospitalized with prolonged diarrhea and should be continued until diarrhea resolves

*Abigerges D et al. J Natl Cancer Inst 1994;86:446–449
Rothenberg ML et al. J Clin Oncol 2001;19:3801–3807
Wadler S et al. J Clin Oncol 1998;16:3169–3178

(continued)

Treatment Modifications

Adverse Event	Dose Modification*
No toxicity	Optional escalation of fluorouracil dosage by 10%
G1 toxicity	Maintain dose
G2 nonhematologic adverse events	Reduce fluorouracil dosage by 20%
G3 hematologic adverse events	
G3/4 nonhematologic adverse events	Reduce fluorouracil dosage by 30%
G4 hematologic adverse events	

*Leucovorin dosage remains constant at 500 mg/m² per dose

Van Cutsem E et al. J Clin Oncol 2001;19:4097–4106

(continued)

Oral care
Prophylaxis and treatment for mucositis/stomatitis
  General advice:
  • Encourage patients to maintain intake of non-alcoholic fluids
  • Evaluate patients for oral pain and provide analgesic medications
  • Consider histamine (H_2-subtype) receptor antagonists (eg, ranitidine, famotidine), or a proton pump inhibitor for epigastric pain
  • *Lactobacillus* sp.-containing probiotics may be beneficial in preventing diarrhea
  • Patients with intact oral mucosa:
  • Clean the mouth, tongue, and gums by brushing after every meal and at bedtime with an ultra-soft toothbrush with fluoride toothpaste
  • Floss teeth gently every day unless contraindicated. If gums bleed and hurt, avoid bleeding or sore areas, but floss other teeth
  • Patients may use saline or commercial bland, non-alcoholic rinses
    ▪ Do not use mouthwashes that contain alcohols
  If mucositis or stomatitis is present:
  • Keep the mouth moist utilizing water, ice chips, sugarless gum, sugar-free hard candies, or a saliva substitute
  • Rinse mouth several times a day to remove debris
    ▪ Use a solution of ¼ teaspoon (1.25 g) each of baking soda and table salt (sodium chloride) in one quart (~950 mL) of warm water. Follow with a plain water rinse
    ▪ Do not use mouthwashes that contain alcohols
  • Foam-tipped swabs (eg, Toothettes®) are useful in moisturizing oral mucosa, but ineffective for cleansing teeth and removing plaque
  • Advise patients who develop mucositis to:
    ▪ Choose foods that are easy to chew and swallow
    ▪ Take small bites of food, chew slowly, and sip liquids with meals
    ▪ Encourage soft, moist foods such as cooked cereals, mashed potatoes, and scrambled eggs
    ▪ For trouble swallowing, soften food with gravies, sauces, broths, yogurt, or other bland liquids
    ▪ Avoid sharp, crunchy foods; hot, spicy or highly acidic foods (eg, citrus fruits and juices); sugary foods; toothpicks; tobacco products; alcoholic drinks

Hand-foot reaction (palmar-plantar erythrodysesthesia, PPE)
For patients who develop a hand-foot reaction, use topical emollients (eg, Aquaphor®), topical or orally administered steroids, antihistamine agents (H_1-receptor antagonists), or pyridoxine
  Pyridoxine may provide relief for discomfort/pain associated with PPE although the mechanism through which this occurs remains unclear
  • The suggested pyridoxine starting dose is 50 mg/day, which may be increased to a maximum of 200 mg/day

Patient Population Studied

Patients with stage II or III colorectal cancer after potentially curative resection, or with advanced colorectal cancer.

Efficacy (N = 301)

Complete response	0.7%
Partial response	14.3%
Stable disease	55.5%
Mean duration of response	9.4 months
Median time to progression	4.7 months
Median survival	12.1 months

Van Cutsem E et al. J Clin Oncol 2001;19:4097–4106

Toxicity (N = 299)

	% All G	% G3	% G4
Nonhematologic			
Stomatitis	55	13	0.3
Diarrhea	48	9.4	1
Nausea	39	—	—
Vomiting	25	—	—
Fatigue	12	—	—
Hand-foot syndrome	7	0.3	—
Increased bilirubin*	—	3	3.3
Hematologic			
Anemia	—	0.7	0.3
Neutropenia	—	9.4	10.4
Thrombocytopenia	—	0	0.3

*G3 and G4 correspond to G2 and G3 in updated National Cancer Institute of Canada Common Toxicity Criteria

Van Cutsem E et al. J Clin Oncol 2001;19:4097–4106

Therapy Monitoring

1. *Before each cycle:* H&P, CBC with differential, CEA, serum electrolytes, creatinine, BUN, and LFTs
2. *Every 2–3 months:* CT scans to assess cancer status

ADJUVANT AND ADVANCED REGIMEN

CAPECITABINE

Twelves C et al. N Engl J Med 2005;352:2696–2704
Van Cutsem E et al. J Clin Oncol 2001;19:4097–4106

Capecitabine 1250 mg/m² per dose; administer orally with water within 30 minutes after a meal twice daily for 28 doses on days 1–14, every 3 weeks (total dosage/cycle = 35,000 mg/m²)

Notes:
- Capecitabine is given for 2 consecutive weeks followed by 1 week without treatment
- Doses are rounded down to approximate a calculated dose using combinations of 500-mg and 150-mg tablets
- In practice, treatment often is begun with capecitabine 1000 mg/m² per dose twice daily for 28 doses on days 1–14 (total dosage/cycle = 28,000 mg/m²). Dosage may be increased during subsequent cycles if initial treatment at a lesser dosage is tolerated

Supportive Care
Antiemetic prophylaxis
Emetogenic potential is **LOW**
See Chapter 39 for antiemetic recommendations

Hematopoietic growth factor (CSF) prophylaxis
Primary prophylaxis is *NOT* indicated
See Chapter 43 for more information

Antimicrobial prophylaxis
Risk of fever and neutropenia is LOW
Antimicrobial primary prophylaxis to be considered:
- Antibacterial—not indicated
- Antifungal—not indicated
- Antiviral—not indicated unless patient previously had an episode of HSV

See Chapter 47 for more information

Diarrhea management
Latent or delayed onset diarrhea*:
Loperamide 4 mg orally initially after the first loose or liquid stool, *then*
Loperamide 2 mg orally every 2 hours during waking hours, *plus*
Loperamide 4 mg orally every 4 hours during hours of sleep
- Continue for at least 12 hours after diarrhea resolves
- Recurrent diarrhea after a 12-hour diarrhea-free interval is treated as a new episode
- Rehydrate orally with fluids and electrolytes during a diarrheal episode
- If diarrhea persists >48 hours despite loperamide, stop loperamide and hospitalize the patient for IV hydration

Persistent diarrhea:
Octreotide 100–150 mcg subcutaneously 3 times daily. Maximum total daily dose is 1500 mcg

Antibiotic therapy during latent or delayed onset diarrhea:
A fluoroquinolone (eg, **Ciprofloxacin** 500 mg orally every 12 hours) if absolute neutrophil count is <500/mm³ with or without accompanying fever in association with diarrhea
- Antibiotics should also be administered if patient is hospitalized with prolonged diarrhea and should be continued until diarrhea resolves

*Abigerges D et al. J Natl Cancer Inst 1994;86:446–449
Rothenberg ML et al. J Clin Oncol 2001;19:3801–3807
Wadler S et al. J Clin Oncol 1998;16:3169–3178

(continued)

Treatment Modifications

Adverse Event	Dose Modification
First occurrence of a G2 toxicity	No dose reduction*
Second occurrence of a given G2 toxicity	Reduce dosage by 25%*
First occurrence of a G3 toxicity	
Third occurrence of a given G2 toxicity	Reduce dosage by 50%*
Second occurrence of a given G3 toxicity	
Any G4 toxicity	
Fourth occurrence of a given G2 toxicity	Discontinue capecitabine
Third occurrence of a given G3 toxicity	
Second occurrence of a given G4 toxicity	
Both G4 hematologic and G4 nonhematologic toxicity	

*Interrupt capecitabine treatment until is toxicity resolves to G ≤1

National Cancer Institute of Canada Common Toxicity Criteria

(continued)

Oral care
Prophylaxis and treatment for mucositis/stomatitis
General advice:
- Encourage patients to maintain intake of non-alcoholic fluids
- Evaluate patients for oral pain and provide analgesic medications
- Consider histamine (H_2-subtype) receptor antagonists (eg, ranitidine, famotidine), or a proton pump inhibitor for epigastric pain
- *Lactobacillus* sp.-containing probiotics may be beneficial in preventing diarrhea

Patients with intact oral mucosa:
- Clean the mouth, tongue, and gums by brushing after every meal and at bedtime with an ultra-soft toothbrush with fluoride toothpaste
- Floss teeth gently every day unless contraindicated. If gums bleed and hurt, avoid bleeding or sore areas, but floss other teeth
- Patients may use saline or commercial bland, non-alcoholic rinses
  - Do not use mouthwashes that contain alcohols

If mucositis or stomatitis is present:
- Keep the mouth moist utilizing water, ice chips, sugarless gum, sugar-free hard candies, or a saliva substitute
- Rinse mouth several times a day to remove debris
  - Use a solution of ¼ teaspoon (1.25 g) each of baking soda and table salt (sodium chloride) in one quart (~950 mL) of warm water. Follow with a plain water rinse
  - Do not use mouthwashes that contain alcohols
- Foam-tipped swabs (eg, Toothettes®) are useful in moisturizing oral mucosa, but ineffective for cleansing teeth and removing plaque
- Advise patients who develop mucositis to:
  - Choose foods that are easy to chew and swallow
  - Take small bites of food, chew slowly, and sip liquids with meals
  - Encourage soft, moist foods such as cooked cereals, mashed potatoes, and scrambled eggs
  - For trouble swallowing, soften food with gravies, sauces, broths, yogurt, or other bland liquids
  - Avoid sharp, crunchy foods; hot, spicy or highly acidic foods (eg, citrus fruits and juices); sugary foods; toothpicks; tobacco products; alcoholic drinks

Hand-foot reaction (palmar-plantar erythrodysesthesia, PPE)
For patients who develop a hand-foot reaction, use topical emollients (eg, Aquaphor®), topical or orally administered steroids, antihistamine agents (H_1-receptor antagonists), or pyridoxine

Pyridoxine may provide relief for discomfort/pain associated with PPE although the mechanism through which this occurs remains unclear
- The suggested pyridoxine starting dose is 50 mg/day, which may be increased to a maximum of 200 mg/day

Toxicity (N = 297)

	% All G	% G3	% G4
Nonhematologic			
Diarrhea	50.2	9.4	1.3
Hand-foot syndrome	48	16.2	0
Nausea	37.7	—	—
Stomatitis	21.9	1	0.3
Vomiting	18.5	—	—
Fatigue	10	—	—
Increased bilirubin[*,†]	—	23.6	4.7
Hematologic			
Anemia	—	2.7	0
Neutropenia	—	0	2
Thrombocytopenia	—	0.7	0.3

*G3 and G4 correspond to G2 and G3 in updated National Cancer Institute of Canada Common Toxicity Criteria

†Eight (10%) patients with G3/4 hyperbilirubinemia also had G3 abnormalities in ALT or AST

Van Cutsem E et al. J Clin Oncol 2001;19:4097–4106

Therapy Monitoring
1. *Before each cycle:* H&P, CBC with differential, CEA, serum electrolytes, creatinine, BUN, and LFTs
2. *Every 2–3 months:* CT scans to assess cancer status in patients presenting with advanced colorectal cancer

Patient Population Studied

Patients receiving first-line treatment for metastatic colorectal cancer and adjuvant therapy for early stage colorectal cancer. Equivalent to bolus fluorouracil 1 leucovorin. At present, the standard regimen for adjuvant therapy is FOLFOX-4 for six months

For advanced disease, this regimen should be considered for special cases; eg, elderly patients

Efficacy (N = 301)

Complete response	0.3%
Partial response	18.6%
Stable disease	56.8%
Mean duration of response	7.2 months
Median time to progression	5.2 months
Median survival	13.2 months

Van Cutsem E et al. J Clin Oncol 2001;19:4097–4106

METASTATIC DISEASE REGIMEN
INFUSIONAL FLUOROURACIL

Hansen RM et al. J Natl Cancer Inst 1996;88:668–674

Fluorouracil 300 mg/m² per day; administer by continuous intravenous infusion in 50–1000 mL 0.9% sodium chloride injection or 5% dextrose injection (total dosage/week = 2100 mg/m²). Treatment is continued indefinitely until toxicity/disease progression

Supportive Care
Antiemetic prophylaxis
Emetogenic potential is **LOW**
See Chapter 39 for antiemetic recommendations

Hematopoietic growth factor (CSF) prophylaxis
Primary prophylaxis is NOT indicated
See Chapter 43 for more information

Antimicrobial prophylaxis
Risk of fever and neutropenia is LOW
   Antimicrobial primary prophylaxis to be considered:
   • Antibacterial—not indicated
   • Antifungal—not indicated
   • Antiviral—not indicated unless patient previously had an episode of HSV
See Chapter 47 for more information

Diarrhea management
Latent or delayed onset diarrhea*:
   Loperamide 4 mg orally initially after the first loose or liquid stool, *then*
   Loperamide 2 mg orally every 2 hours during waking hours, *plus*
   Loperamide 4 mg orally every 4 hours during hours of sleep
   • Continue for at least 12 hours after diarrhea resolves
   • Recurrent diarrhea after a 12-hour diarrhea-free interval is treated as a new episode
   • Rehydrate orally with fluids and electrolytes during a diarrheal episode
   • If diarrhea persists >48 hours despite loperamide, stop loperamide and hospitalize the patient for IV hydration
Persistent diarrhea:
   Octreotide 100–150 mcg subcutaneously 3 times daily. Maximum total daily dose is 1500 mcg
Antibiotic therapy during latent or delayed onset diarrhea:
   A fluoroquinolone (eg, **Ciprofloxacin** 500 mg orally every 12 hours) if absolute neutrophil count is <500/mm³ with or without accompanying fever in association with diarrhea
   • Antibiotics should also be administered if patient is hospitalized with prolonged diarrhea and should be continued until diarrhea resolves

*Abigerges D et al. J Natl Cancer Inst 1994;86:446–449
Rothenberg ML et al. J Clin Oncol 2001;19:3801–3807
Wadler S et al. J Clin Oncol 1998;16:3169–3178

Oral care
Prophylaxis and treatment for mucositis/stomatitis
   General advice:
   • Encourage patients to maintain intake of non-alcoholic fluids
   • Evaluate patients for oral pain and provide analgesic medications
   • Consider histamine (H₂-subtype) receptor antagonists (eg, ranitidine, famotidine), or a proton pump inhibitor for epigastric pain
   • *Lactobacillus* sp.-containing probiotics may be beneficial in preventing diarrhea

(continued)

Patient Population Studied

A study of 159 patients with previously untreated metastatic adenocarcinoma of the colon or rectum

Toxicity (N = 159)
Requiring Treatment Interruption

G2 stomatitis	35%
G3 stomatitis	5%
G2/3 hand-foot syndrome	36%
G3 vomiting and diarrhea	3%
G3/4 hematologic	6%
All toxicities	
None	2%
Mild	15%
Moderate	52%
Severe	27%
Life-threatening	4%
Lethal	1%

(*continued*)

Patients with intact oral mucosa:
- Clean the mouth, tongue, and gums by brushing after every meal and at bedtime with an ultra-soft toothbrush with fluoride toothpaste
- Floss teeth gently every day unless contraindicated. If gums bleed and hurt, avoid bleeding or sore areas, but floss other teeth
- Patients may use saline or commercial bland, non-alcoholic rinses
  - Do not use mouthwashes that contain alcohols

If mucositis or stomatitis is present:
- Keep the mouth moist utilizing water, ice chips, sugarless gum, sugar-free hard candies, or a saliva substitute
- Rinse mouth several times a day to remove debris
  - Use a solution of ¼ teaspoon (1.25 g) each of baking soda and table salt (sodium chloride) in one quart (~950 mL) of warm water. Follow with a plain water rinse
  - Do not use mouthwashes that contain alcohols
- Foam-tipped swabs (eg, Toothettes®) are useful in moisturizing oral mucosa, but ineffective for cleansing teeth and removing plaque
- Advise patients who develop mucositis to:
  - Choose foods that are easy to chew and swallow
  - Take small bites of food, chew slowly, and sip liquids with meals
  - Encourage soft, moist foods such as cooked cereals, mashed potatoes, and scrambled eggs
  - For trouble swallowing, soften food with gravies, sauces, broths, yogurt, or other bland liquids
  - Avoid sharp, crunchy foods; hot, spicy or highly acidic foods (eg, citrus fruits and juices); sugary foods; toothpicks; tobacco products; alcoholic drinks

Hand-foot reaction (palmar-plantar erythrodysesthesia, PPE)
For patients who develop a hand-foot reaction, use topical emollients (eg, Aquaphor®), topical or orally administered steroids, antihistamine agents (H_1-receptor antagonists), or pyridoxine
  Pyridoxine may provide relief for discomfort/pain associated with PPE although the mechanism through which this occurs remains unclear
- The suggested pyridoxine starting dose is 50 mg/day, which may be increased to a maximum of 200 mg/day

Treatment Modifications

Adverse Event	Dose Modification
G2 nonhematologic toxicity	Reduce fluorouracil dosage by 50 mg/m² per day
G3 nonhematologic toxicity	Reduce fluorouracil dosage by 100 mg/m² per day
Hematologic toxicity	No modifications

Therapy Monitoring

1. *Before each cycle:* H&P, CBC with differential, CEA serum electrolytes, and LFTs
2. *Weekly:* CBC with differential count
3. *Every 2–3 months:* CT scans to assess response

Efficacy (N = 159)

Overall response	28%
Complete response	5%
Median survival	13 months

METASTATIC DISEASE REGIMEN
SINGLE-AGENT IRINOTECAN (CPT-11)

Cunningham D et al. Lancet 1998;352:1413–1418

Irinotecan 350 mg/m²; administer intravenously over 90 minutes in 250 mL 5% dextrose injection (D5W) or 0.9% sodium Chloride injection (0.9% NS), on day 1, every 3 weeks (total dosage/cycle = 350 mg/m²)

Note: Reduce dosage to 300 mg/m² for patients ≥70 years of age or whose WHO performance status = 2 (total dosage/4-week cycle = 300 mg/m²)

Alternative

Pitot HC. Oncology 1998;12(8 Suppl 6):48–53

Irinotecan 100–125 mg/m²; administer intravenously over 90 minutes in 250 mL 0.9% NS or D5W every week for 4 consecutive weeks every 6 weeks (total dosage/cycle = 400–500 mg/m²)

Note: Four weeks of treatment followed by 2 weeks without treatment

Supportive Care
Antiemetic prophylaxis
Emetogenic potential is **MODERATE**
See Chapter 39 for antiemetic recommendations

Hematopoietic growth factor (CSF) prophylaxis
Primary prophylaxis is NOT indicated
See Chapter 43 for more information

Antimicrobial prophylaxis
Risk of fever and neutropenia is LOW
  Antimicrobial primary prophylaxis to be considered:
  • Antibacterial—not indicated
  • Antifungal—not indicated
  • Antiviral—not indicated unless patient previously had an episode of HSV
See Chapter 47 for more information

Acute cholinergic syndrome
Atropine sulfate 0.25–1 mg administer subcutaneously or intravenously if abdominal cramping or diarrhea develop during or within 1 hour after irinotecan administration
• If symptoms are severe, add as primary prophylaxis at least 30 min before irinotecan during subsequent cycles
• For irinotecan, acute cholinergic syndrome may be characterized by: abdominal cramping, diarrhea, diaphoresis, hypotension, flushing, bradycardia, rhinitis, increased salivation, meiosis, and lacrimation

Diarrhea management
Latent or delayed onset diarrhea*:
  Loperamide 4 mg orally initially after the first loose or liquid stool, *then*
  Loperamide 2 mg orally every 2 hours during waking hours, *plus*
  Loperamide 4 mg orally every 4 hours during hours of sleep
  • Continue for at least 12 hours after diarrhea resolves
  • Recurrent diarrhea after a 12-hour diarrhea-free interval is treated as a new episode
  • Rehydrate orally with fluids and electrolytes during a diarrheal episode
  • If diarrhea persists >48 hours despite loperamide, stop loperamide and hospitalize the patient for IV hydration
Persistent diarrhea:
  Octreotide 100–150 mcg subcutaneously 3 times daily. Maximum total daily dose is 1500 mcg
Antibiotic therapy during latent or delayed onset diarrhea:
  A fluoroquinolone (eg, **Ciprofloxacin** 500 mg orally every 12 hours) if absolute neutrophil count is <500/mm³ with or without accompanying fever in association with diarrhea
  • Antibiotics should also be administered if patient is hospitalized with prolonged diarrhea and should be continued until diarrhea resolves

*Abigerges D et al. J Natl Cancer Inst 1994;86:446–449
Rothenberg ML et al. J Clin Oncol 2001;19:3801–3807
Wadler S et al. J Clin Oncol 1998;16:3169–3178

(continued)

(*continued*)

Oral care
Prophylaxis and treatment for mucositis/stomatitis
General advice:
- Encourage patients to maintain intake of non-alcoholic fluids
- Evaluate patients for oral pain and provide analgesic medications
- Consider histamine (H$_2$-subtype) receptor antagonists (eg, ranitidine, famotidine), or a proton pump inhibitor for epigastric pain
- *Lactobacillus* sp.-containing probiotics may be beneficial in preventing diarrhea

Patients with intact oral mucosa:
- Clean the mouth, tongue, and gums by brushing after every meal and at bedtime with an ultra-soft toothbrush with fluoride toothpaste
- Floss teeth gently every day unless contraindicated. If gums bleed and hurt, avoid bleeding or sore areas, but floss other teeth
- Patients may use saline or commercial bland, non-alcoholic rinses
  - Do not use mouthwashes that contain alcohols

If mucositis or stomatitis is present:
- Keep the mouth moist utilizing water, ice chips, sugarless gum, sugar-free hard candies, or a saliva substitute
- Rinse mouth several times a day to remove debris
  - Use a solution of ¼ teaspoon (1.25 g) each of baking soda and table salt (sodium chloride) in one quart (~950 mL) of warm water. Follow with a plain water rinse
  - Do not use mouthwashes that contain alcohols
- Foam-tipped swabs (eg, Toothettes®) are useful in moisturizing oral mucosa, but ineffective for cleansing teeth and removing plaque
- Advise patients who develop mucositis to:
  - Choose foods that are easy to chew and swallow
  - Take small bites of food, chew slowly, and sip liquids with meals
  - Encourage soft, moist foods such as cooked cereals, mashed potatoes, and scrambled eggs
  - For trouble swallowing, soften food with gravies, sauces, broths, yogurt, or other bland liquids
  - Avoid sharp, crunchy foods; hot, spicy or highly acidic foods (eg, citrus fruits and juices); sugary foods; toothpicks; tobacco products; alcoholic drinks

Treatment Modifications

(Camptosar, irinotecan hydrochloride injection product label, July 2005. Pharmacia & Upjohn Company, Division of Pfizer, Inc., New York, NY)

Irinotecan—Once Every 3 Weeks

Notes:
- Dose modifications are based on the National Cancer Institute (USA) Common Toxicity Criteria. At: http://ctep.cancer.gov/protocolDevelopment/electronic_applications/ctc.htm [accessed October 11, 2013]
- Before beginning a treatment cycle, patients should have baseline bowel function (similar to that before start of treatment) without antidiarrheal therapy for 24 hours, ANC ≥1500/mm^3, and platelet count ≥100,000/mm^3
- Treatment should be delayed 1–2 weeks to allow for recovery from treatment-related toxicities. If a patient has not recovered after 2 weeks, consider stopping therapy

Toxicity in Previous Cycle	Irinotecan Dosage at the Start of a 3-Week Cycle
Neutropenia/Thrombocytopenia	
G1 ANC (1500–1999/mm^3) or G1 thrombocytopenia	Maintain dose and schedule
G2 ANC (1000–1499/mm^3) or G2 thrombocytopenia	Maintain dose and schedule
G3 ANC (500–999/mm^3) or G3 thrombocytopenia	Reduce dosage by 50 mg/m^2
G4 ANC (<500/mm^3) or G4 thrombocytopenia	Reduce dosage by 50 mg/m^2
Febrile neutropenia	Hold until neutropenia resolves. Resume treatment with irinotecan dosage reduced by 50 mg/m^2

(*continued*)

Treatment Modifications (continued)

Toxicity in Previous Cycle	Irinotecan Dosage at the Start of a 3-Week Cycle
Diarrhea	
G1 (2–3 stools/day > baseline)	Maintain dose and schedule
G2 (4–6 stools/day > baseline)	Maintain dose and schedule
G3 (7–9 stools/day > baseline)	Reduce irinotecan dosage by 50 mg/m²
G4 (≥10 stools/day > baseline)	Reduce irinotecan dosage by 50 mg/m²
Other Nonhematologic Toxicities	
Any G1 toxicity	Maintain dose and schedule
Any G2 toxicity	Maintain dose and schedule
Any G3 toxicity	Reduce dosage by 50 mg/m²
Any G4 toxicity	Reduce dosage by 50 mg/m²

Weekly Irinotecan—4 of Every 6 Weeks

Notes:

- Dose modifications are based on the National Cancer Institute (USA) Common Toxicity Criteria. At: http://ctep.cancer.gov/protocolDevelopment/electronic_applications/ctc.htm [accessed October 11, 2013]
- Before beginning a treatment cycle, patients should have baseline bowel function (similar to that before start of treatment) without antidiarrheal therapy for 24 hours, ANC ≥1500/mm³, and platelet count ≥100,000/mm³
- Treatment should be delayed 1–2 weeks to allow for recovery from treatment-related toxicities. If a patient has not recovered after 2 weeks, consider stopping therapy

Toxicity	Weekly Irinotecan Dosage Based on Intracycle Toxicity	Irinotecan Dosage at Start of a 6-Week Cycle
Neutropenia/Thrombocytopenia		
G1 ANC (1500–1999/mm³) or G1 thrombocytopenia	Maintain dose and schedule	Maintain dose and schedule
G2 ANC (1000–1499/mm³) or G2 thrombocytopenia	Decrease weekly dosage by 25 mg/m²	Maintain dose and schedule
G3 ANC (500–999/mm³) or G3 thrombocytopenia	Omit weekly dose until toxicity G ≤2, then reduce irinotecan dosage by 25 mg/m²	Reduce dosage by 25 mg/m²
G4 ANC (<500/mm³) or G4 thrombocytopenia	Omit weekly dose until toxicity G ≤2, then reduce irinotecan dosage by 50 mg/m²	Reduce dosage by 50 mg/m²
Febrile neutropenia	Omit weekly dose until neutropenia G ≤2, then reduce irinotecan dosage by 50 mg/m²	Reduce dosage by 50 mg/m²
Diarrhea		
G1 (2–3 stools/day > baseline)	Delay treatment until diarrhea resolves to baseline; then resume irinotecan treatment	Maintain dose and schedule
G2 (4–6 stools/day > baseline)	Delay until diarrhea resolves to baseline, then reduce irinotecan dosage by 25 mg/m²	Maintain dose and schedule
G3 (7–9 stools/day > baseline)	Delay until diarrhea resolves to baseline, then reduce irinotecan dosage by 25 mg/m²	Reduce dosage by 25 mg/m²
G4 (≥10 stools/day > baseline)	Delay until diarrhea resolves to baseline, then reduce irinotecan dosage by 50 mg/m²	Reduce dosage by 50 mg/m²

(continued)

Treatment Modifications (continued)

Toxicity	Weekly Irinotecan Dosage Based on Intracycle Toxicity	Irinotecan Dosage at Start of a 6-Week Cycle
Other Nonhematologic Toxicities		
Any G1 toxicity	Maintain dose and schedule	Maintain dose and schedule
Any G2 toxicity	Delay until toxicity resolves to G ≤1, then reduce irinotecan dosage by 25 mg/m²	Maintain dose and schedule
Any G3 toxicity	Delay until toxicity resolves to G ≤2, then reduce irinotecan dosage by 25 mg/m²	Reduce dosage by 25 mg/m²
Any G4 toxicity	Delay until toxicity resolves to G ≤2, then reduce irinotecan dosage by 50 mg/m²	Reduce dosage by 50 mg/m²

Toxicity (N = 183)

Toxicity	% G3/4
Any G3/4 toxicity	79
Nonhematologic	
Diarrhea	22
Nonabdominal pain	19
Asthenia	15
Abdominal pain	14
Nausea	14
Vomiting	14
Neurologic symptoms	12
Cholinergic symptoms	12
Constipation	10
Infection without G3/4 ANC	9
Anorexia	5
Mucositis	2
Cutaneous signs	2
Hematologic	
Leukopenia/neutropenia	22
Anemia	7
Thrombocytopenia	1
Fever/infection with G3 ANC	3

Cunningham D et al. Lancet 1998;352:1413–1418

Patient Population Studied

A study of 189 patients with metastatic colorectal cancer with documented disease progression within 6 months of fluorouracil-based treatment

Efficacy (N = 189)

	Irinotecan	Best Supportive Care
Partial response	4%	0.7%
Partial or minor response	10.5%	4.4%
Median survival	9.2 months	6.5 months

Therapy Monitoring

1. *Before each cycle:* H&P, CBC with differential, CEA, serum electrolytes, and LFTs
2. *Weekly:* CBC with differential count
3. *Every 2–3 months:* CT scans to assess response

METASTATIC DISEASE REGIMEN
IRINOTECAN + BOLUS FLUOROURACIL + LEUCOVORIN (IFL)

Saltz LB et al. N Engl J Med 2000;343:905–914

Irinotecan 125 mg/m² per dose; administer intravenously in 250 mL 5% dextrose injection (D5W) over 90 minutes, given weekly for 4 consecutive weeks (4 doses), every 6 weeks (total dosage/cycle = 500 mg/m²)

Leucovorin calcium 20 mg/m² per dose; administer by intravenous injection over 30 seconds, given weekly for 4 consecutive weeks (4 doses), every 6 weeks (total dosage/cycle = 80 mg/m²)

Fluorouracil 500 mg/m² per dose; administer by intravenous injection over 1–2 minutes after leucovorin, given weekly for 4 consecutive weeks (4 doses), every 6 weeks (total dosage/cycle = 2000 mg/m²)

Supportive Care
Antiemetic prophylaxis
Emetogenic potential is **MODERATE**
See Chapter 39 for antiemetic recommendations

Hematopoietic growth factor (CSF) prophylaxis
Primary prophylaxis is NOT indicated
See Chapter 43 for more information

Antimicrobial prophylaxis
Risk of fever and neutropenia is LOW
Antimicrobial primary prophylaxis to be considered:
- Antibacterial—not indicated
- Antifungal—not indicated
- Antiviral—not indicated unless patient previously had an episode of HSV

See Chapter 47 for more information

Acute cholinergic syndrome
Atropine sulfate 0.25–1 mg administer subcutaneously or intravenously if abdominal cramping or diarrhea develop during or within 1 hour after irinotecan administration
- If symptoms are severe, add as primary prophylaxis at least 30 min before irinotecan during subsequent cycles
- For irinotecan, acute cholinergic syndrome may be characterized by: abdominal cramping, diarrhea, diaphoresis, hypotension, flushing, bradycardia, rhinitis, increased salivation, meiosis, and lacrimation

Diarrhea management
Latent or delayed onset diarrhea*:
Loperamide 4 mg orally initially after the first loose or liquid stool, *then*
Loperamide 2 mg orally every 2 hours during waking hours, *plus*
Loperamide 4 mg orally every 4 hours during hours of sleep
- Continue for at least 12 hours after diarrhea resolves
- Recurrent diarrhea after a 12-hour diarrhea-free interval is treated as a new episode
- Rehydrate orally with fluids and electrolytes during a diarrheal episode
- If diarrhea persists >48 hours despite loperamide, stop loperamide and hospitalize the patient for IV hydration

Persistent diarrhea:
Octreotide 100–150 mcg subcutaneously 3 times daily. Maximum total daily dose is 1500 mcg

Antibiotic therapy during latent or delayed onset diarrhea:
A fluoroquinolone (eg, **Ciprofloxacin** 500 mg orally every 12 hours) if absolute neutrophil count is <500/mm³ with or without accompanying fever in association with diarrhea
- Antibiotics should also be administered if patient is hospitalized with prolonged diarrhea and should be continued until diarrhea resolves

*Abigerges D et al. J Natl Cancer Inst 1994;86:446–449
Rothenberg ML et al. J Clin Oncol 2001;19:3801–3807
Wadler S et al. J Clin Oncol 1998;16:3169–3178

Oral care
Prophylaxis and treatment for mucositis/stomatitis
General advice:
- Encourage patients to maintain intake of non-alcoholic fluids
- Evaluate patients for oral pain and provide analgesic medications
- Consider histamine (H₂-subtype) receptor antagonists (eg, ranitidine, famotidine), or a proton pump inhibitor for epigastric pain
- *Lactobacillus* sp.-containing probiotics may be beneficial in preventing diarrhea

(continued)

(continued)

Patients with intact oral mucosa:
- Clean the mouth, tongue, and gums by brushing after every meal and at bedtime with an ultra-soft toothbrush with fluoride toothpaste
- Floss teeth gently every day unless contraindicated. If gums bleed and hurt, avoid bleeding or sore areas, but floss other teeth
- Patients may use saline or commercial bland, non-alcoholic rinses
  - Do not use mouthwashes that contain alcohols

If mucositis or stomatitis is present:
- Keep the mouth moist utilizing water, ice chips, sugarless gum, sugar-free hard candies, or a saliva substitute
- Rinse mouth several times a day to remove debris
  - Use a solution of ¼ teaspoon (1.25 g) each of baking soda and table salt (sodium chloride) in one quart (~950 mL) of warm water. Follow with a plain water rinse
  - Do not use mouthwashes that contain alcohols
- Foam-tipped swabs (eg, Toothettes®) are useful in moisturizing oral mucosa, but ineffective for cleansing teeth and removing plaque
- Advise patients who develop mucositis to:
  - Choose foods that are easy to chew and swallow
  - Take small bites of food, chew slowly, and sip liquids with meals
  - Encourage soft, moist foods such as cooked cereals, mashed potatoes, and scrambled eggs
  - For trouble swallowing, soften food with gravies, sauces, broths, yogurt, or other bland liquids
  - Avoid sharp, crunchy foods; hot, spicy or highly acidic foods (eg, citrus fruits and juices); sugary foods; toothpicks; tobacco products; alcoholic drinks

Hand-foot reaction (palmar-plantar erythrodysesthesia, PPE)
For patients who develop a hand-foot reaction, use topical emollients (eg, Aquaphor®), topical or orally administered steroids, antihistamine agents (H_1-receptor antagonists), or pyridoxine
  Pyridoxine may provide relief for discomfort/pain associated with PPE although the mechanism through which this occurs remains unclear
- The suggested pyridoxine starting dose is 50 mg/day, which may be increased to a maximum of 200 mg/day

Treatment Modifications

(Camptosar, irinotecan hydrochloride injection product label, July 2005. Pharmacia & Upjohn Company, Division of Pfizer, Inc., New York, NY)

	Dosage Levels		
	Initial	−1	−2
Irinotecan	125 mg/m²	100 mg/m²	75 mg/m²
Leucovorin	Racemic leucovorin calcium 400 mg/m² or levoleucovorin calcium 200 mg/m²		
Fluorouracil	500 mg/m²	400 mg/m²	300 mg/m²

Notes:
- Dose modifications are based on the National Cancer Institute (USA) Common Toxicity Criteria. At: http://ctep.cancer.gov/protocolDevelopment/electronic_applications/ctc.htm [accessed October 11, 2013]
- Before beginning a treatment cycle, patients should have baseline bowel function (similar to that before start of treatment) without antidiarrheal therapy for 24 hours, ANC ≥1500/mm³, and platelet count ≥100,000/mm³
- Treatment should be delayed 1−2 weeks to allow for recovery from treatment-related toxicities. If a patient has not recovered after 2 weeks, consider stopping therapy
- If toxicity occurs despite 2 dose reductions (ie, on level −2) discontinue therapy

(continued)

Treatment Modifications (continued)

Toxicity	Weekly Dosage Based on Intracycle Toxicity	Dosage at the Start of a 6-Week Cycle
Neutropenia/Thrombocytopenia		
G1 ANC (1500–1999/mm³) or G1 thrombocytopenia	Maintain dose and schedule	Maintain dose and schedule
G2 ANC (1000–1499/mm³) or G2 thrombocytopenia	Reduce weekly dosages of irinotecan and fluorouracil by 1 dosages level	Maintain dose and schedule
G3 ANC (500–999/mm³) or G3 thrombocytopenia	Hold treatment until toxicity G ≤2, then reduce weekly dosages of irinotecan and fluorouracil by 1 dosage level	Reduce weekly dosages of irinotecan and fluorouracil by 1 dosage level
G4 ANC (<500/mm³) or G4 thrombocytopenia	Hold treatment until toxicity G ≤2, then reduce weekly dosages of irinotecan and fluorouracil by 2 dosage levels	Reduce weekly dosages of irinotecan and fluorouracil by 2 dosage levels
Febrile neutropenia	Hold treatment until toxicity resolves, then reduce weekly dosage by 1 dosage level	
Diarrhea		
G1 (2–3 stools/day > baseline)	Maintain dose and schedule	Maintain dose and schedule
G2 (4–6 stools/day > baseline)	Hold until diarrhea resolves to baseline, then reduce weekly dosages by 1 level	Maintain dose and schedule
G3 (7–9 stools/day > baseline)	Delay until diarrhea resolves to baseline, then reduce weekly dosages by 1 level	Reduce weekly dosages of irinotecan and fluorouracil by 1 dosage level
G4 (≥10 stools/day > baseline)	Delay until diarrhea resolves to baseline, then reduce weekly dosages by 2 levels	Reduce weekly dosages of irinotecan and fluorouracil by 2 dosage levels
Other Nonhematologic Toxicities		
Any G1 toxicity	Maintain dose and schedule	Maintain dose and schedule
Any G2 toxicity	Hold treatment until toxicity G ≤1, then reduce weekly dosages of irinotecan and fluorouracil by 1 dosage level	Maintain dose and schedule
Any G3 toxicity	Hold treatment until toxicity G ≤1, then reduce weekly dosages of irinotecan and fluorouracil by 1 dosage level	Reduce weekly dosages of irinotecan and fluorouracil by 1 dosage level
Any G4 toxicity	Hold treatment until toxicity G ≤1, then reduce weekly dosages of irinotecan and fluorouracil by 2 dosage levels	Reduce weekly dosages of irinotecan and fluorouracil by 2 dosage levels
G2–4 mucositis	Reduce fluorouracil by 1 dosage level (do not alter irinotecan)	

Goldberg RM et al. J Clin Oncol 2004;22:23–30
Saltz LB et al. N Engl J Med 2000;343:905–914

Efficacy (N = 231)
(Intention-to-Treat Analysis)

Confirmed objective response	39%
Median duration of response	9.2 months
Median progression-free survival	7 months
Median overall survival	14.8 months

Toxicity (N = 225)

	% G3	% G4
Diarrhea	15.1	7.6
Vomiting	5.3	4.4
Mucositis	2.2	0
Neutropenia	29.8	24
Fever/neutropenia		7.1
Fever/infection		1.8
Therapy discontinued because of toxicity		7.6
Drug-related death		0.9

Patient Population Studied

A study of 231 patients with metastatic colorectal cancer who had not previously received chemotherapy except adjuvant therapy that was completed more than 12 months before study entry. Patients had not previously received pelvic radiation

Therapy Monitoring

1. *Before each cycle:* H&P, CBC with differential, CEA, serum electrolytes, and LFTs
2. *Weekly:* CBC with differential count and safety assessment
3. *Every 6 weeks × 4 (24 weeks), then every 12 weeks:* CT scans to assess response

METASTATIC DISEASE REGIMEN
LEUCOVORIN + INFUSIONAL
FLUOROURACIL + IRINOTECAN
(FOLFIRI)

Douillard JY et al. Lancet 2000;355:1041–1047
Tournigand C et al. J Clin Oncol 2004;22:229–237

Common to both alternative regimens (Douillard et al. and Tournigand et al.):
Irinotecan 180 mg/m²; administer intravenously over 90 minutes in 500 mL 5% dextrose injection (D5W) on day 1, every 2 weeks (total dosage/cycle = 180 mg/m²), *plus one of the following alternative regimens:*

Douillard et al. Lancet 2000;355:1041–1047

(Racemic) Leucovorin calcium 200 mg/m² per day; administer intravenously over 1 hour in 25–500 mL 0.9% sodium chloride injection (0.9% NS) or D5W for 2 consecutive days, on days 1 and 2, every 2 weeks (total dosage/cycle = 400 mg/m²) *followed by:*
Fluorouracil 400 mg/m² per day; administer by intravenous injection over 1–2 minutes after leucovorin for 2 consecutive days, on days 1 and 2, every 2 weeks, *followed by:*
Fluorouracil 600 mg/m² per day; administer by continuous intravenous infusion over 22 hours in 100–1000 mL 0.9% NS or D5W for 2 consecutive days, on days 1 and 2, every 2 weeks (total dosage/cycle = 2000 mg/m²)

or

Tournigand et al. J Clin Oncol 2004;22:229–237

Either: (racemic) **Leucovorin calcium** 400 mg/m² *or* **levoleucovorin calcium** 200 mg/m²; administer intravenously over 2 hours in 25–500 mL 0.9% NS or D5W on day 1, every 2 weeks (total dosage/cycle for racemic leucovorin = 400 mg/m², for levoleucovorin = 200 mg/m²), *followed by:*
Fluorouracil 400 mg/m²; administer by intravenous injection over 1–2 minutes after leucovorin on day 1, every 2 weeks, *followed by:*
Fluorouracil 2400 mg/m²; administer by continuous intravenous infusion over 46 hours in 100–1000 mL 0.9% NS or D5W, starting on day 1 every 2 weeks (total dosage/cycle = 2800 mg/m²)
• Infusional fluorouracil dosage may be increased to 3000 mg/m² by continuous intravenous infusion over 46 hours, starting on cycle 3, day 1, and repeated every 2 weeks in patients who do not develop adverse effects G >1 during the first 2 cycles (total dosage/cycle = 3400 mg/m²)

Supportive Care
Antiemetic prophylaxis
Emetogenic potential on day 1 is **MODERATE**
Emetogenic potential on day 2 is **LOW**
See Chapter 39 for antiemetic recommendations

Hematopoietic growth factor (CSF) prophylaxis
Primary prophylaxis is NOT indicated
See Chapter 43 for more information

Antimicrobial prophylaxis
Risk of fever and neutropenia is LOW
Antimicrobial primary prophylaxis to be considered:
• Antibacterial—not indicated
• Antifungal—not indicated
• Antiviral—not indicated unless patient previously had an episode of HSV
See Chapter 47 for more information

Acute cholinergic syndrome
Atropine sulfate 0.25–1 mg administer subcutaneously or intravenously if abdominal cramping or diarrhea develop during or within 1 hour after irinotecan administration
• If symptoms are severe, add as primary prophylaxis at least 30 min before irinotecan during subsequent cycles
• For irinotecan, acute cholinergic syndrome may be characterized by: abdominal cramping, diarrhea, diaphoresis, hypotension, flushing, bradycardia, rhinitis, increased salivation, meiosis, and lacrimation

(continued)

(*continued*)

Diarrhea management

Latent or delayed onset diarrhea*:

Loperamide 4 mg orally initially after the first loose or liquid stool, *then*

Loperamide 2 mg orally every 2 hours during waking hours, *plus*

Loperamide 4 mg orally every 4 hours during hours of sleep

- Continue for at least 12 hours after diarrhea resolves

- Recurrent diarrhea after a 12-hour diarrhea-free interval is treated as a new episode

- Rehydrate orally with fluids and electrolytes during a diarrheal episode

- If diarrhea persists >48 hours despite loperamide, stop loperamide and hospitalize the patient for IV hydration

Persistent diarrhea:

Octreotide 100–150 mcg subcutaneously 3 times daily. Maximum total daily dose is 1500 mcg

Antibiotic therapy during latent or delayed onset diarrhea:

A fluoroquinolone (eg, **Ciprofloxacin** 500 mg orally every 12 hours) if absolute neutrophil count is <500/mm^3 with or without accompanying fever in association with diarrhea

- Antibiotics should also be administered if patient is hospitalized with prolonged diarrhea and should be continued until diarrhea resolves

*Abigerges D et al. J Natl Cancer Inst 1994;86:446–449
Rothenberg ML et al. J Clin Oncol 2001;19:3801–3807
Wadler S et al. J Clin Oncol 1998;16:3169–3178

Oral care

Prophylaxis and treatment for mucositis/stomatitis

General advice:

- Encourage patients to maintain intake of non-alcoholic fluids

- Evaluate patients for oral pain and provide analgesic medications

- Consider histamine (H$_2$-subtype) receptor antagonists (eg, ranitidine, famotidine), or a proton pump inhibitor for epigastric pain

- *Lactobacillus* sp.-containing probiotics may be beneficial in preventing diarrhea

Patients with intact oral mucosa:

- Clean the mouth, tongue, and gums by brushing after every meal and at bedtime with an ultra-soft toothbrush with fluoride toothpaste

- Floss teeth gently every day unless contraindicated. If gums bleed and hurt, avoid bleeding or sore areas, but floss other teeth

- Patients may use saline or commercial bland, non-alcoholic rinses

  ▪ Do not use mouthwashes that contain alcohols

If mucositis or stomatitis is present:

- Keep the mouth moist utilizing water, ice chips, sugarless gum, sugar-free hard candies, or a saliva substitute

- Rinse mouth several times a day to remove debris

  ▪ Use a solution of ¼ teaspoon (1.25 g) each of baking soda and table salt (sodium chloride) in one quart (~950 mL) of warm water. Follow with a plain water rinse

  ▪ Do not use mouthwashes that contain alcohols

- Foam-tipped swabs (eg, Toothettes®) are useful in moisturizing oral mucosa, but ineffective for cleansing teeth and removing plaque

- Advise patients who develop mucositis to:

  ▪ Choose foods that are easy to chew and swallow

  ▪ Take small bites of food, chew slowly, and sip liquids with meals

  ▪ Encourage soft, moist foods such as cooked cereals, mashed potatoes, and scrambled eggs

  ▪ For trouble swallowing, soften food with gravies, sauces, broths, yogurt, or other bland liquids

  ▪ Avoid sharp, crunchy foods; hot, spicy or highly acidic foods (eg, citrus fruits and juices); sugary foods; toothpicks; tobacco products; alcoholic drinks

Hand-foot reaction (palmar-plantar erythrodysesthesia, PPE)

For patients who develop a hand-foot reaction, use topical emollients (eg, Aquaphor®), topical or orally administered steroids, antihistamine agents (H$_1$-receptor antagonists), or pyridoxine

Pyridoxine may provide relief for discomfort/pain associated with PPE although the mechanism through which this occurs remains unclear

- The suggested pyridoxine starting dose is 50 mg/day, which may be increased to a maximum of 200 mg/day

Treatment Modifications

(Camptosar, irinotecan hydrochloride injection product label, July 2005. Pharmacia & Upjohn Company, Division of Pfizer, Inc., New York, NY)

	Dosage Levels		
	Initial	−1	−2
Irinotecan	180 mg/m²	150 mg/m²	120 mg/m²
Leucovorin	Racemic leucovorin calcium 400 mg/m² *or* levoleucovorin calcium 200 mg/m²		
Bolus fluorouracil	400 mg/m²	300 mg/m²	
Infusional fluorouracil	600 mg/m²	480 mg/m²	360 mg/m²
Infusional fluorouracil	2400 mg/m²	2000 mg/m²	1800 mg/m²

Notes:
* Dose modifications are based on the National Cancer Institute (USA) Common Toxicity Criteria. At: http://ctep.cancer.gov/protocolDevelopment/electronic_applications/ctc.htm [accessed October 11, 2013]
* Before beginning a treatment cycle, patients should have baseline bowel function (similar to that before the start of treatment) without antidiarrheal therapy for 24 hours, ANC ≥1500/mm³, and platelet count ≥100,000/mm³
* Treatment should be delayed 1–2 weeks to allow for recovery from treatment-related toxicities. If a patient has not recovered after 2 weeks, consider stopping therapy

If toxicity occurs despite 2 dose reductions (ie, on level −2), discontinue therapy

Toxicity	Modifications for Irinotecan and Fluorouracil
Neutropenia/Thrombocytopenia	
G1 ANC (1500–1999/mm³) or G1 thrombocytopenia	Maintain dose and schedule
G2 ANC (1000–1499/mm³) or G2 thrombocytopenia	Reduce dosages by 1 dosage level
G3 ANC (500–999/mm³) or G3 thrombocytopenia	Hold treatment until toxicity resolves to G ≤2, then reduce dosages by 1 dosage level
G4 ANC (<500/mm³) or G4 thrombocytopenia	Hold treatment until toxicity resolves to G ≤2, then reduce dosages by 2 dosage levels
Febrile neutropenia	Hold treatment until neutropenia resolves, then reduce dosages by 2 dosage levels
Diarrhea	
G1 (2–3 stools/day > baseline)	Maintain dose and schedule
G2 (4–6 stools/day > baseline)	Delay until diarrhea resolves to baseline, then reduce dosage by 1 dosage level
G3 (7–9 stools/day > baseline)	Delay until diarrhea resolves to baseline, then reduce dosage by 1 dosage level
G4 (≥10 stools/day > baseline)	Delay until diarrhea resolves to baseline, then reduce dosage by 2 dosage levels

(continued)

Patient Population Studied

A study of 199 patients with previously untreated advanced colorectal cancer

Efficacy (N* = 169/198)

Confirmed overall response	40.8% (34.8%)†
Complete response	3.6% (3.0%)
Partial response	37.3% (31.8%)
Median time to progression	6.7 months
Median survival	17.4 months

*Evaluable = 169 patients; intention-to-treat = 198 patients. Both totals include patients receiving weekly and 2-weekly regimens
†Percent of evaluable patients (percent of intention-to-treat patients)

Douillard JY et al. Lancet 2000;355:1041–1047

Treatment Modifications (*continued*)

Toxicity	Modifications for Irinotecan and Fluorouracil
Other Nonhematologic Toxicities	
Any G1 toxicity	Maintain dose and schedule
Any G2 toxicity	Hold treatment until toxicity resolves to G ≤1, then reduce dosage by 1 dosage level
Any G3 toxicity	Hold treatment until toxicity resolves to G ≤1, then reduce dosage by 1 dosage level
Any G4 toxicity	Hold treatment until toxicity resolves to G ≤1, then reduce dosage by 2 dosage levels
G2–4 mucositis	Decrease only fluorouracil by 20%

André T et al. Eur J Cancer 1999;35:1343–1347
Douillard JY et al. Lancet 2000;355:1041–1047
Tournigand C et al. J Clin Oncol 2004;22:229–237

Therapy Monitoring

1. *Before each cycle:* H&P, CBC with differential, CEA serum electrolytes, and LFTs
2. *Every 2–3 months:* CT scans to assess response

Toxicity (N = 54)

	% All G	% G3/4
Nonhematologic		
Diarrhea	68.3	13.1
Nausea	58.6	2.1
Alopecia	56.6	—
Asthenia	44.8	6.2
Vomiting	41.4	2.8
Mucositis	38.6	4.1
Cholinergic syndrome	28.3	1.4
Anorexia	17.2	2.1
Pain other than abdominal	9.7	0.7
Nonabdominal pain	8.3	–
Hand-foot syndrome	9	0.7
Hematologic		
Anemia	97.2	2.1
Neutropenia	82.5	46.2
Fever with G3/4 neutropenia	—	3.4
Infection with G3/4 neutropenia	—	2.1

Douillard JY et al. Lancet 2000;355:1041–1047

METASTATIC OR ADJUVANT REGIMEN

LEUCOVORIN + INFUSIONAL FLUOROURACIL + OXALIPLATIN (FOLFOX)

André T et al. N Engl J Med 2004;350:2343–2351
de Gramont A et al. J Clin Oncol 2000;18:2938–2947
Rothenberg ML et al. J Clin Oncol 2003;21:2059–2069
Tournigand C et al. J Clin Oncol 2004;22:229–237

FOLFOX-4 (de Gramont et al., Rothenberg et al., André et al.):
Oxaliplatin 85 mg/m²; administer intravenously over 2 hours in 250 mL 5% dextrose injection (D5W) on day 1, every 2 weeks, concurrently with leucovorin administration (total dosage/cycle = 85 mg/m²)

Note: Oxaliplatin must not be mixed with sodium chloride injection. Therefore, when leucovorin and oxaliplatin are given concurrently via the same administration set tubing, both drugs must be administered in D5W

Leucovorin calcium 200 mg/m² per day; administer intravenously over 2 hours in 25–500 mL D5W for 2 consecutive days, on days 1 and 2, every 2 weeks (total dosage/cycle = 400 mg/m²) *followed by:*
Fluorouracil 400 mg/m² per day; administer by intravenous injection over 1–4 minutes after leucovorin for 2 consecutive days, on days 1 and 2, every 2 weeks, *followed by:*
Fluorouracil 600 mg/m² per day; administer by continuous intravenous infusion over 22 hours in 100–1000 mL 0.9% sodium chloride injection (0.9% NS) or D5W for 2 consecutive days, on days 1 and 2, every 2 weeks (total dosage/cycle = 2000 mg/m²)

or

FOLFOX-6 (Tournigand et al.)
Oxaliplatin 100 mg/m²; administer intravenously over 2 hours in 500 mL D5W on day 1, every 2 weeks, concurrently with leucovorin administration (total dosage/cycle = 100 mg/m²)

Note: Oxaliplatin must not be mixed with sodium chloride injection. Therefore, when leucovorin and oxaliplatin are given concurrently via the same administration set tubing, both drugs must be administered in D5W
Either: **(racemic) Leucovorin calcium** 400 mg/m² or **levoleucovorin calcium** 200 mg/m²; administer intravenously over 2 hours in 25–500 mL 0.9% NS or D5W on day 1, every 2 weeks (total dosage/cycle for racemic leucovorin = 400 mg/m², for levoleucovorin = 200 mg/m²), *followed by:*
Fluorouracil 400 mg/m²; administer by intravenous injection over 1–2 minutes after leucovorin on day 1, every 2 weeks, *followed by:*
Fluorouracil 2400 mg/m²; administer by continuous intravenous infusion over 46 hours in 100–1000 mL 0.9% NS or D5W, starting on day 1 every 2 weeks (total dosage/cycle = 2800 mg/m²)
• Infusional fluorouracil dosage may be increased to 3000 mg/m² by continuous intravenous infusion over 46 hours, starting on cycle 3, day 1, and repeated every 2 weeks in patients who do not develop adverse effects G >1 during the first 2 cycles (total dosage/cycle = 3400 mg/m²)
Note: The fluorouracil loading dose (400 mg/m²) can be omitted for better hematologic tolerance

Supportive Care
Antiemetic prophylaxis
Emetogenic potential on day 1 is **MODERATE**
Emetogenic potential on day 2 is **LOW to MODERATE**
See Chapter 39 for antiemetic recommendations

Hematopoietic growth factor (CSF) prophylaxis
Primary prophylaxis is NOT indicated
See Chapter 43 for more information

Antimicrobial prophylaxis
Risk of fever and neutropenia is LOW
Antimicrobial primary prophylaxis to be considered:
• Antibacterial—not indicated
• Antifungal—not indicated
• Antiviral—not indicated unless patient previously had an episode of HSV
See Chapter 47 for more information

(continued)

Patient Population Studied

Patients with previously untreated advanced colorectal cancer

Treatment Modifications (FOLFOX-4)

Adverse Event	Dose Modification
Any G2/3/4 nonhematologic toxicity	Delay start of next cycle until the severity of all toxicities are G ≤1 and decrease fluorouracil loading dosage from 400 mg/m² to 300 mg/m²
ANC ≤1500/mm³ or platelet count ≤100,000/mm³	Delay start of next cycle until ANC >1500/mm³ *and* platelet count >100,000/mm³
G3/4 nonneurologic	Reduce fluorouracil and oxaliplatin dosages by 20%
G3/4 ANC	Reduce oxaliplatin dosage by 20%
Persistent (≥14 days) paresthesias	Reduce oxaliplatin dosage by 20%
Temporary (7–14 days) painful paresthesias	Reduce oxaliplatin dosage by 20%
Temporary (7–14 days) functional impairment	Reduce oxaliplatin dosage by 20%
Persistent (≥14 days) painful paresthesias	Discontinue oxaliplatin
Persistent (≥14 days) functional impairment	Discontinue oxaliplatin

de Gramont A et al. J Clin Oncol 2000;18:2938–2947

(continued)

Diarrhea management

Latent or delayed onset diarrhea:

Loperamide 4 mg orally initially after the first loose or liquid stool, *then*

Loperamide 2 mg orally every 2 hours during waking hours, *plus*

Loperamide 4 mg orally every 4 hours during hours of sleep

• Continue for at least 12 hours after diarrhea resolves

• Recurrent diarrhea after a 12-hour diarrhea-free interval is treated as a new episode

• Rehydrate orally with fluids and electrolytes during a diarrheal episode

• If diarrhea persists >48 hours despite loperamide, stop loperamide and hospitalize the patient for IV hydration

Persistent diarrhea:

Octreotide 100–150 mcg subcutaneously 3 times daily. Maximum total daily dose is 1500 mcg

Antibiotic therapy during latent or delayed onset diarrhea:

A fluoroquinolone (eg, **Ciprofloxacin** 500 mg orally every 12 hours) if absolute neutrophil count <500/mm³ with or without accompanying fever in association with diarrhea

• Antibiotics should also be administered if patient is hospitalized with prolonged diarrhea and should be continued until diarrhea resolves

*Abigerges D et al. J Natl Cancer Inst 1994;86:446–449
Rothenberg ML et al. J Clin Oncol 2001;19:3801–3807
Wadler S et al. J Clin Oncol 1998;16:3169–3178

Oral care

Prophylaxis and treatment for mucositis/stomatitis

General advice:

• Encourage patients to maintain intake of non-alcoholic fluids

• Evaluate patients for oral pain and provide analgesic medications

• Consider histamine (H$_2$-subtype) receptor antagonists (eg, ranitidine, famotidine), or a proton pump inhibitor for epigastric pain

• *Lactobacillus* sp.-containing probiotics may be beneficial in preventing diarrhea

Patients with intact oral mucosa:

• Clean the mouth, tongue, and gums by brushing after every meal and at bedtime with an ultra-soft toothbrush with fluoride toothpaste

• Floss teeth gently every day unless contraindicated. If gums bleed and hurt, avoid bleeding or sore areas, but floss other teeth

• Patients may use saline or commercial bland, non-alcoholic rinses

 ▪ Do not use mouthwashes that contain alcohols

If mucositis or stomatitis is present:

• Keep the mouth moist utilizing water, ice chips, sugarless gum, sugar-free hard candies, or a saliva substitute

• Rinse mouth several times a day to remove debris

 ▪ Use a solution of ¼ teaspoon (1.25 g) each of baking soda and table salt (sodium chloride) in one quart (~950 mL) of warm water. Follow with a plain water rinse

 ▪ Do not use mouthwashes that contain alcohols

• Foam-tipped swabs (eg, Toothettes®) are useful in moisturizing oral mucosa, but ineffective for cleansing teeth and removing plaque

• Advise patients who develop mucositis to:

 ▪ Choose foods that are easy to chew and swallow

 ▪ Take small bites of food, chew slowly, and sip liquids with meals

 ▪ Encourage soft, moist foods such as cooked cereals, mashed potatoes, and scrambled eggs

 ▪ For trouble swallowing, soften food with gravies, sauces, broths, yogurt, or other bland liquids

 ▪ Avoid sharp, crunchy foods; hot, spicy or highly acidic foods (eg, citrus fruits and juices); sugary foods; toothpicks; tobacco products; alcoholic drinks

Treatment Modifications (FOLFOX-6)

Adverse Event	Dose Modification
ANC ≤1500/mm³ *or* platelet count ≤100,000/mm³ *or* persistent nonhematologic toxicity G ≥2	Delay start of next cycle until ANC >1500/mm³ *and* platelet count >100,000/mm³; omit fluorouracil by intravenous injection
G ≥3 toxicity	Reduce fluorouracil dosage to 2000 mg/m²
G4 ANC, G3/4 thrombocytopenia or G4 diarrhea	Reduce oxaliplatin dosage to 75 mg/m²
G2 paresthesias (persistent paresthesia or dysesthesia without functional impairment)	Reduce oxaliplatin dosage to 75 mg/m²
Persistent G2/3 paresthesia/ dysesthesia	Discontinue oxaliplatin
Persistent painful paresthesia or G3 neurotoxicity (persistent paresthesia or dysesthesia with persistent functional impairment)	Discontinue oxaliplatin

Tournigand C et al. J Clin Oncol 2004;22:229–237

Toxicity (N = 209) (FOLFOX-4)

	% G1	% G2	% G3	% G4
Nonhematologic				
Nausea	44	22.5	5.7	NA
Vomiting	24	24.4	4.3	1.5
Diarrhea	30.6	16.3	8.6	3.3
Mucositis	24.9	12.9	5.3	0.5
Cutaneous	19.6	9.1	0	0
Alopecia	15.8	1.9	NA	NA
Neurologic	20.6	29.2	18.2	NA
Hematologic				
Neutropenia	14.3	14.3	29.7	12
Thrombocytopenia	62.2	11.5	2	0.5
Anemia	59.8	23.5	3.3	0

de Gramont A et al. J Clin Oncol 2000;18:2938–2947

Efficacy (N = 210)

Intent-to-Treat Analysis

Objective response	50%
Complete response	1.4%
Partial response	48.6%
Stable disease	31.9%
Progressive disease	10%
Median survival	16.2 months

de Gramont A et al. J Clin Oncol 2000;18:2938–2947
WHO Criteria

Therapy Monitoring

1. *Before each cycle:* H&P, CBC with differential, CEA serum electrolytes, and LFTs
2. *Every 2–3 months:* CT scans to assess response in patients presenting with advanced colorectal cancer

Toxicity (N = 110) (FOLFOX-6)

	% G1	% G2	% G3	% G4
Nonhematologic				
Nausea	39	25	3	0
Vomiting	22	17	3	0
Diarrhea	28	13	9	2
Mucositis	35	10	1	0
Cutaneous	17	5	2	0
Alopecia	19	9	NA	NA
Neurologic*	26	37	34	NA
Fatigue	17	15	3	0
Hematologic				
Neutropenia	18	20	31	13
Thrombocytopenia	57	21	5	0
Anemia	39	12	3	0

*Neurotoxicity scale:
G1 = Short-lasting paresthesia with complete regression by next cycle
G2 = Persistent paresthesia or dysesthesia without functional impairment
G3 = Persistent functional impairment

Tournigand C et al. J Clin Oncol 2004;22:229–237

METASTATIC DISEASE REGIMEN
LEUCOVORIN + BOLUS FLUOROURACIL + IRINOTECAN (IFL) + BEVACIZUMAB

Hurwitz H et al. N Engl J Med 2004;350:2335–2342

Bevacizumab 5 mg/kg; administer intravenously in 100 mL 0.9% sodium chloride injection (0.9% NS) every 2 weeks (total dosage/6-week cycle = 15 mg/kg)

Note: Administration duration for the initial dose is 90 minutes. If administration is well tolerated, the administration duration may be decreased stepwise during subsequent administrations to 60 minutes and, finally, to a minimum duration of 30 minutes

Irinotecan 125 mg/m² per dose; administer intravenously in 250 mL 5% dextrose injection (D5W) over 90 minutes, weekly for 4 consecutive weeks, every 6 weeks (total dosage/6-week cycle = 500 mg/m²)
Leucovorin calcium 20 mg/m² per dose; administer intravenously over 2 hours in 25–500 mL 0.9% NS or D5W, weekly for 4 consecutive weeks, every 6 weeks (total dosage/6-week cycle = 80 mg/m²), *followed by:*
Fluorouracil 500 mg/m² per dose; administer by intravenous injection over 1–2 minutes, after leucovorin, weekly for 4 consecutive weeks, every 6 weeks (total dosage/cycle = 2000 mg/m²)

Supportive Care
Antiemetic prophylaxis
Emetogenic potential with or without bevacizumab is **MODERATE**
See Chapter 39 for antiemetic recommendations

Hematopoietic growth factor (CSF) prophylaxis
Primary prophylaxis is NOT indicated
See Chapter 43 for more information

Antimicrobial prophylaxis
Risk of fever and neutropenia is LOW
Antimicrobial primary prophylaxis to be considered:
- Antibacterial—not indicated
- Antifungal—not indicated
- Antiviral—not indicated unless patient previously had an episode of HSV
See Chapter 47 for more information

Acute cholinergic syndrome
Atropine sulfate 0.25–1 mg administer subcutaneously or intravenously if abdominal cramping or diarrhea develop during or within 1 hour after irinotecan administration
- If symptoms are severe, add as primary prophylaxis at least 30 min before irinotecan during subsequent cycles
- For irinotecan, acute cholinergic syndrome may be characterized by: abdominal cramping, diarrhea, diaphoresis, hypotension, flushing, bradycardia, rhinitis, increased salivation, meiosis, and lacrimation

Diarrhea management
Latent or delayed onset diarrhea*:
Loperamide 4 mg orally initially after the first loose or liquid stool, *then*
Loperamide 2 mg orally every 2 hours during waking hours, *plus*
Loperamide 4 mg orally every 4 hours during hours of sleep
- Continue for at least 12 hours after diarrhea resolves
- Recurrent diarrhea after a 12-hour diarrhea-free interval is treated as a new episode
- Rehydrate orally with fluids and electrolytes during a diarrheal episode
- If diarrhea persists >48 hours despite loperamide, stop loperamide and hospitalize the patient for IV hydration

(continued)

Patient Population Studied
First-line therapy of metastatic colorectal cancer. Exclusion criteria included prior chemotherapy or biologic therapy for metastatic disease, although adjuvant or radiosensitizing use of fluoropyrimidines with or without leucovorin or levamisole was permitted

Efficacy (N = 402)

Overall response rate	44.8%
Complete response	3.7%
Partial response	41%
Median survival	20.3 months
Progression-free survival	10.6 months

RECIST criteria (Response Evaluation Criteria in Solid Tumors. Therasse P et al. J Natl Cancer Inst 2000;92:205–216)

(continued)

Persistent diarrhea:

Octreotide 100–150 mcg subcutaneously 3 times daily. Maximum total daily dose is 1500 mcg

Antibiotic therapy during latent or delayed onset diarrhea:

A fluoroquinolone (eg, **Ciprofloxacin** 500 mg orally every 12 hours) if absolute neutrophil count is <500/mm³ with or without accompanying fever in association with diarrhea
  • Antibiotics should also be administered if patient is hospitalized with prolonged diarrhea and should be continued until diarrhea resolves

*Abigerges D et al. J Natl Cancer Inst 1994;86:446–449
Rothenberg ML et al. J Clin Oncol 2001;19:3801–3807
Wadler S et al. J Clin Oncol 1998;16:3169–3178

Oral care

Prophylaxis and treatment for mucositis/stomatitis

General advice:

• Encourage patients to maintain intake of non-alcoholic fluids

• Evaluate patients for oral pain and provide analgesic medications

• Consider histamine (H_2-subtype) receptor antagonists (eg, ranitidine, famotidine), or a proton pump inhibitor for epigastric pain

• *Lactobacillus* sp.-containing probiotics may be beneficial in preventing diarrhea

Patients with intact oral mucosa:

• Clean the mouth, tongue, and gums by brushing after every meal and at bedtime with an ultra-soft toothbrush with fluoride toothpaste

• Floss teeth gently every day unless contraindicated. If gums bleed and hurt, avoid bleeding or sore areas, but floss other teeth

• Patients may use saline or commercial bland, non-alcoholic rinses
  ▪ Do not use mouthwashes that contain alcohols

If mucositis or stomatitis is present:

• Keep the mouth moist utilizing water, ice chips, sugarless gum, sugar-free hard candies, or a saliva substitute

• Rinse mouth several times a day to remove debris

▪ Use a solution of ¼ teaspoon (1.25 g) each of baking soda and table salt (sodium chloride) in one quart (~950 mL) of warm water. Follow with a plain water rinse

▪ Do not use mouthwashes that contain alcohols

  • Foam-tipped swabs (eg, Toothettes®) are useful in moisturizing oral mucosa, but ineffective for cleansing teeth and removing plaque

  • Advise patients who develop mucositis to:
    ▪ Choose foods that are easy to chew and swallow
    ▪ Take small bites of food, chew slowly, and sip liquids with meals
    ▪ Encourage soft, moist foods such as cooked cereals, mashed potatoes, and scrambled eggs
    ▪ For trouble swallowing, soften food with gravies, sauces, broths, yogurt, or other bland liquids
    ▪ Avoid sharp, crunchy foods; hot, spicy or highly acidic foods (eg, citrus fruits and juices); sugary foods; toothpicks; tobacco products; alcoholic drinks

Toxicity (N = 393)

Adverse events occurred with greater incidence (≥2%) among patients who received bevacizumab 1 bolus IFL than those who received bolus IFL 1 placebo

Toxicity	% of Patients
Any G3/4 toxicity	85
Cardiovascular	
Any thrombosis	19.4
Deep venous thrombosis	8.9
Pulmonary embolus	3.6
Any hypertension	22.4
G3 hypertension	11
Digestive	
G3/4 diarrhea	32.4
Hematologic	
G3/4 leukopenia	37
Other Toxicities (G1–4)	
Proteinuria	26.5
G2/3 proteinuria	3.1/0.8

Therapy Monitoring

1. *Before each cycle:* H&P, CBC with differential, serum electrolytes, CEA BUN, creatinine, and LFTs. Urine for protein analysis including 24-hour urine for protein if needed

2. *Twice per week initially, then at a minimum of once per week:* Blood pressure

3. *Every 6 weeks for the first 24 weeks:* CT scans to assess response

Treatment Modifications

Adverse Event	Dose Modification
Gastrointestinal perforation, serious bleeding	Discontinue bevacizumab permanently
Wound dehiscence requiring medical intervention	
Nephrotic syndrome	
Hypertensive crisis	
Moderate to severe proteinuria	Hold bevacizumab pending further evaluation (eg, 24-hour urine protein or work-up and treatment of hypertension)
Severe hypertension not controlled with medical management	

Note: Bevacizumab should be suspended at least several weeks before elective surgery and should not be resumed until a surgical incision is fully healed

Information from product label:
http://www.gene.com/gene/products/information/pdf/avastin-prescribing.pdf or http://www.fda.gov/cder/approval/index.htm

Standard intracycle and intercycle dose modifications of irinotecan and fluorouracil, according to the package insert, were permitted in patients with treatment-related adverse events. Suggestions include the following:

(Camptosar, irinotecan hydrochloride injection product label, July 2005. Pharmacia & Upjohn Company, Division of Pfizer, Inc, New York, NY)

	Dosage Levels		
	Initial	**−1**	**−2**
Irinotecan	125 mg/m^2	100 mg/m^2	75 mg/m^2
Leucovorin	20 mg/m^2		
Fluorouracil	500 mg/^{2}	400 mg/m^2	300 mg/m^2

Notes:
- Dose modifications are based on the National Cancer Institute (USA) Common Toxicity Criteria http://ctep.cancer.gov/protocolDevelopment/electronic_applications/ctc.htm [accessed October 11, 2013]
- Before beginning a treatment cycle, patients should have baseline bowel function (present before start of treatment) without antidiarrheal therapy for 24 hours, ANC ≥1500/mm^3, and platelet count ≥100,000/mm^3
- Treatment should be delayed 1–2 weeks to allow for recovery from treatment-related toxicities. If a patient has not recovered after 2 weeks, consider stopping therapy
- If toxicity occurs despite 2 dose reductions (ie, on level −2) discontinue therapy

Toxicity	Weekly Dosage Based on Intracycle Toxicity	Dosage at Start of a 6-Week Cycle
Neutropenia/Thrombocytopenia		
G1 ANC (1500–1999/mm^3) or G1 thrombocytopenia	Maintain dose and schedule	Maintain dose and schedule
G2 ANC (1000–1499/mm^3) or G2 thrombocytopenia	Reduce weekly dosages of irinotecan and leucovorin by 1 dosage level	Maintain dose and schedule
G3 ANC (500–999/mm^3) or G3 thrombocytopenia	Hold treatment until toxicity G ≥2, then reduce weekly dosages of irinotecan and leucovorin by 1 dosage level	Reduce weekly dosages of irinotecan and leucovorin by 1 dosage level
G4 ANC (<500/mm^3) or G4 thrombocytopenia	Hold treatment until toxicity G ≤2, then reduce weekly dosages of irinotecan and leucovorin by 2 dosage levels	Reduce weekly dosages of irinotecan and leucovorinz by 2 dosage levels
Febrile neutropenia	Hold treatment until toxicity resolves, then reduce weekly dosages of irinotecan and leucovorin by 1 dosage level	

(continued)

Treatment Modifications (continued)

Toxicity	Weekly Dosage Based on Intracycle Toxicity	Dosage at Start of a 6-Week Cycle
Diarrhea		
G1 (2–3 stools/day > baseline)	Maintain dose and schedule	Maintain dose and schedule
G2 (4–6 stools/day > baseline)	Hold until diarrhea resolves to baseline, then reduce weekly dosages of irinotecan and leucovorin by 1 dosage level	Maintain dose and schedule
G3 (7–9 stools/day > baseline)	Delay until diarrhea resolves to baseline, then reduce weekly dosages of irinotecan and leucovorin by 1 dosage level	Reduce weekly dosages of irinotecan and leucovorin by 1 dosage level
G4 (≥10 stools/day > baseline)	Delay until diarrhea resolves to baseline, then reduce weekly dosages of irinotecan and leucovorin by 2 dosage levels	Reduce weekly dosages of irinotecan and leucovorin by 2 dosage levels
Other Nonhematologic Toxicities		
Any G1 toxicity	Maintain dose and schedule	Maintain dose and schedule
Any G2 toxicity	Hold treatment until toxicity G ≤1, then reduce weekly dosages of irinotecan and leucovorin by 1 dosage level	Maintain dose and schedule
Any G3 toxicity	Hold treatment until toxicity G ≤1, then reduce weekly dosages of irinotecan and leucovorin by 1 dosage level	Reduce weekly dosages of irinotecan and leucovorin by 1 dosage level
Any G4 toxicity	Hold treatment until toxicity G ≤1, then reduce weekly dosages of irinotecan and leucovorin by 2 dosage levels	Reduce weekly dosage by 2 dosage levels for irinotecan and leucovorin levels
G2–4 mucositis	Reduce fluorouracil by 1 dosage level (do not alter irinotecan)	

Goldberg RM et al. J Clin Oncol 2004;22:23–30
Saltz LB et al. N Engl J Med 2000;343:905–914

METASTATIC DISEASE REGIMEN

CETUXIMAB

Cunningham et al. N Engl J Med 2004;351:337–345
Saltz LB et al. J Clin Oncol 2004;22:1201–1208

Warning: Despite the use of prophylactic antihistamines, severe infusion reactions occur with the administration of cetuximab in about 3% of patients, rarely with fatal outcome (<1 in 1000). Approximately 90% of severe infusion reactions are associated with initial cetuximab administration and are characterized by the rapid onset of airway obstruction (bronchospasm, stridor, hoarseness), urticaria, and/or hypotension. Exercise caution with every cetuximab infusion

Notes:

1. Test doses do not reliably predict hypersensitivity reactions to cetuximab administration and are not recommended
2. Mild to moderate infusion reactions
   - Interrupt or slow the cetuximab infusion rate
   - Permanently decrease administration rate by 50%
   - Give antihistamine prophylaxis before repeated treatments
3. Severe reactions
   - Immediately interrupt cetuximab therapy
   - Administer epinephrine, glucocorticoids, intravenous antihistamines, bronchodilators, and oxygen as needed
   - Permanently discontinue further treatment

Cetuximab premedication:
Administer a H_1-receptor antagonist (eg, diphenhydramine 50 mg) intravenously 30–60 minutes before starting cetuximab administration. Hypersensitivity prophylaxis should be administered for subsequent cetuximab doses based on clinical judgment and presence and severity of infusion reactions during prior exposures

Initial cetuximab dose:
Cetuximab 400 mg/m^2; administer intravenously over 120 minutes (maximum infusion rate = 5 mL/min [10 mg/min]) as a single dose (total initial dosage = 400 mg/m^2), followed after an interval of 1 week by:

Weekly maintenance cetuximab doses:
Cetuximab 250 mg/m^2; administer intravenously over 60 minutes (maximum infusion rate = 5 mL/min [10 mg/min]) every week (total weekly dosage = 250 mg/m^2)

Notes:
- Cetuximab is intended for direct administration and should not be diluted
- Maximum infusion rate = 5 mL (10 mg)/min (300 mL/h, or 600 mg/h)
- Administer cetuximab through a low protein-binding inline filter with pore size = 0.22 μm
- Use 0.9% sodium chloride injection to flush vascular access devices after administration is completed

Supportive Care
Antiemetic prophylaxis
*Emetogenic potential is **LOW***
See Chapter 39 for antiemetic recommendations

Hematopoietic growth factor (CSF) prophylaxis
Primary prophylaxis is NOT indicated
See Chapter 43 for more information

Antimicrobial prophylaxis
Risk of fever and neutropenia is LOW
   Antimicrobial primary prophylaxis to be considered:
   - Antibacterial—not indicated
   - Antifungal—not indicated
   - Antiviral—not indicated unless patient previously had an episode of HSV
See Chapter 47 for more information

(continued)

Patient Population Studied

A study of patients with metastatic colorectal cancer whose tumor expresses EGFR and whose disease had progressed after receiving an irinotecan-containing regimen

Efficacy

	Cetuximab + Irinotecan	Cetuximab
Response	22.9%	10.8%
Progression-free survival	4.1 months	1.5 months

Cunningham et al. N Engl J Med 2004;351:337–345

Toxicity

Toxicity	% G3/4	
	Cetuximab + Irinotecan	Cetuximab Alone
Asthenia/malaise	14	10
Abdominal pain	3	5
Fever	2	0
Infusion reaction	0	4
Acne-like rash	9	5
Nausea/vomiting	7	4

(*continued*)

Diarrhea management

Loperamide 4 mg orally initially after the first loose or liquid stool, *then*

Loperamide 2 mg orally every 2 hours during waking hours, *plus*

Loperamide 4 mg orally every 4 hours during hours of sleep

- Continue for at least 12 hours after diarrhea resolves

- Recurrent diarrhea after a 12-hour diarrhea-free interval is treated as a new episode

- Rehydrate orally with fluids and electrolytes during a diarrheal episode

If diarrhea persists >48 hours despite loperamide, stop loperamide and hospitalize the patient for IV hydration

In the pivotal trial, cetuximab was given alone or in combination with irinotecan. All patients received a 20-mg test dose on day 1, then cetuximab was given at 400 mg/m^2 intravenously as an initial dose, followed by 250 mg/m^2 per week intravenously until disease progression or unacceptable toxicity. Cetuximab was added to irinotecan using the same dose and schedule for irinotecan on which the patient's tumor had previously progressed

Treatment Modifications

(ERBITUX [cetuximab] injection, for intravenous infusion, product label, August 2013. Manufactured by ImClone LLC, a subsidiary of Eli Lilly and Co., Branchburg, NJ. Distributed and Marketed by Bristol-Myers Squibb Company, Princeton, NJ, and Eli Lilly and Company., Indianapolis, IN)

Infusion Reactions

Mild-moderate (G1/2) and nonserious G3/4	Permanently decrease administration rates by 50%
Serious (G3/4)	Immediately and permanently discontinue cetuximab

Severe (G3/4) Dermatologic Toxicity

Occurrence	Cetuximab	Improvement	Cetuximab Dosage
First	Delay infusion 1–2 weeks	Yes	Continue at 250 mg/m^2
		No	Discontinue
Second	Delay infusion 1–2 weeks	Yes	Decrease to 200 mg/m^2
		No	Discontinue
Third	Delay infusion 1–2 weeks	Yes	Decrease to 150 mg/m^2
		No	Discontinue
Fourth	Discontinue		

Information from the product label: http://www.erbitux.com/ (last accessed October 15, 2013)

Therapy Monitoring

1. *Before each cycle:* H&P, CBC with differential, CEA serum electrolytes, BUN, creatinine, and LFTs. Urine for protein analysis including 24-hour urine for protein if needed

2. *Every 6 weeks for the first 24 weeks:* CT scans to assess response

3. Monitor patients for 1 hour after completing cetuximab administration in a setting with resuscitation equipment and other agents necessary to treat anaphylaxis (eg, epinephrine, intravenous glucocorticoids and antihistamines, bronchodilators, and oxygen)
   - Monitor for longer periods to confirm resolution of signs and symptoms of hypersensitivity in patients who require treatment for infusion reactions

4. Interrupt cetuximab for acute onset or worsening of pulmonary symptoms (dyspnea, cough). Permanently discontinue cetuximab for confirmed Interstitial lung disease (ILD occurred in <0.5% of patients receiving cetuximab in clinical trials)

5. Instruct patients to limit sun exposure. Monitor for inflammation and infection involving the skin and nails
   - Dermatologic toxicities, including: acneform rash, skin drying and fissuring, paronychial inflammation, infectious sequelae (eg, *Staphylococcus aureus* sepsis, abscess formation, cellulitis, blepharitis, conjunctivitis, keratitis, cheilitis), and hypertrichosis have occurred in patients receiving cetuximab
   - Acneform rash occurred in 76–88% of patients who received cetuximab in clinical trials; severe acneform rash occurred in 1–17% of patients
   - Acneform rash usually develops within the first 2 weeks after starting therapy and resolves in a majority of the patients after treatment cessation, although in nearly half of patients studied rash continued beyond 28 days after treatment ceased

METASTATIC COLORECTAL CANCER REGIMEN
CETUXIMAB + FOLFOX-4

Bokemeyer C et al. J Clin Oncol 2009;27:663–671
Cunningham D et al. N Engl J Med 2004;351:337–345
de Gramont A et al. J Clin Oncol 2000;18:2938–2947

Warning:

1. Severe infusion reactions occurred with the administration of cetuximab in approximately 3% (17/633) of patients, rarely with fatal outcome (<1 in 1000)
2. Approximately 90% of severe infusion reactions are associated with the first infusion of cetuximab despite the use of prophylactic antihistamines
3. Infusion reactions are characterized by the rapid onset of airway obstruction (bronchospasm, stridor, hoarseness), urticaria, and/or hypotension
4. Caution must be exercised with every cetuximab infusion, as there were patients who experienced their first severe infusion reaction during later infusions
5. Provocative test doses do not reliably predict hypersensitivity reactions to cetuximab administration and are not recommended

Mild to moderate infusion reactions
• Interrupt or slow the cetuximab infusion rate
• Permanently decrease the administration rate by 50%
• Give antihistamine prophylaxis before repeated treatments

Severe reactions
• Immediately interrupt cetuximab therapy
• Administer epinephrine, glucocorticoids, intravenous antihistamines, bronchodilators, and oxygen as needed
• Permanently discontinue further treatment

Cetuximab premedication:
Diphenhydramine 50 mg by intravenous injection before cetuximab administration (other H_1-receptor antagonists may be substituted)

Initial cetuximab dose:
Cetuximab 400 mg/m²; administer intravenously over 120 minutes (maximum infusion rate = 5 mL/min [10 mg/min]) as a single dose (total initial dosage = 400 mg/m²)

Maintenance cetuximab doses:
Cetuximab 250 mg/m²; administer intravenously over 60 minutes (maximum infusion rate = 5 mL/min [10 mg/min]) every week (total weekly dosage = 250 mg/m²)

Notes:
• Cetuximab is intended for direct administration and should not be diluted
• Maximum infusion rate = 5 mL (10 mg)/min (300 mL/h, or 600 mg/h)
• Administer cetuximab through a low protein-binding inline filter with pore size = 0.22 μm
• Use 0.9% sodium chloride injection to flush vascular access devices after administration is completed
See Chapter 40 for more information about antineoplastic use

FOLFOX-4 (de Gramont A et al.):
Oxaliplatin 85 mg/m²; administer intravenously in 250 mL 5% dextrose injection (D5W) over 2 hours concurrently with leucovorin administration, on day 1 every 2 weeks, (total dosage/cycle = 85 mg/m²)
Note: Oxaliplatin must not be mixed with sodium chloride injection. Therefore, when leucovorin and oxaliplatin are given concurrently via a **Y**-connector, both drugs must be administered in D5W
Leucovorin calcium 200 mg/m² per dose; administer intravenously in 25–500 mL D5W over 2 hours on 2 consecutive days, on days 1 and 2, every 2 weeks (total dosage/cycle = 400 mg/m²), *followed by:*
Fluorouracil 400 mg/m² per dose; administer by intravenous injection over 1–2 minutes after leucovorin on 2 consecutive days, on days 1 and 2, every 2 weeks, *followed by:*
Fluorouracil 600 mg/m² per dose; administer by continuous intravenous infusion in 100–1000 mL 0.9% sodium chloride injection (0.9% NS) or D5W over 22 hours on 2 consecutive days, on days 1 and 2, every 2 weeks (total dosage/cycle = 2000 mg/m²)
Note: **Fluorouracil** boluses (400 mg/m² by intravenous injection) may be omitted for better hematologic tolerance

(continued)

(*continued*)

Supportive Care
Antiemetic prophylaxis
Emetogenic potential on days with cetuximab is **MINIMAL**
Emetogenic potential on days with oxaliplatin is **MODERATE**
Emetogenic potential on days with fluorouracil and leucovorin alone is **LOW**
See Chapter 39 for antiemetic recommendations

Hematopoietic growth factor (CSF) prophylaxis
Primary prophylaxis may be indicated
See Chapter 43 for more information

Antimicrobial prophylaxis
Risk of fever and neutropenia is LOW
  Antimicrobial primary prophylaxis to be considered:
  • Antibacterial—not indicated
  • Antifungal—not indicated
  • Antiviral—not indicated unless patient previously had an episode of HSV
See Chapter 47 for more information

Diarrhea management
Latent or delayed onset diarrhea*:
  Loperamide 4 mg orally initially after the first loose or liquid stool, *then*
  Loperamide 2 mg orally every 2 hours during waking hours, *plus*
  Loperamide 4 mg orally every 4 hours during hours of sleep
  • Continue for at least 12 hours after diarrhea resolves
  • Recurrent diarrhea after a 12-hour diarrhea-free interval is treated as a new episode
  • Rehydrate orally with fluids and electrolytes during a diarrheal episode
  • If a patient develops blood or mucus in stool, dehydration, or hemodynamic instability, or if diarrhea persists >48 hours despite loperamide, stop loperamide and hospitalize the patient for IV hydration
  Alternatively, a trial of **Diphenoxylate hydrochloride** 2.5 mg **with Atropine sulfate** 0.025 mg (eg, Lomotil)
  • Initial adult dose is 2 tablets 4 times daily until control has been achieved, after which the dose may be reduced to meet individual requirements. Control may often be maintained with as little as 2 tablets daily
  • Clinical improvement of acute diarrhea is usually observed within 48 hours. If improvement of chronic diarrhea after treatment with a maximum daily dose of 8 tablets is not observed within 10 days, control is unlikely with further administration
Persistent diarrhea:
  Octreotide 100–150 mcg subcutaneously 3 times daily. Maximum total daily dose is 1500 mcg
Antibiotic therapy during latent or delayed onset diarrhea:
  A fluoroquinolone (eg, **Ciprofloxacin** 500 mg orally every 12 hours) if absolute neutrophil count <500/mm^3 with or without accompanying fever in association with diarrhea
  • Antibiotics should also be administered if patient is hospitalized with prolonged diarrhea and should be continued until diarrhea resolves

*Abigerges D et al. J Natl Cancer Inst 1994;86:446–449
Rothenberg ML et al. J Clin Oncol 2001;19:3801–3807
Wadler S et al. J Clin Oncol 1998;16:3169–3178

Hand-foot reaction (palmar-plantar erythrodysesthesia, PPE)
For patients who develop a hand-foot reaction, use topical emollients (eg, Aquaphor®), topical or orally administered steroids, antihistamine agents (H$_1$-receptor antagonists), or pyridoxine
  Pyridoxine may provide relief for discomfort/pain associated with PPE although the mechanism through which this occurs remains unclear
• The suggested pyridoxine starting dose is 50 mg/day, which may be increased to a maximum of 200 mg/day

Patient Population Studied

463 patients with histologically confirmed, first occurrence of a nonresectable, EGFR-expressing metastatic colorectal cancer (mCRC) with a life expectancy of >12 weeks; an Eastern Cooperative Oncology Group Performance Status (ECOG-PS) >2. Patients were ineligible if they had a history of previous exposure to EGFR-targeted therapy or previous chemotherapy (except adjuvant treatment) for mCRC

Efficacy*

	ITT (N = 337)		KRAS WT (N = 134)		KRAS MT (N = 99)	
	F	F + C	F	F + C	F	F + C
Complete Response (%)	0.6	1	1	3	2	0
Partial Response (%)	35	44	36	57	45	33
Progression-free survival (months)	7.2	7.2	7.2	7.7	8.6	5.5
Percent progression-free at 3 months	85	83	78	93	87	78
Percent progression-free at 6 months	59	53	54	66	69	39
Percent progression-free at 9 months	34	34	27	47	42	20
Percent progression-free at 12 months	12	24	13	30	14	6

C, Cetuximab; F, FOLFOX-4 (oxaliplatin, leucovorin, and fluorouracil); ITT, intention to treat; MT, mutant; WT, wild type
*Modified WHO criteria

Therapy Monitoring

1. *Before each cycle:* H&P, CBC with differential, CEA if initially elevated, serum electrolytes, serum magnesium, and LFTs
2. *Every 2–3 months:* CT scans to assess response in patients presenting with advanced colorectal cancer

Treatment Modifications

ERBITUX (Cetuximab) product label, August 2013. Manufactured by ImClone Systems Incorporated, Branchburg, NJ. Distributed and marketed by Bristol-Myers Squibb Company, Princeton, NJ, and Eli Lilly and Company., Indianapolis, IN

Cetuximab Infusion Reactions

Mild/moderate (G1/2)	Permanently decrease administration rates by 50%
Severe (G3/4)	Immediately and permanently discontinue

Cetuximab Dermatologic Toxicity—Severe (G3/4)

Occurrence	Cetuximab	Improvement	Cetuximab Dosage
First	Delay infusion 1–2 weeks	Yes	Continue at 250 mg/m²
		No	Discontinue
Second	Delay infusion 1–2 weeks	Yes	Decrease to 200 mg/m²
		No	Discontinue
Third	Delay infusion 1–2 weeks	Yes	Decrease to 150 mg/m²
		No	Discontinue
Fourth	Discontinue		

Information from the product label: www.erbitux.com/index.aspx (last accessed October 15, 2013)

(*continued*)

Treatment Modifications (*continued*)

Fluorouracil and Oxaliplatin

Any G2/3/4 nonhematologic toxicity	Delay start of next cycle until the severity of all toxicities are G ≤1
ANC ≤1500/mm³ or platelet count ≤100,000/mm³	Delay start of next cycle until ANC >1500/mm³ and platelet count >100,000/mm³
G3/4 Nonneurologic	Reduce fluorouracil and oxaliplatin dosages by 20%
G3/4 ANC	Reduce oxaliplatin dosage by 20%
Persistent (≥14 days) paresthesias	Reduce oxaliplatin dosage by 20%
Temporary (7–14 days) painful paresthesias	
Temporary (7–14 days) functional impairment	
Persistent (≥14 days) painful paresthesias	Discontinue oxaliplatin
Persistent (≥14 days) functional impairment	

Adapted in part from de Gramont A et al. J Clin Oncol 2000;18:2938–2947

Relevant G3/4 Adverse Events Occurring in ≥3% of Patients[*]

G3/4 Adverse Event	FOLFOX-4	Cetuximab + FOLFOX-4
Any G3/4 event	70	78
Neutropenia	34	30
Rash[†]	0.6	11
Diarrhea[†]	7	8
Leukopenia	6	7
Thrombocytopenia	2	4
Fatigue[†]	3	4
Palmar-plantar erythrodysesthesia (PPE)[†]	0.6	4
Peripheral sensory neuropathy[†]	7	4
Anemia[†]	2	4
Composite Categories		
Skin reactions[†,‡]	0.6	18
Infusion-related reactions[§]	2	5

[*]National Cancer Institute (USA) Common Toxicity Criteria, version 2.0. At: http://ctep.cancer.gov/protocolDevelopment/electronic_applications/ctc.htm [accessed October 11, 2013]

[†]No G4 adverse events

[‡]The special adverse event category skin reactions included the following *Medical Dictionary for Regulatory Activities 8.1* terms: acne, acne pustular, cellulitis, dermatitis acneiform, dry skin, erysipelas, erythema, face edema, folliculitis, growth of eyelashes, hair growth abnormal, hypertrichosis, nail bed infection, nail bed inflammation, nail disorder, nail infection, paronychia, pruritus, rash, rash erythematous, rash follicular, rash generalized, rash, macular, rash maculopapular, rash popular, rash pruritic, rash pustular, skin exfoliation, skin hyperpigmentation, skin necrosis, staphylococcal scalded skin syndrome, telangiectasia, wound necrosis, xerosis

[§]The special adverse event category infusion-related reactions included the following *Medical Dictionary for Regulatory Activities 8.1* terms: acute respiratory failure, apnea, asthma, bronchial obstruction, bronchospasm, cyanosis, dyspnea, dyspnea at rest, dyspnea exacerbated, dyspnea exertional, hypoxia, orthopnea, respiratory distress, respiratory failure, chills, hyperpyrexia, pyrexia, acute myocardial infarction, angina pectoris, blood pressure decreased, cardiac failure, cardiopulmonary failure, clonus, convulsion, epilepsy, hypotension, infusion-related reaction, loss of consciousness, myocardial infarction, myocardial ischemia, shock, sudden death and syncope, occurring on the first day of treatment; and anaphylactic reaction, anaphylactic shock, anaphylactoid reaction, anaphylactoid shock, drug hypersensitivity and hypersensitivity, occurring at any time during treatment

Notes: The median duration of cetuximab treatment was 24 weeks, with 84% of patients having a relative dose intensity (RDI) of ≥80%. Similar numbers of patients in both arms had RDIs of ≥80% for oxaliplatin (75% and 80% of patients receiving cetuximab plus FOLFOX-4 and FOLFOX-4, respectively) and FU (67% and 70% of patients, respectively). Reductions and delays in cetuximab dosing were primarily because of skin reactions, and delays in chemotherapy dosing were because of hematologic, GI, or neurologic reactions

METASTATIC COLORECTAL CANCER REGIMEN
CETUXIMAB + FOLFIRI

Van Cutsem E et al. N Engl J Med 2009;360:1408–1417

Warning:

1. Severe infusion reactions occurred with the administration of cetuximab in approximately 3% (17/633) of patients, rarely with fatal outcome (<1 in 1000)

2. Approximately 90% of severe infusion reactions are associated with the first infusion of cetuximab despite the use of prophylactic antihistamines

3. Infusion reactions are characterized by the rapid onset of airway obstruction (bronchospasm, stridor, hoarseness), urticaria, and/or hypotension

4. Caution must be exercised with every cetuximab infusion, as there were patients who experienced their first severe infusion reaction during later infusions

5. Provocative test doses do not reliably predict hypersensitivity reactions to cetuximab administration and are not recommended

Mild to moderate infusion reactions
- Interrupt or slow the cetuximab infusion rate
- Permanently decrease the administration rate by 50%
- Give antihistamine prophylaxis before repeated treatments

Severe reactions
- Immediately interrupt cetuximab therapy
- Administer epinephrine, glucocorticoids, intravenous antihistamines, bronchodilators, and oxygen as needed
- Permanently discontinue further treatment

Cetuximab premedication:
Diphenhydramine 50 mg; administer by intravenous injection before cetuximab administration (other H_1-receptor antagonists may be substituted)

Initial cetuximab dose:
Cetuximab 400 mg/m²; administer intravenously over 120 minutes (maximum infusion rate = 5 mL/min [10 mg/min]) as a single dose (total initial dosage = 400 mg/m²)

Maintenance cetuximab doses:
Cetuximab 250 mg/m²; administer intravenously over 60 minutes (maximum infusion rate = 5 mL/min [10 mg/min]) every week (total weekly dosage = 250 mg/m²)

Notes:
- Cetuximab is intended for direct administration and should not be diluted
- Maximum infusion rate = 5 mL (10 mg)/min (300 mL/h, *or* 600 mg/h)
- Administer cetuximab through a low protein-binding inline filter with pore size = 0.22 μm
- Use 0.9% sodium chloride injection to flush vascular access devices after administration is completed

See Chapter 40 for more information about antineoplastic use

Irinotecan 180 mg/m²; administer intravenously over 90 minutes in 500 mL 5% dextrose injection (D5W) on day 1, every 2 weeks (total dosage/cycle = 180 mg/m²), *plus:*
Either: **(racemic) leucovorin calcium** 400 mg/m² *or* **levoleucovorin calcium** 200 mg/m²; administer intravenously over 2 hours in 25–500 mL 0.9% sodium chloride injection (0.9% NS) or D5W on day 1, every 2 weeks (total dosage/cycle for racemic leucovorin = 400 mg/m², for levoleucovorin = 200 mg/m²), *followed by:*
Fluorouracil 400 mg/m²; administer by intravenous injection over 1–2 minutes after leucovorin on day 1, every 2 weeks, *followed by:*
Fluorouracil 2400 mg/m²; administer by continuous intravenous infusion over 46 hours in 100–1000 mL 0.9% NS or D5W, starting on day 1, every 2 weeks (total dosage/cycle = 2800 mg/m²)

Supportive Care
Antiemetic prophylaxis
Emetogenic potential on day 1 is **MODERATE**
Emetogenic potential on day 2 is **LOW**
See Chapter 39 for antiemetic recommendations

Hematopoietic growth factor (CSF) prophylaxis
Primary prophylaxis is NOT indicated
See Chapter 43 for more information

(continued)

(*continued*)

Antimicrobial prophylaxis
Risk of fever and neutropenia is LOW
   Antimicrobial primary prophylaxis to be considered:
   • Antibacterial—not indicated
   • Antifungal—not indicated
   • Antiviral—not indicated unless patient previously had an episode of HSV
See Chapter 47 for more information

Acute cholinergic syndrome
Atropine sulfate 0.25–1 mg subcutaneously or intravenously if abdominal cramping or diarrhea develop during or within 1 hour after irinotecan administration
• If symptoms are severe, add as primary prophylaxis at least 30 minutes before irinotecan during subsequent cycles
• For irinotecan, acute cholinergic syndrome may be characterized by abdominal cramping, diarrhea, diaphoresis, hypotension, flushing, bradycardia, rhinitis, increased salivation, meiosis, and lacrimation

Diarrhea management
Latent or delayed onset diarrhea*:
   Loperamide 4 mg orally initially after the first loose or liquid stool, *then*
   Loperamide 2 mg orally every 2 hours during waking hours, *plus*
   Loperamide 4 mg orally every 4 hours during hours of sleep
   • Continue for at least 12 hours after diarrhea resolves
   • Recurrent diarrhea after a 12-hour diarrhea-free interval is treated as a new episode
   • Rehydrate orally with fluids and electrolytes during a diarrheal episode
   • If diarrhea persists >48 hours despite loperamide, stop loperamide and hospitalize the patient for IV hydration
Persistent diarrhea:
   Octreotide 100–150 mcg subcutaneously 3 times daily. Maximum total daily dose is 1500 mcg
Antibiotic therapy during latent or delayed onset diarrhea:
   A fluoroquinolone (eg, **Ciprofloxacin** 500 mg orally every 12 hours) if absolute neutrophil count <500/mm^3 with or without accompanying fever in association with diarrhea
   • Antibiotics should also be administered if patient is hospitalized with prolonged diarrhea and should be continued until diarrhea resolves

*Abigerges D et al. J Natl Cancer Inst 1994;86:446–449
Rothenberg ML et al. J Clin Oncol 2001;19:3801–3807
Wadler S et al. J Clin Oncol 1998;16:3169–3178

Hand-foot reaction (palmar-plantar erythrodysesthesia, PPE)
For patients who develop a hand-foot reaction, use topical emollients (eg, Aquaphor®), topical or orally administered steroids, antihistamine agents (H$_1$-receptor antagonists), or pyridoxine
   Pyridoxine may provide relief for discomfort/pain associated with PPE although the mechanism through which this occurs remains unclear
• The suggested pyridoxine starting dose is 50 mg/day, which may be increased to a maximum of 200 mg/day

Patient Population Studied

An open-label, multicenter study, comparing 14-day cycles of cetuximab plus FOLFIRI and FOLFIRI alone, randomized and treated 1198 patients. The primary end point was progression-free survival time. Inclusion criteria included histologically confirmed adenocarcinoma of the colon or rectum, first occurrence of metastatic disease that could not be resected for curative purposes, immunohistochemical evidence of tumor EGFR expression, and Eastern Cooperative Oncology Group (ECOG) Performance Status score of 2 or less. Exclusion criteria were previous exposure to an anti-EGFR therapy or irinotecan-based chemotherapy, previous chemotherapy for metastatic colorectal cancer, adjuvant treatment that was terminated 6 months or less before the start of treatment on trial

Efficacy (N = 1198)

	FOLFIRI (N = 599)	FOLFIRI + Cetuximab (N = 599)
Median progression-free survival	8 months	8.9 months
Median overall survival	18.6 months	19.9 months
Complete response	0.3%	0.5%
Partial response	38.4%	46.4%

Therapy Monitoring

1. *Before each cycle:* H&P, CBC with differential, CEA if initially elevated, serum electrolytes, serum magnesium, and LFTs
2. *Every 2–3 months:* CT scans to assess response in patients presenting with advanced colorectal cancer

Treatment Modifications

(ERBITUX [cetuximab] injection, for intravenous infusion, product label, August 2013. Manufactured by ImClone LLC, a subsidiary of Eli Lilly and Co., Branchburg, NJ. Distributed and Marketed by Bristol-Myers Squibb Company, Princeton, NJ), and Eli Lilly and Company., Indianapolis, IN

Cetuximab Infusion Reactions

Mild/moderate (G1/2)	Permanently decrease administration rates by 50%
Severe (G3/4)	Immediately and permanently discontinue

Cetuximab Dermatologic Toxicity—Severe (G3/4)

Occurrence	Cetuximab	Improvement	Cetuximab Dosage
First	Delay infusion 1–2 weeks	Yes	Continue at 250 mg/m^2
		No	Discontinue
Second	Delay infusion 1–2 weeks	Yes	Decrease to 200 mg/m^2
		No	Discontinue
Third	Delay infusion 1–2 weeks	Yes	Decrease to 150 mg/m^2
		No	Discontinue
Fourth	Discontinue		

Information from the product label: www.erbitux.com/index.aspx (last accessed April 23, 2013)

Irinotecan and Fluorouracil

	Dosage Levels		
	Initial	**−1**	**−2**
Irinotecan	180 mg/m^2	150 mg/m^2	120 mg/m^2
Leucovorin	Racemic leucovorin calcium 400 mg/m^2 *or* levoleucovorin calcium 200 mg/m^2		
Fluorouracil injection	400 mg/m^2	320 mg/m^2	240 mg/m^2
Infusional fluorouracil	2400 mg/m^2	2000 mg/m^2	1600 mg/m^2

Notes:
- Dose modifications are based on the National Cancer Institute (USA) Common Toxicity Criteria. At: http://ctep.cancer.gov/protocolDevelopment/electronic_applications/ctc.htm [accessed October 11, 2013]
- Before beginning a treatment cycle, patients should have baseline bowel function (similar to that before start of treatment) without antidiarrheal therapy for 24 hours, ANC ≥1500/mm^3, and platelet count ≥100,000/mm^3
- Treatment should be delayed 1–2 weeks to allow for recovery from treatment-related toxicities
- If a patient has not recovered after 2 weeks, consider stopping therapy. If toxicity occurs despite 2 dose reductions (ie, on level −2), discontinue therapy

Toxicity	Modifications for Irinotecan and Fluorouracil
Neutropenia/Thrombocytopenia	
G1 ANC (1500–1999/mm^3) or G1 thrombocytopenia (75,000/mm^3 to less than normal limits)	Maintain dose and schedule
G2 ANC (1000–1499/mm^3) or G2 thrombocytopenia (≥50,000 to <75,000/mm^3)	Reduce dosage by 1 dosage level
G3 ANC (500–999/mm^3) or G3 thrombocytopenia (≥10,000 to <50,000/mm^3)	Hold treatment until toxicity resolves to G ≤2, then reduce dosage by 1 dosage level
G4 ANC (<500/mm^3) or G4 thrombocytopenia (<10,000/mm^3)	Hold treatment until toxicity resolves to G ≤2, then reduce dosage by 2 dosage levels
Febrile neutropenia	Hold treatment until neutropenia resolves, then reduce dosage by 2 dosage levels

(continued)

Treatment Modifications (*continued*)

Toxicity	Modifications for Irinotecan and Fluorouracil
Diarrhea	
G1 (2–3 stools/day > baseline)	Maintain dose and schedule
G2 (4–6 stools/day > baseline)	Delay until diarrhea resolves to baseline then reduce dosage by 1 dosage level
G3 (7–9 stools/day > baseline)	Delay until diarrhea resolves to baseline then reduce dosage by 1 dosage level
G4 (≥10 stools/day > baseline)	Delay until diarrhea resolves to baseline then reduce dosage by 2 dosage levels
Other Nonhematologic Toxicities	
Any G1 toxicity	Maintain dose and schedule
Any G2 toxicity	Hold treatment until toxicity resolves to G ≤1, then reduce dosage by 1 dosage level
Any G3 toxicity	Hold treatment until toxicity resolves to G ≤1, then reduce dosage by 1 dosage level
Any G4 toxicity	Hold treatment until toxicity resolves to G ≤1, then reduce dosage by 2 dosage levels
G2–4 mucositis	Decrease only fluorouracil by 20%

André T et al. Eur J Cancer 1999;35:1343–1347
Camptosar, irinotecan hydrochloride injection product label, August 2010. Pharmacia & Upjohn Company, Division of Pfizer, Inc., New York, NY
Douillard JY et al. Lancet 2000;355:1041–1047
Tournigand C et al. J Clin Oncol 2004;22:229–237

Most Common G3/4 Adverse Events and Special Adverse Event Categories in the Safety Population, According to Treatment Group

MedDRA Preferred Term*	FOLFIRI (N = 602)	FOLFIRI + Cetuximab (N = 600)	P-Value
Any	61	79.3	<0.001
Neutropenia[†]	24.6	28.2	0.16
Leukopenia	5.1	7.2	0.15
Diarrhea	10.5	15.7	0.008
Fatigue	4.7	5.3	0.59
Rash	0	8.2	<0.001
Dermatitis acneiform	0	5.3	<0.001
Vomiting	5	4.7	0.80
Special Adverse Events			
Skin reactions			
All	0.2	19.7	<0.001
Acne-like rash	0	16.2	<0.001
Infusion-related reaction	0	2.5	<0.001

*Among the *Medical Dictionary for Regulatory Activities* (MedDRA, version 10.0) preferred terms, no grade 4 reactions were reported for dermatitis acneiform, acne-like rash, or all skin reactions
[†]Grade 3 or 4 febrile neutropenia was reported in 18 of the 600 patients (3.0%) receiving cetuximab plus FOLFIRI and in 13 of the 602 patients (2.2%) receiving FOLFIRI alone

METASTATIC COLORECTAL CANCER REGIMEN

PANITUMUMAB + BEST SUPPORTIVE CARE

Van Cutsem E et al. J Clin Oncol 2007;25:1658–1664

Panitumumab 6 mg/kg; administer intravenously in 0.9% sodium chloride injection (100 mL for doses ≤1000 mg; 150 mL for doses >1000 mg; product concentration should be <10 mg/mL) over 60–90 minutes on day 1, every 2 weeks (total dosage/cycle = 6 mg/kg)

Notes:

- Severe infusion reactions occur in approximately 1% of patients (anaphylactic reactions, bronchospasm, fever, chills, and hypotension). Dose adjustment or discontinuation of panitumumab is warranted depending on the severity of the reaction

- Panitumumab should always be administered by a rate controlling device via a low-protein-binding 0.22-μm inline filter

- Flush line before and after panitumumab with 0.9% sodium chloride injection

- Doses ≤1000 mg should be administered over 60 minutes; >1000 mg should be administered over 90 minutes

  - If tolerated, second and subsequent infusions may be administered over 30 minutes

- The routine use of an antihistamine prior to panitumumab administration is not recommended by the manufacturer; however, doing so may prevent infusion reactions

See Chapter 40 for more information about antineoplastic use

Supportive Care

Antiemetic prophylaxis
Emetogenic potential is **MINIMAL** *to* **LOW**
See Chapter 39 for antiemetic recommendations

Hematopoietic growth factor (CSF) prophylaxis
Primary prophylaxis is NOT indicated
See Chapter 43 for more information

Antimicrobial prophylaxis
Risk of fever and neutropenia is LOW
 Antimicrobial primary prophylaxis to be considered:
  - Antibacterial—not indicated
  - Antifungal—not indicated
  - Antiviral—not indicated unless patient previously had an episode of HSV
See Chapter 47 for more information

Diarrhea management
Loperamide 4 mg; administer orally initially after the first loose or liquid stool, *then*
Loperamide 2 mg; administer orally every 2 hours during waking hours, *plus*
Loperamide 4 mg; administer orally every 4 hours during hours of sleep
- Continue for at least 12 hours after diarrhea resolves
- Recurrent diarrhea after a 12-hour diarrhea free interval is treated as a new episode
- Rehydrate orally with fluids and electrolytes during a diarrheal episode
- If a patient develops blood or mucus in stool, dehydration, or hemodynamic instability, or if diarrhea persists >48 hours despite loperamide, stop loperamide and hospitalize the patient for IV hydration

Alternatively, a trial of **Diphenoxylate hydrochloride** 2.5 mg **with Atropine sulfate** 0.025 mg (eg, Lomotil®)
- Initial adult dose is two tablets four times daily until control has been achieved, after which the dose may be reduced to meet individual requirements. Control may often be maintained with as little as two tablets daily
- Clinical improvement of acute diarrhea is usually observed within 48 hours. If improvement of chronic diarrhea after treatment with a maximum daily dose of 8 tablets is not observed within 10 days, control is unlikely with further administration

(continued)

Patient Population Studied

A study of 463 patients with pathologic diagnosis of metastatic colorectal adenocarcinoma and radiologic documentation of disease progression during or within 6 months following the last administration of fluoropyrimidine, irinotecan, and oxaliplatin. A total of 231 patients were assigned to receive panitumumab + best supportive care (BSC) versus 232 patients assigned to BSC alone. To ensure adequate exposure to prior chemotherapy, average dose-intensity of irinotecan (>65 mg/m² per week) and of oxaliplatin (>30 mg/m² per week) were required. Other key eligibility criteria included: Eastern Cooperative Oncology Group (ECOG) Performance Status score of 0–2, 2 or 3 prior chemotherapy regimens for metastatic colorectal cancer, and 1% or more EGFR-positive membrane staining in evaluated tumor cells (primary or metastatic) by immunohistochemistry

Efficacy* (N = 463)

	Panitumumab + BSC (N = 231)	BSC (N = 232)
Median progression-free survival[†]	8 weeks	7.3 weeks
Mean progression-free survival (SE)[†]	13.8 (0.8) weeks	8.5 (0.5) weeks
Progression-free survival at week 8[†]	49%	30%
Overall survival	No significant difference observed between groups (HR,1.00; 95% CI, 0.82–1.22; P = 0.81)	
Overall response rate[‡]	10%	0%

*Assessed by modified RECIST criteria at weeks 8, 12, 16, 24, 32, 40, and 48, and every 3 months thereafter until disease progression (Response Evaluation Criteria in Solid Tumors. Therasse P et al. J Natl Cancer Inst 2000;92:205-216)
[†]Patients receiving panitumumab had a 46% decrease in the relative progression rate compared with patients receiving BSC (HR, 0.54; 95% CI, 0.44–0.66), and a 95%
CI for the difference in PFS rates favored panitumumab at all scheduled assessments from weeks 8–32; SE = Standard error
[‡]Median time to response was 7.9 (range: 6.7–15.6) weeks and median duration of response was 17.0 (range: 7.9–76.7) weeks; all responses were partial responses

(continued)

Persistent diarrhea:
  Octreotide acetate (solution) 100–150 mcg; administer subcutaneously 3 times daily.
  Maximum total daily dose is 1500 mcg
Antibiotic therapy during latent or delayed onset diarrhea:
  A fluoroquinolone (eg, **Ciprofloxacin** 500 mg orally every 12 hours) if absolute neutrophil
  count <500/mm³ with or without accompanying fever in association with diarrhea
  • Antibiotics should also be administered if patient is hospitalized with prolonged diarrhea
    and should be continued until diarrhea resolves

Toxicities (N = 463)

	Panitumumab + BSC		BSC	
	% All Grades	% G3/4	% All Grades	% G3/4
Patients with at least 1 adverse event	100%	34.5	86	19.2
Erythema	64	5	1	0
Dermatitis acneiform	62	7	1	0
Pruritus	57	2	2	0
Skin exfoliation	24	2	0	0
Fatigue	24	4	15	3
Paronychia	24	1	0	0
Abdominal pain	23	7	17	4.7
Anorexia	22	3.5	18	2
Nausea	22	1	15	0
Diarrhea	21	1	11	0
Rash	20	1	1	0
Skin fissures	20	1	0	0
Constipation	19	3	9	1
Vomiting	18	2	12	1
Dyspnea	14	4.8	13	3
Pyrexia	14	0	12	2
Asthenia	14	3	12	2
Cough	14	0	7	0
Back pain	10	2	7	0
Edema peripheral	10	1	6	0
General physical health deterioration	10	7	3	2.1

Note: In the panitumumab group, 36% of patients had declines in blood magnesium levels versus 1% in the BSC group. Grade 3 or 4 hypomagnesemia occurred in 3% of patients and required magnesium supplementation

Treatment Modifications

Adverse Event	Dose Modification
G1/2 infusion reaction to panitumumab	Decrease infusion rate by 50% for duration of infusion
G3/4 infusion reaction to panitumumab	Immediately and permanently discontinue infusion
G3/4 or intolerable dermatologic reaction to panitumumab	Withhold panitumumab. If toxicity improves to G ≤2 and patient symptomatically improved after withholding no more than 2 doses, resume treatment at 50% of the original dose. If toxicity does not improve to G ≤2 within 1 month, permanently discontinue panitumumab *Note:* **If toxicities do not recur,** subsequent doses of panitumumab may be increased by increments of 25% of original dose until a 6-mg/kg dose is achieved
Recurrence of G3/4 or intolerable dermatologic reaction to panitumumab	Permanently discontinue infusion
Any G2/3/4 nonhematologic toxicity	Delay start of next cycle until the severity of all toxicities are G ≤1
ANC ≤1500/mm³ or platelet count ≤100,000/mm³	Delay start of next cycle until ANC >1500/mm³ and platelet count >100,000/mm³

Therapy Monitoring

1. *Before each cycle:* H&P, CBC with differential, CEA if initially elevated, serum electrolytes, serum magnesium, and LFTs
2. *Every 2–3 months:* CT scans to assess response in patients presenting with advanced colorectal cancer

METASTATIC COLORECTAL CANCER REGIMEN

PANITUMUMAB + FOLFOX-4

de Gramont A et al. J Clin Oncol 2000;18:2938–2947
Douillard J-Y et al. J Clin Oncol 2010;28:4697–4705

Panitumumab 6 mg/kg; administer intravenously in 0.9% sodium chloride injection (100 mL for doses ≤1000 mg; 150 mL for doses >1000 mg; product concentration should be <10 mg/mL) over 60–90 minutes on day 1 before FOLFOX-4 chemotherapy, every 2 weeks (total dosage/cycle = 6 mg/kg)

Notes:
- Severe infusion reactions occur in approximately 1% of patients (anaphylactic reactions, bronchospasm, fever, chills, and hypotension). Dose adjustment or discontinuation of panitumumab is warranted depending on the severity of the reaction
- Panitumumab should always be administered by a rate controlling device via a low-protein-binding 0.22-μm inline filter
- Flush line before and after panitumumab with 0.9% sodium chloride injection
- Doses ≤1000 mg should be administered over 60 minutes; >1000 mg should be administered over 90 minutes
- If tolerated, subsequent infusions may be administered over 30 minutes
- The routine use of an antihistamine prior to panitumumab administration is not recommended by the manufacturer; however, doing so may prevent infusion reactions

FOLFOX-4 (de Gramont A et al.):
Oxaliplatin 85 mg/m²; administer intravenously in 250 mL 5% dextrose injection (D5W) over 2 hours concurrently with leucovorin administration, on day 1, every 2 weeks, (total dosage/cycle = 85 mg/m²)

Note: Oxaliplatin must not be mixed with sodium chloride injection. Therefore, when leucovorin and oxaliplatin are given concurrently via a Y-connector, both drugs must be administered in D5W
Leucovorin calcium 200 mg/m² per dose; administer intravenously in 25–500 mL D5W over 2 hours on 2 consecutive days, on days 1 and 2, every 2 weeks (total dosage/cycle = 400 mg/m²), *followed by:*
Fluorouracil 400 mg/m² per dose; administer by intravenous injection over 1–2 minutes after leucovorin on 2 consecutive days, on days 1 and 2, every 2 weeks, *followed by:*
Fluorouracil 600 mg/m² per dose; administer by continuous intravenous infusion in 100–1000 mL 0.9% sodium chloride injection or D5W over 22 hours on 2 consecutive days, on days 1 and 2, every 2 weeks (total dosage/cycle = 2000 mg/m²)

Note: **Fluorouracil** boluses (400 mg/m² by intravenous injection) may be omitted for better hematologic tolerance

Supportive Care
Antiemetic prophylaxis
Emetogenic potential on day 1 is **MODERATE**
Emetogenic potential on day 2 is **LOW**
See Chapter 39 for antiemetic recommendations

Hematopoietic growth factor (CSF) prophylaxis
Primary prophylaxis is NOT indicated
See Chapter 43 for more information

Antimicrobial prophylaxis
Risk of fever and neutropenia is LOW
  Antimicrobial primary prophylaxis to be considered:
  - Antibacterial—not indicated
  - Antifungal—not indicated
  - Antiviral—not indicated unless patient previously had an episode of HSV
See Chapter 47 for more information

(continued)

Patient Population Studied

An open-label, multicenter, phase III trial comparing the efficacy of panitumumab-FOLFOX-4 with FOLFOX-4 alone in patients with *previously untreated* metastatic colorectal cancer (mCRC) according to tumor *KRAS* status. Patients with Eastern Cooperative Oncology Group Performance Status 0 or 1 versus 2 were randomly assigned (1:1) to receive either panitumumab-FOLFOX-4 or FOLFOX-4. The primary objective of the study was to assess the treatment effect on progression-free survival (PFS) of the addition of panitumumab to FOLFOX-4 as initial therapy for mCRC in patients with wild-type (WT) *KRAS* tumors and also in patients with mutant (MT) *KRAS* tumors. The study was amended to compare PFS (primary end point) and overall survival (secondary end point) according to *KRAS* status before any efficacy analyses

Treatment Modifications

Adverse Event	Dose Modification
G1/2 infusion reaction to panitumumab	Decrease infusion rate by 50% for duration of infusion
G3/4 infusion reaction to panitumumab	Immediately and permanently discontinue infusion
G3/4 or intolerable dermatologic reaction to panitumumab	Withhold panitumumab. If toxicity improves to G ≤2 and patient symptomatically improved after withholding no more than 2 doses, resume treatment at 50% of original dose. If toxicity does not improve to G ≤2 within 1 month, permanently discontinue panitumumab *Note:* **If toxicities do not recur**, subsequent doses of panitumumab may be increased by increments of 25% of original dose until a 6-mg/kg dose is achieved

(continued)

(*continued*)

Diarrhea management

Latent or delayed onset diarrhea*:

Loperamide 4 mg orally initially after the first loose or liquid stool, *then*
Loperamide 2 mg orally every 2 hours during waking hours, *plus*
Loperamide 4 mg orally every 4 hours during hours of sleep

• Continue for at least 12 hours after diarrhea resolves

• Recurrent diarrhea after a 12-hour diarrhea-free interval is treated as a new episode

• Rehydrate orally with fluids and electrolytes during a diarrheal episode

• If diarrhea persists >48 hours despite loperamide, stop loperamide and hospitalize the patient for IV hydration

Persistent diarrhea:

Octreotide 100–150 mcg subcutaneously 3 times daily. Maximum total daily dose is 1500 mcg

Antibiotic therapy during latent or delayed onset diarrhea:

A fluoroquinolone (eg, **Ciprofloxacin** 500 mg orally every 12 hours) if absolute neutrophil count <500/mm³ with or without accompanying fever in association with diarrhea

• Antibiotics should also be administered if patient is hospitalized with prolonged diarrhea and should be continued until diarrhea resolves

*Abigerges D et al. J Natl Cancer Inst 1994;86:446–449
Rothenberg ML et al. J Clin Oncol 2001;19:3801–3807
Wadler S et al. J Clin Oncol 1998;16:3169–3178

Oral care

Prophylaxis and treatment for mucositis/stomatitis

General advice:

• Encourage patients to maintain intake of non-alcoholic fluids

• Evaluate patients for oral pain and provide analgesic medications

• Consider histamine (H$_2$-subtype) receptor antagonists (eg, ranitidine, famotidine), or a proton pump inhibitor for epigastric pain

• *Lactobacillus* sp.-containing probiotics may be beneficial in preventing diarrhea

Patients with intact oral mucosa:

• Clean the mouth, tongue, and gums by brushing after every meal and at bedtime with an ultra-soft toothbrush with fluoride toothpaste

• Floss teeth gently every day unless contraindicated. If gums bleed and hurt, avoid bleeding or sore areas, but floss other teeth

• Patients may use saline or commercial bland, non-alcoholic rinses

▪ Do not use mouthwashes that contain alcohols

If mucositis or stomatitis is present:

• Keep the mouth moist utilizing water, ice chips, sugarless gum, sugar-free hard candies, or a saliva substitute

• Rinse mouth several times a day to remove debris

▪ Use a solution of ¼ teaspoon (1.25 g) each of baking soda and table salt (sodium chloride) in one quart (~950 mL) of warm water. Follow with a plain water rinse

▪ Do not use mouthwashes that contain alcohols

• Foam-tipped swabs (eg, Toothettes®) are useful in moisturizing oral mucosa, but ineffective for cleansing teeth and removing plaque

• Advise patients who develop mucositis to:

▪ Choose foods that are easy to chew and swallow

▪ Take small bites of food, chew slowly, and sip liquids with meals

▪ Encourage soft, moist foods such as cooked cereals, mashed potatoes, and scrambled eggs

▪ For trouble swallowing, soften food with gravies, sauces, broths, yogurt, or other bland liquids

▪ Avoid sharp, crunchy foods; hot, spicy or highly acidic foods (eg, citrus fruits and juices); sugary foods; toothpicks; tobacco products; alcoholic drinks

Treatment Modifications
(*continued*)

Adverse Event	Dose Modification
Recurrence of G3/4 or intolerable dermatologic reaction to panitumumab	Permanently discontinue infusion
Any G2/3/4 nonhematologic toxicity	Delay start of next cycle until the severity of all toxicities are G ≤1
ANC ≤1500/mm³ or platelet count ≤100,000/mm³	Delay start of next cycle until ANC >1500/mm³ and platelet count >100,000/mm³
G3/4 Nonneurologic	Reduce fluorouracil and oxaliplatin dosages by 20%
G3/4 ANC	Reduce oxaliplatin dosage by 20%
Persistent (≥14 days) paresthesias	Reduce oxaliplatin dosage by 20%
Temporary (7–14 days) painful paresthesias	
Temporary (7–14 days) functional impairment	
Persistent (≥14 days) painful paresthesias	Discontinue oxaliplatin
Persistent (≥14 days) functional impairment	

Adapted in part from de Gramont A et al. J Clin Oncol 2000;18:2938–2947

Efficacy (N = 649)*

	Wild-Type KRAS		Mutant KRAS	
	FOLFOX-4 (N = 190)	FOLFOX-4 + Panitumumab (N = 165)	FOLFOX-4 (N = 142)	FOLFOX-4 + Panitumumab (N = 152)
Progression-free survival	8 months	9.6 months	8.8 months	7.3 months
Overall survival	19.7 months	23.9 months	19.3 months	15.5 months
Overall response rate	48%	55%	40%	40%

*RECIST (Response Evaluation Criteria in Solid Tumors. Therasse P et al. J Natl Cancer Inst 2000;92:205-216)

Note: Metastasectomy of any site was attempted in 10.5% of patients treated with panitumumab-FOLFOX-4 and 9.4% of patients treated with FOLFOX-4 with WT *KRAS* status; complete resections were achieved in 8.3% and 7.0% of patients, respectively

Note: Treatment-emergent binding antipanitumumab antibodies were detected in 14 (3.0%) of 470 patients who received panitumumab. Neutralizing antibodies were detected in postdose samples from 2 (0.4%) of 470 patients

Toxicity* (N = 539†)

	% G3/4
Any G3/4 event	82
Neutropenia	40.2
Skin toxicity	33.8
Diarrhea	18.9
Neurologic toxicities	16.3
Hypokalemia	9.5
Fatigue	8.5
Mucositis	7.4
Hypomagnesemia	6.1
Pulmonary embolism	3
Paronychia	2.8
Febrile neutropenia	2.8
Panitumumab infusion-related reaction‡	<1

*NCI Common Terminology Criteria for Adverse Events, v3. At: http://ctep.cancer.gov/protocolDevelopment/electronic_applications/ctc.htm [accessed October 11, 2013]
†Includes patients with wild-type (WT) KRAS and mutant (MT) KRAS who were treated with panitumumab
‡Grade 3 panitumumab-related infusion reactions occurred in 2 patients; both patients received additional panitumumab treatment after premedication

Therapy Monitoring

1. *Before each cycle:* H&P, CBC with differential, CEA if initially elevated, serum electrolytes, serum magnesium, and LFTs
2. *Every 2–3 months:* CT scans to assess response in patients presenting with advanced colorectal cancer

METASTATIC COLORECTAL CANCER REGIMEN
PANITUMUMAB + FOLFIRI

Douillard JY et al. Lancet 2000;355:1041–1047
Peeters M et al. J Clin Oncol 2010;28:4706–4713
Tournigand C et al. J Clin Oncol 2004;22:229–237

Panitumumab 6 mg/kg; administer intravenously in 0.9% sodium chloride injection (100 mL for doses ≤1000 mg; 150 mL for doses >1000 mg; product concentration should be <10 mg/mL) over 60–90 minutes on day 1 before FOLFIRI chemotherapy, every 2 weeks (total dosage/cycle = 6 mg/kg)

Notes:
- Severe infusion reactions occur in approximately 1% of patients (anaphylactic reactions, bronchospasm, fever, chills, and hypotension). Dose adjustment or discontinuation of panitumumab is warranted depending on the severity of the reaction
- Panitumumab should always be administered by a rate-controlling device via a low-protein-binding 0.22-μm inline filter
- Flush line before and after panitumumab with 0.9% sodium chloride injection
- Doses ≤1000 mg should be administered over 60 minutes; >1000 mg should be administered over 90 minutes
- If tolerated, subsequent infusions may be administered over 30 minutes
- The routine use of an antihistamine prior to panitumumab administration is not recommended by the manufacturer; however, doing so may prevent infusion reactions

Irinotecan 180 mg/m^2; administer intravenously over 90 minutes in 500 mL 5% dextrose injection (D5W) on day 1, every 2 weeks (total dosage/cycle = 180 mg/m^2), *plus:*
Either: (**racemic**) **leucovorin calcium** 400 mg/m^2 *or* **levoleucovorin calcium** 200 mg/m^2; administer intravenously over 2 hours in 25–500 mL 0.9% sodium chloride injection (0.9% NS) or D5W on day 1, every 2 weeks (total dosage/cycle for racemic leucovorin = 400 mg/m^2, for levoleucovorin = 200 mg/m^2), *followed by:*
Fluorouracil 400 mg/m^2; administer by intravenous injection over 1–2 minutes after leucovorin on day 1, every 2 weeks, *followed by:*
Fluorouracil 2400 mg/m^2; administer by continuous intravenous infusion over 46 hours in 100–1000 mL 0.9% NS or D5W, starting on day 1, every 2 weeks (total dosage/cycle = 2800 mg/m^2)

Supportive Care
Antiemetic prophylaxis
Emetogenic potential on day 1 is **MODERATE**
Emetogenic potential on day 2 is **LOW**
See Chapter 39 for antiemetic recommendations

Hematopoietic growth factor (CSF) prophylaxis
Primary prophylaxis is NOT indicated
See Chapter 43 for more information

Antimicrobial prophylaxis
Risk of fever and neutropenia is LOW
   Antimicrobial primary prophylaxis to be considered:
   - Antibacterial—not indicated
   - Antifungal—not indicated
   - Antiviral—not indicated unless patient previously had an episode of HSV
See Chapter 47 for more information

Acute cholinergic syndrome
Atropine sulfate 0.25–1 mg subcutaneously or intravenously if abdominal cramping or diarrhea develop during or within 1 hour after irinotecan administration
- If symptoms are severe, add as primary prophylaxis at least 30 minutes before irinotecan during subsequent cycles
- For irinotecan, acute cholinergic syndrome may be characterized by abdominal cramping, diarrhea, diaphoresis, hypotension, flushing, bradycardia, rhinitis, increased salivation, meiosis, and lacrimation

Diarrhea management
Latent or delayed onset diarrhea*:
   Loperamide 4 mg orally initially after the first loose or liquid stool, *then*
   Loperamide 2 mg orally every 2 hours during waking hours, *plus*
   Loperamide 4 mg orally every 4 hours during hours of sleep
   - Continue for at least 12 hours after diarrhea resolves
   - Recurrent diarrhea after a 12-hour diarrhea-free interval is treated as a new episode
   - Rehydrate orally with fluids and electrolytes during a diarrheal episode
   - If diarrhea persists >48 hours despite loperamide, stop loperamide and hospitalize the patient for IV hydration

*Abigerges D et al. J Natl Cancer Inst 1994;86:446–449
Rothenberg ML et al. J Clin Oncol 2001;19:3801–3807
Wadler S et al. J Clin Oncol 1998;16:3169–3178

(continued)

(*continued*)

Persistent diarrhea:
  Octreotide 100–150 mcg subcutaneously 3 times daily. Maximum total daily dose is 1500 mcg

Antibiotic therapy during latent or delayed onset diarrhea:
  A fluoroquinolone (eg, **Ciprofloxacin** 500 mg orally every 12 hours) if absolute neutrophil count <500/mm³ with or without accompanying fever in association with diarrhea
  • Antibiotics should also be administered if patient is hospitalized with prolonged diarrhea and should be continued until diarrhea resolves

Oral care

Prophylaxis and treatment for mucositis/stomatitis

General advice:
  • Encourage patients to maintain intake of non-alcoholic fluids
  • Evaluate patients for oral pain and provide analgesic medications
  • Consider histamine (H₂-subtype) receptor antagonists (eg, ranitidine, famotidine), or a proton pump inhibitor for epigastric pain
  • *Lactobacillus* sp.-containing probiotics may be beneficial in preventing diarrhea

Patients with intact oral mucosa:
  • Clean the mouth, tongue, and gums by brushing after every meal and at bedtime with an ultra-soft toothbrush with fluoride toothpaste
  • Floss teeth gently every day unless contraindicated. If gums bleed and hurt, avoid bleeding or sore areas, but floss other teeth
  • Patients may use saline or commercial bland, non-alcoholic rinses
    ▪ Do not use mouthwashes that contain alcohols

If mucositis or stomatitis is present:
  • Keep the mouth moist utilizing water, ice chips, sugarless gum, sugar-free hard candies, or a saliva substitute
  • Rinse mouth several times a day to remove debris
    ▪ Use a solution of ¼ teaspoon (1.25 g) each of baking soda and table salt (sodium chloride) in one quart (~950 mL) of warm water. Follow with a plain water rinse
    ▪ Do not use mouthwashes that contain alcohols
  • Foam-tipped swabs (eg, Toothettes®) are useful in moisturizing oral mucosa, but ineffective for cleansing teeth and removing plaque
  • Advise patients who develop mucositis to:
    ▪ Choose foods that are easy to chew and swallow
    ▪ Take small bites of food, chew slowly, and sip liquids with meals
    ▪ Encourage soft, moist foods such as cooked cereals, mashed potatoes, and scrambled eggs
    ▪ For trouble swallowing, soften food with gravies, sauces, broths, yogurt, or other bland liquids
    ▪ Avoid sharp, crunchy foods; hot, spicy or highly acidic foods (eg, citrus fruits and juices); sugary foods; toothpicks; tobacco products; alcoholic drinks

Treatment Modifications

Adverse Event	Dose Modification
G1/2 infusion reaction to panitumumab	Decrease infusion rate by 50% for duration of infusion
G3/4 infusion reaction to panitumumab	Immediately and permanently discontinue infusion
G3/4 or intolerable dermatologic reaction to panitumumab	Withhold panitumumab. If toxicity improves to G ≤2 and patient symptomatically improves after withholding no more than 2 doses, resume treatment at 50% of the original dose. If toxicity does not improve to G ≤2 within 1 month, permanently discontinue panitumumab *Note:* **If toxicities do not recur,** subsequent doses of panitumumab may be increased by increments of 25% of original dose until a 6-mg/kg dose is achieved
Recurrence of G3/4 or intolerable dermatologic reaction to panitumumab	Permanently discontinue panitumumab
Any G2/3/4 nonhematologic toxicity	Delay start of next cycle until the severity of all toxicities are G ≤1
ANC ≤1500/mm³ or platelet count ≤100,000/mm³	Delay start of next cycle le until ANC >1500/mm³ and platelet count >100,000/mm³

(*continued*)

Treatment Modifications (continued)

	Dosage Levels		
	Initial	−1	−2
Irinotecan	180 mg/m²	150 mg/m²	120 mg/m²
Leucovorin	Racemic leucovorin calcium 400 mg/m² or levoleucovorin calcium 200 mg/m²		
Fluorouracil injection	400 mg/m²	320 mg/m²	240 mg/m²
Infusional fluorouracil	2400 mg/m²	2000 mg/m²	1600 mg/m²

Notes:
- Dose modifications are based on the National Cancer Institute (USA) Common Toxicity Criteria. At: http://ctep.cancer.gov/protocolDevelopment/electronic_applications/ctc.htm [accessed October 11, 2013]
- Before beginning a treatment cycle, patients should have baseline bowel function (similar to that before start of treatment) without antidiarrheal therapy for 24 hours, ANC ≥1500/mm³, and platelet count ≥100,000/mm³
- Treatment should be delayed 1–2 weeks to allow for recovery from treatment-related toxicities
- If a patient has not recovered after 2 weeks, consider stopping therapy
- If toxicity occurs despite 2 dose reductions (ie, on level −2), discontinue therapy

Toxicity	Modifications for Irinotecan and Fluorouracil
Neutropenia/Thrombocytopenia	
G1 ANC (1500–1999/mm³) or G1 thrombocytopenia (75,000/mm³ to less than normal limits)	Maintain dose and schedule
G2 ANC (1000–1499/mm³) or G2 thrombocytopenia (≥50,000 to <75,000/mm³)	Reduce dosage by 1 dosage level
G3 ANC (500–999/mm³) or G3 thrombocytopenia (≥10,000 to <50,000/mm³)	Hold treatment until toxicity resolves to G ≤2, then reduce dosage by 1 dosage level
G4 ANC (<500/mm³) or G4 thrombocytopenia (<10,000/mm³)	Hold treatment until toxicity resolves to G ≤2, then reduce dosage by 2 dosage levels
Febrile neutropenia	Hold treatment until neutropenia resolves, then reduce dosage by 2 dosage levels
Diarrhea	
G1 (2–3 stools/day > baseline)	Maintain dose and schedule
G2 (4–6 stools/day > baseline)	Delay until diarrhea resolves to baseline then reduce dosage by 1 dosage level
G3 (7–9 stools/day > baseline)	Delay until diarrhea resolves to baseline then reduce dosage by 1 dosage level
G4 (≥10 stools/day > baseline)	Delay until diarrhea resolves to baseline then reduce dosage by 2 dosage levels
Other Nonhematologic Toxicities	
Any G1 toxicity	Maintain dose and schedule
Any G2 toxicity	Hold treatment until toxicity resolves to G ≤1, then reduce dosage by 1 dosage level
Any G3 toxicity	Hold treatment until toxicity resolves to G ≤1, then reduce dosage by 1 dosage level
Any G4 toxicity	Hold treatment until toxicity resolves to G ≤1, then reduce dosage by 2 dosage levels
G2–4 mucositis	Decrease only fluorouracil by 20%

André T et al. Eur J Cancer 1999;35:1343–1347
Camptosar, irinotecan hydrochloride injection product label, July 2005. Pharmacia & Upjohn Company, Division of Pfizer, Inc, New York, NY
Douillard JY et al. Lancet 2000;355:1041–1047
Tournigand C et al. J Clin Oncol 2004;22:229–237

Efficacy (N = 1083)*

	Wild-Type (WT) KRAS		Mutant (MT) KRAS	
	FOLFIRI (N = 294)	FOLFIRI + Panitumumab (N = 303)	FOLFIRI (N = 248)	FOLFIRI + Panitumumab (N = 238)
Progression-free survival	3.9 months	5.9 months	4.9 months	5.0 months
Overall survival	12.5 months	14.5 months	11.1 months	11.8 months
Overall response rate	10%	35%	14%	13%

*RECIST (Response Evaluation Criteria in Solid Tumors. Therasse P et al. J Natl Cancer Inst 2000;92:205-216)

Toxicity* (N = 539†)

	% G3/4
Any G3/4 event	68.6
Skin toxicity	34.5
Neutropenia	16.9
Diarrhea	13.5
Mucositis	8.3
Hypokalemia	5.4
Pulmonary embolism	4.1
Hypomagnesemia	3.7
Dehydration	3.3
Paronychia	2.8
Febrile neutropenia	1.7
Panitumumab infusion-related reaction‡	<1

*NCI CTCAE, National Cancer Institute (USA) Common Terminology Criteria for Adverse Events, version 3. At: http://ctep.cancer.gov/ protocolDevelopment/electronic_applications/ ctc.htm [accessed December 7, 2013]
†Includes patients with WT KRAS and MT KRAS who were treated with panitumumab
‡Grade 3 panitumumab-related infusion reactions occurred in 2 patients; these patients did not receive additional panitumumab treatment

Patient Population Studied

A study of 1186 patients with Eastern Cooperative Oncology Group (ECOG) Performance Status of 0, 1, or 2 and a diagnosis of adenocarcinoma of the colon or rectum. *Only one prior chemotherapy regimen for metastatic colorectal cancer (mCRC) consisting of first-line fluoropyrimidine-based chemotherapy was allowed.* Patients were excluded if they previously received irinotecan or anti-EGFR therapy. Radiographically confirmed disease progression must have occurred during or within 6 months after first-line chemotherapy

Therapy Monitoring

1. *Before each cycle:* H&P, CBC with differential, CEA if initially elevated, serum electrolytes, serum magnesium, and LFTs
2. *Every 2–3 months:* CT scans to assess response in patients presenting with advanced colorectal cancer

SECOND-LINE COLORECTAL CANCER REGIMEN
ZIV-AFLIBERCEPT + FOLFIRI

Van Cutsem E et al. J Clin Oncol 2012;30:3499–3506

ziv-Aflibercept 4 mg/kg; administer intravenously over 60 minutes in a volume of 0.9% sodium chloride injection (0.9% NS) or 5% dextrose injection (D5W) sufficient to produce a concentration within the range 0.6–8 mg/mL on day 1, every 2 weeks (total dosage/cycle = 4 mg/kg), *followed by:*

Irinotecan 180 mg/m²; administer intravenously over 90 minutes in 500 mL D5W on day 1, every 2 weeks (total dosage/cycle = 180 mg/m²), *plus:*

Either: **(racemic) leucovorin calcium** 400 mg/m² *or* **levoleucovorin calcium** 200 mg/m²; administer intravenously in 25–500 mL 0.9% NS or D5W over 2 hours on day 1, every 2 weeks (total dosage/cycle for racemic leucovorin = 400 mg/m², for levoleucovorin = 200 mg/m²), *followed by:*

Fluorouracil 400 mg/m²; administer by intravenous injection over 1–2 minutes after leucovorin on day 1, every 2 weeks, *followed by:*

Fluorouracil 2400 mg/m²; administer by continuous intravenous infusion over 46 hours in 100–1000 mL 0.9% NS or D5W, starting on day 1 every 2 weeks (total dosage/cycle = 2800 mg/m²)

Supportive Care
Antiemetic prophylaxis
Emetogenic potential on day 1 is **MODERATE**
Emetogenic potential on day 2 is **LOW**
See Chapter 39 for antiemetic recommendations

Hematopoietic growth factor (CSF) prophylaxis
Primary prophylaxis is NOT indicated
See Chapter 43 for more information

Antimicrobial prophylaxis
Risk of fever and neutropenia is LOW
   Antimicrobial primary prophylaxis to be considered:
   • Antibacterial—not indicated
   • Antifungal—not indicated
   • Antiviral—not indicated unless patient previously had an episode of HSV
See Chapter 47 for more information

Acute cholinergic syndrome
Atropine sulfate 0.25–1 mg subcutaneously or intravenously if abdominal cramping or diarrhea develop during or within 1 hour after irinotecan administration
• If symptoms are severe, add as primary prophylaxis at least 30 minutes before irinotecan during subsequent cycles
• For irinotecan, acute cholinergic syndrome may be characterized by abdominal cramping, diarrhea, diaphoresis, hypotension, flushing, bradycardia, rhinitis, increased salivation, meiosis, and lacrimation

Diarrhea management
Latent or delayed onset diarrhea*:
   Loperamide 4 mg orally initially after the first loose or liquid stool, *then*
   Loperamide 2 mg orally every 2 hours during waking hours, *plus*
   Loperamide 4 mg orally every 4 hours during hours of sleep
   • Continue for at least 12 hours after diarrhea resolves
   • Recurrent diarrhea after a 12-hour diarrhea-free interval is treated as a new episode
   • Rehydrate orally with fluids and electrolytes during a diarrheal episode
   • If diarrhea persists >48 hours despite loperamide, stop loperamide and hospitalize the patient for IV hydration

Persistent diarrhea:
   Octreotide 100–150 mcg subcutaneously 3 times daily. Maximum total daily dose is 1500 mcg
Antibiotic therapy during latent or delayed onset diarrhea:
   A fluoroquinolone (eg, **Ciprofloxacin** 500 mg orally every 12 hours) if absolute neutrophil count <500/mm³ with or without accompanying fever in association with diarrhea
   • Antibiotics should also be administered if patient is hospitalized with prolonged diarrhea and should be continued until diarrhea resolves

*Abigerges D et al. J Natl Cancer Inst 1994;86:446–449
Rothenberg ML et al. J Clin Oncol 2001;19:3801–3807
Wadler S et al. J Clin Oncol 1998;16:3169–3178

(continued)

(continued)

Oral care
Prophylaxis and treatment for mucositis/stomatitis
General advice:
- Encourage patients to maintain intake of non-alcoholic fluids
- Evaluate patients for oral pain and provide analgesic medications
- Consider histamine (H_2-subtype) receptor antagonists (eg, ranitidine, famotidine), or a proton pump inhibitor for epigastric pain
- *Lactobacillus* sp.-containing probiotics may be beneficial in preventing diarrhea

Patients with intact oral mucosa:
- Clean the mouth, tongue, and gums by brushing after every meal and at bedtime with an ultra-soft toothbrush with fluoride toothpaste
- Floss teeth gently every day unless contraindicated. If gums bleed and hurt, avoid bleeding or sore areas, but floss other teeth
- Patients may use saline or commercial bland, non-alcoholic rinses
  - Do not use mouthwashes that contain alcohols

If mucositis or stomatitis is present:
- Keep the mouth moist utilizing water, ice chips, sugarless gum, sugar-free hard candies, or a saliva substitute
- Rinse mouth several times a day to remove debris
  - Use a solution of ¼ teaspoon (1.25 g) each of baking soda and table salt (sodium chloride) in one quart (~950 mL) of warm water. Follow with a plain water rinse
  - Do not use mouthwashes that contain alcohols
- Foam-tipped swabs (eg, Toothettes®) are useful in moisturizing oral mucosa, but ineffective for cleansing teeth and removing plaque
- Advise patients who develop mucositis to:
  - Choose foods that are easy to chew and swallow
  - Take small bites of food, chew slowly, and sip liquids with meals
  - Encourage soft, moist foods such as cooked cereals, mashed potatoes, and scrambled eggs
  - For trouble swallowing, soften food with gravies, sauces, broths, yogurt, or other bland liquids
  - Avoid sharp, crunchy foods; hot, spicy or highly acidic foods (eg, citrus fruits and juices); sugary foods; toothpicks; tobacco products; alcoholic drinks

Hand-foot reaction (palmar-plantar erythrodysesthesia, PPE)
For patients who develop a hand-foot reaction, use topical emollients (eg, Aquaphor®), topical or orally administered steroids, antihistamine agents (H_1-receptor antagonists), or pyridoxine
Pyridoxine may provide relief for discomfort/pain associated with PPE although the mechanism through which this occurs remains unclear
- The suggested pyridoxine starting dose is 50 mg/day, which may be increased to a maximum of 200 mg/day

Patient Population Studied

Patients with an Eastern Cooperative Oncology Group (ECOG) Performance Status (PS) of 0–2 and histologically or cytologically proven colorectal adenocarcinoma with metastatic disease not amenable to potentially curative treatment were randomly assigned (1:1) to receive either ziv-aflibercept or placebo followed by combination chemotherapy with the FOLFIRI regimen. Although disease progression was to have been documented either during or after completion of a single prior oxaliplatin-containing regimen, patients were not selected for the timing of their progression. Patients who experienced relapse within 6 months of completion of oxaliplatin-based adjuvant therapy were eligible. Prior bevacizumab was permitted, but not prior irinotecan. Patients with a history of major surgery within 28 days were not allowed to participate

Dose Modifications

Note: Adjust each treatment component individually and/or delay cycle (up to 2 weeks) in the event of toxicity

Adverse Event	Dose Modification
Severe hemorrhage	Discontinue ziv-aflibercept
Gastrointestinal perforation	
Compromised wound healing	
Fistula formation	
Hypertensive crisis or hypertensive encephalopathy	
Arterial thromboembolic events	
Nephrotic syndrome or thrombotic microangiopathy (TMA)	
Reversible posterior leukoencephalopathy syndrome (RPLS)	
Recurrent or severe hypertension	Hold ziv-aflibercept until hypertension abates to G $\leq$1, and permanently reduce ziv-aflibercept dosage to 2 mg/kg
Proteinuria of 2 g/24 h	Hold ziv-aflibercept and resume when proteinuria is $\leq$2 g/24 h
Recurrent proteinuria	Hold ziv-aflibercept and resume when proteinuria is $\leq$2 g/24 h, and permanently reduce ziv-aflibercept dosage to 2 mg/kg
Planned surgery	Suspend ziv-aflibercept at least 4 weeks prior to elective surgery

Irinotecan and Fluorouracil

	Dosage Levels		
	Initial	−1	−2
Irinotecan	180 mg/m²	150 mg/m²	120 mg/m²
Leucovorin	Racemic leucovorin calcium 400 mg/m² or levoleucovorin calcium 200 mg/m²		
Fluorouracil injection	400 mg/m²	320 mg/m²	240 mg/m²
Infusional fluorouracil	2400 mg/m²	2000 mg/m²	1600 mg/m²

Notes:
- Dose modifications are based on the NCI CTCAE, National Cancer Institute (USA) Common Terminology Criteria for Adverse Events, version 3. At: http://ctep.cancer.gov/protocolDevelopment/electronic_applications/ctc.htm [accessed December 7, 2013]
- Before beginning a treatment cycle, patients should have baseline bowel function (similar to that before start of treatment) without antidiarrheal therapy for 24 hours, ANC $\geq$1500/mm³, and platelet count $\geq$100,000/mm³
- Treatment should be delayed 1–2 weeks to allow for recovery from treatment-related toxicities
- If a patient has not recovered after 2 weeks of withholding ziv-aflibercept, consider stopping therapy. If toxicity occurs despite 2 dose reductions (ie, on level −2), discontinue therapy

(continued)

Dose Modifications (*continued*)

Toxicity	Modifications for Irinotecan and Fluorouracil
Neutropenia/Thrombocytopenia	
G1 ANC (1500–1999/mm³) or G1 thrombocytopenia (75,000/mm³ to less than normal limits)	Maintain dose and schedule
G2 ANC (1000–1499/mm³) or G2 thrombocytopenia (≥50,000 to <75,000/mm³)	Reduce dosage by 1 dosage level
G3 ANC (500–999/mm³) or G3 thrombocytopenia (≥10,000 to <50,000/mm³)	Hold treatment until toxicity resolves to G ≤2, then reduce dosage by 1 dosage level
G4 ANC (<500/mm³) or G4 thrombocytopenia (<10,000/mm³)	Hold treatment until toxicity resolves to G ≤2, then reduce dosage by 2 dosage levels
Febrile neutropenia	Hold treatment until neutropenia resolves, then reduce dosage by 2 dosage levels
Diarrhea	
G1 (2–3 stools/day > baseline)	Maintain dose and schedule
G2 (4–6 stools/day > baseline)	Delay until diarrhea resolves to baseline, then reduce dosage by 1 dosage level
G3 (7–9 stools/day > baseline)	Delay until diarrhea resolves to baseline, then reduce dosage by 1 dosage level
G4 (≥10 stools/day > baseline)	Delay until diarrhea resolves to baseline, then reduce dosage by 2 dosage levels
Other Nonhematologic Toxicities	
Any G1 toxicity	Maintain dose and schedule
Any G2 toxicity	Hold treatment until toxicity resolves to G ≤1, then reduce dosage by 1 dosage level
Any G3 toxicity	Hold treatment until toxicity resolves to G ≤1, then reduce dosage by 1 dosage level
Any G4 toxicity	Hold treatment until toxicity resolves to G ≤1, then reduce dosage by 2 dosage levels
G2–4 mucositis	Decrease only fluorouracil dosage by 20%

André T et al. Eur J Cancer 1999;35:1343–1347
Camptosar, irinotecan hydrochloride injection product label, July 2005. Pharmacia & Upjohn Company, Division of Pfizer, Inc., New York, NY
Douillard JY et al. Lancet 2000;355:1041–1047
Tournigand C et al. J Clin Oncol 2004;22:229–237

Efficacy		
Survival Measure	Placebo/FOLFIRI	ZIV-Aflibercept/FOLFIRI
Median overall survival (months, 95%CI)	12.06 (11.07–13.10)	13.5 (12.51–14.94)
	P = 0.0032; HR 0.81 (0.71–0.93)	
Overall Survival Probability (95%CI)		
12 months	0.50 (0.46–0.54)	0.56 (0.52–0.60)
18 months	0.30 (0.26–0.34)	0.38 (0.34–0.42)
24 months	0.18 (0.14–0.22)	0.28 (0.23–0.32)
30 months	0.12 (0.08–0.16)	0.22 (0.17–0.26)
Median progression-free survival (months, 95%CI)	4.67 (4.21–5.36)	6.9 (6.51–7.2)
	P<0.001; HR 0.75 (0.66–0.86)	
Best Overall Response		
Overall response	11.1% (8.5–13.8)	19.8% (16.4–23.2)
	P<0.001	
Complete response	0.4%	0
Partial response	10.8%	19.8%
Stable disease	64.9%	65.9%
Progressive disease	21.5%	10.4%
Not evaluable	2.5%	4.0%
Reason for Treatment Discontinuation		
Adverse event	12.1%	26.6%
Disease progression	71.2%	49.8%
Patient request	7.3%	13.6%
Investigator decision	3.4%	3.3%
Metastatic surgery	1.6%	2.0%
Other	1.8%	1.6%
Ongoing treatment	1.8%	2.3%

Toxicity

Adverse Event*	Placebo/FOLFIRI (n = 605)			ziv-Aflibercept/FOLFIRI (n = 611)		
	All Grades (%)	Grade 3 (%)	Grade 4 (%)	All Grades (%)	Grade 3 (%)	Grade 4 (%)
Any	97.9	45.1	17.4	99.2	62.0	21.4
Diarrhea	56.5	7.6	0.2	69.2	19.0	0.3
Asthenic conditions	50.2	10.4	0.2	60.4	16.0	0.8
Stomatitis and ulceration	34.9	5.0	—	54.8	13.6	0.2
Nausea	54	3.0	—	53.4	1.8	—
Infections and infestations	32.7	6.1	0.8	46.2	11.0	1.3
Hypertension	10.7	1.5	—	41.4	19.1	0.2
Hemorrhage	19	1.7	—	37.8	2.8	0.2
Epistaxis	7.4	—	—	27.7	0.2	—
GI and abdominal pains	29.1	3.1	0.2	34	5.1	0.3
Vomiting	33.4	3.5	—	32.9	2.6	0.2
Decreased appetite	23.8	1.7	0.2	31.9	3.4	—
Weight decreased	14.4	0.8	—	31.9	2.6	—
Alopecia	30.1	—	—	26.8	—	—
Dysphonia	3.3	—	—	25.4	0.5	—
Constipation	24.6	1.0	—	22.4	0.8	—
Headache	8.8	0.3	—	22.3	1.6	—
Palmar-plantar erythrodysesthesia syndrome	4.3	0.5	—	11.0	2.8	—
Other anti-VEGF–associated events						
Arterial thromboembolic event	1.5	0.5	—	2.6	0.8	1.0
Venous thromboembolic event	7.3	2.6	3.6	9.3	3.1	4.7
Fistula from GI origin	0.3	0.2	—	1.1	0.3	—
Fistula from other than GI origin	0.2	—	—	0.3	—	—
GI perforation	0.5	0.2	0.2	0.5	0.2	0.3
Biologic abnormalities						
Hematologic						
Anemia	91.1	3.5	0.8	82.3	3.3	0.5
Neutropenia	56.3	19.1	10.4	67.8	23.1	13.6
Neutropenic complications	3.0	1.7	1.2	6.5	4.4	1.3
Thrombocytopenia	33.8	0.8	0.8	47.4	1.7	1.7
Nonhematologic						
Proteinuria	40.7	1.2	—	62.2	7.5	0.3
ALT increased	37.1	2.2	—	47.3	2.5	0.2

*Grades were determined according to National Cancer Institute (USA) Common Terminology Criteria for Adverse Events, version 3.0. At: http://ctep.cancer.gov/protocolDevelopment/electronic_applications/ctc.htm [accessed October 11, 2013]

SECOND-LINE COLORECTAL CANCER REGIMENS

BEVACIZUMAB AFTER FIRST PROGRESSION
BEVACIZUMAB + FOLFIRI

Bevacizumab 5 mg/kg; administer intravenously in 100 mL 0.9% sodium chloride Injection (0.9% NS) every 2 weeks (total dosage/cycle = 15 mg/kg)

Note: Administration duration for the initial dose is 90 minutes. If administration is well tolerated, the administration duration may be decreased stepwise during subsequent administrations to 60 minutes and, finally, to a minimum duration of 30 minutes

FOLFIRI (Tournigand C et al. J Clin Oncol 2004;22:229–237):

Irinotecan 180 mg/m^2; administer intravenously over 90 minutes in 500 mL 5% dextrose injection (D5W) on day 1, every 2 weeks (total dosage/cycle = 180 mg/m^2), *plus:*
Either: (**racemic**) **leucovorin calcium** 400 mg/m^2 *or* **levoleucovorin calcium** 200 mg/m^2; administer intravenously over 2 hours in 25–500 mL 0.9% NS or D5W on day 1, every 2 weeks (total dosage/cycle for racemic leucovorin = 400 mg/m^2, for levoleucovorin = 200 mg/m^2), *followed by:*
Fluorouracil 400 mg/m^2; administer by intravenous injection over 1–2 minutes after leucovorin on day 1, every 2 weeks, *followed by:*
Fluorouracil 2400 mg/m^2; administer by continuous intravenous infusion over 46 hours in 100–1000 mL 0.9% NS or D5W, starting on day 1, every 2 weeks (total dosage/cycle = 2800 mg/m^2)

Supportive Care
Antiemetic prophylaxis
Emetogenic potential on day 1 is **MODERATE**
Emetogenic potential on day 2 is **LOW**
See Chapter 39 for antiemetic recommendations

Hematopoietic growth factor (CSF) prophylaxis
Primary prophylaxis is NOT indicated
See Chapter 43 for more information

Antimicrobial prophylaxis
Risk of fever and neutropenia is LOW
  Antimicrobial primary prophylaxis to be considered:
  • Antibacterial—not indicated
  • Antifungal—not indicated
  • Antiviral—not indicated unless patient previously had an episode of HSV
See Chapter 47 for more information

Acute cholinergic syndrome
Atropine sulfate 0.25–1 mg subcutaneously or intravenously if abdominal cramping or diarrhea develop during or within 1 hour after irinotecan administration
• If symptoms are severe, add as primary prophylaxis at least 30 minutes before irinotecan during subsequent cycles
• For irinotecan, acute cholinergic syndrome may be characterized by: abdominal cramping, diarrhea, diaphoresis, hypotension, flushing, bradycardia, rhinitis, increased salivation, meiosis, and lacrimation

Diarrhea management
Latent or delayed onset diarrhea*:
  Loperamide 4 mg orally initially after the first loose or liquid stool, *then*
  Loperamide 2 mg orally every 2 hours during waking hours, *plus*
  Loperamide 4 mg orally every 4 hours during hours of sleep
  • Continue for at least 12 hours after diarrhea resolves
  • Recurrent diarrhea after a 12-hour diarrhea-free interval is treated as a new episode
  • Rehydrate orally with fluids and electrolytes during a diarrheal episode
  • If diarrhea persists >48 hours despite loperamide, stop loperamide and hospitalize the patient for IV hydration
Persistent diarrhea:
  Octreotide 100–150 mcg subcutaneously 3 times daily. Maximum total daily dose is 1500 mcg
Antibiotic therapy during latent or delayed onset diarrhea:
  A fluoroquinolone (eg, **Ciprofloxacin** 500 mg orally every 12 hours) if absolute neutrophil count <500/mm^3 with or without accompanying fever in association with diarrhea
  • Antibiotics should also be administered if patient is hospitalized with prolonged diarrhea and should be continued until diarrhea resolves

*Abigerges D et al. J Natl Cancer Inst 1994;86:446–449
Rothenberg ML et al. J Clin Oncol 2001;19:3801–3807
Wadler S et al. J Clin Oncol 1998;16:3169–3178

(continued)

(continued)

BEVACIZUMAB + FOLFOX-4

Bevacizumab 5 mg/kg; administer intravenously in 100 mL 0.9% sodium chloride Injection (0.9% NS) every 2 weeks (total dosage/cycle = 15 mg/kg)

Note: Administration duration for the initial dose is 90 minutes. If administration is well tolerated, the administration duration may be decreased stepwise during subsequent administrations to 60 minutes and, finally, to a minimum duration of 30 minutes

FOLFOX-4 *(de Gramont A et al. J Clin Oncol 2000;18:2938–2947):*
Oxaliplatin 85 mg/m^2; administer intravenously in 250 mL 5% dextrose injection (D5W) over 2 hours concurrently with leucovorin administration, on day 1, every 2 weeks, (total dosage/cycle = 85 mg/m^2)

Note: Oxaliplatin must not be mixed with sodium chloride injection. Therefore, when leucovorin and oxaliplatin are given concurrently via a Y-connector, both drugs must be administered in D5W

Leucovorin calcium 200 mg/m^2 per dose; administer intravenously in 25–500 mL D5W over 2 hours on 2 consecutive days, on days 1 and 2, every 2 weeks (total dosage/cycle = 400 mg/m^2), *followed by:*
Fluorouracil 400 mg/m^2 per dose; administer by intravenous injection over 1–2 minutes after leucovorin on 2 consecutive days, on days 1 and 2, every 2 weeks, *followed by:*
Fluorouracil 600 mg/m^2 per dose; administer by continuous intravenous infusion in 100–1000 mL 0.9% NS or D5W over 22 hours on 2 consecutive days, on days 1 and 2, every 2 weeks (total dosage/cycle = 2000 mg/m^2)

Note: **Fluorouracil** boluses (400 mg/m^2 by intravenous injection) may be omitted for better hematologic tolerance

Supportive Care
Antiemetic prophylaxis
Emetogenic potential on days with cetuximab is **MINIMAL**
Emetogenic potential on days with oxaliplatin is **MODERATE**
Emetogenic potential on days with fluorouracil and leucovorin is **LOW**
See Chapter 39 for antiemetic recommendations

Hematopoietic growth factor (CSF) prophylaxis
Primary prophylaxis may be indicated
See Chapter 43 for more information

Antimicrobial prophylaxis
Risk of fever and neutropenia is LOW
   Antimicrobial primary prophylaxis to be considered:
   • Antibacterial—not indicated

   • Antifungal—not indicated

   • Antiviral—not indicated unless patient previously had an episode of HSV
See Chapter 47 for more information

Diarrhea management
Latent or delayed onset diarrhea*:
   Loperamide 4 mg orally initially after the first loose or liquid stool, *then*
   Loperamide 2 mg orally every 2 hours during waking hours, *plus*
   Loperamide 4 mg orally every 4 hours during hours of sleep
   • Continue for at least 12 hours after diarrhea resolves

   • Recurrent diarrhea after a 12-hour diarrhea-free interval is treated as a new episode

   • Rehydrate orally with fluids and electrolytes during a diarrheal episode

   • If a patient develops blood or mucus in stool, dehydration, or hemodynamic instability, or if diarrhea persists >48 hours despite loperamide, stop loperamide and hospitalize the patient for IV hydration
   Alternatively, a trial of **Diphenoxylate hydrochloride** 2.5 mg **with Atropine sulfate** 0.025 mg (eg, Lomotil)
   • Initial adult dose is 2 tablets 4 times daily until control has been achieved, after which the dose may be reduced to meet individual requirements. Control may often be maintained with as little as 2 tablets daily

   • Clinical improvement of acute diarrhea is usually observed within 48 hours. If improvement of chronic diarrhea after treatment with a maximum daily dose of 8 tablets is not observed within 10 days, control is unlikely with further administration

(continued)

(continued)

Persistent diarrhea:
   Octreotide 100–150 mcg subcutaneously 3 times daily. Maximum total daily dose is 1500 mcg
Antibiotic therapy during latent or delayed onset diarrhea:
   A fluoroquinolone (eg, **Ciprofloxacin** 500 mg orally every 12 hours) if absolute neutrophil count <500/mm³ with or without accompanying fever in association with diarrhea
   • Antibiotics should also be administered if patient is hospitalized with prolonged diarrhea and should be continued until diarrhea resolves

*Abigerges D et al. J Natl Cancer Inst 1994;86:446–449
Rothenberg ML et al. J Clin Oncol 2001;19:3801–3807
Wadler S et al. J Clin Oncol 1998;16:3169–3178

Oral care
Prophylaxis and treatment for mucositis/stomatitis
   General advice:
   • Encourage patients to maintain intake of non-alcoholic fluids
   • Evaluate patients for oral pain and provide analgesic medications
   • Consider histamine (H₂-subtype) receptor antagonists (eg, ranitidine, famotidine), or a proton pump inhibitor for epigastric pain
   • *Lactobacillus* sp.-containing probiotics may be beneficial in preventing diarrhea
   Patients with intact oral mucosa:
   • Clean the mouth, tongue, and gums by brushing after every meal and at bedtime with an ultra-soft toothbrush with fluoride toothpaste
   • Floss teeth gently every day unless contraindicated. If gums bleed and hurt, avoid bleeding or sore areas, but floss other teeth
   • Patients may use saline or commercial bland, non-alcoholic rinses
      ▪ Do not use mouthwashes that contain alcohols
   If mucositis or stomatitis is present:
   • Keep the mouth moist utilizing water, ice chips, sugarless gum, sugar-free hard candies, or a saliva substitute
   • Rinse mouth several times a day to remove debris
      ▪ Use a solution of ¼ teaspoon (1.25 g) each of baking soda and table salt (sodium chloride) in one quart (~950 mL) of warm water. Follow with a plain water rinse
      ▪ Do not use mouthwashes that contain alcohols
   • Foam-tipped swabs (eg, Toothettes®) are useful in moisturizing oral mucosa, but ineffective for cleansing teeth and removing plaque
   • Advise patients who develop mucositis to:
      ▪ Choose foods that are easy to chew and swallow
      ▪ Take small bites of food, chew slowly, and sip liquids with meals
      ▪ Encourage soft, moist foods such as cooked cereals, mashed potatoes, and scrambled eggs
      ▪ For trouble swallowing, soften food with gravies, sauces, broths, yogurt, or other bland liquids
      ▪ Avoid sharp, crunchy foods; hot, spicy or highly acidic foods (eg, citrus fruits and juices); sugary foods; toothpicks; tobacco products; alcoholic drinks

Treatment Modifications

Fluorouracil and Oxaliplatin

Any G2/3/4 nonhematologic toxicity	Delay start of next cycle until the severity of all toxicities are G ≤1
ANC ≤1500/mm³ or platelet count ≤100,000/mm³	Delay start of next cycle until ANC >1500/mm³ and platelet count >100,000/mm³
G3/4 Nonneurologic	Reduce fluorouracil and oxaliplatin dosages by 20%
G3/4 ANC	Reduce oxaliplatin dosage by 20%
Persistent (≥14 days) paresthesias	Reduce oxaliplatin dosage by 20%
Temporary (7–14 days) painful paresthesias	
Temporary (7–14 days) functional impairment	
Persistent (≥14 days) painful paresthesias	Discontinue oxaliplatin
Persistent (≥14 days) functional impairment	

Adapted in part from de Gramont A et al. J Clin Oncol 2000;18:2938–2947

(continued)

Treatment Modifications (*continued*)

Irinotecan and Fluorouracil

	Dosage Levels		
	Initial	−1	−2
Irinotecan	180 mg/m²	150 mg/m²	120 mg/m²
Leucovorin	Racemic leucovorin calcium 400 mg/m² or levoleucovorin calcium 200 mg/m²		
Fluorouracil injection	400 mg/m²	320 mg/m²	240 mg/m²
Infusional fluorouracil	2400 mg/m²	2000 mg/m²	1600 mg/m²

Notes:

• Dose modifications are based on the National Cancer Institute (USA) Common Toxicity Criteria. At: http://ctep.cancer.gov/ protocolDevelopment/electronic_applications/ ctc.htm [accessed October 11, 2013]

• Before beginning a treatment cycle, patients should have baseline bowel (similar to that before start of treatment) function without antidiarrheal therapy for 24 hours, ANC ≥1500/mm³, and platelet count ≥100,000/mm³

• Treatment should be delayed 1–2 weeks to allow for recovery from treatment-related toxicities

• If a patient has not recovered after 2 weeks, consider stopping therapy. If toxicity occurs despite 2 dose reductions (ie, on level −2), discontinue therapy

Toxicity	Modifications for Irinotecan and Fluorouracil
Neutropenia/Thrombocytopenia	
G1 ANC (1500–1999/mm³) or G1 thrombocytopenia (75,000/mm³ to less than normal limits)	Maintain dose and schedule
G2 ANC (1000–1499/mm³) or G2 thrombocytopenia (≥50,000 to <75,000/mm³)	Reduce dosage by 1 dosage level
G3 ANC (500–999/mm³) or G3 thrombocytopenia (≥10,000 to <50,000/mm³)	Hold treatment until toxicity resolves to G≤2, then reduce dosage by 1 dosage level
G4 ANC (<500/mm³) or G4 thrombocytopenia (<10,000/mm³)	Hold treatment until toxicity resolves to G≤2, then reduce dosage by 2 dosage levels
Febrile neutropenia	Hold treatment until neutropenia resolves, then reduce dosage by 2 dosage levels
Diarrhea	
G1 (2–3 stools/day > baseline)	Maintain dose and schedule
G2 (4–6 stools/day > baseline)	Delay until diarrhea resolves to baseline then reduce dosage by 1 dosage level
G3 (7–9 stools/day > baseline)	Delay until diarrhea resolves to baseline then reduce dosage by 1 dosage level
G4 (≥10 stools/day > baseline)	Delay until diarrhea resolves to baseline then reduce dosage by 2 dosage levels
Other Nonhematologic Toxicities	
Any G1 toxicity	Maintain dose and schedule
Any G2 toxicity	Hold treatment until toxicity resolves to G ≤1, then reduce dosage by 1 dosage level
Any G3 toxicity	Hold treatment until toxicity resolves to G ≤1, then reduce dosage by 1 dosage level
Any G4 toxicity	Hold treatment until toxicity resolves to G ≤1, then reduce dosage by 2 dosage levels
G2–4 mucositis	Decrease only fluorouracil by 20%

André T et al. Eur J Cancer 1999;35:1343–1347

Camptosar, irinotecan hydrochloride injection product label, July 2005. Pharmacia & Upjohn Company, Division of Pfizer, Inc., New York, NY

Douillard JY et al. Lancet 2000;355:1041–1047

Tournigand C et al. J Clin Oncol 2004;22:229–237

Efficacy

Tumor Response by RECIST*

	Bevacizumab + Chemotherapy (n = 404)	Chemotherapy Alone (n = 406)
Complete response	1 (<1%)	2 (<1%)
Partial response	21 (5%)	14 (3%)
Stable disease	253 (63%)	204 (50%)
Progressive disease	87 (22%)	142 (35%)
Missing/not assessable	42 (10%)	44 (11%)

Data are number (%)
*Includes only those patients with one or more measurable lesion at baseline. (RECIST, Response Evaluation Criteria in Solid Tumors. Therasse P et al. J Natl Cancer Inst 2000;92:205–216)

Response Durations

	Bevacizumab + Chemotherapy (n = 404)	Chemotherapy Alone (n = 406)
Median follow-up (months)	11.1 (6.4–15.6)	9.6 (IQR 5.4–13.9)
Median overall survival (months)	11.2 (95%CI 10.4–12.2)	9.8 (95%CI 8.9–10.7)
	HR 0.81 (95% CI 0.69–0.94); P = 0.0062	
Median progression-free survival (months)	5.7 (5.2–6.2)	4.1 (95% CI 3.7–4.4)
	HR 0.68 (95% CI 0.59–0.78); P <0.0001	
Median overall survival from start of first-line treatment* (months)	23.9 (95% CI 22.2–25.7)	22.5 (21.4–24.5)
	HR 0.90 (95% CI 0.77–1.05); P = 0.17	
Median overall treatment exposure (months)	4.2 (IQR 2.0–7.2)	3.2 months (1.7–5.2)
Treatment duration with bevacizumab (months)	3.9 (1.8–6.9)	N/A

Exploratory Subgroup Analysis According to *KRAS* Status (n = 616)

Progression-free survival KRAS wild type	HR 0.61, 95% CI 0.49–0.77; P <0.0001[†]
Progression-free survival KRAS mutant	HR 0.70, 95% CI 0.56–0.89; P = 0.003[†]
Overall survival KRAS wild type	HR 0.69, 95% CI 0.53–0.90; P = 0.005[†‡]
Overall survival KRAS mutant	HR 0.92, 95% CI 0.71–1.18; P = 0.50[‡]

*Retrospectively documented
[†]Better outcome with bevacizumab
[‡]Treatment by *KRAS* status interaction test was negative for both progression-free survival (*P* = 0.4436) and overall survival (*P* = 0.1266), indicating there is no evidence treatment effect is dependent on *KRAS* mutational status.

Toxicity

Incidence of Grades 3–5 Adverse Events Occurring in ≥2% of Patients Given Chemotherapy with or without Bevacizumab After Disease Progression Following First-Line Bevacizumab-Based Treatment (Safety Population*)

	Bevacizumab + Chemotherapy (n = 401)	Chemotherapy Alone (n = 409)
Neutropenia	65 (16%)	52 (13%)
Leucopenia	16 (4%)	12 (3%)
Asthenia	23 (6%)	17 (4%)
Fatigue	14 (3%)	10 (2%)
Diarrhea	40 (10%)	34 (8%)
Vomiting	14 (3%)	13 (3%)
Nausea	13 (3%)	11 (3%)
Decreased appetite	5 (1%)	9 (2%)
Mucosal inflammation	13 (3%)	4 (1%)
Abdominal pain	15 (4%)	12 (3%)
Polyneuropathy	12 (3%)	6 (1%)
Peripheral neuropathy	5 (1%)	10 (2%)
Hypokalemia	9 (2%)	8 (2%)
Dyspnea	6 (1%)	12 (3%)
Pulmonary embolism	10 (2%)	8 (2%)
Hypertension	7 (2%)	5 (1%)
Bleeding or hemorrhage	8 (2%)	1 (<1%)
Venous thromboembolic events	19 (5%)	12 (3%)
Gastrointestinal perforation	7 (2%)	3 (<1%)
Subileus	8 (2%)	2 (<1%)
Patients who discontinued any treatment because of adverse events	63 (16%)[†]	36 (9%)

*The safety population = 810 patients given ≥1 dose of study drug, including 407 patients in the chemotherapy group and 403 in the chemotherapy plus bevacizumab group. Two patients assigned to chemotherapy plus bevacizumab were not given bevacizumab and for the safety analyses, were assigned to the chemotherapy group
[†]A total of 53 (13%) patients discontinued chemotherapy only or both bevacizumab and chemotherapy and 10 (2%) discontinued bevacizumab

Patient Population Studied

Prospective, randomized, open-label, phase III study that enrolled patients if they had: (a) histologically confirmed, measurable metastatic colorectal cancer; (b) Eastern Cooperative Oncology Group (ECOG) Performance Status 0–2; (c) tumor disease according to RECIST criteria evaluated by investigator up to 4 weeks prior to start of study treatment; (d) previous treatment with bevacizumab plus standard first-line chemotherapy including a fluoropyrimidine plus either oxaliplatin or irinotecan; and (e) they were not candidates for primary metastasectomy. Patients were excluded if they: (a) had a diagnosis of progressive disease for more than 3 months after the last bevacizumab administration; (b) had first-line progression-free survival of less than 3 months; and (c) were given less than 3 months (consecutive) of first-line bevacizumab

LATE-STAGE METASTATIC COLORECTAL CANCER REGIMEN

REGORAFENIB

Grothey A et al. Lancet 2013;381:303–312

Regorafenib 160 mg/day; administer orally for 21 consecutive days, days 1–21, every 28 days (total dose/28-day cycle = 3360 mg)

Notes:
Regorafenib tablets must be stored in the manufacturer's original container at room temperature between 20° and 25°C (68° and 77°F)
- Regorafenib must not be repackaged in other vials or pill boxes
- Regorafenib containers should be tightly closed after doses are removed
- The bottle in which regorafenib is packaged contains a desiccant, which should remain in the container

Regorafenib containers should be labeled to identify the date on which they were first opened
- Any unused regorafenib tablets are to be discarded 28 days after the container was initially opened

Regorafenib should be taken about the same time each day
- If a dose is missed, it should be taken on the same day it was to have been taken; that is, patients should not take more than 1 dose on a single day to make up for 1 or more doses missed on previous days

Tablets should be swallowed whole (no breaking, crushing, or chewing)

Regorafenib is taken with a low-fat breakfast that contains less than 30% fat. Two examples of low-fat breakfasts are:

1. Two slices of white toast with 1 tablespoon of low-fat margarine and 1 tablespoon of jelly, and 8 ounces of skim milk (319 calories and 8.2 g fat); *or*
2. One cup of cereal, 8 ounces of skim milk, 1 slice of toast with jam, apple juice, and 1 cup of coffee or tea (520 calories and 2 g fat)

Supportive Care
Antiemetic prophylaxis
Emetogenic potential on is **MINIMAL–LOW**
See Chapter 39 for antiemetic recommendations

Hematopoietic growth factor (CSF) prophylaxis
Primary prophylaxis is NOT indicated
See Chapter 43 for more information

Antimicrobial prophylaxis
Risk of fever and neutropenia is LOW
Antimicrobial primary prophylaxis to be considered:
- Antibacterial—not indicated
- Antifungal—not indicated
- Antiviral—not indicated, unless patient previously had an episode of HSV

See Chapter 47 for more information

Hand-foot reaction (palmar-plantar erythrodysesthesia, PPE)
For patients who develop a hand-foot reaction, use topical emollients (eg, Aquaphor®), topical or orally administered steroids, antihistamine agents (H_1-receptor antagonists), or pyridoxine
  Pyridoxine may provide relief for discomfort/pain associated with PPE although the mechanism through which this occurs remains unclear
- The suggested pyridoxine starting dose is 50 mg/day, which may be increased to a maximum of 200 mg/day

(continued)

Dose Modifications
Starting Dose = 160 mg Regorafenib

Adverse Event	Dose Modification
First occurrence of G2 hand-foot skin reaction (HFSR) (palmar-plantar erythrodysesthesia [PPE]) of any duration at a regorafenib dose of 160 mg	Reduce regorafenib at a daily dose of 120 mg
G3 HFSR (PPE) at a regorafenib dose of 160 mg	Discontinue therapy for a minimum of 7 days until toxicity resolves to G ≤1 and resume regorafenib at a daily dose of 120 mg
G3/4* adverse reaction at a regorafenib dose of 160 mg (except hepatotoxicity)	Discontinue regorafenib until toxicity resolves to G ≤1 and resume regorafenib at a daily dose of 120 mg
G3 aspartate aminotransferase (AST)/alanine aminotransferase (ALT) elevation at a regorafenib dose of 160 mg	Resume only if the potential benefit outweighs the risk of hepatotoxicity. Resume at a regorafenib at a daily dose of 120 mg
Recurrence of G2 HFSR at the 120 mg dose	Discontinue therapy for a minimum of 7 days until toxicity resolves to G ≤1 and resume regorafenib at a daily dose of 80 mg
G3/4* adverse reaction at the 120 mg dose (except hepatotoxicity)	Discontinue regorafenib until toxicity resolves to G ≤1 and resume regorafenib at a daily dose to 80 mg
G3 HFSR (PPE) at a regorafenib dose of 120 mg	Discontinue therapy for a minimum of 7 days until toxicity resolves to G ≤1 and resume regorafenib at a daily dose of 80 mg
G2 HFSR (PPE) does not improve within 7 days despite dose reduction to 120 mg	

(continued)

(*continued*)

Diarrhea management

Latent or delayed onset diarrhea*:

Loperamide 4 mg; administer orally initially after the first loose or liquid stool, *then*

Loperamide 2 mg; administer orally every 2 hours during waking hours, *plus*

Loperamide 4 mg; administer orally every 4 hours during hours of sleep

- Continue for at least 12 hours after diarrhea resolves
- Recurrent diarrhea after a 12-hour diarrhea free interval is treated as a new episode
- Rehydrate orally with fluids and electrolytes during a diarrheal episode
- If a patient develops blood or mucus in stool, dehydration, or hemodynamic instability, or if diarrhea persists >48 hours despite loperamide, stop loperamide and hospitalize the patient for IV hydration

Alternatively, a trial of **Diphenoxylate hydrochloride** 2.5 mg with **Atropine sulfate** 0.025 mg (eg, Lomotil®)

- Initial adult dose is two tablets four times daily until control has been achieved, after which the dose may be reduced to meet individual requirements. Control may often be maintained with as little as two tablets daily
- Clinical improvement of acute diarrhea is usually observed within 48 hours. If improvement of chronic diarrhea after treatment with a maximum daily dose of 8 tablets is not observed within 10 days, control is unlikely with further administration

Persistent diarrhea:

Octreotide acetate (solution) 100–150 mcg; administer subcutaneously 3 times daily. Maximum total daily dose is 1500 mcg

Antibiotic therapy during latent or delayed onset diarrhea:

A fluoroquinolone (eg, **Ciprofloxacin** 500 mg orally every 12 hours) if absolute neutrophil count <500/mm³ with or without accompanying fever in association with diarrhea

- Antibiotics should also be administered if patient is hospitalized with prolonged diarrhea and should be continued until diarrhea resolves

*Abigerges D et al. J Natl Cancer Inst 1994;86:446–449
Rothenberg ML et al. J Clin Oncol 2001;19:3801–3807
Wadler S et al. J Clin Oncol 1998;16:3169–3178

Oral care

Prophylaxis and treatment for mucositis/stomatitis

General advice:

- Encourage patients to maintain intake of non-alcoholic fluids
- Evaluate patients for oral pain and provide analgesic medications
- Consider histamine (H$_2$-subtype) receptor antagonists (eg, ranitidine, famotidine), or a proton pump inhibitor for epigastric pain
- *Lactobacillus* sp.-containing probiotics may be beneficial in preventing diarrhea

Patients with intact oral mucosa:

- Clean the mouth, tongue, and gums by brushing after every meal and at bedtime with an ultra-soft toothbrush with fluoride toothpaste
- Floss teeth gently every day unless contraindicated. If gums bleed and hurt, avoid bleeding or sore areas, but floss other teeth
- Patients may use saline or commercial bland, non-alcoholic rinses
  - Do not use mouthwashes that contain alcohols

If mucositis or stomatitis is present:

- Keep the mouth moist utilizing water, ice chips, sugarless gum, sugar-free hard candies, or a saliva substitute
- Rinse mouth several times a day to remove debris
  - Use a solution of ¼ teaspoon (1.25 g) each of baking soda and table salt (sodium chloride) in one quart (~950 mL) of warm water. Follow with a plain water rinse
  - Do not use mouthwashes that contain alcohols
- Foam-tipped swabs (eg, Toothettes®) are useful in moisturizing oral mucosa, but ineffective for cleansing teeth and removing plaque
- Advise patients who develop mucositis to:
  - Choose foods that are easy to chew and swallow
  - Take small bites of food, chew slowly, and sip liquids with meals
  - Encourage soft, moist foods such as cooked cereals, mashed potatoes, and scrambled eggs
  - For trouble swallowing, soften food with gravies, sauces, broths, yogurt, or other bland liquids
  - Avoid sharp, crunchy foods; hot, spicy or highly acidic foods (eg, citrus fruits and juices); sugary foods; toothpicks; tobacco products; alcoholic drinks

Dose Modifications (*continued*)

Adverse Event	Dose Modification
Symptomatic G2 hypertension	Discontinue therapy a minimum of 7 days until symptoms resolve to G ≤1 and resume regorafenib at a daily dose of 80 mg
Failure to tolerate 80 mg daily	Permanently discontinue regorafenib
Any occurrence of AST or ALT >20 times the upper limit of normal (ULN)	
Any occurrence of AST or ALT >3 times ULN with concurrent bilirubin >2 times ULN	
Recurrence of AST or ALT >5 times ULN despite dose reduction to 120 mg	

*For any G4 adverse reaction, only resume if the potential benefit outweighs the risks

Adverse Events

- Dose modifications were required in 378 (76%) of 500 patients assigned to receive regorafenib
- 100 patients (20%) required ≥1 dose reduction
- 352 (70%) required ≥1 dose interruption)
- Adverse events were the most common reason for dose modification

Treatment-Related Adverse Events Occurring in ≥5% of Patients in Either Group from Start of Treatment to 30 Days After End of Treatment (Safety Population)

	Regorafenib (n = 500)			Placebo (n = 253)		
	Any Grade	Grade 3	Grade 4	Any Grade	Grade 3	Grade 4
Any event	465 (93%)	253 (51%)	17 (3%)	154 (61%)	31 (12%)	4 (2%)
Clinical Adverse Event						
Fatigue	237 (47%)	46 (9%)	2 (<1%)	71 (28%)	12 (5%)	1 (<1%)
Hand-foot skin reaction	233 (47%)	83 (17%)	0	19 (8%)	1 (<1%)	0
Diarrhea	169 (34%)	35 (7%)	1 (<1%)	21 (8%)	2 (1%)	0
Anorexia	152 (30%)	16 (3%)	0	39 (15%)	7 (3%)	0
Voice changes	147 (29%)	1 (<1%)	0	14 (6%)	0	0
Hypertension	139 (28%)	36 (7%)	0	15 (6%)	2 (1%)	0
Oral mucositis	136 (27%)	15 (3%)	0	9 (4%)	0	0
Rash or desquamation	130 (26%)	29 (6%)	0	10 (4%)	0	0
Nausea	72 (14%)	2 (<1%)	0	28 (11%)	0	0
Weight loss	69 (14%)	0	0	6 (2%)	0	0
Fever	52 (10%)	4 (1%)	0	7 (3%)	0	0
Constipation	42 (8%)	0	0	12 (5%)	0	0
Dry skin	39 (8%)	0	0	7 (3%)	0	0
Alopecia	36 (7%)	0	0	1 (<1%)	0	0
Taste Alteration	35 (7%)	0	0	5 (2%)	0	0
Vomiting	38 (8%)	3 (1%)	0	13 (5%)	0	0
Sensory neuropathy	34 (7%)	2 (<1%)	0	9 (4%)	0	0
Nose bleed	36 (7%)	0	0	5 (2%)	0	0
Dyspnea	28 (6%)	1 (<1%)	0	4 (2%)	0	0
Muscle pain	28 (6%)	2 (<1%)	0	7 (3%)	0	0
Headache	26 (5%)	3 (1%)	0	8 (3%)	0	0
Pain abdomen	25 (5%)	1 (<1%)	0	10 (4%)	0	0

(*continued*)

Adverse Events (continued)

	Regorafenib (N = 500)			Placebo (N = 253)		
	Any Grade	Grade 3	Grade 4	Any Grade	Grade 3	Grade 4
Laboratory Abnormalities						
Thrombocytopenia	63 (13%)	13 (3%)	1 (<1%)	5 (2%)	1 (<1%)	0
Hyperbilirubinemia	45 (9%)	10 (2%)	0	4 (2%)	2 (1%)	0
Proteinuria	35 (7%)	7 (1%)	0	4 (2%)	1 (<1%)	0
Anemia	33 (7%)	12 (2%)	2 (<1%)	6 (2%)	0	0
Hypophosphatemia	25 (5%)	19 (4%)	0	1 (<1%)	1 (<1%)	0

Patient Population Studied

Randomized, placebo-controlled, phase III study involving 114 centers in 16 countries. Patients had to have (a) histologic or cytologic documentation of adenocarcinoma of the colon or rectum; (b) have received locally and currently approved standard therapies; and (c) have disease progression during or within 3 months after the last administration of the last standard therapy or to have stopped standard therapy because of unacceptable toxic effects. Because available standard therapies varied it had to include as many of the following as were licensed: a fluoropyrimidine, oxaliplatin, irinotecan, and bevacizumab; and cetuximab or panitumumab for patients who had *KRAS* wild-type tumors. Eastern Cooperative Oncology Group (ECOG) Performance Status of 0 or 1; life expectancy of at least 3 months

	Regorafenib	Placebo
Median OS (months)*	6.4 (IQR 3.6–11.8)	5.0 (IQR 2.8–10.4)
	HR 0.77, 95% CI 0.64–0.94; P = 0.0052	
OS rate at 3 months	80.3%	72.7%
OS rate at 6 months	52.5%	43.5%
OS rate at 9 months	38.2%	30.8%,
OS rate at 12 months	24.3%	24.0%
Median PFS (months)†	1.9 (IQR 1.6–3.9)	1.7 (IQR 1.4–1.9)
	HR 0.49, 95% CI 0.42–0.58; P<0.0001	
ORR	1.0%	0.4%
CR	0	0
PR	1.0%	0.4%
	P = 0.19	
Disease control‡	207 (41%)	38 (15%)
	(P<0.0001)	
Median duration of SD (months)‡	2.0 (IQR 1.7–4.0)	1.7 (IQR 1.4–1.9)

*Regorafenib showed an apparent benefit in 24 of 25 subgroups, the exception being the group of patients with primary disease in colon and rectum, which was based on only a few events. Compared with placebo, regorafenib had a greater effect on overall survival in the subgroup of patients with colon cancer (HR 0.70, 95% CI 0.56–0.89) than in those with rectal cancer (0.95, 0.63–1.43)

†For PFS, all subgroup analyses significantly favored regorafenib compared with placebo, except for patients from eastern Europe, for whom the difference was not significant. Regorafenib had much the same effect on PFS in patients with colon cancer (HR 0.55, 95% CI 0.45–0.67) and those with rectal cancer (0.45, 95% CI 0.33–0.62)

‡Disease control = PR + SD assessed at least 6 weeks after randomization

RECTAL CANCER REGIMEN
ADJUVANT OR NEOADJUVANT CHEMOTHERAPY + RADIATION

O'Connell MJ et al. N Engl J Med 1994;331:502–507

Chemotherapy Before or After Radiation

Fluorouracil + calcium leucovorin (Roswell Park, Mayo Clinic, or infusional fluorouracil) or FOLFOX
Note: Systemic chemotherapy is usually administered 4 weeks before or after surgery or chemoradiotherapy

Radiation + Chemotherapy

Fluorouracil 225 mg/m^2 per day; administer by continuous intravenous infusion over 24 hours in 50–1000 mL 0.9% sodium chloride injection or 5% dextrose injection, daily throughout radiation therapy (total dosage/week = 1575 mg/m^2)
Radiation therapy 180 cGy per fraction for 25 fractions (total dose = 4500 cGy), directed at the initial pelvic field, followed by a minimum boost of 540 cGy, to the entire tumor bed, the immediately adjacent lymph nodes, and 2 cm of adjacent tissues (the perineum was excluded after it had received 4500 cGy in patients with abdominoperineal resection). A second boost of 360 cGy was allowed to a smaller field in patients with good-to-excellent displacement of the small bowel out of the field

Supportive Care
Antiemetic prophylaxis
Emetogenic potential is **LOW**
See Chapter 39 for antiemetic recommendations

Hematopoietic growth factor (CSF) prophylaxis
Primary prophylaxis is NOT indicated
See Chapter 43 for more information

Antimicrobial prophylaxis
Risk of fever and neutropenia is LOW
   Antimicrobial primary prophylaxis to be considered:
- Antibacterial—not indicated
- Antifungal—not indicated
- Antiviral—not indicated unless patient previously had an episode of HSV

See Chapter 47 for more information

Oral care
Prophylaxis and treatment for mucositis/stomatitis
   General advice:
- Encourage patients to maintain intake of non-alcoholic fluids
- Evaluate patients for oral pain and provide analgesic medications
- Consider histamine (H$_2$-subtype) receptor antagonists (eg, ranitidine, famotidine), or a proton pump inhibitor for epigastric pain
- *Lactobacillus* sp.-containing probiotics may be beneficial in preventing diarrhea

   Patients with intact oral mucosa:
- Clean the mouth, tongue, and gums by brushing after every meal and at bedtime with an ultra-soft toothbrush with fluoride toothpaste
- Floss teeth gently every day unless contraindicated. If gums bleed and hurt, avoid bleeding or sore areas, but floss other teeth
- Patients may use saline or commercial bland, non-alcoholic rinses
  - Do not use mouthwashes that contain alcohols

   If mucositis or stomatitis is present:
- Keep the mouth moist utilizing water, ice chips, sugarless gum, sugar-free hard candies, or a saliva substitute
- Rinse mouth several times a day to remove debris
  - Use a solution of ¼ teaspoon (1.25 g) each of baking soda and table salt (sodium chloride) in one quart (~950 mL) of warm water. Follow with a plain water rinse
  - Do not use mouthwashes that contain alcohols
- Foam-tipped swabs (eg, Toothettes®) are useful in moisturizing oral mucosa, but ineffective for cleansing teeth and removing plaque
- Advise patients who develop mucositis to:
  - Choose foods that are easy to chew and swallow
  - Take small bites of food, chew slowly, and sip liquids with meals
  - Encourage soft, moist foods such as cooked cereals, mashed potatoes, and scrambled eggs
  - For trouble swallowing, soften food with gravies, sauces, broths, yogurt, or other bland liquids
  - Avoid sharp, crunchy foods; hot, spicy or highly acidic foods (eg, citrus fruits and juices); sugary foods; toothpicks; tobacco products; alcoholic drinks

(continued)

(continued)

Hand-foot reaction (palmar-plantar erythrodysesthesia, PPE)
For patients who develop a hand-foot reaction, use topical emollients (eg, Aquaphor®), topical or orally administered steroids, antihistamine agents (H_1-receptor antagonists), or pyridoxine
   Pyridoxine may provide relief for discomfort/pain associated with PPE although the mechanism through which this occurs remains unclear
• The suggested pyridoxine starting dose is 50 mg/day, which may be increased to a maximum of 200 mg/day

Patient Population Studied

A study of patients with surgically resected stage II or III rectal cancer with the inferior edge of tumor at or below the level of sacral promontory or within 12 cm of the anal verge

Efficacy (N = 328)

Bolus fluorouracil for 2 cycles ± semustine before and after RT with fluorouracil by continuous infusion during radiation

4-Year relapse-free survival	63%
4-Year overall survival	70%

O'Connell MJ et al. N Engl J Med 1994;331:502–507

Treatment Modifications

Adverse Event	Dose Modification
G ≥3 Gastrointestinal toxicity	Interrupt radiation treatments. Resume when the toxicities decrease to G ≤2
G ≥3 Hematologic toxicity	
G ≥3 Gastrointestinal toxicity	Interrupt fluorouracil infusion. Resume when the toxicities decrease to G ≤2
G ≥3 Hematologic toxicity	

Therapy Monitoring

1. *Before each cycle and weekly during RT:* H&P, CBC with differential, serum electrolytes, BUN, creatinine, and LFTs
2. *Every 2–3 months:* CT scans to assess response

LOCALLY ADVANCED RECTAL CANCER

CHEMORADIOTHERAPY WITH CAPECITABINE

Hofheinz R-D et al. Lancet Oncol 2012;13:579-588

Adjuvant Therapy
Before radiation therapy:
Capecitabine 1250 mg/m^2 per dose; administer orally twice daily (approximately every 12 hours, within 30 minutes after a meal) for 14 consecutive days, on days 1–14 (28 doses), every 21 days (weeks 1 and 4), for 2 cycles (total dosage/cycle = 35,000 mg/m^2)

Throughout radiation therapy:
Capecitabine 825 mg/m^2 per dose; administer orally twice daily (approximately every 12 hours, within 30 minutes after a meal) continually throughout and coincident with the duration of radiation therapy (weeks 8 through 12 or 13; total dosage/week = 11,550 mg/m^2), *plus:*
Radiotherapy to a total dose of 50.4 Gy delivered in conventional daily 1.8-Gy fractions on 5 days per week, over 5–6 weeks

Notes:
• Radiotherapy and capecitabine are started on the same day and capecitabine is stopped on the last day of radiotherapy
• Three-dimensional conformal techniques with high-energy photons (6–25 MeV) and belly boards were used. The clinical target volume included the entire macroscopic tumor with a minimum margin of 5 cm, the mesorectum (plus 1.0- to 1.5-cm margin lateral to the pelvic brim), and the iliac and presacral lymph nodes up to the L5–S1 junction (or L4–L5 junction in the case of extensive lymph-node involvement)

After radiation therapy:
Capecitabine 1250 mg/m^2 per dose; administer orally twice daily (approximately every 12 hours, within 30 minutes after a meal) for 14 consecutive days, on days 1–14 (28 doses) every 21 days (weeks 15, 18, and 21), for 3 cycles (total dosage/cycle = 35,000 mg/m^2)

Notes:
• Phenytoin and coumarin-derivative anticoagulant doses may need to be reduced when either drug is administered concomitantly with capecitabine. In patients receiving concomitant capecitabine and oral coumarin-derivative anticoagulant therapy, the INR or prothrombin time should be monitored frequently in order to adjust the anticoagulant dose

Supportive Care
Antiemetic prophylaxis
Emetogenic potential with capecitabine alone is **MINIMAL–LOW**
Emetogenic potential during chemoradiotherapy is at least **LOW**
See Chapter 39 for antiemetic recommendations

Hematopoietic growth factor (CSF) prophylaxis
Primary prophylaxis is NOT indicated
See Chapter 43 for more information

Antimicrobial prophylaxis
Risk of fever and neutropenia is LOW
  Antimicrobial primary prophylaxis to be considered:
  • Antibacterial—not indicated
  • Antifungal—not indicated
  • Antiviral—not indicated, unless patient previously had an episode of HSV
See Chapter 47 for more information

Hand-foot reaction (palmar-plantar erythrodysesthesia, PPE)
For patients who develop a hand-foot reaction, use topical emollients (eg, Aquaphor®), topical or orally administered steroids, antihistamine agents (H$_1$-receptor antagonists), or pyridoxine
    Pyridoxine may provide relief for discomfort/pain associated with PPE although the mechanism through which this occurs remains unclear
• The suggested pyridoxine starting dose is 50 mg/day, which may be increased to a maximum of 200 mg/day

(continued)

Treatment Modifications

Adverse Event	Dose Modification
G1 toxicity	Continue capecitabine and maintain dose level
First episode of G2 toxicity	Interrupt capecitabine treatment until adverse effects abate to G ≤1. Then, administer same dose in the next cycle
Second episode of G2 toxicity	Interrupt capecitabine treatment until adverse effects abate to G ≤1. Then, administer 75% dose in the next cycle
Third episode of G2 toxicity	Interrupt capecitabine treatment until adverse effects abate to G ≤1. Then, administer 50% dose in the next cycle
Fourth episode of G2 toxicity	Discontinue therapy
First episode of G3 toxicity	Interrupt capecitabine treatment until adverse effects abate to G ≤1. Then, administer 75% dose in the next cycle
Second episode of G3 toxicity	Interrupt capecitabine treatment until adverse effects abate to G ≤1. Then, administer 50% dose in the next cycle
Third episode of G3 toxicity	Discontinue therapy
First episode of G4 toxicity	Discontinue capecitabine treatment unless continued therapy deemed to be in the patient's best interest. In the latter case, interrupt treatment until adverse effects abate to G ≤1. Then, administer 50% dose in the next cycle

(*continued*)

Diarrhea management

Loperamide 4 mg; administer orally initially after the first loose or liquid stool, *then*

Loperamide 2 mg; administer orally every 2 hours during waking hours, *plus*

Loperamide 4 mg; administer orally every 4 hours during hours of sleep

- Continue for at least 12 hours after diarrhea resolves
- Recurrent diarrhea after a 12-hour diarrhea free interval is treated as a new episode
- Rehydrate orally with fluids and electrolytes during a diarrheal episode
- If a patient develops blood or mucus in stool, dehydration, or hemodynamic instability, or if diarrhea persists >48 hours despite loperamide, stop loperamide and hospitalize the patient for IV hydration

Alternatively, a trial of **Diphenoxylate hydrochloride** 2.5 mg **with Atropine sulfate** 0.025 mg (eg, Lomotil®)

- Initial adult dose is 2 tablets 4 times daily until control has been achieved, after which the dose may be reduced to meet individual requirements. Control may often be maintained with as little as 2 tablets daily
- Clinical improvement of acute diarrhea is usually observed within 48 hours. If improvement of chronic diarrhea after treatment with a maximum daily dose of 8 tablets is not observed within 10 days, control is unlikely with further administration

Rothenberg ML et al. J Clin Oncol 2001;19:3801–3807
Wadler S et al. J Clin Oncol 1998; 16:3169–3178

Oral care

Prophylaxis and treatment for mucositis/stomatitis

General advice:

- Encourage patients to maintain intake of nonalcoholic fluids
- Evaluate patients for oral pain and provide analgesic medications
- Consider histamine (H_2-subtype) receptor antagonists (eg, ranitidine, famotidine), or a proton pump inhibitor for epigastric pain
- *Lactobacillus* sp.-containing probiotics may be beneficial in preventing diarrhea

Patients with intact oral mucosa:

- Clean the mouth, tongue, and gums by brushing after every meal and at bedtime with an ultrasoft toothbrush with fluoride toothpaste
- Floss teeth gently every day unless contraindicated. If gums bleed and hurt, avoid bleeding or sore areas, but floss other teeth
- Patients may use saline or commercial brand, nonalcoholic rinses
  - Do not use mouthwashes that contain alcohols

If mucositis or stomatitis is present:

- Keep the mouth moist utilizing water, ice chips, sugarless gum, sugar-free hard candies, or a saliva substitute
- Rinse mouth several times a day to remove debris
  - Use a solution of ¼ teaspoon (1.25 g) each of baking soda and table salt (sodium chloride) in one quart (~950 mL) of warm water. Follow with a plain water rinse
  - Do not use mouthwashes that contain alcohols
- Foam-tipped swabs (eg, Toothettes®) are useful in moisturizing oral mucosa, but ineffective for cleansing teeth and removing plaque
- Advise patients who develop mucositis to:
  - Choose foods that are easy to chew and swallow
  - Take small bites of food, chew slowly, and sip liquids with meals
  - Encourage soft, moist foods such as cooked cereals, mashed potatoes, and scrambled eggs
  - For trouble swallowing, soften food with gravies, sauces, broths, yogurt, or other bland liquids
  - Avoid sharp, crunchy foods; hot, spicy or highly acidic foods (eg, citrus fruits and juices); sugary foods; toothpicks; tobacco products; alcoholic drinks

Patient Population Studied

A noninferiority, phase 3 trial comparing fluorouracil with capecitabine for perioperative treatment of patients with locally advanced rectal cancer. Patients had histologically confirmed adenocarcinoma of the rectum (defined as a distal tumor border <16 cm from the anal verge, measured by rigid rectoscopy), with no evidence of distant metastases (identified by abdominal ultrasound or CT scan and chest radiograph)

Adjuvant cohort: Had undergone R0 resection (ie, leaving no residual tumor) for $pT3$–4 N_{any} or pT_{any} $N_{positive}$ nonmetastatic rectal cancer. TME was mandatory for tumors in the lower two-thirds of the rectum, with PME being permitted for those in the upper third, provided a distal margin of at least 5 cm without coning was observed

Neoadjuvant cohort: Had to have a clinical $cT3$–4 N_{any} or cT_{any} $N_{positive}$ tumor staged by endoscopic ultrasound, provided the lower border of the tumor was 0–16 cm from the anal verge (measured by rigid rectoscopy) and the primary tumor was deemed R0 resectable by TME or PME on the basis of clinical assessment (pelvic CT or MRI were done at the discretion of the local investigators)

Patient Characteristics (N = 197 Treated with Capecitabine)

Age (range)	65 y (30–85 y)
Sex–male-to-female ratio	129 (65%)/68 (35%)
WHO status	
0	120 (61%)
1	60 (30%)
2	3 (2%)
Missing data	14 (7%)
Tumor category*	
T1 or T2	29 (15%)
T3	150 (76%)
T4	15 (8%)
Missing data	3 (2%)
Nodal category*	
Node negative	78 (40%)
Node positive	112 (57%)
Missing data	7 (4%)

*Clinical or pathologic category

Efficacy*

	Capecitabine (n = 197)	Fluorouracil (n = 195)	p Value
Site of recurrence			
Local	12 (6%)	14 (7%)	0.67[†]
Distant	37 (19%)	54 (28%)	0.04[†]
Deaths			
Total	38 (19%)	55 (28%)	0.04[†]
Disease-related	26 (13%)	37 (19%)	
Other causes	12 (6%)	15 (8%)	
Unknown	0	3 (2%)	

*Data are cumulative number of events (%)
[†]χ^2 test

Treatment Monitoring

1. *Before starting:* History and physical examination, CEA determination, CBC with differential and serum chemistries
2. *During treatment:* CBC with differential and serum chemistries before each treatment cycle
3. *Tumor assessments:* Abdominal computed tomography, magnetic resonance imaging, or ultrasound, at baseline, every 6 months initially, and annually thereafter. CEA levels every 3 months initially and every 6 months thereafter

Toxicity*,†

	Capecitabine (n = 197)			Fluorouracil (n = 195)			p Value[‡]
	G1/2	G3/4	Total	G1/2	G3/4	Total	
Laboratory							
Lowered hemoglobin	58	0	62	49	2	52	0.29
Lowered leucocytes	47	3	50	50	16	68	0.04
Lowered platelets	23	0	23	29	1	32	0.18
Raised creatinine	5	0	5	2	0	2	0.26
Raised bilirubin	6	1	8	1	1	2	0.06
Gastrointestinal							
Nausea	33	2	36	30	0	32	0.63
Vomiting	11	1	14	8	1	9	0.30
Diarrhoea	83	17	104	76	4	85	0.07
Mucositis	11	1	12	15	2	17	0.32
Stomatitis	8	0	8	11	0	12	0.35
Abdominal pain	19	1	23	11	0	14	0.13
Proctitis	26	1	31	9	1	10	<0.001
Other							
Fatigue	50	0	55	27	2	29	0.002
Anorexia	13	0	13	5	1	6	0.10
Alopecia	4	0	4	11	0	11	0.06
Hand-foot skin reaction	56	4	62	3	0	3	<0.001
Radiation dermatitis	22	2	29	32	1	35	0.39

*Data are number of patients or p value
[†]National Cancer Institute (USA) Common Toxicity Criteria, version 2.0. At: http://ctep.cancer.gov/protocolDevelopment/electronic_applications/ctc.htm [accessed December 7, 2013]
[‡]χ^2

ADJUVANT THERAPY
STAGE III COLON CANCER
CAPECITABINE + OXALIPLATIN (XELOX)

Haller DG et al. J Clin Oncol 2011;29:1465–1471

Oxaliplatin 130 mg/m^2; administer intravenously in 250–500 mL 5% dextrose injection over 2 hours on day 1, every 3 weeks, for 8 cycles (total dosage/cycle = 130 mg/m^2), *plus*

Capecitabine 1000 mg/m^2 per dose; administer orally twice daily (approximately every 12 hours, within 30 minutes after a meal) for 14 consecutive days, on days 1–14 (28 doses), every 3 weeks for 8 cycles (total dosage/cycle = 28,000 mg/m^2)

Notes: Capecitabine monotherapy was continued in patients who refused or discontinued oxaliplatin because of toxicity
XELOX was compared to 2 fluorouracil and leucovorin (folinic acid) (FU/FA) regimens given either for 6 cycles over 24 weeks or 4 cycles over 32 weeks (Haller DG et al. J Clin Oncol 2005;23:8671–8678)

Supportive Care
Antiemetic prophylaxis
Emetogenic potential on day 1 is **MODERATE**
Emetogenic potential on days with capecitabine alone is **MINIMAL–LOW**
See Chapter 39 for antiemetic recommendations

Hematopoietic growth factor (CSF) prophylaxis
Primary prophylaxis may be indicated
See Chapter 43 for more information

Antimicrobial prophylaxis
Risk of fever and neutropenia is LOW
  Antimicrobial primary prophylaxis to be considered:
  • Antibacterial—not indicated
  • Antifungal—not indicated
  • Antiviral—not indicated, unless patient previously had an episode of HSV
See Chapter 47 for more information

Hand-foot reaction (palmar-plantar erythrodysesthesia, PPE)
For patients who develop a hand-foot reaction, use topical emollients (eg, Aquaphor®), topical or orally administered steroids, antihistamine agents (H$_1$-receptor antagonists), or pyridoxine
  Pyridoxine may provide relief for discomfort/pain associated with PPE, although the mechanism through which this occurs remains unclear
• The suggested pyridoxine starting dose is 50 mg/day, which may be increased to a maximum of 200 mg/day

Diarrhea management
  Loperamide 4 mg; administer orally initially after the first loose or liquid stool, *then*
  Loperamide 2 mg; administer orally every 2 hours during waking hours, *plus*
  Loperamide 4 mg; administer orally every 4 hours during hours of sleep
  • Continue for at least 12 hours after diarrhea resolves
  • Recurrent diarrhea after a 12-hour diarrhea free interval is treated as a new episode
  • Rehydrate orally with fluids and electrolytes during a diarrheal episode
  • If a patient develops blood or mucus in stool, dehydration, or hemodynamic instability, or if diarrhea persists >48 hours despite loperamide, stop loperamide and hospitalize the patient for IV hydration
  Alternatively, a trial of **Diphenoxylate hydrochloride** 2.5 mg **with Atropine sulfate** 0.025 mg (eg, Lomotil®)
  • Initial adult dose is 2 tablets 4 times daily until control has been achieved, after which the dose may be reduced to meet individual requirements. Control may often be maintained with as little as 2 tablets daily
  • Clinical improvement of acute diarrhea is usually observed within 48 hours. If improvement of chronic diarrhea after treatment with a maximum daily dose of 8 tablets is not observed within 10 days, control is unlikely with further administration

Rothenberg ML et al. J Clin Oncol 2001; 19:3801–3807
Wadler S et al. J Clin Oncol 1998; 16:3169–3178

Oral care
Prophylaxis and treatment for mucositis/stomatitis
  General advice:
  • Encourage patients to maintain intake of nonalcoholic fluids
  • Evaluate patients for oral pain and provide analgesic medications
  • Consider histamine (H$_2$-subtype) receptor antagonists (eg, ranitidine, famotidine), or a proton pump inhibitor for epigastric pain
  • *Lactobacillus* sp.-containing probiotics may be beneficial in preventing diarrhea

(continued)

(*continued*)

Patients with intact oral mucosa:

• Clean the mouth, tongue, and gums by brushing after every meal and at bedtime with an ultrasoft toothbrush with fluoride toothpaste

• Floss teeth gently every day unless contraindicated. If gums bleed and hurt, avoid bleeding or sore areas, but floss other teeth

• Patients may use saline or commercial brand, nonalcoholic rinses

  ▪ Do not use mouthwashes that contain alcohols

If mucositis or stomatitis is present:

• Keep the mouth moist utilizing water, ice chips, sugarless gum, sugar-free hard candies, or a saliva substitute

• Rinse mouth several times a day to remove debris

  ▪ Use a solution of ¼ teaspoon (1.25 g) each of baking soda and table salt (sodium chloride) in one quart (~950 mL) of warm water. Follow with a plain water rinse

  ▪ Do not use mouthwashes that contain alcohols

• Foam-tipped swabs (eg, Toothettes®) are useful in moisturizing oral mucosa, but ineffective for cleansing teeth and removing plaque

• Advise patients who develop mucositis to:

  ▪ Choose foods that are easy to chew and swallow

  ▪ Take small bites of food, chew slowly, and sip liquids with meals

  ▪ Encourage soft, moist foods such as cooked cereals, mashed potatoes, and scrambled eggs

  ▪ For trouble swallowing, soften food with gravies, sauces, broths, yogurt, or other bland liquids

  ▪ Avoid sharp, crunchy foods; hot, spicy or highly acidic foods (eg, citrus fruits and juices); sugary foods; toothpicks; tobacco products; alcoholic drinks

Treatment Modifications

Adverse Event	Dose Modification
ANC nadir <1000/mm³ *or* platelet nadir <50,000/mm³ after treatment	Delay treatment until ANC is ≥1000/mm³ *and* platelet count is ≥50,000/mm³, then decrease oxaliplatin dosage by 25%, and decrease daily capecitabine dosages by 50% during subsequent cycles.* Alternatively, consider using hematopoietic growth factors
Persistent G1/G2 neuropathy	Delay oxaliplatin 1 week. After toxicity resolves, resume oxaliplatin at a dosage decreased to 100 mg/m² during subsequent cycles
"Transient" G3/4 neuropathy (7–14 days)	Hold oxaliplatin. After toxicity resolves, resume oxaliplatin at a dosage decreased to 100 mg/m² during subsequent cycles
Persistent G3/4 neuropathy	Discontinue oxaliplatin
G3/4 diarrhea or stomatitis despite capecitabine dose reductions	Reduce oxaliplatin dosage to 100 mg/m²
G3/4 nonhematologic adverse events other than renal function and neurotoxicity	Reduce oxaliplatin and capecitabine dosages by 25% during subsequent cycles
G2 stomatitis, diarrhea, or nausea	Hold capecitabine; resume capecitabine at full dosage after resolution of toxicity
Second episode of G2 stomatitis, diarrhea, or nausea	Hold capecitabine; resume capecitabine with dosage reduced by 25% after toxicity resolves
Third episode of G2 stomatitis, diarrhea, or nausea	Hold capecitabine; resume capecitabine with dosage reduced by 50% after toxicity resolves
Fourth episode of G2 stomatitis, diarrhea, or nausea	Discontinue capecitabine
G3 stomatitis, diarrhea, or nausea	Hold capecitabine. If G3 toxicity is adequately controlled within 2 days, resume capecitabine at full dosage when toxicity abates to G ≤1. If G3 toxicity takes >2 days to be controlled, resume capecitabine with dosage reduced by 25% after toxicity abates to G ≤1
Second episode of G3 stomatitis, diarrhea, or nausea	Hold capecitabine. If G3 toxicity is controlled adequately within 2 days, then resume capecitabine with dosage reduced by 50% after toxicity abates to G ≤1

(*continued*)

Treatment Modifications (*continued*)

Adverse Event	Dose Modification
Third episode of G3 stomatitis, diarrhea, or nausea	Discontinue capecitabine
G4 stomatitis, diarrhea, or nausea	Discontinue capecitabine. Resume capecitabine with dosage reduced by 50% after toxicity resolves
G1 capecitabine-associated PPE[†]	Begin pyridoxine 50 mg orally 3 times daily and continue capecitabine without dose modification
G2 capecitabine-associated PPE[†]	Begin pyridoxine 50 mg orally 3 times daily and withhold capecitabine. Resume capecitabine with dosage reduced by 15% after toxicity resolves
G3 capecitabine-associated PPE[†]	Begin pyridoxine 50 mg orally 3 times daily and withhold capecitabine. Resume capecitabine with dosage reduced by 30% after toxicity resolves
Recurrent G3 capecitabine-associated PPE[†]	Begin pyridoxine 50 mg orally 3 times daily and withhold capecitabine. Resume capecitabine with dosage reduced by 50% after toxicity resolves

*Treatment delays for unresolved adverse events of >3 weeks duration warrant discontinuation of treatment
[†]PPE, Palmar plantar erythrodysesthesia (hand-foot syndrome)

Efficacy

The authors concluded "The addition of oxaliplatin to capecitabine improves DFS in patients with stage III colon cancer. XELOX is an additional adjuvant treatment option for these patients."

	XELOX	FU/FA
3-year DFS	70.9% (95% CI, 67.9% to 73.9%)	66.5% (95% CI, 63.4% to 69.6%)
4-year DFS	68.4% (95% CI, 65.3% to 71.4%)	62.3% (95% CI, 59.1% to 65.5%)
5-year DFS	66.1% (95% CI, 62.9% to 69.4%)	59.8% (95% CI, 56.4% to 63.1%)
3-year RFS	72.1%	67.5%
4-year RFS	69.7% (95% CI, 66.7% to 72.8%)	63.3% (95% CI, 60.1% to 66.5%)
5-year RFS	67.8% (95% CI, 64.6% to 71.0%)	60.9% (95% CI, 57.6% to 64.2%)
OS*	79.1%	76.1%
	[HR, 0.87; 95% CI, 0.72 to 1.05; $P = 0.1486$]	
5-year OS	77.6% (95% CI, 74.7% to 80.3%)	74.2% (95% CI, 71.3% to 77.2%)

DFS, disease-free survival; FU/FA, Fluorouracil/folinic acid (leucovorin); OS, overall survival; RFS, relapse-free survival; XELOX, capecitabine plus oxaliplatin
*After median follow-up of 57.0 months

Patient Population Studied

Patients with histologically confirmed stage III colon carcinoma (T1-4/N1-2/M0), defined as a tumor located ≥15 cm from the anal verge or above the peritoneal reflection. Surgery with curative intent was performed in all patients ≤8 weeks before random assignment, by which time full recovery from surgery was required

Patient Characteristic (n = 944)

	Percent of Patients
Age – Median (Range)	61 y (22–83 y)
Sex – Male/Female	54%/46%
ECOG performance status	
0	74%
1	25%
Primary tumor classification	
T1-2	11%
T3	74%
T4	15%
TX	<1%
Regional lymph nodes classification	
N0	<1%
N1	65%
N2	35%
Histologic appearance	
Well differentiated	11%
Moderately differentiated	70%
Poorly differentiated	15%
Undetermined/ unknown/data missing	4

Efficacy (Intention to Treat)

End Point	Follow-Up (months)	Number of Patients	Number of Patients with Event	Hazard Ratio (95% CI)	*P* (Log-Rank Test)
DFS	55.0				
XELOX	—	944	295	0.80 (0.69–0.93)	0.0045
FU/FA	—	942	353		
RFS	55.0				
XELOX	—	944	278	0.78 (0.67–0.92)	0.0024
FU/FA	—	942	340		
OS	57.0				
XELOX	—	944	197	0.87 (0.72–1.05)	0.1486
FU/FA	—	942	225		

DFS, disease-free survival; FU/FA, Fluorouracil/folinic acid (leucovorin); OS, overall survival; RFS, relapse-free survival; XELOX, capecitabine plus oxaliplatin;

Efficacy – Multivariate Analysis

Variable	DFS HR (95% CI)	*P*	OS HR (95% CI)	*P*
Stratification				
Treatment (XELOX *vs* FU/FA)				
	0.78 (0.67-0.92)	0.0022	0.88 (0.72–1.06)	0.1836
Lymph nodes (≤3 *vs* >3)				
	0.55 (0.43–0.70)	<0.001	0.48 (0.35–0.64)	<0.001
Baseline CEA (normal *vs* abnormal)				
	0.41 (0.32–0.52)	<0.001	0.41 (0.31–0.54)	<0.001
Region by lymph node interaction				
	0.98 (0.95–1.01)	0.1597	0.98 (0.95-1.01)	0.2231
Prognostic				
Sex (male *vs* female)				
	1.13 (0.96–1.32)	0.1321	1.18 (0.97-1.44)	0.0919
Age (10-year intervals)*				
	1.07 (0.99–1.15)	0.0819	1.17 (1.06–1.28)	0.0016
Time from surgery to randomization (10-day intervals)*				
	1.09 (1.01-1.17)	0.0254	1.10 (1.00–1.21)	0.0395

CEA, carcinoembryonic antigen; CI, confidence interval; DFS, disease-free survival; HR, hazard ratio; FU/FA, Fluorouracil/folinic acid (leucovorin); OS, overall survival; XELOX, capecitabine plus oxaliplatin
*Continuous variable: increase in hazard ratio represents risk increase per pre-defined increment

Treatment Monitoring

1. Before starting treatment: History and physical examination, ECG, CEA determination, CBC with differential, and serum chemistries
2. During treatment: CBC with differential and serum chemistries before each treatment cycle
3. Tumor assessments: Abdominal computed tomography, magnetic resonance imaging, or ultrasound, at baseline, every 6 months for the first 4 years, and annually thereafter. CEA levels every 3 months for the first 3 years and every 6 months thereafter

Toxicity

Most Common Treatment-Related AEs

Schmoll H-J et al. J Clin Oncol 2007;25:102–109

	XELOX (n = 938)		FU/LV (N = 926)	
	Percent of Patients		Percent of Patients	
	All Grades (≥20%)*	Grade 3/4 (≥5%)*	All Grades (≥20%)*	Grade 3/4 (≥5%)*
Patients with at least 1 AE	98%	55%	94%	47%
Neurosensory toxicity	78%	11%	7%	<1%
Nausea	66%	5%	57%	4%
Diarrhea	60%	19%	72%	20%
Vomiting	43%	6%	25%	3%
Fatigue	35%	N/R	34%	N/R
Hand-foot syndrome	29%	5%	10%	<1%
Neutropenia	27%	9%	28%	16%
Thrombocytopenia	N/R	5%	N/R	<1%
Anorexia	24%	N/R	18%	N/R
Stomatitis	21%	<1%	51%	9%
Abdominal pain	17%	2%	18%	2%
Alopecia	4%	N/R	20%	N/R
Dehydration	N/R	3%	N/R	3%
Hypokalemia	N/R	2%	N/R	2%
Febrile neutropenia	N/R	<1%	N/R	4%

AE, adverse event; FU/LV, fluorouracil/leucovorin; N/R, not reported; XELOX, capecitabine and oxaliplatin
*Reported if any grade of AE occurred in >20% or G3/4 occurred in >5% of patients in either treatment arm with some exceptions

(*continued*)

Toxicity (continued)

Analysis of Safety by Age

Schmoll H-J et al. J Clin Oncol 2007;25:102–109

	XELOX		FU/LV	
	Age of Patients			
	<65 Years (n = 583)	≥65 Years (n = 355)	<65 Years (n = 544)	≥65 Years (n = 382)
Patient Condition and Event	%	%	%	%
Patients with AEs	99%	99%	95%	96%
Patients with grade 3/4 AEs	57%	65%	52%	53%
Patients with grade 4 AEs	5%	10%	10%	12%
Patients with serious AEs	17%	30%	23%	26%
Grade 3/4 events				
Diarrhea	17%	23%	20%	21%
Vomiting	7%	6%	3%	3%
Nausea	5%	6%	4%	5%
Dehydration	2%	7%	3%	3%
Stomatitis	<1%	1%	9%	9%
Neutropenia/granulocytopenia	9%	8%	17%	15%
Febrile neutropenia	<1%	<1%	4%	5%
Infections/infestations	2%	5%	4%	5%
Hand-foot syndrome	6%	4%	<1%	<1%
Neurosensory toxicity	12%	10%	<1%	—
Cardiac disorders	1%	2%	1%	2%
Venous thromboembolic events	1%	3%	3%	2%
Patients withdrawn due to AEs	16%	30%	8%	9%

AE, adverse event; FU/LV, fluorouracil/leucovorin; XELOX, capecitabine and oxaliplatin

10. Endometrial Cancer

Maurie Markman, MD

Epidemiology

Incidence: 52,630 (Estimated new cases for 2014 in the United States) 24.3 per 100,000 women per year.

Deaths: Estimated 8,590 in 2014

Median age at diagnosis: 62 years

Stage at Presentation

Localized:	72%	Stage I:	79%
Regional:	16%	Stage II:	12.5%
Distant:	8%	Stage III:	13.3%
Unstaged:	4%	Stage IV:	4%

Modified from Creasman WT et al. J Epidemiol Biostat 2001;6:47–86

Siegel R et al. CA Cancer J Clin 2014;64:9–29

Surveillance, Epidemiology and End Results (SEER) Program, available from http://seer.cancer.gov (accessed in 2013)

Pathology

Endometrioid • Ciliated adenocarcinoma • Secretory adenocarcinoma • Adenocarcinoma with squamous differentiation —Adenosquamous	75–80%
Serous	<10%
Clear cell	4%
Mucinous	1%
Squamous	<1%
Mixed	10%
Undifferentiated	

Kurman RJ, Ellenson LH, Ronnett BM editors. Blaustein's Pathology of the Female Genital Tract. 6th ed: Springer; 2011

Work-up

Stage I	H&P CBC with platelet count Chest x-ray Cervical cytology
Stage II	Consider endocervical curettage or cervical biopsy
Stages III/IV	CA-125 MRI/CT as clinically indicated

Staging

TNM Category	FIGO Stage*	Primary Tumor (T)
TX		Primary tumor cannot be assessed
T0		No evidence of primary tumor
Tis		Carcinoma *in situ* (preinvasive carcinoma)
T1	I	Tumor confined to corpus uteri
T1a	IA	Tumor limited to endometrium or invades less than one-half of the myometrium
T1b	IB	Tumor invades one-half or more of the myometrium
T2	II	Tumor invades stromal connective tissue of the cervix but does not extend beyond uterus†
T3a	IIIA	Tumor involves serosa and/or adnexa (direct extension or metastasis)
T3b	IIIB	Vaginal involvement (direct extension or metastasis) or parametrial involvement
T4	IVA	Tumor invades bladder mucosa and/or bowel mucosa (bullous edema is not sufficient to classify a tumor as T4)

*FIGO staging no longer includes stage 0 (Tis)
†Endocervical glandular involvement only should be considered as stage I and not stage II

TNM Category	FIGO Stage	Regional Lymph Nodes (N)
NX		Regional lymph nodes cannot be assessed
N0		No regional lymph node metastasis
N1	IIIC1	Regional lymph node metastasis to pelvic lymph nodes
N2	IIIC2	Regional lymph node metastasis to para-aortic lymph nodes, with or without positive pelvic lymph nodes

TNM Category	FIGO Stage	Distant Metastasis (M)
M0		No distant metastasis (no pathologic M0; use clinical M to complete stage group)
MI	IVB	Distant metastasis (includes metastasis to inguinal lymph nodes intraperitoneal disease, or lung, liver, or bone. It excludes metastasis to paraaortic lymph nodes, vagina, pelvic serosa, or adnexa)

Histologic Grade (G)

G1	Well differentiated
G2	Moderately differentiated
G3–4	Poorly differentiated or undifferentiated

Staging

Group	T	N	M
0*	Tis	N0	M0
I	T1	N0	M0
I	T1a	N0	M0
IB	T1b	N0	M0
II	T2	N0	M0
III	T3	N0	M0
IIIA	T3a	N0	M0
IIIB	T3b	N0	M0
IIIC1	T1-T3	N1	M0
IIIC2	T1-T3	N2	M0
IVA	T4	Any N	M0
IVB	Any T	Any N	M1

*FIGO no longer includes stage 0 (Tis)

Overall 5-Year Survival: Relative to FIGO Disease Stage

Stage	% Survival
Ia	88.9
Ib	90
Ic	80.7
IIa	79.9
IIb	72.3
IIIa	63.4
IIIb	38.8
IIIc	51.1
IVa	19.9
IVb	17.2

Edge SB, Byrd DR, Compton CC, Fritz AG, Greene FL, Trotti A, eds. *AJCC Cancer Staging Manual.* 7th ed. New York, NY: Springer; 2010.

Expert Opinion

Over the past decade there has been considerable evolution in the management of endometrial cancer. Fortunately, the large majority of patients present with early stage disease, and in these patients surgical resection are undertaken with curative intent. Recent reports have questioned the routine use of postoperative external beam radiation therapy in patients with an intermediate risk of recurrence, and a definitive answer to the role of radiation requires further investigation

However, it is the place of cytotoxic chemotherapy in the treatment of advanced, metastatic, and recurrent endometrial cancer that has undergone the greatest change. Once considered a relatively *chemoresistant* malignancy, it is now recognized that objective responses can be observed in ≥50% of patients with measurable disease[1,2] following treatment with several combination chemotherapy regimens including:

- Cisplatin + doxorubicin
- Cisplatin + doxorubicin + paclitaxel
- Paclitaxel + carboplatin

A number of single agents have documented activity (>15–20% objective response rates) in this malignancy including:

- Paclitaxel
- Doxorubicin
- Topotecan
- Cisplatin
- Carboplatin

Unfortunately, because of the relative rarity of metastatic endometrial cancer, there have been no phase III trials directly comparing the utility of these individual drugs that might help guide routine clinical management

Older randomized trials had revealed the potential for combination chemotherapy to improve objective response rates and progression-free survival in metastatic or recurrent endometrial cancer. The Gynecologic Oncology Group (GOG) 177 trial established doxorubicin + cisplatin followed by paclitaxel (TAP) as the standard for systemic treatment of stage III-IV and recurrent endometrial cancer.[1] However, TAP was associated with substantially more toxicity compared than the comparator arm, doxorubicin + cisplatin (AP). G2/3 neurotoxicity in 39% of patients who received TAP compared with 5% of those given AP, and 24% of patients who received TAP discontinued treatment because of toxicities compared with 9% of patients who received AP. As a result, TAP often was not utilized

An earlier report suggested the activity of a paclitaxel + carboplatin (TC) combination without doxorubicin might be similar to TAP but with less toxicity.[2,3] The TC combination had a high objective response rate in endometrial cancer and a relatively favorable side-effect profile. These results provided the rationale for GOG 209, in which TAP and TC were compared in 1300 women with advanced or recurrent endometrial cancer. Patients were randomly assigned to receive either:

- TAP: Doxorubicin 45 mg/m^2 + cisplatin 50 mg/m^2 (day 1), followed by paclitaxel 160 mg/m^2 (day 2) every 21 days with hematopoietic growth factor support for a maximum of 7 cycles, *or*
- TC: Paclitaxel 175 mg/m^2 + carboplatin AUC = 6 mg/mL/min (day 1) every 21 days for a maximum of 7 cycles
  - Paclitaxel 135 mg/m^2 and carboplatin AUC = 5 mg/mL/min were given to women with a history of pelvic/spine irradiation

Designed as a noninferiority trial, the study had 2 primary objectives:

1. Determine whether TC was therapeutically equivalent (noninferior) to TAP with respect to overall survival
2. Determine whether TC has a more favorable toxicity profile

A test for homogeneity suggested a consistent effect of treatment with TC across all prespecified subgroups. At interim analysis the authors concluded: "TC is not inferior to TAP in terms of PFS and OS….Overall, the toxicity profile favors TC. Thus, TC as prescribed in this study is an acceptable backbone for further trials in combination with 'targeted' therapies."

GOG 209 Interim Analysis

Miller D et al. Randomized phase III noninferiority trial of first-line chemotherapy for metastatic or recurrent endometrial carcinoma: a Gynecologic Oncology Group study [abstract]. Gynecol Oncol 2012;125:771

	TAP	TC	
Interim Efficacy Analysis			
PFS	14 months	14 months	HR = 1.03
OS	38 months	32 months	HR = 1.01

(continued)

(continued)

Expert Opinion (*continued*)

GOG 209 Interim Analysis (*continued*)

Safety/Tolerability

Discontinued therapy for toxicity*	17.6%	11.9%	
Neutropenia and fever	7%	6%	P = 0.01
G1 sensory neuropathy	26%	19%	P <0.01
G3/4 thrombocytopenia	22.8%	12.8%	P <0.001
G3/4 neutropenia	**52.1%**	**79.7%**	**P <0.001**
G3/4 other hematologic	30.6%	21.2%	P <0.001
G3/4 nausea	8.9%	5.6%	P = 0.024
G3/4 vomiting	7.0%	3.5%	P = 0.006
G3/4 diarrhea	5.7%	2.0%	P <0.001
G3/4 stomatitis	1.3%	0.2%	P = 0.019
G3/4 creatinine elevation	1.9%	0.6%	P = 0.044

TAP = Doxorubicin + cisplatin, followed by paclitaxel with growth factor support.
TC = paclitaxel + carboplatin
*About two-thirds of patients in each group completed 7 planned cycles, and another 10% completed 6 cycles. The most common reason for discontinuation was completion of protocol specified therapy

It should also be noted that a combination chemotherapy regimen (cisplatin + doxorubicin) has been demonstrated in a phase III trial to improve survival compared to whole abdominal radiotherapy when employed as initial treatment following surgical cytoreduction in women with stage III and IV (maximum 2-cm residual disease) endometrial cancer.[4] Based on existing data, many clinicians currently elect to employ 4–6 cycles of systemic chemotherapy, followed by local pelvic radiation in women whose major disease manifestations are principally confined to the pelvic region. The intent of the radiation is to reduce the risk of disease local recurrence in this specific clinical setting. Future randomized trials will hopefully define the utility of a combined chemotherapy-plus-radiotherapy approach in advanced and metastatic endometrial cancer

Certain subpopulations of endometrial cancer have long been known to be responsive to therapy with progesterone.[5] Clinical features that would predict for a patient who may respond to this treatment option include:

1. Low-grade cancer (grade 1)
2. Evidence of progesterone receptors within the primary tumor specimen
3. Long disease-free interval (eg, >1–2 years) between the diagnosis of endometrial cancer and documented disease recurrence
4. Nonvisceral metastatic disease

Perhaps the single most important factor to consider in this setting is tumor grade. Patients with high-grade endometrial cancers are unlikely to respond to hormonal manipulation. Conversely, it may be quite reasonable to initially attempt to treat a patient with a low-grade metastatic endometrial cancer with progesterone before administering chemotherapy

Summary:

1. Primary treatment for localized (stages I, II) endometrial cancer is surgery. In appropriately selected patients, postoperative radiation is delivered to reduce the risk of local relapse. For patients unable to undergo surgery (eg, significant preexisting cardiac dysfunction), external beam radiation therapy may substitute as the primary treatment modality
2. In stage III, stage IV, or recurrent endometrial cancer, the current "standard-of-care" should be considered combination chemotherapy following an attempt at optimal surgical resection (principally in the stage III setting). The regimen-of-choice remains to be defined, but options include cisplatin + doxorubicin + paclitaxel, carboplatin + paclitaxel, or cisplatin + doxorubicin
3. Patients unable to receive combination chemotherapy (eg, secondary to clinically relevant preexisting comorbidity) may be treated with one of several previously noted cytotoxic agents with known biological activity in metastatic endometrial cancer
4. In carefully selected patients (criteria described above), prior to the delivery of cytotoxic chemotherapy, treatment with a progesterone agent may reasonably be attempted

[1]Fleming GF et al. J Clin Oncol 2004;22:2159–2166
[2]Sorbe B et al. Int J Gynecol Cancer 2008;18:803–808
[3]Hoskins PJ et al. J Clin Oncol 2001;19:4048–4053
[4]Randall M et al. J Clin Oncol 2006;24:36–44
[5]Thigpen JT et al. J Clin Oncol 1999;17:1736–1774

REGIMEN FOR ADVANCED OR RECURRENT ENDOMETRIAL CARCINOMA
DOXORUBICIN + CISPLATIN (AC)

Randall ME et al. J Clin Oncol 2006;24:36–44

Prehydration for cisplatin: $\geq$1000 mL 0.9% sodium chloride injection (0.9% NS) by intravenous infusion over 2 hours

Note: Encourage patients to increase oral intake of non-alcoholic fluids, and provide electrolyte replacement as needed (potassium, magnesium, sodium)

Doxorubicin 60 mg/m^2; administer by slow intravenous injection over 3–5 minutes on day 1, every 21 days (total dosage/cycle = 60 mg/m^2)
- Maximum allowable total cumulative lifetime doxorubicin dosage = 420 mg/m^2; that is, no more than 7 repeated treatment cycles
- Doxorubicin may be given during hydration for cisplatin

Cisplatin 50 mg/m^2; administer intravenously in 250 mL 0.9% NS over 1 hour after doxorubicin on day 1, every 21 days (total dosage per cycle = 50 mg/m^2)

Supportive Care
Antiemetic prophylaxis
Emetogenic potential: **HIGH. Potential for delayed symptoms**
See Chapter 39 for antiemetic recommendations

Hematopoietic growth factor (CSF) prophylaxis
Primary prophylaxis may be indicated
See Chapter 43 for more information

Antimicrobial prophylaxis
Risk of fever and neutropenia is LOW
   Antimicrobial primary prophylaxis to be considered:
- Antibacterial—not indicated
- Antifungal—not indicated
- Antiviral—not indicated unless patient previously had an episode of HSV

See Chapter 47 for more information

Treatment Modifications

Adverse Event*	Dose Modification
Doxorubicin 60 mg/m^2 *and* ANC <1500/mm^3 *or* platelet count <100,000/mm^3	Reduce doxorubicin dosage to 45 mg/m^{2†}
Doxorubicin 45 mg/m^2 *and* ANC <1500/mm^3 *or* platelet count <100,000/mm^3	Reduce doxorubicin dosage to 30 mg/m^{2†}
Doxorubicin 30 mg/m^2 *and* ANC <1500/mm^3 *or* platelet count <100,000/mm^3	Reduce doxorubicin dosage to 15 mg/m^{2†}
Doxorubicin 15 mg/m^2 *and* ANC <1500/mm^3 *or* platelet count <100,000/mm^3	Discontinue doxorubicin
Treatment interruption caused by myelosuppression exceeding 6 weeks	Discontinue doxorubicin
Decline in cardiac ejection fraction of 20% from baseline, or development of congestive heart failure or other life-threatening cardiac problems	Discontinue doxorubicin; continue cisplatin
Serum creatinine $\geq$2.0 mg/dL ($\geq$177 μmol/L)	Hold cisplatin

*Consider growth factor support for myelosuppression
†Reinstitute dose if myelosuppression resolves

Patient Population Studied

A study of 422 women with stages III or IV endometrial carcinoma with a maximum of 2 cm of postoperative residual disease who were randomly allocated to receive whole abdominal radiation or doxorubicin and cisplatin

Efficacy (N = 194)

Initial Site of Recurrence	No (%)
Pelvis	34 (18%)
Abdomen	27 (14%)
Extraabdominal or liver metastases	34 (18%)

Toxicity (N = 191)

Adverse Events	% of Patients			
Grade	1	2	3	4
Leukopenia	11	23	44	18
Neutropenia	4	4	18	67
Thrombocytopenia	34	15	11	10
Other hematologic	28	31	17	3
Maximum hematologic	4	5	20	69
GI	20	38	13	7
Hepatic	<1	2	1	—
Genitourinary	9	9	2	1
Cardiac	5	12	11	4
Vascular	2	2	<1	1
Pulmonary	4	4	1	<1
Neurologic	25	10	6	1
Pain	8	5	<1	—
Weakness	6	3	3	—
Fatigue	14	11	5	<1
Metabolic	6	8	4	<1
Infection	1	2	4	3
Fever	6	12	4	2
Allergy	—	—	—	—
Dermatologic	10	4	1	<1
Alopecia	6	69	NA	NA

NA, not available

Reason for Treatment Discontinuation (N = 194)*

	N	Percent
Completed treatment	123	63.4
Progression	18	9.3
Patient refusal	14	7.2
Toxicity	33	17.0
Death	4	2.1
Other	2	1.0

*Based on 7 cycles of doxorubicin + cisplatin followed by 1 cycle of cisplatin alone

Therapy Monitoring

1. Physical examination, CBC and differential count, and serum creatinine before each chemotherapy cycle
2. Evaluation of ejection fraction immediately before cycle 6 (or earlier, if clinically indicated)
3. Efficacy assessment every 2 to 3 cycles

REGIMEN FOR ADVANCED OR RECURRENT ENDOMETRIAL CARCINOMA

PACLITAXEL + CARBOPLATIN (TC)

Sorbe B et al. Int J Gynecol Cancer 2008;18:803–808

Premedication for paclitaxel:

Dexamethasone 20 mg per dose; administer orally or intravenously in 10–50 mL 0.9% sodium chloride injection (0.9% NS) or 5% dextrose injection (D5W) for 2 doses, 12–14 hours and 6–7 hours before starting paclitaxel

Diphenhydramine 50 mg, by intravenous injection 30 minutes before starting paclitaxel

Ranitidine 50 mg; administer intravenously over 30–60 minutes, 30 minutes before starting paclitaxel

Paclitaxel 175 mg/m^2; administer intravenously in a volume of 0.9% NS or D5W sufficient to produce a solution with concentration within the range 0.3–1.2 mg/mL over 3 hours on day 1 every 3 weeks (total dosage/cycle = 175 mg/m^2)

Carboplatin* AUC = 5 mg/mL · min; administer intravenously in 50–150 mL D5W over 60 minutes, on day 1, every 3 weeks (total dosage/cycle calculated to produce an AUC = 6 mg/mL · min) (see equation below)

*Carboplatin dose is based on Calvert et al.'s formula to achieve a target area under the plasma concentration versus time curve (AUC) [AUC units = mg/mL · min]

$$\text{Total carboplatin dose (mg)} = \left(\text{target AUC}\right) \times \left(\text{GFR} + 25\right)$$

In practice, creatinine clearance (Clcr) is used in place of glomerular filtration rate (GFR). Clcr can be calculated from the equation of Cockcroft and Gault:

$$\text{For males, Clcr} = \frac{(140 \pm \text{age [years]}) \times \text{body weight [kg]}}{72 \times (\text{serum creatinine [mg/dL]})}$$

$$\text{For females, Clcr} = \frac{(140 - \text{age [years]}) \times \text{body weight [kg]}}{72 \times (\text{serum creatinine [mg/dL]})} \times 0.85$$

Note: On October 8, 2010, the U.S. Food and Drug Administration (FDA) identified a potential safety issue with carboplatin dosing based on recent changes in the measurement of serum creatinine. By the end of 2010, all clinical laboratories in the USA will use the standardized Isotope Dilution Mass Spectrometry (IDMS) method to measure serum creatinine, which could result in an overestimation of the GFR in some patients with normal renal function. A carboplatin dose calculated with an IDMS-measured serum creatinine result using the Calvert formula could exceed an expected exposure (AUC) and result in increased drug-related toxicity

Provided actual GFR measurements are made to assess renal function, carboplatin can be safely dosed according to the Calvert formula described in product labeling

If GFR (or creatinine clearance) is estimated based on serum creatinine measurements by the IDMS method, the FDA recommended for patients with normal renal function capping an estimated GFR at 125 mL/min for any targeted AUC value. No greater estimated GFR values should be used

U.S. FDA. Carboplatin dosing. [online] May 23, 2013. Available from: http://www.fda.gov/AboutFDA/CentersOffices/OfficeofMedicalProductsandTobacco/CDER/ucm228974.htm [accessed February 26, 2014]

Calvert AH et al. J Clin Oncol 1989;7:1748–1756
Cockcroft DW, Gault MH. Nephron 1976;16:31–41
Jodrell DI et al. J Clin Oncol 1992;10:520–528
Sorensen BT et al. Cancer Chemother Pharmacol 1991;28:397–401

(continued)

Patient Population Studied

A prospective, phase II, multicenter study evaluating carboplatin and paclitaxel in the treatment of patients with primary advanced or recurrent endometrial carcinoma. Sixty-six patients were enrolled: 18 with primary advanced tumors and 48 with recurrences. All histologic types and tumor grades were allowed

Efficacy (N = 66)

Complete response	29%
Partial response	38%
Median progression-free survival	14 months
3-Year progression-free survival	18.2%
5-Year progression-free survival	12.5%
Median overall survival	26 months
3-Year overall survival	33.3%
5-Year overall survival	20.3%

Primary Advanced Cases (N = 18)

Complete response	50%
Partial response	33%
Median progression-free survival	14 months
Median survival	19 months

Recurrent Cases (N = 48)

Complete response	21%
Partial response	40%
Median progression-free survival	14 months
Median survival	27 months

Assessment: Clinical examination, gynecologic examination under anesthesia, transvaginal and transabdominal ultrasound, and computerized tomography were used in the evaluation of the tumor status. WHO response criteria were used to evaluate tumor

Note: Prior radiotherapy was not associated with response rate (P = 0.565), PFS rate (P = 0.420), or OS rate (P = 0.637) in this study

(*continued*)

Supportive Care
Antiemetic prophylaxis
Emetogenic potential: **HIGH.** *Potential for delayed symptoms*
See Chapter 39 for antiemetic recommendations

Hematopoietic growth factor (CSF) prophylaxis
Primary prophylaxis may be indicated
See Chapter 43 for more information

Antimicrobial prophylaxis
Risk of fever and neutropenia is LOW
  Antimicrobial primary prophylaxis to be considered:
  • Antibacterial—not indicated
  • Antifungal—not indicated
  • Antiviral—not indicated unless patient previously had an episode of HSV
See Chapter 47 for more information

Toxicity (N = 66)

Adverse Events	% of Patients			
	Grade (%)			
	1	**2**	**3**	**4**
Hematologic				
Anemia	40.9	43.9	—	—
Neutropenia*	25.8	15.2	4.5	3.0
Thrombocytopenia	47	3.0	1.5	3.0
Nonhematologic				
Infection/fever	—	—	—	—
Renal	42.2	—	—	—
Cardiac	7.6	—	—	—
Neurologic†	37.9	31.8	13.6	—
Nausea/vomiting	39.4	16.7	4.5	1.5

*In 6 cases (9.1%), chemotherapy was stopped because of this toxicity
†In 13 cases (19.7%), therapy was prematurely stopped because of this toxicity
In 2 cases, allergic reactions prohibited completion of therapy
NCI CTC, National Cancer Institute (USA) Common Toxicity Criteria, version 2.0. At:
http://ctep.cancer.gov/protocolDevelopment/electronic_applications/ctc.htm [accessed December 7, 2013]

Therapy Monitoring

1. Physical examination, CBC and serum creatinine before each chemotherapy cycle
2. Efficacy assessment every 2–3 cycles

Treatment Modifications

Adverse Event	Dose Modification
At start of a cycle ANC ≤1000/mm³ *or* platelet count ≤100,000/mm³	Delay start of cycle up to 2 weeks until ANC >1000/mm³ *and* platelet count >100,000/mm³
ANC ≤1000/mm³ or platelet count ≤100,000/mm³ for more than 2 weeks but less than 3 weeks after scheduled start of next cycle	Reduce paclitaxel and carboplatin dosages by 20% (140 mg/m² and AUC = 4, respectively)
At start of a cycle ANC ≤1000/mm³ *or* platelet count ≤100,000/mm³ despite dose reduction	Delay start of cycle up to 2 weeks until ANC >1000/mm³ *and* platelet count >100,000/mm³, then administer filgrastim or pegfilgrastim after completing chemotherapy without changing chemotherapy dosages
Serum creatinine >2 mg/dL (>177 µmol/L) or G ≥3 peripheral neuropathy	Delay start of cycle up to 2 weeks; if serum creatinine does not decrease to ≤2 mg/dL (≤177 µmol/L) or G peripheral neuropathy within that 2-week period, discontinue therapy

REGIMEN

PACLITAXEL, DOXORUBICIN, CISPLATIN (TAP)

Fleming GF et al. J Clin Oncol 2004;22:2159–2166

Prehydration for cisplatin: 1000 mL 0.9% sodium chloride injection (0.9% NS); administer intravenously over at least 2 hours

Notes: Encourage patients to increase oral intake of non-alcoholic fluids, and provide electrolyte replacement as needed (potassium, magnesium, sodium)

Doxorubicin may be administered during hydration for cisplatin

Doxorubicin 45 mg/m^2 (maximum single dose = 90 mg); administer by slow intravenous injection over 3–5 minutes on day 1 every 21 days (total dosage/cycle = 45 mg/m^2; maximum dose/cycle = 90 mg)

Followed immediately afterward by:
Cisplatin 50 mg/m^2 (maximum single dose = 100 mg); administer intravenously in 250 mL 0.9% sodium chloride injection (0.9% NS) over 1 hour on day 1 after doxorubicin administration, every 21 days (total dosage/cycle = 50 mg/m^2; maximum dose/cycle = 100 mg)

Paclitaxel 160 mg/m^2 (maximum single dose = 320 mg); administer by intravenous infusion in a volume of 0.9% NS or 5% dextrose injection sufficient to produce a concentration within the range of 0.3–1.2 mg/mL over 3 hours on day 2, every 21 days (total dosage/cycle = 160 mg/m^2; maximum dose/cycle = 320 mg)

Notes:
• No modifications to starting drug doses based on age or history of pelvic radiation therapy
• Women with a BSA >2 m^2 received treatment as if their BSA was equal to only 2 m^2

Supportive Care
Antiemetic prophylaxis
Emetogenic potential on day 1: **HIGH**. *Potential for delayed symptoms*
Emetogenic potential on day 2: **LOW**
See Chapter 39 for antiemetic recommendations

Hematopoietic growth factor (CSF) prophylaxis
Primary prophylaxis is indicated with one of the following:
   Filgrastim (G-CSF) 5 mcg/kg per day, by subcutaneous injection, *or*
   Pegfilgrastim (pegylated filgrastim) 6 mg/0.6 mL, by subcutaneous injection for 1 dose
   • Begin use from 24–72 hours after myelosuppressive chemotherapy is completed
   • For daily filgrastim, continue use until ANC ≥10,000/mm^3 on 2 consecutive daily measurements
See Chapter 43 for more information

Antimicrobial prophylaxis
Risk of fever and neutropenia is LOW
See Chapter 47 for more information

Treatment Modifications

Adverse Event	Dose Modification
G3/4 thrombocytopenia or G4 ANC	Reduce cisplatin and paclitaxel dosages by 20%
G3 peripheral neuropathy	Hold therapy until neuropathy G ≤1. Restart therapy with paclitaxel and cisplatin dosages reduced by 20%
Recurrent G3 neurologic toxicity	Discontinue therapy
LVEF <45% or a fall in LVEF ≥20% from baseline	Discontinue therapy
Toxicity-related delay in administration of >3 weeks	Discontinue therapy

Patient Population Studied

Chemotherapy-naïve women with histologically documented measurable stage III or stage IV or recurrent endometrial carcinoma of any cell type plus a GOG performance status of 0–2

Efficacy (N = 134)

Complete response	22%
Partial response	35%
Median progression-free survival	8.3 months
Median overall survival	15.3 months

Toxicity (N = 131)

	% of Patients		
	G2	G3	G4
Nonhematologic			
Auditory	7	0	0
LVEF	10	2	0
Pulmonary	5	2	0
DVT	1	6	0
Constitutional	31	10	2
Vomiting	23	10	2
Diarrhea	8	8	1
Mucositis or stomatitis	7	1	0
Genitourinary/renal	3	3	1
Metabolic	8	12	7
Sensory neuropathy	27	12	0
Hematologic			
Neutropenia	13	23	36
Thrombocytopenia	21	20	2

Therapy Monitoring

1. *Every cycle:* Pelvic examination and serum electrolytes, calcium, magnesium, BUN, and creatinine
2. *Every other cycle:* Tumor measurements by radiologic examination
3. *Every third cycle:* Left ventricular ejection fraction

11. Esophageal Cancer

Jimmy Hwang, MD and John Marshall, MD

Epidemiology

Incidence: 18,170 (male: 14,660; female: 3,510. Estimated new cases for 2014 in the United States)
7.7 per 100,000 male, 1.8 per 100,000 female
Deaths: Estimated 15,450 in 2014 (male: 12,450; female: 3,000)
Median age at diagnosis*: Squamous cell esophageal carcinoma: 53.4 years
Adenocarcinoma of the esophagus: 62.6 years
Male to female ratio: 3:1 for squamous cell carcinoma and 7:1 for adenocarcinoma
Stage at presentation: Locoregional disease: 50%
Distant metastasis: 50%

*Kelsen DP et al. Textbook of Gastrointestinal Oncology: Principles and Practice. Lippincott Williams & Williams, 2001
Siegel R et al. CA Cancer J Clin 2014;64:9–29
Surveillance, Epidemiology and End Results (SEER) Program, available from http://seer.cancer.gov (accessed in 2013)

Pathology

Upper to midthoracic esophagus:	Predominantly squamous cell carcinoma
Distal esophagus and GE junction:	Predominantly adenocarcinoma
Other rare pathology:	Basaloid-squamous carcinoma (1.9%)* or small cell carcinomas

Especially in white men, the incidence of adenocarcinoma of the GE junction has risen significantly in the United States, whereas that of squamous cell carcinoma has slightly decreased. In the 1960s, squamous cell cancer accounted for 90% or more of esophageal cancer.[†] Data from 1996 suggested that they occur with equal frequency, and in 2004 the trend has changed further so that adenocarcinoma now accounts for at least 75% of esophageal cancers. This is thought to be related to increase in body mass index and Barrett esophagus

*Abe K et al. Am J Surg Pathol 1996;20:453–461
[†]Daly JM et al. National Cancer Data Base Report on Esophageal Carcinoma. Cancer 1996;78:1820–1828

Work-up

1. H&P, esophagogastroduodenoscopy, CBC, serum electrolytes, BUN, creatinine, LFTs and mineral panel, PET scan ± CT scan, of chest and abdomen

2. Endoscopic ultrasound is highly recommended if there is no evidence of distant metastases, with FNA if indicated

3. For locoregional cancer at or above the carina, a bronchoscopy must be considered

4. In selected patients with local-regional GE junction cancer, a laparoscopic staging of the peritoneal cavity may be warranted

5. In patients with locoregional cancer, PET/CT scan is strongly recommended. Suspicious metastatic cancer should be confirmed

6. In addition, for patients with locoregional cancer (stages I–III), a multidisciplinary evaluation is required, including nutritional assessment. The need for supplementation depends on the severity of dysphagia, and the overall nutritional status (>10% weight loss). Enteral nutritional support is preferred (PEG is avoided if surgery is a consideration)

Staging

Primary Tumor (T)		Regional Lymph Nodes (N) (Any periesophageal lymph node from cervical nodes to celiac nodes)		Metastases	
TX	Primary tumor cannot be assessed			M0	No distant metastases
T0	No evidence of primary tumor			M1	Distant metastases
Tis	High-grade dysplasia	NX	Regional lymph nodes cannot be assessed		
T1	Tumor invades lamina propria or submucosa			**Grade**	
T2	Tumor invades muscularis propria	N0	No regional lymph node metastases	1	Well-differentiated
T3	Tumor invades adventitia	N1	1–2 positive regional lymph nodes	2	Moderately differentiated
T4a	Resectable cancer invades adjacent structures such as pleura, pericardium, diaphragm	N2	3–6 positive regional lymph nodes	3	Poorly differentiated
T4b	Unresectable cancer invades adjacent structures such as aorta, vertebral body, trachea	N3	≥7 positive regional lymph nodes	4	Undifferentiated

(continued)

Staging (continued)

Cancer Location

Upper thoracic	20–25 cm from incisors
Middle thoracic	>25–30 cm from incisors
Lower thoracic	>30–40 cm from incisors
Esophagogastric junction	Includes cancers whose epicenter is in the distal thoracic esophagus, esophagogastric junction, or within the proximal 5 cm of the stomach (cardia) that extend into the esophagogastric junction or distal thoracic esophagus (Siewert III). These stomach cancers are stage grouped similarly to adenocarcinoma of the esophagus

Staging Groupings for Esophageal Adenocarcinoma

Stage	T	N	M	G
0	is (HGD*)	0	0	1
IA	1	0	0	1–2
IB	1	0	0	3
	2	0	0	1–2
IIA	2	0	0	3
IIB	3	0	0	Any
	1–2	1	0	Any
IIIA	1–2	2	0	Any
	3	1	0	Any
	4a	0	0	Any
IIIB	3	2	0	Any
	4a	1–2	0	Any
IIIC	4b	Any	0	Any
	Any	3	0	Any
IV	Any	Any	1	Any

*High-grade dysplasia

Staging Groupings for Esophageal Squamous Cell Carcinoma

Stage	T	N	M	G	Location
0	is (HGD*)	0	0	1	Any
IA	1	0	0	1	Any
IB	1	0	0	2–3	Any
	2–3	0	0	1	Lower
IIA	2–3	0	0	1	Upper/middle
	2–3	0	0	2–3	Lower
IIB	2–3	0	0	2–3	Upper/middle
	1–2	1	0	Any	Any
IIIA	1–2	2	0	Any	Any
	3	1	0	Any	Any
	4a	0	0	Any	Any
IIIB	3	2	0	Any	Any
IIIC	4a	1–2	0	Any	Any
	4b	Any	0	Any	Any
	Any	3	0	Any	Any
IV	Any	Any	1	Any	Any

*High grade dysplasia
Edge SB, Byrd DR, Compton CC, Fritz AG, Greene FL, Trotti A, editors. AJCC Cancer Staging Manual. 7th ed. New York: Springer; 2010.

Five-Year Survival Adenocarcinoma

Stage 0	≈82
Stage IA	≈77
Stage IB	≈63
Stage IIA	≈50
Stage IIB	≈40
Stage IIIA	≈25
Stage IIIB	≈18
Stage IIIC	≈14

Rice et al. Ann Surg Oncol 2010;17:1721–1724

Five-Year Survival Squamous Cell Carcinoma

Stage 0	≈71
Stage IA	≈71
Stage IB	≈61
Stage IIA	≈53
Stage IIB	≈41
Stage IIIA	≈25
Stage IIIB	≈18
Stage IIIC	≈14

Rice et al. Ann Surg Oncol 2010;17:1721–1724

Expert Opinion

Management of localized/locally advanced disease:
A distinction must be made between the treatment of localized/locally advanced *esophageal squamous cell carcinoma* and *esophageal adenocarcinoma*

Squamous cell carcinoma:
• Treatment should be surgery or radiation with concurrent chemotherapy
• The role of preoperative or postoperative radiation with concurrent chemotherapy is unclear

Adenocarcinoma:
• Treatment should be multimodality with surgery
  ▪ Preoperative radiation with concurrent chemotherapy, followed by surgery
  ▪ Perioperative chemotherapy (MAGIC: Cunningham D et al. N Engl J Med 2006;355:11–20)
  ▪ Postoperative chemotherapy and radiation (INT 116: Macdonald JS et al. N Engl J Med 2001;345:725–730)

Chemotherapy:
There is no single standard chemotherapy for esophageal cancer
Squamous cell carcinoma:
• No single standard chemotherapy regimen

Adenocarcinoma:
• Tend to be grouped with gastric and gastroesophageal adenocarcinomas
  ▪ Combination chemotherapy with platinum and fluoropyrimidine is the community standard, as defined by the regimen that is most commonly used. In patients with good functional status, a third drug is typically added. Options as that third drug may include trastuzumab (in HER-2 amplified disease); epirubicin (especially in the United Kingdom), and docetaxel
• **Docetaxel, cisplatin, and infusional fluorouracil (DCF)**
  ▪ The "reference standard," but too toxic in the general population to be considered a "community standard"
  ▪ Variations of DCF are under evaluation, but their efficacy compared to DCF is unclear
• The role of **"targeted therapies"** is uncertain
  ▪ **Trastuzumab:** The ToGA study (Van Cutsem et al. J Clin Oncol 2009;27 Suppl:18s [abstract LBA4509], and Bang Y-J et al. Lancet 2010;376:687–697) evaluated the potential role of trastuzumab in *HER-2–positive* gastroesophageal adenocarcinomas. Although the addition of trastuzumab to cisplatin and fluoropyrimidine combinations improved survival, it is possible that the addition of other "third drugs," such as epirubicin or docetaxel, to a platinum and fluoropyrimidine backbone could produce a similar survival benefit in this patient population
  ▪ **EGFR TKIs:** The differences in response rates to EGFR TKIs between esophageal (11%; Ferry DR et al. Clin Cancer Res 2007;13:5869–5875), gastroesophageal junction (9%; Dragovich T et al. J Clin Oncol 2006;24:4922–4927) and gastric adenocarcinomas (zero; Dragovich T et al. J Clin Oncol 2006;24:4922–4927) emphasizes potential differences among these disease locations. In addition, there may be a difference in disease control by histology (Janmaat ML et al. J Clin Oncol 2006;24:1612–1619). It is difficult to project survival in patients with metastatic disease, as available studies allowed both histologies, and many include gastric, gastroesophageal cancers

Palliative approaches include:
• Stents
• Photodynamic therapy
• Radiation
• Chemotherapy

Locoregional cancer defined as:
• Potentially resectable, or
• Unresectable, which includes T4 lesion, supraclavicular adenopathy, and celiac nodal metastasis in patients with upper or mid-thoracic esophageal cancer

REGIMEN

FLUOROURACIL + CISPLATIN + RADIATION

Herskovic A et al. N Engl J Med 1992;326:1593–1598
Minsky BD et al. J Clin Oncol 2002;20:1167–1174 (INT 0123; RTOG 94-05)

Hydration before cisplatin: ≥1000 mL 0.9% sodium chloride injection (0.9% NS); administer intravenously at ≥100 mL/hour before and after cisplatin administration. Also encourage patients to increase oral intake of non-alcoholic fluids. Monitor serum electrolytes and replace as needed (potassium, magnesium, sodium)

Mannitol diuresis: May be given to patients who have received adequate hydration. A dose of 12.5–25 g mannitol can be administered by intravenous injection before cisplatin or prepared as an admixture in the same container as cisplatin. Continued intravenous hydration is essential In an inpatient or "day hospital" setting, additional mannitol can be administered in the form of an infusion: 100–200 mL 20% mannitol injection administered intravenously over 4–8 hours. This can be done either during or immediately after cisplatin, but requires maintenance of adequate intravenous fluid input during and for hours after mannitol administration

Cisplatin 75 mg/m^2; administer intravenously in 50–250 mL of 0.9% NS at a rate of 1 mg/minute, on day 1 during weeks 1, 5, 9, and 13 (total dosage per 28-day cycle [1 dose] = 75 mg/m^2)

Fluorouracil 1000 mg/m^2 per day; administer by continuous intravenous infusion in 500–1000 mL 0.9% NS or 5% dextrose injection over 24 hours for 4 consecutive days on days 1–4 during weeks 1, 5, 9, and 13 (total dosage per 28-day cycle [4 doses] = 4000 mg/m^2)

Radiation 1.8 Gy/day for 5 days/week
Starts concurrently with chemotherapy
Planned cumulative dose = 50.4 Gy (duration of planned treatment is 5 weeks, 3 days)

Supportive Care

Antiemetic prophylaxis
Emetogenic potential on days with cisplatin is **HIGH**. *Potential for delayed symptoms*
Emetogenic potential on days with fluorouracil + radiation and radiation alone is **LOW**
See Chapter 39 for antiemetic recommendations

Hematopoietic growth factor (CSF) prophylaxis
Primary prophylaxis is NOT indicated
See Chapter 43 for more information

Antimicrobial prophylaxis
Risk of fever and neutropenia is LOW
  Antimicrobial primary prophylaxis to be considered:
  • Antibacterial—not indicated
  • Antifungal—not indicated
  • Antiviral—not indicated unless patient previously had an episode of HSV
See Chapter 47 for more information

Patient Population Studied

A clinical trial of 236 patients with AJCC clinical stage T1–4 N0–1 M0 primary squamous cell or adenocarcinoma of the cervical, mid, or distal esophagus selected for a nonsurgical (definitive chemoradiation) approach. Patients received combined modality therapy consisting of chemotherapy with concurrent radiation therapy. Patients were randomized to receive either 64.8 Gy or 50.4 Gy. The higher radiation dose did not increase survival or local/regional control

Notes

1. Doses for this regimen and other data based on Minsky et al
2. Patients who cannot tolerate cisplatin are treated with carboplatin (AUC = 5 mg/mL • min)

Therapy Monitoring

1. *Weekly:* H&P
2. *Before each cycle:* CBC with differential and serum electrolytes, BUN, creatinine, and magnesium
3. *Response evaluation:* 5–6 weeks after completion of therapy

Efficacy (N = 109)

Median duration of response	4.2 months
Alive/no failure	25%
Locoregional failure at 2 years	52%
Distant failure	16%
Treatment-related death	2%

Toxicity (N = 109/99)

Grade	% Acute Toxicities	% Late Toxicities
1	1	20
2	26	22
3	43	24
4	26	13
5	2	0

Maximum toxicity per patient based on RTOG morbidity scale. N = 109 for acute toxicity and 99 for late toxicity

Treatment Modifications

Adverse Event	Dose Modification
G3/4 toxicity	A minimum 1-week treatment delay. Resume when toxicity is grade ≤2. Continue radiation if toxicity is unrelated to radiation therapy (RT)
If during weeks 1, 5, 9, or 13, day 1: ANC ≥2000/mm^3 but <3000/mm^3 or platelets ≥75,000/mm^3 but <100,000/mm^3	Reduce cisplatin and fluorouracil dosages by 25%; continue RT
If during weeks 1, 5, 9, or 13, day 1: ANC <2000/mm^3 or platelets <75,000/mm^3	Hold chemotherapy and RT until toxicity resolves, then reduce cisplatin and fluorouracil dosages by 50%
ANC <1000/mm^3 or platelets ≤75,000/mm^3 between cycles on days chemotherapy is not administered	Reduce cisplatin and fluorouracil dosages by 50%
Serum creatinine = 1.6–2.0 mg/dL (141–177 µmol/L)	Reduce cisplatin dosage by 50%
Creatinine >2.0 mg/dL (>177 µmol/L	Discontinue cisplatin; continue RT
G3/4 stomatitis during fluorouracil treatment	Do not administer additional fluorouracil during that cycle. Reduce all subsequent fluorouracil dosages by 25%
G3/4 stomatitis on days chemotherapy not administered	Reduce all subsequent fluorouracil dosages by 25%
G ≥3 RT-related toxicity	Hold RT, and resume when toxicity is G ≤2

REGIMEN

WEEKLY IRINOTECAN + CISPLATIN + CONCURRENT RADIOTHERAPY

Ilson DH et al. J Clin Oncol 2003;21:2926–2932
Enzinger PC et al. Proc Am Soc Clin Oncol 2006;24:194s [abstract 4064]

Weeks 1 to 5: Induction chemotherapy therapy once weekly on weeks 1, 2, 4, and 5; rest on week 3

Hydration with cisplatin: ≥1000 mL 0.9% sodium chloride injection (0.9% NS) or 5% dextrose/0.45% sodium chloride injection (D5W/0.45% NS); administer intravenously over 2–4 hours as tolerated before starting cisplatin administration. Also, encourage patients to increase oral intake of non-alcoholic fluids. Monitor serum electrolytes and replace as needed (potassium, magnesium, sodium)

Cisplatin 30 mg/m² per dose; administer intravenously in 50–500 mL 0.9% NS over 30 minutes for 4 doses on weeks 1, 2, 4, and 5 (total dosage during induction = 120 mg/m²), *followed by:*
Irinotecan 65 mg/m² per dose; administer intravenously in 250 mL 0.9% NS or 5% dextrose injection (D5W) over 30 minutes for 4 doses after cisplatin, during weeks 1, 2, 4, and 5 (total dosage during induction = 260 mg/m²)

Supportive Care
Antiemetic prophylaxis
Emetogenic potential is **HIGH**
See Chapter 39 for antiemetic recommendations

Hematopoietic growth factor (CSF) prophylaxis
Primary prophylaxis is NOT indicated
See Chapter 43 for more information

Antimicrobial prophylaxis
Risk of fever and neutropenia is LOW
 Antimicrobial primary prophylaxis to be considered:
 • Antibacterial—not indicated
 • Antifungal—not indicated
 • Antiviral—not indicated unless patient previously had an episode of HSV
See Chapter 47 for more information

Acute cholinergic syndrome
Atropine sulfate 0.25–1 mg administered subcutaneously or intravenously if abdominal cramping or diarrhea develop during or within 1 hour after irinotecan administration
• If symptoms are severe, add as primary prophylaxis at least 30 minutes before irinotecan during subsequent cycles
• For irinotecan, acute cholinergic syndrome is characterized by abdominal cramping, diarrhea, diaphoresis, hypotension, flushing, bradycardia, rhinitis, increased salivation, meiosis, and lacrimation

Weeks 6 and 7: Two-week rest period
Weeks 8 to 14: Chemoradiotherapy:
  Chemotherapy—weekly each Monday of weeks 8, 9, 11, and 12
  Radiation therapy—1.8 Gy daily; total dose of 50.4 Gy

Hydration with cisplatin: ≥1000 mL 0.9% NS or D5W/0.45% NS; administer intravenously over 2–4 hours as tolerated before starting cisplatin administration. Also, encourage patients to increase oral intake of non-alcoholic fluids. Monitor serum electrolytes and replace as needed (potassium, magnesium, sodium)
Cisplatin 30 mg/m² per dose; administer intravenously in 50–500 mL 0.9% NS over 30 minutes for 4 doses during weeks 8, 9, 11, and 12 (total dosage during induction = 120 mg/m²), *followed by:*
Irinotecan 65 mg/m² per dose; administer intravenously in 250 mL 0.9% NS or D5W over 30 minutes for 4 doses after cisplatin, during weeks 8, 9, 11, and 12 (total dosage during induction = 260 mg/m²)

Supportive Care
Antiemetic prophylaxis
Emetogenic potential is **HIGH**
See Chapter 39 for antiemetic recommendations

Hematopoietic growth factor (CSF) prophylaxis
Primary prophylaxis is NOT indicated
See Chapter 43 for more information

Antimicrobial prophylaxis
Risk of fever and neutropenia is LOW
 Antimicrobial primary prophylaxis to be considered:
 • Antibacterial—not indicated
 • Antifungal—not indicated
 • Antiviral—not indicated unless patient previously had an episode of HSV
See Chapter 47 for more information

(continued)

(*continued*)

Thromboprophylaxis
Low-dose **warfarin** 1 mg/day; administer orally beginning 3 days before the initiation of combined chemoradiotherapy and continuing until 4 weeks after completion of combined chemoradiotherapy

Acute cholinergic syndrome
Atropine sulfate 0.25–1 mg subcutaneously if abdominal cramping or diarrhea develop within 1 hour after irinotecan infusion
• If symptoms are severe, add as primary prophylaxis during subsequent cycles
• For irinotecan, acute cholinergic syndrome is characterized by abdominal cramps, diarrhea, diaphoresis, hypotension, bradycardia, rhinitis, increased salivation, visual disturbances, and lacrimation

Radiation therapy (notes):
• Delivered with megavoltage equipment (15 MV) using a multiple-field technique. Patients treated 5 days per week at 1.8 Gy/day to a total dose of 50.4 Gy
• All fields treated each day
• Portal films of at least 2 fields obtained each week or more often if needed
• Treatment delivered to 4 fields (anterior-posterior, posterior-anterior, and opposed laterals) such that dose does not vary by more than 5% over the entire target volume
• Dose prescribed to the isodose line to cover the volume at risk
• Use lung inhomogeneity corrections
• Superior and inferior borders of the radiation field should be 5 cm beyond the primary tumor
• Lateral, anterior, and posterior borders of the field should be ≥2 cm beyond the borders of the primary tumor
• Tumor size defined by EUS, barium swallow or CT scan (whichever is larger)
• Primary and regional lymph nodes included in radiation field

Week 18: Surgery after 4-week rest period

Treatment Modifications

Adverse Event	Dose Modifications*
During Induction Chemotherapy	
WBC <2000/mm^3, ANC <1000/mm^3, platelet count <75,000/mm^3, serum creatinine >1.6 mg/dL (>141 μmol/L), or G3/4 diarrheal toxicity	Delay chemotherapy until WBC ≥2000/mm^3, ANC ≥1000/mm^3, platelet count ≥75,000/mm^3, serum creatinine ≤1.6 mg/dL (≤141 μmol/L), and diarrheal toxicity G ≤2
If the fourth treatment (week 5) of induction therapy is delayed more than 1 week because of hematologic or diarrheal toxicity	Do not administer fourth treatment (week 5) of induction therapy (shortened to 3 treatment weeks); proceed to combined chemoradiotherapy after a minimum 2-week rest period
WBC <2000/mm^3, ANC <1000/mm^3, platelet count <75,000/mm^3, serum creatinine >1.6 mg/dL (>141 μmol/L), or G3/4 diarrheal toxicity after the second treatment (week 2)	Reduce irinotecan dosage to 50 mg/m^2 · dose to permit delivery of a third and final induction course
Serum creatinine >1.6 mg/dL (<141 μmol/L) but ≤2 mg/dL (≤177 μmol/L)	Reduce cisplatin dosage to 15 mg/m^2 · dose
During Chemoradiotherapy	
Serum creatinine >1.6 mg/dL (>141 μmol/L) but ≤2 mg/dL (≤177 μmol/L)	Reduce cisplatin dosage to 15 mg/m^2 · dose

Note: Do not reduce irinotecan dosage during combined chemoradiotherapy

Patient Population Studied

Squamous cell carcinoma, adenocarcinoma, or poorly differentiated non–small cell carcinoma of the esophagus, which was locally advanced. Staged by computed tomography (CT) scan and endoscopic ultrasound (EUS). Included clinical stages II to III disease ($T_1 N_1 M_0$, $T_{2-4} N_{0-1} M_0$). Patients with T1N0 disease excluded. For tumors of the gastroesophageal junction, at least 50% of the tumor had to involve the distal esophagus

Efficacy*
(N = 19)

All Patients

CCR[†] or PCR[‡]	6/19 (32%) (95% confidence interval, 13–55%)[§]
Median OS	25 months (range: 8.6–35.2 months); 8 (42%) alive and free of disease at a median follow-up of 21 months
Patients with CCR or PCR	4/6 free of disease at a median follow-up of 26.7 months
Patients with viable cancer at surgery	4/10 free of disease at a median follow-up of 19.2 months
Documented recurrent disease	6 patients—3 recurrences of distant disease only; 3 first site of recurrence locoregionally (anastomotic recurrence, n = 1; mediastinal nodal recurrence, n = 2)

Dysphagia at Baseline (N = 16)

Resolved	10/16 (62%)
Improved	3/16 (19%)
No change or worsening	3/16 (19%)

Surgical Resection Not Undertaken (4/19; 21%)

Metastatic disease in abdominal lymph nodes outside radiotherapy field	2 (11%)
Clinical complete response (negative posttreatment endoscopy with negative biopsy); 1 durable 34+ months after therapy initiated	2 (11%)
Death of probable locally recurrent disease, with fatal hematemesis, 2 years after initiation of therapy	1 (7%)

Surgical Resection Undertaken (15/19; 79%)

Complete resections with negative margins	14 (73%)
PCR	4 (21%)
Evidence of down-staging at surgery	11 (58%)

Surgical Complications

Anastomotic leak	4/15 (27%)
Wound infection	3/15 (20%)
Postoperative death	1/15 (7%) (Protracted postoperative complications including diaphragmatic wound dehiscence)

*Modified WHO
[†]CCR: Clinical complete response
[‡]PCR: Pathologic complete response
[§]Seen at all irinotecan dose levels, including 2 PCR in 3 patients at 40 mg/m² · dose, 2 CCR at 50 mg/m² · dose and 65 mg/m² · dose, and 2 PCR in 6 patients treated at 80 mg/m² · dose

Therapy Monitoring

1. Complete blood counts with differential leukocyte counts at least weekly
2. LFTs, serum BUN, and creatinine before each chemotherapy administration
3. Assessment of response after induction chemotherapy and after chemoradiotherapy

Adverse Event (N = 19)

Toxicity	Grade (%)			
	1	2	3	4
Induction Chemotherapy				
Hematologic Toxicity				
WBC	42	21	11	0
Absolute neutrophil count	21	5	32	0
Platelets	5	0	0	0
Hemoglobin	16	11	0	0
Nonhematologic Toxicity				
Diarrhea	68	26	5	0
Nausea	42	5	0	0
Vomiting	21	5	0	0
Stomatitis	5	0	0	0
Fatigue	63	21	0	0
Pulmonary/cough, dyspnea	5	5	0	0
Constipation	26	0	0	0
Alopecia	5	0	—	—
Dermatologic	11	0	0	0
Chemoradiotherapy				
Hematologic Toxicity				
WBC	84	53	26	0
Absolute neutrophil count	53	16	21	0
Platelets	58	11	5	0
Hemoglobin	37	21	5	0
Nonhematologic Toxicity				
Diarrhea	32	21	0	0
Esophagitis	32	5	0	0
Nausea	58	0	0	0
Vomiting	21	0	0	0
Stomatitis	21	0	0	0
Fatigue	58	11	0	0
Thrombosis	0	0	5	16
Alopecia	11	5	—	—
Pulmonary/dyspnea	0	21	5	0
Dermatologic	11	0	0	0
Hypomagnesemia	11	5	5	0
Hypotension	0	5	0	0
Anorexia	11	0	0	0
Dehydration	0	5	0	0

CTCAE

REGIMEN

OXALIPLATIN + PROTRACTED INFUSION FLUOROURACIL AND EXTERNAL BEAM RADIATION THERAPY (EBRT) PRIOR TO SURGERY

Leichman L et al. Proc Am Soc Clin Oncol 2009;27:205s [abstract 4513]

Neoadjuvant combined modality therapy:

Oxaliplatin 85 mg/m^2 per dose; administer intravenously in 250–500 mL 5% dextrose injection (D5W) over 2 hours for 3 doses on days 1, 15, and 29 (total dosage/course = 255 mg/m^2)

Protracted infusion fluorouracil 180 mg/m^2 per day; administer by continuous intravenous infusion in 50–1000 mL 0.9% sodium chloride injection (0.9% NS) or D5W over 24 hours for 35 consecutive days, days 8–43 (total dosage/35-day course = 6300 mg/m^2)

External beam radiation therapy 180 cGy/day starting day 8, on 5 days/week for 25 fractions, to a total dose 4500 cGy

Esophagectomy:

Two to 4 weeks after completing neoadjuvant combined modality therapy

Adjuvant chemotherapy (optional after recovery from surgery):

Oxaliplatin 85 mg/m^2 per dose; administer intravenously in 250–500 mL D5W over 2 hours for 3 doses on days 1, 15, and 29 (total dosage/course = 255 mg/m^2)

Protracted infusion fluorouracil 180 mg/m^2 per day; administer by continuous intravenous infusion in 50–1000 mL 0.9% NS or D5W over 24 hours for 35 consecutive days, days 8–43 (total dosage/35-day course = 6300 mg/m^2)

Note: Postoperative chemotherapy was not given to all patients; not given to patients with pathologic complete response. In study reported, <50% received postoperative chemotherapy. The investigators recommended completing *all* therapy before surgery

Supportive Care

Antiemetic prophylaxis

Emetogenic potential on days with oxaliplatin is **MODERATE**, *on days with fluorouracil without EBRT is* **LOW**, *and on days with fluorouracil + EBRT is* **LOW–MODERATE**

See Chapter 39 for antiemetic recommendations

Hematopoietic growth factor (CSF) prophylaxis

Primary prophylaxis is NOT indicated

See Chapter 43 for more information

Antimicrobial prophylaxis

Risk of fever and neutropenia is LOW

Antimicrobial primary prophylaxis to be considered:

- Antibacterial—not indicated
- Antifungal—not indicated
- Antiviral—not indicated unless patient previously had an episode of HSV

See Chapter 47 for more information

Patient Population Studied

Clinical stages II/III esophageal adenocarcinoma, Zubrod PS ≤2 and tumor <2 cm into the gastric cardia

Treatment Modifications

Adverse Event	Dose Modifications*
Inadequate hematologic recovery at time of oxaliplatin administration (absolute neutrophil count <1500/mm^3 or platelet count <10,0000/mm^3)	Delay therapy 1 week
Persistent G2 or any G3 neuropathy	Reduced oxaliplatin dosage by 25%

Adverse Event (N = 90)

Toxicity Grade (G)	Percent of Patients
Any G3 toxicity	43%
Any G4 toxicity	18%
Any G gastrointestinal toxicity	39%
Any G flu-like/fatigue	22%
Any G pulmonary toxicity	17%
Any G hematologic toxicity	16%
Any G mucositis toxicity	14%
Any G neurologic toxicity	3%
Death due to protocol*	4.5%

*Two a result of neoadjuvant combined modality therapy, two to surgery

Efficacy (N = 90)

Patients undergoing surgery	77 (86%)
Pathologic complete response	30 (33%)
Cancer in situ or T1N0M0	9 (10%)

Therapy Monitoring

1. Complete blood counts with differential leukocyte counts at least weekly
2. LFTs, serum BUN, and creatinine before each chemotherapy administration
3. Assessment of response after neoadjuvant combined modality therapy and after surgery

ADVANCED ESOPHAGEAL *OR* JUNCTIONAL CANCER PRE-OPERATIVE CHEMORADIOTHERAPY REGIMEN
CARBOPLATIN + PACLITAXEL + CONCURRENT RADIOTHERAPY

van Hagen P et al. N Engl J Med 2012;366:2074–2084

Hypersensitivity prophylaxis before paclitaxel:

Dexamethasone 20 mg per dose; administer orally for 2 doses: the first dose between 12 and 14 hours before starting paclitaxel, and a second dose 6–7 hours before starting paclitaxel

• Alternatively, give **Dexamethasone** 10 mg; administer intravenously 30 minutes before starting paclitaxel

Diphenhydramine 50 mg; administer by intravenous injection 30 minutes before starting paclitaxel

Ranitidine 50 mg; administer intravenously in 25–100 mL of 0.9% sodium chloride injection (0.9% NS) or 5% dextrose injection (D5W), over 15–30 minutes, 30–60 minutes before starting paclitaxel

Paclitaxel 50 mg/m² per dose; administer intravenously diluted in 0.9% NS or D5W to a concentration within the range 0.3–1.2 mg/mL over 60 minutes before carboplatin for 5 doses on days 1, 8, 15, 22, and 29 (total dosage/course = 250 mg/m²), *with:*

Carboplatin AUC = 2 mg/mL · min* per dose; administer intravenously diluted in 0.9% NS or D5W to a concentration >0.5 mg/mL over 60 minutes after paclitaxel for 5 doses on days 1, 8, 15, 22, and 29 (total course includes 5 doses each calculated to produce an AUC = 2 mg/mL · min*)

*Carboplatin dose is based on a formula described by Calvert et al. to achieve a target area under the plasma concentration versus time curve (AUC)

$$\text{Total carboplatin dose (mg)} = (\text{target AUC}) \times (\text{GFR} + 25)$$

In practice, creatinine clearance (Clcr) is used in place of glomerular filtration rate (GFR). Clcr can be estimated from the equation of Cockcroft and Gault, thus:

$$\text{For males, Clcr} = \frac{(140 - \text{age [years]}) \times (\text{body weight [kg]})}{72 \times (\text{serum creatinine [mg/dL]})}$$

$$\text{For females, Clcr} = \frac{(140 - \text{age [years]}) \times (\text{body weight [kg]})}{72 \times (\text{serum creatinine [mg/dL]})} \times 0.85$$

Calvert AH et al. J Clin Oncol 1989;7:1748–1756
Cockcroft DW, Gault MH. Nephron 1976;16:31–41
Jodrell DI et al. J Clin Oncol 1992;10:520–528
Sorensen BT et al. Cancer Chemother Pharmacol 1991;28:397–401

Note: On October 8, 2010, the U.S. Food and Drug Administration (FDA) identified a potential safety issue with carboplatin dosing based on recent changes in the measurement of serum creatinine. By the end of 2010, all clinical laboratories in the United States began using the standardized isotope dilution mass spectrometry (IDMS) method to measure serum creatinine, which could result in an overestimation of the GFR in some patients with normal renal function. A carboplatin dose calculated with an IDMS-measured serum creatinine result using the Calvert formula could exceed an expected exposure (AUC) and result in increased drug-related toxicity

Provided actual GFR measurements are made to assess renal function, carboplatin can be safely dosed according to the Calvert formula described in product labeling

If GFR (or creatinine clearance) is estimated based on serum creatinine measurements by the IDMS method, the FDA recommends for patients with normal renal function capping an estimated GFR at 125 mL/min for any targeted AUC value. No greater estimated GFR values should be used

U.S. Food and Drug Administration (FDA) Carboplatin dosing. [online] October 8, 2010. Available from: http://www.fda.gov/AboutFDA/CentersOffices/OfficeofMedicalProductsandTobacco/CDER/ucm228974.htm [accessed February 26, 2014]

Radiation Therapy
External beam radiation, using 3D conformal radiation technique

Fractionation Schedule
Administer a total dose of 41.4 Gy in 23 fractions of 1.8 Gy, 5 fractions per week, starting the first day of the first cycle of chemotherapy

Position of the Patient
Supine position. Assess reproducibility by orthogonal laser beams

(continued)

(continued)

Definitions of Target Volumes and Critical Structures
Define gross tumor volume (GTV) as the primary tumor and any enlarged regional lymph nodes, and draw on each relevant CT slice. Use available information including physical examination, endoscopy, EUS, and CT-thorax/abdomen to determine the GTV. The planning target volume (PTV) should provide a proximal and distal margin of 4 cm. In case of tumor extension into the stomach, use a distal margin of 3 cm. Provide a 2-cm radial margin around the GTV to include the area of subclinical involvement around the GTV and to compensate for tumor motion and setup variations. Contour both lungs. Contour the heart on all slices; include the infundibulum of the right ventricle and the apex of both atria in its cranial border and exclude the great vessels as much as possible. Define the caudal border as the lowest part of the left ventricle's inferior wall that is distinguishable from the liver. Contour the spinal canal to represent the spinal cord

Simulation Procedure
Prior to the start of the irradiation make a planning CT scan from the cricoid to L1 vertebra with a slice thickness of 5 mm, with the patient in treatment position. Determine the isocenter at the planning CT

Radiation Technique
Use a multiple-field technique. Give treatment with a combination of anterior/posterior, oblique or lateral field. Use customized blocks or a multileaf collimator to shape the treatment fields. Have all patients undergo 3D planning. Use beams-eye-view (BEV) to ensure optimal target volume coverage and optimal normal tissue sparing. Choose the most appropriate technical solutions (eg, beam quality, field arrangement, conformal therapy planning) as long as they comply with ICRU 50/62 safety margins and homogeneity requirements

Normal Tissue Tolerance
Obtain Dose-Volume- Histograms (DVHs) of both lungs, the heart, and spinal cord for all patients. Use DVHs primarily to document normal tissue damage. Use DVHs to help select the most appropriate treatment plan. Minimize the risks for severe pneumonitis for patients by the use of BEV planning and field-shaping (with optimal sparing of both lungs). Do not exceed spinal cord tolerance (50 Gy)

External Beam Equipment
Use megavoltage equipment with photon energies ≥6 MV. Use a multileaf collimator or individually shaped blocks to shape the irradiation portal according to the planning target volume

Dose Specification
Specify the prescription dose at the ICRU 50/62 reference point, which will be the isocenter for most patients. Ensure the daily prescription dose will be 1.8 Gy at the ICRU reference point and ensure the 95% isodose encompasses the entire planning target volume (PTV). Do not exceed the prescription dose by >7% (ICRU 50/62 guidelines) at the maximum to the PTV. Use tissue density inhomogeneity correction

Treatment Verification
Obtain portal images during the first fraction of all fields. On indication repeat portal images

Note: The median time between the end of chemoradiotherapy and surgery was 6.6 weeks (inter quartile range: 5.7 to 7.9)

Supportive Care
Antiemetic prophylaxis
Emetogenic potential is **HIGH** *on days with chemotherapy with potential for delayed symptoms*
Emetogenic potential with radiation therapy alone is **LOW–MODERATE**
See Chapter 39 for antiemetic recommendations

Hematopoietic growth factor (CSF) prophylaxis
Primary prophylaxis is NOT indicated
See Chapter 43 for more information

Antimicrobial prophylaxis
Risk of fever and neutropenia is LOW
  Antimicrobial primary prophylaxis to be considered:
  • Antibacterial—not indicated
  • Antifungal—not indicated
  • Antiviral—not indicated unless patient previously had an episode of HSV
See Chapter 47 for more information

Dose Modification

Adverse Event	Treatment Modification
WBC <1000/mm³ and/or platelets <50,000/mm³ on days 8, 15, 22, and 29	Delay chemotherapy by 1 week until WBC count is >1000/mm³ and platelet count is >50,000/mm³
Febrile neutropenia (ANC <500/mm³ and fever >38.5°C [>101.3°F])	Hold chemotherapy
Severe bleeding requiring ≥2 platelet transfusions	Hold chemotherapy
Hypersensitivity: Mild symptoms (eg flushing, rash, pruritus)	Complete paclitaxel infusion. Supervise at bedside. No treatment required
Hypersensitivity: Moderate symptoms (eg rash, flushing, mild dyspnea, chest discomfort, mild hypotension)	Stop paclitaxel infusion, give IV antihistamine (clemastine 2 mg or diphenhydramine 50 mg IV, or equivalent antihistamine) and dexamethasone (10 mg IV). After symptoms abate, resume paclitaxel infusion at a rate of 20 mL/hour for 15 minutes, then 50 mL/hour for 15 minutes. Then, if symptoms of hypersensitivity do not recur, at full dose-rate until infusion is completed
Hypersensitivity: Severe symptoms (one or more of the following): respiratory distress requiring treatment, generalized urticaria, angioedema, hypotension requiring therapy	Stop paclitaxel infusion, give IV antihistamine and steroid as above. Add epinephrine or bronchodilators if indicated, discontinue therapy
Creatinine ≤1.5 × the upper limit of normal on the day of retreatment	Continue therapy
Creatinine is >1.5 × the upper limit of normal	Establish intravenous hydration the evening preceding treatment at a flow rate sufficient to correct volume deficits and produce a urine flow ≥50 mL/hour. Repeat serum creatinine measurement in the morning. If repeated serum creatinine result is ≤1.5 × the upper limit of normal → proceed with treatment. Stop chemotherapy if the repeated serum creatinine result is >1.5 × the upper limit of normal
Mucositis with oral ulcers or protracted vomiting despite antiemetic premedication	Delay chemotherapy one week
G ≤2 neurotoxicity	Continue therapy
G >2 neurotoxicity	Discontinue chemotherapy
Asymptomatic bradycardia or isolated and asymptomatic ventricular extrasystoles	Continue therapy under continuous cardiac monitoring
First-degree AV block	Continue therapy under continuous cardiac monitoring
Symptomatic arrhythmia or AV block (except first degree) or other heart blocks	Continue therapy under continuous cardiac monitoring. Stop paclitaxel, manage arrhythmia according to standard practice, until patient goes off protocol.
G4 radiation induced esophagitis	Hold both chemotherapy and radiotherapy until the esophagitis is G ≤3

Efficacy

	Chemoradiotherapy + Surgery (N = 161)	Surgery Alone (N = 161)	P
R0 resection achieved	148 (92%)	111 (69%)	<0.001
Median number of lymph nodes resected	15	18	0.77
≥1 positive lymph node in resection specimen	50 (31%)	120 (75%)	<0.001
Median disease-free survival	Not reached	24.2 months	<0.001 HR, 0.498 95% CI 0.357–0.693
Median overall survival (ITT)	49.4 months	24.0 months	0.003 HR, 0.657 95% CI 0.495–0.871
1-Year overall survival rate	82%	70%	HR, 0.665 95% CI 0.500–0.884
2-Year overall survival rate	67%	50%	
3-Year overall survival rate	58%	44%	
5-Year overall survival rate	47%	34%	

Toxicity

Adverse Events During Neoadjuvant Chemoradiotherapy and After Surgery*

Event	Chemoradiotherapy and Surgery (N = 171)	Surgery Alone (N = 186)
Postoperative Events		
Event	Number of Patients (%)†	
Pulmonary complications‡	78/168 (46)	82/186 (44)
Cardiac complications§	36/168 (21)	31/186 (17)
Chylothorax	17/168 (10)	11/186 (6)
Mediastinitis	5/168 (3)	12/186 (6)
Anastomotic leakage	36/161 (22)	48/161 (30)
Death		
In hospital	6/168 (4)	8/186 (4)
After 30 days	4/168 (2)	5/186 (3)

Events During Chemoradiotherapy

Event	Number of Patients (%)	
	Any Grade	Grade ≥3
Anorexia	51 (30)	9 (5)
Alopecia	25 (15)	—
Constipation	47 (27)	1 (1)
Diarrhea	30 (18)	2 (1)
Esophageal perforation	1 (1)	1 (1)
Esophagitis	32 (19)	2 (1)
Fatigue	115 (67)	5 (3)
Nausea	91 (53)	2 (1)
Neurotoxic effects	25 (15)	—
Vomiting	43 (25)	1 (1)
Leukopenia	103 (60)	11 (6)
Neutropenia	16 (9)	4 (2)
Thrombocytopenia	92 (54)	1 (1)

*Adverse events according to NCI CTCAE, National Cancer Institute (USA) Common Terminology Criteria for Adverse Events, version 3. At: http://ctep.cancer.gov/protocolDevelopment/electronic_applications/ctc.htm [accessed December 7, 2013]
†168/171 patients treated with chemoradiotherapy underwent surgery
‡Includes pneumonia (isolation of pathogen from sputum culture and a new or progressive infiltrate on CXR), serious atelectasis (lobar collapse on chest radiograph), pneumothorax (collection of air, requiring drainage), pleural effusion (collection of fluid, requiring drainage), pulmonary embolus (detected on spiral CT or V/Q mismatch on scintigraphy), and acute respiratory failure (partial pressure of arterial oxygen <60 mm Hg while breathing ambient air)
§Including arrhythmia (any change in rhythm requiring treatment), myocardial infarction, and left ventricular failure (marked pulmonary edema on CXR)

Patient Population Studied

Patients with histologically confirmed, potentially curable squamous-cell carcinoma, adenocarcinoma, or large-cell undifferentiated carcinoma of the esophagus or esophagogastric junction (ie, tumors involving both the cardia and the esophagus on endoscopy) were eligible for inclusion in the study. The upper border of the tumor had to be ≥3 cm below the upper esophageal sphincter. Patients who had proximal gastric tumors with minimal invasion of the esophagus were excluded. The length and width of the tumor could not exceed 8 cm and 5 cm, respectively. Only patients with tumors of clinical stage T1N1 or T2-3N0-1 and no clinical evidence of metastatic spread (M0), according to the International Union against Cancer tumor–node–metastasis (TNM) classification, were enrolled. Eligible patients had a World Health Organization performance status score ≤2 and had lost ≤10% of body weight

Treatment Monitoring

1. Tumor assessment every 2 cycles
2. CBC with differential and serum creatinine: weekly while receiving chemotherapy; and at completion of chemoradiotherapy
3. During the first year after treatment completed, see patients every 3 months. In the second year, every 6 months, and then at the end of each year until 5 years after treatment

ADVANCED ESOPHAGEAL (and GASTRIC) CANCER FIRST-LINE THERAPY REGIMEN
CISPLATIN + CAPECITABINE

Kang Y-K et al. Ann Oncol 2009;20:666–673

Hydration before cisplatin: 1000 mL 0.9% sodium chloride injection (0.9% NS); administer intravenously over a minimum of 1 hour before commencing cisplatin administration

Cisplatin 80 mg/m^2; administer intravenously in 50–500 mL 0.9% NS over 2 hours on day 1, every 3 weeks (total dosage/cycle = 80 mg/m^2)

Hydration after cisplatin: ≥1000 mL 0.9% NS; administer intravenously over a minimum of 2 hours. Monitor and replace magnesium and other electrolytes as needed. Encourage patients to increase their intake of nonalcoholic fluids

Capecitabine 1000 mg/m^2 per dose; administer orally twice daily with water within 30 minutes after a meal for 14 consecutive days (28 doses) on days 1–14, every 3 weeks (total dosage/cycle = 28,000 mg/m^2)

Supportive Care
Antiemetic prophylaxis
Emetogenic potential on day 1 is **HIGH**. *Potential for delayed symptoms*
Emetogenic potential with capecitabine alone is **MINIMAL–LOW**
See Chapter 39 for antiemetic recommendations

Hematopoietic growth factor (CSF) prophylaxis
Primary prophylaxis may be indicated
See Chapter 43 for more information

Antimicrobial prophylaxis
Risk of fever and neutropenia is LOW
Antimicrobial primary prophylaxis to be considered:
- Antibacterial—not indicated
- Antifungal—not indicated
- Antiviral—not indicated unless patient previously had an episode of HSV

See Chapter 47 for more information

Oral care
Risk of mucositis/stomatitis is HIGH
General advice:
- Encourage patients to maintain intake of non-alcoholic fluids
- Evaluate patients for oral pain and provide analgesic medications
- Consider histamine (H$_2$-subtype) receptor antagonists (eg, ranitidine, famotidine), or a proton pump inhibitor for epigastric pain
- Probiotics containing *Lactobacillus* sp. may be beneficial in preventing diarrhea

Patients with intact oral mucosa:
- Clean the mouth, tongue, and gums by brushing after every meal and at bedtime with an ultrasoft toothbrush with fluoride toothpaste
- Floss teeth gently every day unless contraindicated. If gums bleed and hurt, avoid bleeding or sore areas, but floss other teeth
- Patients may use saline or commercial bland, nonalcoholic rinses
  - Do not use mouthwashes that contain alcohols

If mucositis or stomatitis is present:
- Keep the mouth moist utilizing water, ice chips, sugarless gum, sugar-free hard candies, or a saliva substitute
- Rinse mouth several times a day to remove debris
  - Use a solution of ¼ teaspoon (1.25 g) each of baking soda and table salt (sodium chloride) in 1 quart (~950 mL) of warm water. Follow with a plain-water rinse
  - Do not use mouthwashes that contain alcohols
- Foam-tipped swabs (eg, Toothettes) are useful in moisturizing oral mucosa, but ineffective for cleansing teeth and removing plaque
- Advise patients who develop mucositis to:
  - Choose foods that are easy to chew and swallow
  - Take small bites of food, chew slowly, and sip liquids with meals
  - Encourage soft, moist foods such as cooked cereals, mashed potatoes, and scrambled eggs
  - For trouble swallowing, soften food with gravies, sauces, broths, yogurt, or other bland liquids
  - Avoid sharp, crunchy foods; hot, spicy or highly acidic foods (eg, citrus fruits and juices); sugary foods; toothpicks; tobacco products; alcoholic drinks

Treatment Modifications

Adverse Event	Dose Modification
ANC nadir <1000/mm³ or platelet nadir <50,000/mm³ after treatment	Delay treatment until ANC ≥1000/mm³ *and* platelet ≥50,000/mm³, then decrease cisplatin dosage by 25%, and decrease daily capecitabine dosages by 50% during subsequent cycles*. Alternatively, consider using hematopoietic growth factors
Serum creatinine >1.5 mg/dL (>133 μmol/L), but <3 mg/dL (<265 μmol/L) *or* creatinine clearance >40 mL/min but <60 mL/min (>0.66 mL/s, but <1 mL/s)	Delay treatment until serum creatinine ≤1.5 mg/dL (≤133 μmol/L), then decrease cisplatin dosage by 50%*
Serum creatinine >3 mg/dL (>265 μmol/L) *or* creatinine clearance <40 mL/min (<0.66 mL/s)	Stop cisplatin
Persistent G2 neuropathy	Hold cisplatin until toxicity resolves to G ≤1; reduce dose by 25% for subsequent cycles
Transient G3/4 neuropathy (duration 7–14 days)	Hold cisplatin. Resume cisplatin after toxicity resolves with dosage reduced by 25% for subsequent cycles
Persistent G3/4 neuropathy	Discontinue cisplatin
G3/4 nonhematologic adverse events other than renal function and neurotoxicity	Reduce cisplatin and capecitabine dosages by 25% for subsequent cycles
G2 stomatitis, diarrhea, or nausea	Hold capecitabine; resume capecitabine at full dosage after resolution of toxicity
Second episode of G2 stomatitis, diarrhea, or nausea	Hold capecitabine; resume capecitabine with dosage reduced by 25% after resolution of toxicity
Third episode of G2 stomatitis, diarrhea, or nausea	Hold capecitabine; resume capecitabine with dosage reduced by 50% after resolution of toxicity
Fourth episode of G2 stomatitis, diarrhea, or nausea	Discontinue capecitabine
G3 stomatitis, diarrhea, or nausea, first episode	Hold capecitabine; if G3 toxicity is adequately controlled within 2 days, resume capecitabine at full dosage when toxicity resolves to G ≤1. If G3 toxicity takes >2 days to be controlled, resume capecitabine with dosage reduced by 25% after toxicity resolves to G ≤1
Second episode of G3 stomatitis, diarrhea, or nausea	Hold capecitabine; if G3 toxicity is controlled adequately within 2 days, then resume capecitabine with dosage reduced by 50% after toxicity resolves to G ≤1
Third episode of G3 stomatitis, diarrhea, or nausea	Discontinue capecitabine
G4 stomatitis, diarrhea, or nausea	Withhold capecitabine. Resume capecitabine with dosage reduced by 50% after toxicity resolves
G1 capecitabine-associated PPE[†]	Begin pyridoxine 50 mg orally 3 times daily and continue capecitabine without dose modification
G2 capecitabine-associated PPE[†]	Begin pyridoxine 50 mg orally 3 times daily and withhold capecitabine. Resume capecitabine with dosage reduced by 15% after toxicity resolves
G3 capecitabine-associated PPE[†]	Begin pyridoxine 50 mg orally 3 times daily and withhold capecitabine. Resume capecitabine with dosage reduced by 30% after toxicity resolves
Recurrent G3 capecitabine-associated PPE[†]	Begin pyridoxine 50 mg orally 3 times daily and withhold capecitabine. Resume capecitabine with dosage reduced by 50% after toxicity resolves

*Treatment delays for unresolved adverse events of >3 weeks duration warrant discontinuation of treatment
†PPE, Palmar plantar erythrodysesthesia (hand-foot syndrome)

Efficacy

	Capecitabine + Cisplatin	Fluorouracil + Cisplatin	Hazard Ratio (95%CI)	P Value
Median progression-free survival	5.6 months	5.0 months	0.81 (0.63–1.04)	<0.001*
Median overall survival	10.5 months	9.3 months	0.85 (0.64–1.13)	0.008*
Objective response rate	46 (38–55)†	32 (24–41)†	1.80 (1.11–2.94)‡	0.020
Complete response	2%	3%		
Partial response	44%	29%		
Mean time to response	3.7 months	3.8 months	1.61 (1.10–2.35)	0.015
Median duration of response	7.6 months	6.2 months	0.88 (0.56–1.36)	0.554

*For noninferiority versus 1.25
†95% CI in parentheses
‡Odds ratio (95% CI)

Patient Population Studied

Patients with histologically confirmed measurable advanced gastric cancer, a Karnofsky performance status of seventy or more, no previous chemotherapy other than neoadjuvant or adjuvant regimens, no radiotherapy to target lesions, and adequate hepatic, cardiac, and renal function, the latter defined as an estimated creatinine clearance $\geq$60 mL/min estimated with the Cockcroft and Gault formula

Treatment Monitoring

1. Tumor assessment every 2 cycles
2. CBC with differential before the start of a new cycle

Toxicity

Treatment-Related Adverse Events (in >15% of patients) by NCI-CTC*

No. (%) of Patients

Adverse Event	Capecitabine + Cisplatin (N = 156)				Fluorouracil + Cisplatin (N = 155)			
	G1	G2	G3	G4	G1	G2	G3	G4
Nausea	49 (31)	35 (22)	3 (2)	—	44 (28)	37 (24)	4 (3)	—
Vomiting	32 (21)	33 (21)	10 (6)	1 (<1)	31 (20)	47 (30)	13 (8)	—
Diarrhea	9 (6)	14 (9)	7 (4)	1 (<1)	11 (7)	6 (4)	6 (4)	1 (<1)
Stomatitis	11 (7)	4 (3)	3 (2)	—	15 (10)	16 (10)	10 (6)	—
Neutropenia	2 (1)	24 (15)	22 (14)	3 (2)	2 (1)	15 (10)	23 (15)	6 (4)
Leucopenia	3 (2)	15 (10)	4 (3)	—	4 (3)	16 (10)	4 (3)	2 (1)
Anorexia	23 (15)	18 (12)	3 (2)	—	23 (15)	19 (12)	1 (<1)	—
Fatigue	15 (10)	8 (5)	1 (<1)	—	11 (7)	3 (2)	1 (<1)	—
Asthenia	10 (6)	9 (6)	3 (2)	—	14 (9)	12 (8)	1 (<1)	—
Hand-foot syndrome	20 (13)	8 (5)	6 (4)	—	5 (3)	1 (<1)	—	—

*NCI, CTC, National Cancer Institute (USA) Common Toxicity Criteria, version 2.0. At: http://ctep.cancer.gov/protocolDevelopment/electronic_applications/ctc.htm [accessed December 7, 2013]

REGIMEN

IRINOTECAN + CISPLATIN

Ilson DH et al. J Clin Oncol 1999;17:3270–3275

Hydration before cisplatin: 5% dextrose/0.9% sodium chloride injection (D5W/0.9% NS) or 0.9% NS ≥500 mL; administer intravenously over a minimum of 1 hour. Also encourage patients to increase oral intake of non-alcoholic fluids. Monitor serum electrolytes and replace as needed (potassium, magnesium, sodium)

Cisplatin 25–30 mg/m² per dose; administer intravenously in 25–100 mL 0.9% sodium chloride injection (0.9% NS) over 30–60 minutes weekly for 4 consecutive weeks (4 doses) on days 1, 8, 15, and 22, followed by 20 days (days 23–42) without cisplatin (total dosage/cycle = 100–120 mg/m²) *followed by:*

Irinotecan 50–65 mg/m² per dose; administer intravenously in a volume of 5% dextrose injection (D5W) sufficient to produce a solution with concentration of 0.12–2.8 mg/mL over 30 minutes, weekly, for 4 consecutive weeks (4 doses) on days 1, 8, 15, and 22, followed by 20 days (days 23–42) without irinotecan (total dosage/cycle = 200–260 mg/m²)

Supportive Care

Antiemetic prophylaxis

Emetogenic potential on days of chemotherapy is **HIGH**. *Potential for delayed symptoms*
See Chapter 39 for antiemetic recommendations

Hematopoietic growth factor (CSF) prophylaxis

Primary prophylaxis is NOT indicated
See Chapter 43 for more information

Antimicrobial prophylaxis

Risk of fever and neutropenia is LOW
Antimicrobial primary prophylaxis to be considered:
- Antibacterial—not indicated
- Antifungal—not indicated
- Antiviral—not indicated unless patient previously had an episode of HSV

See Chapter 47 for more information

Acute cholinergic syndrome

Atropine sulfate 0.25–1 mg administer subcutaneously or intravenously if abdominal cramping or diarrhea develop during or within 1 hour after irinotecan administration

- If symptoms are severe, add as primary prophylaxis at least 30 minutes before irinotecan during subsequent cycles
- For irinotecan, acute cholinergic syndrome may be characterized by: abdominal cramping, diarrhea, diaphoresis, hypotension, flushing, bradycardia, rhinitis, increased salivation, meiosis, and lacrimation

Diarrhea management

Latent or delayed onset diarrhea*:
Loperamide 4 mg orally initially after the first loose or liquid stool, *then*
Loperamide 2 mg orally every 2 hours during waking hours, *plus*
Loperamide 4 mg orally every 4 hours during hours of sleep

- Continue for at least 12 hours after diarrhea resolves
- Recurrent diarrhea after a 12-hour diarrhea free interval is treated as a new episode
- Rehydrate orally with fluids and electrolytes during a diarrheal episode
- If diarrhea persists >48 hours despite loperamide, stop loperamide and hospitalize the patient for IV hydration

Persistent diarrhea:
Octreotide 100–150 mcg subcutaneously 3 times daily. Maximum total daily dose is 1500 mcg

Antibiotic therapy during latent or delayed onset diarrhea:
Ciprofloxacin 500 mg orally every 12 hours if absolute neutrophil count <500/mm³ with or without accompanying fever in association with diarrhea

- Antibiotics should also be administered if patient is hospitalized with prolonged diarrhea and should be continued until diarrhea resolves

*Rothenberg ML et al. J Clin Oncol 2001;19:3801–3807; Wadler S et al. J Clin Oncol 1998;16:3169–3178

(*continued*)

Patient Population Studied

A study of 35 patients with advanced (unresectable or metastatic) esophageal adenocarcinoma or squamous cell carcinoma with good performance status

Efficacy (N = 35)

Complete response	6%
Partial response	51%
Minor response	20%
Stable disease	20%
Disease progression	3%
Median duration of response	4.2 months

Treatment Modifications

Adverse Event	Dose Modification
G3/4 diarrhea or mucositis	Reduce irinotecan dosage by 10 mg/m² per dose
G4 fatigue >3 days	
On the day of retreatment if ANC <1000/mm³, WBC <3000/mm³, or platelet <100,000/mm³	Hold treatment until ANC ≥1000/mm³, WBC ≥3000/mm³, *and* platelet ≥100,000/mm³ No dosage reductions for treatment delays ≤1 week. Reduce irinotecan dosage by 10 mg/m² per dose if treatment is delayed >2 weeks, for febrile neutropenia, or for bleeding from thrombocytopenia
If blood counts on day 22 do not permit administering the fourth week of planned chemotherapy	Shorten treatment to a 5-week cycle: 3 consecutive weeks of treatment (days 1, 8, and 15), followed by 20 consecutive days without chemotherapy (days 16–35)
Serum creatinine >1.7 mg/dL (>150 μmol/L), but <2.0 mg/dL (<177 μmol/L)	Reduce cisplatin dosage to 15 mg/m² per dose
G ≥2 diarrhea or mucositis on treatment days	Hold treatment for 1 week

Note: If toxicities warrant holding either drug, both drugs are held
One-week treatment delays are common owing to leukocyte counts <3000/mm³ and ANC <1000/mm³ on treatment days

(*continued*)

Oral care

- Encourage patients to maintain intake of non-alcoholic fluids

If mucositis or stomatitis is present:

- Rinse mouth several times a day with ¼ teaspoon (1.25 g) each of baking soda and table salt in one quart of warm water. Follow with a plain water rinse
  - Do not use mouthwashes that contain alcohols

Toxicity (N = 35)

	% G1/2	% G3/4
Hematologic		
Neutropenia	43	46
Anemia	69	31
Thrombocytopenia	57	0
Nonhematologic		
Diarrhea	74	11
Fatigue	97	3
Nausea	94	6
Vomiting	45	3
Cardiac	0	3
Renal	60	3
Pulmonary/dyspnea	52	0
Neurosensory	54	0
Neurocerebellar	0	3
Skin	43	0
Stomatitis	20	0
Increased bilirubin	3	0

NCI, CTC, National Cancer Institute (USA) Common Toxicity Criteria, version 2.0. At: http://ctep.cancer.gov/protocolDevelopment/electronic_applications/ctc.htm [accessed December 7, 2013]
Reported as percent of patients experiencing toxicity at any time during therapy

Therapy Monitoring

1. *Pretreatment:* Complete H&P, 12-lead ECG, CBC, PT, PTT, serum electrolytes, BUN, creatinine, mineral panel and LFTs, urinalysis, chest x-ray, ± double-contrast barium esophagram, and chest and abdominal CT

2. *Before each cycle:* CBC and serum electrolytes, magnesium BUN, creatinine, mineral panel, and LFTs, with weekly intracycle CBC and serum creatinine

3. *Response evaluation:* After the first and second cycles and after every second cycle thereafter

Notes

Alternate infusion schedule of 2 weeks on and 1 week off may be better for some patients (days 1 and 8 every 21 days)

REGIMEN

EPIRUBICIN + CISPLATIN + FLUOROURACIL (ECF)

Findlay M et al. Ann Oncol 1994;5:609–616
Ross P et al. J Clin Oncol 2002;20:1996–2004

All chemotherapy is given through a central vascular access device

Warfarin 1 mg/day; administer orally continuously (prophylaxis against vascular access device occlusion)

Epirubicin 50 mg/m²; administer by intravenous injection over 3–5 minutes just before cisplatin on day 1 every 3 weeks for up to 8 cycles (total dosage/3-week cycle = 50 mg/m²)

Hydration before cisplatin: 1000 mL 0.9% sodium chloride injection (0.9% NS); administer intravenously over 80 minutes (~750 mL/hour) with:

Furosemide 40 mg; administer orally or intravenously, followed by 500 mL 0.9% NS; administer intravenously over 40 minutes (~750 mL/hour)

Cisplatin 60 mg/m²; administer intravenously in 1000 mL 0.9% NS with mannitol 20 g over 4 hours on day 1, every 3 weeks for up to 8 cycles (total cisplatin dosage/3-week cycle = 60 mg/m²) *followed by:*

Hydration after cisplatin: 1000 mL 0.9% NS; administer intravenously over 6 hours (~167 mL/hour)

Fluorouracil 200 mg/m² per day; administer by continuous intravenous infusion in 500–1000 mL 0.9% NS or 5% dextrose injection over 24 hours, daily, for up to 24 weeks, starting on the same day as the first dose of epirubicin and cisplatin (total dosage/3-week cycle = 4200 mg/m²)

General hydration: Encourage patients to increase oral intake of non-alcoholic fluids. Monitor serum electrolytes and replace as needed (potassium, magnesium, sodium)

Supportive Care

Antiemetic prophylaxis

Emetogenic potential on day 1 is **HIGH**. *Potential for delayed symptoms*

Emetogenic potential on days with fluorouracil alone is **LOW**

See Chapter 39 for antiemetic recommendations

Hematopoietic growth factor (CSF) prophylaxis

Primary prophylaxis is NOT indicated

See Chapter 43 for more information

Antimicrobial prophylaxis

Risk of fever and neutropenia is LOW

Antimicrobial primary prophylaxis to be considered:

- Antibacterial—not indicated
- Antifungal—not indicated
- Antiviral—not indicated unless patient previously had an episode of HSV

See Chapter 47 for more information

Hand-foot reaction (palmar-plantar erythrodysesthesia, PPE)

Use topical emollients (eg, Aquaphor®), topical or orally administered steroids, antihistamines, or pyridoxine 50 to 200 mg/day

Diarrhea management

Latent or delayed-onset diarrhea*:

Loperamide 4 mg; administer orally initially after the first loose or liquid stool, *then*

Loperamide 2 mg every 2 hours while awake; every 4 hours during sleep

Alternatively, a trial of **Diphenoxylate hydrochloride** 2.5 mg **with Atropine sulfate** 0.025 mg (eg, Lomotil®) two tablets four times daily until control has been achieved.

Persistent diarrhea:

Octreotide acetate (solution) 100–150 mcg; administer subcutaneously 3 times daily.

Antibiotic therapy during latent or delayed-onset diarrhea:

A fluoroquinolone (eg, **Ciprofloxacin** 500 mg orally every 12 hours) if absolute neutrophil count <500/mm³

*Abigerges D et al. J Natl Cancer Inst 1994;86:446–449
Rothenberg ML et al. J Clin Oncol 2001;19:3801–3807
Wadler S et al. J Clin Oncol 1998; 16:3169–3178

Patient Population Studied

A study of 429 (290 + 139) previously untreated patients with good performance status and locally advanced or metastatic adenocarcinoma or squamous cell carcinoma of the esophagus

Efficacy (N = 278/128)

Complete response	11%*	12%†
Partial response	32%*	59%†
Stable disease	23%*	
Disease progression/died	29%*	10%†
Median failure-free survival	7 months	

*Ross P et al. J Clin Oncol 2002;20:1996–2004; N = 278
†Findlay M et al. Ann Oncol 1994;5:609–616; N = 128

Toxicity (N = 272/139)

	% G1/2/3/4		% G3/4	
Hematologic				
Leukopenia	62*	—	13*	21†
Neutropenia	67*	—	32*	—
Thrombocytopenia	15*	—	4*	8†
Anemia	73*	—	9*	—
Nonhematologic				
Mucositis/ stomatitis	55*	24†	5*	7†
Plantar-palmar erythema	30*	27†	1*	1†
Nausea	81*	—	10*	
Vomiting	—	58†	—	13†
Diarrhea	44*	26†	6*	4†
Alopecia	87*	100†	—	—
Lethargy	89*	—	18*	—
Infection	38*	19†	6*	6†
Fever	14*	—	1*	—
Reduced GFR	—	73†	—	5†
Increased serum creatinine	—	18†	—	1†

*NCI CTC, National Cancer Institute (USA) Common Toxicity Criteria, version 2.0. At: http://ctep.cancer.gov/protocolDevelopment/electronic_applications/ctc.htm [accessed December 7, 2013] (Ross P et al. J Clin Oncol 2002;20:1996–2004; N = 272)
†WHO criteria (Findlay M et al. Ann Oncol 1994;5: 609–616; N = 139)

Treatment Modifications

Adverse Event	Dose Modification
Palmar/plantar erythema (PPE)	Add oral pyridoxine 50 mg 3 times daily. If PPE does not improve, discontinue fluorouracil for 1 week, then restart at fluorouracil 150 mg/m^2 per day (25% decrease)
G1/2 mucositis or diarrhea	Hold fluorouracil until toxicity resolves, then restart at fluorouracil 150 mg/m^2 per day (25% reduction)
G3/4 mucositis or diarrhea	Hold fluorouracil until toxicity resolves, then restart at fluorouracil 100 mg/m^2 per day (50% reduction)
Creatinine clearance ≥60 mL/min (≥1 mL/s)[†]	Cisplatin 60 mg/m^2 (100%)
Creatinine clearance 40–60 mL/min (0.66–1 mL/s)[†]	Cisplatin X mg/m^2 where X = absolute value of creatinine clearance
Creatinine clearance <40 mL/min (<1 mL/s)[†]	Hold cisplatin
EF[*] ≥50%	Epirubicin 50 mg/m^2 per dose
EF[*] <50%	Not eligible to receive epirubicin
First episode of ANC <2000/mm^3 *or* platelets <100,000/mm^3 on the day of epirubicin + cisplatin treatment	Delay treatment for 1 week, or until ANC is ≥2000/mm^3 *and* platelet count is ≥100,000/mm^3
Second episode of ANC <2000/mm^3 *or* platelets <100,000/mm^3 on the day of epirubicin + cisplatin treatment, or febrile neutropenia after previous treatment	Delay treatment until ANC is ≥2000/mm^3 and platelet count is ≥100,000/mm^3 then reduce epirubicin dosage to 38.5 mg/m^2 per dose (25% reduction) in subsequent cycles

*Obtain baseline multigated cardiac scan to determine left ventricular ejection fraction (EF) for evidence of cardiovascular disease
†Creatinine clearance as a measure of glomerular filtration rate (GFR)

Therapy Monitoring

1. *Before each chemotherapy cycle:* CBC with differential, platelet count, serum electrolytes, magnesium BUN, creatinine, LFTs, and mineral panel
2. *Response evaluation:* After cycles 3, 6, and 8, CT scan and endoscopy
3. Obtain a baseline multigated cardiac scan to determine left ventricular ejection fraction for evidence of cardiovascular disease

REGIMEN

FLUOROURACIL + CISPLATIN

Bleiberg H et al. Eur J Cancer 1997;33:1216–1220

Hydration before cisplatin: ≥1000 mL 0.9% sodium chloride injection (0.9% NS); administer intravenously at ≥100 mL/hour before and after cisplatin administration. Also encourage patients to increase oral intake of non-alcoholic fluids. Monitor serum electrolytes and replace as needed (potassium, magnesium, sodium)

Cisplatin 75–100 mg/m²; administer intravenously in 250 mL 0.9% NS over 60 minutes, given on day 1 every 3 weeks (total dosage/cycle = 75–100 mg/m²)

Take home: Potassium and magnesium oral supplements to use as needed, guided by laboratory monitoring

Fluorouracil 750–1000 mg/m² per day; administer by continuous intravenous infusion in 2000 mL 0.9% NS or 5% dextrose injection over 24 hours on days 1–5 every 3 weeks (total dosage/cycle = 3750–5000 mg/m²)

Supportive Care

Antiemetic prophylaxis

Emetogenic potential on day 1 is **HIGH***. Potential for delayed symptoms*

Emetogenic potential on days with fluorouracil alone is **LOW**

See Chapter 39 for antiemetic recommendations

Hematopoietic growth factor (CSF) prophylaxis

Primary prophylaxis may be indicated

See Chapter 43 for more information

Antimicrobial prophylaxis

Risk of fever and neutropenia is LOW

   Antimicrobial primary prophylaxis to be considered:

   • Antibacterial—not indicated

   • Antifungal—not indicated

   • Antiviral—not indicated unless patient previously had an episode of HSV

See Chapter 47 for more information

Oral care

   • Encourage patients to maintain intake of non-alcoholic fluids

   If mucositis or stomatitis is present:

   • Rinse mouth several times a day with ¼ teaspoon (1.25 g) each of baking soda and table salt in one quart of warm water. Follow with a plain water rinse

     ■ Do not use mouthwashes that contain alcohols

Diarrhea management

Latent or delayed-onset diarrhea*:

Loperamide 4 mg; administer orally initially after the first loose or liquid stool, *then*

Loperamide 2 mg every 2 hours while awake; every 4 hours during sleep

Alternatively, a trial of **Diphenoxylate hydrochloride** 2.5 mg **with Atropine sulfate** 0.025 mg (eg, Lomotil®) two tablets four times daily until control has been achieved.

Persistent diarrhea:

Octreotide acetate (solution) 100–150 mcg; administer subcutaneously 3 times daily.

Antibiotic therapy during latent or delayed-onset diarrhea:

A fluoroquinolone (eg, **Ciprofloxacin** 500 mg orally every 12 hours) if absolute neutrophil count <500/mm³

*Abigerges D et al. J Natl Cancer Inst 1994;86:446–449; Rothenberg ML et al. J Clin Oncol 2001;19:3801–3807; Wadler S et al. J Clin Oncol 1998;16:3169–3178

Patient Population Studied

A study of 44 patients with advanced squamous cell carcinoma of the esophagus

Therapy Monitoring

1. *Before each cycle:* H&P, chest x-ray, CBC with differential, serum electrolytes, BUN, creatinine, and mineral panel

2. *Response evaluation:* Every 2 cycles

Notes

1. This regimen should be used in selected patients with good performance status

2. Also used for metastatic adenocarcinoma of the distal esophagus and GE junction

3. Patients who cannot tolerate cisplatin can be treated with carboplatin (AUC = 5 mg/mL · min)

Treatment Modifications

Adverse Event	Dose Modification
ANC nadir <1000/mm³ or platelet nadir <50,000/mm³ after treatment	Delay treatment until ANC >1000/mm³ *and* platelet >50,0000/mm³, then decrease cisplatin dosage by 25% and decrease daily fluorouracil dosages by 50% in subsequent cycles*
Serum creatinine >1.5 mg/dL (133 μmol/L), but <3 mg/dL (265 μmol/L) *or* creatinine clearance >40 mL/min, but <60 mL/min	Delay treatment until serum creatinine <1.5 mg/dL (133 μmol/L), then decrease cisplatin dosage by 50%*
Serum creatinine >3 mg/dL (265 μmol/L) *or* creatinine clearance <40 mL/min	Stop cisplatin
G >2 Stomatitis or diarrhea	Decrease fluorouracil dosage by 50%

*Treatment delays for unresolved adverse events of ≥3 weeks warrant discontinuation of treatment

Efficacy (N = 34)

Complete response	3%
Partial response	32%
Stable disease	29%
Disease progression	18%
Early death	15%
Median failure free survival	7 months

Toxicity (N = 44)

	% G3/4
Hematologic	
Leukopenia	14
Thrombocytopenia	14
Nonhematologic	
Nausea/vomiting*	27
Vascular thrombosis	9
Mucositis	5
Diarrhea	2

*The high rate of nausea and vomiting observed in the original 1997 study should be reduced considerably by using currently available serotonin receptor (5-HT₃) antagonist and other antiemetics
WHO criteria

REGIMEN

DOCETAXEL + CISPLATIN + FLUOROURACIL (DCF)

Ajani JA et al. Proc Am Soc Clin Oncol 2003;22:249 [abstract 999]

Docetaxel 75 mg/m²; administer intravenously in a volume of 0.9% sodium chloride injection (0.9% NS) or 5% dextrose injection (D5W) sufficient to produce a solution with concentration within the range 0.3–0.74 mg/mL over 60 minutes, given on day 1 every 3 weeks (total dosage/cycle = 75 mg/m²)

Hydration with cisplatin: ≥1000 mL 0.9% NS; administer intravenously at ≥100 mL/hour before and after cisplatin administration. Also encourage patients to increase oral intake of non-alcoholic fluids. Monitor serum electrolytes and replace as needed (potassium, magnesium, sodium)

Cisplatin 75 mg/m²; administer intravenously in 25–250 mL of 0.9% NS over 15–60 minutes, given on day 1 every 3 weeks (total dosage/cycle = 75 mg/m²)

Fluorouracil 750 mg/m² per day; administer by continuous intravenous infusion in 250–1000 mL of 0.9% NS or D5W over 24 hours for 5 consecutive days, on days 1–5 every 3 weeks (total dosage/cycle = 3750 mg/m²)

Supportive Care

Antiemetic prophylaxis

Emetogenic potential on day 1 is **HIGH***. Potential for delayed symptoms*

Emetogenic potential on days 2–5 is **LOW**

See Chapter 39 for antiemetic recommendations

Hematopoietic growth factor (CSF) prophylaxis

Primary prophylaxis is indicated with one of the following:

Filgrastim (G-CSF) 5 mcg/kg per day, by subcutaneous injection, or

Pegfilgrastim (pegylated filgrastim) 6 mg/0.6 mL, by subcutaneous injection for one dose

- Begin use from 24–72 h after myelosuppressive chemotherapy is completed
- Continue daily Filgrastim use until ANC ≥ 10,000/mm³ on two measurements separated temporally by ≥12 hours
- Discontinue daily Filgrastim use at least 24 hours before administering myelosuppressive treatment. Do not administer Pegfilgrastim within 14 days before administering myelosuppressive treatment

See Chapter 43 for more information

Antimicrobial prophylaxis

Risk of fever and neutropenia is INTERMEDIATE

Antimicrobial primary prophylaxis to be considered:

- Antibacterial—consider a fluoroquinolone or no prophylaxis; *P. jirovecii* prophylaxis is recommended (eg, cotrimoxazole)
- Antifungal—consider concomitant use of cotrimoxazole during periods of neutropenia, and in anticipation of mucositis
- Antiviral—anti-herpes antivirals (eg, acyclovir, famciclovir, valacyclovir)

See Chapter 47 for more information

Oral care

Risk of mucositis/stomatitis is HIGH

General advice:

- Encourage patients to maintain intake of non-alcoholic fluids
- Evaluate patients for oral pain and provide analgesic medications
- Consider histamine (H₂-subtype) receptor antagonists (eg, ranitidine, famotidine), or a proton pump inhibitor for epigastric pain
- *Lactobacillus* sp.-containing probiotics may be beneficial in preventing diarrhea

Patients with intact oral mucosa:

- Clean the mouth, tongue, and gums by brushing after every meal and at bedtime with an ultra-soft toothbrush with fluoride toothpaste
- Floss teeth gently every day unless contraindicated. If gums bleed and hurt, avoid bleeding or sore areas, but floss other teeth
- Patients may use saline or commercial bland, non-alcoholic rinses
  - Do not use mouthwashes that contain alcohols

(continued)

Treatment Modifications

Adverse Event	Dose Modification
G3/4 hematologic adverse events	Use hematopoietic growth factors or decrease doses of docetaxel, cisplatin, and fluorouracil by 25% for subsequent cycles
G3/4 nonhematologic adverse events	Reduce doses of docetaxel, cisplatin, and fluorouracil by 25% for subsequent cycles

Patient Population Studied

A study of 115 patients with metastatic or locally unresectable gastric or gastroesophageal junction adenocarcinoma and measurable or evaluable disease

Toxicity (N = 115)

	% Patients
Any G3/4 adverse events	82
Complicated neutropenia	30
Death rate from all causes within 30 days after the last treatment	11.7

Efficacy (N = 115)

Overall response rate	39%
One year survival	44%
Time to progression	5.2 months
Median overall survival	10.2 months

(*continued*)

If mucositis or stomatitis is present:
- Keep the mouth moist utilizing water, ice chips, sugarless gum, sugar-free hard candies, or a saliva substitute
- Rinse mouth several times a day to remove debris
  - Use a solution of ¼ teaspoon (1.25 g) each of baking soda and table salt (sodium chloride) in one quart (~950 mL) of warm water. Follow with a plain water rinse
  - Do not use mouthwashes that contain alcohols
- Foam-tipped swabs (eg, Toothettes®) are useful in moisturizing oral mucosa, but ineffective for cleansing teeth and removing plaque
- Advise patients who develop mucositis to:
  - Choose foods that are easy to chew and swallow
  - Take small bites of food, chew slowly, and sip liquids with meals
  - Encourage soft, moist foods such as cooked cereals, mashed potatoes, and scrambled eggs
  - For trouble swallowing, soften food with gravies, sauces, broths, yogurt, or other bland liquids
  - Avoid sharp, crunchy foods; hot, spicy or highly acidic foods (eg, citrus fruits and juices); sugary foods; toothpicks; tobacco products; alcoholic drinks

Diarrhea management
Latent or delayed-onset diarrhea*:
Loperamide 4 mg; administer orally initially after the first loose or liquid stool, *then*
Loperamide 2 mg; administer orally every 2 hours during waking hours, *plus*
Loperamide 4 mg; administer orally every 4 hours during hours of sleep
- Continue for at least 12 hours after diarrhea resolves
- Recurrent diarrhea after a 12-hour diarrhea-free interval is treated as a new episode
- Rehydrate orally with fluids and electrolytes during a diarrheal episode
- If a patient develops blood or mucus in stool, dehydration, or hemodynamic instability, or if diarrhea persists >48 hours despite loperamide, stop loperamide and hospitalize the patient for IV hydration

Alternatively, a trial of **Diphenoxylate hydrochloride** 2.5 mg **with Atropine sulfate** 0.025 mg (eg, Lomotil®)
- Initial adult dose is two tablets four times daily until control has been achieved, after which the dose may be reduced to meet individual requirements. Control may often be maintained with as little as two tablets daily
- Clinical improvement of acute diarrhea is usually observed within 48 hours. If improvement in chronic diarrhea after treatment with a maximum daily dose of 8 tablets is not observed within 10 days, control is unlikely with further administration

Persistent diarrhea:
Octreotide acetate (solution) 100–150 mcg; administer subcutaneously 3 times daily. Maximum total daily dose is 1500 mcg

Antibiotic therapy during latent or delayed-onset diarrhea:
A fluoroquinolone (eg, **Ciprofloxacin** 500 mg orally every 12 hours) if absolute neutrophil count <500/mm^3 with or without accompanying fever in association with diarrhea
- Antibiotics should also be administered if patient is hospitalized with prolonged diarrhea and should be continued until diarrhea resolves

*Abigerges D et al. J Natl Cancer Inst 1994;86:446–449
Rothenberg ML et al. J Clin Oncol 2001;19:3801–3807
Wadler S et al. J Clin Oncol 1998;16:3169–3178

Therapy Monitoring

1. *Before each cycle:* H&P, CBC with differential, serum electrolytes, BUN, creatinine, and mineral panel
2. *Response evaluation:* Every 2 cycles

Notes

1. Reported DCF data reflects interim analysis
2. This regimen is not recommended for patients with WHO/ECOG performance status >1
3. For patients who cannot tolerate cisplatin, DCF is not recommended; however, substitutes such as oxaliplatin or carboplatin have been used
4. Primary prophylaxis with filgrastim or pegfilgrastim may also be considered for qualifying patients

REGIMEN

OXALIPLATIN + FLUOROURACIL + LEUCOVORIN (FOLFOX)

Mauer AM et al. Ann Oncol 2005;16:1320–1325

Oxaliplatin 85 mg/m²; administer intravenously in 250–500 mL 5% dextrose injection (D5W) over 2 hours on day 1, every 14 days (total dosage/cycle = 85 mg/m²)

Leucovorin 500 mg/m² per day; administer by intravenous infusion in 10–500 mL 0.9% sodium chloride injection (0.9% NS) or D5W over 2 hours for 2 doses on days 1 and 2, every 14 days (total dosage/cycle = 1000 mg/m²); *followed each day by:*

Fluorouracil 400 mg/m² per day; administer by intravenous push or infusion in 10–100 mL 0.9% NS or D5W over 2–15 minutes for 2 doses on days 1 and 2, every 14 days; *followed immediately afterward by:*

Fluorouracil 600 mg/m² per day; administer by continuous intravenous infusion over 22 hours in 50–1000 mL 0.9% NS or D5W for 2 doses on days 1 and 2, every 14 days (total dosage/cycle = 2000 mg/m²)

Note:
• Patients were counseled to avoid exposure to cold liquids or air because the acute neurotoxicity encountered with oxaliplatin appears to be exacerbated by exposure to cold

Supportive Care
Antiemetic prophylaxis
Emetogenic potential on day 1 is HIGH
Emetogenic potential on day 2 is LOW
See Chapter 39 for antiemetic recommendations

Hematopoietic growth factor (CSF) prophylaxis
Primary prophylaxis is NOT indicated
See Chapter 43 for more information

Antimicrobial prophylaxis
Risk of fever and neutropenia is LOW
  Antimicrobial primary prophylaxis to be considered:
  • Antibacterial—not indicated
  • Antifungal—not indicated
  • Antiviral—not indicated unless patient previously had an episode of HSV
See Chapter 47 for more information

Oral care
  • Encourage patients to maintain intake of non-alcoholic fluids
  If mucositis or stomatitis is present:
  • Rinse mouth several times a day with ¼ teaspoon (1.25 g) each of baking soda and table salt in one quart of warm water. Follow with a plain water rinse
    ▪ Do not use mouthwashes that contain alcohols

Diarrhea management
Latent or delayed-onset diarrhea:
  Loperamide 4 mg; administer orally initially after the first loose or liquid stool, then **Loperamide** 2 mg every 2 hours while awake; every 4 hours during sleep
  Alternatively, a trial of **Diphenoxylate hydrochloride** 2.5 mg with **Atropine sulfate** 0.025 mg (eg, Lomotil®) two tablets four times daily until control has been achieved.

Persistent diarrhea:
  Octreotide acetate (solution) 100–150 mcg; administer subcutaneously 3 times daily.

Antibiotic therapy during latent or delayed-onset diarrhea:
A fluoroquinolone (eg, **Ciprofloxacin** 500 mg orally every 12 hours) if absolute neutrophil count <500/mm³

*Abigerges D et al. J Natl Cancer Inst 1994;86:446–449
Rothenberg ML et al. J Clin Oncol 2001;19:3801–3807
Wadler S et al. J Clin Oncol 1998;16:3169–3178

Patient Population Studied

Recurrent or metastatic cancer of the esophagus or gastric cardia. Prior treatment with a single chemotherapy regimen and radiotherapy allowed. Eastern Cooperative Oncology Group (ECOG) performance status of 0, 1, or 2. Laboratory measures required at study entry: creatinine ≤1.5 times the institutional upper limit of normal or creatinine clearance ≥50 mL/min; bilirubin ≤1.5 mg/dL; and glutamic–oxaloacetic transaminase less than 2 times the institutional limit of normal

Adverse Events (N = 35)

Hematologic Toxicity

Toxicity Grade	G1	G2	G3	G4	G5
Leukopenia	6	14	7	1	0
Neutropenia	2	3	12	10	1
Thrombocytopenia	14	2	2	1	0
Anemia	17	9	3	0	0

Nonhematologic Toxicity

Toxicity Grade	G1	G2	G3	G4	G5
Fatigue	14	15	2	1	—
Vomiting	9	7	1	0	—
Stomatitis	5	4	0	0	–
Anorexia	13	5	2	0	—
Diarrhea	6	3	4	0	—
Laryngodysesthesia	0	0	0	0	—
Neuropathy, motor	3	0	0	0	—
Neuropathy, sensory	13	8	1	0	—
Respiratory	0	4	1	0	—
Infection	1	1	1	0	—
Creatinine elevation	0	0	0	1*	—

*Reversible renal insufficiency secondary to oxaliplatin-induced hemolysis
NCI CTC, National Cancer Institute (USA) Common Toxicity Criteria, version 2.0. At: http://ctep.cancer.gov/protocolDevelopment/electronic_applications/ctc.htm [accessed December 7, 2013]

Treatment Modifications

Adverse Event	Dose Modifications*
Inadequate hematologic recovery by day 15 (ANC <1500/mm³ *or* platelet count <100,000/mm³)	Delay therapy 1 week
G4 neutropenia or thrombocytopenia	Reduce oxaliplatin and fluorouracil dosages 25% in subsequent cycle
G3/4 stomatitis or diarrhea	Reduce oxaliplatin and fluorouracil dosages by 25% in the subsequent cycle after recovery to baseline
Persistent G2 or any G3 neuropathy	Reduce oxaliplatin dosages by 25%
Febrile or prolonged neutropenia	Administer prophylactic granulocyte colony stimulating factor in subsequent cycles

*Based on the worst toxicity observed during the previous course

Therapy Monitoring

1. Complete blood counts with differential leukocyte counts at least weekly
2. LFTs, serum BUN, and creatinine before each cycle of chemotherapy
3. Assessment of response after every 4 cycles of therapy

Efficacy (N = 35)*

	Number (%)
Complete response	1 (2.5%)
Partial response	13 (37%)
Overall RR, all patients†	40% (95% CI, 24–57%)
Overall RR, chemotherapy-naïve patients	45% (95% CI, 27–64%)
Overall RR, previously treated patients	0 (95% CI, 0–53%)
Stable disease (≥4 cycles of chemotherapy)	10 (29%)
Progressive disease	10 (29%)
Not evaluated	1 (2.5%)
Median PFS, all patients	4.6 months (95% CI, 2.2–6.8)
Median PFS, chemotherapy-naïve patients	4.9 months‡
Median PFS, previously treated patients	1.7 months‡
1-Year PFS probability	0.15
Median OS, all patients	7.1 months (95% CI, 5.9–10.9)
Median OS, chemotherapy-naïve patients	7.6 months§
Median OS, previously treated patients	2.1 months§
1-Year survival probability	0.31 (95% CI, 0.17–0.47)
2-Year survival probability	0.11

*WHO Criteria
†Histology of responding patients: adenocarcinoma (13) adenosquamous (1)
‡$p = 0.0009$; log rank test
§$p = 0.011$; log-rank test

REGIMEN

EPIRUBICIN + OXALIPLATIN + CAPECITABINE (EOC, EOX)

Cunningham D et al. N Engl J Med 2008;358:36–46
Cunningham D et al. N Engl J Med 2010;362:858–859
Sumpter K et al. Br J Cancer 2005;92:1976–1983

Epirubicin 50 mg/m^2; administer by intravenous injection over 3–20 minutes on day 1, every 3 weeks, for a maximum of 8 cycles (total dosage/cycle = 50 mg/m^2)

Oxaliplatin 130 mg/m^2; administer intravenously in 250–500 mL 5% dextrose injection over 2 hours on day 1, every 3 weeks, for a maximum of 8 cycles (total dosage/cycle = 130 mg/m^2)

Capecitabine 625 mg/m^2 per dose; administer orally with water within 30 minutes after a meal twice daily, continually during a 3-week cycle for a maximum of 8 cycles (daily dosage = 1250 mg/m^2; total dosage/cycle = 26,250 mg/m^2)

Supportive Care

Antiemetic prophylaxis
Emetogenic potential on day 1 is **MODERATE**
Emetogenic potential on days with capecitabine alone is **LOW**
See Chapter 39 for antiemetic recommendations

Hematopoietic growth factor (CSF) prophylaxis
Primary prophylaxis is NOT indicated
See Chapter 43 for more information

Antimicrobial prophylaxis
Risk of fever and neutropenia is LOW
Antimicrobial primary prophylaxis to be considered:
- Antibacterial—not indicated
- Antifungal—not indicated
- Antiviral—not indicated unless patient previously had an episode of HSV

See Chapter 47 for more information

Thromboprophylaxis
Low-dose **warfarin** 1 mg/day; administer orally

Hand-foot reaction (palmar-plantar erythrodysesthesia, PPE)
Use topical emollients (eg, Aquaphor®), topical or orally administered steroids, antihistamines, or pyridoxine 50 to 200 mg/day

Diarrhea management
Latent or delayed-onset diarrhea*:
Loperamide 4 mg; administer orally initially after the first loose or liquid stool, *then*
Loperamide 2 mg every 2 hours while awake; every 4 hours during sleep
Alternatively, a trial of **Diphenoxylate hydrochloride** 2.5 mg with **Atropine sulfate** 0.025 mg (eg, Lomotil®) two tablets four times daily until control has been achieved.

Persistent diarrhea:
Octreotide acetate (solution) 100–150 mcg; administer subcutaneously 3 times daily.

Antibiotic therapy during latent or delayed-onset diarrhea:
A fluoroquinolone (eg, **Ciprofloxacin** 500 mg orally every 12 hours) if absolute neutrophil count <500/mm^3

*Abigerges D et al. J Natl Cancer Inst 1994;86:446–449
Rothenberg ML et al. J Clin Oncol 2001;19:3801–3807
Wadler S et al. J Clin Oncol 1998;16:3169–3178

Treatment Modifications

Adverse Event	Dose Modifications
Inadequate hematologic recovery (ANC <1000/mm^3 *or* platelet count <75,000/mm^3) on day 1 of repeated cycles	Delay oxaliplatin 1 week
G2–4 thrombocytopenia or G3/4 neutropenia in previous cycle	Delay start of oxaliplatin until toxicity is resolved, then reduce oxaliplatin dosage to 100 mg/m^2 in subsequent cycles

(continued)

Patient Population Studied

Adenocarcinoma, squamous cell carcinoma, or undifferentiated carcinoma of the esophagus, gastroesophageal junction, or stomach that was locally advanced (inoperable) or metastatic. Eastern Cooperative Oncology Group performance status of 0–2. Major exclusion criteria were previous chemotherapy or radiotherapy (unless the latter was adjuvant treatment with relapse outside the radiotherapy field)

Efficacy

Compete response	3.9%
Partial response	44%
Median progression-free survival	7 months
1-Year survival rate	46.8%
Median survival	11.2 months
Median survival—metastatic disease	10 months

Adverse Events
(N = 227–232)

	% All Grades	% G3/4
Hematologic Toxicities		
Anemia	64.1	8.6
Thrombocytopenia	21.1	5.2
Neutropenia	62.9	27.6
Febrile neutropenia	9.8	7.8
Nonhematologic Toxicities		
Diarrhea	61.7	11.9
Stomatitis	38.1	2.2
Hand-foot syndrome	39.3	3.1
Nausea and vomiting	78.9	11.4
Peripheral neuropathy	83.7	4.4
Lethargy	96.1	24.9
Alopecia	74.2	28.8
Thromboembolism	7.5	NA
Death within 60 days	6.1	

Treatment Modifications (*continued*)

Adverse Event	Dose Modifications
G2 stomatitis, diarrhea, or nausea	Hold capecitabine; resume capecitabine at full dose after resolution of toxicity
Second episode of G2 stomatitis, diarrhea, or nausea	Hold capecitabine; resume capecitabine with dosage reduced by 25% after resolution of toxicity
Third episode of G2 stomatitis, diarrhea, or nausea	Hold capecitabine; resume capecitabine with dosage reduced by 50% after resolution of toxicity
Fourth episode of G2 stomatitis, diarrhea, or nausea	Discontinue capecitabine
G3 stomatitis, diarrhea, or nausea	Hold capecitabine; if G3 toxicity is adequately controlled within 2 days, resume capecitabine at full dosage when toxicity resolves to G ≤1. If G3 toxicity takes >2 days to be controlled, then resume capecitabine with dosage reduced by 25% after toxicity resolves to G ≤1
Second episode of G3 stomatitis, diarrhea, or nausea	Hold capecitabine; if G3 toxicity controlled adequately within 2 days then resume capecitabine with dosage reduced by 50% after toxicity resolves to G ≤1
Third episode of G3 stomatitis, diarrhea, or nausea	Discontinue capecitabine
G4 stomatitis, diarrhea, or nausea	Withhold capecitabine. Resume capecitabine with dosage reduced by 50% after toxicity resolves
G1 capecitabine-associated PPE*	Begin pyridoxine 50 mg orally 3 times daily and continue capecitabine without dose modification
G2 capecitabine-associated PPE*	Begin pyridoxine 50 mg orally 3 times daily and withhold capecitabine. Resume capecitabine with dosage reduced by 15% after toxicity resolves
G3 capecitabine-associated PPE*	Begin pyridoxine 50 mg orally 3 times daily and withhold capecitabine. Resume capecitabine with dosage reduced by 30% after toxicity resolves
Recurrent G3 capecitabine-associated PPE*	Begin pyridoxine 50 mg orally 3 times daily and withhold capecitabine. Resume capecitabine with dosage reduced by 50% after toxicity resolves
Persistent G1 or G2 neuropathy	Delay oxaliplatin 1 week. Resume oxaliplatin after toxicity resolves at a dosage decreased to 100 mg/m^2 during subsequent cycles
G3/4 neuropathy	Hold oxaliplatin
"Transient" G3/4 neuropathy (duration, 7–14 days)	Hold oxaliplatin. Resume oxaliplatin after toxicity resolves at a dosage decreased to 100 mg/m^2 during subsequent cycles
Persistent G3/4 neuropathy	Discontinue oxaliplatin[†]
Laryngeal dysesthesia	Administer subsequent oxaliplatin infusions over a 6-hour period
G3/4 diarrhea or stomatitis despite capecitabine dose reductions	Reduce oxaliplatin dosage to 100 mg/m^2

*PPE, Palmar plantar erythrodysesthesia (hand-foot syndrome)
[†]Consider substituting carboplatin

Therapy Monitoring

1. Complete blood counts with differential leukocyte counts at least weekly
2. LFTs, serum BUN, and creatinine before each cycle of chemotherapy
3. Assessment of response after every 4 cycles of therapy

REGIMEN

IRINOTECAN + FLUOROURACIL + LEUCOVORIN (FOLFIRI)

Dank M et al. Ann Oncol 2008;19:1450–1457
Pozzo C et al. Ann Oncol 2004;15:1773–1781

Irinotecan 80 mg/m² per dose; administer intravenously in 250 mL 0.9% sodium chloride injection (0.9% NS) or 5% dextrose injection (D5W) over 30 minutes for 6 weekly doses on days 1, 8, 15, 22, 29, and 36, every 7 weeks (total dosage during induction = 480 mg/m²), *followed by:*
Leucovorin 500 mg/m² per dose; administer intravenously in 25–500 mL 0.9% NS or D5W over 2 hours for 6 weekly doses on days 1, 8, 15, 22, 29, and 36, every 7 weeks (total dosage/cycle = 3000 mg/m²), *followed by*
Fluorouracil 2000 mg/m² per dose; administer by continuous intravenous infusion over 22 hours in 50–1000 mL 0.9% NS or D5W for 6 weekly doses on days 1, 8, 15, 22, 29, and 36, every 7 weeks (total dosage/cycle = 12,000 mg/m²)

Supportive Care
Antiemetic prophylaxis
Emetogenic potential is **MODERATE**
See Chapter 39 for antiemetic recommendations

Hematopoietic growth factor (CSF) prophylaxis
Primary prophylaxis is NOT indicated
- **Filgrastim** (G-CSF) 5 mcg/kg per day, by subcutaneous injection from day 4 until ANC recovery (>1000/mm³) was recommended for treatment and secondary prophylaxis in patients who developed febrile neutropenia, neutropenia and infection, or neutropenia G ≥3 of >7 days duration during a previous cycle

See Chapter 43 for more information

Antimicrobial prophylaxis
Risk of fever and neutropenia is LOW
  Antimicrobial primary prophylaxis to be considered:
- Antibacterial—not indicated
- Antifungal—not indicated
- Antiviral—not indicated unless patient previously had an episode of HSV

See Chapter 47 for more information

Acute cholinergic syndrome
Atropine sulfate 0.25–1 mg; administer subcutaneously or intravenously if abdominal cramping or diarrhea develop during or within 1 hour after irinotecan administration
- If symptoms are severe, add as primary prophylaxis at least 30 minutes before irinotecan during subsequent cycles
- For irinotecan, acute cholinergic syndrome may be characterized by abdominal cramping, diarrhea, diaphoresis, hypotension, flushing, bradycardia, rhinitis, increased salivation, meiosis, and lacrimation

Diarrhea management
Latent or delayed onset diarrhea*:
  Loperamide 4 mg orally initially after the first loose or liquid stool, *then*
  Loperamide 2 mg orally every 2 hours during waking hours, *plus*
  Loperamide 4 mg orally every 4 hours during hours of sleep
- Continue for at least 12 hours after diarrhea resolves
- Recurrent diarrhea after a 12-hour diarrhea-free interval is treated as a new episode
- Rehydrate orally with fluids and electrolytes during a diarrheal episode
- If diarrhea persists >48 hours despite loperamide, stop loperamide and hospitalize the patient for IV hydration

Persistent diarrhea:
  Octreotide 100–150 mcg subcutaneously 3 times daily. Maximum total daily dose is 1500 mcg

Concomitant diarrhea and vomiting, fever, or Karnofsky performance status <70%:
- Hospitalize the patient for IV hydration

Antibiotic therapy during latent or delayed-onset diarrhea:
  Ciprofloxacin 500 mg orally every 12 hours if absolute neutrophil count is <500/mm³ with or without accompanying fever in association with diarrhea
- Antibiotics should also be administered if patient is hospitalized with prolonged diarrhea and should be continued until diarrhea resolves

*Rothenberg ML et al. J Clin Oncol 2001;19:3801–3807; Wadler S et al. J Clin Oncol 1998;16:3169–3178

Oral care
- Encourage patients to maintain intake of non-alcoholic fluids
  If mucositis or stomatitis is present:
- Rinse mouth several times a day with ¼ teaspoon (1.25 g) each of baking soda and table salt in one quart of warm water. Follow with a plain water rinse
  - Do not use mouthwashes that contain alcohols

Treatment Modifications

Dose Levels

Irinotecan

Level 0	80 mg/m²
Level −1	65 mg/m²
Level −2	50 mg/m²

Fluorouracil

Level 0	2000 mg/m²
Level −1	1750 mg/m²
Level −2	1500 mg/m²

Adverse Event	Dose Modifications*
Inadequate hematologic recovery by start of next cycle (ANC <1500/mm³ or platelet count <100,000/mm³)	Delay start of next treatment cycle up to 2 weeks
G >1 diarrhea	Delay start of next treatment cycle up to 2 weeks; treat as needed
Persistent G ≥1 toxicity after a 2-week delay or recurrent toxicity after more than 2-dose reductions, or G4 stomatitis or G3/4 peripheral neurotoxicity/ototoxicity	Discontinue therapy
Any toxicity G >2 except alopecia and anemia	Reduce irinotecan and fluorouracil dosages by 1 dose level
Second episode of isolated febrile neutropenia or G3/4 neutropenia lasting >7 days, despite filgrastim	Reduce irinotecan by 1 dose level
G3 stomatitis lasting >48 hours	Reduce fluorouracil by 1 dose level
G4 diarrhea, diarrhea with concomitant grade 3/4 neutropenia without fever, or diarrhea with fever or infection	Administer oral fluoroquinolones; reduce irinotecan and/or fluorouracil by 1 dose level
G2–4 acute cholinergic syndrome	Reduce irinotecan dosage by 1 dose level; administer atropine during subsequent cycles
Delayed diarrhea	Reduce irinotecan and/or fluorouracil 1 dose by level; administer loperamide
Febrile neutropenia, neutropenia and infection, or neutropenia G3/4 lasting more than 7 days	Administer filgrastim in subsequent cycles starting on day 4 and continue until ANC >1000/mm³

Patient Population Studied

Adenocarcinoma (including diffuse type, intestinal type and linitis) of the esophagogastric junction, with measurable or evaluable metastatic disease or locally recurrent disease with 1 or more measurable lymph node. A Karnofsky performance status (KPS) >70%. Must have finished prior radiotherapy and surgery 6 and 3 weeks, respectively. Previous adjuvant or neoadjuvant chemotherapy was allowed if completed >12 months before first relapse

Efficacy*

Response rate	31.8%
Median time to treatment failure†	4 months
Median time to progression	5 months
Median response duration	7.6 months
Median overall survival	9 months

*WHO Criteria
†TTF was influenced by the discontinuation of therapy. The majority of these discontinuations occurred within the first 2 months of treatment. The most frequent causes of discontinuation were asthenia, diarrhea, and infection

Adverse Event*

Toxicity	% All Grades	% G3/4
Hematologic		
Leukopenia	64.5	16.3
Neutropenia	66.1	24.8
Febrile neutropenia, neutropenia, and infection	4.8	4.8
Anemia	88	11.4
Thrombocytopenia	9	1.8
Gastrointestinal		
Anorexia	16.2	3
Diarrhea	63.5	21.6
Nausea	50.9	4.8
Stomatitis	15.6	2.4
Vomiting	39.5	6.6
Hepatic		
AST elevated	27.2	2.5
ALT elevated	29.7	3.2
AP elevated	52.9	5.2
Hyperbilirubinemia	12.3	8.4
Neurologic		
Altered hearing	1.2	—
Sensory	5.4	—
Skin		
Alopecia	15.6	—
Local toxicity	12.6	1.2
Other		
Asthenia	38.3	7.2
Cholinergic syndrome	13.2	—
Creatinine elevation	9.3	0.6
Fever in absence of infection	14.4	1.8
Infection	7.2	3

*National Cancer Institute of Canada–Clinical Trials Group Expanded Common Toxicity Criteria

Therapy Monitoring

1. Complete blood counts with differential leukocyte counts at least weekly
2. LFTs, serum BUN, and creatinine before each cycle of chemotherapy
3. Assessment of response every 7–8 weeks

REGIMEN
CISPLATIN + CAPECITABINE ± TRASTUZUMAB

Bang Y-J et al. Lancet 2010;376:687–697

Hydration with cisplatin: ≥1000 mL 0.9% sodium chloride injection (0.9% NS); administer intravenously at ≥100 mL/hour before and after cisplatin administration. Also, encourage patients to increase oral intake of non-alcoholic fluids. Monitor serum electrolytes and replace as needed (potassium, magnesium, sodium)

Cisplatin 80 mg/m^2; administer intravenously in 100–250 mL 0.9% NS over 60 minutes on day 1, every 3 weeks, for 6 cycles (total dosage/cycle = 80 mg/m^2)

Capecitabine 1000 mg/m^2 per dose; administer orally twice daily (approximately every 12 hours) with water within 30 minutes after a meal for 28 doses on days 1–14, every 3 weeks, for 6 cycles (total dosage/cycle = 28,000 mg/m^2)

Trastuzumab

• **Initial dose: Trastuzumab** 8 mg/kg; administer intravenously in 250 mL 0.9% NS over 90 minutes (total dosage during cycle 1 = 8 mg/kg), *followed after 3 weeks by:*

• **Subsequent doses: Trastuzumab** 6 mg/kg per dose; administer intravenously in 250 mL 0.9% NS over 30–90 minutes (total dosage/cycle = 6 mg/kg)

Notes: Trastuzumab treatment continues every 3 weeks until disease progression, unacceptable toxicities, or patient withdrawal

An optimal sequence for drug administration is suggested by experimental evidence, but has not been proved in clinical trials (Li X-L. Cancer Invest 2010;28:1038–1047)

Supportive Care
Antiemetic prophylaxis
Emetogenic potential on day 1 is **HIGH**
Emetogenic potential on days with capecitabine alone is **LOW**
See Chapter 39 for antiemetic recommendations

Hematopoietic growth factor (CSF) prophylaxis
Primary prophylaxis is NOT indicated
See Chapter 43 for more information

Antimicrobial prophylaxis
Risk of fever and neutropenia is LOW
  Antimicrobial primary prophylaxis to be considered:
  • Antibacterial—not indicated
  • Antifungal—not indicated
  • Antiviral—not indicated unless patient previously had an episode of HSV
See Chapter 47 for more information

Trastuzumab infusion reactions:
• A symptom complex most commonly consisting of chills and/or fever may occur in as many as 40% of patients during the first infusion of trastuzumab. These symptoms occur infrequently with subsequent trastuzumab infusions. Other signs and/or symptoms may include nausea, vomiting, pain (in some cases at tumor sites), rigors, headache, dizziness, dyspnea, hypotension, rash, and asthenia. Although the symptoms are usually mild to moderate in severity, infrequently, trastuzumab may need to be discontinued

• When such a symptom complex is observed, it can be treated with or without reduction in the rate of trastuzumab infusion, and:

  ▪ **Acetaminophen** 650 mg; administer orally

  ▪ **Diphenhydramine** 25–50 mg administer orally or by intravenous injection, and

  ▪ **Meperidine** 12.5–25 mg; administer by intravenous injection every 10 minutes if needed for shaking chills (generally, cumulative doses >50 mg are not needed; use with caution in persons with moderate or more severely impaired renal function)

Treatment plan notes:
• LVEF assessment (MUGA or echocardiography) every 3 months in patients receiving trastuzumab

Hand-foot reaction (palmar-plantar erythrodysesthesia, PPE)
Use topical emollients (eg, Aquaphor®), topical or orally administered steroids, antihistamines, or pyridoxine 50 to 200 mg/day

(continued)

Patient Population Studied

Patients with measurable or nonmeasurable histologically confirmed inoperable locally advanced, recurrent, or metastatic adenocarcinoma of the stomach or gastroesophageal junction with defined HER2+ status who had not previously received treatment for metastatic disease. New immunohistochemistry scoring criteria (Hofmann M et al. Histopathology 2008;52:797–805) determined eligibility. Patients whose tumor samples scored 3+ on immunohistochemical staining for HER2 or if samples were FISH positive (HER2:CEP17 ratio ≥2) were eligible to participate

(continued)

Diarrhea management

Latent or delayed onset-diarrhea*:

Loperamide 4 mg; administer orally initially after the first loose or liquid stool, *then*
Loperamide 2 mg every 2 hours while awake; every 4 hours during sleep
Alternatively, a trial of **Diphenoxylate hydrochloride** 2.5 mg **with Atropine sulfate** 0.025 mg (eg, Lomotil®) two tablets four times daily until control achieved.

Persistent diarrhea:

Octreotide acetate (solution) 100–150 mcg; administer subcutaneously 3 times daily.

Antibiotic therapy during latent or delayed-onset diarrhea:

A fluoroquinolone (eg, **Ciprofloxacin** 500 mg orally every 12 hours) if absolute neutrophil count $<500/mm^3$

*Abigerges D et al. J Natl Cancer Inst 1994;86:446–449
Rothenberg ML et al. J Clin Oncol 2001;19:3801–3807
Wadler S et al. J Clin Oncol 1998;16:3169–3178

Oral care

- Encourage patients to maintain intake of non-alcoholic fluids

If mucositis or stomatitis is present:

- Rinse mouth several times a day with ¼ teaspoon (1.25 g) each of baking soda and table salt in one quart of warm water. Follow with a plain water rinse
  - Do not use mouthwashes that contain alcohols

Therapy Monitoring

1. LVEF assessments at baseline and at least every 12 weeks
2. Complete blood counts and leukocyte differential counts at least weekly
3. LFTs, serum BUN, and creatinine before each cycle of chemotherapy
4. Assessment of response every 6 weeks

Treatment Modifications

Adverse Event	Dose Modifications*
Inadequate hematologic recovery by day 21 (absolute neutrophil count $<1500/mm^3$ *or* platelet count $<100,000/mm^3$)	Delay cisplatin and capecitabine for 1 week or until myelosuppression resolves
Recurrent treatment delay because of myelosuppression	Delay cisplatin and capecitabine for 1 week *or* until myelosuppression resolves, *then* decrease cisplatin and capecitabine dosage by 25% during subsequent treatments
Capecitabine	
G2 stomatitis, diarrhea, or nausea	Hold capecitabine; resume capecitabine at full dose after resolution of toxicity
Second episode of G2 stomatitis, diarrhea, or nausea	Hold capecitabine; resume capecitabine with dosage reduced by 25% after resolution of toxicity
Third episode of G2 stomatitis, diarrhea, or nausea	Hold capecitabine; resume capecitabine with dosage reduced by 50% after resolution of toxicity
Fourth episode of G2 stomatitis, diarrhea, or nausea	Discontinue capecitabine
G3 stomatitis, diarrhea, or nausea	Hold capecitabine; if G3 toxicity is adequately controlled within 2 days, then on resolution of toxicity to G ≤2, resume capecitabine at full dosage. If G3 toxicity takes >2 days to be controlled, then on resolution of toxicity to G ≤2, resume capecitabine with dosage decreased by 25%
Second episode of G3 stomatitis, diarrhea, or nausea	Hold capecitabine; if G3 toxicity is adequately controlled within 2 days, then on resolution of toxicity to G ≤2, resume capecitabine with dosage reduced by 50%
Third episode of G3 stomatitis, diarrhea, or nausea	Discontinue capecitabine
G4 stomatitis, diarrhea, or nausea	Discontinue capecitabine or on resolution of toxicity resume capecitabine with dosage reduced by 50%
G1 capecitabine-associated plantar palmar erythema (PPE)	Begin pyridoxine 50 mg 3 times daily and continue capecitabine without dose modification
G2 capecitabine-associated PPE	Begin pyridoxine 50 mg 3 times daily; withhold capecitabine until symptoms resolve, then resume capecitabine with dosage reduced by 15%

(continued)

Treatment Modifications (*continued*)

Adverse Event	Dose Modifications*
G3 capecitabine-associated PPE	Begin pyridoxine 50 mg 3 times daily; withhold capecitabine until symptoms resolve, then resume capecitabine with dosage reduced by 30%
Recurrent G3 capecitabine-associated PPE	Begin pyridoxine 50 mg 3 times daily; withhold capecitabine until symptoms resolve, then resume capecitabine with dosage reduced by 50%

Cisplatin

Reduction in creatinine clearance* to ≤60% of on study value	Delay therapy 1 week. If creatinine clearance does not recover to pretreatment values, then consider reducing cisplatin dose
Creatinine clearance* 40 to 60 mL/min (0.66–1 mL/s)	Consider reducing cisplatin so that dose in milligrams equals the creatinine clearance* value in mL/min†
Creatinine clearance* <40 mL/min (<0.66 mL/s)	Hold cisplatin
Clinically significant ototoxicity	Discontinue cisplatin
Persistent (>14 days) peripheral neuropathy without functional impairment	Decrease cisplatin dose by 50%
Clinically significant sensory loss—persistent (>14 days) peripheral neuropathy with functional impairment	Discontinue cisplatin

Trastuzumab

Trastuzumab toxicity was managed by treatment interruptions

*Creatinine clearance used as a measure of glomerular filtration rate
†This also applies to patients with creatinine clearance (GFR) of 40 to 60 mL/min at the outset of treatment

Efficacy

	Chemotherapy + Trastuzumab (N = 294)	Chemotherapy Alone (N = 290)
Median overall survival	13.8 months (95% CI, 12–16 months)	11.1 months (95% CI, 10–13 months)
Median PFS	6.7 months (95% CI, 6–8 months)*	5.5 months (95% CI, 5–6 months)†
Duration of response	6.9 months (95% CI, 6–8 months)*	4.8 months (95% CI, 4–6 months)†
Overall tumor response rate	139 (47%)	100 (35%)
CR	16 (5%)	7 (2%)
PR	123 (42%)	93 (32%)

*N = 139
†N = 100

Post-hoc exploratory analysis

	High HER2 Expression (IHC 2+ & FISH+ or IHC 3+)		Low HER2 Expression (IHC 0 or 1+ and FISH+)	
	Chemotherapy + Trastuzumab	Chemotherapy Alone	Chemotherapy + Trastuzumab	Chemotherapy Alone
Hazard ratio	0.65 (95% CI, 0.51–0.83)		1.07 (95% CI, 0.70–1.62)	
Median OS	16.0 months	11.8 months	10 months	8.7 months

IHC, HER2 immunohistochemistry
There was evidence of a significant interaction test (p = 0.036) between treatment and the 2 HER2 subgroups (high HER2 expression vs. low HER2 expression)

Adverse Events

(NCI-CTCAE, National Cancer Institute (USA) Common Terminology Criteria for Adverse Events, version 3.0 and serious adverse events according to International Conference on Harmonisation guidelines). Available at: http://ctep.cancer.gov/protocolDevelopment/electronic_applications/ctc.htm [accessed December 7, 2013]

Adverse events of all grades (>5%) and G3/4 (≥1%) plus adverse events of any grade with >5% difference between groups

	Trastuzumab + Chemotherapy (N = 294)		Chemotherapy Alone (N = 290)	
	All Grades	G3/4	All Grades	G3/4
Any adverse event	292 (99%)	201 (68%)	284 (98%)	198 (68%)
Gastrointestinal Disorders				
Nausea	197 (67%)	22 (7%)	184 (63%)	21 (7%)
Vomiting	147 (50%)	18 (6%)	134 (46%)	22 (8%)
Diarrhea	109 (37%)	27 (9%)	80 (28%)	11 (4%)
Constipation	75 (26%)	2 (1%)	93 (32%)	5 (2%)
Stomatitis	72 (24%)	2 (1%)	43 (15%)	6 (2%)
Abdominal pain	66 (22%)	7 (2%)	56 (19%)	5 (2%)
Dysphagia	19 (6%)	7 (2%)	10 (3%)	1 (<1%)
Blood and Lymphatic System Disorders				
Neutropenia	157 (53%)	79 (27%)	165 (57%)	88 (30%)
Anemia	81 (28%)	36 (12%)	61 (21%)	30 (10%)
Thrombocytopenia	47 (16%)	14 (5%)	33 (11%)	8 (3%)
Febrile neutropenia	15 (5%)	15 (5%)	8 (3%)	8 (3%)
General, Metabolic, and Other Disorders				
Anorexia	135 (46%)	19 (6%)	133 (46%)	18 (6%)
Fatigue	102 (35%)	12 (4%)	82 (28%)	7 (2%)
Hand-foot syndrome	75 (26%)	4 (1%)	64 (22%)	5 (2%)
Weight decreased	69 (23%)	6 (2%)	40 (14%)	7 (2%)
Asthenia	55 (19%)	14 (5%)	53 (18%)	10 (3%)
Fever	54 (18%)	3 (1%)	36 (12%)	0
Renal impairment	47 (16%)	2 (1%)	39 (13%)	3 (1%)
Mucosal inflammation	37 (13%)	6 (2%)	18 (6%)	2 (1%)
Nasopharyngitis	37 (13%)	0	17 (6%)	0
Chills	23 (8%)	1 (<1%)	0	0
Hypokalemia	22 (7%)	13 (4%)	13 (4%)	7 (2%)
Dehydration	18 (6%)	7 (2%)	16 (6%)	5 (2%)
Dyspnea	9 (3%)	1 (<1%)	16 (6%)	5 (2%)

Serious Adverse Events

	Trastuzumab + Chemotherapy (N = 294)	Chemotherapy Alone (N = 290)
Serious adverse events	95 (32%)	81 (28%)
Adverse events leading to dose modifications or treatment interruption	246 (84%)	237 (82%)
60-day mortality	15 deaths (5%)	20 deaths (7%)
Treatment-related mortality	10 deaths (3%)	3 deaths (1%)
Severe infusion reactions (G ≥3; eg, allergic reaction or hypersensitivity, chills, arthralgia, dyspnea)	17 (6%)	NR
Cardiac adverse events	17 (6%)	18 (6%)
G3/4	4 patients, 9 events	9 patients, 9 events
Cardiac dysfunction (LVEF decrease ≥10%, or decrease to absolute LVEF <50%)	11 (5%)*	2 (1%)†

*N = 237
†N = 187

12. Gastric Cancer

Jonas W. Feilchenfeldt, MD and Manish A. Shah, MD

Epidemiology

Incidence: 22,220 (male: 13,730; female: 8,490. Estimated new cases for 2014 in the United States)
10.4 per 100,000 male, 5.3 per 100,000 female
The incidence of gastric cancer varies with different geographic regions

Deaths: Estimated 10,990 in 2014 (male: 6,720; female: 4,270)

Median age: 69 years

Male to female ratio: ~2:1

Stage at Presentation

Localized	24%
Regional	30%
Distant	35%

Kamangar F et al. J Clin Oncol 2006;24:2137–2150
Siegel R et al. CA Cancer J Clin 2014;64:9–29
Surveillance, Epidemiology and End Results (SEER) Program, available from http://seer.cancer.gov (accessed in 2013)

Work-up

1. Multidisciplinary evaluation
2. History and physical examination
3. CBC and chemistry profile
4. CT abdomen with contrast; CT/ultrasound pelvis in women pelvis
5. Chest imaging*
6. Esophagogastroduodenoscopy (EGD)
7. PET-CT or PET scan (optional)
8. Endoscopic ultrasound (EUS) (optional)
9. *Helicobacter pylori* test[†] (optional)

*A combined CT scan of chest and abdomen is a pragmatic option
[†]Chey WD et al. Am J Gastroenterol 2007;102:1808–1825

Locoregional (M0):

1. Medically fit (medically able to tolerate major abdominal surgery), potentially resectable
2. Medically fit (medically able to tolerate major abdominal surgery), unresectable
3. Medically unfit. Laparoscopy is performed to evaluate for peritoneal spread when considering chemoradiation or surgery. Laparoscopy is not indicated if a palliative resection is planned

Stage IV (M1):

1. No further work-up necessary

Note: PET-CT may have a role for monitoring chemotherapy response

Pathology

Borrman Classification

Gross appearance is the basis for the first classification system of stomach cancers. Any of the 4 types may coexist:

Type I: Polypoid
Type II: Fungating
Type III: Ulcerated
Type IV: Infiltrative

Lauren Classification

Pattern of local invasion based on histologic features:

1. Intestinal: composed of cohesive neoplastic cells that form glands and tubular structures
2. Diffuse: scattered neoplastic cells that invade individually with minimal intercellular cohesion
3. Unclassified

World Health Organization Classification

1. Intraepithelial neoplasia—adenoma
2. Carcinoma
3. Adenocarcinoma (intestinal type, diffuse type)
4. Papillary adenocarcinoma
5. Tubular adenocarcinoma
6. Mucinous adenocarcinoma
7. Signet ring cell carcinoma
8. Adenosquamous carcinoma
9. Squamous cell carcinoma
10. Undifferentiated carcinoma
11. Others

Stemmermann GN et al. Gastric cancer: pathology. In: Kelsen DP et al. eds. Gastrointestinal Oncology: Principles and Practice. Baltimore, MD: Lippincott Williams & Wilkins, 2008:257–274

Pathologic Staging

Primary Tumor (T)

TX	Primary tumor cannot be assessed
T0	No evidence of primary tumor
Tis	Carcinoma *in situ*: intraepithelial tumor without invasion of the lamina propria
T1	Tumor invades lamina propria, muscularis mucosae, or submucosa
T1a	Tumor invades lamina propria or muscularis mucosae
T1b	Tumor invades submucosa
T2	Tumor invades muscularis propria
T3	Tumor penetrates subserosal connective tissue without invasion of visceral peritoneum or adjacent structures[*,†,‡]
T4	Tumor invades serosa (visceral peritoneum) or adjacent structures[†,‡]
T4a	Tumor invades serosa (visceral peritoneum)
T4b	Tumor invades adjacent structures

*A tumor may penetrate the muscularis propria with extension into the gastrocolic or gastrohepatic ligaments, or into the greater or lesser omentum, without perforation of the visceral peritoneum covering these structures. In this case, the tumor is classified T3. If there is perforation of the visceral peritoneum covering the gastric ligaments or the omentum, the tumor should be classified T4
†The adjacent structures of the stomach include the spleen, transverse colon, liver, diaphragm, pancreas, abdominal wall, adrenal gland, kidney, small intestine, and retroperitoneum
‡Intramural extension to the duodenum or esophagus is classified by the depth of the greatest invasion in any of these sites, including the stomach

Regional Lymph Nodes (N)

NX	Regional lymph node(s) cannot be assessed
N0	No regional lymph node metastasis*
N1	Metastasis in 1 to 2 regional lymph nodes
N2	Metastasis in 3 to 6 regional lymph nodes
N3	Metastasis in 7 or more regional lymph nodes
N3a	Metastasis in 7 to 15 regional lymph nodes
N3b	Metastasis in 16 or more regional lymph nodes

*A designation of pN0 should be used if all examined lymph nodes are negative, regardless of the total number removed and examined

Distant Metastasis (M)

	No distant metastasis (no pathologic M0; use clinical M to complete stage group)
M1	Distant metastasis

Staging

Group	T	N	M
0	Tis	N0	M0
IA	T1	N0	M0
IB	T2	N0	M0
	T1	N1	M0
IIA	T3	N0	M0
	T2	N1	M0
	T1	N2	M0
IIB	T4a	N0	M0
	T3	N1	M0
	T2	N2	M0
	T1	N3	M0
IIIA	T4a	N1	M0
	T3	N2	M0
	T2	N3	M0
IIIB	T4b	N0	M0
	T4b	N1	M0
	T4a	N2	M0
	T3	N3	M0
IIIC	T4b	N2	M0
	T4b	N3	M0
	T4a	N3	M0
IV	Any T	Any N	M1

Edge SB, Byrd DR, Compton CC, Fritz AG, Greene FL, Trotti A, editors. AJCC Cancer Staging Manual. 7th ed. New York: Springer; 2010
Washington K. Ann Surg Oncol 2010;17:3077–3079

Treatment and Survival by Stage

Stage	Treatment	5-Year Survival Rate
Stage 0 (in situ)	Surgery	>90%
Stage IA	Surgery	60–80%
Stage IB	Surgery ± adjuvant therapy	50–60%
Stage II	Surgery + adjuvant therapy	30–50%
Stage IIIA	Surgery + adjuvant therapy	~20% (distal tumors)
Stage IIIB	Surgery + adjuvant therapy	~10%
Stage IV	Palliative chemotherapy, radiation therapy	~5%

Expert Opinion

1. Diffuse gastric histology and peritoneal spread may adversely affect the motility of the gastrointestinal tract. Consider promotility agents

2. Common sites of metastatic spread:

   Lymphatic: M1 lymph nodes include paraaortic nodes. Supradiaphragmatic and mediastinal nodes may also be involved. Rare involvement of the left supraclavicular nodes occurs via the thoracic duct

   Blood-borne hematogenous: Distant metastases to the liver, lungs, bone, and skin. Either hematogenous spread or neoplastic seeding of the peritoneum, mesentery, and omentum can result in massive bilateral involvement of the ovaries (Krukenberg tumor)

3. For locally advanced, non-metastatic disease, several studies demonstrate benefit with adjuvant therapy:
   - perioperative chemotherapy
   - post-operative chemoradiation
   - post-operative chemotherapy (preferred in Asia)

4. All tumors should be examined for HER2 status. HER2 positive patients should receive cisplatin/capecitabine and trastuzumab based therapy

5. In second line, either single agent docetaxel or single agent irinotecan can be administered

Bonin SR et al. Gastric cancer. In: Pazdur R et al. eds. Cancer Management: A Multidisciplinary Approach, 7th ed. The Oncology Group, 2003:259–270
D' Angelica M et al. Patterns of initial recurrence in completely resected gastric adenocarcinoma. Ann Surg 2004;240:808–816

6. **New tool for treatment monitoring: 18-fluorodeoxyglucose-PET**

   a. Although no data exist to routinely perform a PET-CT for staging purposes, the MUNICON trial points to a role of PET in predicting response to treatment in localized disease

   b. The trial included 119 patients with locally advanced adenocarcinoma of the esophagogastric junction who underwent staging with PET prior to initiating treatment. PET was repeated after 2 weeks of chemotherapy. Tumors with a decrease of 35% of standard uptake values (SUVs) were considered "responders." Difference of overall survival between responders and nonresponders was significant at censured follow-up of 2.3 years

Lordick F et al. Lancet Oncol 2007;8:797–805

7. A study reporting poor prognostic factors in locally advanced and metastatic esophagogastric cancer analyzed prognostic factors based on three randomized trials (N = 1080):

Ross P et al. J Clin Oncol 2002;20:1996–2004
Tebbutt NC et al. Ann Oncol 2002;13:1568–1575
Webb A et al. J Clin Oncol 1997;15:261–267

Multivariate Baseline Prognostic Model			
Factors	Hazard Ratio	99% CI	p-Value
Performance status 2–3	1.575	1.251–1.981	<0.0001
Liver metastasis	1.409	1.139–1.743	<0.0001
Peritoneal metastasis	1.329	1.013–1.743	0.007
Alkaline phosphatase ≥100 units/L	1.412	1.136–1.755	<0.0001

Multivariate Logistic Regression Model for Tumor Response to Chemotherapy			
Factors	Risk Ratio	99% CI	p-Value
Performance Status 2–3	0.469	0.280–0.787	<0.001
Peritoneal metastasis	0.475	0.254–0.889	0.002
Alkaline phosphatase ≥100 units/L	0.655	0.433–0.992	0.009

Chau I et al. J Clin Oncol 2004;22:2395–2403

Surgical Options

Resectable Tumors

1. Tis or T1* limited to mucosa (T1a)
   - Gastrectomy (endoscopic resection in experienced centers)

2. T1b-T3[†]
   - Distal gastrectomy
   - Subtotal gastrectomy (preferred for distal gastric cancers)
   - Total gastrectomy

   Notes:
   - Gastric resection should encompass the regional lymph nodes (D1), with a desired goal of removing/examining ≥15 lymph nodes[‡§]
   - Consider placing a feeding jejunostomy tube especially if postoperative chemoradiation appears a likely recommendation

Criteria of unresectability
Locoregionally advanced

1. Level 3 or 4 lymph node highly suspicious on imaging or confirmed by biopsy

2. Invasion or encasement of major vascular structures

3. Distant metastasis or peritoneal seeding (including positive peritoneal cytology)

*Soetikno R et al. J Clin Oncol 2005;23:4490–4498
[†]Ito H et al. J Am Coll Surg 2004;199:880–886
[‡]Hartgrink HH et al. J Clin Oncol 2004;22:2069–2077
[§]Schwarz RE et al. Ann Surg Oncol 2007;14:317–328

ADJUVANT CHEMORADIATION REGIMEN

FLUOROURACIL + LEUCOVORIN + RADIATION

Macdonald JS et al. N Engl J Med 2001;345:725–730

Following curative surgery, patients receive 5 cycles of chemotherapy and concomitant radiotherapy spanning cycles 2 and 3 (based on a regimen described by Poon MA et al. J Clin Oncol 1989;7:1407–1418)

Cycle 1, neoadjuvant chemotherapy only:
Leucovorin 20 mg/m² per day; administer intravenously in 25–100 mL of 0.9% sodium chloride injection (0.9% NS) or 5% dextrose injection (D5W) over 5–15 minutes for 5 consecutive days on days 1–5 (total dosage/cycle = 100 mg/m²)
Fluorouracil 425 mg/m² per day; administer intravenously in 25–100 mL 0.9% NS or D5W over 5–30 minutes after leucovorin for 5 consecutive days on days 1–5 (total dosage/cycle = 2125 mg/m²)

Cycles 2 and 3, chemotherapy plus radiation:
Starts 28 days after the start of cycle 1 (ie, day 29)
Leucovorin 20 mg/m² per day; administer intravenously in 25–100 mL of 0.9% NS or D5W over 5–15 minutes for 4 consecutive days on days 1–4 during the first week of radiation therapy (total dosage during the first week of combined chemoradiation = 80 mg/m²)
Fluorouracil 400 mg/m² per day; administer intravenously in 25–100 mL of 0.9% NS or D5W over 5–30 minutes after leucovorin for 4 consecutive days on days 1–4 during the first week of radiation therapy (total dosage during first week of combined chemoradiation = 1600 mg/m²)
Radiation 180 cGy/day for 5 days/week for 5 consecutive weeks (total dose 4500 cGy in twenty-five 180-cGy fractions)

• Radiation fields must be evaluated carefully
• One-third of patients require field adjustments (INT-0116 study)

Leucovorin 20 mg/m² per day; administer intravenously in 25–100 mL of 0.9% NS or D5W over 5–15 minutes for 3 consecutive days on days 3–5 during the fifth week of radiation therapy (total dosage during the fifth week of combined chemoradiation = 60 mg/m²)
Fluorouracil 400 mg/m² per day; administer intravenously in 25–100 mL of 0.9% NS or D5W over 5–30 minutes after leucovorin for 3 consecutive days on days 3–5 during the fifth week of radiation therapy (total dosage during the fifth week of combined chemoradiation = 1200 mg/m²)

Cycles 4 and 5, chemotherapy only:
Starts 1 month after completing radiation therapy
Leucovorin 20 mg/m² per day; administer intravenously in 25–100 mL of 0.9% NS or D5W over 5–15 minutes on days 1–5, every 4 weeks for 2 cycles (total dosage/cycle = 100 mg/m²)
Fluorouracil 425 mg/m² per day; administer intravenously in 25–100 mL of 0.9% NS or D5W over 5–30 minutes after leucovorin on days 1–5 every 4 weeks, for 2 cycles (total dosage/cycle = 2125 mg/m²)

Supportive Care
Antiemetic prophylaxis
Emetogenic potential is **LOW** for chemotherapy alone
Emetogenic potential is at least **MODERATE** during chemoradiation
See Chapter 39 for antiemetic recommendations

Hematopoietic growth factor (CSF) prophylaxis
Primary prophylaxis is NOT indicated
See Chapter 43 for more information

Antimicrobial prophylaxis
Risk of fever and neutropenia is LOW
 Antimicrobial primary prophylaxis to be considered:
 • Antibacterial—not indicated
 • Antifungal—not indicated
 • Antiviral—not indicated unless patient previously had an episode of HSV
See Chapter 47 for more information

(continued)

Patient Population Studied

A study of 556 evaluable patients with stage IB-IV M0 gastric cancer who had undergone curative surgery were randomly assigned to receive adjuvant chemoradiation or observation alone. Patients had completely recovered from resection and were no longer losing weight

Efficacy (N = 281)*

Median overall survival	36 months
3-Year disease-free survival	48%
Median relapse free survival	30 months
Local recurrence	19%
Regional relapse†	65%
Distant Relapses	33%

*Intention-to-treat analysis
†Typically, abdominal carcinomatosis

Therapy Monitoring

1. *Prior to each cycle:* Interval history with emphasis on clinical toxicities, physical examination, CBC with differential, serum creatinine, and LFTs
2. *Response evaluation:* Clinical follow-up at 3-months intervals for 2 years, then at 6-months intervals for 3 years, and yearly thereafter. Follow-up consists of physical examination, CBC, liver function tests, chest radiography, and CT as clinically indicated

Cessation of Chemoradiotherapy (N = 281)

Reason	No. of Patients (%)
Protocol treatment completed	181 (64)
Toxic effects	49 (17)
Patient declined further treatment	23 (8)
Progression of disease	13 (5)
Death	3 (1)
Other	12 (4)

(*continued*)

Oral care

Prophylaxis and treatment for mucositis/stomatitis

General advice:
- Encourage patients to maintain intake of non-alcoholic fluids
- Evaluate patients for oral pain and provide analgesic medications
- Consider histamine (H_2-subtype) receptor antagonists (eg, ranitidine, famotidine), or a proton pump inhibitor for epigastric pain
- *Lactobacillus* sp.-containing probiotics may be beneficial in preventing diarrhea

Patients with intact oral mucosa:
- Clean the mouth, tongue, and gums by brushing after every meal and at bedtime with an ultra-soft toothbrush with fluoride toothpaste
- Floss teeth gently every day unless contraindicated. If gums bleed and hurt, avoid bleeding or sore areas, but floss other teeth
- Patients may use saline or commercial bland, non-alcoholic rinses
  - Do not use mouthwashes that contain alcohols

If mucositis or stomatitis is present:
- Keep the mouth moist utilizing water, ice chips, sugarless gum, sugar-free hard candies, or a saliva substitute
- Rinse mouth several times a day to remove debris
  - Use a solution of ¼ teaspoon (1.25 g) each of baking soda and table salt (sodium chloride) in one quart (~950 mL) of warm water. Follow with a plain water rinse
  - Do not use mouthwashes that contain alcohols
- Foam-tipped swabs (eg, Toothettes®) are useful in moisturizing oral mucosa, but ineffective for cleansing teeth and removing plaque
- Advise patients who develop mucositis to:
  - Choose foods that are easy to chew and swallow
  - Take small bites of food, chew slowly, and sip liquids with meals
  - Encourage soft, moist foods such as cooked cereals, mashed potatoes, and scrambled eggs
  - For trouble swallowing, soften food with gravies, sauces, broths, yogurt, or other bland liquids
  - Avoid sharp, crunchy foods; hot, spicy or highly acidic foods (eg, citrus fruits and juices); sugary foods; toothpicks; tobacco products; alcoholic drinks

Hand-foot reaction (palmar-plantar erythrodysesthesia, PPE)
For patients who develop a hand-foot reaction, use topical emollients (eg, Aquaphor®), topical or orally administered steroids, antihistamine agents (H_1-receptor antagonists), or pyridoxine
  Pyridoxine may provide relief for discomfort/pain associated with PPE, although the mechanism through which this occurs remains unclear
- The suggested pyridoxine starting dose is 50 mg/day, which may be increased to a maximum of 200 mg/day

Toxicity (N = 273) (Grade ≥3)	No. of Patients (%)
Hematologic	148 (54)
Gastrointestinal	89 (33)
Influenza-like symptoms	25 (9)
Infection	16 (6)
Neurologic	12 (4)
Cardiovascular	11 (4)
Pain	9 (3)
Metabolic	5 (2)
Hepatic	4 (1)
Lung-related	3 (1)
Death*	3 (1)

*One patient died from a cardiac event, 1 from pulmonary fibrosis, and 1 from sepsis complicating myelosuppression

Treatment Modifications

Dose modification as clinically indicated based on the most significant toxicity
Recommendations apply to all 5 chemotherapy cycles

Dosage level −1	Fluorouracil 350 mg/m²
Dosage level −2	Fluorouracil 300 mg/m²

Adverse Event	Dose Modification
Myelosuppression/ Thrombocytopenia	Consider reducing chemotherapy doses during subsequent cycles
Hand-foot syndrome (palmar-plantar erythrodysesthesia)	Interrupt fluorouracil therapy until symptoms resolve. Reduce fluorouracil dosage or discontinue fluorouracil
Mucositis	Interrupt fluorouracil therapy until symptoms resolve. Reduce fluorouracil dosage or discontinue fluorouracil
Diarrhea	Interrupt fluorouracil therapy until symptoms resolve. Reduce fluorouracil dosage or discontinue fluorouracil

ADJUVANT REGIMEN PRE- AND POSTOPERATIVE

EPIRUBICIN (E) + CISPLATIN (C) + FLUOROURACIL (F)

Cunningham D et al. N Engl J Med 2006;355:11–20. Comment in: N Engl J Med 2006;355:76–77, N Engl J Med 2006;355:1386–1388, ACP J Club 2007;146:2, Nat Clin Pract Oncol 2007;4:76–77

Pre- and postoperative chemotherapy: Administer 3–4 cycles of the chemotherapy regimen neoadjuvantly, with the last cycle given 3–6 weeks before surgery. Give 3–4 cycles of the chemotherapy regimen adjuvantly starting 6–12 weeks after surgery

Prior to starting chemotherapy: In patients with a history of ischemic heart disease measure left ventricular ejection fraction by multiple gated acquisition (MUGA) scanning or echocardiography. Omit epirubicin if the left ventricular ejection fraction is <50%

Epirubicin 50 mg/m^2; administer intravenously over 3–20 minutes on day 1 every 3 weeks (total dosage/cycle = 50 mg/m^2)
Hydration before cisplatin: ≥1000 mL 0.9% sodium chloride injection (0.9% NS); administer intravenously over a minimum of 3 hours
Mannitol 12.5–25 g; administer by intravenous injection or intravenous infusion over 5–15 minutes before starting cisplatin

- Mannitol may be given to patients who have received adequate hydration. Continued intravenous hydration is essential to ensure diuresis
- Mannitol may be prepared as an admixture (in the same container) with cisplatin

Cisplatin 60 mg/m^2; administer intravenously in 100–500 mL 0.9% NS over 30–60 minutes on day 1 every 3 weeks (total dosage/cycle = 60 mg/m^2)

Hydration after cisplatin: ≥1000 mL 0.9% NS; administer intravenously over a minimum of 3 hours. Encourage increased oral fluid intake. Goal is to achieve a urine output of ≥100 mL/hour. Monitor and replace magnesium and other electrolytes as needed
Fluorouracil 200 mg/m^2 per day; administer by continuous intravenous infusion over 24 hours in 50–1000 mL 0.9% NS or 5% dextrose injection for 21 consecutive days, on days 1–21 (total dosage/cycle = 4200 mg/m^2)

Supportive Care
Antiemetic prophylaxis
Emetogenic potential on day 1 is **HIGH**. *Potential for delayed emetic symptoms*
Emetogenic potential on days 2–21 is **LOW**
See Chapter 39 for antiemetic recommendations

Hematopoietic growth factor (CSF) prophylaxis
Primary prophylaxis may be indicated
See Chapter 43 for more information

Antimicrobial prophylaxis
Risk of fever and neutropenia is LOW
Antimicrobial primary prophylaxis to be considered:
- Antibacterial—not indicated
- Antifungal—not indicated
- Antiviral—not indicated unless patient previously had an episode of HSV
See Chapter 47 for more information

Diarrhea management
Latent or delayed-onset diarrhea:
Loperamide 4 mg; administer orally initially after the first loose or liquid stool, *then*
Loperamide 2 mg; administer orally every 2 hours during waking hours, *plus*
Loperamide 4 mg; administer orally every 4 hours during hours of sleep
- Continue for at least 12 hours after diarrhea resolves
- Recurrent diarrhea after a 12-hour diarrhea-free interval is treated as a new episode
- Rehydrate orally with fluids and electrolytes during a diarrheal episode
- If a patient develops blood or mucus in stool, dehydration, or hemodynamic instability, or if diarrhea persists >48 hours despite loperamide, stop loperamide and hospitalize the patient for IV hydration

(continued)

Treatment Modifications

Adverse Event	Dose Modification
Myelosuppression/thrombocytopenia	Consider reducing chemotherapy dosages during subsequent cycles
Hand-foot syndrome (palmar-plantar erythrodysesthesia)	Interrupt fluorouracil therapy until symptoms resolve. Reduce fluorouracil dosage or discontinue fluorouracil
Mucositis	Interrupt fluorouracil therapy until symptoms resolve. Reduce fluorouracil dosage or discontinue fluorouracil
Diarrhea	Interrupt fluorouracil therapy until symptoms resolve. Reduce fluorouracil dosage or discontinue fluorouracil
Reduction in creatinine clearance* to ≤60% of on study value	Delay therapy 1 week. If creatinine clearance does not recover to pretreatment values, then consider reducing cisplatin dosage
Creatinine clearance* 40–60 mL/min (0.66–1 mL/s)	Consider decreasing the amount of cisplatin administered, so the cisplatin dose in milligrams equals the creatinine clearance* value in mL/min†
Creatinine clearance* <40 mL/min (<0.66 mL/s)	Hold cisplatin
Left ventricular fraction less than 50%	Omit or discontinue epirubicin
Clinically significant ototoxicity	Discontinue cisplatin
Clinically significant sensory loss	Discontinue cisplatin

*Creatinine clearance is used as a measure of glomerular filtration rate (GFR)
†This also applies to patients with creatinine clearance (GFR) = 40–60 mL/min (0.66–1 mL/s) before starting or restarting treatment

(continued)

Alternatively, a trial of **Diphenoxylate hydrochloride** 2.5 mg **with Atropine sulfate** 0.025 mg (eg, Lomotil®)
- Initial adult dose is two tablets four times daily until control has been achieved, after which the dose may be reduced to meet individual requirements. Control may often be maintained with as little as two tablets daily
- Clinical improvement of acute diarrhea is usually observed within 48 hours. If improvement of chronic diarrhea after treatment with a maximum daily dose of 8 tablets is not observed within 10 days, control is unlikely with further administration

*Rothenberg ML et al. J Clin Oncol 2001;19:3801–3807
Wadler S et al. J Clin Oncol 1998;16:3169–3178

Oral care
Prophylaxis and treatment for mucositis/stomatitis
General advice:
- Encourage patients to maintain intake of non-alcoholic fluids
- Evaluate patients for oral pain and provide analgesic medications
- Consider histamine (H_2-subtype) receptor antagonists (eg, ranitidine, famotidine), or a proton pump inhibitor for epigastric pain
- *Lactobacillus* sp.-containing probiotics may be beneficial in preventing diarrhea

Patients with intact oral mucosa:
- Clean the mouth, tongue, and gums by brushing after every meal and at bedtime with an ultra-soft toothbrush with fluoride toothpaste
- Floss teeth gently every day unless contraindicated. If gums bleed and hurt, avoid bleeding or sore areas, but floss other teeth
- Patients may use saline or commercial bland, non-alcoholic rinses
  - Do not use mouthwashes that contain alcohols

If mucositis or stomatitis is present:
- Keep the mouth moist utilizing water, ice chips, sugarless gum, sugar-free hard candies, or a saliva substitute
- Rinse mouth several times a day to remove debris
  - Use a solution of ¼ teaspoon (1.25 g) each of baking soda and table salt (sodium chloride) in one quart (~950 mL) of warm water. Follow with a plain water rinse
  - Do not use mouthwashes that contain alcohols
- Foam-tipped swabs (eg, Toothettes®) are useful in moisturizing oral mucosa, but ineffective for cleansing teeth and removing plaque
- Advise patients who develop mucositis to:
  - Choose foods that are easy to chew and swallow
  - Take small bites of food, chew slowly, and sip liquids with meals
  - Encourage soft, moist foods such as cooked cereals, mashed potatoes, and scrambled eggs
  - For trouble swallowing, soften food with gravies, sauces, broths, yogurt, or other bland liquids
  - Avoid sharp, crunchy foods; hot, spicy or highly acidic foods (eg, citrus fruits and juices); sugary foods; toothpicks; tobacco products; alcoholic drinks

Hand-foot reaction (palmar-plantar erythrodysesthesia, PPE)
For patients who develop a hand-foot reaction, use topical emollients (eg, Aquaphor®), topical or orally administered steroids, antihistamine agents (H_1-receptor antagonists), or pyridoxine Pyridoxine may provide relief for discomfort/pain associated with PPE although the mechanism through which this occurs remains unclear
- The suggested pyridoxine starting dose is 50 mg/day, which may be increased to a maximum of 200 mg/day

Therapy Monitoring

1. *Before each cycle:* CBC with differential, blood urea nitrogen, electrolytes, serum creatinine, and LFTs
2. In patients with a history of ischemic heart disease, evaluate serially left ventricular ejection fraction with MUGA scanning or echocardiography

Patient Population Studied

Clinical trial of 503 patients with operable GI cancers (distal esophagus, GE junction, or gastric) randomly assigned to surgery only or perioperative chemotherapy consisting of 3 cycles of chemotherapy with the ECF regimen followed after 3–6 weeks by surgery, and then another 3 cycles of chemotherapy initiated 6–12 weeks after surgery. The surgical control arm underwent a surgical intervention within 6 weeks after randomization. The trial demonstrated significantly improved progression-free and overall survival in the chemotherapy arm

Toxicity

	Preoperative % G3/4	Postoperative % G3/4
Neutropenia	23.8	27.8
Leukopenia	11.5	11.1
Anemia	4.7	0.7
Thrombo-cytopenia	0.4	3.0
Nausea	6.4	12.3
Vomiting	5.6	10.1
Stomatitis	4.3	3.6
Diarrhea	2.6	3.6
Skin effects	3.4	1.5
Neurologic effects	3.8	3.6

Chemotherapy Administration/Tolerance

Completed preoperative chemotherapy	86% of patients initially assigned to chemotherapy (215/250); 90.7% of those who started chemotherapy (215/237)*
Began postoperative chemotherapy	54.8% of patients initially assigned to chemotherapy (137/250); 65.6% of those who had surgical resection (137/209)†
Completed postoperative chemotherapy	41.6% of patients initially assigned to chemotherapy; 75.9% of those who started (104/137)

*Reasons for not completing 3 preoperative cycles (N = 250): toxic effects (12 patients), patient request (3), problems with a Hickman catheter (3), early cancer-related death (2), and other (2)
†Reasons for not starting postoperative chemotherapy (N = 209) after completing the first 3 cycles were disease progression or early death (37 patients), patient choice (11), postoperative complications (10), problems with a Hickman catheter (4), previous toxic effects (3), lack of response to preoperative treatment (2), and worsening coexisting disease (2)

Efficacy

Surgical and Pathologic Results

Variable	Perioperative-Chemotherapy Group (N = 250)	Surgery Group (N = 253)
Extent of Resection According to Surgeon		
Curative Surgery	69.3%	66.4%
Palliative Surgery	18%	28%
D1 resection (distal + total)	17.8%	18.5%
D2 resection (distal + total)	42.5%	40.4%
Pathology Reports		
Tumor stage (all patients)		
T1	15.7%	8.3
T2	36.0%	28.5
T3	43.6%	54.9%
T4	4.7%	8.3%
Nodal status (patients with gastric cancer)		
N0	31.3%	26.9
N1	53.3%	43.6%
N2	14.1%	21.8%
N4	1.5%	7.7%

Progression-Free Survival and Overall Survival

Months	0	12	24	36	48	60	72
Progression-free Survival							
ECF → S → ECF (N = 250)	100%	64%	40%	27%	19%	13%	9.2%*
S (N = 253)	100%	49%	23%	17%	11%	6%	3.2%
Overall Survival							
ECF → S → ECF (N = 250)	100%	67%	44%	32%	21%	15%	11%*
S (N = 253)	100%	61%	32%	20%	12%	7.1%	3.6%

ECF, Epirubicin + cisplatin + fluorouracil; S, surgery
*Statistically significant

ADJUVANT REGIMEN

ADJUVANT CAPECITABINE AND OXALIPLATIN FOR GASTRIC CANCER AFTER D2 GASTRECTOMY

Bang Y-J et al. Lancet 2012;379:315–321

Capecitabine 1000 mg/m^2 per dose; administer orally twice daily for 14 consecutive days, on days 1–14, every 3 weeks for 8 cycles (total dosage/cycle = 28,000 mg/m^2), *plus*:

Oxaliplatin 130 mg/m^2; administer intravenously in 250–500 mL 5% dextrose injection over 2 hours on day 1, every 3 weeks, for 8 cycles (total dosage/cycle = 130 mg/m^2)

Supportive Care
Antiemetic prophylaxis
Emetogenic potential on Day 1 is **MODERATE**
Emetogenic potential on days with capecitabine alone is **MINIMAL–LOW**
See Chapter 39 for antiemetic recommendations

Hematopoietic growth factor (CSF) prophylaxis
Primary prophylaxis may be indicated
See Chapter 43 for more information

Antimicrobial prophylaxis
Risk of fever and neutropenia is LOW
  Antimicrobial primary prophylaxis to be considered:
  • Antibacterial—not indicated
  • Antifungal—not indicated
  • Antiviral—not indicated, unless patient previously had an episode of HSV
See Chapter 47 for more information

Hand-foot reaction (palmar-plantar erythrodysesthesia, PPE)
For patients who develop a hand-foot reaction, use topical emollients (eg, Aquaphor®), topical or orally administered steroids, antihistamine agents (H$_1$-receptor antagonists), or pyridoxine
  Pyridoxine may provide relief for discomfort/pain associated with PPE, although the mechanism through which this occurs remains unclear
• The suggested pyridoxine starting dose is 50 mg/day, which may be increased to a maximum of 200 mg/day

Diarrhea management
  Loperamide 4 mg; administer orally initially after the first loose or liquid stool, *then*
  Loperamide 2 mg; administer orally every 2 hours during waking hours, *plus*
  Loperamide 4 mg; administer orally every 4 hours during hours of sleep
  • Continue for at least 12 hours after diarrhea resolves
  • Recurrent diarrhea after a 12-hour diarrhea-free interval is treated as a new episode
  • Rehydrate orally with fluids and electrolytes during a diarrheal episode
  • If a patient develops blood or mucus in stool, dehydration, or hemodynamic instability, or if diarrhea persists >48 hours despite loperamide, stop loperamide and hospitalize the patient for IV hydration
  Alternatively, a trial of **Diphenoxylate hydrochloride** 2.5 mg **with Atropine sulfate** 0.025 mg (eg, Lomotil®)
  • Initial adult dose is two tablets four times daily until control has been achieved, after which the dose may be reduced to meet individual requirements. Control may often be maintained with as little as two tablets daily
  • Clinical improvement of acute diarrhea is usually observed within 48 hours. If improvement of chronic diarrhea after treatment with a maximum daily dose of 8 tablets is not observed within 10 days, control is unlikely with further administration

Rothenberg ML et al. J Clin Oncol 2001;19:3801–3807
Wadler S et al. J Clin Oncol 1998;16:3169–3178

Oral care
Prophylaxis and treatment for mucositis/stomatitis
  General advice:
  • Encourage patients to maintain intake of non-alcoholic fluids
  • Evaluate patients for oral pain and provide analgesic medications
  • Consider histamine (H$_2$-subtype) receptor antagonists (eg, ranitidine, famotidine), or a proton pump inhibitor for epigastric pain
  • *Lactobacillus* sp.-containing probiotics may be beneficial in preventing diarrhea
  Patients with intact oral mucosa:
  • Clean the mouth, tongue, and gums by brushing after every meal and at bedtime with an ultra-soft toothbrush with fluoride toothpaste
  • Floss teeth gently every day unless contraindicated. If gums bleed and hurt, avoid bleeding or sore areas, but floss other teeth
  • Patients may use saline or commercial bland, non-alcoholic rinses
    ▪ Do not use mouthwashes that contain alcohols

(continued)

(continued)

If mucositis or stomatitis is present:
- Keep the mouth moist utilizing water, ice chips, sugarless gum, sugar-free hard candies, or a saliva substitute
- Rinse mouth several times a day to remove debris
  - Use a solution of ¼ teaspoon (1.25 g) each of baking soda and table salt (sodium chloride) in one quart (~950 mL) of warm water. Follow with a plain water rinse
  - Do not use mouthwashes that contain alcohols
- Foam-tipped swabs (eg, Toothettes®) are useful in moisturizing oral mucosa, but ineffective for cleansing teeth and removing plaque
- Advise patients who develop mucositis to:
  - Choose foods that are easy to chew and swallow
  - Take small bites of food, chew slowly, and sip liquids with meals
  - Encourage soft, moist foods such as cooked cereals, mashed potatoes, and scrambled eggs
  - For trouble swallowing, soften food with gravies, sauces, broths, yogurt, or other bland liquids
  - Avoid sharp, crunchy foods; hot, spicy or highly acidic foods (eg, citrus fruits and juices); sugary foods; toothpicks; tobacco products; alcoholic drinks

Treatment Modifications

Adverse Event	Dose Modification
ANC nadir $<1000/mm^3$ *or* platelet nadir $<50,000/mm^3$ after treatment	Delay treatment until ANC $\geq 1000/mm^3$ *and* platelet $\geq 50,000/mm^3$, then decrease oxaliplatin dosage by 25%, and decrease daily capecitabine dosages by 50% during subsequent cycles*. Alternately consider using hematopoietic growth factors
Persistent G1/G2 neuropathy	Delay oxaliplatin 1 week. Resume oxaliplatin after toxicity resolves at a dosage decreased to $100 mg/m^2$ during subsequent cycles
"Transient" G3/4 neuropathy (7–14 days duration)	Hold oxaliplatin. Resume oxaliplatin after toxicity resolves at a dosage decreased to $100 mg/m^2$ during subsequent cycles
Persistent G3/4 neuropathy	Discontinue oxaliplatin
G3/4 diarrhea or stomatitis despite capecitabine dose reductions	Reduce oxaliplatin dosage to $100 mg/m^2$
G3/4 nonhematologic adverse events other than renal function and neurotoxicity	Reduce cisplatin and capecitabine dosages by 25% for subsequent cycles
G2 stomatitis, diarrhea, or nausea	Hold capecitabine; resume capecitabine at full dosage after resolution of toxicity
Second episode of G2 stomatitis, diarrhea, or nausea	Hold capecitabine; resume capecitabine with dosage reduced by 25% after resolution of toxicity
Third episode of G2 stomatitis, diarrhea, or nausea	Hold capecitabine; resume capecitabine with dosage reduced by 50% after resolution of toxicity
Fourth episode of G2 stomatitis, diarrhea, or nausea	Discontinue capecitabine
G3 stomatitis, diarrhea, or nausea	Hold capecitabine. If G3 toxicity is adequately controlled within 2 days, resume capecitabine at full dosage when toxicity resolves to G ≤ 1. If G3 toxicity takes >2 days to be controlled, resume capecitabine with dosage reduced by 25% after toxicity resolves to G ≤ 1
Second episode of G3 stomatitis, diarrhea, or nausea	Hold capecitabine; if G3 toxicity is controlled adequately within 2 days, then resume capecitabine with dosage reduced by 50% after toxicity resolves to G ≤ 1
Third episode of G3 stomatitis, diarrhea, or nausea	Discontinue capecitabine
G4 stomatitis, diarrhea, or nausea	Withhold capecitabine. Resume capecitabine with dosage reduced by 50% after toxicity resolves
G1 capecitabine-associated PPE[†]	Begin pyridoxine 50 mg orally 3 times daily and continue capecitabine without dose modification
G2 capecitabine-associated PPE[†]	Begin pyridoxine 50 mg orally 3 times daily and withhold capecitabine. Resume capecitabine with dosage reduced by 15% after toxicity resolves
G3 capecitabine-associated PPE[†]	Begin pyridoxine 50 mg orally 3 times daily and withhold capecitabine. Resume capecitabine with dosage reduced by 30% after toxicity resolves
Recurrent G3 capecitabine-associated PPE[†]	Continue pyridoxine 50 mg orally 3 times daily and withhold capecitabine. Resume capecitabine with dosage reduced by 50% after toxicity resolves

*Treatment delays for unresolved adverse events of >3 weeks duration warrant discontinuation of treatment
[†]PPE, palmar plantar erythrodysesthesia (hand-foot syndrome)

Efficacy

[Study Compared Adjuvant CAPE-OX After Surgery vs Surgery Only]

	Surgery Only (N = 515)	Surgery + CAPE-OX (N = 520)
Relapsed, developed a new gastric cancer, or died by time of data cutoff	163 (32%)	106 (20%)
3-year disease-free survival (DFS)	59% (95% CI, 53–64)	74% (95% CI, 69–79)
	HR 0.56, 95% CI 0.44–0.72; p <0.0001	
3-year DFS, stage II	71% (95% CI, 64–78)	85% (95% CI, 79–90)
3-year DFS, stage IIIa	51% (95% CI, 42–60)	66% (95% CI, 57–75)
3-year DFS stage IIIb	33% (95% CI, 15–51)	61% (95% CI, 48–73)
Deaths by time of data cutoff	85 (17%)	65 (13%)
3-year overall survival	78% (95% CI, 74–83)	83% (95% CI, 79–87)
	HR 0.72, 95% CI 0.52–1.00; p = 0.0493	
Recurrence or new gastric cancer	155 (30%)	96 (18%)
Peritoneal recurrence	56 (11%)	47 (9%)
Locoregional recurrence	44 (8.5%)	21 (4%)
Recurrence at distant sites	78 (15%)	49 (9.4%)

CAPE-OX, capecitabine and oxaliplatin

Toxicity

Adverse events reported by ≥10% of patients (safety population*)

Capecitabine and Oxaliplatin (N = 496)

	All Grades	Grades 3/4
Patients with ≥1 adverse event	490 (99%)	279 (56%)
Nausea	326 (66%)	39 (8%)
Neutropenia	300 (60%)	107 (22%)
Decreased appetite	294 (59%)	23 (5%)
Peripheral neuropathy	277 (56%)	12 (2%)
Diarrhea	236 (48%)	9 (2%)
Vomiting	191 (39%)	37 (7%)
Fatigue	156 (31%)	23 (5%)
Thrombo-cytopenia	130 (26%)	40 (8%)
Hand–foot syndrome	93 (19%)	5 (1%)
Asthenia	87 (18%)	10 (2%)
Abdominal pain	85 (17%)	8 (2%)
Constipation	63 (13%)	1 (<1%)
Dizziness	64 (13%)	3 (<1%)
Stomatitis, all	59 (12%)	3 (<1%)
Weight decreased	59 (12%)	1 (<1%)
Peripheral sensory neuropathy	50 (10%)	3 (<1%)

Data are n (%)
*Patients who received ≥1 dose of capecitabine or oxaliplatin

Treatment Monitoring

1. *Before each cycle:* Physical examination with attention to clinical toxicities, CBC with differential, serum magnesium, and LFTs
2. *Efficacy Assessments:* Every two cycles

Patient Population Studied

Patients with histologically confirmed gastric adenocarcinoma without evidence of metastatic disease. Only patients whose tumors were American Joint Committee on Cancer/Union Internationale Contre le Cancer (AJCC/UICC) stage II (T2N1, T1N2, T3N0), IIIA (T3N1, T2N2, T4N0), or IIIB (T3N2) were eligible. All patients had curative D2 gastrectomy and achieved R0 resection ≤6 weeks before randomization. At least 15 lymph nodes were examined. All surgeons were experienced (>50 procedures per year), standard operating procedures were predefined, and surgery was photographed

Patient Characteristics (N = 520)

Age (years)	56.1 (11.1)
Men	373 (72%)
Karnofsky performance status 90–100	90%
Time since surgery (months)	1.14 (0.17)
AJCC/UICC stage	
IB	1 (<1%)
II	253 (49%)
IIIA	193 (37%)
IIIB	73 (14%)
IV	0
Tumor stage	
T1	8 (2%)
T2	282 (54%)
T3	227 (44%)
T4	3 (1%)
Tumor location	
Antrum [lower third]	237 (46%)
Body [middle third]	166 (32%)
Body and antrum	31 (6%)
Fundus [upper third]	46 (9%)
Fundus and body	10 (2%)
Gastro-oesophageal junction	15 (3%)
Whole gastric	6 (1%)
Other [multiple localizations]	9 (2%)
Lymph nodes examined	45.0 (17.4)
Nodal status	
N0	47 (9%)
N1	313 (60%)
N2	160 (31%)

Data are mean (SD), n (%), or median (interquartile range); AJCC/UICC, American Joint Cancer Committee/Union Internationale Contre le Cancer

ADVANCED DISEASE REGIMEN

EPIRUBICIN + CISPLATIN + FLUOROURACIL (ECF)

Webb A et al. J Clin Oncol 1997;15:261–267

Epirubicin 50 mg/m²; administer by intravenous injection over 3–20 minutes on day 1, every 3 weeks, for a maximum of 8 cycles (total dosage/3-week cycle = 50 mg/m²)

Hydration before cisplatin: ≥1000 mL 0.9% sodium chloride injection (0.9% NS); administer intravenously over a minimum of 3–4 hours. Monitor and replace magnesium/electrolytes as needed

Mannitol diuresis: **Mannitol** may be given to patients who have received adequate hydration. A bolus dose of 12.5 g mannitol can be administered as an intravenous injection before starting cisplatin or in the same container as cisplatin. Continued hydration is essential

Cisplatin 60 mg/m²; administer intravenously in 100–500 mL of 0.9% NS over 30–60 minutes on day 1, every 3 weeks, for a maximum of 8 cycles (total dosage/3-week cycle = 60 mg/m²)

Hydration after cisplatin: ≥1000 mL 0.9% NS; administer intravenously over a minimum of 3–4 hours. Also, encourage increased oral intake of non-alcoholic fluids. Goal is to achieve a urine output of ≥100 mL/hour

Fluorouracil 200 mg/m² by continuous intravenous infusion in 50–1000 mL 0.9% NS, or 5% dextrose injection over 24 hours, starting on cycle 1, day 1, continuously for a maximum duration of 6 months (total dosage/3-week cycle = 4200 mg/m²)

Supportive Care

Antiemetic prophylaxis
Emetogenic potential on day 1 is **HIGH**. *Potential for delayed emetic symptoms*
Emetogenic potential on days 2–21 is **LOW**
See Chapter 39 for antiemetic recommendations

Hematopoietic growth factor (CSF) prophylaxis
Primary prophylaxis may be indicated
See Chapter 43 for more information

Antimicrobial prophylaxis
Risk of fever and neutropenia is LOW
  Antimicrobial primary prophylaxis to be considered:
  • Antibacterial—not indicated
  • Antifungal—not indicated
  • Antiviral—not indicated unless patient previously had an episode of HSV
See Chapter 47 for more information

Diarrhea management
Latent or delayed-onset diarrhea*:
  Loperamide 4 mg; administer orally initially after the first loose or liquid stool, *then*
  Loperamide 2 mg; administer orally every 2 hours during waking hours, *plus*
  Loperamide 4 mg; administer orally every 4 hours during hours of sleep
  • Continue for at least 12 hours after diarrhea resolves
  • Recurrent diarrhea after a 12-hour diarrhea-free interval is treated as a new episode
  • Rehydrate orally with fluids and electrolytes during a diarrheal episode
  • If a patient develops blood or mucus in stool, dehydration, or hemodynamic instability, or if diarrhea persists >48 hours despite loperamide, stop loperamide and hospitalize the patient for IV hydration

(continued)

Efficacy (N = 111–126)

	N = 111	N = 126 (Intent to Treat)
Complete response	6%	5.5%
Partial response	39%	34%
Stable disease	21%	18%
Progressive disease	20%	17%

Insufficient Treatment

Early death	6%
Toxic death	1%
Toxicity	3.5%
Patient request	3.5%

Symptomatic Response

Dysphagia	70%
Weight loss	81%
Anorexia	65%
Reflux	74%
Vomiting	77%
Nausea	57%
Pain	79%

Survival and Failure-Free Survival

Median survival	8.9 months
1-Year survival	36%
2-Year survival	11%
Median failure-free survival	7.4 months

WHO criteria

Patient Population Studied

A trial of 274 patients with previously untreated advanced esophagogastric cancer randomized to receive epirubicin, cisplatin, and fluorouracil (ECF; N = 137) compared with fluorouracil, doxorubicin, and methotrexate (FAMTX; N = 137). The ECF regimen resulted in a survival and response advantage, tolerable toxicity, and better quality of life, and cost-effectiveness

(continued)

Alternatively, a trial of **Diphenoxylate hydrochloride** 2.5 mg **with Atropine sulfate** 0.025 mg (eg, Lomotil®)
- Initial adult dose is two tablets four times daily until control has been achieved, after which the dose may be reduced to meet individual requirements. Control may often be maintained with as little as two tablets daily
- Clinical improvement of acute diarrhea is usually observed within 48 hours. If improvement of chronic diarrhea after treatment with a maximum daily dose of 8 tablets is not observed within 10 days, control is unlikely with further administration

*Rothenberg ML et al. J Clin Oncol 2001;19:3801–3807
Wadler S et al. J Clin Oncol 1998;16:3169–3178

Oral care
Prophylaxis and treatment for mucositis/stomatitis
General advice:
- Encourage patients to maintain intake of non-alcoholic fluids

If mucositis or stomatitis is present:
- Use a solution of ¼ teaspoon (1.25 g) each of baking soda and table salt (sodium chloride) in one quart (~950 mL) of warm water. Follow with a plain water rinse
- Do not use mouthwashes that contain alcohols

Hand-foot reaction (palmar-plantar erythrodysesthesia, PPE)
For patients who develop a hand-foot reaction, use topical emollients (eg, Aquaphor®), topical or orally administered steroids, antihistamine agents (H_1-receptor antagonists), or pyridoxine

Pyridoxine may provide relief; starting dose is 50 mg/day, which may be increased to a maximum of 200 mg/day

Treatment Modifications

Adverse Event	Dose Modification
Plantar/palmar erythema (PPE)	Give pyridoxine 50 mg orally 3 times daily. If PPE does not improve, hold fluorouracil for 1 week, then resume with fluorouracil 150 mg/m² per day by continuous infusion
G ≤1/2 mucositis or diarrhea	Interrupt chemotherapy until mucositis and diarrhea resolve, then resume fluorouracil with daily dosage reduced by 50 mg/m²
G3/4 mucositis or diarrhea	Interrupt chemotherapy until mucositis and diarrhea resolve, then resume fluorouracil with daily dosage reduced by 100 mg/m²
Creatinine clearance 40–60 mL/min (0.66–1 mL/s)	Reduce cisplatin so that dose in milligrams equals the creatinine clearance value in mL/min
Creatinine clearance <40 mL/min (<0.66 mL/s)	Hold cisplatin
Day 1 WBC <2000/mm³ *or* platelet count <100,000/mm³	Delay cisplatin and epirubicin for 1 week or until myelosuppression resolves
Second treatment delay because of myelosuppression	Delay cisplatin and epirubicin for 1 week, or until myelosuppression resolves, then decrease epirubicin dosage by 25% during subsequent treatments
Sepsis during an episode of neutropenia	

Findlay M et al. Ann Oncol 194;5:609–616

Toxicity

	% All Grades	% G3/4
Hematologic		
Leukopenia	61	12
Neutropenia	68	36*
Thrombocytopenia	10	4
Anemia	68	8
Nonhematologic		
Mucositis	49	6
Plantar-palmar erythema	31	3
Nausea/vomiting	88	17
Diarrhea	38	6
Infection	40	8
Renal	12	1
Peripheral neuropathy	20	—
Alopecia	93 (56†)	—

*Treatment-related death in 1 patient caused by sepsis during a period of neutropenia
†G2 alopecia, pronounced or total hair loss
National Cancer Institute (USA) Common Toxicity Criteria, version 2.0. Available at: http://ctep.cancer.gov/protocolDevelopment/electronic_applications/ctc.htm [accessed October 25, 2013]

Therapy Monitoring

1. *Before each cycle:* Physical examination with attention to clinical toxicities, CBC with differential, serum sodium, potassium, magnesium, creatinine, BUN, and LFTs
2. *Before repeated cisplatin treatments:* Monitor serum creatinine with estimated creatinine clearance (CrCl), or measure CrCl with either a 12- or a 24-hour urine collection

Note: Prior to starting chemotherapy: In patients with a history of ischemic heart disease, measure left ventricular ejection fraction by multiple gated acquisition (MUGA) scanning or echocardiography. Omit epirubicin if the left ventricular ejection fraction is <50%

ADVANCED DISEASE REGIMEN
DOCETAXEL + CISPLATIN + FLUOROURACIL (DCF)

van Cutsem E et al. J Clin Oncol 2006;24:4991–4997

Docetaxel 75 mg/m²; administer intravenously diluted in a volume of 0.9% sodium chloride injection (0.9% NS) or 5% dextrose injection (D5W) sufficient to produce a docetaxel concentration within the range 0.3–0.74 mg/mL over 60 minutes on day 1, every 3 weeks (total dosage/cycle = 75 mg/m²)

Hydration before cisplatin: ≥1000 mL 0.9% NS; administer intravenously over a minimum of 3 hours
Mannitol 12.5–25 g; administer by intravenous injection or infusion over 5–15 minutes before starting cisplatin. Mannitol may be given to patients who have received adequate hydration. Continued intravenous hydration is essential to insure diuresis. Mannitol may be prepared as an admixture (in the same container) with cisplatin
Cisplatin 75 mg/m²; administer intravenously in 100–250 mL 0.9% NS over 1–3 hours on day 1, every 3 weeks (total dosage/cycle = 75 mg/m²)

Hydration after cisplatin: ≥1000 mL 0.9% NS; administer intravenously over a minimum of 3 hours. Encourage increased oral intake of non-alcoholic fluids. Goal is to achieve a urine output of ≥100 mL/hour. Monitor and replace magnesium and other electrolytes as needed
Fluorouracil 750 mg/m² per day; administer by continuous intravenous infusion in 50–1000 mL 0.9% NS or D5W over 24 hours for 5 consecutive days, on days 1–5, every 3 weeks (total dosage/cycle = 3750 mg/m²)

Supportive Care
Antiemetic prophylaxis
Emetogenic potential on day 1 is **HIGH**. *Potential for delayed emetic symptoms*
Emetogenic potential on days 2–5 is **LOW**
See Chapter 39 for antiemetic recommendations

Hematopoietic growth factor (CSF) prophylaxis
Primary prophylaxis is indicated with one of the following:
Filgrastim (G-CSF) 5 mcg/kg per day by subcutaneous injection, *or*
Pegfilgrastim (pegylated filgrastim) 6 mg/0.6 mL by subcutaneous injection for 1 dose
- Begin use from 24–72 hours after myelosuppressive chemotherapy is completed

See Chapter 43 for more information

Antimicrobial prophylaxis
Risk of fever and neutropenia is LOW
Antimicrobial primary prophylaxis to be considered:
- Antibacterial—not indicated
- Antifungal—not indicated
- Antiviral—not indicated unless patient previously had an episode of HSV

See Chapter 47 for more information

Diarrhea management
Latent or delayed-onset diarrhea*:
Loperamide 4 mg; administer orally initially after the first loose or liquid stool, *then*
Loperamide 2 mg; administer orally every 2 hours during waking hours, *plus*
Loperamide 4 mg; administer orally every 4 hours during hours of sleep
- Continue for at least 12 hours after diarrhea resolves
- Recurrent diarrhea after a 12-hour diarrhea-free interval is treated as a new episode
- Rehydrate orally with fluids and electrolytes during a diarrheal episode
- If a patient develops blood or mucus in stool, dehydration, or hemodynamic instability, or if diarrhea persists >48 hours despite loperamide, stop loperamide and hospitalize the patient for IV hydration

Alternatively, a trial of **Diphenoxylate hydrochloride** 2.5 mg **with Atropine sulfate** 0.025 mg (eg, Lomotil®)
- Initial adult dose is two tablets four times daily until control has been achieved, after which the dose may be reduced to meet individual requirements. Control may often be maintained with as little as two tablets daily

(continued)

Treatment Modifications

- Cycle delays occurred in 64% of patients. Dose reductions occurred in 41% of patients
- Fluorouracil dose was most commonly reduced in comparison with docetaxel and cisplatin

Dosage Level		
Docetaxel	Level −1	55 mg/m²
Cisplatin	Level −1	60 mg/m²
Fluorouracil	Level −1	500 mg/m² per day for 5 days

Adverse Event	Dose Modification
G3/4 diarrhea or stomatitis	Reduce fluorouracil by 1 dose level
Reduction in creatinine clearance* to <60% of on-study value	Delay therapy 1 week. If creatinine clearance does not recover to pretreatment values, then reduce cisplatin by 1 dose level
Creatinine clearance* 40–60 mL/min (0.66–1 mL/s)	Consider decreasing the amount of cisplatin administered, so the cisplatin dose in milligrams equals the creatinine clearance* value in mL/min†
Creatinine clearance* <40 mL/min (<0.66 mL/s)	Hold cisplatin
Peripheral neuropathy	Delay therapy 1 week. If symptoms do not resolve to G ≤1, reduce cisplatin and or docetaxel by 1 dose level
G3/4 peripheral neurotoxicity or ototoxicity	Discontinue therapy

*Creatinine clearance is used as a measure of glomerular filtration rate (GFR)
†This also applies to patients with creatinine clearance (GFR) of 40–60 mL/min (0.66–1 mL/s) before starting or restarting treatment
Note: Other dose modifications as clinically indicated based on the most significant toxicity

(*continued*)

- Clinical improvement of acute diarrhea is usually observed within 48 hours. If improvement of chronic diarrhea after treatment with a maximum daily dose of 8 tablets is not observed within 10 days, control is unlikely with further administration

*Rothenberg ML et al. J Clin Oncol 2001;19:3801–3807
Wadler S et al. J Clin Oncol 1998;16:3169–3178

Oral care

Prophylaxis and treatment for mucositis/stomatitis

General advice:

- Encourage patients to maintain intake of non-alcoholic fluids
- Evaluate patients for oral pain and provide analgesic medications
- Consider histamine (H_2-subtype) receptor antagonists (eg, ranitidine, famotidine), or a proton pump inhibitor for epigastric pain
- *Lactobacillus* sp.-containing probiotics may be beneficial in preventing diarrhea

Patients with intact oral mucosa:

- Clean the mouth, tongue, and gums by brushing after every meal and at bedtime with an ultra-soft toothbrush with fluoride toothpaste
- Floss teeth gently every day unless contraindicated. If gums bleed and hurt, avoid bleeding or sore areas, but floss other teeth
- Patients may use saline or commercial bland, non-alcoholic rinses
  - Do not use mouthwashes that contain alcohols

If mucositis or stomatitis is present:

- Keep the mouth moist utilizing water, ice chips, sugarless gum, sugar-free hard candies, or a saliva substitute
- Rinse mouth several times a day to remove debris
  - Use a solution of ¼ teaspoon (1.25 g) each of baking soda and table salt (sodium chloride) in one quart (~950 mL) of warm water. Follow with a plain water rinse
  - Do not use mouthwashes that contain alcohols
- Foam-tipped swabs (eg, Toothettes®) are useful in moisturizing oral mucosa, but ineffective for cleansing teeth and removing plaque
- Advise patients who develop mucositis to:
  - Choose foods that are easy to chew and swallow
  - Take small bites of food, chew slowly, and sip liquids with meals
  - Encourage soft, moist foods such as cooked cereals, mashed potatoes, and scrambled eggs
  - For trouble swallowing, soften food with gravies, sauces, broths, yogurt, or other bland liquids
  - Avoid sharp, crunchy foods; hot, spicy or highly acidic foods (eg, citrus fruits and juices); sugary foods; toothpicks; tobacco products; alcoholic drinks

Efficacy

Response Rate

Overall response rate	36.7% (95% CI, 30.3–43.4%)
Complete response	2%
Partial response	35%
No change/stable disease	30%
Progressive disease	17%
Not assessable	16%

Progression-free and Overall Survival

Time to disease progression	5.6 months (95% CI, 4.9–5.9 months)
Median overall survival	9.2 months (95% CI, 8.4–10.6 months)
Patients alive at 1 year	40%
Patients alive at 2 years	18%

WHO Criteria

Patient Population Studied

A trial of 445 evaluable patients with metastatic or locally recurrent, unresectable gastric carcinoma randomly assigned to receive DCF or cisplatin and fluorouracil (CF). The DCF regimen resulted in a significantly longer time to progression, survival and higher response rate than CF, but G3/4 adverse events were significant in both arms

Toxicity (N = 221)

Adverse Events	% G3/4	% All Grades
Hematologic Toxicities		
Neutropenia	82	95
Leukopenia	65	96
Anemia	18	97
Thrombocytopenia	8	25
Febrile neutropenia or infection with neutropenia	—	29
Nonhematologic Toxicities		
Lethargy*	19	56
Infection	13	17
Neurosensory	8	38
Stomatitis	21	59
Diarrhea	19	75
Nausea	14	72
Vomiting	14	61
Anorexia	10	45
Death Rate		
Death rate from all causes within 30 days after last chemotherapy	10.4%	

*The most common adverse event leading to cycle delay

Notes:

- Cycle delays occurred in 64% of patients
- Dose reductions occurred in 41% of patients
- Of patients who withdrew consent, 46% had a G3/4 adverse event in the last cycle before withdrawing consent

National Cancer Institute (USA) Common Toxicity Criteria, version 2.0. Available at: http://ctep.cancer.gov/protocolDevelopment/electronic_applications/ctc.htm [accessed October 25, 2013]

Therapy Monitoring

1. *Before each cycle:* Physical examination, CBC with differential, serum electrolytes, magnesium, calcium, creatinine, BUN, and LFTs
2. *Response evaluation:* Every 2 cycles

ADVANCED DISEASE REGIMENS

EPIRUBICIN (E), CISPLATIN (C), FLUOROURACIL (F), OXALIPLATIN (O), CAPECITABINE (X)
ECF, ECX, EOF, AND EOX

Cunningham D et al. N Engl J Med 2008;358:36–46. Comment in: N Engl J Med 2008;358:1965, Nat Clin Pract Gastroenterol Hepatol 2008;5:414–415, N Engl J Med 2010;362:858–859

REAL-2 study conclusion: Capecitabine and oxaliplatin are as effective as fluorouracil and cisplatin, respectively, in patients with previously untreated esophagogastric cancer

ECF Regimen
Epirubicin 50 mg/m^2; administer intravenously over 3–20 minutes on day 1 before cisplatin, every 3 weeks, for a maximum of 8 cycles (total dosage/cycle = 50 mg/m^2)

Hydration before cisplatin: ≥1000 mL 0.9% sodium chloride injection (0.9% NS); administer intravenously over a minimum of 3 hours
Cisplatin 60 mg/m^2; administer intravenously in 100–500 mL 0.9% NS over 30–60 minutes on day 1, every 3 weeks, for a maximum of 8 cycles (total dosage/cycle = 60 mg/m^2)

Hydration after cisplatin: ≥1000 mL 0.9% NS; administer intravenously over a minimum of 3 hours. Encourage increased oral fluid intake. Goal is to achieve a urine output ≥100 mL/hour. Monitor and replace magnesium and other electrolytes as needed
Fluorouracil 200 mg/m^2 per day; administer by continuous intravenous infusion over 24 hours in 50–1000 mL 0.9% NS or 5% dextrose injection (D5W) for 21 consecutive days, on days 1–21, every 3 weeks, for a maximum of 8 cycles (total dosage/cycle = 4200 mg/m^2)

ECX Regimen
Epirubicin 50 mg/m^2; administer intravenously over 3–20 minutes on day 1 before cisplatin, every 3 weeks, for a maximum of 8 cycles (total dosage/cycle = 50 mg/m^2)

Hydration before cisplatin: ≥1000 mL 0.9% NS; administer intravenously over a minimum of 3 hours
Cisplatin 60 mg/m^2; administer intravenously in 100–500 mL 0.9% NS over 30–60 minutes on day 1, every 3 weeks, for a maximum of 8 cycles (total dosage/cycle = 60 mg/m^2)

Hydration after cisplatin: ≥1000 mL 0.9% NS; administer intravenously over a minimum of 3 hours. Encourage increased oral fluid intake. Goal is to achieve a urine output ≥100 mL/hour. Monitor and replace magnesium and other electrolytes as needed
Capecitabine 625 mg/m^2 per dose; administer orally, twice daily for 21 consecutive days, on days 1–21, every 3 weeks, for a maximum of 8 cycles (total dosage/cycle = 26,250 mg/m^2)
• The first 80 patients received capecitabine 500 mg/m^2 per dose, twice daily

EOF Regimen
Epirubicin 50 mg/m^2; administer intravenously over 3–20 minutes on day 1 before oxaliplatin, every 3 weeks, for a maximum of 8 cycles (total dosage/cycle = 50 mg/m^2)
Oxaliplatin 130 mg/m^2; administer intravenously in 250 mL D5W over 2 hours on day 1, every 3 weeks, for a maximum of 8 cycles (total dosage/cycle = 130 mg/m^2)
Note: Oxaliplatin must not be mixed with sodium chloride solutions

Fluorouracil 200 mg/m^2 per day; administer by continuous intravenous infusion in 50–1000 mL 0.9% NS or D5W over 24 hours for 21 consecutive days, on days 1–21, for a maximum of 8 cycles (total dosage/cycle = 4200 mg/m^2)

EOX Regimen
Epirubicin 50 mg/m^2; administer intravenously over 3–20 minutes on day 1 before oxaliplatin, every 3 weeks, for a maximum of 8 cycles (total dosage/cycle = 50 mg/m^2)
Oxaliplatin 130 mg/m^2; administer intravenously in 250 mL D5W over 2 hours on day 1, every 3 weeks, for a maximum of 8 cycles (total dosage/cycle = 130 mg/m^2)
Note: Oxaliplatin must not be mixed with sodium chloride solutions

Capecitabine 625 mg/m^2 per dose; administer orally, twice daily for 21 consecutive days, on days 1–21, every 3 weeks, for a maximum of 8 cycles (total dosage/cycle = 26,250 mg/m^2)
• The first 80 patients received capecitabine 500 mg/m^2 per dose, twice daily

(continued)

Treatment Modifications

Adverse Event	Dose Modification
Plantar-palmar erythema (PPE)	Give pyridoxine 50 mg orally 3 times daily. If PPE does not improve, hold fluorouracil or capecitabine for 1 week, then resume treatment at 75% of the dosage at which symptoms occurred
G1/2 mucositis or diarrhea	Interrupt chemotherapy until mucositis and diarrhea resolve, then resume fluorouracil or capecitabine at 75% of the dosage at which symptoms occurred
G3/4 mucositis or diarrhea	Interrupt chemotherapy until mucositis and diarrhea resolve, then resume fluorouracil or capecitabine at 50% of the dosage at which symptoms occurred
Creatinine clearance* 40–60 mL/min (0.66–1 mL/s)	Decrease the amount of cisplatin administered, so the cisplatin dose in milligrams equals the creatinine clearance* value in mL/min[†]
Creatinine clearance* <40 mL/min (<0.66 mL/s)	Hold cisplatin
Day 1 WBC <2000/mm^3 or platelet count <100,000/mm^3	Delay cisplatin, oxaliplatin, and epirubicin for 1 week or until myelosuppression resolves
Second treatment delay caused by myelosuppression	Delay cisplatin, oxaliplatin, and epirubicin for 1 week, or until myelosuppression resolves, then decrease cisplatin, oxaliplatin, and epirubicin dosages by 25% during subsequent treatments
Sepsis during an episode of neutropenia	
Peripheral neuropathy	Delay therapy 1 week. If symptoms do not resolve to G ≤1, reduce cisplatin or oxaliplatin dosage by 25%

*Creatinine clearance is used as a measure of glomerular filtration rate (GFR)
[†]This also applies to patients with creatinine clearance (GFR) of 40–60 mL/min before starting or restarting treatment

Findlay M et al. Ann Oncol 1994;5:609–616

(*continued*)

Supportive Care

Antiemetic prophylaxis for ECF and ECX regimens

*Emetogenic potential on day 1 is **HIGH**. Potential for delayed emetic symptoms*

Emetogenic potential on days 2–21 is LOW

Antiemetic prophylaxis for ECF and ECX regimens

*Emetogenic potential on day 1 is **MODERATE***

Emetogenic potential on days 2–21 is LOW

See Chapter 39 for antiemetic recommendations

Hematopoietic growth factor (CSF) prophylaxis

Primary prophylaxis may be indicated

See Chapter 43 for more information

Antimicrobial prophylaxis

Risk of fever and neutropenia is LOW

See Chapter 47 for more information

Diarrhea management

Latent or delayed-onset diarrhea*:

Loperamide 4 mg; administer orally initially after the first loose or liquid stool, *then*

Loperamide 2 mg; administer orally every 2 hours during waking hours, *plus*

Loperamide 4 mg; administer orally every 4 hours during hours of sleep

- Continue for at least 12 hours after diarrhea resolves
- Recurrent diarrhea after a 12-hour diarrhea-free interval is treated as a new episode
- Rehydrate orally with fluids and electrolytes during a diarrheal episode
- If a patient develops blood or mucus in stool, dehydration, or hemodynamic instability, or if diarrhea persists >48 hours despite loperamide, stop loperamide and hospitalize the patient for IV hydration

Alternatively, a trial of **Diphenoxylate hydrochloride** 2.5 mg **with Atropine sulfate** 0.025 mg (eg, Lomotil®)

- Initial adult dose is two tablets four times daily until control has been achieved, after which the dose may be reduced to meet individual requirements. Control may often be maintained with as little as two tablets daily

*Rothenberg ML et al. J Clin Oncol 2001;19:3801–3807
Wadler S et al. J Clin Oncol 1998;16:3169–3178

Oral care

Prophylaxis and treatment for mucositis/stomatitis

General advice:

- Encourage patients to maintain intake of non-alcoholic fluids
- Evaluate patients for oral pain and provide analgesic medications

If mucositis or stomatitis is present:

- Use a solution of ¼ teaspoon (1.25 g) each of baking soda and table salt (sodium chloride) in one quart (~950 mL) of warm water. Follow with a plain water rinse
- Do not use mouthwashes that contain alcohols

Hand-foot reaction (palmar-plantar erythrodysesthesia, PPE)

For patients who develop a hand-foot reaction, use topical emollients (eg, Aquaphor®), topical or orally administered steroids, antihistamine agents (H_1-receptor antagonists), or pyridoxine

Pyridoxine may provide relief; starting dose is 50 mg/day, which may be increased to a maximum of 200 mg/day

Treatment Modifications (Per Protocol-Patients)

Variable	ECF	ECX	EOF	EOX
Number of patients	250	243	236	239
Total number of cycles delivered	1310	1400	1288	1295
Median number of cycles	6	6	6	6
Fluoro-pyrimidines (percent dose)	88.4	88.4	88.3	88.1
Platinating agents (percent dose)	90.5	92.3	91.7	91.6
Epirubicin (percent dose)	92.6	89.2*	93.0	91.9
Percentage of patients with a delay	92.6	60.1	47.9	50.2
Mean number of days delayed per patient	7.7	11.2	5.8*	7.4

*Statistically significant difference from ECF

Efficacy

Analysis of Efficacy (Intention-to-Treat Population)

Variable	ECF	ECX	EOF	EOX
No. of patients	263	250	245	244
Overall survival	9.9 months	9.9 months	9.3 months	11.2 months
1-Year survival	37.7 (31.8–43.6)	40.8 (34.7–46.9)	40.4 (34.2–46.5)	46.8 (40.4–52.9)
PFS	6.2 months	6.7 months	6.5 months	7.0 months
Responses				
Complete (%)	4.1	4.2	2.6	3.9
Partial (%)	36.6	42.2	39.8	44.0
p-Value (vs. ECF)	—	0.2	0.69	0.11

Response Evaluation Criteria in Solid Tumors (RECIST; Therasse P et al. J Natl Cancer Inst 2000;92:205–216)

Toxicities

Regimen (Total Patients)	ECF (234)		ECX (234)		EOF (225)		EOX (227)	
	Grades (%)							
Adverse Events	All	3/4	All	3/4	All	3/4	All	3/4
Anemia	78.4	13.1	79.5	10.5	65.8	6.5*	64.2	8.6
Thrombocytopenia	14.5	4.7	17.0	4.8	13.4	4.3	21.1	5.2
Neutropenia	73.6	41.7	85.6	51.1*	68.4	29.9*	62.9	27.6*
Febrile neutropenia	13.2	9.3	10.5	6.7	11.5	8.5	9.8	7.8
Diarrhea	39.3	2.6	41.9	5.1	62.7	10.7*	61.7	11.9*
Stomatitis	50.9	1.3	39.3	1.7	44.4	4.4*	38.1	2.2
Hand-foot syndrome	29.8	4.3	45.9	10.3*	28.9	2.7	39.3	3.1
Nausea and vomiting	79.1	10.2	82.1	7.7	83.1	13.8	78.9	11.4
Peripheral neuropathy	30.0	0.4	36.3	1.7	79.6	8.4*	83.7	4.4*
Lethargy	89.7	16.6	92.7	15.5	90.2	12.9	96.1	24.9*
Alopecia†	81.5	—	82.5	—	75.4	—	74.2	—
Thromboembolism‡	16.9	NA	13.3	NA	7.7*	NA	7.5*	NA
Death§	7.2		5.6		5.7		6.1	

*Statistically significant for the comparison with the ECF group
†Highest grade of alopecia was G2
‡A diagnosis of thromboembolism was made only in the per-protocol population
§Death within 60 days after randomization was evaluated only in the intention-to-treat population
National Cancer Institute (USA) Common Toxicity Criteria, version 2.0, were used in grading adverse events. Available at: http://ctep.cancer.gov/protocolDevelopment/electronic_applications/ctc.htm [accessed October 25, 2013]

Patient Population Studied

The REAL-2 study was a trial of 1002 patients with previously untreated advanced esophagogastric cancer who were randomly assigned to 1 of 4 combination chemotherapy regimens, including epirubicin, cisplatin, and fluorouracil (ECF; N = 263); epirubicin, cisplatin, and capecitabine (ECX; N = 250); epirubicin, oxaliplatin, and fluorouracil (EOF; N = 245); and epirubicin, oxaliplatin, and capecitabine (EOX; N = 244). The primary endpoint was noninferiority in overall survival for the triplet therapies containing capecitabine or fluorouracil, and for those containing oxaliplatin or cisplatin. Progression-free survival and response rates did not differ significantly among the regimens. Adverse effects associated with capecitabine and fluorouracil were similar. In comparison with cisplatin, oxaliplatin-containing regimens had less associated G3 or G4 neutropenia, alopecia, renal toxicity, and thromboembolism but higher rates of G3 or G4 diarrhea and peripheral neuropathy. The investigators concluded capecitabine and oxaliplatin are as effective as fluorouracil and cisplatin, respectively, in patients with previously untreated esophagogastric cancer

Therapy Monitoring

1. *Before each cycle:* Physical examination, CBC and differential counts, clotting analysis, LFTs, serum creatinine and (estimated or measured) creatinine clearance

2. In patients with a history of ischemic heart disease, measure left ventricular ejection fraction by MUGA scanning or echocardiography prior to starting therapy and at intervals thereafter

3. Baseline chest radiography and computed tomography of the chest, abdomen, and pelvis, with or without upper gastrointestinal endoscopy within 28 days before treatment commences

Note: Prior to starting therapy: In patients with a history of ischemic heart disease, measure left ventricular ejection fraction by multiple gated acquisition (MUGA) scanning or echocardiography. Omit epirubicin if the left ventricular ejection fraction is <50%

ADVANCED DISEASE REGIMEN

IRINOTECAN + CISPLATIN

Ajani JA et al. Cancer 2002;94:641–646

Irinotecan 65 mg/m^2; administer intravenously by intravenous infusion diluted in 5% dextrose injection (D5W) to a concentration within the range 0.12–2.8 mg/mL over 90 minutes every week for 4 consecutive weeks, weeks 1–4, every 6 weeks (total dosage/cycle = 260 mg/m^2)

Hydration before cisplatin: ≥1000 mL 0.9% sodium chloride injection (0.9% NS); administer intravenously over a minimum of 3 hours
Cisplatin 30 mg/m^2; administer intravenously in 100–500 mL 0.9% NS over 60 minutes, every week after irinotecan for 4 consecutive weeks, weeks 1–4, every 6 weeks (total dosage/cycle = 120 mg/m^2)

Hydration after cisplatin: ≥1000 mL 0.9% NS; administer intravenously over a minimum of 3 hours. Encourage increased oral fluid intake. Goal is to achieve a urine output of ≥100 mL/hour. Monitor and replace magnesium and other electrolytes as needed
Note: Irinotecan and cisplatin are administered weekly for 4 consecutive weeks followed by a recovery period of 2 weeks without treatment

Supportive Care
Antiemetic prophylaxis
Emetogenic potential: **HIGH**. *Potential for delayed emetic symptoms*
See Chapter 39 for antiemetic recommendations

Hematopoietic growth factor (CSF) prophylaxis
Primary prophylaxis may be indicated
See Chapter 43 for more information

Antimicrobial prophylaxis
Risk of fever and neutropenia is LOW
  Antimicrobial primary prophylaxis to be considered:
  • Antibacterial—not indicated
  • Antifungal—not indicated
  • Antiviral—not indicated unless patient previously had an episode of HSV
See Chapter 47 for more information

Diarrhea management
Latent or delayed-onset diarrhea*:
  Loperamide 4 mg orally initially, then 2 mg orally every 2 hours during waking hours, *plus*
  Loperamide 4 mg orally every 4 hours during hours of sleep
  • Continue for at least 12 hours after diarrhea resolves
  • Recurrent diarrhea after a 12-hour diarrhea-free interval is treated as a new episode
  • If diarrhea persists >48 hours despite loperamide, stop loperamide and hospitalize patient for IV hydration
Persistent diarrhea:
  Octreotide 100–150 mcg subcutaneously 3 times daily. Maximum total daily dose = 1500 mcg
Antibiotic therapy during latent or delayed onset diarrhea:
  Ciprofloxacin 500 mg orally every 12 hours if absolute neutrophil count <500/mm^3 with or without accompanying fever in association with diarrhea
  • Antibiotics should also be administered if patient is hospitalized with prolonged diarrhea and should be continued until diarrhea resolves

*Rothenberg ML et al. J Clin Oncol 2001;19:3801–3807; Wadler S et al. J Clin Oncol 1998;16:3169–3178

Acute cholinergic syndrome
Atropine sulfate 0.25–1 mg subcutaneously
• If symptoms are severe, add as primary prophylaxis during subsequent cycles
• For irinotecan, acute cholinergic syndrome is characterized by abdominal cramps, diarrhea, diaphoresis, hypotension, bradycardia, rhinitis, increased salivation, visual disturbances, and lacrimation

Patient Population Studied

A phase II trial of 36 evaluable patients with advanced untreated gastric or gastroesophageal junction carcinoma

Efficacy (N = 36)

Complete response	11%
Partial response	47%
Minor response	14%
Progressive disease	22%
Stable disease	6%
Median time to progression	24 weeks (95% CI, 16–32 weeks)
Median survival	9 months (95% CI, 7.5–10.5 months)

Toxicity (N = 36)

	% G1	% G2	% G3	% G4
Nonhematologic Toxicity				
Diarrhea	27	21	17	5
Fatigue	13	16	27	14
Myalgia	13	2	2	0
Nausea	18	32	15	1
Emesis	22	19	4	2
Neuropathy	6	2	0	0
Alopecia	36	33	0	0
Dizziness	1	2	0	0
Hematologic Toxicity				
Neutropenia	15	18	12	15
Febrile neutropenia	0	3	4	0

Note: One treatment-related death occurred in an elderly patient associated with neutropenia, sepsis, and multiple organ failure

Treatment Modifications

First modification	Consider changing the administration schedule to day 1 and day 8, every 21 days
Subsequent modifications	

Cisplatin	Initial dose level	30 mg/m²
	First dose reduction	20 mg/m²
Irinotecan	Initial dose level	65 mg/m²
	First dose reduction	50 mg/m²
	Second dose reduction	40 mg/m²

Adverse Event	Dose Modification
If on cycle day 1, WBC <3000/mm³, ANC <1000/mm³, platelet count <100,000/mm³, serum creatinine >1.5 mg/dL (>133 μmol/L), and nonhematologic toxicity G ≥2	Hold irinotecan and cisplatin for 1 week, then resume treatment when WBC ≥3000/mm³, ANC ≥1000/mm³, platelet count ≥100,000/mm³, serum creatinine <1.5 mg/dL (<133 μmol/L), and nonhematologic toxicity G ≤1
If on cycle day 1, a second episode of nonhematologic adverse event G ≥2 nonhematologic adverse event, or serum creatinine ≥1.8 mg/dL (≥159 μmol/L)	Hold cisplatin and irinotecan for 1 week, then resume at cisplatin dose decreased by one level if serum creatinine is <1.5 mg/dL (<133 μmol/L)
G4 neutropenia (with or without fever)	Add primary prophylaxis with filgrastim during all subsequent cycles
Febrile neutropenia despite filgrastim support	Hold treatment until adverse event resolves, then resume chemotherapy with irinotecan or cisplatin dosage reduced by 1 dose level
G3/4 nonhematologic adverse events (except nausea or vomiting), G3/4 diarrhea despite loperamide, G4 ANC, or thrombocytopenia during cycle 1	
Reduction in creatinine clearance* to ≤60% of on-study value	Delay therapy for 1 week. If creatinine clearance does not recover to pretreatment values, consider reducing cisplatin dosage
Creatinine clearance* 40–60 mL/min (0.66–1 mL/s)	Consider decreasing the amount of cisplatin administered, so the cisplatin dose in milligrams equals the creatinine clearance* value in mL/min†
Creatinine clearance* <40 mL/min (<0.66 mL/s)	Hold cisplatin
Peripheral neuropathy	Delay therapy for 1 week. If symptoms do not resolve to G ≤1, reduce cisplatin dose by 25%
G3/4 peripheral neurotoxicity or ototoxicity	Discontinue therapy

*Creatinine clearance is used as a measure of glomerular filtration rate (GFR)
†This also applies to patients with creatinine clearance (GFR) = 40–60 mL/min (0.66–1 mL/s) before starting or restarting treatment

Modified from Ajani JA et al. Cancer 2002;94:641–646 and Saltz LB et al. J Clin Oncol 1998;16:3858–3865

Therapy Monitoring

1. *Cycle 1:* CBC with differential, serum electrolytes, magnesium, calcium, creatinine, BUN, and LFTs on days 1 and 22
2. *Before repeated cycles:* Physical examination, CBC with differential, serum electrolytes, magnesium, calcium, creatinine, BUN, and LFTs

ADVANCED DISEASE REGIMEN

CISPLATIN + FLUOROURACIL (FUP)

Vanhoefer U et al. J Clin Oncol 2000;18:2648–2657

Fluorouracil 1000 mg/m²; administer by continuous intravenous infusion in 50–1000 mL 0.9% sodium chloride injection (0.9% NS) or 5% dextrose injection (D5W) over 24 hours for 5 consecutive days, on days 1–5, every 28 days (total dosage/cycle = 5000 mg/m²)

Hydration before cisplatin: ≥1000 mL 0.9% NS; administer intravenously over a minimum of 3 hours

Optional mannitol diuresis: **Mannitol** 12.5–25 g; administer by intravenous injection or infusion over 5–15 minutes before starting cisplatin

- Mannitol may be given to patients who have received adequate hydration
- Mannitol may be prepared as an admixture (in the same container) with cisplatin

Cisplatin 100 mg/m²; administer intravenously in 100–500 mL of 0.9% NS over 1 hour on day 2, every 28 days (total dosage/cycle = 100 mg/m²)

Hydration after cisplatin: ≥1000 mL 0.9% NS; administer intravenously over a minimum of 3 hours. Encourage increased oral fluid intake. Goal is to achieve a urine output of ≥100 mL/hour. Monitor and replace magnesium and other electrolytes as needed

Optional mannitol diuresis: **Mannitol** 20–50 g; administer intravenously over 2–5 hours after cisplatin

- Administer through a hydrophilic inline filter with pore size ≤5 μm to prevent infusion of mannitol crystals
- Continuing intravenous administration of fluids is essential for effective diuresis, particularly if mannitol is administered before, during, or after cisplatin

Supportive Care
Antiemetic prophylaxis
*Emetogenic potential on days 1 and 3–5 is **LOW***
*Emetogenic potential on day 2 is **HIGH**. Potential for delayed emetic symptoms*
See Chapter 39 for antiemetic recommendations

Hematopoietic growth factor (CSF) prophylaxis
Primary prophylaxis is NOT indicated
See Chapter 43 for more information

Antimicrobial prophylaxis
Risk of fever and neutropenia is LOW
  Antimicrobial primary prophylaxis to be considered:
  - Antibacterial—not indicated
  - Antifungal—not indicated
  - Antiviral—not indicated unless patient previously had an episode of HSV
See Chapter 47 for more information

Diarrhea management
Latent or delayed-onset diarrhea:
  Loperamide 4 mg; administer orally initially after the first loose or liquid stool, *then*
  Loperamide 2 mg; administer orally every 2 hours during waking hours, *plus*
  Loperamide 4 mg; administer orally every 4 hours during hours of sleep
- Continue for at least 12 hours after diarrhea resolves
- Recurrent diarrhea after a 12-hour diarrhea-free interval is treated as a new episode
- Rehydrate orally with fluids and electrolytes during a diarrheal episode
- If a patient develops blood or mucus in stool, dehydration, or hemodynamic instability, or if diarrhea persists >48 hours despite loperamide, stop loperamide and hospitalize the patient for IV hydration

Alternatively, a trial of **Diphenoxylate hydrochloride** 2.5 mg **with Atropine sulfate** 0.025 mg (eg, Lomotil®)
- Initial adult dose is two tablets four times daily until control has been achieved, after which the dose may be reduced to meet individual requirements. Control may often be maintained with as little as two tablets daily

(continued)

Efficacy

Eligible Patients with Measurable Disease (N = 81)	
Partial response	20% (95% CI, 11.5–30)
No change	43%
Progressive disease	21%
Early death	6%*
Not assessable	10%

Intention-to-Treat Analyses (N = 134)	
Progression-free survival	4.1 months (95% CI, 3.8–5.4 months)
Median survival	7.2 months (95% CI, 6.3–9.0 months)
Probability at 1 year for survival	27% (95% CI, 19–35%)

*Disease, 1%; toxicity, 1%; other, 4%
WHO Response Criteria

Toxicity (N = 127)

Adverse Event	% Patients with G3 or G4
Leukopenia	17
Neutropenia	35
Thrombocytopenia	9
Infection	5
Nausea/vomiting	26
Mucositis	12
Diarrhea	6
Renal	2
Peripheral neuropathy	<1
Alopecia	16
Treatment-related death in 2 patients	

WHO criteria

(*continued*)

- Clinical improvement of acute diarrhea is usually observed within 48 hours. If improvement of chronic diarrhea after treatment with a maximum daily dose of 8 tablets is not observed within 10 days, control is unlikely with further administration

*Rothenberg ML et al. J Clin Oncol 2001;19:3801–3807
Wadler S et al. J Clin Oncol 1998;16:3169–3178

Oral care
Prophylaxis and treatment for mucositis/stomatitis
General advice:

- Encourage patients to maintain intake of non-alcoholic fluids
- Evaluate patients for oral pain and provide analgesic medications
- Consider histamine (H_2-subtype) receptor antagonists (eg, ranitidine, famotidine), or a proton pump inhibitor for epigastric pain
- *Lactobacillus* sp.-containing probiotics may be beneficial in preventing diarrhea

Patients with intact oral mucosa:

- Clean the mouth, tongue, and gums by brushing after every meal and at bedtime with an ultra-soft toothbrush with fluoride toothpaste
- Floss teeth gently every day unless contraindicated. If gums bleed and hurt, avoid bleeding or sore areas, but floss other teeth
- Patients may use saline or commercial bland, non-alcoholic rinses
  - Do not use mouthwashes that contain alcohols

If mucositis or stomatitis is present:

- Keep the mouth moist utilizing water, ice chips, sugarless gum, sugar-free hard candies, or a saliva substitute
- Rinse mouth several times a day to remove debris
  - Use a solution of ¼ teaspoon (1.25 g) each of baking soda and table salt (sodium chloride) in one quart (~950 mL) of warm water. Follow with a plain water rinse
  - Do not use mouthwashes that contain alcohols
- Foam-tipped swabs (eg, Toothettes®) are useful in moisturizing oral mucosa, but ineffective for cleansing teeth and removing plaque
- Advise patients who develop mucositis to:
  - Choose foods that are easy to chew and swallow
  - Take small bites of food, chew slowly, and sip liquids with meals
  - Encourage soft, moist foods such as cooked cereals, mashed potatoes, and scrambled eggs
  - For trouble swallowing, soften food with gravies, sauces, broths, yogurt, or other bland liquids
  - Avoid sharp, crunchy foods; hot, spicy or highly acidic foods (eg, citrus fruits and juices); sugary foods; toothpicks; tobacco products; alcoholic drinks

Patient Population

The EORTC trial 40902 of 245 eligible patients with advanced adenocarcinoma of the stomach randomized to receive sequential high-dose methotrexate, fluorouracil, and doxorubicin (FAMTX) versus etoposide, leucovorin, and fluorouracil (ELF) versus infusional fluorouracil and cisplatin (FUP). The overall response rate in patients with measurable disease was 12% (FAMTX), 9% (ELF), and 20% (FUP)

Therapy Monitoring

1. *Before each cycle:* Physical examination, CBC with differential, serum electrolytes, magnesium, calcium, creatinine, BUN, and LFTs
2. *Response evaluation:* Every 2 cycles

Treatment Modifications

Dosage Levels

Cisplatin	Initial dosage	100 mg/m²
	Level −1	75 mg/m²
	Level −2	50 mg/m²
Fluorouracil	Initial dosage	1000 mg/m² per day for 5 days
	Level −1	800 mg/m² per day for 5 days
	Level −2	600 mg/m² per day for 5 days

Adverse Event	Dose Modification
Plantar-palmar erythema (PPE)	Give pyridoxine 50 mg orally 3 times daily. If PPE does not improve, hold fluorouracil for 1 week, then resume fluorouracil at 1 dose level less than that at which symptoms occurred
G1/2 mucositis or diarrhea	Interrupt chemotherapy until mucositis and diarrhea resolve, then resume fluorouracil at 1 dose level less than that at which symptoms occurred
G3/4 mucositis or diarrhea	Interrupt chemotherapy until mucositis and diarrhea resolve, then resume fluorouracil at 2 dose levels less than that at which symptoms occurred
Reduction in creatinine clearance* to ≤60% of on-study measurement	Delay therapy for 1 week. If creatinine clearance does not recover to pretreatment values, then decrease cisplatin dosage by 1 dose level
Creatinine clearance* 40–60 mL/min (0.66–1 mL/s)	Consider decreasing the amount of cisplatin administered, so the cisplatin dose in milligrams equals the creatinine clearance* value in mL/min†
Creatinine clearance* <40 mL/min (<0.66 mL/s)	Hold cisplatin
Peripheral neuropathy	Delay therapy for 1 week. If symptoms do not resolve to G ≤1, reduce cisplatin by 1 dose level
G3/4 peripheral neurotoxicity or ototoxicity	Discontinue therapy

Other modifications as clinically indicated based on the most significant toxicity
*Creatinine clearance is used as measure of glomerular filtration rate (GFR)
†This also applies to patients with creatinine clearance (GFR) of 40–60 mL/min (0.66–1 mL/s) before starting or restarting treatment

ADVANCED DISEASE REGIMENS
CISPLATIN + FLUOROURACIL (CF)
IRINOTECAN + FLUOROURACIL (IF)

Dank M et al. Ann Oncol 2008;19:1450–1457

Cisplatin + Fluorouracil (CF):

Hydration before cisplatin: ≥1000 mL 0.9% sodium chloride injection (0.9% NS); administer intravenously over a minimum of 3 hours

Optional mannitol diuresis: **Mannitol** 12.5–25 g; administer by intravenous injection or infusion over 5–15 minutes before starting cisplatin

• Mannitol may be given to patients who have received adequate hydration

• Mannitol may be prepared as an admixture (in the same container) with cisplatin

Cisplatin 100 mg/m²; administer intravenously in 100–500 mL 0.9% NS over 1–3 hours on day 1, every 28 days (total dosage/cycle = 100 mg/m²)

Hydration after cisplatin: ≥1000 mL 0.9% NS; administer intravenously over a minimum of 3 hours. Encourage increased oral fluid intake. Goal is to achieve a urine output of ≥100 mL/hour. Monitor and replace magnesium and other electrolytes as needed

Optional mannitol diuresis: **Mannitol** 20–50 g; administer intravenously over 2–5 hours after cisplatin

• Administer through a hydrophilic inline filter with pore size ≤5 μm to prevent infusion of mannitol crystals

• Continuing intravenous fluid administration is essential for effective diuresis, particularly if mannitol is administered before, during, or after cisplatin

Fluorouracil 1000 mg/m² per day; administer by continuous intravenous infusion in 50–1000 mL 0.9% NS or 5% dextrose injection over 24 hours for 5 consecutive days, on days 1–5, every 28 days (total dosage/cycle = 5000 mg/m²)

Supportive Care
Antiemetic prophylaxis
Emetogenic potential on day 1 is **HIGH**. *Potential for delayed emetic symptoms*
Emetogenic potential on days 2–5 is **LOW**
See Chapter 39 for antiemetic recommendations

Hematopoietic growth factor (CSF) prophylaxis
Primary prophylaxis may be indicated
See Chapter 43 for more information

Antimicrobial prophylaxis
Risk of fever and neutropenia is LOW
　Antimicrobial primary prophylaxis to be considered:
　• Antibacterial—not indicated
　• Antifungal—not indicated
　• Antiviral—not indicated unless patient previously had an episode of HSV
See Chapter 47 for more information

Irinotecan + Fluorouracil (IF):

Note: IF provides a platinum-free frontline treatment alternative for metastatic gastric cancer

Irinotecan 80 mg/m² per dose; administer intravenously diluted in D5W to a concentration within the range 0.12–2.8 mg/mL over 30 minutes, weekly, for 6 consecutive weeks followed by a 1-week rest (total dosage/7-week cycle = 480 mg/m²), *followed by:*
Leucovorin 500 mg/m² per dose; administer intravenously in 25–250 mL 0.9% NS
or D5W over 2 hours, weekly, for 6 consecutive weeks followed by a 1-week rest
(total dosage/7-week cycle = 3000 mg/m²), *followed by:*
Fluorouracil 2000 mg/m² per dose; administer intravenously in 50–1000 mL 0.9% NS or D5W over 22 hours, weekly, for 6 consecutive weeks followed by a 1-week rest
(total dosage/7-week cycle = 12,000 mg/m²)

Supportive Care
Antiemetic prophylaxis
Emetogenic potential: **MODERATE**
See Chapter 39 for antiemetic recommendations

Hematopoietic growth factor (CSF) prophylaxis
Primary prophylaxis is NOT indicated
See Chapter 43 for more information

(continued)

(continued)

Antimicrobial prophylaxis
Risk of fever and neutropenia is LOW
> *Antimicrobial primary prophylaxis to be considered:*
> • Antibacterial—not indicated
> • Antifungal—not indicated
> • Antiviral—not indicated unless patient previously had an episode of HSV

See Chapter 47 for more information

Acute cholinergic syndrome associated with irinotecan
Atropine sulfate 0.25–1 mg subcutaneously
• If symptoms are severe, add as primary prophylaxis during subsequent cycles
• For irinotecan, acute cholinergic syndrome is characterized by: abdominal cramps, diarrhea, diaphoresis, hypotension, bradycardia, rhinitis, increased salivation, visual disturbances, and lacrimation

Supportive Care for both CF and IF regimens:
Diarrhea management
Latent or delayed-onset diarrhea*:
> **Loperamide** 4 mg; administer orally initially after the first loose or liquid stool, *then*
> **Loperamide** 2 mg; administer orally every 2 hours during waking hours, *plus*
> **Loperamide** 4 mg; administer orally every 4 hours during hours of sleep
> • Continue for at least 12 hours after diarrhea resolves
> • Recurrent diarrhea after a 12-hour diarrhea-free interval is treated as a new episode
> • Rehydrate orally with fluids and electrolytes during a diarrheal episode
> • If a patient develops blood or mucus in stool, dehydration, or hemodynamic instability, or if diarrhea persists >48 hours despite loperamide, stop loperamide and hospitalize the patient for IV hydration

> Alternatively, a trial of **Diphenoxylate hydrochloride** 2.5 mg **with Atropine sulfate** 0.025 mg (eg, Lomotil®)
> • Initial adult dose is two tablets four times daily until control has been achieved, after which the dose may be reduced to meet individual requirements. Control may often be maintained with as little as two tablets daily
> • Clinical improvement of acute diarrhea is usually observed within 48 hours. If improvement of chronic diarrhea after treatment with a maximum daily dose of 8 tablets is not observed within 10 days, control is unlikely with further administration

Persistent diarrhea:
> **Octreotide** acetate (solution) 100–150 mcg; administer subcutaneously 3 times daily. Maximum total daily dose is 1500 mcg

Antibiotic therapy during latent or delayed-onset diarrhea:
> A fluoroquinolone (eg, **Ciprofloxacin** 500 mg orally every 12 hours) if absolute neutrophil count <500/mm^3 with or without accompanying fever in association with diarrhea
> • Antibiotics should also be administered if patient is hospitalized with prolonged diarrhea and should be continued until diarrhea resolves

*Abigerges D et al. J Natl Cancer Inst 1994;86:446–449
Rothenberg ML et al. J Clin Oncol 2001;19:3801–3807
Wadler S et al. J Clin Oncol 1998;16:3169–3178

Oral care
Prophylaxis and treatment for mucositis/stomatitis
> *General advice:*
> • Encourage patients to maintain intake of non-alcoholic fluids
> • Evaluate patients for oral pain and provide analgesic medications
> • Consider histamine (H$_2$-subtype) receptor antagonists (eg, ranitidine, famotidine), or a proton pump inhibitor for epigastric pain
> • *Lactobacillus* sp.-containing probiotics may be beneficial in preventing diarrhea
> *Patients with intact oral mucosa:*
> • Clean the mouth, tongue, and gums by brushing after every meal and at bedtime with an ultra-soft toothbrush with fluoride toothpaste
> • Floss teeth gently every day unless contraindicated. If gums bleed and hurt, avoid bleeding or sore areas, but floss other teeth
> • Patients may use saline or commercial bland, non-alcoholic rinses
>   ▪ Do not use mouthwashes that contain alcohols
> *If mucositis or stomatitis is present:*
> • Keep the mouth moist utilizing water, ice chips, sugarless gum, sugar-free hard candies, or a saliva substitute
> • Rinse mouth several times a day to remove debris
>   ▪ Use a solution of ¼ teaspoon (1.25 g) each of baking soda and table salt (sodium chloride) in one quart (~950 mL) of warm water. Follow with a plain water rinse
>   ▪ Do not use mouthwashes that contain alcohols

(continued)

(continued)

- Foam-tipped swabs (eg, Toothettes®) are useful in moisturizing oral mucosa, but ineffective for cleansing teeth and removing plaque
- Advise patients who develop mucositis to:
  - Choose foods that are easy to chew and swallow
  - Take small bites of food, chew slowly, and sip liquids with meals
  - Encourage soft, moist foods such as cooked cereals, mashed potatoes, and scrambled eggs
  - For trouble swallowing, soften food with gravies, sauces, broths, yogurt, or other bland liquids
  - Avoid sharp, crunchy foods; hot, spicy or highly acidic foods (eg, citrus fruits and juices); sugary foods; toothpicks; tobacco products; alcoholic drinks

Hand-foot reaction (palmar-plantar erythrodysesthesia, PPE)
For patients who develop a hand-foot reaction, use topical emollients (eg, Aquaphor®), topical or orally administered steroids, antihistamine agents (H_1-receptor antagonists), or pyridoxine
　Pyridoxine may provide relief for discomfort/pain associated with PPE, although the mechanism through which this occurs remains unclear
- The suggested pyridoxine starting dose is 50 mg/day, which may be increased to a maximum of 200 mg/day

Efficacy (N = 333)

	IF	CF
Full-analysis Population	**N = 170**	**N = 163**
Time to tumor progression	5.0 months	4.2 months
6-months progression free survival	38%	31%
Response rate (ERCC)	31.8%	25.8%
Duration of response	7.6 months	7.4 months
Time to treatment failure	4.0 months	3.4 months
Median overall survival	9.0 months	8.7 months
Probability for survival at 1 year	37%	31%
Per-protocol Population		
Time to tumor progression	5.1 months	5.1 months

ERCC External Radiological Review Committee
WHO Criteria

Patient Population

A trial of 333 patients with advanced adenocarcinoma of the stomach or esophagogastric junction randomized to receive irinotecan and fluorouracil (IF arm, 170 patients) versus cisplatin and fluorouracil (CF arm, 163 patients). The overall response rate in patients with measurable disease was 31.8% (IF) versus 25.8% (CF)

Monitoring

1. *Before each cycle:* Physical examination, CBC with differential, serum electrolytes, magnesium, calcium, creatinine, BUN, and LFTs
2. *Response evaluation:* Every 8 weeks

Toxicity

	IF (N = 127)		CF (N = 166)	
	% G1/2	% G3/4	% G1/2	% G3/4
Gastrointestinal				
Anorexia	13.2	3.0	16.9	4.2
Diarrhea	41.9	21.6	28.3	7.2
Stomatitis	13.2	2.4	24.7	16.9
Nausea	46.1	4.8	50.0	9.0
Vomiting	32.9	6.6	36.2	8.4
Hematologic				
Leukopenia	48.2	16.3	51.6	24.5
Neutropenia	41.3	24.8	27.4	51.6
Febrile neutropenia	—	4.8	—	10.2
Anemia	76.6	11.4	76.1	17.2
Thrombocytopenia	7.2	1.8	22.7	11.7
Infection	—	3.0	—	4.8

(continued)

Toxicity (continued)

	IF (N = 127)		CF (N = 166)	
	% G1/2	% G3/4	% G1/2	% G3/4
Neurological				
Altered hearing	1.2	—	9.6	1.2
Sensory	5.4	—	10.9	3.0
Hepatic				
AST elevated	24.7	2.5	27.7	1.3
ALT elevated	26.5	3.2	16.0	—
AP elevated	47.7	5.2	48.4	6.5
Hyperbilirubinemia	3.9	8.4	8.3	4.5
Other				
Asthenia	31.3	7.2	32	6.6
Creatinine increased	8.7	0.6	24.2	1.9
Cholinergic syndrome	13.2	—	—	—
Fever in absence of infection	12.6	1.8	7.8	1.8
Infection	4.2	3.0	3.6	4.8

AST, Aspartate aminotransferase; ALT, alanine aminotransferase; AP, alkaline phosphatase
NCI of Canada Clinical Trials Group Common Toxicity Criteria

Treatment Modifications

Dosage Levels

Cisplatin

Initial dosage	100 mg/m^2
First reduction	75 mg/m^2
Second reduction	50 mg/m^2

Irinotecan

Initial dosage	80 mg/m^2
First reduction	65 mg/m^2
Second reduction	50 mg/m^2

Fluorouracil

	CF regimen (CIV over 24 h, days 1–5)	IF regimen (IV over 22 h, day 1)
Initial dosage	1000 mg/m^2 · day	2000 mg/m^2
First reduction	800 mg/m^2 · day	1750 mg/m^2
Second reduction	600 mg/m^2 · day	1500 mg/m^2

CIV, continuous intravenous infusion

(continued)

Treatment Modifications (continued)

Treatment Modifications for Cisplatin + Fluorouracil (CF)

Adverse Event	Modification
ANC <1000/mm³, *or* platelet count <100,000/mm³, *or* diarrhea on day 1 of any cycle	Delay treatment for up to 2 weeks until ANC ≥1000/mm³, platelet count is ≥100,000/mm³, and diarrhea resolves. Resume treatment with cisplatin or fluorouracil dosages decreased by 1 dosage level if ANC recovers within 2 weeks after the planned retreatment date. If toxicity does not resolve within 2 weeks, permanently discontinue treatment
G4 neutropenia with or without fever	Give filgrastim during subsequent cycles from day 6 until ANC recovers to 5,000/mm³ on a single measurement, or is >1000/mm³ on two measurements separated by ≥1 day. Consider decreasing the cisplatin dosage by 1 dosage level during subsequent cycles
Febrile neutropenia, *or* neutropenia and infection, *or* G3/4 neutropenia for >7 days	Give filgrastim during subsequent cycles from day 6 until ANC recovers to ≥5,000/mm³ on a single measurement, or is >1000/mm³ on two measurements separated by ≥1 day
G1/2 mucositis/stomatitis	Withhold treatment until mucositis/stomatitis resolves, then resume treatment. Consider decreasing fluorouracil dosage by 1 dosage level
G3 mucositis/stomatitis of >48 hours duration	Withhold treatment until mucositis/stomatitis resolves, then resume treatment with fluorouracil dosage decreased by 1 dosage level
G4 mucositis/stomatitis	Permanently discontinue treatment
G1 diarrhea (2–3 stools/day > baseline)	Maintain cisplatin and fluorouracil dosages and schedules. Treat with loperamide or other antidiarrheal agents
G2 diarrhea (4–6 stools/day > baseline)	Withhold treatment and treat with loperamide or other antidiarrheal agents until diarrhea resolves to baseline. Then resume treatment with fluorouracil dosage decreased by 1 dosage level
G3 diarrhea (7–9 stools/day > baseline)	Withhold treatment and treat with loperamide or other antidiarrheal agents until diarrhea resolves to baseline. Then resume treatment with fluorouracil dosage decreased by 1 dosage level
G4 diarrhea (≥10 stools/day > baseline)	Withhold treatment and treat with loperamide or other antidiarrheal agents until diarrhea resolves to baseline. Then resume treatment with fluorouracil dosage decreased by 2 dosage levels
If on day 1 of a cycle, serum creatinine is >1.8 mg/dL (>159 μmol/L), or other non-hematological adverse event G ≥2	Withhold cisplatin for 1 week. Then, if serum creatinine has decreased to <1.5 mg/dL (<133 μmol/L), resume treatment with cisplatin dosage decreased by 1 dosage level
Decrease in creatinine clearance to ≤60% of on-study value*	Delay treatment for 1 week. If creatinine clearance does not recover to pre-treatment values, resume treatment with cisplatin dosage decreased by 1 dosage level
Creatinine clearance <40 mL/min (<0.66 mL/s)	Withhold cisplatin
G2 peripheral neuropathy	Delay treatment for 1 week. If neuropathy has not abated to G ≤1 after a 1-week delay, resume treatment with cisplatin dosage decreased by 1 dosage level
G3/4 peripheral neuropathy or ototoxicity	Permanently discontinue treatment
Concomitant vomiting with diarrhea, fever, or decreased performance status	Hospitalization for intravenous hydration and supportive care
G1 palmar-plantar erythrodysesthesia (PPE, hand-foot syndrome)	Give pyridoxine 50 mg orally 3 times daily. Continue fluorouracil without modification
G2/3 PPE	Give pyridoxine 50 mg orally 3 times daily. After PPE signs and symptoms resolve, resume fluorouracil at 1 dosage level less than that at which symptoms occurred
Recurrent G3 PPE (at dosage level –1)	Continue pyridoxine 50 mg orally 3 times daily. After PPE signs and symptoms resolve, resume fluorouracil at 1 dosage level less than that at which symptoms occurred
>2 Dosage reductions required	Permanently discontinue treatment

(continued)

Treatment Modifications (continued)

Treatment Modifications for Irinotecan + Fluorouracil (IF)

Adverse Event	Modification
ANC <1500/mm³, platelet count <100,000/mm³, or diarrhea G >1	Delay treatment for up to 2 weeks. Resume treatment with irinotecan and fluorouracil dosages decreased by 1 dosage level if ANC recovers to ≥1500/mm³, platelet count is ≥100,000/mm³, and diarrhea resolves within 2 weeks after the planned retreatment date
G4 neutropenia with or without fever	Give filgrastim on the days between repeated treatments, but discontinue filgrastim at least 24 hours before resuming treatment. Consider decreasing the irinotecan dosage by 1 dosage level during subsequent cycles
G3/4 neutropenia (duration >7 days)	Withhold treatment until neutropenia has resolved. Resume treatment with irinotecan dosage decreased by 1 dosage level. Give filgrastim on the days between repeated treatments, but discontinue filgrastim at least 24 hours before resuming treatment
Febrile neutropenia	Withhold treatment until fever and neutropenia are resolved, then resume treatment at the same dosages previously given. Consider secondary prophylaxis with filgrastim on the days between repeated treatments, but discontinue filgrastim at least 24 hours before resuming treatment
Febrile neutropenia, second episode despite filgrastim use	Withhold treatment until fever and neutropenia are resolved, then resume treatment with irinotecan dosage decreased by 1 dosage level. Continue filgrastim on the days between repeated treatments, but discontinue filgrastim at least 24 hours before resuming treatment
G1/2 mucositis/stomatitis	Withhold treatment until mucositis/stomatitis resolves, then resume treatment. Consider decreasing fluorouracil dosage by 1 dosage level
G1 diarrhea (2–3 stools/day > baseline)	Maintain irinotecan and fluorouracil dosages and schedules. Treat with loperamide or other antidiarrheal agents
G2 diarrhea (4–6 stools/day > baseline)	Withhold treatment and treat with loperamide or other antidiarrheal agents until diarrhea resolves to baseline. Then resume treatment with irinotecan dosage decreased by 1 dosage level
G3 diarrhea (7–9 stools/day > baseline)	
G4 diarrhea (≥10 stools/day > baseline)	Withhold treatment and treat with loperamide or other antidiarrheal agents until diarrhea resolves to baseline. Then resume treatment with irinotecan dosage decreased by 2 dosage levels
Diarrhea persisting >48 h, despite loperamide	Hospitalization, broad-spectrum antibiotic treatment (eg, a fluoroquinolone), and replace loperamide with alternative antidiarrheal agents
G3/4 neutropenia with diarrhea, *or* diarrhea with fever or infection	Withhold treatment until toxicities have resolved then resume treatment with irinotecan and/or fluorouracil dosages decreased by 1 dosage level
Diarrhea concomitant with vomiting, fever, or decreased performance status (Karnofsky scale <70%; ECOG>2)	Hospitalization for intravenous hydration and supportive care
G3 mucositis/stomatitis of >48 hours duration	Withhold treatment until mucositis/stomatitis resolves, then resume treatment with fluorouracil dosage decreased by 1 dosage level
G4 mucositis/stomatitis	Discontinue treatment
G1 palmar-plantar erythrodysesthesia (PPE, hand-foot syndrome)	Give pyridoxine 50 mg orally 3 times daily. Continue fluorouracil without modification
G2/3 PPE	Give pyridoxine 50 mg orally 3 times daily. After PPE signs and symptoms resolve, resume fluorouracil at 1 dosage level less than that at which symptoms occurred
Recurrent G3 PPE (recurrence at dosage level −1)	Continue pyridoxine 50 mg orally 3 times daily. After PPE signs and symptoms resolve, resume fluorouracil at 1 dosage level less than that at which symptoms occurred
>2 Dosage reductions required	Permanently discontinue treatment

Other Non-hematological Toxicities (CF and IF regimens)

Any G1 toxicity not specifically addressed above	Continue treatment at the same dosages and on the same schedules
Any G2/3 toxicity not specifically addressed above	Withhold treatment until toxicity resolves to G ≤1 or for up to 2 weeks. Then, resume treatment with the dosages of suspected contributing agents decreased by 1 dosage level or 25%. If toxicity does not resolve to G ≤1 within 2 weeks, discontinue treatment
Any G4 toxicity not specifically addressed above	Withhold treatment until toxicity resolves to G ≤1 or for up to 2 weeks. Then, resume treatment with the dosages of suspected contributing agents decreased by 2 dosage levels or 50%. If toxicity does not resolve to G ≤1 within 2 weeks, discontinue treatment

Other modifications as clinically indicated based on the most significant toxicity
*Creatinine clearance is used as measure of glomerular filtration rate

Ajani JA et al. Cancer 2002;94:641–646 and Saltz LB et al. J Clin Oncol 1998;16:3858–3865
Pozzo C et al. Ann Oncol 2004;15:1773–1781

ADVANCED DISEASE REGIMEN

HER2-POSITIVE ADVANCED GASTRIC CANCER
CISPLATIN + TRASTUZUMAB WITH CAPECITABINE *OR* FLUOROURACIL

Bang Y-J et al. Lancet 2010;376:687–697

Either:

Capecitabine 1000 mg/m^2 per dose; administer orally twice daily for 14 consecutive days, on days 1–14 (28 doses), every 3 weeks for 6 cycles, (total dosage/cycle = 28,000 mg/m^2)
OR

Fluorouracil 800 mg/m^2 per day; administer by continuous intravenous infusion in 50–1000 mL 0.9% sodium chloride injection (0.9% NS) or 5% dextrose injection over 24 hours for 5 consecutive days, on days 1–5, every 3 weeks, for 6 cycles (total dosage/cycle = 4000 mg/m^2)
With:

Hydration before cisplatin: 1000 mL 0.9% NS; administer intravenously over a minimum of 1 hour before commencing cisplatin administration
(optional) **Mannitol** 12.5–25 g; administer by intravenous injection or intravenous infusion over 5–15 minutes before starting cisplatin

- Mannitol may be given to patients who have received adequate hydration. Continued hydration is essential to ensure diuresis

- Mannitol may be prepared as an admixture (in the same container) with cisplatin

Cisplatin 80 mg/m^2; administer intravenously in 50–500 mL 0.9% NS over 30–60 minutes on day 1, every 3 weeks, for 6 cycles (total dosage/cycle = 80 mg/m^2)

Hydration after cisplatin: ≥1000 mL 0.9% NS; administer intravenously over a minimum of 2 hours. Monitor and replace magnesium and other electrolytes as needed. Encourage patients to increase their intake of non-alcoholic fluids

Trastuzumab: Administer intravenously in 250 mL 0.9% NS every 3 weeks for 6 cycles

Loading Dose: **Trastuzumab** 8 mg/kg; administer over 90 minutes as a loading dose on cycle 1, day 1 only (total dosage during the 1st cycle = 8 mg/kg), *then:*

Maintenance Doses: **Trastuzumab** 6 mg/kg; administer over 30 minutes on day 1, every 21 days for 5 cycles (total dosage/cycle = 6 mg/kg)

Note: Assess left ventricular ejection fraction (LVEF) prior to initiating trastuzumab and at regular intervals during treatment
Crossover to trastuzumab at the time of disease progression was not allowed

Supportive Care
Antiemetic prophylaxis
Emetogenic potential on days with cisplatin is **HIGH**. *Potential for delayed emetic symptoms*
Emetogenic potential on days with capecitabine or fluorouracil is **LOW**
Emetogenic potential on days with trastuzumab alone is **MINIMAL–LOW**
See Chapter 39 for antiemetic recommendations

Hematopoietic growth factor (CSF) prophylaxis
Primary prophylaxis may be indicated
See Chapter 43 for more information

Antimicrobial prophylaxis
Risk of fever and neutropenia is LOW
Antimicrobial primary prophylaxis to be considered:
- Antibacterial—not indicated

- Antifungal—not indicated

- Antiviral—not indicated, unless patient previously had an episode of HSV

See Chapter 47 for more information

Diarrhea management
Latent or delayed-onset diarrhea*:
Loperamide 4 mg; administer orally initially after the first loose or liquid stool, *then*
Loperamide 2 mg; administer orally every 2 hours during waking hours, *plus*
Loperamide 4 mg; administer orally every 4 hours during hours of sleep
- Continue for at least 12 hours after diarrhea resolves

- Recurrent diarrhea after a 12-hour diarrhea-free interval is treated as a new episode

- Rehydrate orally with fluids and electrolytes during a diarrheal episode

- If a patient develops blood or mucus in stool, dehydration, or hemodynamic instability, or if diarrhea persists >48 hours despite loperamide, stop loperamide and hospitalize the patient for IV hydration

(continued)

(*continued*)

Alternatively, a trial of **Diphenoxylate hydrochloride** 2.5 mg **with Atropine sulfate** 0.025 mg (eg, Lomotil®)
- Initial adult dose is two tablets four times daily until control has been achieved, after which the dose may be reduced to meet individual requirements. Control may often be maintained with as little as two tablets daily
- Clinical improvement of acute diarrhea is usually observed within 48 hours. If improvement of chronic diarrhea after treatment with a maximum daily dose of 8 tablets is not observed within 10 days, control is unlikely with further administration

*Rothenberg ML et al. J Clin Oncol 2001;19:3801–3807
Wadler S et al. J Clin Oncol 1998;16:3169–3178

Trastuzumab infusion reactions
- A symptom complex most commonly consisting of chills and/or fever may occur in as many as 40% of patients during the first infusion of trastuzumab. These symptoms occur infrequently with subsequent trastuzumab infusions. Other signs and/or symptoms may include nausea, vomiting, pain (in some cases at tumor sites), rigors, headache, dizziness, dyspnea, hypotension, rash, and asthenia. Although the symptoms are usually mild to moderate in severity, infrequently, trastuzumab may need to be discontinued
- When such a symptom complex is observed, it can be treated with or without reduction in the rate of trastuzumab infusion, and:
  - **Acetaminophen** 650 mg; administer orally
  - **Diphenhydramine** 25–50 mg administer orally or by intravenous injection, and
  - **Meperidine** 12.5–25 mg; administer by intravenous injection every 10 minutes if needed for shaking chills (generally, cumulative doses >50 mg are not needed; use with caution in persons with moderate or more severely impaired renal function)

Hand-foot reaction (palmar-plantar erythrodysesthesia, PPE)
For patients who develop a hand-foot reaction, use topical emollients (eg, Aquaphor®), topical or orally administered steroids, antihistamine agents (H_1-receptor antagonists), or pyridoxine
  Pyridoxine may provide relief for discomfort/pain associated with PPE, although the mechanism through which this occurs remains unclear
- The suggested pyridoxine starting dose is 50 mg/day, which may be increased to a maximum of 200 mg/day

Oral care
Prophylaxis and treatment for mucositis/stomatitis
General advice:
- Encourage patients to maintain intake of non-alcoholic fluids
- Evaluate patients for oral pain and provide analgesic medications
- Consider histamine (H_2-subtype) receptor antagonists (eg, ranitidine, famotidine), or a proton pump inhibitor for epigastric pain
- *Lactobacillus* sp.-containing probiotics may be beneficial in preventing diarrhea

Patients with intact oral mucosa:
- Clean the mouth, tongue, and gums by brushing after every meal and at bedtime with an ultra-soft toothbrush with fluoride toothpaste
- Floss teeth gently every day unless contraindicated. If gums bleed and hurt, avoid bleeding or sore areas, but floss other teeth
- Patients may use saline or commercial bland, non-alcoholic rinses
  - Do not use mouthwashes that contain alcohols

If mucositis or stomatitis is present:
- Keep the mouth moist utilizing water, ice chips, sugarless gum, sugar-free hard candies, or a saliva substitute
- Rinse mouth several times a day to remove debris
  - Use a solution of ¼ teaspoon (1.25 g) each of baking soda and table salt (sodium chloride) in one quart (~950 mL) of warm water. Follow with a plain water rinse
  - Do not use mouthwashes that contain alcohols
- Foam-tipped swabs (eg, Toothettes®) are useful in moisturizing oral mucosa, but ineffective for cleansing teeth and removing plaque

Advise patients who develop mucositis to:
- Choose foods that are easy to chew and swallow
- Take small bites of food, chew slowly, and sip liquids with meals
- Encourage soft, moist foods such as cooked cereals, mashed potatoes, and scrambled eggs
- For trouble swallowing, soften food with gravies, sauces, broths, yogurt, or other bland liquids
- Avoid sharp, crunchy foods; hot, spicy or highly acidic foods (eg, citrus fruits and juices); sugary foods; toothpicks; tobacco products; alcoholic drinks

Treatment Modifications

Adverse Event	Dose Modification
ANC nadir <1000/mm^3 *or* platelet nadir <50,000/mm^3 after treatment	Delay treatment until ANC ≥1000/mm^3 *and* platelet ≥50,000/mm^3, then decrease cisplatin dosage by 25%, and decrease daily capecitabine or fluorouracil dosages by 50% during subsequent cycles*. Alternatively, consider using hematopoietic growth factors
Serum creatinine >1.5 mg/dL (>133 μmol/L), but <3 mg/dL (<265 μmol/L) *or* creatinine clearance >40 mL/min (>0.66 mL/s) but <60 mL/min (<1 mL/s)	Delay treatment until serum creatinine ≤1.5 mg/dL (≤133 μmol/L), then decrease cisplatin dosage by 50%*
Serum creatinine >3 mg/dL (>265 μmol/L) *or* creatinine clearance <40 mL/min (<0.66 mL/s)	Stop cisplatin
Persistent G2 neuropathy	Hold cisplatin until toxicity resolves to G ≤1; reduce cisplatin dosage by 25% for subsequent cycles
Transient G3/4 neuropathy (duration 7–14 days)	Hold cisplatin. Resume cisplatin after toxicity resolves with dosage reduced by 25% for subsequent cycles
Persistent G3/4 neuropathy	Discontinue cisplatin
G3/4 nonhematologic adverse events other than renal function and neurotoxicity	Reduce cisplatin and capecitabine dosages by 25% for subsequent cycles
G2 stomatitis, diarrhea, or nausea	Hold capecitabine or fluorouracil; resume capecitabine or fluorouracil at full dosage after resolution of toxicity
Second episode of G2 stomatitis, diarrhea, or nausea	Hold capecitabine or fluorouracil; resume capecitabine or fluorouracil with dosage reduced by 25% after resolution of toxicity
Third episode of G2 stomatitis, diarrhea, or nausea	Hold capecitabine or fluorouracil; resume capecitabine or fluorouracil with dosage reduced by 50% after resolution of toxicity
Fourth episode of G2 stomatitis, diarrhea, or nausea	Discontinue capecitabine or fluorouracil
G3 stomatitis, diarrhea, or nausea	Hold capecitabine or fluorouracil; if G3 toxicity is adequately controlled within 2 days, resume capecitabine at full dosage when toxicity resolves to G ≤1
G3 stomatitis, diarrhea, or nausea	Hold capecitabine or fluorouracil; if G3 toxicity takes >2 days to be controlled, resume capecitabine or fluorouracil with dosage reduced by 25% after toxicity resolves to G ≤1
Second episode of G3 stomatitis, diarrhea, or nausea	Hold capecitabine or fluorouracil; if G3 toxicity is controlled adequately within 2 days, then resume capecitabine or fluorouracil with dosage reduced by 50% after toxicity resolves to G ≤1
Third episode of G3 stomatitis, diarrhea, or nausea	Discontinue capecitabine or fluorouracil
G4 stomatitis, diarrhea, or nausea	Discontinue capecitabine or fluorouracil. Resume capecitabine or fluorouracil with dosage reduced by 50% after toxicity resolves
G1 capecitabine-associated PPE[†]	Begin pyridoxine 50 mg orally 3 times daily and continue capecitabine without dose modification
G2 capecitabine-associated PPE[†]	Begin pyridoxine 50 mg orally 3 times daily and withhold capecitabine. Resume capecitabine with dosage reduced by 15% after toxicity resolves

(continued)

Patient Population Studied

Patients with histologically confirmed inoperable locally advanced, recurrent, or metastatic adenocarcinoma of the stomach or gastro-esophageal junction. Tumors were centrally tested for HER2 status with immunohistochemistry and fluorescence *in situ* hybridization. Patients were eligible if their tumor samples were scored as 3+ on immunohistochemistry or if they were FISH positive (HER2:CEP17 ratio ≥2). Major exclusion criteria included a history of cardiac disease

Patient Characteristics
Trastuzumab + Chemotherapy
(N = 293)

Age (years)	59.4 (10.8)
ECOG performance status	
0–1	264 (90%)
2	30 (10%)
Men	226 (77%)
Ethnic origin	
Black	1 (<1%)
White	115 (39%)
Asian	151 (51%)
Other	27 (9%)
Chemotherapy regimen	
Capecitabine and cisplatin	256 (87%)
Fluorouracil and cisplatin	38 (13%)
Primary tumor site	
Stomach	236 (80%)
Gastro-esophageal junction	58 (20%)
Type of gastric cancer	
Intestinal	225 (77%)
Diffuse	26 (9%)
Mixed	42 (14%)
Extent of disease at study entry	
Locally advanced	10 (3%)
Metastatic	284 (97%)

(continued)

Treatment Modifications (continued)

Adverse Event	Dose Modification
G3 capecitabine-associated PPE[†]	Begin pyridoxine 50 mg orally 3 times daily and withhold capecitabine. Resume capecitabine with dosage reduced by 30% after toxicity resolves
Recurrent G3 capecitabine-associated PPE[†]	Continue pyridoxine 50 mg orally 3 times daily and withhold capecitabine. Resume capecitabine with dosage reduced by 50% after toxicity resolves
Mild or moderate infusion reaction due to trastuzumab	Decrease the rate of trastuzumab infusion
Infusion reaction characterized by dyspnea or clinically significant hypotension	Interrupt the trastuzumab infusion. Monitor patients until symptoms completely resolve. After symptoms resolve restart the infusion at a slower rate
Severe or life-threatening infusion reactions due to trastuzumab—anaphylaxis, angioedema, interstitial pneumonitis, or acute respiratory distress syndrome	Discontinue trastuzumab
≥16% absolute decrease in LVEF from pretreatment values	Withhold trastuzumab dosing for at least 4 weeks. Trastuzumab may be resumed if, within 4–8 weeks, the LVEF returns to normal limits and the absolute decrease from baseline is ≤15%
LVEF below institutional limits of normal and ≥10% absolute decrease in LVEF from pretreatment values	
Persistent (>8 weeks) LVEF decline or suspension of trastuzumab dosing on more than 3 occasions for cardiomyopathy	Permanently discontinue trastuzumab

*Treatment delays for unresolved adverse events of >3 weeks duration warrant discontinuation of treatment
[†]PPE, Palmar plantar erythrodysesthesia (hand-foot syndrome)

Patient Population Studied (continued)

Metastatic sites per patient[†]	
1–2	152 (52%)
>2	141 (48%)
Previous radiotherapy	5 (2%)
Previous anthracycline therapy	2 (1%)
Previous chemotherapy	27 (9%)[‡]
Previous gastrectomy	71 (24%)
HER2 status	
FISH positive/IHC 0	23 (8%)
FISH positive/IHC 1+	38 (13%)
FISH positive/IHC 2+	80 (27%)
FISH positive/IHC 3+	131 (45%)
FISH negative/IHC 3+	9 (3%)
FISH positive/IHC no result	5 (2%)
FISH no result/IHC 3+	8 (3%)

Data are mean (SD) or number (%)
HER2, human epidermal growth factor receptor 2 (also known as ERBB2); FISH, fluorescence *in situ* hybridization; IHC, immunohistochemistry

Efficacy

	Trastuzumab + Chemotherapy (N = 294)	Chemotherapy Alone (N = 290)	HR (95% CI)	p value
Median OS* (in months, 95% CI)	13.8 (12–16)	11.1 (10–13)	0.74 (0.60–0.91)	0.0046
Median PFS (in months, 95% CI)	6.7 (6–8)	5.5 (5–6)	0.71 (0.59–0.85)[†] 0.71 (0.59–0.86)[‡]	0.0002[†] 0.0004[‡]
Median TTP (in months, 95% CI)	7.1 (6–8)	5.6 (5–6)	0.70 (0.58–0.85)[†] 0.69 (0.57–0.84)[‡]	0.0003[†] 0.0003[‡]
Median DOR (in months, 95% CI)	6.9 (6–8) (N = 139)	4.8 (4–6) (N = 100)	0.54 (0.40–0.73)[†] 0.53 (0.39–0.73)[‡]	<0.0001[†] <0.0001[‡]
			OR (95% CI)	**p value**
ORR	139 (47%)	100 (35%)	1.70 (1.22–2.38)	0.0017[§]
CR	16 (5%)	7 (2%)	2.33 (0.94–5.74)	0.0599[§]
PR	123 (42%)	93 (32%)	1.52 (1.09–2.14)	0.0145[§]
SD	93 (32%)	101 (35%)		
PD	35 (12%)	53 (18%)		
Missing	27 (9%)	36 (12%)		

CR, complete response; DOR, duration of response; HR, hazard ratio; OR, odds ratio; ORR, overall response rate; OS, overall survival; PD, progressive disease; PFS, progression-free survival; PR, partial response; SD, stable disease; TTP, time to progression
Data are median (95% CI) or number (%)
*A treatment effect could not be excluded in any of the predefined subgroups; the overall HR of 0.74 included the 95% CI for all subgroups, apart from the non-measurable disease subgroup. These results must be interpreted with caution because of the small numbers of events within some subgroups
[†]Non-stratified effect size
[‡]Stratified effect size
[§]χ^2 test

Toxicity

Adverse events of all grades (>5%), grades 3 or 4 (≥1%), plus adverse events of any grade with >5% difference between groups

	Trastuzumab + Chemotherapy (n = 294)		Chemotherapy Alone (n = 290)	
	All Grades	**Grades 3 or 4**	**All Grades**	**Grades 3 or 4**
Any adverse event	292 (99%)	201 (68%)	284 (98%)	198 (68%)
Gastrointestinal disorders				
Nausea	197 (67%)	22 (7%)	184 (63%)	21 (7%)
Vomiting	147 (50%)	18 (6%)	134 (46%)	22 (8%)
Diarrhea	109 (37%)	27 (9%)	80 (28%)	11 (4%)
Constipation	75 (26%)	2 (1%)	93 (32%)	5 (2%)
Stomatitis	72 (24%)	2 (1%)	43 (15%)	6 (2%)
Abdominal pain	66 (22%)	7 (2%)	56 (19%)	5 (2%)
Dysphagia	19 (6%)	7 (2%)	10 (3%)	1 (<1%)
Blood and lymphatic system disorders				
Neutropenia	157 (53%)	79 (27%)	165 (57%)	88 (30%)
Anemia	81 (28%)	36 (12%)	61 (21%)	30 (10%)
Thrombocytopenia	47 (16%)	14 (5%)	33 (11%)	8 (3%)
Febrile neutropenia	15 (5%)	15 (5%)	8 (3%)	8 (3%)
General, metabolic, and other disorders				
Anorexia	135 (46%)	19 (6%)	133 (46%)	18 (6%)
Fatigue	102 (35%)	12 (4%)	82 (28%)	7 (2%)
Hand-foot syndrome	75 (26%)	4 (1%)	64 (22%)	5 (2%)
Weight decreased	69 (23%)	6 (2%)	40 (14%)	7 (2%)
Asthenia	55 (19%)	14 (5%)	53 (18%)	10 (3%)
Pyrexia	54 (18%)	3 (1%)	36 (12%)	0
Renal impairment	47 (16%)	2 (1%)	39 (13%)	3 (1%)
Mucosal inflammation	37 (13%)	6 (2%)	18 (6%)	2 (1%)
Nasopharyngitis	37 (13%)	0	17 (6%)	0
Chills	23 (8%)	1 (<1%)	0	0
Hypokalemia	22 (7%)	13 (4%)	13 (4%)	7 (2%)
Dehydration	18 (6%)	7 (2%)	16 (6%)	5 (2%)
Dyspnea	9 (3%)	1 (<1%)	16 (6%)	5 (2%)

Treatment Monitoring

1. CBC with differential, serum electrolytes, magnesium and calcium, BUN, and creatinine before the start of a new cycle
2. Tumor assessment every two cycles
3. LVEF assessment (MUGA or echocardiography) every 3 months in patients receiving trastuzumab

ADVANCED DISEASE REGIMENS

SINGLE-AGENT DOCETAXEL *OR* SINGLE-AGENT IRINOTECAN IN SECOND LINE

Kang JH et al. J Clin Oncol 2012;30:1513–1518

Docetaxel 60 mg/m²; administer intravenously in a volume of 0.9% sodium chloride injection or 5% dextrose injection (D5W) sufficient to produce a docetaxel concentration within the range 0.3–0.74 mg/mL over 60 minutes on day 1, every 3 weeks (total dosage/cycle = 60 mg/m²)
OR
Irinotecan 150 mg/m²; administer intravenously in 500 mL D5W over 90 minutes on day 1, every 2 weeks (total dosage/cycle = 150 mg/m²)

Supportive Care
Antiemetic prophylaxis
Emetogenic potential with docetaxel is **LOW**
Emetogenic potential with irinotecan is **MODERATE**
See Chapter 39 for antiemetic recommendations

Hematopoietic growth factor (CSF) prophylaxis
Primary prophylaxis may be indicated
See Chapter 43 for more information

Antimicrobial prophylaxis
Risk of fever and neutropenia is LOW
   Antimicrobial primary prophylaxis to be considered:
   • Antibacterial—not indicated
   • Antifungal—not indicated
   • Antiviral—not indicated, unless patient previously had an episode of HSV
See Chapter 47 for more information

Acute cholinergic syndrome
Atropine sulfate 0.25–1 mg; administer subcutaneously or intravenously if abdominal cramping or diarrhea develops during or within 1 hour after irinotecan administration
• If symptoms are severe, add as primary prophylaxis at least 30 min before irinotecan during subsequent cycles
• For irinotecan, acute cholinergic syndrome may be characterized by abdominal cramping, diarrhea, diaphoresis, hypotension, flushing, bradycardia, rhinitis, increased salivation, meiosis, and lacrimation

Diarrhea management
Latent or delayed-onset diarrhea*:
   Loperamide 4 mg; administer orally initially after the first loose or liquid stool, *then*
   Loperamide 2 mg; administer orally every 2 hours during waking hours, *plus*
   Loperamide 4 mg; administer orally every 4 hours during hours of sleep
   • Continue for at least 12 hours after diarrhea resolves
   • Recurrent diarrhea after a 12-hour diarrhea-free interval is treated as a new episode
   • Rehydrate orally with fluids and electrolytes during a diarrheal episode
   • If a patient develops blood or mucus in stool, dehydration, or hemodynamic instability, or if diarrhea persists >48 hours despite loperamide, stop loperamide and hospitalize the patient for IV hydration
   Alternatively, a trial of **Diphenoxylate hydrochloride** 2.5 mg **with Atropine sulfate** 0.025 mg (eg, Lomotil®)
   • Initial adult dose is two tablets four times daily until control has been achieved, after which the dose may be reduced to meet individual requirements. Control may often be maintained with as little as two tablets daily
   • Clinical improvement of acute diarrhea is usually observed within 48 hours. If improvement of chronic diarrhea after treatment with a maximum daily dose of 8 tablets is not observed within 10 days, control is unlikely with further administration
Persistent diarrhea:
   Octreotide acetate (solution) 100–150 mcg; administer subcutaneously 3 times daily. Maximum total daily dose is 1500 mcg
Antibiotic therapy during latent or delayed-onset diarrhea:
   A fluoroquinolone (eg, **Ciprofloxacin** 500 mg orally every 12 hours) if absolute neutrophil count <500/mm³ with or without accompanying fever in association with diarrhea
   • Antibiotics should also be administered if patient is hospitalized with prolonged diarrhea and should be continued until diarrhea resolves

*Abigerges D et al. J Natl Cancer Inst 1994;86:446–449
Rothenberg ML et al. J Clin Oncol 2001;19:3801–3807
Wadler S et al. J Clin Oncol 1998;16:3169–3178

(continued)

(*continued*)

Oral care
Prophylaxis and treatment for mucositis/stomatitis

General advice:
- Encourage patients to maintain intake of non-alcoholic fluids
- Evaluate patients for oral pain and provide analgesic medications
- Consider histamine (H_2-subtype) receptor antagonists (eg, ranitidine, famotidine), or a proton pump inhibitor for epigastric pain
- *Lactobacillus* sp.-containing probiotics may be beneficial in preventing diarrhea

Patients with intact oral mucosa:
- Clean the mouth, tongue, and gums by brushing after every meal and at bedtime with an ultra-soft toothbrush with fluoride toothpaste
- Floss teeth gently every day unless contraindicated. If gums bleed and hurt, avoid bleeding or sore areas, but floss other teeth
- Patients may use saline or commercial bland, non-alcoholic rinses
  - Do not use mouthwashes that contain alcohols

If mucositis or stomatitis is present:
- Keep the mouth moist utilizing water, ice chips, sugarless gum, sugar-free hard candies, or a saliva substitute
- Rinse mouth several times a day to remove debris
  - Use a solution of ¼ teaspoon (1.25 g) each of baking soda and table salt (sodium chloride) in one quart (~950 mL) of warm water. Follow with a plain water rinse
  - Do not use mouthwashes that contain alcohols
- Foam-tipped swabs (eg, Toothettes®) are useful in moisturizing oral mucosa, but ineffective for cleansing teeth and removing plaque
- Advise patients who develop mucositis to:
  - Choose foods that are easy to chew and swallow
  - Take small bites of food, chew slowly, and sip liquids with meals
  - Encourage soft, moist foods such as cooked cereals, mashed potatoes, and scrambled eggs
  - For trouble swallowing, soften food with gravies, sauces, broths, yogurt, or other bland liquids
  - Avoid sharp, crunchy foods; hot, spicy or highly acidic foods (eg, citrus fruits and juices); sugary foods; toothpicks; tobacco products; alcoholic drinks

Toxicity

Maximum Grade Adverse Events per Patient

Adverse Event	Docetaxel (N = 66)		Irinotecan (N = 60)		Best Supportive Care (N = 62)	
	% All G	% G3/4	% All G	% G3/4	% All G	% G3/4
Neutropenia	62%	15%	58%	18%	13%	2%
Anemia	76%	30%	77%	32%	61%	23%
Thrombocytopenia	24%	2%	22%	3%	5%	0%
Fatigue	38%	26%	22%	10%	40%	27%
Anorexia	17%	6%	33%	5%	47%	10%
Nausea	21%	5%	32%	3%	32%	6%
Diarrhea	14%	3%	15%	8%	18%	5%
Stomatitis	15%	3%	18%	5%	5%	2%

Treatment Modifications

Docetaxel

Adverse Event	Dose Modification
G4 neutropenia for >7 days, alone, or accompanied by fever >38°C (>100.4°F)	Reduce docetaxel dosage by 25% in all subsequent treatments
G4 thrombocytopenia	After platelet count recovers, resume docetaxel with dosage decreased by 25%
G4 vomiting not controlled by antiemetics	Reduce docetaxel dosage by 25%
G ≥3 diarrhea	
G ≥3 neuropathy	Discontinue therapy

Irinotecan

	Dosage Levels		
	Initial	**−1**	**−2**
Irinotecan	150 mg/m²	120 mg/m²	90 mg/m²

Notes:

• Dose modifications are based on National Cancer Institute (USA) Common Terminology Criteria for Adverse Events, version 3.0. Available at: http://ctep.cancer.gov/protocolDevelopment/electronic_applications/ctc.htm [accessed December 7, 2013]

• Before beginning a treatment cycle, patients should have baseline bowel function without antidiarrheal therapy for 24 hours, ANC ≥1500/mm³, and platelet count ≥100,000/mm³

• Treatment should be delayed 1–2 weeks to allow for recovery from treatment-related toxicities

• If a patient has not recovered after 2 weeks, consider stopping therapy. If toxicity occurs despite 2 dose reductions (ie, on level −2), discontinue therapy

Adverse Event	Dose Modifications
Neutropenia/Thrombocytopenia	
G1 ANC (1500–1999/mm³) or G1 thrombocytopenia (75,000/mm³ to less than normal limits)	Maintain dose and schedule
G2 ANC (1000–1499/mm³) or G2 thrombocytopenia (≥50,000 to <75,000/mm³)	Reduce dosage by 1 dosage level
G3 ANC (500–999/mm³) or G3 thrombocytopenia (≥10,000 to <50,000/mm³)	Hold treatment until toxicity resolves to G ≤2, then reduce dosage by 1 dosage level
G4 ANC (<500/mm³) or G4 thrombocytopenia (<10,000/mm³)	Hold treatment until toxicity resolves to G ≤2, then reduce dosage by 2 dosage levels
Febrile neutropenia	Hold treatment until neutropenia resolves, then reduce dosage by 2 dosage levels
Diarrhea	
G1 (2–3 stools/day greater than baseline)	Maintain dose and schedule
G2 or G3 (4–9stools/day greater than baseline)	Delay until diarrhea resolves to baseline, then reduce dosage by 1 dosage level
G4 (≥10 stools/day greater than baseline)	Delay until diarrhea resolves to baseline, then reduce dosage by 2 dosage levels
Other Nonhematologic Toxicities	
Any G1 toxicity	Maintain dose and schedule
Any G2 or G3 toxicity	Hold treatment until toxicity resolves to G ≤1, then reduce dosage by 1 dosage level
Any G4 toxicity	Hold treatment until toxicity resolves to G ≤1, then reduce dosage by 2 dosage levels

André T et al. Eur J Cancer 1999;35:1343–1347

Camptosar®, irinotecan hydrochloride injection product label, July 2005. Pharmacia & Upjohn Company, Division of Pfizer, Inc, New York, NY

Douillard JY et al. Lancet 2000;355:1041–1047

Tournigand C et al. J Clin Oncol 2004;22:229–237

Patient Population Studied

Patients with histologically confirmed advanced gastric cancer who had not received benefit after one or two chemotherapy regimens for metastatic disease consisting of either fluoropyrimidine- or platinum-based chemotherapy, or a fluoropyrimidine and platinum combination. Exclusion criteria included more than two prior chemotherapy regimens or prior exposure to both taxanes and irinotecan

Patient Characteristics (N = 133)

Characteristic	Number (%)
Age, years − Median (Range)	56 (31–83)
Sex − Male/Female	93 (70%)/ 40 (30%)
Number of prior chemotherapy regimens	
1	100 (75%)
2	33 (25%)
Prior surgery	29 (22%)
Prior adjuvant treatment	20 (15%)
Response to prior chemotherapy	
No	79 (59%)
Yes	54 (41%)
ECOG performance status	
0	72 (54%)
1	61 (46%)
Number of metastatic sites	
1	42 (32%)
≥2	91 (68%)
Involved sites	
Peritoneum	56 (42%)
Liver	30 (23%)
Lymph node	50 (38%)
Lung	12 (9%)
Bone	10 (8%)
Interval from last chemotherapy	
<3	101 months
≥3	32 months

Efficacy

	Docetaxel N = 66* N = 42†	Irinotecan N = 60* N = 50†	BSC N = 62	
Partial response	7/42	5/50		
Stable disease	18/42	21/50		
Median duration of therapy (95%CI)	4.4 months (3.8–4.9)	4.2 months (3.4–5.0)		
Median overall survival (95%CI)	5.3 months (4.1–6.5)		3.8 months (3.1–4.5)	HR = 0.657 (0.485–0.891) one-sided P = 0.007
Median overall survival (95%CI)	5.2 months (3.8–6.6)	6.5 months (4.5–8.5)		two-sided P = 0.116

BSC, best supportive care; CI, confidence interval; HR, hazard ratio
*Number of patients treated with docetaxel or irinotecan or given BSC
†Number of patients who had measurable disease

Univariate Analyses for Survival

Clinical Parameter	HR	95% CI	P
Age			
≤ Median (56 years)	1	—	0.686
>Median	1.063	0.789 to 1.433	
Sex			
Male	1	—	0.267
Female	0.831	0.599 to 1.152	
Number of prior chemotherapy regimens			
1	1	—	<0.001
2	2.044	1.440 to 2.901	
Response to prior therapy			
No	1	—	0.123
Yes	0.784	0.576 to 1.068	
ECOG performance status			
0	1	—	<0.001
1	2.022	1.494 to 2.736	
No. of metastatic sites			
1	1	—	0.173
≥2	1.239	0.911 to 1.686	
Interval from last therapy, months			
<3	1	—	0.030
≥3	0.682	0.483 to 0.964	

HR, hazard ratio

Treatment Monitoring

1. CBC with differential, serum electrolytes, magnesium and calcium, BUN, creatinine, and liver function tests before the start of a new cycle
2. Tumor assessment every two cycles

13. Gestational Trophoblastic Neoplasia

John R. Lurain, MD

Epidemiology

Incidence:*

Hydatidiform mole: 1 in 1000–2000 pregnancies (United States and Europe)

Choriocarcinoma: 1 in 20,000–40,000 pregnancies (United States and Europe)

Gestational trophoblastic neoplasia (GTN) lesions are nearly always disorders of the reproductive years. The incidence is higher in women <20 years and >40 years

*The reported incidence of hydatidiform mole and choriocarcinoma varies widely throughout the world, being greatest in Asia, Africa, and Latin America, and substantially lower in North America and Europe

Lurain JR. Am J Obstet Gynecol 2010;203:531–539

Pathology

Hydatidiform Mole

Benign (80%)
Complete hydatidiform mole
Partial hydatidiform mole

GTN (20%)
Invasive mole (18%)
Choriocarcinoma (2%)*
Placental site trophoblastic tumor (rare)
Epithelioid trophoblastic tumors (rare)

*Note: Half of all choriocarcinomas occur in association with nonmolar pregnancies

Gestational Trophoblastic Neoplasia

- Potential for local invasion and metastases
- Most commonly develops after a molar pregnancy, but can arise de novo after any gestational experience: spontaneous or induced abortion, ectopic pregnancy, or preterm or term pregnancy
- The most common sites of metastases are lungs (80%), brain (10%) liver (10%), and vagina (~5%)

Hancock BW et al. Gestational Trophoblastic Disease, 3rd ed, 2009

Work-up

Once a diagnosis of GTN has been made, it is necessary to determine the extent of disease

Once the initial work-up is completed, patients are categorized (see Staging below)

1. H&P
2. Serum hCG

Note: For staging purposes, the hCG level that is important is that obtained immediately before instituting treatment and not the hCG obtained at the time of the previous molar evacuation

3. CBC, LFT, serum electrolytes, BUN, creatinine, PTT, and PT
4. Chest x-ray
5. CT of chest, abdomen, and pelvis
6. MRI brain (especially in patients with lung lesions. Asymptomatic patients with a normal chest x-ray are unlikely to have brain metastasis)
7. TSH, T_4 (elevations of thyroid tests are not common in patients with GTN but can occur mostly in association with hydatidiform mole)

Lurain JR. American J Obstet Gynecol 2011;204:11–18

Staging

FIGO Anatomic Staging System for GTN

Stage	Extent of GTN
I:	Confined to the uterus
II:	Extends outside the uterus, but is limited to the genital structures (adnexa, vagina, broad ligament)
III:	Extends to the lungs, with or without known genital tract involvement
IV:	All other metastatic sites

(continued)

Staging *(continued)*

FIGO Scoring System* (Modified WHO Scoring System)

[*Note:* This scoring system does not apply to patients with placental-site trophoblastic tumors]

Prognostic Factor	0	1	2	4
Age (years)	≤39	>39	—	—
Antecedent pregnancy	Hydatidiform mole	Abortion	Term pregnancy	—
Interval from index pregnancy	<4 months	4–6 months	7–12 months	>12 months
Pretreatment hCG level (IU/L)	<1000	1000–10,000	>10,000–100,000	>100,000
Largest tumor size including uterus	—	3–4 cm	≥5 cm	—
Sites of metastases	Lung[†]	Spleen, kidney	GI tract	Brain, liver
Number of metastases identified[†]	0	1–4	5–8	>8
Previous ineffective chemotherapy	—	—	Single drug	≥2 drugs

*FIGO staging system includes a modification of the WHO prognostic index score for risk assessment
[†]Chest x-ray is used to count the number of metastases for risk score assessment

Note: Total score for a patient is obtained by adding individual scores for each prognostic factor

Total Score	Risk
0–6	Low risk
≥7	High risk

Both **FIGO Anatomic Staging System** and the **Modified WHO score should be** used. By convention, the FIGO stage is depicted by a Roman numeral and is followed by the Modified WHO Score depicted by an Arabic numeral. The 2 values are separated by a colon (eg, III:9)

Kohorn EI:. Int J Gynecol Cancer 2001;11:73–77
Ngan HYS et al. Int J Gynaecol Obstet 2003;83:175–177

Survival

GTN can be cured predictably even in the presence of widespread metastases. Overall survival is >95%, with survival rates approaching 100% for stage I and stages II/III with WHO score <7 and 80–90% for stage IV or WHO score >7 disease

Expert Opinion

Nonmetastatic GTN

1. Patients with nonmetastatic GTN (FIGO stage I) should be treated with single-agent methotrexate or dactinomycin chemotherapy. Several different outpatient chemotherapy protocols have been used, yielding excellent and fairly comparable results. Hysterectomy may be used as part of primary therapy in patients who no longer desire to preserve fertility

2. Cure is anticipated in 100% of patients with nonmetastatic GTN. Approximately 85–90% of patients will be cured by the initial single-agent chemotherapy regimen. Most of the remaining patients will be placed into permanent remission with an alternate single agent. Multiagent chemotherapy is needed in approximately 2%, and hysterectomy is required in fewer than 5% of patients to achieve cure

    a. Methotrexate given intravenously for 5 days every 2 weeks* results in the highest primary remission rate of approximately 90%

    b. Methotrexate + leucovorin (folinic acid) given over 8 days every two weeks[†-§] is reported to have decreased toxicity (especially stomatitis), but is also more expensive, less convenient, and associated with a more frequent need for a change in chemotherapy (20–25%) to achieve remission

(continued)

Expert Opinion (continued)

c. Methotrexate 30–50 mg/m² by intramuscular injection once weekly

   Methotrexate 100 mg/m² per dose by intravenous injection over 5–30 seconds, followed by:

   Methotrexate 200 mg/m² by intravenous infusion in 25–1000 mL 0.9% NS or D5W over 12 hours

   Leucovorin 15 mg/dose by intramuscular injection or orally every 12 hours for 4 doses starting 24 hours after beginning the methotrexate

   • These treatment protocols are NOT recommended because of the lower primary remission rates of 53–70% and the more frequent need for multiagent chemotherapy to achieve remission

d. Dactinomycin given on a 5-day regimen every 2 weeks[**] or once every 2 weeks[††] are acceptable alternatives to methotrexate

   • Dactinomycin generally causes more nausea and alopecia than methotrexate and produces vesicant injury if extravasation into perivascular tissues occurs. Therefore, dactinomycin is most often used as secondary therapy in the presence of methotrexate resistance or as primary therapy when patients have hepatic or renal compromise or effusions contraindicating the use of methotrexate

Low-Risk Metastatic GTN

1. Patients categorized as having low-risk metastatic GTN (FIGO stages II and III, score <7) can usually be treated successfully with sequential single-agent chemotherapy[*], with:

   • A 5-day methotrexate or dactinomycin regimen[€]

   • An 8-day methotrexate and leucovorin regimen

2. When resistance to sequential single-agent chemotherapy develops, multiagent chemotherapy as for high-risk disease should be given. Hysterectomy may become necessary to eradicate persistent, chemotherapy-resistant disease in the uterus, or it may be performed as adjuvant treatment coincident with the initiation of chemotherapy to shorten the duration of treatment if fertility preservation is not desired

3. Cure rate for low-risk metastatic GTN approaches 100%. Because approximately 30–50% of patients in this category develop resistance to the first chemotherapeutic agent, it is important to carefully monitor patients for evidence of drug resistance so that a change in chemotherapy can be made at the earliest possible time. Eventually, 5–15% of patients treated with sequential single-agent chemotherapy will require multiagent chemotherapy or surgery to achieve remission

High-Risk Metastatic GTN

1. Patients with high-risk metastatic GTN (FIGO stage IV or score ≥7) should be treated initially with multiagent chemotherapy with or without adjuvant surgery or radiation therapy. The EMA/CO protocol, or some variation of it, is currently the treatment of choice for high-risk metastatic GTN because of low toxicity allowing adherence to treatment schedule and relatively high complete response rates of 70–80%[‡,§§]

2. When central nervous system metastases are present, whole-brain irradiation (3000 cGy in 200-cGy fractions), or surgical excision with stereotactic irradiation in selected patients, is usually given simultaneously with the initiation of systemic chemotherapy. During radiotherapy, the methotrexate infusion dosage in the EMA/CO protocol is increased to 1000 mg/m² and 30 mg of leucovorin is given every 12 hours for 3 days starting 32 hours after the methotrexate infusion began. Reported cure rates with brain metastases are 50–80%, depending on patient symptoms as well as number, size, and location of brain lesions

3. Adjuvant surgical procedures, especially hysterectomy and pulmonary resection for chemotherapy-resistant disease, as well as procedures to control hemorrhage, are important components in the management of high-risk GTN. Almost 50% of high-risk patients treated with EMA/CO will require 1 or more operations in order to affect cure

4. Cure rates for high-risk metastatic GTN of 80–90% are now achievable with intensive multimodality treatment with EMA/CO chemotherapy, along with adjuvant radiotherapy or surgery when indicated. Approximately 30% of high-risk patients will fail to benefit not achieve a complete response from first-line therapy or relapse from remission. Salvage therapy with platinum-containing drug combinations, such as:

   Etoposide + cisplatin/etoposide + methotrexate + dactinomycin (EP/EMA),

   Bleomycin + etoposide + cisplatin (BEP),

   Etoposide + ifosfamide + cisplatin (VIP), or ifosfamide + carboplatin + etoposide (ICE), and

   Paclitaxel + cisplatin alternating with paclitaxel + etoposide (TP/TE),

   often in conjunction with surgical resection of sites of persistent tumor, will result in cure of most of these high-risk patients with resistant disease

[*]Chapman-Davis E et al. Gynecol Oncol 2012;125:572–575

[†]McNeish IA et al. J Clin Oncol 2002;20;1838–1844

[‡]Khan F et al. Br J Cancer 2003;89:2197–2201

[§]Growden WB et al. Gynecol Oncol 2009;112:353–357

[€]Osborne RJ et al. J Clin Oncol 2011;29:825–831

[**]Osathanondh R et al. Cancer 1975;36:863–866

[††]Petrilli ES et al. Cancer 1987;60:2173–2176

[‡‡]Lurain JR et al. J Reprod Med 2010;55:199–207

[§§]Lurain JR, Schink JC. J Reprod Med 2012;57:219–224

REGIMEN FOR LOW-RISK GTN

METHOTREXATE

Lurain JR, Elfstrand EP. Am J Obstet Gynecol 1995;172:574–579
Roberts JP, Lurain JR. Am J Obstet Gynecol 1996;174:1917–1924

Methotrexate 0.4 mg/kg (maximum daily dose = 25 mg) per day; administer by intravenous injection daily for 5 consecutive days on days 1–5, every 2 weeks (total dosage/14-day cycle = 2 mg/kg, maximum dose/14-day cycle = 125 mg)

Recommendations:

1. Administer treatment courses as often as toxicity permits, usually every 14 days
2. Encourage increased oral fluid intake or, if NPO, give parenteral hydration
3. Avoid drugs that can alter methotrexate elimination, such as nonsteroidal antiinflammatory drugs, omeprazole (and possibly other proton pump inhibitors), penicillins, probenecid, and salicylates
4. Administer 2 additional cycles after the first normal hCG level

Note: Determination of GFR before treatment does not predict for methotrexate clearance and potential toxicity, but serum creatinine that is within normal limits and a GFR >60 mL/min are generally accepted as adequate renal function

Supportive Care
Antiemetic prophylaxis
Emetogenic potential on days 1–5: **MINIMAL**
See Chapter 39 for antiemetic recommendations

Hematopoietic growth factor (CSF) prophylaxis
Primary prophylaxis is NOT indicated
See Chapter 43 for more information

Antimicrobial prophylaxis
Risk of fever and neutropenia is LOW
See Chapter 47 for more information

Oral care
Prophylaxis and treatment for mucositis/stomatitis
  General advice:
- Encourage patients to maintain intake of non-alcoholic fluids
  - Do not use mouthwashes that contain alcohols

  If mucositis or stomatitis is present:
- Rinse mouth several times a day to remove debris
  - Use a solution of ¼ teaspoon (1.25 g) each of baking soda and table salt (sodium chloride) in one quart (~950 mL) of warm water. Follow with a plain water rinse
  - Do not use mouthwashes that contain alcohols

Therapy Monitoring

1. *Every other week:* PE, CBC with differential, serum electrolytes, LFTs, serum creatinine, BUN, and hCG
2. *Methotrexate levels:* Not routinely performed
3. *Complete remission:* Three consecutive weekly hCG levels within normal range
4. *Resistance to treatment:* hCG plateau over 2 consecutive treatments or a hCG rise after any treatment
5. *Following remission:* hCG levels are obtained monthly for 12 months, and every 3 months during the second year

Patient Population Studied

Retrospective review of 253 patients with nonmetastatic gestational trophoblastic tumors (invasive mole [209] or choriocarcinoma [44]) treated from 1962 to 1990. Antecedent pregnancy was hydatidiform mole (230), abortion (16), and term or preterm delivery (7). A mean of 4.7 courses (range: 1–7) of single-agent methotrexate was administered

Efficacy (N = 253)

Treatment	% Complete Response
Methotrexate alone	89.3*
Methotrexate + dactinomycin	8.7
Multiagent chemotherapy or surgery	2.0
Survival	100

*Six patients (2.4%) had a relapse 1–9 months after achieving a complete response. All were placed into a permanent remission with additional chemotherapy

Toxicity (N = 253)

Stomatitis	G3 (16 patients) mild to moderate (many)
Conjunctivitis	3 patients
Pleuritic/peritoneal pain	3 patients
Hair loss	None
Nausea/vomiting	Not common
Toxicity requiring dose reduction	11 patients (4.3%)
Toxicity requiring change in therapy*	12 patients (4.7%)

*Reasons: G3 stomatitis (5), rash and stomatitis (4); prolonged neutropenia (2), elevated LFTs (1)

Treatment Modifications

Adverse Event	Dose Modification
G ≤1 toxicity	Continue therapy if easy to manage
G2 toxicity	Consider a 20% reduction in methotrexate dosage
G ≥3 toxicity	Discontinue methotrexate and institute other therapy

REGIMEN FOR LOW-RISK GTN
METHOTREXATE WITH LEUCOVORIN

Bagshawe KD et al. Br J Obstet Gynaecol 1989;96:795–802
Berkowitz RS et al. Gynecol Oncol 1986;23:111–118
Wong LC et al. Am J Obstet Gynecol 1985;152:59–62

Methotrexate 1 mg/kg (maximum daily dose = 50 mg) per dose; administer by intramuscular injection for 4 doses on days 1, 3, 5, and 7, every 2 weeks (total dosage/14-day cycle = 4 mg/kg, or a maximum total dose of 200 mg)

Leucovorin calcium 0.1 mg/kg; administer orally or by intramuscular injection for 4 doses on days 2, 4, 6, and 8, at 30 hours after each dose of methotrexate, every 2 weeks (total dosage/cycle = 0.4 mg/kg)

Notes:

1. Administer treatment courses as often as toxicity permits after a minimum rest period of 7 days (usually every 14 days)
2. Encourage increased oral fluid intake or, if NPO, give parenteral hydration
3. Avoid drugs that can alter methotrexate elimination, such as nonsteroidal antiinflammatory drugs, omeprazole (and possibly other proton pump inhibitors), penicillins, probenecid, and salicylates
4. Administer 2 additional cycles after the first normal hCG level

Supportive Care
Antiemetic prophylaxis
Emetogenic potential on days 1, 3, 5, and 7: **MINIMAL**
See Chapter 39 for antiemetic recommendations

Hematopoietic growth factor (CSF) prophylaxis
Primary prophylaxis is NOT indicated
See Chapter 43 for more information

Antimicrobial prophylaxis
Risk of fever and neutropenia is LOW
Antimicrobial primary prophylaxis to be considered:
• Antibacterial—not indicated
• Antifungal—not indicated
• Antiviral—not indicated unless patient previously had an episode of HSV

See Chapter 47 for more information

Patient Population Studied

Patients with low-risk GTN

Efficacy (N = 348)

Outcome	% of Patients
Changed treatment for drug resistance	20
Relapsed	4
Survival	99.7

One death attributed to concurrent non-Hodgkin lymphoma
Bagshawe KD et al. Br J Obstet Gynaecol 1989;96:795–802

Treatment Modifications

Adverse Event	Dose Modification
G ≤1 toxicity	Continue therapy if easy to manage
G2 toxicity including LFTs	Consider a 20% reduction in methotrexate dosage
G ≥3 toxicity including LFTs	Discontinue methotrexate and institute other therapy

Toxicity (N = 185)

Toxicity	% of Patients
Hepatotoxicity; normalized in 1 week	14.1
Granulocytopenia without infection or need for antibiotics	5.9; no secondary infections
Thrombocytopenia without need for platelets	1.6; without infections
Pleuritic chest pain	3.1
Nausea/vomiting	1; requiring intravenous therapy
Alopecia	0
Toxicity requiring change in therapy*	6

Berkowitz RS et al. Gynecol Oncol 1986;23:111–118
Bagshawe KD et al. Br J Obstet Gynaecol 1989;96:795–802

Therapy Monitoring

1. *Every morning before methotrexate:* CBC and LFTs
2. *Every other week:* PE, CBC with differential, serum electrolytes, LFTs, serum creatinine, BUN, and hCG
3. *Methotrexate levels:* Not routinely performed
4. *Complete remission:* Three consecutive weekly hCG levels within normal range
5. *Resistance to treatment:* hCG plateau over 2 consecutive treatments or a hCG rise after any treatment
6. *Following remission:* hCG levels are obtained monthly for 12 months and every 3 months during the second year

REGIMEN FOR LOW-RISK GTN

DACTINOMYCIN

Osathanondh R et al. Cancer 1975;36:863–866

Dactinomycin 12 mcg/kg per day; administer by intravenous injection over 1–2 minutes for 5 consecutive days on days 1–5, every 2 weeks (total dosage/cycle = 60 mcg/kg)

Notes:
1. Therapy was reinstituted only when and if the human chorionic gonadotropin (hCG) level reached a plateau for 2 consecutive weeks, or again increased
2. Patients who did not respond after 2 consecutive cycles were classified as having resistant disease

Alternate regimen:
Dactinomycin 1.25 mg/m²; administer by intravenous injection over 1–2 minutes, on day 1 every 2 weeks (total dosage/cycle = 1.25 mg/m²)

Petrilli ES et al. Cancer 1987;60:2173–2176

Note: This is an acceptable regimen for the treatment of nonmetastatic postmolar GTN, but should not be used for metastatic disease, known choriocarcinoma or as secondary therapy to treat methotrexate-resistant disease

Supportive Care
Antiemetic prophylaxis—first regimen
Emetogenic potential on days 1–5: **MODERATE**

Antiemetic prophylaxis—alternate regimen
Emetogenic potential: **MODERATE**
See Chapter 39 for antiemetic recommendations

Hematopoietic growth factor (CSF) prophylaxis
Primary prophylaxis may be indicated
See Chapter 43 for more information

Antimicrobial prophylaxis
Risk of fever and neutropenia is LOW
   Antimicrobial primary prophylaxis to be considered:
   • Antibacterial—not indicated
   • Antifungal—not indicated
   • Antiviral—not indicated unless patient previously had an episode of HSV
See Chapter 47 for more information

Efficacy (N = 70*)

	Nonmetastatic GTN (N = 31)			Metastatic GTN (N = 39)		
	Non-CCA	CCA	Total	Non-CCA	CCA	Total
CR†	93%	100%	94%	76%	56%	67%

*CCA, choriocarcinoma
†CR (complete response) = hCG in normal range for 3 consecutive weeks off therapy

Treatment Modifications

Adverse Event	Dose Modification
WBC <3000/mm³	Hold dactinomycin until WBC >3000/mm³
ANC <1500/mm³	Hold dactinomycin until ANC >1500/mm³
Platelet count <100,000/mm³	Hold dactinomycin until platelet >100,000/mm³
Hepatotoxicity before or during treatment (LFTs ≥3 × ULN)	Hold dactinomycin until LFTs ≤1.5 × ULN
Increasing hCG level	Discontinue dactinomycin
Plateau in hCG levels after 2 cycles of dactinomycin	Discontinue dactinomycin

Patient Population Studied

A study of 70 patients (previously untreated) with nonmetastatic (31) and metastatic (39) gestational trophoblastic disease accrued from 1965 to 1973

Toxicity (N = 32)

Toxicity	% of Patients
Hematologic	
WBC <2500/mm³	25
ANC <1500/mm³	38
Platelets <100,000/mm³	16
Nonhematologic	
SGOT (AST) >50 units/L	22
Nausea and vomiting	66
Stomatitis	38
Skin rash	34
Alopecia	44

Goldstein DP et al. Obstet Gynecol 1972;39:341–345

Therapy Monitoring

1. *Every other week:* PE, CBC with differential, serum electrolytes, LFTs, serum creatinine, BUN, and hCG
2. *Complete remission:* Three consecutive weekly hCG levels within normal range
3. *Resistance to treatment:* hCG plateau over 2 consecutive treatments or a hCG rise after any treatment
4. *Following remission:* hCG levels are obtained monthly for 12 months and every 3 months during the second year

Notes

1. In current practice, dactinomycin is most frequently used as secondary therapy after the development of methotrexate resistance, rather than as primary therapy, because it causes more nausea and alopecia than methotrexate and produces local tissue injury if extravasation occurs while administered
2. Appropriate as primary therapy for patients with liver or renal disease or with large effusions that are relative contraindications to methotrexate

REGIMEN FOR HIGH-RISK GTN

ETOPOSIDE + METHOTREXATE + DACTINOMYCIN + CYCLOPHOSPHAMIDE + VINCRISTINE (EMA/CO)

Bower M et al. J Clin Oncol 1997;15:2636–2643
Escobar PF et al. Gynecol Oncol 2003;91:552–557
Kim SJ et al. Gynecol Oncol 1998;71:247–253
Lu W-G et al. Int J Gynecol Cancer 2008;18:357–362
Turan T et al. Int J Gynecol Cancer 2006;16:1432–1438

EMA component (days 1–3):
Dactinomycin 0.5 mg (fixed dose) per day; administer by intravenous injection over 1–2 minutes for 2 consecutive days on days 1 and 2, every 2 weeks (total dose/cycle = 1 mg)
Etoposide 100 mg/m^2 per day; administer intravenously diluted in 0.9% sodium chloride injection (0.9% NS) to a concentration within the range of 0.2–0.4 mg/mL over 60 minutes for 2 consecutive days on days 1 and 2, every 2 weeks (total dosage/cycle = 200 mg/m^2)
Methotrexate 100 mg/m^2; administer intravenously by injection or in 25 mL 0.9% NS or 5% dextrose injection (D5W) over 5 minutes, given on day 1, *followed immediately afterward by:*
Methotrexate 200 mg/m^2; administer intravenously in ≥1000 mL 0.9% NS over 12 hours on day 1, every 2 weeks (total dosage/cycle = 300 mg/m^2)
Note: See dose adjustment for patients with documented CNS metastases, below
Leucovorin calcium 15 mg; administer orally or by intramuscular injection every 12 hours for 4 doses on days 2 and 3, beginning 24 hours after the start of methotrexate infusion, every 2 weeks (total dose/cycle = 60 mg). *Note:* See dose adjustment for CNS metastases below

CO component (day 8):
Vincristine 0.8 mg/m^2 (maximum dose, 2 mg); administer by intravenous injection over 1–2 minutes, given on day 8, every 2 weeks (total dosage/cycle = 0.8 mg/m^2; maximum dose/cycle = 2 mg)
Cyclophosphamide 600 mg/m^2; administer intravenously in 250 mL 0.9% NS over 30 minutes, given on day 8, every 2 weeks (total dosage/cycle = 600 mg/m^2)

CNS treatment for patients with documented cranial metastases:
3000-cGy whole-brain radiation; administer in fifteen 200-cGy fractions given 5 times per week for 3 weeks
Dexamethasone as needed, 4 mg; administer orally every 6 hours while radiation is administered, tapering over 2–4 weeks after the completion of radiation
Alternative approach: Surgical excision followed by stereotactic radiation

Methotrexate 1000 mg/m^2; administer by continuous intravenous infusion over 24 hours in 1000 mL 0.9% NS on day 1, every 2 weeks (total dosage/cycle = 1000 mg/m^2)
Leucovorin calcium 30 mg; administer orally, intramuscularly, or intravenously every 12 hours for 6 doses on days 2–4, beginning 32 hours after the start of methotrexate infusion, every 2 weeks (total dose/cycle = 180 mg)

Note: During CNS therapy, the methotrexate regimen given during the *EMA component* is replaced with **Methotrexate** 1000 mg/m^2 by continuous intravenous infusion over 24 hours *for 2–3 cycles,* and the leucovorin calcium dose is increased to 30 mg/dose

Encourage increased oral fluid intake or, if NPO, give parenteral hydration

Duration of therapy:
Repeat EMA alternating weekly with CO to serologic remission (serum hCG <5 IU/L), then administer for an additional 4–8 weeks (2–4 cycles) of therapy. In the report by Escobar et al. of 45 high-risk GTT patients, 4–7 cycles were administered with a mean of 5.5 cycles

Supportive Care
Antiemetic prophylaxis—EMA/CO
Emetogenic potential on days 1 and 2: **MODERATE–HIGH**

Antiemetic prophylaxis—during methotrexate for CNS treatment
Emetogenic potential: **MODERATE**
See Chapter 39 for antiemetic recommendations

Hematopoietic growth factor (CSF) prophylaxis
Primary prophylaxis is NOT indicated
See Chapter 43 for more information

(continued)

Treatment Modifications

Adverse Event	Dose Modification
WBC <3000/mm^3, platelets <100,000/mm^3, or liver transaminases >1.5 × ULN	Hold therapy until WBC ≥3000/mm^3, platelets ≥100,000/mm^3, and liver transaminases ≤ 1.5 × ULN
More than 1 treatment delay for WBC <3000/mm^3	Administer filgrastim 300 mcg/day subcutaneously on days 9–14 of all subsequent cycles
Hgb <10 g/dL	Transfuse as needed and administer erythropoietin
Peripheral neuropathy G > 2	Discontinue vincristine

Patient Population Studied

Women with high-risk GTN. Almost one-half had received prior chemotherapy

(continued)

Antimicrobial prophylaxis
Risk of fever and neutropenia is LOW
Antimicrobial primary prophylaxis to be considered:
- Antibacterial—not indicated
- Antifungal—not indicated
- Antiviral—not indicated unless patient previously had an episode of HSV

See Chapter 47 for more information

Efficacy (N = 272)

All Patients		Prior Therapy	
		No	Yes
Complete response	78.3%*	78%	79%
Progressive disease	17.2%†	14%	21%
Early deaths	4.5%	8%	—
Cumulative overall 5-year survival rate	86%		
Disease-specific 5-year survival rate	88%		

*Sixteen of 213 patients suffered relapse after attaining a complete response
†Forty-seven patients developed resistance to EMA/CO. Sixteen of 21 (76%) patients without prior therapy and 17/26 (65%) patients with prior therapy underwent successful salvage treatment and were alive and in remission at the time of publication

Bower M et al. J Clin Oncol 1997;15:2636–2643

(N = 45)

All Patients		Prior Therapy	
		No	Yes
Initial complete response	71%	76%	65%
Successful salvage therapy	20%*	—	—
Died of disease	9%	—	—
Survival†	91%	92%	90%

*All achieved remission with cisplatin-based therapy
†Median follow-up 36 months

Escobar PF et al. Gynecol Oncol 2003;91:552–557

Toxicity (N = 257 cycles)

	% Cycles		
	G1	G2	G3
Anemia	0.8	8.5	5.8
Neutropenia	6.6	5.4	1.6
Thrombocytopenia	1.6	—	—
Alopecia	All patients		

Gastrointestinal toxicity (nausea, vomiting, diarrhea, and stomatitis) occurred in some patients, but was G3 requiring hospitalization in only 1 patient

Bower M et al. J Clin Oncol 1997;15:2636–2643

(N = 272):
Two cases of AML FAB subtypes M1 and M5

Escobar PF et al. Gynecol Oncol 2003;91:552–557

Therapy Monitoring

1. *Every other week:* PE, CBC with differential, serum electrolytes, LFTs, serum creatinine, BUN, and hCG
2. *Methotrexate levels:* Not routinely performed
3. *Complete remission:* Three consecutive weekly hCG levels within normal range
4. *Resistance to treatment:* hCG plateau over 2 consecutive treatments or a hCG rise after any treatment
5. *Following remission:* hCG levels are obtained monthly for 12 months and every 3 months during the second year

REGIMEN FOR REFRACTORY GTN

ETOPOSIDE + METHOTREXATE + DACTINOMYCIN/ETOPOSIDE + CISPLATIN (EP/EMA)

Lurain JR, Bahareh N. Gynecol Oncol 2005;97:618–623 *(discussion only, the regimen is not described)*
Mao Y et al. Int J Gynaecol Obstet 2007;98:44–47
Newlands ES et al. J Clin Oncol 2000;18:854–859

EP component (day 1)
Etoposide 150 mg/m^2; administer intravenously diluted in 0.9% sodium chloride injection (0.9% NS) or 5% dextrose injection (D5W) to a concentration within the range of 0.2–0.4 mg/mL over 60 minutes, on day 1, every 2 weeks
Cisplatin 25 mg/m^2; administer intravenously in 1000 mL 0.9% NS over 4 hours every 4 hours for 3 doses (total duration of continuous infusion is 12 hours) on day 1, every 2 weeks (total dosage/2-week cycle = 75 mg/m^2)
Hydration after cisplatin: Encourage increased oral intake of nonalcoholic fluids if possible. Monitor and replace magnesium, potassium, and other electrolytes as needed

EMA component (days 8–10)
Dactinomycin 0.5 mg (fixed dose); administer by intravenous injection over 1–2 minutes, on day 8 every 2 weeks (total dose/2-week cycle = 0.5 mg)
Etoposide 100 mg/m^2; administer intravenously in 0.9% NS or D5W to a concentration within the range of 0.2–0.4 mg/mL over 60 minutes, on day 8, every 2 weeks (total dosage/2-week cycle = 250 mg/m^2 [sum of EP + EMA regimens])
Methotrexate 100 mg/m^2; administer intravenously by injection or in 25 mL 0.9% NS or D5W over 5 minutes, given on day 8, *followed immediately afterward by:*
Methotrexate 200 mg/m^2; administer intravenously in ≥1000 mL 0.9% NS over 12 hours on day 8 every 2 weeks (total dosage/2-week cycle = 300 mg/m^2)

Leucovorin calcium 15 mg; administer orally, intravenously, or by intramuscular injection every 12 hours for 4 doses on days 9 and 10, beginning 24 hours after the start of methotrexate infusion, every 2 weeks (total dose/cycle = 60 mg)

Recommendations:
1. EP and EMA components of treatment are alternated at weekly intervals
2. Encourage increased oral fluid intake or, if NPO, give parenteral hydration
3. Avoid concomitant use of drugs that can alter methotrexate elimination, such as nonsteroidal antiinflammatory drugs, omeprazole (and perhaps other proton pump inhibitors), penicillins, probenecid, and salicylates

Supportive Care
Antiemetic prophylaxis—EP regimen
*Emetogenic potential: **HIGH**. Potential for delayed symptoms*

Antiemetic prophylaxis—EMA regimen
*Emetogenic potential: **MODERATE***
See Chapter 39 for antiemetic recommendations

Hematopoietic growth factor (CSF) prophylaxis
Primary prophylaxis is indicated:
Filgrastim (G-CSF) 5 mcg/kg per day by subcutaneous injection
- Begin use on day 9 (24 hours after myelosuppressive chemotherapy is completed)
- Discontinue use at least 24 hours before myelosuppressive treatment resumes
See Chapter 43 for more information

Antimicrobial prophylaxis
Risk of fever and neutropenia is LOW
Antimicrobial primary prophylaxis to be considered:
- Antibacterial—not indicated
- Antifungal—not indicated
- Antiviral—not indicated unless patient previously had an episode of HSV
See Chapter 47 for more information

Treatment Modifications

Adverse Event	Dose Modification
WBC count <2000/mm^3, *and* platelet count <75,000/mm^3	Hold therapy until WBC count ≥2000/mm^3 *and* platelet count ≥75,000/mm^3
Serum creatinine >1.5 × ULN	Measure or estimate creatinine clearance (CrCl) and reduce cisplatin dose by the same percentage as the reduction in CrCl from baseline
G ≥2 mucositis	Double the dose of leucovorin and double the duration of administration (8 doses) before considering methotrexate dose reduction
Any treatment delay for WBC count <2000/mm^3	Administer filgrastim 300 mcg/day, subcutaneously on days 9–14 of all subsequent cycles

Patient Population Studied

A study of 42 women with high-risk GTN refractory to or relapsing after EMA/CO chemotherapy. Patients either (1) had improvement while receiving EMA/CO but a persistently low hCG level or (2) developed a reelevation of hCG after having a complete response to prior treatment with EMA/CO

Efficacy

Response	Alive in Remission
hCG Plateau on EMA/CO* (n = 22)	
—	21 (95%)
Resistant to or Relapsed After EMA/CO† (n = 12)	
12 (100%)	9 (75%)
Placental Site Trophoblastic Tumor (n = 8)	
—	4 (50%)
All Patients (N = 42)	
—	34 (81%)

*hCG sufficiently close to normal range, but not possible to evaluate response
†>1 log decline in hCG

Surgical Procedures in Patients Receiving EP/EMA

Operation	Effect on hCG Response		
	Decreased	None	Not assessed
Hysterectomy	2	4	4
Thoracotomy	1	3	5
Craniotomy	2	0	1
Total	5 (23%)	7 (32%)	10 (45%)

Toxicity*

	% G3	% G4
Hematologic (n = 25)		
Anemia	20	—
Leukopenia	48	20
Thrombocytopenia	24	16

Ten patients (40%) had multiple G3/4 toxicities

	% G3	% G4
Nonhematologic (n = 22)		
Elevated BUN	32%	9%

*Complete results on patients treated before 1988 were no longer available. In the 42 patients:
• Treatment delays because of myelosuppression were observed in 37/42 patients (88%)
• Dose reductions were required in 16/42 patients (38%)
• Filgrastim was administered to 13/42 patients (31%)

NCI, CTC, National Cancer Institute (USA) Common Toxicity Criteria, version 2.0. At: http://ctep.cancer.gov/protocolDevelopment/electronic_applications/ctc.htm [accessed December 7, 2013]

Therapy Monitoring

1. *Every other week*: PE, CBC with differential, serum electrolytes, LFTs, serum creatinine, BUN, and hCG
2. *Methotrexate levels:* Not routinely performed
3. *Complete remission*: Three consecutive weekly hCG levels within normal range
4. *Resistance to treatment:* hCG plateau over 2 consecutive treatments or a hCG rise after any treatment
5. *Following remission:* hCG levels are obtained monthly for 12 months, and every 3 months during the second year

SALVAGE REGIMEN FOR RELAPSED GTN AND PSTT

PACLITAXEL + CISPLATIN/PACLITAXEL + ETOPOSIDE (TP/TE)

Wang J et al. Ann Oncol 2008;19:1578–1583

Day 1: TP component
Primary prophylaxis against hypersensitivity reactions to paclitaxel:
Dexamethasone 20 mg/dose; administer orally for 2 doses every 6 hours, starting approximately 12 hours before paclitaxel administration begins
Cimetidine 300 mg (or equivalent histaminergic receptor [H_2 subtype] antagonist); administer intravenously over 15–30 minutes + **diphenhydramine** 25–50 mg (or equivalent H_1 receptor antagonist); administer intravenously 30–60 minutes before starting paclitaxel administration
Paclitaxel 135 mg/m²; administer intravenously in a volume of 0.9% sodium chloride injection (0.9% NS) or 5% dextrose injection (D5W) sufficient to produce a solution with concentration within the range 0.3–1.2 mg/mL over 3 hours (total dosage/cycle for TP + TE = 270 mg/m²)
Hydration before cisplatin: Administer intravenously ≥1000 mL 0.9% NS over a minimum of 2–4 hours
Cisplatin 60–75 mg/m² with 12.5 g **mannitol**; administer intravenously in 1000 mL 0.9% NS after paclitaxel over 2–3 hours (total dosage/cycle = 60–75 mg/m²)
Hydration after cisplatin: Administer intravenously ≥1000 mL 0.9% NS over a minimum of 2–4 hours. Also encourage increased oral intake of non-alcoholic fluids. Monitor and replace magnesium and other electrolytes as needed

Day 15: TE component
Primary prophylaxis against hypersensitivity reactions to paclitaxel:
Dexamethasone 20 mg/dose; administer orally for 2 doses every 6 hours, starting approximately 12 hours before paclitaxel administration begins
Cimetidine 300 mg (or equivalent H_2 receptor antagonist); administer intravenously over 15–30 minutes + **diphenhydramine** 25–50 mg (or equivalent H_1 receptor antagonist); administer intravenously 30–60 minutes before starting paclitaxel administration
Paclitaxel 135 mg/m²; administer intravenously in a volume of 0.9% NS or D5W sufficient to produce a solution with concentration within the range 0.3–1.2 mg/mL over 3 hours, *followed by:*
Etoposide 150 mg/m²; administer intravenously diluted in 0.9% NS to a concentration within the range of 0.2–0.4 mg/mL over at least 60 minutes (total dosage/cycle = 150 mg/m²)

Supportive Care
Antiemetic prophylaxis
Emetogenic potential on day 1: **HIGH**. *Potential for delayed symptoms after cisplatin*
Emetogenic potential on day 15: **LOW**
See Chapter 39 for antiemetic recommendations

Hematopoietic growth factor (CSF) prophylaxis
Primary prophylaxis is indicated:
>   **Filgrastim** (G-CSF) 5 mcg/kg per day by subcutaneous injection,
- Begin use at least 24 hours after myelosuppressive chemotherapy is completed
- Discontinue use at least 24 hours before resuming myelosuppressive chemotherapy, or for a postnadir ANC ≥10,000/mm³
See Chapter 43 for more information

Antimicrobial prophylaxis
Risk of fever and neutropenia is LOW
Antimicrobial primary prophylaxis to be considered:
- Antibacterial—not indicated
- Antifungal—not indicated
- Antiviral—not indicated unless patient previously had an episode of HSV

See Chapter 47 for more information
Recommendations:
1. TP and TE components of treatment are alternated at 2-week intervals
2. Encourage increased oral fluid intake or, if NPO, give parenteral hydration
3. *Duration of therapy:* Repeat TP alternating with TE to serologic remission (serum hCG <5 IU/L), then administer for an additional 8–16 weeks (2–4 cycles) of therapy

Treatment Modifications

Adverse Event	Dose Modification
WBC count <3000/mm³ *and* platelet count <100,000/mm³	Hold therapy until WBC count ≥3000/mm³ *and* platelet count ≥100,000/mm³
Serum creatinine >1.5 mg/dL (>133 μmol/L)	Measure or estimate creatinine clearance (CrCl) and reduce cisplatin dose by the same percentage as the reduction in CrCl from baseline
Platelet nadir <50,000/mm³	Decrease doses of all drugs by 20%
Peripheral neuropathy G >2	Discontinue therapy or possibly substitute docetaxel 60 mg/m² for paclitaxel

Patient Population Studied

A trial in which 24 women with relapsed/refractory GTN or placental site trophoblastic tumor (PSTT) were treated with TP/TE: 16 had failed to benefit from previous chemotherapy, including 6 who had received cisplatin-containing regimens and 8 who had prior treatment-induced toxic effects

Efficacy (N = 24)

Category	Complete Response	Partial Response	Alive in Remission
Relapsed disease (N = 16)	3 (19%)	5 (31%)*	7 (44%)*
Prior treatment Toxic (N = 8)[†]	2 (25%)	2 (25%)[§]	6 (75%)[‡]
Total (N = 24)	5 (21%)	7 (29%)	13 (54%)

*Median follow-up = 25 months; 4 patients with PR entered remission/cured with subsequent surgery and/or chemotherapy
[†]Four not assessable for response because hCG already normal or close to normal at start
[‡]Median follow-up = 19 months
[§]Two patients (1 PR and 1 not assessable for response) entered remission/cured with subsequent surgery and/or chemotherapy

Toxicity (N = 24)

	% G1	% G2	% G3	% G4
Neutropenia			42	
Thrombocytopenia			13	
Anemia	8			
Neuropathy	17		4	
Nausea	13			

Therapy Monitoring

1. *Every other week:* Physical examination, CBC with differential, serum electrolytes, LFTs, serum creatinine, BUN, and hCG
2. *Complete remission:* Three consecutive weekly hCG levels within normal range
3. *Resistance to treatment:* hCG plateau over 2 consecutive treatments or a hCG rise after any treatment
4. *Following remission:* hCG levels are obtained monthly for 12 months and every 3 months during the second year

14. Head and Neck Cancers

Pol Specenier, MD, PhD and JB Vermorken, MD, PhD

Epidemiology

Incidence: Tongue 13,590 (male: 9,720; female: 3,870. Estimated new cases for 2014 in the United States)

Mouth 11,920 (male: 7,150; female: 4,770. Estimated new cases for 2014 in the United States)

Pharynx 14,410 (male:11,550; female: 2,860. Estimated new cases for 2014 in the United States)

Larynx 12,630 (male: 10,000; female: 2,630. Estimated new cases for 2014 in the United States)

Deaths: Tongue estimated 2,150 in 2014 (male: 1,450; female: 700)

Mouth estimated 2,070 in 2014 (male: 1,130; female: 940)

Pharynx estimated 2,540 in 2013 (male: 1,900; female: 640)

Larynx estimated 3,610 (male: 2,870 female: 740)

Median age: Oral cavity and pharynx 62 years

Tongue 61 years

Larynx 65 years

Male to female ratio: 2.5:1

Siegel R et al. CA Cancer J Clin 2014;64:9–29

Surveillance, Epidemiology and End Results (SEER) Program, available from http://seer.cancer.gov (accessed in 2013)

Pathology

1. Squamous carcinomas (90%)
2. Lymphomas
3. Salivary gland tumors (adenocarcinoma, adenoid cystic carcinoma, mucoepidermoid carcinoma)
4. Sarcomas
5. Melanomas

Work-up

1. History and physical examination
2. ENT examination
3. Laryngoscopy with biopsy of suspicious lesions
4. CT and/or MRI of the head and neck
5. X-ray or CT of chest (to rule out metastatic disease or second primary tumor)
6. Needle biopsy of lymph node not associated with obvious primary tumor

Organ Site Specific Work-up

a. Ethmoid sinus: H&P, CT and/or MRI, CXR, pathology review if diagnosis with incomplete excision

b. Maxillary sinus: H&P, Head and neck CT with contrast ± MRI, CXR, dental/prosthetic consultation as indicated

c. Salivary glands: H&P, CT/MRI, CXR, pathology review

d. Lip, oral cavity: H&P, CT/MRI, parorex, biopsy, preanesthesia studies, dental evaluation

e. Hypopharynx: H&P, biopsy, CXR or chest CT, CT with contrast or MRI of primary and neck, examination under anesthesia with laryngoscopy/esophagoscopy, preanesthesia studies, dental evaluation, multidisciplinary consultation as indicated

f. Glottic larynx: Same work up as for hypopharynx + CT scan with contrast and thin cuts of the larynx or MRI of primary, speech and swallowing studies

Staging

Primary Tumor (T)
- Differs for each site
- For larynx and hypopharynx cancers, vocal cord paralysis indicates at least T3
- Local invasion of adjacent structures indicates T4

Regional Lymph Nodes (N)

NX	Regional lymph nodes cannot be assessed
N0	No regional lymph node metastasis
N1	Metastasis in a single ipsilateral lymph node, 3 cm or less in greatest dimension
N2	Metastasis in a single ipsilateral lymph node, more than 3 cm but not more than 6 cm in greatest dimension, or in multiple ipsilateral lymph nodes, none more than 6 cm in greatest dimension, or in bilateral or contralateral lymph nodes, none more than 6 cm in greatest dimension
N2a	Metastasis in a single ipsilateral lymph node, more than 3 cm but not more than 6 cm in greatest dimension
N2b	Metastasis in multiple ipsilateral lymph nodes, none more than 6 cm in greatest dimension
N2c	Metastasis in bilateral or contralateral lymph nodes, none more than 6 cm in greatest dimension
N3	Metastasis in a lymph node, more than 6 cm in greatest dimension

Distant Metastasis (M)

M0	No distant metastasis
M1	Distant metastasis

Staging Groups
(Cancers of Oral Cavity, Oropharynx, Hypopharynx, and Larynx*)

	T (Primary)	N	M
Stage 0	Tis	N0	M0
Stage I	T1	N0	M0
Stage II	T2	N0	M0
Stage III	T3	N0	M0
	T1	N1	M0
	T2	N1	M0
	T3	N1	M0
Stage IVA	T4a	N0	M0
	T4a	N1	M0
	T1	N2	M0
	T2	N2	M0
	T3	N2	M0
	T4a	N2	M0
Stage IVB	T4b	Any N	M0
	Any T	N3	M0
Stage IVC	Any T	Any N	M1

*The same for all primary sites, except nasopharynx

Edge SB, Byrd DR, Compton CC, Fritz AG, Greene FL, Trotti A, editors. AJCC Cancer Staging Manual. 7th ed. New York: Springer; 2010

Larynx: 5-Year Relative Survival by Stage at Diagnosis for All Races, Both Sexes

Stage at Diagnosis	5-Year Relative Survival (%)
Localized (confined to primary site)	76.1
Regional (spread to regional lymph nodes)	42.8
Distant (cancer has metastasized)	35.3

Oral Cavity and Pharynx: 5-Year Relative Survival by Stage at Diagnosis for All Races, Both Sexes

Stage at Diagnosis	5-Year Relative Survival (%)
Localized (confined to primary site)	82.7
Regional (spread to regional lymph nodes)	59.2
Distant (cancer has metastasized)	36.3

Tongue: 5-Year Relative Survival by Stage at Diagnosis for All Races, Both Sexes

Stage at Diagnosis	5-Year Relative Survival (%)
Localized (confined to primary site)	78.0
Regional (spread to regional lymph nodes)	60.9
Distant (cancer has metastasized)	35.2

Surveillance, Epidemiology and End Results (SEER) Program, available from http://seer.cancer.gov (accessed in 2013)

Expert Opinion

Treatment

General: All patients should have access to a *multidisciplinary team* with expertise in all aspects of care for patients with head and neck cancer including:

1. Head and neck surgery
2. Radiation oncology
3. Medical oncology
4. Reconstructive surgery
5. Dentistry
6. Speech and swallowing therapy
7. Diagnostic radiology
8. Pathology
9. Nutrition support
10. Social work

Smoking cessation counseling is indicated

Resectable versus unresectable disease: The tumor is considered unresectable when a (team of) surgeons with particular expertise in head and neck cancer has serious doubts about the ability to remove the gross tumor with a reasonable likelihood of local control, even with the addition of adjuvant chemoradiation

Postoperative chemoradiation: Postoperative cisplatin-based chemoradiation using *cisplatin 100 mg/m² every 3 weeks* is superior to irradiation alone in patients with adverse risk factors in the resection specimen. Postoperative chemoradiation is:

1. Indicated in patients with extracapsular nodal spread and/or positive surgical margins
2. To be considered in patients with:
   - pT3 or pT4 primary
   - N2 or N3 nodal disease
   - Perineural invasion
   - Vascular tumor embolism

Postoperative chemoradiation should be started within 6 weeks after surgery. But note, combined modality treatment is associated with a substantial increase in adverse effects

Organ preservation: In some patients with resectable disease a combination of chemotherapy and definitive irradiation can spare a functional organ without sacrificing the probability of cure. Each patient should be evaluated by the multidisciplinary team in order to offer to a patient the best options

Definitive nonsurgical treatment for patients with unresectable disease or as organ preservation:
- *Concurrent chemoradiation using cisplatin 100 mg/m² every 3 weeks for 3 doses should still be considered the standard regimen*
- Cetuximab with irradiation can be used in patients who cannot tolerate cisplatin-based chemotherapy
- PET-CT imaging 12 weeks after the end of chemoradiation may help to select patients with initial N2 or N3 disease who achieved a complete response from combined modality treatment for whom elective neck dissection is unnecessary
- *Salvage surgery* is indicated in patients with residual tumor at the *primary site* whenever the disease is resectable at that time
- *Neck dissection* is indicated in cases of residual *disease in the neck*

Considerations in patients undergoing chemoradiation:
1. All patients for whom chemoradiation is planned should be evaluated and treated by a dentist before the start of treatment
2. Follow patients closely during chemoradiation with special attention to:
   - Hydration
   - Nutritional status
   - Electrolyte balance
3. Tube feeding is indicated in cases of a 10% decrease of body weight. Some centers prefer prophylactic tube feeding before the start of chemoradiation
4. Swallowing exercises during and after treatment are strongly advocated in order to diminish the risk of permanent disturbance of oral food intake
5. Adequate analgesic therapy often including opioids may be required

(continued)

Expert Opinion (continued)

Induction chemotherapy:

1. **TPF (docetaxel + cisplatin + fluorouracil)** *is to be considered the current standard induction chemotherapy regimen in cases where induction chemotherapy is considered appropriate*

2. Induction chemotherapy reduces the risk of distant metastases but should not be considered standard treatment pending the results of ongoing randomized phase III trials

3. Induction chemotherapy may be an option for specific patient categories

Recurrent/metastatic disease: Active single agents include:

1. Cisplatin
2. Carboplatin
3. Paclitaxel
4. Docetaxel
5. Fluorouracil
6. Methotrexate
7. Ifosfamide
8. Bleomycin
9. Cetuximab

Consideration in recurrent/metastatic disease:

1. Response rates with single cytotoxic agents range from 15–30% in nonrandomized trials

2. In randomized comparisons *platinum-based combination chemotherapy regimens (in particular cisplatin plus infusional fluorouracil) induce higher response rates than single-agent chemotherapy but at the cost of increased toxicity*

3. Addition of a taxane to cisplatin and fluorouracil doublet increases response rates but also adds to toxicity

4. The addition of cetuximab to cisplatin and fluorouracil improves survival without a significant increase in serious toxicities. *The combination of cisplatin + fluorouracil + cetuximab, therefore, is the preferred regimen in patients who are most likely to benefit from combination chemotherapy*

5. Single agent chemotherapy is still an option in patients with a decreased performance status or in a frail condition:
   - Weekly methotrexate is the best-studied regimen for that indication
   - Taxanes may be adequate alternatives

6. Outcomes with second-line chemotherapy are generally disappointing

7. Single-agent cetuximab is a reasonable option in patients with platinum-refractory disease who did not receive cetuximab as part of their initial treatment for recurrent/metastatic disease

8. Selected patients with a locoregional relapse may be salvaged by surgery or re-irradiation
   - Metastatic disease outside the head/neck area is present in only 10% at presentation, but 20% of those treated for cure with surgery and/or radiation or with chemoradiation develop metastatic disease outside the locoregional area, commonly concurrent with a locoregional recurrence
   - Patients cured of the initial tumor have a 2–6% per year incidence of second primary tumors, commonly diagnosed in the upper aerodigestive tract

Thyroid function: Patients who received thyroid gland irradiation are prone to the development of hypothyroidism. Thyroid stimulating hormone should be followed every 6–12 months for the lifetime of affected patients

Bernier J et al. N Engl J Med 2004;350:1945–1952
Bernier J et al. Head Neck 2005;27:843–850
Forastiere AA et al. N Engl J Med 2003;349:2091–2098
Haddad RI, Shin DM. N Engl J Med 2008;359:1143–1154
Lefebvre JL. Lancet Oncol 2006;7:745–755
Posner MR et al. N Engl J Med 2007;357:1705–1715
Specenier PM, Vermorken JB. Target Oncol 2007;2:73–88
Vermorken JB et al. Cancer 2008;112:2710–2719
Vermorken JB et al. N Engl J Med 2007;357:1695–1704
Vermorken JB et al. N Engl J Med 2008;359:1116–1127

CONCOMITANT CHEMORADIATION REGIMENS

CISPLATIN WITH RADIATION THERAPY

Adelstein DJ et al. J Clin Oncol 2003;21:92–98
Forastiere AA et al. N Engl J Med 2003;349:2091–2098

Pretreatment:
Dental evaluation; percutaneous feeding tube; nutrition evaluation

Chemoradiation

As noted in the Expert Opinion section: Concurrent chemoradiation using cisplatin every 3 weeks for 3 doses should still be considered the standard regimen

Hydration before, during, and after cisplatin administration ± mannitol:
- *Pre-cisplatin hydration* with 1000 mL 0.9% sodium chloride injection (0.9% NS); administer with potassium and magnesium supplementation as needed based on pretreatment laboratory results
- *Mannitol diuresis:* May be given to patients who have received adequate hydration. A dose of **mannitol 12.5–25 g** may be administered by intravenous injection or a short infusion before or during cisplatin administration, or prepared as an admixture with cisplatin. Continued intravenous hydration is essential
- *Continued mannitol diuresis:* In an inpatient or day-hospital setting, one may administer additional mannitol in the form of an intravenous infusion: **mannitol 10–40 g**; administer intravenously over 1–4 hours. This can be done either during or immediately after cisplatin, but requires maintenance of adequate intravenously administered fluids during and for hours after mannitol administration
- *Post-cisplatin hydration* with ≥1000 mL 0.9% NS; administer with potassium and magnesium supplementation as needed based on measured values

Cisplatin 100 mg/m²; administer intravenously in 50–1000 mL 0.9% NS over 60 minutes on day 1, every 3 weeks for 3 cycles during radiation (total dosage/cycle = 100 mg/m²)
Radiation therapy at least 70 Gy to primary site and clinically positive nodes given in daily (Monday–Friday) fractions of 2 Gy/day over 7 weeks; at least 50 Gy to entire neck

Supportive Care
Antiemetic prophylaxis
Emetogenic potential on day 1 is **HIGH**. *Potential for delayed symptoms*
See Chapter 39 for antiemetic recommendations

Hematopoietic growth factor (CSF) prophylaxis
Primary prophylaxis is *NOT* indicated
See Chapter 43 for more information

Antimicrobial prophylaxis
Risk of fever and neutropenia is LOW
  Antimicrobial primary prophylaxis to be considered:
  - Antibacterial—not indicated
  - Antifungal—not indicated
  - Antiviral—not indicated unless patient previously had an episode of HSV
See Chapter 47 for more information

Oral care (mucositis prophylaxis and management)
Risk of mucositis/stomatitis is HIGH
  General advice:
  - Encourage patients to maintain intake of non-alcoholic fluids
  - Evaluate patients for oral pain and provide analgesic medications
  - Consider histamine (H₂-subtype) receptor antagonists (eg, ranitidine, famotidine), or a proton pump inhibitor for epigastric pain
  - *Lactobacillus* sp.-containing probiotics may be beneficial in preventing diarrhea
  Patients with intact oral mucosa:
  - Clean the mouth, tongue, and gums by brushing after every meal and at bedtime with an ultra-soft toothbrush with fluoride toothpaste
  - Floss teeth gently every day unless contraindicated. If gums bleed and hurt, avoid bleeding or sore areas, but floss other teeth

(continued)

Treatment Modifications

Adverse Event	Dose Modification*
Creatinine clearance <50 mL/min (<0.83 mL/s)	Ineligible for therapy
Day 1, 22, or 43 ANC <1500/mm³ or platelets <100,000/mm³	Delay cisplatin until ANC >1500/mm³ *and* platelets >100,000/mm³, for up to 3 weeks. Discontinue cisplatin if recovery has not occurred after a 3-week delay
ANC nadir <500/mm³	Reduce cisplatin dosage to 75 mg/m²
Platelet nadir <25,000/mm³	
G1 neurotoxicity or ototoxicity	
Serum creatinine 1.5–2.0 mg/dL (133–177 μmol/L)	Hold cisplatin†, then reduce dosage to 75 mg/m²
ANC nadir <500/mm³ with a cisplatin dosage of 75 mg/m²	Reduce cisplatin dosage to 50 mg/m²
Platelet nadir <25,000/mm³ with a cisplatin dosage of 75 mg/m²	
G2 neurotoxicity or ototoxicity	
Serum creatinine 2.1–3.0 mg/dL (186–265 μmol/L)	Hold cisplatin†, then reduce dosage to 50 mg/m²
ANC nadir <500/mm³ with a cisplatin dosage of 50 mg/m²	Discontinue cisplatin
Platelet nadir <25,000/mm³ with a cisplatin dosage of 50 mg/m²	
Serum creatinine >3.0 mg/dL (>265 μmol/L)	
G3/4 neurotoxicity or ototoxicity	

*The use of colony-stimulating factors is discouraged
†Hold cisplatin dosage until serum creatinine <1.5 mg/dL (<133 μmol/L) or within 0.2 mg/dL (17.7 μmol/L) of baseline

(continued)

- Patients may use saline or commercial bland, non-alcoholic rinses
  - Do not use mouthwashes that contain alcohols

If mucositis or stomatitis is present:

- Keep the mouth moist utilizing water, ice chips, sugarless gum, sugar-free hard candies, or a saliva substitute
- Rinse mouth several times a day to remove debris
  - Use a solution of ¼ teaspoon (1.25 g) each of baking soda and table salt (sodium chloride) in one quart (~950 mL) of warm water. Follow with a plain water rinse
  - Do not use mouthwashes that contain alcohols
- Foam-tipped swabs (eg, Toothettes®) are useful in moisturizing oral mucosa, but ineffective for cleansing teeth and removing plaque
- Advise patients who develop mucositis to:
  - Choose foods that are easy to chew and swallow
  - Take small bites of food, chew slowly, and sip liquids with meals
  - Encourage soft, moist foods such as cooked cereals, mashed potatoes, and scrambled eggs
  - For trouble swallowing, soften food with gravies, sauces, broths, yogurt, or other bland liquids
  - Avoid sharp, crunchy foods; hot, spicy or highly acidic foods (eg, citrus fruits and juices); sugary foods; toothpicks; tobacco products; alcoholic drinks

Efficacy

Larynx Preservation Regimen (N = 172)*

Complete response	90.6%
Laryngeal preservation at median 3.8 years follow-up	84%
2-Year estimated overall survival	74%
2-Year estimated laryngectomy-free survival[†]	66%
2-Year estimated disease-free survival	61%
5-Year estimated overall survival	54%
5-Year estimated laryngectomy-free survival[†]	45%
5-Year estimated disease-free survival	36%
Percent receiving >95% of planned RT dose	91%
Moderate[‡] or worse speech impairment at 2 year[§]	11%
Moderate[‡] or worse speech impairment at 1 year[§]	6%
Able to swallow only soft foods or liquids at 1 year	23%
Able to swallow only soft foods or liquids at 2 years	15%
Unable to swallow at 1 year	3%

*Forastiere AA et al. N Engl J Med 2003;349:2091–2098
[†]Composite endpoint on which the sample size of the trial was predicated. Either laryngectomy or death from any cause constituted treatment failure
[‡]Difficulty in pronouncing some words and being understood on the telephone
[§]*Note:* Information on speech and swallowing was available from only 78% of patients who were disease-free and had an intact larynx

Efficacy

Patients with Unresectable Squamous Cell Head and Neck Cancer (N = 87)*

Complete response	40.2%
3-Year overall survival	37%
Median Survival	19.1 months
3-Year disease-specific survival	51%
Compliance	85.1%
Distant metastasis as first site of recurrence	21.8%

*Adelstein DJ et al. J Clin Oncol 2003;21:92–98

Patient Population Studied

Organ preservation: Patients with previously untreated stage III or stage IV squamous cell carcinoma of the glottic or supraglottic larynx, the surgical treatment of which would require total laryngectomy. The disease had to be considered curable with surgery and postoperative radiation therapy. Karnofsky performance status (PS) at least 60%; adequate organ function; creatinine clearance at least 50 mL/min (≥0.83 mL/s)
Unresectable: Patients with stages III/IV unresectable squamous cancer excluding nasopharyngeal cancer, or cancers of the paranasal sinuses or parotid glands. ECOG PS 0–1, adequate organ function

Toxicity (N = 266)

Organ Preservation (n = 171);
Unresectable (n = 95)

Toxicity	% G3/4/5 Toxicity	
	Organ Preservation	Unresectable
Hematologic Leukopenia Anemia Thrombocy-topenia	47	42 18 3
Mucosal	43	45
Pharyngeal/ esophageal	35	—
Nausea or vomiting	20	16
Laryngeal	18	—
Dermatologic*	7	7
Infection	4	—
Renal/ genitourinary	4	8
Neurologic	5	—
Other (not specified)	40	—
G5 toxicity	5	4

*Within radiation field

Therapy Monitoring

1. *Before cisplatin and weekly after treatment:* CBC with differential, serum electrolytes, calcium, and magnesium
2. *Weekly follow-up recommended during therapy:* Attention to signs and symptoms of dehydration as supplemental hydration and nutritional support often are required
3. *Every 4–6 months:* Thyroid function studies

CONCOMITANT CHEMORADIATION REGIMENS

CISPLATIN + PACLITAXEL WITH RADIATION THERAPY

Garden AS et al. Preliminary results of RTOG 97–03. J Clin Oncol 2004;22:2856–2864

Pretreatment:
Dental evaluation; percutaneous feeding tube; nutrition evaluation

Premedication:
Dexamethasone 8–20 mg; administer by intravenous injection or short intravenous infusion 30 minutes before paclitaxel
Diphenhydramine 50 mg; administer by intravenous injection 30–60 minutes before paclitaxel
Ranitidine 50 mg; administer intravenously over 5–20 minutes, 30–60 minutes before paclitaxel
Paclitaxel 30 mg/m^2 per dose; administer intravenously in a volume of 0.9% sodium chloride injection (0.9% NS), or 5% dextrose injection (D5W) sufficient to produce a concentration within the range 0.3–1.2 mg/mL over 3–24 hours weekly, on day 1, for 7 consecutive weeks (total dosage/7-week cycle = 210 mg/m^2)
Optional: **Dexamethasone** 4 mg; administer orally every 6 hours for 4 doses following paclitaxel with glucose monitoring if indicated
Cisplatin 20 mg/m^2 per dose; administer intravenously in 100–1000 mL 0.9% NS over 15–60 minutes weekly on day 2, for 7 consecutive weeks (total dosage/7-week cycle = 140 mg/m^2)
Radiation at least 70 Gy to primary site and clinically positive nodes given in daily (Monday–Friday) fractions of 2 Gy/day over 7 weeks

Supportive Care
Antiemetic prophylaxis
Emetogenic potential on days with paclitaxel is **LOW**
Emetogenic potential on days with cisplatin is **HIGH**
See Chapter 39 for antiemetic recommendations

Hematopoietic growth factor (CSF) prophylaxis
Primary prophylaxis is NOT indicated
See Chapter 43 for more information

Antimicrobial prophylaxis
Risk of fever and neutropenia is LOW
   Antimicrobial primary prophylaxis to be considered:
   • Antibacterial—not indicated
   • Antifungal—consider use during neutropenia and for anticipated mucositis
   • Antiviral—not indicated unless patient previously had an episode of HSV
See Chapter 47 for more information

Oral care (mucositis prophylaxis and management)
Risk of mucositis/stomatitis is MODERATE
   General advice:
   • Encourage patients to maintain intake of non-alcoholic fluids
   • Evaluate patients for oral pain and provide analgesic medications
   • Consider histamine (H$_2$-subtype) receptor antagonists (eg, ranitidine, famotidine), or a proton pump inhibitor for epigastric pain
   • *Lactobacillus* sp.-containing probiotics may be beneficial in preventing diarrhea
   Patients with intact oral mucosa:
   • Clean the mouth, tongue, and gums by brushing after every meal and at bedtime with an ultra-soft toothbrush with fluoride toothpaste
   • Floss teeth gently every day unless contraindicated. If gums bleed and hurt, avoid bleeding or sore areas, but floss other teeth
   • Patients may use saline or commercial bland, non-alcoholic rinses
      ▪ Do not use mouthwashes that contain alcohols

(continued)

Toxicity (N = 77)

	% G3/4
Nonhematologic	84
Hematologic	39
Mucositis	10 (G4)
Skin	3 (G4)

% Late Grade 4 Toxicities* (N = 72)

Bone	4.2
Mucous membrane	1.4
Pharynx and esophagus	1.4
Larynx	1.4
Spinal cord	1.4
Skin	0
Subcutaneous tissue	0

*No grade 5 toxicities

Treatment Modifications

Adverse Event	Dose Modification
Creatinine clearance <50 mL/min (<0.83 mL/s)	Ineligible for therapy
ANC <1000/mm^3 or platelets <75,000/mm^3 at the time of chemotherapy administration	Delay chemotherapy until ANC >1000/mm^3 and platelets >75,000/mm^3. Discontinue chemotherapy if recovery has not occurred after a 3-week delay
Serum creatinine >1.5 mg/dL (>133 μmol/L) or 20% higher than baseline value if baseline was >1.5 mg/dL	Hold cisplatin dosage until serum creatinine <1.5 mg/dL (<133 μmol/L) or within 0.2 mg/dL (17.7 mol/L) of baseline
G2 neurotoxicity or ototoxicity	Hold cisplatin and paclitaxel until neurotoxicity resolves to G ≤1
G3/4 neurotoxicity or ototoxicity	Discontinue chemotherapy

(continued)

If mucositis or stomatitis is present:

- Keep the mouth moist utilizing water, ice chips, sugarless gum, sugar-free hard candies, or a saliva substitute
- Rinse mouth several times a day to remove debris
  - Use a solution of ¼ teaspoon (1.25 g) each of baking soda and table salt (sodium chloride) in one quart (~950 mL) of warm water. Follow with a plain water rinse
  - Do not use mouthwashes that contain alcohols
- Foam-tipped swabs (eg, Toothettes®) are useful in moisturizing oral mucosa, but ineffective for cleansing teeth and removing plaque
- Advise patients who develop mucositis to:
  - Choose foods that are easy to chew and swallow
  - Take small bites of food, chew slowly, and sip liquids with meals
  - Encourage soft, moist foods such as cooked cereals, mashed potatoes, and scrambled eggs
  - For trouble swallowing, soften food with gravies, sauces, broths, yogurt, or other bland liquids
  - Avoid sharp, crunchy foods; hot, spicy or highly acidic foods (eg, citrus fruits and juices); sugary foods; toothpicks; tobacco products; alcoholic drinks

Efficacy (N = 77)

Complete response	82%
Estimated 2-year disease-free survival	51.3%
Estimated 2-year overall survival	66.6%

Patient Population Studied

A study of 77 patients with stage III or stage IV M0 squamous cancer of oral cavity, oropharynx, or hypopharynx, previously untreated, assigned to 1 of 3 arms in a randomized phase II RTOG trial. ECOG PS at least 70% and adequate organ function are required

Therapy Monitoring

1. *Weekly:* CBC with differential, serum electrolytes, calcium, and magnesium. Weekly follow-up recommended during therapy with attention to signs and symptoms of dehydration because supplemental hydration and nutritional support are often required
2. *Every 4–6 months:* Thyroid function studies

CONCOMITANT CHEMORADIATION REGIMENS

CARBOPLATIN + FLUOROURACIL WITH RADIATION THERAPY

Calais G et al. J Natl Cancer Inst 1999;91:2081–2086

Pretreatment:
Dental evaluation; percutaneous feeding tube; nutrition evaluation
Carboplatin 70 mg/m² per day; administer intravenously in 50–100 mL 5% dextrose injection (D5W) or 0.9% sodium chloride injection (0.9% NS) over 15–30 minutes for 4 consecutive days, given on days 1–4, every 3 weeks (total dosage/cycle = 280 mg/m²)
Fluorouracil 600 mg/m² per day; administer by continuous intravenous infusion in 50–1000 mL 0.9% NS or D5W over 24 hours for 4 consecutive days, given on days 1–4, every 3 weeks (total dosage/cycle = 2400 mg/m²)
Radiation 2 Gy/day, 5 fractions per week to tumor and clinically positive nodes to a total dose of 70 Gy

Supportive Care
Antiemetic prophylaxis
Emetogenic potential is **MODERATE**
See Chapter 39 for antiemetic recommendations

Hematopoietic growth factor (CSF) prophylaxis
Primary prophylaxis is NOT indicated
See Chapter 43 for more information

Antimicrobial prophylaxis
Risk of fever and neutropenia is LOW
Antimicrobial primary prophylaxis to be considered:
- Antibacterial—not indicated
- Antifungal—not indicated
- Antiviral—not indicated unless patient previously had an episode of HSV
See Chapter 47 for more information

Diarrhea management
Latent or delayed onset diarrhea*:
Loperamide 4 mg orally initially after the first loose or liquid stool, *then*
Loperamide 2 mg orally every 2 hours during waking hours, *plus*
Loperamide 4 mg orally every 4 hours during hours of sleep
- Continue for at least 12 hours after diarrhea resolves
- Recurrent diarrhea after a 12-hour diarrhea-free interval is treated as a new episode
- Rehydrate orally with fluids and electrolytes during a diarrheal episode
- If diarrhea persists >48 hours despite loperamide, stop loperamide and hospitalize the patient for IV hydration

Persistent diarrhea:
Octreotide 100–150 mcg subcutaneously 3 times daily. Maximum total daily dose is 1500 mcg
Antibiotic therapy during latent or delayed onset diarrhea:
A fluoroquinolone (eg, **Ciprofloxacin** 500 mg orally every 12 hours) if absolute neutrophil count <500/mm³ with or without accompanying fever in association with diarrhea
- Antibiotics should also be administered if patient is hospitalized with prolonged diarrhea and should be continued until diarrhea resolves

*Rothenberg ML et al. J Clin Oncol 2001;19:3801–3807
Abigerges D et al. J Natl Cancer Inst 1994;86:446–449
Wadler S et al. J Clin Oncol 1998;16:3169–178

Oral care (mucositis prophylaxis and management)
Risk of mucositis/stomatitis is HIGH
General advice:
- Encourage patients to maintain intake of non-alcoholic fluids
- Evaluate patients for oral pain and provide analgesic medications

(continued)

Patient Population Studied

A study of 109 patients with previously untreated stage III or stage IV squamous cell carcinoma of the oropharynx without evidence of distant metastases. Patients were assigned to the chemoradiation arm of a randomized phase III trial with Karnofsky PS at least 60% and adequate organ function

Efficacy (N = 109)

Locoregional control	66%
3-Year overall survival	51%
3-Year disease-free survival	42%
Median survival	29.2 months

Therapy Monitoring

1. *Weekly:* CBC with differential, serum electrolytes, calcium, and magnesium. Weekly follow-up recommended during therapy with attention to signs and symptoms of dehydration because supplemental hydration and nutritional support are often required
2. *Every 4–6 months:* Thyroid function studies

(*continued*)

- Consider histamine (H$_2$-subtype) receptor antagonists (eg, ranitidine, famotidine), or a proton pump inhibitor for epigastric pain
- *Lactobacillus* sp.-containing probiotics may be beneficial in preventing diarrhea

Patients with intact oral mucosa:

- Clean the mouth, tongue, and gums by brushing after every meal and at bedtime with an ultra-soft toothbrush with fluoride toothpaste
- Floss teeth gently every day unless contraindicated. If gums bleed and hurt, avoid bleeding or sore areas, but floss other teeth
- Patients may use saline or commercial bland, non-alcoholic rinses
  - Do not use mouthwashes that contain alcohols

If mucositis or stomatitis is present:

- Keep the mouth moist utilizing water, ice chips, sugarless gum, sugar-free hard candies, or a saliva substitute
- Rinse mouth several times a day to remove debris
  - Use a solution of ¼ teaspoon (1.25 g) each of baking soda and table salt (sodium chloride) in one quart (~950 mL) of warm water. Follow with a plain water rinse
  - Do not use mouthwashes that contain alcohols
- Foam-tipped swabs (eg, Toothettes®) are useful in moisturizing oral mucosa, but ineffective for cleansing teeth and removing plaque
- Advise patients who develop mucositis to:
  - Choose foods that are easy to chew and swallow
  - Take small bites of food, chew slowly, and sip liquids with meals
  - Encourage soft, moist foods such as cooked cereals, mashed potatoes, and scrambled eggs
  - For trouble swallowing, soften food with gravies, sauces, broths, yogurt, or other bland liquids
  - Avoid sharp, crunchy foods; hot, spicy or highly acidic foods (eg, citrus fruits and juices); sugary foods; toothpicks; tobacco products; alcoholic drinks

Toxicity (N = 109)

	% of Patients
Acute Nonhematologic Toxicity	
G3/4 mucositis	71
Erythema/pruritis/dry desquamation	44
Moist desquamation	23
Weight loss >10% body mass	14
Need for feeding tube	36
G5 toxicities	0.9
Acute Hematologic Toxicity	
G3/4 neutropenia	4
G3/4 thrombocytopenia	6
G3/4 anemia	3
Late Toxicities	
G3/4 xerostomia	10
Severe cervical fibrosis	12

Treatment Modifications

Adverse Event	Dose Modification
Creatinine clearance <50 mL/min (<0.83 mL/s)	Ineligible for therapy
ANC <1000/mm³ *or* platelets <75,000/mm³ at time of chemotherapy administration	Delay chemotherapy until ANC >1000/mm³ *and* platelets >75,000/mm³
G ≥2 neurotoxicity	Hold carboplatin until neurotoxicity resolves to G ≤1
G3/4 neurotoxicity	Discontinue carboplatin
G ≥2 diarrhea (4–6 stools/day > baseline)	Delay until diarrhea resolves to baseline
G ≥2 mucositis	Delay chemotherapy until toxicity resolves to G ≤1
G ≥2 nonhematologic toxicity	

CONCOMITANT CHEMORADIATION REGIMEN

CISPLATIN WITH RADIATION THERAPY FOLLOWED BY CISPLATIN + FLUOROURACIL

Al-Sarraf M et al. J Clin Oncol 1998;16:1310–1317

Pretreatment:
Dental evaluation; percutaneous feeding tube; nutrition evaluation

Hydration before, during, and after cisplatin administration ± *mannitol:*
- *Pre-cisplatin hydration* with 1000 mL 0.9% sodium chloride injection (0.9% NS); administer intravenously with potassium and magnesium supplementation as needed based on pretreatment laboratory results
- *Mannitol diuresis:* May be given to patients who have received adequate hydration. A dose of **mannitol 12.5–25 g** may be administered by intravenous injection or a short intravenous infusion before or during cisplatin administration, or prepared as an admixture with cisplatin. Continued intravenous hydration is essential
- *Continued mannitol diuresis:* In an inpatient or day-hospital setting, one may administer additional mannitol in the form of an intravenous infusion: **mannitol 10–40 g**; administer intravenously over 1–4 hours. This can be done either during or immediately after cisplatin, but requires maintenance of adequate intravenously administered fluids during and for hours after mannitol administration
- *Post-cisplatin hydration* with ≥1000 mL 0.9% NS; administer intravenously with potassium and magnesium supplementation as needed based on measured values

During radiation therapy:
Cisplatin 100 mg/m² per dose; administer intravenously in 25–1000 mL 0.9% NS over 15–20 minutes every 21 days for 3 cycles, given on days 1, 22, and 43 of radiation therapy (total dosage/cycle = 100 mg/m²)
Radiation 1.8–2 Gy/day, 5 fractions per week to tumor and clinically positive nodes to a total dose of 70 Gy. A total of 50 Gy to entire neck is recommended

After radiation therapy:
Note: Start 4 weeks after radiation therapy or the last dose of cisplatin, regardless of response to cisplatin + radiation
Cisplatin 80 mg/m² per dose; administer intravenously in 25–1000 mL 0.9% NS over 15–30 minutes every 4 weeks for 3 cycles, given on days 71, 99, and 127 (total dosage/cycle = 80 mg/m²)
Fluorouracil 1000 mg/m² per day; administer by continuous intravenous infusion in 100–1000 mL 0.9% NS or 5% dextrose injection over 24 hours for 4 consecutive days every 4 weeks for 3 cycles (96-hour infusion; on days 71–74, 99–102, and 127–130) (total dosage/cycle = 4000 mg/m²)

Supportive Care
Antiemetic prophylaxis
Emetogenic potential during radiation therapy on days with cisplatin is **HIGH**. *Potential for delayed symptoms*
Emetogenic potential after radiation therapy on days with cisplatin is **HIGH**. *Potential for delayed symptoms*
Emetogenic potential after radiation therapy on days with fluorouracil alone is **LOW**
See Chapter 39 for antiemetic recommendations

Hematopoietic growth factor (CSF) prophylaxis
Primary prophylaxis is NOT indicated
See Chapter 43 for more information

Antimicrobial prophylaxis
Risk of fever and neutropenia is LOW
Antimicrobial primary prophylaxis to be considered:
- Antibacterial—not indicated
- Antifungal—not indicated
- Antiviral—not indicated unless patient previously had an episode of HSV

See Chapter 47 for more information

(continued)

Treatment Modifications

Adverse Event	Dose Modification
ANC <2000/mm³ or platelet count <100,000/mm³	Hold chemotherapy until ANC ≥2000/mm³ *and* platelet count ≥100,000/mm³
ANC nadir ≥1500/mm³ *or* platelet count nadir ≥75,000/mm³	No dose modification
ANC nadir 1000–1499/mm³ *and/or* platelet nadir 50,000–74,999/mm³	Reduce cisplatin dosage to 80 mg/m²
ANC nadir <1000/mm³ *and/or* platelet nadir <50,000/mm³	Hold chemotherapy until ANC >2000/mm³ *and* platelet >100,000/mm³ and then reduce cisplatin dosage to 60 mg/m²
Serum creatinine ≤2.0 mg/dL (≤177 µmol/L) *or* creatinine clearance ≥60 mL/min (≥1.00 mL/s)	No dose modification
Serum creatinine 2.1–4 mg/dL (186–354 µmol/L) *or* creatinine clearance 40–59 mL/min (0.66–0.98 mL/s)	Hold cisplatin dosage until serum creatinine <1.5 mg/dL (<133 µmol/L), then reduce cisplatin dosage to 80 mg/m²
Serum creatinine >4 mg/dL (>354 µmol/L) *or* creatinine clearance <40 mL/min (<0.66 mL/s)	Discontinue cisplatin
G ≥2 diarrhea (4–6 stools/day > baseline)	Hold fluorouracil until diarrhea resolves to baseline
G ≥2 mucositis	Hold fluorouracil until toxicity resolves to G ≤1
G ≥2 neurotoxicity	Hold cisplatin until neurotoxicity resolves to G ≤1
G3/4 neurotoxicity	Discontinue cisplatin

CISPLATIN WITH RADIATION THERAPY FOLLOWED BY CISPLATIN + FLUOROURACIL

(*continued*)

Diarrhea management

Latent or delayed onset diarrhea*:

Loperamide 4 mg orally initially after the first loose or liquid stool, *then*

Loperamide 2 mg orally every 2 hours during waking hours, *plus*

Loperamide 4 mg orally every 4 hours during hours of sleep

- Continue for at least 12 hours after diarrhea resolves
- Recurrent diarrhea after a 12-hour diarrhea free interval is treated as a new episode
- Rehydrate orally with fluids and electrolytes during a diarrheal episode
- If diarrhea persists >48 hours despite loperamide, stop loperamide and hospitalize the patient for IV hydration

Persistent diarrhea:

Octreotide 100–150 mcg subcutaneously 3 times daily. Maximum total daily dose is 1500 mcg

Antibiotic therapy during latent or delayed onset diarrhea:

A fluoroquinolone (eg, **Ciprofloxacin** 500 mg orally every 12 hours) if absolute neutrophil count <500/mm^3 with or without accompanying fever in association with diarrhea

- Antibiotics should also be administered if patient is hospitalized with prolonged diarrhea and should be continued until diarrhea resolves

*Rothenberg ML et al. J Clin Oncol 2001;19:3801–3807

Abigerges D et al. J Natl Cancer Inst 1994;86:446–449

Wadler S et al. J Clin Oncol 1998;16:3169–3178

Oral care (mucositis prophylaxis and management)

Risk of mucositis/stomatitis is MODERATE–HIGH

General advice:

- Encourage patients to maintain intake of non-alcoholic fluids
- Evaluate patients for oral pain and provide analgesic medications
- Consider histamine (H$_2$-subtype) receptor antagonists (eg, ranitidine, famotidine), or a proton pump inhibitor for epigastric pain
- *Lactobacillus* sp.-containing probiotics may be beneficial in preventing diarrhea

Patients with intact oral mucosa:

- Clean the mouth, tongue, and gums by brushing after every meal and at bedtime with an ultra-soft toothbrush with fluoride toothpaste
- Floss teeth gently every day unless contraindicated. If gums bleed and hurt, avoid bleeding or sore areas, but floss other teeth
- Patients may use saline or commercial bland, non-alcoholic rinses
  - Do not use mouthwashes that contain alcohols

If mucositis or stomatitis is present:

- Keep the mouth moist utilizing water, ice chips, sugarless gum, sugar-free hard candies, or a saliva substitute
- Rinse mouth several times a day to remove debris
  - Use a solution of ¼ teaspoon (1.25 g) each of baking soda and table salt (sodium chloride) in one quart (~950 mL) of warm water. Follow with a plain water rinse
  - Do not use mouthwashes that contain alcohols
- Foam-tipped swabs (eg, Toothettes®) are useful in moisturizing oral mucosa, but ineffective for cleansing teeth and removing plaque
- Advise patients who develop mucositis to:
  - Choose foods that are easy to chew and swallow
  - Take small bites of food, chew slowly, and sip liquids with meals
  - Encourage soft, moist foods such as cooked cereals, mashed potatoes, and scrambled eggs
  - For trouble swallowing, soften food with gravies, sauces, broths, yogurt, or other bland liquids
  - Avoid sharp, crunchy foods; hot, spicy or highly acidic foods (eg, citrus fruits and juices); sugary foods; toothpicks; tobacco products; alcoholic drinks

Patient Population Studied

A study of 78 patients with stage III or stage IV nasopharyngeal cancer without evidence of systemic metastasis and no history of previous radiation therapy or chemotherapy. Patients were randomized to the combined modality arm of a 2-arm randomized phase III trial

Efficacy (N = 78)

Complete remission	49%
3-Year overall survival	78%
Median overall survival	>2.7 years
Estimated 3-year progression-free survival	69%

Therapy Monitoring

1. *Weekly:* CBC with differential, serum electrolytes, calcium, and magnesium. Weekly follow-up recommended during therapy with attention to signs and symptoms of dehydration, as supplemental hydration and nutritional support are often required

2. *For 2 days, starting the day after cisplatin administration, and as needed:* Serum electrolytes and magnesium

3. *Every 4–6 months:* Thyroid function studies

Toxicity (N = 78/53)

	% G3/4 Toxicities	
	Chemotherapy + Radiation (N = 78)	Adjuvant Chemotherapy (N = 53)
Hematologic		
Anemia	0	5.7
Leukopenia	29.5	22.6
Granulocytopenia	6.4	3.8
Thrombocytopenia	1.3	0
Nonhematologic		
Stomatitis	37.2	20.8
Nausea	17.9	9.4
Vomiting	14.1	1.9
Impaired hearing	11.5	11.3
Weight loss	6.4	0
Infection	2.6	1.9
Renal	0	0
Desquamation, RT field	2.6	N/A

No grade 5 toxicities with either part of regimen

ADVANCED DISEASE
INDUCTION CHEMOTHERAPY FOLLOWED BY CHEMORADIATION
DOCETAXEL + CISPLATIN + FLUOROURACIL (TPF) *OR*
CISPLATIN + FLUOROURACIL (PF)

Posner MR et al. N Engl J Med 2007;357:1705–1715

Induction Chemotherapy
(Three cycles of TPF or PF)

As noted in the Expert Opinion section: **TPF (docetaxel + cisplatin + fluorouracil)** is to be considered the current standard induction chemotherapy regimen in cases where induction chemotherapy is considered appropriate

Hydration before, during, and after cisplatin administration ± mannitol:
- *Pre-cisplatin hydration* with 1000 mL 0.9% sodium chloride injection (0.9% NS); administer intravenously with potassium and magnesium supplementation as needed based on pretreatment laboratory results
- *Mannitol diuresis:* May be given to patients who have received adequate hydration. A dose of **mannitol 12.5–25 g** may be administered by intravenous injection or a short intravenous infusion before or during cisplatin administration, or prepared as an admixture with cisplatin. Continued intravenous hydration is essential
- *Continued mannitol diuresis:* In an inpatient or day-hospital setting, one may administer additional mannitol in the form of an intravenous infusion: **mannitol 10–40 g;** administer intravenously over 1–4 hours. This can be done either during or immediately after cisplatin, but requires maintenance of adequate intravenously administered fluids during and for hours after mannitol administration
- *Post-cisplatin hydration* with ≥1000 mL 0.9% NS; administer intravenously with potassium and magnesium supplementation as needed based on measured values

TPF induction chemotherapy:
Dexamethasone 8 mg/dose; administer orally or intravenously twice daily for 6 doses starting the day before docetaxel administration (total dose/cycle = 48 mg)
- As prophylaxis against docetaxel-related hypersensitivity reactions, skin toxic effects, and fluid retention

Docetaxel 75 mg/m²; administer intravenously in a volume of 0.9% NS or 5% dextrose injection (D5W) sufficient to produce a docetaxel concentration within the range 0.3–0.74 mg/mL over 60 minutes on day 1, every 21 days for 3 cycles (total dosage/cycle = 75 mg/m²), *followed by:*
Cisplatin 100 mg/m²; administer intravenously in 50–1000 mL 0.9% NS over 0.5–3 hours on day 1, every 21 days for 3 cycles (total dosage/cycle = 100 mg/m²), *followed by:*
Fluorouracil 1000 mg/m² per day; administer in 50–1000 mL 0.9% NS or D5W by continuous intravenous infusion over 24 hours for 4 consecutive days, on days 1–4, every 21 days for 3 cycles (total dosage/cycle = 4000 mg/m²)
Prophylactic antibiotics days 5–14

or

PF induction chemotherapy:
Cisplatin 100 mg/m²; administer intravenously in 50–1000 mL 0.9% NS over 0.5–3 hours on day 1, every 21 days for 3 cycles (total dosage/cycle = 100 mg/m²), *followed by*
Fluorouracil 1000 mg/m² per day; administer intravenously in 50–1000 mL 0.9% NS or D5W by continuous infusion over 24 hours for 5 consecutive days, days 1–5, every 21 days for 3 cycles (total dosage/cycle = 5000 mg/m²)

Note: Induction chemotherapy is discontinued in case of (a) disease progression; (b) a reduction in tumor after 2 cycles <25% (WHO) or <30% (RECIST); or (c) unacceptable toxicity

Supportive Care for Patients Receiving Either TPF or PF Chemotherapies
Antiemetic prophylaxis
Emetogenic potential on day 1 is **HIGH**. *Potential for delayed symptoms*
Emetogenic potential on days with fluorouracil alone is **LOW**
See Chapter 39 for antiemetic recommendations

(continued)

(continued)

Diarrhea management
Latent or delayed onset diarrhea*:
Loperamide 4 mg orally initially after the first loose or liquid stool, *then*
Loperamide 2 mg orally every 2 hours during waking hours, *plus*
Loperamide 4 mg orally every 4 hours during hours of sleep
• Continue for at least 12 hours after diarrhea resolves
• Recurrent diarrhea after a 12-hour diarrhea-free interval is treated as a new episode
• Rehydrate orally with fluids and electrolytes during a diarrheal episode
• If a patient develops blood or mucus in stool, dehydration, or hemodynamic instability, or if diarrhea persists >48 hours despite loperamide, stop loperamide and hospitalize the patient for IV hydration

Persistent diarrhea:
Octreotide 100–150 mcg subcutaneously 3 times daily. Maximum total daily dose is 1500 mcg
Antibiotic therapy during latent or delayed onset diarrhea:
A fluoroquinolone (eg, **Ciprofloxacin** 500 mg orally every 12 hours) if absolute neutrophil count <500/mm^3 with or without accompanying fever in association with diarrhea
Antibiotics should also be administered if patient is hospitalized with
• prolonged diarrhea and should be continued until diarrhea resolves

*Rothenberg ML et al. J Clin Oncol 2001;19:3801–3807
Abigerges D et al. J Natl Cancer Inst 1994;86:446–449
Wadler S et al. J Clin Oncol 1998;16:3169–3178

Oral care
Risk of mucositis/stomatitis is HIGH
General advice:
• Encourage patients to maintain intake of non-alcoholic fluids
• Evaluate patients for oral pain and provide analgesic medications
• Consider histamine (H$_2$-subtype) receptor antagonists (eg, ranitidine, famotidine), or a proton pump inhibitor for epigastric pain
• *Lactobacillus* sp.-containing probiotics may be beneficial in preventing diarrhea

Patients with intact oral mucosa:
• Clean the mouth, tongue, and gums by brushing after every meal and at bedtime with an ultra-soft toothbrush with fluoride toothpaste
• Floss teeth gently every day unless contraindicated. If gums bleed and hurt, avoid bleeding or sore areas, but floss other teeth
• Patients may use saline or commercial bland, non-alcoholic rinses
  ▪ Do not use mouthwashes that contain alcohols

If mucositis or stomatitis is present:
• Keep the mouth moist utilizing water, ice chips, sugarless gum, sugar-free hard candies, or a saliva substitute
• Rinse mouth several times a day to remove debris
  ▪ Use a solution of ¼ teaspoon (1.25 g) each of baking soda and table salt (sodium chloride) in one quart (~950 mL) of warm water. Follow with a plain water rinse
  ▪ Do not use mouthwashes that contain alcohols
• Foam-tipped swabs (eg, Toothettes®) are useful in moisturizing oral mucosa, but ineffective for cleansing teeth and removing plaque
• Advise patients who develop mucositis to:
  ▪ Choose foods that are easy to chew and swallow
  ▪ Take small bites of food, chew slowly, and sip liquids with meals
  ▪ Encourage soft, moist foods such as cooked cereals, mashed potatoes, and scrambled eggs
  ▪ For trouble swallowing, soften food with gravies, sauces, broths, yogurt, or other bland liquids
  ▪ Avoid sharp, crunchy foods; hot, spicy or highly acidic foods (eg, citrus fruits and juices); sugary foods; toothpicks; tobacco products; alcoholic drinks

(continued)

(continued)

For Patients Who Receive TPF Chemotherapy
Hematopoietic growth factor (CSF) prophylaxis
Primary prophylaxis is indicated with 1 of the following:

   Filgrastim (G-CSF) 5 mcg/kg per day by subcutaneous injection, *or*
   Pegfilgrastim (pegylated filgrastim) 6 mg/0.6 mL by subcutaneous injection for 1 dose
   • Begin use from 24–72 hours after myelosuppressive chemotherapy is completed

See Chapter 43 for more information

Antimicrobial prophylaxis
Risk of fever and neutropenia is INTERMEDIATE
   Antimicrobial primary prophylaxis to be considered:
   • Antibacterial—consider a fluoroquinolone or no prophylaxis
      ▪ Posner et al gave antibiotic prophylaxis to patients who received the TPF regimen for 10 days starting on cycle day 5. Choice of antibiotics was not specified
   • Antifungal—consider use during neutropenia and for anticipated mucositis
   • Antiviral—antiherpes antivirals (eg, acyclovir)
See Chapter 47 for more information

For Patients Who Receive PF Chemotherapy
Hematopoietic growth factor (CSF) prophylaxis
Primary prophylaxis is NOT indicated
See Chapter 43 for more information

Antimicrobial prophylaxis
Risk of fever and neutropenia is LOW
   Antimicrobial primary prophylaxis to be considered:
   • Antibacterial—not indicated
      ▪ Posner et al gave antibiotic prophylaxis only to patients who received the TPF regimen: patients who received the PF regimen did not receive antimicrobial primary prophylaxis
   • Antifungal—not indicated
   • Antiviral—not indicated unless patient previously had an episode of HSV
See Chapter 47 for more information

Chemoradiation

(Follows Induction Chemotherapy)

Seven weeks of chemoradiation: Starting between days 22 and 56 of induction chemotherapy cycle 3 (3–8 weeks after the start of cycle 3 of induction chemotherapy)

Radiotherapy:
70–74 Gy to primary tumor in 5 daily fractions/week of 2 Gy/fraction
At least 50 Gy to uninvolved lymph nodes
At least 60–74 Gy to involved lymph nodes
Concurrent chemotherapy:
Carboplatin* (calculated dose) AUC = 1.5 mg/mL · min per dose; administer intravenously diluted to concentrations as low as 0.5 mg/mL with either D5W or 0.9% NS over 1 hour, once weekly for up to 7 doses during the course of radiotherapy (total dose/week calculated to produce a target AUC = 1.5 mg/mL · min)

*Carboplatin dose is based on a formula described by Calvert et al. to achieve a target area under the plasma concentration versus time curve (AUC)

$$\text{Total Carboplatin Dose (mg)} = (\text{target AUC}) \times (\text{GFR} + 25)$$

(continued)

(*continued*)

In practice, creatinine clearance (Clcr) is used in place of glomerular filtration rate (GFR). Clcr can be estimated from the equation of Cockcroft and Gault, thus:

$$\text{For males, Clcr} = \frac{(140 - \text{age [years]}) \times (\text{body weight [kg]})}{72 \times (\text{serum creatinine [mg/dL]})}$$

$$\text{For females, Clcr} = \frac{(140 - \text{age [years]}) \times (\text{body weight [kg]})}{72 \times (\text{serum creatinine [mg/dL]})} \times 0.85$$

Calvert AH et al. J Clin Oncol 1989;7:1748–1756
Cockcroft DW , Gault MH. Nephron 1976;16:31–41
Jodrell DI et al. J Clin Oncol 1992;10:520–528
Sorensen BT et al. Cancer Chemother Pharmacol 1991;28:397–401

Note: On October 8, 2010, the U.S. FDA identified a potential safety issue with carboplatin dosing based on recent changes in the measurement of serum creatinine. By the end of 2010, all clinical laboratories in the United States were required to use the standardized Isotope Dilution Mass Spectrometry (IDMS) method to measure serum creatinine, which can result in an overestimation of the GFR in some patients with normal renal function. A carboplatin dose calculated with an IDMS-measured serum creatinine result using the Calvert formula can exceed an expected exposure (AUC) and result in increased drug-related toxicity

Provided actual GFR measurements are made to assess renal function, carboplatin can be safely dosed according to the Calvert formula described in product labeling

If GFR (or creatinine clearance) is estimated based on serum creatinine measurements by the IDMS method, the FDA recommended for patients with normal renal function capping an estimated GFR at 125 mL/min for any targeted AUC value. No greater estimated GFR values should be used

U.S. FDA. Carboplatin dosing. [online] Available from: http://www.fda.gov/AboutFDA/CentersOffices/OfficeofMedicalProductsandTobacco/CDER/ucm228974.htm [accessed February 26, 2014]

Supportive Care
Antiemetic prophylaxis
Emetogenic potential on days when carboplatin is administered is **MODERATE**
See Chapter 39 for antiemetic recommendations

Hematopoietic growth factor (CSF) prophylaxis
Primary prophylaxis is NOT indicated
See Chapter 43 for more information

Antimicrobial prophylaxis
Risk of fever and neutropenia is LOW
   Antimicrobial primary prophylaxis to be considered:
   • Antibacterial—not indicated

   • Antifungal—not indicated

   • Antiviral—not indicated unless patient previously had an episode of HSV

See Chapter 47 for more information

Dose Modification

Adverse Event	Dose Modifications
G3/4 hematologic toxicity	Hold chemotherapy up to 2 weeks until toxicity resolves to G ≤1. If toxicity does not resolve to G ≤1 within 2 weeks, then discontinue therapy
G3/4 nonhematologic toxicity other than alopecia, fatigue, malaise, and nail changes (exceptions: neurotoxicity, ototoxicity, and mucositis as detailed below)	Hold chemotherapy up to 2 weeks until toxicity resolves to G ≤1. If toxicity does not resolve to G ≤1 within 2 weeks, then discontinue therapy
G3/4 neurotoxicity or ototoxicity	Discontinue therapy
G4 mucositis and diarrhea	Discontinue therapy
Febrile neutropenia or infection	Administer filgrastim during subsequent cycles
Delay in ANC recovery beyond day 28	
G4 neutropenia ≥7 days	
ANC <2000/mm^3; platelet count <100,000/mm^3; or hemoglobin <10 g/dL)	Withhold start of RT
Incomplete resolution of mucositis	

Efficacy*

	TPF[†] (N = 255)	PF[†] (N = 246)	Hazard Ratio or P-Value
ORR after induction chemotherapy	72%	64%	P = 0.07
CR rate after induction chemotherapy	17%	15%	P = 0.66
Median PFS, months	36	13	0.71 (0.56–0.90)
Estimated 2-year PFS	53%	42%	P = 0.01
Estimated 3-year PFS	49%	37%	—
Median OS, months	71	30	0.7 (0.54–0.90)
Estimated 2-year OS	67%	55%	—
Estimated 3-year OS	62%	48%	P = 0.002
Median OS resectable tumors, months	NR	42	P = 0.007
Median OS unresectable tumors, months	40	21	P = 0.06
Loco-regional failure	30%	38%	P = 0.04

CR, complete response; ORR, overall response rate; OS, overall survival; PFS, progression-free survival
*WHO Criteria
[†]TPF, Docetaxel + cisplatin + fluorouracil; PF, cisplatin + fluorouracil

Surgery

(Elective Neck Dissection)
Elective neck dissection 6–12 weeks after end of chemoradiation for patients with initial N2 disease and a partial response to induction chemotherapy, N3 disease, or residual disease after chemoradiation

Patient Population Studied

A study of 539 patients with measurable, nonmetastatic, stage III or IV, histologically proven, previously untreated squamous cell carcinoma of the oral cavity, larynx, oropharynx, or hypopharynx with a tumor deemed to be unresectable (because of tumor fixation, involvement of the nasopharynx, or fixed lymph nodes), or of low surgical curability on basis of advanced tumor stage (3 or 4) or regional node stage (2–3, except T1N2), or if a patient was a candidate for organ preservation. WHO performance status 0 or 1. Adequate organ function and age ≥18 years

Therapy Monitoring

1. *Pretreatment evaluation:* Medical history and tumor assessment by clinical evaluation and imaging studies
2. *Toxicity assessment:* Weekly during treatment with chemotherapy
3. *Tumor assessment:* After cycles 2 and 3; then, 6–12 weeks after chemoradiation

Toxicity		
	TPF*	PF*
Adverse Events During Induction Chemotherapy	% G3/4 (N = 251)	% G3/4 (N = 243)
Anemia	12	9
Thrombocytopenia	4	11
Neutropenia	83	56
Febrile neutropenia	12	7
Neutropenia and infection	12	8
Mucositis	21	27
Esophagitis, dysphagia, or odynophagia	13	9
Anorexia	12	12
Nausea	14	14
Vomiting	8	10
Diarrhea	7	3
Infection	6	5
Lethargy	5	10
Adverse Events During Chemoradiation	% G3/4 N = 202	% G3/4 N = 184
Mucositis	37	38
Esophagitis, dysphagia, or odynophagia	23	24
Anorexia	11	15
Nausea	6	6
Vomiting	3	5
Diarrhea	0	2
Infection	9	7
Lethargy	6	6

*TPF, Docetaxel + cisplatin + fluorouracil; PF, cisplatin + fluorouracil

ADVANCED DISEASE
INDUCTION CHEMOTHERAPY FOLLOWED BY RADIOTHERAPY

DOCETAXEL + CISPLATIN + FLUOROURACIL (TPF) *OR*

CISPLATIN + FLUOROURACIL (PF)

Vermorken JB et al. N Engl J Med 2007;357:1695–1704

Induction Chemotherapy

(Three Cycles of TPF or PF)

As noted in the Expert Opinion section: **TPF (docetaxel + cisplatin + fluorouracil)** is to be considered the current standard induction chemotherapy regimen in cases where induction chemotherapy is considered appropriate

Hydration before, during, and after cisplatin administration ± mannitol:
- *Pre-cisplatin hydration* with 1000 mL 0.9% sodium chloride injection (0.9% NS); administer intravenously with potassium and magnesium supplementation as needed based on pretreatment laboratory results
- *Mannitol diuresis:* May be given to patients who have received adequate hydration. A dose of **mannitol** 12.5–25 g may be administered by intravenous injection or a short infusion before or during cisplatin administration, or prepared as an admixture with cisplatin. Continued intravenous hydration is essential
- *Continued mannitol diuresis:* In an inpatient or day-hospital setting, one may administer additional mannitol in the form of an intravenous infusion: **mannitol** 10–40 g; administer intravenously over 1–4 hours. This can be done either during or immediately after cisplatin, but requires maintenance of adequate intravenously administered fluids during and for hours after mannitol administration
- *Post-cisplatin hydration* with ≥1000 mL 0.9% NS; administer intravenously with potassium and magnesium supplementation as needed based on measured values

Docetaxel + Cisplatin + Fluorouracil (TPF)

Premedication:
Dexamethasone 8 mg/dose; administer orally or intravenously twice daily for 6 doses starting the day before docetaxel administration (total dose/cycle = 48 mg)
- As prophylaxis against docetaxel-related hypersensitivity reactions, skin toxic effects, and fluid retention

Induction chemotherapy:
Docetaxel 75 mg/m²; administer intravenously in a volume of 0.9% NS or 5% dextrose injection (D5W) sufficient to produce a docetaxel concentration within the range 0.3–0.74 mg/mL over 60 minutes on day 1, every 3 weeks for up to 4 cycles (total dosage/cycle = 75 mg/m²), *followed by:*
Cisplatin 75 mg/m²; administer intravenously in 50–1000 mL 0.9% NS over 60 minutes on day 1, every 3 weeks for up to 4 cycles (total dosage/cycle = 75 mg/m²), *followed by:*
Fluorouracil 750 mg/m² per day; administer in 50–1000 mL 0.9% NS or D5W by continuous intravenous infusion over 24 hours for 5 consecutive days, on days 1–5, every 3 weeks for up to 4 cycles (total dosage/cycle = 3750 mg/m²)

or

Cisplatin + Fluorouracil (PF)

Induction chemotherapy:
Cisplatin 100 mg/m²; administer intravenously in 50–1000 mL 0.9% NS over 60 minutes on day 1, every 3 weeks for up to 4 cycles (total dosage/cycle = 100 mg/m²), *followed by:*
Fluorouracil 1000 mg/m² per day; administer in 50–1000 mL 0.9% NS or D5W by continuous intravenous infusion over 24 hours for 5 consecutive days, on days 1–5, every 3 weeks for up to 4 cycles (total dosage/cycle = 5000 mg/m²)

Supportive Care for Patients Receiving Either TPF or PF Chemotherapies
Antiemetic prophylaxis
Emetogenic potential on day 1 is **HIGH**. *Potential for delayed symptoms*
Emetogenic potential on days with fluorouracil alone is **LOW**
See Chapter 39 for antiemetic recommendations

Diarrhea management
Latent or delayed onset diarrhea*:
   Loperamide 4 mg orally initially after the first loose or liquid stool, *then*
   Loperamide 2 mg orally every 2 hours during waking hours, *plus*
   Loperamide 4 mg orally every 4 hours during hours of sleep
   - Continue for at least 12 hours after diarrhea resolves
   - Recurrent diarrhea after a 12-hour diarrhea-free interval is treated as a new episode
   - Rehydrate orally with fluids and electrolytes during a diarrheal episode

(continued)

(*continued*)

- If a patient develops blood or mucus in stool, dehydration, or hemodynamic instability, or if diarrhea persists >48 hours despite loperamide, stop loperamide and hospitalize the patient for IV hydration

Persistent diarrhea:

Octreotide 100–150 mcg subcutaneously 3 times daily. Maximum total daily dose is 1500 mcg

Antibiotic therapy during latent or delayed onset diarrhea:

- A fluoroquinolone (eg, **Ciprofloxacin** 500 mg orally every 12 hours) if absolute neutrophil count <500/mm³ with or without accompanying fever in association with diarrhea
- Antibiotics should also be administered if patient is hospitalized with prolonged diarrhea and should be continued until diarrhea resolves

*Rothenberg ML et al. J Clin Oncol 2001;19:3801–3807
Abigerges D et al. J Natl Cancer Inst 1994;86:446–449
Wadler S et al. J Clin Oncol 1998;16:3169–3178

Oral care

Risk of mucositis/stomatitis is MODERATE

General advice:

- Encourage patients to maintain intake of non-alcoholic fluids
- Evaluate patients for oral pain and provide analgesic medications
- Consider histamine (H₂-subtype) receptor antagonists (eg, ranitidine, famotidine), or a proton pump inhibitor for epigastric pain
- *Lactobacillus* sp.-containing probiotics may be beneficial in preventing diarrhea

Patients with intact oral mucosa:

- Clean the mouth, tongue, and gums by brushing after every meal and at bedtime with an ultra-soft toothbrush with fluoride toothpaste
- Floss teeth gently every day unless contraindicated. If gums bleed and hurt, avoid bleeding or sore areas, but floss other teeth
- Patients may use saline or commercial bland, non-alcoholic rinses
  - Do not use mouthwashes that contain alcohols

If mucositis or stomatitis is present:

- Keep the mouth moist utilizing water, ice chips, sugarless gum, sugar-free hard candies, or a saliva substitute
- Rinse mouth several times a day to remove debris
  - Use a solution of ¼ teaspoon (1.25 g) each of baking soda and table salt (sodium chloride) in one quart (~950 mL) of warm water. Follow with a plain water rinse
  - Do not use mouthwashes that contain alcohols
- Foam-tipped swabs (eg, Toothettes®) are useful in moisturizing oral mucosa, but ineffective for cleansing teeth and removing plaque
- Advise patients who develop mucositis to:
  - Choose foods that are easy to chew and swallow
  - Take small bites of food, chew slowly, and sip liquids with meals
  - Encourage soft, moist foods such as cooked cereals, mashed potatoes, and scrambled eggs
  - For trouble swallowing, soften food with gravies, sauces, broths, yogurt, or other bland liquids
  - Avoid sharp, crunchy foods; hot, spicy or highly acidic foods (eg, citrus fruits and juices); sugary foods; toothpicks; tobacco products; alcoholic drinks

For Patients Who Receive TPF Chemotherapy

Hematopoietic growth factor (CSF) prophylaxis

Primary prophylaxis may be indicated

- Particularly in patients who do not receive antibiotic prophylaxis

See Chapter 43 for more information

(*continued*)

Radiotherapy

Starting within 4–7 weeks after completion of chemotherapy

Radiotherapy: Conventional fractionation (66–70 Gy) or
Accelerated irradiation (70 Gy]) or
Hyperfractionated irradiation (74 Gy)

Surgery

(Elective Neck Dissection)

Elective neck dissection can be considered before radiotherapy and again 3 months after the completion of radiotherapy

Dose Modification

Adverse Event	Dose Modification
G3/4 hematologic toxicity	Hold chemotherapy up to 2 weeks until toxicity resolves to G ≤1. If toxicity has not resolved to G ≤1 within 2 weeks, discontinue therapy
G3/4 nonhematologic toxicity other than alopecia, fatigue, malaise, and nail changes (exceptions: neurotoxicity, ototoxicity and mucositis as detailed below)	
G3/4 neurotoxicity or ototoxicity	Discontinue therapy
G4 mucositis and diarrhea	
Febrile neutropenia or infection	Administer filgrastim in subsequent cycles
Delay in ANC recovery beyond day 28	
G4 neutropenia ≥7 days	
ANC <2000/mm³, platelet count <100,000/mm³, or hemoglobin <10 g/dL	Withhold start of RT
Incomplete resolution of mucositis	

Patient Population Studied

A study of 358 patients with measurable, nonmetastatic stages III or IV, histologically or cytologically proven, previously untreated squamous cell carcinoma of the oral cavity, larynx, oropharynx, or hypopharynx, with a tumor considered to be unresectable by a multidisciplinary team. WHO performance status 0 or 1, adequate organ function, and ages 18–70 years

(*continued*)

Antimicrobial prophylaxis
Risk of fever and neutropenia is INTERMEDIATE
Antimicrobial primary prophylaxis to be considered:
- Antibacterial—consider a fluoroquinolone or no prophylaxis
  - Vermorken et al gave antibiotic prophylaxis to patients who received the TPF regimen from cycle days 5–15
- Antifungal—consider use during neutropenia and for anticipated mucositis
- Antiviral—not indicated unless patient previously had an episode of HSV

See Chapter 47 for more information

For Patients Who Receive PF Chemotherapy
Hematopoietic growth factor (CSF) prophylaxis
Primary prophylaxis is NOT indicated
See Chapter 43 for more information

Antimicrobial prophylaxis
Risk of fever and neutropenia is LOW
Antimicrobial primary prophylaxis to be considered:
- Antibacterial—not indicated
  - Vermorken et al gave antibiotic prophylaxis only to patients who received the TPF regimen
- Antifungal—not indicated
- Antiviral—not indicated unless patient previously had an episode of HSV

See Chapter 47 for more information

Efficacy

	TPF* (N = 181)	PF* (N = 177)
Median progression-free survival, months	11	8.2
Estimated 3-year progression-free survival	17%	14%
Median overall survival, months	18.8	14.5
Estimated 3-year overall survival	37%	26%
Overall response rate after induction chemotherapy	68%	54%
Complete response rate after induction chemotherapy	8.5%	6.6%

*TPF, Docetaxel + cisplatin + fluorouracil; PF, cisplatin + fluorouracil

Therapy Monitoring

1. *Day 1 of each cycle:* Medical history and physical exam, CBC with differential, LFTs, electrolytes, BUN, and creatinine
2. *At end of cycles 2 and 4:* Diagnostic imaging

Toxicity

Adverse Events During Induction Chemotherapy	TPF* % G3/4 N = 179	PF* % G3/4 N = 173
Anemia	9.2	12.8
Thrombocytopenia	5.2	17.9
Neutropenia	76.9	52.5
Leukopenia	41.6	22.9
Febrile neutropenia	5.2	2.8
Infection	6.9	6.1
Alopecia	11.6	0
Stomatitis	4.6	11.2
Esophagitis, dysphagia, or odynophagia	0.6	0
Anorexia	0.6	3.4
Nausea	0.6	6.7
Vomiting	0.6	4.5
Diarrhea	2.9	3.4
Constipation	0	0.6
Lethargy	2.9	1.7
Weight loss	0	0.6
Gastrointestinal pain	0	0.6
Neurotoxicity	0.6	0.6
Hearing loss	0	2.8
Local toxic effect	0.6	0.6
Toxic deaths	2.3	5.5

*TPF, Docetaxel + cisplatin + fluorouracil; PF, cisplatin + fluorouracil

ADVANCED DISEASE
CHEMORADIATION IN UNRESECTABLE DISEASE

CISPLATIN ALONE *OR*
CISPLATIN + FLUOROURACIL

Adelstein DJ et al. J Clin Oncol 2003;21:92–98

Chemoradiation

As noted in the Expert Opinion section: Chemoradiation concurrent with cisplatin 100 mg/m² every 3 weeks × 3 doses should still be considered the standard regimen

Hydration before, during, and after cisplatin administration ± mannitol:
- *Pre-cisplatin hydration* with 1000 mL 0.9% sodium chloride injection (0.9% NS); administer intravenously with potassium and magnesium supplementation as needed based on pretreatment laboratory results
- *Mannitol diuresis:* May be given to patients who have received adequate hydration. A dose of **mannitol** 12.5–25 g may be administered by intravenous injection or a short infusion before or during cisplatin administration, or prepared as an admixture with cisplatin. Continued intravenous hydration is essential
- *Continued mannitol diuresis:* In an inpatient or day-hospital setting, one may administer additional mannitol in the form of an intravenous infusion: **mannitol** 10–40 g; administer intravenously over 1–4 hours. This can be done either during or immediately after cisplatin, but requires maintenance of adequate intravenously administered fluids during and for hours after mannitol administration
- *Post-cisplatin hydration* with ≥1000 mL 0.9% NS; administer intravenously with potassium and magnesium supplementation as needed based on measured values

Cisplatin 100 mg/m²; administer intravenously in 50–1000 mL 0.9% NS over 60 minutes on day 1, every 3 weeks for 3 cycles during radiation (total dosage/cycle = 100 mg/m²)
Radiation therapy administered to a total dose of 70 Gy given continually in single, daily, 2-Gy fractions over 7 weeks

Supportive Care
Antiemetic prophylaxis
Emetogenic potential on day 1 is **HIGH**. Potential for delayed symptoms
See Chapter 39 for antiemetic recommendations

Hematopoietic growth factor (CSF) prophylaxis
Primary prophylaxis is NOT indicated
See Chapter 43 for more information

Antimicrobial prophylaxis
Risk of fever and neutropenia is LOW
Antimicrobial primary prophylaxis to be considered:
- Antibacterial—not indicated
- Antifungal—not indicated
- Antiviral—not indicated unless patient previously had an episode of HSV
See Chapter 47 for more information

or

Cisplatin 75 mg/m²; administer intravenously in 50–1000 mL 0.9% NS over 60 minutes on day 1, every 4 weeks for 3 cycles during radiation (total dosage/cycle = 75 mg/m²), *followed by:*
Fluorouracil 1000 mg/m² per day; administer in 50–1000 mL 0.9% NS or D5W by continuous intravenous infusion over 24 hours for 4 consecutive days, on days 1–4, every 4 weeks for 3 cycles during radiation (total dosage/cycle = 4000 mg/m²)

Concurrent radiation therapy, at a rate of 2 Gy/day, split as follows:
- *First chemotherapy cycle:* A total of 30 Gy administered as 15 daily fractions of 2 Gy/fraction, 5 days/week, starting on day 1 of cycle 1

(continued)

Patient Population Studied

A study of 295 patients with a histologically confirmed diagnosis of squamous cell or undifferentiated stage III or IV, nonmetastatic, carcinoma of the head and neck, excluding tumors originating in the nasopharynx, paranasal sinus, or parotid gland Unresectability was predefined for each tumor site as follows:
- *Hypopharynx:* tumor extension across the midline of the posterior pharyngeal wall or fixed to the cervical spine
- *Larynx:* direct extension into surrounding muscle or skin or greater than 3 cm subglottic extension
- *Oral cavity:* functional reconstruction not possible
- *Base of tongue:* extension into the root of tongue or refusal of total glossectomy
- *Tonsil:* extension into the pterygoid region as manifested by clinical trismus or demonstrated radiographically, or tumor extension across the midline of the pharyngeal wall or direct invasion into the soft tissue of the neck

Adequate organ function and an ECOG performance score ≤1 were required

Dose Modification

Note: It is anticipated that radiation therapy will continue despite the development of significant mucositis and or myelosuppression

Adverse Event	Dose Modification
G3/4 hematologic toxicity	Hold chemotherapy for up to 3 weeks until toxicity resolves to G ≤1. If toxicity has not resolved to G ≤1 within 3 weeks, do not administer next cycle
G3/4 nonhematologic toxicity other than alopecia, fatigue, malaise, and nail changes (exceptions: neurotoxicity, ototoxicity, and mucositis as detailed below)	
G3/4 neurotoxicity or ototoxicity	Discontinue chemotherapy
G4 mucositis	

(*continued*)

- *Third chemotherapy cycle:* A total of 30–40 Gy administered as 15–20 daily fractions of 2 Gy/fraction, 5 days/week, starting on day 1 of cycle 3
- Administer 30–40 Gy for a total dose of 60–70 Gy depending on response

Note: The radiation therapy break is planned to allow for the possibility of surgical resection in patients whose disease is rendered resectable after the first 2 courses of chemotherapy and the first 30 Gy of radiation. Patients who do not achieve a complete response after the first 2 courses of chemotherapy and the first 30 Gy of radiation, or whose disease remains unresectable complete chemoradiation without surgery

As a result of the break, almost 7 additional weeks were required to complete treatment

Supportive Care
Antiemetic prophylaxis
Emetogenic potential on day 1 is **HIGH**. *Potential for delayed symptoms*
Emetogenic potential on days with fluorouracil ± *RT is* **LOW–MODERATE**
See Chapter 39 for antiemetic recommendations

Hematopoietic growth factor (CSF) prophylaxis
Primary prophylaxis is NOT indicated
See Chapter 43 for more information

Antimicrobial prophylaxis
Risk of fever and neutropenia is LOW
Antimicrobial primary prophylaxis to be considered:
- Antibacterial—not indicated
- Antifungal—not indicated
- Antiviral—not indicated unless patient previously had an episode of HSV

See Chapter 47 for more information

Oral care
Risk of mucositis/stomatitis is **HIGH**
General advice:
- Encourage patients to maintain intake of non-alcoholic fluids
- Evaluate patients for oral pain and provide analgesic medications
- Consider histamine (H_2-subtype) receptor antagonists (eg, ranitidine, famotidine), or a proton pump inhibitor for epigastric pain
- *Lactobacillus* sp.-containing probiotics may be beneficial in preventing diarrhea

Patients with intact oral mucosa:
- Clean the mouth, tongue, and gums by brushing after every meal and at bedtime with an ultra-soft toothbrush with fluoride toothpaste
- Floss teeth gently every day unless contraindicated. If gums bleed and hurt, avoid bleeding or sore areas, but floss other teeth
- Patients may use saline or commercial bland, non-alcoholic rinses
  - Do not use mouthwashes that contain alcohols

If mucositis or stomatitis is present:
- Keep the mouth moist utilizing water, ice chips, sugarless gum, sugar-free hard candies, or a saliva substitute
- Rinse mouth several times a day to remove debris
  - Use a solution of ¼ teaspoon (1.25 g) each of baking soda and table salt (sodium chloride) in one quart (~950 mL) of warm water. Follow with a plain water rinse
  - Do not use mouthwashes that contain alcohols
- Foam-tipped swabs (eg, Toothettes®) are useful in moisturizing oral mucosa, but ineffective for cleansing teeth and removing plaque
- Advise patients who develop mucositis to:
  - Choose foods that are easy to chew and swallow
  - Take small bites of food, chew slowly, and sip liquids with meals
  - Encourage soft, moist foods such as cooked cereals, mashed potatoes, and scrambled eggs
  - For trouble swallowing, soften food with gravies, sauces, broths, yogurt, or other bland liquids
  - Avoid sharp, crunchy foods; hot, spicy or highly acidic foods (eg, citrus fruits and juices); sugary foods; toothpicks; tobacco products; alcoholic drinks

Efficacy

	Cisplatin + Radiation N = 95	Cisplatin + Fluorouracil + Radiation N = 94
Complete response rate	40.2%	49.4%*
Estimated 3-year survival	37%	27%
Median overall survival, months	19.1	13.8
Disease-specific survival rates	51%	41%

*Includes patients undergoing mid-course surgical resection

G3–5 Toxicity

	Cisplatin + Radiation N = 95	Cisplatin + Fluorouracil + Radiation N = 94	p-Value
Nausea/vomiting	15	8	
Mucositis/dysphagia	43	44	
Leukopenia	40	29	<0.001
Thrombocytopenia	3	3	
Anemia	17	18	
Renal	8	0	0.01
Skin	7	2	
Feeding tube	49	48	
Toxic death	4	2	
All G3–5	85	72	0.02
Treatment regimen compliance*	85.1%	73%	0.05

*As measured by treatment completion

Therapy Monitoring

1. *Day 1 of each cycle:* Medical history and physical exam, CBC with differential, LFTs, electrolytes, BUN, and creatinine
2. *Diagnostic imaging:* At treatment completion and 3 months later

CHEMORADIATION WITH CISPLATIN IN UNRESECTABLE DISEASE

CHEMORADIATION FOR LARYNX PRESERVATION
CISPLATIN WITH RADIATION THERAPY

Forastiere AA et al. N Engl J Med 2003;349:2091–2098

As noted in the Expert Opinion section: Concurrent chemoradiation using cisplatin 100 mg/m² every 3 weeks × 3 doses should still be considered the standard regimen

Chemoradiation

Hydration before, during, and after cisplatin administration ± mannitol:
- *Pre-cisplatin hydration* with 1000 mL 0.9% sodium chloride injection (0.9% NS); administer intravenously with potassium and magnesium supplementation as needed based on pretreatment laboratory results
- *Mannitol diuresis:* May be given to patients who have received adequate hydration. A dose of **mannitol** 12.5–25 g may be administered by intravenous injection or a short infusion before or during cisplatin administration, or prepared as an admixture with cisplatin. Continued intravenous hydration is essential
- *Continued mannitol diuresis:* In an inpatient or day-hospital setting, one may administer additional mannitol in the form of an intravenous infusion: **mannitol** 10–40 g; administer intravenously over 1–4 hours. This can be done either during or immediately after cisplatin, but requires maintenance of adequate intravenously administered fluids during and for hours after mannitol administration
- *Post-cisplatin hydration* with ≥1000 mL 0.9% NS; administer intravenously with potassium and magnesium supplementation as needed based on measured values

Cisplatin 100 mg/m²; administer intravenously in 50–1000 mL 0.9% NS over 60 minutes on day 1, every 3 weeks for 3 cycles during radiation (total dosage/cycle = 100 mg/m²)

Radiotherapy 70 Gy given in 35 fractions of 2 Gy/fraction over 7 weeks to the primary tumor and clinically positive nodes; 50 Gy in fractions of 2 Gy to the entire neck

Supportive Care
Antiemetic prophylaxis
Emetogenic potential on days with cisplatin is **HIGH**. *Potential for delayed symptoms*
See Chapter 39 for antiemetic recommendations

Hematopoietic growth factor (CSF) prophylaxis
Primary prophylaxis is NOT indicated
See Chapter 43 for more information

Antimicrobial prophylaxis
Risk of fever and neutropenia is LOW
Antimicrobial primary prophylaxis to be considered:
- Antibacterial—not indicated
- Antifungal—not indicated
- Antiviral—not indicated unless patient previously had an episode of HSV
See Chapter 47 for more information

Oral care
Risk of mucositis/stomatitis is HIGH
General advice:
- Encourage patients to maintain intake of non-alcoholic fluids
- Evaluate patients for oral pain and provide analgesic medications
- Consider histamine (H$_2$-subtype) receptor antagonists (eg, ranitidine, famotidine), or a proton pump inhibitor for epigastric pain
- *Lactobacillus* sp.-containing probiotics may be beneficial in preventing diarrhea

Patients with intact oral mucosa:
- Clean the mouth, tongue, and gums by brushing after every meal and at bedtime with an ultra-soft toothbrush with fluoride toothpaste
- Floss teeth gently every day unless contraindicated. If gums bleed and hurt, avoid bleeding or sore areas, but floss other teeth
- Patients may use saline or commercial bland, non-alcoholic rinses
  - Do not use mouthwashes that contain alcohols

(continued)

(continued)

If mucositis or stomatitis is present:
- Keep the mouth moist utilizing water, ice chips, sugarless gum, sugar-free hard candies, or a saliva substitute
- Rinse mouth several times a day to remove debris
  - Use a solution of ¼ teaspoon (1.25 g) each of baking soda and table salt (sodium chloride) in one quart (~950 mL) of warm water. Follow with a plain water rinse
  - Do not use mouthwashes that contain alcohols
- Foam-tipped swabs (eg, Toothettes®) are useful in moisturizing oral mucosa, but ineffective for cleansing teeth and removing plaque
- Advise patients who develop mucositis to:
  - Choose foods that are easy to chew and swallow
  - Take small bites of food, chew slowly, and sip liquids with meals
  - Encourage soft, moist foods such as cooked cereals, mashed potatoes, and scrambled eggs
  - For trouble swallowing, soften food with gravies, sauces, broths, yogurt, or other bland liquids
  - Avoid sharp, crunchy foods; hot, spicy or highly acidic foods (eg, citrus fruits and juices); sugary foods; toothpicks; tobacco products; alcoholic drinks

Induction Chemotherapy Followed By Radiotherapy

Cisplatin 100 mg/m²; administer intravenously in 50–1000 mL 0.9% NS over 60 minutes on day 1, every 3 weeks for 3 cycles (total dosage/cycle = 100 mg/m²), *followed by:*

Fluorouracil 1000 mg/m² per day; administer in 50–1000 mL 0.9% NS or D5W by continuous intravenous infusion over 24 hours for 5 consecutive days on days 1–5, every 3 weeks for 3 cycles (total dosage/cycle = 5000 mg/m²)

After 2 cycles of cisplatin + fluorouracil, evaluate extent of response and disease status in the neck with indirect laryngoscopy and CT imaging of the neck
- If evaluation reveals a complete or partial response of the primary tumor and no sign of progression in the neck, a third course of cisplatin plus fluorouracil is given, followed by radiotherapy
- If evaluation reveals less than partial response of the primary tumor or with progression in the neck, laryngectomy followed by adjuvant radiotherapy is recommended

Radiotherapy, 70 Gy given in 35 fractions of 2 Gy/fraction over 7 weeks to the primary tumor and clinically positive nodes; 50 Gy in fractions of 2 Gy to the entire neck

Supportive Care
Antiemetic prophylaxis
Emetogenic potential on days with cisplatin is **HIGH**. *Potential for delayed symptoms*
Emetogenic potential on days with fluorouracil alone is **LOW**
See Chapter 39 for antiemetic recommendations

Hematopoietic growth factor (CSF) prophylaxis
Primary prophylaxis is NOT indicated
See Chapter 43 for more information

Antimicrobial prophylaxis
Risk of fever and neutropenia is LOW
Antimicrobial primary prophylaxis to be considered:
- Antibacterial—not indicated
- Antifungal—not indicated
- Antiviral—not indicated unless patient previously had an episode of HSV

See Chapter 47 for more information

Oral care
Risk of mucositis/stomatitis is HIGH
General advice:
- Encourage patients to maintain intake of non-alcoholic fluids
- Evaluate patients for oral pain and provide analgesic medications
- Consider histamine (H₂-subtype) receptor antagonists (eg, ranitidine, famotidine), or a proton pump inhibitor for epigastric pain
- *Lactobacillus* sp.-containing probiotics may be beneficial in preventing diarrhea

Patients with intact oral mucosa:
- Clean the mouth, tongue, and gums by brushing after every meal and at bedtime with an ultra-soft toothbrush with fluoride toothpaste
- Floss teeth gently every day unless contraindicated. If gums bleed and hurt, avoid bleeding or sore areas, but floss other teeth
- Patients may use saline or commercial bland, non-alcoholic rinses
  - Do not use mouthwashes that contain alcohols

(continued)

(*continued*)

If mucosis or stomatitis is present:
- Keep the mouth moist utilizing water, ice chips, sugarless gum, sugar-free hard candies, or a saliva substitute
- Rinse mouth several times a day to remove debris
  - Use a solution of ¼ teaspoon (1.25 g) each of baking soda and table salt (sodium chloride) in one quart (~950 mL) of warm water. Follow with a plain water rinse
  - Do not use mouthwashes that contain alcohols
- Foam-tipped swabs (eg, Toothettes®) are useful in moisturizing oral mucosa, but ineffective for cleansing teeth and removing plaque
- Advise patients who develop mucositis to:
  - Choose foods that are easy to chew and swallow
  - Take small bites of food, chew slowly, and sip liquids with meals
  - Encourage soft, moist foods such as cooked cereals, mashed potatoes, and scrambled eggs
  - For trouble swallowing, soften food with gravies, sauces, broths, yogurt, or other bland liquids
  - Avoid sharp, crunchy foods; hot, spicy or highly acidic foods (eg, citrus fruits and juices); sugary foods; toothpicks; tobacco products; alcoholic drinks

Surgery

Patients with either a single lymph node ≥3 cm or with multiple lymph node metastases on initial clinical staging of the neck should undergo neck dissection 8 weeks after completing radiotherapy. Laryngectomy should be performed in patients who had histologically proven persistent or recurrent carcinoma after the completion of treatment, or who had an inadequate response after 2 courses of induction chemotherapy

Toxicity

G3/4 Toxicity

	Induction Chemotherapy (Cisplatin + Fluorouracil) → RT (N = 168)		Radiotherapy Alone (N = 156)		Chemoradiation (Cisplatin + RT) (N = 171)	
	% G3	% G4	% G3	% G4	% G3	% G4
Hematologic	26	26	8	6.5	37	10
Infection	2.5	2.5	1	—	4	—
Mucositis	16	4	23	1	37	5
Pharyngeal/esophageal	—	—	19	—	35	—
Laryngeal	—	—	13	0.5	17	1
Radiation dermatitis	—	—	10	—	6	1
Nausea/vomiting	12	2	—	—	16	1
Renal/genitourinary	2	—	1	—	3.5	0.5
Neurologic	2.5	0.5	—	—	5	0.5
Other	12	4	10	1	34	6.5
Overall maximal	37	29	42	8	58	19

Note: Deaths caused by treatment occurred in 3% of the group assigned to induction cisplatin plus fluorouracil followed by radiotherapy, 3% of the group assigned to RT alone, and 5% percent of the group assigned to radiotherapy with concurrent cisplatin

Patient Population Studied

A study of 547 patients with biopsy-proven, previously untreated, stage III or IV squamous cell carcinoma of the larynx for whom surgical treatment would require total laryngectomy. Excluded were patients with large T4 tumors, defined as tumors penetrating through the cartilage or extending >1 cm into the base of tongue, and patients with a stage T1 primary tumor. Karnofsky performance score of ≥60 and adequate organ function were required

Dose Modification

Note: It is anticipated that radiation therapy will continue despite the development of significant mucositis and or myelosuppression

Adverse Event	Dose Modification
G3/4 hematologic toxicity	Hold chemotherapy up to 3 weeks until toxicity resolves to G ≤1. If toxicity has not resolved to G ≤1 within 3 weeks, do not administer next cycle
G3/4 nonhematologic toxicity other than alopecia, fatigue, malaise, and nail changes (exceptions: neurotoxicity, ototoxicity and mucositis as detailed below)	
G3/4 neurotoxicity or ototoxicity	Discontinue chemotherapy
G4 mucositis	

Efficacy			
	Induction Chemotherapy (Cisplatin + Fluorouracil) → RT (N = 168)	Radiotherapy Alone (N = 156)	Chemoradiation (Cisplatin + RT) (N = 171)
Larynx Preservation Rate			
at 2 years	84%	67%	72%
Estimated Laryngectomy-free Survival			
at 2 years	59%	53%	66%
at 5 years	43%	38%	45%
Estimated Overall Survival			
at 2 years	76%	75%	74%
at 5 years	55%	56%	54%
Estimated Disease-free Survival			
at 2 years	52%	44%	61%
at 5 years	38%	27%	36%

Therapy Monitoring

1. *Day 1 of each cycle:* Medical history and physical exam, CBC with differential, LFTs, electrolytes, BUN, and creatinine
2. *Posttreatment reevaluation:* 8 weeks after the completion of therapy by examination of the head and neck and CT imaging. If persistent disease is suspected, perform the examination while the patient is under anesthesia so that direct laryngoscopy can be performed
3. *Scheduled follow-up visits:* Complete examination of the head and neck, with evaluation for late toxicity

HIGH-RISK PATIENTS

POSTOPERATIVE CHEMORADIATION WITH CISPLATIN

Bernier J et al. N Engl J Med 2004;350:1945–1952
Cooper JS et al. N Engl J Med 2004;350:1937–1944

Chemoradiation

Note: Among high-risk patients with resected head and neck cancer, the chemoradiation therapy regimen described significantly improved the rates of local and regional control and disease-free survival. However, compared to RT alone, chemoradiation is associated with a substantial increase in adverse effects

Hydration before, during, and after cisplatin administration ± mannitol:

• *Pre-cisplatin hydration* with 1000 mL 0.9% sodium chloride injection (0.9% NS); administer intravenously with potassium and magnesium supplementation as needed based on pretreatment laboratory results

• *Mannitol diuresis:* May be given to patients who have received adequate hydration. A dose of **mannitol** 12.5–25 g may be administered by intravenous injection or a short infusion before or during cisplatin administration, or prepared as an admixture with cisplatin. Continued intravenous hydration is essential

• *Continued mannitol diuresis:* In an inpatient or day-hospital setting, one may administer additional mannitol in the form of an intravenous infusion: **mannitol** 10–40 g; administer intravenously over 1–4 hours. This can be done either during or immediately after cisplatin, but requires maintenance of adequate intravenously administered fluids during and for hours after mannitol administration

• *Post-cisplatin hydration* with ≥1000 mL 0.9% NS; administer intravenously with potassium and magnesium supplementation as needed based on measured values

Cisplatin 100 mg/m²; administer intravenously in 50–1000 mL 0.9% NS over 60 minutes on day 1, every 3 weeks for 3 cycles during radiation (total dosage/cycle = 100 mg/m²)
Radiotherapy 60–66 Gy in 30–33 fractions of 2 Gy/fraction given continually over 6–6.6 weeks

Supportive Care
Antiemetic prophylaxis
Emetogenic potential on days with cisplatin is **HIGH**. *Potential for delayed symptoms*
See Chapter 39 for antiemetic recommendations

Hematopoietic growth factor (CSF) prophylaxis
Primary prophylaxis is NOT indicated
See Chapter 43 for more information

Antimicrobial prophylaxis
Risk of fever and neutropenia is LOW
  Antimicrobial primary prophylaxis to be considered:
  • Antibacterial—not indicated
  • Antifungal—not indicated
  • Antiviral—not indicated unless patient previously had an episode of HSV
See Chapter 47 for more information

Diarrhea management
Latent or delayed onset diarrhea*:
  Loperamide 4 mg orally initially after the first loose or liquid stool, *then*
  Loperamide 2 mg orally every 2 hours during waking hours, *plus*
  Loperamide 4 mg orally every 4 hours during hours of sleep

  • Continue for at least 12 hours after diarrhea resolves
  • Recurrent diarrhea after a 12-hour diarrhea-free interval is treated as a new episode
  • Rehydrate orally with fluids and electrolytes during a diarrheal episode
  • If a patient develops blood or mucus in stool, dehydration, or hemodynamic instability, or if diarrhea persists >48 hours despite loperamide, stop loperamide and hospitalize the patient for IV hydration

Persistent diarrhea:
  Octreotide 100–150 mcg subcutaneously 3 times daily. Maximum total daily dose is 1500 mcg

Antibiotic therapy during latent or delayed onset diarrhea:
  A fluoroquinolone (eg, **Ciprofloxacin** 500 mg orally every 12 hours) if absolute neutrophil count <500/mm³ with or without accompanying fever in association with diarrhea
  • Antibiotics should also be administered if patient is hospitalized with prolonged diarrhea and should be continued until diarrhea resolves

*Rothenberg ML et al. J Clin Oncol 2001;19:3801–3807
Abigerges D et al. J Natl Cancer Inst 1994;86:446–449
Wadler S et al. J Clin Oncol 1998;16:3169–31378

(continued)

(continued)

Oral care
Risk of mucositis/stomatitis is HIGH
  General advice:
- Encourage patients to maintain intake of non-alcoholic fluids
- Evaluate patients for oral pain and provide analgesic medications
- Consider histamine (H_2-subtype) receptor antagonists (eg, ranitidine, famotidine), or a proton pump inhibitor for epigastric pain
- *Lactobacillus* sp.-containing probiotics may be beneficial in preventing diarrhea

Patients with intact oral mucosa:
- Clean the mouth, tongue, and gums by brushing after every meal and at bedtime with an ultra-soft toothbrush with fluoride toothpaste
- Floss teeth gently every day unless contraindicated. If gums bleed and hurt, avoid bleeding or sore areas, but floss other teeth
- Patients may use saline or commercial bland, non-alcoholic rinses
  - Do not use mouthwashes that contain alcohols

If mucositis or stomatitis is present:
- Keep the mouth moist utilizing water, ice chips, sugarless gum, sugar-free hard candies, or a saliva substitute
- Rinse mouth several times a day to remove debris
  - Use a solution of ¼ teaspoon (1.25 g) each of baking soda and table salt (sodium chloride) in one quart (~950 mL) of warm water. Follow with a plain water rinse
  - Do not use mouthwashes that contain alcohols
- Foam-tipped swabs (eg, Toothettes®) are useful in moisturizing oral mucosa, but ineffective for cleansing teeth and removing plaque
- Advise patients who develop mucositis to:
  - Choose foods that are easy to chew and swallow
  - Take small bites of food, chew slowly, and sip liquids with meals
  - Encourage soft, moist foods such as cooked cereals, mashed potatoes, and scrambled eggs
  - For trouble swallowing, soften food with gravies, sauces, broths, yogurt, or other bland liquids
  - Avoid sharp, crunchy foods; hot, spicy or highly acidic foods (eg, citrus fruits and juices); sugary foods; toothpicks; tobacco products; alcoholic drinks

Patient Population Studied

EORTC 22931
A study of 334 patients with previously untreated, histologically proven, squamous cell carcinoma of the oral cavity, oropharynx, hypopharynx, or larynx with: (a) tumor stage pT3 or pT4 and any nodal stage except T3N0 of the larynx with negative resection margins, (b) N2/N3 disease, (c) T1/2N1/N2 disease with extranodal spread, (d) positive section margins, (e) perineural involvement, (f) vascular involvement, or (g) oral cavity or oropharyngeal tumors with involvement of lymph nodes at levels IV or V. Adequate organ function, WHO performance status of 0–2, and age ≥18 years

RTOG 9501/Intergroup
A study of 459 patients with squamous cell carcinoma of the oral cavity, oropharynx, larynx, or hypopharynx, who underwent macroscopically complete resection but had at least 1 high-risk characteristic defined as: (a) invasion of at least 2 lymph nodes, (b) extracapsular extension of nodal disease, or (c) microscopically involved mucosal margins of resection. Adequate organ function and Karnofsky performance status of ≥60 were required

Dose Modification

Note: Continuity of radiotherapy should be maintained if at all possible. Keep to a minimum interruptions resulting from treatment-related adverse effects

Adverse Event	Dose Modification
On day 12 of any cycle, ANC <1000/mm³ *or* platelet count <75,000/mm³	Hold cisplatin until ANC >1000/mm³ *and* platelet count >75,000/mm³
G1/2 neurotoxicity	Reduce cisplatin dosage to 60 mg/m²
G3/4 neurotoxicity or ototoxicity	Discontinue cisplatin
Creatinine clearance 40–50 mL/min (0.66–0.83 mL/s)	Reduce cisplatin dosage to 75 mg/m²
Creatinine clearance <40 mL/min (<0.66 mL/s)	Discontinue cisplatin

Efficacy

EORTC* (Bernier J et al. N Engl J Med 2004;350:1945–1952)

	Radiotherapy	Chemoradiation
Median progression-free survival, months[‡]	23	55
Median overall survival, months	32	72
Estimate of 5-year		
Progression-free survival	36%	47%
Overall survival	40%	53%
Cumulative incidence of loco-regional relapse	31%	18%

RTOG/INTERGROUP[†] (Cooper JS et al. N Engl J Med 2004;350:1937–1944)

	Radiotherapy N = 210	Chemoradiation N = 206
Estimated 2-year rate of local regional control[‡]	72%	82%
First site of treatment failure		
Local regional recurrence	29%	16%
Distant metastasis	23%	20%
Overall survival	No significant difference Hazard ratio for death = 0.84; 95% CI = 0.65–1.09; P = 0.19	

*Median follow up was 60 months
[†]Median follow up was 46 months
[‡]Primary end point. *Note:* Only 8 local and regional recurrences were observed beyond 2 years

G3/4 Toxicity*

	Radiotherapy	Chemoradiation
Acute toxicity	N = 209 (%)	N = 204 (%)
Hematologic	<1	38
Anemia	0	3
Mucous membrane	18	30
Pharynx and esophagus	15	25
Larynx	1	3
Salivary gland	1	2
Nausea/vomiting	0	20
Upper GI tract	3	16
Diarrhea	0	1
Skin	10	7
Subcutaneous	0	1
Infection	<1	6

(continued)

Therapy Monitoring

1. *Day 1 of each cisplatin treatment:* Medical history and physical exam, CBC with differential, LFTs, electrolytes, BUN, and creatinine
2. *Posttreatment reevaluation:* 8 weeks after the completion of therapy by examination of the head and neck and CT imaging. If persistent disease is suspected, perform the examination while the patient is under anesthesia so that direct laryngoscopy can be performed
3. *Scheduled follow-up visits:* Complete examination of the head and neck, with evaluation for late toxicity

G3/4 Toxicity* (continued)

	Radiotherapy	Chemoradiation
Acute toxicity	N = 209 (%)	N = 204 (%)
Neurologic	0	5
Genitourinary	0	3
Renal	0	3
Hepatic	0	1
Respiratory	0	<1
Bone	<1	<1
All others	2	15
Any G3/4	34	76
Late toxicity	N = 208	N = 201
Hematologic	<1	1
Mucous membrane	2	2
Pharynx and esophagus	6	7
Larynx	2	2
Salivary gland	2	3
Upper GI tract	<1	1
Skin	1	2
Subcutaneous	3	1
Neurologic	1	1
Joint	1	<1
Bone	1	3
All others	3	2
Any G3/4	17	20
Number of treatment related deaths	0	4

*RTOG/Intergroup (Cooper JS et al. N Engl J Med 2004;350:1937–1944)

HIGH-RISK PATIENTS

POSTOPERATIVE CHEMORADIATION
WITH CISPLATIN + FLUOROURACIL

Fietkau R et al. Proc Am Soc Clin Oncol 2006;24(18S, Part 1 of 2):281s (abstract 5507)

Chemoradiation

Hydration before, during, and after cisplatin administration:
- *Pre-cisplatin hydration* with 500–1000 mL 0.9% sodium chloride injection (0.9% NS); administer intravenously with potassium and magnesium supplementation as needed based on pretreatment laboratory results
- *Post-cisplatin hydration* with 500–1000 mL 0.9% NS; administer intravenously with potassium and magnesium supplementation as needed based on measured values

Cisplatin 20 mg/m² per day; administer intravenously in 50–1000 mL 0.9% NS over 60 minutes for 5 consecutive days, on days 1–5, every 4 weeks for 2 cycles during radiation (total dosage/cycle = 100 mg/m²), *and*
Fluorouracil 600 mg/m² per day; administer in 50–1000 mL 0.9% NS or D5W by continuous intravenous infusion over 24 hours for 5 consecutive days, on days 1–5, every 4 weeks for 2 cycles during radiation (total dosage/cycle = 3000 mg/m²)
Radiotherapy (50 Gy in case of pN0, 56 Gy in case of pN+ without extracapsular spread, 64 Gy in case of pN+ with extracapsular spread)

Supportive Care
Antiemetic prophylaxis
Emetogenic potential on days with cisplatin is **HIGH**. *Potential for delayed symptoms*
Emetogenic potential on days with fluorouracil alone is **LOW**
See Chapter 39 for antiemetic recommendations

Hematopoietic growth factor (CSF) prophylaxis
Primary prophylaxis is NOT indicated
See Chapter 43 for more information

Antimicrobial prophylaxis
Risk of fever and neutropenia is LOW
Antimicrobial primary prophylaxis to be considered:
- Antibacterial—not indicated
- Antifungal—not indicated
- Antiviral—not indicated unless patient previously had an episode of HSV

See Chapter 47 for more information

Diarrhea management
Latent or delayed onset diarrhea*:
Loperamide 4 mg orally initially after the first loose or liquid stool, *then*
Loperamide 2 mg orally every 2 hours during waking hours, *plus*
Loperamide 4 mg orally every 4 hours during hours of sleep
- Continue for at least 12 hours after diarrhea resolves
- Recurrent diarrhea after a 12-hour diarrhea-free interval is treated as a new episode
- Rehydrate orally with fluids and electrolytes during a diarrheal episode
- If a patient develops blood or mucus in stool, dehydration, or hemodynamic instability, or if diarrhea persists >48 hours despite loperamide, stop loperamide and hospitalize the patient for IV hydration

Persistent diarrhea:
Octreotide 100–150 mcg subcutaneously 3 times daily. Maximum total daily dose is 1500 mcg
Antibiotic therapy during latent or delayed onset diarrhea:
A fluoroquinolone (eg, **Ciprofloxacin** 500 mg orally every 12 hours) if absolute neutrophil count <500/mm³ with or without accompanying fever in association with diarrhea
- Antibiotics should also be administered if patient is hospitalized with prolonged diarrhea and should be continued until diarrhea resolves

*Rothenberg ML et al. J Clin Oncol 2001;19:3801–3807
Abigerges D et al. J Natl Cancer Inst 1994;86:446–449
Wadler S et al. J Clin Oncol 1998;16:3169–3178

Oral care
Risk of mucositis/stomatitis during chemoradiation is MODERATE–HIGH
General advice:
- Encourage patients to maintain intake of non-alcoholic fluids
- Evaluate patients for oral pain and provide analgesic medications

(continued)

(continued)

- Consider histamine (H$_2$-subtype) receptor antagonists (eg, ranitidine, famotidine), or a proton pump inhibitor for epigastric pain
- *Lactobacillus* sp.-containing probiotics may be beneficial in preventing diarrhea

Patients with intact oral mucosa:
- Clean the mouth, tongue, and gums by brushing after every meal and at bedtime with an ultra-soft toothbrush with fluoride toothpaste
- Floss teeth gently every day unless contraindicated. If gums bleed and hurt, avoid bleeding or sore areas, but floss other teeth
- Patients may use saline or commercial bland, non-alcoholic rinses
  - Do not use mouthwashes that contain alcohols

If mucositis or stomatitis is present:
- Keep the mouth moist utilizing water, ice chips, sugarless gum, sugar-free hard candies, or a saliva substitute
- Rinse mouth several times a day to remove debris
  - Use a solution of ¼ teaspoon (1.25 g) each of baking soda and table salt (sodium chloride) in one quart (~950 mL) of warm water. Follow with a plain water rinse
  - Do not use mouthwashes that contain alcohols
- Foam-tipped swabs (eg, Toothettes®) are useful in moisturizing oral mucosa, but ineffective for cleansing teeth and removing plaque
- Advise patients who develop mucositis to:
  - Choose foods that are easy to chew and swallow
  - Take small bites of food, chew slowly, and sip liquids with meals
  - Encourage soft, moist foods such as cooked cereals, mashed potatoes, and scrambled eggs
  - For trouble swallowing, soften food with gravies, sauces, broths, yogurt, or other bland liquids
  - Avoid sharp, crunchy foods; hot, spicy or highly acidic foods (eg, citrus fruits and juices); sugary foods; toothpicks; tobacco products; alcoholic drinks

Patient Population Studied

A study of 440 patients with pTR1, PT4, or ≥3 positive lymph nodes, or extracapsular spread and no macroscopic residual tumor

Dose Modification

Note: Continuity of radiotherapy should be maintained if at all possible. Keep to a minimum interruptions resulting from treatment-related adverse effects

Adverse Event	Dose Modification
G3/4 hematologic toxicity attributable to chemotherapy	Hold chemotherapy
G3/4 nonhematologic toxicity other than alopecia, fatigue, malaise, and nail changes attributable to chemotherapy (exception: mucositis as detailed below)	
G4 mucositis	Discontinue therapy

G3/4 Toxicity (%)

Adverse Event	Radiotherapy	Chemoradiation
Mucositis	12.6	20.8
Dermatitis	8.9	13.1
Leukopenia	0	4.4
Thrombocytopenia	0	1.7
Serum creatinine >1.5 × upper limit of normal range	1.2	6.4
Infections	6.9	8.8

Efficacy

	Radiotherapy	Chemoradiation
5-Year locoregional control	61.9%	83.3%
5-Year rate free of distant metastases	68%	70%
5-Year disease survival	50.1%	62.4%
5-Year survival	48.6%	58.1%

Therapy Monitoring

1. *Days 1 and 29:* Medical history and physical exam, CBC with differential, LFTs, electrolytes, BUN, and creatinine
2. *Posttreatment reevaluation:* 8 weeks after the completion of therapy by examination of the head and neck and CT imaging. If persistent disease is suspected, perform the examination while the patient is under anesthesia so that direct laryngoscopy can be performed
3. *Scheduled follow-up visits:* Complete examination of the head and neck, with evaluation for late toxicity

INITIAL OR METASTATIC DISEASE REGIMEN
CETUXIMAB ± RADIATION

Bonner JA et al. N Engl J Med 2006;354:567–578

Premedication:

Diphenhydramine 50 mg (or an equivalent [H_1] antihistamine); administer by intravenous injection or as a short infusion 30 minutes prior to cetuximab administration

Note: Severe infusion reactions can occur with the administration of cetuximab Approximately 90% of severe reactions were associated with the first infusion despite the use of prophylactic antihistamines

Initial dose:

Cetuximab 400 mg/m²; administer intravenously over 120 minutes (maximum infusion rate = 5 mL [10 mg] per min) 1 week prior to radiation therapy

Maintenance doses:

Cetuximab 250 mg/m² per dose; administer intravenously over 60 minutes (maximum infusion rate = 5 mL [10 mg] per min), weekly ± **radiation**

Note: If administering radiation, administer cetuximab weekly for the duration of radiation

Radiation Regimens Used in the Randomized Trial

Regimen	Total Radiation Dose	Once-Daily Fractions	Twice-Daily Fractions
Once daily	70.0 Gy 35 fractions	2.0 Gy/fraction 5 fractions/week 7 weeks	Not applicable
Twice daily	72.0–76.8 Gy 60–64 fractions	Not applicable	1.2 Gy/fraction; 10 fractions/week for 6.0–6.5 weeks
Concomitant boost	72.0 Gy 42 fractions	32.4 Gy 1.8 Gy/fraction 5 fractions/week for 3.6 weeks	*Morning dose:* 21.6 Gy; 1.8 Gy/fraction; 5 fractions/week; 2.4 weeks *Afternoon dose:* 18.0 Gy; 1.5 Gy/fraction; 5 fractions/week; 2.4 weeks

Supportive Care
Antiemetic prophylaxis
Emetogenic potential with cetuximab is **MINIMAL**
See Chapter 39 for antiemetic recommendations

Hematopoietic growth factor (CSF) prophylaxis
Primary prophylaxis is NOT indicated
See Chapter 43 for more information

Antimicrobial prophylaxis
Risk of fever and neutropenia is LOW
  Antimicrobial primary prophylaxis to be considered:
  • Antibacterial—not indicated
  • Antifungal—not indicated
  • Antiviral—not indicated unless patient previously had an episode of HSV
See Chapter 47 for more information

Oral care
Risk of mucositis/stomatitis is HIGH
  General advice:
  • Encourage patients to maintain intake of non-alcoholic fluids
  • Evaluate patients for oral pain and provide analgesic medications
  • Consider histamine (H_2-subtype) receptor antagonists (eg, ranitidine, famotidine), or a proton pump inhibitor for epigastric pain
  • *Lactobacillus* sp.-containing probiotics may be beneficial in preventing diarrhea
  Patients with intact oral mucosa:
  • Clean the mouth, tongue, and gums by brushing after every meal and at bedtime with an ultra-soft toothbrush with fluoride toothpaste
  • Floss teeth gently every day unless contraindicated. If gums bleed and hurt, avoid bleeding or sore areas, but floss other teeth
  • Patients may use saline or commercial bland, non-alcoholic rinses
    ▪ Do not use mouthwashes that contain alcohols
  If mucositis or stomatitis is present:
  • Keep the mouth moist utilizing water, ice chips, sugarless gum, sugar-free hard candies, or a saliva substitute
  • Rinse mouth several times a day to remove debris
    ▪ Use a solution of ¼ teaspoon (1.25 g) each of baking soda and table salt (sodium chloride) in one quart (~950 mL) of warm water. Follow with a plain water rinse
    ▪ Do not use mouthwashes that contain alcohols

(continued)

(*continued*)

- Foam-tipped swabs (eg, Toothettes®) are useful in moisturizing oral mucosa, but ineffective for cleansing teeth and removing plaque
- Advise patients who develop mucositis to:
  - Choose foods that are easy to chew and swallow
  - Take small bites of food, chew slowly, and sip liquids with meals
  - Encourage soft, moist foods such as cooked cereals, mashed potatoes, and scrambled eggs
  - For trouble swallowing, soften food with gravies, sauces, broths, yogurt, or other bland liquids
  - Avoid sharp, crunchy foods; hot, spicy or highly acidic foods (eg, citrus fruits and juices); sugary foods; toothpicks; tobacco products; alcoholic drinks

Dose Modification

Infusion Reaction Severity	Cetuximab Dosage
G1/2	Reduce dosage by 50%
G3/4	Discontinue cetuximab

Severe Acneiform Rash*	Cetuximab	Subsequent Treatment Modifications by Outcome	
		Improvement	No improvement
First occurrence	Delay repeated treatment for 1–2 weeks	Resume with cetuximab 250 mg/m² weekly	Discontinue cetuximab
Second occurrence		Resume with cetuximab 200 mg/m² weekly	
Third occurrence		Resume with cetuximab 150 mg/m² weekly	
Fourth occurrence		Discontinue cetuximab	

*In patients with mild and moderate skin toxicity treatment should continue without dose modification

Efficacy (N = 211)

	Radiotherapy Alone (N = 213)	Radiotherapy Plus Cetuximab (N = 211)
Locoregional Control		
Median duration (months)	14.9	24.4
Median Duration of Locoregional Control According to Site (Months)		
Oropharynx	23	49
Larynx	11.9	12.9
Hypopharynx	10.3	12.5
Median Duration of Locoregional Control According to Stage		
Stage III	16.2	38.9
Stage IV	13.5	20.9
Progression-Free Survival		
Median duration (months)	12.4	17.1
Rate at 2 years (%)	37	46
Overall Survival (OS)		
Median duration (months)	29.3	49
Median Duration of OS According to Site		
Oropharynx	30.3	>66
Larynx	31.6	32.8
Hypopharynx	13.5	13.7

Patient Population Studied

A study of 424 patients with stage III or IV nonmetastatic measurable squamous cell carcinoma of the oropharynx, hypopharynx, or larynx who were randomly assigned to receive high-dose radiotherapy alone (n = 213) or high-dose radiotherapy plus cetuximab (n = 211)

Therapy Monitoring

Weekly: CBC with differential, serum electrolytes, calcium, and magnesium weekly during radiation

(*continued*)

Efficacy (N = 211) (continued)

Median Duration of OS According to Stage		
Stage III	42.9	55.2
Stage IV	24.2	47.4
Median Duration of OS According to Radiotherapy Regimen (Months)		
Once daily	15.3	18.9
Twice daily	53.3	58.9
Concomitant boost	31	>66

Toxicity (N = 208)

Adverse Event	Radiotherapy Alone (N = 212)		Radiotherapy Plus Cetuximab (N = 208)	
	% All Grades	% G3–5	% All Grades	% G3–5
Mucositis	94	52	93	56
Acneiform rash*	10	1	87	17
Radiation dermatitis	90	18	86	23
Weight loss	72	7	84	11
Xerostomia	71	3	72	5
Dysphagia	63	30	65	26
Asthenia	49	5	56	4
Nausea	37	2	49	2
Constipation	30	5	35	5
Taste perversion	28	0	29	0
Vomiting	23	4	29	2
Pain	28	7	28	6
Anorexia	23	2	27	2
Fever	13	1	26	1
Pharyngitis	19	4	26	3
Dehydration	19	8	25	6
Oral candidiasis	22	0	20	0
Coughing	19	0	20	<1
Voice alteration	22	0	19	2
Diarrhea	13	1	19	2
Headache	8	<1	19	<1
Pruritus	4	0	16	0
Infusion reaction*	2	0	15	3
Insomnia	14	0	15	0
Dyspepsia	9	1	14	0
Increased sputum	15	1	13	<1
Infection	9	1	13	1
Anxiety	9	1	11	<1
Chills	5	0	11	0
Anemia	13	6	3	1

*With the exception of acneiform rash and infusion-related events, the incidence rates of G3–5 reactions were similar in the 2 treatment groups

Note: Four patients discontinued cetuximab because of hypersensitivity reactions after the test dose or first dose

Notes

1. *Indications:*

Cetuximab, in combination with radiation therapy, is indicated for the treatment of locally or regional advanced squamous cell carcinoma of the head and neck

Bonner JA et al. N Engl J Med 2006;354:567–578

Cetuximab as a single agent is indicated for the treatment of patients with recurrent or metastatic squamous cell carcinoma of the head and neck after prior platinum based therapy has failed

Trigo J et al. Proc Am Soc Clin Oncol 2004;23:488s [abstract 5502]

Evaluated the efficacy of cetuximab monotherapy in 103 patients with platinum-refractory, recurrent or metastatic squamous cell carcinoma of the head and neck in a multicenter phase II study. An initial dose of cetuximab 400 mg/m² was followed by cetuximab 250 mg/m² weekly, until disease progression, with an option to switch to cetuximab plus the same platinum agent on which patients' disease had previously progressed after disease progression occurred with cetuximab monotherapy. Drug-related adverse events in >10% of patients included skin rash/acne 80% (1% G3), fatigue 24% (4% G3), fever/chills 19% (2% G3), nail changes 15% (all G1/2), and nausea 13% (1% G3). There was 1 treatment-related death as a result of a hypersensitivity reaction in a patient for whom mechanical ventilation was not suitable. Preliminary efficacy data were as follows: 5 CR, 12 PR, 38 SD, 47 PD, and 1 not assessable, for an overall objective response rate of 16.5% (95% CI, 9.9–25.1%). The disease control rate was 53.4% (95% CI, 43.3–63.3%). Median TTP and median survival were 85 days and 175 days, respectively

METASTATIC DISEASE REGIMEN

METHOTREXATE
(See also CISPLATIN + FLUOROURACIL AND CARBOPLATIN + FLUOROURACIL)

Note: These 3 regimens were compared in a randomized trial. The Efficacy and Toxicity tables provide the comparative data

Forastiere AA et al. J Clin Oncol 1992;10:1245–1251

Methotrexate 40 mg/m²; administer by intravenous injection over 15–30 seconds, or as a short infusion in 10–100 mL 0.9% sodium chloride injection or 5% dextrose injection over 5–15 minutes every week, continually (total dosage/week = 40 mg/m²)

Note: Increase methotrexate dosage to 50 mg/m² weekly if patients experience only grade 0 (zero) mucositis or myelosuppression after 40 mg/m² per week

Supportive Care
Antiemetic prophylaxis
*Emetogenic potential is **MINIMAL***
See Chapter 39 for antiemetic recommendations

Hematopoietic growth factor (CSF) prophylaxis
Primary prophylaxis is NOT indicated
See Chapter 43 for more information

Antimicrobial prophylaxis
Risk of fever and neutropenia is LOW
   Antimicrobial primary prophylaxis to be considered:
   • Antibacterial—not indicated
   • Antifungal—not indicated
   • Antiviral—not indicated unless patient previously had an episode of HSV
See Chapter 47 for more information

Oral care (mucositis prophylaxis and management)
   General advice:
   • Encourage patients to maintain intake of non-alcoholic fluids
   • Evaluate patients for oral pain and provide analgesic medications
   • Consider histamine (H₂-subtype) receptor antagonists (eg, ranitidine, famotidine), or a proton pump inhibitor for epigastric pain
   • *Lactobacillus* sp.-containing probiotics may be beneficial in preventing diarrhea
   Patients with intact oral mucosa:
   • Clean the mouth, tongue, and gums by brushing after every meal and at bedtime with an ultra-soft toothbrush with fluoride toothpaste
   • Floss teeth gently every day unless contraindicated. If gums bleed and hurt, avoid bleeding or sore areas, but floss other teeth
   • Patients may use saline or commercial bland, non-alcoholic rinses
      ▪ Do not use mouthwashes that contain alcohols
   If mucositis or stomatitis is present:
   • Keep the mouth moist utilizing water, ice chips, sugarless gum, sugar-free hard candies, or a saliva substitute
   • Rinse mouth several times a day to remove debris
      ▪ Use a solution of ¼ teaspoon (1.25 g) each of baking soda and table salt (sodium chloride) in one quart (~950 mL) of warm water. Follow with a plain water rinse
      ▪ Do not use mouthwashes that contain alcohols
   • Foam-tipped swabs (eg, Toothettes®) are useful in moisturizing oral mucosa, but ineffective for cleansing teeth and removing plaque
   • Advise patients who develop mucositis to:
      ▪ Choose foods that are easy to chew and swallow
      ▪ Take small bites of food, chew slowly, and sip liquids with meals
      ▪ Encourage soft, moist foods such as cooked cereals, mashed potatoes, and scrambled eggs
      ▪ For trouble swallowing, soften food with gravies, sauces, broths, yogurt, or other bland liquids
      ▪ Avoid sharp, crunchy foods; hot, spicy or highly acidic foods (eg, citrus fruits and juices); sugary foods; toothpicks; tobacco products; alcoholic drinks

Patient Population Studied

A randomized comparison of 3 treatments: (a) single-agent methotrexate; (b) cisplatin plus fluorouracil; and (c) carboplatin plus fluorouracil. The study enrolled 277 patients with recurrent and metastatic squamous cell carcinoma of the head and neck. The primary objective was to compare separately the response rates of each regimen. Eligible patients had histologically proven squamous cell carcinoma of the head and neck that was either recurrent after attempted cure with surgery and radiation therapy or newly diagnosed disease with distant metastases. Patients with recurrent disease had not previously received chemotherapy for treatment of the recurrence, although they could have received induction chemotherapy ≥6 months before study entry. All patients were required to have measurable disease; a life expectancy of at least 12 weeks; a performance status of 0, 1, or 2 on the SWOG criteria; and a 24-hour creatinine clearance >50 mL/min (>0.83 mL/s)

Treatment Modifications

Adverse Event	Dose Modification
G ≥ 2 Hematologic or nonhematologic toxicity	Reduce methotrexate dosage by 10 mg/m²

Therapy Monitoring

Weekly: CBC with differential. Serum creatinine and LFTs as needed

Notes

Median duration of therapy is 8 weeks

Efficacy*

	Methotrexate (N = 87)	Cisplatin + Fluorouracil (N = 85)	Carboplatin + Fluorouracil (N = 86)
Complete response	2	6	2
Partial response	8	26	19
Stable disease/no response	50	37	42
Increasing disease	32	16	25
Assumed no response[†]	8	15	12

*WHO criteria
[†]Early death or not assessable

Toxicity*

	Methotrexate (N = 87)		Cisplatin + Fluorouracil (N = 85)		Carboplatin + Fluorouracil (N = 86)	
	% G1/2	% G3/4	% G1/2	% G3/4	% G1/2	% G3/4
Hematologic Toxicity						
Anemia	25.3	3.4	55.3	4.7	41.9	14
Granulocytopenia	8	6.9	31.8	8.2	20.9	2.3
Leukopenia	28.7	16.1	42.4	30.6	50	11.6
Thrombocytopenia	9.2	5.7	12.9	5.9	18.6	12.8
Nonhematologic Toxicity						
Diarrhea	3	0	12	2	6	2
Stomatitis	34	10	19	14	28	15
Nausea/vomiting	38	8	68	8	48	6
Peripheral neuropathy	0	0	5	1	2	0
Ototoxicity	2	0	8	4	2	0
Renal	3	3	18	9	1	1
% G5 toxicity	1.1		1.1		1.2	

*SWOG Criteria
[†]Lower rates are expected with current antiemetics

METASTATIC DISEASE REGIMEN

CISPLATIN + FLUOROURACIL

(See also Methotrexate and Carboplatin + Fluorouracil)

Note: These 3 regimens were compared in a randomized trial. The Efficacy and Toxicity tables provide the comparative data

Forastiere AA et al. J Clin Oncol 1992;10:1245–1251

Hydration before, during, and after cisplatin administration ± mannitol:

• *Pre-cisplatin hydration* with 1000 mL 0.9% sodium chloride injection (0.9% NS); administer intravenously with potassium and magnesium supplementation as needed based on pretreatment laboratory results

• *Mannitol diuresis:* May be given to patients who have received adequate hydration. A dose of **mannitol** 12.5–25 g may be administered by intravenous injection or a short infusion before or during cisplatin administration, or prepared as an admixture with cisplatin. Continued intravenous hydration is essential

• *Continued mannitol diuresis:* In an inpatient or day-hospital setting, one may administer additional mannitol in the form of an intravenous infusion: **mannitol** 10–40 g; administer intravenously over 1–4 hours. This can be done either during or immediately after cisplatin, but requires maintenance of adequate intravenously administered fluids during and for hours after mannitol administration

• Post-cisplatin hydration with ≥1000 mL 0.9% NS; administer intravenously with potassium and magnesium supplementation as needed based on measured values

Cisplatin 100 mg/m²; administer intravenously in 25–250 mL of 0.9% NS over 15–30 minutes, given on day 1 every 21 days (total dosage/cycle = 100 mg/m²)
Fluorouracil 1000 mg/m² per day; administer by continuous intravenous infusion in 100–1000 mL 0.9% NS or 5% dextrose injection over 24 hours for 4 consecutive days (96-hour infusion), given on days 1–4 every 21 days (total dosage/cycle = 4000 mg/m²)

Supportive Care
Antiemetic prophylaxis
Emetogenic potential on days with cisplatin is **HIGH***. Potential for delayed symptoms*
Emetogenic potential on days with fluorouracil alone is **LOW**
See Chapter 39 for antiemetic recommendations

Hematopoietic growth factor (CSF) prophylaxis
Primary prophylaxis is NOT indicated
See Chapter 43 for more information

Antimicrobial prophylaxis
Risk of fever and neutropenia is LOW
  Antimicrobial primary prophylaxis to be considered:
  • Antibacterial—not indicated
  • Antifungal—not indicated
  • Antiviral—not indicated unless patient previously had an episode of HSV
See Chapter 47 for more information

Diarrhea management
Latent or delayed onset diarrhea*:
  Loperamide 4 mg orally initially after the first loose or liquid stool, *then*
  Loperamide 2 mg orally every 2 hours during waking hours, *plus*
  Loperamide 4 mg orally every 4 hours during hours of sleep
  • Continue for at least 12 hours after diarrhea resolves
  • Recurrent diarrhea after a 12-hour diarrhea-free interval is treated as a new episode
  • Rehydrate orally with fluids and electrolytes during a diarrheal episode
  • If a patient develops blood or mucus in stool, dehydration, or hemodynamic instability, or if diarrhea persists >48 hours despite loperamide, stop loperamide and hospitalize the patient for IV hydration

Persistent diarrhea:
  Octreotide 100–150 mcg subcutaneously 3 times daily. Maximum total daily dose is 1500 mcg

(continued)

Treatment Modifications

Adverse Event	Dose Modification
G ≥2 Mucosal or skin toxicity	Reduce fluorouracil dosage by 20%
G ≥2 Diarrhea (4–6 stools/day > baseline)	Hold fluorouracil until diarrhea resolves to baseline
G3 myelosuppression	Reduce cisplatin dosage by 25%. Do not change fluorouracil dosage
G4 myelosuppression	Reduce cisplatin dosage by 40%. Do not change fluorouracil dosage
Creatinine clearance <50 mL/min (<0.83 mL/s)	Do not administer therapy
Serum creatinine >1.5 mg/dL (>133 μmol/L) or 20% higher than baseline if >1.5 mg/dL (>133 μmol/L)	Hold cisplatin dose until serum creatinine <1.5 mg/dL (<133 μmol/L) or within 0.2 mg/dL (17.7 μmol/L) of baseline
Serum creatinine 1.5–2.0 mg/dL (133–177 μmol/L) immediately before a cycle	Hold cisplatin*, then reduce cisplatin dosage by 25% during subsequent cycles
Serum creatinine 2.1–3.0 mg/dL (186–265 μmol/L) immediately before a cycle	Hold cisplatin*, then reduce cisplatin dosage by 50% during subsequent cycles
Serum creatinine >3.0 mg/dL (>265 μmol/L) immediately before a cycle	Hold cisplatin
G2 neurotoxicity or ototoxicity	Hold cisplatin until neurotoxicity resolves to G ≤1
G3/4 neurotoxicity or ototoxicity	Discontinue chemotherapy

*Hold cisplatin until serum creatinine <1.5 mg/dL (<133 μmol/L), or within 0.2 mg/dL (17.7 μmol/L) of baseline

(*continued*)

Antibiotic therapy during latent or delayed onset diarrhea:
A fluoroquinolone (eg, **Ciprofloxacin** 500 mg orally every 12 hours) if absolute neutrophil count $<500/mm^3$ with or without accompanying fever in association with diarrhea
- Antibiotics should also be administered if patient is hospitalized with prolonged diarrhea and should be continued until diarrhea resolves

*Rothenberg ML et al. J Clin Oncol 2001;19:3801–3807
Abigerges D et al. J Natl Cancer Inst 1994;86:446–449
Wadler S et al. J Clin Oncol 1998;16:3169–3178

Oral care (mucositis prophylaxis and management)
General advice:
- Encourage patients to maintain intake of non-alcoholic fluids
- Evaluate patients for oral pain and provide analgesic medications
- Consider histamine (H_2-subtype) receptor antagonists (eg, ranitidine, famotidine), or a proton pump inhibitor for epigastric pain
- *Lactobacillus* sp.-containing probiotics may be beneficial in preventing diarrhea

Patients with intact oral mucosa:
- Clean the mouth, tongue, and gums by brushing after every meal and at bedtime with an ultra-soft toothbrush with fluoride toothpaste
- Floss teeth gently every day unless contraindicated. If gums bleed and hurt, avoid bleeding or sore areas, but floss other teeth
- Patients may use saline or commercial bland, non-alcoholic rinses
  - Do not use mouthwashes that contain alcohols

If mucositis or stomatitis is present:
- Keep the mouth moist utilizing water, ice chips, sugarless gum, sugar-free hard candies, or a saliva substitute
- Rinse mouth several times a day to remove debris
  - Use a solution of ¼ teaspoon (1.25 g) each of baking soda and table salt (sodium chloride) in one quart (~950 mL) of warm water. Follow with a plain water rinse
  - Do not use mouthwashes that contain alcohols
- Foam-tipped swabs (eg, Toothettes®) are useful in moisturizing oral mucosa, but ineffective for cleansing teeth and removing plaque
- Advise patients who develop mucositis to:
  - Choose foods that are easy to chew and swallow
  - Take small bites of food, chew slowly, and sip liquids with meals
  - Encourage soft, moist foods such as cooked cereals, mashed potatoes, and scrambled eggs
  - For trouble swallowing, soften food with gravies, sauces, broths, yogurt, or other bland liquids
  - Avoid sharp, crunchy foods; hot, spicy or highly acidic foods (eg, citrus fruits and juices); sugary foods; toothpicks; tobacco products; alcoholic drinks

Patient Population Studied

A randomized comparison of 3 treatments: (a) single-agent methotrexate; (b) cisplatin plus fluorouracil; and (c) carboplatin plus fluorouracil. The study enrolled 277 patients with recurrent and metastatic squamous cell carcinoma of the head and neck. The primary objective was to compare separately the response rates of each regimen. Eligible patients had histologically proven squamous cell carcinoma of the head and neck that was either recurrent after attempted cure with surgery and radiation therapy or newly diagnosed disease with distant metastases. Patients with recurrent disease had not previously received chemotherapy for treatment of the recurrence, although they could have received induction chemotherapy ≥6 months before study entry. All patients were required to have measurable disease; a life expectancy of at least 12 weeks; a performance status of 0, 1, or 2 on the SWOG criteria; and a 24-hour creatinine clearance >50 mL/min (>0.83 mL/s)

Therapy Monitoring

1. *Before each cycle:* PE, CBC, LFTs, serum electrolytes, calcium, and magnesium
2. *One week after treatment:* Serum electrolytes, calcium, and magnesium
3. *Weekly follow-up recommended during at least the first cycle:* Attention to signs and symptoms of dehydration as supplemental hydration is often required

Efficacy*

	Methotrexate (N = 87)	Cisplatin + Fluorouracil (N = 85)	Carboplatin + Fluorouracil (N = 86)
Complete response	2	6	2
Partial response	8	26	19
Stable disease/no response	50	37	42
Increasing disease	32	16	25
Assumed no response[†]	8	15	12

*WHO Criteria
[†]Early death or not assessable

Toxicity*

	Methotrexate (N = 87)		Cisplatin + Fluorouracil (N = 85)		Carboplatin + Fluorouracil (N = 86)	
	% G1/2	% G3/4	% G1/2	% G3/4	% G1/2	% G3/4
Hematologic Toxicity						
Anemia	25.3	3.4	55.3	4.7	41.9	14
Granulocytopenia	8	6.9	31.8	8.2	20.9	2.3
Leukopenia	28.7	16.1	42.4	30.6	50	11.6
Thrombocytopenia	9.2	5.7	12.9	5.9	18.6	12.8
Nonhematologic Toxicity						
Diarrhea	3	0	12	2	6	2
Stomatitis	34	10	19	14	28	15
Nausea/vomiting†	38	8	68	8	48	6
Peripheral neuropathy	0	0	5	1	2	0
Ototoxicity	2	0	8	4	2	0
Renal	3	3	18	9	1	1
% G5 toxicity	1.1		1.1		1.2	

*SWOG Criteria
†Lower rates are expected with current antiemetics

METASTATIC DISEASE REGIMEN
CARBOPLATIN + FLUOROURACIL

(See also Methotrexate and Cisplatin + Fluorouracil)

Note: These 3 regimens were compared in a randomized trial. The Efficacy and Toxicity tables provide the comparative data

Forastiere AA et al. J Clin Oncol 1992;10:1245–1251

Carboplatin 300 mg/m^2; administer intravenously in 50–500 mL 5% dextrose injection (D5W) or 0.9% sodium chloride injection (0.9% NS) over at least 15 minutes, given on day 1, every 28 days (total dosage/cycle = 300 mg/m^2)

Fluorouracil 1000 mg/m^2 per day; administer by continuous intravenous infusion in 100–1000 mL 0.9% NS or D5W over 24 hours for 4 consecutive days (96-hour infusion), given on days 1–4, every 28 days (total dosage/cycle = 4000 mg/m^2)

Supportive Care
Antiemetic prophylaxis
Emetogenic potential on days with carboplatin is **HIGH**. *Potential for delayed symptoms*
Emetogenic potential on days with fluorouracil alone is **LOW**
See Chapter 39 for antiemetic recommendations

Hematopoietic growth factor (CSF) prophylaxis
Primary prophylaxis is NOT indicated
See Chapter 43 for more information

Antimicrobial prophylaxis
Risk of fever and neutropenia is LOW
   Antimicrobial primary prophylaxis to be considered:
   • Antibacterial—not indicated
   • Antifungal—not indicated
   • Antiviral—not indicated unless patient previously had an episode of HSV
See Chapter 47 for more information

Diarrhea management
Latent or delayed onset diarrhea*:
   Loperamide 4 mg orally initially after the first loose or liquid stool, *then*
   Loperamide 2 mg orally every 2 hours during waking hours, *plus*
   Loperamide 4 mg orally every 4 hours during hours of sleep
   • Continue for at least 12 hours after diarrhea resolves
   • Recurrent diarrhea after a 12-hour diarrhea-free interval is treated as a new episode
   • Rehydrate orally with fluids and electrolytes during a diarrheal episode
   • If a patient develops blood or mucus in stool, dehydration, or hemodynamic instability, or if diarrhea persists >48 hours despite loperamide, stop loperamide and hospitalize the patient for IV hydration

Persistent diarrhea:
   Octreotide 100–150 mcg subcutaneously 3 times daily. Maximum total daily dose is 1500 mcg

Antibiotic therapy during latent or delayed onset diarrhea:
   A fluoroquinolone (eg, **Ciprofloxacin** 500 mg orally every 12 hours) if absolute neutrophil count <500/mm^3 with or without accompanying fever in association with diarrhea
   • Antibiotics should also be administered if patient is hospitalized with prolonged diarrhea and should be continued until diarrhea resolves

*Rothenberg ML et al. J Clin Oncol 2001;19:3801–3807
Abigerges D et al. J Natl Cancer Inst 1994;86:446–449
Wadler S et al. J Clin Oncol 1998;16:3169–3178

(continued)

Patient Population Studied

A randomized comparison of 3 treatments: (a) single-agent methotrexate, (b) cisplatin plus fluorouracil, and (c) carboplatin plus fluorouracil. The study enrolled 277 patients with recurrent and metastatic squamous cell carcinoma of the head and neck. The primary objective was to compare separately the response rates of each regimen. Eligible patients had histologically proven squamous cell carcinoma of the head and neck that was either recurrent after attempted cure with surgery and radiation therapy or newly diagnosed disease with distant metastases. Patients with recurrent disease had not previously received chemotherapy for treatment of the recurrence, although they could have received induction chemotherapy ≥6 months before study entry. All patients were required to have measurable disease; a life expectancy of at least 12 weeks; a performance status of 0, 1, or 2 on the SWOG criteria; and a 24-hour creatinine clearance >50 mL/min (>0.83 mL/s)

Treatment Modifications

Adverse Event	Dose Modification
G ≥2 mucosal or skin toxicity	Reduce fluorouracil dosage by 20%
G ≥2 diarrhea (4–6 stools/day > baseline)	Hold fluorouracil until diarrhea resolves
G3/4 toxicity myelosuppression	Reduce carboplatin dosage by 20%. Do not change fluorouracil dosage
G0/1 myelosuppression	Increase carboplatin dosage by 20% to 360 mg/m^2 on the same administration schedule

(*continued*)

Oral care (mucositis prophylaxis and management)

General advice:

- Encourage patients to maintain intake of non-alcoholic fluids
- Evaluate patients for oral pain and provide analgesic medications
- Consider histamine (H_2-subtype) receptor antagonists (eg, ranitidine, famotidine), or a proton pump inhibitor for epigastric pain
- *Lactobacillus* sp.-containing probiotics may be beneficial in preventing diarrhea

Patients with intact oral mucosa:

- Clean the mouth, tongue, and gums by brushing after every meal and at bedtime with an ultra-soft toothbrush with fluoride toothpaste
- Floss teeth gently every day unless contraindicated. If gums bleed and hurt, avoid bleeding or sore areas, but floss other teeth
- Patients may use saline or commercial bland, non-alcoholic rinses
  - Do not use mouthwashes that contain alcohols

If mucositis or stomatitis is present:

- Keep the mouth moist utilizing water, ice chips, sugarless gum, sugar-free hard candies, or a saliva substitute
- Rinse mouth several times a day to remove debris
  - Use a solution of ¼ teaspoon (1.25 g) each of baking soda and table salt (sodium chloride) in one quart (~950 mL) of warm water. Follow with a plain water rinse
  - Do not use mouthwashes that contain alcohols
- Foam-tipped swabs (eg, Toothettes®) are useful in moisturizing oral mucosa, but ineffective for cleansing teeth and removing plaque
- Advise patients who develop mucositis to:
  - Choose foods that are easy to chew and swallow
  - Take small bites of food, chew slowly, and sip liquids with meals
  - Encourage soft, moist foods such as cooked cereals, mashed potatoes, and scrambled eggs
  - For trouble swallowing, soften food with gravies, sauces, broths, yogurt, or other bland liquids
  - Avoid sharp, crunchy foods; hot, spicy or highly acidic foods (eg, citrus fruits and juices); sugary foods; toothpicks; tobacco products; alcoholic drinks

Therapy Monitoring

1. *Weekly:* PE, CBC, serum electrolytes, LFTs calcium, and magnesium
2. *Weekly follow-up recommended during at least the first cycle:* Attention to signs and symptoms of dehydration as supplemental hydration is often required

Efficacy*

	Methotrexate (N = 87)	Cisplatin + Fluorouracil (N = 85)	Carboplatin + Fluorouracil (N = 86)
Complete response	2	6	2
Partial response	8	26	19
Stable disease/no response	50	37	42
Increasing disease	32	16	25
Assumed no response[†]	8	15	12

*WHO criteria
[†]Early death or not assessable

	Toxicity*					
	Methotrexate (N = 87)		Cisplatin + Fluorouracil (N = 85)		Carboplatin + Fluorouracil (N = 86)	
	% G1/2	% G3/4	% G1/2	% G3/4	% G1/2	% G3/4
Hematologic Toxicity						
Anemia	25.3	3.4	55.3	4.7	41.9	14
Granulocytopenia	8	6.9	31.8	8.2	20.9	2.3
Leukopenia	28.7	16.1	42.4	30.6	50	11.6
Thrombocytopenia	9.2	5.7	12.9	5.9	18.6	12.8
Nonhematologic Toxicity						
Diarrhea	3	0	12	2	6	2
Stomatitis	34	10	19	14	28	15
Nausea/vomiting†	38	8	68	8	48	6
Peripheral neuropathy	0	0	5	1	2	0
Ototoxicity	2	0	8	4	2	0
Renal	3	3	18	9	1	1
% G5 toxicity	1.1		1.1		1.2	

*SWOG Criteria
†Lower rates are expected with current antiemetics

METASTATIC DISEASE REGIMEN

CISPLATIN

Jacobs C et al. J Clin Oncol 1992;10:257–263

Hydration before, during, and after cisplatin administration ± mannitol:

- *Pre-cisplatin hydration* with 1000 mL 0.9% sodium chloride injection (0.9% NS); administer intravenously with potassium and magnesium supplementation as needed based on pretreatment laboratory results
- *Mannitol diuresis:* May be given to patients who have received adequate hydration. A dose of **mannitol** 12.5–25 g may be administered by intravenous injection or a short infusion before or during cisplatin administration, or prepared as an admixture with cisplatin. Continued intravenous hydration is essential
- *Continued mannitol diuresis:* In an inpatient or day-hospital setting, one may administer additional mannitol in the form of an intravenous infusion: **mannitol** 10–40 g; administer intravenously over 1–4 hours. This can be done either during or immediately after cisplatin, but requires maintenance of adequate intravenously administered fluids during and for hours after mannitol administration
- *Post-cisplatin hydration* with ≥1000 mL 0.9% NS; administer intravenously with potassium and magnesium supplementation as needed based on measured values

Cisplatin 100 mg/m²; administer intravenously in 25–250 mL of 0.9% NS over 15–20 minutes every 21 days (total dosage/cycle = 100 mg/m²)

Supportive Care

Antiemetic prophylaxis
Emetogenic potential is **HIGH**. Potential for delayed symptoms
See Chapter 39 for antiemetic recommendations

Hematopoietic growth factor (CSF) prophylaxis
Primary prophylaxis is *NOT* indicated
See Chapter 43 for more information

Antimicrobial prophylaxis
Risk of fever and neutropenia is LOW
Antimicrobial primary prophylaxis to be considered:
- Antibacterial—not indicated
- Antifungal—consider use during neutropenia and for anticipated mucositis
- Antiviral—not indicated unless patient previously had an episode of HSV

See Chapter 47 for more information

Patient Population Studied

A study of 84 patients with unresectable recurrent disease or newly diagnosed distant metastatic disease who had received no prior chemotherapy, who were randomized to the cisplatin alone arm of a 3-arm phase III randomized trial. WHO performance status <4 and good organ function were required. Thirty-six percent had performance status of 2 or 3

Efficacy (N = 83)

Complete response	3.6%
Partial response	13.3%
Median duration of response	2 months
Median survival	5.7 months

Toxicity (N = 83)

	% G1/2	% G3/4
Hematologic		
Neutropenia	35	1
Thrombocytopenia	11	1
Anemia (Hgb <8 g/dL)	NR	11
Nonhematologic		
Vomiting	54	18
Diarrhea	17	0
Mucositis	3	2
Ototoxicity	3	1
Magnesium <1.5 mg/dL		= 22%
Creatinine >2 mg/dL (>177 μmol/L)		= 14%
G >1 cardiovascular toxicity		= 5%
Alopecia		= 4%

Therapy Monitoring

1. *Weekly:* CBC with differential
2. *Before each cycle:* serum electrolytes, creatinine, calcium, magnesium, and liver function tests

Treatment Modifications

Adverse Event	Dose Modification
Creatinine clearance <50 mL/min (<0.83 mL/s)	Ineligible for therapy
Day 1 ANC <1500/mm³ or platelets <100,000/mm³	Delay cisplatin until ANC >1500/mm³ *and* platelets >100,000/mm³ for up to 3 weeks. Discontinue cisplatin if recovery has not occurred after a 3-week delay
ANC nadir <500/mm³	Reduce dosage to 75 mg/m²
Platelet nadir <25,000/mm³	
G1 neurotoxicity or ototoxicity	
Serum creatinine 1.5–2.0 mg/dL (133–177 μmol/L)	Hold cisplatin*, then reduce dosage to 75 mg/m²
ANC nadir <500/mm³ with a cisplatin dosage of 75 mg/m²	Reduce dosage to 50 mg/m²
Platelet nadir <25,000/mm³ with a cisplatin dosage of 75 mg/m²	
G2 neurotoxicity or ototoxicity	
Serum creatinine 2.1–3.0 mg/dL (186–265 μmol/L)	Hold cisplatin*, then reduce cisplatin dosage to 50 mg/m²
ANC nadir <500/mm³ with a cisplatin dosage of 50 mg/m²	Discontinue cisplatin
Platelet nadir <25,000/mm³ with a cisplatin dosage of 50 mg/m²	
Serum creatinine >3.0 mg/dL (>265 μmol/L)	
G3/4 neurotoxicity or ototoxicity	

*Hold cisplatin until serum creatinine <1.5 mg/dL (<133 μmol/L) or within 0.2 mg/dL (17.7 μmol/L) of baseline

METASTATIC DISEASE REGIMEN
DOCETAXEL

Catimel G et al. Ann Oncol 1994;5:533–537

Premedication:
Dexamethasone 8 mg; administer orally twice daily for 3 days (6 doses), starting the day before docetaxel administration (total dose/cycle = 48 mg)
optional **Diphenhydramine** 25–50 mg; administer by intravenous injection 30–60 minutes before docetaxel
Docetaxel 100 mg/m²; administer intravenously after dilution in a volume of 0.9% sodium chloride injection or 5% dextrose injection sufficient to produce a final docetaxel concentration within the range 0.3–0.74 mg/mL over 60 minutes every 21 days (total dosage/cycle = 100 mg/m²)

Supportive Care
Antiemetic prophylaxis
*Emetogenic potential is **LOW***
See Chapter 39 for antiemetic recommendations

Hematopoietic growth factor (CSF) prophylaxis
Primary prophylaxis is NOT indicated
See Chapter 43 for more information

Antimicrobial prophylaxis
Risk of fever and neutropenia is LOW
  Antimicrobial primary prophylaxis to be considered:
  • Antibacterial—not indicated
  • Antifungal—consider use during neutropenia and for anticipated mucositis
  • Antiviral—not indicated unless patient previously had an episode of HSV
See Chapter 47 for more information

Oral care (mucositis prophylaxis and management)
Risk of mucositis/stomatitis is MODERATE
  General advice:
  • Encourage patients to maintain intake of non-alcoholic fluids
  • Evaluate patients for oral pain and provide analgesic medications
  • Consider histamine (H₂-subtype) receptor antagonists (eg, ranitidine, famotidine), or a proton pump inhibitor for epigastric pain
  • *Lactobacillus* sp.-containing probiotics may be beneficial in preventing diarrhea
  Patients with intact oral mucosa:
  • Clean the mouth, tongue, and gums by brushing after every meal and at bedtime with an ultra-soft toothbrush with fluoride toothpaste
  • Floss teeth gently every day unless contraindicated. If gums bleed and hurt, avoid bleeding or sore areas, but floss other teeth
  • Patients may use saline or commercial bland, non-alcoholic rinses
    ▪ Do not use mouthwashes that contain alcohols
  If mucositis or stomatitis is present:
  • Keep the mouth moist utilizing water, ice chips, sugarless gum, sugar-free hard candies, or a saliva substitute
  • Rinse mouth several times a day to remove debris
    ▪ Use a solution of ¼ teaspoon (1.25 g) each of baking soda and table salt (sodium chloride) in one quart (~950 mL) of warm water. Follow with a plain water rinse
    ▪ Do not use mouthwashes that contain alcohols
  • Foam-tipped swabs (eg, Toothettes®) are useful in moisturizing oral mucosa, but ineffective for cleansing teeth and removing plaque

(continued)

Patient Population Studied

A trial of 40 patients with unresectable recurrent disease following attempted cure with surgery and/or radiation therapy (may have received neoadjuvant chemotherapy) or newly diagnosed with distant metastases treated in a phase II trial. Performance status WHO ≤2, age <75 years, and adequate organ function were required

Efficacy (N = 37)

Complete response	5.4%
Partial response	27%
Stable disease	35%
Median duration of response	6.5 months

Toxicity (N = 39 Patients/166 Cycles)

	G1/2 (% Cycles)	G3/4 (% Cycles)
Hematologic		
Leukopenia	23 (43)	74 (48)
Neutropenia	5 (20)	87 (61)
Anemia	74 (61)	5 (1)
Thrombocytopenia	13 (5)	0 (0)
Nonhematologic		
Skin toxicity	46	7.5
Asthenia	46	23
Peripheral neuropathy	41	—
Nausea	33	2.5
Edema	30.7	—
Vomiting	28.5	2.5
Stomatitis	25.6	13
Diarrhea	25.6	2.5
Phlebitis	23	—
Hypersensitivity	20.5	2.5
Myalgia	13	—

(continued)

- Advise patients who develop mucositis to:
  - Choose foods that are easy to chew and swallow
  - Take small bites of food, chew slowly, and sip liquids with meals
  - Encourage soft, moist foods such as cooked cereals, mashed potatoes, and scrambled eggs
  - For trouble swallowing, soften food with gravies, sauces, broths, yogurt, or other bland liquids
  - Avoid sharp, crunchy foods; hot, spicy or highly acidic foods (eg, citrus fruits and juices); sugary foods; toothpicks; tobacco products; alcoholic drinks

Treatment Modifications

Adverse Event	Dose Modification
G ≥2 cutaneous toxicity without recovery to G ≤1 at time of retreatment	Reduce docetaxel dosage 25%
G ≥2 peripheral neuropathy without recovery to G ≤1 at time of retreatment	
G4 granulocytopenia lasting more than 7 days or associated with fever >38.5°C (>101.3°F)	
G3/4 nonhematologic toxicity	

Therapy Monitoring

1. *Weekly:* CBC with differential
2. *During dexamethasone:* monitor glucose if indicated

METASTATIC DISEASE REGIMEN

GEFITINIB *OR* ERLOTINIB
(ORAL EPIDERMAL GROWTH FACTOR INHIBITORS)

Cohen EEW et al. J Clin Oncol 2003;21:1980–1987
Soulieres D et al. J Clin Oncol 2004;22:77–85

Gefitinib 500 mg; administer orally once daily, continually (total dose/week = 3500 mg)

or

Erlotinib 150 mg; administer orally once daily, continually (total dose/week = 1050 mg)
Note: Patients unable to swallow tablets or those with silicone-based feeding tubes may dissolve gefitinib or erlotinib tablets in water

Supportive Care
Antiemetic prophylaxis
*Emetogenic potential is **MINIMAL***
See Chapter 39 for antiemetic recommendations

Hematopoietic growth factor (CSF) prophylaxis
Primary prophylaxis is NOT indicated
See Chapter 43 for more information

Antimicrobial prophylaxis
Risk of fever and neutropenia is LOW
  Antimicrobial primary prophylaxis to be considered:
  • Antibacterial—not indicated
  • Antifungal—consider use during neutropenia and for anticipated mucositis
  • Antiviral—not indicated unless patient previously had an episode of HSV
See Chapter 47 for more information

Patient Population Studied

Gefitinib: 52 patients with recurrent or metastatic disease considered ineligible for curative surgery or radiation therapy who had received ≤1 prior systemic therapy. Performance status ECOG ≤2 and adequate organ function were required
Erlotinib: 115 patients with locally recurrent and/or metastatic head and neck squamous cell carcinoma regardless of their HER1/EGFR status. ECOG performance status 0–2

Efficacy (N = 47/115)

	Gefitinib (N = 47)	Erlotinib (N = 115)
Complete response	2.1%	0
Partial response	8.5%	4.3%
Stable disease	42.6%	38.3%
Median duration of response	1.6 months	
Median time to progression	3.4 months	9.6 weeks
Median survival	8.1 months	6 months
1-Year survival	29.2%	20%

Treatment Modifications

Adverse Event	Dose Modification
Gefitinib	
G2 Skin rash, nausea, or diarrhea	Hold gefitinib until toxicity G ≤1
Repeat G2 skin rash, nausea, or diarrhea	Reduce gefitinib dose to 250 mg/day
Other nonhematologic G2 toxicities	Hold gefitinib until toxicity G ≤1, then reduce dose to 250 mg/day
Any G3/4 toxicity	Hold gefitinib until toxicity resolves to G ≤1, then resume with dose reduced to 250 mg daily
Toxicity not resolved to G ≤1 after interrupting treatment for 2 weeks, or a second dose reduction indicated	Discontinue treatment
Erlotinib	
G2 skin rash	Hold erlotinib until toxicity G ≤1
Repeat G2 skin rash	Reduce erlotinib dose to 100 mg/day
Other nonhematologic G2/3 toxicities	Hold erlotinib until toxicity G ≤1, then reduce erlotinib dose to 100 mg/day
G4 toxicity	Discontinue erlotinib
Treatment for 4 weeks at the same daily dose without adverse effects attributed to erlotinib	Escalate the daily dose in 50-mg/day increments to a maximum daily dose of 250 mg (stepwise increases from 150 mg/day to 200 mg/day to 250 mg/day)

Toxicity (N = 50/115)	Gefitinib (N = 50)		Erlotinib (N = 115)	
	% G1/2	% G3/4	% G1/2	% G3/4
Skin rash	48	0	34	6
Diarrhea	44	6	17	2
Anorexia	20	6		
Nausea	14	4	9	0
Vomiting	12	0	N/A	
Dyspnea	6	0	N/A	
Keratitis	4	0	N/A	
↑AST	12	0		
↑ALT	4	0	24	2
↑Alkaline phosphatase	4	0		
↑Creatinine	2	0	10	
Hypercalcemia	14	6		

Therapy Monitoring

1. *Every 8 weeks:* Tumor response evaluation
2. *Shortness of breath:* Stop gefitinib and evaluate for pneumonitis

Notes

Protocol for managing rash:
- Mild soap and lukewarm water to wash affected area
- Moisturize area with mild lotion
- Limit direct sun exposure. Use a sunscreen appropriate for sensitive skin (SPF15 or higher)
- Avoid over-the-counter acne treatments
- Avoid applying cosmetic products

METASTATIC DISEASE REGIMEN

DOCETAXEL + CISPLATIN

Glisson BS et al. J Clin Oncol 2002;20:1593–1599

Premedication:
Dexamethasone 8 mg; administer orally or intravenously twice daily for 3 days starting the day before docetaxel infusion (total dose/cycle = 48 mg)

Hydration before, during, and after cisplatin administration ± mannitol:
- *Pre-cisplatin hydration* with 1000 mL 0.9% sodium chloride injection (0.9% NS); administer intravenously with potassium and magnesium supplementation as needed based on pretreatment laboratory results
- *Mannitol diuresis:* May be given to patients who have received adequate hydration. A dose of **mannitol** 12.5–25 g may be administered by intravenous injection or a short infusion before or during cisplatin administration, or prepared as an admixture with cisplatin. Continued intravenous hydration is essential
- *Continued mannitol diuresis:* In an inpatient or day-hospital setting, one may administer additional mannitol in the form of an intravenous infusion: **mannitol** 10–40 g; administer intravenously over 1–4 hours. This can be done either during or immediately after cisplatin, but requires maintenance of adequate intravenously administered fluids during and for hours after mannitol administration
- *Post-cisplatin hydration* with ≥1000 mL 0.9% NS; administer intravenously with potassium and magnesium supplementation as needed based on measured values

Docetaxel 75 mg/m²; administer intravenously diluted in a volume of 0.9% NS or 5% dextrose injection sufficient to produce a docetaxel concentration within the range 0.3–0.74 mg/mL over 60 minutes, on day 1, every 21 days (total dosage/cycle = 75 mg/m²), *followed by*
Cisplatin 75 mg/m²; administer intravenously in 25–250 mL 0.9% NS over 30 minutes on day 1, every 21 days (total dosage/cycle = 75 mg/m²)

Supportive Care
Antiemetic prophylaxis
Emetogenic potential is **HIGH**. *Potential for delayed symptoms*
See Chapter 39 for antiemetic recommendations

Hematopoietic growth factor (CSF) prophylaxis
Primary prophylaxis is NOT indicated
See Chapter 43 for more information

Antimicrobial prophylaxis
Risk of fever and neutropenia is LOW
   Antimicrobial primary prophylaxis to be considered:
   - Antibacterial—not indicated
   - Antifungal—not indicated
   - Antiviral—not indicated unless patient previously had an episode of HSV
See Chapter 47 for more information

Oral care (mucositis prophylaxis and management)
Risk of mucositis/stomatitis is LOW–MODERATE
   General advice:
   - Encourage patients to maintain intake of non-alcoholic fluids
   - Evaluate patients for oral pain and provide analgesic medications
   - Consider histamine (H$_2$-subtype) receptor antagonists (eg, ranitidine, famotidine), or a proton pump inhibitor for epigastric pain
   - *Lactobacillus* sp.-containing probiotics may be beneficial in preventing diarrhea
   Patients with intact oral mucosa:
   - Clean the mouth, tongue, and gums by brushing after every meal and at bedtime with an ultra-soft toothbrush with fluoride toothpaste
   - Floss teeth gently every day unless contraindicated. If gums bleed and hurt, avoid bleeding or sore areas, but floss other teeth
   - Patients may use saline or commercial bland, non-alcoholic rinses
     - Do not use mouthwashes that contain alcohols

(continued)

Treatment Modifications

Adverse Event	Dose Modification
ANC <1500/mm³ *or* platelets <100,000/mm³ at the time of chemotherapy administration	Delay chemotherapy until ANC > 1500/mm³ *and* platelets >100,000/mm³. Discontinue if recovery has not occurred after a 3-week delay
Creatinine clearance <50 mL/min (<0.83 mL/s)	Do not administer therapy
Serum creatinine >1.5 mg/dL (>133 μmol/L) or 20% higher than baseline value if baseline was >1.5 mg/dL (>133 μmol/L)	Hold cisplatin until serum creatinine <1.5 mg/dL (<133 μmol/L) or within 0.2 mg/dL (17.7 μmol/L) of baseline
Serum creatinine 1.5–2.0 mg/dL (133–177 μmol/L) immediately before a cycle	Hold cisplatin*, then reduce cisplatin dosage by 25% during subsequent cycles
Serum creatinine 2.1–3.0 mg/dL (186–265 μmol/L) immediately before a cycle	Hold cisplatin*, then reduce cisplatin dosage by 50% during subsequent cycles
Serum creatinine >3.0 mg/dL (>265 μmol/L) immediately before a cycle	Hold cisplatin
G2 neurotoxicity or ototoxicity	Hold cisplatin until neurotoxicity resolves to G ≤1
G3/4 neurotoxicity or ototoxicity	Discontinue chemotherapy

*Hold cisplatin until serum creatinine <1.5 mg/dL (<133 μmol/L) or within 0.2 mg/dL (17.7 μmol/L) of baseline

(continued)

If mucositis or stomatitis is present:

- Keep the mouth moist utilizing water, ice chips, sugarless gum, sugar-free hard candies, or a saliva substitute
- Rinse mouth several times a day to remove debris
  - Use a solution of ¼ teaspoon (1.25 g) each of baking soda and table salt (sodium chloride) in one quart (~950 mL) of warm water. Follow with a plain water rinse
  - Do not use mouthwashes that contain alcohols
- Foam-tipped swabs (eg, Toothettes®) are useful in moisturizing oral mucosa, but ineffective for cleansing teeth and removing plaque
- Advise patients who develop mucositis to:
  - Choose foods that are easy to chew and swallow
  - Take small bites of food, chew slowly, and sip liquids with meals
  - Encourage soft, moist foods such as cooked cereals, mashed potatoes, and scrambled eggs
  - For trouble swallowing, soften food with gravies, sauces, broths, yogurt, or other bland liquids
  - Avoid sharp, crunchy foods; hot, spicy or highly acidic foods (eg, citrus fruits and juices); sugary foods; toothpicks; tobacco products; alcoholic drinks

Patient Population Studied

A study of 36 patients with recurrent disease or disease deemed incurable, who had not previously received chemotherapy for recurrent disease and had never received a taxane, were entered in a multicenter phase II trial. Performance status ECOG 0–1 and adequate organ function were required, including creatinine clearance ≥50 mL/min (≥0.83 mL/s)

Efficacy (N = 36)

Complete response	6%
Partial response	34%
Stable disease	34%
Median duration of response	4.9 months
Median time to response	5 weeks
Median time to treatment failure	3 months
Median survival	9.6 months
1-Year survival	28%
2-Year survival	19%

Toxicity (N = 35/36)

	% G1/2	% G3/4
Hematologic (N = 35)		
Neutropenia	NR	80
Thrombocytopenia	NR	3
Anemia	NR	14
Nonhematologic (N = 36)		
Nausea	56	11
Asthenia	53	25
Stomatitis	44	3
Vomiting	41	8
Neurosensory	39	3
Diarrhea	38	6
Infection	27	17
Skin	19	0
Neurosensory, hearing	17	0
Pulmonary	14	8
Allergy	14	8
Neuromotor	14	3
Hypotension	14	0
G5 toxicity	2.8%	

NR, Not reported
National Cancer Institute Common Toxicity Criteria

Therapy Monitoring

1. *Weekly:* CBC with differential
2. *Before each cycle:* Serum electrolytes, creatinine, calcium, magnesium, LFTs, and urinalysis
3. *During dexamethasone:* monitor glucose if indicated

METASTATIC DISEASE REGIMEN
PACLITAXEL + CARBOPLATIN

Pivot X et al. Oncology 2001;60:66–71

Premedication:

Prednisone 60 mg; administer orally twice daily for a total of 4 doses, starting the day before chemotherapy (total dose/cycle = 240 mg), *or*

Dexamethasone 20 mg/dose; administer orally for 2 doses at 12–14 hours and 6–7 hours before starting paclitaxel administration (total dose/cycle = 40 mg), *or*

Dexamethasone 20 mg; administer intravenously 30 minutes before starting paclitaxel administration (total dose/cycle = 20 mg)

Cimetidine 300 mg (*or* **Ranitidine** 50 mg *or* **Famotidine** 20 mg or an equivalent histamine receptor [H2]-subtype antagonist); administer intravenously over 15–30 minutes, 30–60 minutes before paclitaxel

Diphenhydramine 50 mg; administer by intravenous injection, 30–60 minutes before paclitaxel

Paclitaxel 175 mg/m²; administer by intravenous infusion in a volume of 0.9% NS or D5W sufficient to produce a concentration within the range 0.3–1.2 mg/mL over 3 hours on day 1, every 21 days (total dosage/cycle = 175 mg/m²), *followed by:*

Carboplatin (calculated dose) AUC = 6 mg/mL · min; administer by intravenous infusion in 500 mL of 0.9% NS over 2 hours on day 1, every 21 days (total dosage/cycle calculated to produce an AUC of 6 mg/mL · min)

An equation for calculating carboplatin doses developed by Chatelut et al accounts for inter-individual carboplatin clearance (CL) based on patient-specific factors for weight, age, and sex (Chatelut E et al. J Natl Cancer Inst 1995;87:573–580):

$$\text{CL(females)} = (0.134 \times \text{wt}) + \frac{\left[(218 \times \text{wt}) \times (1 - 0.00457 \times \text{age}) \times 0.686\right]}{\text{serum creatinine}}$$

$$\text{CL(males)} = (0.134 \times \text{wt}) + \frac{\left[(218 \times \text{wt}) \times (1 - 0.00457 \times \text{age})\right]}{\text{serum creatinine}}$$

Weight is expressed in kilogram units, age in years, serum creatinine in micromoles/L (micromoles/L = mg/dL × 88.4), and the value for sex is 0 (zero) for males and 1 (one) for females

A carboplatin dose (in milligrams) is calculated from a target area under the plasma concentration versus time curve (AUC) and a value for carboplatin clearance (CL) appropriate for a female or male patient:

$$\text{Carboplatin dose (mg)} = \text{CL (mL/min)} \times \text{AUC (mg} \cdot \text{min/mL)}$$

Supportive Care
Antiemetic prophylaxis

Emetogenic potential is **HIGH**. *Potential for delayed symptoms*

See Chapter 39 for antiemetic recommendations

Hematopoietic growth factor (CSF) prophylaxis

Primary prophylaxis is indicated with one of the following:

Filgrastim (G-CSF) 5 mcg/kg per day, by subcutaneous injection, *or*

Pegfilgrastim (pegylated filgrastim) 6 mg/0.6 mL, by subcutaneous injection for one dose

- Begin use from 24–72 h after myelosuppressive chemotherapy is completed
- Continue daily Filgrastim use until ANC ≥10,000/mm³ on two measurements separated temporally by ≥12 hours
- Discontinue daily Filgrastim use at least 24 hours before administering myelosuppressive treatment. Do not administer Pegfilgrastim within 14 days before administering myelosuppressive treatment

See Chapter 43 for more information

Antimicrobial prophylaxis

Risk of fever and neutropenia is INTERMEDIATE

Antimicrobial primary prophylaxis to be considered:

- Antibacterial—consider a fluoroquinolone or no prophylaxis
- Antifungal—consider concomitant use of cotrimoxazole during periods of neutropenia, and in anticipation of mucositis
- Antiviral—not indicated, unless patient previously had an episode of HSV

See Chapter 47 for more information

Oral care

Risk of mucositis/stomatitis is MODERATE

General advice:

- Encourage patients to maintain intake of non-alcoholic fluids
- Evaluate patients for oral pain and provide analgesic medications

(continued)

(*continued*)

- Consider histamine (H$_2$-subtype) receptor antagonists (eg, ranitidine, famotidine), or a proton pump inhibitor for epigastric pain
- *Lactobacillus* sp.-containing probiotics may be beneficial in preventing diarrhea

Patients with intact oral mucosa:
- Clean the mouth, tongue, and gums by brushing after every meal and at bedtime with an ultra-soft toothbrush with fluoride toothpaste
- Floss teeth gently every day unless contraindicated. If gums bleed and hurt, avoid bleeding or sore areas, but floss other teeth
- Patients may use saline or commercial bland, non-alcoholic rinses
  - Do not use mouthwashes that contain alcohols

If mucositis or stomatitis is present:
- Keep the mouth moist utilizing water, ice chips, sugarless gum, sugar-free hard candies, or a saliva substitute
- Rinse mouth several times a day to remove debris
  - Use a solution of ¼ teaspoon (1.25 g) each of baking soda and table salt (sodium chloride) in one quart (~950 mL) of warm water. Follow with a plain water rinse
  - Do not use mouthwashes that contain alcohols
- Foam-tipped swabs (eg, Toothettes®) are useful in moisturizing oral mucosa, but ineffective for cleansing teeth and removing plaque
- Advise patients who develop mucositis to:
  - Choose foods that are easy to chew and swallow
  - Take small bites of food, chew slowly, and sip liquids with meals
  - Encourage soft, moist foods such as cooked cereals, mashed potatoes, and scrambled eggs
  - For trouble swallowing, soften food with gravies, sauces, broths, yogurt, or other bland liquids
  - Avoid sharp, crunchy foods; hot, spicy or highly acidic foods (eg, citrus fruits and juices); sugary foods; toothpicks; tobacco products; alcoholic drinks

Patient Population Studied

A study of 27 patients with unresectable recurrent disease or distant metastatic disease. Previous radiation treatment and concomitant or induction chemoradiation were allowed. ECOG performance status 0–2 and adequate organ function were required, including creatinine clearance ≥45 mL/min (≥0.75 mL/s)

Efficacy (N = 27)

Complete response	7.4%
Partial response	22.2%
Stable disease	11.1%
Median duration of response	4.4 months
Median survival	7.2 months

SWOG Criteria

Toxicity (N = 27)

	% G2	% G3/4
Hematologic		
Anemia	40.7	11.1
Neutropenia	14.8	62.9
Febrile neutropenia	—	18.5
Thrombocytopenia	11.1	14.8
Nonhematologic		
Alopecia	29.6	44.4
Neurotoxicity (neuropathy)	11.1	7.4
Mucositis	11.1	7.4
Nausea/vomiting	7.4	7.4
Cardiotoxicity		3.7
G5 toxicity	3.7%*	

*One patient with neutropenia and sepsis
National Cancer Institute Common Toxicity Criteria

Therapy Monitoring

1. *Before each cycle:* CBC with differential, serum electrolytes, calcium, magnesium, and LFTs
2. *Weekly:* CBC with differential

Treatment Modifications

Adverse Event	Dose Modification
G3/4 mucositis	Reduce paclitaxel dosage by 20%
G3 thrombocytopenia	Reduce paclitaxel dosage by 20%
G4 thrombocytopenia	Reduce paclitaxel dosage by 50%
G4 neutropenia >5 days	Reduce paclitaxel dosage by 20%
ANC <1500/mm^3 or platelets <100,000/mm^3 at the time of chemotherapy administration	Delay chemotherapy until ANC >1500/mm^3 *and* platelets >100,000/mm^3. Discontinue chemotherapy if recovery has not occurred after a 2-week delay
Creatinine clearance (Clcr) <45 mL/min (<0.75 mL/s)	Delay treatment until Clcr >45 mL/min (>0.75 mL/s). Discontinue therapy if has not recovered by 6 weeks
G2 neurotoxicity	Hold paclitaxel until neurotoxicity resolves to G ≤1
G 3/4 neurotoxicity	Discontinue chemotherapy

RECURRENT/METASTATIC DISEASE

PLATINUM-REFRACTORY TUMORS SINGLE-AGENT CETUXIMAB

Vermorken JB et al. J Clin Oncol 2007;25:2171–2177

Cetuximab premedication:
Diphenhydramine 50 mg; administer by intravenous injection or infusion before cetuximab administration (other H_1-receptor antagonists may be substituted)

Initial cetuximab dose:
Cetuximab 400 mg/m²; administer intravenously over 120 minutes (maximum infusion rate = 5 mL [10 mg] per min) as a single loading dose (total initial dosage = 400 mg/m²)

Maintenance cetuximab doses:
Cetuximab 250 mg/m² per dose; administer intravenously over 60 minutes (maximum infusion rate = 5 mL [10 mg] per min) every week, continually (total weekly dosage = 250 mg/m²)

Notes:
Cetuximab is intended for direct administration and should not be diluted
Maximum infusion rate = 5 mL (10 mg)/min
Administer cetuximab through a low protein-binding inline filter with pore size = 0.22 μm
Use 0.9% sodium chloride injection to flush vascular access devices after administration is completed

Note: Continue cetuximab single-agent therapy for at least 6 weeks. If tumors appear to respond to treatment and disease stability (SD) is attained, treatment may be continued until progressive disease (PD), clinical deterioration, or unacceptable adverse events are observed

Supportive Care
Antiemetic prophylaxis
*Emetogenic potential is **MINIMAL***
See Chapter 39 for antiemetic recommendations

Hematopoietic growth factor (CSF) prophylaxis
Primary prophylaxis is NOT indicated
See Chapter 43 for more information

Antimicrobial prophylaxis
Risk of fever and neutropenia is LOW
 Antimicrobial primary prophylaxis to be considered:
 • Antibacterial—not indicated
 • Antifungal—not indicated
 • Antiviral—not indicated unless patient previously had an episode of HSV
See Chapter 47 for more information

Dose Modifications

Adverse Event	Treatment Modifications
Progressive disease, clinical deterioration, or unacceptable toxicity	Discontinue treatment
First occurrence G3 skin toxicity	Hold cetuximab up to 2 weeks
Second occurrence G3 skin toxicity	Reduce cetuximab dosage to 200 mg/m²
Third occurrence G3 skin toxicity	Reduce cetuximab dosage to 150 mg/m²
Fourth occurrence G3 skin toxicity	Discontinue cetuximab

Efficacy (N = 103)

Overall response rate	0
Complete response rate	13%
Stable disease	33%
Progressive disease	37%
Disease not assessable	18%
Median time to progression	70 days
Median overall survival	178 days

Toxicity (N = 103)*

Adverse Event	% All Grades	% G3/4
Rash	49	1
Acne	26	0
Asthenia	24	4
Nail disorder	16	0
Dry skin	14	0
Fever	14	1
Nausea	13	1
Vomiting	11	2
Dyspnea	5	4
Infusion-related reactions	6	1
Treatment-related death	1 Patient	

*Common Toxicity Criteria, version 2.0, (U.S.) National Cancer Institute

Patient Population Studied

A study of 103 patients with measurable metastatic and/or recurrent histologically proven squamous cell carcinoma of the head and neck with documented disease progression within 30 days after a minimum of 2 cycles and a maximum of 6 cycles of chemotherapy: cisplatin-based (≥60 mg/m² per cycle) or carboplatin-based (≥300 mg/m², or dose based on target AUC ≥4 mg/mL · min per cycle). Adequate organ function, a Karnofsky performance status ≥60, and age ≥18 years were required

Therapy Monitoring

1. *Pretreatment evaluation:* Medical history and tumor assessment by clinical evaluation and imaging studies
2. *Response evaluation:* Every 6 weeks

RECURRENT/METASTATIC DISEASE: PLATINUM-REFRACTORY TUMORS

CISPLATIN- *OR* CARBOPLATIN-BASED CHEMOTHERAPY + CETUXIMAB

Baselga J et al. J Clin Oncol 2005;23:5568–5577

Cetuximab premedication:
Diphenhydramine 50 mg; administer by intravenous injection or infusion before cetuximab administration (other H_1-receptor antagonists may be substituted)

Initial cetuximab dose:
Cetuximab 400 mg/m²; administer intravenously over 120 minutes (maximum infusion rate = 5 mL [10 mg] per min) as a single loading dose (total initial dosage = 400 mg/m²)

Maintenance cetuximab doses:
Cetuximab 250 mg/m² per dose; administer intravenously over 60 minutes (maximum infusion rate = 5 mL [10 mg] per min) every week, continually (total weekly dosage = 250 mg/m²)

Notes:
Cetuximab is intended for direct administration and should not be diluted
Maximum infusion rate = 5 mL (10 mg) per minute
Administer cetuximab through a low protein-binding inline filter with pore size = 0.22 μm
Use 0.9% sodium chloride injection to flush vascular access devices after administration is completed
One hour after completing cetuximab administration, either cisplatin *or* carboplatin is given

Note: In the study reported by Baselga et al, carboplatin or cisplatin were administered at the same doses, routes of administration, and every 3- or 4-week schedules utilized in the regimens subjects had received during which they developed disease progression

Suggested Cisplatin and Carboplatin Regimens

(Vermorken JB et al. N Engl J Med 2008;359:1116–1127)

Cisplatin + Fluorouracil Regimen

Hydration before, during, and after cisplatin administration ± mannitol:
• *Pre-cisplatin hydration* with 1000 mL 0.9% sodium chloride injection (0.9% NS); administer intravenously with potassium and magnesium supplementation as needed based on pretreatment laboratory results
• *Mannitol diuresis:* May be given to patients who have received adequate hydration. A dose of **mannitol** 12.5–25 g may be administered by intravenous injection or a short infusion before or during cisplatin administration, or prepared as an admixture with cisplatin. Continued intravenous hydration is essential
• *Continued mannitol diuresis:* In an inpatient or day-hospital setting, one may administer additional mannitol in the form of an intravenous infusion: **mannitol** 10–40 g; administer intravenously over 1–4 hours. This can be done either during or immediately after cisplatin, but requires maintenance of adequate intravenously administered fluids during and for hours after mannitol administration
• *Post-cisplatin hydration* with ≥1000 mL 0.9% NS; administer intravenously with potassium and magnesium supplementation as needed based on measured values

Cisplatin 100 mg/m²; administer intravenously in 50–1000 mL 0.9% NS over 60 minutes on day 1 at least one hour after completing cetuximab doses, every 3 weeks (total dosage/cycle = 100 mg/m²), *followed by:*

Fluorouracil 1000 mg/m² per day; administer in 50–1000 mL 0.9% NS or D5W by continuous intravenous infusion over 24 hours for 4 consecutive days on days 1–4, every 3 weeks (total dosage/cycle = 4000 mg/m²)

Carboplatin + Fluorouracil Regimen

Carboplatin* (calculated dose) AUC = 5 mg/mL · min per dose; administer by intravenous infusion diluted to concentrations as low as 0.5 mg/mL with either D5W or 0.9% NS over 1 hour, on day 1 at least one hour after completing cetuximab doses, every 3 weeks (total dose/cycle calculated to produce a target AUC = 5 mg/mL · min), *followed by:*

Fluorouracil 1000 mg/m² per day; administer in 50–1000 mL 0.9% NS or D5W by continuous intravenous infusion over 24 hours for 4 consecutive days, on days 1–4, every 21 days for 4 cycles (total dosage/cycle = 4000 mg/m²)

*Carboplatin dose is based on a formula described by Calvert et al. to achieve a target area under the plasma concentration versus time curve (AUC)

$$\text{Total Carboplatin Dose (mg)} = (\text{target AUC}) \times (\text{GFR} + 25)$$

(continued)

(continued)

In practice, creatinine clearance (Clcr) is used in place of glomerular filtration rate (GFR). Clcr can be estimated from the equation of Cockcroft and Gault, thus:

$$\text{For males, Clcr} = \frac{(140 - \text{age [years]}) \times (\text{body weight [kg]})}{72 \times (\text{serum creatinine [mg/dL]})}$$

$$\text{For females, Clcr} = \frac{(140 - \text{age [years]}) \times (\text{body weight [kg]})}{72 \times (\text{serum creatinine [mg/dL]})} \times 0.85$$

Calvert AH et al. J Clin Oncol 1989;7:1748–1756
Cockcroft DW , Gault MH. Nephron 1976;16:31–41
Jodrell DI et al. J Clin Oncol 1992;10:520–528
Sorensen BT et al. Cancer ChemotherPharmacol 1991;28:397–401

Note: On October 8, 2010, the U.S. FDA identified a potential safety issue with carboplatin dosing based on recent changes in the measurement of serum creatinine. By the end of 2010, all clinical laboratories in the United States were required to use the standardized Isotope Dilution Mass Spectrometry (IDMS) method to measure serum creatinine, which can result in an overestimation of the GFR in some patients with normal renal function. A carboplatin dose calculated with an IDMS-measured serum creatinine result using the Calvert formula can exceed an expected exposure (AUC) and result in increased drug-related toxicity

Provided actual GFR measurements are made to assess renal function, carboplatin can be safely dosed according to the Calvert formula described in product labeling

If GFR (or creatinine clearance) is estimated based on serum creatinine measurements by the IDMS method, the FDA recommends, for patients with normal renal function, capping an estimated GFR at 125 mL/min for any targeted AUC value. No greater estimated GFR values should be used

U.S. FDA. Carboplatin dosing. [online] October 8, 2010. Available from: http://www.fda.gov/AboutFDA/CentersOffices/OfficeofMedicalProductsandTobacco/CDER/ucm228974.htm [accessed February 26, 2014]

Supportive Care
Antiemetic prophylaxis
Emetogenic potential on days with cetuximab alone is **MINIMAL**
Emetogenic potential on days with cisplatin or carboplatin is **HIGH**. *Potential for delayed symptoms*
Emetogenic potential on days with fluorouracil alone is **LOW**
See Chapter 39 for antiemetic recommendations

Hematopoietic growth factor (CSF) prophylaxis
Primary prophylaxis is NOT indicated
See Chapter 43 for more information

Antimicrobial prophylaxis
Risk of fever and neutropenia is LOW
 Antimicrobial primary prophylaxis to be considered:
- Antibacterial—not indicated
- Antifungal—not indicated
- Antiviral—not indicated unless patient previously had an episode of HSV

See Chapter 47 for more information

Oral care
Risk of mucositis/stomatitis is MODERATE
 General advice:
- Encourage patients to maintain intake of non-alcoholic fluids
- Evaluate patients for oral pain and provide analgesic medications
- Consider histamine (H_2-subtype) receptor antagonists (eg, ranitidine, famotidine), or a proton pump inhibitor for epigastric pain
- *Lactobacillus* sp.-containing probiotics may be beneficial in preventing diarrhea

 Patients with intact oral mucosa:
- Clean the mouth, tongue, and gums by brushing after every meal and at bedtime with an ultra-soft toothbrush with fluoride toothpaste
- Floss teeth gently every day unless contraindicated. If gums bleed and hurt, avoid bleeding or sore areas, but floss other teeth
- Patients may use saline or commercial bland, non-alcoholic rinses
  - Do not use mouthwashes that contain alcohols

(continued)

(*continued*)

If mucositis or stomatitis is present:
- Keep the mouth moist utilizing water, ice chips, sugarless gum, sugar-free hard candies, or a saliva substitute
- Rinse mouth several times a day to remove debris
  - Use a solution of ¼ teaspoon (1.25 g) each of baking soda and table salt (sodium chloride) in one quart (~950 mL) of warm water. Follow with a plain water rinse
  - Do not use mouthwashes that contain alcohols
- Foam-tipped swabs (eg, Toothettes®) are useful in moisturizing oral mucosa, but ineffective for cleansing teeth and removing plaque
- Advise patients who develop mucositis to:
  - Choose foods that are easy to chew and swallow
  - Take small bites of food, chew slowly, and sip liquids with meals
  - Encourage soft, moist foods such as cooked cereals, mashed potatoes, and scrambled eggs
  - For trouble swallowing, soften food with gravies, sauces, broths, yogurt, or other bland liquids
  - Avoid sharp, crunchy foods; hot, spicy or highly acidic foods (eg, citrus fruits and juices); sugary foods; toothpicks; tobacco products; alcoholic drinks

Patient Population Studied

A study of 98 patients with measurable, stage III or IV squamous cell carcinoma of the head and neck, who were not candidates for local therapy, with disease progression after a minimum of 2 and a maximum of 4 cycles of cisplatin- or carboplatin-based chemotherapy. Adequate organ function, a Karnofsky performance status of ≥60, and age ≥18 years were required

Efficacy (N = 96)

Overall response rate	10%
Complete response rate	0
Partial response rate	10%
Stable disease	43%
Progressive disease	28%
Not assessable	19%

Median overall survival, days	183
Median time to progression, days	85

Toxicity (N = 96)*

Adverse Event	% All Grades	% G3/4
Skin reactions	80	3
Acne-like rash	72	3
Asthenia	65	19
Mucositis	18	2
Diarrhea	16	0
Fever	40	3
Nausea/vomiting	57	6
Respiratory disorder	32	13
Hypersensitivity reactions	3	0
Heart failure	2	0
Thromboembolism	2	2
Bleeding	24	8

*Common Toxicity Criteria, version 2.0, (U.S.) National Cancer Institute

Therapy Monitoring

1. *Pretreatment evaluation:* Medical history and tumor assessment by clinical evaluation and imaging studies
2. *Response evaluation:* Every 6 weeks

Treatment Modifications

Adverse Event	Dose Modification
First occurrence G3 skin toxicity	Hold cetuximab up to 2 weeks
Second occurrence G3 skin toxicity	Reduce cetuximab dosage to 200 mg/m²
Third occurrence G3 skin toxicity	Reduce cetuximab dosage to 150 mg/m²
Fourth occurrence G3 skin toxicity	Discontinue cetuximab
G ≥2 mucosal or skin toxicity	Reduce fluorouracil dosage by 20%
G ≥2 diarrhea (4–6 stools/day greater than baseline)	Hold fluorouracil until diarrhea resolves to baseline
G3 myelosuppression	Reduce cisplatin dosage by 25% or carboplatin dosage by 20%. Do not change fluorouracil dosage
G4 myelosuppression	Reduce cisplatin dosage by 40% or carboplatin dosage by 20%. Do not change fluorouracil dosage
Creatinine clearance <50 mL/min (<0.83 mL/s)	Do not administer therapy
Serum creatinine >1.5 mg/dL (>133 μmol/L), or 20% greater than baseline if baseline was >1.5 mg/dL	Hold cisplatin dosage until serum creatinine <1.5 mg/dL (<133 μmol/L) or within 0.2 mg/dL (17.7 μmol/L) of baseline
Serum creatinine 1.5–2.0 mg/dL (133–177 μmol/L) immediately before a cycle	Hold cisplatin*, then reduce cisplatin dosage by 25% during subsequent cycles
Serum creatinine 2.1–3.0 mg/dL (186–265 μmol/L) immediately before a cycle	Hold cisplatin*, then reduce cisplatin dosage by 50% during subsequent cycles
Serum creatinine >3.0 mg/dL (>265 μmol/L) immediately before a cycle	Hold cisplatin
G2 neurotoxicity or ototoxicity	Hold cisplatin until neurotoxicity resolves to G ≤1
G3/4 neurotoxicity or ototoxicity	Discontinue chemotherapy
G ≥3 nausea/vomiting despite use of a serotonin (5HT₃) receptor antagonist + dexamethasone + aprepitant, consistent with published guidelines (see Chapter 39)	Reduce cisplatin dosage or carboplatin dose, or discontinue the platinating agent

*Hold cisplatin until serum creatinine <1.5 mg/dL or within 0.2 mg/dL of baseline

RECURRENT/METASTATIC DISEASE: ADVANCED DISEASE

CISPLATIN + PACLITAXEL
CISPLATIN + FLUOROURACIL

Gibson MK et al. J Clin Oncol 2005;23:3562–3567

Cisplatin + Paclitaxel

Premedication for paclitaxel
Dexamethasone 20 mg/dose; administer orally or intravenously for 2 doses at 12–14 hours and 6–7 hours before starting paclitaxel (total dose/cycle = 40 mg), *or*
Dexamethasone 20 mg; administer intravenously 30 minutes before administering paclitaxel (total dose/cycle = 20 mg)

plus

Diphenhydramine 50 mg; administer intravenously 30 minutes before administering paclitaxel
Cimetidine 300 mg (*or* **Ranitidine** 50 mg *or* **Famotidine** 20 mg *or* an equivalent histamine receptor [H_2]-subtype antagonist); administer intravenously in 20–50 mL 0.9% sodium chloride injection (0.9% NS) or 5% dextrose injection (D5W) over 15–20 minutes, 30 minutes before administering paclitaxel

Hydration before, during, and after cisplatin administration ± mannitol:
* *Pre-cisplatin hydration* with 1000 mL 0.9% NS; administer intravenously with potassium and magnesium supplementation as needed based on pretreatment laboratory results
* *Mannitol diuresis:* May be given to patients who have received adequate hydration. A dose of **mannitol** 12.5–25 g may be administered by intravenous injection or a short infusion before or during cisplatin administration, or prepared as an admixture with cisplatin. Continued intravenous hydration is essential
* *Continued mannitol diuresis:* In an inpatient or day-hospital setting, one may administer additional mannitol in the form of an intravenous infusion: **mannitol** 10–40 g; administer intravenously over 1–4 hours. This can be done either during or immediately after cisplatin, but requires maintenance of adequate intravenously administered fluids during and for hours after mannitol administration
* *Post-cisplatin hydration* with ≥1000 mL 0.9% NS; administer intravenously with potassium and magnesium supplementation as needed based on measured values

Paclitaxel 175 mg/mg; administer intravenously in a volume of 0.9% NS or D5W sufficient to produce a concentration within the range 0.3–1.2 mg/mL over 3 hours on day 1, every 21 days (total dosage/cycle = 175 mg/m²), *followed by:*
Cisplatin 75 mg/m²; administer intravenously in 50–1000 mL 0.9% NS over 60 minutes on day 1, every 21 days (total dosage/cycle = 75 mg/m²)

Notes: Treatment is continued for at least 6 cycles in patients who continue to respond
Carboplatin (target AUC = 6 mg/mL · min) may be substituted for cisplatin in patients who develop G ≥2 neuropathy or renal impairment (creatinine clearance <50 mL/min [<0.83 mL/s])

Supportive Care
Antiemetic prophylaxis
Emetogenic potential on day 1 is **HIGH**. *Potential for delayed symptoms*
See Chapter 39 for antiemetic recommendations

Hematopoietic growth factor (CSF) prophylaxis
Primary prophylaxis is NOT indicated
See Chapter 43 for more information

Antimicrobial prophylaxis
Risk of fever and neutropenia is LOW
   Antimicrobial primary prophylaxis to be considered:
   * Antibacterial—not indicated
   * Antifungal—not indicated
   * Antiviral—not indicated unless patient previously had an episode of HSV
See Chapter 47 for more information

Cisplatin + Fluorouracil

Hydration before, during, and after cisplatin administration ± mannitol:
* *Pre-cisplatin hydration* with 1000 mL 0.9% sodium chloride injection (0.9% NS); administer intravenously with potassium and magnesium supplementation as needed based on pretreatment laboratory results
* *Mannitol diuresis:* May be given to patients who have received adequate hydration. A dose of **mannitol** 12.5–25 g may be administered by intravenous injection or a short infusion before or during cisplatin administration, or prepared as an admixture with cisplatin. Continued intravenous hydration is essential

(continued)

(*continued*)

- *Continued mannitol diuresis:* In an inpatient or day-hospital setting, one may administer additional mannitol in the form of an intravenous infusion: **mannitol** 10–40 g; administer intravenously over 1–4 hours. This can be done either during or immediately after cisplatin, but requires maintenance of adequate intravenously administered fluids during and for hours after mannitol administration

- *Post-cisplatin hydration* with ≥1000 mL 0.9% NS; administer intravenously with potassium and magnesium supplementation as needed based on measured values

Cisplatin 100 mg/m²; administer intravenously in 50–1000 mL 0.9% NS over 60 minutes on day 1, every 21 days (total dosage/cycle = 100 mg/m²)

Fluorouracil 1000 mg/m² per day; administer in 50–1000 mL 0.9% NS or 5% dextrose injection by continuous intravenous infusion over 24 hours for 4 consecutive days, on days 1–4, every 21 days (total dosage/cycle = 4000 mg/m²)

Notes: Treatment is continued for at least 6 cycles in patients who continue to respond. Carboplatin (target AUC = 6 mg/mL · min) may be substituted for cisplatin in patients who develop G ≥2 neuropathy or renal impairment (creatinine clearance <50 mL/min [<0.83 mL/s])

Supportive Care

Antiemetic prophylaxis

Emetogenic potential on days with cisplatin or carboplatin is **HIGH**. *Potential for delayed symptoms*

Emetogenic potential on days with fluorouracil alone is **LOW**

See Chapter 39 for antiemetic recommendations

Hematopoietic growth factor (CSF) prophylaxis

Primary prophylaxis may be indicated

See Chapter 43 for more information

Antimicrobial prophylaxis

Risk of fever and neutropenia is LOW

Antimicrobial primary prophylaxis to be considered:

- Antibacterial—consider a fluoroquinolone or no prophylaxis

- Antifungal—not indicated

- Antiviral—not indicated unless patient previously had an episode of HSV

See Chapter 47 for more information

Diarrhea management

Latent or delayed onset diarrhea*:

Loperamide 4 mg orally initially after the first loose or liquid stool, *then*

Loperamide 2 mg orally every 2 hours during waking hours, *plus*

Loperamide 4 mg orally every 4 hours during hours of sleep

- Continue for at least 12 hours after diarrhea resolves

- Recurrent diarrhea after a 12-hour diarrhea-free interval is treated as a new episode

- Rehydrate orally with fluids and electrolytes during a diarrheal episode

- If a patient develops blood or mucus in stool, dehydration, or hemodynamic instability, or if diarrhea persists >48 hours despite loperamide, stop loperamide and hospitalize the patient for IV hydration

Persistent diarrhea:

Octreotide 100–150 mcg subcutaneously 3 times daily. Maximum total daily dose is 1500 mcg

Antibiotic therapy during latent or delayed onset diarrhea:

A fluoroquinolone (eg, **Ciprofloxacin** 500 mg orally every 12 hours) if absolute neutrophil count <500/mm³ with or without accompanying fever in association with diarrhea

- Antibiotics should also be administered if patient is hospitalized with prolonged diarrhea and should be continued until diarrhea resolves

*Rothenberg ML et al. J Clin Oncol 2001;19:3801–3807
Abigerges D et al. J Natl Cancer Inst 1994;86:446–449
Wadler S et al. J Clin Oncol 1998;16:3169–3178

Oral care

Risk of mucositis/stomatitis is HIGH

General advice:

- Encourage patients to maintain intake of non-alcoholic fluids

- Evaluate patients for oral pain and provide analgesic medications

- Consider histamine (H₂-subtype) receptor antagonists (eg, ranitidine, famotidine), or a proton pump inhibitor for epigastric pain

- *Lactobacillus* sp.-containing probiotics may be beneficial in preventing diarrhea

(*continued*)

(continued)

Patients with intact oral mucosa:

• Clean the mouth, tongue, and gums by brushing after every meal and at bedtime with an ultra-soft toothbrush with fluoride toothpaste

• Floss teeth gently every day unless contraindicated. If gums bleed and hurt, avoid bleeding or sore areas, but floss other teeth

• Patients may use saline or commercial bland, non-alcoholic rinses

  ▪ Do not use mouthwashes that contain alcohols

If mucositis or stomatitis is present:

• Keep the mouth moist utilizing water, ice chips, sugarless gum, sugar-free hard candies, or a saliva substitute

• Rinse mouth several times a day to remove debris

  ▪ Use a solution of ¼ teaspoon (1.25 g) each of baking soda and table salt (sodium chloride) in one quart (~950 mL) of warm water. Follow with a plain water rinse

  ▪ Do not use mouthwashes that contain alcohols

• Foam-tipped swabs (eg, Toothettes®) are useful in moisturizing oral mucosa, but ineffective for cleansing teeth and removing plaque

• Advise patients who develop mucositis to:

  ▪ Choose foods that are easy to chew and swallow

  ▪ Take small bites of food, chew slowly, and sip liquids with meals

  ▪ Encourage soft, moist foods such as cooked cereals, mashed potatoes, and scrambled eggs

  ▪ For trouble swallowing, soften food with gravies, sauces, broths, yogurt, or other bland liquids

  ▪ Avoid sharp, crunchy foods; hot, spicy or highly acidic foods (eg, citrus fruits and juices); sugary foods; toothpicks; tobacco products; alcoholic drinks

Patient Population Studied

A study of 218 patients with measurable or assessable histologically confirmed squamous cell carcinoma of the head and neck (excluding nasopharyngeal carcinoma) not curable with surgery or radiation. Prior chemotherapy for recurrent disease was not allowed. Prior chemotherapy delivered as part of initial curative therapy was allowed; treatment with paclitaxel or fluorouracil had to be completed more than 12 months before study entry and treatment with cisplatin had to be completed more than 6 months before study entry. Age ≥18 years, adequate organ function, and ECOG performance status ≤1 were required

Therapy Monitoring

1. *Pretreatment evaluation:* Medical history and tumor assessment by clinical evaluation and imaging studies

2. *Response evaluation:* Every 2 cycles

Efficacy

	Cisplatin + Fluorouracil	Cisplatin + Paclitaxel
Complete response	6.7%	7%
Partial response	23.1%	19%
Stable disease	55.8%	54%
Progressive disease	3.8%	6%
Not assessable	10.6%	14%
Median overall survival, months	8.7	8.1
1-Year survival	41.4%	32.4%

	Toxicity			Dose Modifications	
	Cisplatin + Fluorouracil	Cisplatin + Paclitaxel		Adverse Event	Dose Modification
Adverse Event	% G3/4/5 N = 106	% G3/4/5 N = 108		G4 toxicity	Withhold treatment until G ≤1
Anemia	33	13		G2 hepatic toxicity	Withhold treatment until G ≤1
Thrombocytopenia	23	4		G3 hepatic toxicity	Withhold treatment until G ≤1, then reduce paclitaxel dosage by 20%
Neutropenia	67	55			
Leukopenia	63	35			
Infection	21*	13*		Neutrophil count <1500/mm³	Withhold treatment until ANC is ≥1500/mm³
Genitourinary	3	1			
Stomatitis	31	0		Platelet count <100,000/mm³	Withhold treatment until platelet count is ≥100,000/mm³
Mucositis	1	0			
Diarrhea	6	1			
Nausea	19	18		Nadir thrombocytopenia G4	Reduce dosages of all agents by 20%
Vomiting	18	10			
Fatigue	9	7		G4 neutropenia ≥5 days	Reduce dosages of all agents by 20%
Decreased performance status	1	2			
Hemorrhage	2†	1†		Febrile neutropenia requiring hospitalization and antibiotics	Reduce dosages of all agents by 20%
Cardiac	3†	4			
Metabolic	15	10			
Dehydration	5	4		G ≥2 mucosal or skin toxicity	Reduce fluorouracil dosage by 20%
Liver	1	3			
Hypotension	2	5		G3 mucositis	Reduce paclitaxel and fluorouracil dosages by 20%
Neurosensory	4	5			
Neuromotor	3	4		G ≥2 diarrhea (4–6 stools/day greater than baseline)	Hold fluorouracil until diarrhea resolves to baseline
Toxic deaths	7	5			

*Includes 4% G5 toxicities
†Includes 1% G5 toxicities

Adverse Event	Dose Modification
Creatinine clearance ≤50 mL/min (≤0.83 mL/s)	Replace cisplatin with carboplatin AUC = 6 mg/mL · min
G2 neuropathy	Replace cisplatin with carboplatin AUC = 6 mg/mL · min; do not alter paclitaxel dosage
G2 neuropathy lasting ≥1 cycle after substituting carboplatin for cisplatin	Reduce paclitaxel dosages by 20%
G3 neuropathy	Discontinue therapy

RECURRENT/METASTATIC DISEASE

CISPLATIN *OR* CARBOPLATIN WITH FLUOROURACIL + CETUXIMAB

Vermorken JB et al. N Engl J Med 2008;359:1116–1127

Cetuximab premedication:
Diphenhydramine 50 mg; administer by intravenous injection or infusion before cetuximab administration (other H_1-receptor antagonists may be substituted)

Initial cetuximab dose:
Cetuximab 400 mg/m²; administer intravenously over 120 minutes (maximum infusion rate = 5 mL [10 mg] per min) as a single loading dose (total initial dosage = 400 mg/m²)

Maintenance cetuximab doses:
Cetuximab 250 mg/m² per dose; administer intravenously over 60 minutes (maximum infusion rate = 5 mL [10 mg] per min) every week (total weekly dosage = 250 mg/m²)

Notes:
Cetuximab is intended for direct administration and should not be diluted
Maximum infusion rate = 5 mL (10 mg)/min
Administer cetuximab through a low protein-binding inline filter with pore size = 0.22 μm
Use 0.9% sodium chloride injection to flush vascular access devices after administration is completed
One hour after completing cetuximab administration, either cisplatin *or* carboplatin is given

Cisplatin-Containing Regimen

Hydration before, during, and after cisplatin administration ± mannitol:

- *Pre-cisplatin hydration* with 1000 mL 0.9% sodium chloride injection (0.9% NS); administer intravenously with potassium and magnesium supplementation as needed based on pretreatment laboratory results

- *Mannitol diuresis:* May be given to patients who have received adequate hydration. A dose of **mannitol 12.5–25 g** may be administered by intravenous injection or a short infusion before or during cisplatin administration, or prepared as an admixture with cisplatin. Continued intravenous hydration is essential

- *Continued mannitol diuresis:* In an inpatient or day-hospital setting, one may administer additional mannitol in the form of an intravenous infusion: **mannitol 10–40 g**; administer intravenously over 1–4 hours. This can be done either during or immediately after cisplatin, but requires maintenance of adequate intravenously administered fluids during and for hours after mannitol administration

- *Post-cisplatin hydration* with ≥1000 mL 0.9% NS; administer intravenously with potassium and magnesium supplementation as needed based on measured values

Cisplatin 100 mg/m²; administer intravenously in 50–1000 mL 0.9% NS over 60 minutes on day 1, every 3 weeks (total dosage/cycle = 100 mg/m²), *followed by:*

Fluorouracil 1000 mg/m² per day; administer in 50–1000 mL 0.9% NS or D5W by continuous intravenous infusion over 24 hours for 4 consecutive days, on days 1–4, every 3 weeks (total dosage/cycle = 4000 mg/m²)

Carboplatin-Containing Regimen

Carboplatin* (calculated dose) AUC = 5 mg/mL · min per dose; administer by intravenous infusion diluted to concentrations as low as 0.5 mg/mL with either D5W or 0.9% NS over 1 hour, on day 1, every 3 weeks (total dose/cycle calculated to produce a target AUC = 5 mg/mL · min), *followed by:*

Fluorouracil 1000 mg/m² per day; administer in 50–1000 mL 0.9% NS or D5W by continuous intravenous infusion over 24 hours for 4 consecutive days, on days 1–4, every 3 weeks for 4 cycles (total dosage/cycle = 4000 mg/m²)

*Carboplatin dose is based on a formula described by Calvert et al. to achieve a target area under the plasma concentration versus time curve (AUC)

$$\text{Total Carboplatin Dose (mg)} = (\text{target AUC}) \times (\text{GFR} + 25)$$

In practice, creatinine clearance (Clcr) is used in place of glomerular filtration rate (GFR). Clcr can be estimated from the equation of Cockcroft and Gault, thus:

$$\text{For males, Clcr} = \frac{(140 - \text{age [years]}) \times (\text{body weight [kg]})}{72 \times (\text{serum creatinine [mg/dL]})}$$

(continued)

(*continued*)

$$\text{For females, Clcr} = \frac{(140 - \text{age [years]}) \times (\text{body weight [kg]})}{72 \times (\text{serum creatinine [mg/dL]})} \times 0.85$$

Calvert AH et al. J Clin Oncol 1989;7:1748–1756
Cockcroft DW , Gault MH. Nephron 1976;16:31–41
Jodrell DI et al. J Clin Oncol 1992;10:520–528
Sorensen BT et al. Cancer Chemother Pharmacol 1991;28:397–401

Note: On October 8, 2010, the U.S. FDA identified a potential safety issue with carboplatin dosing based on recent changes in the measurement of serum creatinine. By the end of 2010, all clinical laboratories in the United States were required to use the standardized Isotope Dilution Mass Spectrometry (IDMS) method to measure serum creatinine, which can result in an overestimation of the GFR in some patients with normal renal function. A carboplatin dose calculated with an IDMS-measured serum creatinine result using the Calvert formula can exceed an expected exposure (AUC) and result in increased drug-related toxicity

Provided actual GFR measurements are made to assess renal function, carboplatin can be safely dosed according to the Calvert formula described in product labeling

If GFR (or creatinine clearance) is estimated based on serum creatinine measurements by the IDMS method, the FDA recommends, for patients with normal renal function, capping an estimated GFR at 125 mL/min for any targeted AUC value. No greater estimated GFR values should be used

U.S. FDA. Carboplatin dosing. [online] October 8, 2010. Available from: http://www.fda.gov/AboutFDA/CentersOffices/OfficeofMedicalProductsandTobacco/CDER/ucm228974.htm [accessed February 26, 2014]

Treatment duration:
Until evidence of disease progression or unacceptable toxicity for a maximum of 6 cycles of chemotherapy. Cetuximab may be continued as a single agent until unacceptable toxicity or disease progression

Supportive Care
Antiemetic prophylaxis
Emetogenic potential on days with cetuximab alone is **MINIMAL**
Emetogenic potential on days with cisplatin or carboplatin is **HIGH**. *Potential for delayed symptoms*
Emetogenic potential on days with fluorouracil alone is **LOW**
See Chapter 39 for antiemetic recommendations

Hematopoietic growth factor (CSF) prophylaxis
Primary prophylaxis is NOT indicated
See Chapter 43 for more information

Antimicrobial prophylaxis
Risk of fever and neutropenia is LOW
Antimicrobial primary prophylaxis to be considered:
- Antibacterial—not indicated
- Antifungal—not indicated
- Antiviral—not indicated unless patient previously had an episode of HSV
See Chapter 47 for more information

Diarrhea management
Latent or delayed onset diarrhea:
Loperamide 4 mg orally initially after the first loose or liquid stool, *then*
Loperamide 2 mg orally every 2 hours during waking hours, *plus*
Loperamide 4 mg orally every 4 hours during hours of sleep
- Continue for at least 12 hours after diarrhea resolves
- Recurrent diarrhea after a 12-hour diarrhea free interval is treated as a new episode
- Rehydrate orally with fluids and electrolytes during a diarrheal episode
- If a patient develops blood or mucus in stool, dehydration, or hemodynamic instability, or if diarrhea persists >48 hours despite loperamide, stop loperamide and hospitalize the patient for IV hydration
Alternatively, a trial of **Diphenoxylate hydrochloride** 2.5 mg with **Atropine sulfate** 0.025 mg (eg, Lomotil®)
- Initial adult dose is two tablets four times daily until control has been achieved, after which the dose may be reduced to meet individual requirements. Control may often be maintained with as little as two tablets daily
- Clinical improvement of acute diarrhea is usually observed within 48 hours. If improvement of chronic diarrhea after treatment with a maximum daily dose of 8 tablets is not observed within 10 days, control is unlikely with further administration

(*continued*)

(*continued*)

Persistent diarrhea:
  Octreotide 100–150 mcg subcutaneously 3 times daily. Maximum total daily dose is 1500 mcg
Antibiotic therapy during latent or delayed onset diarrhea:
  A fluoroquinolone (eg, **Ciprofloxacin** 500 mg orally every 12 hours) if absolute neutrophil count <500/mm³ with or without accompanying fever in association with diarrhea
  • Antibiotics should also be administered if patient is hospitalized with prolonged diarrhea and should be continued until diarrhea resolves

*Rothenberg ML et al. J Clin Oncol 2001;19:3801–3807
Wadler S et al. J Clin Oncol 1998;16:3169–31178
Abigerges D et al. J Natl Cancer Inst 1994;86:446-449

Oral care
Risk of mucositis/stomatitis is HIGH
  General advice:
  • Encourage patients to maintain intake of non-alcoholic fluids
  • Evaluate patients for oral pain and provide analgesic medications
  • Consider histamine (H_2-subtype) receptor antagonists (eg, ranitidine, famotidine), or a proton pump inhibitor for epigastric pain
  • *Lactobacillus* sp.-containing probiotics may be beneficial in preventing diarrhea
  Patients with intact oral mucosa:
  • Clean the mouth, tongue, and gums by brushing after every meal and at bedtime with an ultra-soft toothbrush with fluoride toothpaste
  • Floss teeth gently every day unless contraindicated. If gums bleed and hurt, avoid bleeding or sore areas, but floss other teeth
  • Patients may use saline or commercial bland, non-alcoholic rinses
    ▪ Do not use mouthwashes that contain alcohols
  If mucositis or stomatitis is present:
  • Keep the mouth moist utilizing water, ice chips, sugarless gum, sugar-free hard candies, or a saliva substitute
  • Rinse mouth several times a day to remove debris
    ▪ Use a solution of ¼ teaspoon (1.25 g) each of baking soda and table salt (sodium chloride) in one quart (~950 mL) of warm water. Follow with a plain water rinse
    ▪ Do not use mouthwashes that contain alcohols
  • Foam-tipped swabs (eg, Toothettes®) are useful in moisturizing oral mucosa, but ineffective for cleansing teeth and removing plaque
  • Advise patients who develop mucositis to:
    ▪ Choose foods that are easy to chew and swallow
    ▪ Take small bites of food, chew slowly, and sip liquids with meals
    ▪ Encourage soft, moist foods such as cooked cereals, mashed potatoes, and scrambled eggs
    ▪ For trouble swallowing, soften food with gravies, sauces, broths, yogurt, or other bland liquids
    ▪ Avoid sharp, crunchy foods; hot, spicy or highly acidic foods (eg, citrus fruits and juices); sugary foods; toothpicks; tobacco products; alcoholic drinks

Patient Population Studied

A study of 442 patients with measurable histologically or cytologically confirmed recurrent and/or metastatic squamous cell carcinoma of the head and neck (except nasopharyngeal carcinoma) that was not curable with surgery or radiation. Prior chemotherapy for recurrent disease was not allowed. Prior chemotherapy delivered as part of initial curative therapy was allowed provided it was completed at least 6 months before study entry. Age ≥18 years, adequate organ function, and Karnofsky performance status of ≥70 were required

Efficacy
(PF Comparator = The Same Chemotherapy Without Cetuximab)*

	PFC† (N = 222)	PF† (N = 220)	Hazard Ratio (p-Value)
Median overall survival, months	10.1	7.4	0.8 (0.04)
Median progression-free survival, months	5.6	3.3	0.54 (<0.001)
Median time to treatment failure, months	4.8	3	0.59 (<0.001)
Median duration of response, months	5.6	4.7	0.76 (0.21)
	PFC (N = 222)	PF (N = 220)	Odds Ratio (p-Value)
Overall response rate	36%	20%	2.23 (<0.001)

*WHO
†PFC, Cisplatin or carboplatin with fluorouracil + cetuximab; PF, cisplatin or carboplatin with + fluorouracil

Treatment Modifications

Adverse Event	Dose Modification
First occurrence G3 skin toxicity	Hold cetuximab up to 2 weeks
Second occurrence G3 skin toxicity	Reduce cetuximab dosage to 200 mg/m²
Third occurrence G3 skin toxicity	Reduce cetuximab dosage to 150 mg/m²
Fourth occurrence G3 skin toxicity	Discontinue cetuximab
G ≥2 mucosal or skin toxicity	Reduce fluorouracil dosage 20%
G ≥2 diarrhea (4–6 stools/day greater than baseline)	Hold fluorouracil until diarrhea resolves to baseline
Creatinine clearance ≤50 mL/min (≤0.83 mL/s)	Replace cisplatin with carboplatin AUC = 5 mg/mL·min
G3 myelosuppression	Reduce cisplatin dosage by 25% or carboplatin dosage by 20%. Do not change fluorouracil dosage
G4 myelosuppression	Reduce cisplatin dosage by 40% or carboplatin dosage by 20%. Do not change fluorouracil dosage
Creatinine clearance <50 mL/min (<0.83 mL/s)	Do not administer therapy
Serum creatinine >1.5 mg/dL (>133 μmol/L) or 20% higher than baseline if baseline was >1.5 mg/dL	Hold cisplatin dosage until serum creatinine <1.5 mg/dL (<133 μmol/L) or within 0.2 mg/dL (17.7 μmol/L) of baseline
Serum creatinine 1.5–2.0 mg/dL (133–177 μmol/L) immediately before a cycle	Hold cisplatin*, then reduce cisplatin dosage by 25% during subsequent cycles
Serum creatinine 2.1–3.0 mg/dL (186–265 μmol/L) immediately before a cycle	Hold cisplatin*, then reduce cisplatin dosage by 50% during subsequent cycles
Serum creatinine >3.0 mg/dL immediately before a cycle	Hold cisplatin
G2 neurotoxicity or ototoxicity	Hold cisplatin until neurotoxicity resolves to G ≤1
G3/4 neurotoxicity or ototoxicity	Discontinue chemotherapy
G ≥3 nausea/vomiting despite use of a serotonin (5-HT₃) receptor antagonist + dexamethasone + aprepitant, consistent with published guidelines (see Chapter 39)	Reduce cisplatin dosage or carboplatin dose, or discontinue the platinating agent

*Hold cisplatin until serum creatinine <1.5 mg/dL (<133 μmol/L) or within 0.2 mg/dL (17.7 μmol/L) of baseline

Toxicity

(PF Comparator = The Same Chemotherapy Without Cetuximab)*

Adverse Event	PFC† % G3/4 (N = 219)	PF† % G3/4 (N = 215)
Anemia	13	19
Thrombocytopenia	11	11
Neutropenia	22	23
Leukopenia	9	9
Febrile neutropenia	5	5
Sepsis	4	<1
Skin reactions	9	<1
Pneumonia	4	2
Dyspnea	4	8
Respiratory failure	<1	2
Anorexia	5	1
Vomiting	5	3
Asthenia	5	6
Decreased performance status	1	2
Tumor hemorrhage	1	3
Cardiac events	7	4
Hypomagnesemia	5	1
Hypocalcemia	4	1
Hypokalemia	7	5

*NCI, CTC, National Cancer Institute (USA) Common Toxicity Criteria and Common Terminology Criteria for Adverse Events, all versions. Available at: http://ctep.cancer.gov/protocolDevelopment/electronic_applications/ctc.htm [accessed December 7, 2013]
†PFC, Cisplatin or carboplatin with fluorouracil + cetuximab; PF, cisplatin or carboplatin with fluorouracil

Therapy Monitoring

1. *Pretreatment evaluation:* Medical history and tumor assessment by clinical evaluation and imaging studies
2. *Response evaluation:* Every 2 cycles

RECURRENT/METASTATIC DISEASE

WEEKLY DOCETAXEL

Guardiola E et al. Eur J Cancer 2004;40:2071–2076

Premedication for docetaxel
Dexamethasone 8 mg/dose; administer orally for 3 doses at 12 hours, 3 hours, and 1 hour before starting docetaxel (total dose/cycle = 24 mg)

Docetaxel 40 mg/m²; administer intravenously in a volume of 0.9% sodium chloride injection or 5% dextrose injection sufficient to produce a docetaxel concentration within the range 0.3–0.74 mg/mL over 60 minutes every 7 days (total dosage/week = 40 mg/m²)

Supportive Care
Antiemetic prophylaxis
Emetogenic potential is **LOW**
See Chapter 39 for antiemetic recommendations

Hematopoietic growth factor (CSF) prophylaxis
Primary prophylaxis is NOT indicated
See Chapter 43 for more information

Antimicrobial prophylaxis
Risk of fever and neutropenia is LOW
   Antimicrobial primary prophylaxis to be considered:
   • Antibacterial—not indicated
   • Antifungal—not indicated
   • Antiviral—not indicated unless patient previously had an episode of HSV
See Chapter 47 for more information

Diarrhea management
Latent or delayed onset diarrhea*:
   Loperamide 4 mg orally initially after the first loose or liquid stool, *then*
   Loperamide 2 mg orally every 2 hours during waking hours, *plus*
   Loperamide 4 mg orally every 4 hours during hours of sleep
   • Continue for at least 12 hours after diarrhea resolves
   • Recurrent diarrhea after a 12-hour diarrhea free interval is treated as a new episode
   • Rehydrate orally with fluids and electrolytes during a diarrheal episode
   • If a patient develops blood or mucus in stool, dehydration, or hemodynamic instability, or if diarrhea persists >48 hours despite loperamide, stop loperamide and hospitalize the patient for IV hydration
   Alternatively, a trial of **Diphenoxylate hydrochloride** 2.5 mg with **Atropine sulfate** 0.025 mg (eg, Lomotil®)
   • Initial adult dose is two tablets four times daily until control has been achieved, after which the dose may be reduced to meet individual requirements. Control may often be maintained with as little as two tablets daily
   • Clinical improvement of acute diarrhea is usually observed within 48 hours. If improvement of chronic diarrhea after treatment with a maximum daily dose of 8 tablets is not observed within 10 days, control is unlikely with further administration
Persistent diarrhea:
   Octreotide 100–150 mcg subcutaneously 3 times daily. Maximum total daily dose is 1500 mcg
Antibiotic therapy during latent or delayed onset diarrhea:
   A fluoroquinolone (eg, **Ciprofloxacin** 500 mg orally every 12 hours) if absolute neutrophil count <500/mm3 with or without accompanying fever in association with diarrhea
   • Antibiotics should also be administered if patient is hospitalized with prolonged diarrhea and should be continued until diarrhea resolves

*Rothenberg ML et al. J Clin Oncol 2001;19:3801–3807
Abigerges D et al. J Natl Cancer Inst 1994;86:446–449
Wadler S et al. J Clin Oncol 1998;16:3169–3178

(continued)

Patient Population Studied

A study of 57 patients with measurable recurrent and/or metastatic squamous cell carcinoma of the head and neck. Excluded were patients with adenocarcinoma, undifferentiated nasopharyngeal carcinoma, or known brain metastasis. Prior chemotherapy for recurrent disease was not allowed. Prior chemotherapy delivered as part of initial curative therapy was allowed. Age ≥18 years, adequate organ function, and performance status ≤2 were required

Efficacy (Comparator = Weekly Methotrexate)*

	Docetaxel (N = 37)	Methotrexate (N = 20)
Overall response rate	27%	15%
Median time to progression, months	1.97	1.5
Median overall survival, months	3.7	3.9

*WHO

Dose Modifications

Adverse Event	Dose Modification
G4 toxicity	Withhold treatment until G ≤1
Neutrophil count <1500/mm³	Withhold treatment until ANC is ≥1500/mm³
Platelet count <100,000/mm³	Withhold treatment until platelet count is ≥100,000/mm³
G3 mucositis	Reduce docetaxel dosage by 20%
G2 neuropathy	Reduce docetaxel dosage by 20%
G3 neuropathy	Discontinue therapy

Therapy Monitoring

1. *Pretreatment evaluation:* Medical history and tumor assessment by clinical evaluation and imaging studies
2. *Toxicity:* Assess weekly
3. *Response evaluation:* Every 2 cycles

(*continued*)

Oral care (prophylaxis and management of mucositis)

General advice:

- Encourage patients to maintain intake of non-alcoholic fluids
- Evaluate patients for oral pain and provide analgesic medications
- Consider histamine (H_2-subtype) receptor antagonists (eg, ranitidine, famotidine), or a proton pump inhibitor for epigastric pain
- *Lactobacillus* sp.-containing probiotics may be beneficial in preventing diarrhea

Patients with intact oral mucosa:

- Clean the mouth, tongue, and gums by brushing after every meal and at bedtime with an ultra-soft toothbrush with fluoride toothpaste
- Floss teeth gently every day unless contraindicated. If gums bleed and hurt, avoid bleeding or sore areas, but floss other teeth
- Patients may use saline or commercial bland, non-alcoholic rinses
  - Do not use mouthwashes that contain alcohols

If mucositis or stomatitis is present:

- Keep the mouth moist utilizing water, ice chips, sugarless gum, sugar-free hard candies, or a saliva substitute
- Rinse mouth several times a day to remove debris
  - Use a solution of ¼ teaspoon (1.25 g) each of baking soda and table salt (sodium chloride) in one quart (~950 mL) of warm water. Follow with a plain water rinse
  - Do not use mouthwashes that contain alcohols
- Foam-tipped swabs (eg, Toothettes®) are useful in moisturizing oral mucosa, but ineffective for cleansing teeth and removing plaque
- Advise patients who develop mucositis to:
  - Choose foods that are easy to chew and swallow
  - Take small bites of food, chew slowly, and sip liquids with meals
  - Encourage soft, moist foods such as cooked cereals, mashed potatoes, and scrambled eggs
  - For trouble swallowing, soften food with gravies, sauces, broths, yogurt, or other bland liquids
  - Avoid sharp, crunchy foods; hot, spicy or highly acidic foods (eg, citrus fruits and juices); sugary foods; toothpicks; tobacco products; alcoholic drinks

Toxicity (Comparator = Weekly Methotrexate)[*]

Adverse Event	Docetaxel		Methotrexate	
	% G1/2	% G3/4	% G1/2	% G3/4
	(N = 37)		(N = 20)	
Anemia	25	19	10	15
Thrombocytopenia	0	0	0	0
Neutropenia	6	12.5	10	5
	(N = 32)		(N = 20)	
Mucositis	28	9	30	5
Diarrhea	19	0	5	5
Constipation	9	0	5	0
Nausea/vomiting	16	0	5	0
Neurologic	19	0	0	0
Edema	9	0	0	0
Cutaneous	19	0	42	0
Alopecia	3	9	5	0
Ungual	0	9	0	0

[*]NCI Common Toxicity Criteria and UICC

RECURRENT/METASTATIC DISEASE
METHOTREXATE *OR*
CISPLATIN + FLUOROURACIL *OR*
CARBOPLATIN + FLUOROURACIL

Forastiere AA et al. J Clin Oncol 1992;10:1245–1251

Note: Combination chemotherapy (cisplatin + fluorouracil or carboplatin + fluorouracil) resulted in improved response rates but was associated with increased toxicity and no improvement in overall survival

Note: Other regimens for cisplatin + fluorouracil or carboplatin + fluorouracil can be found in other areas of this chapter

Methotrexate

Methotrexate 40 mg/m²; administer intravenously in 25–500 mL of 0.9% sodium chloride injection (0.9% NS) or 5% dextrose injection (D5W) over 1 hour every 7 days (total dosage/week = 40 mg/m²)

Supportive Care for Patients Receiving Weekly Methotrexate
Antiemetic prophylaxis
Emetogenic potential is **MINIMAL**
See Chapter 39 for antiemetic recommendations

Hematopoietic growth factor (CSF) prophylaxis
Primary prophylaxis is NOT indicated
See Chapter 43 for more information

Antimicrobial prophylaxis
Risk of fever and neutropenia is LOW
   Antimicrobial primary prophylaxis to be considered:
   • Antibacterial—not indicated

   • Antifungal—not indicated

   • Antiviral—not indicated unless patient previously had an episode of HSV
See Chapter 47 for more information

Oral care
Risk of mucositis/stomatitis is LOW–MODERATE
   General advice:
   • Encourage patients to maintain intake of non-alcoholic fluids

   • Evaluate patients for oral pain and provide analgesic medications

   • Consider histamine (H$_2$-subtype) receptor antagonists (eg, ranitidine, famotidine), or a proton pump inhibitor for epigastric pain

   • *Lactobacillus* sp.-containing probiotics may be beneficial in preventing diarrhea
   Patients with intact oral mucosa:
   • Clean the mouth, tongue, and gums by brushing after every meal and at bedtime with an ultra-soft toothbrush with fluoride toothpaste

   • Floss teeth gently every day unless contraindicated. If gums bleed and hurt, avoid bleeding or sore areas, but floss other teeth

   • Patients may use saline or commercial bland, non-alcoholic rinses
     ▪ Do not use mouthwashes that contain alcohols
   If mucositis or stomatitis is present:
   • Keep the mouth moist utilizing water, ice chips, sugarless gum, sugar-free hard candies, or a saliva substitute

   • Rinse mouth several times a day to remove debris

   • Use a solution of ¼ teaspoon (1.25 g) each of baking soda and table salt (sodium chloride) in one quart (~950 mL) of warm water. Follow with a plain water rinse
     ▪ Do not use mouthwashes that contain alcohols
   • Foam-tipped swabs (eg, Toothettes®) are useful in moisturizing oral mucosa, but ineffective for cleansing teeth and removing plaque

   • Advise patients who develop mucositis to:
     ▪ Choose foods that are easy to chew and swallow

     ▪ Take small bites of food, chew slowly, and sip liquids with meals

     ▪ Encourage soft, moist foods such as cooked cereals, mashed potatoes, and scrambled eggs

     ▪ For trouble swallowing, soften food with gravies, sauces, broths, yogurt, or other bland liquids

     ▪ Avoid sharp, crunchy foods; hot, spicy or highly acidic foods (eg, citrus fruits and juices); sugary foods; toothpicks; tobacco products; alcoholic drinks

(continued)

Cisplatin + Fluorouracil

Hydration before, during, and after cisplatin administration ± mannitol:

- *Pre-cisplatin hydration* with 1000 mL 0.9% NS; administer intravenously with potassium and magnesium supplementation as needed based on pretreatment laboratory results
- *Mannitol diuresis:* May be given to patients who have received adequate hydration. A dose of **mannitol** 12.5–25 g may be administered by intravenous injection or a short infusion before or during cisplatin administration, or prepared as an admixture with cisplatin. Continued intravenous hydration is essential
- *Continued mannitol diuresis:* In an inpatient or day-hospital setting, one may administer additional mannitol in the form of an intravenous infusion: **mannitol** 10–40 g; administer intravenously over 1–4 hours. This can be done either during or immediately after cisplatin, but requires maintenance of adequate intravenously administered fluids during and for hours after mannitol administration
- *Post-cisplatin hydration* with ≥1000 mL 0.9% NS; administer intravenously with potassium and magnesium supplementation as needed based on measured values

Cisplatin 100 mg/m²; administer intravenously in 25–250 mL 0.9% NS over 15–30 minutes on day 1, every 21 days (total dosage/cycle = 100 mg/m²)

Fluorouracil 1000 mg/m² per day; administer in 50–1000 mL 0.9% NS or D5W by continuous intravenous infusion over 24 hours for 4 consecutive days, on days 1–4, every 21 days (total dosage/cycle = 4000 mg/m²)

Carboplatin + Fluorouracil

Carboplatin 300 mg/m²; administer by intravenous infusion diluted to concentrations as low as 0.5 mg/mL with either D5W or 0.9% NS over at least 15 minutes on day 1, every 28 days (total dosage/cycle = 300 mg/m²)

Fluorouracil 1000 mg/m² per day; administer in 50–1000 mL 0.9% NS or D5W by continuous intravenous infusion over 24 hours for 4 consecutive days, on days 1–4, every 28 days (total dosage/cycle = 4000 mg/m²)

Supportive Care for Patients Receiving Fluorouracil with Either Cisplatin or Carboplatin

Antiemetic prophylaxis

Emetogenic potential on days with cisplatin or carboplatin is **HIGH**. *Potential for delayed symptoms*

Emetogenic potential on days with fluorouracil alone is **LOW**

See Chapter 39 for antiemetic recommendations

Hematopoietic growth factor (CSF) prophylaxis

Primary prophylaxis is NOT indicated

See Chapter 43 for more information

Antimicrobial prophylaxis

Risk of fever and neutropenia is LOW

   Antimicrobial primary prophylaxis to be considered:

   - Antibacterial—not indicated
   - Antifungal—not indicated
   - Antiviral—not indicated unless patient previously had an episode of HSV

See Chapter 47 for more information

Diarrhea management

Latent or delayed onset diarrhea*:

   Loperamide 4 mg orally initially after the first loose or liquid stool, *then*

   Loperamide 2 mg orally every 2 hours during waking hours, *plus*

   Loperamide 4 mg orally every 4 hours during hours of sleep

   - Continue for at least 12 hours after diarrhea resolves
   - Recurrent diarrhea after a 12-hour diarrhea-free interval is treated as a new episode
   - Rehydrate orally with fluids and electrolytes during a diarrheal episode
   - If a patient develops blood or mucus in stool, dehydration, or hemodynamic instability, or if diarrhea persists >48 hours despite loperamide, stop loperamide and hospitalize the patient for IV hydration

Persistent diarrhea:

   Octreotide 100–150 mcg subcutaneously 3 times daily. Maximum total daily dose is 1500 mcg

Antibiotic therapy during latent or delayed onset diarrhea:

   A fluoroquinolone (eg, **Ciprofloxacin** 500 mg orally every 12 hours) if absolute neutrophil count <500/mm³ with or without accompanying fever in association with diarrhea

   - Antibiotics should also be administered if patient is hospitalized with prolonged diarrhea and should be continued until diarrhea resolves

*Rothenberg ML et al. J Clin Oncol 2001;19:3801–3807
Abigerges D et al. J Natl Cancer Inst 1994;86:446–449
Wadler S et al. J Clin Oncol 1998;16:3169–3178

(*continued*)

(continued)

Oral care
Risk of mucositis/stomatitis is HIGH
  General advice:
- Encourage patients to maintain intake of non-alcoholic fluids
- Evaluate patients for oral pain and provide analgesic medications
- Consider histamine (H_2-subtype) receptor antagonists (eg, ranitidine, famotidine), or a proton pump inhibitor for epigastric pain
- *Lactobacillus* sp.-containing probiotics may be beneficial in preventing diarrhea

Patients with intact oral mucosa:
- Clean the mouth, tongue, and gums by brushing after every meal and at bedtime with an ultra-soft toothbrush with fluoride toothpaste
- Floss teeth gently every day unless contraindicated. If gums bleed and hurt, avoid bleeding or sore areas, but floss other teeth
- Patients may use saline or commercial bland, non-alcoholic rinses
  - Do not use mouthwashes that contain alcohols

If mucositis or stomatitis is present:
- Keep the mouth moist utilizing water, ice chips, sugarless gum, sugar-free hard candies, or a saliva substitute
- Rinse mouth several times a day to remove debris
  - Use a solution of ¼ teaspoon (1.25 g) each of baking soda and table salt (sodium chloride) in one quart (~950 mL) of warm water. Follow with a plain water rinse
  - Do not use mouthwashes that contain alcohols
- Foam-tipped swabs (eg, Toothettes®) are useful in moisturizing oral mucosa, but ineffective for cleansing teeth and removing plaque
- Advise patients who develop mucositis to:
  - Choose foods that are easy to chew and swallow
  - Take small bites of food, chew slowly, and sip liquids with meals
  - Encourage soft, moist foods such as cooked cereals, mashed potatoes, and scrambled eggs
  - For trouble swallowing, soften food with gravies, sauces, broths, yogurt, or other bland liquids
  - Avoid sharp, crunchy foods; hot, spicy or highly acidic foods (eg, citrus fruits and juices); sugary foods; toothpicks; tobacco products; alcoholic drinks

Patient Population Studied

A study of 261 eligible patients with histologically proven locally recurrent or metastatic squamous cell carcinoma of the head and neck. Prior chemotherapy for recurrent or metastatic disease was not allowed. Prior induction chemotherapy as part of the initial treatment was allowed provided it was completed at least 6 months before enrollment. Adequate organ function, life expectancy ≥12 weeks, and a performance status 0–2 according to SWOG criteria were required

Toxicity*

Toxicity	PF (N = 85)[†] % G1/2	% G3/4	CF (N = 86)[†] % G1/2	% G3/4	MTX (N = 87)[†] % G1/2	% G3/4
Anemia	47	4	36	12	22	3
Granulocytopenia	27	7	18	2	7	6
Leukopenia	35	26	43	10	25	14
Thrombocytopenia	11	5	16	11	8	5
Diarrhea	12	2	6	2	3	0
Stomatitis	19	14	28	15	34	10
Nausea/vomiting	68	8	48	6	38	8
Peripheral neuropathy	5	1	2	0	0	0
Ototoxicity	8	4	2	0	2	0
Renal	18	9	1	1	3	3

*SWOG criteria
[†]PF, Cisplatin + fluorouracil; CF, carboplatin + fluorouracil; MTX, methotrexate

Dose Modification

Adverse Event	Dose Modification
G0 mucositis or myelosuppression	Increase methotrexate dosage to 50 mg/m^2 weekly
G ≥2 toxicity including stomatitis and dermatitis	Reduce methotrexate dosage by 10 mg/m^2 weekly
G ≥2 mucosal or skin toxicity	Reduce fluorouracil dosage by 20%
G ≥2 diarrhea (4–6 stools/day greater than baseline)	Hold fluorouracil until diarrhea resolves to baseline
G3 myelosuppression	Reduce cisplatin dosage by 25% or carboplatin dosage by 20%. Do not change fluorouracil dosage
G4 myelosuppression	Reduce cisplatin dosage by 40% or carboplatin dosage by 20%. Do not change fluorouracil dosage
Creatinine clearance <50 mL/min (<0.83 mL/s)	Do not administer therapy
Serum creatinine >1.5 mg/dL (>133 μmol/L) or 20% higher than baseline if baseline was >1.5 mg/dL	Hold cisplatin dosage until serum creatinine <1.5 mg/dL (<133 μmol/L) or within 0.2 mg/dL (17.7 μmol/L) of baseline
Serum creatinine 1.5–2.0 mg/dL (133–177 μmol/L) immediately before a cycle	Hold cisplatin*, then reduce cisplatin dosage by 25% during subsequent cycles
Serum creatinine 2.1–3.0 mg/dL (186–265 μmol/L) immediately before a cycle	Hold cisplatin*, then reduce cisplatin dosage by 50% during subsequent cycles
Serum creatinine >3.0 mg/dL (>265 μmol/L) immediately before a cycle	Hold cisplatin
G2 neurotoxicity or ototoxicity	Hold cisplatin until neurotoxicity resolves to G ≤1
G3/4 neurotoxicity or ototoxicity	Discontinue chemotherapy
G0/1 myelosuppression	Increase carboplatin dosage by 20% to 360 mg/m^2 on the same administration schedule

*Hold cisplatin until serum creatinine is <1.5 mg/dL (<133 μmol/L) or within 0.2 mg/dL (17.7 μmol/L) of baseline

Therapy Monitoring

1. *Pretreatment evaluation:* Medical history and tumor assessment by clinical evaluation and imaging studies
2. *Toxicity:* Assess weekly during at least the first cycle with attention to signs and symptoms of dehydration as supplemental hydration is often required
3. *Laboratory analyses:* Weekly CBC, serum electrolytes, LFTs, calcium, and magnesium
4. *Response evaluation:* Every 6–8 weeks

Efficacy

	PF* (N = 87)	CF* (N = 86)	MTX* (N = 88)
Overall response rate	32%[†]	21%[†]	10%[†]
Complete response rate	6%	2%	2%
Progressive disease	16%	25%	32%
Median response duration, months	4.2	5.1	4.1
Median survival, months	6.6	5	5.6
Patients alive at 9 months	31%	30%	27%

*PF, Cisplatin + fluorouracil; CF, carboplatin + fluorouracil; MTX, methotrexate
[†]PF vs. MTX (*P* <0.001); CF vs. MTX (*P* = 0.05)

15. Hepatocellular Carcinoma

Tim Greten, MD, PhD and Nadine Abi-Jaoudeh, MD

Epidemiology

Incidence*: 16 cases per 100,000 population

worldwide: 626,000 cases per year

Deaths (worldwide): 598,000 per year

Median age* (Asia and Western Europe): 50–60 years

Male to female ratio: ~2.4:1

Stage at presentation

Stage A: 35%

Stage B: 25%

Stage C: 10%

Stage D: 30%

*The incidence and age of hepatocellular carcinoma vary widely according to geographic location. The distribution also differs among ethnic groups and regions within the same country

Forner et al. Lancet 2012;379:1245–1255
Llovet JM et al. J Natl Cancer Inst 2008;100:698–711
Parkin DM et al. CA Cancer J Clin 2005;55:74–108

Work-up

1. Alpha-fetoprotein (AFP)
2. Liver function test (see Child-Pugh classification)
3. Ultrasound and abdominal/chest spiral CT and/or dynamic liver MRI
4. Specific clinical scenarios such as selection for liver transplantation may also require bone scintigraphy to exclude bone metastases, but there are no robust data supporting the cost-efficiency of this policy

Diagnostic Criteria for HCC: Non-invasive criteria (Restricted to cirrhotic patients)
1. Radiological criteria: (arterial hypervascularization/washout in portal phase)

   Two coincident imaging techniques, nodule <2 cm

   One imaging technique, nodule >2 cm
2. Combined criteria: one imaging technique associated with AFP

   Focal lesion >2 cm with arterial hypervascularization

Bruix J, Sherman M. Hepatology 2005;42:1208–1236
Forner A et al. Hepatology 2008;47:97–104

Pathology

Hepatocellular carcinoma	99%
Fibrolamellar hepatocellular carcinoma	<1%

Nakashima T, Kojiro M. Hepatocellular Carcinoma. Tokyo, Japan: Springer Verlag, 1987

Staging

Primary Tumor (T)

TX	Primary tumor cannot be assessed
T0	No evidence of primary tumor
T1	Solitary tumor without vascular invasion
T2	Solitary tumor with vascular invasion or multiple tumors none more than 5 cm
T3a	Multiple tumors more than 5 cm
T3b	Single tumor or multiple tumors of any size involving a major branch of the portal vein or hepatic vein
T4	Tumor(s) with direct invasion of adjacent organs other than the gallbladder or with perforation of visceral peritoneum

Regional Lymph Nodes (N)

NX	Regional lymph nodes cannot be assessed
N0	No regional lymph node metastasis
N1	Regional lymph node metastasis

Distant Metastasis (M)

M0	No distant metastasis (no pathologic M0; use clinical M to complete stage group)
M1	Distant metastasis

Staging

	T	N	M
I	T1	N0	M0
II	T2	N0	M0
IIIA	T3a	N0	M0
IIIB	T3b	N0	M0
IIIC	T4	N0	M0
IVA	any T	N1	M0
IVB	any T	any N	M1

Edge SB, Byrd DR, Compton CC, Fritz AG, Greene FL, Trotti A, editors. AJCC Cancer Staging Manual. 7th ed. New York: Springer; 2010

Child-Pugh Classification

Measure	Score*		
	1 Point	**2 Points**	**3 Points**
Ascites	Absent	Slight	Moderate
Serum bilirubin	<2.0 mg/dL (<34.2 mmol/L)	2.0–3.0 mg/dL (34.2–51.3 mmol/L)	>3.0 mg/dL (>51.3 mmol/L)
Serum albumin	>3.5 g/dL	2.8–3.5 g/dL	<2.8 g/dL
Prothrombin time (seconds prolonged)	<4	4–6	>6
Encephalopathy grade	None	1–2	3–4

*Child-Pugh A: 5 or 6 points; Child-Pugh B: 7–9 points; Child-Pugh C: >9 points

Survival (BCLC Staging)

Stage	3-Year Survival
Stage 0-A	40–70%
Stage B	50%
Stage C	10%
Stage D	0

Llovet JM et al. J Natl Cancer Inst 2008;100:698–711
Llovet JM et al. Lancet 2003;362:1907–1917

Barcelona Clinic Liver Cancer (BCLC) Classification

	Tumor Status	Child-Pugh Classification	Performance Status
Stage 0 Very Early Stage	Single HCC <2 cm; Carcinoma *in situ*	A	0
Stage A Early Stage	Single HCC or 3 nodules <3 cm	A–B	0
Stage B Intermediate Stage	Large/multinodular. Without vascular invasion or extrahepatic spread	A–B	0
Stage C Advanced Stage	Any size with vascular invasion or extrahepatic spread. [N1M1]	A–B	1–2
Stage D Terminal Stage	Any size	C	3–4

Llovet JM et al. J Natl Cancer Inst 2008;100:698–711

Expert Opinion

TREATMENT ACCORDING TO STAGE

European Association for the Study of the Liver (EASL)/European Organization for Research and Treatment of Cancer (EORTC) Guidelines J. Hepatol 2012;56:908–943

1. *Stage 0–A*

   Patients diagnosed at an early stage (BCLC A) should be considered for one of the options that can achieve complete response: resection, liver transplantation from cadaveric or live donor, and percutaneous ablation by ethanol injection or radiofrequency

2. *Stage B*

   Chemoembolization

3. *Stage C*

   Sorafenib

4. *Stage D*

   Symptomatic treatment

Hepatocellular Carcinoma—BCLC Staging and Treatment Strategy

Adapted from Forner et al, Lancet 2012;379:1245–1255

Very Early Stage (0) Single <2 cm Child-Pugh A, PS 0	Early Stage (A) Single HCC or three nodules <3 cm Child-Pugh A–B, PS 0	Intermediate Stage (B) Large or multinodular Child-Pugh A–B, PS 0	Advanced Stage (C) Portal invasion, Extrahepatic spread Child-Pugh A–B, PS 1–2	Terminal Stage (D) Advanced disease Child-Pugh C, PS 3–4
↓	↓ ↓			
Potential candidate for liver transplantation*	Single 3 nodules ≤3 cm			
↓ ↓	Yes			
No* Yes*	↓			
↓	Portal pressure, bilirubin [indocyanine green retention rate]†	↓	↓	↓
Portal pressure, bilirubin [indocyanine green retention rate]†				
↓ ↓	↓ ↓			
↓ Normal Increased	Normal Increased			
↓	↓			
Associated Diseases	Associated Diseases			
↓ ↓ ↓	↓ ↓ ↓			
No Yes	No Yes			
↓ ↓	↓ ↓			
Ablation* Resection* Liver Transplant Ablation	Resection Liver Transplant Ablation	Chemoembolization	Sorafenib	Best Supportive Care
Curative Treatments		Palliative Treatments		Best Supportive Care

*Very Early Stage (BCLC0) patients are considered for resection only if transplant available. If transplant not an option, ablation first-line option and surgery justified only in patients with contraindication to ablation or in whom ablation fails. If patients eligible for transplant, then strategy of transplantation depending on risk of recurrence as per tumor pathology favors resection as the first-line approach. Analysis of resected tumor would distinguish BCLC 0 with marginal risk of recurrence (no need to transplant) and more advanced disease with microscopic vascular invasion or satellites that favor transplantation because of high risk of recurrence

†Selection of candidates for resection: In Japan it often relies on indocyanine green retention rate, whereas portal pressure and bilirubin are variables used in Europe and the USA. Clinically relevant portal hypertension defined as a hepatic vein pressure gradient >10 mm Hg, but also confirmed by esophageal varices or splenomegaly with a platelet count <100 × 10⁹/L. Bruix and Sherman, Hepatology 2011;53:1020–1022; Llovet et al. Semin Liver Dis 2005;25:181–200

(continued)

Expert Opinion (continued)

Therapeutic Strategies/Options
Adapted from Forner A et al. Lancet 2012;379:1245–1255

Procedure/Treatment	Benefit	Level of Evidence	Comment
Surgical Treatments			
Surgical resection	Increased survival	3ii A	• Treatment of choice in 5–10% without cirrhosis and one tumor. High rate of CRs; potential for cure • 5-year survival: ~70% without portal hypertension and normal bilirubin; 50% with portal hypertension; <50% if bilirubin increased
Adjuvant treatments	Controversial	1 A–D	• Tumor recurrence 70% at 5 y. Includes early (true) recurrence, usually in first 2 years > resection, and late (*de novo*) tumors • No effective neo-adjuvant or adjuvant treatments
Liver transplantation	Increased survival	3ii A	• Most effective option to prevent intrahepatic recurrence; recurrence rate <25%. One tumor ≤5 cm or ≤3 cm without vascular invasion or extra-hepatic spread ~75% 4-year survival; <15% recurrence rates • Can offer to patients treated with resection but with a high risk of recurrence according to pathologic analysis
Adjuvant treatments	Treatment response	3 Diii	• If transplant donors wait >6 months, trans-arterial chemoembolization and ablation are done, even though effectiveness is unproven
Loco-Regional Treatments—Image-Guided Tumor Ablation			
Percutaneous treatment [injection of chemicals (ethanol, acetic acid) or temperature modification (radiofrequency (RFA), microwave, laser)]	Increased survival	3ii A	• First-line technique now radiofrequency ablation (RFA) • Both ethanol and RFA highly effective in HCC <2 cm, but effectiveness of ethanol falls in 2–5 cm tumors • Effectiveness limited by (1) tumor size—ablation not recommended for tumors >5 cm; and (2) tumor location—with RFA avoid tumors located in subcapsular region, vicinity of major blood vessels or biliary tree, near to bowel or heart • Side-effects more frequent after RFA • Better disease control with RFA than ethanol could translate into better outcomes
Radiofrequency ablation (RFA)	Increased survival	1ii A	
Other modalities		2 D	
Combined modalities	Treatment response	3ii D	
Loco-Regional Treatments—Image-Guided Transcatheter Tumor Treatment			
Chemoembolization	Increased survival	1ii A	• Best candidates patients with compensated Child-Pugh A with asymptomatic multifocal or large hepatocellular tumors not amenable to resection (BCLC stage B) • >50% of patients have objective response that translates into improved in survival • Portal vein thrombosis, even if segmental, predicts poor tolerability and worse outcome
Radioembolization [Internal radiotherapy, ^{131}I, ^{90}Y]	Treatment response	3ii Diii	• Anti-tumor activity but survival benefit not proven • Role not yet defined
Systemic Treatments			
Sorafenib	↑ survival	1i A	• Non-curative treatment that improves survival
Hormonal compounds [Tamoxifen, Octreotide, Antiandrogen, Seocalcitiol]	No survival benefit	1i A	• Completely ineffective
Systemic chemotherapy		1i A	• Marginal activity; frequently toxic
Immunotherapy		1ii A	

Evidence-based classification adapted from the National Cancer Institute
1 = Randomized controlled trial or meta-analysis [1i = Double-blinded, 1ii = Non-blinded]; 2 = Non-randomized controlled trial; 3 = Case series [3i = Population-based, 3ii = Non-population-based, consecutive, 3iii = Non-population-based, non-consecutive]. A = Survival endpoint. B = Cause-specific mortality. C = Quality of life. D = Indirect surrogates [Di = Disease-free survival, Dii = Progression-free survival, Diii = Tumor response]

(*continued*)

Expert Opinion (continued)

Surgical Resection
- Best candidates patients with small solitary tumors and well-preserved liver function
- Tumor recurrence 70% at 5 years. Includes true recurrence, usually within the first 2 years after resection, and *de novo* tumors
- "Early" (true) recurrence: Microvascular invasion, poor histological differentiation, satellites, and multifocal disease predict early recurrence
- Late (*de novo*) recurrence: Depends mainly on carcinogenic effect of underlying chronic liver disease. Estimated by liver function variables related to inflammatoryactivity, evolutionary stage, or both
- No effective neo-adjuvantor adjuvant treatment options to reduce risk of recurrenceare available

Bruix and Sherman. Hepatology 2011;53:1020–1022
Imamura et al. J Hepatol 2003;38:2000–2007
Llovet et al. Semin Liver Dis 2005;25:181–200
Sala et al. Liver Transpl 2004;10:1294–1300

Liver Transplantation
- Most beneficial for patients deemed poor candidates for resection, especially those within Milano criteria (solitary tumor ≤5 cm and up to three nodules ≤3 cm)
- Donor shortage limits applicability
- Excellent results achieved in era with prompt availability of organs. Shortage of donors has imposed delay before transplantation, and tumor can progress and impede transplantation. Delays impair effectiveness of transplantation when considered according to intention
- When waiting >6 months, ablation and trans-arterial chemoembolization are done, even though effectiveness is unproven
- No role for systemic chemotherapy prior to transplantation

Bismuth et al. Ann Surg 1993;218:145–151
Clavien et al. Lancet Oncol 2011;2045:70175–70179
Freeman et al. Am J Transplant 2006;6:1416–1421
Jonas et al. Hepatology 2001;33:1080–1086
Mazzaferro et al. N Engl J Med 1996;334:693–699

Percutaneous Ablation
- Induces tumor necrosis by injection of chemicals (eg, ethanol, acetic acid) or temperature modification (ablation by radio frequency (RFA), microwave, or laser)
  Note: Cryoablation resulted in shock and hepatic failure, and laser is not yet approved by the FDA
- Most ablation procedures done percutaneously, but can also done intraoperatively
- First-line technique is now radiofrequency ablation (RFA). Both ethanol injection and RFA highly effective in HCC <2 cm, but effectiveness of ethanol falls in 2–5 cm tumors
- Effectiveness limited by
  1. Tumor size: All ablation not recommended for tumors >5 cm
  2. Tumor location: With RFA avoid some tumors located in subcapsular region, vicinity of major blood vessels or biliary tree, near to bowel or heart
- Better disease control with RFA than ethanol could translate into better outcomes
- Side-effects more frequent after RFA
- Survival > ablation in Child-Pugh A patients is 50–75% at 5 years, paralleling surgical resection. Has challenged resection as the first-line treatment in patients with small solitary HCCs. Ablation nearly 100% effective in HCCs <2 cm and survival almost identical after resection or ablation
- RFA is associated with less treatment-associated morbidity than resection

Chen et al. Ann Surg 2006;243:321–328
Cho et al. Hepatology 2009;49:453–459
Germani et al. J Hepatol 2010;52:380–388
Huang et al. Ann Surg 2005;242:36–42
Huang et al. Ann Surg 2010;252:903–912
Lencioni. Hepatology 2010;52:762–773
Orlando et al. Am J Gastroenterol 2009;104:514–524
Tateishi et al. Cancer 2005;103:1201–1209

(continued)

Expert Opinion (continued)

Image-Guided Transcatheter Tumor Treatment—Chemoembolization

- Best candidates for trans-arterial chemoembolization are patients with compensated Child-Pugh A with asymptomatic multifocal or large hepatocellular carcinomas not amenable to resection (ie, BCLC stage B)
- >50% of patients have an objective response, and this translates into improvement in survival
- After initial success with transarterial chemoembolization, treated tumors re-vascularize and can be re-treated. However, in the long term, control is lost
- Median survival in old series almost 2 years but with better selection and optimum treatment, median survival >3 years
- Portal vein thrombosis, even if segmental, is a predictor of poor tolerability and impaired outcome
- No standard regimen established
- Extra systemic therapy between/following TACE procedures failed to improve outcome and is not recommended

Lammer et al. Cardiovasc Intervent Radiol 2010;33:41–52
Lin et al. Gastroenterology 1988;94:453–456
Llovet et al. Lancet 2002;359:1734–1739
Pelletier et al. J Hepatol 1990;11:181–184

Image-Guided Transcatheter Tumor Treatment—Radioembolization

- Radioembolization with yttrium-90 (Yt^{90})-labeled spheres has anti-tumor activity. There are no randomized controlled trials comparing this option with any other established treatment. A retrospective comparison to chemoembolization (TACE) found that radioembolization and chemoembolization had similar survival rates; however, radioembolization had longer time to progression and less toxicity than chemoembolization [Salem R et al. Gastroenterology 2011;140:497–507]

Hilgard et al. Hepatology 2010;52:1741–1749
Salem et al. Gastroenterology 2010;138:52–64
Sangro et al. Hepatology 2011;54:868–878

Systemic Treatment—Sorafenib

- 602 patients in a multicenter, randomized, double-blind placebo-controlled trial
- Median OS in sorafenib group 10.7 months (95% CI 9.4–13.3) versus 7.9 months (6.8–9.1) in placebo group (hazard ratio 0.69, 95% CI 0.55–0.87; p = 0.0001)
- Median PFS 5.5 months for sorafenib versus 2.8 months for placebo (0.58, 0.45–0.74; p <0.001)
- No difference in median time to symptomatic progression (4.1 months vs 4.9 months; p = 0.77)
- Overall incidence of treatment-related adverse events (predominantly grade 1 or 2 in severity) 80% in sorafenib group and 52% in placebo group
- Findings have been replicated by a randomized controlled trial in Asia
- These results have established sorafenib as the standard of care for advanced HCC

Cheng et al. Lancet Oncol 2009;10:25–34
Llovet et al. N Engl J Med 2008;359:378–390

EXTRAHEPATIC COLLATERAL VESSELS SUPPLYING HEPATOCELLULAR CARCINOMAS

Kim HC et al. Radiographics 2005;25(Suppl 1):S25–S39

- Extra-hepatic collateral arteries commonly supply hepatocellular carcinomas especially if the tumors are large or peripherally located
- Development of these vessels can interfere with effective tumor control with transcatheter arterial chemoembolization (TACE)
- When both the hepatic artery and extra-hepatic collateral vessels supply a tumor, additional extra-hepatic collateral vessel chemoembolization should be attempted to increase the therapeutic efficacy of TACE
- Extrahepatic collateral vessels originated from thirteen different sources (see Table): Considering the broad contact between the liver and the diaphragm, it is not surprising that diaphragmatic blood supplies, including the inferior phrenic, internal mammary, and intercostal arteries, are major sources of collateral circulation. Exophytic growth and extra-capsular HCC infiltration can cause omental adhesion. Direct contact or invasion into other organs, including the stomach, colon, adrenal gland, and kidney, may create blood supply to the tumor from these organs

(continued)

Expert Opinion (continued)

• Extrahepatic collateral vessels suspected when:
1. A tumor grows exophytically or invades adjacent organs
2. A tumor is in contact with the ligaments and bare area of the liver
3. A hypertrophied extrahepatic collateral vessel is observed on a computed tomographic (CT) scan
4. A peripheral defect of iodized oil retention within a tumor is seen during chemoembolization or on a follow-up CT scan
5. A local recurrence develops at the peripheral portion of the treated tumor during follow-up
6. A sustained elevation in serum α-fetoprotein level is noted despite adequate embolization of the hepatic artery

• Outcomes:
1. 2104 such vessels observed in 1622 sessions in 860 (27%) patients
2. TACE performed via 1556 extrahepatic collateral vessels (74%) in 732 patients in 1281 sessions
3. Multiple extrahepatic collateral vessels embolized in 221 patients (two vessels in 186 patients, three vessels in 27, four vessels in six, and five vessels in two)

Extra-Hepatic Collateral Vessels Supplying HCC in 3179 Patients

Collateral Vessel	Observed Vessels	Embolized Vessels*
Right inferior phrenic artery	1026	864 (84)
Omental branch	306	176 (58)
Adrenal artery	188	152 (81)
Intercostal and subcostal artery	128	83 (65)
Cystic artery	89	82 (92)
Left inferior phrenic artery	78	58 (74)
Right internal mammary artery	76	59 (78)
Renal or renal capsular artery	70	29 (41)
Branch of superior mesenteric artery	48	20 (42)
Left gastric artery	46	12 (26)
Right gastric artery	23	5 (22)
Left internal mammary artery	21	14 (67)
Lumbar artery	5	2 (40)
Total	2104	1556

*Percentages in parentheses

REGIMEN

CHEMOEMBOLIZATION WITH DOXORUBICIN

Llovet JM et al. Lancet 2002;359:1734–1739

Doxorubicin dose adjusted to serum bilirubin concentration (see table below) prepared as an emulsion with 10 mL of ethiodized oil injection administered intra-arterially followed by mechanical obstruction achieved by intra-arterial injection of gelatin sponge fragments suspended in radiologic contrast media until flow stagnation occurred. Chemoembolization was performed at baseline, repeated 2 months and 6 months later, and then every 6 months until disease progression observed

Notes:
• Doxorubicin dosage was based on serum total bilirubin concentration as per the table below:

Total Bilirubin		Doxorubicin Dosage
(µmol/L)	(mg/dL)	
<25.6	<1.5	75 mg/m^2
25.6–51.3	1.5–3	50 mg/m^2
51.3–85.5	3–5	25 mg/m^2

• Extra-hepatic arterial supply of HCC is important. See section on **Extrahepatic collateral vessels supplying hepatocellular carcinomas** [Kim HC, Chung JW, Lee W, Jae HJ, Park JH, Radiographics 2005;25(Suppl 1):S25–S39]
• The mean numbers of treatment sessions were 3.08 (95% CI 2.4–3.5; range 0–7) for embolization and 2.8 (2.3–3.2; 1–8) for chemoembolization (p = 0.5)

GENERAL GUIDELINES

Prior to embolization:
• **Hydration**
  ▪ Start intravenous **hydration** with 0.9% sodium chloride injection (0.9% NS)
  ▪ Continuous 0.9% NS 100 mL/h beginning a minimum of 6 hours prior to procedure
• **Antibiotic prophylaxis** not always required but may be considered with the first doses given before embolization:
  ▪ **Metronidazole** 500 mg; administer intravenously prior to procedure followed by 500 mg every 12 hours × 3 doses, *plus*
  ▪ **Cefazolin** 1000 mg; administer intravenously prior to procedure followed by **Cefazolin** 500 mg; administer intravenously every 8 hours × 5 doses
• **Antiemetic primary prophylaxis**
  Give a serotonin receptor (5HT$_3$) antagonist plus a high-potency glucocorticoid
  ▪ **Ondansetron** 16 mg; administer intravenously or 24 mg orally, *plus*
  ▪ **Dexamethasone** 10–12 mg; administer intravenously or orally 30–60 minutes before the procedure

Post-embolization syndrome:
• The triad of abdominal pain, vomiting, and fever that frequently occurs 24–72 hours after chemoembolization is commonly referred to as post-embolization syndrome
• Post-embolization syndrome uniformly responds to supportive care including analgesics and antiemetics
• Use care administering acetaminophen (paracetamol) and non-steroidal anti-inflammatory drugs in patients with liver cirrhosis

After embolization:
• Continue intravenous **hydration** with 0.9% NS or another clinically appropriate fluid until patient resumes adequate oral fluid intake
• Provide **analgesic support** with parenterally administered opioid medications (**morphine, hydromorphone, fentanyl**) after chemoembolization until patient is able to continue analgesic treatment with oral products
• Continue **antiemetic prophylaxis** with a 5HT$_3$ antagonist plus a high-potency glucocorticoid:
  ▪ **Ondansetron** 8 mg; administer intravenously or orally every 8 hours, *plus*
  ▪ **Dexamethasone** 8 mg; administer intravenously or orally every 8 hours for 2–3 days
• **Filgrastim** (G-CSF) 5 mcg/kg per day; administer by subcutaneous injection
  ▪ May be used for patients who develop an ANC <500/mm^3, neutropenia and fever, or documented infections during neutropenia
  ▪ Discontinue filgrastim at least 24 hours before a chemoembolization procedure

Patient Population Studied

A total of 903 patients were screened and 791 excluded due to early HCC, advanced liver disease, vascular invasion, extra-hepatic spread, and end-stage cancer. 112 patients with intermediate BCLC stage (stage B or C) randomized to conservative treatment (n = 35), embolization (n = 37), or chemoembolization (n = 40)

Patient Characteristics

	Embolization (n = 37)	Chemoembolization (n = 40)	Control (n = 35)
Demography			
Age, years*	64 (62–67)	63 (61–66)	66 (64–68)
M/F	30/17 [81%/19%]	32/8 [80%/20%]	23/12 [66%/34%]
Cause of Cirrhosis			
Hepatitis C virus	30 (81%)	33 (82%)	32 (91%)
Hepatitis B virus	2 (5%)	4 (10%)	1 (3%)
Alcohol	4 (11%)	3 (8%)	1 (3%)
Other	1 (3%)	—	1 (3%)
Tumor-Related Symptoms			
Ascites	9 (24%)	6 (15%)	11 (31%)
Abdominal pain	7 (19%)	3 (8%)	3 (9%)
Constitutional syndrome	1 (3%)	1 (2%)	4 (11%)
Biochemistry			
Serum bilirubin (mmol/L)*	22.2 (18.8–27.4)	20.5 (18.8–23.9)	25.6 (22.2–29.1)
Prothrombin activity (%)*	81 (75–87)	82 (77–87)	77 (71–83)
Serum albumin (g/L)*	35 (33–37)	35 (33–37)	35 (33–37)
γ-glutamyltranspeptidase*,‡	113 (70–156)	112 (85–139)	101 (66–137)
Alkaline phosphatase*,‡	233 (203–263)	220 (182–258)	257 (202–311)
Distribution of α-fetoprotein Concentrations			
<10 mg/L	15	15	11
10–100 mg/L	9	18	16
>100 mg/L	13	7	8
Tumor Stage			
Solitary (66%)†	9 (24%)	13 (32%)	8 (23%)
Multinodular	27 (73%)	26 (65%)	27 (77%)
Two nodules	6	7	8
More than two nodules	21	19	19
Diffuse	1 (3%)	1 (3%)	—

(continued)

Treatment Modifications

Doxorubicin dosage modifications were based on serum total bilirubin concentrations before treatment

Patient Population Studied (continued)

	Embolization (n = 37)	Chemoembolization (n = 40)	Control (n = 35)
Disease Characteristics			
Diameter main nodule (mm)*	52 (46–60)	49 (40–58)	44 (39–49)
Bilobar disease	18 (49%)	19 (47%)	18 (51%)
Child-Pugh class A/B	27/10	31/9	21/14
Okuda Stage I/II	24/13	27/13	22/13
BCLC Stage B/C	28/9	35/5	27/8
Performance Status			
0	28	35	27
1	7	4	4
2	2	1	4

Data are numbers of patients unless otherwise indicated
*Mean (95% CI)
†Solitary tumors with or without satellites
‡(IU/L)

Efficacy

1. Chemoembolization induced objective responses sustained for at least 6 months in 35% (14) of cases, and was associated with a significantly lower rate of portal vein invasion than conservative treatment

2. Probability of portal vein invasion reduced from 58% in control to 17% in patients with chemoembolization

3. Survival probabilities at 1 year and 2 years were 75% and 50% for embolization, and 82% and 63% for chemoembolization

4. Patients who achieved objective responses sustained for at least 6 months had probabilities of survival at 1, 2, and 3 years of 96%, 77%, and 47%, respectively (p = 0.002 compared with patients with treatment failure, and p = 0.006 vs control group)

5. Treatment allocation was the sole baseline variable independently related to survival (odds ratio 0.45 [95% CI 0.25–0.81], p = 0.02) in the Cox's regression model. Inclusion of treatment response identified this variable as an independent predictor (odds ratio 0.59 [0.44–0.81], p = 0.0007) together with constitutional syndrome (0.46 [0.25–0.86], p = 0.04)

6. There were no differences in intention-to-treat survival between non-responders and the control group (1-year survival 65% vs 63%; 2-year survival 41% vs 26%, p = 0.3)

	Embolization (n = 37)	Chemoembolization (n = 40)*	Control (n = 35)*
Mean follow-up, month	21.7	21.2	14.5
Mean follow-up, 95% CI	17.5–26.0	17.3–25.1	10.6–18.4
Probability of survival at 1 year	75%	82%	63%
Probability of survival at 2 years	50%	63%	27%
Probability of survival at 3 years	29%	29%	17%
Mean survival, months	25.3	28.7	17.9
Mean survival, 95% CI	20.3–30.2	23.6–33.7	13.1–22.7

(continued)

Efficacy (continued)

	Embolization (n = 37)	Chemoembolization (n = 40)*	Control (n = 35)*
Assessment of Response in 102 Patients Who Survived for at Least 5 Months			
Objective responses	16†	14†	
Probability of portal-vein invasion at 2 years	—	17%	58%
		p = 0.005	

*Survival was significantly better in the chemoembolization group than in the control group (p = 0.009)
†Embolization vs control, p = 0.001; chemoembolization vs control, p = 0.004

Causes of Death

	Embolization (n = 37)	Chemoembolization (n = 40)	Control (n = 35)	Total (n = 112)
Deaths	25 (67%)	21 (52%)	25 (71%)	71 (63%)
Cause of Death				
Tumor progression	20	14	23	57
Hepatic failure with SD*	4	5	2	11
Other	1†	2‡	0	3

*SD, stable disease
†Neoplasm of lung
‡Neoplasm of tongue and treatment-related death (septic shock)

Reasons for Treatment Discontinuation Among Patients Who Received Embolization*

	Embolization (n = 37)	Chemoembolization (n = 40)	Both Groups (n = 77)
Reason			
Tumor progression (portal thrombosis, extra-hepatic spread, or performance status >2)	15	9	24
Liver failure without tumor progression	3	2	5
Technical problems (arterial hepatic obstruction, collateral or hepatofugal blood flow, low ejection fraction)	3	8	11
Adverse events (leucopenia, ischemic biliary stricture, transient ischemic attack, allergic dermatitis)	1	4	5
Patient's decision	2	4	6
Death on treatment	4	3	7
Other (lung cancer, percutaneous ethanol injection)	2	0	2
Treatment discontinuation	29 (78%)	31 (77%)	60 (78%)
Active treatment at end of follow-up	8 (22%)	9 (23%)	17 (22%)

*There were no significant differences between groups

Toxicity (N = 40)

Adverse Event	Number of Patients
Cholecystitis	2
Leukopenia	2
Ischemic biliary stricture	1
Hepatic infarction	1
Spontaneous bacterial peritonitis	1
Bacteremia	1
Septic shock	1
Allergic dermatitis	1
Severe alopecia	1

Other complications associated with TACE procedures in general:
- Hepatic artery occlusion: 4%
- Damage to the hepatic artery: pseudoaneurysm (rare), occlusion, and dissection
- Treatment was discontinued in 60 (78%) patients

Therapy Monitoring

1. Days 7 and 14 after TACE and then monthly: CBC and LFTs
2. Response assessment using computed tomography (CT) every 3 months

REGIMEN

CHEMOEMBOLIZATION WITH CISPLATIN

Lo C-M et al. Hepatology 2002;35:1164–1171

Chemoembolization: Cisplatin (1 mg/mL) emulsified with ethiodized oil injection in equivalent volumes (1:1)
- Administer cisplatin intra-arterially via the left or right hepatic artery as appropriate for tumor vascularization. If selective catheterization is not possible, the cisplatin emulsion is injected into the hepatic artery, distal to the gastroduodenal artery
- The emulsion is injected slowly under fluoroscopic monitoring to a maximum volume of 60 mL ($\leq$30 mg cisplatin) at a controlled rate to prevent retrograde flow, followed by mechanical obstruction achieved by intra-arterial injection of gelatin sponge pellets 1 mm in diameter mixed with gentamicin 40 mg
- Chemoembolization is repeated every 2–3 months until comorbid pathologies, adverse events, or disease progression are observed

Notes:
- Extra-hepatic arterial supply of HCC is important. See section on **Extrahepatic collateral vessels supplying hepatocellular carcinomas** [Kim HC, Chung JW, Lee W, Jae HJ, Park JH. Radiographics 2005;25(Suppl 1):S25–S39]
- Forty patients assigned to the chemoembolization group received a total of 192 courses of chemoembolization, with each patient receiving a median of 4.5 courses (range, 1–15). Ninety-four courses (49%) of the chemoembolization were performed by selective injection into the right or left hepatic artery. The median volume of cisplatin-ethiodized oil emulsion injected in 1 course was 20 mL (range, 2–60), and the dosage was significantly related to the tumor size ($r = 0.70$; $P < 0.001$)

Two patients were scheduled for continuation of chemoembolization as of the date of the latest follow-up. The remaining 38 patients had treatment stopped because of progressive disease (12 patients), death (7 patients), poor liver function (6 patients), adverse effects (6 patients), patient refusal (3 patients), arteriovenous shunting (2 patients), and hepatic artery thrombosis (2 patients)

The most common clinical adverse effect was a self-limiting syndrome consisting of fever, abdominal pain, and vomiting. The median hospital stay for each course of treatment was 2 days (range, 1–21)

GENERAL GUIDELINES

Prior to embolization:
- **Hydration**
  - Start intravenous **hydration** with 0.9% sodium chloride injection (0.9% NS)
  - Continuous 0.9% NS 100 mL/h beginning a minimum of 6 hours prior to procedure
- **Antibiotic prophylaxis** not always required but may be considered with the first doses given before embolization:
  - **Metronidazole** 500 mg; administer intravenously prior to procedure followed by **Metronidazole** 500 mg; administer intravenously every 12 hours × 3 doses, *plus*
  - **Cefazolin** 1000 mg; administer intravenously prior to procedure followed by **Cefazolin** 500 mg; administer intravenously every 8 hours × 5 doses
- **Antiemetic primary prophylaxis**

  Give a serotonin receptor ($5HT_3$) antagonist plus a high-potency glucocorticoid
  - **Ondansetron** 16 mg; administer intravenously or 24 mg orally, *plus*
  - **Dexamethasone** 10–12 mg; administer intravenously or orally 30–60 minutes before the procedure

Post-embolization syndrome:
- The triad of abdominal pain, vomiting, and fever that frequently occurs 24–72 hours after chemoembolization is commonly referred to as post-embolization syndrome
- Post-embolization syndrome uniformly responds to supportive care including analgesics and antiemetics
- Use care administering acetaminophen (paracetamol) and non-steroidal anti-inflammatory drugs in patients with liver cirrhosis

After embolization:
- Continue intravenous **hydration** with 0.9% NS or another clinically appropriate fluid until patient resumes adequate oral fluid intake
- Provide **analgesic support** with parenterally administered opioid medications (**morphine, hydromorphone, fentanyl**) after chemoembolization until patient is able to continue analgesic treatment with oral products
- Continue **antiemetic prophylaxis** with a $5HT_3$ antagonist plus a high-potency glucocorticoid:
  - **Ondansetron** 8 mg; administer intravenously or orally every 8 hours, *plus*
  - **Dexamethasone** 8 mg; administer intravenously or orally every 8 hours for 2–3 days
- **Filgrastim** (G-CSF) 5 mcg/kg per day; administer by subcutaneous injection
  - May be used for patients who develop an ANC <500/mm³, neutropenia and fever, or documented infections during neutropenia
  - Discontinue filgrastim at least 24 hours before a chemoembolization procedure

Treatment Modifications

Withhold or discontinue chemoembolization for:
• Hepatic artery thrombosis
• Main portal vein thrombosis
• Arteriovenous shunting
• Hepatic encephalopathy
• Ascites not controlled by diuretics
• Variceal bleeding within the last 3 months
• Serum total bilirubin >50 μmol/L (>2.9 mg/dL)
• Serum albumin <28 g/L (<2.8 g/dL)
• Prothrombin time 4 seconds > control

Patient Population Studied

A study of 80 patients with Okuda Stages I–II HCC and no contraindications for chemoembolization; 40 assigned to chemoembolization and 39 assigned to control

Baseline Characteristics of the Study Patients According to the Treatment Group

	Chemoembolization (N = 40)	Control (N = 39)
Age (y)*	62 (53–69)	63 (53–70)
Sex (men/women)	36/4	34/5
Serum hepatitis B surface antigen (positive/negative)	34/6	29/10
Serum creatinine, μmol/L*	92 (82–102)	87 (78–98)
Serum total bilirubin, μmol/L*	14 (10–21)	13 (11–23)
Serum albumin, g/L*	38 (32–42)	37 (33–40)
Serum alanine aminotransferase, U/L*	51 (38–83)	53 (35–88)
Prothrombin time, s*	11.5 (10.9–12.4)	11.5 (10.8–12.5)
Serum α-fetoprotein, ng/mL*	505 (55–5, 874)	500 (58–24, 458)
Serum α-fetoprotein (ng/mL; <20/20–500/>500)	6/14/20	8/12/19
Indocyanine green retention at 15 minutes (%)*	24 (6–33)	18 (6–38)
ECOG performance status rating (0/1/2/3)	20/16/3/1	14/19/4/2
Presenting symptom (asymptomatic/ symptomatic)	12/28	10/29
Diameter of largest tumor mass, cm*	7 (4–14)	7 (5–11)
Number of tumors (solitary/multinodular)	17/23	15/24
Portal vein obstruction (right/left/main)†	6/3/0	7/5/0
Okuda stage (I/II)	19/21	18/21

Note: P >0.05 for all variables when the 2 groups are compared
*Values are medians, with interquartile ranges shown in parentheses
†Assessed by computed tomography

Efficacy

Patients with Measurable Disease*

	Chemoembolization (N = 28)	Control (N = 18)
Objective response	39%	6%
	P = 0.014	
Complete response	(0)	(0)
Major responses	11/28 (39.3)	1 (5.55%)
Minor response	6/28 (21.4%)	2 (11.1%)
Stabilization	7/28 (25%)	6 (33.3%)
Progression	4/28 (14.3%)	9 (50%)

Patients with Measurable AFP†

	Chemoembolization (N = 29)	Control (N = 21)
Objective response in α-FP	21/29 (72.4%)	2/21 (9.5%)
	P <0.001	
Complete response in α-FP	9/29 (31%)	0/21 (0)
Major responses α-FP	12/29 (41.4%)	2/21 (9.5%)
Minor response in α-FP	0/29 (0)	0/21 (0)
Stabilization of α-FP	1/29 (3.4%)	1/21 (4.8%)
Progression of α-FP	7/29 (24.1%)	18/21 (85.7%)

All Patients

	Chemoembolization	Control
1-Year survival	57%[‡]	32%[‡]
2-Year survival	31%[‡]	11%[‡]
3-Year survival	26%[*,‡]	3%[‡]

*Patients who survived more than 3 months and had a measurable tumor on computed tomographic scan
†Patients with a baseline serum α-fetoprotein level >20 ng/mL who survived more than 3 months
‡Relative risk of death in the chemoembolization group was 0.50; 95% CI, 0.31–0.81; p <005

Univariate Analysis of Prognostic Variables for Survival

Characteristics	Number of Patients	Probability of Survival (%)			P
		12 Months	24 Months	36 Months	
Study treatment					
Chemoembolization	40	57	31	26	0.002
Control	39	32	11	3	
Sex					
Men	70	44	20	15	NS (0.720)
Women	9	56	33	11	

(*continued*)

		\multicolumn{3}{c}{Probability of Survival (%)}	

<table>
<thead>
<tr><th rowspan="2">Characteristics</th><th rowspan="2">Number of Patients</th><th colspan="3">Probability of Survival (%)</th><th rowspan="2">P</th></tr>
<tr><th>12 Months</th><th>24 Months</th><th>36 Months</th></tr>
</thead>
<tbody>
<tr><td colspan="6">Age (y)</td></tr>
<tr><td>≤60</td><td>34</td><td>35</td><td>15</td><td>12</td><td rowspan="2">NS (0.274)</td></tr>
<tr><td>>60</td><td>45</td><td>52</td><td>26</td><td>17</td></tr>
<tr><td colspan="6">ECOG performance status rating</td></tr>
<tr><td>0</td><td>34</td><td>43</td><td>18</td><td>9</td><td rowspan="2">NS (0.384)</td></tr>
<tr><td>1–3</td><td>45</td><td>46</td><td>23</td><td>19</td></tr>
<tr><td colspan="6">Presenting symptom</td></tr>
<tr><td>Asymptomatic</td><td>22</td><td>77</td><td>43</td><td>29</td><td rowspan="2">0.004</td></tr>
<tr><td>Symptomatic</td><td>57</td><td>33</td><td>13</td><td>9</td></tr>
<tr><td colspan="6">Tumor size (cm)</td></tr>
<tr><td>≤5</td><td>26</td><td>65</td><td>39</td><td>27</td><td rowspan="2">0.019</td></tr>
<tr><td>>5</td><td>50</td><td>37</td><td>13</td><td>9</td></tr>
<tr><td colspan="6">Tumor number</td></tr>
<tr><td>Single</td><td>32</td><td>55</td><td>29</td><td>16</td><td rowspan="2">NS (0.225)</td></tr>
<tr><td>Multiple</td><td>47</td><td>39</td><td>16</td><td>14</td></tr>
<tr><td colspan="6">Unilobar portal vein obstruction</td></tr>
<tr><td>Negative</td><td>58</td><td>60</td><td>27</td><td>18</td><td rowspan="2"><0.001</td></tr>
<tr><td>Positive</td><td>21</td><td>5</td><td>5</td><td>5</td></tr>
<tr><td colspan="6">Okuda stage</td></tr>
<tr><td>I</td><td>37</td><td>61</td><td>35</td><td>23</td><td rowspan="2">0.003</td></tr>
<tr><td>II</td><td>42</td><td>31</td><td>10</td><td>7</td></tr>
<tr><td colspan="6">Serum albumin (g/L)</td></tr>
<tr><td>≤37</td><td>40</td><td>44</td><td>16</td><td>10</td><td rowspan="2">NS (0.341)</td></tr>
<tr><td>>37</td><td>39</td><td>46</td><td>27</td><td>19</td></tr>
<tr><td colspan="6">Serum bilirubin (μmol/L)</td></tr>
<tr><td>≤14</td><td>41</td><td>41</td><td>23</td><td>18</td><td rowspan="2">NS (0.967)</td></tr>
<tr><td>>14</td><td>38</td><td>49</td><td>19</td><td>11</td></tr>
<tr><td colspan="6">% Indocyanine green retention at 15 minutes</td></tr>
<tr><td>≤20</td><td>38</td><td>39</td><td>20</td><td>17</td><td rowspan="2">NS (0.635)</td></tr>
<tr><td>>20</td><td>41</td><td>50</td><td>23</td><td>13</td></tr>
<tr><td colspan="6">α-Fetoprotein (ng/mL)</td></tr>
<tr><td>≤500</td><td>40</td><td>54</td><td>32</td><td>19</td><td rowspan="2">NS (0.059)</td></tr>
<tr><td>>500</td><td>39</td><td>36</td><td>10</td><td>10</td></tr>
</tbody>
</table>

Efficacy (continued)

(continued)

Efficacy (continued)

Comparison of Survival Between the Chemoembolization and Control Groups Stratified by Baseline Prognostic Variables*

	Chemoembolization	Control	P
Presenting symptom			
Asymptomatic	25.4 (17.5)	16.6 (2.5)	0.039
Symptomatic	11.2 (2.6)	5.2 (1.4)	0.019
Unilobar portal vein obstruction			
Negative	18.0 (3.5)	9.2 (5.6)	0.008
Positive	5.1 (2.2)	2.6 (2.3)	NS (0.406)
Tumor size (cm)			
≤5	29.8 (12.2)	11.5 (3.0)	0.003
>5	11.2 (1.8)	5.3 (1.4)	NS (0.115)
Okuda stage			
I	25.4 (9.1)	11.5 (5.8)	0.016
II	9.2 (4.1)	5.2 (1.5)	0.040

*Values are median survival times in months with standard errors in parentheses

Comparison of Liver Function as Assessed by the Serum Bilirubin Level, Serum Albumin Level, and Indocyanine Green Retention Rate at 15 Minutes

	Chemoembolization Group		Control Group		
	Number of Patients	Median (Interquartile Range)	Number of Patients	Median (Interquartile Range)	P
Bilirubin (μmol/L)					
3 Months	34	15 (10–31)	24	21 (14–42)	0.038
6 Months	24	14 (11–24)	13	17 (10–28)	0.987
9 Months	19	16 (10–20)	7	18 (12–32)	0.385
12 Months	17	13 (9–23)	9	15 (11–30)	0.517
Albumin (g/L)					
3 Months	34	36 (31–40)	24	32 (26–37)	0.073
6 Months	24	35 (31–39)	13	35 (28–38)	0.425
9 Months	19	35 (31–37)	7	33 (28–36)	0.223
12 Months	17	33 (31–39)	9	34 (27–39)	0.499
Indocyanine green retention at 15 minutes (%)					
3 Months	32	25 (14–43)	25	36 (20–52)	0.169
6 Months	25	25 (18–38)	13	26 (17–51)	0.433
9 Months	22	25 (20–34)	10	28 (15–48)	0.405
12 Months	17	26 (13–34)	9	32 (22–47)	0.146

Toxicity
(N = 40 Patients/192 Courses)

	Number (%) Cycles
Fevers ≥38°C (≥100.4°F)*	63 (32.8)
Abdominal pain*	50 (26%)
Vomiting*	32 (16.7%)
Ascites	10 (5.2%)
Gastrointestinal bleeding	8 (4.2%)
Bleeding at femoral puncture	3 (1.6%)
Encephalopathy	3 (1.6%)
Ruptured tumor	2 (1%)
Pleural effusion	2 (1%)
Liver abscess	1 (0.5%)
Hematuria	1 (0.5%)
Hypotension	1 (0.5%)
Bradycardia	1 (0.5%)

*The most common clinical adverse effect was a self-limiting syndrome consisting of fever, abdominal pain, and vomiting. The median hospital stay for each course of treatment was 2 days (range, 1–21)

Therapy Monitoring

1. Days 7 and 14 after TACE and then monthly: CBC and LFTs
2. Response assessment using computed tomography (CT) every 3 months

REGIMEN

DEB-TACE: TRANSARTERIAL CHEMOEMBOLIZATION (TACE) USING DRUG-ELUTING BEADS (DEB)

Lammer J et al. Cardiovasc Intervent Radiol 2010;33:41–52

Transarterial chemoembolization using drug-eluting beads (DEB), an embolizing device that slowly releases chemotherapy to decrease systemic toxicity

Pretreatment approach:
- A baseline angiography of the celiac trunk, superior mesenteric artery, and hepatic artery is performed using a peripheral arterial approach
- Antibiotic prophylaxis is not required but may be considered

Note: Extra-hepatic arterial supply of HCC is important. See section on **Extrahepatic collateral vessels supplying hepatocellular carcinomas** [Kim HC, Chung JW, Lee W, Jae HJ, Park JH. Radiographics 2005;25(Suppl 1):S25–S39]

Drug-eluting beads (DEB) [BioCompatibles Ltd., UK] with a diameter ranging between 300 and 700 micrometers are loaded with **doxorubicin** and mixed with an equal volume of contrast media. Additional unloaded spheres are used to complete the embolization procedure

Doxorubicin 150 mg (bilirubin <1.5 mg/dL; <25.7 μmol/L)

Loading process to obtain a final loading dose of 150 mg doxorubicin per two 2-mL vials of beads:
- Begin about 2 hours before the TACE is planned
- Reconstitute a vial containing doxorubicin 50 mg with 2 mL of sterile water for injection. Mix well to obtain a clear red doxorubicin solution with concentration = 25 mg/mL
- Remove as much of the solution as possible from a vial of beads using a syringe with a small-gauge needle
- Using a syringe and needle, add 2 mL of reconstituted doxorubicin solution directly to the vial of beads
- Agitate the beads in the doxorubicin solution occasionally to encourage mixing. The dark red color of the suspension should become slightly pink and the beads, which are initially blue, should become red, indicating that doxorubicin has been loaded into the beads
  Note: Although the solution retains a red color, the doxorubicin will be loaded. Loading will take a minimum of 20 minutes for the smallest beads and up to 120 minutes for the largest beads
- Prior to use, transfer the beads loaded with doxorubicin to a syringe and add an equal volume of non-ionic contrast media. Invert the syringe gently to obtain an even suspension of beads

Note: Beads should only be loaded with doxorubicin HCl; liposomal formulations of doxorubicin are not suitable for loading into beads. A dose of up to 37.5 mg doxorubicin per mL of beads can be loaded. The maximum recommended total dose of doxorubicin per procedure is 150 mg. Beads loaded with doxorubicin may be stored for up to 24 hours at 2°–8°C (35.6°–46.4°F) in the presence or absence of non-ionic contrast media. Two hours of dwell time for 500–700 μmol DEB has been reported to allow for loading of more than 90% of 100 mg doxorubicin in the beads (Lewis AL et al. J Vasc Interv Radiol 2006;17:1335–1343)

TACE Procedure:
- The vascular network associated with the lesion is carefully evaluated using high-resolution imaging prior to beginning the embolization procedure
- **Highly selective catheterization** is performed with a 3-French microcatheter in order to obtain complete obstruction of the nourishing arteries and avoid damage to non-tumoral liver
- Beads are available in a range of sizes and care should be taken to choose the appropriate size of the bead that best matches the pathology (ie, vascular target/vessel size) and provides the desired clinical outcome
- A delivery catheter is chosen based on the size of the target vessel. Beads can tolerate temporary compression of 20–30% in order to facilitate passage through a delivery catheter

(continued)

Patient Population Studied

A trial in which 212 patients with Child-Pugh A/B cirrhosis (76% male, 59% HCV) with HCC unsuitable for resection without portal invasion or extra-hepatic spread and less than 50% liver involvement received chemoembolization with doxorubicin loaded DEB at doses adjusted for bilirubin and body surface (range: 47–150 mg). Patients were excluded if they had another primary tumor, advanced liver disease (bilirubin levels >3 mg/dL, AST or ALT >5 × upper limit of normal or >250 U/L), advanced tumoral disease (vascular invasion or extrahepatic spread, or diffuse HCC, defined as >50% liver involvement), or contraindications for doxorubicin administration. In this international, multicenter, prospective, randomized single-blind, phase II study patients were randomized to receive doxorubicin with DC Bead or conventional TACE defined as 50–75 mg/m² doxorubicin emulsified in ethiodized oil followed by particle embolization with an embolic agent of choice

Therapy Monitoring

1. Days 7 and 14 after TACE and then monthly: CBC and LFTs
2. Response assessment using computed tomography (CT) every 3 months

(*continued*)

- The delivery catheter is introduced into the target vessel according to standard techniques. The catheter tip is positioned as close as possible to the treatment site to avoid inadvertent occlusion of normal vessels
- Because the beads are not radiopaque, monitoring the embolization under fluoroscopic visualization necessitates adding contrast medium to the DEB suspension
- Care should be taken to ensure proper suspension of the beads in the contrast medium to enhance distribution during injection
- Beads are drawn into a syringe and slowly injected
- After completion of the treatment, the catheter is removed while maintaining gentle suction so as not to dislodge beads still within the catheter lumen
- The embolization end point will be to achieve complete occlusion of the neovascularity, avoiding, however, complete stasis in the afferent artery, which could lead to endothelial damage and subsequent thrombosis precluding future treatments

Note: Treatment is given at 2-monthly intervals, with a maximum of three chemoembolization (at baseline, 2 months, and 4 months) with a 6-month follow-up

GENERAL GUIDELINES

Prior to embolization:
- **Hydration**
  - Start intravenous **hydration** with 0.9% sodium chloride injection (0.9% NS)
  - Continuous 0.9% NS 100 mL/h beginning a minimum of 6 hours prior to procedure
- **Antibiotic prophylaxis** not always required but may be considered with the first doses given before embolization:
  - **Metronidazole** 500 mg; administer intravenously prior to the procedure followed by **Metronidazole** 500 mg; administer intravenously every 12 hours × 3 doses, *plus*
  - **Cefazolin** 1000 mg; administer intravenously prior to the procedure followed by **Cefazolin** 500 mg; administer intravenously every 8 hours × 5 doses
- **Antiemetic primary prophylaxis**
  Give a serotonin receptor ($5HT_3$) antagonist plus a high-potency glucocorticoid
  - **Ondansetron** 16 mg; administer intravenously *or* 24 mg orally, *plus*
  - **Dexamethasone** 10–12 mg; administer intravenously or orally 30–60 minutes before the procedure

Post-embolization syndrome:
- The triad of abdominal pain, vomiting, and fever that frequently occurs 24–72 hours after chemoembolization is commonly referred to as post-embolization syndrome
- Post-embolization syndrome uniformly responds to supportive care including analgesics and antiemetics
- Use care administering acetaminophen (paracetamol) and non-steroidal anti-inflammatory drugs in patients with liver cirrhosis

After embolization:
- Continue intravenous **hydration** with 0.9% NS or another clinically appropriate fluid until patient resumes adequate oral fluid intake
- Provide **analgesic support** with parenterally administered opioid medications (**morphine, hydromorphone, fentanyl**) after chemoembolization until the patient is able to continue analgesic treatment with oral products
- Continue **antiemetic prophylaxis** with a $5HT_3$ antagonist plus a high-potency glucocorticoid:
  - **Ondansetron** 8 mg; administer intravenously or orally every 8 hours, *plus*
  - **Dexamethasone** 8 mg; administer intravenously or orally every 8 hours for 2–3 days
- **Filgrastim** (G-CSF) 5 mcg/kg per day; administer by subcutaneous injection
  - May be used for patients who develop an ANC <500/mm³, neutropenia and fever, or documented infections during neutropenia
  - Discontinue filgrastim at least 24 hours before a chemoembolization procedure

Efficacy

Response Rates

Tumor Response Rate at 6 Months	DC Bead (N = 93)*	cTACE (N = 108)*
Objective response	48/93 (51.6%)	47/108 (43.5%)
	one-sided P = 0.11†	
Complete response	25/93 (26.9%)	24/108 (22.2%)
Partial response	23/93 (24.7%)	23/108 (21.3%)
Stable disease	11/93 (11.8%)	9/108 (8.3%)
Disease control rate	59/93 (63.4%)	56/108 (51.9%)
	two-sided P = 0.11	
Progressive disease	30/93 (32.3%)	44/108 (40.7%)
Advanced disease patients‡		
Objective response, advanced disease‡	32/61 (52.4%)	25/72 (34.7)
	Chi-square P = 0.038	
Complete response, advanced disease‡	15/61 (24.5%)	10/72 (13.9%)
	Chi-square P = 0.091	
Disease control rate, advanced disease‡	38/61 (63.5%)	32/72 (44.4%)
	Chi-square P = 0.026	
Disease control rate, Child-Pugh B	21/33 (63%)	13/41 (32%)
Disease control rate, ECOG 1	19/30 (63%)	21/66 (32%)
Disease control rate, bilobar	51/86 (59%)	46/94 (49%)
Disease control rate, recurrent disease	17/23 (73%)	13/24 (54%)

*4 DC Bead patients and 8 cTACE patients withdrew prior to the first MRI scan. Reasons for these withdrawals were AEs (four DC Bead and four cTACE), withdrawn consent (two cTACE), and post consent ineligibility (two cTACE)
†The hypothesis of superiority was not met. The difference between groups in favor of DC Bead was 8.1% (two-sided 95% repeated confidence interval (RCI), −4.8 to 22.6%)
‡Advanced disease = 67% of patients with Child-Pugh B, ECOG 1, bilobar or recurrent disease

Toxicity

Incidence of Serious Adverse Events* within 30 Days of a Procedure Analysis by Stratification (Safety Population)

	Number of Patients/Total (%) Number of Events	
	DC Bead (N = 93)	cTACE (N = 108)
Treatment-related SAEs within 30 days of a procedure [primary safety endpoint]	19 (20.4%) 28 events	21 (19.4%) 24 events
	P = 0.86	
	Number of Patients/Total (%)	
Stratification factor	DC Bead (N = 93)	cTACE (N = 108)
All patients	22/93 (23.7)	32/108 (29.6)
Child-Pugh A	19/77 (24.7)	26/89 (29.2)
Child-Pugh B	3/16 (18.8)	6/19 (31.6)
ECOG 0	17/74 (23.0)	23/80 (28.8)
ECOG 1	5/19 (26.3)	9/28 (32.1)
Unilobar	12/52 (23.1)	18/63 (28.6)
Bilobar	10/41 (24.4)	14/45 (31.1)
No prior curative treatments	19/82 (23.2)	28/95 (29.5)
Recurrent disease	3/11 (27.3)	4/13 (30.8)

*Note: Serious adverse events were defined as events: (1) resulting in death; (2) that were immediately life-threatening; (3) resulting in permanent or significant disability/incapacity; (4) requiring or extending inpatient hospitalization; or (5) congenital anomaly/birth defects. Analysis of treatment groups overall: chi-square test P = 0.34; difference in incidence rates, −6.0%; 95% CI, −18.2 to 6.2

Effects of Systemic Doxorubicin

Events/SWOG Toxicity Grade	DC Bead (N = 93)		cTACE (N = 108)	
	Number of Events	Number of Patients	Number of Events	Number of Patients
	12	11 (11.8%)	40	28 (25.9%)
All doxorubicin-related events	Incidence = −14.1%; 95% CI, −24.7% to −3.5%; P = 0.012			
Alopecia	1	1 (1%)	23	22 (20.4%)
Grade 1	1		12	
Grade 2	0		11	
Marrow suppression	5	5 (5.4%)	8	6 (5.6%)
Grade 1	2		1	
Grade 2	2		1	
Grade 3	1		4	
Grade 4	0		2	
Mucositis	4	4 (4.3%)	7	6 (5.6%)
Grade 1	4		5	
Grade 2	0		1	
Grade 3	0		1	
Skin discoloration	2	2 (2.2%)	2	2 (1.9%)
Grade 1	1		0	
Grade 2	1		2	
Post-embolization syndrome	35	23 (24.7%)	43	28 (25.9%)

REGIMEN

SORAFENIB

Llovet JM et al. N Engl J Med 2008;359:378–90
Cheng et al. Lancet Oncol 2009;10:25–34

Sorafenib 400 mg per dose; administer orally, twice daily, continually
(total dose/week = 5600 mg)

Supportive Care
Antiemetic prophylaxis
Emetogenic potential: **LOW**
See Chapter 39 for antiemetic recommendations

Hematopoietic growth factor (CSF) prophylaxis
Primary prophylaxis is NOT indicated
See Chapter 43 for more information

Antimicrobial prophylaxis
Risk of fever and neutropenia is LOW
  Antimicrobial primary prophylaxis to be considered:
  • Antibacterial—not indicated
  • Antifungal—not indicated
  • Antiviral—not indicated, unless patient previously had an episode of HSV
See Chapter 47 for more information

Diarrhea management
Latent or delayed-onset diarrhea*:
  Loperamide 4 mg orally initially after the first loose or liquid stool, *then*
  Loperamide 2 mg orally every 2 hours during waking hours, *plus*
  Loperamide 4 mg orally every 4 hours during hours of sleep
  • Continue for at least 12 hours after diarrhea resolves
  • Recurrent diarrhea after a 12-hour diarrhea-free interval is treated as a new episode
  • Rehydrate orally with fluids and electrolytes during a diarrheal episode
  • If a patient develops blood or mucus in stool, dehydration, or hemodynamic instability, or if diarrhea persists >48 hours despite loperamide, stop loperamide and hospitalize the patient for IV hydration
  Alternatively, a trial of **Diphenoxylate hydrochloride** 2.5 mg **with Atropine sulfate** 0.025 mg (eg, Lomotil®)
  • Initial adult dose is two tablets four times daily until control has been achieved, after which the dose may be reduced to meet individual requirements. Control may often be maintained with as little as two tablets daily
  • Clinical improvement of acute diarrhea is usually observed within 48 hours. If improvement of chronic diarrhea after treatment with a maximum daily dose of 8 tablets is not observed within 10 days, control is unlikely with further administration
Persistent diarrhea:
  Octreotide 100–150 mcg subcutaneously 3 times daily. Maximum total daily dose is 1500 mcg
Antibiotic therapy during latent or delayed-onset diarrhea:
  A fluoroquinolone (eg, **Ciprofloxacin** 500 mg orally every 12 hours) if absolute neutrophil count <500/mm³ with or without accompanying fever in association with diarrhea
  • Antibiotics should also be administered if patient is hospitalized with prolonged diarrhea and should be continued until diarrhea resolves

*Abigerges D et al. J Natl Cancer Inst 1994;86:446–449
Rothenberg ML et al. J Clin Oncol 2001;19:3801–3807
Wadler S et al. J Clin Oncol 1998;16:3169–3178

Patient Population Studied

Llovet JM et al. N Engl J Med 2008;359:378–390

Multicenter, phase 3, double-blind, placebo-controlled trial. Six hundred two patients with advanced hepatocellular carcinoma who had not previously received systemic treatment were randomly assigned to receive either sorafenib (n = 299) or placebo (n = 303). The study population consisted of patients with advanced-stage hepatocellular carcinoma. Patients were classified as having advanced disease if they were not eligible or had disease progression after surgical or locoregional therapies. Eligibility criteria also included (a) Eastern Cooperative Oncology Group performance status score ≤2; (b) Child-Pugh liver function class A; (c) prothrombin time international normalized ratio ≤2.3 or prothrombin time ≤6 sec greater than control; (d) albumin, ≥2.8 g/dL; (e) total bilirubin ≤3 mg/dL (≤51.3 micromol/L); and (f) alanine aminotransferase and aspartate aminotransferase ≤5 times the upper limit of the normal range

Cheng et al. Lancet Oncol 2009;10:25–34

Patients with advanced (unresectable or metastatic) hepatocellular carcinoma who had not received previous systemic therapy were eligible for this trial. Eligibility criteria also included ECOG PS of 0/1/2; Child-Pugh liver function class A; and a life expectancy ≥12 weeks; albumin concentration of at least 28 g/L; total bilirubin concentration of 51.3 μmol/L or less; alanine aminotransferase concentration of five times the upper limit of normal (ULN) or less. Patients who had received previous local therapy, such as surgery, radiotherapy, hepatic arterial embolization, chemoembolization, radiofrequency ablation, percutaneous injection, or cryoablation, were eligible for enrolment in the study, provided that either the target lesion increased in size by 25% or more, or the target lesion had not been treated with local therapy. Furthermore, the local therapy must have been stopped at least 4 weeks before study entry. Patients with recurrent disease after previous resection were considered eligible for the study. Exclusion criteria included previous or concomitant systemic therapy (including new, molecularly targeted therapies)

(continued)

Patient Population Studied (*continued*)

Demographic and Baseline Characteristics of the Patients (Intention-to-Treat Population)*

Llovet JM et al. N Engl J Med 2008;359:378–390

Variable	Sorafenib (N = 299)	Placebo (N = 303)
Age, y	64.9 ± 11.2	66.3 ± 10.2
Sex, no. (%) Male/Female	260 (87)/39 (13)	264 (87)/39 (13)
Region, no. (%)		
Europe and Australasia	263 (88)	263 (87)
North America	27 (9)	29 (10)
Central and South America	9 (3)	11 (4)
Cause of disease, no. (%)		
Hepatitis C only	87 (29)	82 (27)
Alcohol only	79 (26)	80 (26)
Hepatitis B only	56 (19)	55 (18)
Unknown	49 (16)	56 (19)
Other	28 (9)	29 (10)
ECOG performance status, 0/1/2 no. (%)	161(54)/114(38)/24(8)	164(54)/117(39)/22(7)
BCLC stage, B (intermediate)/ C (advanced) no. (%)	54(18)/244(82)‡	51(17)/252(83)
Macroscopic vascular invasion, no. (%)	108 (36)	123 (41)
Extrahepatic spread, no. (%)	159 (53)	150 (50)
Lymph nodes, no. (%)	89 (30	65 (21)
Lung, no. (%)	67 (22)	58 (19)
Macroscopic vascular invasion, extra-hepatic spread, or both, Absent/Present, no. (%)	90 (30)/209 (70)	91 (30)/212 (70)
Child-Pugh class, A/B, no. (%)	284 (95)/14 (5)	297 (98)/6 (2)
Biochemical analysis		
Albumin, g/dL, Median (Range)	3.9 (2.7–5.3)	4.0 (2.5–5.1)
Total bilirubin, mg/dL, Median (Range)†	07. (0.1–16.4)	0.7 (0.2–6.1)
Alpha-fetoprotein, ng/mL—Median (Range)	44.3 ($0–208 \times 10^4$)	99.0 ($0–5 \times 10^5$)
Previous therapy, no. (%)§		
Surgical resection	57 (19)	62 (20)
Locoregional therapy		
Transarterial chemoembolization	86 (29)	90 (30)
Percutaneous ethanol injection	28 (9)	20 (7)
Radiofrequency ablation	17 (6)	12 (4)
Radiotherapy ϵ	13 (4)	15 (5)

(*continued*)

Patient Population Studied (*continued*)

Variable	Sorafenib (N = 299)	Placebo (N = 303)
Systemic anticancer therapy		
Hormonal therapy	7 (2)	8 (3)
Cytotoxic chemotherapy	1 (<1)	1 (<1)
Concomitant systemic antiviral therapy, no. (%)	6 (2)	2 (1)

*Plus–minus values are means ± SD. None of the differences between the two study groups were significant (P ≥0.05)

†To convert the values for bilirubin to micromoles per liter, multiply by 17.1. BCLC denotes

‡One patient in the sorafenib group had a BCLC score of D and a Child-Pugh class of C

§Patients may have received more than one type of therapy. There was no significant difference between groups in the number of patients who had received previous palliative or curative therapy or previous adjuvant or neoadjuvant therapy (P ≥0.05)

¶Radiotherapy was applied to extrahepatic metastatic lesions in all patients except five in the sorafenib group and three in the placebo group

Dose Modifications

Adverse Event	Dose Modification
G3/4 or persistent G2 drug-related adverse event	Decrease sorafenib to 400 mg daily*
G3/4 or persistent G2 drug-related adverse event on 400 mg daily	Decrease sorafenib to 400 mg every other day
G3/4 or persistent G2 drug-related adverse event on 400 mg every other day	Discontinue sorafenib

*A recent study in patients with thyroid cancer reduced doses initially from 400/400 daily to 400/200 each day before reducing the dose to 400 daily (Brose MS et al. Proc Am Soc Clin Oncol Annual Meeting 2013 [Abstract 4])

Efficacy

Llovet JM et al. N Engl J Med 2008;359:378–390

Outcome	Sorafenib	Placebo	HR/p-value
Median overall survival, months [95% CI]	10.7 months [9.4–13.3]	7.9 months [6.8–9.1]	0.69 (0.55–0.87) <0.001
1-year survival rate	44%	33%	0.009
Time to symptomatic progression*, median [95% CI]	4.1 Months [3.5–4.8]	4.9 months [4.2–6.3]	1.08 (0.88–1.31) 0.77
Time to radiologic progression, median [95% CI]	5.5 months [4.1–6.9]	2.8 months [2.7–3.9]	0.58 (0.45–0.74) <0.001
Level of Response†			
Complete response	0	0	NA
Partial response	2%	1%	0.05
Stable disease	71%	67%	0.17
Disease control rate‡	43%	32%	0

*Symptomatic progression was defined as a decrease of 4 or more points from the baseline score on the Functional Assessment of Cancer Therapy–Hepatobiliary Symptom Index 8 (FHSI8), deterioration to a score of 4 in Eastern Cooperative Group performance status, or death, whichever occurred first

†Response was measured according to RECIST

‡Percentage of patients with CR/PR/SD according to RECIST maintained for 28 days

(*continued*)

Efficacy (continued)

Cheng et al. Lancet Oncol 2009;10:25–34

	Sorafenib Group (n = 150)	Placebo Group (n = 76)
Complete response	0 (0)	0 (0)
Partial response	5 (3.3)	1 (1.3)
Stable disease	81 (54.0)	21 (27.6)
Progressive disease	46 (30.7)	41 (54.0)
Not assessable	18 (12.0)	13 (17.1)
DCR*, n (%; 95% CI)	53 (35.3; 27.7–43.6)	12 (15.8; 8.4–26.0)
Median overall survival	6.5 mos (95% CI, 5.56–7.56)	4.2 mos (95% CI, 3.75–5.46)
	HR 0.68 [95% CI, 0.50–0.93]; p = 0.014	
6-month overall survival	53.3%	36.7%
Median time to progression	2.8 mos [95% CI, 2.63–3.58]	1.4 mos [95% CI, 1.35–1.55]
	HR 0.57 [95% CI, 0.42–0.79]; p = 0.0005	
TTSP as assessed by the FHSI-8†	3.5 mos [95% CI, 2.80–4.24]	3.4 mos [95% CI, 2.40–4.08]
	HR 0.90 [95% CI 0.67–1.22]; p = 0.50	

*DCR (disease control rate) = proportion of patients who had the best response of complete response, partial response, or stable disease, maintained ≥4 weeks
†Time To Symptomatic Progression was defined as deterioration to ECOG PS 4 status or a change from baseline score on the 8-item, symptom-focused Functional Assessment of Cancer Therapy–Hepatobiliary Symptom Index (FHSI-8) questionnaire, associated with a deterioration of symptoms

Toxicity

Incidence of Drug-Related Adverse Events (Safety Population)*

Llovet JM et al. N Engl J Med 2008;359:378–390

Adverse Event	Sorafenib (N = 297)			Placebo (N = 302)			P Value	
	Any G	G3	G4	Any G	G3	G4	Any G	G3/4
	Percent							
Overall incidence	80			52				
Constitutional symptoms								
Fatigue	22	3	1	`6	3	<1	0.07	1.00
Weight loss	9	2	0	1	0	0	<0.001	0.03
Dermatologic events								
Alopecia	14	0	0	2	0	0	<0.001	NA
Dry skin	8	0	0	4	0	0	0.04	NA
Hand–foot skin reaction	21	8	0	3	<1	0	<0.001	<0.001
Pruritus	8	0	0	7	<1	0	0.65	1.0
Rash or desquamation	16	1	0	11	0	0	0.12	0.12
Other	5	1	0	1	0	0	<0.001	0.12

(continued)

Toxicity (*continued*)

Adverse Event	Sorafenib (N = 297)			Placebo (N = 302)			P Value	
	Any G	G3	G4	Any G	G3	G4	Any G	G3/4
	Percent							
Gastrointestinal events								
Anorexia	14	<1	0	3	1	0	<0.001	1.00
Diarrhea	39	8	0	11	2	0	<0.001	<0.001
Nausea	11	<1	0	8	1	0	0.16	0.62
Vomiting	5	1	0	3	1	0	0.14	0.68
Voice changes	6	0	0	1	0	0	<0.001	NA
Hypertension	5	2	0	2	1	0	0.05	0.28
Liver dysfunction	<1	<1	0	0	0	0	0.50	0.50
Abdominal pain not otherwise specified	8	2	0	3	1	0	0.007	0.17
Bleeding	7	1	0	4	1	<1	0.07	1.00

	Sorafenib (N = 297)	Placebo (N = 302)
Rate of discontinuation	38%	37%
Dose reductions due to adverse events‡	26%	7%
Dose interruptions due to adverse events	44%	30%

NA, denotes not applicable
*Listed are adverse events, as defined by the National Cancer Institute Common Terminology Criteria (version 3.0), that occurred in at least 5% of patients in either study group
†The most frequent adverse events leading to discontinuation of sorafenib were gastrointestinal events (6%), fatigue (5%), and liver dysfunction (5%). Drug-related adverse events leading to permanent treatment discontinuation occurred in 34 patients in the sorafenib group (11%) and 15 patients in the placebo group (5%)
‡The most frequent adverse events leading to dose reductions of sorafenib were diarrhea (8%), hand–foot skin reaction (5%), and rash or desquamation (3%)

Drug-related Adverse Events, Dose Reductions, and Discontinuations

Cheng et al. Lancet Oncol 2009;10:25–34

Drug-related, n (%)*	Sorafenib Group (n = 149)		Placebo Group (n = 75)	
	All	Grade 3/4	All	Grade 3/4
HFSR	67 (45.0)	16 (10.7)	2 (2.7)	0 (0)
Diarrhea	38 (25.5)	9 (6.0)	4 (5.3)	0 (0)
Alopecia	37 (24.8)	—	1 (1.3)	—
Fatigue	30 (20.1)	5 (3.4)	6 (8.0)	1 (1.3)
Rash/desquamation	30 (20.1)	1 (0.7)	5 (6.7)	0 (0)
Hypertension	28 (18.8)	3 (2.0)	1 (1.3)	0 (0)
Anorexia	19 (12.8)	0 (0)	2 (2.7)	0 (0)
Nausea	17 (11.4)	1 (0.7)	8 (10.7)	1 (1.3)

(*continued*)

Toxicity (*continued*)

	Sorafenib Group (n = 149)		Placebo Group (n = 75)	
	All	Grade 3/4	All	Grade 3/4
Dose reduction, n (%)†	46 (30.9)		2 (2.7)	
HFSR	17 (11.4)	—	0 (0)	—
Diarrhea	11 (7.4)	—	0 (0)	—
Discontinuation, n (%)‡	29 (19.5)		10 (13.3)	
Hemorrhage, upper GI	4 (2.7)	—	3 (4.0)	—
Ascites	4 (2.7)	—	2 (2.7)	—
Fatigue	4 (2.7)	—	0 (0)	—
Liver dysfunction	1 (0.7)	—	2 (2.7)	

HFSR, hand-foot skin reaction; GI, gastrointestinal tract
*Drug-related adverse events in ≥10% of patients in any study group
†Adverse events causing dose reduction ≥5% of patients in any study group
‡Adverse events causing discontinuation ≥2.5% of patients in any study group

Therapy Monitoring

At screening and every 6 weeks: Tumor measurements by computed tomography or magnetic resonance imaging

16. HIV-Related Malignancies

Bruce J. Dezube, MD

Kaposi Sarcoma (KS)

Epidemiology of KS

Incidence/100,000	
United States	
Males:	2.1
Females:	0.11
Africa	
Males:	39.3
Females:	21.8

Stage at Presentation in HAART Era (Based on ACTG* Modified TIS Staging)
Poor risk: 25%
Good risk: 75%

*ACTG: AIDS Clinical Trials Group
Deaths caused by AIDS since advent of HAART
have decreased by more than 50%

Nasti G et al. J Clin Oncol 2003;21:2876–2882

Pathology

1. All KS is caused by human herpesvirus 8 (HHV-8), also called the Kaposi sarcoma-associated herpesvirus (KSHV), a gamma herpesvirus first identified in 1994
2. Pathology shows a highly vascular tumor with spindle-shaped cells staining positive for KSHV

Moore PS, Chang Y. N Engl J Med 1995;332:1181–1185

Work-up

1. Biopsy to confirm diagnosis
2. HIV serology
3. CD4 and HIV-1 viral load
4. Assessment of tumor extent:
   - Physical examination of the skin and lymph nodes
   - Chest x-ray
   - Chest CT scan not routinely indicated unless x-ray is abnormal
   - For GI symptoms, work-up as indicated
   - Fecal occult blood testing

Di Lorenzo G et al. Lancet Oncol 2007;8:167–176

Staging (Validated ACTG TIS Staging for AIDS-KS)*

Good Risk: Stage 0 (Stage 0: All criteria below must be satisfied)	Poor Risk: Stage 1 (Stage 1: If any of the criteria are present)
Tumor (T)	
Confined to skin and/or lymph nodes	Tumor-associated edema or ulceration Extensive oral KS Gastrointestinal KS KS in other nonnodal viscera
Immune System (I)*	
CD4 cells >150/mm³	CD4 cells <150/mm³
Systemic Illness (S)	

• No history of opportunistic infection or thrush
• No B symptoms persisting >2 weeks, including
  1. Unexplained fever
  2. Night sweats
  3. >10% involuntary weight loss
  4. Diarrhea
• Performance status >70 (Karnofsky scale)
	• History of opportunistic infections, thrush, or both
	• B symptoms present
	
	• Performance status <70 (Karnofsky scale)
	• Other HIV-related illness (eg, neurologic disease, lymphoma)

Staging example:
A patient with KS restricted to the skin, CD4 count of 10 cells/mm³, and a history of *Pneumocystis jirovecii* (formerly, *P. carinii*) pneumonia would be $T_0 I_1 S_1$

*According to the AIDS Clinical Trials Group (ACTG). Staging takes into account tumor extent (T), immune status (I), and systemic illness (S)

Notes:
1. In the HAART era, immune status may not be prognostically predictive. However, in patients with resistant HIV, immune status may be relevant
2. In the HAART era, poor prognosis is $T_1 S_1$. All other stages are considered good prognosis

Krown SE et al. J Clin Oncol 1997;15:3085–3092
Nasti G et al. J Clin Oncol 2003;21:2876–2882

Survival

Stage	3-Year Survival (%)
$T_0 S_0$	88
$T_1 S_0$	80
$T_0 S_1$	81
$T_1 S_1$	53

Nasti G et al. J Clin Oncol 2003;21:2876–2882

Expert Opinion

Kaposi sarcoma, as an AIDS-presenting manifestation in antiretroviral therapy (ART) naïve patients, often responds to ART. However, not all patients achieve lesion resolution with ART. In addition to ART, radiotherapy or surgery can be used to treat isolated lesions

Systemic chemotherapy may be required if lesions do not regress with primary ART therapy, diffuse involvement of a large portion of an extremity or in widespread, bulky, or rapidly progressive disease with visceral organ involvement. Early systemic chemotherapy may help to suppress or prevent immune reconstitution inflammatory syndrome (IRIS)-associated flares

Despite the lack of randomized trials demonstrating superiority, pegylated liposomal doxorubicin can be used as first-line therapy of choice unless there is a cardiac contraindication. For patients who progressed while receiving pegylated liposomal doxorubicin or for those who do not respond there are several options for second-line therapy including the use of paclitaxel

KS REGIMEN (HIV REGIMENS)

HIGHLY ACTIVE ANTIRETROVIRAL THERAPY (HAART)

HAART should be considered as fundamental oncologic care in patients with AIDS-KS. Unless there is some overwhelming reason not to administer it, HAART should be given in essentially all AIDS-KS patients

Antiretroviral drugs are classified according to the type of compound and the part of the viral life cycle that a drug inhibits. The HAART regimen generally comprises a combination of 3 or more drugs from at least 2 different classes as defined by these criteria. The treatment goal is potent inhibition of HIV replication to levels <50 copies HIV mRNA/μL. HAART should be considered part of the fundamental oncologic therapy for AIDS-KS

Guidelines for the use of antiretroviral therapy can be found at www.aidsinfo.nih.gov (U.S. Department of Health and Human Services)

or

Thompson MA et al. JAMA 2012;308:387–402 (International Antiviral Society-USA panel)

Note: In patients for whom chemotherapy is planned, avoid zidovudine if possible, as it may aggravate myelosuppression

Efficacy

1. For initial therapy of KS, a trial of HAART is reasonable in many cases. Up to 74% of treatment-naïve cases (ie, never previously treated for either HIV or KS) can have a substantial tumor response to HAART
2. Responses may be seen within 3–6 months
3. Patients most likely to respond are those with:
   - Minimal tumor burden
   - HIV viral load suppression to very low levels
   - CD4 cell increases $\geq$150 cells/mm^3 above pretreatment levels
4. Response durations can be long-lasting, although progressive diseases may occur early
5. Beware of KS flare as a result of immune reconstitution inflammatory syndrome (IRIS). Such flares are treated with chemotherapy

Treatment Modifications

Antiretroviral drugs should be managed by physicians with expertise in the care of patients with HIV disease. Certain drug combinations can be antagonistic and should not be used. Dose modifications must be done with caution because inadequate plasma drug levels increase the potential to develop resistant mutant HIV. At least 3 medications are required for HAART: If toxicity requiring dosing cessation is ascribed to 1 medication, patients should be instructed to stop all medications to avoid resistance

Patient Population Studied

Patients without previous HIV or KS therapy

Therapy Monitoring

1. *Monthly for first 3 months:* Clinical evaluation, assessment of tumor burden, HIV-1 viral loads, immunologic assessment (CD4 cells) CBC with differential, liver function tests, BUN, creatinine, amylase, and lipase
2. *Every 3 months after first 3 months (if clinically improving):* Clinical evaluation, assessment of tumor burden, viral titers, immunologic assessment (CD4 cells), CBC with differential, liver function tests, BUN, creatinine, amylase, and lipase

KS REGIMEN

LOCAL THERAPY: RADIATION THERAPY, INTRALESIONAL THERAPY, CRYOTHERAPY (LIQUID NITROGEN, ALITRETINOIN GEL (TOPICAL ALL-*TRANS*-RETINOIC ACID)), PHOTODYNAMIC THERAPY

Von Roenn JH. Hematol Oncol Clin North Am 2003;17:747–762
Ramirez-Amador et al. Oral Oncol 2002;38:460–467

Important to administer HAART to all patients

Radiation therapy:
Dosing varies; radiation therapy may be more toxic in HIV patients

Intralesional therapy:
Vinblastine 0.1 mL of 0.1 mg/mL (or 0.2 mg/mL per 1 cm² of lesion surface area); administer intralesionally every 1–2 weeks,

or

3% Sodium tetradecyl sulfate (Sotradecol) injection 0.1–0.3 mL; administer intralesionally every 1–2 weeks

Cryotherapy (liquid nitrogen):
Liquid nitrogen is effective for treatment of small cosmetically disturbing lesions, particularly in the face. Liquid nitrogen is applied to the lesion to achieve a thaw time of approximately 40 seconds. High response rates lasting from 6 weeks to 6 months have been reported. Treatment-related hypopigmentation may be cosmetically unacceptable, particularly in dark-skinned patients

Alitretinoin gel:
Alitretinoin 0.1% gel; apply topically to affected areas 3–5 times per day; avoid application to normal skin and mucosal surfaces

Supportive Care (for therapy listed above):
Antiemetic prophylaxis
Emetogenic potential: **MINIMAL**
See Chapter 39 for antiemetic recommendations

Hematopoietic growth factor (CSF) prophylaxis
Primary prophylaxis is NOT indicated
See Chapter 43 for more information

Antimicrobial prophylaxis
Risk of fever and neutropenia is LOW
  Antimicrobial primary prophylaxis to be considered:
  • Antibacterial—not indicated
  • Antifungal—not indicated
  • Antiviral—not indicated unless patient previously had an episode of HSV
See Chapter 47 for more information

Photodynamic therapy:
Photodynamic therapy utilizes the activation by light of a photosensitizing drug that preferentially accumulates in tumor tissue, such as Kaposi sarcoma. Drugs that have been used include **porfimer sodium** (Photofrin) and **thiazine compounds** (methylene blue and toluidine blue)

Note: Limited role for surgical resection

Toxicity

Radiation therapy:
Burning sensation during treatment; chronic lymphedema

Intralesional injections:
Painful

Cryotherapy:
Avoid in dark-skinned patients; permanently destroys melanocytes, leaving a white spot

Alitretinoin gel:
Can cause local irritation

Photodynamic therapy:
Erythema and edema in the treatment field

Patient Population Studied

Most studies were conducted before the widespread use of HAART in patients with minimal disease

Efficacy

1. Rarely useful except with limited disease
2. Local recurrence is common
3. Patients who benefit favorably from HAART may have better long-term outcome in terms of tumor recurrence
4. Patients who derive no benefit from HAART are likely to have new tumors or recurrent tumors relatively quickly in the treatment fields

Radiation therapy:
For limited disease, can be effective

Intralesional injections:
Useful for small lesions of cosmetic import. Not feasible for multiple lesions

Cryotherapy:
Not feasible for multiple lesions

Alitretinoin gel:
Reported response rate up to 40% May be most useful for patients with minimal disease

Photodynamic therapy:
Effective palliative treatment for limited disease

Treatment Modifications

1. HIV infection may render certain tissues more vulnerable to toxic effects of radiation
2. Radiation therapy of oral disease should be reserved for symptomatic oral KS because of the high incidence of radiation-induced mucositis

Therapy Monitoring

Monitor for efficacy; no specific monitoring required

KS REGIMEN

DAUNORUBICIN CITRATE LIPOSOME INJECTION (LIPOSOMAL DAUNORUBICIN)

Gill PS et al. J Clin Oncol 1996;14:2353–2364

Important to administer HAART to all patients

Daunorubicin citrate liposome injection 40 mg/m²; administer intravenously in a volume of 5% dextrose injection equivalent to the volume of liposomal daunorubicin over 60 minutes every 2 weeks (total dosage/cycle = 40 mg/m²)

Ancillary medications: Secondary prophylaxis for neutropenia at discretion of investigator

Pegfilgrastim 6 mg; administer subcutaneously starting 24–48 hours after chemotherapy is completed. Most patients do not require growth factor support (eg, pegfilgrastim). Filgrastim may be used as an alternative

Supportive Care
Antiemetic prophylaxis
Emetogenic potential: LOW
See Chapter 39 for antiemetic recommendations

Hematopoietic growth factor (CSF) prophylaxis
Primary prophylaxis is NOT indicated
See Chapter 43 for more information

Antimicrobial prophylaxis
Risk of fever and neutropenia is LOW
  Antimicrobial primary prophylaxis to be considered:
  • Antibacterial—not indicated
  • Antifungal—not indicated
  • Antiviral—not indicated unless patient previously had an episode of HSV
See Chapter 47 for more information

Patient Population Studied

Advanced AIDS-KS pre-HAART. A prospective randomized phase III trial of 232 patients randomly assigned to receive liposomal daunorubicin 40 mg/m² or a combination chemotherapy regimen of doxorubicin 10 mg/m², bleomycin 15 units, and vincristine 1 mg (ABV). Both regimens were administered every 2 weeks

Efficacy (N = 116)

Complete response	2.6%
Partial response	22.4%
Median response duration	175 days
Median survival	369 days

Treatment Modifications

Treatment proceeds as planned if pretreatment ANC is ≥750/mm³ and platelet count ≥75,000/mm³

Adverse Event	Dose Modification
ANC ≤750/mm³	Delay liposomal daunorubicin until ANC recovery above this level. Consider adding pegfilgrastim during subsequent cycles
Cardiac toxicity (≥20% reduction in ejection fraction)	Discontinue therapy
Pulmonary toxicity	Discontinue therapy
Liver dysfunction*	Dosage modifications indicated, but not specified

*DaunoXome (daunorubicin citrate liposome injection) labeling indicates dose modifications for increased bilirubin, but some protease inhibitors (eg, indinavir, atazanavir) cause mild hyperbilirubinemia; dose adjustment may not be required in this setting

Toxicity (N = 116)

	% G1/2	% G3/4
Hematologic*		
Neutropenia	12/55	36/15
Leukopenia	12/79	33/5
Thrombocytopenia	93/12	0/1
Anemia	62/55	9/2
Nonhematologic		
Fatigue	43	6
Fever	42	5
Diarrhea	34	4
Nausea	51	3
Vomiting	20	3
Abdominal pain	20	3
Dyspnea	23	3
Headache	22	3
Anorexia	21	2
Cough	26	2
Neuropathy	12	1
Alopecia	8	
Back pain/flushing/chest tightness	14	
Reduced ejection fraction†	0	

*Some patients experienced toxicity on ≥1 cycle
†Occurred within 5 minutes of infusion; subsided if discontinued; did not recur if resumed at slower rate

Therapy Monitoring

1. *Before therapy:* CBC with differential, LFTs, BUN, serum creatinine, and ejection fraction
2. *Before each cycle:* CBC with differential LFTs. BUN and serum creatinine
3. *Cumulative daunorubicin or doxorubicin dosage ≥500 mg/m²:* Ejection fraction

Notes

1. Trial conducted in the pre-HAART era. Of patients, 95% received antiretroviral drugs as monotherapy or 2 drugs concurrent with liposomal daunorubicin
2. Chronic therapy may be required; patients responding to HAART may have long-term progression-free survival and require fewer (eg, 4–6) cycles of chemotherapy

KS REGIMEN

DOXORUBICIN HCl LIPOSOME INJECTION (LIPOSOMAL DOXORUBICIN)

Northfelt DW et al. J Clin Oncol 1998;16:2445–2451

Important to administer HAART to all patients

Doxorubicin HCl liposome injection 20 mg/m^2; administer intravenously in 250 mL 5% dextrose injection over 60 minutes every 3 weeks (total dosage/cycle = 20 mg/m^2)

Premedication: Generally not required

Supportive Care
Antiemetic prophylaxis
Emetogenic potential: **LOW**
See Chapter 39 for antiemetic recommendations

Hematopoietic growth factor (CSF) prophylaxis
Primary prophylaxis may be indicated with 1 of the following:
Filgrastim (G-CSF) 5 mcg/kg per day by subcutaneous injection, *or*
Pegfilgrastim (pegylated filgrastim) 6 mg/0.6 mL by subcutaneous injection for 1 dose
• Begin use from 24–72 hours after myelosuppressive chemotherapy is completed
• Most patients do not require growth factor support
See Chapter 43 for more information

Antimicrobial prophylaxis
Risk of fever and neutropenia is LOW
Antimicrobial primary prophylaxis to be considered:
• Antibacterial—not indicated
• Antifungal—not indicated
• Antiviral—not indicated unless patient previously had an episode of HSV
See Chapter 47 for more information

Hand-foot reaction (palmar-plantar erythrodysesthesia, PPE)
For patients who develop a hand-foot reaction, use topical emollients (eg, Aquaphor®), topical or orally administered steroids, antihistamine agents (H$_1$-receptor antagonists), or pyridoxine
  Pyridoxine may provide relief for discomfort/pain associated with PPE although the mechanism through which this occurs remains unclear
• The suggested pyridoxine starting dose is 50 mg/day, which may be increased to a maximum of 200 mg/day
• Patients who develop G1/2 PPE while receiving doxorubicin HCl liposome injection may receive a fixed daily dose of pyridoxine 200 mg. This may allow for treatment to be completed without dosage reduction, treatment delay, or recurrence of PPE

Oral care
Prophylaxis and treatment for mucositis/stomatitis
  General advice:
• Encourage patients to maintain intake of non-alcoholic fluids
• Evaluate patients for oral pain and provide analgesic medications
• Consider histamine (H$_2$-subtype) receptor antagonists (eg, ranitidine, famotidine), or a proton pump inhibitor for epigastric pain
• *Lactobacillus* sp.-containing probiotics may be beneficial in preventing diarrhea
  Patients with intact oral mucosa:
• Clean the mouth, tongue, and gums by brushing after every meal and at bedtime with an ultra-soft toothbrush with fluoride toothpaste
• Floss teeth gently every day unless contraindicated. If gums bleed and hurt, avoid bleeding or sore areas, but floss other teeth
• Patients may use saline or commercial bland, non-alcoholic rinses
  ▪ Do not use mouthwashes that contain alcohols

(continued)

Patient Population Studied

A trial of 258 patients pre-HAART with advanced AIDS-KS randomly assigned to either pegylated-liposomal doxorubicin 20 mg/m^2 or a doxorubicin, bleomycin, and vincristine (ABV) regimen. Both regimens were administered every 14 days for 6 cycles

Efficacy* (N = 133)

Complete response	0.8%
Partial response	45.1%
• Flattening of lesions	37%
• Decreased sum of products of largest perpendicular diameters	6%
• Reduced number and flattening of lesions	1%
• Reduced size and flattening of lesions	1%
Median response duration	90 days
Median survival	160 days

*Modified AIDS Clinical Trials Group

Treatment Modifications

Adverse Event	Dose Modification
G3 toxicity other than granulocytopenia	Delay treatment for up to 14 days
ANC <750/mm^3 on cycle day 1	Delay treatment until ANC recovers
Palmar-plantar erythrodysesthesia	Delay treatment. May require dosage reductions

Although Doxil (doxorubicin HCl liposome injection) product labeling indicates dose modifications for increased bilirubin, some protease inhibitors (eg, indinavir, atazanavir) cause a mild hyperbilirubinemia, in which cases, dose adjustment may not be necessary

(continued)

If mucositis or stomatitis is present:

- Keep the mouth moist utilizing water, ice chips, sugarless gum, sugar-free hard candies, or a saliva substitute
- Rinse mouth several times a day to remove debris
  - Use a solution of ¼ teaspoon (1.25 g) each of baking soda and table salt (sodium chloride) in one quart (~950 mL) of warm water. Follow with a plain water rinse
  - Do not use mouthwashes that contain alcohols
- Foam-tipped swabs (eg, Toothettes®) are useful in moisturizing oral mucosa, but ineffective for cleansing teeth and removing plaque
- Advise patients who develop mucositis to:
  - Choose foods that are easy to chew and swallow
  - Take small bites of food, chew slowly, and sip liquids with meals
  - Encourage soft, moist foods such as cooked cereals, mashed potatoes, and scrambled eggs
  - For trouble swallowing, soften food with gravies, sauces, broths, yogurt, or other bland liquids
  - Avoid sharp, crunchy foods; hot, spicy or highly acidic foods (eg, citrus fruits and juices); sugary foods; toothpicks; tobacco products; alcoholic drinks

Toxicity (N = 133)[*][†]

	% G3/4
At least one G3/4 toxicity	92
Hematologic	
Leukopenia[‡]	36
ANC $<500/mm^3$	6
Febrile with ANC $<500/mm^3$	0
Anemia	9.8
Thrombocytopenia	3
Septic episodes	6
Nonhematologic	
Nausea or vomiting	15
Mucositis/stomatitis	5
Peripheral neuropathy	6
Alopecia	1
Palmar-plantar erythrodysesthesia	4
Infusion-related reactions[§]	4.5
Cardiac ejection fraction decreased ≥20% from baseline (n = 47)[ϵ]	2 patients

[*]WHO Criteria
[†]Percent of patients experiencing G3/4 toxicity
[‡]44% received G-CSF or GM-CSF
[§]Flushing, chest pain, dyspnea, difficulty swallowing, hypotension, back pain
[ϵ]One death because of cardiomyopathy

Therapy Monitoring

1. *Before therapy:* CBC with differential, LFTs, BUN and serum creatinine, and cardiac ejection fraction
2. *Before each cycle:* CBC with differential, LFTs, BUN, serum creatinine, and response assessment
3. *Cumulative daunorubicin or doxorubicin dosage ≥ 500 mg/m²:* Ejection fraction

Notes

1. Trial conducted in the pre-HAART era
2. Chronic therapy may be required; patients responding to HAART may have long-term progression-free survival and require fewer (eg, 4–6 cycles) of chemotherapy

REGIMEN

PACLITAXEL (TAXOL)

Gill PS et al. J Clin Oncol 1999;17:1876–1883
Saville MW et al. Lancet 1995;346:26–28

Important to administer HAART to all patients

Premedication: Primary prophylaxis against hypersensitivity reactions from paclitaxel:
Dexamethasone 20 mg; administer intravenously prior to paclitaxel (reduce to 8 mg if no hypersensitivity reactions occur during cycle 1), *plus:*
Diphenhydramine 50 mg; administer by intravenous injection 30 minutes before paclitaxel, *and:*
Ranitidine 50 mg or an equivalent dose of an alternative histamine (H_2) receptor antagonist; administer intravenously in 25–100 mL 0.9% sodium chloride injection (0.9% NS) or 5% dextrose injection (D5W) over 5–30 minutes, 30 minutes before paclitaxel
Paclitaxel 135 mg/m²; administer intravenously, in a volume of 0.9% NS or D5W sufficient to produce a concentration within the range of 0.3–1.2 mg/mL, over 3 hours every 21 days (total dosage/cycle = 135 mg/m²)

or

Premedication: Primary prophylaxis against hypersensitivity reactions from paclitaxel:
Dexamethasone 10 mg/dose for 2 doses; administer orally, 14 and 7 hours prior to paclitaxel, *plus*
Diphenhydramine 50 mg; administer by intravenous injection 30 minutes before paclitaxel, *and:*
Ranitidine 50 mg; administer intravenously in 25–100 mL 0.9% sodium chloride injection or 5% dextrose injection over 5–30 minutes, 30 minutes before paclitaxel
Paclitaxel 100 mg/m²; administer intravenously in a volume of 0.9% NS or D5W sufficient to produce a concentration within the range of 0.3–1.2 mg/mL, over 3 hours every 21 days (total dosage/cycle = 100 mg/m²)

Supportive Care

Antiemetic prophylaxis
Emetogenic potential: **MINIMAL**
See Chapter 39 for antiemetic recommendations

Hematopoietic growth factor (CSF) prophylaxis
Primary prophylaxis may be indicated with 1 of the following:
  Filgrastim (G-CSF) 5 mcg/kg per day by subcutaneous injection, *or*
  Pegfilgrastim (pegylated filgrastim) 6 mg/0.6 mL by subcutaneous injection for 1 dose
  • Begin use from 24–72 hours after myelosuppressive chemotherapy is completed
  • Most patients do not require growth factor support
See Chapter 43 for more information

Antimicrobial prophylaxis
Risk of fever and neutropenia is LOW
  Antimicrobial primary prophylaxis to be considered:
  • Antibacterial—not indicated
  • Antifungal—not indicated
  • Antiviral—not indicated, unless patient previously had an episode of herpes simplex virus
See Chapter 47 for more information

Oral care
Prophylaxis and treatment for mucositis/stomatitis
  General advice:
  • Encourage patients to maintain intake of non-alcoholic fluids
  • Evaluate patients for oral pain and provide analgesic medications
  • Consider histamine (H_2-subtype) receptor antagonists (eg, ranitidine, famotidine), or a proton pump inhibitor for epigastric pain
  • *Lactobacillus* sp.-containing probiotics may be beneficial in preventing diarrhea
  Patients with intact oral mucosa:
  • Clean the mouth, tongue, and gums by brushing after every meal and at bedtime with an ultra-soft toothbrush with fluoride toothpaste
  • Floss teeth gently every day unless contraindicated. If gums bleed and hurt, avoid bleeding or sore areas, but floss other teeth
  • Patients may use saline or commercial bland, non-alcoholic rinses
    ▪ Do not use mouthwashes that contain alcohols

(continued)

Patient Population Studied

Data from phase-II trials with advanced KS in highly immunosuppressed patients treated pre-HAART

Efficacy

Objective responses (Saville et al.)	71%
Objective responses (Gill et al.)	59%
Median response duration (Saville et al.)	2.5 months
Median duration of response (Gill et al.)	10.4 months

Treatment Modifications

Adverse Event	Dose Modification
G4 hematologic toxicity	Decrease paclitaxel dosage by 25%

Saville MW et al. Lancet 1995;346:26–28

Adverse Event	Dose Modification
Cycle, day 1 ANC <1000/mm³, or platelet count <50,000/mm³	Delay treatment until ANC >1000/mm³, and platelet count >50,000/mm³
ANC <500/mm³ for 7 days	Reduce paclitaxel dosage by 20%
G1/2 peripheral neuropathy*	Reduce paclitaxel dosage by 20%
G3/4 peripheral neuropathy*	Discontinue therapy
Total bilirubin >3.0 mg/dL (>51.3 μmol/L)	Delay treatment until bilirubin <3.0 mg/dL (<51.3 μmol/L), then reduce dosage by 20%
Liver transaminases >5 times the upper limit of normal range	Delay treatment until liver transaminases <3 times the upper limit of normal, then reduce dosage by 20%

*Increased neuropathy reported when using stavudine

Gill PS et al. J Clin Oncol 1999;17:1876–1883

(*continued*)

If mucositis or stomatitis is present:
- Keep the mouth moist utilizing water, ice chips, sugarless gum, sugar-free hard candies, or a saliva substitute
- Rinse mouth several times a day to remove debris
  - Use a solution of ¼ teaspoon (1.25 g) each of baking soda and table salt (sodium chloride) in one quart (~950 mL) of warm water. Follow with a plain water rinse
  - Do not use mouthwashes that contain alcohols
- Foam-tipped swabs (eg, Toothettes®) are useful in moisturizing oral mucosa, but ineffective for cleansing teeth and removing plaque
- Advise patients who develop mucositis to:
  - Choose foods that are easy to chew and swallow
  - Take small bites of food, chew slowly, and sip liquids with meals
  - Encourage soft, moist foods such as cooked cereals, mashed potatoes, and scrambled eggs
  - For trouble swallowing, soften food with gravies, sauces, broths, yogurt, or other bland liquids
  - Avoid sharp, crunchy foods; hot, spicy or highly acidic foods (eg, citrus fruits and juices); sugary foods; toothpicks; tobacco products; alcoholic drinks

Therapy Monitoring

Before each cycle: CBC with differential, LFTs, BUN, serum creatinine, and physical examination with careful attention to peripheral nerves

Notes

1. Chronic therapy may be required
2. Active in patients who did not benefit from other therapies

Toxicity

	% G1/2	% G3/4
Neutropenia*	—	61
Diarrhea	—	12
Fever	—	11
Nausea	—	6
Peripheral neuropathy	45	4
Rash	—	2

Alopecia: Common; complete in 10%

*Growth factors not used routinely

Saville MW et al. Lancet 1995;346:26–28 (N = 20) (NCI CTC)

	% G1/2*	% G3	%G4
Hematologic			
Neutropenia[†]	33	25	36
Anemia	45	22	5
Thrombocytopenia	25	4	2
Nonhematologic			
Alopecia	78	9	—
Fatigue	50	23	2
Rash ± pruritus	9	0	—
Myalgia	21	16	—
Nausea/vomiting	57	13	0
Diarrhea	57	14	2
Neuropathy	45	2	0
Mucositis	18	2	0
Elevated AST	35	5	0

*Includes patients with unknown grades
[†]Although 50% of patients were on G-CSF on entry

Gill PS et al. J Clin Oncol 1999;17:1876–1883 (N = 56) (Southwest Oncology Group Toxicity Criteria)
Welles L et al. J Clin Oncol 1998;16:1112–1121

KS REGIMEN

INTERFERON ALFA-2B

Krown SE. Curr Opin Oncol 2001;13:374–381
Krown SE et al. J Interferon Cytokine Res 2002;22:295–303
Von Roenn JH. Hematol Oncol Clin North Am 2003;17:747–762

Important to administer HAART to all patients

Premedications:

1. Primary antipyretic prophylaxis:

   Acetaminophen 650–1000 mg; administer orally,

   or

   Ibuprofen 400–600 mg; administer orally starting 1 hour before interferon, then every 4–6 hours as needed

2. Secondary antiemetic prophylaxis:

   If required for treating emetic symptoms, use as primary prophylaxis with subsequent interferon doses.
   See Chapter 39 for antiemetic recommendations

Low dose: **Interferon alfa-2b** 1 million IU once daily; administer subcutaneously or intramuscularly with antiretroviral therapy

Intermediate dose: **Interferon alfa-2b** 10 million IU once daily; administer subcutaneously or intramuscularly with antiretroviral therapy

Supportive Care

Antiemetic prophylaxis
Emetogenic potential: **MINIMAL**
See Chapter 39 for antiemetic recommendations

Hematopoietic growth factor (CSF) prophylaxis
Primary prophylaxis is NOT indicated
See Chapter 43 for more information

Antimicrobial prophylaxis
Risk of fever and neutropenia is LOW
Antimicrobial primary prophylaxis to be considered:
- Antibacterial—not indicated
- Antifungal—not indicated
- Antiviral—not indicated unless patient previously had an episode of HSV

See Chapter 47 for more information

Treatment Modifications

Adverse Event	Dose Modification
G ≤2 constitutional symptoms	Administer analgesics, antihistamines, antiemetics, antidiarrheal agents, and other supportive measures, including hematopoietic growth factors
G3 constitutional and CNS toxicities; elevations in AST, and thrombocytopenia	Interrupt interferon alfa-2b dosing
G2 cardiac toxicity, stomatitis, and renal, bladder, pulmonary, allergic, or mucocutaneous toxicities	Interrupt interferon alfa-2b dosing
Recurrent toxicities or development of major opportunistic infection after dosage reduction	Discontinue interferon alfa-2b administration

Patient Population Studied

Patients with HIV-related KS

Efficacy

- Response rates to interferon as a single agent vary from 20% to 60%
- Multiple studies combining interferon and zidovudine reported response rates of 40% or higher

	Low-Dose Group*	Intermediate-Dose Group[†]
CR/CCR/PR[‡]	40%	55%
Complete response[‡]	3%	9%
Clinical Complete response[‡]	11%	12%
Partial response[‡]	26%	33%
Stable disease	37%	27%
Progressive disease	17%	3%
Not evaluable	5%	15%
Median time to response	24.6 weeks	40 weeks
Estimated median response duration	110 weeks	110 weeks

*Interferon alfa-2b 1 million IU once daily; administer by subcutaneous injection with **didanosine** 125–200 mg administer orally every 12 hours
[†]Interferon alfa-2b 10 million IU once daily; administer by subcutaneous injection with **didanosine** 125–200 mg administer orally every 12 hours
[‡]CR, no residual lesion, confirmed by biopsy; CCR, no residual lesion without biopsy confirmation; PR, 50% reduction in size, number or nodularity of cutaneous lesions, or complete resolution of cutaneous lesions with persistent tumor-associated edema

Krown SE et al. J Interferon Cytokine Res 2002;22:295–303

Toxicity

Low-dose group: 35 patients treated with interferon alfa-2b 1 million units; administer subcutaneously or intramuscularly once daily with didanosine* 125–200 mg orally every 12 hours

Intermediate-dose group: 33 patients treated with interferon alfa-2b 10 million units; administer subcutaneously or intramuscularly once daily with didanosine* 125–200 mg orally every 12 hours

*125 mg if weight <60 kg; 200 mg if weight ≥60 kg. Other antiretroviral therapies were subsequently substituted for or added to didanosine

	Low-Dose Group*	Intermediate-Dose Group[†]
	% G3/4	% G3/4
Neutropenia	3	21
Hyperamylasemia[‡]	9	18
Anemia	<10	<10
Thrombocytopenia	<10	<10
Elevated LFT	<10	<10
Hypertriglyceridemia	<10	<10

*Interferon alfa-2b** 1 million IU, subcutaneously or intramuscularly once daily with **didanosine** 125–200 mg, orally every 12 hours
[†]**Interferon alfa-2b** 10 million IU, subcutaneously or intramuscularly once daily with **didanosine** 125–200 mg, orally every 12 hours
[‡]Difference between low and intermediate doses is significant

Notes:
- Grades 2/3 chills, fatigue, and fever occurred significantly more often in the intermediate-dose group than in the low-dose group
- Additional adverse events included cough, dyspnea, headache, anorexia, myalgias, and rash
- The majority of treatment withdrawals occur in the first 4 months of treatment, after which discontinuation of therapy because of toxicity is unusual

Krown SE et al. J Interferon Cytokine Res 2002;22:295–303

Therapy Monitoring

1. *Every 2 weeks initially, then once per month:* CBC with differential and serum electrolytes, BUN, creatinine, LFTs, and mineral panel
2. *Response evaluation:* Patients are evaluated for response every 4–8 weeks

Notes

1. In the era of HAART and with the advent of liposomal chemotherapy (Doxil, DaunoXome), interferon alfa has a very limited role in KS management
2. Combine interferon alfa-2b with HAART for best outcome
3. Patients with CD4 counts ≥200/mm^3 have better responses than those whose CD4 counts are <200/mm^3
4. High interferon alfa-2b doses may be associated with better efficacy, but because of the complexity of interactions regarding the status of underlying HIV disease and response potential, not all patients require high doses

HIV-Related Lymphoma (ARL)

Epidemiology

Incidence
- 43 cases/10,000 person-years in HIV-positive individuals
- Approximately 3% of HIV-infected patients develop ARL as the AIDS-defining diagnosis
- 10–15% of patients with AIDS develop ARL
- Since the advent of HAART, ARL has decreased by 50% owing to CD4 cell preservation; however, incidence within CD4 strata has not been changed by HAART

Stage at presentation
- More than 60% have advanced stages III–IV disease with B-cell symptoms
- Extranodal involvement common
- Among HIV-infected patients with non-Hodgkin lymphoma (NHL), 80% of NHL are aggressive; by comparison, 30% of non–HIV-associated lymphomas are aggressive

Besson C et al. Blood 2001;98:2339–2344

Pathology

Distribution of histologic subtypes tracks with CD4 cells and has been influenced by HAART-induced immune preservation. Specifically, since HAART, fewer immunoblastic subtypes are seen
1. Diffuse large B-cell lymphoma (DLBCL): 70%
   - Centroblastic: 20–30% associated with Epstein-Barr virus (EBV)
   - Immunoblastic: 80% associated with EBV
   - Primary central nervous system lymphoma: 100% associated with EBV
2. Burkitt lymphoma: 20%
   - 0–50% associated with EBV
3. Other (eg, primary effusion lymphoma [PEL], plasmablastic lymphoma [PBL], often of the oral cavity): 10%
   - 70% associated with EBV

Jaffe ES, Harris NL, Stein H, Vardiman JW. World Health Organization Classification of Tumors: Pathology & Genetics: Tumors of Haematopoietic and Lymphoid Tissues. Lyon, France: IARC Press, 2001:351

Work-up

1. Assessment of hematologic and biochemical parameters
2. CT scans of chest, abdomen, and pelvis
3. Bone marrow biopsy
4. Lumbar puncture for cytology and cell count
5. CD4 cell count
6. FDG-PET scans are very useful, if available

If primary brain lymphoma is suspected:
1. Brain biopsy is the gold standard
2. Must rule out peripheral disease
3. Slit-lamp exam of optic nerve
4. Minimally invasive diagnosis combining FDG-PET (or SPECT) with assessment of EBV presence in the CSF by polymerase chain reaction can be used in some cases rather than biopsy
   - If both tests are positive: 100% positive predictive value for primary brain lymphoma
   - If both tests are negative: 100% negative predictive value for brain lymphoma
   - If these tests are discordant: Biopsy is required to establish the diagnosis

Antinori A et al. J Clin Oncol 1999;17:554–560
Levine AM. Semin Oncol 1990;17:104–112

Staging

Ann Arbor Staging System for Lymphomas

Stage	Description
I	Single lymph node region
IE	Single extralymphatic organ or site
II	Two or more lymph node regions on the same side of the diaphragm
IIE	Single extranodal site + adjacent nodes
III	Nodal regions on both sides of the diaphragm (III)
IIIE	Nodal regions on both sides of the diaphragm + single extranodal site
IIIS	Nodal regions on both sides of the diaphragm + involvement of spleen
IIISE	Nodal regions on both sides of the diaphragm + single extranodal site + involvement of spleen
IV	Diffuse or disseminated involvement of one or more extralymphatic organs Bone marrow involvement Liver involvement Brain involvement

Absence of associated symptoms is designated A
Presence of symptoms is designated B. B symptoms include unexplained fevers, >10% unexplained weight loss, sweats

Survival

Overall survival is generally poor in most reports, but has improved since the advent of HAART:
1. *Diffuse large B-cell lymphoma (DLCBL):*
   - Pre-HAART 4–18 months
   - Since HAART 21 months
   - Recent phase II trial of dose-adjusted (DA)-EPOCH demonstrated survival equivalent to non-AIDS, bcl-2–negative DLBCL
2. *PEL:* Median survival approximately 4–6 months with therapy
3. *PBL:* Initial reports suggested poor survival as a result of low CR, but clinical heterogeneity of these cases is becoming more evident, and some may have favorable outcome
4. CD4 cell count is the primary prognostic determinant

Besson C et al. Blood 2001;98:2339–2344
Castillo J et al. Am J Hematol 2008;83:804–809

REGIMEN

ETOPOSIDE + PREDNISONE + VINCRISTINE + CYCLOPHOSPHAMIDE + DOXORUBICIN ± RITUXIMAB (DOSE-ADJUSTED EPOCH ± R: DA-EPOCH ± R)

Little RF et al. Blood 2003;101:4653–4659

Important Note: Most specialists recommend continuing HAART for patients already on a stable regimen. However, in some centers, HAART is suspended until all cycles are completed, and then optimized on/after day 6 of final cycle

Premedication for Rituximab—All Cycles
Acetaminophen 650 mg; administer orally 30–60 minutes before starting rituximab, *plus*
Diphenhydramine 25 mg; administer intravenously 30–60 minutes before starting rituximab

Rituximab 375 mg/m²; administer intravenously in 0.9% sodium chloride injection (0.9% NS) or 5% dextrose injection (D5W), diluted to a concentration within the range 1–4 mg/mL, day 1 every 21 days for a maximum of 6 cycles (total dosage/cycle = 375 mg/m²)

Note: Caution is advised particularly if patient's CD4 count is <50/mm³

Rituximab administration:
• Infuse initially at 50 mg/hour. If hypersensitivity or infusion reactions do not occur during the first 30 minutes, increase the rate by 50 mg/hour every 30 minutes as tolerated to a maximum rate of 400 mg/hour. During subsequent treatments if previous rituximab administration was well tolerated, start at 100 mg/hour and increase by 100 mg/hour every 30 minutes as tolerated to a maximum rate of 400 mg/hour

Interrupt rituximab administration for fever, chills, edema, congestion of the head and neck mucosa, hypertension, and other serious adverse events. Resume rituximab administration after adverse events abate

Etoposide 50 mg/m² per day; administer by continuous intravenous infusion over 24 hours,* for 4 consecutive days, on days 1–4, every 21 days, for a maximum of 6 cycles (total dosage/cycle = 200 mg/m²)

Doxorubicin 10 mg/m² per day; administer by continuous intravenous infusion over 24 hours,* for 4 consecutive days, on days 1–4, every 21 days, for a maximum of 6 cycles (total dosage/cycle = 40 mg/m²)

Vincristine 0.4 mg/m² per day; administer by continuous intravenous infusion over 24 hours,* for 4 consecutive days, on days 1–4, every 21 days, for a maximum of 6 cycles (total dosage/cycle = 1.6 mg/m²)

*Note: See Special Instructions below for preparing a 3-in-1 admixture with etoposide, doxorubicin, and vincristine

Prednisone 60 mg/m² per day; administer orally for 5 consecutive days, on days 1–5 every 21 days for a maximum of 6 cycles (total dosage/cycle = 300 mg/m²)

Cyclophosphamide; administer intravenously in 100 mL 0.9% NS or D5W over 30 minutes on day 5 after completing etoposide + doxorubicin + vincristine administration, every 21 days for a maximum of 6 cycles (total initial dosage/cycle = 187–375 mg/m²)

Note: Baseline CD4+ lymphocyte count determines cycle 1 cyclophosphamide dosage

Baseline CD4 + Count	Cyclophosphamide Dosage
<100/mm³	187 mg/m²
≥100/mm³	375 mg/m²

Note: After cycle 1, cyclophosphamide dosage is increased or decreased in increments of 187 mg/m² (to a maximum 750 mg/m²) to achieve an ANC nadir of ≅500/mm³

(continued)

Treatment Modifications

Adverse Event	Dose Modification
ANC nadir during previous cycle ≥500/mm³	Increase cyclophosphamide dosage in increments of 187 mg/m² per cycle to a maximum of 750 mg/m² per cycle
ANC nadir during previous cycle <500/mm³	Reduce cyclophosphamide dosage by 187 mg/m²
Platelet count nadir during previous cycle <25,000/mm³	Reduce cyclophosphamide dosage by 187 mg/m²

Patient Population Studied

Phase II trial of 39 patients with previously untreated ARL. Median CD4 cells/mm³: 198 (range: 3–1182). Median potential follow-up of 53 months

Efficacy (without Rituximab)

Complete response	74%
Partial response	13%
Complete response (CD4+ cells >100/mm³)	87%
Complete response (CD4+ cells ≤100/mm³)	56%
At 53 Months' Potential Follow-up	
Disease-free survival of patients achieving a CR	92%
Overall survival	60%
Overall survival (CD4+ cells >100/mm³)	87%
Overall survival (CD4+ cells ≤100/mm³)	16%

(continued)
Supportive Care
Antiemetic prophylaxis
Emetogenic potential on Days 1–4 is **MINIMAL**
Emetogenic potential on Day 5 is **MODERATE**
See Chapter 39 for antiemetic recommendations

Hematopoietic growth factor (CSF) prophylaxis
Primary prophylaxis is indicated with one of the following:
   Filgrastim (G-CSF) 5 mcg/kg per day, by subcutaneous injection, or
   Pegfilgrastim (pegylated filgrastim) 6 mg/0.6 mL, by subcutaneous injection for one dose
   • Begin use from 24–72 h after myelosuppressive chemotherapy is completed
   • Continue daily Filgrastim use until ANC ≥5000/mm³ after the leukocyte nadir
   • Discontinue daily Filgrastim use at least 24 hours before administering myelosuppressive treatment. Do not administer Pegfilgrastim within 14 days before administering myelosuppressive treatment
See Chapter 43 for more information

Antimicrobial prophylaxis
Risk of fever and neutropenia is INTERMEDIATE
Antimicrobial primary prophylaxis to be considered:
   • Antibacterial—consider a fluoroquinolone or no prophylaxis; *P. jirovecii* prophylaxis is recommended (eg, cotrimoxazole)
   • Antifungal—consider concomitant use of cotrimoxazole during periods of neutropenia, and in anticipation of mucositis
   • Antiviral—anti-herpes antivirals (eg, acyclovir, famciclovir, valacyclovir)
See Chapter 47 for more information

Additional prophylaxis
Add a **proton pump inhibitor** during prednisone use to prevent gastritis and duodenitis
Give **stool softeners and/or laxatives** during and after vincristine administration

CNS therapy
CNS prophylaxis:
Cytarabine 50 mg per dose; administer intrathecally in a volume of **preservative-free** 0.9% sodium chloride injection equivalent to the amount of CSF removed (eg, 3–10 mL) via lumbar puncture, intraventricular catheter or reservoir (eg, Ommaya) once weekly for 4 consecutive weeks (total dose/4-week course = 200 mg)
or
Methotrexate 12 mg per dose; administer intrathecally in a volume of **preservative-free** 0.9% sodium chloride injection equivalent to the amount of CSF removed via lumbar puncture, intraventricular catheter, or reservoir on days 1 and 5, every 21 days, during cycles 3, 4, 5, and 6 (total dose/cycle = 24 mg)

CNS treatment (confirmed CNS disease)*:
Methotrexate 6 mg per dose, *plus*
Cytarabine 30 mg per dose, *plus*
Hydrocortisone 15 mg per dose
Induction: All 3 drugs are given together twice weekly for at least 4 consecutive weeks, or for 2 weeks after CSF specimens show no evidence of lymphoma. Administer intrathecally in a volume of **preservative-free** 0.9% sodium chloride injection equivalent to the amount of CSF removed via lumbar puncture, intraventricular catheter, or reservoir. Total doses/week: **methotrexate** = 12 mg; **cytarabine** = 60 mg; **hydrocortisone** = 30 mg

Consolidation: All 3 drugs are given together once weekly for 6 weeks. Administer intrathecally in a volume of **preservative-free** 0.9% sodium chloride injection equivalent to the amount of CSF removed via intraventricular catheter or reservoir. Total doses/week: **methotrexate** = 6 mg; **cytarabine** = 30 mg; **hydrocortisone** = 15 mg

Maintenance: All 3 drugs are given together, once monthly for 6 months. Administer intrathecally in a volume of **preservative-free** 0.9% sodium chloride injection equivalent to the amount of CSF removed. Total doses/month: **methotrexate** = 6 mg; **cytarabine** = 30 mg; **hydrocortisone** = 15 mg

**Note:* Monotherapy with methotrexate or cytarabine may be feasible in patients with sensitive disease

(continued)

Toxicity*† (N = 209 Cycles/39 Patients)

	% of Cycles
Hematologic	
G4 neutropenia (ANC <500/mm³)	30†
Febrile neutropenia	13
G3/4 anemia	17
G3/4 thrombocytopenia	21
Nonhematologic	
G3/4 constipation	3
G3/4 stomatitis	3
G3 neuropathy	2 patients

*ECOG criteria
†Despite filgrastim 5 mcg/kg per day

Therapy Monitoring
1. *Day 1 each cycle:* CBC with differential count, LFTs, BUN, and serum creatinine
2. *Twice-weekly during chemotherapy:* CBC with differential
3. *Cycle 4 and at end of cycle 6:* CD4+ cell count (modify prophylaxis or therapy for opportunistic infections in response to findings)
4. *After cycles 4 and 6:* Tumor restaging
5. *End of cycle 6:* Viral load
6. *Every 3 months thereafter:* CD4+ cell count and viral load as baseline to starting/resuming HAART

Note
Carriers of hepatitis B receiving rituximab should be monitored closely for clinical and laboratory signs of active HBV infection and for signs of hepatitis during and for up to several months following rituximab therapy

(continued)

CNS treatment (confirmed CNS disease)*:
Cytarabine liposome injection (DepoCyt) may be given as an alternative. The advantage of DepoCyt is that less frequent administrations are necessary

Induction: Cytarabine liposome injection 50 mg; administer intrathecally (intraventricular or lumbar puncture) every 14 days for 2 doses (weeks 1 and 3)

Consolidation therapy: Cytarabine liposome injection 50 mg; administer intrathecally (intraventricular or lumbar puncture) every 14 days for 3 doses (weeks 5, 7, and 9) followed by 1 additional dose at week 13

Maintenance: Cytarabine liposome injection 50 mg; administer intrathecally every 28 days for 4 doses (weeks 17, 21, 25, and 29)

Patients should receive **dexamethasone** 4 mg twice daily; administer either orally or intravenously, for 5 consecutive days, beginning on the day of cytarabine liposome injection
- DepoCyt product labeling includes a **Boxed Warning** indicating chemical arachnoiditis occurs commonly in association with DepoCyt use, characterized by nausea, vomiting, headache, and fever
- If left untreated, chemical arachnoiditis may be fatal
- The incidence and severity of chemical arachnoiditis symptoms can be reduced by a brief course of dexamethasone begun at the time DepoCyt is administered

Special Instructions

General instructions:
To prepare a 3-in-1 admixture with etoposide + doxorubicin + vincristine, dilute all 3 drug products in 0.9% sodium chloride injection (0.9% NS) as follows:

Total Dose of Etoposide	Volume of 0.9% NS
≤130 mg	500 mL
>130 mg	1000 mL

Etoposide (base) + doxorubicin + vincristine 3-in-1 admixtures:
Etoposide 50 mg/m^2, doxorubicin hydrochloride 10 mg/m^2, and vincristine sulfate 0.4 mg/m^2 admixtures diluted in 0.9% NS to produce a final etoposide concentration <250 mcg/mL, in polyolefin-lined infusion bags are stable and compatible for 72 hours at 23°–25°C (73.4°–77°F), and at 31°–33°C (87.8°–91.4°F) when protected from exposure to light

Wolfe JL et al. Am J Health Syst Pharm 1999;56:985–989

Etoposide Phosphate + doxorubicin + vincristine 3-in-1 admixtures:
Etoposide phosphate, doxorubicin hydrochloride, and vincristine sulfate admixtures diluted in 0.9% NS, to produce a final etoposide concentration <250 mcg/mL in polyolefin-lined infusion bags are stable and compatible for up to 124 hours at 2°–6°C (35.6°–42.8°F) and 35°–40°C (95°–104°F) in the dark and under fluorescent light. In admixtures stored at 35°–40°C (95°–104°F) and exposed to light, the initial drug concentrations decreased slightly, but remain within acceptable concentrations

Yuan P et al. Am J Health Syst Pharm 2001;58:594–598

A 3-in-1 admixture does not prevent microbial growth after exposure to bacterial and fungal contamination. With respect to product sterility, expiration dating should be determined by the aseptic techniques used in preparation and local and national guidelines

REGIMEN

CYCLOPHOSPHAMIDE + DOXORUBICIN + VINCRISTINE + PREDNISONE (CHOP) ± RITUXIMAB (CHOP ± RITUXIMAB)

Kaplan DL et al. Blood 2005;106:1538–1543

Important to note that most specialists recommend continuing HAART for patients already on a stable regimen. However, in some centers, HAART is suspended until all cycles are completed and then optimized on/after day 6 of final cycle

Rituximab premedication

Acetaminophen 650 mg; administer orally 30 minutes before rituximab

Diphenhydramine 50 mg; administer by intravenous injection 30 minutes before rituximab

Rituximab 375 mg/m²; administer intravenously in 0.9% sodium chloride injection (0.9% NS) or 5% dextrose injection (D5W), diluted to a concentration within the range 1–4 mg/mL, on day 1, every 21 days, for a maximum of 6 cycles (total dosage/cycle = 375 mg/m²)

Note: Caution is advised particularly if a patient's CD4+ cell count is <50/mm³

Notes on rituximab administration:

- Infuse initially at 50 mg/hour. If hypersensitivity or infusion reactions do not occur during the first 30 minutes, increase the rate by 50 mg/hour every 30 minutes as tolerated to a maximum rate of 400 mg/hour. During subsequent treatments, if previous rituximab administration was well tolerated, start at 100 mg/hour and increase by 100 mg/hour every 30 minutes as tolerated to a maximum rate of 400 mg/hour

- Interrupt rituximab administration for fever, chills, edema, congestion of the head and neck mucosa, hypertension, and other serious adverse events. Resume rituximab administration after adverse events abate

Cyclophosphamide 750 mg/m²; administer intravenously in 100 mL of 0.9% NS or D5W over 30 minutes, on day 1, every 21 days (total dosage/cycle = 750 mg/m²)

Doxorubicin 50 mg/m²; administer by slow intravenous injection over 3–5 minutes, on day 1, every 21 days (total dosage/cycle = 50 mg/m²)

Vincristine 1.2 mg/m²; administer by slow intravenous injection over 1–2 minutes, on day 1, every 21 days (total dosage/cycle = 1.2 mg/m²)

Prednisone 100 mg/day; administer orally for 5 consecutive days, on days 1–5, every 21 days (total dose/cycle = 500 mg)

Supportive Care

Antiemetic prophylaxis

Emetogenic potential: **HIGH**. *Potential for delayed symptoms*

See Chapter 39 for antiemetic recommendations

Hematopoietic growth factor (CSF) prophylaxis

Primary prophylaxis is indicated with one of the following:

Filgrastim (G-CSF) 5 mcg/kg per day; administer by subcutaneous injection, *or*

Pegfilgrastim (pegylated filgrastim) 6 mg/0.6 mL; administer by subcutaneous injection for 1 dose

- Begin use from 24–72 hours after myelosuppressive chemotherapy is completed

See Chapter 43 for more information

Antimicrobial prophylaxis

Risk of fever and neutropenia is INTERMEDIATE

Antimicrobial primary prophylaxis to be considered:

- Antibacterial

  ▪ Consider a fluoroquinolone during expected periods of neutropenia, or no prophylaxis

  ▪ *P. jirovecii* prophylaxis is recommended

    ○ Cotrimoxazole (trimethoprim 80 mg and sulfamethoxazole 400 mg) once daily

    or

    ○ Aerosolized pentamidine once monthly

  ▪ *Mycobacterium avium/intracellulare* complex prophylaxis for patients with CD4+ counts <100/mm³

    ○ Azithromycin 1200 mg/dose; administer orally once weekly

(continued)

Patient Population Studied

A 2:1 randomization trial with 95 patients randomized to receive the CHOP-rituximab arm and 47 patients the CHOP arm. Median CD4+ lymphocyte count was 133 cells/mm³; 79% of patients had stages III/IV disease

Efficacy (N = 47)

47 Patients Treated with CHOP

Complete response	50%
Median time to response	9 weeks

Treatment Modifications

Adverse Event	Dose Modification
ANC <1000/mm³ for 3 consecutive days or febrile neutropenia	Administer pegfilgrastim in subsequent cycles if not already given in cycle 1; reduce cyclophosphamide and doxorubicin dosages by 25%
Platelet count <75,000/mm³	Reduce cyclophosphamide and doxorubicin dosages by 25%

Toxicity* (N = 47)

	% Patients
G3/4 neutropenia	17
Fever and ANC <100/mm³	8.5
Death caused by infection	2

*National Cancer Institute (USA) Common Toxicity Criteria, version 2.0. Available at: http://ctep.cancer.gov/protocolDevelopment/electronic_applications/ctc.htm [accessed December 7, 2013]

(continued)

Note: Fluoroquinolone prophylaxis therapy is particularly important for patients treated with combination rituximab and chemotherapy.
- Antifungal—not indicated
- Antiviral—not indicated, unless patient previously had an episode of herpes simplex virus infection

See Chapter 47 for more information

Additional prophylaxis
Add a **proton pump inhibitor** during prednisone use to prevent gastritis and duodenitis
Give **stool softeners** and/or laxatives during and after vincristine administration

Therapy Monitoring

1. *Day 1 of each cycle:* CBC with differential count
2. *Twice-weekly during chemotherapy:* CBC with differential
3. *Every 2 cycles:* Tumor restaging

Note

Carriers of hepatitis B receiving rituximab should be monitored closely for clinical and laboratory signs of active hepatitis B virus infection and for signs of hepatitis during and for several months following rituximab therapy

17. Leukemia, Acute Lymphoblastic (ADULT)

Michael M. Boyiadzis, MD, MHSc, Ivan Aksentijevich, MD, and Judith Karp, MD

Epidemiology

Incidence: 6,020 (male: 3,140; female: 2,880. Estimated new cases for 2014 in the United States)
1.7 per 100,000 male and female per year (1.9 per 100,000 male, 1.5 per 100,000 female)

Deaths: Estimated 1,440 in 2014 (male: 810; female: 630)

Median age: B-cell lymphoblastic leukemia/lymphoma: 12 years
T-cell lymphoblastic leukemia/lymphoma: 18 years
Lymphoblastic leukemia/lymphoma unknown lineage: 12 years
Age-specific incidence patterns are characterized by a peak between the ages of 2 and 4 years and again during the sixth decade

Male to female ratio: 1.33

Dores GM. Blood 2012;119:34–43
Siegel R et al. CA Cancer J Clin 2014;64:9–29
Surveillance, Epidemiology and End Results (SEER) Program, available from http://seer.cancer.gov (accessed in 2013)

Work-up

1. H&P
2. CBC, leukocyte differential, platelets, electrolytes, liver function tests, PT, PTT, fibrinogen, LDH, uric acid
3. Bone marrow biopsy/aspirate
4. HLA typing for patients who are candidates for allogeneic hematopoietic cell transplantation
5. Cardiac scan if prior cardiac history or prior anthracycline use
6. CT/MRI of head if neurologic symptoms
7. CT chest for T-ALL patients

Pathology

Common Chromosomal and Molecular Abnormalities in ALL

Cytogentics	Gene	Frequency in Adults	Frequency in Children
Hyperdiploidy	–	7%	25%
Hypodiploidy	–	2%	1%
t(9;22)(q34;q11) Philadelphia chromosome (Ph)	BCR-ABL1	25%	3%
t(12;21)(p13;q22)	TEL-AML1	2%	22%
t(v;11q23), e.., t(4;11), t(9;11), t11;19)	MLL	10%	8%
t(1;19)	E2A-PBX1	3%	5%
t(5;14)(q31;q32)	IL3-IGH	<1%	<1%
t(8;14), t(2;8), t(8;22)	c-MYC	4%	2%
t(1;14)(p32;q11)	TAL-1*	12%	7%
t(10;14)(q24;q11)	HOX11*	8%	1%
t(5;14)(q35;q32)	HOX11L2*	1%	3%

*Abnormalities observed exclusively in T-cell lineage ALL; all other occur exclusively or predominately in B-cell linage ALL

Prognostic Factors for Risk Stratification of Adult ALL	
Characteristics	**High Risk Factors**
Age	>35 years
Leukocytosis	>30,000 mm^3 (B lineage) >100,000 mm^3 (T lineage)
Karyotype	t(9;22), t(4;11) (q21;q23), complex, hypodiploid
Therapy response	Time to morphology CR >4weeks Persistent minimal residual disease (MRD)

Expert Opinion

Treatment regimens for acute lymphoblastic leukemia (ALL) have evolved empirically into complex schemes that use numerous agents in various doses, combinations, and schedules, and few of the individual components have been tested rigorously in randomized trials. However, the backbone of chemotherapy for ALL remains the sequence of induction, consolidation, and maintenance

Remission induction: Most regimens include steroids, vincristine, an anthracycline, and usually asparaginase. Cyclophosphamide and cytarabine are often added. The combination of these agents results in CR rate to 80–90%; thus, treating physicians should use a regimen with which they are familiar and have experience in providing supportive care. See table below for different adult ALL regimens

Consolidation: Eradication of minimal residual disease during hematologic remission is the primary aim of the consolidation phase. It is difficult to assess the value of individual components of treatment because the number, schedule, and combination of antineoplastic drugs vary considerably among studies. Consolidation therapy typically consists of several cycles of treatment similar to, but often less intensive than, the drugs, dosages, and administration schedules given during induction, and consolidation usually is better tolerated than induction

Maintenance: Maintenance therapies are important for patients not undergoing allogeneic hematopoietic cell transplantation (allo-HCT). Maintenance regimens consist of combinations of mercaptopurine, methotrexate, vincristine, and steroids given continually for 2–3 years. Patients with the genetic defect of thiopurine methyltransferase (TPMT) are more sensitive to myelosuppressive effects of mercaptopurine and should be consider for testing for TPMT gene polymorphisms

Myeloablative allo-HCT should be considered for adult patients with ALL in first clinical remission (CR) for all disease risk groups. Allo-HCT provides a significant improvement in overall and leukemia-free survival in younger patients (ages <35 years), standard risk, patients with Philadelphia chromosome (Ph)-negative ALL compared with less-intensive chemotherapy regimens. In older (ages >35 years) patients with standard risk, Ph-negative ALL, a higher treatment related mortality diminishes the significant survival advantage with allo-HCT

Cooperative group analysis have consistently demonstrated superior outcomes for adolescent and young adult (AYA) patients with ALL when treated with pediatric versus adult ALL regimens. Thus AYA patients should be treated with pediatric-based treatment protocols in clinical trials

Note: Mature B-cell ALL: Patients with mature B-cell ALL (Burkitt cell leukemia, L3) experience improvement in survival rate when high doses of cyclophosphamide, methotrexate, and cytarabine are incorporated early in treatment. The probability of leukemia-free survival improved with standard ALL induction from 35% to 60–70% with these agents. No maintenance therapy is given to patients with mature B-cell ALL since relapse occurs early and most patients are cured after approximately 1.5 years

Philadelphia chromosome-positive acute lymphoblastic leukemia: Patients with Philadelphia chromosome-positive acute lymphoblastic leukemia (Ph+ ALL) are a distinct disease subgroup comprising 20–30% of adults. Chemotherapy regimens that have combined tyrosine kinase inhibitors (TKIs) offer enhanced CR rates and a greater opportunity for patients to proceed to allo-HCT. The potential benefits of allo-HCT in patients with Ph+ ALL have been described in several studies. For patients who receive allo-HCT DFS and OS always appear better than would be expected with chemotherapy alone. For patients who are too old or unfit for allo-HCT, TKIs should be continued without interruption in addition to whatever components of standard maintenance therapy can be tolerated

Patients with relapsed ALL have a poor prognosis with standard salvage therapy. Response rates to salvage chemotherapy range from 30–70% but are generally short-lived with a median survival of 6 months. Patients in second CR should be considered for allo-HCT

Studies in adults with ALL have demonstrated the strong correlation between minimal residual disease (MRD) and risks of relapse. The timing of MRD assessment varies depending on the ALL regimen protocol being used, and may occur during or after completion of initial induction therapy. For MRD evaluation by multicolor flow cytometry, sampling of bone marrow mononuclear cells is preferred over peripheral blood samples. For MRD evaluation by RQ-PCR, sampling of bone marrow mononuclear cells is preferred. The minimal limit of assay sensitivity (to declare MRD negativity) should be <1 × 10^4, <0.01%)

(continued)

Expert Opinion (continued)

Results of Clinical Trials in Adult ALL

Rowe JM. Br J Haematol 2009;144:468–483

Study	Year	N	Median Age (Range [Years])	SCT	CR Rate	Early Death	Survival
CALGB 9111, USA	1998	198	35 (16–83)	Ph+	85%	8%	40% (3 years)
Larson RA et al. Blood 1998;92:1556–1564							
LALA 87, France	2000	572	33 (15–60)	PO	76%	9%	27% (10 years)
Thiebaut A et al. Hematol Oncol Clin North Am 2000;1353–1366							
NILG 08/96, Italy	2001	121	35 (15–74)	PR	84%	8%	48% (5 years)
Bassan R et al. Hematol J 2001;2:117–126							
GMALL 05/93, Germany	2001	1163	35 (15–65)	PR	83%	NR	35% (5 years)
Goekbuget N et al. Blood 2001;98 [abstract 3338]							
JALSG-ALL93, Japan	2002	263	31 (15–59)	PO	78%	6%	30% (6 years)
Takeuchi J et al. Leukemia 2002;16:1259–1266							
UCLA, USA	2002	84	27 (16–59)	PR	93%	1%	47% (5 years)
Linker C et al. J Clin Oncol 2002;20:2464–2471							
Sweden	2002	153	42 (16–82)	PR	75%	NR	28% (5 years)
Hallböök H et al. Br J Haematol 2002;118:748–754							
GIMEMA 0288, Italy	2002	767	28 (12–60)	—	82%	11%	27% (9 years)
Annino L et al. Blood 2002;99:863–871							
MD Anderson, USA	2004	288	40 (15–92)	Ph+	92%	5%	38% (5 years)
Kantarjian H et al. Cancer 2004;101:2788–2801							
EORTC ALL-3, Europe	2004	340	33 (14–79)	PO	74%	NR	36%* (6 years)
Labar B et al. Haematologica 2004;89:809–817							
LALA 94, France	2004	922	33 (15–55)	PR	84%	5%	36% (5 years)
Thomas X et al. J Clin Oncol 2004;22:4075–4086							
GOELAL02, France	2004	198	33 (15–59)	HR	86%	2%	41% (6 years)
Hunault M et al. Blood 2004;104:3028–3037							
MRC XII/ECOG E 2993, UK-USA	2005	1521	31 (15–64)	PO	91%	4Æ8%	38% (5 years)
Rowe JM et al. Blood 2005;106:3760–3767							
GIMEMA 0496, Italy	2005	450	16–60	NR	80%	NR	33% (5 years)
Mancini M et al. Blood 2001;98:[abstract 3492]							
Pethema ALL-93, Spain	2005	222	27 (15–50)	HR	82%	6%	34% (5 years)
Ribera J-M et al. Haematologica 2005;90:1346–1356							
PALG 4–2002, Poland	2008	131	26 (17–60)	PO	90%	NR	43% (3 years)
Holowiecki J et al. Br J Haematol 2008;142:227–237							

(continued)

Results of Clinical Trials in Adult ALL (continued)

Study	Year	N	Median Age (Range [Years])	SCT	CR Rate	Early Death	Survival
Total of all studies (using weighted mean)		7393			84%	7%	35%

Ph+, SCT in Philadelphia chromosome positive-ALL; PO, prospective SCT in all patients with donors; PR, SCT according to prospective risk model; HR, prospective SCT in a study for high-risk patients only; NR, not reported

Central nervous system involvement: Up to 10% of adults with ALL present with CNS involvement at the time of diagnosis. The cumulative risk of CNS leukemia in patients who do not receive prophylaxis can be as high as 50%. Factors associated with increased risks for CNS leukemia in adults include mature B-cell immunophenotype, T-cell immunophenotype, high presenting WBC count, and elevated serum LDH levels. CNS involvement should be evaluated by lumbar puncture at the appropriate timing in accordance with the specific treatment protocol used and when LP is performed intrathecal therapy administered concomitantly. Adult patients with ALL and CNS involvement at diagnosis require CNS-directed therapy starting at the same time as induction therapy. Treatment and prophylaxis of CNS involvement may consist of intrathecally administered methotrexate either alone or combined with intrathecally administered cytarabine or corticosteroids and/or intravenously administered high-dose cytarabine, high-dose cytarabine methotrexate. With the incorporation of adequate systemic chemotherapy and intrathecal chemotherapy regimens, it is possible to avoid the use of upfront cranial irradiation except for cases of overt CNS leukemia at presentation and reserve the use of irradiation for salvage therapy settings. Allo-HCT is indicated in patients with isolated CNS relapse and is probably the only curative approach for some patients, because of the high risk of occult marrow contamination at the time of CNS progression

Bassan R, Hoelzer D. J Clin Oncol 2011;29:532–543
Fielding AK. Blood 2010;116:3409–3417
Fielding AK. Hematol Oncol Clin North Am 2011;25:1255–1279
Gökbuget N, Hoelzer D. Semin Hematol 2009;46:64–75
Oliansky DM et al. Biol Blood Marrow Transplant 2012;18:18–36
Rowe JM. Br J HaematolBr J Hematol 2009;144:468–483
Rowe JM. Br J HaematolBr J Hematol 2010;150:389–405

PROPHYLAXIS AGAINST TUMOR LYSIS SYNDROME

HYDRATION, URINARY ALKALINIZATION, AND ALLOPURINOL ADMINISTRATION

Hydration with 2500–3000 mL/m^2 per day as tolerated; administer intravenously to maintain urine output ≥100 mL/m^2 per hour (or ≥2 mL/kg per hour in persons whose body weight is <50 kg)

Urinary alkalinization with **sodium bicarbonate** injection added to intravenously administered fluids

- The amount of sodium bicarbonate added to intravenously administered fluids should produce a solution with sodium content not greater than the concentration of sodium in 0.9% sodium chloride injection (≤154 mEq/L):

Sodium Bicarbonate is Added to a Solution to Increase Urine pH within a Range 6.5 to ≤7

Base Solution Sodium Content	Sodium Bicarbonate Additive	Total Sodium Content
0.45% Sodium Chloride Injection (0.45% NS)		
77 mEq/L	50–75 mEq	127–152 mEq/L
0.2% Sodium Chloride Injection (0.2% NS)		
34 mEq/L	100–125 mEq	134–159 mEq/L
5% Dextrose injection (D5W)		
0	125–150 mEq	125–150 mEq/L
D5W/0.45% NS		
77 mEq/L	50–75 mEq	127–152 mEq/L
D5W/0.2% NS		
34 mEq/L	100–125 mEq	134–159 mEq/L

Notes:
- Hydration rate may be decreased at the completion of chemotherapy administration
- Urinary alkalization increases the solubility and excretion of uric acid and its oxypurine precursors (hypoxanthine and xanthine) and helps avoid uric acid crystallization in renal tubules; however, alkalinization is not uniformly recommended because:
  1. It favors precipitation of calcium phosphate in renal tubules, a concern in patients with concomitant hyperphosphatemia
  2. A metabolic alkalemia may result from the administration of bicarbonate that can worsen the neurologic manifestations of hypocalcemia
- Discontinue sodium bicarbonate administration (while continuing hydration) if serum bicarbonate concentration is >30 mEq/L (>30 mmol/L) or urine pH >7.5

Allopurinol
- Administer orally or intravenously starting 12 hours to 3 days (preferably, 2–3 days) before starting cytoreductive chemotherapy
- Hyperuricemia develops within 24 to 48 hours after initiating chemotherapy when the excretory capacity of the renal tubules for uric acid is exceeded
- In the presence of an acid pH, uric acid crystals form in the renal tubules, leading to intraluminal renal tubular obstruction, an acute renal obstructive uropathy, and renal dysfunction
- *Initial dosage*
  Allopurinol 100 mg/m^2 per dose; administer orally every 8 hours (maximum daily dose = 800 mg), *or*
  Allopurinol 3.3 mg/kg per dose; administer orally every 8 hours (maximum daily dose = 800 mg), *or*
  Allopurinol 200–400 mg/m^2 per day; administer intravenously (maximum daily dose = 600 mg) in a volume of 5% dextrose injection or 0.9% sodium chloride injection sufficient to yield a concentration not greater than 6 mg/mL. The duration for administering individual doses should be informed by the volume to be given
  - Allopurinol may be administered as a single daily dose, or the total daily dose may be divided equally for administration at 6-, 8-, or 12-hour intervals
- **Maintenance doses** should be based on serum uric acid determinations performed approximately 48 hours after initiation of allopurinol therapy, and periodically thereafter
- Continue administering allopurinol until leukemic blasts have been cleared from the peripheral blood

(continued)

(continued)

Notes:
- Allopurinol dose adjustments for impaired renal function:

Creatinine Clearance	Oral Allopurinol Dose
10–20 mL/min (0.17–0.33 mL/s)	200 mg/day
3–10 mL/min (0.05–0.17 mL/s)	100 mg/day
<3 mL/min (<0.05 mL/s)	100 mg every 36–48 hours

- Allopurinol does not remove uric acid already present
- The incidence of allergic reactions is increased in patients receiving amoxicillin, ampicillin, or thiazide diuretics

Rasburicase
- Rasburicase is recombinant urate oxidase (uricase) produced by genetically modified *Saccharomyces cerevisiae* that express urate oxidase cDNA cloned from a strain of *Aspergillus flavus*
- Uricase enzymes catalyze uric acid oxidation to allantoin, which is at least 5-times more soluble than uric acid
- Rational utilization
  - Rasburicase should be considered among initial interventions against hyperuricemia in patients with high peripheral WBC counts, rapidly increasing blasts counts, high uric acid, or with evidence of impaired renal function; that is:

Burkitt leukemia	
WBC count ≥100,000/mm^3	
WBC count <100,000/mm^3 + LDH ≥2 × ULN	
WBC count <100,000/mm^3 + LDH <2 × ULN +	acute kidney injury *or* normal renal function + uric acid > ULN, *or* potassium > ULN, *or* phosphorus > ULN
ULN, upper limit of normal	

See Chapter 46, *Oncologic Emergencies*

Rasburicase 0.2 mg/kg per dose intravenously in a total volume of 50 mL 0.9% sodium chloride injection over 30 minutes once daily for up to 5 consecutive days is often used, but much less is usually sufficient (See Chapter 46, Oncologic Emergencies) (dosage and administration recommendations published in U.S. Food and Drug Administration product labeling, January 2011)
- Rasburicase has demonstrated effectiveness in prophylaxis and treatment for hyperuricemia and acute increases in uric acid associated with cytoreductive therapies at dosages <0.2 mg/kg based on body weight, with fixed doses, and after administration of from 1–3 doses

See Chapter 46 for more information

Cairo MS, Bishop M. Br J Haematol 2004;127:3–11
Cairo MS et al. Br J Haematol 2010;149:578–586
Coiffier B et al. J Clin Oncol 2008;26:2767–2778
Klinenberg JR et al. Ann Intern Med 1965;62:639–647

REGIMEN

LARSON REGIMEN

Larson RA et al. Blood 1998;92:1556–1564

Course I, Induction (1 course, 4 weeks in duration)

Treatment Stratified by Patient Age

<60 years	≥60 years
Cyclophosphamide 1200 mg/m²; administer intravenously in 100–250 mL 0.9% sodium chloride injection (0.9% NS) or 5% dextrose injection (D5W) over 15–30 minutes on day 1 (total dosage/course = 1200 mg/m²) **Daunorubicin** 45 mg/m² per day; administer by intravenous injection over 3–5 minutes for 3 consecutive days, on days 1–3 (total dosage/course = 135 mg/m²) **Prednisone** 60 mg/m² per day; administer orally, continually, for 21 consecutive days, on days 1–21 (total dosage/course = 1260 mg/m²)	**Cyclophosphamide** 800 mg/m²; administer intravenously in 100–250 mL 0.9% sodium chloride injection (0.9% NS) or 5% dextrose injection (D5W) over 15–30 minutes on day 1 (total dosage/course = 800 mg/m²) **Daunorubicin** 30 mg/m² per day; administer by intravenous injection over 3–5 minutes for 3 consecutive days, on days 1–3 (total dosage/course = 90 mg/m²) **Prednisone** 60 mg/m² per day; administer orally, continually, for 7 consecutive days, on days 1–7 (total dosage/course = 420 mg/m²)

All Patients

Vincristine 2 mg per dose; administer by intravenous injection over 1–2 minutes for 4 doses, on days 1, 8, 15, and 22 (total dose/course = 8 mg)

Asparaginase 6000 IU/m² per dose; administer intramuscularly, or intravenously in 10–50 mL 0.9% NS or D5W over at least 30 minutes for 6 doses, on days 5, 8, 11, 15, 18, and 22 (total dosage/course = 36,000 IU/m²)

Filgrastim 5 mcg/kg per day; administer by subcutaneous injection for at least 7 consecutive days. Start on day 4, at least 12 hours after the last dose of daunorubicin, and continue after the ANC nadir until the ANC is ≥1000/mm³ on 2 consecutive days (measurements ≥24 hours apart)

Supportive Care
Antiemetic prophylaxis
Emetogenic potential on day 1 is **HIGH**. *Potential for delayed symptoms*
Emetogenic potential on days 2 and 3 is **MODERATE**
Emetogenic potential on days with asparaginase ± vincristine is **MINIMAL**
See Chapter 39 for antiemetic recommendations

Hematopoietic growth factor (CSF) prophylaxis
Primary prophylaxis is indicated with:
    Filgrastim (G-CSF) 5 mcg/kg per day, by subcutaneous injection
- Begin use on day 4
- Continue daily filgrastim use for at least 7 days, and until ANC ≥1000/mm³ on 2 measurements separated temporally by ≥24 hours
- Discontinue daily filgrastim use at least 24 hours before administering myelosuppressive treatment

See Chapter 43 for more information

Antimicrobial prophylaxis
Risk of fever and neutropenia is HIGH
Antimicrobial primary prophylaxis is recommended:
- Antibacterial—consider fluoroquinolone prophylaxis; *Pneumocystis jirovecii* prophylaxis is recommended (eg, cotrimoxazole)
- Antifungal—recommended
- Antiviral—antiherpes antivirals (eg, acyclovir, famciclovir, valacyclovir)

See Chapter 47 for more information

(continued)

Patient Population Studied

102 patients (median age 35 years) with newly diagnosed ALL

Efficacy (N = 102)

Induction Course

Complete CR (n = 97*)	90%
≥60 years (n = 21)	81%
<60 years (n = 76)	89%
Refractory disease (n = 102)	8%
Died during induction (n = 102)	5%
DFS, median	2.3 years
DFS Ph+ patients, median	0.8 years
Overall survival, median	2.4 years

*Among 102 patients randomly assigned to receive filgrastim during induction and early intensification courses, 97 patients were eligible for comparisons with patients who did not receive filgrastim

(continued)

(*continued*)

Courses IIA and IIB, early intensification (2 courses, each is 4 weeks in duration)

Methotrexate 15 mg; administer intrathecally via lumbar puncture in 3–15 mL *preservative-free* 0.9% sodium chloride injection (PF 0.9% NS) on day 1, every 4 weeks for 2 courses (total dose/course = 15 mg)

Cyclophosphamide 1000 mg/m²; administer intravenously in 100–250 mL 0.9% NS or D5W over 15–30 minutes on day 1, every 4 weeks for 2 courses (total dosage/course = 1000 mg/m²)

Mercaptopurine 60 mg/m² per day, administer orally, continually, for 14 consecutive days, days 1–14, every 4 weeks for 2 courses (total dosage/course = 840 mg/m²)

Cytarabine 75 mg/m² per dose; administer by subcutaneous injection for 8 doses on days 1–4 and days 8–11, every 4 weeks for 2 courses (total dosage/course = 600 mg/m²)

Vincristine 2 mg per dose; administer by intravenous injection over 1–2 minutes for 2 doses, on days 15 and 22, every 4 weeks for 2 courses (total dose/course = 4 mg)

Asparaginase 6000 IU/m² per dose; administer intramuscularly, or intravenously in 10–50 mL 0.9% NS or D5W over at least 30 minutes for 4 doses, on days 15, 18, 22, and 25, every 4 weeks for 2 courses (total dosage/course = 24,000 IU/m²)

Filgrastim 5 mcg/kg per day; administer by subcutaneous injection for at least 14 consecutive days. Start on day 2, and continue after the ANC nadir until the ANC is ≥5000/mm³ on 2 consecutive days (measurements ≥24 hours apart)

Note: In all cases, filgrastim should be discontinued at least 2 days before cyclophosphamide administration resumed on the first day of the second early intensification course

Supportive Care
Antiemetic prophylaxis
Emetogenic potential on Day 1 is **MODERATE**
Emetogenic potential on days with cytarabine is **LOW**
Emetogenic potential on days with mercaptopurine alone is **MINIMAL–LOW**
Emetogenic potential on days with asparaginase ± vincristine is **MINIMAL**
See Chapter 39 for antiemetic recommendations

Hematopoietic growth factor (CSF) prophylaxis
Primary prophylaxis is indicated with:
  Filgrastim (G-CSF) 5 mcg/kg per day, by subcutaneous injection
  • Begin use on day 2
  • Continue daily filgrastim use for at least 14 days, and until ANC ≥5000/mm³ on 2 measurements separated temporally by ≥24 hours
  • Priority was given to starting the second course (Course IIB) 28 days after the first began
    ▪ For patients whose ANC recovers to ≥1000/mm³ and platelet count ≥50,000/mm³ 28 days after starting the first course (Course IIA), the second course of therapy began on the 29th day of Course IIA even if they had not yet recovered an ANC ≥5000/mm³ by day 27
  • Discontinue daily filgrastim use at least 2 days before restarting myelosuppressive treatment
See Chapter 43 for more information

Antimicrobial prophylaxis
Risk of fever and neutropenia is HIGH
  Antimicrobial primary prophylaxis is recommended:
  • Antibacterial—consider fluoroquinolone prophylaxis; *P. jirovecii* prophylaxis is recommended (eg, cotrimoxazole)
  • Antifungal—recommended
  • Antiviral—antiherpes antivirals (eg, acyclovir, famciclovir, valacyclovir)
See Chapter 47 for more information

Course III, CNS prophylaxis and interim maintenance (1 course, 12 weeks in duration)

Cranial irradiation 2400 cGy (total dose), delivered during 12 consecutive days, days 1–12
Methotrexate 15 mg per dose; administer intrathecally via lumbar puncture in 3–15 mL preservative-free 0.9% sodium chloride injection for 5 doses, on days 1, 8, 15, 22, and 29 (total dose/course = 75 mg)

(*continued*)

Efficacy (N = 102) (*continued*)
Adverse Effects of Remission Induction

	Grades 3 & 4 or Grade 5 Toxicity
WBC (<1000/mm³)	98
Platelets (<25,000/mm³)	97
Hemoglobin (<6.5 g/dL)	93
Infection	78
Nausea	23
Bilirubin (>1.5 times NL)	44
Transaminase (>5 times NL)	35
Malaise/fatigue (PS >2)	16
Motor neuropathy	18
Pain	21
Hyperglycemia (>250 mg/dL)	33
Hypofibrinogenemia (<0.5 times NL)	26

Adverse Effects of Intensification and Maintenance

Grades 3 & 4 Toxicities	Intensification	Maintenance
Leucopenia	97	75
Thrombocytopenia	84	32
Anemia	84	26
Hemorrhage	4	0
Infection	49	25
Nausea/vomiting	17	8
Stomatitis	9	7
Diarrhea	3	1
Hepatic	28	30
Pulmonary	5	4
Cardiac	1	6
Genitourinary	2	1
CNS	13	6
Peripheral nervous system	12	7
Skin	1	2
Allergy	1	1

Data from 197 newly diagnosed ALL patients who were treated with the same chemotherapy regimen but did not receive filgrastim Larson RA et al. Blood 1995;85:2025–2037

(continued)

Mercaptopurine 60 mg/m² per day; administer orally, continually, for 70 consecutive days, days 1–70 (total dosage/course = 4200 mg/m²)

Methotrexate 20 mg/m² per dose; administer orally, for 5 doses, on days 36, 43, 50, 57, and 64 (total dosage/course = 100 mg/m²)

Supportive Care
Antiemetic prophylaxis
Emetogenic potential is MINIMAL–LOW
See Chapter 39 for antiemetic recommendations

Hematopoietic growth factor (CSF) prophylaxis
Primary prophylaxis is NOT indicated
See Chapter 43 for more information

Antimicrobial prophylaxis
Risk of fever and neutropenia is HIGH
Antimicrobial primary prophylaxis is recommended:
- Antibacterial—*P. jirovecii* prophylaxis is recommended (eg, cotrimoxazole)
- Antifungal—recommended
- Antiviral—antiherpes antivirals (eg, acyclovir, famciclovir, valacyclovir)

See Chapter 47 for more information

Course IV, late intensification (1 course, 8 weeks in duration)

Doxorubicin 30 mg/m² per dose; administer by intravenous injection over 3–5 minutes for 3 doses, on days 1, 8, and 15 (total dosage/course = 90 mg/m²)

Vincristine 2 mg per dose; administer by intravenous injection over 1–2 minutes for 3 doses, on days 1, 8, and 15 (total dose/course = 6 mg)

Dexamethasone 10 mg/m² per day; administer orally, continually, for 14 consecutive days, days 1–14 (total dosage/course = 140 mg/m²)

Cyclophosphamide 1000 mg/m²; administer intravenously in 100–250 mL 0.9% NS or D5W over 15–30 minutes on day 29 (total dosage/course = 1000 mg/m²)

Thioguanine 60 mg/m² per day; administer orally, continually, for 14 consecutive days, days 29–42 (total dosage/course = 840 mg/m²)

Cytarabine 75 mg/m² per dose; administer by subcutaneous injection for 8 doses on days 29–32 and days 36–39 (total dosage/course = 600 mg/m²)

Supportive Care
Antiemetic prophylaxis
Emetogenic potential on Days 1, 8, 15, and 29 is MODERATE
Emetogenic potential on Days 30–32 and 36–39 is LOW
Emetogenic potential on days with thioguanine alone is MINIMAL–LOW
See Chapter 39 for antiemetic recommendations

Hematopoietic growth factor (CSF) prophylaxis
Primary prophylaxis may be indicated
- *During the intervals between doses of doxorubicin, and the interval from days 16 through 28*
- Discontinue daily filgrastim use at least 24 hours before administering myelosuppressive treatment

See Chapter 43 for more information

Antimicrobial prophylaxis
Risk of fever and neutropenia is HIGH
Antimicrobial primary prophylaxis is recommended:
- Antibacterial—consider fluoroquinolone prophylaxis; *P. jirovecii* prophylaxis is recommended (eg, cotrimoxazole)
- Antifungal—recommended
- Antiviral—antiherpes antivirals (eg, acyclovir, famciclovir, valacyclovir)

See Chapter 47 for more information

(continued)

Therapy Monitoring

1. CBC with differential daily during and after chemotherapy until recovery of ANC >500/mm³. Platelets every day while in hospital until patients no longer require platelet transfusions

2. Serum electrolytes, mineral panel, and uric acid, at least daily during active treatment until the risk of tumor lysis is past

3. Amylase and fibrinogen levels prior to asparaginase administration. If fibrinogen level is <100 mg/dL (<1 g/L) consider prophylactic administration of cryoprecipitate

4. Bone marrow aspirate and biopsy at day 29 of the initial induction course. After a patient achieves a CR, bone marrow biopsy and aspirate should be performed at the end of each consolidation cycle (or at the very least, every other cycle), and every 3 months during maintenance therapy

Treatment Modifications

Adverse Events	Treatment Modifications
Creatinine 1.5–2 mg/dL (133–177 µmol/L)	Reduce methotrexate dosage by 25%
Creatinine >2 mg/dL (>177 µmol/L)	Reduce methotrexate dosage by 50%
Creatinine >3 mg/dL (>265 µmol/L)	Reduce daunorubicin dosage by 50%
Total bilirubin 3–5 mg/dL (51–86 µmol/L)	Reduce daunorubicin dosage by 50% Reduce methotrexate dosage by 25%
Total bilirubin >3 mg/dL (>51 µmol/L)	Reduce vincristine dosage by 50%
Total bilirubin >5 mg/dL (>86 µmol/L)	Hold daunorubicin Hold methotrexate

(continued)

Course V, prolonged maintenance (courses are 4 weeks in duration and are repeated until 24 months after diagnosis)
Vincristine 2 mg per dose; administer by intravenous injection over 1–2 minutes, on day 1, every 4 weeks (total dose/course = 2 mg)
Prednisone 60 mg/m^2 per day; administer orally, continually, for 5 consecutive days, on days 1–5, every 4 weeks (total dosage/course = 300 mg/m^2)
Mercaptopurine 60 mg/m^2 per day; administer orally, continually, for 28 consecutive days, days 1–28, every 4 weeks (total dosage/course = 1680 mg/m^2)
Methotrexate 20 mg/m^2 per dose; administer orally, for 4 doses, on days 1, 8, 15, and 22, every 4 weeks (total dosage/course = 80 mg/m^2)

Supportive Care
Antiemetic prophylaxis
Emetogenic potential is **MINIMAL–LOW**
See Chapter 39 for antiemetic recommendations

Hematopoietic growth factor (CSF) prophylaxis
Primary prophylaxis is NOT indicated
See Chapter 43 for more information

Antimicrobial prophylaxis
Risk of fever and neutropenia is HIGH
 Antimicrobial primary prophylaxis is recommended:
 • Antibacterial—*P. jirovecii* prophylaxis is recommended (eg, cotrimoxazole)
 • Antifungal—recommended
 • Antiviral—antiherpes antivirals (eg, acyclovir, famciclovir, valacyclovir)
See Chapter 47 for more information

Asparaginase Toxicity Management
Stock W et al. Leuk Lymphoma 2011;52:2237–2253

Toxicity	Grade 2	Grade 3	Grade 4
Hypersensitivity Urticaria, wheezing, laryngospasm, hypotension, etc.	For urticaria without bronchospasm, hypotension, edema, or need for parenteral intervention, continue asparaginase	For wheezing or other symptomatic bronchospasm with or without urticaria, indicated parenteral intervention, angioedema, or hypotension, discontinue asparaginase. If erwinia asparaginase is available, replace pegaspargase with erwinia asparaginase	For life-threatening consequences or indicated urgent intervention, discontinue asparaginase. If erwinia asparaginase is available, replace pegaspargase with erwinia asparaginase
Hypertriglyceridemia	If serum triglyceride level <1000 mg/dL (<11.3 mmol/L), continue asparaginase but follow patient closely for evolving pancreatitis	Hold asparaginase for triglyceride >1000 mg/dL (>11.3 mmol/L); follow closely for pancreatitis; resume asparaginase at prior dose level after patient's triglyceride level returns to normal range	Hold asparaginase for triglyceride >1000 mg/dL (>11.3 mmol/L); follow closely for pancreatitis; resume asparaginase at prior dose level after patient's triglyceride level returns to normal range
Hyperglycemia, ketoacidosis	Continue asparaginase for uncomplicated hyperglycemia	For hyperglycemia requiring insulin therapy, hold asparaginase (and glucocorticoid therapy) until blood glucose regulated with insulin; resume asparaginase at prior dose level	For hyperglycemia with life-threatening consequences or indicated urgent intervention, hold asparaginase (and glucocorticoid therapy) until blood glucose is regulated with insulin; resume asparaginase and do not make up for missed doses
Hyperammonemia-related fatigue	Continue asparaginase	Reduce asparaginase dose by 25%; resume full dose when toxicity is grade ≤2; make up for missed doses	Reduce asparaginase dose 50%; resume full dose when toxicity grade 2; make up for missed doses
Pancreatitis	Continue asparaginase for asymptomatic amylase or lipase elevation >3 × ULN (chemical pancreatitis) or only radiologic abnormalities; observe closely for rising amylase or lipase levels	Continue pegaspargase for non-symptomatic chemical pancreatitis but observe patient closely for development of symptomatic pancreatitis for early treatment. Hold native asparaginase for amylase or lipase elevation >3 × ULN until enzyme levels stabilize or are declining. Permanently discontinue asparaginase for symptomatic pancreatitis	Permanently discontinue all asparaginase for clinical pancreatitis (vomiting, severe abdominal pain) with amylase or lipase elevation >3 × ULN for >3 days and/or development of pancreatic pseudocyst

(continued)

Asparaginase Toxicity Management (continued)

Toxicity	Grade 2	Grade 3	Grade 4
Increased hepatic transaminases	For alanine or glutamine aminotransferase elevation >3–5 × ULN, continue asparaginase	For alanine or glutamine aminotransferase elevation >5–20 × ULN, delay next dose of asparaginase until transaminasemia is grade <2	For alanine or glutamine aminotransferase elevation >20 × ULN, discontinue asparaginase if toxicity reduction to grade <2 takes >1 week
Hyperbilirubinemia	Continue asparaginase if direct bilirubin <3.0 mg/dL (<51 μmol/L)	If direct bilirubin is 3.1–5.0 mg/dL (53–86 μmol/L), hold asparaginase and resume when direct bilirubin is <2.0 mg/dL Consider switching to native asparaginase	If direct bilirubin is >5.0 mg/dL (>86 μmol/L), discontinue all asparaginase and do not make up for missed doses
Non-CNS thrombosis	For abnormal laboratory findings without clinical correlates, continue asparaginase	Withhold asparaginase until acute toxicity and clinical signs resolve and anticoagulant therapy is stable or completed. Do not withhold asparaginase for abnormal laboratory findings without a clinical correlate	Withhold asparaginase until acute toxicity and clinical signs resolve and anticoagulant therapy is stable or completed
Non-CNS hemorrhage	For bleeding in conjunction, with hypofibrinogenemia, withhold asparaginase until bleeding is grade ≤1. Do not withhold asparaginase for abnormal laboratory findings without a clinical correlate	Withhold asparaginase until bleeding is grade ≤1, until acute toxicity and clinical signs resolve, and coagulant replacement therapy is stable or completed	Withhold asparaginase until bleeding is grade ≤1, until acute toxicity and clinical signs resolve, and coagulant replacement therapy is stable or completed
CNS thrombosis	For abnormal laboratory findings without a clinical correlate, continue asparaginase	Discontinue all asparaginase; if CNS symptoms and signs are fully resolved and significant asparaginase remains to be administered, may resume asparaginase therapy at a lower dose and/or longer intervals between doses	Permanently discontinue all asparaginase
CNS hemorrhage	Discontinue asparaginase; do not withhold asparaginase for abnormal laboratory findings without a clinical correlate	Discontinue all asparaginase; if CNS symptoms and signs are fully resolved and significant asparaginase remains to be administered, may resume asparaginase therapy at a lower dose and/or longer intervals between doses	Permanently discontinue all asparaginase

Grade according to the National Cancer Institute Common Terminology Criteria for Advance Events version 4, with the exception of pancreatitis

Notes

1. An additional group of 96 patients in a study reported by Larson et al. (Blood 1998;92:1556–1564) did not receive filgrastim after assignment to treatment. The median time to recover neutrophils ≥1000/mm^3 during the remission induction course was 16 days for patients assigned to receive filgrastim and 22 days for patients assigned to placebo. Patients who received filgrastim had significantly shorter durations of neutropenia and thrombocytopenia and fewer days in hospital compared with patients who received placebo

2. Among patients assigned to receive filgrastim, more achieved CR and fewer experienced death during remission induction than those who received placebo. Overall toxicity was not lessened by the use of filgrastim. After a median follow-up of 4.7 years there was no significant difference in the overall survival between the two groups

3. Larson et al. (Blood 1995:85:2025–2037) performed lumbar puncture at diagnosis of ALL only in symptomatic patients. Patients with CNS leukemia should receive intrathecal therapy via lumbar puncture or an intraventricular reservoir (eg, Ommaya) weekly until CNS clearance with Methotrexate 15 mg + Hydrocortisone sodium succinate 50 mg per dose; administer intrathecally once weekly, alternating with: Cytarabine 100 mg + Hydrocortisone sodium succinate 50 mg per dose; administer intrathecally once weekly

   • Doses may be given in a volume of 0.9% Sodium Chloride Injection WITHOUT antimicrobial preservatives (preservative-free) equal to the volume of CSF removed for chemical or cytological evaluations

   • Intrathecal chemotherapy is given twice weekly; alternating doses of either methotrexate + hydrocortisone or cytarabine + hydrocortisone

   • Alternating intrathecal chemotherapy doses are separated by at least 3 days

4. Patients should continue systemic treatment as specified in the regimen

REGIMEN

HYPER-CVAD

Kantarjian H et al. Cancer 2004;101:2788–2801
Kantarjian HM et al. J Clin Oncol 2000;18:547–561

Dose-intensive chemotherapy
The dose-intensive phase consists of 8 cycles of hyper-CVAD alternating with high-dose methotrexate and cytarabine every 3–4 weeks (when the WBC count is >3000/mm³ and platelet count is >60,000/mm³)

Hyper-CVAD (cycles 1, 3, 5, and 7)
Cyclophosphamide 300 mg/m² per dose; administer intravenously over 3 hours in 500 mL 0.9% sodium chloride injection (0.9% NS) or 5% dextrose injection (D5W) every 12 hours for 6 doses on days 1–3, for 4 cycles, cycles 1, 3, 5, and 7 (total dosage/cycle = 1800 mg/m²)

Mesna 600 mg/m² per 24 hours; administer by continuous intravenous infusion in 1000 mL 0.9% NS for approximately 69 hours for 4 cycles, cycles 1, 3, 5, and 7 (total dosage/cycle ~1725 mg/m²)
• Mesna administration starts concurrently with cyclophosphamide on day 1 and continues until 6 hours after the last dose of cyclophosphamide is completed (69 hours)

Vincristine 2 mg/dose; administer by intravenous injection over 1–2 minutes for 2 doses, on days 4 and 11, for 4 cycles, cycles 1, 3, 5, and 7 (total dose/cycle = 4 mg)

Doxorubicin 50 mg/m²; administer intravenously via central venous access in 25–250 mL 0.9% NS or D5W over 2 hours on day 4, for 4 cycles, cycles 1, 3, 5, and 7 (total dosage/cycle = 50 mg/m²)

Dexamethasone 40 mg per day; administer orally, or intravenously in 25–150 mL 0.9% NS or D5W over 15–30 minutes for 8 doses, on days 1–4 and days 11–14, for 4 cycles, cycles 1, 3, 5, and 7 (total dose/cycle = 320 mg)

Supportive Care
Antiemetic prophylaxis
Emetogenic potential on Days 1–4 is **MODERATE**
Emetogenic potential on Days 11 is **MINIMAL**
See Chapter 39 for antiemetic recommendations

Hematopoietic growth factor (CSF) prophylaxis
Primary prophylaxis is indicated with:
  Filgrastim (G-CSF) 5 mcg/kg per dose; administer by subcutaneous injection every 12 hours, starting on day 5 (24 hours after doxorubicin)
  • Continue filgrastim administration until postnadir WBC count >3000/mm³ and platelet count is >60,000/mm³. If platelet recovery is delayed, filgrastim is continued until the WBC count >30,000/mm³
  • Discontinue daily filgrastim use at least 24 hours before administering myelosuppressive treatment
See Chapter 43 for more information

Antimicrobial prophylaxis
Risk of fever and neutropenia is HIGH
  Antimicrobial primary prophylaxis is recommended:
  • Antibacterial—consider fluoroquinolone prophylaxis; *P. jirovecii* prophylaxis is recommended (eg, cotrimoxazole)
  • Antifungal—recommended
  • Antiviral—antiherpes antivirals (eg, acyclovir, famciclovir, valacyclovir)
See Chapter 47 for more information

(continued)

Patient Population Studied

288 newly diagnosed ALL patients (median age: 40 years)

Efficacy (N = 288)

CR	92%
CR <30 years	99%
CR >60 years	80%
Resistant disease	3%
Died during induction	5%
5-Year estimated survival rate	38%
5-Year CR rate	38%
CR for Ph+ ALL	91%
5-Year survival for Ph+ ALL	12%

(*continued*)

High-dose methotrexate + cytarabine (cycles 2, 4, 6, and 8)
Hydration: with a solution containing a total amount of sodium not >0.9% NS (ie, ≤154 mEq sodium/1000 mL) by intravenous infusion during methotrexate administration and for at least 24 hours afterward

- Commence fluid administration 2–12 hours before starting methotrexate, depending on patient's fluid status
- Urine output should be at least 100 mL/hour before starting methotrexate infusion
- Maintain hydration at a rate that maintains urine output ≥100 mL/hour until the serum methotrexate concentration is <0.1 μmol/L
- Urine pH should be increased within the range ≥7.0 to ≤8.0 to enhance methotrexate solubility and ensure elimination
- Adverse effects attributable to methotrexate are related to systemic methotrexate concentrations *and* the duration for which concentrations are maintained

Sodium bicarbonate 50–150 mEq/1000 mL is added to parenteral hydration solutions to maintain urine pH ≥7.0 to ≤8.0

Base Solution Sodium Content	Sodium Bicarbonate Additive	Total Sodium Content
0.45% Sodium Chloride Injection (0.45% NS)		
77 mEq/L	50–75 mEq	127–152 mEq/L
0.2% Sodium Chloride Injection (0.2% NS)		
34 mEq/L	100–125 mEq	134–159 mEq/L
5% Dextrose injection (D5W)		
0	125–150 mEq	125–150 mEq/L
D5W/0.45% NS		
77 mEq/L	50–75 mEq	127–152 mEq/L
D5W/0.2% NS		
34 mEq/L	100–125 mEq	134–159 mEq/L

Methotrexate 200 mg/m^2; administer intravenously over 2 hours, on day 1, *followed by:*
Methotrexate 800 mg/m^2; administer intravenously over 24 hours, on day 1, for 4 cycles, cycles 2, 4, 6, and 8 (total dosage/cycle, bolus + infusion = 1000 mg/m^2)

Note: For logistical practicality and efficiency, parenteral admixtures containing methotrexate may include a portion or all of the fluid and sodium bicarbonate needed to meet hydration and urinary alkalinization requirements during methotrexate administration

Leucovorin calcium 15 mg per dose; administer intravenously in 25–250 mL 0.9% NS or D5W over 15–30 minutes, starting 48 hours after methotrexate administration began (22 hours after methotrexate administration ends), every 6 hours for 8 doses (total dosage/cycle = 120 mg)

(*continued*)

Dose Modifications During the Induction Phase

Adverse Effect	Dose Modification
Total bilirubin >2 mg/dL (>34 μmol/L)	Reduce vincristine doses to 1 mg
Total bilirubin 2–3 mg/dL (34–51 μmol/L)	Reduce doxorubicin dosage by 25%
Total bilirubin 3–4 mg/dL (51–68 μmol/L)	Reduce doxorubicin dosage by 50%
Total bilirubin 3–5 mg/dL (51–86 μmol/L)	Reduce methotrexate dosage by 25%
Total bilirubin >4mg/dL (>68 μmol/L)	Reduce doxorubicin dosage by 75%
Total bilirubin >5 mg/dL (>86 μmol/L)	Hold methotrexate
Creatinine 1.5–2 mg/dL (133–177 μmol/L)	Reduce methotrexate dosage by 25%
Bilirubin level 3–5 mg/dL (51–86 μmol/L)	Reduce MTX dose by 25%
Bilirubin >5 mg/dL (>86 μmol/L)	Hold MTX
Creatinine >2 mg/dL (>177 μmol/L)	Reduce methotrexate dosage by 50% Reduce cytarabine dosage to 1000 mg/m^2

(continued)

Note: If serum methotrexate concentrations are:

Hours After *Starting* Methotrexate	Methotrexate Concentration	Leucovorin Regimen
Hour 24	>20 μmol/L (>2 × 10^{-5} mol/L)	Increase **leucovorin** dosages to 50 mg/dose; administer intravenously in 25–250 mL 0.9% NS or D5W over 15–30 minutes every 6 hours until serum methotrexate concentrations are <0.1 μmol/L (<1 × 10^{-7} mol/L)
Hour 48	>1 μmol/L (>1 × 10^{-6} mol/L)	
Hour 72	>0.1 μmol/L (>1 × 10^{-7} mol/L, or >100 nmol/L)	

Cytarabine
Patient ages <60 years: **Cytarabine** 3000 mg/m^2 per dose; administer intravenously in 50–500 mL 0.9% NS or D5W over 2 hours every 12 hours for 4 doses on days 2 and 3, for 4 cycles, cycles 2, 4, 6, and 8 (total dosage/cycle [not including intrathecal cytarabine] = 12,000 mg/m^2)
Patient ages ≥60 years: **Cytarabine** 1000 mg/m^2 per dose; administer intravenously in 50–500 mL 0.9% NS or D5W over 2 hours every 12 hours for 4 doses on days 2 and 3, for 4 cycles, cycles 2, 4, 6, and 8 (total dosage/cycle [not including intrathecal cytarabine] = 4000 mg/m^2)

Methylprednisolone 50 mg; administer intravenously twice daily for 6 doses, on days 1–3 (total dose/cycle = 300 mg)

Filgrastim 5 mcg/kg per dose; administer subcutaneously, every 12 hours, starting on day 4 (24 hours after the last dose of chemotherapy) and continue until postnadir WBC count >3000/mm^3 and platelet count is >60,000/mm^3. If platelet recovery is delayed, filgrastim is continued until the WBC count >30,000/mm^3

Supportive Care
Antiemetic prophylaxis
Emetogenic potential on Days 1–3 is **MODERATE**
See Chapter 39 for antiemetic recommendations

Hematopoietic growth factor (CSF) prophylaxis
Primary prophylaxis is indicated with:
Filgrastim (G-CSF) 5 mcg/kg per dose; administer by subcutaneous injection every 12 hours, starting on day 4 (24 hours after the last dose of cytarabine)
- Continue filgrastim administration until postnadir WBC count >3000/mm^3 and platelet count is >60,000/mm^3. If platelet recovery is delayed, filgrastim is continued until the WBC count >30,000/mm^3
- Discontinue daily filgrastim use at least 24 hours before administering myelosuppressive treatment

See Chapter 43 for more information

Antimicrobial prophylaxis
Risk of fever and neutropenia is HIGH
Antimicrobial primary prophylaxis is recommended:
- Antibacterial—consider fluoroquinolone prophylaxis; *P. jirovecii* prophylaxis is recommended (eg, cotrimoxazole)
- Antifungal—recommended
- Antiviral—antiherpes antivirals (eg, acyclovir, famciclovir, valacyclovir)

See Chapter 47 for more information

(continued)

Toxicity (N = 288)

Induction Chemotherapy (First Course of Hyper-CVAD Therapy)

Myelosuppression	
Median time to ANC >1000/mm^3	19 days
Median time to platelets >100,000/mm^3	22 days
Hospitalization	54%
Sepsis	11%
Pneumonia	16%
Fungal infection	4%
Fever of unknown origin	37%
Neurotoxicity	64%
Moderate–severe mucositis	4%
Moderate–severe diarrhea	3%
Disseminated intravascular coagulopathy	3%
Induction deaths	5%

Consolidation Courses (Second Course of Hyper-CVAD Therapy)

Pneumonia	4%
Hospitalization	16%
Neurotoxicity	7%
Mucositis	1%
Diarrhea	1%
Sepsis	10%
Fever of unknown origin	8%

(continued)

(*continued*)

Keratitis prophylaxis
Steroid ophthalmic drops (prednisolone 1% or dexamethasone 0.1%) administer by intraocular instillation daily until 24 hours after high-dose cytarabine is completed

Maintenance phase
Mercaptopurine 50 mg/dose; administer orally on an empty stomach, continually, 3 times daily for 2 years (total dose/4 weeks = 4200 mg)
Methotrexate 20 mg/m² per dose; administer orally, once weekly for 2 years (total dosage/4 weeks = 80 mg/m²)
Vincristine 2 mg; administer by intravenous injection over 1–2 minutes, once monthly for 2 years (total dose/month = 2 mg)
Prednisone 200 mg per day; administer orally, continually, for 5 consecutive days every month, starting on the day vincristine is given (total dose/month = 1000 mg)

Supportive Care
Antiemetic prophylaxis
*Emetogenic potential is **MINIMAL–LOW***
See Chapter 39 for antiemetic recommendations

Hematopoietic growth factor (CSF) prophylaxis
Primary prophylaxis is NOT indicated
See Chapter 43 for more information

Antimicrobial prophylaxis
Risk of fever and neutropenia is HIGH
   Antimicrobial primary prophylaxis is recommended:
- Antibacterial—consider fluoroquinolone prophylaxis; *P. jirovecii* prophylaxis is recommended (eg, cotrimoxazole)
- Antifungal—recommended
- Antiviral—antiherpes antivirals (eg, acyclovir, famciclovir, valacyclovir)

See Chapter 47 for more information

Toxicity (N = 288) (*continued*)

High-Dose Methotrexate + Cytarabine Therapy	
Sepsis	8%
Pneumonia	5%
Fever of unknown origin	22%
Neurotoxicity	5%
Minor infections	4%
Hospitalization	36
Mucositis	4%
Rash and desquamation of palms and feet	2%
Diarrhea	1%

Therapy Monitoring

1. CBC with differential daily during and after chemotherapy until recovery of ANC >500/mm³. Platelets every day while in hospital until patient no longer requires platelet transfusions
2. Serum electrolytes, mineral panel, and uric acid, at least daily during active treatment until the risk of tumor lysis is past
3. Bone marrow aspirate and biopsy at day 29 of the initial induction course. After patient achieves a CR, bone marrow biopsy and aspirate should be performed at the end of each consolidation cycle (or at the very least, every other cycle), and every 3 months during maintenance therapy

Notes

1. In the studies reported by Kantarjian et al. (J Clin Oncol 2000;18:547–561), patients underwent a diagnostic LP on day 2 of the first course of treatment

   a. Patients with CNS disease at the time of diagnosis receive intrathecal therapy with:

      • **Methotrexate;** administer intrathecally 12 mg/dose via lumbar puncture *or* 6 mg/dose intraventricularly via indwelling ventricular reservoir catheter (eg, Ommaya) twice weekly until cerebrospinal fluid cell counts normalize and cytology becomes negative for malignant disease, *then:*

      • **Methotrexate;** administer intrathecally 12 mg/dose via lumbar puncture *or* 6 mg/dose intraventricularly via indwelling ventricular reservoir catheter on day 2 of each remaining treatment cycle, plus

      • **Cytarabine** 100 mg/dose; administer intrathecally via lumbar puncture *or* intraventricularly via indwelling ventricular reservoir catheter on day 8 of each remaining treatment cycle

   b. Patients with cranial nerve root involvement received radiation 24–30 Gy in 10–12 fractions to the base of the skull or whole brain

   c. Patients with no evidence of CNS disease should receive intrathecal prophylaxis based on prognostic factors for CNS leukemia

CNS Prophylaxis

Risk Factors	Risk Categories		
	High	Low	Unknown
LDH	>600 units/L	Within normal limits	unknown
Proliferative index (% S+G$_2$M)	≥14%		
Histology	Mature B-cell ALL	Not applicable	

Regimen for Intrathecal Prophylaxis	Administration Schedule by Risk Category		
	High Risk	Unknown Risk	Low Risk
Methotrexate; administer intrathecally 12 mg/dose via lumbar puncture *or* 6 mg/dose intraventricularly (via Ommaya reservoir) on day 2 of each cycle indicated, *plus* **Cytarabine** 100 mg administer; intrathecally via lumbar puncture or intraventricularly on day 8 of each cycle indicated	For 8 cycles, cycles 1–8	For 4 cycles, cycles 1–4	For 2 cycles, cycles 1 & 2

2. Patients with mature B-cell ALL received no maintenance therapy

3. Patients who receive high-dose cytarabine need to be closely monitored for changes in renal function. Renal dysfunction is highly correlated with increased risk of cerebellar toxicity associated with cytarabine. Patients need to be monitored for nystagmus, dysmetria, and ataxia before each cytarabine dose

4. Hyper-CVDA+Rituximab (Thomas DA et al. J Clin Oncol 2010;28:3880–3889): two hundred eighty-two adolescents and adults with de novo Philadelphia chromosome (Ph)–negative precursor B-lineage ALL were treated with standard or modified hyper-CVAD regimens. The latter incorporated standard-dose rituximab if CD20 expression ≥20%. The complete remission (CR) rate was 95% with 3-year rates of CR duration (CRD) and survival (OS) of 60% and 50%, respectively. In the younger (age <60 years) CD20-positive subset, rates of CRD and OS were superior with the modified hyper-CVAD and rituximab regimens compared with standard hyper-CVAD (70% *v* 38%; *P* <.001% and 75% *v* 47%, *P* = .003). In contrast, rates of CRD and OS for CD20-negative counterparts treated with modified versus standard hyper-CVAD regimens were similar (72% *v* 68%, *P* = not significant [NS] and 64% *v* 65%, *P* = NS, respectively). Older patients with CD20-positive ALL did not benefit from rituximab-based chemoimmunotherapy (rates of CRD 45% *v* 50%, *P* = NS and OS 28% *v* 32%, *P* = NS, respectively), related in part to deaths in CR. The incorporation of rituximab into the hyper-CVAD regimen improve outcome for younger patients with CD20-positive Ph-negative precursor B-lineage ALL.

REGIMEN

LINKER REGIMEN

Linker C et al. J Clin Oncol 2002;20:2464–2471

Treatment consisted of a total of 7 courses given in the order 1A → 1B → 1C → 2A → 2B → 2C → 3C, followed by maintenance chemotherapy

Induction (course 1A): DVP/Asp

Daunorubicin 60 mg/m^2 per day; administer by intravenous injection over 3–5 minutes for 3 consecutive days, on days 1–3 (total dosage/course after 3 doses = 180 mg/m^2)
Note: If day 14 bone marrow evaluation reveals residual leukemia, give a fourth dose of daunorubicin on day 15 (total dosage/course after 4 doses = 240 mg/m^2)

Vincristine
   Patient age ≤40 years: **Vincristine** 1.4 mg/m^2 per dose; administer by intravenous injection over 1–2 minutes for 4 doses on days 1, 8, 15, and 22 (total dosage/course = 5.6 mg/m^2)
   Patient age >40 years: **Vincristine** 1.4 mg/m^2 per dose (maximum single dose = 2 mg), administer by intravenous injection over 1–2 minutes for 4 doses on days 1, 8, 15, and 22 (total dosage/course = 5.6 mg/m^2; maximum dose/course = 8 mg)

Prednisone 60 mg/m^2 per day; administer orally, continually, for 28 consecutive days, on days 1–28 (total dosage/course = 1680 mg/m^2)

Asparaginase 6000 IU/m^2 per day; administer intramuscularly, or intravenously in 10–50 mL 0.9% sodium chloride injection or 5% dextrose injection over at least 30 minutes for 12 consecutive days on days 17–28 (total dosage/course = 72,000 IU/m^2)

CNS Prophylaxis and Treatment

1. Patients received CNS prophylaxis with methotrexate administered intrathecally during the initial diagnostic lumbar puncture. Five additional doses began with the first course of postremission chemotherapy with repeated doses delivered at weekly intervals as tolerated

2. Patients with CNS disease at diagnosis received intensified CNS therapy: 10 intrathecal treatments, and cranial irradiation 18 Gy was given after bone marrow remission was achieved

Methotrexate 12 mg per dose; administer intrathecally via lumbar puncture in 3–12 mL preservative-free 0.9% sodium chloride injection

	Prophylaxis	Treatment
Methotrexate (12 mg/dose)		
Total number of doses	6*	10*
Total dose/all courses	72 mg	120 mg
Cranial irradiation	None	1800 cGy after bone marrow CR

*First dose is given at the start of Induction Course 1A
Second and subsequent doses start concurrently with post-CR chemotherapy, and continue on a weekly schedule

(continued)

Patient Population Studied

84 newly diagnosed ALL adult patients (median age 27 years)

Efficacy (N = 84)

Induction	

Complete remission (CR)
   1 Treatment-related
      death
   5 Patients had resistant
      disease
	93%

5-Year event-free survival	48% ± 13%
Overall survival	47%
5-Year event-free survival for patients achieving remission	52%
5-Year DFS for patients achieving remission	54%

(*continued*)

Supportive Care
Antiemetic prophylaxis
Emetogenic potential on days when daunorubicin is given is **MODERATE–HIGH**
Emetogenic potential on days when vincristine or asparaginase ± vincristine are given is **MINIMAL**
See Chapter 39 for antiemetic recommendations

Hematopoietic growth factor (CSF) prophylaxis
Primary prophylaxis is indicated with:
    Filgrastim (G-CSF) 5 mcg/kg per day, by subcutaneous injection
- If only 3 doses of daunorubicin are given, begin filgrastim use on day 14. If a fourth dose of daunorubicin is given (on day 15) postpone instituting filgrastim use until 24 hours after daunorubicin was administered
- Continue daily filgrastim use until ANC >1500/mm³ on two measurements separated temporally by ≥24 hours
- Discontinue daily filgrastim use at least 24 hours before commencing the next course of myelosuppressive treatment

See Chapter 43 for more information

Antimicrobial prophylaxis
Risk of fever and neutropenia is HIGH
    Antimicrobial primary prophylaxis is recommended:
- Antibacterial—consider fluoroquinolone prophylaxis; *P. jirovecii* prophylaxis is recommended (eg, cotrimoxazole)
- Antifungal—recommended
- Antiviral—antiherpes antivirals (eg, acyclovir, famciclovir, valacyclovir)

See Chapter 47 for more information

Consolidation (courses 1B and 2B): high-dose cytarabine + etoposide (HDAC/etoposide)

Cytarabine 2000 mg/m² per day; administer intravenously in 100–1000 mL 0.9% sodium chloride injection (0.9% NS) or 5% dextrose injection (D5W) over 2 hours for 4 consecutive days on days 1–4 (total dosage/course = 8000 mg/m²)

Etoposide 500 mg/m² per day; administer intravenously diluted in 0.9% NS or D5W to a concentration within the range of 0.2–0.4 mg/mL over 3 hours for 4 consecutive days on days 1–4 (total dosage/course = 2000 mg/m²)

Supportive Care
Antiemetic prophylaxis
Emetogenic potential is at least **MODERATE**
See Chapter 39 for antiemetic recommendations

Hematopoietic growth factor (CSF) prophylaxis
Primary prophylaxis is indicated with one of the following:
    Filgrastim (G-CSF) 5 mcg/kg per day, by subcutaneous injection, *or*
    Pegfilgrastim (pegylated filgrastim) 6 mg/0.6 mL, by subcutaneous injection for 1 dose
- Begin use from 24–72 hours after myelosuppressive chemotherapy is completed
- Continue daily filgrastim use until ANC >1500/mm³ on 2 measurements separated temporally by ≥24 hours
- Discontinue daily Filgrastim use at least 24 hours before commencing the next course of myelosuppressive treatment. Do not administer pegfilgrastim within 14 days before administering myelosuppressive treatment

See Chapter 43 for more information

Antimicrobial prophylaxis
Risk of fever and neutropenia is HIGH
    Antimicrobial primary prophylaxis is recommended:
- Antibacterial—consider fluoroquinolone prophylaxis; *P. jirovecii* prophylaxis is recommended (eg, cotrimoxazole)
- Antifungal—recommended
- Antiviral—antiherpes antivirals (eg, acyclovir, famciclovir, valacyclovir)

See Chapter 47 for more information

Therapy Monitoring

1. CBC with differential daily during and after chemotherapy until recovery of ANC >500/mm³. Platelets every day while in hospital until patients no longer require platelet transfusions
2. Electrolytes, mineral panel, and uric acid at least daily during active treatment until the risk of tumor lysis is past
3. Amylase and fibrinogen levels prior to asparaginase administration. If fibrinogen level is <100 mg/dL (<1 g/L) consider prophylactic administration of cryoprecipitate
4. Bone marrow aspirate and biopsy at day 29 of the initial induction course. After a patient achieves a CR, bone marrow biopsy and aspirate should be performed at the end of each consolidation cycle (or at the very least, every other cycle), and every 3 months during maintenance therapy

(*continued*)

(*continued*)

Keratitis prophylaxis
Steroid ophthalmic drops (prednisolone 1% or dexamethasone 0.1%); administer by intraocular instillation daily until 24 hours after high-dose cytarabine is completed

Consolidation (course 2A): DVP/Asp
Daunorubicin 60 mg/m² per day; administer by intravenous injection over 3–5 minutes for 3 consecutive days on days 1–3 (total dosage/course = 180 mg/m²)

Vincristine
Patients age ≤40 years: **Vincristine** 1.4 mg/m² per dose; administer by intravenous injection over 1–2 minutes for 3 doses on days 1, 8, and 15 (total dosage/course = 4.2 mg/m²)
Patients age >40 years: **Vincristine** 1.4 mg/m² per dose (maximum single dose = 2 mg); administer by intravenous injection over 1–2 minutes for 3 doses on days 1, 8, and 15 (total dosage/course = 4.2 mg/m²; maximum dose/course = 6 mg)

Prednisone 60 mg/m² per day; administer orally, continually, for 21 consecutive days on days 1–21 (total dosage/course = 1260 mg/m²)

Asparaginase 12,000 IU/m² per dose; administer intramuscularly, or intravenously in 10–50 mL 0.9% sodium chloride injection or 5% dextrose injection over at least 30 minutes, for 3 doses/week (eg, Monday, Wednesday, and Friday), for a total of 6 doses during 2 consecutive weeks (total dosage/course = 72,000 IU/m²)

Supportive Care
Antiemetic prophylaxis
Emetogenic potential on days when daunorubicin is given is **MODERATE–HIGH**
Emetogenic potential on days when vincristine or asparaginase ± vincristine are given is **MINIMAL**
See Chapter 39 for antiemetic recommendations

Hematopoietic growth factor (CSF) prophylaxis
Primary prophylaxis is indicated with one of the following:
Filgrastim (G-CSF) 5 mcg/kg per day, by subcutaneous injection, *or*
Pegfilgrastim (pegylated filgrastim) 6 mg/0.6 mL by subcutaneous injection for 1 dose
• Begin use from 24–72 hours after myelosuppressive chemotherapy is completed
• Continue daily filgrastim use until ANC >1500/mm³ on 2 measurements separated temporally by ≥24 hours
• Discontinue daily filgrastim use at least 24 hours before commencing the next course of myelosuppressive treatment. Do not administer pegfilgrastim within 14 days before administering myelosuppressive treatment
See Chapter 43 for more information

Antimicrobial prophylaxis
Risk of fever and neutropenia is HIGH
Antimicrobial primary prophylaxis is recommended:
• Antibacterial—consider fluoroquinolone prophylaxis; *P. jirovecii* prophylaxis is recommended (eg, cotrimoxazole)
• Antifungal—recommended
• Antiviral—antiherpes antivirals (eg, acyclovir, famciclovir, valacyclovir)
See Chapter 47 for more information

Consolidation (courses 1C, 2C, and 3C): high-dose methotrexate + mercaptopurine
Hydration with methotrexate:
Administer 1500–3000 mL/m² per day. Use a solution containing a total amount of sodium not greater than 0.9% sodium chloride injection (ie, 154 mEq/1000 mL); administer by intravenous infusion during methotrexate administration and for at least 24 hours afterward
• Commence fluid administration 2–12 hours before starting methotrexate, depending upon a patient's fluid status
• Urine output should be at least 100 mL/hour before starting methotrexate infusion
• Maintain hydration at a rate that maintains urine output of at least 100 mL/hour until the serum methotrexate concentration is <0.05 µmol/L
• Adverse effects attributable to methotrexate are related to systemic methotrexate concentrations *and* the duration for which concentrations are maintained

(*continued*)

Treatment Modifications

Adverse Events	Treatment Modifications
Creatinine 1.5–2 mg/dL (133–177 µmol/L)	Reduce methotrexate dosage by 25%
Creatinine >2 mg/dL (>177 µmol/L)	Reduce methotrexate dosage by 50%
Creatinine >3 mg/dL (>265 µmol/L)	Reduce daunorubicin dosage by 50%
Total bilirubin 3–5 mg/dL (51–86 µmol/L)	Reduce daunorubicin dosage by 50% Reduce methotrexate dosage by 25%
Total bilirubin >3 mg/dL (>51 µmol/L)	Reduce vincristine dosage by 50%
Total bilirubin >5 mg/dL (>86 µmol/L)	Hold daunorubicin Hold methotrexate

(continued)

Sodium bicarbonate 50–150 mEq/1000 mL is added to parenteral
hydration solutions to maintain urine pH ≥7.0 to ≤8.0

Base Solution Sodium Content	Sodium Bicarbonate Additive	Total Sodium Content
0.45% Sodium Chloride Injection (0.45% NS)		
77 mEq/L	50–75 mEq	125–152 mEq/L
0.2% Sodium Chloride Injection (0.2% NS)		
34 mEq/L	100–125 mEq	134–159 mEq/L
5% Dextrose Injection (D5W)		
0	125–150 mEq	125–150 mEq/L
D5W/0.45% NS		
77 mEq/L	50–75 mEq	125–152 mEq/L
D5W/0.2% NS		
34 mEq/L	100–125 mEq	134–159 mEq/L

Methotrexate 220 mg/m²; administer intravenously over 1 hour (loading dose, or *bolus*),
every 2 weeks on days 1 and 15, *followed by*

Methotrexate 60 mg/m² per hour; administer by continuous intravenous infusion for
36 hours, every 2 weeks on days 1 and 15 (total dosage/administration event, bolus +
infusion = 2380 mg/m²; total dosage/course = 4760 mg/m²)

Note: For logistical practicality and efficiency, parenteral admixtures containing methotrexate
may include a portion or all of the fluid and sodium bicarbonate needed to meet hydration and
urinary alkalinization requirements during methotrexate administration

Leucovorin calcium 50 mg/m² per dose; administer intravenously in 25–250 mL 0.9% NS
or D5W over 15–30 minutes starting immediately after methotrexate is completed (37 hours
after methotrexate administration began), every 6 hours for 3 doses, every 2 weeks on days 2
and 16, *and then:*

Leucovorin calcium 50 mg/dose; administer orally starting 6 hours after the last intravenously
administered dose of leucovorin. Continue administration every 6 hours until serum methotrexate
concentrations are <0.05 μmol/L (<5 × 10⁻⁸ mol/L, or <50 nmol/L), every 2 weeks

Mercaptopurine 75 mg/m² per day; administer orally, continually, for 28 consecutive days
on days 1–28 (total dosage/course = 2100 mg/m²)

Supportive Care
Antiemetic prophylaxis
Emetogenic potential on days when methotrexate is given is **MODERATE**
Emetogenic potential on days when mercaptopurine alone is given is **MINIMAL–LOW**
See Chapter 39 for antiemetic recommendations

Hematopoietic growth factor (CSF) prophylaxis
Primary prophylaxis is NOT indicated
See Chapter 43 for more information

Antimicrobial prophylaxis
Risk of fever and neutropenia is HIGH
  Antimicrobial primary prophylaxis is recommended:
  • Antibacterial—consider fluoroquinolone prophylaxis; *P. jirovecii* prophylaxis is
    recommended (eg, cotrimoxazole)
  • Antifungal—recommended
  • Antiviral—antiherpes antivirals (eg, acyclovir, famciclovir, valacyclovir)
See Chapter 47 for more information

(continued)

(continued)

Maintenance Therapy

Mercaptopurine 75 mg/m^2 per day; administer orally, continually, until complete remission is sustained for 30 months (total dosage/week = 525 mg/m^2)

Methotrexate 20 mg/m^2 per dose; administer orally once weekly until complete remission is sustained for 30 months (total dosage/week = 20 mg/m^2)

Supportive Care
Antiemetic prophylaxis
Emetogenic potential is **MINIMAL–LOW**
See Chapter 39 for antiemetic recommendations

Hematopoietic growth factor (CSF) prophylaxis
Primary prophylaxis is NOT indicated
See Chapter 43 for more information

Antimicrobial prophylaxis
Risk of fever and neutropenia is HIGH
  Antimicrobial primary prophylaxis is recommended:
  • Antibacterial—*P. jirovecii* prophylaxis is recommended (eg, cotrimoxazole)
  • Antifungal—not indicated
  • Antiviral—antiherpes antivirals (eg, acyclovir, famciclovir, valacyclovir)
See Chapter 47 for more information

Adverse Effects
Median Number of Days to Hematologic Recovery

	Courses			
	Induction 1A DVP/Asp n = 84	1B HDAC/Etoposide n = 79	2A DVP/Asp n = 59	2B HDAC/Etoposide n = 53
ANC >500/mm^3	18	19	16	20
ANC >1000/mm^3	23	20	17	20
No. of days with ANC <500/mm^3	14	12	5	12
Platelets				
>20,000/mm^3	15	19	1	22
>50,000/mm^3	18	21	20	27
>100,000/mm^3	22	24	29	29
No. of platelet transfusions	4	3	0	4
No. of RBC transfusions	6	7	2	6

11 Patients experienced a peak serum total bilirubin >3 mg/dL, 1 had a peak total bilirubin >10 mg/dL

Asparaginase Toxicity Management

Stock W et al. Leuk Lymphoma 2011;52:2237–2253

Toxicity	Grade 2	Grade 3	Grade 4
Hypersensitivity Urticaria, wheezing, laryngospasm, hypotension, etc.	For urticaria without bronchospasm, hypotension, edema, or need for parenteral intervention, continue asparaginase	For wheezing or other symptomatic bronchospasm with or without urticaria, indicated parenteral intervention, angioedema, or hypotension, discontinue asparaginase. If erwinia asparaginase is available, replace pegaspargase with erwinia asparaginase	For life-threatening consequences or indicated urgent intervention, discontinue asparaginase. If erwinia asparaginase is available, replace pegaspargase with erwinia asparaginase
Hypertriglyceridemia	If serum triglyceride level <1000 mg/dL (<11.3 mmol/L), continue asparaginase but follow patient closely for evolving pancreatitis	Hold asparaginase for triglyceride >1000 mg/dL (>11.3 mmol/L); follow closely for pancreatitis; resume asparaginase at prior dose level after patient's triglyceride level returns to normal range	Hold asparaginase for triglyceride >1000 mg/dL (>11.3 mmol/L); follow closely for pancreatitis; resume asparaginase at prior dose level after patient's triglyceride level returns to normal range
Hyperglycemia, ketoacidosis	Continue asparaginase for uncomplicated hyperglycemia	For hyperglycemia requiring insulin therapy, hold asparaginase (and glucocorticoid therapy) until blood glucose regulated with insulin; resume asparaginase at prior dose level	For hyperglycemia with life-threatening consequences or indicated urgent intervention, hold asparaginase (and glucocorticoid therapy) until blood glucose is regulated with insulin; resume asparaginase and do not make up for missed doses
Hyperammonemia-related fatigue	Continue asparaginase	Reduce asparaginase dose by 25%; resume full dose when toxicity is grade ≤2; make up for missed doses	Reduce asparaginase dose 50%; resume full dose when toxicity grade 2; make up for missed doses
Pancreatitis	Continue asparaginase for asymptomatic amylase or lipase elevation >3 × ULN (chemical pancreatitis) or only radiologic abnormalities; observe closely for rising amylase or lipase levels	Continue pegaspargase for non-symptomatic chemical pancreatitis but observe patient closely for development of symptomatic pancreatitis for early treatment. Hold native asparaginase for amylase or lipase elevation >3 × ULN until enzyme levels stabilize or are declining. Permanently discontinue asparaginase for symptomatic pancreatitis	Permanently discontinue all asparaginase for clinical pancreatitis (vomiting, severe abdominal pain) with amylase or lipase elevation >3 × ULN for >3 days and/or development of pancreatic pseudocyst
Increased hepatic transaminases	For alanine or glutamine aminotransferase elevation >3–5 × ULN, continue asparaginase	For alanine or glutamine aminotransferase elevation >5–20 × ULN, delay next dose of asparaginase until transaminasemia is grade <2	For alanine or glutamine aminotransferase elevation >20 × ULN, discontinue asparaginase if toxicity reduction to grade <2 takes >1 week
Hyperbilirubinemia	Continue asparaginase if direct bilirubin <3.0 mg/dL (<51 μmol/L)	If direct bilirubin is 3.1–5.0 mg/dL (53–86 μmol/L), hold asparaginase and resume when direct bilirubin is <2.0 mg/dL Consider switching to native asparaginase	If direct bilirubin is >5.0 mg/dL (>86 μmol/L), discontinue all asparaginase and do not make up for missed doses
Non-CNS thrombosis	For abnormal laboratory findings without clinical correlates, continue asparaginase	Withhold asparaginase until acute toxicity and clinical signs resolve and anticoagulant therapy is stable or completed. Do not withhold asparaginase for abnormal laboratory findings without a clinical correlate	Withhold asparaginase until acute toxicity and clinical signs resolve and anticoagulant therapy is stable or completed
Non-CNS hemorrhage	For bleeding in conjunction, with hypofibrinogenemia, withhold asparaginase until bleeding is grade ≤1. Do not withhold asparaginase for abnormal laboratory findings without a clinical correlate	Withhold asparaginase until bleeding is grade ≤1, until acute toxicity and clinical signs resolve, and coagulant replacement therapy is stable or completed	Withhold asparaginase until bleeding is grade ≤1, until acute toxicity and clinical signs resolve, and coagulant replacement therapy is stable or completed

(continued)

Asparaginase Toxicity Management (*continued*)

Toxicity	Grade 2	Grade 3	Grade 4
CNS thrombosis	For abnormal laboratory findings without a clinical correlate, continue asparaginase	Discontinue all asparaginase; if CNS symptoms and signs are fully resolved and significant asparaginase remains to be administered, may resume asparaginase therapy at a lower dose and/or longer intervals between doses	Permanently discontinue all asparaginase
CNS hemorrhage	Discontinue asparaginase; do not withhold asparaginase for abnormal laboratory findings without a clinical correlate	Discontinue all asparaginase; if CNS symptoms and signs are fully resolved and significant asparaginase remains to be administered, may resume asparaginase therapy at a lower dose and/or longer intervals between doses	Permanently discontinue all asparaginase

Grade according to the National Cancer Institute Common Terminology Criteria for Advance Events version 4, with the exception of pancreatitis

REGIMEN

ALL TRIAL: MRC UKALL XII/ECOG E2993

Rowe JM et al. Blood 2005;106:3760–3767

Induction therapy

Induction—Phase 1 (weeks 1–4)

Daunorubicin 60 mg/m² per dose; administer by intravenous injection over 3–5 minutes for 4 doses on days 1, 8, 15, and 22 (total dosage/4-week course = 240 mg/m²)

Vincristine 1.4 mg/m² per dose; administer by intravenous injection over 1–2 minutes for 4 doses on days 1, 8, 15, and 22 (total dosage/4-week course = 5.6 mg/m²)

Prednisone 60 mg/m² per day; administer orally, continually, for 28 consecutive days on days 1 to 28 (total dosage/4-week course = 1680 mg/m²)
• Daily prednisone doses may be given in a single dose or ≥2 divided doses

Methotrexate 12.5 mg; administer intrathecally in 3–12 mL preservative-free 0.9% sodium chloride injection on day 15 (total dose/4-week course = 12.5 mg)

Asparaginase 10,000 IU/dose; administer intramuscularly, or intravenously in 10–50 mL 0.9% sodium chloride injection (0.9% NS) or 5% dextrose injection (D5W) for 12 consecutive days, on days 17 to 28 (total dose/4-week course = 120,000 IU)

Induction—Phase 2 (weeks 5–8)
(Regardless of whether residual leukemia is present at the end of phase 1)

Cyclophosphamide 650 mg/m²; administer intravenously in 100–1000 mL 0.9% NS or D5W over 15–60 min for 3 doses on days 1, 15, and 29 (total dosage/4-week course = 1950 mg/m²)

Cytarabine 75 mg/m² per dose; administer intravenously in 25–250 mL 0.9% NS or D5W over 15–60 min for 16 doses on days 1–4, 8–11, 15–18, and 22–25 (total dosage/4-week course = 1200 mg/m²)

Mercaptopurine 60 mg/m² per day; administer orally, continually, for 28 consecutive days on days 1 to 28 (total dosage/4-week course = 1680 mg/m²)

Methotrexate 12.5 mg per dose; administer intrathecally in 3–12 mL preservative-free 0.9% sodium chloride injection for 4 doses on days 1, 8, 15, and 22 (total dose/4-week course = 50 mg)

Notes: A diagnostic spinal tap was performed on all patients. If CNS leukemia was present at diagnosis, methotrexate was administered intrathecally via lumbar puncture or through a ventricular reservoir (eg, Ommaya) every week until blast cells were no longer present in the spinal fluid. In addition, 2400 cGy of cranial irradiation and 1200 cGy to the spinal cord were administered concurrently during induction, phase 2. For patients with CNS leukemia at presentation, intrathecal methotrexate was not administered during phase 2

Intensification therapy

Hydration for methotrexate: 6–18 hours before the anticipated start of methotrexate, start intravenous hydration containing sodium bicarbonate (NaHCO₃) to alkalinize a patient's urine to pH ≥7.0, but ≤8.0, at a rate that achieves a urine output ≥100 mL/hour
Options recommended to initially produce an alkaline urine, include:

Fluid	Administration Rate	Sodium Bicarbonate Content (per 1000 mL)
0.45% NS		50–75 mEq
0.2% NS		100–125 mEq
D5W/0.45% NS	150–250 mL/hour	50–75 mEq
D5W/0.2% NS		100–125 mEq
D5W		150 mEq

D5W, 5% Dextrose injection; NS, sodium chloride injection

Notes: Urine alkalinization to pH ≥7.0 to ≤8.0 and urine output ≥100 mL/hour often initially require more NaHCO₃ and more rapid hydration rates than will be required to maintain either or both parameters after they are achieved

(continued)

Population Studied

Of patients from 15 to 59 years of age newly diagnosed with ALL, 1521 received identical induction therapy, irrespective of risk assessment, including central nervous system (CNS) prophylaxis and treatment of CNS disease, if present at diagnosis. Philadelphia chromosome (Ph)-positive patients were considered the highest risk group. Patients who were Ph-negative were considered at high risk if any of the following were present: age ≥35 years; time to CR >4 weeks or WBC count >30 × 10⁹/L for B-lineage ALL and >100 × 10⁹/L for T-lineage ALL. Ph-negative patients who had none of these risk factors were considered at standard risk. After induction therapy, all patients younger than 50 years of age who had a human leukocyte antigen (HLA)–compatible sibling were assigned to undergo allogeneic transplantation. All other patients were randomly assigned between autologous transplantation and standard consolidation/maintenance therapy. Patients who were Ph-positive were offered a search for a matched unrelated donor if they did not have a histocompatible family donor

(*continued*)

The amount of sodium bicarbonate added to intravenously administered fluids should produce a solution with sodium content not greater than the concentration of sodium in 0.9% sodium chloride injection ($\leq$154 mEq/L)

Methotrexate 3000 mg/m²; administer intravenously in one of the solutions identified above in admixture with 25–75 mEq NaHCO₃ over 4 hours after urine pH $\geq$7.0 to $\leq$8.0 and urine output >100 mL/hour are confirmed for 3 doses on days 1, 8, and 22 (total dosage/ course = 9000 mg/m²)
- Temporarily interrupt hydration while methotrexate is administered
  - The methotrexate product should contain volume and sodium bicarbonate content equivalent to what was being given in intravenous hydration to maintain urine pH $\geq$7.0 to $\leq$8.0 and output >100 mL/hour
- Order daily serum methotrexate levels timed to start 24 hours after methotrexate administration begins and continue daily measurements until the serum methotrexate level is $\leq$0.05 μmol/L
- Continue hydration with urine alkalinization (pH $\geq$7.0 to $\leq$8.0) until serum methotrexate level is $\leq$0.05 μmol/L

Leucovorin calcium 100 mg/m² per dose (preferred), or **levoleucovorin calcium** 50 mg/m² per dose; administer intravenously in 25–250 mL 0.9% NS or D5W over 10–30 minutes every 6 hours starting 24 hours after methotrexate administration began, and continue for at least 6 doses or until serum methotrexate concentrations are $\leq$0.5 μmol/L, whichever occurs later

When the methotrexate level is <0.5 μmol/L, parenterally administered leucovorin or levoleucovorin may be replaced with leucovorin administered orally (10 mg/m², or a fixed 25-mg dose for patients whose body surface area is <2.5 m²), until the serum methotrexate level is $\leq$0.05 μmol/L

Asparaginase 10,000 IU/dose; administer intramuscularly, or intravenously in 10–50 mL 0.9% NS or D5W intravenously or intramuscularly for 3 doses on days 2, 9, and 23 (total dose/course = 30,000 IU)

Consolidation therapy
Cytarabine 50 mg/dose; administer intrathecally in 3–12 mL preservative-free 0.9% sodium chloride injection weekly for 4 weeks, *with:*
Cranial irradiation 2400 cGy
Consolidation—Cycle 1
Cytarabine 75 mg/m² per day; administer intravenously in 25–250 mL 0.9% NS or D5W over 15–60 minutes for 5 consecutive days on days 1–5 (total dosage/cycle = 375 mg/m²)
Etoposide 100 mg/m² per day; administer intravenously in a volume of 0.9% NS or D5W sufficient to produce a concentration within the range, 0.2–0.4 mg/mL over at least 60 minutes for 5 consecutive days on days 1–5 (total dosage/cycle = 500 mg/m²)
Vincristine 1.4 mg/m² per dose; administer intravenously over 1–2 minutes for 4 doses on days 1, 8, 15, and 22 (total dosage/cycle = 5.6 mg/m²)
Dexamethasone 10 mg/m² per day; administer orally, continually, for 28 consecutive days on days 1 to 28 (total dosage/cycle = 280 mg/m²)
Consolidation—Cycle 2 (starts 4 weeks after cycle 1)
Cytarabine 75 mg/m² per day; administer intravenously in 25–250 mL 0.9% NS or D5W over 15–60 minutes for 5 consecutive days on days 1–5 (total dosage/cycle = 375 mg/m²)
Etoposide 100 mg/m² per day; administer intravenously in a volume of 0.9% NS or D5W sufficient to produce a concentration within the range, 0.2–0.4 mg/mL over at least 60 minutes for 5 consecutive days on days 1–5 (total dosage/cycle = 500 mg/m²)
Consolidation—Cycle 3 (starts 4 weeks after cycle 2)
Daunorubicin 25 mg/m² per dose; administer by intravenous injection over 3–5 minutes for 4 doses on days 1, 8, 15, and 22 (total dosage/4-week course = 100 mg/m²)
Cyclophosphamide 650 mg/m²; administer intravenously in 100–1000 mL 0.9% NS or D5W over 15–60 min on day 29 (total dosage/4-week course = 650 mg/m²)
Cytarabine 75 mg/m² per dose; administer intravenously in 25–250 mL 0.9% NS or D5W over 15–60 minutes for 8 doses on days 31–34 and 38–41 (total dosage/4-week course = 600 mg/m²)
Thioguanine 60 mg/m² per day; administer orally, continually, for 14 consecutive days on days 29–42 (total dosage/4-week course = 840 mg/m²)

(*continued*)

(continued)

Consolidation—Cycle 4 (8 weeks after the conclusion of cycle 3)
Cytarabine 75 mg/m² per day; administer intravenously in 25–250 mL 0.9% NS or D5W over 15–60 minutes for 5 consecutive days on days 1–5 (total dosage/cycle = 375 mg/m²)
Etoposide 100 mg/m² per day; administer intravenously in a volume of 0.9% NS or D5W sufficient to produce a concentration within the range, 0.2–0.4 mg/mL over at least 60 minutes for 5 consecutive days on days 1–5 (total dosage/cycle = 500 mg/m²)

Maintenance therapy (continues for a total of 2.5 years after the start of intensification therapy)
Cytarabine 50 mg/dose; administer intrathecally in 3–12 mL preservative-free 0.9% sodium chloride injection on 4 occasions 3 months apart during maintenance therapy (total of 4 doses = 200 mg)
Vincristine 1.4 mg/m²; administer by intravenous injection over 1–2 minutes every 3 months (total dosage/3-month period = 1.4 mg/m²)
Prednisone 60 mg/m²; administer orally for 5 consecutive days every 3 months (total dosage/3-month period = 300 mg/m²)
Mercaptopurine 75 mg/m²; administer orally, continually each day (total dosage/week = 525 mg/m²)
Methotrexate 20 mg/m²; administer orally or intravenously once a week (total dosage/week = 20 mg/m²)

Supportive Care
Antiemetic Prophylaxis During Induction–Phase 1
Emetogenic potential on days 1, 8, and 15 is **MODERATE**
Emetogenic potential on days with asparaginase (days 17–28) is **MINIMAL**

Antiemetic Prophylaxis During Induction–Phase 2
Emetogenic potential on days with cyclophosphamide (days 1, 15, and 29) is **MODERATE**
Emetogenic potential on days with cytarabine without cyclophosphamide is **LOW**
Emetogenic potential on days with mercaptopurine alone is **MINIMAL–LOW**

Antiemetic Prophylaxis During Intensification
Emetogenic potential on days with methotrexate (days 1, 8, and 22) is **MODERATE**
Emetogenic potential on days with asparaginase (days 2, 9, and 23) is **MINIMAL**

Antiemetic Prophylaxis During Consolidation, Cycle 1
Emetogenic potential on days 1–5 is **LOW**
Emetogenic potential on days 8 and 15 is **MINIMAL**

Antiemetic Prophylaxis During Consolidation, Cycle 2
Emetogenic potential on days 1–5 is **LOW**

Antiemetic Prophylaxis During Consolidation, Cycle 3
Emetogenic potential on days 1, 8, 15, and 29 is **MODERATE**
Emetogenic potential on days with cytarabine is **LOW**
Emetogenic potential on days with thioguanine alone is **LOW**

Antiemetic Prophylaxis During Consolidation, Cycle 4
Emetogenic potential on days 1–5 is **LOW**

Antiemetic Prophylaxis During Maintenance
Emetogenic potential on days methotrexate is given is **MINIMAL–LOW**
Emetogenic potential all other days is **MINIMAL**
See Chapter 39 for antiemetic recommendations

Hematopoietic growth factor (CSF) prophylaxis
Primary prophylaxis is NOT indicated
See Chapter 43 for more information

Antimicrobial prophylaxis
Risk of fever and neutropenia is HIGH
  Antimicrobial primary prophylaxis is recommended:
  • Antibacterial—consider fluoroquinolone prophylaxis; *Pneumocystis jirovecii* prophylaxis is recommended (eg, cotrimoxazole)
  • Antifungal—recommended
  • Antiviral—antiherpes antivirals (eg, acyclovir, famciclovir, valacyclovir)
See Chapter 47 for more information

Efficacy

	No.	CR, %	5-Year Survival, %	5-Year Survival for Patients in CR, %
All patients	1521	91	38	41
Ph+	293	83	25	28
Ph−	1153	93	41	44
Standard risk*	533	97	54	57
High risk*	590	90	29	35
Unknown risk	30	84	23	

*Risk stratification at diagnosis based on age and WBC count only

Overall survival (OS) rates at 5 years in this study were 38% for all patients, 41% for Ph-negative patients, and 25% for Ph-positive patients

In subsequent reports (Goldstone AH et al. Blood 2008;111:1827–1833), the 5 year OS in 1913 ALL patients was 39% and 43% for patients with Ph-negative ALL. In Ph-positive patients (Fielding AK et al. Blood 2009;113:4489–4496), the OS was 44% after sib allo-HSCT, 36% after MUD, and 19% after chemotherapy

Toxicity

Overall mortality rates for induction therapy were 4.7% (54 of 1153 patients) for Ph-negative patients and 5.5% (16 of 293 patients) for Ph-positive patients. Twenty-nine patients died of infection, most significantly caused by *Aspergillus* (7 patients). Five patients died of hemorrhage (3 pulmonary, 2 cerebral), 2 patients died of thromboses (possibly related to asparaginase), and 1 patient died from tumor lysis. The remaining 10 patients died of causes described as multiorgan failure, which might also have been related to an infectious etiology

Treatment Modifications

Adverse Events	Treatment Modifications
Creatinine 1.5–2 mg/dL (133–177 μmol/L)	Reduce methotrexate dosage by 25%
Creatinine >2 mg/dL (>177 μmol/L)	Reduce methotrexate dosage by 50%
Creatinine >3 mg/dL (>265 μmol/L)	Reduce daunorubicin dosage by 50%
Total bilirubin 3–5 mg/dL (51–86 μmol/L)	Reduce daunorubicin dosage by 50% Reduce methotrexate dosage by 25%
Total bilirubin >3 mg/dL (>51 μmol/L)	Reduce vincristine dosage by 50%
Total bilirubin >5 mg/dL (>86 μmol/L)	Hold daunorubicin Hold methotrexate

Asparaginase Toxicity Management

Stock W et al. Leuk Lymphoma 2011;52:2237–2253

Toxicity	Grade 2	Grade 3	Grade 4
Hypersensitivity Urticaria, wheezing, laryngospasm, hypotension, etc.	For urticaria without bronchospasm, hypotension, edema, or need for parenteral intervention, continue asparaginase	For wheezing or other symptomatic bronchospasm with or without urticaria, indicated parenteral intervention, angioedema, or hypotension, discontinue asparaginase. If erwinia asparaginase is available, replace pegaspargase with erwinia asparaginase	For life-threatening consequences or indicated urgent intervention, discontinue asparaginase. If erwinia asparaginase is available, replace pegaspargase with erwinia asparaginase
Hypertriglyceridemia	If serum triglyceride level <1000 mg/dL (<11.3 mmol/L), continue asparaginase but follow patient closely for evolving pancreatitis	Hold asparaginase for triglyceride >1000 mg/dL (>11.3 mmol/L); follow closely for pancreatitis; resume asparaginase at prior dose level after patient's triglyceride level returns to normal range	Hold asparaginase for triglyceride >1000 mg/dL (>11.3 mmol/L); follow closely for pancreatitis; resume asparaginase at prior dose level after patient's triglyceride level returns to normal range
Hyperglycemia, ketoacidosis	Continue asparaginase for uncomplicated hyperglycemia	For hyperglycemia requiring insulin therapy, hold asparaginase (and glucocorticoid therapy) until blood glucose regulated with insulin; resume asparaginase at prior dose level	For hyperglycemia with life-threatening consequences or indicated urgent intervention, hold asparaginase (and glucocorticoid therapy) until blood glucose is regulated with insulin; resume asparaginase and do not make up for missed doses
Hyperammonemia-related fatigue	Continue asparaginase	Reduce asparaginase dose by 25%; resume full dose when toxicity is grade ≤2; make up for missed doses	Reduce asparaginase dose 50%; resume full dose when toxicity grade 2; make up for missed doses
Pancreatitis	Continue asparaginase for asymptomatic amylase or lipase elevation >3 × ULN (chemical pancreatitis) or only radiologic abnormalities; observe closely for rising amylase or lipase levels	Continue pegaspargase for non-symptomatic chemical pancreatitis but observe patient closely for development of symptomatic pancreatitis for early treatment. Hold native asparaginase for amylase or lipase elevation >3 × ULN until enzyme levels stabilize or are declining. Permanently discontinue asparaginase for symptomatic pancreatitis	Permanently discontinue all asparaginase for clinical pancreatitis (vomiting, severe abdominal pain) with amylase or lipase elevation >3 × ULN for >3 days and/or development of pancreatic pseudocyst
Increased hepatic transaminases	For alanine or glutamine aminotransferase elevation >3–5 × ULN, continue asparaginase	For alanine or glutamine aminotransferase elevation >5–20 × ULN, delay next dose of asparaginase until transaminasemia is grade <2	For alanine or glutamine aminotransferase elevation >20 × ULN, discontinue asparaginase if toxicity reduction to grade <2 takes >1 week
Hyperbilirubinemia	Continue asparaginase if direct bilirubin <3.0 mg/dL (<51 μmol/L)	If direct bilirubin is 3.1–5.0 mg/dL (53–86 μmol/L), hold asparaginase and resume when direct bilirubin is <2.0 mg/dL Consider switching to native asparaginase	If direct bilirubin is >5.0 mg/dL (>86 μmol/L), discontinue all asparaginase and do not make up for missed doses
Non-CNS thrombosis	For abnormal laboratory findings without clinical correlates, continue asparaginase	Withhold asparaginase until acute toxicity and clinical signs resolve and anticoagulant therapy is stable or completed. Do not withhold asparaginase for abnormal laboratory findings without a clinical correlate	Withhold asparaginase until acute toxicity and clinical signs resolve and anticoagulant therapy is stable or completed
Non-CNS hemorrhage	For bleeding in conjunction, with hypofibrinogenemia, withhold asparaginase until bleeding is grade ≤1. Do not withhold asparaginase for abnormal laboratory findings without a clinical correlate	Withhold asparaginase until bleeding is grade ≤1, until acute toxicity and clinical signs resolve, and coagulant replacement therapy is stable or completed	Withhold asparaginase until bleeding is grade ≤1, until acute toxicity and clinical signs resolve, and coagulant replacement therapy is stable or completed

(continued)

Asparaginase Toxicity Management (continued)

Toxicity	Grade 2	Grade 3	Grade 4
CNS thrombosis	For abnormal laboratory findings without a clinical correlate, continue asparaginase	Discontinue all asparaginase; if CNS symptoms and signs are fully resolved and significant asparaginase remains to be administered, may resume asparaginase therapy at a lower dose and/ or longer intervals between doses	Permanently discontinue all asparaginase
CNS hemorrhage	Discontinue asparaginase; do not withhold asparaginase for abnormal laboratory findings without a clinical correlate	Discontinue all asparaginase; if CNS symptoms and signs are fully resolved and significant asparaginase remains to be administered, may resume asparaginase therapy at a lower dose and/ or longer intervals between doses	Permanently discontinue all asparaginase

Grade according to the National Cancer Institute Common Terminology Criteria for Advance Events version 4, with the exception of pancreatitis

Monitoring Therapy

1. CBC with differential daily during and after chemotherapy until recovery of ANC >500/mm³. Platelets every day while in hospital until patient no longer requires platelet transfusions
2. Metabolic panel and uric acid, at least daily during active treatment until the risk of tumor lysis is past
3. Amylase and fibrinogen levels prior to asparaginase administration. If fibrinogen level is <100 mg/dL (<1 g/L) consider prophylactic administration of cryoprecipitate
4. Bone marrow aspirate and biopsy after phase 1 and phase 2 of induction therapy. After a patient achieves a CR, bone marrow biopsy and aspirate should be performed at the end of each consolidation cycle (or at the very least, every other cycle), and every 3 months during maintenance therapy

Notes: A diagnostic spinal tap was performed on all patients

If CNS leukemia was present at diagnosis, methotrexate administered intrathecally via lumbar puncture or through a ventricular reservoir (eg, Ommaya) was given weekly until blast cells were no longer present in the spinal fluid. In addition, 2400 cGy of cranial irradiation and 1200 cGy to the spinal cord were administered concurrently during phase 2. For patients with CNS leukemia at presentation, intrathecal methotrexate was not administered during phase 2

In a subsequent analysis (Fielding AK et al. Blood 2007;109:944–950) of the MRC UKALL XII/ECOG E2993 study, among 1372 patients with ALL who entered remission, 609 (44%) relapsed at a median of 11 months after the start of treatment. Most (556 [91%]) patients relapsed within the bone marrow, the sole site of relapse in most (90%) of those patients. A group of 45 (8%) patients relapsed solely at extramedullary sites

Most patients (81%) relapsed within 2 years after diagnosis, although a significant minority (19%) relapsed >2 years after diagnosis. Of the 440 chemotherapy-treated patients, 349 relapsed within 2 years after diagnosis, and 87 relapsed later. Those on chemotherapy who relapsed within 2 years can be considered "relapses on therapy" because the duration of therapy was set to be 18 months from the point of initiation of the consolidation therapy (ie, 23 months)

The median survival after relapse was 24 weeks. Survival at 1 year was 22% (95% CI = 18–25%), and 7% (95% CI = 4–9%) at 5 years. Only 42 of 609 patients who relapsed remain alive without further relapse

Factors predicting a good outcome after salvage therapy were young age (OS of 12% in patients <20 years vs. OS of 3% in patients >50 years; 2P <0.001) and short duration of first remission (CR1) (OS of 11% in those with a CR1 >2 years vs. OS of 5% in those with a CR1 <2 years; 2P <0.001). Patients treated with HSCT had a superior OS (15% [95% CI = 0–35%] for autograft [n = 13], 16% [95% CI = 7–26%] for matched unrelated donor transplantation [n = 65], and 23% [95% CI = 10–36%] for sibling allograft [n = 42]) to those receiving chemotherapy alone (n = 182) whose OS was only 4% (95% CI = 1–7%) at 5 years

REGIMEN
LIPOSOMAL VINCRISTINE SULFATE

O'Brien S et al. J Clin Oncol 2013;31:676–683

Vincristine sulfate liposome injection 2.25 mg/m^2 per dose; administer intravenously in (total volume [q.s.]) 100 mL 0.9% sodium chloride or 5% dextrose injection over 60 minutes for 4 doses on days 1, 8, 15, and 22, every 28 days (total dosage/cycle = 9 mg/m^2)
- Liposomal vincristine sulfate doses are calculated from actual body surface area, and are not capitated

Supportive Care
Antiemetic prophylaxis
Emetogenic potential is MINIMAL
See Chapter 39 for antiemetic recommendations

Hematopoietic growth factor (CSF) prophylaxis
Primary prophylaxis is NOT indicated
See Chapter 43 for more information

Antimicrobial prophylaxis
Risk of fever and neutropenia is LOW
Antimicrobial primary prophylaxis to be considered:
- Antibacterial—not indicated
- Antifungal—not indicated
- Antiviral—not indicated unless patient previously had an episode of HSV

See Chapter 47 for more information

Patient Population Studied

Sixty-five adults (median age: 31 years; range: 19–83 years) with Ph-negative ALL in second or greater relapse, or whose disease had progressed following 2 or more leukemia therapies

Efficacy

CR/CRi rate was 20% and overall response rate was 35%

Median OS, overall, 4.6 months (range: <1 month to >25 months), and 7.7 months (range: 2.4 to >23.3 months) among patients who achieved a CR/CRi.

Therapy Monitoring

CBC with differential leukocyte count, renal and hepatic function tests prior to each dose of liposomal vincristine sulfate

Bone marrow biopsy on day 28 of treatment courses 1 and 2 and every second treatment course thereafter

Treatment Modifications

G ≥3 adverse effects (severe symptoms; limiting self-care activities of daily living [ADL]*) or persistent G2 (moderate symptoms; limiting instrumental ADL)† peripheral neuropathy:	Interrupt vinCRIstine sulfate LIPOSOME If the peripheral neuropathy remains at G ≥3, discontinue liposomal vincristine sulfate If the peripheral neuropathy recovers to G ≤2, continue treatment with liposomal vincristine sulfate dosage decreased to 2 mg/m^2 per dose
Persistent G2 peripheral neuropathy after the first dose reduction to 2 mg/m^2	Interrupt liposomal vincristine sulfate for up to 7 days If the peripheral neuropathy increases to G ≥3, discontinue liposomal vincristine sulfate If peripheral neuropathy recovers to G ≤1, continue treatment with liposomal vincristine sulfate dosage decreased to 1.825 mg/m^2 per dose
Persistent G ≥2 peripheral neuropathy after a second dose reduction to 1.825 mg/m^2	Interrupt liposomal vincristine sulfate for up to 7 days If the peripheral increases to G ≥3, discontinue liposomal vincristine sulfate If the toxicity recovers to G ≤1, continue treatment with liposomal vincristine sulfate dosage decreased to 1.5 mg/m^2 per dose

If neutropenia, thrombocytopenia, or anemia G ≥3 develop, consider dose modification or reduction as well as supportive care measures.

Reduce liposomal vincristine sulfate dosages or interrupt treatment for hepatic toxicity

Severity grading for adverse events is based on the National Cancer Institute (NCI) Common Terminology Criteria for Adverse Events (CTCAE) v3.0. Available at: http://ctep.cancer.gov/protocolDevelopment/electronic_applications/ctc.htm [accessed December 7, 2013]
*Self-care ADL refers to bathing, dressing and undressing, feeding self, using the toilet, taking medications, and not bedridden
†Instrumental ADL refers to preparing meals, shopping for groceries and clothes, using telephone, managing money, etc.

Toxicity

	All Grades %	G3 %	G4 %
Any treatment-related adverse event	82	39	19
Nervous system disorders	63	19	2
Neuropathy peripheral	29	15	0
Hypoesthesia	25	2	0
Paraesthesia	20	2	0
Areflexia	9	2	0
Hyporeflexia	8	0	0
GI disorders	51	12	0
Constipation	34	3	0
Nausea	22	0	0
Vomiting	11	0	0
Abdominal pain	9	3	0
Diarrhea	6	2	0
Blood and lymphatic system disorders	29	9	12
Neutropenia	17	8	8
Anemia	12	5	0
Thrombocytopenia	9	2	5
Febrile neutropenia	8	3	0
General disorders and administration site conditions	25	8	0
Fatigue	11	3	0
Asthenia	9	3	0
Pyrexia	9	2	0
Metabolism and nutrition disorders	22	6	3
Decreased appetite	12	2	0
Tumor lysis syndrome	8	2	3
Investigations	19	8	2
Weight decreased	11		

Notes:
- Liposomal vincristine sulfate is a vinca alkaloid indicated for the treatment of adult patients with Philadelphia chromosome-negative (Ph−) acute lymphoblastic leukemia (ALL) in second or subsequent relapse, or whose disease has progressed following 2 or more antileukemia therapies
- Liposomal vincristine sulfate is contraindicated in patients with demyelinating conditions including Charcot-Marie-Tooth syndrome
- Neurologic toxicity: Monitor patients for peripheral, motor, and sensory, central and autonomic neuropathy, and reduce, interrupt, or discontinue treatment if signs or symptoms present
  - Patients with preexisting severe neuropathy should be treated with liposomal vincristine sulfate only after careful risk-benefit assessment

REGIMEN

NELARABINE

Gökbuget N et al. Blood 2011;118:3504–3511

Nelarabine 1500 mg/m² per dose; administer intravenously (without dilution) over 2 hours for 3 doses on days 1, 3, and 5, every 21 days (total dosage/cycle = 4500 mg/m²)

Supportive Care
Antiemetic prophylaxis
Emetogenic potential is **MINIMAL**
See Chapter 39 for antiemetic recommendations

Hematopoietic growth factor (CSF) prophylaxis
Primary prophylaxis is NOT indicated
See Chapter 43 for more information

Antimicrobial prophylaxis
Risk of fever and neutropenia is LOW
   Antimicrobial primary prophylaxis to be considered:
   • Antibacterial—not indicated
   • Antifungal—not indicated
   • Antiviral—not indicated unless patient previously had an episode of HSV
See Chapter 47 for more information

Patient Population Studied

Study of 126 relapsed/refractory patients (85% T-cell acute lymphoblastic leukemia (T-ALL),15% T-cell lymphoblastic lymphoma), median age 33 years (range: 18–81 years) treated with nelarabine

Treatment Modifications

Nelarabine administration should be discontinued for neurologic adverse reactions of NCI Common Terminology Criteria for Adverse Events grades ≥2. Treatment may be delayed for other toxicities

Therapy Monitoring

1. Weekly and before a treatment cycle: CBC with differential, renal, and hepatic function
2. Response evaluation: bone marrow biopsy every 2 cycles

Efficacy (N = 126)

	Result after Cycle 1 (%)	Overall Result after 1–3 Cycles (%)
CR	32	36
PR	19	10
Failure	47	52
Death on therapy	1	1
Withdrawal	2	2

Toxicity

Hematologic	G 3–4 (%)
Leukopenia	41
Granulocytopenia	37
Thrombocytopenia	17

• Patients with CR after 1 cycle (N = 36) tended to have a better 3-year survival (32% ± 8%) compared with those who later achieved a CR (N = 9; 11% ± 10%; P = 0.06)
• The probability of survival after 1 year was 24% (SE ± 3%) and after 3 years 12% (SE ± 3%) with a median survival of 6 months
• The 3-year survival of patients with failure or PR after nelarabine (N = 81) compared with patients who achieved a CR (N = 45) was 4% (SE ± 2%) versus 28% (SE ± 7%), respectively (P <0.0001)
• A total of 36 of 45 patients (80%) who achieved a CR after nelarabine subsequently received stem cell transplantation (SCT) in continuous CR. Four patients died in CR (11%) related to transplantation (GVHD N = 1, infection N = 3) and 20 patients relapsed (56%). The probability of survival 3 years after transplantation in 36 patients transplanted in CR after nelarabine is 31% (SE ± 8%), and the relapse-free survival at 3 years is 37% (SE ± 9%). The median time to relapse after SCT was 4 months (range: 1–24) months. In patients alive after SCT, the median survival was 41 months (range: 13–85 months)
• Survival probability at 3 years was 36% (SE ± 8%) in the 36 patients transplanted in CR after nelarabine. In comparison, CR patients without transplantation in CR after nelarabine (N = 9) survival probability was zero and failure or PR was 4% (SE ± 2%; N = 81) after 3 years (P <0.0001)

Neurotoxicity

	Incidence, N (%) of Cycles	G 1	G 2	G 3	G 4
		Number of Cycles			
Cognitive disturbance	9 (4)	3	0	1	5
Confusion	9 (4)	3	0	3	3
Consciousness impaired	1 (0.5)	0	0	1	0
Dizziness	13 (6)	7	2	2	2
Fatigue	1 (0.5)	1	0		0
Guillain-Barré–like syndrome	1 (0.5)	0	0	1	0
Hallucination	4 (2)	0	0	2	2
Insomnia	2 (1)	1	0	1	0
Memory impaired	7 (3)	2	1	1	3
Mood alteration	12 (6)	7	1	4	0
Neuropathy increased	5 (2)	2	2	1	0
Restlessness	4 (2)	1	2	0	1
Somnolence	1 (0.5)	0	0	1	0
Tremor	4 (2)	1	1	2	0

- Neurologic toxicities of any degree were observed after 26 cycles (13%) in 20 patients (16%). The majority of events were G1 or G2. In 4% of the cycles (N = 4) and 7% of the patients (N = 9), G3/4 neurotoxicities were observed
- In 1 patient, treatment had to be stopped because of a Guillain-Barré–like syndrome with tetraparesis, hallucinations, and reduced vigilance, which developed at day 3 of the first cycle. The symptoms improved slowly after nelarabine was withdrawn

Notes

- Nelarabine is indicated for the treatment of patients with T-cell acute lymphoblastic leukemia and T-cell lymphoblastic lymphoma whose disease has not responded to or has relapsed following treatment with at least 2 chemotherapy regimens
- Severe neurologic adverse reactions have been reported with the use of nelarabine, including altered mental states, such as severe somnolence, central nervous system effects, such as convulsions, and peripheral neuropathy, ranging from numbness and paresthesias to motor weakness and paralysis. There have also been reports of adverse reactions associated with demyelination, and ascending peripheral neuropathies similar to Guillain-Barré syndrome

  Full recovery from adverse reactions has not always occurred with cessation of therapy with nelarabine. Close monitoring for neurologic adverse reactions is strongly recommended
- DeAngelo DJ et al. (Blood 2007;109: 5136–5142) also reported their experience with 26 refractory/relapsed patients with T-cell acute lymphoblastic leukemia (T-ALL) and 13 patients with T-cell lymphoblastic lymphoma whose median age was 34 years (range: 16–66 years). Treatment consisted of **nelarabine** 1500 mg/m² per dose intravenously over 2 hours for 3 doses on days 1, 3, and 5, every 21 days (total dosage/ cycle = 4500 mg/m²). The investigators reported a complete remission rate of 31% (95% confidence interval [CI], 17%, 48%), and an overall response of 41% (95% CI, 26%, 58%). The principal toxicities were G3 or G4 neutropenia and thrombocytopenia, which occurred in 37% and 26% of patients, respectively. Only one G4 neurologic adverse event occurred, a reversible depressed level of consciousness. The median disease-free survival (DFS) was 20 weeks (95% CI, 11%, 56%), and the median overall survival was 20 weeks (95% CI, 13%, 36%). The 1-year overall survival was 28% (95% CI, 15%, 43%)

18. Leukemia, Acute Myeloid

Michael M. Boyiadzis, MD, MHSc, Ivan Aksentijevich, MD, and Judith Karp, MD

Epidemiology

Incidence: 18,860 (male: 11,530; female: 7,330. Estimated new cases for 2014 in the United States)

3.7 per 100,000 male and female per year (4.5 per 100,000 male, 3.1 per 100,000 female)

Deaths: Estimated 10,460 in 2014 (male: 6,010; female: 4,450)

Median age: 67 years (median age for acute promyelocytic leukemia: 40 years)

Male to female ratio: 1.48

Dores GM. Blood 2012;119:34–43

Siegel R et al. CA Cancer J Clin 2014;64:9–29

Surveillance, Epidemiology and End Results (SEER) Program, available from http://seer.cancer.gov (accessed in 2013)

Work-up

- H&P
- CBC and leukocyte differential counts, platelets, electrolytes, liver function tests, PT, PTT, INR, fibrinogen, LDH, uric acid
- Bone marrow biopsy with cytogenetics, immunophenotyping, and molecular studies (including c-KIT, FLT3-ITD, NPM, CEBPA)
- HLA typing for patients who are candidates for allogeneic hematopoietic stem cell transplantation
- Cardiac scan if prior cardiac history or prior anthracycline use
- Lumbar puncture if neurologic symptoms (LP should be performed if a mass/lesion is not detected on imaging studies)

Pathology

WHO Classification of Acute Myeloid Leukemia

1. **AML with recurrent genetic abnormalities**
   - AML with t(8;21)(q22;q22) (RUNX1-RUNX1T1)
   - AML with inv(16)(p13.1q22) or t(16;16)(p13.1;q22) (CBFB-MYH11)
   - APL with t(15;17)(q22;q12); PML-RARA
   - AML with t(9;11)(p22;q23); MLLT3-MLL
   - AML with t(6;9)(p23;q34); DEK-NUP214
   - AML with inv(3)(q21q26.2) or t(3;3) (q21;q26.2); RPN1-EVI1
   - AML (megakaryoblastic) with t(1;22) (p13;q13); RBM15-MKL1
   - AML with mutated NPM1
   - AML with mutated CEBPA
2. **AML with MDS-related features**
3. **Therapy-related AML**
4. **AML not otherwise specified**
   - AML minimal with differentiation
   - AML without maturation
   - AML with maturation
   - Acute myelomonocytic leukemia
   - Acute monoblastic and monocytic leukemia
   - Acute erythroid leukemia
   - Acute megakaryoblastic leukemia
   - Acute basophilic leukemia
   - Acute panmyelosis with myelofibrosis
5. **Myeloid proliferation related to Down syndrome**
   - Transient abnormal myelopoiesis
   - Myeloid leukemia associated with Down syndrome

Swerdlow SH et al., eds. WHO Classification of Tumours of Haematopoietic and Lymphoid Tissues, 4th ed. Lyon, France: International Agency for Research on Cancer Press; 2008

Response Criteria for Acute Myeloid Leukemia

Morphologic leukemia-free state

Bone marrow <5% blasts in an aspirate with spicules

No blasts or Auer rods or persistence of extramedullary disease

Complete remission

Patient achieves a morphologic leukemia-free state, *and*

Absolute neutrophil count >1000/mm³

Platelets ≥100,000/mm³

No residual evidence of extramedullary disease

Morphologic CR–patient independent of transfusions

Cytogenetic CR–cytogenetics normal (in those with previously abnormal cytogenetics)

Molecular CR–negative molecular studies in patients with APL or Ph+ leukemia

Patients who fail to achieve a complete response are considered treatment failures

Relapse following a complete response is defined as reappearance of leukemic blasts in the peripheral blood or the finding of more than 5% blasts in the bone marrow, not attributable to another cause

Cheson BD et al. J Clin Oncol 2003;21:4642–4649

Risk Stratification

Risk Status	Cytogenetics	Molecular Abnormalities
Better-risk	inv(16) or t(16;16) t(8;21) t(15;17)	normal cytogenetics with NPM1 mutation or isolated CEBPA mutation in the absence of FLT3-ITD
Intermediate risk	normal cytogenetics +8 t(9;11) other nondefined	t(8;21), inv (16), t(16;16) with c-kit mutation
Poor risk	complex −5,5q−,−7,7q− 11q23 –non t(9;11) inv(3), t(3;3) t(6;9) t(9;22)	normal cytogenetics with flt3-itd mutation

O'Donnell MR et al. J Natl Compr Canc Netw 2011;9:280–317

Expert Opinion

Acute Myeloid Leukemia

- Three days of an anthracycline and 7 days of cytarabine (the "3+7" induction regimen) currently remains the standard for newly diagnosed patients with AML (excluding APL) who can tolerate intensive chemotherapy. Bone marrow biopsy/aspirate should be performed 7–10 days after completion of therapy. If the bone marrow is hypoplastic (defined as cellularity <10–20% and residual blasts <5–10%), a repeated bone marrow should be performed until count recovery when the remission status can be assessed. If the bone marrow has residual blasts, then a second course of therapy can be administered; this can be identical to the first induction course, escalation to high-dose cytarabine or non–cross-resistant antileukemic regimens (eg, mitoxantrone and etoposide). Young patients without comorbidities who are refractory to initial induction regimens should be considered for allogeneic hematopoietic cell transplantation (HCT) using a myeloablative regimen

- The choice of postremission therapy must be determined by the prognostic group, most importantly, the cytogenetics/molecular studies at presentation. In patients with favorable cytogenetics/molecular studies intensive postremission therapy should be administered. The use of peripheral autologous hematopoietic cell transplantation should be considered in experienced centers that have demonstrated a consistently low morbidity and therapy-related mortality

- Postremission with intensive therapy should be considered in patients with core-binding factor AML (CBF-AML) characterized by t(8;21)(q22;q22); *RUNX1-RUNX1T1* and inv(16)(p13.1q22) or t(16;16)(p13.1;q22); and *CBFB-MYH11* (activating *KIT* mutations are found in approximately one-third of CBF-AML, and are associated with a significantly inferior outcome in most but not all studies; a clinical trial or allo-HCT should be consider for these patients). Similar to CBF-AML, repetitive cycles of high-dose cytarabine is a reasonable first-line strategy in patients with normal karyotype and mutated NPM1 or CEBPA^dm without FLT3-ITD

- In patients with AML with intermediate-risk cytogenetics, allo-HCT should be considered if a HLA-matched donor is available. There is no added benefit in receiving additional high-dose postremission therapy prior to allo-HCT if there is no delay in the HCT. Allo-HCT should also be considered in patients with cytogenetically normal karyotype whose leukemic cells have FLT-3 ITD. For patients with poor cytogenetics or molecular abnormalities, patients with prior myelodysplasia allo-HCT should also be considered

- Older patients with good performance status, minimal comorbidity, and good risk cytogenetics or molecular mutations, may benefit from standard therapies regardless of chronologic age. Patients deemed unfit to received intensive chemotherapy may be managed by one of the following options: best supportive care, subcutaneously administered cytarabine, azacitidine, decitabine, or clofarabine. Patients in first relapse after a CR duration >6–12 months can be retreated with either the induction regimen they last received or a high-dose cytarabine-containing regimen; after a second CR, patients should be considered for an allo-HCT. For patients in first relapse after a short CR duration (<6 months) a non–cross-resistant antileukemic regimen should be used, and, after a second CR, patients should be considered for an allo-HCT

(continued)

Expert Opinion (continued)

Evaluation for CNS Leukemia

- Leptomeningeal involvement is much less frequent (<5%) in AML than in ALL; thus, routine lumbar puncture is not recommended during routine diagnostic work-up. However, if neurologic symptoms are present at diagnosis, an initial MRI/CT should be first performed to rule out bleeding or mass effect. If the lumbar puncture is positive, intrathecal chemotherapy with cytarabine or methotrexate is recommended, concurrent with induction chemotherapy. Intrathecal chemotherapy is given twice per week until cerebrospinal fluid cytology shows no blasts, and then weekly for 4–6 weeks. Liposomal cytarabine has a longer half-life than conventional formulations (cytarabine injection; Cytarabine for Injection, USP) and offers the benefit of less-frequent (once weekly) administration. Screening for occult CNS should be considered in AML patients in remission with M4 or M5 morphology, biphenotypic leukemia, or WBC >100,000/mm^3 at diagnosis

Acute promyelocytic leukemia (APL)

- APL is a medical emergency primarily because of bleeding, which continues to represent a major cause of early death. Once the diagnosis is suspected on the basis of clinical findings and the peripheral blood smear (even without waiting for a bone marrow examination), and before the diagnosis is confirmed by cytogenetic or molecular studies, tretinoin (all *trans*-retinoic acid; ATRA) should be given emergently, both to resolve the coagulopathy as well as to initiate induction therapy

- The concurrent administration of tretinoin plus cytotoxic chemotherapy produces a complete remission (CR) in 80–95% of patients of all ages with APL. Tretinoin plus anthracyclines either alone or with cytarabine for induction (in high risk patients, WBC>10,000/mm^3) is the current standard of care. The combination of all-trans retinoic acid + arsenic trioxide has provided the opportunity to minimize and even eliminate standard cytotoxic chemotherapy from initial treatment regimens without compromising the excellent outcomes achieved by anthracycline-containing protocols

- The goal of consolidation therapy for APL is the conversion of a morphologic and cytogenetic remission into a durable molecular remission. Molecular remission often requires at least 2 cycles of consolidation

- Two or 3 cycles of an anthracycline, either daunorubicin or idarubicin, are administered until a molecular CR is achieved. Tretinoin is also given for 1 to 2 weeks with each cycle of consolidation. In patients with high-risk disease (WBC >10,000/mm^3), either intermediate- or high-dose cytarabine may be administered. The choice of regimen should be influenced by risk group, age, and cardiovascular risk. Patients should be treated according to regimens established from large clinical trials, and one should use a regimen consistently through all components not mixing induction from one trial with consolidation from a different trial

- Mercaptopurine + methotrexate have been used as maintenance therapy, which continues for 1–2 years. The addition of tretinoin in maintenance improved disease-free survival and relapse rates. However, as consolidation regimens have evolved to incorporate tretinoin or arsenic trioxide, the role of these agents in maintenance needs to be defined, especially in low-risk patients who achieve molecular CR after consolidation

- Bone marrow biopsy should be done after peripheral blood counts recover from induction therapy to determine whether a CR by morphology has been achieved. Monitoring RT-PCR for the PML-RAR-α fusion transcript to document molecular remission should be performed on a marrow sample at completion of consolidation. Subsequent monitoring of patients by PCR can be done with peripheral blood at a minimum of every 2 months for 2 years to detect molecular relapse

Adès L et al. J Clin Oncol 2006;24:5703–5710
Powell BL et al. Blood 2010;116:3751–3757
Sanz MA et al. Blood 2010;115:5137–5146

Supportive Care
Hyperleukocytosis in AML

- The frequency of hyperleukocytosis (conventionally and arbitrarily defined as a WBC count >100,000/mm^3) ranges from 5% to 13% in adult patients with AML

- Symptoms may arise from the involvement of any organ, but intracranial hemorrhages and respiratory failure account for the majority of deaths. In many patients, leukostasis becomes evident a few days after diagnosis, and sometimes after the first leukocytoreduction. Clinical deterioration and death may occur after the blast count has been significantly reduced, which suggests that although leukocytoreduction is an important step in the management of leukostasis, additional measures are needed to prevent leukostasis-related deaths

Treatment

- Prompt leukocytoreduction, initiation of chemotherapy, and supportive care

- Leukocytoreduction can be achieved by the use of hydroxyurea. Hydroxyurea should be started immediately in all patients with hyperleukocytotic AML. Hydroxyurea given at dosages up to 50–60 mg/kg per day orally until WBCs are <10,000–20,000/mm^3

- Leukopheresis is also an option for the initial management of hyperleukocytosis. The disadvantage of leukopheresis is that it requires the placement of a large caliber central venous catheter in patients who may be thrombocytopenic and coagulopathic, and it may also worsen their thrombocytopenia. There are no guidelines that identify the absolute WBC count to be achieved by leukopheresis that correlates with reversal of the signs and symptoms of leukostasis

PROPHYLAXIS AGAINST TUMOR LYSIS SYNDROME

HYDRATION + URINARY ALKALINIZATION + ADMINISTRATION OF ALLOPURINOL

Hydration with 2500–3000 mL/m^2 per day as tolerated; administer intravenously to maintain urine output ≥100 mL/hour (or ≥2 mL/kg per hour in persons whose body weight is <50 kg)

Urinary alkalinization with sodium bicarbonate injection added to intravenously administered fluids
- The amount of sodium bicarbonate added to intravenously administered fluids should produce a solution with sodium content not greater than the concentration of sodium in 0.9% sodium chloride injection (≤154 mEq/L):

Sodium Bicarbonate is Added to a Solution to Increase Urine pH within a Range 6.0 to ≤7

Base Solution Sodium Content	Sodium Bicarbonate Additive	Total Sodium Content
0.45% Sodium Chloride Injection (0.45% NS)		
77 mEq/L	50–75 mEq	127–152 mEq/L
0.2% Sodium Chloride Injection (0.2% NS)		
34 mEq/L	100–125 mEq	134–159 mEq/L
5% Dextrose Injection (D5W)		
0	125–150 mEq	125–150 mEq/L
D5W/0.45% NS		
77 mEq/L	50–75 mEq	127–152 mEq/L
D5W/0.2% NS		
34 mEq/L	100–125 mEq	134–159 mEq/L

Notes:
- Hydration rate may be decreased at the completion of chemotherapy administration
- Urinary alkalization increases the solubility and excretion of uric acid and its oxypurine precursors (hypoxanthine and xanthine) and helps avoid uric acid crystallization in renal tubules; however, alkalinization is not uniformly recommended because:
  1. It favors precipitation of calcium/phosphate in renal tubules, a concern in patients with concomitant hyperphosphatemia
  2. A metabolic alkalemia may result from the administration of bicarbonate that can worsen the neurologic manifestations of hypocalcemia

Allopurinol
- Administer orally or intravenously starting 12 hours to 3 days (preferably 2–3 days) before starting cytoreductive chemotherapy
- Hyperuricemia develops within 24–48 hours after initiating chemotherapy when the excretory capacity of the renal tubules is exceeded
- In the presence of an acid pH, uric acid crystals form in the renal tubules, leading to intraluminal renal tubular obstruction, an acute renal obstructive uropathy, and renal dysfunction

Initial dosage
- Allopurinol 100 mg/m^2 per dose; administer orally every 8 hours (maximum daily dose = 800 mg), *or*
- Allopurinol 3.3 mg/kg per dose; administer orally every 8 hours (maximum daily dose = 800 mg), *or*
- Allopurinol 200–400 mg/m^2 per day; administer intravenously (maximum daily dose = 600 mg) in a volume of 5% dextrose injection or 0.9% sodium chloride injection sufficient to yield a concentration not greater than 6 mg/mL. The duration for administering individual doses should be informed by the volume to be given
  - Allopurinol may be administered as a single daily dose, or the total daily dose may be divided equally for administration at 6-, 8-, or 12-hour intervals
- **Maintenance doses** should be based on serum uric acid determinations performed approximately 48 hours after initiation of allopurinol therapy, and periodically thereafter
- Continue administering allopurinol until leukemic blasts have been cleared from the peripheral blood

(continued)

(continued)

Notes:
• Allopurinol dose adjustments for impaired renal function:

Creatinine Clearance	Oral Allopurinol Dose
10–20 mL/min (0.17–0.33 mL/s)	200 mg/day
3–10 mL/min (0.05–0.17 mL/s)	100 mg/day
<3 mL/min (<0.05 mL/s)	100 mg every 36–48 hours

• The incidence of allergic reactions is increased in patients receiving amoxicillin, ampicillin, or thiazide diuretics

Rasburicase is recombinant urate oxidase (uricase) produced by genetically modified *Saccharomyces cerevisiae* that express urate oxidase cDNA cloned from a strain of *Aspergillus flavus*

• Uricase enzymes catalyze uric acid oxidation to allantoin, which is at least 5 times more soluble than uric acid

Rasburicase should be considered among initial interventions against hyperuricemia in patients with high peripheral WBC counts, rapidly increasing blasts counts, high uric acid, or with evidence of impaired renal function; that is:

WBC ≥100,000/mm^3	
WBC ≥25, 000 to <100,000/mm^3 *or* WBC <25,000/mm^3 + LDH ≥2× ULN	+ acute kidney injury *or* + normal renal function uric acid >ULN potassium or phosphorus >ULN

ULN, upper limit of normal

See Chapter 46, *Oncologic Emergencies*

Rasburicase 0.2 mg/kg per dose intravenously in a total volume of 50 mL 0.9% sodium chloride injection over 30 minutes once daily for up to 5 consecutive days is often used, but much less is usually sufficient (See Chapter 46, Oncologic Emergencies) (dosage and administration recommendations published in U.S. Food and Drug Administration product labeling, January 2011)

• Rasburicase has demonstrated effectiveness in prophylaxis and treatment for hyperuricemia and acute increases in uric acid associated with cytoreductive therapies at dosages <0.2 mg/kg based on body weight, with fixed doses, and after administration of from 1–3 doses

Cairo MS et al. Br J Haematol 2010;149:578–586
Coiffier B et al. J Clin Oncol 2008;26:2767–2778
Döhner H et al. Blood 2010;115:453–474
Döhner H, Gaidzik VI. Hematology Am Soc Hematol Educ Program 2011;2011:36–42
O'Donnell MR et al. J Natl Compr Canc Netw 2011;9:280–317
Rowe JM, Tallman MS. Blood 2010;116:3147–3156
Sanz MA et al. Blood 2009;113:1875–1891
Tallman MS, Altman JK. Blood 2009;114:5126–5135

INDUCTION THERAPY FOR PREVIOUSLY UNTREATED ACUTE MYELOGENOUS LEUKEMIA REGIMEN

CYTARABINE + DAUNORUBICIN

Fernandez HF et al. N Engl J Med 2009;361:1249–1259

Cytarabine 100 mg/m² per day; administer by continuous intravenous infusion in 100–1000 mL 0.9% sodium chloride injection or 5% dextrose injection over 24 hours for 7 consecutive days on days 1–7 (total dosage/cycle = 700 mg/m²)

Daunorubicin 60–90 mg/m² per day; administer by intravenous injection over 3–5 minutes for 3 consecutive days on days 1–3 (total dosage/cycle = 180–270 mg/m²)

Supportive Care

Antiemetic prophylaxis

Emetogenic potential on days 1–3 is **MODERATE**

Emetogenic potential on days 4–7 is **LOW**

See Chapter 39 for antiemetic recommendations

Hematopoietic growth factor (CSF) should be considered in patients with severe infection or in elderly patients or in patients with slow bone marrow recovery. Begin use after bone marrow aplasia is confirmed and continue use until ANC recovers

Primary prophylaxis is indicated with one of the following:

Filgrastim (G-CSF) 5 mcg/kg per day; administer by subcutaneous injection, *or*

Sargramostim (GM-CSF) 250 mcg/m² per day; administer by subcutaneous injection

See Chapter 43 for more information

Antimicrobial prophylaxis

Risk of fever and neutropenia is HIGH

Antimicrobial primary prophylaxis is recommended:

- Antibacterial—consider fluoroquinolone prophylaxis; *P. jirovecii* prophylaxis is recommended (eg, cotrimoxazole)

- Antifungal—recommended

- Antiviral—antiherpes antivirals (eg, acyclovir, famciclovir, valacyclovir)

See Chapter 47 for more information

Patient Population Studied

Study of 657 patients who had untreated AML (ages: 17–60 years) who were randomized to receive 3 once-daily doses of daunorubicin at either the standard dose (45 mg/m² of body-surface area per day) or a high dose (90 mg/m² per day), combined with 7 daily doses of cytarabine 100 mg/m² per day by continuous intravenous infusion

Efficacy

Induction therapy: 57% in the standard-dose group *vs.* 71% in the high-dose group

In the standard-dose group, patients younger than the age of 50 years had a CR of 59.4% in comparison with CR of 74.3% in the high-dose group

High-dose daunorubicin (90 mg/m² per day) did not provide benefit in patients older than the age of 50 years or those with unfavorable cytogenetic profile

The median overall survival was 15.7 months in the standard-dose group and 23.7 months in the high-dose group

Toxicity

Adverse Events	Standard Dose (45 mg/ m² · day) N = 318		High Dose (90 mg/ m² · day) N = 315	
	G3	G4	G3	G4
Low hemoglobin	67	11	63	13
Low Blood Count				
Leukocytes	2	95	<1	98
Neutrophils	3	93	18	80
Platelets	16	81	18	80
Transfusions Required				
Platelets	55	5	57	6
PRBC	59	1	59	<1
Fatigue	5	<1	3	3
Fever	5	1	5	3
Rash or desquamation	5	<1	5	0
Anorexia	4	4	5	5
Nausea	6	<1	5	0
Hemorrhage with G3/4 low platelet count	8	1	10	1
Febrile neutropenia	32	3	31	4
Infection with G3/4 neutropenia	40	7	39	<1
Dyspnea	4	2	<1	3
Cardiac event*	5	2	4	3

*A reduced left ventricular ejection fraction was reported in none of 318 patients in the standard group and in 4 of 315 patients in the high-dose group

Notes: The death rates during induction therapy were 4.5% in the standard-dose group and 5.5% in the high-dose group (P = 0.60). Causes of death were infection (14 patients), pulmonary failure (6 patients), cardiac failure (4 patients), hemorrhage (3 patients), hypotension (2 patients), and ileus (1 patient)

Treatment Modifications

Adverse Events	Treatment Modifications
Creatinine >3 mg/dL (>265 μmol/L)	Reduce daunorubicin dosage by 50%
Total bilirubin 2.5–5 mg/dL (42.8–85.5 μmol/L)	
Total bilirubin >5 mg/dL (>85.5 μmol/L)	Hold daunorubicin

Therapy Monitoring

1. CBC with differential daily during induction chemotherapy and following therapy until neutrophil recovery (>500/mm^3) and patients achieve independence from platelet transfusions
2. Electrolytes, mineral panel, liver function tests daily, and uric acid at least daily during active treatment until risk of tumor lysis is past
3. Bone marrow aspirate/biopsy 7–10 days after chemotherapy is completed

INDUCTION THERAPY FOR PREVIOUSLY UNTREATED ACUTE MYELOGENOUS LEUKEMIA REGIMEN

CYTARABINE + IDARUBICIN

Vogler WR et al. J Clin Oncol 1992;10:1103–1111

Cytarabine 100 mg/m² per day; administer by continuous intravenous infusion in 100–1000 mL 0.9% sodium chloride injection (0.9% NS) or 5% dextrose injection (D5W) over 24 hours for 7 consecutive days, on days 1–7 (total dosage/cycle = 700 mg/m²)

Idarubicin 12 mg/m² per day; administer intravenously diluted to a concentration >0.01 mg/mL with 0.9% NS or D5W over 15–30 minutes for 3 consecutive days, on days 1–3 (total dosage/cycle = 36 mg/m²)

Supportive Care
Antiemetic prophylaxis
Emetogenic potential on Days 1–3 is **MODERATE**
Emetogenic potential on Days 4–7 is **LOW**
See Chapter 39 for antiemetic recommendations

Hematopoietic growth factor (CSF) should be considered in patients with severe infection or in elderly patients or in patients with slow bone marrow recovery. Begin use after bone marrow aplasia is confirmed and continue use until ANC recovers

Primary prophylaxis is indicated with one of the following:
    Filgrastim (G-CSF) 5 mcg/kg per day by subcutaneous injection, *or*
    Sargramostim (GM-CSF) 250 mcg/m² per day by subcutaneous injection
See Chapter 43 for more information

Antimicrobial prophylaxis
Risk of fever and neutropenia is HIGH
    Antimicrobial primary prophylaxis is recommended:
- Antibacterial—consider fluoroquinolone prophylaxis; *P. jirovecii* prophylaxis is recommended (eg, cotrimoxazole)
- Antifungal—recommended
- Antiviral—antiherpes antivirals (eg, acyclovir, famciclovir, valacyclovir)

See Chapter 47 for more information

Patient Population Studied

Study of 111 patients (median age: 60 years) with newly diagnosed AML

Efficacy (N = 105)

Induction CR 69%, Number in CR with 1 course: 77 %
Median time to CR: 42 days
Response by age group
Ages   15–50 years (N = 29): 86%
            51–60 years (N = 24): 71%
            >60 years (N = 52): 63%

Toxicity (N = 105)

Adverse Events	G1/2 %	G3/4 %
Nausea and vomiting	76	6
Diarrhea	57	16
Mucositis	43	7
Total bilirubin	36	9
SGOT (AST)	47	5
Alkaline phosphatase	52	5
Creatinine	29	2
Skin rash	41	5
Cardiac	5	11
Hair loss	37	40

	Mean Duration of Aplasia (Days)
WBC <1000/mm³	31.2
Platelets <50,000/mm³	35.1

Therapy Monitoring

1. CBC with differential daily during induction chemotherapy and following therapy until neutrophil recovery (>500/mm³), and until patients achieve independence from platelet transfusions
2. Electrolytes, mineral panel, liver function tests daily, and uric acid at least daily during active treatment until risk of tumor lysis is past
3. Bone marrow aspirate/biopsy 7–10 days after chemotherapy is completed

Treatment Modifications

Adverse Events	Treatment Modifications
Creatinine >3 mg/dL (>265 µmol/L)	Reduce idarubicin dosage by 50%
Total bilirubin 2.6–5 mg/dL (44.5–85.5 µmol/L)	Reduce idarubicin dosage by 50%
Total bilirubin >5 mg/dL (>85.5 µmol/L)	Hold idarubicin

INTENSIVE POSTREMISSION CHEMOTHERAPY IN ADULTS WITH ACUTE MYELOID LEUKEMIA REGIMEN

HIGH-DOSE CYTARABINE

Mayer RJ et al. N Engl J Med 1994;331:896–903

Cytarabine 3000 mg/m² per dose; administer intravenously in 100–1000 mL 0.9% sodium chloride injection or 5% dextrose injection over 3 hours, every 12 hours for 6 doses (2 doses/day) on days 1, 3, and 5, every 28 days for 4 cycles (total dosage/cycle = 18,000 mg/m²)

Notes: Repeated cycles were initiated no sooner than 28 days after a previously administered cycle, or 1 week after patients achieved postnadir ANC >1500/mm³ and platelet counts >100,000/mm³, with the expectation the maximal interval between consecutive cycles would be ≤35 days

Supportive Care
Antiemetic prophylaxis
Emetogenic potential on days of treatment is **MODERATE–HIGH**
See Chapter 39 for antiemetic recommendations

Hematopoietic growth factor (CSF) should be considered in patients with severe infection or in elderly patients or in patients with slow bone marrow recovery. Begin use after bone marrow aplasia is confirmed and continue use until ANC recovers

Primary prophylaxis is indicated with one of the following:
Filgrastim (G-CSF) 5 mcg/kg per day by subcutaneous injection, *or*
Sargramostim (GM-CSF) 250 mcg/m² per day by subcutaneous injection
See Chapter 43 for more information

Antimicrobial prophylaxis
Risk of fever and neutropenia is HIGH
Antimicrobial primary prophylaxis is recommended:
- Antibacterial—consider fluoroquinolone prophylaxis; *P. jirovecii* prophylaxis is recommended (eg, cotrimoxazole)
- Antifungal—recommended
- Antiviral—antiherpes antivirals (eg, acyclovir, famciclovir, valacyclovir)

See Chapter 47 for more information

Keratitis prophylaxis
Steroid ophthalmic drops (prednisolone 1% or dexamethasone 0.1%) administer by intraocular instillation daily until 24 hours after high-dose cytarabine is completed

Patient Population Studied

Study of 596 patients in CR after induction chemotherapy (daunorubicin + cytarabine) who were randomly assigned to receive 4 cycles of cytarabine on one of three 5-day dosage schedules: low-dose or moderate-dose cytarabine administered by continuous intravenous infusion, or high-dose cytarabine administered intravenously intermittently

Efficacy

The likelihood of remaining alive and disease-free (DFS) after 4 years was 21% among subjects who received low-dose continuous infusion cytarabine, 25% in the moderate-dose group, and 39% among those who received high-dose cytarabine

The probability of remaining alive (survival) for 4 years after randomization was 31% for the group assigned to receive low-dose continuous infusion cytarabine, 35% for the group assigned to receive moderate-dose intermittent infusions, and 46% among patient who received high-dose cytarabine

The probability of remaining in continuous complete remission after 4 years among patients ≤60 years of age was 24% in the low-dose group, 29% in the moderate-dose group, and 44% in the high-dose group

In contrast, for patients older than 60 years of age, the probability of remaining disease-free after 4 years was ≤16% in each group

Subsequent analysis showed a disease-free survival rate of 60% for patients with good-risk cytogenetics, 30% with intermediate-risk cytogenetics, and 12% with poor-risk cytogenetics in patients who received high-dose cytarabine

Bloomfield CD et al. Cancer Res 1998;58:4173–4179

Treatment Modifications

Adverse Events	Treatment Modifications	
Neurologic toxicity	Hold cytarabine. Patients who develop CNS symptoms should not receive subsequent high-dose cytarabine	
The risk of neurotoxicity with high-dose cytarabine therapy is directly related to renal function throughout therapy	**Serum Creatinine**	**Cytarabine Dosage**
	<1.5 mg/dL (<133 μmol/L)	2000 mg/m²
	1.5–1.9 mg/dL (133–168 μmol/L), or an increase from baseline by 0.5–1.2 mg/dL (44–106 μmol/L)	1000 mg/m²
	≥2 mg/dL (≥177 μmol/L), or an increase of >1.2 mg/dL (>106 μmol/L)	100 mg/m² per day by continuous intravenous infusion over 24 hours for up to 6 days
In patients exhibiting rapidly rising creatinine as a result of tumor lysis	Hold cytarabine	

Toxicity

% of Patients Who Received 4 Planned Cycles	Cytarabine Regimens		
	LD CIVI	MD CIVI	High-Dose
All patients	76%	74%	56%
Patients, ages ≤60 years	78%	76%	62%

Cytarabine Regimens	Cycles During Which Patients Were Hospitalized	Serious CNS Toxicity	Deaths During Remission
LD CIVI	16%	0	1%
MD CIVI	59%	0	6%
High-Dose	71%	12%	5%

LD CIVI, Cytarabine 100 mg/m² per day by continuous intravenous infusion over 24 hours for 5 consecutive days on days 1–5; MD CIVI, cytarabine 400 mg/m² per day by continuous intravenous infusion over 24 hours for 5 consecutive days on days 1–5; High-Dose, 3000 mg/m² per dose by intravenous infusion over 3 hours, twice daily on days 1, 3, and 5, for 6 doses

Therapy Monitoring

1. CBC with differential and platelet counts daily during chemotherapy; electrolytes, LFTs, and mineral panel, daily during chemotherapy

2. *Outpatient monitoring postchemotherapy:* CBC with differential, platelets, and electrolytes, 2–3 times weekly until counts recovery

3. *Between cycles:* Bone marrow biopsy/aspirate if peripheral blood counts are abnormal, or patients failure to recover counts after therapy. Bone marrow biopsy after recovery of counts following the last course of therapy

Notes:

1. This trial of postremission therapy for AML demonstrated a significant dose–response effect for cytarabine. Patients 60 years of age or younger who received high-dose cytarabine were more likely to remain in remission and to survive longer than patients in the same age group who received lower doses. Serious CNS abnormalities were reported only in the group given high-dose cytarabine, and were especially common in patients older than 60 years of age

2. Patients who receive high-dose cytarabine need to be closely monitored for changes in renal function. Renal dysfunction is highly correlated with an increased risk of cerebellar toxicity. Patients need to be monitored for nystagmus, dysmetria, and ataxia before each dose of cytarabine

ACUTE PROMYELOCYTIC LEUKEMIA (APL) INDUCTION REGIMEN

TRETINOIN (ALL *TRANS*-RETINOIC ACID) + IDARUBICIN

Sanz MA et al. Blood 2010;115:5137–5146

Tretinoin 22.5 mg/m^2 per dose; administer orally every 12 hours until hematologic CR (total dosage/week = 315 mg/m^2)

Idarubicin 12 mg/m^2 per dose; administer intravenously diluted to a concentration >0.01 mg/mL in 0.9% sodium chloride injection or 5% dextrose injection over 15–30 minutes for 4 doses on days 2, 4, 6, and 8 (total dosage/induction course = 48 mg/m^2)

Supportive Care
Antiemetic prophylaxis
Emetogenic potential on days with tretinoin alone is **MINIMAL–LOW**
Emetogenic potential on days with idarubicin is **MODERATE**
See Chapter 39 for antiemetic recommendations

Hematopoietic growth factor (CSF) prophylaxis
Primary prophylaxis is NOT indicated
See Chapter 43 for more information

Antimicrobial prophylaxis
Risk of fever and neutropenia is HIGH
  Antimicrobial primary prophylaxis is recommended:
  • Antibacterial—consider fluoroquinolone prophylaxis; *P. jirovecii* prophylaxis is recommended (eg, cotrimoxazole)
  • Antifungal—recommended
  • Antiviral—antiherpes antivirals (eg, acyclovir, famciclovir, valacyclovir)
See Chapter 47 for more information

Toxicity

Causes of induction deaths*
Hemorrhage: 3.7%
Infection: 1.5%
Differentiation syndrome: 1%

*Hemorrhage and infection accounted for most of the deaths during induction therapy (15 and 6 patients, respectively). Deaths caused by hemorrhage were caused by intracranial (12 patients, 80%), pulmonary (2 patients, 13%), and gastrointestinal hemorrhages (1 patient, 7%). Differentiation syndrome and acute myocardial infarction were contributing causes of death in 4 and 2 patients, respectively. The remaining 3 deaths were attributable to massive suprahepatic thrombosis, myocarditis, and cardiac failure, each of which occurred in 1 patient

Therapy Monitoring

1. CBC 2- to 3-times daily until resolution of coagulopathy, then daily
2. Fibrinogen, PT, and PPT, twice daily until resolution of coagulopathy, then daily
3. Electrolytes, mineral panel, and uric acid, at least daily during active treatment until risk of tumor lysis is past
4. Bone marrow biopsy should be done once the peripheral blood counts recover from induction to determine whether a CR by morphology has been achieved

Patient Population Studied

Study of 437 consecutive patients with genetic diagnosis of APL

Efficacy

Of 402 evaluable patients, 372 achieved morphologic CR (92.5%)*
The median time interval to CR was 39 days (range: 18–81 days)
Patients with WBC counts >10,000/mm^3 and >50,000/mm^3 had a poorer response rates (83% and 73%, respectively) compared with those with low- and intermediate-risk patients (99% and 96%, respectively; P <0.001)

*The median time to reach neutrophil counts >1000/mm^3 and platelet counts >50,000/mm^3 was 24 days (range: 6–72 days) and 19 days (range: 4–80 days), respectively

Treatment Modifications

Adverse Events	Treatment Modifications
Creatinine >3 mg/dL (>265 μmol/L)	Reduce idarubicin dosage by 50%
Total bilirubin 2.6–5 mg/dL (44.5–85.5 μmol/L)	Reduce idarubicin dosage by 50%
Total bilirubin >5 mg/dL (>85.5 μmol/L)	Hold idarubicin
ATRA syndrome	Hold ATRA and treat with dexamethasone 10 mg intravenously every 12 hours for 3–5 days, then decrease the dexamethasone dose and administration schedule (taper) over a week to discontinue. Restart ATRA when symptoms and signs improve

Notes:

1. ATRA (all *trans*-retinoic acid) syndrome occurs in patients with APL after treatment initiation. It is characterized by fever, peripheral edema, pulmonary infiltrates, hypoxemia, respiratory distress, hypotension, renal and hepatic dysfunction, and serositis, resulting in pleural and pericardial effusions. Considering that this complex of symptoms is not specific to the use of retinoic acid but may occur during therapy with agents such as arsenic trioxide it is now referred as the "APL differentiation syndrome"

   Early recognition and aggressive management with dexamethasone (10 mg; administer intravenously every 12 hours for ≥3 days) has been effective in most patients. If the symptoms or signs are severe, ATRA is discontinued and resumed at resolution of symptoms and signs, but under the cover of steroids, because the syndrome may recur. Tretinoin can be restarted in most cases

2. Disseminated intravascular coagulation (DIC) is frequently present at diagnosis in patients with APL, or occurs soon after the initiation of cytotoxic chemotherapy. This complication constitutes a medical emergency, because, if left untreated, it can cause pulmonary or cerebrovascular hemorrhage in up to 40% of patients with a 10–20% incidence of early hemorrhagic death. Tretinoin therapy appears to shorten the duration of the coagulopathy

3. Platelets are transfused to maintain platelet counts >30,000–50,000/mm³, and cryoprecipitate is administered to maintain the fibrinogen level >150 mg/dL (>1.5 g/L). Both products should be transfused multiple times a day if necessary to maintain respective levels during the first week therapy or longer until coagulopathy resolves

ACUTE PROMYELOCYTIC LEUKEMIA (APL) INDUCTION REGIMEN

TRETINOIN (ALL *TRANS*-RETINOIC ACID; ATRA) + ARSENIC TRIOXIDE

Lo-Coco F et al. N Engl J Med 2013;369:111–121
Comment in: N Engl J Med 2013;369:186–187

(Supplementary materials published online)

Induction:
Arsenic trioxide 0.15 mg/kg per day; administer intravenously in 100–250 mL 0.9% sodium chloride injection (0.9% NS) or 5% dextrose injection (D5W) over 2 hours, daily, continually, until hematological complete remission (HCR) *or* a maximum of 60 days (total dosage/week = 1.05 mg/kg); *plus*
Tretinoin 22.5 mg/m² per dose; administer orally twice daily, continually, until HCR *or* for a maximum of 60 days (total dosage/week = 315 mg/m²)

Consolidation:
Arsenic trioxide 0.15 mg/kg per dose; administer intravenously in 100–250 mL 0.9% NS or D5W over 2 hours for 5 days/week, weekly for 4 consecutive weeks (weeks 1–4, 9–12, 17–20, and 25–28), followed by 4 consecutive weeks without arsenic trioxide treatment, for a total of 4 courses (total dosage/week = 0.75 mg/kg; total dosage/4-week course = 3 mg/kg); *plus*
Tretinoin 22.5 mg/m² per dose; administer orally twice daily for 2 consecutive weeks (28 doses during weeks 1–2, 5–6, 9–10, 13–14, 17–18, 21–22, and 25–26) followed by 2 consecutive weeks without tretinoin treatment for a total of 7 courses (total dosage/week = 315 mg/m²; total dosage/2-week course = 630 mg/m²)

Supportive Care
Antiemetic prophylaxis
Emetogenic potential when arsenic trioxide is administered is **MODERATE**
Emetogenic potential when tretinoin alone is administered is **MINIMAL–LOW**
See Chapter 39 for antiemetic recommendations

Hematopoietic growth factor (CSF) prophylaxis
Primary prophylaxis is NOT indicated
See Chapter 43 for more information

Risk of fever and neutropenia is INTERMEDIATE
Antimicrobial primary prophylaxis to be considered:
- Antibacterial—consider a fluoroquinolone or no prophylaxis; *Pneumocystis jirovecii* prophylaxis is recommended (eg, cotrimoxazole)
- Antifungal—consider concomitant use of cotrimoxazole during periods of neutropenia
- Antiviral—antiherpes antivirals (eg, acyclovir, famciclovir, valacyclovir)

See Chapter 47 for more information

Toxicity

The differentiation syndrome, including moderate and severe forms, developed in 15 patients in the group who received tretinoin (ATRA)–arsenic trioxide (19%) and in 13 patients in the ATRA–chemotherapy group (16%) (P = 0.62)

Four patients in the ATRA–chemotherapy group died during induction therapy: 2 from differentiation syndrome, 1 from ischemic stroke, and 1 from bronchopneumonia

Grades 3 or 4 neutropenia lasting >15 days and G3 or G4 thrombocytopenia lasting >15 days occurred with significantly greater frequency during induction therapy and after each consolidation course in the ATRA–chemotherapy group than in the ATRA–arsenic trioxide group

A total of 43 of 68 patients in the ATRA–arsenic trioxide group (63%) and 4 of 69 patients in the ATRA–chemotherapy group (6%) had G3 or G4 hepatic toxic effects during induction or consolidation therapy or during maintenance therapy (only patients in the ATRA–chemotherapy group) (P <0.001)

Prolongation of the QTc interval occurred in 12 patients in the ATRA–arsenic trioxide group (16%) and in no patients in the ATRA–chemotherapy group (P <0.001)

Patient Population Studied

A phase 3, multicenter trial comparing ATRA plus chemotherapy with ATRA plus arsenic trioxide in patients with APL classified as low-to-intermediate risk (white-cell count, ≤10,000/mm³). Patients (18–71 years of age), were randomly assigned to receive either ATRA plus arsenic trioxide for induction and consolidation therapy or standard ATRA–idarubicin induction therapy followed by 3 cycles of consolidation therapy with ATRA, plus chemotherapy and maintenance therapy with low-dose chemotherapy and ATRA

Efficacy

	ATRA–Arsenic Trioxide Group (n = 77)	ATRA–Chemotherapy Group (n = 79)
Hematologic complete remission*	100%	95%
Two-year event-free survival rates†	97%	86%

*The median time to hematologic complete remission was 32 days (range: 22 to 68 days) in the ATRA–arsenic trioxide group and 35 days (range: 26 to 63 days) in the ATRA–chemotherapy group
†Two-year event-free survival rates were 97% in the ATRA–arsenic trioxide group and 86% in the ATRA–chemotherapy group (95% confidence interval for the difference, 2 to 22 percentage points; P <0.001 for noninferiority and P = 0.02 for superiority of ATRA–arsenic trioxide). Overall survival was also better with ATRA–arsenic trioxide (P = 0.02)

Treatment Modifications

QT prolongation QTc interval >450 msec for men and >460 msec for women	Withhold arsenic trioxide and replete electrolytes 1. After QTc normalizes, resume arsenic trioxide with dosage decreased by 50%: arsenic trioxide 0.075 mg/kg per day 2. If no further QTc prolongation occurs at the reduced dosage, escalate arsenic trioxide dosage to 0.11 mg/kg per day 3. If QTc prolongation does not occur after escalation to 0.11 mg/kg per day, arsenic trioxide dosage may again be escalated to 0.15 mg/kg per day (full dose)
Grades 3–4 hepatotoxicity (serum total bilirubin, AST, alkaline phosphatase)	Temporarily discontinue ATRA and/or arsenic trioxide After serum bilirubin, SGOT, and alkaline phosphatase decrease to <4× the upper limit of their normal ranges (ULN), treatment with ATRA and/or arsenic trioxide may resume at 50% of the dosages previously given for 7 days If toxicity does not recur during the 7 days after resuming ATRA and arsenic trioxide, drug administration may resume at full dosages If hepatotoxicity recurs, the drugs are permanently discontinued
Grades 3–4 nonhematologic toxicity	Withhold ATRA and arsenic trioxide until toxicities remit to G <2, then resume treatment with both agents at decreased dosages according to a pre-defined table of dose reduction

	Dosages	
Dose Levels	**Arsenic Trioxide (mg/kg per day)**	**Tretinoin (ATRA) (mg/m² per dose, Twice Daily)**
0 (starting dose)	0.15	22.5
−1	0.11	18.75
−2	0.10	12.5
−3	0.075	10

Therapy Monitoring

1. CBC, 2 to 3 times daily until resolution of coagulopathy, then daily
2. Fibrinogen, PT, and PTT, twice daily until resolution of coagulopathy, then daily
3. Electrolytes, mineral panel, and uric acid, at least daily during active treatment until risk of tumor lysis is past
4. Bone marrow biopsy should be done after peripheral blood counts recovers from induction to determine whether a CR by morphology has been achieved. Patients often remain molecularly positive at the end of induction even when their marrow shows morphologic remission
5. Arsenic trioxide monitoring
   Prior to initialing therapy: ECG for QTc interval assessment
   Serum electrolytes and creatinine

During therapy: maintain serum potassium concentration >4 mEq/L (>4 mmol/L)
   Maintain serum magnesium concentration >0.74 mmol/L (>1.8 mg/dL, >1.48 mEq/L)
ECG weekly during induction

Notes:
Hu et al reported long-term follow-up (median: 70 months) for 85 patients with APL treated with ATRA + arsenic trioxide. Among 80 of 85 patients (94.1%) who achieved CR with a median of 27 days (range: 15–38 days), 5 experienced early deaths within 15 days after starting induction therapy as a result of intracranial hemorrhage (3 patients), retinoic acid syndrome (1 patient), or disseminated intravascular coagulation (1 patient)

Kaplan-Meier estimates of the 5-year event-free survival and overall survival (OS) for all patients were 89.2% ± 3.4% and 91.7% ± 3.0%, respectively, and the 5-year relapse-free survival and OS for patients who achieved CR (n = 80) were 94.8% ± 2.5% and 97.4% ± 1.8%, respectively

Hu J et al. Proc Natl Acad Sci USA 2009;106: 3342–3347
Shen Z-X et al. Proc Natl Acad Sci USA 2004;101: 5328–5335

ACUTE PROMYELOCYTIC LEUKEMIA (APL) RELAPSED PATIENTS REGIMEN

ARSENIC TRIOXIDE

Soignet SL et al. J Clin Oncol 2001;19:3852–3860

Arsenic trioxide 0.15 mg/kg per day; administer intravenously in 100–250 mL 5% dextrose injection (D5W) or 0.9% sodium chloride injection (0.9% NS) over 2 hours until bone marrow remission or to a cumulative maximum of 60 doses (total dosage/week = 1.05 mg/kg; maximum dosage during induction = 9 mg/kg [60 doses])

or

Arsenic trioxide 0.15 mg/kg per dose administer intravenously in 100–250 mL D5W or 0.9% NS over 2 hours for 5 days/week (eg, Monday through Friday) until bone marrow remission or to a cumulative maximum of 60 doses (total dosage/week = 0.75 mg/kg; maximum dosage during induction = 9 mg/kg [60 doses])

Supportive Care
Antiemetic prophylaxis
Emetogenic potential is **MODERATE**
See Chapter 39 for antiemetic recommendations

Hematopoietic growth factor (CSF) prophylaxis
Primary prophylaxis is NOT indicated
See Chapter 43 for more information

Risk of fever and neutropenia is INTERMEDIATE
Antimicrobial primary prophylaxis to be considered:
- Antibacterial—consider a fluoroquinolone or no prophylaxis; *P. jirovecii* prophylaxis is recommended (eg, cotrimoxazole)
- Antifungal—consider concomitant use of cotrimoxazole during periods of neutropenia
- Antiviral—antiherpes antivirals (eg, acyclovir, famciclovir, valacyclovir)

See Chapter 47 for more information

Toxicity (N = 40)

Adverse Events	All Grades	G4
Nausea	75%	—
Vomiting	58%	—
Diarrhea	53%	—
Sore throat	40%	—
Abdominal pain	38%	8%
Cough	65%	—
Dyspnea	38%	10%
Headache	60%	3%
Insomnia	43%	3%
Dermatitis	43%	—
Hypokalemia	50%	13%
Hyperglycemia	45%	13%
Tachycardia	55%	—
Fatigue	63%	—
Fever	63%	—
QTc prolongation	40%	—
APL syndrome*	25%	—
Peripheral neuropathy	43%	—

There were no treatment-related deaths
*Treatment with arsenic trioxide for remission induction is associated with the development of symptoms identical to retinoic acid syndrome. Considering the complex of symptoms is not specific to the use of retinoic acid, it is now referred as the APL syndrome

Patient Population Studied

Study of 40 patients with either relapsed and/or refractory acute promyelocytic leukemia

Efficacy

CR: 85%
Median time to clinical CR: 59 days

Treatment Modifications

Adverse Events	Treatment Modifications
APL syndrome	Hold arsenic trioxide and treat with dexamethasone 10 mg intravenously every 12 hours for 3–5 days, then decrease the dexamethasone dose and schedule (taper) over a week to discontinue. Restart arsenic trioxide when symptoms and signs improve
Drug-related toxicity G ≥3, or nonhematologic toxicity G4	Hold therapy until resolution of the toxic event or recovery to baseline. Restart treatment at 50% of the preceding dose on the same administration schedule. If the toxic event does not recur within 3 days after restarting at a reduced dosage, continue treatment at the original dosage. If the same toxicity recurs, discontinue arsenic trioxide

Therapy Monitoring

1. CBC twice weekly, or more frequently based on transfusion requirements
2. Chemistry, LFTs, and electrolytes, twice weekly
3. Bone marrow
4. EKG daily for 7 days to assure QTc stability, then monitor weekly

Notes:
Careful monitoring to maintain serum electrolytes in the upper range of normal will lessen the risk of cardiac arrhythmias:
Calcium ≥2.25 mmol/L (≥4.5 mEq/L, ≥9 mg/dL)
Potassium ≥4 mmol/L (≥4 mEq/L)
Magnesium ≥0.9 mmol/L (≥1.8 mEq/L, ≥2.2 mg/dL)

19. Leukemia, Chronic Lymphocytic

Patricia Kropf, MD and Kenneth Foon, MD

Epidemiology

Incidence: 15,720 (male: 9,100; female: 6,620. Estimated new cases for 2014 in the United States) 4.3 per 100,000 male and female per year (5.9 per 100,000 male, 3.1 per 100,000 female)

Deaths: Estimated 4,600 in 2014 (male: 2,800; female: 1,800)

Median age: 70 years

Male to female ratio: 1.3:1

Stage at Presentation (Rai):

Stage 0:   31%
Stage I/II: 59%
Stages III/IV: 10%

Siegel R et al. CA Cancer J Clin 2014;64:9–29
Surveillance, Epidemiology and End Results (SEER) Program, available from http://seer.cancer.gov (accessed in 2013)

Work-up

Essential

1. Medical history and PE: attention to node-bearing areas, including the Waldeyer ring, and to size of liver and spleen
2. Performance status
3. B-symptoms
4. Laboratory work-up: CBC with differential, LDH, comprehensive metabolic panel
5. Hepatitis B testing if CD20 monoclonal antibody contemplated
6. MUGA scan/echocardiogram if anthracycline-based regimen is indicated
7. Pregnancy testing in women of child-bearing age (if chemotherapy planned)
8. Unilateral bone marrow biopsy + aspirate

Useful in certain circumstances

1. Quantitative immunoglobulins
2. β_2-Microglobulin
3. Reticulocyte count, haptoglobin, direct Coombs test
4. Uric acid
5. Chest, abdomen, and pelvis CT scans prior to initiation of therapy

Informative for prognostic and/or therapy determination

1. Cytogenetics/FISH analysis to detect: t(11q;v), +12, del(11q), del(13q), del(17p)
2. Determination of CD38 and Zap 70 expression
3. Immunoglobulin heavy-chain variable gene (IGHV) mutation status

Diagnosis

NCI-working group diagnostic criteria

1. Absolute lymphocytosis in the peripheral blood with a count of $\geq 5 \times 10^9$ B lymphocytes and cells morphologically mature in appearance
2. The clonality of the B cells must be confirmed by flow cytometry
3. The monoclonal B-cell lymphocytes express low levels of surface immunoglobulins, simultaneously with CD5, CD23, CD19, and CD20

Hallek M et al. Blood 2008;111:5446–5456

Prognosis

Poor risk factors

1. Advanced clinical stage
2. Rapid lymphocyte doubling time (<6 months)
3. Diffuse bone marrow involvement
4. High LDH, β_2-microglobulin
5. 17p and 11q deletions (normal karyotype and trisomy 12 have an intermediate prognosis, while 13q deletion has a good prognosis)*
6. Expression of CD38 (>30%)
7. Unmutated IGHV genes
8. Zap-70 expression (>30%)

*Döhner H et al. N Engl J Med 2000;343:1910–1916

Staging and Survival

Kay NE et al. Hematology Am Soc Hematol Educ Program 2002:193–213

Rai	Lymphocytosis	Lymph Node Enlargement	Spleen/Liver Enlargement	Hemoglobin <11 g/dL	Platelets <100,000/mm³	Survival Years
0	Yes	No	No	No	No	>13
I	Yes	Yes	No	No	No	8
II	Yes	±	Yes	No	No	6
III	Yes	±	±	Yes*	No	4
IV	Yes	±	±	±	Yes*	2

*Not immune-related

Expert Opinion

Chronic lymphocytic leukemia (CLL) is one of the most common leukemias in the Western world, characterized by the monoclonal proliferation of mature B lymphocytes in the blood, lymph nodes, and marrow. The diagnosis requires a count of over 5000 circulating CLL type cells per cubic millimeter. The median overall survival in patients with CLL is about 10 years. The individual prognosis, however, is extremely variable. In some patients, the disease runs an indolent course and life expectancy is near normal, while in others, the disease progresses rapidly with an aggressive clinical course resulting in refractory disease and shortened overall survival. The diagnosis of CLL does not imply the need for treatment; rather, a number of indications justify the need for patient-specific therapy

Treatment by Stage:
- Asymptomatic early stage disease (Rai 0, Binet A) should be monitored without therapy unless there is evidence of disease progression
- Intermediate (stages I and II) and high risk (stages III and IV) according to the modified Rai classification or at Binet stage B or C usually benefit from the initiation of treatment. Some of these patients (in particular, Rai intermediate risk or Binet stage B) can be monitored without therapy until they have evidence for progressive or symptomatic disease

Indications for treatment include:
- Evidence of progressive marrow failure as manifested by the development or worsening anemia (hemoglobin <11 g/dL) and/or thrombocytopenia (platelets $<100 \times 10^9$/L)
- Constitutional symptoms: A minimum of any one of the following disease-related symptoms must be present:
  a. Unintentional weight loss ≥10% within the previous 6 months
  b. Significant fatigue; that is, Eastern Cooperative Oncology Group performance status 2 or worse (cannot work or unable to perform usual activities)
  c. Fevers >100.5°F (>38.0°C) for ≥2 weeks without other evidence of infection
  d. Night sweats for more than 1 month without evidence of infection
- Massive, progressive, or symptomatic splenomegaly
- Massive, progressive, or symptomatic lymphadenopathy
- Autoimmune hemolytic anemia and/or thrombocytopenia that is poorly responsive to corticosteroids or other second-line treatments (splenectomy, intravenous immunoglobulin, and/or immunosuppressive agents, rituximab, or alemtuzumab)
- Rapidly increasing lymphocytosis with an increase of >50% over 2 months or lymphocyte doubling time of <6 months[1]

Note: Recurrent bacterial infections are very common in patients with CLL, but we do not view this as a reason to treat the underlying CLL unless any of the above mentioned criteria for initiating therapy exist. We would first attempt therapy with intravenous gamma globulin (IVIG) monthly for the prevention of recurrent bacterial infections. If IVIG is not successful in preventing recurrent bacterial infections then we would initiate therapy

Isolated hypogammaglobulinemia, or monoclonal or oligoclonal paraproteinemia do not constitute a basis for initiating therapy. Patients with CLL may present with a markedly elevated leukocyte count; however, the symptoms associated with leukocyte aggregates that develop in patients with acute leukemia rarely occur in patients with CLL. Therefore, the absolute lymphocyte count should not be used as the sole indicator for initiating treatment

Therapy: There are multiple treatment options available for patients with CLL, however, there is not one treatment that is considered the "standard of care" for all patients. The choice of therapy depends upon patient characteristics including age, performance status, and the expected clinical course based upon disease risk factors

(continued)

Expert Opinion (continued)

Choice of Therapy

- Patient characteristics, such as age and performance status, allow practioners to define the goal of therapy. Data suggest that improved therapies lead to improved overall survival.[2] In addition, research has shown that obtaining minimal residual disease improves survival.[3] Complete response is the most beneficial response with respect to long-term disease control, and complete responses are seen in about 50–80% of patients treated with chemoimmunotherapies, albeit at increased toxicity

- In young, fit patients, the goal of therapy is a complete response. We recommend fludarabine, cyclophosphamide, rituximab (FCR), or bendamustine and rituximab (BR) as frontline therapy, given for 6 cycles, based on high complete remission rates and improved progression-free survival.[4,5,6,7] Alternative options include low-dose fludarabine, and cyclophosphamide with high-dose rituximab (FCR-Lite)[8] or pentostatin, cyclophosphamide, rituximab (PCR)[9]. Both regimens are associated with superb efficacy data and perhaps less toxicity, although phase III data directly comparing the regimens are lacking. Recently, long-term results of the FCR-lite regimen were released revealing that patients treated with this regimen enjoyed a median progression-free survival of 5.8 years (the median overall survival has not yet been reached).[10] In young, fit patients with del (17p) or del (11q), we recommend FCR as initial therapy or treatment on a clinical trial. In addition, such patients should be considered for an allogeneic transplant in first remission. Patients who harbor del (17p) or del (11q) are at high risk of not responding to initial therapy or relapsing soon thereafter

- In older patients, such as those over 70 years of age, or in unfit patients who cannot tolerate aggressive therapy, the goal is the palliation of symptoms using a treatment regimen with a favorable toxicity profile. In such cases, we recommend treatment with single agent chlorambucil[11], which is palliative and has an acceptable toxicity profile. Other options include bendamustine with or without rituximab, single agent rituximab or ofatumumab[12,13,14]

- In determining the most appropriate treatment for patients with CLL, one must take into account the anticipated progression rate based on disease characteristics. To date, there are no data showing that in patients with aggressive disease, early intervention positively impacts survival. Therefore, even in the context of high risk features, we advocate an approach of "expectant observation." High risk features includes those patients with chromosomal del 11q, 17p deletion, lymphocyte doubling time <12 months, unmutated immunoglobulin heavy chain variable region genes, ZAP-70 (>20% positive), and CD38 (>30% positive)[1,15]

- With respect to stem cell transplant, transplant in the treatment of CLL continues to be defined. Due to the high relapse rates following autologous hematopoietic stem cell transplant (auto-HSCT) we believe that auto-HSCT for CLL should only be offered in the context of a clinical trial and should be considered early during the patient's clinical course, thus avoiding multiple therapies that may impair the ability to harvest the patient's stem cells or damage the patient's stem cells

- With respect to allogeneic stem cell transplant, an allogeneic transplant should only be considered in patients with exceptionally poor cytogenetics such as those patients who harbor del (17p) or del (11q), or those who are resistant to conventional therapy with fludarabine-based regimens. An allogeneic transplant is generally limited to younger patients (age <60) with a good performance status[16,17,18]

- Therapy of CLL may change dramatically in the next few years as highly active small molecules that target the B-cell receptor and BCL-2 should be approved. Lenalidomide, a small molecule with potent immunomodulatory activity, has activity in CLL and may also be approved for treatment of CLL in the near future[19]

[1]Hallek M et al. Blood 2008;111:5446–5456
[2]Abrisqueta P et al. Blood 2009;114:4916–4921
[3]Moreton P et al. J Clin Oncol 2005;23:2971–2979
[4]Hallek M et al. Lancet 2010;376:1164–1174
[5]Badoux X et al. Blood 2011;117:3016–3024
[6]Knauf WU et al. J Clin Oncol 2009;27(26):4378
[7]Fischer K et al. J Clin Oncol 2012 Sep;30(26):3209–3216
[8]Foon KA et al. J Clin Oncol 2009;27:498–503
[9]Samaniego F et al. Blood 2008;112–309
[10]Foon KA et al. Blood 2012;119:3184–3185
[11]Rai KR et al. N Engl J Med 2000;343:1750–1757
[12]Coiffier B et al. Blood 2008;111(3):1094
[13]Wierda WG et al. J Clin Oncol. 2010;28(10):1749
[14]Chowdhury O et al. Br J Haematol 2011 Nov;155(4):519–521
[15]Döhner H et al. NEJM 2000;343:1910–1916
[16]Dreger P et al. Leukemia 2007;21:12–17
[17]Boyiadzis M et al. Expert Opin Biol Ther 2007;7:1789–1797
[18]Delgado J et al. Blood 2009;114:2581–2588
[19]Badoux XC et al. Blood 2011;118 Abstract 98

CLL REGIMEN

FLUDARABINE + CYCLOPHOSPHAMIDE + RITUXIMAB (FCR)

Hallek M et al. Lancet 2010;376:1164–1174

Prophylaxis Against Tumor Lysis Syndrome—Cycle 1
Allopurinol 300 mg/day; administer orally or intravenously for 7 consecutive days, days 1–7

Premedication for rituximab—All Cycles
Acetaminophen 650 mg; administer orally 30–60 minutes before starting rituximab, *plus*
Diphenhydramine 25 mg; administer intravenously 30–60 minutes before starting rituximab

4-Week Cycles

Cycle 1	Cycles 2–6
Rituximab 375 mg/m^2; administer intravenously on day 0 (total dosage/cycle = 375 mg/m^2)	**Rituximab** 500 mg/m^2; administer intravenously on day 1 (total dosage/cycle = 500 mg/m^2)

Rituximab is diluted in 0.9% sodium chloride injection (0.9% NS) or 5% dextrose injection (D5W) to a concentration within the range of 1–4 mg/mL.

Notes on rituximab administration:
- During a first cycle, initiate rituximab infusion at a rate of 50 mg/hour. If hypersensitivity or infusion reactions do not occur during the first 30 minutes, the administration rate may be increased by 50 mg/hour every 30 minutes as tolerated, to a maximum rate of 400 mg/hour. Subsequently, if previous administration was well tolerated, start at 100 mg/hour, and escalate the rate as tolerated in increments of 100 mg/hour every 30 minutes to a maximum rate of 400 mg/hour
- Interrupt rituximab administration for fever, chills, edema, congestion of the head and neck mucosa, hypotension, and other serious adverse events. Resume rituximab administration at a slower rate after adverse events abate

Cycles 1–6

Cyclophosphamide 250 mg/m^2 per day; administer intravenously in 25–250 mL 0.9% NS or D5W over 10–30 minutes daily for 3 consecutive days on days 1–3 (total dosage/cycle = 750 mg/m^2)

Fludarabine 25 mg/m^2 per day; administer by intravenous infusion in 100–125 mL 0.9% NS or D5W over 20–30 minutes daily for 3 consecutive days on days 1–3 (total dosage/cycle = 75 mg/m^2)

- Fludarabine and cyclophosphamide administration begin 1 day after completing rituximab administration only during the first cycle
- During cycles 2–6, the day on which rituximab is given (day 1) and the first day on which fludarabine and cyclophosphamide are administered coincide

Supportive Care
Antiemetic prophylaxis
Emetogenic potential on Cycle 1, Day 0 is LOW
Emetogenic potential on Cycle 1, Days 1–3 is MODERATE
Emetogenic potential on Cycles 2–6, Days 1–3 is MODERATE
See Chapter 39 for antiemetic recommendations

Hematopoietic growth factor (CSF) prophylaxis
Primary prophylaxis is indicated with one of the following:
    Filgrastim (G-CSF) 5 mcg/kg per day by subcutaneous injection, *or*
    Pegfilgrastim (pegylated filgrastim) 6 mg/0.6 mL by subcutaneous injection for 1 dose
    - Begin use from 24–72 hours after myelosuppressive chemotherapy is completed
See Chapter 43 for more information

(continued)

Patient Population Studied

Study of 408 treatment naïve patients (ages: 30–81 years) with active chronic lymphocytic leukemia

Efficacy (N = 408)

Overall response	90%
Complete response	44%
Progression-free survival	median 51.8 months
Overall survival at 3 years	87%

Adverse Events (N = 404)
Toxicities Associated with FCR

	Grade 3 or Grade 4 %
Neutropenia	34
Thrombocytopenia	7
Anemia	5
Autoimmune hemolytic anemia	<1
Infections, total	25

Treatment Modifications

ANC ≤1000/mm^3 or platelet ≤80,000/mm^3 after the first treatment cycle	Treatment postponed until toxicity resolves. If delay >1 week, restart treatment with dose reduction of the cyclophosphamide dosage to 200 mg/m^2 per day and fludarabine dosage to 20 mg/m^2 per day. If further dose reduction is needed reduce the cyclophosphamide dosage to 150 mg/m^2 per day and fludarabine dosage to 15 mg/m^2 per day The rituximab dose is not reduced
Major infection	Reduce cyclophosphamide dosage to 200 mg/m^2 per day and fludarabine dosage to 20 mg/m^2 per day. If further dose reduction is needed reduce the cyclophosphamide dosage to 150 mg/m^2 per day and fludarabine dosage to 15 mg/m^2 per day The rituximab dose is not reduced

(continued)

Antimicrobial prophylaxis

Risk of fever and neutropenia is INTERMEDIATE

Antimicrobial primary prophylaxis to be considered:

- Antibacterial—consider a fluoroquinolone or no prophylaxis; *P. jirovecii* prophylaxis is recommended (eg, cotrimoxazole)

- Antifungal—consider concomitant use with a broad-spectrum antibacterial (eg, cotrimoxazole) and during periods of neutropenia

- Antiviral—antiherpes antivirals (eg, acyclovir, famciclovir, valacyclovir)

See Chapter 47 for more information

Infusion reactions associated with rituximab

Fevers, chills, and rigors

1. Interrupt rituximab administration for severe symptoms, and give:

- **Acetaminophen** 650 mg; administer orally for fever. For persistent or recurrent symptoms, repeat administration every 4–6 hours as needed during rituximab administration

- **Diphenhydramine** 25–50 mg; administer orally or by intravenous injection for pruritus, hypotension, or angioedema. For persistent or recurrent symptoms, repeat administration every 4–6 hours as needed during rituximab administration

- **Meperidine** 12.5–25 mg; administer by intravenous injection every 10–20 minutes as needed for shaking chills (generally, cumulative doses >100 mg are not needed; use repeated doses with caution in persons with moderate or more severely impaired renal function)

2. If rituximab administration was interrupted, resume infusion at a slower rate than the maximum rate previously attempted. Rate escalation may be reattempted at smaller incremental steps with close monitoring. Do not exceed the maximum recommended rate of 400 mg/hour

Dyspnea or wheezing without allergic findings (urticaria, or tongue or laryngeal edema)

1. Interrupt rituximab administration immediately

2. Give **hydrocortisone** 100 mg by intravenous injection (or an alternative steroid with equivalent glucocorticoid potency)

3. Give a **histamine (H$_2$)-receptor antagonist** (ranitidine 50 mg, cimetidine 300 mg, or famotidine 20 mg) intravenously over 15–30 minutes

After symptoms resolve, resume rituximab administration at 25 mg/hour with close monitoring. Do not increase the administration rate

Therapy Monitoring

1. *Prior to each cycle:* CBC with differential and serum electrolytes, BUN, creatinine, and LFTs

2. *Response evaluation:* every 2–3 cycles

ALTERNATIVE REGIMEN

FLUDARABINE + CYCLOPHOSPHAMIDE WITH HIGH-DOSE RITUXIMAB

Foon KA et al. J Clin Oncol 2009;27:498–503
Foon KA et al. Blood 2012;119:3184–3185

4-Week Cycles

Cycle 1	Cycles 2–6
Rituximab 375 mg/m^2; administer intravenously on day 1, *plus* **Rituximab** 500 mg/m^2; administer intravenously on day 14 (total dosage during the first cycle = 875 mg/m^2)	**Rituximab** 500 mg/m^2; administer intravenously on days 1 and 14 (total dosage/cycle = 1000 mg/m^2)

Rituximab is diluted in 0.9% sodium chloride injection (0.9% NS) or 5% dextrose injection (D5W) to a concentration within the range of 1–4 mg/mL

Notes on rituximab administration:
- During a first cycle, initiate rituximab infusion at a rate of 50 mg/hour. If hypersensitivity or infusion reactions do not occur during the first 30 minutes, the administration rate may be increased by 50 mg/hour every 30 minutes as tolerated, to a maximum rate of 400 mg/hour. Subsequently, if previous administration was well tolerated, start at 100 mg/hour, and escalate the rate as tolerated in increments of 100 mg/hour every 30 minutes to a maximum rate of 400 mg/hour
- Interrupt rituximab administration for fever, chills, edema, congestion of the head and neck mucosa, hypotension, and other serious adverse events. Resume rituximab administration at a slower rate after adverse events abate

Cycle 1	Cycles 2–6
Cyclophosphamide 150 mg/m^2 per day; administer intravenously in 25–250 mL 0.9% NS or D5W over 15–60 minutes daily for 3 consecutive days on days 2–4 (total dosage during cycle 1 = 450 mg/m^2)	**Cyclophosphamide** 150 mg/m^2 per day; administer intravenously in 25–250 mL 0.9% NS or D5W over 15–60 minutes daily for 3 consecutive days on days 1–3 (total dosage/cycle = 450 mg/m^2)
Fludarabine 20 mg/m^2 per day; administer by intravenous infusion in 100–125 mL 0.9% NS or D5W over 30 minutes, daily for 3 consecutive days on days 2–4 (total dosage during cycle 1 = 60 mg/m^2)	**Fludarabine** 20 mg/m^2 per day; administer by intravenous infusion in 100–125 mL 0.9% NS or D5W over 30 minutes, daily for 3 consecutive days on days 1–3 (total dosage/cycle = 60 mg/m^2)

After 6 cycles of combined chemoimmunotherapy, rituximab 500 mg/m^2 was administered once every 3 months until relapse

Supportive Care
Antiemetic prophylaxis
Emetogenic potential on Cycle 1, Day 1 is **LOW**
Emetogenic potential on Cycle 1, Days 2–4 is **MODERATE**
Emetogenic potential on Cycles 2–6, Days 1–3 is **MODERATE**
See Chapter 39 for antiemetic recommendations

Hematopoietic growth factor (CSF) prophylaxis
Primary prophylaxis is indicated with one of the following:
    Filgrastim (G-CSF) 5 mcg/kg per day by subcutaneous injection, *or*
    Pegfilgrastim (pegylated filgrastim) 6 mg/0.6 mL by subcutaneous injection for 1 dose
    - Begin use from 24–72 hours after myelosuppressive chemotherapy is completed
See Chapter 43 for more information

(continued)

Patient Population Studied

Study of 50 patients (median age: 58 years) with active chronic lymphocytic leukemia

Efficacy (N = 48)

Complete response	77%
Partial response	23%

Median duration of complete response: 22.3 months (range: 5.2–42.3 months)

(continued)

Antimicrobial prophylaxis

Risk of fever and neutropenia is INTERMEDIATE

Antimicrobial primary prophylaxis to be considered:

- Antibacterial—consider a fluoroquinolone or no prophylaxis; *P. jirovecii* prophylaxis is recommended (eg, cotrimoxazole)

- Antifungal—consider concomitant use with a broad-spectrum antibacterial (eg, cotrimoxazole) and during periods of neutropenia

- Antiviral—antiherpes antivirals (eg, acyclovir, famciclovir, valacyclovir)

See Chapter 47 for more information

Infusion reactions associated with rituximab

Fevers, chills, and rigors

1. Interrupt rituximab administration for severe symptoms, and give:

- **Acetaminophen** 650 mg; administer orally for fever. For persistent or recurrent symptoms, repeat administration every 4–6 hours as needed during rituximab administration

- **Diphenhydramine** 25–50 mg; administer orally or by intravenous injection for pruritus, hypotension, or angioedema. For persistent or recurrent symptoms, repeat administration every 4–6 hours as needed during rituximab administration

- **Meperidine** 12.5–25 mg; administer by intravenous injection every 10–20 minutes as needed for shaking chills (generally, cumulative doses >100 mg are not needed; use repeated doses with caution in persons with moderate or more severely impaired renal function)

2. If rituximab administration was interrupted, resume infusion at a slower rate than the maximum rate previously attempted. Rate escalation may be reattempted at smaller incremental steps with close monitoring. Do not exceed the maximum recommended rate of 400 mg/hour

Dyspnea or wheezing without allergic findings (urticaria, or tongue or laryngeal edema)

1. Interrupt rituximab administration immediately

2. Give **hydrocortisone** 100 mg by intravenous injection (or an alternative steroid with equivalent glucocorticoid potency)

3. Give a **histamine (H$_2$)-receptor antagonist** (ranitidine 50 mg, cimetidine 300 mg, or famotidine 20 mg) intravenously over 15–30 minutes

After symptoms resolve, resume rituximab administration at 25 mg/hour with close monitoring. Do not increase the administration rate

CLL REGIMEN

CHLORAMBUCIL

Rai KR et al. N Engl J Med 2000;343:1750–1757

Premedication: **Allopurinol** 300 mg/day; administer orally for 9 consecutive days, starting the day before chlorambucil is administered, every 28 days
• Continue use during the first 3 cycles
• Use may continue for additional cycles if clinically appropriate

Chlorambucil 40 mg/m²; administer orally on day 1 (single dose), every 28 days for a maximum of 12 cycles (total dosage/cycle = 40 mg/m²)

Alternative Chlorambucil Regimens
Dighiero G et al. N Engl J Med 1998;338:1506–1514
    Chlorambucil 0.3 mg/kg per day; administer orally for 5 consecutive days on days 1–5, every 28 days (total dosage/28-day cycle = 1.5 mg/kg), *or*
    Chlorambucil 0.1 mg/kg per day; administer orally continually for 28 consecutive days on days 1–28, every 28 days (total dosage/28-day cycle = 2.8 mg/kg)
    • Continue treatment until clinical resistance develops

Supportive Care
Antiemetic prophylaxis
Emetogenic potential is LOW
See Chapter 39 for antiemetic recommendations

Hematopoietic growth factor (CSF) prophylaxis
Primary prophylaxis is NOT indicated
See Chapter 43 for more information

Antimicrobial prophylaxis
Risk of fever and neutropenia is INTERMEDIATE
    Antimicrobial primary prophylaxis to be considered:
    • Antibacterial—consider a fluoroquinolone or no prophylaxis; *P. jirovecii* prophylaxis is recommended (eg, cotrimoxazole)
    • Antifungal—not indicated
    • Antiviral—antiherpes antivirals (eg, acyclovir, famciclovir, valacyclovir)
See Chapter 47 for more information

Patient Population Studied

Study of 181 previously untreated patients with stages I–IV CLL

Efficacy (N = 181)

Complete response	4%
Partial response	33%
Stable or progressive disease	63%
Median duration of response	14 months
Median survival	56 months

Toxicity (N = 178)

(CALGB Expanded Common Toxicity Criteria)

Toxicity	% Patients with G3/4
Thrombocytopenia	14
Neutropenia	19
Infection	9
Any G3/4 toxicity	44

Grade 3, Severe side effect; Grade 4, life-threatening side effect

Treatment Modification

Adverse Event	Treatment Modification
Hematologic toxicity G ≥3	Reduce chlorambucil dose 25%. For recurrent hematologic toxicity (G ≥3), further reduce chlorambucil dose an additional 25%. May cautiously re-escalate dose in subsequent cycles
Nonhematologic toxicity G ≥3	Reduce chlorambucil dose 25%. May cautiously re-escalate dose in subsequent cycles

Toxicity N = 161

Percentage of Patients with Hematologic Toxicity

	% G3 or G4
Neutropenia	23
Thrombocytopenia	19

Percentage of Patients with Nonhematologic Toxicity During Any Cycle

	% G1/2	% G3/4
Infection	4.3	1.9
Fatigue	7.5	1.2
Nausea/vomiting	34.8	1.8
Diarrhea	8.7	1.2
Rash	6.8	2.5
Hypersensitivity	3.8	1.2

Therapy Monitoring

1. *Prior to each cycle:* CBC with differential and serum electrolytes, BUN, creatinine, and LFTs
2. *Response evaluation:* every 2–3 cycles

Notes

1. Recommended as frontline therapy
2. Chlorambucil may be combined with rituximab

CLL REGIMEN
BENDAMUSTINE + RITUXIMAB

Fisher K et al. J Clin Oncol 2011;29:3559–3566

Premedication for Rituximab—All Cycles
Acetaminophen 650 mg orally 30–60 minutes before starting rituximab, *plus*
Diphenhydramine 25 mg intravenously 30–60 minutes before starting rituximab

4-Week Cycles

Cycle 1	Cycles 2–6
Rituximab 375 mg/m²; administer intravenously on day 0 (total dosage/cycle = 375 mg/m²)	**Rituximab** 500 mg/m²; administer intravenously on day 1 (total dosage/cycle = 500 mg/m²)

Rituximab is diluted in 0.9% sodium chloride injection (0.9% NS) or 5% dextrose injection (D5W) to a concentration within the range of 1–4 mg/mL

Notes on rituximab administration:
- During the first cycle, initiate rituximab infusion at a rate of 50 mg/hour. If hypersensitivity or infusion reactions do not occur during the first 30 minutes, the administration rate may be increased in 50-mg/hour increments every 30 minutes as tolerated, to a maximum rate of 400 mg/hour. Subsequently, if previous administration was well tolerated, start at 100 mg/hour, and escalate the rate as tolerated in increments of 100 mg/hour every 30 minutes to a maximum rate of 400 mg/hour
- Interrupt rituximab administration for fever, chills, edema, congestion of the head and neck mucosa, hypotension, and other serious adverse events. Resume rituximab administration at a slower rate after adverse events abate

Bendamustine HCl 70 mg/m² per day; administer intravenously in a volume of 0.9% NS or D2.5W/0.45% sodium chloride injection sufficient to produce a solution within the concentration range 0.2–0.6 mg/mL, over 30 minutes for 2 consecutive days, on days 1 and 2, every 4 weeks for up to 6 cycles depending on response and toxicity (total dosage/cycle = 140 mg/m²)

Supportive Care
Antiemetic prophylaxis
Emetogenic potential with rituximab alone is **MINIMAL**
Emetogenic potential on days with bendamustine is **MODERATE**
See Chapter 39 for antiemetic recommendations

Hematopoietic growth factor (CSF) prophylaxis
Primary prophylaxis is **NOT** *indicated*
See Chapter 43 for more information

Antimicrobial prophylaxis
Risk of fever and neutropenia is INTERMEDIATE
  Antimicrobial primary prophylaxis to be considered:
  - Antibacterial—consider a fluoroquinolone or no prophylaxis; *Pneumocystis jirovecii* prophylaxis is recommended (eg, cotrimoxazole)
  - Antifungal—consider use during neutropenia
  - Antiviral—antiherpes antivirals (eg, acyclovir, famciclovir, valacyclovir)
See Chapter 47 for more information

Dose Modifications

G4 hematologic toxicity or G ≥2 nonhematologic toxicities during second and subsequent cycles	Delay retreatment with bendamustine until ANC is ≥1000/mm³ and platelet count is ≥75,000/mm³, and nonhematologic toxicities remit to G ≤1, then resume bendamustine at 50 mg/m² per day on days 1 and 2, every 4 weeks. Consider reescalating bendamustine dosage to 70 mg/m² per dose only if G4 hematologic or G ≥2 nonhematologic toxicities do not recur after at least 1 cycle at 50 mg/m² per day on days 1 and 2
Recurrence of G4 hematologic toxicity or G ≥2 nonhematologic toxicities with bendamustine at 50 mg/m² per dose	Delay retreatment with bendamustine until ANC is ≥1000/mm³ and platelet count is ≥75,000/mm³, and nonhematologic toxicities remit to G ≤1, then resume bendamustine at 25 mg/m² per day on days 1 and 2, every 4 weeks. Consider reescalating bendamustine dosage to 50 mg/m² per dose only if G4 hematologic or G ≥2 nonhematologic toxicities do not recur after at least 1 cycle at 25 mg/m² per day on days 1 and 2

Efficacy

Factor	No. of Patients	OS Median (months)	P	PFS Median (months)	P	EFS Median (months)	P
All patients	78	33.9	—	15.197	—	14.7	—
Genetic subgroup							
17p deletion	14	16.3	0.007	6.8	0.19	4.8	0.044
11q deletion*	15	NR		15.9		15.9	
Trisomy 12†	5	20.5		16.9		10.7	
13q deletion‡	19	41.0		17.5		17.5	
No abnormalities according to the hierarchical model§	16	33.9		16.7		13.8	
IGVH status							
Unmutated	49	25.6	0.009	13.8	0.025	13.2	0.013
Mutated	23	NR		17.5		17.5	
Binet stage							
A	13	NR	0.93	17.5	0.7	15.9	0.831
B	24	33.9		14.7		14.7	
C	34	NR		15.2		13.8	
No. of previous therapies							
≤2	56	36.2	0.02	16.5	0.07	15.2	0.198
>2	18	24.0		11.6		11.6	

EFS, event-free survival; NR, not reached at time of analysis; OS, overall survival; PFS, progression-free survival
*Not including 17p deletion
†Not including 17p deletion or 11q deletion
‡Not including 17p deletion, 11q deletion, or trisomy 12
§Not including 17p deletion, 11q deletion, 13q deletion, or trisomy 12

Toxicity

Adverse events according to patients (n = 78)	Grade 3 No.	%	Grade 4 No.	%
Total patients with at least 1 G3 or G4 event	21	26.9	19	24.4
Hematologic toxicity	19	24.4	20	25.6
Leukopenia	8	10.3	6	7.7
Neutropenia	7	9.0	11	14.1
Thrombocytopenia	11	14.1	11	14.1
Anemia	9	11.5	4	5.1
Tumor lysis syndrome	0	0	0	0
Hemolysis	2	2.6	0	0
Allergic reaction	2	2.6	0	0
Infections	10	12.8	0	0
Other nonhematologic toxicities	9	11.5	2	2

Patient Population Studied

Seventy-eight patients with relapsed and/or refractory CLL; 22 patients had fludarabine refractory disease; 14 patients had deletion of 17p

Monitoring Therapy

1. Prior to each cycle: CBC with differential and serum electrolytes, BUN, creatinine, and liver function tests
2. A response assessment may be performed after 2 cycles and/or at the completion of therapy. This may include peripheral blood flow cytometry and/or a bone marrow biopsy and aspirate

CLL REGIMEN

OFATUMUMAB

Coiffier B et al. Blood 2008;111:1094–1100

Premedications before each ofatumumab dose:

Acetaminophen 1000 mg; administer orally 30 minutes to 2 hours before starting ofatumumab

Cetirizine 10 mg (or equivalent H_1 receptor antagonist); administer orally 30 minutes to 2 hours before starting ofatumumab

Prednisolone 100 mg (or another glucocorticoid at an equipotent dose); administer intravenously 30 minutes to 2 hours before starting ofatumumab

• Prednisolone 100 mg (*or glucocorticoid equivalent*) should be given prior to ofatumumab during weeks 1, 2, and 9

• Glucocorticoid doses may be gradually decreased during weeks 3–8 if an infusion reaction G ≥3 did not occur with preceding ofatumumab doses

• For doses 10–12, give prednisolone 50–100 mg/dose (*or glucocorticoid equivalent*) if an infusion reaction G ≥3 did not occur with preceding ofatumumab doses

Initial Ofatumumab Dose (week 1):

Ofatumumab 300 mg; administer intravenously in a total volume of 1000 mL 0.9% sodium chloride injection (0.9% NS), *followed 1 week later by:*

Subsequent Ofatumumab Doses (weeks 2–8, 12, 16, 20, and 24):

Ofatumumab 2000 mg/dose; administer intravenously in a total volume of 1000 mL 0.9% NS, weekly for 7 consecutive weeks (weeks 2–8), *followed 4 weeks later by:*

Ofatumumab 2000 mg/dose; administer intravenously in a total volume of 1000 mL 0.9% NS every 4 weeks for 4 doses (weeks 12, 16, 20, and 24)

Ofatumumab administration rates:

Initial dose (Ofatumumab 0.3 mg/mL)

Interval After Starting Administration	Administration Rate	
	(mL/h)	(mg/h)
0–30 min	12	3.6
31–60 min	25	7.5
61–90 min	50	15
91–120 min	100	30
>120 min	200	60

Second dose (Ofatumumab 2 mg/mL)

Interval After Starting Administration	Administration Rate	
	(mL/h)	(mg/h)
0–30 min	12	24
31–60 min	25	50
61–90 min	50	100
91–120 min	100	200
>120 min	200	400

(continued)

Treatment Modification

Adverse Event	Treatment Modification
Grade 4 infusion reaction	Do not resume the infusion
Grades 1, 2, or 3 infusion reactions	If an infusion reaction resolves or remains G ≤2, resume the infusion with the following modifications according to the initial grade of the infusion reaction • G1 or G2: Infuse at 50% of the previous infusion rate • G3: Infuse at 12 mL/hour After resuming the infusion the rate may be increased according to the recommended ofatumumab administration rates (above), based on patient tolerance

Efficacy (N = 33)

Objective Response Rate (%)

Cohort A	1(33)
Cohort B	0
Cohort C	13(50)

Patient Population Studied

Thirty-three patients with relapsed or refractory B-cell CLL who had already received treatment with rituximab.

Patients received once weekly infusions of ofatumumab. Patients were divided into 3 cohorts based on the dose of ofatumumab:

A. One 100-mg dose followed after 1 week by 3 weekly 500-mg doses; N = 3

B. One 300-mg dose followed after 1 week by 3 weekly 1000-mg doses; N = 3

C. One 500-mg dose followed after 1 week by 3 weekly 2000-mg doses; N = 27

(continued)

Doses 3–12 (Ofatumumab 2 mg/mL)

Interval After Starting Administration	Administration Rate	
	(mL/h)	(mg/h)
0–30 min	25	50
31–60 min	50	100
61–90 min	100	200
91–120 min	200	400
>120 min	400	800

Supportive Care

Antiemetic prophylaxis
Emetogenic potential is MINIMAL
See Chapter 39 for antiemetic recommendations

Hematopoietic growth factor (CSF) prophylaxis
Primary prophylaxis is NOT indicated
See Chapter 43 for more information

Risk of Fever and Neutropenia is HIGH
   Antimicrobial primary prophylaxis is recommended:
   • Antibacterial—*Pneumocystis jirovecii* prophylaxis is recommended (eg, cotrimoxazole)
   • Antifungal—recommended
   • Antiviral—antiherpes antivirals (eg, acyclovir)
See Chapter 47 for more information

Toxicities

Grades 3 and 4 adverse events according to NCI Common Terminology Criteria for Adverse Events (CTCAE), version 3.0

	No. of Patients	No. of Events
Total no. subjects with G3 or G4 adverse events	10	18
Thrombocytopenia	3	4
Neutropenia	2	2
Anemia, NOS	1	1
Infection	3	3
Pyrexia	2	2
Pain NOS	1	1
Nervous system disorders	2	2
Angina	1	1
Cytolytic hepatitis	1	1
Hypoxia	1	1

Infusion-related toxicities decreased with time

Other Treatment-Related Events	% G1/2	% G3/4
Infections	28	27
Septicemia	4	11
CMV reactivation	3	4
Neutropenia	30% during weeks 5/6	
Thrombocytopenia	In first 2 weeks	

Monitoring Therapy

1. *Every week:* PE, CBC with differential, serum electrolytes, and creatinine
2. *Response evaluation:* after the sixth weekly infusion (lab work and physical exam only) and at the completion of therapy

Notes

1. Progressive multifocal leukoencephalopathy (PML), including fatal PML, can occur with ofatumumab. Consider PML in any patient with new onset of or changes in preexisting neurologic signs or symptoms. Discontinue ofatumumab if PML is suspected and initiate evaluation including neurologic consult, brain MRI and lumbar puncture
2. Hepatitis B Infection (HBV) and reactivation may occur in patients following treatment with ofatumumab. Screen patients at high risk for HBV prior to initiating therapy. Closely monitor carriers of hepatitis B for clinical and laboratory signs of active HBV during treatment and for 12 months following the last infusion of ofatumumab

CLL REGIMEN

FLUDARABINE + RITUXIMAB

Byrd JC et al. Blood 2003;101:6–14
Woyach JA et al. J Clin Oncol 2011;29:1349–1355

Premedication:
Allopurinol 300 mg/day; administer orally for 14 consecutive days on days 1–14
Acetaminophen 650 mg; administer orally 30 minutes before rituximab
Diphenhydramine 50 mg; administer by intravenous injection 30 minutes before rituximab

Fludarabine 25 mg/m^2 per day; administer by intravenous infusion in 100–125 mL 5% dextrose injection (D5W) or 0.9% sodium chloride injection (0.9% NS) over 20–30 minutes for 5 consecutive day on days 1–5, every 28 days for 6 cycles (total dosage/cycle = 125 mg/m^2)

Cycle 1: Rituximab 375 mg/m^2 per dose; administer by intravenous infusion in a volume of D5W or 0.9% NS sufficient to produce a concentration within the range 1–4 mg/mL for 2 doses on days 1 and 4 (total dosage/cycle 1 = 750 mg/m^2)

Cycles 2–6: Rituximab 375 mg/m^2; administer by intravenous infusion in a volume of D5W or 0.9% NS sufficient to produce a concentration within the range 1–4 mg/mL on day 1, every 28 days for 5 cycles (total dosage/cycle = 375 mg/m^2)

Supportive Care
Antiemetic prophylaxis
Emetogenic potential is **MINIMAL**
See Chapter 39 for antiemetic recommendations

Hematopoietic growth factor (CSF) prophylaxis
Primary prophylaxis may be indicated
See Chapter 43 for more information

Antimicrobial prophylaxis
Risk of fever and neutropenia is INTERMEDIATE
Antimicrobial primary prophylaxis to be considered:
- Antibacterial—consider a fluoroquinolone or no prophylaxis; *P. jirovecii* prophylaxis is recommended (eg, cotrimoxazole)
- Antifungal—consider concomitant use with cotrimoxazole, during periods of neutropenia
- Antiviral—antiherpes antivirals (eg, acyclovir, famciclovir, valacyclovir)

See Chapter 47 for more information

Infusion reactions associated with rituximab
Fevers, chills, and rigors

1. Interrupt rituximab administration for severe symptoms, and give:
   - **Acetaminophen** 650 mg; administer orally for fever. For persistent or recurrent symptoms, repeat administration every 4–6 hours as needed during rituximab administration
   - **Diphenhydramine** 25–50 mg; administer orally or by intravenous injection for pruritus, hypotension, or angioedema. For persistent or recurrent symptoms, repeat administration every 4–6 hours as needed during rituximab administration
   - **Meperidine** 12.5–25 mg; administer by intravenous injection every 10–20 minutes as needed for shaking chills (generally, cumulative doses >100 mg are not needed; use repeated doses with caution in persons with moderate or more severely impaired renal function)
2. If rituximab administration was interrupted, resume infusion at a slower rate than the maximum rate previously attempted. Rate escalation may be reattempted at smaller incremental steps with close monitoring. Do not exceed the maximum recommended rate of 400 mg/hour

Dyspnea or wheezing without allergic findings (urticaria, or tongue or laryngeal edema)

1. Interrupt rituximab administration immediately
2. Give **hydrocortisone** 100 mg by intravenous injection (or an alternative steroid with equivalent glucocorticoid potency)
3. Give a **histamine (H$_2$) receptor antagonist** (ranitidine 50 mg, cimetidine 300 mg, or famotidine 20 mg) intravenously over 15–30 minutes

After symptoms resolve, resume rituximab administration at 25 mg/hours with close monitoring. Do not increase the administration rate

Patient Population Studied
Study of 104 previously untreated patients with symptomatic CLL

Efficacy (N = 104)

Overall response rate	84%
Complete response rate	38%
Estimated 5-year progression-free survival	28%
Median overall survival	85 months

Adverse Events (N = 51)
Hematologic Toxicity (Modified NCI Criteria for CLL)

Toxicity	% G1/2	% G3/4
Neutropenia	8	76
Thrombocytopenia	47	20
Anemia	65	4
Infection	43	20

Nonhematologic Toxicity (NCI CTC)

Toxicity	% G1/2	% G3/4
Nausea	48	0
Vomiting	16	0
Myalgias	28	0
Fatigue/malaise	62	0
Dyspnea/hypoxemia*	12	14
Hypotension*	10	6
Fever*	32	0
Chills/rigors*	36	0
G3/4 pulmonary toxicity	3 cases	
Thrombocytopenic purpura	1 case	
Pure red cell aplasia	1 case	

*Infusion-related toxicities occurred in 100% of patients during the first administration of rituximab. Usually G1/2, although 20% experienced G3/4. Only 2 patients (4%) experienced infusion-related adverse events during a second administration

Treatment Modifications

Adverse Event	Treatment Modification
Fludarabine-Related Toxicities	
G3 neutropenia, thrombocytopenia, or anemia	Delay treatment until recovery to within 20% of baseline, then resume treatment with dosage of fludarabine reduced by 25%
G4 neutropenia, thrombocytopenia, or anemia	Delay treatment until recovery to within 20% of baseline, then resume treatment with dosage of fludarabine reduced by 50%
Infection without G3/4 neutropenia	Hold treatment until infection resolves, then restart at the same dosages
Evidence of autoimmune hemolytic anemia or thrombocytopenia	Replace rituximab and fludarabine with alternative treatment as appropriate
Grade ≥2 nonhematologic adverse events attributable to fludarabine, except nausea, vomiting, fatigue, diarrhea, infusion-related fever, or chills	Reduce fludarabine dosage by 50%
G3/4, or irreversible G2 nonhematologic toxicity	Reduce fludarabine dosage by 50%, or consider withdrawing fludarabine

Therapy Monitoring

1. *Before each cycle:* CBC with differential and serum electrolytes, creatinine, and LFTs
2. *Response evaluation:* every 3 cycles

Note

Recommended as initial therapy for patients with CLL. This regimen is increasingly used in combination with cyclophosphamide

CLL REGIMEN

PENTOSTATIN + CYCLOPHOSPHAMIDE + RITUXIMAB

Lamanna N et al. J Clin Oncol 2006;24:1575–1581

Hydration: ≥1500 mL 0.9% sodium chloride injection (0.9% NS) at ≥100 mL/hour before cyclophosphamide every 21 days

Premedication:
Allopurinol 300 mg/day administer orally for 9 consecutive days, starting the day before chemotherapy treatment begins, every 21 days
• Continue use during the first 2 cycles
• Use may continue for additional cycles if clinically appropriate

Cycles 1–6:
Cyclophosphamide 600 mg/m²; administer by intravenous infusion in 50–150 mL 5% dextrose injection (D5W) or 0.9% NS over 15–60 minutes, on day 1, every 3 weeks for up to 6 cycles (total dosage/cycle = 600 mg/m²), *followed by:*

Pentostatin 4 mg/m²; administer by intravenous infusion in 25–50 mL D5W or 0.9% NS, over 20–30 minutes, on day 1, every 3 weeks for up to 6 cycles (total dosage/cycle = 4 mg/m²)

Cycles 2–6:
Rituximab 375/m²; administer by intravenous infusion in a volume of D5W or 0.9% NS sufficient to produce a concentration within the range 1–4 mg/mL, on day 1 of cycles 2–6 after pentostatin administration is completed, every three weeks for 5 cycles (total dosage/cycle = 375 mg/m²)

Filgrastim; administer by subcutaneous injection, daily, starting on cycle day 3 and continuing until patient achieves a single postnadir ANC >5000/mm³, or an ANC >1500/ mm³ on 2 consecutive days

Filgrastim doses are based on a patient's body weight as follows:

Body Weight	Filgrastim Dose
≤70 kg	300 mcg/day
>70 kg	480 mcg/day

Supportive Care
Antiemetic prophylaxis
Emetogenic potential is **MODERATE**
See Chapter 39 for antiemetic recommendations

Hematopoietic growth factor (CSF) prophylaxis
Primary prophylaxis is indicated with one of the following:
  Filgrastim (G-CSF) 5 mcg/kg per day by subcutaneous injection, *or*
  Pegfilgrastim (pegylated filgrastim) 6 mg/0.6 mL by subcutaneous injection for 1 dose
  • Begin use from 24–72 hours after myelosuppressive chemotherapy is completed
See Chapter 43 for more information

Antimicrobial prophylaxis
Risk of fever and neutropenia is INTERMEDIATE
  Antimicrobial primary prophylaxis to be considered:
  • Antibacterial—consider a fluoroquinolone or no prophylaxis; *P. jirovecii* prophylaxis is recommended (eg, cotrimoxazole)
  • Antifungal—consider concomitant use with cotrimoxazole, during periods of neutropenia
  • Antiviral—antiherpes antivirals (eg, acyclovir, famciclovir, valacyclovir)
See Chapter 47 for more information

(continued)

Treatment Modifications

Adverse Event	Treatment Modification
Serum creatinine >2 mg/dL (>177 μmol/L) or increased by 20% above baseline	Hold treatment until serum creatinine ≤2 mg/dL (≤177 μmol/L) or is <20% greater than baseline result, or creatinine clearance ≥50 mL/min (≥0.83 mL/s)
G2 toxicity	Hold drug until G ≤1 then restart at same dose
Repeated G2 toxicity	Hold drug until G ≤1 then restart at with all drug dosages decreased by 25%
G3/4 toxicity	Hold drug until G ≤1 then restart with all drug dosages decreased by 25–50%
Patient whose disease does not achieve at least a PR after 3 cycles	Therapy considered ineffective and discontinued

Efficacy (N = 32)

Complete response	25%
Partial response	47%
Stable disease	3%
Median response duration	25 months
Median survival	44 months

(continued)

Infusion reactions associated with rituximab

Fevers, chills, and rigors

1. Interrupt rituximab administration for severe symptoms, and give:

   • **Acetaminophen** 650 mg; administer orally for fever. For persistent or recurrent symptoms, repeat administration every 4–6 hours as needed during rituximab administration

   • **Diphenhydramine** 25–50 mg; administer orally or by intravenous injection for pruritus, hypotension, or angioedema. For persistent or recurrent symptoms, repeat administration every 4–6 hours as needed during rituximab administration

   • **Meperidine** 12.5–25 mg; administer by intravenous injection every 10–20 minutes as needed for shaking chills (generally, cumulative doses >100 mg are not needed; use repeated doses with caution in persons with moderate or more severely impaired renal function)

2. If rituximab administration was interrupted, resume infusion at a slower rate than the maximum rate previously attempted. Rate escalation may be reattempted at smaller incremental steps with close monitoring. Do not exceed the maximum recommended rate of 400 mg/hour

Dyspnea or wheezing without allergic findings (urticaria, or tongue or laryngeal edema)

1. Interrupt rituximab administration immediately

2. Give **hydrocortisone** 100 mg by intravenous injection (or an alternative steroid with equivalent glucocorticoid potency)

3. Give a **histamine (H_2)-receptor antagonist** (ranitidine 50 mg, cimetidine 300 mg, or famotidine 20 mg) intravenously over 15–30 minutes

4. After symptoms resolve, resume rituximab administration at 25 mg/hour with close monitoring. Do not increase the administration rate

Patient Population Studied

Study of 32 previously treated patients with CLL. Patients had previously received from 1–7 regimens (median: 2). In 32% of patients, disease was refractory to prior fludarabine

Toxicity (N = 32)
Hematologic Toxicity
(NCI Working Group Guidelines)

Toxicity	% G3/4
Anemia	9
Thrombocytopenia	16
Neutropenia	53

Nonhematologic Toxicity
(NCI CTC)

Toxicity	% G3/4
Infection	28
Nausea	3
Vomiting	0
Constipation	0
Hepatic toxicity	0
Renal toxicity	0
Neurotoxicity	0

Therapy Monitoring

1. *Before each cycle:* CBC with differential and serum electrolytes, BUN, creatinine, and LFTs

2. *Response evaluation:* every 3 cycles

CLL REGIMEN
IBRUTINIB

Byrd JC et al. N Engl J Med 2013;369:32–42

Ibrutinib 420 mg/day orally, continually (total dose/week = 2940 mg)
Note: Administration with food increases ibrutinib exposure approximately 2-fold compared with administration after overnight fasting (IMBRUVICA [ibrutinib] capsules, for oral use; November 2013 product label. Janssen Biotech, Inc. Horsham, PA-C, USA)

Supportive Care
Antiemetic prophylaxis
Emetogenic potential is **LOW**
See Chapter 39 for antiemetic recommendations

Hematopoietic growth factor (CSF) prophylaxis
Primary prophylaxis is **NOT** *indicated*
See Chapter 43 for more information

Antimicrobial prophylaxis
Risk of fever and neutropenia is LOW
Antimicrobial primary prophylaxis to be considered:
- Antibacterial—not indicated
- Antifungal—not indicated
- Antiviral—not indicated unless patient previously had an episode of HSV

See Chapter 47 for more information

Diarrhea management
Latent or delayed-onset diarrhea*:
Loperamide 4 mg; administer orally initially after the first loose or liquid stool, *then*
Loperamide 2 mg every 2 hours while awake; every 4 hours during sleep
Alternatively, a trial of **Diphenoxylate hydrochloride** 2.5 mg **with Atropine sulfate** 0.025 mg (eg, Lomotil®) two tablets four times daily until control has been achieved

Persistent diarrhea:
Octreotide acetate (solution) 100–150 mcg; administer subcutaneously 3 times daily

Antibiotic therapy during latent or delayed-onset diarrhea:
A fluoroquinolone (eg, **Ciprofloxacin** 500 mg orally every 12 hours) if absolute neutrophil count $<500/mm^3$

*Rothenberg ML et al. J Clin Oncol 2001;19:3801–3807
Wadler S et al. J Clin Oncol 1998;16:3169–3178
Abigerges D et al. J Natl Cancer Inst 1994;86:446–449

Oral care
Encourage patients to maintain intake of non-alcoholic fluids
If mucositis or stomatitis is present:
- Rinse mouth several times a day with 1/4 teaspoon (1.25 g) each of baking soda and table salt in one quart of warm water. Follow with a plain water rinse
- Do not use mouthwashes that contain alcohols

Patient Population Studied
Byrd JC et al. N Engl J Med 2013;369:32–42

Patients with a diagnosis of relapsed or refractory CLL or small lymphocytic lymphoma, defined according to the International Workshop on Chronic Lymphocytic Leukemia and World Health Organization classifications. Those enrolled were deemed to be in need of treatment. The first and second cohorts were required to have received ≥2 previous therapies, including a purine analog. A third cohort included patients with high-risk disease that did not respond to a chemoimmunotherapy regimen or whose disease progressed within 24 months after completion of the regimen

Treatment Monitoring
1. *Before treatment:* physical examination; CBC with differential; assessment of serum chemistry; and bone marrow aspiration and biopsy as indicated
2. *Assessment of efficacy:* Every 2 to 3 cycles

Efficacy (N = 85)

Byrd JC et al. N Engl J Med 2013;369:32–42

Subgroup	Number	ORR (95% CI)*
All patients	85	71% (60–80)
Dose		
420 mg	51	71% (56–82)
840 mg	34	71% (52–85)
Age		
<70 years	55	69% (55–81)
≥70 years	30	73% (54–88)
Rai stage at baseline		
0 (low-risk) I, or II (intermediate-risk)	29	69% (49–85)
III or IV (high risk)	55	71% (57–82)
Previous chemotherapy		
<3 Regimens	27	74% (54–89)
≥3 Regimens	58	69% (56–81)
17p13.1 deletion		
Positive	28	68% (48–84)
Negative	52	71% (57–83)
11q22.3 deletion		
Positive	31	77% (59–90)
Negative	49	65% (50–78)
IGHV (immunoglobulin variable-region heavy-chain gene)		
Mutated	12	33% (10–65)
Unmutated	69	77% (65–86)
β_2-Microglobulin		
≤3 mg/L	39	72% (55–85)
>3 mg/L	41	68% (52–82)

*Only patients who received ibrutinib and had at least one post-baseline assessment

Dose Modification

Toxicity Occurrence	CLL Dose Modification After Recovery Starting Dose = 420 mg
First	Restart at 420 mg daily
Second	Restart at 280 mg daily
Third	Restart at 140 mg daily
Fourth	Discontinue ibrutinib

Interrupt ibrutinib therapy for any Grade 3 or greater nonhematological, Grade 3 or greater neutropenia with infection or fever, or Grade 4 hematological toxicities. Once the symptoms of the toxicity have resolved to Grade 1 or baseline (recovery), ibrutinib therapy may be reinitiated at the starting dose. If the toxicity reoccurs, reduce dose by one capsule (140 mg per day). A second reduction of dose by 140 mg may be considered as needed. If these toxicities persist or recur following two dose reductions, discontinue ibrutinib

Toxicity (N = 48)*

System Organ		All Grades (%)	Grade 3 or 4 (%)
Gastrointestinal disorders	Diarrhea	63	4
	Constipation	23	2
	Nausea	21	2
	Stomatitis	21	0
	Vomiting	19	2
	Abdominal pain	15	0
	Dyspepsia	13	0
Infections and infestations	Upper respiratory tract infection	48	2
	Sinusitis	21	6
	Skin infection	17	6
	Pneumonia	10	8
	Urinary tract infection	10	0
General disorders and administrative site conditions	Fatigue	31	4
	Pyrexia	25	2
	Peripheral edema	23	0
	Asthenia	13	4
	Chills	13	0
Skin and subcutaneous tissue disorders	Bruising	54	2
	Rash	27	0
	Petechiae	17	0
Respiratory, thoracic and mediastinal disorders	Cough	19	0
	Oropharyngeal pain	15	0
	Dyspnea	10	0
Musculoskeletal and connective tissue disorders	Musculoskeletal pain	27	6
	Arthralgia	23	0
	Musclespasms	19	2
Nervous system disorders	Dizziness	21	0
	Headache	19	2
	Peripheral neuropathy	10	0
Metabolism and nutrition disorders	Decreased appetite	17	2
Neoplasms benign, malignant, unspecified	Second malignancies	10	0
Injury, poisoning, and procedural complications	Laceration	10	2
Psychiatric disorders	Anxiety	10	0
	Insomnia	10	0
Vascular disorders	Hypertension	17	8

Treatment-Emergent Decrease of Hemoglobin, Platelets, or Neutrophils in Patients with CLL (N = 48)

	Percent of Patients (N = 48)	
	All Grades (%)	Grade 3 or 4 (%)
Platelets decreased	71	10
Neutrophils decreased	54	27
Hemoglobin decreased	44	0

CLL REGIMEN

OBINUTUZUMAB + CHLORAMBUCIL

Goede et al. N Engl J Med 2014;370:1101–1110

Chlorambucil 650 0.5 mg/kg; administer orally on days 1 and 15 of each 28-day cycle (total dose per cycle: 1 mg/kg)

Obinutuzumab administer as an intravenous infusion in 100–250 mL of 0.9% normal saline (NS) to a final concentration of 0.4–4 mg/mL every 28 days as follows:

Day 1, Cycle 1:	100 mg	Administer at 25 mg/hr over 4 hours. Do not increase the infusion rate
Day 2, Cycle 1:	900 mg	Administer at 50 mg/hr. The rate of the infusion can be escalated in increments of 50 mg/hr every 30 minutes to a maximum rate of 400 mg/hr
Days 8 and 15, Cycle 1:	1000 mg	Infusions can be started at a rate of 100 mg/hr and increased by 100 mg/hr increments every 30 minutes to a maximum of 400 mg/hr
Day 1, Cycles 2–6:	1000 mg	

Premedicate with glucocorticoid acetaminophen and anti-histamine

Premedication for Obinutuzumab Infusion to Reduce Infusion-Related Reactions (IRR)

Day of Treatment Cycle	Patients Requiring Premedication	Premedication	Administration
Cycle 1: Day 1, Day 2	All patients	Intravenous glucocorticoid: 20 mg dexamethasone or 80 mg methylprednisolone*	Completed at least 1 hour prior to obinutuzumab infusion
		650–1000 mg acetaminophen	At least 30 minutes before obinutuzumab infusion
		Anti-histamine (eg, diphenhydramine 50 mg)	
Cycle 1: Day 8, Day 15 Cycles 2–6: Day 1	All patients	650–1000 mg acetaminophen	≥30 minutes before obinutuzumab infusion
	IRR (≥G1) with previous infusion	Anti-histamine (eg, diphenhydramine 50 mg)	≥30 minutes before obinutuzumab infusion
	G3 IRR with previous infusion OR lymphocyte count >25 × 10⁹/L prior to next treatment	Intravenous glucocorticoid: 20 mg dexamethasone or 80 mg methylprednisolone*	Completed ≥1 hour prior to obinutuzumab infusion

*Hydrocortisone not recommended; has not been effective in reducing rate of infusion reactions
Adapted from: gene.com/download/pdf/gazyva_prescribing.pdf

Notes:

• Hepatitis B Virus (HBV) reactivation, in some cases resulting in fulminant hepatitis, hepatic failure, and death, can occur in patients receiving CD20-directed cytolytic antibodies, including obinutuzumab. Screen all patients for HBV infection before treatment initiation. Monitor HBV positive patients during and after treatment with obinutuzumab. Discontinue obinutuzumab and concomitant medications in the event of HBV reactivation

• Progressive multifocal leukoencephalopathy (PML), including fatal PML, can occur in patients receiving obinutuzumab

• Obinutuzumab can cause severe and life-threatening infusion reactions. Symptoms may include hypotension, tachycardia, dyspnea, and respiratory symptoms (eg, bronchospasm, larynx and throat irritation, wheezing, laryngeal edema). Other common symptoms include nausea, vomiting, diarrhea, hypertension, flushing, headache, pyrexia, and chills

• *Two-thirds of patients experienced a reaction to the first 1000 mg infused of obinutuzumab. Infusion reactions can also occur with subsequent infusions*

• Premedicate patients before each infusion. Closely monitor patients during the entire infusion. Infusion reactions occur within 24 hours of receiving obinutuzumab

• Hypotension may occur as an infusion reaction. Consider withholding antihypertensive treatments for 12 hours prior to and during each obinutuzumab infusion, and for the first hour after administration until blood pressure is stable

Dose Modifications

Adverse Event	Dose Adjustment
G1/2 obinituzumab infusion reactions	Interrupt or reduce the rate of the infusion and manage symptoms
G3 obinituzumab infusion reactions	Interrupt obinituzumab until resolution of symptoms
G4 obinituzumab infusion reactions including but not limited to anaphylaxis, acute life-threatening respiratory symptoms, or other life-threatening infusion reactions	Stop the obinituzumab infusion. Permanently discontinue obinituzumab
Patient who develops PML	Discontinue obinituzumab therapy and consider discontinuation or reduction of any concomitant chemotherapy or immunosuppressive therapy
G3/4 neutropenia	Strongly recommended to receive antimicrobial prophylaxis throughout the treatment period. Antiviral and antifungal prophylaxis should be considered

Efficacy

Metric	Obinutuzumab + Chlorambucil [O + C]	Rituximab + Chlorambucil [R + C]	Chlorambucil-Alone [CA]
ORR 3 months > the end of treatment	77.3–78.4%	65.1–65.7%	31.4%
	O + C vs R + C: P <0.001		
	O + C vs CA: P < 0.001		
	R + C vs CA: P <0.001		
CR 3 months > the end of treatment	55–57.7	58.1–58.4	—
PR 3 months > the end of treatment	20.7–22.3	7.0–7.3	31.4
Median PFS	26.7 months	16.3 months	11.1 months
	O + C vs CA: HR for progression or death, 0.18; 95% CI, 0.13–0.24; P <0.001		
	R + C vs CA: HR, 0.44; 95% CI, 0.34–0.57; P <0.001		
Median PFS	26.7 months	15.2 months	
	O + C vs R + C: HR, 0.39; 95% CI, 0.31–0.49; P <0.001		
Rate negative MRD in bone marrow	19.5%	2.6%	
	O + C vs R + C: P <0.001		
Rate negative MRD in peripheral blood	37.7%	3.3%	
	O + C vs R + C: P <0.001		
Rates of death	8–9%	12%	20%,
	O + C vs CA: HR for death, 0.41; 95% CI, 0.23–0.74; P = 0.002		
	O + C vs R + C: HR, 0.66; 95% CI, 0.41–1.06; P = 0.08		

CI, confidence interval; CR, complete response; HR, hazard ratio; MRD, minimal residual disease; ORR, overall response rates; PFS, progression-free survival; PR, partial response

Toxicity

Adverse Events of Grade 3 or Higher, Safety Population*

| | Obinutuzumab–Chlorambucil vs. Chlorambucil Alone | | Obinutuzumab–Chlorambucil vs. Rituximab–Chlorambucil | |
| | Obinutuzumab–Chlorambucil (N = 241) | Chlorambucil Alone (N = 116) | Obinutuzumab–Chlorambucil (N = 336) | Rituximab–Chlorambucil (N = 321) |
Event	Number of Patients (percent)			
Any event	175 (73)	58 (50)	235 (70)	177 (55)
Infusion-related reactions	51 (21)	—	67 (20)	12 (4)
Neutropenia	84 (35)	18 (16)	111 (33)	91 (28)
Anemia	11 (5)	5 (4)	14 (4)	12 (4)
Thrombocytopenia	27 (11)	5 (4)	35 (10)	10 (3)
Leukopenia	13 (5)	0	15 (4)	3 (1)
Infections	27 (11)	16 (14)	40 (12)	44 (14)
Pneumonia	8 (3)	4 (3)	13 (4)	17 (5)
Febrile neutropenia	4 (2)	5 (4)	8 (2)	4 (1)

*The safety population included all patients who received at least one dose of study medication. Shown are adverse events of grade 3, 4, or 5 with an incidence of 3% or higher in any treatment group, irrespective of whether the event was considered related or unrelated to treatment by the investigators

Patient Population Studied

Open-label study that enrolled patients with CD20-positive CLL that was diagnosed according to the criteria of the International Workshop on Chronic Lymphocytic Leukemia. Previously untreated patients requiring treatment (ie, those with Binet stage C or symptomatic disease) were included. Enrolled patients were required to have a clinically meaningful burden of coexisting conditions, as reflected by a score higher than 6 on the Cumulative Illness Rating Scale (CIRS) (range, 0 to 56, with higher scores indicating worse health status) or a creatinine clearance of 30 to 69 mL per minute as assessed with the use of the Cockcroft–Gault formula

Treatment Modifications

1. *Before treatment:* physical examination; CBC with differential; assessment of serum chemistry; and bone marrow aspiration and biopsy as indicated
2. *Assessment of efficacy:* Every 2 to 3 cycles

20. Leukemia, Chronic Myelogenous

Michael W.N. Deininger, MD, PhD and Brian J. Druker, MD

Epidemiology

Incidence: 5,980 (male: 3,130; female: 2,850.
Estimated new cases for 2014 in the United States)
Deaths: Estimated 810 in 2014 (male: 550; female: 260)
Median age: 65 years
Male to female ratio: 1.7:1

Phase at presentation:
Chronic phase: 85–90%
Accelerated phase and blast crisis: 10–15%

Cervantes F et al. Haematologica 1999;84:324–327
O'Brien SG et al. N Engl J Med 2003;348:994–1004
Siegel R et al. CA Cancer J Clin 2014;64:9–29
Surveillance, Epidemiology and End Results (SEER) Program, available from http://seer.cancer.gov (accessed in 2013)

Pathology

Peripheral blood findings at diagnosis: median (range)

1. *WBC:* 174,000/mm^3 (15–850/mm^3)
2. *Hemoglobin:* 10.3 g/dL (4.9–16.6 g/dL)
3. *Platelet count:* 430,000/mm^3 (17–3182/mm^3)
4. Left-shifted white cell differential, basophilia, and eosinophilia
5. *Blasts:* <15%—chronic phase

Bone marrow findings at diagnosis

1. Increased cellularity
2. Increased myeloid-to-erythroid ratio with full myeloid maturation
3. Blasts <15%—chronic phase
4. Basophilia
5. Megakaryocyte hyperplasia
6. Reticulin fibrosis

Cytogenetics and molecular diagnostics

1. Philadelphia (Ph) chromosome including variant translocations (90%)
2. *BCR-ABL* translocation by FISH (95%)*
3. *BCR-ABL* transcripts by RT-PCR (95%)*
4. Chromosomal abnormalities in addition to the Ph chromosome (clonal evolution)[†]:

    (Associated with disease progression, usually absent in the chronic phase at diagnosis)

Trisomy 8	52.9%
Second Philadelphia chromosome	50.7%
Isochromosome 17	35.8%
Trisomy 19	24.3%

*Approximately 5% of patients with morphologically and clinically typical CML are negative for BCR-ABL by FISH and RT-PCR; these patients constitute a heterogeneous group with a poorer prognosis that is usually unresponsive to imatinib. The data given here do not apply to this group of patients
[†]Clonal evolution is associated with a less-favorable response to standard drug therapy (imatinib), regardless of disease phase, but is not an independent prognostic variable. In patients treated with nonimatinib therapies, isochromosome 17 is an adverse prognostic factor in multivariate analysis

Deininger MWN. Semin Hematol 2003;40(2 Suppl 2):50–55
Johansson B et al. Acta Haematol 2002;107:76–94
Mitelman F. Leuk Lymphoma 1993;11(Suppl 1):11–15
Savage DG et al. Br J Haematol 1997;96:111–116
Thiele J et al. Leuk Lymphoma 2000;36:295–308

Work-up

History and physical examination

1. CBC and leukocyte differential counts, platelets, electrolytes, liver function tests
2. HLA typing for patients who are candidates for allogeneic hematopoietic cell transplantation
3. Bone marrow aspirate and biopsy (bone marrow cytogenetics can detect chromosomal abnormalities other than Ph chromosome that are not detectable using peripheral blood)
4. BCR-ABL1 transcript levels by quantitative reverse transcriptase polymerase reaction (QPCR) before initiation of treatment.
5. If collection of bone marrow is not feasible, fluorescence in situ hybridization (FISH) on a peripheral blood specimen with dual probes for BCR and ABL1 genes

Classification of Disease: Phases of Disease

Chronic phase:
1. Bone marrow and peripheral blood blasts <15%
2. Peripheral blood promyelocytes and blasts combined <30%
3. Peripheral blood basophils <20%
4. Platelets >100,000/mm^3

Accelerated phase:
1. Bone marrow and peripheral blood blasts 15–30%
2. Peripheral blood promyelocytes + blasts ≥30% (but blasts alone <30%)
3. Peripheral blood basophils ≥20%
4. Platelets ≤100,000/mm^3 (unless related to therapy)

Blast crisis:
1. Bone marrow or peripheral blood blasts ≥30%
2. Myeloid immunophenotype: MPO-positive
3. Lymphoid immunophenotype: TdT-positive

Cytogenetic abnormalities in addition to the Philadelphia chromosome (typically, isochromosome 17, trisomy 8, trisomy 19, second Ph chromosome) are considered indicative of accelerated phase by some authors, even in the absence of other defining criteria. Adverse prognostic significance is best documented for isochromosome 17

Johansson B et al. Acta Haematol 2002;107:76–94
Talpaz M et al. Blood 2002;99:1928–1937

CML Extras

Calculation of Relative Risk

Adapted from Hasford J et al. Blood 2011;118:686–692

Study		Calculation	Risk Definition by Calculation
Sokal et al. 1984*		Exp 0.0116 × (age − 43.4)	Low risk: <0.8
	+	0.0345 × (spleen − 7.51)	
	+	0.188 × [(platelet count ÷ 700)^2 − 0.563]	Intermediate risk: 0.8–1.2
	+	0.0887 × (myeloblasts − 2.10)	High risk: >1.2
Euro Hasford et al. 1998†		0.666 when age ≥50 y	Low risk: ≤780
	+	(0.042 × spleen)	
	+	1.0956 when platelet count >1500 × 10^{9}L	Intermediate risk: 781–1480
	+	(0.0584 × myeloblast)	
	+	0.20399 when basophils >3%	High risk: >1480
	+	(0.0413 × eosinophils) × 100	
EUTOS Hasford et al. 2011‡		Spleen × 4	Low risk: ≤87
	+	Basophils × 7	High risk: >87

Calculation of the risk requires use of clinical and hematologic data at diagnosis, prior to any treatment:
- Age is given in years
- Spleen is given in centimeters below the costal margin (maximum distance)
- Myeloblasts, eosinophils, and basophils are given in percent of peripheral blood differential

Relative risk for the Sokal calculation is expressed as exponential of the total; that for the Hasford calculation is expressed as the total × 1000

To calculate Sokal and Euro risk score, go to:
http://www.leukemia-net.org/content/leukemias/cml/cml_score/index_eng.html
To calculate EUTOS risk score, go to:
http://www.leukemia-net.org/content/leukemias/cml/eutos_score/index_eng.html

*Sokal et al. Blood 1984;63:789–799. Risk according to Sokal et al. defined based on patients treated with conventional chemotherapy.
†Hasford et al. J Natl Cancer Inst. 1998;90:850–858. Risk according to Hasford et al. defined based on patients treated with rIFNα-based regimens
‡Hasford J et al. Blood 2011;118:686–692. Risk according to EUTOS score derived from patients treated with imatinib

(continued)

CML Extras (*continued*)

**Approximate relationship between response, the putative
number of leukemic cells, and the level of BCR-ABL transcripts**
[Adapted from Baccarani M et al. Blood 2006;108:1809–1820]

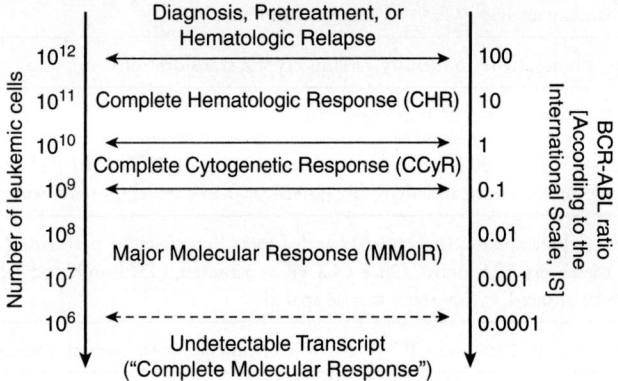

Response Definitions and Monitoring

Adapted from Baccarani et al. Blood 2013;122:872–884

	Complete Hematologic Response (CHR)*	Cytogenetic Response (CyR)†	Molecular Response (MolR)‡
Definitions	• Normalization of blood counts: ■ Platelet count <450,000/mm³ ■ WBC <10,000/mm³; ■ Differential without immature granulocytes and <5% basophils • Spleen not palpable • Disappearance of CML symptoms	Percent of 20 marrow metaphases with Philadelphia chromosome (Ph) detected by karyotyping: • Complete (CCyR)* = 0% • Partial/Major (MCyR) = 1–35% • Minor CyR = 36%–65% • Minimal CyR = 66%–95% • None = >95%	"Complete (CMR, CMolR)" = Transcript not detectable§ Major (MMolR)* = ≥3 $\log_{10}$ reduction in *BCR-ABL1* transcripts (≤0.10% IS)
Monitoring	• Check CBC every 2 weeks until CHR achieved and confirmed • Once CHR achieved check CBC every 3 months unless otherwise required	• Check CyR at 3, 6, 12 months and then at least every 6 months until CCyR achieved and confirmed • Once CCyR achieved check every 12 months	• Check every 3 months • Perform mutational analysis in case of failure, suboptimal response, or >5-fold increase in transcript level

*Complete HR, complete CCyR, and major MolR should be confirmed on at least 2 occasions

†CyR is evaluated by morphologic cytogenetics of at least 20 marrow metaphases. FISH of peripheral blood cells should be used only if marrow metaphases cannot be obtained

‡MolR is assessed on peripheral blood cells. Following quantitative real time PCR (qRT-PCR) analysis, the *BCR-ABL1*/control gene transcript ratio is determined using the International Scale (IS) standardized baseline. The international scale for measuring MolR is that proposed by Hughes et al. Blood 2006;108:28–37

§There is no universal definition of complete molecular response (CMR, CMolR). Some of the studies used define CMR as a negative (undetectable) result on a nested PCR assay; however, this is problematic owing to test variability. Others suggest that CMR be defined as undetectable *BCR-ABL1* mRNA in 2 consecutive samples with a 4.5-log detection limit. This definition may become inadequate once sensitivity increases beyond the 4.5-log levels. It may be best to indicate test sensitivity and avoid the term CMR

(*continued*)

CML Extras (continued)

Recommendations for Cytogenetic and Molecular Monitoring

Adapted from Baccarani et al. Blood 2013;122:872–884

At diagnosis	Chromosome banding analysis (CBA) of marrow cell metaphases
	FISH in case of Ph negativity to identify variant, cryptic translocations
	Qualitative PCR (identification of transcript type)
During treatment	Quantitative real-time PCR (RQ-PCR) for the determination of *BCR-ABL1* transcripts level on the international scale, to be performed every 3 months until an MMR (BCR-ABL $\leq$0.1%, or MR$^{3.0}$) has been achieved, then every 3–6 months *and/or*
	CBA of marrow cell metaphases (at least 20 banded metaphases), to be performed at 3, 6, and 12 months until a CCyR has been achieved, then every 12 months. Once a CCyR is achieved, FISH on blood cells can be done. If adequate molecular monitoring can be ensured, cytogenetics can be spared
Failure, progression	RQ-PCR, mutational analysis, and CBA of marrow cell metaphases. Immunophenotyping in BP
Warning	Molecular and cytogenetic tests to be performed more frequently. CBA of marrow cell metaphases recommended in case of myelodysplasia or CCA/Ph$^-$ with chromosome 7 involvement

CCA/Ph$^-$ clonal chromosome abnormalities in Ph$^-$ cells; FISH, fluorescence in situ hybridization

Note: The responses can be assessed either with molecular tests alone or with cytogenetic tests alone, depending on the local laboratory facilities, but whenever possible, both cytogenetic and molecular tests are recommended until a CCyR and an MMR are achieved. Then RQ-PCR alone may be sufficient. Mutational analysis by conventional Sanger sequencing is recommended in case of progression, failure, and warning. In case of failure, warning, and development of myelodysplastic features (unexpected leucopenia, thrombocytopenia, or anemia), CBA of marrow cell metaphases is recommended

Definition of the Response to TKIs (Any TKI) as First-Line Treatment
[Previously Untreated Patients in Early Chronic Phase (ECP) CML]

Adapted from Baccarani et al. Blood 2013;122:872–884

Time	Failure*	Warning†	Optimal
Diagnosis/Baseline	NA	High risk *or* CCA/Ph$^+$, major route‡	NA
3 months on TKI treatment	No CHR *and/or* Ph$^+$ >95%	BCR-ABL1 >10% *and/or* Ph$^+$ 36–95%	BCR-ABL1 $\leq$10% *and/or* Ph$^+$ $\leq$35%
6 months on TKI treatment	BCR-ABL1 >10% *and/or* Ph$^+$ >35%	BCR-ABL1 1–10% *and/or* Ph$^+$ 1–35%	BCR-ABL1 <1% *and/or* Ph$^+$ 0%
12 months on TKI treatment	BCR-ABL1 >1% *and/or* Ph$^+$ >0%	BCR-ABL1 >0.1–1%	BCR-ABL1 $\leq$0.1%
Then, and at any time	Loss of CHR Loss of CCyR Confirmed loss of MMR§ New mutation CCA/Ph$^+$	CCA/Ph$^-$ ($-$7 or 7q$-$)	BCR-ABL1 $\leq$0.1%

CCA, clonal chromosomal abnormalities; CCyR, complete cytogenetic response, Philadelphia chromosome (Ph) not detected by karyotyping in 20/20 marrow metaphases; CHR, complete hematologic response; CyR, cytogenetic response; NA, not applicable

*Failure implies patient should be moved to other treatments when available

†Warning implies that the characteristics of the disease and the response to treatment require more frequent monitoring to permit timely changes in therapy in case of treatment failure. Such patients may become eligible for other treatments

‡Major route abnormalities include trisomy 8, trisomy Ph ($+$der(22)t(9;22)(q34;q11)), isochromosome 17 (i(17)(q10)), trisomy 19 and ider(22)(q10)t(9;22)(q34;q11)

§To be confirmed on 2 occasions, at least 1 of which with BCR-ABL $\geq$1%

(continued)

CML Extras (continued)

Definitions of the Response to Second-Line Therapy in Case of Failure of Imatinib
Adapted from Baccarani et al. Blood 2013;122:872–884

	Failure	Warning	Optimal
Diagnosis/Baseline	NA	No CHR or loss of CHR on imatinib or Lack of CyR to first-line TKI or High risk	NA
3 months on TKI treatment	No CHR or Ph+ >95% or New mutations	BCR-ABL1 >10% and/or Ph+ 65–95%	BCR-ABL1 ≤10% and/or Ph+ <65%
6 months on TKI treatment	BCR-ABL1 >10% and/or Ph+ >65% and/or New mutations	Ph+ 35–65%	BCR-ABL1 ≤10% and/or Ph+ <35%
12 months on TKI treatment	BCR-ABL1 >10% and/or Ph+ >35% and/or New mutations	BCR-ABL1 1–10% and/or Ph+ 1–35%	BCR-ABL1 <1% and/or Ph+ 0
Then, and at any time	Loss of CHR or Loss of CCyR or PCyR New mutations Confirmed loss of MMR* CCA/Ph+	CCA/Ph− (−7 or 7q−) or BCR-ABL1 >0.1%	BCR-ABL1 ≤0.1%

CCA/Ph+, clonal chromosome abnormalities in Ph+ cells; CCA/Ph−, clonal chromosome abnormalities in Ph− cells; MMR, BCR-ABL1 ≥0.1% = MR3.0 or better; NA, not applicable

*In 2 consecutive tests, of which 1 with a BCR-ABL transcripts level ≥1%

Note: These definitions are mainly based on data reported for nilotinib and dasatinib, but can be used provisionally also for bosutinib and ponatinib, until more data are available. These definitions cannot apply to the evaluation of the response to third-line treatment.

Rates of CCyR and MMR
Adapted from Mealing et al. Exp Hematol Oncol 2013;2:5

Study	Dasatinib			Nilotinib 600 mg			Nilotinib 800 mg			Imatinib 400 mg			Imatinib 800 mg		
Percent with Complete Cytogenic Response (CCyR) at 6, 12, and 18 Months															
Time (Months)	6	12	18	6	12	18	6	12	18	6	12	18	6	12	18
DASISION	73	85	85*							59	73	82*			
ENESTnd				67	80	85	63	78	82	45	65	74			
Baccarani et al.										50	58		52	64	74
German CML										22	50	67	34	63	
Cortes et al.										45	66		57	70	
ISTAHIT										20	82		44	69	
SPIRIT										50	58		69	65	
S0325 Intergroup†											67			85	

(continued)

CML Extras (*continued*)

Rates of CCyR and MMR (*continued*)

	Dasatinib	Nilotinib 600 mg	Nilotinib 800 mg	Imatinib 400 mg	Imatinib 800 mg
Baccarani et al.				33	40
DASISION	46			28	
ENESTnd		44	43	22	
German CML				31	55
Cortes et al.				40	46
SPIRIT				38	49
S0325 Intergroup[†]				36	53

Percent with Major Molecular Response (MMR) at 12 Months

*24 months

[†]Based on blood specimens collected 295–406 days after randomization (if a patient's molecular response was tested more than once during that interval, only the result obtained closest to day 365 was included in this analysis)

- Baccarani et al: Baccarani et al. Blood 2009;113:4497–4504
- Cortes et al: Cotes JE et al. J Clin Oncol 2010;28:424–430
- DASISION: Kantarijan HM et al. N Engl J Med 2010;362:2260–2270; Kantarijan HM et al. Blood 2012;119:1123–1129
- ENESTnd: Saglio G et al. N Engl J Med 2010;362:2251–2259; Larson RA et al. Leukemia, 2012;26:2197–2203; Hughes TP et al. Blood 2013 Dec 11 [Epub ahead of print]; Larson RA et al. Leukemia 2012;26:2197–2203
- German CML: German CML-Study IV-Hehlmann R et al. J Clin Oncol 2013 Dec 2 [Epub ahead of print]
- ISTAHIT: Petzer AL et al. Haematologica 2010;95:908–913
- SPIRIT: Preudhomme C et al. N Engl J Med 2010;363:2511–2521
- S0325 Intergroup: Deininger et al. Br J Hematol 2014;164:223–232

Expert Opinion

FDA-Approved Indications and Usage

1. Imatinib is approved for:
   - *Newly diagnosed adult* and pediatric patients with CML* in chronic phase
   - Patients with CML in blast crisis (BC), accelerated phase (AP), or in chronic phase (CP) after failure of interferon-α therapy
   - Adult patients with relapsed or refractory Philadelphia chromosome-positive acute lymphoblastic leukemia (Ph[+] ALL)
   - Pediatric patients with Ph[+] ALL in combination with chemotherapy

2. Dasatinib is approved for:
   - *Newly diagnosed adults* with CML in chronic phase
   - Adults with chronic-, accelerated-, or myeloid or lymphoid blast-phase CML with resistance or intolerance to prior therapy that included imatinib
   - Adults with Ph[+] ALL with resistance or intolerance to prior therapy

3. Nilotinib is approved for:
   - *Newly diagnosed adults* with CML in chronic phase
   - Adults with chronic- or accelerated-phase CML with resistance or intolerance to prior therapy that included imatinib

4. Bosutinib is approved for:
   - Adult patients with chronic-, accelerated-, or blast-phase CML with resistance or intolerance to prior therapy

5. Ponatinib is approved for:
   - T315I-positive CML (chronic phase, accelerated phase, or blast phase) or T315I-positive Ph[+] ALL
   - Chronic-phase, accelerated-phase, or blast-phase CML or Ph[+] ALL for whom no other tyrosine-kinase inhibitor therapy is indicated

6. Omacetaxine Mepesuccinate is approved for:
   - Adult patients with chronic- or accelerated-phase CML with resistance and/or intolerance to 2 or more tyrosine kinase inhibitors (TKIs)

*According to the WHO, chronic myeloid leukemia (CML) is defined by the presence of the Ph chromosome or the BCR-ABL fusion gene in the context of a myeloproliferative neoplasm. Therefore the qualification "Ph chromosome-positive CML" is unnecessary

(*continued*)

Expert Opinion (*continued*)

Treatment options:

1. In the opinion of some, imatinib remains the standard drug therapy regimen for the initial treatment of all phases of CML. Other agents are considered second-line and are reserved for patients who are intolerant of or whose disease is resistant to imatinib. In the opinion of others, nilotinib and dasatinib represent better first-line options than imatinib. But everyone agrees that the availability of 3 first-line therapies provides clinicians with a range of options for managing intolerance and resistance

2. Although imatinib is an excellent therapy, it is not perfect: with 8 years of follow-up, 16% of IRIS patients discontinued treatment for insufficient efficacy and 6% for adverse events. These outcomes led many to ask whether first-line use of more potent tyrosine kinase inhibitors (TKIs), such as dasatinib and nilotinib, could reduce the rate of failures. Promising results in single-arm studies with both dasatinib and nilotinib led to randomized trials comparing dasatinib to imatinib (**Da**satinib versus imatinib study in treatment **naïve** CML patients [**DASISION**] study) and nilotinib to imatinib (Evaluating **n**ilotinib **e**fficacy and **s**afety in clinical **t**rials of **n**ewly **d**iagnosed Ph-positive CML patients [**ENESTnd**] study). Both studies found dasatinib and nilotinib superior to imatinib with respect to:
   - Complete cytogenetic responses (CCyR)
   - Major molecular responses (MMR), and
   - Complete molecular responses (CMR)

   These observations led to their approval for first-line therapy of CML-CP

3. Dasatinib and nilotinib provide several advantages
   - Response milestones are achieved sooner and in a greater proportion of patients
   - Progression to advanced disease is reduced (statistically significant for nilotinib)

   However, the numerical advantages are slight, overall survival is not significantly different, and some late side effects have been observed for the second-generation inhibitors (nilotinib: peripheral occlusive arterial disease, POADs; dasatinib: pulmonary hypertension). Thus, longer follow-up will be necessary, before a general recommendation can be made

4. Dasatinib and nilotinib control the majority of BCR-ABL1 mutations that confer resistance to imatinib, with partially complementary exceptions. The choice between dasatinib and nilotinib can be partially rationalized based on BCR-ABL genotype (kinase domain mutation analysis) and patient history (side-effects profile). However, the 2 agents have not been compared in a prospective study. Patients with the T315I mutation of BCR-ABL do not respond to either agent

5. Bosutinib is active against several BCR-ABL1 mutants that confer resistance to nilotinib and dasatinib, and is approved for the treatment of adult patients with chronic-, accelerated-, or blast-phase CML with resistance or intolerance to prior therapy

6. The most problematic point mutation is the BCR-ABL^{T315I} "gatekeeper" mutation. BCR-ABL^{T315I} is insensitive to imatinib, dasatinib, nilotinib, and bosutinib

7. Ponatinib was demonstrated to have in vitro activity against BCR-ABL1^{T315I} and other resistant mutants. However, certain T315I-inclusive compound mutants exhibit high-level resistance. The extent to which T315I-inclusive compound mutations (eg, BCR-ABL1$^{E255V/T315I}$) reduce the effectiveness of ponatinib remains to be established. Ponatinib has demonstrated considerable clinical activity in patients with and without BCR-ABL^{T315I}, especially in the chronic phase of CML, but safety concerns prevents its use in second-line therapy, except in the case of BCR-ABL^{T315I}

8. Interferon-α may be considered in exceptional cases, but is generally ineffective in patients with disease resistant to tyrosine kinase inhibitors

9. Hydroxyurea is used for lowering excessively high white blood cell counts if the diagnosis is uncertain, and in the case of intolerance or resistance to tyrosine kinase inhibitors. Hydroxyurea is considered a palliative regimen, as it does not usually induce lasting responses

10. Although the Sokal score was developed in patients treated with chemotherapy, it also predicts the likelihood of achieving a complete cytogenetic response to imatinib (91% vs. 84% vs. 69% at 48 months for low-, intermediate-, and high-risk patients, respectively). Complete cytogenetic response is associated with a favorable outcome

11. The definitions of disease phases given above were used in the clinical trials of imatinib that led to regulatory approval. They are widely, but not universally, accepted

12. AML- or ALL-type chemotherapy is indicated for tyrosine kinase inhibitor-resistant CML in myeloid and lymphoid blast crisis, respectively. No data from controlled trials are available that demonstrate superiority of one regimen over another. All efforts should be made to proceed to allogeneic hematopoietic cell transplantation as soon as possible. Complete hematologic remission is achieved in 40–60% of patients

Cortes J et al. Am J Hematol 2013;88:350–354
Cortes J et al. Blood 2012;120:2573–2580
Cortes JE et al. N Engl J Med 2012;367:2075–2088
Derderian PM et al. Am J Med 1993;94:69–74
Druker BJ et al. N Engl J Med 2006;355:2408–2417
Jabbour E et al. Blood 2011;117:1822–1827
Jabbour E et al. Blood 2011;118:4541–4546
Kantarjian H et al. N Engl J Med 2006;354:2542–2551
Kantarjian HM et al. Lancet Oncol 2011;12:841–851
Kantarjian HM et al. Am J Med 1987;83:445–454
Kantarjian HM et al. Blood 2012;119:1123–1129
Kantarjian HM et al. N Engl J Med 2010;362:2260–2270
Khoury HJ et al. Blood 2012;119:3403–3412
Saglio G et al. N Engl J Med 2010;362:2251–2259
Talpaz M et al. N Engl J Med 2006;354:2531–2541

CML REGIMEN

IMATINIB

Deininger MWN et al. J Clin Oncol 2003;21:1637–1647

Chronic phase CML:
Initial dose:
Imatinib 400 mg/day; administer orally, continually, with the largest meal of the day (total dose/week = 2800 mg)
Dose escalation:
Escalate to **Imatinib** 600 mg/day; administer orally, continually, with the largest meal of the day (total dose/week = 4200 mg), if patient has not reached:

1. Complete hematologic response at 3 months, *or*
2. <95% Ph-negative metaphases at 6 months, *or*
3. <35% Ph-negative metaphases at 12 months

Accelerated phase and blast crisis CML
Initial dose:
Imatinib 600 mg/day; administer orally, continually, with the largest meal of the day (total dose/week = 4200 mg)

Supportive Care
Antiemetic prophylaxis
Emetogenic potential is **MINIMAL–LOW**
See Chapter 39 for antiemetic recommendations

Hematopoietic growth factor (CSF) prophylaxis
Primary prophylaxis is NOT indicated
See Chapter 43 for more information

Antimicrobial prophylaxis
Risk of fever and neutropenia is LOW
Antimicrobial primary prophylaxis to be considered:
• Antibacterial—not indicated
• Antifungal—not indicated
• Antiviral—not indicated, unless patient previously had an episode of HSV
See Chapter 47 for more information

Efficacy
(Chronic phase, N = 553)*

Complete hematologic response	98%
Complete cytogenetic response	87%
Partial cytogenetic response (1–35% Ph⁺ metaphases)	5%
Freedom from progression to accelerated phase or blast crisis	93%

*Projected rates at 60 months

Druker BJ et al. N Engl J Med 2006;355:2408–2417

Treatment Modifications

Hematologic Toxicity
(No Modifications for Anemia)

G1/2	No dose modifications
G3	Hold imatinib until toxicity resolves to grade 1*, then restart at 400 mg/day
Recurrent G3	Hold imatinib until toxicity resolves to grade 1, then restart at 300 mg/day
G4	Withhold imatinib until toxicity resolves to grade 1, then restart at 300 mg/day
Recurrent G4	Hold imatinib until toxicity resolves to grade 1, then restart at 300 mg/day†

Nonhematologic Toxicity

G1	No dose modifications
G2/3	Hold imatinib until toxicity resolves to grade 1, then restart at 400 mg/day
Recurrent G2/3	Hold imatinib until toxicity resolves to grade 1, then restart at 300 mg/day
G4	Hold imatinib until toxicity resolves to grade 1, then restart at 300 mg/day
Recurrent G4	Discontinue imatinib

*Consider filgrastim for persistent neutropenia
†No dose reduction to <300 mg/day

Deininger MWN et al. J Clin Oncol 2003;21: 1637–1647

Therapy Monitoring

1. *CBC:* Weekly; every 2 weeks after achievement of complete hematologic response; every 4–6 weeks after achievement of a complete cytogenetic response
2. *Blood chemistry:* Weekly; every 4–8 weeks after achievement of complete hematologic response
3. *Bone marrow cytogenetics:* Every 3 months until complete cytogenetic response, then at 12- to 24-month intervals
4. *Quantitative RT-PCR for BCR-ABL from peripheral blood or bone marrow:* Every 3–6 months after achievement of complete cytogenetic response

Patient Population Studied

Study of 553 patients with newly diagnosed CML in chronic phase

Toxicity
(In >10% of patients, N = 553)

Toxicity	% G1/2	% G3/4
Superficial edema	54.6	0.9
Thrombocytopenia	48.8	7.8
Neutropenia	46.5	14.3
Nausea	43	0.7
Anemia	41.5	3.1
Increased liver transaminases	38.1	5.1
Muscle cramps	37	1.3
Musculoskeletal pain	33.8	2.7
Rash	31.9	2.0
Fatigue	33.4	1.1
Diarrhea	31	1.8
Headache	30.8	0.4
Joint pain	25.9	2.4
Abdominal pain	24.6	2.4
Nasopharyngitis	22.0	—
Myalgia	19.9	1.5
Hemorrhage	20.2	0.7
Vomiting	15.4	1.5
Dyspepsia	16.2	—
Pharyngolaryngeal pain	15.8	0.2
Cough	14.3	0.2
Dizziness	13.6	0.9
Upper respiratory infection	14.3	0.2
Weight gain	12.5	0.9
Pyrexia	12.4	0.7
Insomnia	12.2	—

O'Brien SG et al. N Engl J Med 2003;348:994–1004

Notes

In patients who develop disease progression while receiving imatinib, the option of allogeneic stem cell transplantation should be reevaluated

CML REGIMEN

DASATINIB

Shah NP et al. J Clin Oncol 2008;26:3204–3212

Chronic phase CML:
Initial dose:
Dasatinib 100 mg/day; administer orally, continually, with or without a meal (total dose/week = 700 mg)
Dose escalation:
Escalate to **dasatinib** 140 mg/day; administer orally, continually, with or without a meal in case of insufficient response (total dose/week = 980 mg)

Accelerated phase and blast crisis CML:
Initial dose:
Dasatinib 140 mg/day; administer orally, continually, with or without meal (total dose/week = 980 mg)
Dose escalation:
Escalate to **dasatinib** 180 mg/day; administer orally, continually, with or without a meal in case of insufficient response (total dose/week = 1260 mg)

Supportive Care
Antiemetic prophylaxis
Emetogenic potential is **MINIMAL–LOW**
See Chapter 39 for antiemetic recommendations

Hematopoietic growth factor (CSF) prophylaxis
Primary prophylaxis is NOT indicated
See Chapter 43 for more information

Antimicrobial prophylaxis
Risk of fever and neutropenia is LOW
  Antimicrobial primary prophylaxis to be considered:
  • Antibacterial—not indicated
  • Antifungal—not indicated
  • Antiviral—not indicated, unless patient previously had an episode of HSV
See Chapter 47 for more information

Toxicity (In >10% of patients, N = 166)

Toxicity	% G1/2	% G3/4
Anemia	79	10
Leukocytopenia	43	16
Neutropenia	30	33
Thrombocytopenia	38	22
Fluid retention	20	1
Superficial edema	14	0
Pleural effusion	6	1
Headache	30	<1
Diarrhea	23	<1
Fatigue	19	1
Nausea	15	<1
Rash	10	1
Myalgia	11	0
Dyspnea	9	1
Peripheral edema	10	0

Shah NP et al. J Clin Oncol 2008;26:3204–3212

Patient Population Studied

Study of 166 patients with CML in chronic phase resistant to or intolerant of imatinib

Therapy Monitoring

1. *CBC:* Weekly; every 2 weeks after achievement of complete hematologic response; every 4–6 weeks after achievement of complete cytogenetic response
2. *Blood chemistry:* Weekly; every 4–8 weeks after achievement of complete hematologic response
3. *Bone marrow cytogenetics:* Every 3 months until complete cytogenetic response, then at 12–24 months intervals
4. *Quantitative RT-PCR for BCR-ABL from peripheral blood or bone marrow:* Every 3–6 months after achievement of complete cytogenetic response

Efficacy (Chronic phase, N = 166)

Complete hematologic response*	90%
Complete cytogenetic response[†]	41%
Partial cytogenetic response[†] (1–35% Ph+ metaphases)	18%
Freedom from progression to accelerated phase or blast crisis	93%

*51% of patients were in CHR at entry
[†]20% of patients were in major cytogenetic response at entry

Shah NP et al. J Clin Oncol 2008;26:3204–3212

Treatment Modifications

Hematologic Toxicity: Chronic Phase
(No Modifications for Anemia)

G1/2	No dose modifications
ANC <500/mm³*	Hold dasatinib until ANC ≥1000/mm³ Recovery within 7 days: resume at 100 mg/day Recovery within >7 days or first recurrence: resume at 80 mg/day Second recurrence: discontinue
Platelet count <50,000/mm³	Hold dasatinib until platelet count is ≥50,000/mm³ Recovery within ≤7 days: resume at 100 mg/day Recovery within >7 days or first recurrence: resume at 80 mg/day Second recurrence: discontinue drug
Platelet count <25,000/mm³	Hold dasatinib until platelet count is ≥50,000/mm³ and resume at 80 mg/day First recurrence: Hold dasatinib until platelet count is ≥50,000/mm³ and resume at 80 mg/day Second recurrence: discontinue drug

Hematologic Toxicity: Accelerated or Blastic Phase

G1–3	No dose modifications
G4—first occurrence	If cytopenia is unrelated to leukemia (bone marrow assessment), hold dasatinib until recovery to platelet count ≥20,000/mm³ and ANC ≥1000/mm³ and resume at 140 mg/day†
G4—second occurrence	Hold dasatinib until recovery to platelet count ≥20,000/mm³ and ANC ≥1000/mm³, and resume at 100 mg/day
G4—third occurrence	Hold dasatinib until recovery to platelet count ≥20,000/mm³ and ANC ≥1000/mm³, and resume at 80 mg/day

Nonhematologic Toxicity

G1	No dose modifications
G2/3	Hold dasatinib until toxicity resolves to grade 1, then restart at 100 mg/day
Recurrent G2/3	Hold dasatinib until toxicity resolves to grade 1, then restart at 80 mg/day
G4	Hold dasatinib until toxicity resolves to grade 1, then restart at 80 mg/day
Recurrent G4	Discontinue dasatinib

*Consider filgrastim for persistent neutropenia
†Consider dose escalation to 180 mg/day in case of leukemia-related cytopenia
http://packageinserts.bms.com/pi/pi_sprycel.pdf (last accessed Dec. 19, 2011)

CML REGIMEN

NILOTINIB

le Coutre P et al. Blood 2008;111:1834–1839

Chronic phase CML:
Nilotinib 400 mg; administer orally twice daily, continually, at least 2 hours after the last and 1 hour before the next meal

Accelerated phase CML:
Nilotinib 400 mg; administer orally twice daily, continually, at least 2 hours after the last and 1 hour before the next meal

Note: Dose escalation is not indicated

Supportive Care

Antiemetic prophylaxis
*Emetogenic potential is **MINIMAL–LOW***
See Chapter 39 for antiemetic recommendations

Hematopoietic growth factor (CSF) prophylaxis
Primary prophylaxis is NOT indicated
See Chapter 43 for more information

Antimicrobial prophylaxis
Risk of fever and neutropenia is LOW
Antimicrobial primary prophylaxis to be considered:
- Antibacterial—not indicated
- Antifungal—not indicated
- Antiviral—not indicated, unless patient previously had an episode of HSV

See Chapter 47 for more information

Patient Population Studied

Study of 280 patients with CML in chronic phase resistant to or intolerant of nilotinib

Toxicity
(In >10% of patients, N = 280)

Toxicity	% G1/2	% G3/4
Thrombocytopenia	NR	29
Neutropenia	NR	29
Rash	25	3
Pruritus	23	1
Headache	17	2
Fatigue	18	1
Constipation	12	0
Diarrhea	9	2
Vomiting	11	<1
Nausea	23	1

LeCoutre P et al. Blood 2008;111:1834–1839

Therapy Monitoring

1. *CBC:* Weekly; every 2 weeks after achievement of complete hematologic response; every 4–6 weeks after achievement of complete cytogenetic response
2. *Blood chemistry:* Weekly; every 4–8 weeks after achievement of complete hematologic response
3. *Bone marrow cytogenetics:* Every 3 months until complete cytogenetic response, then at 12–24-month intervals
4. *Quantitative RT-PCR for BCR-ABL from peripheral blood or bone marrow:* Every 3–6 months after achievement of complete cytogenetic response

Efficacy
(Chronic phase, N = 280)

Complete hematologic response*	74%
Complete cytogenetic response*	31%
Partial cytogenetic response* (1–35% Ph+ metaphases)	16%

*Only patients without response at baseline
le Coutre P et al. Blood 2008;111:1834–1839

Notes

1. Hypokalemia and hypophosphatemia should be corrected before initiating nilotinib therapy and serum electrolyte levels monitored during nilotinib treatment
2. EKG monitoring for QT prolongation is indicated at baseline, within 7 days after initiating therapy or changing the dose, and periodically thereafter
3. The Fridericia correction of the QT interval (QTcF) should be used for all calculations

Treatment Modifications

Hematologic Toxicity
(No Modifications for Anemia)

G1/2	No dose modifications
G3/4	Hold nilotinib until toxicity resolves to grade 2 Recovery within 2 weeks: restart at 400 mg twice daily Recovery within >2 weeks: restart at 400 mg/day

Nonhematologic Toxicity (Noncardiac)

G1/2	No dose modifications
G3/4	Hold nilotinib until toxicity resolves to grade 1, then restart at 400 mg/day If tolerated, consider re-escalation to 400 mg twice daily

QT Prolongation

| QTcF >480 msec | Hold nilotinib and correct any hypokalemia and/or hypomagnesemia
QTcF <450 msec and within 20 msec of baseline within 2 weeks: resume at 400 mg twice daily
QTcF 450–480 msec: resume at 400 mg/day; if recurrence of QTcF >480 msec, discontinue nilotinib |

http://www.pharma.us.novartis.com/product/pi/pdf/tasigna.pdf (last accessed, Dec. 19, 2011)

REFRACTORY PHILADELPHIA CHROMOSOME-POSITIVE CML REGIMEN

PONATINIB (ICLUSIG)

Cortes JE et al. N Engl J Med 2012;367:2075–2088

Ponatinib hydrochloride 45 mg/day; administer orally with or without food, continually for 28 consecutive days, on days 1–28, every 4 weeks (total dose/28-day cycle = 1260 mg)

Notes:
- On the basis of safety, pharmacokinetic, and pharmacodynamic data, 45 mg of ponatinib was determined to be the maximum tolerated dose
- The optimal dose of ponatinib has not been identified. In clinical trials, the starting dose of ponatinib was 45 mg administered orally once daily. However, 59% of the patients required dose reductions to 30 mg or 15 mg once daily during the course of therapy
- More safety information will become available with additional analysis and follow-up
- *Start dosing with 45 mg once daily. Consider reducing the dose of ponatinib for CP CML and AP CML patients who have achieved a major cytogenetic response*
- *The recommended dose should be reduced to 30 mg once daily when administering ponatinib with strong CYP3A subfamily inhibitors*

Supportive Care
Antiemetic prophylaxis
Emetogenic potential is **MINIMAL**
See Chapter 39 for antiemetic recommendations

Hematopoietic growth factor (CSF) prophylaxis
Primary prophylaxis is NOT indicated
See Chapter 43 for more information

Antimicrobial prophylaxis
Risk of fever and neutropenia is LOW
Antimicrobial primary prophylaxis to be considered:
- Antibacterial—not indicated
- Antifungal—not indicated
- Antiviral—not indicated unless patient previously had an episode of HSV

See Chapter 47 for more information

United States Food and Drug Administration (US FDA)
Safety Announcement, 12-20-2013

The U.S. Food and Drug Administration (FDA) is requiring several new safety measures for the leukemia drug Iclusig (ponatinib) to address the risk of life-threatening blood clots and severe narrowing of blood vessels. Once these new safety measures are in place, the manufacturer of Iclusig is expected to resume marketing to appropriate patients. Healthcare professionals should review these additional safety measures and carefully consider them when evaluating the risks and benefits of Iclusig for each patient

The required safety measures involve label changes to narrow the indication, provide additional warnings and precautions about the risk of blood clots and severe narrowing of blood vessels, revise recommendations about dosage and administration of Iclusig, and update the patient Medication Guide. We are also requiring a risk evaluation and mitigation strategy (REMS). In addition, the manufacturer of Iclusig, ARIAD Pharmaceuticals, must conduct postmarket investigations to further characterize the drug's safety and dosing

On October 31, 2013, FDA requested and ARIAD agreed to voluntarily suspend marketing of Iclusig. FDA's request resulted from FDA's investigation, which revealed a steady increase in the number of serious vascular occlusion events identified through continued safety monitoring of the drug. This observation represented a significant change in the safety profile of Iclusig as the proportion of patients on the drug experiencing vascular occlusion events such as blood clots and severe narrowing of blood vessels was significantly greater than the proportion reported at the time of its approval in December 2012

During the marketing suspension, Iclusig treatment has been available through single patient or emergency investigational new drug applications (INDs). Patients should continue to receive Iclusig under their authorized IND until marketing of Iclusig is resumed. FDA is working closely with ARIAD on the new safety measures and anticipates these will be in place by the end of January 2014. Once that process is complete, patients being treated under these INDs can be transitioned back to receiving the marketed Iclusig product. In more detail, the new safety measures for Iclusig include the following:
- The indications for use are limited to:
  - Treatment of adult patients with T315I-positive chronic myeloid leukemia (chronic phase, accelerated phase, or blast phase) or T315I-positive Philadelphia chromosome-positive acute lymphoblastic leukemia (Ph$^+$ ALL)
  - Treatment of adult patients with chronic phase, accelerated phase, or blast phase chronic myeloid leukemia or Ph$^+$ ALL for whom no other tyrosine kinase inhibitor (TKI) therapy is indicated
- The *Warnings and Precautions* in the label are revised to describe the vascular occlusion events. This includes a description of the observed arterial and venous thrombosis and occlusions that have occurred in at least 27%—more than 1 in every 4—of patients treated with Iclusig

(continued)

(continued)

- The *Dosage and Administration* recommendations are revised to state that the optimal dose of Iclusig has not been identified. The recommended starting dose remains 45 mg administered orally once daily with or without food; however, additional information is included regarding dose decreases and discontinuations
- The patient Medication Guide is revised to include additional safety information consistent with the safety information in the revised drug label
- The Iclusig REMS will inform prescribers about the approved indications for use and the serious risk of vascular occlusion and thromboembolism associated with the drug
- We urge healthcare professionals and patients to report side effects involving Iclusig to the FDA MedWatch program, using the information in the "Contact FDA" box at the bottom of this page

European Medicines Agency Recommendations
November 22, 2013

Following a review of the data on the risk of occlusive vascular events with Iclusig, the European Medicines Agency has concluded that healthcare professionals may continue to use ponatinib in its authorized indication with increased caution. The Agency has made the following recommendations:

- Iclusig should not be used in patients with a history of heart attack or stroke, unless the potential benefits of treatment outweigh the risks
- The cardiovascular status of patients should be assessed and cardiovascular risk factors actively managed before starting treatment with Iclusig. Cardiovascular status should continue to be monitored and optimized during treatment
- Hypertension should be controlled during treatment with Iclusig and healthcare professionals should consider interrupting treatment if hypertension is not controlled
- Patients should be monitored for evidence of vascular occlusion or thromboembolism, and treatment should be interrupted immediately if this occurs

The recommendations are based on a review of data from clinical studies, including 2 ongoing studies (a phase I dose-finding study and a pivotal phase II study), which showed a higher incidence of arterial and venous thrombotic events in patients treated with Iclusig than was observed at the time of marketing authorization. In the phase I study, preliminary analysis of follow-up data from September 2013 showed a rate of serious occlusive vascular events of 22% (18 out of 81 patients) while in a preliminary analysis of data from the phase II study the rate was 13.8% (62 out of 449 patients). Median treatment duration was 2.7 years in the phase I study and 1.3 years in the phase II study

In addition, in a recently discontinued phase III study that compared Iclusig with imatinib with a median treatment duration of 3 months, there was a higher number of occlusive vascular events reported in the Iclusig arm, although the data from this study are still preliminary

The reported events from the studies include cardiovascular, cerebrovascular, peripheral vascular and venous thrombotic events. These events were seen in patients with and without risk factors but were seen more frequently in older patients and patients with a history of ischaemia (such as heart attacks) and strokes, high blood pressure, diabetes or blood fat disorders

Changes in Prescribing Information for Iclusig (Ponatinib) as of 12/2013
in Accordance with FDA Guidelines:

Boxed Warning
WARNING: VASCULAR OCCLUSION, HEART FAILURE, and HEPATOTOXICITY
Vascular Occlusion:
- Arterial and venous thrombosis and occlusions have occurred in at least 27% of Iclusig-treated patients, including fatal myocardial infarction, stroke, stenosis of large arterial vessels of the brain, severe peripheral vascular disease, and the need for urgent revascularization procedures. Patients with and without cardiovascular risk factors, including patients age 50 years or younger, experienced these events
- Monitor for evidence of thromboembolism and vascular occlusion. Interrupt or stop Iclusig immediately for vascular occlusion. A benefit–risk consideration should guide a decision to restart Iclusig therapy

Heart Failure:
- Heart failure, including fatalities, occurred in 8% of Iclusig-treated patients. Monitor cardiac function. Interrupt or stop Iclusig for new or worsening heart failure

Hepatotoxicity:
- Hepatotoxicity, liver failure and death have occurred in Iclusig-treated patients. Monitor hepatic function. Interrupt Iclusig if hepatotoxicity is suspected

1. Indications and Usage

Iclusig (ponatinib) is a kinase inhibitor indicated for the:
- Treatment of adult patients with T315I-positive chronic myeloid leukemia (CML) (chronic phase, accelerated phase, or blast phase) and T315I-positive Philadelphia chromosome-positive acute lymphoblastic leukemia (Ph+ ALL)
- Treatment of adult patients with chronic phase, accelerated phase, or blast phase chronic myeloid leukemia or Ph+ ALL for whom no other tyrosine kinase inhibitor (TKI) therapy is indicated

These indications are based upon response rate. There are no trials verifying an improvement in disease-related symptoms or increased survival with Iclusig

(continued)

(*continued*)

2. Dosage and Administration

2.1. Recommended Dosing

- The optimal dose of Iclusig has not been identified. In clinical trials, the starting dose of Iclusig was 45 mg administered orally once daily. However, 59% of the patients required dose reductions to 30 mg or 15 mg once daily during the course of therapy
- Start dosing with 45 mg once daily. Consider reducing the dose of Iclusig for CP CML and AP CML patients who have achieved a major cytogenetic response
- Consider discontinuing Iclusig if response has not occurred by 3 months (90 days)
- Iclusig may be taken with or without food. Tablets should be swallowed whole

3. Warnings and Precautions

3.1. Vascular Occlusion

Arterial and venous thrombosis and occlusions, including fatal myocardial infarction, stroke, stenosis of large arterial vessels of the brain, severe peripheral vascular disease, and the need for urgent revascularization procedures have occurred in at least 27% of Iclusig-treated patients from the phase 1 and phase 2 trials. Iclusig can cause fatal and life-threatening vascular occlusion within 2 weeks of starting treatment. Iclusig can also cause recurrent or multisite vascular occlusion

In the dose-escalation (phase 1) clinical trial, 48% (31/65) of patients with CML or Ph$^+$ ALL developed vascular occlusive events. The median time to onset of the first vascular occlusion event was 5 months. Iclusig can cause fatal and life-threatening vascular occlusion in patients treated at dose levels as low as 15 mg per day

Patients with and without cardiovascular risk factors, including patients age 50 years or younger, experienced these events. Vascular occlusion adverse events were more frequent with increasing age and in patients with prior history of ischemia, hypertension, diabetes, or hyperlipidemia (see Table)

Vascular Occlusion Incidence in Iclusig-Treated Patients in Phase II Trial According to Risk Categories

	Prior History of Ischemia, Hypertension, Diabetes, or Hyperlipidemia	No History of Ischemia, Hypertension, Diabetes, or Hyperlipidemia
Age: 49 or younger	18% (6/33)	12% (13/112)
Age: 50 to 74 years	33% (50/152)	18% (20/114)
Age: 75 and older	56% (14/25)	46% (6/13)
All age groups	33% (70/210)	16% (39/239)
Total	24% (109/449)	

Arterial Occlusion and Thrombosis

Arterial occlusion and thrombosis occurred in at least 20% (91/449) of Iclusig-treated patients with some patients experiencing events of more than 1 type. Patients have required revascularization procedures (cerebrovascular, coronary, and peripheral arterial) because of vascular occlusion from Iclusig

Cardiac vascular occlusion, including fatal and life-threatening myocardial infarction and coronary artery occlusion has occurred in 12% (55/449) of Iclusig-treated patients, Patients have developed heart failure concurrent or subsequent to themyocardial ischemic event

Cerebrovascular occlusion, including fatal stroke has occurred in 6% (27/449) of Iclusig-treated patients. Iclusig can cause stenosis over multiple segments in major arterial vessels that supply the brain (eg, carotid, vertebral, middle cerebralartery)

Peripheral arterial occlusive events, including fatal mesenteric artery occlusion and life-threatening peripheral arterial disease have occurred in 8% (36/449) of Iclusig-treated patients. Patients have developed digital or distal extremity necrosis and have required amputations

Clinicians should consider whether the benefits of Iclusig treatment are expected to exceed the risks of therapy. *In patients suspected of developing arterial thrombotic events, interrupt or stop Iclusig. A benefit—risk consideration should guide a decision to restart Iclusig therapy*

Venous Thromboembolism

Venous thromboembolic events occurred in 5% (23/449) of Iclusig-treated patients, including deep venous thrombosis (8 patients), pulmonary embolism (6 patients), superficial thrombophlebitis (3 patients), and retinal vein thrombosis (2 patients). *Consider dose modification or discontinuation of Iclusig in patients who develop serious venous thromboembolism*

3.2. Heart Failure

Fatal and serious heart failure or left ventricular dysfunction occurred in 5% of Iclusig-treated patients (N = 22). Eight percent of patients (N = 35) experienced any grade of heart failure or left ventricular dysfunction. Monitor patients for signs or symptoms consistent with heart failure and treat as clinically indicated, including interruption of Iclusig. *Consider discontinuation of Iclusig in patients who develop serious heart failure*

(*continued*)

(continued)

3.3. Hypertension

Treatment-emergent hypertension occurred in 67% of patients (300/449). Eight patients (2%) treated with Iclusig in clinical trials experienced treatment-emergent symptomatic hypertension as a serious adverse reaction, including hypertensivecrisis. Patients may require urgent clinical intervention for hypertension associated with confusion, headache, chest pain, or shortness of breath. In patients with baseline systolic BP <140 mm Hg and baseline diastolic BP <90 mm Hg, 78% (220/282) experienced treatment-emergent hypertension; 49% (139/282) developed Stage 1 hypertension (defined as systolic BP ≥140 mm Hg or diastolic BP ≥90 mm Hg) while 29% developed Stage 2 hypertension (defined as systolic BP ≥160 mm Hg or diastolic BP ≥100 mm Hg). In 131 patients with Stage 1 hypertension at baseline, 61% (80/131) developed Stage 2 hypertension. *Monitor and manage blood pressure elevations during Iclusig use and treat hypertension to normalize blood pressure. Interrupt, dose reduce, or stop Iclusig if hypertension is not medically controlled*

3.4. Neuropathy

Peripheral and cranial neuropathy have occurred in Iclusig-treated patients. Overall, 13% (59/449) of Iclusig-treated patients experienced a peripheral neuropathy event of any grade (2%, grade 3/4). In clinical trials, the most common peripheral neuropathies reported were peripheral neuropathy (4%, 18/449), paresthesia (4%, 17/449), hypoesthesia (2%, 11/449), and hyperesthesia (1%, 5/449). Cranial neuropathy developed in 1% (6/449) of Iclusig-treated patients (<1% grade 3/4)

Of the patients who developed neuropathy, 31% (20/65) developed neuropathy during the first month of treatment. Monitor patients for symptoms of neuropathy, such as hypoesthesia, hyperesthesia, paresthesia, discomfort, a burning sensation, neuropathic pain or weakness. *Consider interrupting Iclusig and evaluate if neuropathy is suspected*

3.5. Ocular Toxicity

Serious ocular toxicities leading to blindness or blurred vision have occurred in Iclusig-treated patients. Retinal toxicities including macular edema, retinal vein occlusion, and retinal hemorrhage occurred in 3% of Iclusig-treated patients

Conjunctival or corneal irritation, dry eye, or eye pain occurred in 13% of patients. Visual blurring occurred in 6% of the patients. Other ocular toxicities include cataracts, glaucoma, iritis, iridocyclitis, and ulcerative keratitis. *Conduct comprehensive eye exams at baseline and periodically during treatment*

Treatment Modifications

Adverse Event	Treatment Modification
1st arterial thrombotic event	Interrupt and consider discontinuation of ponatinib
2nd arterial thrombotic event	Discontinue ponatinib
1st episode of G3/4 hepatotoxicity	Interrupt and then reduce or discontinue ponatinib
2nd episode of G3/4 hepatotoxicity	Discontinue ponatinib
First occurrence of ANC <1 × 10⁹/L or platelet <50 × 10⁹/L	Interrupt ponatinib and resume initial 45 mg dose after recovery to ANC $\geq 1.5 \times 10^9$/L and platelet $\geq 75 \times 10^9$/L
Second occurrence of ANC <1 × 10⁹/L or platelet <50 × 10⁹/L	Interrupt ponatinib and resume at 30 mg after recovery to ANC $\geq 1.5 \times 10^9$/L and platelet $\geq 75 \times 10^9$/L
Third occurrence of ANC <1 × 10⁹/L or platelet <50 × 10⁹/L	Interrupt ponatinib and resume at 15 mg after recovery to ANC $\geq 1.5 \times 10^9$/L and platelet $\geq 75 \times 10^9$/L
Elevation of liver transaminase >3 × ULN (G ≥2) at a ponatinib dose of 45 mg	Discontinue ponatinib and monitor hepatic function. Resume ponatinib at 30 mg after recovery to G ≤1 (<3 × ULN)
Elevation of liver transaminase >3 × ULN (G ≥2) at a ponatinib dose of 30 mg	Discontinue ponatinib and monitor hepatic function. Resume ponatinib at 15 mg after recovery to G ≤1 (<3 × ULN)
Elevation of liver transaminase >3 × ULN (G ≥2) at a ponatinib dose of 15 mg	Discontinue ponatinib
Elevation of liver transaminase >3 × ULN (G ≥2) concurrent with an elevation of bilirubin >2 × ULN and alkaline phosphatase <2 × ULN	Discontinue ponatinib
Asymptomatic G1/2 elevation of serum lipase	Consider interruption or dose reduction of ponatinib
Asymptomatic G3/4 elevation of lipase (>2 × ULN) or asymptomatic radiologic pancreatitis (G2 pancreatitis) at a ponatinib dose of 45 mg	Interrupt ponatinib and resume at 30 mg after recovery to G ≤1 (<1.5 × ULN)
Asymptomatic G3/4 elevation of lipase (>2 × ULN) or asymptomatic radiologic pancreatitis (G2 pancreatitis) at a ponatinib dose of 30 mg	Interrupt ponatinib and resume at 15 mg after recovery to G ≤1 (<1.5 × ULN)
Asymptomatic G3/4 elevation of lipase (>2 × ULN) or asymptomatic radiologic pancreatitis (G2 pancreatitis) at a ponatinib dose of 15 mg	Discontinue ponatinib

(continued)

Treatment Modifications (*continued*)

Adverse Event	Treatment Modification
Symptomatic G3 pancreatitis at a ponatinib dose of 45 mg	Interrupt ponatinib and resume at 30 mg after complete resolution of symptoms and after recovery of lipase elevation to G ≤1
Symptomatic G3 pancreatitis at a ponatinib dose of 30 mg	Interrupt ponatinib and resume at 15 mg after complete resolution of symptoms and after recovery of lipase elevation to G ≤1
Symptomatic G3 pancreatitis at a ponatinib dose of 15 mg	Discontinue ponatinib
G4 pancreatitis	Discontinue ponatinib

Notes:
Arterial Thrombosis: Cardiovascular, cerebrovascular, and peripheral vascular thrombosis, including fatal myocardial infarction and stroke have occurred in ponatinib-treated patients. In clinical trials, serious arterial thrombosis occurred in 8% of ponatinib-treated patients. Interrupt and consider discontinuation of ponatinib in patients who develop arterial thrombotic events
Hepatic Toxicity: Hepatotoxicity, liver failure and death have occurred in ponatinib-treated patients. Monitor hepatic function prior to and during treatment. Interrupt and then reduce or discontinue ponatinib for hepatotoxicity

Efficacy

	Philadelphia Chromosome–Positive CML		
	Chronic Phase (N = 43)	Accelerated Phase (N = 9)	Blast Phase (N = 8)
Received treatment	43 (100)	9 (100)	8 (100)
Continuing treatment at time of analysis	33 (77)	2 (22)	0
Median follow up (range, weeks)	73 (7–140)	13 (2–121)	
Discontinued treatment	10 (23)	7 (78)	8 (100)
Documented progressive disease	3 (7)	1 (11)	5 (62)
Adverse event	5 (12)	3 (33)	0
Death	0	1 (11)	1 (12)
Withdrawal of consent	1 (2)	1 (11)	0
Administrative decision	1 (2)	1 (11)	2 (25)

	Chronic-Phase CML				Accelerated-Phase CML, Blast-Phase CML, and PH-Positive ALL (N = 22)			
	Mutation (Number of Patients)				Mutation (Number of Patients)			
Variable	All (43)*	T315I (12)	Other (15)	None (13)	All (22)†	T315I (7)	Other (8)	None (5)
Complete hematologic response	42 (98)‡	12 (100)	14 (93)	13 (100)	NA	NA	NA	NA
Major hematologic response	NA	NA	NA	NA	8 (36)	2 (29)	2 (25)	3 (60)
Major cytogenetic response	31 (72)§	11 (92)	10 (67)	8 (62)	7 (32)	2 (29)	3 (38)	2 (40)
Complete cytogenetic response	27 (63)	9 (75)	10 (67)	6 (46)	3 (14)	1 (14)	0	2 (40)
Partial cytogenetic response	4 (9)	2 (17)	0	2 (15)	4 (18)	1 (14)	3 (38)	0
Major molecular response⁶	19 (44)	8 (67)	8 (53)	2 (15)	2 (9)	2 (29)	0	0
Molecular response 4⁶	9 (21)	3 (25)	6 (40)	0	0	0	0	0
Molecular response 4.5⁶	3 (7)	0	3 (20)	0	0	0	0	0

NA denotes not applicable
*Sequencing data were not available for 3 patients with chronic-phase CML; all 3 had a complete hematologic response, 2 had a major cytogenetic response (both complete), and 1 had a major molecular response
†Sequencing data were not available for 1 patient with accelerated-phase CML and 1 patient with blast-phase CML; the former patient had a major hematologic response
‡Of these patients, 26 had a complete hematologic response at baseline, and all 26 remained in complete hematologic response during the study
§At baseline, 1 patient had a complete hematologic response and a molecular relapse. This patient had a major molecular response during the study. Eight patients had a partial cytogenetic response at entry; of these patients, 7 had a complete cytogenetic response during the study, and 1 maintained a partial cytogenetic response
⁶Molecular response 4 was defined as at least a 4-log reduction, or a transcript ratio of BCR-ABL to ABL ≤0.01% (expressed as a percentage on the International Scale) in peripheral blood, as measured on quantitative reverse-transcriptase–polymerase-chain-reaction assay. Molecular response 4.5 indicates that the ratio is <0.0032%

Toxicity

Most Frequent Treatment-Related Adverse Events (AEs)*
Treatment-Related Adverse Events Total Study Population (N = 81)

	Any Grade	G ≥3	Serious
	Number of Patients (Percent)		
Nonhematologic Event			
Rash†	26 (32)	1 (1)	0
Arthralgia	14 (17)	1 (1)	0
Increased lipase	12 (15)‡	6 (7)	0
Fatigue	11 (14)	1 (1)	0
Acneiform dermatitis	11 (14)	1 (1)	0
Dry skin	11 (14)	0	0
Nausea	11 (14)	0	0
Headache	10 (12)	0	0
Hypertriglyceridemia	10 (12)	0	0
Myalgia	10 (12)	0	0
Pancreatitis§	11 (14)	4 (5)	8 (10)
Abdominal pain	8 (10)	1 (1)	0
Increased alanine aminotransferase	8 (10)	1 (1)	0
Increased aspartate aminotransferase	7 (9)	1 (1)	0
Abdominal distention	3 (4)	1 (1)	0
Increased amylase	3 (4)	2 (2)	0
Chills	3 (4)	1 (1)	0
Dyspnea	3 (4)	1 (1)	0
Prolonged QT interval	3 (4)	2 (2)	1 (1)
Erythema nodosum	2 (2)	1 (1)	0
Increased creatine kinase	1 (1)	1 (1)	0
Congestive cardiac failure	1 (1)	1 (1)	1 (1)
Decreased ejection fraction	1 (1)	1 (1)	1 (1)
Fluid retention	1 (1)	1 (1)	0
Interstitial lung disease	1 (1)	1 (1)	1 (1)
Melanoma	1 (1)	1 (1)	0
Migraine	1 (1)	1 (1)	0
Pain	1 (1)	1 (1)	0
Accidental overdose	1 (1)	0	1 (1)
Cardiomyopathy	1 (1)	0	1 (1)
Hematologic Event			
Thrombocytopenia	22 (27)	16 (20)	1 (1)
Neutropenia	10 (12)	8 (10)	0
Anemia	8 (10)	2 (2)	0
Lymphopenia	3 (4)	1 (1)	0
Decreased white-cell count	3 (4)	1 (1)	0

*Treatment-related AEs were graded by the NCI Common Terminology Criteria for Adverse Events (v.3) and defined as events investigators deemed to have a possible, probable, or definite relationship to ponatinib. Listed are treatment-related AEs reported in ≥10% of patients, along with any G ≥3 or serious events
†Rash includes erythematous and papular rash
‡A G1 increase in the lipase level deemed probably not related to ponatinib occurred in 1 patient
§Included in this category is 1 patient who had 3 events of pancreatitis (all G2; all serious) that were deemed to either not related or probably not related to ponatinib. One event was changed to G3 and possibly related to ponatinib after the database cutoff

Patient Population Studied

Patients with a diagnosis of CML whose disease had relapsed or was resistant to standard care, or for which no standard care was available or acceptable. Ph-positive disease was classified and characterized as relapsed or refractory disease on the basis of standard criteria. In addition, patients were required to have an Eastern Cooperative Oncology Group performance status of 2 or lower

Treatment Monitoring

1. Complete blood counts (CBCs) and leukocyte differential counts should be performed weekly during the first 3 cycles, then every second week during subsequent cycles
2. Serum ALT, AST, alkaline phosphatase, lipase, and (pancreatic) amylase at baseline and weekly during the first 2 cycles, then every second week during subsequent cycles

REFRACTORY PHILADELPHIA CHROMOSOME–POSITIVE CML REGIMEN

BOSUTINIB

Khoury HJ et al. Blood 2012;119:3403–3412

Bosutinib 500 mg/day; administer orally with food, continually (total dose/week = 3500 mg)

Notes:

1. If a dose is missed by more than 12 hours, the patient should skip the dose and resume taking the usual prescribed dose on the following day

2. Consider dose escalation from 500 mg daily to 600 mg once daily with food in patients who do not reach complete hematologic response (CHR) by week 8 or a complete cytogenetic response (CCyR) by week 12, and who did not have G ≥3 adverse reactions

3. *Use in Hepatic Impairment:* In patients with pre-existing mild, moderate, and severe hepatic impairment (Child-Pugh classes A, B, and C, respectively), the recommended dose of bosutinib is 200 mg daily. A daily dose of 200 mg in patients with hepatic impairment is predicted to result in systemic exposure (area under the concentration curve; AUC) similar to the AUC seen in patients with normal hepatic function receiving 500 mg daily. However, there are no clinical data for efficacy at the dose of 200 mg once daily in patients with hepatic impairment and CML

4. *Concomitant Use With CYP3A Inhibitors:* Avoid the concomitant use of strong or moderate CYP3A subfamily and/or P-glycoprotein (P-gp, ABCB1, MDR1) inhibitors with bosutinib as an increase in bosutinib plasma concentration is expected

   a. Strong CYP3A inhibitors include: boceprevir, clarithromycin, conivaptan, indinavir, itraconazole, ketoconazole, nefazodone, nelfinavir, posaconazole, ritonavir, saquinavir, telaprevir, voriconazole, and telithromycin

   b. Moderate CYP3A inhibitors include: amprenavir, aprepitant, atazanavir, ciprofloxacin, crizotinib, darunavir, diltiazem, erythromycin, fluconazole, fosamprenavir, grapefruit products, imatinib, and verapamil

5. *Concomitant Use With CYP3A Inducers:* Avoid the concomitant use of strong or moderate CYP3A inducers with bosutinib as a large reduction in exposure is expected

   a. Strong CYP3A inducers include: carbamazepine, phenobarbital, phenytoin, rifabutin, rifampin, and St. John's Wort

   b. Moderate CYP3A inducers include: bosentan, efavirenz, etravirine, modafinil, and nafcillin

Supportive Care

Antiemetic prophylaxis

Emetogenic potential is **MINIMAL–LOW**

See Chapter 39 for antiemetic recommendations

Hematopoietic growth factor (CSF) prophylaxis

Primary prophylaxis is NOT indicated

See Chapter 43 for more information

Antimicrobial prophylaxis

Risk of fever and neutropenia is LOW

Antimicrobial primary prophylaxis to be considered:

• Antibacterial—not indicated

• Antifungal—not indicated

• Antiviral—not indicated, unless patient previously had an episode of HSV

See Chapter 47 for more information

Treatment Modifications

Adverse Event	Treatment Modification
AST/ALT >5 × ULN	Withhold bosutinib until AST/ALT ≤2.5 × ULN, then resume use at 400 mg once daily
AST/ALT >5 × ULN >4 weeks	Discontinue bosutinib
AST/ALT ≤3 × ULN concurrently with bilirubin elevations >2 × ULN and alkaline phosphatase <2 × ULN (Hy's law case definition)	Discontinue bosutinib
G3/4 diarrhea (≥7 stools/day over baseline/ pretreatment)	Withhold bosutinib until recovery to G ≤1 and resume at 400 mg once daily
Other G3/4 nonhematologic toxicity	Withhold bosutinib until recovery to G ≤1, then resume use at 400 mg once daily. If clinically appropriate, consider re-escalating the dose of bosutinib to 500 mg once daily
1st episode of ANC <1000 × 10⁶/L or platelets <50,000 × 10⁶/L with recovery in <2 weeks	Withhold bosutinib until ANC ≥1000 × 10⁶/L and platelets ≥50,000 × 10⁶/L Resume treatment with bosutinib at the same dose
2nd episode of ANC <1000 × 10⁶/L or platelets <50,000 × 10⁶/L with recovery in <2 weeks	Withhold bosutinib until ANC ≥1000 × 10⁶/L and platelets ≥50,000 × 10⁶/L then resume bosutinib at a dose 100 mg less than the dose previously administered
ANC <1000 × 10⁶/L or platelets <50,000 × 10⁶/L with recovery in <2 weeks	Withhold bosutinib until ANC ≥1000 × 10⁶/L and platelets ≥50,000 × 10⁶/L, then resume bosutinib use at a dose 100 mg less than the dose previously administered
Fluid retention (pericardial effusion, pleural effusion, pulmonary edema, and/or peripheral edema)	Monitor and manage patients using standards of care. Interrupt, decrease the dose, or discontinue bosutinib as necessary

Efficacy

Response, n (%)	IM + DAS Resistant (n = 37)	IM + DAS Intolerant (n = 50)	IM + NI Resistant (n = 27)	IM + DAS + NI (n = 4)*	Total (n = 118)
Median follow-up, mo Median follow-up, (range)	20 (2.7–51.3)	34.5 (0.3–56.2)	23 (7.1–54)	34.5 (22.8–40)	28.5 (0.3–56.2)
Hematologic Response†					
Evaluable patients	37	49	26	4	116
Complete response	23 (62)	39 (80)	20 (77)	3 (75)	85 (73)
Hematologic Response Among Patients with no Baseline CHR					
Evaluable patients	22	24	20	2	68
Complete response	11 (50)	16 (67)	15 (75)	2 (100)	44 (65)
Cytogenetic Response‡					
Evaluable patients	35	43	26	4	108
Major response	11 (31)	13 (30)	9 (35)	2 (50)	35 (32)
Complete response	5 (14)	12 (28)	7 (27)	2 (50)	26 (24)
Partial response	6 (17)	1 (2)	2 (8)	0	9 (8)
Minor response	0	4 (9)	2 (8)	0	6 (6)
Molecular response§					
Evaluable patients	35	48	19	3	105
Major response	1 (3)	12 (25)	2 (11)	1 (33)	16 (15)
Complete response	0	9 (19)	2 (11)	1 (33)	12 (11)

DAS, dasatinib; IM, imatinib; NI, nilotinib; CHR, complete hematologic response
*Includes 3 patients who previously received all 3 inhibitors and 1 patient with NI intolerance
†Evaluable patients had a baseline disease assessment. Patients with CHR at baseline were evaluable for hematologic response and were considered responders if they maintained their response at 2 consecutive postbaseline assessments ≥4 weeks apart
‡Evaluable patients had a baseline disease assessment. Patients with CCyR at baseline were considered nonresponders for assessment of cytogenetic response
§Because of logistical constraints, patients from sites in China, India, Russia, and South Africa were not assessed for molecular response. MMR indicates ≥3 log reduction from standardized baseline Bcr-Abl: Abl ratio, and CMR, undetectable Bcr-Abl, with a sensitivity of ≥5 log. Molecular response was not assessed according to the International Scale

(continued)

Patient Population Studied

Study patients represented a subpopulation of adults with a confirmed diagnosis of Ph$^+$ chronic-phase CML who previously received treatment with imatinib followed by dasatinib and/or nilotinib. All had an Eastern Cooperative Oncology Group performance status of 0 or 1, and no allogeneic hematopoietic stem cell transplantation within 3 months before starting study treatment. All patients had previously received imatinib and developed primary or acquired resistance or intolerance to imatinib, and had also received and developed resistance or intolerance to dasatinib and/or nilotinib. Resistance was defined as failure to achieve or maintain any of the following with previously administered treatments: hematologic improvement within 4 weeks, CHR after 12 weeks, any cytogenetic response by 24 weeks, or MCyR by 12 months. Acquired resistance was defined as loss of a MCyR or any hematologic response. Patients could also have resistance related to Bcr-Abl mutations. Intolerance was defined as an inability to take a protein kinase inhibitor because of drug-related G4 hematologic toxicity lasting more than 7 days, drug-related G3/4 nonhematologic toxicity, persistent G2 toxicity that did not respond to dose reduction and medical management, or loss of previously attained response on lower doses of protein kinase inhibitor therapy with an inability to receive a higher dose because of drug-related toxicity at higher doses

Phase 1/2, open-label, multicenter, 2-part study. The phase 1 (part 1) dose-escalation study enrolled patients with chronic phase CML previously treated with only imatinib. It determined the part 2 starting dose of bosutinib 500 mg/day, despite not reaching a study-defined maximum tolerated dose. Part 2 of the study evaluated the efficacy and safety of bosutinib across multiple patient subpopulations, including those with chronic-phase CML who had been previously treated with imatinib and dasatinib and/or nilotinib. The primary analysis in the subpopulation of patients with chronic-phase CML previously treated with multiple protein kinase inhibitors was MCyR by 24 weeks

Efficacy (continued)

Response by Baseline Mutation Status

Mutation Status	n	Cumulative Response, n/n Evaluable (%)	
		CHR	MCyR
No mutation	44	34/44 (77)	15/43 (35)
Any mutation	39	26/39 (67)	11/35 (31)
>1 mutation	9	3/9 (33)	2/9 (22)
Mutation type*			
P-loop†	14	9/14 (64)	4/13 (31)
G250E	6	3/6	0/5
Y253H	6	5/6	4/6
E255K	1	0/1	0/1
E255V	1	1/1	0/1
Non–P-loop†	29	18/29 (62)	9/26 (35)
M244V	3	3/3	2/3
V299L	2	1/2	0/2
Q300R	1	1/1	1/1
T315I	7	2/7	0/6
F317L	8	4/8	1/7
N336S	1	1/1	0/1
M351T	1	1/1	0/1
F359C	2	2/2	½
F359I	2	2/2	2/2
F359V	2	0/2	½
L387F	1	1/1	0/1
H396R	1	0/1	0/1
E453A	1	1/1	0/0
C475V	1	1/1	1/1
F486S	1	0/1	0/1

*Patients with >1 mutation may be counted in both the P-loop and non–P-loop categories
†P-loop mutations include those from positions 248 to 255
‡Non–P-loop mutations include those from positions 244 to 247 and >255

Treatment Monitoring

1. Complete blood counts (CBCs) and leukocyte differential counts should be performed weekly during the first month after starting bosutinib, and at least monthly thereafter

2. Serum hepatic enzymes monthly during the first 3 months after starting bosutinib, and as clinically indicated thereafter. Increase the frequency of monitoring if hepatic transaminases increase after starting treatment

Toxicity

Dose interruptions and reductions resulting from AEs were required for 63% and 48% of patients, respectively. Twenty-four (20%) patients discontinued bosutinib because of AEs as shown in Table

	IM + DAS Resistant (n = 37)	IM + DAS Intolerant (n = 50)	IM + NI Resistant (n = 27)	IM + DAS + NI (n = 4)*	Total (n = 118)
Reason, n (%)					
Discontinued treatment	31 (84)	34 (68)	16 (59)	3 (75)	84 (71)
Unsatisfactory response	12 (32)	7 (14)	5 (19)	1 (25)	25 (21)
Adverse event†	**6 (16)**	**15 (30)**	**3 (11)**	**0**	**24 (20)**
Disease progression	8 (22)	4 (8)	6 (22)	2 (50)	20 (17)
Death	2 (5)	2 (4)	0	0	4 (3)
Patient request	0	2 (4)	1 (4)	0	3 (3)
Lost to follow-up	2 (5)	0	0	0	2 (2)
Investigator request	0	0	1 (4)	0	1 (1)
Protocol violation	0	1 (2)	0	0	1 (1)
Other‡	1 (3)	3 (6)	0	0	4 (3)

DAS, dasatinib; IM, imatinib; NI, nilotinib
*Includes 3 patients who previously received all 3 inhibitors and 1 patient with NI intolerance
†AEs most frequently leading to discontinuation included thrombocytopenia (4%), neutropenia (3%), and elevated ALT (3%). Of note, 6 patients were in MCyR at the time that they discontinued treatment because of an AE
‡Includes patient noncompliance (n = 2), lack of finances (n = 1), and started chemotherapy for gastric adenocarcinoma (n = 1)

Treatment-Related AEs Occurring in >10% of Patients

AE	All Grades, n (%)	Grade 3/4, n (%)
Diarrhea	96 (81)	10 (8)
Nausea	51 (43)	0
Vomiting	38 (32)	1 (1)
Rash	26 (22)	5 (4)
Fatigue	21 (18)	1 (1)
Abdominal pain	18 (15)	0
Headache	16 (14)	1 (1)
Upper abdominal pain	15 (13)	0
Pruritus	12 (10)	1 (1)

(continued)

Toxicity (continued)

Laboratory Abnormalities Reported by >20% of Patients on Therapy

	At Baseline		On Therapy	
	All G, n (%)	G3/4, n (%)	All G, n (%)	G3/4, n (%)
Laboratory Abnormality				
Anemia	66 (56)	1 (1)	99 (84)	10 (8)
Thrombocytopenia*	20 (17)	1 (1)	69 (58)	30 (25)
Elevated ALT*	12 (10)	0	58 (49)	8 (7)
Neutropenia*	23 (19)	4 (3)	54 (46)	23 (19)
↑ Creatinine	13 (11)	0	50 (42)	1 (1)
↑ AST	15 (13)	0	48 (41)	4 (3)
Hypocalcemia	8 (7)	1 (1)	44 (37)	6 (5)
↑ Alkaline phosphatase	12 (10)	0	41 (35)	0
Hypophosphatemia	8 (7)	0	37 (31)	3 (2)
Hyperglycemia	15 (13)	0	36 (31)	1 (1)
Low bicarbonate	4 (3)	0	36 (31)	0
Hypermagnesemia	11 (9)	9 (8)	34 (29)	14 (12)
↑ PTT	16 (14)	0	30 (25)	1 (1)
↑ Lipase	7 (6)	0	28 (24)	8 (7)
Hyperkalemia	3 (3)	1 (1)	27 (23)	0

*Dose interruptions and reductions resulting from AEs were required for 63% and 48% of patients, respectively. AEs most frequently leading to discontinuation included thrombocytopenia (4%), neutropenia (3%), and elevated ALT (3%)

Reason Dasatinib Intolerant	Number Dasatinib Intolerant	Same G3/4 AE with Bosutinib as with Dasatinib	Discontinued Bosutinib Because of Same AE with Bosutinib as with Dasatinib
Any AE*	50	11 (22)	4 (8)
Hematologic events	20	8 (40)	2 (10)
Thrombocytopenia	8	6 (75)	1 (13)
Pancytopenia	5	0	0
Neutropenia	4	4 (100)	1 (25)
Cardiovascular events	3	0[‡]	1 (33)
Gastrointestinal events	6	0[‡]	0
Diarrhea	3	0[‡]	0
Musculoskeletal events	4	0[‡]	0
Respiratory events	23	3 (13)	1 (4)
Pleural effusion	19	2 (11)[†]	0[†]
Dyspnea	3	1 (33)	1 (33)
Skin disorders	5	0[‡]	0

*Includes all AEs with ≥3 patients categorized as intolerant on prior dasatinib
[†]Two patients had G3/4 pleural effusions on bosutinib (at days 597 and 967 of treatment), but neither discontinued bosutinib because of a pleural effusion
[‡]No patient with dasatinib intolerance related to cardiovascular events, gastrointestinal events, musculoskeletal events, or skin disorders experienced the same toxicity as a G3/4 AE on bosutinib

REFRACTORY PHILADELPHIA CHROMOSOME–POSITIVE CML REGIMEN

Chronic or accelerated phase chronic CML with resistance and/or intolerance to 2 or more tyrosine kinase inhibitors (TKIs)

OMACETAXINE MEPESUCCINATE

Cortes J et al. Am J Hematol 2013;88:350–354
Cortes J et al. Blood 2012;120:2573–2580

Omacetaxine mepesuccinate 1.25 mg/m² per dose by subcutaneous injection:
Induction regimen schedule
Doses are given twice daily for 14 consecutive days, on days 1–14, every 28 days until patients achieve a hematologic response (total dosage/28-day cycle = 35 mg/m²)

Maintenance regimen schedule
Doses are given twice daily for 7 consecutive days, on days 1–7, every 28 days for as long as patients experience clinical benefit from treatment (total dosage/28-day cycle = 17.5 mg/m²)

Supportive Care
Antiemetic prophylaxis
Emetogenic potential is **LOW**
See Chapter 39 for antiemetic recommendations

Hematopoietic growth factor (CSF) prophylaxis
Primary prophylaxis may be indicated
See Chapter 43 for more information

Antimicrobial prophylaxis
Risk of fever and neutropenia is LOW
  Antimicrobial primary prophylaxis to be considered:
  • Antibacterial—not indicated
  • Antifungal—not indicated
  • Antiviral—not indicated unless patient previously had an episode of HSV
See Chapter 47 for more information

Treatment Modifications

G4 neutropenia (ANC <0.5 × 10⁹/L) or G3 thrombocytopenia (<50 × 10⁹/L) during a cycle	Delay start of next cycle until ANC ≥1 × 10⁹/L and platelet count ≥50 × 10⁹/L. Also, for the next cycle, reduce the number of dosing days by 2 days (eg, to 12 or 5 days)
G3/4 non-hematologic toxicity	Interrupt and/or delay omacetaxine mepesuccinate until toxicity is G ≤1. Also, for the next cycle, reduce the number of dosing days by 2 days (eg, to 12 or 5 days)
G2 AE unresponsive to supportive care	Interrupt treatment until G ≤1 then resume omacetaxine mepesuccinate at full dose
G ≥3 AE unresponsive to supportive care	Interrupt treatment until G ≤1 then resume omacetaxine mepesuccinate reducing the number of treatment days by 2 in subsequent cycles

Patient Population Studied

The efficacy of omacetaxine mepesuccinate was evaluated using a combined cohort of adult patients with CML from 2 trials. The combined cohort consisted of patients who had received 2 or more approved TKIs and had, at a minimum, documented evidence of resistance or intolerance to dasatinib and/or nilotinib. Resistance was defined as 1 of the following: no complete hematologic response (CHR) by 12 weeks (whether lost or never achieved); or no cytogenetic response by 24 weeks (ie, 100% Ph-positive [Ph⁺]) (whether lost or never achieved); or no major cytogenetic response (MCyR) by 52 weeks (ie, ≥35% Ph⁺) (whether lost or never achieved); or progressive leukocytosis. Intolerance was defined as 1 of the following: (a) G3/4 nonhematologic toxicity that did not resolve with adequate intervention; (b) G4 hematologic toxicity lasting more than 7 days; or (c) any G ≥2 toxicity unacceptable to the patient. Patients with NYHA class III or IV heart disease, active ischemia, or other uncontrolled cardiac conditions were excluded

A total of 76 patients with chronic phase CML were included in the efficacy analysis. The demographics were: median age 59 years, 30% were 65 years of age or older. All had previously received 2 or more TKIs, including imatinib. Thirty-six (47%) patients had failed treatment with imatinib, dasatinib, and nilotinib. Most patients had also received prior non-TKI treatments, most commonly hydroxyurea (54%), interferon (30%), and/or cytarabine (29%)

Toxicity

Adverse Reactions Occurring in at Least 10% of Patients
(Chronic Myeloid Leukemia–Chronic Phase)

Adverse Reaction	Number (%) of Patients (N = 108)	
	All Reactions	G3/4 Reactions
Patients with ≥1 commonly occurring adverse reaction	107 (99)	94 (87)
Blood and Lymphatic System Disorders		
Thrombocytopenia	80 (74)	72 (67)
Anemia	66 (61)	39 (36)
Neutropenia	54 (50)	49 (45)
Lymphopenia	18 (17)	17 (16)
Bone marrow failure	11 (10)	11 (10)
Febrile neutropenia	11 (10)	11 (10)
Gastrointestinal Disorders		
Diarrhea	45 (42)	1 (1)
Nausea	35 (32)	1 (1)
Constipation	16 (15)	0
Abdominal pain, upper	15 (14)	0
Vomiting	13 (12)	0
General Disorders and Administration Site Conditions		
Fatigue	28 (26)	5 (5)
Pyrexia	26 (24)	1 (1)
Asthenia	25 (23)	1 (1)
Edema peripheral	14 (13)	0
Infusion and injection site–related reactions	37 (34)	0
Infections and Infestations		
Bacterial, viral, fungal, and nonspecified infections	50 (46)	12 (11)
Musculoskeletal and Connective Tissue Disorders		
Arthralgia	20 (19)	1 (1)
Pain in Extremity	14 (13)	1 (1)
Back pain	12 (11)	2 (2)
Nervous System Disorders		
Headache	20 (19)	1 (1)
Psychiatric Disorders		
Insomnia	11 (10)	0
Respiratory, Thoracic and Mediastinal Disorders		
Cough	17 (16)	1 (1)
Epistaxis	16 (15)	1 (1)
Skin and Subcutaneous Tissue Disorders		
Alopecia	16 (15)	0
Rash	11 (10)	0

Notes:
Safety data were evaluated in 163 patients, including 108 patients with CML-CP and 55 patients with CML-AP who received at least 1 dose of omacetaxine mepesuccinate and an additional 4 patients with CML-CP from another open-label, single-arm trial. Ten deaths were reported within 30 days after the last omacetaxine mepesuccinate dose. Four of these were attributed to progressive disease, 4 to cerebral hemorrhage, 1 to multiorgan failure, and 1 to unknown causes

Efficacy

The accelerated FDA approval was based on combined data from 2 open-label single-arm trials enrolling patients with CML in chronic phase (CML-CP) or in accelerated phase (CML-AP). The efficacy population included 76 patients with CML-CP who had received 2 or more prior TKIs, including imatinib

Efficacy Results for Patients with CP CML

The efficacy end point was based on MCyR

	Patients (N = 76)
Primary Response—MCyR	
Total with MCyR, n (%)	14 (18.4)
95% confidence interval	(10.5%–29%)
Cytogenetic Response, n (%)	
Confirmed complete	6 (7.9)
Confirmed partial	3 (3.9)
Mean time to MCyR onset (N = 14)	3.5 months
Median duration of MCyR (N = 14)	12.5 months (Kaplan-Meier estimate)

Cytogenetic response evaluation is based on standard cytogenetic analysis (at least 20 metaphases)
Complete: no Ph+ cells; Partial: >0 to 35% Ph+ cells

Treatment Monitoring

1. Complete blood counts (CBCs) should be performed weekly during induction and initial maintenance cycles
2. After initial maintenance cycles, monitor CBCs every 2 weeks, or as clinically indicated
3. Monitor blood glucose concentrations frequently, especially in patients with diabetes or risk factors for diabetes

CML REGIMEN

HYDROXYUREA

Hehlmann R et al. Blood 1994;84:4064–4077

Starting dose: **Hydroxyurea** 40 mg/kg; administer orally after meals, continually, as a single daily dose or divided into 2 doses (total dosage/week [initially] = 280 mg/kg)

1. Optimal dose is determined **empirically**, with very frequent monitoring of CBC (eg, every 3 days)

2. A dose of 1000–2000 mg/day is frequently sufficient for patients with WBC <100,000/mm^3. With higher WBCs and a need to rapidly lower WBC, hydroxyurea 6000–8000 mg/day may be required initially

3. Total daily dose depends on disease activity and is extremely variable (range: hydroxyurea 500–15,000 mg/day)

4. Therapeutic goal is normalization of the WBC (target: 5000–10,000/mm^3). This may require significantly higher or lower doses than the initial dose. If response is insufficient, aggressiveness of dose escalation must match aggressiveness of the disease. Frequent monitoring of WBC is mandatory during changes to the regimen

   a. Slowly rising WBC or failure to achieve therapeutic target: increase total daily hydroxyurea dose 25–50%, assess effect after 5–7 days before further escalation

   b. Rapidly rising WBC: increase total daily hydroxyurea dose by 50–100%, assess effect of dose increase for 3 days before further dose escalation

5. Very high doses carry a risk of prolonged aplasia

Supportive Care

Antiemetic prophylaxis
*Emetogenic potential is **MINIMAL–LOW***
See Chapter 39 for antiemetic recommendations

Hematopoietic growth factor (CSF) prophylaxis
Primary prophylaxis is NOT indicated
See Chapter 43 for more information

Antimicrobial prophylaxis
Risk of fever and neutropenia is LOW
   Antimicrobial primary prophylaxis to be considered:
   • Antibacterial—not indicated
   • Antifungal—not indicated
   • Antiviral—not indicated, unless patient previously had an episode of HSV
See Chapter 47 for more information

Patient Population Studied

Study of 194 patients with newly diagnosed CML in chronic phase

Efficacy (N = 194)

5-year survival: 45%

Toxicity*

Hematologic side effects

1. Neutropenia and anemia are common, whereas thrombocytopenia is rare

2. Cytopenias are usually rapidly reversible (within 3–4 days)

3. High doses and/or failure to interrupt treatment despite cytopenia may result in prolonged aplasia

Relatively common nonhematologic side effects

1. Gastrointestinal symptoms (stomatitis, anorexia, nausea, vomiting, diarrhea)

2. Acute skin reactions (rash, ulceration, dermatomyositis-like changes, erythema)

Rare, nonhematologic side effects

1. Chronic skin reactions (hyperpigmentation, atrophy of skin and nails, skin cancer, alopecia)

2. Headache, drowsiness, convulsions

3. Fever, chills, asthenia

4. Renal and hepatic impairment

Important note: A comprehensive and detailed analysis of nonhematologic toxicity from a controlled trial is not available

Therapy Monitoring

1. *CBC:* At least weekly at first, then every 2–4 weeks after achieving stable blood counts

2. *Blood chemistry profile:* Every 6 months

3. *Bone marrow morphology and cytogenetics:* Every 6 months

Treatment Modifications

Hematological Toxicity

G1	No dose modifications. G1 WBC or ANC are acceptable or even desirable
G2 or G3	Hold hydroxyurea until toxicity resolves to G1, then restart at 75% of initial dose
Recurrent G2/3	Hold hydroxyurea until toxicity resolves to G1, then restart at 50% of initial dose
G4	Hold hydroxyurea until toxicity resolves to G1, then restart at 25% of initial dose
Recurrent G4	Hold hydroxyurea until toxicity resolves to G1, then restart at 50% of the previous dose

Nonhematologic Toxicity

G1	No dose modifications
G2/3	Hold hydroxyurea until toxicity resolves to G1, then restart at initial dose
Recurrent G2/3	Hold hydroxyurea until toxicity resolves to G1, then restart at 75% of initial dose
G4	Hold hydroxyurea until toxicity resolves to G1, then restart at 50% of dose previously administered
Recurrent G4	Discontinue hydroxyurea

Notes

1. Hydroxyurea is the drug of choice when a rapid reduction of the white cell count is clinically mandated, but the diagnosis of BCR-ABL-positive CML has not been established

2. Hydroxyurea may be indicated in cases of imatinib intolerance or resistance

CML REGIMEN

INTERFERON ALFA

Baccarani M et al. Blood 2002;99:1527–1535
Hehlmann R et al. Blood 1994;84:4064–4077

Premedication:
Acetaminophen 500–650 mg/dose; administer orally, every 4 to 6 hours as needed

Target dose of Interferon alfa:
Interferon alfa-2a 5 million IU/m^2 per day; administer subcutaneously, continually (preferably at bedtime) (total dosage/week = 35 million IU/m^2)

or

Interferon alfa-2b 5 million IU/m^2 per day; administer subcutaneously, continually (preferably at bedtime) (total dosage/week = 35 million IU/m^2)

Typical dose of Interferon alfa:
5 million IU/m^2 per day. To increase tolerability, interferon alfa should be started at low doses (eg, 1.5 million IU/m^2 per day), with gradual increases over several weeks until the target dose is achieved

Supportive Care
Antiemetic prophylaxis
Emetogenic potential is **MINIMAL–LOW**
See Chapter 39 for antiemetic recommendations

Hematopoietic growth factor (CSF) prophylaxis
Primary prophylaxis is NOT indicated
See Chapter 43 for more information

Antimicrobial prophylaxis
Risk of fever and neutropenia is LOW
Antimicrobial primary prophylaxis to be considered:
- Antibacterial—not indicated
- Antifungal—not indicated
- Antiviral—not indicated, unless patient previously had an episode of HSV

See Chapter 47 for more information

Notes

Interferon alfa is reserved for patients who are intolerant of imatinib, nilotinib, and dasatinib. Patients whose disease is resistant to these drugs usually do not respond to interferon alfa

On October 1, 2007, Hoffmann-La Roche, Inc. (Nutley, NJ) announced interferon alfa-2a (Roferon-A®) would be discontinued from the U.S. market

In 1989, interferon alfa-2a received orphan drug designation from the U.S. Food and Drug Administration for the treatment of chronic myelogenous leukemia and other oncological diseases

Patient Population Studied

Patients with newly diagnosed CML in chronic phase:
n = 263
(Baccarani M et al. Blood 2002;99:1527–1535)

n = 194
(Hehlmann R et al. Blood 1994;84:4064–4077)

Efficacy (N = 263)

Complete or partial hematologic response	74%
Complete cytogenetic response	7.6%
Partial cytogenetic response	10.3%
5-year survival	65%

Baccarani M et al. Blood 2002;99:1527–1535

Treatment Modifications

The practical management of patients receiving interferon alfa is complex. The simplified dose modification schema shown below is only a minimal guideline

Nonhematologic Toxicity

G1	No dose reduction
G2	Reduce interferon alfa dosage by 25%
G3/4	Stop interferon alfa. Restart at 50% of the previously administered dose after toxicity resolves. If resumption is tolerated, increase to 75% of the dose that produced G3/4 toxicity

Hematologic Toxicity

G1/2	No dose reduction
G3	Reduce interferon alfa dosage in 25% decrements until abates to grade <3
G4	Stop interferon alfa. Restart at a dosage decreased by 50% when toxicity resolves; increase dosage to 75% of the dose that produced G4 toxicity if tolerated

Modified from: O'Brien S et al. Leuk Lymphoma 1996;23:247–252

Toxicity

Toxicity	% (All Grades)
Fever	92
Asthenia or fatigue	88
Myalgia	68
Chills	63
Anorexia	48
Arthralgia/bone pain	47
Headache	44
Nausea, vomiting	37
Diarrhea	37
Depression	28
Cough	19
Hair changes	18
Skin rashes	18
Decreased mental status	16
Sweating	15
Dizziness	11
Sleep disturbances	11
Paresthesia	8
Dyspnea	8
Cardiac dysrhythmia	7
Involuntary movements	7
Dry skin	7
Pruritus	7
Visual disturbances	6

Roferon-A (interferon alfa-2a, recombinant) product label, October 2004. Hoffmann-La Roche Inc., Nutley, NJ

Therapy Monitoring

1. *CBC:* Weekly; every 3–4 weeks after achievement of complete hematologic response, if counts are stable; every 4–6 weeks after achievement of complete cytogenetic response
2. *Blood chemistry:* Twice weekly; every 4–6 weeks after achievement of complete hematologic response
3. *Bone marrow cytogenetics:* Every 6 months; every 6–12 months after achievement of complete cytogenetic response
4. *Quantitative RT-PCR for BCR-ABL from peripheral blood or bone marrow:* Every 3 months

21. Leukemia, Hairy Cell

Martin S. Tallman, MD

Epidemiology

Incidence: 2% of all leukemia (approximately 600–800 new patients per year in the United States)

Median age: 52 years

Male to female ratio: Approximately 4:1

Bernstein L et al. Cancer Res 1990;50:3605–3609
Staines A, Cartwright RA. Br J Haematol 1993;85:714–717

Pathology

Peripheral blood findings at diagnosis
1. Pancytopenia: 50%
2. "Leukemic" phase with a WBC >1000/mm^3: 10–20%
3. Monocytopenia
4. Hairy cells identified in most patients, but the number is usually low and may be difficult to identify in the peripheral blood because of low numbers and staining technique

Bone marrow findings at diagnosis
1. Hypercellularity
2. Hairy cell infiltration: diffuse, patchy, or interstitial

   Diffuse infiltration: Often results in complete effacement of bone marrow

   Patchy infiltration: Subtle small clusters of hairy cells present focally or throughout the bone marrow

   Interstitial Infiltration: Hairy cells do not form well-defined discreet aggregates, but merge almost imperceptibly with surrounding normal hematopoietic tissue
3. Hairy cell nuclei are usually round, oval, or indented, and are widely separated from each other by abundant, clear or lightly eosinophilic cytoplasm. Rarely hairy cells can be convoluted or spindle shaped
4. Extravasated blood cells create blood lakes in the bone marrow similar to those observed in the spleen
5. Mast cells are often numerous
6. Reticulin stain of the bone marrow almost always shows moderate to marked increase in reticulin fibers
7. Approximately 10–20% of patients show a hypocellular bone marrow

Immunophenotyping, cytogenetics, and molecular diagnostic studies
1. *Cytochemical studies:* Tartrate-resistant acid phosphatase (**TRAP**) stain. However, TRAP is not specific for HCL
2. *Hairy cell immunophenotype:* CD19(+), CD20(+), CD22(+), CD79B(+), CD5(−), CD10(−), CD11C(+), CD25 Sub(+), FMC(+), CD103(+), CD45(+)
3. *Clonal cytogenetics:* Abnormalities in approximately two-thirds of patients. Chromosomes 1, 2, 5, 6, 11, 14, 19, and 20 are most frequently involved. Chromosome 5 is altered in approximately 40%, most commonly as a trisomy 5, pericentric inversion, and interstitial deletions involving band 5q13. However, the identification of cytogenetic abnormalities in a patient with a definite diagnosis of HCL is usually not important as it does not influence, as far as is currently determined, prognosis or therapy

(continued)

Work-up

1. H&P
2. CBC with differential, serum electrolytes, BUN, creatinine, LFTs, and uric acid
3. Bone marrow aspirate and biopsy for tartrate-resistant acid phosphatase (TRAP) (although TRAP is not required for the diagnosis, has been largely abandoned, and has been supplanted by immunophenotyping) and morphologic review; immunophenotyping by flow cytometry with B-cell–associated antibodies, including CD20, CD79A, or DBA.44

Tallman MS et al. Hairy cell leukemia. In: Hoffman, ed. Hematology: Basic Principles and Practice, 3rd ed. Philadelphia, Churchill Livingstone, 2000:1363–1372

Pathology (continued)

Bartl R et al. Am J Clin Pathol 1983;79:531–545
Brunning RD et al. Atlas of Tumor Pathology, 3rd Series, Fascicle 9. Washington DC, AFIP, 1994; pp 277–278
Burke JS et al. Am J Clin Pathol 1978;70:876–884
Burke JS et al. Semin Oncol 1984;11:334–346
Cornfield DB et al. Am J Hematol 2001;67:223–226
Ellison DJ et al. Blood 1994;84:4310–4315
Flandrin G et al. Semin Oncol 1984;11(4 Suppl 2):458–471
Golomb HM et al. Ann Intern Med 1978;89(Part 1):677–683
Haglund U et al. Blood 1994;83:2637–2645
Hakimian D et al. Blood 1993;82:1798–1802
Hanson CA et al. Am J Surg Pathol 1989;13:671–679
Hounieu H et al. Am J Clin Pathol 1992;98:26–33
Katayama I. Hematol Oncol Clin North Am 1988;2:585–602
Kluin-Nelemans HC et al. Blood 1994;84:3134–3141
Kroft SH et al. Blood Rev 1995;9:234–250
Lee WM, Beckstead JH. Cancer 1982;50:2207–2210
Robbins BA et al. Blood 1993;82:1277–1287
Sausville JE et al. Am J Clin Pathol 2003;119:213–217
Turner A, Kjeldsberg CR. Medicine (Baltimore) 1978;57:477–499
Wheaton S et al. Blood 1996;87:1556–1560
Yam LT et al. N Engl J Med 1971;284:357–360

Differential Diagnosis

Other small B-cell lymphoproliferative disorders associated with splenomegaly:

1. Prolymphocytic leukemia
   a. Marked elevation in the WBC
   b. Characteristic morphology of the prolymphocytes
   c. Different immunophenotypic profile
2. Splenic marginal zone lymphoma (splenic lymphoma with villous lymphocytes)
   a. Cells do not usually exhibit TRAP positivity
   b. Bone marrow infiltrates are demarcated sharply
   c. Different immunophenotypic profile; CD103(−)
3. HCL variant
   a. Morphologic features between hairy cells and prolymphocytes
   b. Usually associated with leukocytosis/lack of monocytopenia
   c. Absence of CD25 expression
4. Systemic mastocytosis
   a. Mast cells are negative for B-cell markers, and positive for tryptase

Catovsky D et al. Semin Oncol 1984;11:362–369
Cawley JC et al. Leuk Res 1980;4:547–559
de Totero D et al. Blood 1993;82:528–535
Galton DA et al. Br J Haematol 1974;27:7–23
Horny HP et al. Am J Clin Pathol 1988;89:335–340
Isaacson PG et al. Blood 1994;84:3828–3834
Kroft SH et al. Blood Rev 1995;9:234–250
Matutes E et al. Blood 1994;83:1558–1562
Matutes E et al. Leukemia 2001;15:184–186
Melo JV et al. Br J Haematol 1986;63:377–387
Melo JV et al. Br J Haematol 1987;65:23–29
Mulligan SP et al. Br J Haematol 1991;78:206–209
Sainati L et al. Blood 1990;76:157–162
Troussard X et al. Br J Haematol 1996;93:731–736

Prognosis

Therapy with purine analogs: pentostatin (2'-deoxycoformycin) or cladribine (2-chlorodeoxyadenosine)

Complete remission	70–90%
Peripheral remission	10–20%
No response	5–10%
Relapse rate	5–25%
Estimated 5-year survival rate	85–90%
5–10-year survival rate	80–90%

Catovsky D et al. Leuk Lymphoma 1994;14:109–113
Dearden CE et al. Br J Haematol 1999;106:515–519
Flinn IW et al. Blood 2000;96:2981–2986
Goodman GR et al. J Clin Oncol 2003;21:891–896
Grever M et al. J Clin Oncol 1995;13:974–982
Hoffman MA et al. J Clin Oncol 1997;15:1138–1142
Jehn U et al. Ann Hematol 1999;78:139–144
Kraut EH et al. Blood 1994;84:4061–4063
Saven A et al. Blood 1998;92:1918–1926
Tallman MS et al. Blood 1992;80:2203–2209
Tallman MS et al. Blood 1996;88:1954–1959

Expert Opinion

A diagnosis of HCL by itself is not necessarily an indication to initiate treatment. If a patient is maintaining safe peripheral blood counts, the conservative approach is to "watch and wait" until counts decrease

Treatment is indicated when a patient has developed life-threatening cytopenias (absolute neutrophil count <1000/mm^3, hemoglobin <11 g/dL, or platelet count <100,000/mm^3), or in the presence of symptomatic splenomegaly or constitutional symptoms attributable to the disease

There is no clear advantage to either purine analog as initial treatment for patients with previously untreated HCL with respect to long-term outcome. The ease of administration of cladribine, which requires only a single course of therapy, may offer some advantages

Patients should be followed closely during treatment and for several months after completion of therapy, with special attention to appropriate surveillance and treatment for infection resulting from myelosuppression. An improvement in peripheral blood counts after purine nucleoside analog treatment may require weeks and sometimes months. Bone marrow biopsy to confirm a complete response is usually performed 3 months after the completion of therapy. However, if the peripheral blood counts return to normal, splenomegaly resolves and the patient is asymptomatic, one can argue not to carry out another bone marrow biopsy as the results will likely not influence further therapy. Even if the marrow demonstrates a small amount of HCL, further therapy is not indicated outside the context of a clinical trial exploring the potential benefits of additional therapy for residual disease

For patients who do not respond to initial therapy with a purine analog, the suggested therapeutic option is treatment with a different purine analog. However, the lack of excellent response to one purine analog is exceedingly uncommon and would prompt a reevaluation of the diagnosis

If relapse is suspected, the bone marrow should be reexamined before restarting therapy. In patients who achieved an initial, durable complete response to a purine analog lasting longer than 1 year, a reasonable course of action would be to retreat the patient either with the same agent or an alternative purine analog. If there was an initial remission of short duration (eg, <1 year), a repeated course of the original therapy is unlikely to result in a second remission of equivalent or longer duration. Retreatment with a second cycle of cladribine or pentostatin leads to a second complete remission in up to 70% of patients

The anti-CD20 antibody rituximab has been evaluated in patients with relapsed/refractory HCL and should be considered in patients who are not eligible to enroll in a clinical trial. Clinical trials using the truncated *Pseudomonas* exotoxin-linked recombinant anti-CD22 antibody (BL22) have shown high response rates in patients with previously treated HCL

Estey EH et al. Blood 1992;79:882–887
Grever MR. Blood 2010;115:21–28
Kreitman RJ et al. J Clin Oncol 2009;27:2983–2990
Kreitman RJ et al. N Engl J Med 2001;345:241–247
Saven A et al. Blood 1998;92:1918–1926
Tallman MS et al. Blood 1992;80:2203–2209
Tallman MS, Polliack A. Leuk Lymphoma 2009;50(Suppl 1):2–7

REGIMEN

CLADRIBINE (2-CHLORO-2'-DEOXYADENOSINE, 2-CDA)

Chacko J et al. Br J Haematol 1999;105:1145–1146
Cheson BD et al. J Clin Oncol 1998;16:3007–3015
Lauria F et al. Blood 1997;89:1838–1839
Robak T et al. Leuk Lymphoma 1996;22:107–111
Tallman MS et al. Blood 1992;80:2203–2209
Tallman MS et al. Blood 1996;88:1954–1959

Cladribine 0.1 mg/kg per day; administer by continuous intravenous infusion in 100–500 mL 0.9% sodium chloride injection, (0.9% NS), over 24 hours for 7 consecutive days (total dosage/cycle = 0.7 mg/kg)

or

Cladribine 0.14 mg/kg per day; administer intravenously in 100–500 mL of 0.9% NS over 2 hours for 5 consecutive days (total dosage/cycle = 0.7 mg/kg)

or

Cladribine 0.15 mg/kg per dose; administer intravenously in 100–500 mL 0.9% NS over 3 hours once weekly for 6 consecutive weeks (total dosage/cycle = 0.9 mg/kg)

Chacko J et al. Br J Haematol 1999;105:1145–1146
Lauria F et al. Blood 1997;89:1838–1839

Supportive Care
Antiemetic prophylaxis
See Chapter 39 for antiemetic recommendations
Emetogenic potential is **MINIMAL**
See Chapter 39 for antiemetic recommendations

Hematopoietic growth factor (CSF) prophylaxis
Primary prophylaxis is not indicated

Antimicrobial prophylaxis
Risk of fever and neutropenia is INTERMEDIATE
Antimicrobial primary prophylaxis is not clearly indicated. However, the following can be considered:
• Antibacterial—consider a fluoroquinolone during neutropenia *or*
• Antifungal—consider use during neutropenia
• Antiviral—antiherpes antivirals (eg, acyclovir) as patients may develop herpes viral infections as a result of their underlying disease even without the influence of purine analog therapy
See Chapter 47 for more information

Optional: **Allopurinol** 300 mg/day; administer orally, beginning on the first day of cladribine administration and continue for 2 weeks. Tumor lysis is uncommon and allopurinol need not be routinely administered. In addition, cutaneous disorders have occasionally been reported when cladribine used with allopurinol

Therapy Monitoring

1. Every other day for the week of therapy, then weekly for the next 7 weeks: CBC and serum electrolytes, BUN, creatinine, LFTs, and uric acid
2. *Three months after the completion of therapy:* Bone marrow aspirate and biopsy
3. *Long-term follow-up:* CBC every 3–6 months for 2 years, and then every 6 months for 3 years

Treatment Modifications

Cladribine Dose	No Modification
Platelet count <15,000/mm³	Administer platelets
Symptomatic anemia or hemoglobin <7 g/dL	Administer packed red blood cells

Patient Population Studied

Patients with newly diagnosed as well as relapsed and refractory disease

Efficacy

Complete remission rate	75–90%
Partial remission rate	5–20%
Relapse rate	5–50%

Toxicity (N = 895)

Cheson BD et al. J Clin Oncol 1998;16:3007–3015

	% G1	% G2	% G3	% G4
All Toxicities				
Maximum grade	21	20	22	6
Nonhematologic Toxicities				
Maximum grade	14	18	17	4
Hemorrhage	2	2	0.6	0.6
Nausea/vomiting	14	4	0.5	0.3
Infection	1	13	13	3
Pulmonary	3	2	0.7	0.7
Skin	8	5	4	0.5
Neurologic Toxicities				
Maximum grade	18	6	1	0.1
Motor	8	3	1	0
Headache	11	2	0.3	0
Constipation	5	1	0	0.1

Hematologic Toxicities

ANC <1000/mm³ or >50% decrease from baseline, or platelet count <100,000/mm³ or >50% decrease from baseline*	66%
Fever >38.3°C (101°F)*	48%
Peripheral vein chemical phlebitis*	12%

*Tallman MS et al. Blood 1992;80:2203–2209 (N = 26)

Notes

Cladribine may be administered to patients with relapsed or refractory disease

REGIMEN

PENTOSTATIN
(2'-DEOXYCOFORMYCIN, DCF)

Grever M et al. J Clin Oncol 1995;13:974–982

Hydration: 5% Dextrose/0.9% sodium chloride injection or 5% dextrose/0.45% sodium chloride injection; administer intravenously 1000 mL before and at least 500 mL after pentostatin administration

Pentostatin 4 mg/m^2; administer intravenously over 20–30 minutes in 25–50 mL 0.9% sodium chloride injection (0.9% NS) or 5% dextrose injection (D5W) every 2 weeks until complete remission (total dosage per 2-week course = 4 mg/m^2)
then
Pentostatin 4 mg/m^2; administer intravenously over 20–30 minutes in 25–50 mL 0.9% NS or D5W every 2 weeks for 2 courses (total dosage per 2-week course = 4 mg/m^2)

Supportive Care
Antiemetic prophylaxis
Emetogenic potential is **MINIMAL**
See Chapter 39 for antiemetic recommendations

Hematopoietic growth factor (CSF) prophylaxis
Primary prophylaxis should be considered in patients with:
ANC <500/mm^3 or in patients with history of recurrent episodes of fever and neutropenia
  Pegfilgrastim (pegylated filgrastim) 6 mg/0.6 mL by subcutaneous injection for 1 dose
  • Begin use from 24–72 hours after myelosuppressive chemotherapy is completed

Antimicrobial prophylaxis
Risk of fever and neutropenia is INTERMEDIATE
  Antimicrobial primary prophylaxis is not clearly indicated
  • Antibacterial—no prophylaxis
  • Antifungal—no prophylaxis
  • Antiviral—antiherpes antivirals (eg, acyclovir) as patients may develop herpes viral infections as a result of their underlying disease even without the influence of purine analog therapy

Allopurinol: Tumor lysis is uncommon and allopurinol need not be routinely administered

Patient Population Studied

Study of 154 patients with previously untreated hairy cell leukemia

Efficacy

Complete remission rate	70–80%
Partial remission rate	5–20%
Relapse rate	10–25%

Treatment Modifications

Toxicity	Treatment Modification
Serum creatinine >20% over baseline	Hold pentostatin until serum creatinine returns to baseline or creatinine clearance on a 24-hour urine collection is >50 mL/min (>0.83 mL/s)
New or suspected infection	Hold pentostatin until successful therapy being administered
G2 nonhematologic toxicity	Reduce pentostatin by 33% after toxicity G ≤1
G3 nonhematologic toxicity	Reduce pentostatin by 50% after toxicity G ≤1
G4 nonhematologic toxicity	Discontinue pentostatin

Therapy Monitoring

1. *Two to 3 times per week during therapy:* CBC and serum electrolytes, BUN, creatinine, LFTs, and uric acid
2. *Three months after the completion of therapy:* Bone marrow aspirate and biopsy
3. *Long-term follow-up:* CBC every 3–6 months for 2 years, and then every 6 months for 3 years

Toxicity (N = 154)

Toxicity	% G3	% G4
Allergy/rash	2.6	0
Nausea/vomiting/anorexia	12	0
Chills/fever	1.3	0
Diarrhea	1.3	0
Neurologic	0.7	0
Hepatic	0.7	0
Renal	0.7	0
Anemia	0.7	0
Granulocytopenia (G4)	5.2	14
Thrombocytopenia	2.6	0

Suspected infection during induction	53%
Systemic antibiotics during induction	27%

REGIMEN

RITUXIMAB

Hagberg H, Lundholm L. Br J Haematol 2001;115:609–611
Lauria F et al. Haematologica 2001;86:1046–1050
Nieva J et al. Blood 2003;102:810–813

Premedication:

1. **Acetaminophen** 650–1000 mg; administer orally, 30–60 minutes before rituximab
2. **Diphenhydramine** 25–50 mg; administer orally or by intravenous injection 30–60 minutes before rituximab

Rituximab 375 mg/m² per week; administer intravenously in 0.9% sodium chloride injection (0.9% NS) or 5% dextrose injection (D5W) diluted to a concentration within the range of 1–4 mg/mL for 4 consecutive weeks (total dosage per 4-week course = 1500 mg/m²)

or

Rituximab 375 mg/m² per week; administer intravenously in 0.9% NS or D5W diluted to a concentration within the range of 1–4 mg/mL for 8 consecutive weeks with an additional 4 weekly doses (maximum of 12 doses) if a patient does not achieve a complete remission, but shows signs of continual improvement (total dosage per 8-week and 12-week courses = 3000 mg/m² and 4500 mg/m², respectively)

Thomas DA et al. Blood 2003;102:3906–3911

Rituximab infusion rates:
First dose: Start at an initial rate of 50 mg/hour. If hypersensitivity or infusion reactions do not occur during the first 30 minutes, increase the rate by 50 mg/hour every 30 minutes, to a maximum rate of 400 mg/hour
Subsequent doses: If previous administration was well tolerated, start at 100 mg/hour, and, if tolerated, increase by 100 mg/hour every 30 minutes, to a maximum rate of 400 mg/hour

Supportive Care
Antiemetic prophylaxis
Emetogenic potential is **MINIMAL**
See Chapter 39 for antiemetic recommendations

Hematopoietic growth factor (CSF) prophylaxis
Primary prophylaxis is NOT indicated
See Chapter 43 for more information

Antimicrobial prophylaxis
Risk of fever and neutropenia is LOW
  Antimicrobial primary prophylaxis to be considered:
  • Antibacterial—*P. jirovecii* prophylaxis is recommended (eg, cotrimoxazole)
  • Antifungal—not indicated
  • Antiviral—not indicated, unless patient previously had an episode of HSV
See Chapter 47 for more information

Optional: **Allopurinol** 300 mg/day; administer orally, beginning on the first day of rituximab administration and continuing for 2 weeks. Tumor lysis is uncommon and allopurinol need not be routinely administered

Patient Population Studied

Relapsed or refractory HCL

Efficacy

Thomas DA et al. Blood 2003;102:3906–3911

Overall response rate	80%
Complete response rate	53%
Partial response rate	27%*
No response	20%

*Includes 2 additional patients who achieved complete remission by hematologic parameters but had residual marrow disease (1–5% hairy cells)
Duration of response: With median follow-up of 32 months, 5 of 12 patients had progression of disease at 8, 12, 18, 23, and 39 months from the start of therapy

Toxicity (N = 15)

Thomas DA et al. Blood 2003;102:3906–3911

Toxicity	No. of Patients	G	Dose No.
Fever and chills	9	1	1
Nausea and vomiting	4	1	1, 2
Hypotension*	1	1	1
Palpitations*	1	2	1, 2
Shortness of breath*	1	2	1
Myalgia	1	3	All 8
Fatigue	2	1, 2	1, 2
Back pain	1	1	1
Rash	1	1	1
Infection	0	—	—

*Infusional events associated with the first dose. Rapid resolution occurred with temporary cessation of the infusion

Therapy Monitoring

1. *Weekly prior to each dose of rituximab:* CBC
2. *One to 3 months after the completion of therapy:* Bone marrow aspirate and biopsy with immunophenotyping
3. *Long-term follow-up:* CBC every 3–6 months for 2 years, and then every 6 months for 3 years

Treatment Modifications

Fever, chills, hypotension, and other toxicities:
Slow or interrupt rituximab administration

Severe hypersensitivity reactions:
1. Interrupt administration
2. **Diphenhydramine** 25–50 mg; administration by intravenous injection is recommended
3. Additional treatment with diphenhydramine, bronchodilators, intravenous hydrocortisone, and/or intravenous hydration may be indicated
4. Resume infusion at a 50% reduction in rate when symptoms have completely resolved
5. Medications for the treatment of hypersensitivity reactions should be available for immediate use in the event of a reaction during administration (eg, intravenous fluids, epinephrine, antihistamines, glucocorticoids, and O_2)
6. In many cases, the infusion can be resumed at a 50% reduction in rate when symptoms have completely resolved

Notes

1. Patients requiring close monitoring during first and all subsequent infusions include those with preexisting cardiac and pulmonary conditions, prior clinically significant cardiopulmonary adverse events, or circulating malignant cells >25,000/mm^3 with or without evidence of high tumor burden
2. No clear benefit of 12 doses versus 4 doses

22. Lung Cancer

Enriqueta Felip, MD, PhD and Rafael Rosell, MD

Epidemiology

Incidence: 224,210 (male: 116,000; female: 108,210. Estimated new cases for 2014 in the United States)
61.4 per 100,000 male and female per year (74.3 per 100,000 men, 51.9 per 100,000 women)
Deaths: Estimated 159,260 in 2014 (male: 86,930; female: 72,330)
Median age: 61.4 years
Male-to-female ratio: ~1:1

Stage at Presentation
Localized (confined to primary site): 15%
Regional (spread to regional lymph nodes): 22%
Distant (cancer has metastasized): 57%

Siegel R et al. CA Cancer J Clin 2014;64:9–29
Surveillance, Epidemiology and End Results (SEER) Program, available from http://seer.cancer.gov (accessed in 2013)
Weir HK et al. J Natl Cancer Inst 2003;95:1276–1299

Pathology

Lung cancer is divided into 2 major classes:

1. Non–small cell lung cancer (NSCLC): 75–85%
   • Squamous cell carcinoma
   • Adenocarcinoma
   • Large-cell carcinoma

2. Small cell lung cancer (SCLC) 15–25%

Brambilla E et al. Eur Respir J 2001;18:1059–1068

Non–Small Cell Lung Cancer (NSCLC)

Work-up

1. History and physical examination including performance status and weight loss
2. Chest x-ray, PA and lateral
3. CT scan of chest and upper abdomen including adrenals
4. CBC, serum electrolytes, BUN, creatinine, calcium, magnesium, and LFTs
5. CT scan and/or MRI of brain if neurologic history or examination is abnormal
6. Bone scan if there is bone pain, elevated calcium level, or elevated alkaline phosphatase level
7. Assessment of perioperative risks for potential candidates for surgery, including pulmonary function tests (PFTs)

Stages I–II
    a. Bronchoscopy
    b. FDG-PET scan

Stages IIIA–IIIB
    a. Bronchoscopy
    b. FDG-PET scan
    c. MRI of the chest in superior sulcus tumors
    d. MRI of brain
    e. Bone scan
    f. Mediastinal lymph node biopsy if CT scan shows nodes >1 cm
    Invasive tests: Mediastinoscopy, thoracoscopy, transbronchial needle aspiration, and endoscopic ultrasound and needle aspiration

Stage IV
    Biopsy for otherwise potentially resectable patient with isolated adrenal mass or liver lesion

Staging

Primary Tumor (T)

TX	Primary tumor cannot be assessed
T0	No evidence of primary tumor
Tis	Tis Carcinoma in situ
T1	Tumor ≤3 cm in greatest dimension, surrounded by lung or visceral pleura, without bronchoscopic evidence of invasion more proximal than the lobar bronchus (ie, not in the main bronchus)*
T1a	Tumor ≤2 cm in greatest dimension
T1b	Tumor >2 cm but ≤3 cm in greatest dimension
T2	Tumor >3 cm but ≤7 cm or tumor with any of the following features (T2 tumors with these features are classified T2a if ≤5 cm) Involves main bronchus, ≥2 cm distal to the carina Invades visceral pleura (PL1 or PL2) Associated with atelectasis or obstructive pneumonitis that extends to the hilar region but does not involve the entire lung
T2a	Tumor >3 cm but ≤5 cm in greatest dimension
T2b	Tumor >5 cm but ≤7 cm in greatest dimension
T3	Tumor >7 cm or one that directly invades any of the following: parietal pleural (PL3) chest wall (including superior sulcus tumors), diaphragm, phrenic nerve, mediastinal pleura, parietal pericardium; or tumor in the main bronchus (<2 cm distal to the carina* but without involvement of the carina; or associated atelectasis or obstructive pneumonitis of the entire lung or separate tumor nodule(s) in the same lobe
T4	Tumor of any size that invades any of the following: mediastinum, heart, great vessels, trachea, recurrent laryngeal nerve, esophagus, vertebral body, carina, separate tumor nodule(s) in a different ipsilateral lobe

*The uncommon superficial spreading tumor of any size with its invasive component limited to the bronchial wall, which may extend proximally to the main bronchus, is also classified as T1a

Distant Metastases (M)

M0	No distant metastasis (no pathologic M0; use clinical M to complete stage group)
M1	Distant metastasis
M1a	Separate tumor nodule(s) in a contralateral lobe; tumor with pleural nodules or malignant pleural (or pericardial) effusion*
M1b	Distant metastasis

*Most pleural (and pericardial) effusions with lung cancer are caused by tumor. In a few patients, however, multiple cytopathologic examinations of pleural (pericardial) fluid are negative for tumor, and the fluid is nonbloody and is not an exudate. Where these elements and clinical judgement dictate that the effusion is not related to the tumor, the effusion should be excluded as a staging element and the patient should be classified as M0

Regional Lymph Nodes (N)

NX	Regional lymph nodes cannot be assessed
N0	No regional lymph node metastasis
N1	Metastasis in ipsilateral peribronchial and/or ipsilateral hilar lymph nodes and intrapulmonary nodes, including involvement by direct extension
N2	Metastasis in ipsilateral mediastinal and/or subcarinal lymph node(s)
N3	Metastasis in contralateral mediastinal, contralateral hilar, ipsilateral or contralateral scalene, or supraclavicular lymph node(s)

Staging Groups

Group	T	N	M
Occult	TX	N0	M0
0	Tis	N0	M0
IA	T1a	N0	M0
	T1b	N0	M0
IB	T1a	N0	M0
	T2b	N0	M0
IIA	T1a	N1	M0
	T1b	N1	M0
	T2a	N1	M0
IIB	T2b	N1	M0
	T3	N0	M0
IIIA	T1a	N2	M0
	T1b	N2	M0
	T2a	N2	M0
	T2b	N2	M0
	T3	N1	M0
	T3	N2	M0
	T4	N0	M0
	T4	N1	M0
IIIB	T1a	N3	M0
	T1b	N3	M0
	T2a	N3	M0
	T2b	N3	M0
	T3	N3	M0
	T4	N2	M0
	T4	N3	M0
IV	Any T	Any N	M1a
	Any T	Any N	M1b

Edge SB, Byrd DR, Compton CC, Fritz AG, Greene FL, Trotti A, editors. AJCC Cancer Staging Manual. 7th ed. New York: Springer; 2010

5-Year Relative Survival Rates

All stages	15%
Stage I	56%
Stage II	32%
Stage III	9%
Stage IV	2%

More information at http://www.seer.cancer.gov

Expert Opinion

1. Surgery is the standard treatment in stages I–II disease. Radiation therapy should be considered in medically inoperable stages I–II disease (inadequate pulmonary function tests or comorbid diseases)

2. Four cycles of adjuvant cisplatin-based chemotherapy (a doublet combination) is recommended in patients with pathologic stages II–III. Cisplatin-based chemotherapy may be considered in selected patients with stage IB disease (tumor size >4 cm)

3. Preoperative chemotherapy is the treatment of choice for resectable stage IIIA disease. Platinum-based chemotherapy and thoracic radiation therapy is the standard treatment for unresectable stage III. Concurrent chemoradiation appears to be better than sequential chemoradiation

4. Platinum-based chemotherapy prolongs survival, improves symptom control, and yields superior quality of life in stage IV disease. First-line chemotherapy should be a 2-drug combination regimen. No specific new agent–platinum combination is clearly superior (cisplatin or carboplatin in combination with any of the following: paclitaxel, docetaxel, gemcitabine, vinorelbine). Non–platinum-containing regimens may be used as alternatives to platinum-based combinations

5. For elderly patients or patients with ECOG PS (performance status) 2, available data support the use of single-agent chemotherapy as first-line treatment

6. Docetaxel, pemetrexed, or erlotinib treatment should be considered in patients with advanced NSCLC who experience disease progression after first-line chemotherapy

7. Gefitinib, erlotinib and afatinib are three options available for patients whose tumors harbor EGFR mutations

Pfister DG et al. J Clin Oncol 2004;22:330–353
Winton TL et al. N Engl J Med 2005;352:2589–2597

REGIMEN

PACLITAXEL + CARBOPLATIN

Kelly K et al. J Clin Oncol 2001;19:3210–3218

Premedication (primary prophylaxis against hypersensitivity reactions from paclitaxel):
Dexamethasone 20 mg/dose for 2 doses; administer orally the evening before and the morning of chemotherapy prior to paclitaxel, *plus*:
Diphenhydramine 50 mg for 1 dose; administer by intravenous injection 30 minutes before paclitaxel, *and*:
Ranitidine 50 mg or **cimetidine** 300 mg for 1 dose; administer intravenously in 25–100 mL 0.9% sodium chloride injection (0.9% NS) or 5% dextrose injection (D5W) over 5–30 minutes, 30 minutes before paclitaxel
Paclitaxel 225 mg/m^2; administer intravenously in a volume of 0.9% NS or D5W sufficient to produce a solution with concentration within the range 0.3–1.2 mg/mL over 3 hours on day 1, every 3 weeks (total dosage/cycle = 225 mg/m^2)
Carboplatin (calculated dose) AUC = 6 mg/mL · min; administer intravenously in 50–150 mL D5W over 15–30 minutes, on day 1, every 3 weeks (total dosage/cycle calculated to produce an AUC = 6 mg/mL · min) (see equation below)

Supportive Care

Antiemetic prophylaxis
Emetogenic potential: **HIGH**. *Potential for delayed symptoms*
See Chapter 39 for antiemetic recommendations

Hematopoietic growth factor (CSF) prophylaxis
Primary prophylaxis is indicated with one of the following:
Filgrastim (G-CSF) 5 mcg/kg per day by subcutaneous injection, *or*
  Pegfilgrastim (pegylated filgrastim) 6 mg/0.6 mL by subcutaneous injection for 1 dose
  • Begin use from 24–72 hours after myelosuppressive chemotherapy is completed
  • Continue filgrastim until ANC >10,000/mm^3 on 2 consecutive daily measurements
See Chapter 43 for more information

Antimicrobial prophylaxis
Risk of fever and neutropenia is LOW
  Antimicrobial primary prophylaxis to be considered:
  • Antibacterial—not indicated
  • Antifungal—not indicated
  • Antiviral—not indicated unless patient previously had an episode of HSV
See Chapter 47 for more information

Additional Supportive Care
Dexamethasone 8 mg/dose orally every 12 hours for 6 doses after chemotherapy if G ≥2 arthralgias/myalgias occur
Add a **proton pump inhibitor** during dexamethasone use to prevent gastritis and duodenitis

---

Note: Carboplatin dose is based on Calvert's formula to achieve a target area under the plasma concentration versus time curve (AUC) [AUC units = mg/mL · min]

$$\text{Total carboplatin dose (mg)} = (\text{Target AUC}) \times (\text{GFR} + 25)$$

In practice, creatinine clearance (Clcr) is used in place of glomerular filtration rate (GFR). Clcr can be calculated from the equation of Cockcroft and Gault:

$$\text{For males, Clcr} = \frac{(140 - \text{age [years]}) \times \text{body weight (kg)}}{72 \times (\text{Serum creatinine [mg/dL]})}$$

$$\text{For females, Clcr} = \frac{(140 - \text{age [years]}) \times \text{body weight (kg)}}{72 \times (\text{Serum creatinine [mg/dL]})} \times 0.85$$

Calvert AH et al. J Clin Oncol 1989;7:1748–1756
Cockcroft DW , Gault MH. Nephron 1976;16:31–41
Jodrell DI et al. J Clin Oncol 1992;10:520–528
Sorensen BT et al. Cancer Chemother Pharmacol 1991;28:397–401

(continued)

Treatment Modifications

Adverse Event	Dose Modification
ANC nadir <500/mm^3, platelet nadir <50,000/mm^3, or febrile neutropenia	Reduce carboplatin dosage to AUC = 5 if previous cycle dose was AUC = 6; or to AUC = 4 if previous cycle dose was AUC = 5
ANC nadir <500/mm^3, platelet nadir <50,000/mm^3, or febrile neutropenia after 2 carboplatin dose reductions (AUC in previous cycle = 4)	Reduce paclitaxel dosage to 200 mg/m^2, and decrease carboplatin dosage to AUC = 3
Day 1 ANC <1500/mm^3 or platelets <100,000/mm^3	Delay chemotherapy until ANC >1500/mm^3 and platelets >100,000/mm^3, for maximum delay of 2 weeks
Delay of >2 weeks in reaching ANC >1500/mm^3 and platelet nadir >100,000/mm^3	Discontinue therapy
G2 neurotoxicity	Reduce paclitaxel dosage to 200 mg/m^2
G3 neurotoxicity	Reduce paclitaxel dosage to 175 mg/m^2
G2 arthralgia/myalgia despite dexamethasone prophylaxis	Reduce paclitaxel dosage to 200 mg/m^2
G3 arthralgia/myalgia despite dexamethasone prophylaxis	Reduce paclitaxel dosage to 175 mg/m^2
G ≥2 AST or G ≥3 total bilirubin	Hold paclitaxel
Moderate hypersensitivity	Patient may be retreated
Severe hypersensitivity	Discontinue therapy
Chest pain or arrhythmia during chemotherapy	Immediately stop chemotherapy and evaluate the patient
Symptomatic arrhythmias, or ≥2-degree AV block, or an ischemic event	Discontinue therapy

(*continued*)

Note: A carboplatin dose calculated with an IDMS-measured serum creatinine result using the Calvert formula could exceed an expected exposure (AUC) and result in increased drug-related toxicity. The FDA recommends capping an estimated GFR at 125 mL/min for any targeted AUC value. No greater estimated GFR values should be used [online] May 23, 2013. Available from: http://www.fda.gov/AboutFDA/CentersOffices/OfficeofMedicalProductsandTobacco/CDER/ucm228974.htm [accessed February 26, 2014]

Patient Population Studied

A randomized comparison with vinorelbine + cisplatin in 206 patients with advanced, previously untreated NSCLC

Efficacy (N = 203)*

Response rate (CR + PR)	25%
Median progression-free survival	4 months
Median survival	8.6 months
1-year survival	38%
2-year survival	15%

*WHO criteria

Toxicity (N = 203)*

Adverse Event	% G3	% G4
Hematologic		
Leukopenia	26	5
Neutropenia	21	36
Thrombocytopenia	10	0
Anemia	11	2
Nonhematologic		
Nausea	7	0
Sensory neuropathy	13	0
Vomiting	4	0
Dehydration	4	0
Fatigue	8	0
Hyponatremia	3	0
Weakness (motor neuropathy)	8	0
Respiratory infection/ neutropenia	1	0

*NCI CTC, National Cancer Institute (USA) Common Toxicity Criteria, version 2.0. Available at: http://ctep.cancer.gov/protocolDevelopment/electronic_applications/ctc.htm [accessed December 7, 2013]

Therapy Monitoring

1. *Before each cycle:* H&P, PS evaluation, CBC with differential, LFTs, BUN, and creatinine
2. *Every week:* CBC with differential and platelet count
3. *Response evaluation:* Every 2–3 cycles

REGIMEN

PACLITAXEL + CISPLATIN

Rosell R et al. Ann Oncol 2002;13:1539–1549

Premedication (primary prophylaxis against hypersensitivity reactions from paclitaxel):
Dexamethasone 20 mg/dose for 2 doses; administer orally the evening before and the morning of chemotherapy before paclitaxel, *plus*:
Diphenhydramine 50 mg; administer by intravenous injection, 30 minutes before paclitaxel, *and*:
Ranitidine 50 mg or **cimetidine** 300 mg; administer intravenously in 25–100 mL 0.9% sodium chloride injection (0.9% NS) or 5% dextrose injection (D5W) over 5–30 minutes, 30 minutes before paclitaxel
Paclitaxel 200 mg/m²; administer intravenously in a volume of 0.9% NS or D5W sufficient to produce a solution with concentration within the range 0.3–1.2 mg/mL over 3 hours on day 1, every 21 days (total dosage/cycle = 200 mg/m²)

Hydration before cisplatin: Administer by intravenous infusion ≥1000 mL 0.9% NS over a minimum of 2–4 hours
Cisplatin 80 mg/m²; administer intravenously in 100–250 mL 0.9% NS over 30 minutes, on day 1, every 21 days (total dosage/cycle = 80 mg/m²)
Hydration after cisplatin: Administer by intravenous infusion ≥1000 mL 0.9% NS over a minimum of 2–4 hours. Encourage patients to increase oral intake of non-alcoholic fluids. Monitor serum electrolytes and replace as needed (potassium, magnesium, sodium)

Supportive Care
Antiemetic prophylaxis
Emetogenic potential: **HIGH**. *Potential for delayed symptoms*
See Chapter 39 for antiemetic recommendations

Hematopoietic growth factor (CSF) prophylaxis
Primary prophylaxis is indicated with one of the following:
  Filgrastim (G-CSF) 5 mcg/kg per day by subcutaneous injection, *or*
  Pegfilgrastim (pegylated filgrastim) 6 mg/0.6 mL by subcutaneous injection for 1 dose
  • Begin use from 24–72 hours after myelosuppressive chemotherapy is completed
  • Continue filgrastim until ANC >10,000/mm³ on 2 consecutive daily measurements
See Chapter 43 for more information

Antimicrobial prophylaxis
Risk of fever and neutropenia is LOW
  Antimicrobial primary prophylaxis to be considered:
  • Antibacterial—not indicated
  • Antifungal—not indicated
  • Antiviral—not indicated unless patient previously had an episode of HSV
See Chapter 47 for more information

Additional Supportive Care
Dexamethasone 8 mg/dose orally every 12 hours for 6 doses after chemotherapy if G ≥2 arthralgias/myalgias occur
Add a **proton pump inhibitor** during dexamethasone use to prevent gastritis and duodenitis

Toxicity (N = 302)

Hematologic	
	% G3/4
Neutropenia	51
Leukopenia	16
Anemia	9
Infections	5
Febrile neutropenia	4
Thrombocytopenia	2

Nonhematologic	
	% Severe
Nausea/vomiting	14
Asthenia	10
Arthralgia/myalgia	9
Peripheral neuropathy*	7
Diarrhea	2
Hypersensitivity	1
Renal*	1

*Grade 3

Patient Population Studied

A randomized comparison with paclitaxel + carboplatin in 309 patients with advanced (Stages III/IV) NSCLC not previously treated

Efficacy (N = 284)*

Complete Response	1%
Partial Response	27%
Median progression-free survival†	4.2 months
Median survival†	9.8 months
Estimated 1-year survival	38%
2-Year survival	15%

*WHO criteria
†Intention-to-treat analysis

Treatment Modifications

Dose escalations are not permitted. Dosage reductions are based on toxicity encountered during a previous cycle

Adverse Event	Dose Modification
G ≥2 arthralgias/myalgias	Add dexamethasone as secondary prophylaxis
Day 1 ANC <1500/mm^3 or platelet count <100,000/mm^3	Delay therapy until ANC >1500/mm^3 and platelet count >100,000/mm^3. If >2-week delay, the decision to retreat is based on caregiver's discretion
Febrile neutropenia	Reduce cisplatin and paclitaxel dosages by 25%
Bleeding associated with thrombocytopenia	
Serum creatinine 1.6–2.0 mg/dL (141–177 μmol/L)	Reduce cisplatin dosage by 25%
Serum creatinine >2.0 mg/dL (>177 μmol/L)	Hold cisplatin until serum creatinine ≤2.0 mg/dL (≤177 μmol/L)
G3/4 neurotoxicity	Delay therapy until G ≤2
Moderate hypersensitivity reactions	Decision to retreat based on severity and caregiver's discretion
Severe hypersensitivity reactions	Stop treatment
Symptomatic arrhythmias or AV block ≥ second-degree, or documented ischemic event	
G ≥2 AST (SGOT) or G ≥3 total bilirubin	Stop paclitaxel

Therapy Monitoring

1. *Before each cycle:* H&P, PS evaluation, CBC with differential, serum electrolytes, magnesium, LFTs, BUN, and creatinine
2. *Every week:* CBC with differential and platelet count
3. *Response evaluation:* Every 2–3 cycles

REGIMEN

GEMCITABINE + CISPLATIN

Sandler AB et al. J Clin Oncol 2000;18:122–130

Gemcitabine 1000 mg/m²; administer intravenously in 50–250 mL 0.9% sodium chloride injection (0.9% NS) over 30–60 minutes, on days 1, 8, and 15, every 28 days (total dosage/cycle = 3000 mg/m²). On day 1, administer after or during hydration for cisplatin and follow with cisplatin

Hydration before cisplatin: ≥1000 mL 0.9% NS; administer intravenously over a minimum of 2–4 hours

Cisplatin 100 mg/m²; administer intravenously in 100–250 mL 0.9% NS over 30–120 minutes, on day 1 every 28 days (total dosage/cycle = 100 mg/m²)

Hydration after cisplatin: ≥1000 mL 0.9% NS; administer intravenously over a minimum of 2–4 hours. Also encourage patients to increase oral intake of non-alcoholic fluids. Monitor serum electrolytes and replace as needed (potassium, magnesium, sodium)

Supportive Care

Antiemetic prophylaxis
Emetogenic potential on day 1 is **HIGH**. *Potential for delayed symptoms*
Emetogenic potential on days 8 and 15 is **LOW**
See Chapter 39 for antiemetic recommendations

Hematopoietic growth factor (CSF) prophylaxis
Primary prophylaxis is NOT indicated
See Chapter 43 for more information

Antimicrobial prophylaxis
Risk of fever and neutropenia is LOW
Antimicrobial primary prophylaxis to be considered:
- Antibacterial—not indicated
- Antifungal—not indicated
- Antiviral—not indicated unless patient previously had an episode of HSV

See Chapter 47 for more information

Patient Population Studied

A randomized comparison with single-agent cisplatin in 260 patients with advanced (Stages III/IV) previously untreated NSCLC

Efficacy (N = 260)

Complete response	1.2%
Partial response	29.2%
Estimated median progression-free survival	5.6 months
Estimated median survival	9.1 months
Estimated 1-year survival	39%

Toxicity (N = 260)*

	% G3	% G4
Hematologic		
Granulocytopenia	21.5	35.3
Thrombocytopenia	25	25.4
Anemia	21.9	3.1
Febrile neutropenia	4.6% of patients	
Platelet transfusions	20.4% of patients	
Erythrocyte transfusions	37.7% of patients	
Nonhematologic		
Nausea	25	2
Vomiting	11	12
Increased creatinine	4.4	0.4
Neurologic (hearing)	5.6	0.4
Neurologic (motor)	11.5	0
Dyspnea	4	3
Increased transaminases	2	1
Increased bilirubin	0.8	0.8

*WHO criteria

Treatment Modifications

Adverse Event	Dose Modification
ANC <1500/mm³, or platelets <100,000/mm³	Hold chemotherapy until ANC >1500/mm³ and platelets >100,000/mm³
Febrile granulocytopenia that requires antibiotics	Reduce cisplatin and gemcitabine dosages by 25% in subsequent cycles
Bleeding associated with thrombocytopenia	
Intracycle: G1/2 nonhematologic toxicity or G1–3 nausea or vomiting	100% gemcitabine dosage on days 8 and 15
Intracycle: G3 nonhematologic toxicity, except nausea, vomiting, and alopecia	Reduce gemcitabine dosage by 25% on days 8 and 15, or hold treatment at clinician's discretion
Intracycle: G4 nonhematologic toxicity	Hold gemcitabine
Day 1 serum creatinine 1.6–2.0 mg/dL (141–177 μmol/L)	Reduce cisplatin dosage by 25%
Day 1 serum creatinine >2.0 mg/dL (>177 μmol/L)	Hold cisplatin until serum creatinine ≤2.0 mg/dL (≤177 μmol/L)
G3/4 neurotoxicity	Delay treatment until toxicity resolves to G1
Treatment delay >2 weeks	Discontinue therapy according to clinician's discretion

Therapy Monitoring

1. *Each cycle on day 1:* H&P, performance status reevaluation, CBC with differential and platelet count, serum electrolytes, magnesium, serum creatinine, hepatic transaminases, and bilirubin
2. *Cycle days 8 and 15:* CBC with differential and platelet count
3. *Response evaluation:* Every 2–3 cycles

REGIMEN

DOCETAXEL + CISPLATIN

Fossella F et al. J Clin Oncol 2003;21:3016–3024

Prophylaxis for fluid retention and hypersensitivity reactions from docetaxel:
Dexamethasone 8 mg/dose; administer orally twice daily for 3 days, starting the day before docetaxel is administered (total dose/cycle = 48 mg)

Hydration before cisplatin: ≥1000 mL 0.9% sodium chloride injection (0.9% NS); administer intravenously over a minimum of 2–4 hours
Docetaxel 75 mg/m²; administer intravenously in a volume of 0.9% NS or 5% dextrose injection (D5W) sufficient to produce a solution with concentration within the range 0.3–0.74 mg/mL over 1 hour on day 1, every 3 weeks (total dosage/cycle = 75 mg/m²), *followed immediately by:*
Cisplatin 75 mg/m²; administer intravenously in 100–250 mL 0.9% NS over 1 hour on day 1, every 3 weeks (total dosage/cycle = 75 mg/m²)

Hydration after cisplatin: ≥1000 mL 0.9% NS; administer intravenously over a minimum of 2–4 hours. Encourage patients to increase oral intake of non-alcoholic fluids. Monitor serum electrolytes and replace as needed (potassium, magnesium, sodium)

Supportive Care
Antiemetic prophylaxis
Emetogenic potential: **HIGH**. *Potential for delayed symptoms*
See Chapter 39 for antiemetic recommendations

Hematopoietic growth factor (CSF) prophylaxis
Primary prophylaxis is indicated with one of the following:
Filgrastim (G-CSF) 5 mcg/kg per day by subcutaneous injection, *or*
Pegfilgrastim (pegylated filgrastim) 6 mg/0.6 mL by subcutaneous injection for 1 dose
• Begin use from 24–72 hours after myelosuppressive chemotherapy is completed
• Continue filgrastim until ANC >10,000/mm³ on 2 consecutive daily measurements
See Chapter 43 for more information

Antimicrobial prophylaxis
Risk of fever and neutropenia is LOW
Antimicrobial primary prophylaxis to be considered:
• Antibacterial—not indicated
• Antifungal—not indicated
• Antiviral—not indicated unless patient previously had an episode of HSV
See Chapter 47 for more information

Patient Population Studied

A multicenter, international, prospective, open-label, randomized phase III comparison with vinorelbine + cisplatin in 408 patients with locally advanced or recurrent (Stage IIIB) or metastatic (Stage IV) NSCLC

Efficacy (N = 408)

Complete response	2.0%
Partial response	29.7%
Overall median survival	11.3 months
1-year survival	46%
2-year survival	21%

Therapy Monitoring

1. *Each cycle on day 1:* H&P, PS evaluation, CBC with differential, serum electrolytes, magnesium, BUN, creatinine, and LFTs
2. *Every week:* CBC with differential and platelet count
3. *Response evaluation:* Every 2–3 cycles

Toxicity (N = 406)*

Toxicity†	% G3/4
Hematologic	
Leukopenia	42.8
Neutropenia	74.8
Thrombocytopenia	2.7
Anemia	6.9
Erythrocyte transfusions	10.3% of patients
Nonhematologic	
Infection	8.4
Asthenia	12.3
Nausea	9.9
Pulmonary	9.6
Pain	7.9
Vomiting	7.9
Diarrhea	6.7
Anorexia	5.4

*NCI CTC, National Cancer Institute (USA) Common Toxicity Criteria, version 2.0. Available at: http://ctep.cancer.gov/protocolDevelopment/electronic_applications/ctc.htm [accessed December 7, 2013]
†G3/4 adverse event in >5% of patients

Treatment Modifications

Adverse Event	Dose Modification
ANC <1500/mm³ or platelet count <100,000/mm³	Hold chemotherapy until ANC >1500/mm³ and platelets >100,000/mm³
Febrile granulocytopenia that requires antibiotics Bleeding associated with thrombocytopenia	Reduce cisplatin and docetaxel dosages by 25% during subsequent cycles*
Day 1 serum creatinine 1.6–2.0 mg/dL (141–177 μmol/L)	Reduce cisplatin dosage* by 25%
Day 1 serum creatinine >2.0 mg/dL (>177 μmol/L)	Hold cisplatin until serum creatinine ≤2.0 mg/dL (≤177 μmol/L)
G3/4 neurotoxicity	Delay treatment
Treatment delay ≥2 weeks	Discontinue therapy or according to clinician's criteria

*A maximum of 2 docetaxel or cisplatin dosage reductions are permitted

REGIMEN

VINORELBINE + CISPLATIN

Wozniak AJ et al. J Clin Oncol 1998;16:2459–2465

Vinorelbine 25 mg/m²; administer intravenously in a volume of 0.9% sodium chloride injection (0.9% NS) or 5% dextrose injection (D5W) sufficient to produce a solution with concentration within the range 0.5–3 mg/mL over 6–10 minutes, once weekly for 4 weeks (total dosage/cycle = 100 mg/m²)

Hydration before cisplatin: ≥1000 mL 0.9% NS; administer intravenously over a minimum of 2–4 hours

Cisplatin 100 mg/m²; administer intravenously in 100–250 mL 0.9% NS over 1 hour on day 1, every 4 weeks (total dosage/cycle = 100 mg/m²)

Hydration after cisplatin: ≥1000 mL 0.9% NS; administer intravenously over a minimum of 2–4 hours. Encourage patients to increase oral intake of non-alcoholic fluids. Monitor serum electrolytes and replace as needed (potassium, magnesium, sodium)

Supportive Care
Antiemetic prophylaxis
Emetogenic potential: **HIGH.** *Potential for delayed symptoms*
See Chapter 39 for antiemetic recommendations

Hematopoietic growth factor (CSF) prophylaxis
Primary prophylaxis may be indicated
See Chapter 43 for more information

Antimicrobial prophylaxis
Risk of fever and neutropenia is LOW
Antimicrobial primary prophylaxis to be considered:
• Antibacterial—not indicated
• Antifungal—not indicated
• Antiviral—not indicated unless patient previously had an episode of HSV
See Chapter 47 for more information

Patient Population Studied

A randomized comparison with cisplatin of 206 patients with advanced previously untreated NSCLC

Efficacy

Complete response	2%
Partial response	24%
Median progression-free survival	4 months
Median survival	8 months
1-Year survival	36%
2-Year survival	12%

Toxicity (N = 204)*

Hematologic		
	% G3	% G4
Granulocytopenia	22	59
Thrombocytopenia	4	1
Anemia	21	3
Nonhematologic		
	% G3/4	
Fever/sepsis with granulocytopenia	10	
Nausea/vomiting	20	
Malaise/weakness	15	
Constipation	3	
Diarrhea	3	
Electrolyte imbalance	6	
Hearing	4	
Vision	1	
Neurologic (peripheral)	2	
Neurologic (central)	2	
Renal	5	
Phlebitis/thrombosis	3	

*SWOG criteria

Treatment Modifications

Treatment day ANC must be ≥1500/mm³ and platelets ≥100,000/mm³ to treat on schedule at 100% dosages

Adverse Event	Dose Modification
Treatment day ANC 1000–1499/mm³ or platelets 75,000–99,999/mm³	Reduce cisplatin and vinorelbine dosages by 50%
Treatment day ANC <1000 or platelets <75,000/mm³	Hold cisplatin* and vinorelbine
Treatment delay >2 weeks but <3 weeks	Reduce subsequent cisplatin and vinorelbine dosages by 50%
Fever or sepsis with neutropenia in any cycle	
ANC nadir <500/mm³ or platelet nadir <50,000/mm³	Reduce cisplatin dosage by 50% in subsequent cycles
Serum creatinine ≥1.6 mg/dL (≥141 μmol/L), but creatinine clearance ≥50 mL/min (≥0.83 mL/s)	Reduce cisplatin dosage by 50%
Creatinine clearance <50 mL/min (<0.83 mL/s)	Hold cisplatin*
Serum total bilirubin 2.1–3.0 mg/dL (35.9–51.3 μmol/L)	Reduce vinorelbine dosage by 50%
Serum total bilirubin >3.0 mg/dL (>51.3 μmol/L)	Reduce vinorelbine dosage by 75%
Treatment delay >4 weeks	Discontinue therapy

*If cisplatin treatment is held for any period of time, reduce cisplatin dosage 50% when treatment resumes

Therapy Monitoring

1. *Before repeated cycles:* H&P, PS evaluation, Serum creatinine and calculated creatinine clearance; serum electrolytes, magnesium, hepatic transaminases, and bilirubin
2. *Weekly:* CBC with differential and platelet count
3. *Response evaluation:* Every 2–3 cycles

REGIMEN

CISPLATIN + PEMETREXED

Scagliotti GV et al. J Clin Oncol 2008; 26:3543–3551

Ancillary medications:
Folic acid 350–1000 mcg/day; administer orally beginning 1–2 weeks before the first dose of pemetrexed and continuing until 3 weeks after the last dose of pemetrexed
Cyanocobalamin (vitamin B$_{12}$) 1000 mcg; administer intramuscularly every 9 weeks, beginning 1–2 weeks before the first dose of pemetrexed
Dexamethasone 4 mg; administer orally twice daily for 3 consecutive days, starting the day before pemetrexed administration to decrease the risk and severity of severe skin rash associated with pemetrexed

Hydration before cisplatin: ≥1000 mL 0.9% sodium chloride injection (0.9% NS); administer intravenously over a minimum of 2–4 hours
Pemetrexed 500 mg/m^2; administer intravenously in 100 mL 0.9% NS over 10 minutes on day 1 every 21 days for a maximum of 6 cycles (unless there was earlier evidence of disease progression or intolerance of the study treatment) (total dosage/cycle = 500 mg/m^2)
Cisplatin 75 mg/m^2; administer intravenously in 100–250 mL 0.9% NS over 1 hour on day 1, every 21 days for a maximum of 6 cycles (unless there was earlier evidence of disease progression or intolerance of the study treatment) (total dosage/cycle = 75 mg/m^2)

Hydration after cisplatin: ≥1000 mL 0.9% NS; administer intravenously over a minimum of 2–4 hours

Supportive Care
Antiemetic prophylaxis
Emetogenic potential: **HIGH**. *Potential for delayed symptoms*
See Chapter 39 for antiemetic recommendations

Hematopoietic growth factor (CSF) prophylaxis
Primary prophylaxis is NOT indicated
See Chapter 43 for more information

Antimicrobial prophylaxis
Risk of fever and neutropenia is LOW
Antimicrobial primary prophylaxis to be considered:
• Antibacterial—not indicated
• Antifungal—not indicated
• Antiviral—not indicated unless patient previously had an episode of HSV
See Chapter 47 for more information

Treatment Modifications

Adverse Event	Dose Modification
Day 1 dose reduction of pemetrexed, or cisplatin required	Reduced dose is administered during subsequent treatment cycles
Patients with 2 dose reductions on day 1 who experience toxicity requiring a third dose reduction	Discontinue therapy
Toxicity G ≥2	Delay start of next cycle up to 42 days

Toxicity* (N = 839)

Toxicity	% G3/4
Neutropenia	15.1%
Anemia	5.6%
Thrombocytopenia	4.1%
Febrile neutropenia	1.3%
Nausea	7.2%
Vomiting	6.1%
Fatigue	6.7%
Alopecia, any grade	11.9%
Dehydration, any grade	3.6%

*NCI CTC, National Cancer Institute (USA) Common Toxicity Criteria, version 2.0. Available at: http://ctep.cancer.gov/protocolDevelopment/electronic_applications/ctc.htm [accessed December 7, 2013]

Patient Population Studied

Noninferiority, phase III, randomized study comparing the overall survival between treatment arms in 1725 chemotherapy-naïve patients with histologically or cytologically confirmed NSCLC, classified as stage IIIB not amenable to curative treatment or stage IV and an Eastern Cooperative Oncology Group (ECOG) performance status of 0–1. A total of 862 patients were treated with cisplatin + pemetrexed

Efficacy (N = 862)

Objective response rate*	30.6%
Duration of response	4.5 months
Median overall survival	10.3 months
Median progression-free survival	4.8 months
1-year survival	43.5%
2-year survival	18.9%

*RECIST

Therapy Monitoring

Baseline, every other cycle, and then every 6 weeks:
History and physical examination; assessment by imaging techniques

NSCLC WITH ALK GENE REARRANGEMENT REGIMEN

CRIZOTINIB

Kwak EL et al. N Engl J Med 2010;363:1693–1703
Shaw AT et al. Lancet Oncol 2011;12:1004–1012

Crizotinib 250 mg/dose; administer orally twice daily, continually, with or without food (total dose/week = 3500 mg; total dose/28-day cycle = 14,000 mg)

Supportive Care
Antiemetic prophylaxis
Emetogenic potential is at least **MODERATE**
See Chapter 39 for antiemetic recommendations

Hematopoietic growth factor (CSF) prophylaxis
Primary prophylaxis is NOT indicated
See Chapter 43 for more information

Antimicrobial prophylaxis
Risk of fever and neutropenia is LOW
  Antimicrobial primary prophylaxis to be considered:
  • Antibacterial—not indicated
  • Antifungal—not indicated
  • Antiviral—not indicated unless patient previously had an episode of HSV
See Chapter 47 for more information

Diarrhea management
Latent or delayed onset diarrhea*:
  Loperamide 4 mg orally initially after the first loose or liquid stool, *then*
  Loperamide 2 mg orally every 2 hours during waking hours, *plus*
  Loperamide 4 mg orally every 4 hours during hours of sleep
  • Continue for at least 12 hours after diarrhea resolves
  • Recurrent diarrhea after a 12-hour diarrhea-free interval is treated as a new episode
  • Rehydrate orally with fluids and electrolytes during a diarrheal episode
  • If a patient develops blood or mucus in stool, dehydration, or hemodynamic instability, or if diarrhea persists >48 hours despite loperamide, stop loperamide and hospitalize the patient for IV hydration
  Alternatively, a trial of **Diphenoxylate hydrochloride** 2.5 mg **with Atropine sulfate** 0.025 mg (eg, Lomotil)
  • Initial adult dose is 2 tablets 4 times daily until control has been achieved, after which the dose may be reduced to meet individual requirements. Control may often be maintained with as little as 2 tablets daily
  • Clinical improvement of acute diarrhea is usually observed within 48 hours. If improvement of chronic diarrhea after treatment with a maximum daily dose of 8 tablets is not observed within 10 days, control is unlikely with further administration
Persistent diarrhea:
  Octreotide 100–150 mcg subcutaneously 3 times daily. Maximum total daily dose is 1500 mcg
Antibiotic therapy during latent or delayed onset diarrhea:
  A fluoroquinolone (eg, **Ciprofloxacin** 500 mg orally every 12 hours) if absolute neutrophil count <500/mm³ with or without accompanying fever in association with diarrhea
  • Antibiotics should also be administered if patient is hospitalized with prolonged diarrhea and should be continued until diarrhea resolves

*Abigerges D et al. J Natl Cancer Inst 1994;86:446–449
Rothenberg ML et al. J Clin Oncol 2001;19:3801–3807
Wadler S et al. J Clin Oncol 1998;16:3169–3178

(continued)

Dose Adjustments

Adverse Event	Dose Modification
Hematologic Toxicity*	
G3 hematologic toxicity	Withhold until recovery to G ≤2, then resume at the same dose schedule
G4 hematologic toxicity	Withhold until recovery to G ≤2, then resume at 200 mg twice daily
G4 hematologic toxicity at a dose of 200 mg twice daily	Withhold until recovery to G ≤2, then resume at 250 mg once daily
G4 hematologic toxicity at a dose of 250 mg once daily	Permanently discontinue crizotinib
Non-hematologic Toxicity	
G3/4 alanine aminotransferase (ALT) or aspartate aminotransferase (AST) elevation with G ≤1 total bilirubin	Withhold until recovery to G ≤1 or baseline, then resume at 200 mg twice daily
G3/4 ALT or AST elevation with G ≤1 total bilirubin on a dose of 200 mg twice daily	Withhold until recovery to G ≤1 or baseline, then resume 250 mg once daily
G3/4 ALT or AST elevation with G ≤1 total bilirubin on a dose of 250 mg once daily	Permanently discontinue crizotinib
G2/3/4 ALT or AST elevation with concurrent G2/3/4 total bilirubin elevation (in the absence of cholestasis or hemolysis)	Permanently discontinue crizotinib
Any Grade pneumonitis[†]	Permanently discontinue crizotinib
G3 QTc prolongation	Withhold until recovery to G ≤1, then resume at 200 mg twice daily
G3 QTc prolongation on a dose of 200 mg twice daily	Withhold until recovery to G ≤1 or baseline, then resume 250 mg once daily
G3 QTc prolongation on a dose of 250 mg once daily	Permanently discontinue crizotinib
Grade 4 QTc prolongation	Permanently discontinue crizotinib

*Except lymphopenia (unless associated with clinical events, eg, opportunistic infections)
[†]Not attributable to NSCLC progression, other pulmonary disease, infection, or radiation effect

(*continued*)

Notes:

1. Detection of ALK-positive NSCLC using an FDA-approved test indicated for this use is necessary for selection of patients for treatment with crizotinib

2. Assessment for ALK-positive NSCLC should be performed by laboratories with demonstrated proficiency in the specific technology being utilized. Improper assay performance can lead to unreliable test results

Drugs That May Increase Crizotinib Plasma Concentrations
Coadministration of crizotinib with strong CYP3A inhibitors increases crizotinib plasma concentrations

- Avoid concomitant use of strong CYP3A inhibitors, including but not limited to atazanavir, clarithromycin, indinavir, itraconazole, ketoconazole, nefazodone, nelfinavir, ritonavir, saquinavir, telithromycin, troleandomycin, and voriconazole

- Avoid grapefruit or grapefruit juice which may increase plasma concentrations of crizotinib

- Exercise caution with concomitant use of moderate CYP3A inhibitors

Drugs That May Decrease Crizotinib Plasma Concentrations
Coadministration of crizotinib with strong CYP3A inducers decreases crizotinib plasma concentrations

- Avoid concurrent use of strong CYP3A inducers, including but not limited to carbamazepine, phenobarbital, phenytoin, rifabutin, rifampin, and St. John's Wort

Patient Population Studied

Eighty-two patients with advanced ALK-positive NSCLC who had received crizotinib in the phase 1 clinical trial. For all patients, ALK positivity was confirmed by fluorescence in situ hybridization (FISH). ALK FISH was done before trial enrolment, using the initial diagnostic or surgical specimen, or a repeat biopsy specimen obtained for the purposes of genetic testing. These patients were mainly young (median age: 51 years [range: 25–78 years]), never smokers with adenocarcinoma histology. Among the 82 patients, 50 (61%) were enrolled at U.S. study sites, 26 (32%) at the Korean site, and the remaining 6 (7%) in Australia. Because the protocol placed no restriction on the number of previous therapies, the number varied widely among patients, ranging from 0 to 7 previous lines (median: 2) of therapy for metastatic disease. Seventy-three (89%) of 82 patients had received at least 1 previous therapy for metastatic disease. An additional 36 patients with advanced, ALK-positive NSCLC who had not received crizotinib were identified through retrospective and prospective screening efforts

Efficacy

	ALK(+) Patients*	ALK(+) Patients[†]	ALK(+) Controls[‡]	ALK(+) Patients[§]	ALK(−) EGFR(+) Patients[ᶜ]	Crizotinib-naïve, ALK(+) Controls**	Wild-type Controls[††]
Number of patients	82	30	23	56	63	36	253
Median OS [95% CI][‡]	NR [17 mo–NR][§§]	NR [14 mo–NR]	6 mo [4–17 mo]	NR [17 mo–NR]	24 mo [15–34 mo]	20 mo [13–26 mo]	15 mo [13–17 mo]
		—		—		HR 0.77, 95% CI 0.50–1.19; p = 0.244	
1-year OS [95% CI]	74% [63–82%]	70% [50–83%]	44% [23–64%]	71% [58–81%]	74% [61–83]	72% [54-84%]	
2-year OS [95% CI]	54% [40–66%]	55% [33–72%]	12% [2–30%]	57% [40–71%]	52% [38–65%]	36% [19-54%]	
		HR 0.36, 95% CI 0.17–0.75; p = 0.004		P = 0.786		—	

Mo, Months; NR, not reached; OS, overall survival
*Patients with advanced, ALK-positive NSCLC who had enrolled on the multicenter phase 1 clinical trial of crizotinib. Median follow-up was 18 months (IQR 16–22)
[†]ALK-positive patients given crizotinib in the second- or third-line setting
[‡]ALK+ controls given any second-line therapy
[§]Fifty-six crizotinib-treated, ALK+ patients; 20 (36%) of the 56 crizotinib-treated patients received 3 to 7 previous lines of therapy. This could overestimate the survival benefit associated with crizotinib
[ᶜ]Sixty-three ALK-negative, EGFR-positive patients given EGFR TKI therapy
**Thirty-six crizotinib-naïve, ALK-positive controls
[††]Two hundred fifty-three wild-type controls
[‡]Median OS from date of first crizotinib dose in months
[§§]OS did not differ based on age (≤50 years vs. >50 years, p = 0.692), sex (p = 0.975), smoking history (never vs. any smoking, p = 0.857), or ethnic origin (Asian vs. non-Asian, p = 0.857)

Toxicity

Adapted from XALKORI (crizotinib) Capsules, oral; 05/2013 product label. Pfizer Labs, Division of Pfizer Inc., New York, NY

Adverse Reactions in ≥10% of Patients with Locally Advanced or Metastatic ALK-Positive NSCLC Enrolled in 2 Studies*

Adverse Event	Treatment Emergent N = 255		Treatment Related N = 255	
	All G, n (%)	G3/4, n (%)	All G, n (%)	G3/4, n (%)
Eye Disorders				
Vision Disorder†	163 (64%)	0	159 (62%)	0
Gastrointestinal Disorders				
Nausea	145 (57%)	2 (<1%)	136 (53%)	0
Diarrhea	124 (49%)	1 (<1%)	109 (43%)	0
Vomiting	116 (45%)	3 (1%)	101 (40%)	0
Constipation	98 (38%)	2 (<1%)	69 (27%)	1 (<1%)
Esophageal disorder‡	51 (20%)	3 (1%)	29 (11%)	0
Abdominal pain§	40 (16%)	1 (<1%)	20 (8%)	0
Stomatitis⁋	27 (11%)	1 (<1%)	15 (6%)	1 (<1%)
General Disorders				
Edema**	97 (38%)	2 (<1%)	72 (28%)	0
Fatigue	80 (31%)	6 (2%)	51 (20%)	4 (2%)
Chest pain/discomfort††	30 (12%)	1 (<1%)	3 (1%)	0
Fever	30 (12%)	1 (<1%)	2 (<1%)	0
Infections and Infestations				
Upper respiratory infection‡‡	50 (20%)	1 (<1%)	4 (2%)	0
Investigations				
↑Alanine aminotransferase	38 (15%)	17 (7%)	34 (13%)	14 (5%)
↑Aspartate aminotransferase	29 (11%)	7 (3%)	24 (9%)	5 (2%)
Metabolism and Nutrition				
Decreased appetite	69 (27%)	3 (1%)	49 (19%)	0
Musculoskeletal				
Arthralgia	29 (11%)	3 (1%)	4 (2%)	0
Back pain	28 (11%)	0	2 (<1%)	0
Nervous System Disorders				
Dizziness§§	60 (24%)	0	42 (16%)	0
Neuropathy⁋⁋	58 (23%)	1 (<1%)	34 (13%)***	1 (<1%)
Headache	34 (13%)	1 (<1%)	10 (4%)	0
Dysgeusia	33 (13%)	0	30 (12%)	0
Psychiatric Disorders				
Insomnia	30 (12%)	0	8 (3%)	0
Respiratory Disorders				
Dyspnea	57 (22%)	16 (6%)	5 (2%)	3 (1%)
Cough	54 (21%)	3 (1%)	9 (4%)	0
Skin Disorders				
Rash	41 (16%)	0	25 (10%)	0

(continued)

Treatment Monitoring

1. *Monthly and as clinically indicated:* Complete blood counts (CBC) including differential white blood cell counts and liver function tests
2. *If G3/4 clinical or laboratory abnormalities are observed or if fever or infection occurs:* Frequent monitoring of complete blood counts (CBC) including differential white blood cell counts and liver function tests
3. Consider periodic monitoring with electrocardiograms (ECGs) and electrolytes in patients with congestive heart failure, bradyarrhythmias, electrolyte abnormalities, or who are taking medications that are known to prolong the QT interval

Toxicity *(continued)*

Adverse Event	Treatment Emergent N = 255		Treatment Related N = 255	
	All G, n (%)	G3/4, n (%)	All G, n (%)	G3/4, n (%)
Cardiovascular				
G1/2 bradycardia	12 (5%)			
Hematologic Toxicities				
G3/4 neutropenia	5.2%			
G3/4 thrombocytopenia	0.4%			
G3/4 lymphopenia	11.4%			

*One study used NCI Common Terminology Criteria for Adverse Events (CTCAE) v4.0; the other used CTCAE v3.0. All CTCAE versions available at: http://ctep.cancer.gov/protocolDevelopment/electronic_applications/ctc.htm [accessed December 7, 2013]

†Includes diplopia, photopsia, photophobia, vision blurred, visual field defect, visual impairment, vitreous floaters, visual brightness, and visual acuity reduced. Consider ophthalmologic evaluation, particularly if patients experience photopsia or experience new or increased vitreous floaters. Severe or worsening vitreous floaters and/or photopsia could also be signs of a retinal hole or pending retinal detachment

‡Includes dyspepsia, dysphagia, epigastric discomfort/pain/burning, esophagitis, esophageal obstruction/pain/ spasm/ulcer, gastroesophageal reflux, odynophagia, and reflux esophagitis

§Includes abdominal discomfort, abdominal pain, abdominal pain upper, and abdominal tenderness

¶Includes mouth ulceration, glossodynia, glossitis, cheilitis, mucosal inflammation, oropharyngeal pain/discomfort, oral pain, and stomatitis

**Includes edema, edema localized, and peripheral edema

††Includes chest pain, chest discomfort, and musculoskeletal chest pain

‡‡Includes nasopharyngitis, rhinitis, pharyngitis, and upper respiratory tract infection

§§Includes balance disorder, dizziness, and presyncope

¶¶Includes burning sensation, dysesthesia, hyperesthesia, hypoesthesia, neuralgia, paresthesia, peripheral neuropathy, peripheral motor neuropathy, and peripheral sensory neuropathy

***Although most events were G1, G2 motor neuropathy and G3 peripheral neuropathy were reported in 1 patient each

ADVANCED NSCLC REGIMEN

WEEKLY *nab*-PACLITAXEL + CARBOPLATIN

Socinski MA et al. J Clin Oncol 2012;30:2055–2062

Paclitaxel protein-bound particles for injectable suspension (*nab*-paclitaxel) 100 mg/m^2 per dose; administer intravenously over 30 minutes, once weekly for 3 doses, on days 1, 8, and 15 every 3 weeks (total dosage/cycle = 300 mg/m^2)

Carboplatin [calculated dose] AUC = 6 mg/mL · min*; administer intravenously diluted to concentrations as low as 0.5 mg/mL with either 5% dextrose injection or 0.9% sodium chloride injection over 15–30 minutes on day 1, every 3 weeks (total dosage/cycle calculated to produce an AUC = 6 mg/mL · min)

*Carboplatin dose is based on a formula described by Calvert et al. to achieve a target area under the plasma concentration versus time curve (AUC)

Recommendations for Initial *nab*-paclitaxel Dosage in Hepatically Impaired Patients

	SGOT (AST) Levels		Total Bilirubin Levels	*nab*-Paclitaxel Dosage*
Mild	<10 × ULN	*and*	> ULN to ≤1.25 × ULN	100 mg/m^2
Moderate	<10 × ULN		1.26–2 × ULN	75 mg/m^2
Severe	<10 × ULN		2.01–5 × ULN	50 mg/m^{2†}
	>10 × ULN	*or*	>5 × ULN	Do not administer

*A need for dosage adjustments during repeated treatment cycles should be based on individual tolerance for previous treatment
†Increase dose to 75 mg/m^2 during subsequent courses, as tolerated

$$\text{Total carboplatin dose (mg)} = (\text{Target AUC}) \times (\text{GFR} + 25)$$

In practice, creatinine clearance (Clcr) is used in place of glomerular filtration rate (GFR). Clcr can be estimated from the equation of Cockcroft and Gault, thus:

$$\text{For males, Clcr} = \frac{(140 - \text{age [years]}) \times \text{body weight (kg)}}{72 \times (\text{Serum creatinine [mg/dL]})}$$

$$\text{For females, Clcr} = \frac{(140 - \text{age [years]}) \times \text{body weight (kg)}}{72 \times (\text{Serum creatinine [mg/dL]})} \times 0.85$$

Calvert AH et al. J Clin Oncol 1989;7:1748–1756
Cockcroft DW, Gault MH. Nephron 1976;16:31–41
Jodrell DI et al. J Clin Oncol 1992;10:520–528
Sorensen BT et al. Cancer Chemother Pharmacol 1991;28:397–401

Note: On October 8, 2010, the U.S. Food and Drug Administration (FDA) identified a potential safety issue with carboplatin dosing based on recent changes in the measurement of serum creatinine. By the end of 2010, all clinical laboratories in the United States began using the standardized isotope dilution mass spectrometry (IDMS) method to measure serum creatinine, which could result in an overestimation of the GFR in some patients with normal renal function. A carboplatin dose calculated with an IDMS-measured serum creatinine result using the Calvert formula could exceed an expected exposure (AUC) and result in increased drug-related toxicity

Provided actual GFR measurements are made to assess renal function, carboplatin can be safely dosed according to the Calvert formula described in product labeling

If GFR (or creatinine clearance) is estimated based on serum creatinine measurements by the IDMS method, the FDA recommends for patients with normal renal function capping an estimated GFR at 125 mL/min for any targeted AUC value. No greater estimated GFR values should be used

U.S. FDA. Carboplatin dosing. [online] October 8, 2010. Available from: http://www.fda.gov/AboutFDA/CentersOffices/OfficeofMedicalProductsandTobacco/CDER/ucm228974.htm [accessed February 26, 2014]

(continued)

DOSE ADJUSTMENTS

Adapted in part from Abraxane for Injectable Suspension (paclitaxel protein-bound particles for injectable suspension) (albumin-bound); October 2012 product label. Celgene Corporation, Summit, NJ

Adverse Event	Treatment Modification
On day 1 of a cycle, ANC <1500/mm^3 or platelet count <100,000/mm^3	Withhold *nab*-paclitaxel and carboplatin until ANC ≥1500/mm^3 and platelet count ≥100,000/mm^3
On day 8 of a cycle, ANC <500/mm^3 or platelet count <50,000/mm^3	Withhold *nab*-paclitaxel and carboplatin until ANC ≥500/mm^3 and platelet count ≥50,000/mm^3
On day 15 of a cycle, ANC <500/mm^3 or platelet count <50,000/mm^3	Withhold *nab*-paclitaxel and carboplatin until ANC ≥500/mm^3 and platelet count ≥50,000/mm^3
Fever and neutropenia (ANC <500/mm^3 with fever >38°C [>100.4°F]), or Delay of next cycle >7 days for ANC <1500/mm^3, or ANC <500/mm^3 >7 days at a weekly *nab*-paclitaxel dose of 100 mg/m^2 and carboplatin dose of AUC = 6 mg/mL · min	Reduce weekly *nab*-paclitaxel dose to 75 mg/m^2 and carboplatin dose to AUC = 4.5 mg/mL · min every 3 weeks
Fever and neutropenia (ANC <500/mm^3 with fever >38°C [>100.4°F]), or Delay of next cycle >7 days for ANC <1500/mm^3, or ANC <500/mm^3 >7 days at a weekly *nab*-paclitaxel dose of 75 mg/m^2 and carboplatin dose of AUC = 4.5 mg/mL · min	Reduce weekly *nab*-paclitaxel dose to 50 mg/m^2 and carboplatin dose to AUC = 3 mg/mL · min every 3 weeks

(continued)

(continued)

Supportive Care

Antiemetic prophylaxis

Emetogenic potential on with nab-paclitaxel alone is **LOW**

Emetogenic potential on days with carboplatin alone is **MODERATE–HIGH**. *Potential for delayed symptoms*

See Chapter 39 for antiemetic recommendations

Hematopoietic growth factor (CSF) prophylaxis

Primary prophylaxis may be indicated

See Chapter 43 for more information

Antimicrobial prophylaxis

Risk of fever and neutropenia is LOW

Antimicrobial primary prophylaxis to be considered:

- Antibacterial—not indicated
- Antifungal—not indicated
- Antiviral—not indicated unless patient previously had an episode of HSV

See Chapter 47 for more information

Toxicity

Most Common Treatment-Related G ≥3 Adverse Events According to NCI CTCAE

	nab-PC (%) (N = 514)		Sb-PC (%) (N = 524)		
	G3	G4	G3	G4	P
Hematologic Adverse Events					
Neutropenia	33	14	32	26	<0.001*
Thrombocytopenia	13	5	7	2	<0.00†
Anemia	22	5	6	<1	<0.001†
Febrile neutropenia	<1	<1	1	<1	N/S
Nonhematologic Adverse Events					
Fatigue	4	<1	6	<1	N/S
Sensory neuropathy	3	0	11	<1	<0.001*
Anorexia	2	0	<1	0	N/S
Nausea	<1	0	<1	0	N/S
Myalgia	<1	0	2	0	0.011*
Arthralgia	0	0	2	0	0.008*

N/S, Not significant; nab-PC, 130-nm albumin-bound paclitaxel + carboplatin; NCI CTCAE, National Cancer Institute Common Terminology Criteria for Adverse Events; sb-PC, conventional (solvent-based) paclitaxel + carboplatin
*P<0.05 in favor of *nab*-PC
†P<0.05 in favor of sb-PC

Patient Population Studied

Patients with histologically/cytologically confirmed nonresectable stage IIIB (± pleural effusion) or stage IV NSCLC, Eastern Cooperative Oncology Group performance status of 0–1, who had not previously received treatment for metastatic disease and had no radiotherapy within 4 weeks before enrollment. Prior adjuvant chemotherapy was allowed if it had been completed 12 months prior to enrollment. Patients with CNS metastases and those with neuropathy G ≥1 were excluded

Dose Adjustments *(continued)*

Adverse Event	Treatment Modification
Fever and neutropenia (ANC <500/mm³ with fever >38°C [>100.4°F]), or Delay of next cycle >7 days for ANC <1500/mm³, or ANC <500/mm³ >7 days at a weekly *nab*-paclitaxel dose of 50 mg/m² and carboplatin dose of AUC = 3 mg/mL • min	Discontinue *nab*-paclitaxel and carboplatin
Platelet count <50,000/mm³ at a weekly *nab*-paclitaxel dose of 100 mg/m² and carboplatin dose of AUC >6 mg/mL • min	Reduce weekly *nab*-paclitaxel dose to 75 mg/m² and carboplatin dose to AUC = 4.5 mg/mL • min every 3 weeks
Platelet count <50,000/mm³ at a weekly *nab*-paclitaxel dose of 75 mg/m² and carboplatin dose of AUC = 4.5 mg/mL • min	Discontinue *nab*-paclitaxel and carboplatin
G3/4 sensory neuropathy at a weekly *nab*-paclitaxel dose of 100 mg/m² and carboplatin dose of AUC = 6 mg/mL • min	Withhold *nab*-paclitaxel and carboplatin until toxicity G ≤1, then reduce weekly *nab*-paclitaxel dose to 75 mg/m² and carboplatin dose to AUC = 4.5 mg/mL • min every three weeks
G3/4 sensory neuropathy at a weekly *nab*-paclitaxel dose of 75 mg/m² and carboplatin dose of AUC = 4.5 mg/mL • min	Withhold *nab*-paclitaxel and carboplatin until toxicity G ≤1, then reduce weekly *nab*-paclitaxel dose to 50 mg/m² and carboplatin dose to AUC = 3.0 mg/mL • min every 3 weeks
G3/4 sensory neuropathy at a weekly *nab*-paclitaxel dose of 50 mg/m² and carboplatin dose of AUC = 3 mg/mL • min	Discontinue *nab*-paclitaxel and carboplatin

Efficacy

Response Rates for the Intent-to-Treat Population and Histologic Subset Based on Independent Radiologic Assessment

	nab-PC		sb-PC				
	%	95% CI	%	95% CI	RR Ratio	95% CI	P
Intent-to-treat	N = 521		N = 531				
Overall response	33%	28.6–36.7%	25%	21.2–28.5%	1.313	1.082–1.593	0.005
Complete response	0		<1%				
Partial response	33%		25%				
Stable disease	20%		24%				
Progressive disease	16%		16%				
Squamous subset	N = 229		N = 221				
Overall response	41	34.7–47.4%	24	18.8–30.1%	1.680	1.271–2.221	<0.001
Nonsquamous subset	N = 292		N = 310				
Overall response	26	21.0–31.1	25	20.3–30.0	1.034	0.788–1.358	0.808

Progression-free Survival (PFS) and Overall Survival (OS)

	nab-PC		sb-PC				
	Months	95% CI	Months	95% CI	HR	95% CI	P
Median PFS	6.3	5.6–7.0	5.8	5.6–6.7	0.902	0.767–1.060	0.214
Median OS, ITT	12.1	10.8–12.9	11.2	10.3–12.6	0.922	0.797–1.066	0.271
Median OS, squamous subset	10.7	9.4–12.5	9.5	8.6–11.6	0.890	0.719–1.101	0.284
Median OS, nonsquamous subset	13.1		13.0		0.950		
Median OS, <70 years	11.4		11.3		0.999		
Median OS, ≥70 years	19.9		10.4		0.583		0.009

HR, Hazard ratio; nab-PC, 130-nm albumin-bound paclitaxel + carboplatin; RR ratio, response rate ratio; sb-PC, conventional (solvent-based) paclitaxel + carboplatin

Treatment Monitoring

1. *Monthly and as clinically indicated:* Complete blood counts (CBC) including differential white blood cell counts and liver function tests
2. *If G3/4 clinical or laboratory abnormalities are observed or if fever or infection occurs:* Frequent monitoring of complete blood counts (CBC) including differential white blood cell counts and liver function tests

ADVANCED-STAGE NON–SMALL CELL LUNG CANCER (CHEMOTHERAPY-NAÏVE) REGIMEN

CISPLATIN + PEMETREXED

Scagliotti VG et al. J Clin Oncol 2008;26:3543–3551

Ancillary medications:
Folic acid 350–1000 mcg per day orally beginning 1–2 weeks before the first dose of pemetrexed and continuing until 3 weeks after the last dose of pemetrexed

Cyanocobalamin (vitamin B_{12}) 1000 mcg intramuscularly every 9 weeks, beginning 1–2 weeks before the first dose of pemetrexed

Dexamethasone 4 mg orally twice daily for 3 consecutive days, starting the day before pemetrexed administration to decrease the risk and severity of severe skin rash associated with pemetrexed

Hydration before cisplatin: ≥1000 mL 0.9% sodium chloride injection (0.9% NS) by intravenous infusion over a minimum of 2–4 hours

Pemetrexed disodium 500 mg/m² intravenously in 100 mL 0.9% NS over 10 minutes on day 1 every 3 weeks for a maximum of 6 cycles (unless there was earlier evidence of disease progression or intolerance of the study treatment) (total dosage/cycle: = 500 mg/m²)

Cisplatin 75 mg/m² intravenously in 100–250 mL 0.9% NS over 1 hour on day 1 every 3 weeks for a maximum of 6 cycles (unless there was earlier evidence of disease progression or intolerance of the study treatment) (total dosage/cycle = 75 mg/m²)

Hydration after cisplatin: ≥1000 mL 0.9% NS by intravenous infusion over a minimum of 2–4 hours

Supportive Care

Antiemetic prophylaxis
Emetogenic potential is **HIGH**. *Potential for delayed symptoms*
See Chapter 39 for antiemetic recommendations

Hematopoietic growth factor (CSF) prophylaxis
Primary prophylaxis is NOT indicated
See Chapter 43 for more information

Antimicrobial prophylaxis
Risk of fever and neutropenia is LOW
  Antimicrobial primary prophylaxis to be considered:
  • Antibacterial—not indicated
  • Antifungal—not indicated
  • Antiviral—not indicated unless patient previously had an episode of HSV
See Chapter 47 for more information

Patient Population Studied

Chemotherapy-naïve patients with histologically or cytologically confirmed NSCLC who were classified as stage IIIB not amenable to curative treatment or stage IV, and an Eastern Cooperative Oncology Group performance status of 0 or 1. Prior radiation therapy was permitted if it was completed at least 4 weeks before study treatment and patients had fully recovered from its acute effects. Exclusion criteria included peripheral neuropathy NCI CTC G ≥1

Treatment Modifications

Adapted in part from Alimta (pemetrexed for injection) Lyophilized Powder, for Solution for Intravenous Use; 05/2013 product label. Lilly USA, LLC, Indianapolis, IN

Nadir ANC <500/mm³ and nadir platelets ≥50,000/mm³	75% of previous pemetrexed dose and 75% of previous cisplatin dose
Nadir platelets <50,000/mm³ without bleeding regardless of nadir ANC	75% of previous pemetrexed dose and 75% of previous cisplatin dose
Nadir platelets <50,000/mm³ with bleeding*, regardless of nadir ANC	50% of previous pemetrexed dose and 50% of previous cisplatin dose
Any G3/4 toxicities except mucositis	Withhold treatment until toxicity resolves to the same or less than pretreatment status. Resume treatment with 75% of the previously administered pemetrexed and cisplatin dosages
Any G3/4 toxicities except mucositis after two dose reductions	Discontinue therapy
Any diarrhea requiring hospitalization (irrespective of grade) or G3/4 diarrhea	Withhold treatment until toxicity resolves to the same or less than pretreatment status. Then, resume treatment with 75% of the previously administered pemetrexed and cisplatin dosages
Any diarrhea requiring hospitalization (irrespective of grade) or G3/4 diarrhea after 2 dose reductions	Discontinue therapy
G3/4 mucositis	Withhold treatment until toxicity resolves to the same or less than pretreatment status. Then, resume treatment with pemetrexed dosage decreased by 50% and the same cisplatin dosage (100%) previously given

(continued)

Efficacy

	Cisplatin + Pemetrexed		Cisplatin + Gemcitabine		HR [95% CI]	P
Objective response rates	30.6%		28.2%		—	—
Duration of response	4.5 mo		5.1 mo		—	—
PFS, all patients	4.8 mo	4.6–5.3	5.1 mo	4.6–5.5	1.04 [0.94–1.15]	—
PFS, nonsquamous (L-C + Adeno)	5.3 mo	4.8–5.7	4.7 mo	4.4–5.4	0.90 [0.79–1.02]	—
PFS, squamous cell carcinoma	4.4 mo	4.1–4.9	5.5 mo	4.6–5.9	1.36 [1.12–1.65]	—
OS, all patients	10.3 mo	9.8–11.2	10.3	9.6–10.9	0.94 [0.84–1.05]	—
Survival at 12 months	43.5%		41.9%		—	—
Survival at 24 months	18.9%		14.0%		—	—
OS, nonsquamous (L-C + Adeno)	11.8 mo	10.4–13.2	10.4 mo	9.6–11.2	0.81 [0.70–0.94]	0.005
OS, large cell carcinoma	10.4 mo	—	6.7 mo	—	0.67 [0.48–0.96]	—
OS, adenocarcinoma	12.6 mo	—	10.9 mo	—	0.84 [0.71–0.99]	—
OS, squamous cell carcinoma	9.4 mo	8.4–10.2	10.8 mo	9.5–12.1	1.23 [1.00–1.51]	0.05
No generic/cytologic diagnosis	8.6 mo	—	9.2 mo	—	1.08 [0.81–1.45]	0.586

Survival Based on Baseline Patient and Disease Characteristics

Age <65 years	10.3	9.6–11.3	10.3 mo	9.6–11.3	0.97 [0.84–1.11]	—
Age ≥65 years	10.1	9.2–12.0	10.2 mo	8.5–11.2	0.88 [0.73–1.06]	—
Male	9.6	8.8–10.2	9.9 mo	9.1–10.6	0.98 [0.86–1.11]	—
Female	13.3	12.3–15.0	11.4 mo	10.2–12.7	0.84 [0.68–1.03]	—
Former/current smoker	10.0	9.4–11.1	10.3 mo	9.5–10.9	0.93 [0.81–1.05]	—
Never smoker	15.9	13.8–20.2	15.3 mo	12.1–22.9	1.00 [0.71–1.41]	—
Stage IIIB	11.9	10.0–14.2	11.3 mo	9.6–13.1	0.89 [0.71–1.12]	—
Stage IV	10.0	9.3–10.8	10.1 mo	9.3–10.8	0.95 [0.84–1.08]	—
ECOG PS 0	13.4	11.9–14.9	12.2 mo	11.3–13.4	0.91 [0.75–1.10]	—
ECOG PS 1	9.1	8.1–9.9	9.0 mo	8.3–9.8	0.95 [0.83–1.09]	—

Adeno, Adenocarcinoma; ECOG PS, Eastern Cooperative Group Performance Status; HR, hazard ratio; L-C, large cell; mo, months; OS, overall survival; PFS, progression-free survival

Treatment Modifications
(*continued*)

G3/4 mucositis after 2 dose reductions	Discontinue therapy
G1 neurotoxicity	Continue pemetrexed and cisplatin treatment at 100% of the previously administered dosages
G2 neurotoxicity	Withhold treatment until toxicity resolves to the same or less than pretreatment status. Then, resume treatment with the same pemetrexed dosage (100%) previously given and cisplatin dosage decreased by 50%
G3/4 neurotoxicity	Discontinue therapy

*These criteria meet the NCI Common Toxicity Criteria (CTC, 1998) version 2.0 definition of G ≥2 bleeding

Toxicity

	Cisplatin + Pemetrexed	Cisplatin + Gemcitabine	P
G3/4 neutropenia,	15%	27%	≤0.001
G3/4 anemia	6%	10%	≤0.001
G3/4 thrombocytopenia	4%	13%	≤0.001
Febrile neutropenia	1%	4%	0.002
Alopecia (all grades)	12%	21%	<0.001
G3/4 nausea	7%	4%	0.004
Transfusions	16.4%	28.9%	<0.001
RBC transfusions	16.1%	27.3%	<0.001
Platelet transfusions	1.8%	4.5%	0.002
Erythropoietin administration	10.4%	18.1%	<0.001
Granulocyte-colony stimulating factor administration	3.1%	6.1%	0.004
Deaths attributed to drug toxicity	1.0%	0.7%	

Treatment Monitoring

1. *Monthly and as clinically indicated:* Complete blood counts (CBC) including differential white blood cell counts and liver function tests
2. *If G3/4 clinical or laboratory abnormalities are observed or if fever or infection occurs:* Frequent monitoring of complete blood counts (CBC) including differential white blood cell counts and liver function tests

REGIMEN

DOCETAXEL

Shepherd FA et al. J Clin Oncol 2000;18:2095–2103

Prophylaxis for fluid retention and hypersensitivity reactions from docetaxel:
Dexamethasone 8 mg/dose; administer orally twice daily for 3 days, starting the day before docetaxel is administered (total dose/cycle = 48 mg)
Docetaxel 75 mg/m^2; administer intravenously in a volume of 0.9% sodium chloride injection or 5% dextrose injection sufficient to produce a solution with concentration within the range 0.3–0.74 mg/mL over 1 hour on day 1, every 3 weeks (total dosage/cycle = 75 mg/m^2)

Supportive Care
Antiemetic prophylaxis
Emetogenic potential: LOW
See Chapter 39 for antiemetic recommendations

Hematopoietic growth factor (CSF) prophylaxis
Primary prophylaxis is NOT indicated
See Chapter 43 for more information

Antimicrobial prophylaxis
Risk of fever and neutropenia is LOW
  Antimicrobial primary prophylaxis to be considered:
  • Antibacterial—not indicated
  • Antifungal—not indicated
  • Antiviral—not indicated unless patient previously had an episode of HSV
See Chapter 47 for more information

Patient Population Studied

A randomized comparison with best supportive care of 55 patients with advanced (Stages III/IV) NSCLC previously treated with platinum-containing chemotherapy

Efficacy (N = 55)

Complete response	—
Partial response	7.1%
Median survival	7.5 months
1-Year survival	37%

Toxicity (N = 55)

	% G3/4
Neutropenia	67.3
Anemia	5.5
Febrile neutropenia	1.8
Thrombocytopenia	0
Pulmonary	20
Asthenia	18.2
Infection	5.5
Nausea	3.6
Vomiting	3.6
Diarrhea	1.8
Neuromotor	1.8
Neurosensory	1.8

Treatment Modifications

Adverse Event	Dose Modification
G4 neutropenia for >7 days, alone, or accompanied by fever >38°C (>100.4°F)	Reduce docetaxel dosage by 25% in all subsequent treatments
G4 thrombocytopenia	Resume docetaxel after platelet count recovers with docetaxel dosage decreased by 25%
G4 vomiting not controlled by antiemetics	Reduce docetaxel dosage by 25%
G ≥3 diarrhea	
G ≥3 neuropathy	Discontinue therapy

Therapy Monitoring

1. *Before treatment:* H&P, PS evaluation, CBC with differential, and LFTs
2. *Weekly:* CBC with differential and platelet count
3. *Response evaluation:* Every 2–3 cycles

REGIMEN

VINORELBINE (ELDERLY PATIENTS)

Gridelli C et al. J Natl Cancer Inst 2003;95:362–372

Vinorelbine 30 mg/m² per dose; administer intravenously in a volume of 0.9% sodium chloride injection or 5% dextrose injection sufficient to produce a solution with concentration within the range 0.5–3 mg/mL over 6–10 minutes for 2 doses, on days 1 and 8 every 3 weeks for a maximum of 6 cycles (total dosage/cycle = 60 mg/m²)

Supportive Care
Antiemetic prophylaxis
Emetogenic potential is **MINIMAL**
See Chapter 39 for antiemetic recommendations

Hematopoietic growth factor (CSF) prophylaxis
Primary prophylaxis is NOT indicated
See Chapter 43 for more information

Antimicrobial prophylaxis
Risk of fever and neutropenia is LOW
  Antimicrobial primary prophylaxis to be considered:
  • Antibacterial—not indicated
  • Antifungal—not indicated
  • Antiviral—not indicated unless patient previously had an episode of HSV
See Chapter 47 for more information

Patient Population Studied

A randomized comparison of gemcitabine + vinorelbine in 233 patients ages 70 years and older with advanced (Stages IIIB/IV) untreated NSCLC

Efficacy
(Intent-to-Treat, N = 233)

Response rate	18%
Median survival	36 weeks
6-month survival	60%
Estimated 1-year survival	38%

Toxicity (N = 229)*

	% G3	% G4
Hematologic		
Anemia	3	<1
Neutropenia	14	11
Thrombocytopenia	<1	—
Infection	3	—
Bleeding	1	—
Nonhematologic		
Nausea/vomiting	<1	—
Mucositis	1	—
Fatigue	7	—
Fever	2	—
Cardiac	1	<1
Pulmonary	1	—
Hepatic	<1	—
Constipation	3	<1
Peripheral neuropathy	1	—
Central neurotoxicity	—	<1

*WHO criteria

Treatment Modifications

Adverse Event	Dose Modification
Days 1 and 8 ANC ≥1500/mm³, platelet count ≥100,000/mm³, and no organ toxicity (other than alopecia)	Vinorelbine given at 100% dosage
Days 1 and 8 ANC <1500/mm³, platelet count <100,000/mm³, or organ toxicity (other than alopecia)	Delay treatment for up to 2 weeks
Serum total bilirubin 2.1–3.0 mg/dL (35.9–51.3 μmol/L)	Reduce vinorelbine dosage by 50%
Serum total bilirubin >3.0 mg/dL (51.3 μmol/L)	Reduce vinorelbine dosage by 75%

Therapy Monitoring

1. *Days 1 and 8:* CBC with differential and platelet count. Serum electrolytes, BUN, creatinine, and LFTs
2. *Weekly:* CBC with differential and platelet count
3. *Response evaluation:* Every 2–3 cycles

MAINTENANCE THERAPY—ADVANCED NSCLC REGIMEN

MAINTENANCE PEMETREXED

Ciuleanu T et al. Lancet 2009;374:1432-1440

Ancillary medications:
Folic acid 350–1000 mcg per day; administer orally beginning 1–2 weeks before the first dose of pemetrexed and continuing until 3 weeks after the last dose of pemetrexed
Cyanocobalamin (vitamin B_{12}) 1000 mcg; administer intramuscularly every 9 weeks, beginning 1 to 2 weeks before the first dose of pemetrexed
Dexamethasone 4 mg; administer orally twice daily for 3 consecutive days (6 doses), starting the day before pemetrexed administration to decrease the risk and severity of severe skin rash associated with pemetrexed (total dose/cycle = 24 mg)

Pemetrexed disodium 500 mg/m²; administer intravenously in 100 mL 0.9% sodium chloride injection over 10 minutes on day 1, every 21 days until disease progression (total dosage/cycle = 500 mg/m²), *plus*

Best Supportive Care
Supportive Care
Antiemetic prophylaxis
Emetogenic potential is **LOW**
See Chapter 39 for antiemetic recommendations

Hematopoietic growth factor (CSF) prophylaxis
Primary prophylaxis is NOT indicated
See Chapter 43 for more information

Antimicrobial prophylaxis
Risk of fever and neutropenia is LOW
> *Antimicrobial primary prophylaxis to be considered:*
> • Antibacterial—not indicated
> • Antifungal—not indicated
> • Antiviral—not indicated unless patient previously had an episode of HSV

See Chapter 47 for more information

Treatment Modifications

Adapted in part from Alimta (pemetrexed for injection) Lyophilized Powder, for Solution for Intravenous Use; 05/2013 product label. Lilly USA, LLC, Indianapolis, IN

Nadir ANC <500/mm³ and nadir platelets ≥50,000/mm³	75% of the previous pemetrexed dose
Nadir platelets <50,000/mm³ without bleeding regardless of nadir ANC	75% of the previous pemetrexed dose
Nadir platelets <50,000/mm³ with bleeding*, regardless of nadir ANC	50% of the previous pemetrexed dose
Any G3/4 toxicities except mucositis	Withhold treatment until toxicity resolves to the same or less than pretreatment status. Then, resume treatment with pemetrexed dosage decreased by 75%
Any G3/4 toxicities except mucositis after two dose reductions	Discontinue therapy
Any diarrhea requiring hospitalization (irrespective of grade) or G3/4 diarrhea	Withhold treatment until toxicity resolves to the same or less than pretreatment status. Then, resume treatment with pemetrexed dosage decreased by 75%

(continued)

Patient Population Studied

Patients were enrolled no earlier than 21 days and no later than 42 days after the first day of their last cycle of induction therapy. Inclusion criteria included an Eastern Cooperative Oncology Group performance status of 0 or 1, histologic or cytologic diagnosis of stage IIIB (with pleural effusion, positive supraclavicular lymph nodes, or both) or stage IV non–small cell lung cancer before induction therapy, and adequate organ function. Patients must not have progressed during four 21-day cycles of 1 of the following 6 initial doublet chemotherapy regimens: gemcitabine + carboplatin, gemcitabine + cisplatin, paclitaxel + carboplatin, paclitaxel + cisplatin, docetaxel + carboplatin, or docetaxel + cisplatin. Induction regimens did not include pemetrexed. Previous radiotherapy was completed ≥4 weeks before study enrollment

Patient Characteristics

Sex	
Men	73%
Women	27%
Disease Stage	
IIIB	18%
IV	82%
Smoking status	
Smoker	73%
Never-smoker	26%
ECOG* Performance Status	
0	40%
1	60%
Histologies	
Nonsquamous	74%
Adenocarcinoma	50%
Large cell	2%
Other or indeterminate	21%
Squamous	26%
Induction regimen	
Docetaxel-carboplatin	5%
Docetaxel-cisplatin	2%
Paclitaxel-carboplatin	30%
Paclitaxel-cisplatin	6%
Gemcitabine-carboplatin	24%
Gemcitabine-cisplatin	33%

*Eastern Cooperative Oncology Group

Treatment Modifications (continued)

Any diarrhea requiring hospitalization (irrespective of grade) or G3/4 diarrhea after 2 dose reductions	Discontinue therapy
G3/4 mucositis	Withhold treatment until toxicity resolves to the same or less than pretreatment status. Then, resume treatment with pemetrexed dosage decreased by 50%
G3/4 mucositis after 2 dose reductions	Discontinue therapy

*These criteria meet the National Cancer Institute Common Toxicity Criteria, version 2.0 (1998) definition of bleeding G ≥2. Available at: http://ctep.cancer.gov/protocolDevelopment/electronic_applications/ctc.htm [accessed December 7, 2013]

Treatment Monitoring

1. *Monthly and as clinically indicated:* Complete blood counts (CBC) including differential white blood cell counts and liver function tests
2. *If G3/4 clinical or laboratory abnormalities are observed or if fever or infection occurs:* Frequent monitoring of complete blood counts (CBC) including differential white blood cell counts and liver function tests

Efficacy

	Median PFS*,† (months, 95% CI)		HR (95% CI) p value	Median OS (months, 95% CI)		HR (95% CI) p value	Patients with CR+PR+SD (%)		p Value
	PMTX	Placebo		PMTX	Placebo		PMTX	Placebo	
Overall population	4.3 (4.1-4.7)	2.6 (1.7–2.8)	0.50 (0.42–0.61) <0.0001	13.4 (11.9–15.9)	10.6 (8.7–12.0)	0.79 (0.65–0.95) 0.012	228 (52%)	74 (33%)	<0.0001
Nonsquamous (n = 481)‡	4.5 (4.2–5.6)	2.6 (1.6–2.8)	0.44 (0.36–0.55) <0.0001	15.5 (13.2–18.1)	10.3 (8.1–12.0)	0.70 (0.56–0.88) 0.002	188 (58%)	51 (33%)	<0.0001
Adenocarcinoma (n = 328)	4.7 (4.2–6.1)	2.6 (1.6–2.8)	0.45 (0.35–0.59) <0.0001	16.8 (14.0–19.7)	11.5 (9.1–15.3)	0.73 (0.56–0.96) 0.026	136 (61%)	35 (33%)	<0.0001
Large cell (n = 20)	3.5 (1.6–6.9)	2.1 (1.4–2.9)	0.40 (0.13–1.22) 0.109	8.4 (6.4–10.3)	7.9 (4.1–13.2)	0.98 (0.36–2.65) 0.964	5 (46%)	3 (33%)	0.670
Other (n = 133)	4.2 (3.1–5.6)	2.8 (1.5–3.6)	0.43 (0.28–0.68) 0.0002	11.3 (9.5–18.3)	7.7 (6.6–11.0)	0.61 (0.40–0.94) 0.025	47 (51%)	13 (32%)	0.041
Squamous (n = 182)	2.8 (2.4–4.0)	2.6 (1.6–3.2)	0.69 (0.49–0.98) 0.039	9.9 (7.5–11.5)	10.8 (8.5–13.2)	1.07 (0.77–1.50) 0.678	40 (35%)	23 (35%)	>0.999

CR, Complete response; HR, hazard ratio; OS, overall survival; PFS ,progression-free survival; PMTX, pemetrexed; PR, partial response; SD, stable disease
*Investigator-assessed PFS in intention-to-treat population
†PFS based on independently reviewed population (N = 581: pemetrexed = 387, placebo = 194)
‡Nonsquamous histology included patients with adenocarcinoma, large cell carcinoma, and other or unknown histology (ie, all patients without a diagnosis of predominantly squamous cell carcinoma)

Toxicity*

	Pemetrexed		Placebo	
	All Grades	G3/4	All Grades	G3/4
Hematologic Toxicities				
Neutropenia[†]	26 (6%)	13 (3%)	0	0
Anemia	67 (15%)	12 (3%)	12 (5%)	1 (<1%)
Leukopenia	27 (6%)	7 (2%)	3 (1%)	1 (<1%)
Nonhematologic Toxicities				
ALT	42 (10%)	1 (<1%)	8 (4%)	0
AST	36 (8%)	0	8 (4%)	0
Fatigue[†]	108 (24%)	22 (5%)	23 (10%)	1 (<1%)
Anorexia	82 (19%)	8 (2%)	11 (5%)	0
Infection	23 (5%)	7 (2%)	4 (2%)	0
Diarrhea	23 (5%)	2 (<1%)	6 (3%)	0
Nausea	83 (19%)	4 (<1%)	12 (5%)	1 (<1%)
Vomiting	38 (9%)	1 (<1%)	3 (1%)	0
Sensory neuropathy	39 (9%)	3 (<1%)	9 (4%)	0
Mucositis/stomatitis	31 (7%)	3 (<1%)	4 (2%)	0
Rash	9 (2%)	1 (<1%)	2 (<1%)	0

ALT, Alanine aminotransferase; AST, aspartate aminotransferase
*A cutoff of 5% was used for inclusion of all events for which the investigator considered a possible link with pemetrexed
[†]P<0.05 for grade 3 or 4 rates of neutropenia and fatigue between study groups

NSCLC REGIMEN
PATIENTS WITH TUMORS HARBORING EGFR MUTATIONS

GEFITINIB

Maemondo M et al. N Engl J Med 2010;362:2380–2388

Gefitinib 250 mg per day; administer orally with or without food, continually (total dose/week = 1750 mg)*

*Gefitinib availability in the United States is limited to participation in the Iressa Access Program. Postmarket Drug Safety Information for Patients and Providers may be acquired online from the U.S. Food and Drug Administration at http://www.fda.gov/Drugs/DrugSafety/PostmarketDrugSafetyInformationforPatientsandProviders/ucm110476.htm (last accessed June 7, 2013) or from AstraZeneca

Supportive Care
Antiemetic prophylaxis
Emetogenic potential is **MINIMAL-LOW**
See Chapter 39 for antiemetic recommendations

Hematopoietic growth factor (CSF) prophylaxis
Primary prophylaxis is NOT indicated
See Chapter 43 for more information

Antimicrobial prophylaxis
Risk of fever and neutropenia is LOW
Antimicrobial primary prophylaxis to be considered:
- Antibacterial—not indicated
- Antifungal—not indicated
- Antiviral—not indicated unless patient previously had an episode of HSV
See Chapter 47 for more information

Diarrhea management
Latent or delayed onset diarrhea:
Loperamide 4 mg orally initially after the first loose or liquid stool, *then*
Loperamide 2 mg orally every 2 hours during waking hours, *plus*
Loperamide 4 mg orally every 4 hours during hours of sleep
- Continue for at least 12 hours after diarrhea resolves
- Recurrent diarrhea after a 12-hour diarrhea-free interval is treated as a new episode
- Rehydrate orally with fluids and electrolytes during a diarrheal episode
- If a patient develops blood or mucus in stool, dehydration, or hemodynamic instability, or if diarrhea persists >48 hours despite loperamide, stop loperamide and hospitalize the patient for IV hydration

Alternatively, a trial of **Diphenoxylate hydrochloride** 2.5 mg with **Atropine sulfate** 0.025 mg (eg, Lomotil)
- Initial adult dose is 2 tablets 4 times daily until control has been achieved, after which the dose may be reduced to meet individual requirements. Control may often be maintained with as little as 2 tablets daily
- Clinical improvement of acute diarrhea is usually observed within 48 hours. If improvement of chronic diarrhea after treatment with a maximum daily dose of 8 tablets is not observed within 10 days, control is unlikely with further administration

Persistent diarrhea:
Octreotide 100–150 mcg subcutaneously 3 times daily. Maximum total daily dose is 1500 mcg

Antibiotic therapy during latent or delayed onset diarrhea:
A fluoroquinolone (eg, **Ciprofloxacin** 500 mg orally every 12 hours) if absolute neutrophil count <500/mm³ with or without accompanying fever in association with diarrhea
- Antibiotics should also be administered if patient is hospitalized with prolonged diarrhea and should be continued until diarrhea resolves

*Abigerges D et al. J Natl Cancer Inst 1994;86:446–449
Rothenberg ML et al. J Clin Oncol 2001;19:3801–3807
Wadler S et al. J Clin Oncol 1998;16:3169–3178

Patient Population Studied

Patients with advanced NSCLC (stage IIIB or IV, or postoperative relapse) harboring *sensitive EGFR mutations*, which excludes the resistant EGFR mutation T790M (threonine at amino acid 790 is substituted by methionine), without a previous history of chemotherapy, and ages ≤75 years

Patient Characteristics

Sex	Number (%)
Male	42 (36.8)
Female	72 (63.2)

Age (years)	
Mean	63.9 ± 7.7
Range	43–75

Smoking Status	
Never smoked	75 (65.8)
Previous or current smoker	39 (34.2)

ECOG performance status score	
0	54 (47.4)
1	59 (51.8)
2	1 (0.9)

Histologic diagnosis	
Adenocarcinoma	103 (90.4)
Large cell carcinoma	1 (0.9)
Adenosquamous carcinoma	2 (1.8)
Squamous cell carcinoma	3 (2.6)
Other	5 (4.4)

Clinical stage	
IIIB	15 (13.2)
IV	88 (77.2)
Postoperative relapse	11 (9.6)

Type of EGFR mutation	
Exon 19 deletion	58 (50.9)
L858R	49 (43.0)
Other	7 (6.1)

Dose Adjustments

Summary of product characteristics for IRESSA 250-mg film-coated tablets. Available at: http://www.iressa.com/ [accessed March 21, 2014]

Acute onset of new or progressive pulmonary symptoms, such as dyspnea, cough, or fever	Interrupt treatment with gefitinib pending diagnostic evaluation
Interstitial lung disease (ILD)	Discontinue gefitinib and institute appropriate treatment as necessary
Hepatic failure or gastrointestinal perforation	Discontinue gefitinib
Dehydration, severe bullous, blistering or exfoliative skin conditions, or acute worsening ocular disorders	Interrupt or discontinue gefitinib
G1/2 diarrhea	Interrupt gefitinib temporarily and institute loperamide therapy. Resume gefitinib if symptoms resolve to G ≤1
G3/4 diarrhea	Discontinue or interrupt gefitinib temporarily. Institute symptomatic therapy. If the patient is receiving benefit from gefitinib, and treatment is interrupted only temporarily, resume gefitinib only if symptoms resolve to G ≤1
G3/4 diarrhea despite loperamide	Discontinue gefitinib
G1/2 skin reaction	Interrupt gefitinib temporarily and institute symptomatic therapy; resume gefitinib if symptoms resolve to G ≤1
G3/4 skin reaction	Discontinue or interrupt gefitinib temporarily. Institute symptomatic therapy. If the patient is receiving benefit from gefitinib, and treatment is interrupted only temporarily, resume gefitinib only if symptoms resolve to G ≤1
Total bilirubin >3 × ULN and/or transaminases a >5 × ULN in the setting of normal pretreatment values	Interrupt or discontinue gefitinib

Notes: Gefitinib plasma concentrations may increased by administration concurrently with potent inhibitors of CYP3A4 activity (eg, clarithromycin, itraconazole, ketoconazole, posaconazole, protease inhibitors, telithromycin, voriconazole). The increase may be clinically relevant as adverse reactions are related to dose and exposure. Patients who receive gefitinib concomitantly with potent CYP3A4 inhibitors should be closely monitored for adverse reactions referable to gefitinib
Gefitinib systemic concentrations also may be increased in individuals with CYP2D6 poor metabolizer genotypes

Toxicity*

	Gefitinib (N = 114)					Carboplatin + Paclitaxel (N = 113)					
	Number of Patients				# (%)	Number of Patients				# (%)	
Toxic Effect	G1	G2	G3	G4	G ≥3	G1	G2	G3	G4	G ≥3	P for G ≥3
Diarrhea	32	6	1	0	1 (0.9)	7	0	0	0	0	<0.001
Appetite loss	7	4	6	0	6 (5.3)	39	18	7	0	7	<0.001
Fatigue	8	1	3	0	3 (2.6)	19	11	1	0	1 (0.9)	0.002
Rash	38	37	6	0	6 (5.3	8	14	3	0	3 (2.7)	<0.001
Neuropathy (sensory)	0	1	0	0	0	28	27	7	0	7 (6.2)	<0.001
Arthralgia	1	2	1	0	1 (0.9)	25	21	8	0	8 (7.1)	<0.001
Pneumonitis	3	0	2	1†	3 (2.6)	0	0	0	0	0	0.02
↑ Aminotransferase	20	13	29	1	30 (26)	31	5	0	1	1 (0.9)	<0.001
Neutropenia	5	1	0	1	1 (0.9)	4	9	37	37	74 (66)	<0.001
Anemia	19	2	0	0	0	35	32	6	0	6 (5.3)	<0.001
Thrombocytopenia	8	0	0	0	0	25	3	3	1	4 (3.5)	<0.001
Any	17	44	43	4†	47 (41)	4	25	41	40	81 (72)	<0.001

*Grades are based on the National Cancer Institute Common Terminology Criteria for Adverse Events, version 3.0. Available at: http://ctep.cancer.gov/protocolDevelopment/electronic_applications/ctc.htm [accessed December 7, 2013]
†One patient experienced a grade 5 toxic effect

Efficacy

Response to Treatment in the Intention-to-Treat Population According to Treatment Group*

	Gefitinib (N = 114)	Carboplatin + Paclitaxel (N = 114)	
	Number of Patients (%)		P
Complete response	5 (4.4)	0	<0.001
Partial response	79 (69.3)	35 (30.7)	<0.001
Complete or partial response	84 (73.7)	35 (30.7)	<0.001
Stable disease	18 (15.8)	56 (49.1)	<0.001
Progressive disease	11 (9.6)	16 (14.0)	<0.001
Response could not be evaluated	1 (0.9)	7 (6.1)	

	Gefitinib (N = 114)	Carboplatin + Paclitaxel (N = 114)	HR [95%CI]; P Value
Median progression-free survival (interim analysis)	10.4 months	5.5 months	0.36 [0.25–0.51]; <0.001
Median progression-free survival (final analysis)	10.8 months	5.4 months	0.30 [0.22–0.41]; <0.001
1-year progression-free survival rate	42.1%	3.2%	
2-year progression-free survival rate	8.4%	0%	
Median overall survival*	30.5 months	23.6 months	
2-year survival rate	61.4%	46.7%	P = 0.31

	Men	Women	HR [95%CI]; P Value
Median progression-free survival	6.5 months	6.0 months	0.68 [0.51–0.92; 0.01

	Exon 19 Deletion	L858R Point Mutation	P Value
Median progression-free survival	11.5 months	10.8 months	0.90
Response rate	82.8%)	67.3%)	

*Neither sex nor clinical stage had a significant effect on overall survival

Treatment Monitoring

1. _Weekly, then monthly, then every 3 months:_ History and physical exam, pulse O_2
2. _Weekly, then monthly, then every 3 months:_ Serum creatinine, LFTs

NSCLC REGIMEN
PATIENTS WITH TUMORS HARBORING EGFR MUTATIONS
ERLOTINIB

Rosell R et al. Lancet Oncol 2012;13:239–246

Erlotinib 150 mg per day; administer orally at least 1 hour before or 2 hours after food, continually (total dose/week = 1050 mg)

Supportive Care
Antiemetic prophylaxis
*Emetogenic potential is **MINIMAL-LOW***
See Chapter 39 for antiemetic recommendations

Hematopoietic growth factor (CSF) prophylaxis
Primary prophylaxis is NOT indicated
See Chapter 43 for more information

Antimicrobial prophylaxis
Risk of fever and neutropenia is LOW
  Antimicrobial primary prophylaxis to be considered:
  • Antibacterial—not indicated
  • Antifungal—not indicated
  • Antiviral—not indicated unless patient previously had an episode of HSV
See Chapter 47 for more information

Diarrhea management
Latent or delayed onset diarrhea*:
Loperamide 4 mg orally initially after the first loose or liquid stool, *then*
Loperamide 2 mg orally every 2 hours during waking hours, *plus*
Loperamide 4 mg orally every 4 hours during hours of sleep
• Continue for at least 12 hours after diarrhea resolves
• Recurrent diarrhea after a 12-hour diarrhea-free interval is treated as a new episode
• Rehydrate orally with fluids and electrolytes during a diarrheal episode
• If a patient develops blood or mucus in stool, dehydration, or hemodynamic instability, or if diarrhea persists >48 hours despite loperamide, stop loperamide and hospitalize the patient for IV hydration
Alternatively, a trial of **Diphenoxylate hydrochloride** 2.5 mg **with Atropine sulfate** 0.025 mg (eg, Lomotil)
• Initial adult dose is 2 tablets 4 times daily until control has been achieved, after which the dose may be reduced to meet individual requirements. Control may often be maintained with as little as 2 tablets daily
• Clinical improvement of acute diarrhea is usually observed within 48 hours. If improvement of chronic diarrhea after treatment with a maximum daily dose of 8 tablets is not observed within 10 days, control is unlikely with further administration
Persistent diarrhea:
Octreotide 100–150 mcg subcutaneously 3 times daily. Maximum total daily dose is 1500 mcg
Antibiotic therapy during latent or delayed onset diarrhea:
A fluoroquinolone (eg, **Ciprofloxacin** 500 mg orally every 12 hours) if absolute neutrophil count <500/mm^3 with or without accompanying fever in association with diarrhea
• Antibiotics should also be administered if patient is hospitalized with prolonged diarrhea and should be continued until diarrhea resolves

*Abigerges D et al. J Natl Cancer Inst 1994;86:446–449
Rothenberg ML et al. J Clin Oncol 2001;19:3801–3807
Wadler S et al. J Clin Oncol 1998;16:3169–178

Patient Population Studied

Eligibility criteria included histologic diagnosis of stage IIIB (with pleural effusion) or stage IV NSCLC (based on the sixth TNM staging system), presence of activating EGFR mutations (exon 19 deletion or L858R mutation in exon 21), and no history of chemotherapy for metastatic disease (neoadjuvant or adjuvant chemotherapy was allowed if it ended ≥6 months before study entry). Patients with asymptomatic, stable brain metastases were eligible to participate

Baseline Demographic and Clinical Characteristics of the Intention-to-Treat Population Randomized to Erlotinib (n = 86)

Sex, female	58 (67%)
Age, Years	
Mean (SD)	63.44 (10.95)
Median (range, IQR)	65 (24–82, 56–72)
Smoking Status	
Never smoked	57 (66%)
Previous smoker	22 (26%)
Current smoker	7 (8%)
Eastern Cooperative Oncology Group (ECOG) Performance Status	
0	27 (31%)
1	47 (55%)
2	12 (14%)
Histologic Diagnosis	
Adenocarcinoma	82 (95%)
Bronchoalveolar adenocarcinoma	0
Large cell carcinoma	3 (3%)
Squamous cell carcinoma	1 (1%)
Other*	0
Clinical Stage	
N3 (not candidate for thoracic radiotherapy)	1 (1%)
IIIA	1 (1%)
IIIB (malignant pleural effusion)	6 (7%)
IV	78 (91%)

(continued)

Efficacy

	Erlotinib N = 86	Chemotherapy N = 87	HR (95% CI) P value
Median follow-up (months)	18.9 (10.7–29.0*)	14.4 (7.1–24.8*)	—
Median duration of treatment (months)	8.2 (0.3–32.9)	2.8 (0.7–5.1)	—
Median number of chemotherapy cycles administered	4 (1–6)	4 (2–4)	—
Median PFS (preplanned interim analysis) (months)	9.4 (7.9–12.3)	5.2 (4.4–5.8)	0.42 (0.27–0.64) p <0.0001
Median PFS (final analysis) (months)	9.7 (8.4–12.3)	5.2 (4.5–5.8)	0.37 (0.25–0.54) p <0.0001
1-year PFS (95% CI)	40% (28–52)	10% (4–20)	
2-year PFS (95% CI)	11% (5–26)	0% (NA†)	
Median PFS (months)			
ECOG PS 0	23.9 (9.7–NA†)	6 (4.3–8.0)	p = 0.0006
ECOG PS 1	8.8 (7.5–10.8)	5.0 (4.1–5.5)	p <0.0001
ECOG PS 2	8.3 (1.0–16.4)	4.4 (0.3–6.0)	p = 0.191
Never smokers	9.7 (8.3–15.5)	5.1 (4.4–5.6)	0.24 (0.15–0.39) p <0.0001
Current	8.7 (5.7–15.8)	4.2 (1.0–15.4)	—
Previous smokers	10.7 (2.7–13.8)	8.0 (1.2–NA)	—
Exon 19 deletion	11.0 (8.8–16.4)	4.6 (4.1–5.6)	0.30 (0.18–0.50) p <0.0001
L858R mutation	8.4 (5.2–10.8)	6.0 (4.9–6.8)	0.55 (0.29–1.02) p = 0.0539
Intention-to-treat population			
	N = 86	N = 87	—
CR	2 (2%)	—	—
PR	48 (56%)	13 (15%)	—
Per-protocol population			
	N = 77 (90%)	N = 73 (84%)	—
CR	2 (3%)	—	—
PR	47 (61%)	13 (18%)	7.5 (3.6–15.6)† p <0.0001
Median overall survival (months)‡	19.3 (14.7–26.8)	19.5 (16.1–NA)	1.04 (0.65–1.68) p = 0.87

95% CI, 95% Confidence interval; CR, complete response; ECOG PS, Eastern Cooperative Oncology Group Performance Status; NA, not assessable; PFS, progression-free survival; PR, partial response
*IQR, interquartile range in parentheses
†Odds ratio
‡Sixty-six (76%) of 87 patients in the standard chemotherapy group crossed over to receive EGFR tyrosine kinase inhibitors, primarily erlotinib

Patient Population Studied
(continued)

Bone Metastasis	
Yes	28 (33%)
No	58 (67%)
Brain Metastasis	
Yes	9 (10%)
No	77 (90%)
Type of *EGFR* Mutation	
Deletion of exon 19	57 (66%)
L858R mutation in exon 21	29 (34%)

*Four undifferentiated carcinomas, 1 pleomorphic carcinoma, and 1 adenosquamous carcinoma

Treatment Monitoring

1. *Weekly, then monthly, then every 3 months:* History and physical exam, pulse O$_2$
2. *Weekly, then monthly, then every 3 months:* Serum creatinine
   - Especially in patient at risk of dehydration
3. *Weekly, then monthly, then every 3 months:* LFTs
   - More frequent monitoring in patients with biliary obstruction or hepatic impairment

Dose Adjustments

Adapted in part from: Tarceva (erlotinib) tablets, for oral use; 05/2013 product label. Genentech USA, Inc., 1 DNA Way, South San Francisco, CA

Acute onset of new or progressive pulmonary symptoms, such as dyspnea, cough or fever	Interrupt treatment with erlotinib pending diagnostic evaluation
Interstitial lung disease (ILD)	Discontinue erlotinib and institute appropriate treatment as necessary
Hepatic failure or gastrointestinal perforation	Discontinue erlotinib
Dehydration, severe bullous, blistering or exfoliative skin conditions, or acute worsening ocular disorders	Interrupt or discontinue erlotinib
G1/2 diarrhea	Interrupt erlotinib temporarily and institute loperamide therapy. Resume erlotinib at same dose or with a dose reduction in 50-mg increments
G3/4 diarrhea	Interrupt erlotinib temporarily and institute loperamide therapy. Resume erlotinib with a dose reduction in 50-mg increments
G3/4 diarrhea despite loperamide	Discontinue erlotinib
G1/2 skin reaction	Interrupt erlotinib temporarily and institute symptomatic therapy. Resume erlotinib at same dose or with a dose reduction in 50-mg increments
G3/4 skin reaction	Interrupt erlotinib temporarily and institute symptomatic therapy. Resume erlotinib with a dose reduction in 50-mg increments
Total bilirubin $>3 \times$ ULN and/or transaminases $>5 \times$ ULN in the setting of normal pretreatment values	Interrupt or discontinue erlotinib

Notes: In patients who are taking erlotinib with a strong CYP3A4 inhibitor such as, but not limited to, atazanavir, clarithromycin, indinavir, itraconazole, ketoconazole, nefazodone, nelfinavir, ritonavir, saquinavir, telithromycin, troleandomycin (TAO), voriconazole, or grapefruit products, a dose reduction should be considered if severe adverse reactions occur. Similarly, in patients who are taking erlotinib with an inhibitor of both CYP3A4 and CYP1A2 like ciprofloxacin, a dose reduction of erlotinib should be considered if severe adverse reactions occur

Toxicity

Common Adverse Events in the Safety Population*

	Erlotinib (n = 84)			Standard Chemotherapy (n = 82)			P Value for G3/4 0.0086
	G1/2	G3	G4	G1/2	G3	G4	
Fatigue	43 (51%)	5 (6%)	0	43 (52%)	16 (20%)	0	—
Rash	56 (67%)	11 (13%)	0	4 (5%)	0	0	0.0007
Diarrhea	44 (52%)	4 (5%)	0	15 (18%)	0	0	0.1206
Appetite loss	26 (31%)	0	0	26 (32%)	2 (2%)	0	0.2425
Alopecia	12 (14%)	0	0	—	2 (2%)	0	0.2425
Neuropathy	7 (8%)	0	1 (1%)	11 (13%)	1 (1%)	0	1.0000
Arthralgia	8 (10%)	0	0	—	1 (1%)	0	1.0000
Aminotransferase rise	3 (4%)	0	0	—	0	0	0.4970
Pneumonitis	0	1 (1%)	0	0	1 (1%)	0	1.0000
Anemia	9 (11%)	0	1 (1%)	—	—	—	0.3644
Neutropenia	0	0	0	15 (18%)	12 (15%)	6 (7%)	<0.0001
Thrombocytopenia	1 (1%)	0	0	1 (1%)	6 (7%)	6 (7%)	0.0003
Febrile neutropenia	0	0	0	1 (1%)	1 (1%)	2 (2%)	0.1183

*Adverse events were assessed according to the National Cancer Institute (USA) Common Terminology Criteria for Adverse Events, version 3.0. Available at: http://ctep.cancer.gov/protocolDevelopment/electronic_applications/ctc.htm [accessed December 7, 2013]

	Erlotinib (n = 84)	Standard Chemotherapy (n = 82)
Toxicity *(continued)*		
Safety Data		
Any adverse event (all grades)	82 (98%)	81 (99%)
Treatment-related adverse event (all grades)	78 (93%)	78 (95%)
Grade 3 or 4 adverse event	38 (45%)	55 (67%)
Dose reduction because of adverse event	18 (21%)	23 (28%)
Dose reduction because of drug-related adverse event	18 (21%)	21 (26%)
Discontinuation because of an adverse event	11 (13%)	19 (23%)
Discontinuation because of drug-related adverse event	5 (6%)	16 (20%)
Any severe adverse event	27 (32%)	25 (30%)
Treatment-related severe adverse event	5 (6%)	16 (20%)
Treatment-related death[†]	1 (1%)	2 (2%)
Interstitial lung disease-like events	1 (1%)	1 (1%)

*The safety analysis included all patients who were randomly allocated to treatment groups and received at least 1 dose of study drug
[†]One patient in the erlotinib group experienced hepatotoxicity, 2 patients in the chemotherapy group had cerebrovascular accidents (1 after a grade 5 infection)

NSCLC REGIMEN
PATIENTS WITH TUMORS HARBORING EGFR MUTATIONS

AFATINIB

Yang JC et al. Lancet Oncol 2012;13:539–548
Katakami N et al. J Clin Oncol 2013;31:3335–3341
Wu YL et al. Lancet Oncol 2014;15:213–222

Note: In the US afatinib is approved for first-line treatment of patients with metastatic non-small cell lung cancer (NSCLC) whose tumors have epidermal growth factor receptor (EGFR) exon 19 deletions or exon 21 (L858R) substitution mutations as detected by an FDA-approved test

Afatinib 40 mg orally, once daily

Notes:
- Instruct patient to take afatinib >1 hour before and >2 hours after a meal
- For patients who require therapy with a P-glycoprotein (Pgp) inhibitor, reduce the afatinib daily dose by 10 mg if not tolerated
- For patients who require chronic therapy with a Pgp inducer, increase afatinib daily dose by 10 mg as tolerated
- Increase dose to 50 mg per day if no rash, diarrhea, mucositis, or any other treatment-related adverse event >G1 in the first 21 days of treatment. In the study by Wu et al 38 of 239 (15.9%) patients had dose escalated

Diarrhea management
Latent or delayed onset diarrhea:
   Loperamide 4 mg orally initially after the first loose or liquid stool, *then*
   Loperamide 2 mg orally every 2 hours during waking hours, *plus*
   Loperamide 4 mg orally every 4 hours during hours of sleep
- Continue for at least 12 hours after diarrhea resolves
- Recurrent diarrhea after a 12-hour diarrhea-free interval is treated as a new episode
- Rehydrate orally with fluids and electrolytes during a diarrheal episode
- If a patient develops blood or mucus in stool, dehydration, or hemodynamic instability, or if diarrhea persists >48 hours despite loperamide, stop loperamide and hospitalize the patient for IV hydration

Alternatively, a trial of **Diphenoxylate hydrochloride** 2.5 mg **with Atropine sulfate** 0.025 mg (eg, Lomotil)
- Initial adult dose is 2 tablets 4 times daily until control has been achieved, after which the dose may be reduced to meet individual requirements. Control may often be maintained with as little as 2 tablets daily
- Clinical improvement of acute diarrhea is usually observed within 48 hours. If improvement of chronic diarrhea after treatment with a maximum daily dose of 8 tablets is not observed within 10 days, control is unlikely with further administration

Persistent diarrhea:
   Octreotide 100–150 mcg subcutaneously 3 times daily. Maximum total daily dose is 1500 mcg
Antibiotic therapy during latent or delayed onset diarrhea:
   A fluoroquinolone (eg, **Ciprofloxacin** 500 mg orally every 12 hours) if absolute neutrophil count <500/mm^3 with or without accompanying fever in association with diarrhea
- Antibiotics should also be administered if patient is hospitalized with prolonged diarrhea and should be continued until diarrhea resolves

*Abigerges D et al. J Natl Cancer Inst 1994;86:446–449
Rothenberg ML et al. J Clin Oncol 2001;19:3801–3807
Wadler S et al. J Clin Oncol 1998;16:3169–178

Treatment Modifications

Adverse Event	Dose Modification
Any NCI CTCAE* toxicity ≥G3	Withhold afatinib. Resume treatment when the adverse reaction fully resolves, returns to baseline, or improves to G ≤1. Reinstitute afatinib at a dose that is 10 mg per day less than the dose at which the adverse reaction occurred
G ≥2 diarrhea persisting for ≥2 consecutive days while taking anti-diarrheal medication	
G ≥2 cutaneous reactions lasting ≥7 days or intolerable	
G ≥2 renal dysfunction	
Life-threatening bullous, blistering, or exfoliative skin lesions	Discontinue afatinib
Confirmed interstitial lung disease (ILD)	
Severe drug-induced hepatic impairment	
Persistent ulcerative keratitis	
Symptomatic left ventricular dysfunction	
Severe or intolerable adverse reaction occurring at a dose of 20 mg per day	

*National Cancer Institute Common Terminology Criteria for Adverse Events, v 3.0
Note: In study by Wu et al 122 of 182 (67.0%) patients were still receiving the starting dose of afatinib 40 mg at the end of treatment; while 67 of 239 (28.0%) had their dose reduced to 30 mg, and ten (4.2%) had further reductions to 20 mg

Patient Population Studied

Randomized, open-label, phase 3 trial at 36 centers in China, Thailand, and South Korea. Eligible patients had pathologically confirmed and previously untreated stage IIIB (with pleural effusion) or IV lung adenocarcinoma according to American Joint Committee on Cancer criteria and ECOG PS of 0 or 1, Tumor tissue had to be EGFR mutation-positive at the screening stage. Twenty-nine mutations, including common ones (Leu858Arg, exon 19 deletions) were detected.

Efficacy

Afatinib group (N = 242)

Best overall tumor response [data are n (%)]

	Independent Review	Investigator Review
Disease control	224 (92.6%)	225 (93.0%)
Objective response	162 (66.9%)	180 (74.4%)
Complete response	3 (1.2%)	0 (0%)
Partial response	159 (65.7%)	180 (74.4%)
Stable disease	52 (21.5%)	45 (18.6%)
Progressive disease	9 (3.7%)	10 (4.1%)
Not evaluable*	9 (3.7%)	7 (2.9%)

Progression-free survival, response duration and overall survival in months [95%CI]

Median duration of treatment	398 days	
Median progression-free survival	11.0 [9.7–13.7)]	13.7 [11.5–13.9]
Median progression-free survival exon 19 deletions and Leu858Arg	11.0 [9.7–13.7]	13.8 [12.5–14.4]
Median duration of response	9.7 [8.3–12.5]	—
Median duration disease control	11.1 [9.7–13.8]	—
Median overall survival	22.1 [20.0–not estim]	—

*Withdrew with insufficient data for RECIST assessment after baseline. For the independent/investigator review reasons for withdrawal were: withdrawal of consent (1/1), adverse event (4/3), non-compliance with protocol (3/3), and classed as progressive disease but insufficient imaging for central review (1/0)

Therapy Monitoring

1. Before each 28-day cycle: CBC with differential, LFTs, BUN, and creatinine
2. Response evaluation: Every 2 cycles. Continue treatment until disease progression or unacceptable toxicity

Toxicity

Most Common Treatment-related Adverse Events (N = 239)*

	All Grades	Grade 1–2	Grade 3	Grade 4
Total	236 (98.7%)	150 (62.8%)	82 (34.3%)	3 (1.3%)
Symptomatic adverse events				
Diarrhea	211 (88.3%)	198 (82.8%)	13 (5.4%)	0 (0%)
Rash or acne*	193 (80.8%)	158 (66.1%)	34 (14.2%)	1 (0.4%)
Stomatitis or mucositis*	124 (51.9%)	111 (46.4%)	13 (5.4%)	0 (0.0%)
Paronychia	78 (32.6%)	78 (32.6%)	0 (0%)	0 (0%)
Epistaxis	30 (12.6%)	29 (12.1%)	1 (0.4%)	0 (0%)
Pruritus	26 (10.9%)	25 (10.5%)	1 (0.4%)	0 (0%)
Decreased appetite	24 (10.0%)	21 (8.8%)	3 (1.3%)	0 (0%)
Fatigue*	24 (10.0%)	23 (9.6%)	1 (0.4%)	0 (0%)
Vomiting	23 (9.6%)	21 (8.8%)	2 (0.8%)	0 (0%)
Nausea	18 (7.5%)	18 (7.5%)	0 (0%)	0 (0%)
Constipation	4 (1.7%)	4 (1.7%)	0 (0%)	0 (0%)
Laboratory or hematological adverse events as reported by investigator not based on laboratory data				
↑Alanine aminotransferase	48 (20.1%)	44 (18.4%)	4 (1.7%)	0 (0%)
↑Aspartate aminotransferase	36 (15.1%)	35 (14.6%)	1 (0.4%)	0 (0%)
Anemia	13 (5.4%)	12 (5.0%)	1 (0.4%)	0 (0%)
Neutropenia	5 (2.1%)	4 (1.7%)	1 (0.4%)	0 (0%)
Thrombocytopenia	2 (0.8%)	1 (0.4%)	1 (0.4%)	0 (0%)

*Data are n (%). Events are included if reported for more than 10% of patients at G1–2 or more than 1% of patients for G3–5 in any treatment group. In addition, one sudden death (G5) occurred that was considered related to treatment

REGIMEN

PEMETREXED

Hanna N et al. J Clin Oncol 2004;22:1589–1597

Folic acid 350–1000 mcg per day; administer orally beginning 1–2 weeks before the first dose of pemetrexed and continuing until 3 weeks after the last dose of pemetrexed

Cyanocobalamin (vitamin B$_{12}$) 1000 mcg; administer intramuscularly every 9 weeks, beginning 1–2 weeks before the first dose of pemetrexed

Dexamethasone 4 mg/dose; administer orally twice daily for 3 consecutive days (6 doses), starting the day before pemetrexed administration to decrease the risk and severity of severe skin rash associated with pemetrexed (total dose/cycle = 24 mg)

Pemetrexed 500 mg/m^2; administer intravenously in 100 mL 0.9% sodium chloride injection over 10 minutes on day 1, every 21 days (total dosage/cycle = 500 mg/m^2)

Supportive Care

Antiemetic prophylaxis
Emetogenic potential: LOW
See Chapter 39 for antiemetic recommendations

Hematopoietic growth factor (CSF) prophylaxis
Primary prophylaxis is NOT indicated
See Chapter 43 for more information

Antimicrobial prophylaxis
Risk of fever and neutropenia is LOW
  Antimicrobial primary prophylaxis to be considered:
  • Antibacterial—not indicated
  • Antifungal—not indicated
  • Antiviral—not indicated unless patient previously had an episode of HSV
See Chapter 47 for more information

Patient Population Studied

A study of 283 patients with stages III–IV NSCLC

Efficacy (N = 265)

Overall response rate	9.1%
1-year overall survival	29.7%
Median survival time	8.3 months
Median progression-free survival	2.9 months
Median time to progression	3.4 months
Median duration of response	4.6 months

Toxicity (N = 265)*

	% Any G	% G3/4
Hematologic		
Neutropenia	Not given	5.3
Febrile neutropenia	Not given	1.9
Neutropenia with infection	Not given	0
Anemia	Not given	4.2
Thrombocytopenia	Not given	1.9
Nonhematologic		
Fatigue	34	5.3
Nausea	30.9	2.6
Vomiting	16.2	1.5
Pulmonary	0.8	0
Neurosensory	4.9	0
Stomatitis	14.7	1.1
Alopecia	6.4	0
Diarrhea	12.8	0.4
Rash	14	0.8
Weight loss	1.1	0
Edema	4.5	0

*NCI CTC, National Cancer Institute (USA) Common Toxicity Criteria, version 2.0. Available at: http://ctep.cancer.gov/protocolDevelopment/electronic_applications/ctc.htm [accessed December 7, 2013]

Treatment Modifications

Adverse Event	Dose Modification
G3 hematologic toxicities	Hold therapy until toxicity returns to baseline, then reduce pemetrexed dosage by 25%
G4 hematologic toxicities (thrombocytopenia)	Hold therapy until toxicity returns to baseline, then reduce pemetrexed dosage by 50%
Increased serum creatinine to 1.6–2 mg/dL (141–177 µmol/L)	Reduce pemetrexed dosage by 25%
Serum creatinine increased to ≤2 mg/dL (≤177 µmol/L)	Hold pemetrexed until serum creatinine <1.5 mg/dL (<133 µmol/L), then resume with pemetrexed dosage reduced by 25%
G ≥2 diarrhea	Hold pemetrexed until toxicity resolves to G <2, then resume with pemetrexed dosage reduced by 25%
G3/4 mucositis	Reduce pemetrexed dosage by 50%
Increased liver transaminases	Hold therapy until toxicity resolves, then resume with pemetrexed dosage reduced by 25%
Other G ≥3 nonhematologic toxicities (except nausea, vomiting, elevated transaminases, and alopecia)	Delay treatment until toxicity resolves to baseline, then resume with pemetrexed dosage reduced by 25% from previous dose level

Note: If a patient requires 3 dose reductions, discontinue pemetrexed

Therapy Monitoring

1. *Before each 21-day cycle:* CBC with differential, LFTs, BUN, and creatinine
2. *Weekly:* CBC with differential
3. *Response evaluation every 2 cycles:* Continue treatment until disease progression or unacceptable toxicity
4. *Every 2–3 months:* Consider plasma homocysteine levels. (High homocysteine concentrations are a sensitive indicator of folate deficiency and may predict pemetrexed toxicity)

Notes

In the study reported by Hanna et al. (J Clin Oncol 2004;22:1589–1597), 288 patients were treated with docetaxel 75 mg/m^2 by intravenous infusion every 21 days. Treatment with docetaxel resulted in clinically equivalent efficacy outcomes, but had significantly greater side effects compared with pemetrexed

REGIMEN

PACLITAXEL + CARBOPLATIN + BEVACIZUMAB

Johnson DH et al. J Clin Oncol 2004;22:2184–2191
Sandler AB et al. N Engl J Med 2006;355:2542–2550

Premedication (primary prophylaxis against hypersensitivity reactions from paclitaxel):
Dexamethasone 20 mg/dose for 2 doses; administer orally the evening before and the morning of chemotherapy prior to paclitaxel, *plus:*
Diphenhydramine 50 mg; administer by intravenous injection 30 minutes before paclitaxel, *and:*
Ranitidine 50 mg or **cimetidine** 300 mg; administer intravenously in 25–100 mL 0.9% sodium chloride injection (0.9% NS) or 5% dextrose injection (D5W) over 5–30 minutes, 30 minutes before paclitaxel
Paclitaxel 200 mg/m^2; administer intravenously in a volume of 0.9% NS or D5W sufficient to produce a solution with concentration within the range 0.3–1.2 mg/mL over 3 hours on day 1, every 3 weeks (total dosage/cycle = 200 mg/m^2)
Carboplatin (calculated dose) AUC = 6 mg/mL · min; administer intravenously diluted in D5W or 0.9% NS to a concentration as low as 0.5 mg/mL over 15–30 minutes on day 1, 60 minutes after completing paclitaxel, every 3 weeks (total dosage/cycle calculated to produce an AUC = 6 mg/mL · min) (see equation below)
Bevacizumab 15 mg/kg; administer intravenously in 100 mL 0.9% NS every 3 weeks on day 1, (total dosage/cycle = 15 mg/kg)

Note: Administration duration for the initial bevacizumab dose is 90 minutes. If administration is well tolerated, the administration duration may be decreased stepwise during subsequent administrations to 60 minutes and, finally, to a minimum duration of 30 minutes

Supportive Care
Antiemetic prophylaxis
Emetogenic potential: **HIGH**. *Potential for delayed symptoms*
See Chapter 39 for antiemetic recommendations

Hematopoietic growth factor (CSF) prophylaxis
Primary prophylaxis may be indicated
See Chapter 43 for more information

Antimicrobial prophylaxis
Risk of fever and neutropenia is LOW
  Antimicrobial primary prophylaxis to be considered:
  • Antibacterial—not indicated
  • Antifungal—not indicated
  • Antiviral—not indicated unless patient previously had an episode of HSV
See Chapter 47 for more information

Additional Supportive Care
Dexamethasone 8 mg/dose orally every 12 hours for 6 doses after chemotherapy if G ≥2 arthralgias/myalgias occur
Add a **proton pump inhibitor** during dexamethasone use to prevent gastritis and duodenitis

Note: Carboplatin dose is based on Calvert's formula to achieve a target area under the plasma concentration versus time curve (AUC) (AUC units = mg/mL · min)

$$\text{Total carboplatin dose (mg)} = (\text{target AUC}) \times (\text{GFR} + 25)$$

In practice, creatinine clearance (Clcr) is used in place of glomerular filtration rate (GFR). Clcr can be calculated from the equation of Cockcroft and Gault:

$$\text{For males, Clcr} = \frac{(140 - \text{age [years]}) \times \text{body weight (kg)}}{72 \times (\text{Serum creatinine [mg/dL]})}$$

$$\text{For females, Clcr} = \frac{(140 - \text{age [years]}) \times \text{body weight (kg)}}{72 \times (\text{Serum creatinine [mg/dL]})} \times 0.85$$

Calvert AH et al. J Clin Oncol 1989;7:1748–1756
Cockcroft DW, Gault MH. Nephron 1976;16:31–41
Jodrell DI et al. J Clin Oncol 1992;10:520–528
Sorensen BT et al. Cancer Chemother Pharmacol 1991;28:397–401

Treatment Modifications

Adverse Event	Dose Modification
ANC nadir <500/mm^3, platelet nadir <50,000/mm^3, or febrile neutropenia	Reduce carboplatin dosage to AUC = 5 if previous cycle dose was AUC = 6; or to AUC = 4 if previous cycle dose was AUC = 5
ANC nadir <500/mm^3, platelet nadir <50,000/mm^3, or febrile neutropenia after 2 carboplatin dose reductions (AUC in previous cycle = 4)	Reduce paclitaxel dosage to 200 mg/m^2, and decrease carboplatin dosage to AUC = 3
Day 1 ANC <1500/mm^3 or platelet <100,000/mm3	Delay chemotherapy until ANC >1500/mm^3 and platelet >100,000/mm^3, for maximum delay of 2 weeks
Delay of >2 weeks in reaching ANC >1500/mm^3 and platelet >100,000/mm3	Discontinue therapy
G2 neurotoxicity	Reduce paclitaxel dosage to 200 mg/m^2
G3 neurotoxicity	Reduce paclitaxel dosage to 175 mg/m^2
G2 arthralgia/myalgia despite dexamethasone prophylaxis	Reduce paclitaxel dosage to 200 mg/m^2
G3 arthralgia/myalgia despite dexamethasone prophylaxis	Reduce paclitaxel dosage to 175 mg/m^2
G ≥2 AST or ≥G3 bilirubin	Hold paclitaxel
Moderate hypersensitivity	Patient may be retreated
Severe hypersensitivity	Discontinue therapy
Chest pain or arrhythmia during chemotherapy	Immediately stop chemotherapy and evaluate the patient
Symptomatic arrhythmias, or ≥2-degree AV block, or an ischemic event	Discontinue therapy

Patient Population Studied

A study of 855 patients with advanced, previously untreated stage IIIB (pleural or pericardial effusion only) NSCLC (nonsquamous histologies). A randomized comparison with paclitaxel + carboplatin. ECOG PS 0 (40%) or 1 (60%). INR <1.5 and PTT no greater than upper limit normal. No history of thrombotic or hemorrhagic disorders. No gross hemoptysis defined as one-half teaspoon or more of bright red blood per day. Brain metastases were not allowed; 43% were age ≥65 years, and 28% had ≥5% weight loss

Efficacy (N = 357)

Overall response	27.2%
Complete response	1.4%
Partial response	25.8%
6-month progression-free survival	55%
12-month progression-free survival	14.6%
Median survival	12.5 months
1-year survival	51.9%
2-year survival	22.1%

Toxicity (N = 420)

Hematologic

Toxicity	% G4
Neutropenia	24*
Fever + neutropenia	3.3*
Thrombocytopenia	1.4
Anemia	0

Nonhematologic

	% ≥G3
Hemorrhage	4.5*
Hemoptysis	1.9*
CNS	1*
Gastrointestinal	1.2
Other	1
Hypertension	6*
Venous thrombosis	3.8
Arterial thrombosis	1.9

Treatment-Related Deaths

Hemoptysis	5 (1.2%)
Gastrointestinal bleeding	2 (0.5%)
Fever + neutropenia	1 (0.25%)

*These values were statistically worse than those with paclitaxel + carboplatin alone

Therapy Monitoring

1. *Every week:* CBC with differential and platelet count
2. *Response evaluation:* Every 2–3 cycles

Notes

1. Compared with paclitaxel + carboplatin, overall survival advantage is confined to men; not seen in women ($P = 0.8$), despite statistically significant advantage for progression-free survival and response rate in women
2. Bevacizumab is associated with a small increase in serious bleeding, including hemoptysis. In a phase II trial, apparent risk factors for life-threatening hemorrhages included baseline hemoptysis brain metastases, anticoagulant therapy, and squamous histology (Johnson DH et al. J Clin Oncol 2004;22:2184–2191)
3. This therapy is the ECOG reference standard for first-line treatment of advanced NSCLC and is recommended by NCCN. Confirmatory trials have yet to be performed
4. Only patients with nonsquamous histologies were included in this study

Small Cell Lung Cancer (SCLC)

Work-up

General work-up

1. History and physical examination
2. Complete blood count, liver and renal function tests, LDH, and serum electrolytes with special attention to serum sodium
3. Chest x-ray
4. CT scan of chest and upper abdomen including adrenals
5. Brain MRI (or CT scan)
6. Bone scan
7. FDG-PET scan (optional)

Individualized work-up

1. Bone marrow biopsy in selected patients
2. Pulmonary function tests and cardiac function assessment if thoracic radiation therapy is going to be performed
3. If a patient presents with pleural effusion, a diagnostic thoracocentesis is recommended. Consider thoracoscopy if thoracocentesis is inconclusive
4. Plain-film x-rays of bone scan abnormalities

Staging

Limited disease	Disease confined to ipsilateral hemithorax within a single radiation port
Extensive disease	Disease beyond ipsilateral hemithorax or obvious metastatic disease

Østerlind K et al. Cancer Treat Rep 1983;67:3–9

Five-Year Survival for Each Stage

Limited Disease	
Median survival	14–20 months
2-year survival	40%

Extensive Disease	
Median survival	8–12 months
2-year survival	5%

More information at http://www.seer.cancer.gov

Expert Opinion

Treatment of limited disease

1. Etoposide + cisplatin combination for 4–6 cycles is the regimen of choice to combine with concurrent chest radiation therapy
2. Chest radiation therapy increases local control and survival. Several studies suggest starting chest radiotherapy early
3. Prophylactic cranial irradiation is indicated in patients with complete remission; it reduces the risk of cerebral metastases and improves survival

Treatment of extensive disease

1. Etoposide + platinum or cyclophosphamide + doxorubicin regimens for 4–6 cycles
2. Prophylactic cranial irradiation should be considered in patients with response after chemotherapy

Second-line chemotherapy for both limited and extensive disease

1. Patients who relapse after a response to first-line chemotherapy should be considered for second-line chemotherapy with topotecan

REGIMEN

ETOPOSIDE + CISPLATIN WITH CONCURRENT THORACIC RADIATION THERAPY

Turrisi AT et al. N Engl J Med 1999;340:265–271

Hydration before cisplatin: ≥1000 mL 0.9% sodium chloride injection (0.9% NS); administer intravenously over a minimum of 2–4 hours

Cisplatin 60 mg/m^2; administer intravenously in 50–150 mL 0.9% NS over 60 minutes, on day 1, every 3 weeks for 4 cycles (total dosage/cycle = 60 mg/m^2)

Hydration after cisplatin: ≥1000 mL 0.9% NS; administer intravenously over a minimum of 2–4 hours. Encourage patients to increase oral intake of non-alcoholic fluids. Monitor serum electrolytes and replace as needed (potassium, magnesium, sodium)

Etoposide 120 mg/m^2 per dose; administer intravenously, diluted in 0.9% NS or 5% dextrose injection to a concentration within the range of 0.2–0.4 mg/mL over 60 minutes, for 3 consecutive days, on days 1, 2, and 3, every 3 weeks for 4 cycles (total dosage/cycle = 360 mg/m^2)

Thoracic RT begins concurrently with the first cycle of chemotherapy to a total dose of 45 Gy delivered as:

1. Once daily in 1.8-Gy fractions for 25 treatments over 5 weeks, *or*

2. Twice daily in 1.5-Gy fractions for 30 treatments over 3 weeks

Prophylactic cranial RT is offered to patients who achieve a CR after completing systemic chemotherapy

Supportive Care

Antiemetic prophylaxis

*Emetogenic potential on day 1 is **HIGH**. Potential for delayed symptoms*

*Emetogenic potential on days 2 and 3 is **LOW***

See Chapter 39 for antiemetic recommendations

Hematopoietic growth factor (CSF) prophylaxis

Primary prophylaxis is NOT indicated

See Chapter 43 for more information

Antimicrobial prophylaxis

Risk of fever and neutropenia is LOW

Antimicrobial primary prophylaxis to be considered:

• Antibacterial—not indicated

• Antifungal—not indicated

• Antiviral—not indicated unless patient previously had an episode of HSV

See Chapter 47 for more information

Patient Population Studied

A study of 417 patients with previously untreated limited SCLC. A randomized comparison between twice-daily and once-daily thoracic radiation therapy, both combined with etoposide and cisplatin given at fixed dosages

Therapy Monitoring

1. *Before each cycle:* H&P, CBC with differential, LFTs, BUN, creatinine, and serum electrolytes

2. *Response evaluation:* Evaluate therapy at the end of treatment

Efficacy (N = 206/211)

	RT Fractionation	
	Once Daily (N = 206)	Twice Daily (N = 211)
Complete response	49%	56%
Partial response	38%	31%
Local failure	52%	36%
Median survival	19 months	23 months
2-year survival	41%	47%
5-year survival	16%	26%

Treatment Modifications

Adverse Event	Dose Modification
G4 toxicities, febrile neutropenia, documented infection, or thrombocytopenia with bleeding during cycles 3 and 4	Reduce etoposide dosage by 25%
Serum creatinine = 1.6–2.5 mg/dL (141–221 μmol/L) during cycles 3 and 4	Reduce cisplatin dosage by 25%
Platelets ≤50,000/mm^3	Interrupt radiation therapy
G2 weight loss (≥4.5 kg or ≥10 pounds)	Interrupt radiation therapy
Hospitalization for febrile neutropenia or sepsis	Interrupt radiation therapy
Difficulty swallowing	Do not interrupt radiation therapy*
Fever with low ANC	Do not interrupt radiation therapy*

*In general, interruptions of thoracic radiation therapy are discouraged

Note: DO NOT modify chemotherapy during the first 2 cycles

Toxicity (N = 206/211)

Toxicity	% G3	% G4	% G5
Once-Daily RT (N = 206)			
Overall toxicity	23	63	2
Esophagitis	11	5	0
Granulocytopenia	15	60	0
Thrombocytopenia	16	8	0
Anemia	23	3	0
Infection	6	1	1
Vomiting	8	2	0
Pulmonary effects	3	0.5	0.5
Weight loss	3	0	0
Twice-Daily RT (N = 211)			
Overall toxicity	25	62	3
Esophagitis	27	5	0
Granulocytopenia	21	59	0
Thrombocytopenia	13	8	0
Anemia	23	5	0
Infection	6	2	1
Vomiting	8	1	0
Pulmonary effects	4	1	1
Weight loss	2	0	0

REGIMEN

TOPOTECAN

von Pawel J et al. J Clin Oncol 1999;17:658–667

Topotecan HCl 1.5 mg/m^2 per day; administer intravenously in 50–250 mL 0.9% sodium chloride injection or 5% dextrose injection over 30 minutes, for 5 consecutive days, on days 1 through 5, every 21 days (total dosage/cycle = 7.5 mg/m^2)

Supportive Care
Antiemetic prophylaxis
Emetogenic potential on days 1–5 is **LOW**
See Chapter 39 for antiemetic recommendations

Hematopoietic growth factor (CSF) prophylaxis
Primary prophylaxis is indicated with one of the following:
   Filgrastim (G-CSF) 5 mcg/kg per day by subcutaneous injection, *or*
   Pegfilgrastim (pegylated filgrastim) 6 mg/0.6 mL by subcutaneous injection for 1 dose
   • Begin use from 24–72 hours after myelosuppressive chemotherapy is completed
   • Continue filgrastim until ANC >10,000/mm^3 on 2 consecutive daily measurements
See Chapter 43 for more information

Antimicrobial prophylaxis
Risk of fever and neutropenia is LOW
Antimicrobial primary prophylaxis to be considered:
   • Antibacterial—not indicated
   • Antifungal—not indicated
   • Antiviral—not indicated unless patient previously had an episode of HSV
See Chapter 47 for more information

Patient Population Studied

A study of 107 patients with SCLC and disease progression at least 60 days after having completed first-line chemotherapy. A randomized comparison with combination chemotherapy, including cyclophosphamide, doxorubicin, and vincristine

Efficacy (N = 107)

Intention-to-treat response rate	24.3%*
Median survival	25 weeks
6-month survival	46.7%
1-year survival	14.2%

*Partial responses

Toxicity (N = 107)*

	% G3/4
Neutropenia	88
Thrombocytopenia	58
Anemia	42
Nausea	3.7
Fatigue	4.7
Vomiting	1.9
Stomatitis	1.9
Fever†	1.9
Diarrhea	0.9
Worsening LVEF: 2 of 26 patients (7.7%)	

*NCI CTC, National Cancer Institute (USA) Common Toxicity Criteria, version 2.0. Available at: http://ctep.cancer.gov/protocolDevelopment/electronic_applications/ctc.htm [accessed December 7, 2013]
†Excludes patients with febrile neutropenia

Treatment Modifications

Adverse Event	Dose Modification
Day 1 ANC <1000/mm^3, platelets <100,000/mm^3	Delay treatment until ANC >1000/mm^3, platelets >100,000/mm^3
Toxicity G <2 during the previous cycle	Increase topotecan dosage to a maximum daily dose of 2 mg/m^2 during repeated cycles (ie, first cycle escalated to 1.75 mg/m^2 · d for 5 days; second cycle escalated to 2 mg/m^2 · d for 5 days)
G4 neutropenia with fever or infection, or of duration ≥7 days	Decrease daily topotecan dosage from the previous cycle by 0.25 mg/m^{2*}
G3 neutropenia during the preceding cycle persisting after day 21	
G4 thrombocytopenia	
G3/4 nonhematologic toxicity, excluding grade 3 nausea	Decrease daily topotecan dosage from the previous cycle by 0.25 mg/m^2 or discontinue treatment*
Treatment delay >2 weeks	Discontinue treatment

*The minimum permissible daily topotecan dosage is 1 mg/m^2 per day for 5 days

Therapy Monitoring

1. *Before day 1 chemotherapy:* CBC with differential, LFTs, serum BUN, and creatinine and electrolytes
2. *Weekly:* CBC with differential
3. *Day 15:* LFTs, serum BUN, and creatinine
4. *Before starting and after completing treatment:* ECG and multiple-gated acquisition or echocardiogram assessment of left ventricular ejection fraction (LVEF)
5. *Response evaluation:* Every 2–3 cycles

Notes

Patients with objective responses continue treatment until disease progression or unacceptable toxicity, or for 6 additional cycles after maximal response

23. Lymphoma, Hodgkin

Michael Fuchs, MD, Dennis A. Eichenauer, MD, and Volker Diehl, MD

Epidemiology

Incidence: 9,190 (male: 5,070; female: 4,120. Estimated new cases for 2014 in the United States) 3.2 per 100,000 males; 2.4 per 100,000 females

Deaths: Estimated 1,180 in 2014 (male: 670; female: 510)

Median age: 38 years

Male to female ratio: 1.2:1

Siegel R et al. CA Cancer J Clin 2014;64:9–29

Surveillance, Epidemiology and End Results (SEER) Program, available from http://seer.cancer.gov (accessed in 2013)

Pathology

Since 1944, several classifications have been proposed for Hodgkin lymphoma (HL). Currently, the World Health Organization (WHO) Classification of Hematologic Malignancies is used:

1. Lymphocyte predominant, nodular (NLPHL) (5%)
2. Classic
   a. Lymphocyte-rich (LRCHL) (5%)
   b. Nodular sclerosis (NSHL) (60–80%)
   c. Mixed cellularity (MCHL) (15–30%)
   d. Lymphocyte depleted (LDHL) (1%)
   e. Unclassifiable (<1%)

Jaffe ES, Harris NL, Stein H, Vardiman JW, eds. World Health Organization Classification of Tumours. Pathology and Genetics of Tumours of Haematopoietic and Lymphoid Tissues. Lyon, France: IARC Press, 2001

Work-up

1. History and physical exam
2. Laboratory tests: CBC with differential, ESR, electrolytes, albumin, liver function tests, mineral panel, LDH
3. HIV and hepatitis B and C serologies as clinically indicated
4. Chest x-ray (PA and lateral)
5. CT scan of chest, abdomen, and pelvis (and neck in selected cases)
6. Positron emission tomography (PET) scan if clinically indicated (equivocal CT)
7. Bone marrow aspirate and biopsy
8. Pulmonary function tests
9. Echocardiogram or MUGA scan to determine cardiac ejection fraction
10. Excisional lymph node biopsy to completely assess lymph node architecture is required at initial diagnosis. Fine-needle aspiration biopsy alone is not desirable for the initial diagnosis of lymphoma
11. Fertility counseling, if appropriate

Five-Year Survival Rate

NLPHL	90% (10 years)
Classic HL	70–80%

Jaffe ES, Harris NL, Stein H, Vardiman JW, eds. World Health Organization Classification of Tumours. Pathology and Genetics of Tumours of Haematopoietic and Lymphoid Tissues. Lyon, France: IARC Press, 2001

Staging

Ann Arbor Staging Classification for Hodgkin and Non-Hodgkin Lymphomas

Stage	Description
I	Involvement of a single lymph node region (I) or involvement of a single extralymphatic organ or site (IE)
II	Involvement of 2 or more lymph node regions or lymphatic structures on the same side of the diaphragm alone (II) or with involvement of limited, contiguous extralymphatic organ or tissue (IIE)
III	Involvement of lymph node regions on both sides of the diaphragm (III), which may include the spleen (IIIS), or limited, contiguous extralymphatic organ or site (IIIE), or both (IIIES)
IV	Diffuse or disseminated foci of involvement of one or more extralymphatic organs or tissues with or without associated lymphatic involvement

Abbreviations

A	Asymptomatic
B	Unexplained persistent or recurrent fever with temperature higher than 38°C (100.4°F) or recurrent drenching night sweats within 1 month or unexplained loss of >10% body weight within 6 months
E	Limited direct extension into extralymphatic organ from adjacent lymph node

Carbone PP et al. Cancer Res 1971;31:1860–1861

(continued)

Staging (continued)

Criteria that predict an unfavorable prognosis in *limited-stage HL* differ among study groups
Patients with one or more of these factors are considered to have an unfavorable prognosis

Factor	EORTC	GHSG	NCIC	Stanford
Age (years)	≥50	—	≥40	—
Histology	—	—	MC/LD	—
ESR/B-symptoms	≥30 mm with any B ≥50 mm without B	≥30 mm with any B ≥50 mm without B	≥50 mm or any B	Any B
Mediastinal mass	MTR ≥0.35	MMR >0.33	10 cm or MMR >0.33	MMR >0.33
Number of nodal sites	≥4	≥3	≥4	—
E-lesions	—	Present	—	—

EORTC, European Organization for Research and Treatment of Cancer; GHSG, German Hodgkin *Lymphoma* Study Group; NCIC, National *Cancer* Institute of *Canada*

For patients with *advanced stage HL* the German Hodgkin *Lymphoma* Study Group (*GHSG*) has developed the following prognostic score model:

Number of Factors	Percent of the Population	Estimated Freedom from Disease Progression at 5 Years
0	7%	84%
1	22%	77%
2	29%	67%
3	23%	60%
4	12%	51%
5+	7%	42%

Factors: Stage IV; male sex; age >45 years; hemoglobin <10.5 g/dL; WBC ≥15,000/mm³; lymphocytes <8% or <600/mm³; albumin <4 g/dL

Hasenclever D, Diehl V. N Engl J Med 1998;339: 1506–1514

Expert Opinion

The treatment of adult patients with HL should be stage adapted with respect to age and additional factors such as comorbidities

1. **Patients with early favorable stage HL**
   - Combined modality treatment with a chemotherapy regimen such as ABVD followed by involved-field radiotherapy (IF-RT) is considered the treatment of choice[*,†] with a 5-year event-free survival rate (EFS) of 98% (data from the H8F trial of the EORTC)
2. **Patients with stage IA nodular lymphocyte predominant Hodgkin Lymphoma (NLPHL)**
   - Local radiotherapy is widely accepted as the standard treatment due to the excellent prognosis of this subgroup of patients[‡]
3. **Patients with early unfavorable (intermediate) stage HL**
   - Combined modality treatment, for example, 4–6 cycles of ABVD followed by IF-RT[§]
   - Despite excellent initial remission rates, approximately 15% of patients relapse within 5 years. Thus, an intensification of chemotherapy might improve results. Several ongoing studies are addressing this issue
4. **Patients with advanced stage HL**
   - *Low-risk patients:* IPS <3 risk factors → FDG-PET might help to identify patients for whom 6–8 cycles of ABVD ± IF-RT is sufficient to achieve a cure
   - *High-risk patients:* IPS >3 risk factors → intensive chemotherapy such as dose-escalated BEACOPP is be the treatment of choice.[∈] For patients with advanced HL, eight cycles of BEACOPPescalated are no longer standard of care. The final analysis of the GHSG HD15 trial has shown that six cycles of BEACOPPescalated followed by localized RT of PET-positive residual lymphoma larger than 2.5 cm represent the optimal treatment for these patients
   - The impact of radiotherapy after effective chemotherapy if a CR is achieved is doubtful. Therefore radiotherapy should be restricted to patients in whom FDG-PET scan demonstrates positive lesions after the end of chemotherapy

(continued)

Expert Opinion (*continued*)

5. The following protocols may be considered in the management of patients with Hodgkin lymphoma:

First-line protocols for newly diagnosed Hodgkin lymphoma

1. ABVD
2. Stanford V
3. BEACOPP

Salvage/induction protocols

4. DHAP
5. ICE
6. IGEV
7. GVD
8. Dexa-BEAM
9. IVE

High-dose/conditioning protocols

10. BEAM
11. CBV

Palliative protocols (regimens/drugs)

12. Brentuximab vedotin
13. Gemcitabine
14. Vinorelbine
15. Bendamustine

*Several studies have demonstrated FDG-PET to be a good prognostic predictor when performed after the first or second cycle of chemotherapy. However, because almost all studies were retrospective analyses, it is necessary to prove the value of FDG-PET for tailoring therapy within a large prospective trial. Trials addressing this issue are ongoing

†Patients older than 60 years of age should not receive dose-escalated BEACOPP because of an increased rate of toxicity. These patients should be treated with 6–8 cycles of ABVD followed by radiotherapy in case of residual lymphomas

‡HL patients who relapse or do not respond to primary treatment require an adequate salvage therapy. For most of them, high-dose chemotherapy (HDCT) followed by autologous stem cell transplantation (ASCT) is the treatment of choice. The best regimen for reinduction therapy has not yet been defined

§Patients with contraindications to undergo ASCT or with multiple relapses should either receive a classical palliative treatment with drugs such as gemcitabine or vinorelbine, or be enrolled in clinical trials evaluating novel approaches

ᶜASCT still has to be regarded as an experimental approach as it is associated with high relapse and mortality rates. It should only be considered for patients younger than 30 years of age who are in a good general condition

Bonadonna G, Bonfante V, Viviani S, Di Russo A, Villani F, Valagussa P. ABVD plus subtotal nodal versus involved-field radiotherapy in early-stage Hodgkin's disease: long-term results. J Clin Oncol 2004;22:2835–2841

Diehl V, Franklin J, Pfreundschuh M et al. Standard and increased-dose BEACOPP chemotherapy compared with COPP-ABVD for advanced Hodgkin's disease. N Engl J Med 2003;348:2386–2395

Engert A, Schiller P, Josting A et al. Involved-field radiotherapy is equally effective and less toxic compared with extended-field radiotherapy after four cycles of chemotherapy in patients with early-stage unfavorable Hodgkin's lymphoma: results of the HD8 trial of the German Hodgkin's Lymphoma Study Group. J Clin Oncol 2003;21:3601–3608

Nogova L, Reineke T, Eich HT et al. Extended field radiotherapy, combined modality treatment or involved field radiotherapy for patients with stage IA lymphocyte-predominant Hodgkin's lymphoma: a retrospective analysis from the German Hodgkin Study Group (GHSG). Ann Oncol 2005;16:1683–1687

Noordijk EM, Carde P, Dupouy N et al. Combined-modality therapy for clinical stage I or II Hodgkin's lymphoma: long-term results of the European Organisation for Research and Treatment of Cancer H7 randomized controlled trials. J Clin Oncol 2006;24:3128–3135

REGIMEN FOR NEWLY DIAGNOSED HODGKIN LYMPHOMA

DOXORUBICIN (Adriamycin), BLEOMYCIN, VINBLASTINE, DACARBAZINE (ABVD)

Bonadonna G et al. Cancer 1975;36:252–259
Canellos GP et al. New Engl J Med 1992;327:1478–1484
Duggan DB et al. J Clin Oncol 2003;21:607–614
Hoskins PJ et al. J Clin Oncol 2009;27:5390–5396

Doxorubicin 25 mg/m² per dose; administer by intravenous injection over 3–5 minutes for 2 doses on days 1 and 15, every 28 days (total dosage/cycle = 50 mg/m²)

Bleomycin 10 units/m² per dose; administer intravenously by slow injection over 10 minutes for 2 doses on days 1 and 15, every 28 days (total dosage/cycle = 20 units/m²)

Vinblastine 6 mg/m² per dose; administer by intravenous injection over 1–2 minutes for 2 doses on days 1 and 15, every 28 days (total dosage/cycle = 12 mg/m²)

Dacarbazine 150 mg/m² per dose; administer intravenously in 100–250 mL 0.9% sodium chloride injection or 5% dextrose injection over 15–30 minutes for 5 consecutive days on days 1–5, every 28 days (total dosage/cycle = 750 mg/m²)

Note: There is evidence that ABVD can be given without any dose modification on time irrespective of the peripheral blood count (Evens AM et al. Br J Haematol 2007;137:545–552)

Supportive Care
Antiemetic prophylaxis
Emetogenic potential on Days 1–5 is **HIGH**
Emetogenic potential on Day 15 is **MODERATE**
See Chapter 39 for antiemetic recommendations

Hematopoietic growth factor (CSF) prophylaxis
Primary prophylaxis is indicated with:
Filgrastim (G-CSF) 5 mcg/kg per day, by subcutaneous injection
- Begin use 24–72 h after myelosuppressive chemotherapy is completed
- G-CSF use with bleomycin-containing regimens for Hodgkin's disease has been associated with an increased rate of pulmonary toxicity

See Chapter 43 for more information

Antimicrobial prophylaxis
Risk of fever and neutropenia is LOW
  Antimicrobial primary prophylaxis to be considered:
  - Antibacterial—*P. jirovecii* prophylaxis is recommended (eg, cotrimoxazole)

See Chapter 47 for more information

Treatment Modifications

Adverse Event*	Dose Modification
WBC 3,999–3,000/mm³ or platelet count 129,000–100,000/mm³	Reduce doxorubicin and vinblastine dosages by 50%
WBC 2,999–2,000/mm³ or platelet count 99,000–80,000/mm³	Reduce dacarbazine dosage by 50%. Reduce doxorubicin and vinblastine dosages by 75%
WBC 1,999–1,500/mm³ or platelet count 79,000–50,000/mm³	Reduce dacarbazine dosage by 75%. Hold doxorubicin and vinblastine
WBC <1,500/mm³ or platelet count <50,000/mm³	Hold doxorubicin, vinblastine, and dacarbazine
Clinical or radiologic evidence of pulmonary fibrosis or DLCO <50% pretreatment value	Discontinue bleomycin
Moderate-to-severe renal function impairment (creatinine clearance <50 mL/min [<0.83 mL/s])	Discontinue bleomycin until creatinine clearance improves to ≥50 mL/min

*Refers to values on days 1 or 15

Therapy Monitoring

1. *Semiweekly and before each cycle:* CBC with differential
2. *Before each cycle:* Physical exam, chest x-ray
3. *After second and each subsequent cycle:* DLCO
4. *Response evaluation:* CT of chest, abdomen, and pelvis every 2 cycles starting after cycle 4. FDG-PET scan at conclusion of therapy to document extent of remission. Bone marrow biopsy (if disease existed before therapy) performed 1 month after completing the sixth cycle

Patient Population Studied

Hoskins PJ et al. J Clin Oncol 2009;27:5390–5396

Multicenter, prospective, randomized controlled trial compared the efficacy and toxicity of 2 chemotherapy regimens, ABVD and Stanford V, in advanced Hodgkin lymphoma

Baseline Demographic and Clinical Characteristics

Characteristic	ABVD (n = 261) Number (%)	Stanford V (n = 259) Number (%)	Total (N = 520) Number (%)
Age, median (range)	35 years (18–60)	34 years (18–67)	35 years (18–67)
Male sex	154 (59%)	154 (59%)	308 (59%)
Stage			
I to II	119 (46%)	134 (52%)	253 (49%)
III	81 (31%)	72 (28%)	153 (29%)
IV	61 (23%)	53 (20%)	114 (22%)
"B" symptoms present	184 (73%)	185 (75%)	369 (74%)

(continued)

Patient Population Studied (continued)
Baseline Demographic and Clinical Characteristics

Characteristic	Treatment Arm		Total (N = 520) Number (%)
	ABVD (n = 261) Number (%)	Stanford V (n = 259) Number (%)	
Bulky disease present	94 (41%)	93 (42%)	187 (41%)
Hasenclever score			
0–1	77 (31%)	90 (36%)	167 (34%)
2–3	136 (55%)	122 (50%)	258 (52%)
4–7	33 (13%)	36 (15%)	69 (14%)
Unknown	15	11	26
Histology			
LP	2 (1%)	6 (3%)	8 (2%)
MC	21 (10%)	20 (10%)	41 (10%)
NS	190 (88%)	178 (86%)	368 (87%)
Other	3 (1%)	3 (1%)	6 (1%)
Not reviewed	45	52	97

LP, lymphocyte predominant; MC, mixed cellularity; NS nodular sclerosing

Efficacy

Response	Treatment Arm		Total Number (%)
	ABVD Number (%)	Stanford V Number (%)	
At completion of chemotherapy			
CR	89 (38%)	62 (27%)	151 (33%)
Cru	39 (17%)	21 (9%)	60 (13%)
PR	88 (38%)	133 (58%)	221 (48%)
SD	7 (3%)	7 (3%)	14 (3%)
PD/relapse	9 (4%)	5 (2%)	14 (3%)
Death	1	0	1 (0%)
Unknown	19	20	39
Total	252	248	500
CR/CRu rate*	128/233 (55%)	83/228 (36%)	$P < 0.0001$
At treatment completion			
ORR	228 (92%)	218 (91%)	
CR	113 (46%)	104 (44%)	217 (45%)
CRu	52 (21%)	33 (14%)	85 (17%)
PR	63 (25%)	81 (34%)	144 (30%)
SD	6 (2%)	6 (2%)	12 (2%)
PD/relapse	12 (5%)	15 (6%)	27 (6%)
Death	2 (1%)	0	2 (0)
Unknown	4	9	13
Total	252	248	500
CR/CRu rate†	165/248 (67%)	137/239 (57%)	$P = 0.036$
Estimated 5-year PFS	76%	74%	
5-year OS rates	90%	92%	HR = 0.76; 95% CI, 0.41−1.38; $P = 0.37$

CR, complete response rate; Cru, complete remission unconfirmed; ORR, overall response rate = CR + Cru + PR; PFS, progression-free survival; PR, partial response rate
Note: Treatment completion indicates completion of chemotherapy and radiotherapy

Hoskins PJ et al. J Clin Oncol 2009;27:5390–5396

Toxicity
ABVD

Toxicity	Number of Patients (%)
During initial treatment (N = 412)	
Pulmonary*	101 (24.5%)
Cardiac*	27 (6.6)
Hematologic†	262 (63.6%)
Anorexia†	1 (0.2%)
Fatigue†	7 (1.7%)
Hypotension†	0
After completion of treatment (N = 300)	
Pulmonary*	25 (8.3%)
Cardiac*	10 (3.3%)
Hematologic†	15 (5%)

*G ≥2 dyspnea, partial pressure of oxygen/carbon dioxide, diffusing capacity for carbon monoxide, fibrosis, acute respiratory distress syndrome, noninfectious pneumonitis, cardiac function, or arrhythmia, all of which would result in dose modification or elimination of doxorubicin or bleomycin
†Maximum toxicity G ≥3, severe, life-threatening, or fatal
Note: there were 9 deaths during initial therapy

Duggan DB et al. J Clin Oncol 2003;21:607–614

REGIMEN FOR NEWLY DIAGNOSED HODGKIN LYMPHOMA

STANFORD V

Bartlett NL et al. J Clin Oncol 1995;13:1080–1088

Doxorubicin 25 mg/m^2 per dose; administer by intravenous injection over 3–5 minutes for 2 doses on days 1 and 15, every 28 days, for 3 cycles (total dosage/cycle = 50 mg/m^2)
Vinblastine 6 mg/m^2 per dose; administer by intravenous injection over 1–2 minutes for 2 doses on days 1 and 15, every 28 days, for 3 cycles (total dosage/cycle = 12 mg/m^2)

Note: For patients ≥50 years of age, during the third cycle, decrease vinblastine dosage to 4 mg/m^2 per dose for 2 doses on days 1 and 15 (total dose during the third cycle = 8 mg/m^2)

Mechlorethamine 6 mg/m^2; administer by intravenous injection over 1–2 minutes on day 1, every 28 days for 3 cycles (total dosage/cycle = 6 mg/m^2)
Vincristine 1.4 mg/m^2 per dose; administer (maximum single dose = 2 mg) by intravenous injection over 1–2 minutes for 2 doses on days 8 and 22, every 28 days, for 3 cycles (total dosage/cycle = 2.8 mg/m^2; maximum dose/cycle = 4 mg)

Note: For patients ≥50 years of age, during the third cycle, decrease vincristine dosage to 1 mg/m^2 per dose (maximum single dose = 2 mg) for 2 doses on days 8 and 22 (total dosage during the third cycle = 2 mg/m^2; maximum dose during the third cycle = 4 mg)

Bleomycin 5 units/m^2 per dose; administer by slow intravenous injection over 10 minutes for 2 doses on days 8 and 22, every 28 days, for 3 cycles (total dosage/cycle = 10 units/m^2)
Etoposide 60 mg/m^2 per day; administer intravenously, diluted in 0.9% sodium chloride injection or 5% dextrose injection to a concentration within the range 0.2–0.4 mg/mL over 1 hour for 2 doses on days 15 and 16, every 28 days, for 3 cycles (total dosage/cycle = 120 mg/m^2)
Prednisone 40 mg/m^2 per dose; administer orally every other day (days 1, 3, 5, and so on) for 14 doses, every 28 days

Note: Prednisone dosage is tapered by 10 mg/dose every other day starting on day 14 of the third cycle (total dosage/28-day cycle = 560 mg/m^2 until tapering begins)

Consolidative irradiation, starting 2 weeks after the completion of chemotherapy. Administer 36 Gy to sites of initial tumor bulk defined as disease ≥5 cm in horizontal diameter. The treatment port for patients with bulky mediastinal HL is referred to as a modified mantle and is restricted to the mediastinum and bilateral hilar and supraclavicular regions. Extension of HL to contiguous extralymphatic sites, usually associated with bulky disease is also included in the port. Limit doses to the lung and pleura to 16.5 Gy delivered in 0.75- to 0.9-Gy fractions; pericardial and subcarinal blocks should be placed at 15 Gy and 30 Gy, respectively

Supportive Care
Antiemetic prophylaxis
Emetogenic potential on Day 1 is **HIGH**
Emetogenic potential on Days 8 and 22 is **MINIMAL**
Emetogenic potential on Day 15 is **MODERATE**
Emetogenic potential on Day 16 is **LOW**
See Chapter 39 for antiemetic recommendations

Hematopoietic growth factor (CSF) prophylaxis
Primary prophylaxis is indicated with:
   Filgrastim (G-CSF) 5 mcg/kg per day, by subcutaneous injection
   • Begin use 24–72 h after myelosuppressive chemotherapy is completed
   • G-CSF use with bleomycin-containing regimens for Hodgkin's disease has been associated with an increased rate of pulmonary toxicity
See Chapter 43 for more information

(continued)

Treatment Modifications

Adverse Event	Dose Modification
ANC <1000/mm^3	Reduce doxorubicin, vinblastine, mechlorethamine, and etoposide dosages by 35%
ANC <500/mm^3	Delay treatment 1 week then reduce doxorubicin, vinblastine, mechlorethamine, and etoposide dosages by 35%
Dose reduction or dose delay	Administer filgrastim 5 mcg/kg · day subcutaneously on days 3–13 and 16–26
Clinical or radiologic evidence of pulmonary fibrosis or DLCO <50% pretreatment value	Discontinue bleomycin
Moderate-to-severe renal function impairment (creatinine clearance <50 mL/min [<0.83 mL/s])	Discontinue bleomycin until creatinine clearance improves to ≥50 mL/min (≥0.83 mL/s)

(*continued*)

Antimicrobial prophylaxis

Risk of fever and neutropenia is INTERMEDIATE

Antimicrobial primary prophylaxis to be considered:

- Antibacterial—consider a fluoroquinolone or no prophylaxis; *P. jirovecii* prophylaxis is recommended (eg, cotrimoxazole)
- Antifungal—consider use during neutropenia and for anticipated mucositis
- Antiviral—antiherpes antivirals (eg, acyclovir)

Note: Although the primary report recommended daily ketoconazole, imidazole and triazole antifungals are highly potent cytochrome P450 (CYP3A subfamily) inhibitors that may interfere with drug metabolism. It may be prudent to withhold these drugs the day before, the day of, and the day after doxorubicin, vinblastine, vincristine, and etoposide are administered

See Chapter 47 for more information

Steroid-associated gastritis

Add a **proton pump inhibitor** concurrent with steroid use to prevent gastritis and duodenitis

Patient Population Studied

Patients between 15 and 60 years of age with either advanced-stage (III or IV) HL or stage II with bulky mediastinal involvement were treated with 3 cycles of chemotherapy followed by consolidative radiation to sites of initial bulky (>5 cm) disease

Toxicity (N = 60)

Toxicities Requiring Hospitalization

Fever/neutropenia	17%
Obstipation/ileus	11%
DVT	3%
Pneumonitis	2%
Palpitations	2%
Phlebitis	2%

Overall Toxicities

	% Any Grade	% G3/4
Neutropenia	82	45
Anemia	60	34
Nausea/vomiting	52	9
Sensory neuropathy	71	11
Motor neuropathy	34	8
Autonomic neuropathy	46	12
Phlebitis	38	
Myalgias/arthralgias	24	
Aseptic necrosis femoral head	2	

Therapy Monitoring

1. *Weekly:* CBC with differential
2. *Before every cycle:* CBC with differential, alkaline phosphatase and LDH, chest x-ray; DLCO after second and each subsequent cycle
3. *Response evaluation after completion of therapy:* CT of chest, abdomen, and pelvis after 2 cycles of chemotherapy and before the start of radiation therapy or after 3 cycles of chemotherapy. FDG-PET scan at conclusion of therapy to document extent of remission. Bone marrow biopsy (if disease existed before therapy) performed 1 month after completing therapy

Efficacy (N = 65)

Stage at Diagnosis	Status at 3 Years Failure-Free Survival
II (n = 21)	100
III (n = 20)	92
IV (n = 24)	76
Progression while on therapy	0

Four of 28 patients had positive gallium scans with mediastinal uptake. None had relapsed 6–42 months after consolidative mediastinal RT

Failure-free survival (FFS) time was calculated from the initial date of treatment until disease progression, relapse, death from any cause, or last follow-up evaluation

The 3 year overall survival and FFS were 96% and 87% respectively

The 3 year FFS for stage III to IV patients combined was 82%

Note

Stanford V is widely used, but requires radiation therapy in all patients with attendant late complications

REGIMEN FOR NEWLY DIAGNOSED HODGKIN LYMPHOMA

BLEOMYCIN, ETOPOSIDE, DOXORUBICIN (Adriamycin), CYCLOPHOSPHAMIDE, VINCRISTINE (Oncovin), PROCARBAZINE, PREDNISONE (BEACOPP)

Diehl V et al. J Clin Oncol 1998;16:3810–3821. Erratum in: N Engl J Med 2005;353:744
Diehl V et al. N Engl J Med 2003;348:2386–2395

BEACOPP

Doxorubicin 25 mg/m^2; administer by intravenous injection over 3–5 minutes on day 1, every 21 days (total dosage/cycle = 25 mg/m^2)

Cyclophosphamide 650 mg/m^2; administer intravenously in 25–250 mL 0.9% sodium chloride injection (0.9% NS) or 5% dextrose injection (D5W) over 10–30 minutes on day 1, every 21 days (total dosage/cycle = 650 mg/m^2)

Etoposide 100 mg/m^2 per day; administer intravenously, diluted in 0.9% NS or D5W to a concentration within the range 0.2–0.4 mg/mL over 1 hour for 3 consecutive days, on days 1, 2, and 3, every 21 days (total dosage/cycle = 300 mg/m^2)

Procarbazine 100 mg/m^2 per day; administer orally for 7 consecutive days on days 1–7, every 21 days (total dosage/cycle = 700 mg/m^2)

Prednisone 40 mg/m^2 per day; administer orally for 14 consecutive days on days 1–14, every 21 days (total dosage/cycle = 560 mg/m^2)

Bleomycin 10 units/m^2; administer by slow intravenous injection over 10 minutes on day 8, every 21 days (total dosage/cycle = 10 units/m^2)

Vincristine 1.4 mg/m^2 (maximum single dose = 2 mg); administer by intravenous injection over 1–3 minutes on day 8, every 21 days (total dosage/cycle = 1.4 mg/m^2; maximum dose/cycle = 2 mg)

Dose-Escalated BEACOPP

Doxorubicin 35 mg/m^2; administer by intravenous injection over 3–5 minutes on day 1, every 21 days (total dosage/cycle = 35 mg/m^2)

Cyclophosphamide 1250 mg/m^2; administer intravenously in 100–1000 mL 0.9% NS or D5W over 10–30 minutes on day 1, every 21 days (total dosage/cycle = 1250 mg/m^2)

Etoposide 200 mg/m^2 per day; administer intravenously, diluted in 0.9% NS or D5W to a concentration within the range 0.2–0.4 mg/mL, over 1 hour for 3 consecutive days, on days 1, 2, and 3, every 21 days (total dosage/cycle = 600 mg/m^2)

Procarbazine 100 mg/m^2 per day; administer orally for 7 consecutive days on days 1–7, every 21 days (total dosage/cycle = 700 mg/m^2)

Prednisone 40 mg/m^2 per day; administer orally for 14 consecutive days on days 1–14, every 21 days (total dosage/cycle = 560 mg/m^2)

Bleomycin 10 units/m^2; administer by slow intravenous injection over 10 minutes on day 8, every 21 days (total dosage/cycle = 10 units/m^2)

Vincristine 1.4 mg/m^2 (maximum single dose = 2 mg); administer by intravenous injection over 1–3 minutes on day 8, every 21 days (total dosage/cycle = 1.4 mg/m^2; maximum dose/cycle = 2 mg)

Special instructions:
Procarbazine is a weak monoamine oxidase inhibitor. Concurrent use of sympathomimetic or tricyclic antidepressant drugs and ingestion of tyramine-rich foods may produce severe hypertensive episodes in a patient receiving procarbazine

Anonymous. Med Lett Drugs Ther 1989;31:11–12
Da Prada M et al. J Neural Transm Suppl 1988;26:31–56
McCabe BJ. J Am Diet Assoc 1986;86:1059–1064

(continued)

Treatment Modifications

Adverse Event	Dose Modification
BEACOPP and Dose-Escalated BEACOPP	
WBC <2500/mm^3 or platelet count <80,000/mm^3	Delay cycle until WBC >2500/mm^3 and platelet count >80,000/mm^3; if delayed >2 weeks, reduce dosage of doxorubicin, cyclophosphamide, etoposide, and procarbazine by 25%
Clinical or radiologic evidence of pulmonary fibrosis or DLCO <50% pretreatment value	Discontinue bleomycin
Moderate to severe impairment renal function (creatinine clearance <50 mL/min [<0.83 mL/s])	Discontinue bleomycin until creatinine clearance improves to ≥50 mL/min (≥0.83 mL/s)
Dose-Escalated BEACOPP	
Any G4 toxicity or a 2-week postponement in start of next cycle per above guidelines	Stepwise reduction of cyclophosphamide and etoposide dosages by 25% of the difference between the escalated dosage and standard BEACOPP; immediate reduction to standard BEACOPP dosages if G4 toxicity occurs in 2 successive cycles

(continued)

Supportive Care

Antiemetic prophylaxis
Emetogenic potential on Day 1 is **HIGH**
Emetogenic potential on Days 2–7 is **MODERATE**
Emetogenic potential on Day 8 is **MINIMAL**
See Chapter 39 for antiemetic recommendations

Hematopoietic growth factor (CSF) prophylaxis
Primary prophylaxis is indicated with:
   Filgrastim (G-CSF) 300 mcg/day (patients with body weight <75 kg) or 480 mcg/day (body weight ≥75 kg) by subcutaneous injection starting on day 8 and continuing until WBC ≥1000/mm³ on 3 consecutive days
   • G-CSF use with bleomycin-containing regimens for Hodgkin's disease has been associated with an increased rate of pulmonary toxicity
See Chapter 43 for more information

Antimicrobial prophylaxis
Risk of fever and neutropenia is INTERMEDIATE
   Antimicrobial primary prophylaxis to be considered:
   • Antibacterial—consider a fluoroquinolone or no prophylaxis; *P. jirovecii* prophylaxis is recommended (eg, cotrimoxazole)
   • Antifungal—consider use during neutropenia and for anticipated mucositis
   • Antiviral—antiherpes antivirals (eg, acyclovir)
See Chapter 47 for more information

Steroid-associated gastritis
Add a **proton pump inhibitor** concurrent with steroid use to prevent gastritis and duodenitis

Toxicity (N = 1140; 854 Cycles)

Toxicity	% G3/4	
	BEACOPP	Dose-Escalated BEACOPP
Leukopenia	73%	98%
Thrombocytopenia	9%	70%
Anemia	17%	66%
Infection	16%	22%
Nausea	12%	20%
Mucositis	2%	8%
Respiratory tract effects	5%	4%

Patient Population Studied

Phase III multicenter trial of 935 patients with advanced stage HL, ages 16–65 years. Patients were randomized to receive 8 cycles of BEACOPP or dose-escalated BEACOPP. An additional 260 patients were randomized to standard treatment with COPP/ABVD. This arm was prematurely closed because of the superiority of the BEACOPP arms in terms of FFTF. Radiation therapy was planned to sites of initial bulky disease (>5 cm)

Efficacy (N = 323)

	BEACOPP	Dose-Escalated BEACOPP
Complete remission	88%	96%
Early progression	8%	2%
FFTF at 5 years	76%	87%
OS at 5 years	88%	91%

Therapy Monitoring

1. *Weekly:* CBC with differential
2. *Before each cycle:* PE, CBC with differential, BUN, creatinine, LFTs, and LDH
3. *After the second and each subsequent cycle:* DLCO
4. *Response evaluation after completion of therapy:* CT of chest, abdomen, and pelvis every 2 cycles starting after cycle 4. FDG-PET scan at conclusion of therapy to document extent of remission. Bone marrow biopsy (if disease existed before therapy) performed 1 month after completing the sixth cycle

Notes

1. Approximately 70% of all patients received radiation therapy after chemotherapy had been completed. However, subsequent studies have demonstrated that the percentage of patients that require radiation can be decreased. The latest interim analysis from the HD15 trial showed that only 12% of patients require additional radiotherapy. RT can be restricted to patients who continue to have areas that are positive by PET scan after the completion of chemotherapy (Kobe C et al. Blood 2008;112:3989–3994)

2. Patients older than 60 years of age should not receive dose-escalated BEACOPP because of an increased rate of toxicity

SALVAGE/INDUCTION REGIMEN HODGKIN LYMPHOMA

DEXAMETHASONE + CYTARABINE (Ara-C) + CISPLATIN (DHAP)

Josting A et al. Ann Oncol 2002;13:1628–1635

Hydration: Administer 0.9% sodium chloride injection (0.9% NS); administer by continuous intravenous infusion at 200–250 mL/h starting 6 hours before cisplatin. Monitor and replace magnesium and other electrolytes as needed

Dexamethasone 40 mg/day; administer intravenously in 10–100 mL 0.9% NS or 5% dextrose injection (D5W) over 15–30 minutes for 4 consecutive days on days 1–4, every 14 days (total dose/cycle = 160 mg)

Cisplatin 100 mg/m^2; administer by continuous intravenous infusion over 24 hours in 100–1000 mL 0.9% NS on day 1, every 14 days (total dosage/cycle = 100 mg/m^2)

Cytarabine 2000 mg/m^2 per dose; administer intravenously in 25–250 mL 0.9% NS or D5W over 3 hours every 12 hours for 2 doses on day 2, every 14 days (total dosage/cycle = 4000 mg/m^2)

Supportive Care

Glucocorticoid eye drops; for example, **dexamethasone sodium phosphate** 0.1% ophthalmic drops; administer 2 drops by instillation into both eyes every 6 hours starting just before cytarabine administration begins, and continuing for 2 days after the last dose of cytarabine

• Steroid eye drops are given to prevent and mitigate conjunctivitis associated with cytarabine excretion in tears

Antiemetic prophylaxis
Emetogenic potential on day 1 is **HIGH**
Emetogenic potential on day 2 is **MODERATE–HIGH**
See Chapter 39 for antiemetic recommendations

Hematopoietic growth factor (CSF) prophylaxis
Primary prophylaxis is indicated with:

Filgrastim (G-CSF) 5 mcg/kg per day by subcutaneous injection starting 24 hours after the last dose of cytarabine, and continuing until WBC ≥2500/mm^3 for 3 consecutive days
See Chapter 43 for more information

Antimicrobial prophylaxis
Risk of fever and neutropenia is LOW
Antimicrobial primary prophylaxis to be considered:
• Antibacterial—*P. jirovecii* prophylaxis is recommended (eg, cotrimoxazole)
• Antifungal—not indicated
• Antiviral—not indicated unless patient previously had an episode of HSV
See Chapter 47 for more information

Treatment Modifications

Adverse Event	Dose Modification
ANC <2500/mm^3 or platelets <80,000/mm^3	Delay start of cycle 2 until ANC >2500/mm^3 and platelets >80,000/mm^3

Otherwise, no treatment modifications specified as part of this tumor-reducing program before autologous stem cell transplantation

Patient Population Studied

Phase II multicenter trial, 102 patients with refractory or relapsed HL; age range: 21–64 years. Eleven patients had received COPP/ABVD, ABVD, BEACOPP, or similar regimens as frontline chemotherapy

Definitions

Primary progressive or refractory	Disease progression during first-line chemotherapy, or only transient response (CR or PR lasting ≤90 days) after induction treatment
Progressive disease	(a) ≥5% increase from nadir in the sum of the products of the greatest perpendicular diameters of any previously identified abnormal lymph node for partial responders or nonresponders; (b) appearance of any new lesion during or ≤90 days after the end of therapy
Relapsed HD	Complete disappearance of all detectable clinical and radiographic evidence of disease and disappearance of all disease-related symptoms if present before therapy for ≥3 months
Early relapse	CR lasting ≥3 months to 12 months
CR in late relapses	CR must last ≥12 months

Efficacy

	Complete Response	Partial Response	Treatment Failure
All patients	21%	67%	12%
Late relapse	26%	65%	9%
Early relapse	17%	76%	7%
Multiple relapse	23%	69%	8%
Progressive disease	12%	53%	35%

Note: Using the chi-square test for independence, remission status (relapsed HL vs. progressive HL) and stage at relapse (stages I/II vs. stages III/IV) were significant factors for response to DHAP

Toxicity		
	Number of Courses = 201	
Toxicity	**WHO G3**	**WHO G4**
Leukocytopenia*	50 (25%)	86 (43%)
Thrombocytopenia†	42 (21%)	97 (48%)‡
Anemia§	33 (16%)	1 (0.5%)
Mucositis	0 (0)	0 (0)
Infection⁽	2 (1%)	0 (0)
Nausea/vomiting	49 (24%)	3 (2%)
Renal	0 (0)	0 (0)
Neurotoxicity	1 (0.5%)	0 (0)
Ototoxicity	2 (1%)	0 (0)

*Duration of WHO grade 3 leukocytopenia: median 1.1 days (range: 0–6 days)
†Mean number of platelet transfusions: 0.4 (range: 0–4) transfusions
‡Duration of WHO grade 4 thrombocytopenia: median 1.4 days (range: 0–11 days)
§Mean number of red blood cell units transfused: 0.5 (range: 0–4) units
⁽Days with fever ≥38°C (≥100.4°F): 0.3 days (range: 0–8 days); neither severe infections nor treatment-related deaths occurred

Therapy Monitoring

1. *Semiweekly and before each cycle:* CBC with differential
2. *Before each cycle:* Physical exam
3. *Response evaluation:* CT of all initially involved sites. Bone marrow biopsy if BM-involvement before start of therapy

Notes

1. Stem cell mobilization for autologous stem cell transplantation was performed after the first and, if necessary, the second cycle
2. High-dose chemotherapy and autologous stem cell transplantation was performed after 2 cycles, if patients achieved at least partial remission

SALVAGE/INDUCTION REGIMEN HODGKIN LYMPHOMA

IFOSFAMIDE + CARBOPLATIN + ETOPOSIDE (ICE)

Moskowitz CH et al. Blood 2001;97:616–623

Etoposide 100 mg/m² per day; administer intravenously, diluted in 0.9% sodium chloride injection (0.9% NS) to a concentration within the range of 0.2–0.4 mg/mL, over 60 minutes for 3 consecutive days, on days 1–3, every 2 weeks (total dosage/cycle = 300 mg/m²)

Carboplatin (calculated dose) AUC = 5 mg/mL • min* (maximum absolute dose/cycle = 800 mg); administer intravenously in 100–500 mL 5% dextrose injection (D5W) or 0.9% NS over 15–30 minutes on day 2, every 2 weeks (total dosage/cycle calculated to produce an AUC = 5 mg/mL • min; maximum absolute dose/cycle = 800 mg)

Ifosfamide 5000 mg/m²; administer intravenously in 0.9% NS or D5W to a concentration within the range of 0.6–20 mg/mL, prepared as an admixture (in the same container) with **mesna** 5000 mg/m²; administer by continuous intravenous infusion over 24 hours on day 2, every 2 weeks (total dosage/cycle for ifosfamide = 5000 mg/m² and for mesna = 5000 mg/m²)

*Carboplatin dose is based on Calvert et al's formula to achieve a target area under the plasma concentration versus time curve (AUC) (AUC units = mg/mL • min)

$$\text{Total carboplatin dose (mg)} = (\text{target AUC}) \times (\text{GFR} + 25)$$

In practice, creatinine clearance (Clcr) is used in place of glomerular filtration rate (GFR). Clcr can be calculated from the equation of Cockcroft and Gault:

$$\text{For males, Clcr} = \frac{(140 - \text{age [years]}) \times \text{body weight (kg)}}{72 \times (\text{serum creatinine [mg/dL]})}$$

$$\text{For females, Clcr} = \frac{(140 - \text{age [years]}) \times \text{body weight (kg)}}{72 \times (\text{serum creatinine [mg/dL]})} \times 0.85$$

Calvert AH et al. J Clin Oncol 1989;7:1748–1756
Cockcroft DW, Gault MH. Nephron 1976;16:31–41
Jodrell DI et al. J Clin Oncol 1992;10:520–528
Sorensen BT et al. Cancer Chemother Pharmacol 1991;28:397–401

Note: A carboplatin dose calculated with an IDMS-measured serum creatinine result using the Calvert formula could exceed an expected exposure (AUC) and result in increased drug-related toxicity. The FDA recommends capping an estimated GFR at 125 mL/min for any targeted AUC value. No greater estimated GFR values should be used [online] May 23, 2013. Available from: http://www.fda.gov/AboutFDA/CentersOffices/OfficeofMedicalProductsandTobacco/CDER/ucm228974.htm [accessed February 26, 2014].

Supportive Care

Antiemetic prophylaxis
Emetogenic potential on days 1 and 3 is **LOW**
Emetogenic potential on day 2 is **MODERATE–HIGH**
See Chapter 39 for antiemetic recommendations

Hematopoietic growth factor (CSF) prophylaxis
Primary prophylaxis is indicated with:
    Filgrastim (G-CSF) 5 mcg/kg per day by subcutaneous injection on days 5–12 (except during peripheral blood progenitor cells mobilization)

Antimicrobial prophylaxis
Risk of fever and neutropenia is INTERMEDIATE
    Antimicrobial primary prophylaxis to be considered:
- Antibacterial—consider a fluoroquinolone or no prophylaxis; *P. jirovecii* prophylaxis is recommended (eg, cotrimoxazole)
- Antifungal—consider use during neutropenia and for anticipated mucositis
- Antiviral—antiherpes antivirals (eg, acyclovir)

See Chapter 47 for more information

(continued)

Treatment Modifications

Adverse Event	Dose Modification
ANC <1000/mm³ or platelet count <50,000/mm³	Delay next cycle until ANC ≥1000/mm³ and platelet count ≥50,000/mm³

Patient Population Studied

Phase II single-center trial of 65 patients with relapsed or primary refractory HL after chemotherapy/combined modality therapy; age range: 12–59 years

Efficacy

	Percent of Patients Receiving ICE	Event-Free at a Median Follow-up of 43 Months
Complete response	26	82%*
Partial response	58	59%*
Minor response	3	
Progressive disease	12	Median survival = 5 months

*$P = 0.10$

(continued)

Accelerated fractionation involved field radiotherapy (IFRT):
- Of the 57 patients with chemosensitive disease, 41 received IFRT
- Administered to patients who had nodal sites of disease that measured ≥5 cm prior to the start of ICE chemotherapy or who had residual disease after receiving ICE chemotherapy
- IFRT started within 2 weeks after successful collection of stem cells
- IFRT dose was 18,000–36,000 cGy administered in ten to twenty 180-cGy fractions twice daily (minimal 7-hour interval between fractions) within a period of 5–10 days

Notes:
- Patients who underwent prior radiotherapy to a dose above standard tolerance for a specific site had reduced-dose IFRT or no radiotherapy

Toxicity

Toxicity	Number of Patients
Gram-negative sepsis and neutropenia	1
Pneumonitis and death from aspiration pneumonia and acute respiratory distress syndrome*,†	1
Marantic endocarditis with cerebral emboli and subsequent multisystem organ failure*,†	1
Upper airway bleeding from a tracheal tear that resolved spontaneously†	1
ICE administration delayed beyond planned 14-day interval	40 (62%)
Scheduling difficulty	21 (32%)
Thrombocytopenia	17 (26%)
Infection	2 (3%)

Median Dose Intensities

Ifosfamide	2187 mg/m² per week (87.5%)
Carboplatin	AUC 2.187 mg/mL · min per week (87.5%)
Etoposide	43.5 mg/m² per week (87.5%)

*No evidence of HL at time of death
†Toxicity not thought to be caused by chemotherapy

Therapy Monitoring

1. *Semi-weekly and before each cycle:* CBC with differential
2. *Before each cycle:* Physical exam
3. *Response evaluation:* CT of all initially involved sites. Bone marrow biopsy if BM involvement before start of therapy

Notes

1. Stem cell mobilization for autologous stem cell transplantation was performed after the second cycle of ICE using filgrastim (10 mcg/kg per day) beginning on day 5, and continuing until the completion of leukapheresis. Leukapheresis was initiated when the white blood cell count was greater than 5000/mm³
2. Patients who achieved CR, PR, or a minor response received high-dose chemotherapy and autologous stem cell transplantation

SALVAGE/INDUCTION REGIMEN HODGKIN LYMPHOMA

IFOSFAMIDE + GEMCITABINE, + VINORELBINE (IGEV)

Santoro A et al. Haematologica 2007;92:35–41

Hyperhydration during ifosfamide:
Administer 2000 mL 0.9% sodium chloride injection (0.9% NS) per day by intravenous infusion concurrently with ifosfamide administration, for 4 consecutive days, on days 1–4, every 3 weeks
- If feasible, continue maintenance intravenous hydration during intervals between ifosfamide administration. Encourage oral fluid ingestion. Monitor daily weight, or if implemented in an inpatient setting, monitor fluid input and output. Replace electrolytes as medically appropriate

Ifosfamide 2000 mg/m² per day; administer intravenously, diluted in 0.9% NS or 5% dextrose injection (D5W) to a concentration within the range of 0.6–20 mg/mL, over 2 hours for 4 consecutive days, on days 1–4, every 3 weeks (total dosage/cycle = 8000 mg/m²)

Mesna 2600 mg/m² per day; administer intravenously for 4 consecutive days, on days 1–4, every 3 weeks (total dosage/cycle = 10,400 mg/m²)
- Mesna utilization strategies, include:

   1. Mesna 2600 mg/m² per day; administer by continuous intravenous infusion in 50–1000 mL 0.9% NS or D5W over 12 hours starting simultaneously with ifosfamide

   2. Mesna 650 mg/m² per dose; administer intravenously in 25–100 mL 0.9% NS or D5W over 15–30 minutes every 3 hours for 4 doses each day. The first dose is given when ifosfamide commences (ie, hours 0, 3, 6, and 9)

   3. Mesna 650 mg/m²; administer intravenously in 25–100 mL 0.9% NS or D5W over 15–30 minutes coincident with the start of ifosfamide administration (hour 0), then mesna 800 mg orally every 3–4 hours for an additional 3 doses (every 3 hours: at hours 3, 6, and 9; every 4 hours: at hours 4, 8, and 12; the regimen results in a different total mesna dose/cycle)

Gemcitabine 800 mg/m² per dose; administer intravenously, diluted in 0.9% NS to a concentration as low as 0.1 mg/mL over 30 minutes, for 2 doses on days 1 and 4, every 3 weeks (total dosage/cycle = 1600 mg/m²), *followed by:*

Vinorelbine 20 mg/m²; administer intravenously, diluted in 0.9% NS or D5W to a concentration between 1.5 and 3 mg/mL, over 6–10 minutes, on day 1, every 3 weeks (total dosage/cycle = 20 mg/m²)

Prednisolone 100 mg/day; administer orally, or by intravenous injection or intravenous infusion over 10–30 minutes for 4 consecutive days, on days 1–4, every 3 weeks (total dose/cycle = 400 mg)
- Alternatively, give **prednisone** orally at the same dose and administration schedule, and for the same duration

Supportive Care
Antiemetic prophylaxis
Emetogenic potential on days 1–4 is **MODERATE**
See Chapter 39 for antiemetic recommendations

Hematopoietic growth factor (CSF) prophylaxis
Primary prophylaxis is indicated with:
   Filgrastim (G-CSF) 5 mcg/kg per day, by subcutaneous injection on days 7–12, or until apheresis in the course of mobilization commences

Antimicrobial prophylaxis
Risk of fever and neutropenia is INTERMEDIATE
   Antimicrobial primary prophylaxis to be considered:
- Antibacterial—consider a fluoroquinolone or no prophylaxis; *P. jirovecii* prophylaxis is recommended (eg, cotrimoxazole)
- Antifungal—consider use during neutropenia and for anticipated mucositis
- Antiviral—antiherpes antivirals (eg, acyclovir)

See Chapter 47 for more information

Treatment Modifications
None specified as part of this regimen often used as a preparative regimen

Patient Population Studied
Phase II multicenter trial; 91 patients with refractory or relapsed HL; age range: 17–59 years. Nodular sclerosis was the most frequent histologic subtype (74.7%). A high percentage of patients had B symptoms (59.3%), extranodal involvement (47.2%), more than 3 involved sites (45.1%), and/or bulky disease (45.1%)

Efficacy

Response	Proportion
CR	54%
PR	27%
PD	10%

Response Rate According to Disease Status

	CR	PR	IF
Refractory	33.3%	27.8%	38.9%
Relapse	67.3%	27.3%	5.4%

Response Rate According to Prior RT

Prior radiotherapy	60%	30.9%	9.1%
No prior radiotherapy	44.4%	22.2%	33.3%

CR, Complete response; PR, partial response; IF, induction failure

Notes:
- Stem cell mobilization was performed at various time points (66% after cycle 3)
- High-dose chemotherapy and autologous stem cell transplantation was performed after 4 IGEV cycles
- Overall, 64 of 74 (86%) patients in complete or partial remission after IGEV proceeded to single (29 cases) or tandem (35 cases) high-dose chemotherapy with PBSC support

Toxicity

Delayed cycles		4.2%
Cycles with dose reductions		8.6%
Cycles with infection		3.5%
Toxicity	**G3**	**G4**

Hematologic Toxicity

Neutropenia	22.7%	5.7%
Thrombocytopenia	15.3%	4.8%
Anemia	16.6%	1.6%

Nonhematologic Toxicity

Mucositis	1.9%	0.3%
Nausea	3.2%	0
Cystitis	0.3%	0

Therapy Monitoring

1. *Semi-weekly and before each cycle:* CBC with differential
2. *Before each cycle:* Physical exam
3. *Response evaluation:* CT of all initially involved sites. Bone marrow biopsy if BM involvement before start of therapy

SALVAGE/INDUCTION REGIMEN HODGKIN LYMPHOMA

GEMCITABINE + VINORELBINE, + DOXORUBICIN, LIPOSOMAL (GVD)

Bartlett NL et al. Ann Oncol 2007;18:1071–1079

Hypersensitivity prophylaxis:
Patients who experienced an acute infusion-related reaction to doxorubicin HCl liposome injection (liposomal doxorubicin), defined as flushing, shortness of breath, facial swelling, chills, back pain, or tightness in the chest or throat, should receive 30–60 minutes before all subsequent liposomal doxorubicin doses:

- **Diphenhydramine** 50 mg; administer by intravenous injection
- **Ranitidine** 150 mg (or another histamine subtype H_2 receptor antagonist); administer orally, or 50 mg by intravenous infusion
- **Hydrocortisone** 100 mg; administer by intravenous injection or intravenous infusion

For patients who had NOT received an autologous hematopoietic stem cell transplantation (ASCT):
Vinorelbine 20 mg/m^2 per dose; administer intravenously, diluted in 0.9% sodium chloride injection (0.9% NS) or 5% dextrose injection (D5W) to a concentration between 1.5 and 3 mg/mL, over 6–10 minutes, for 2 doses on days 1 and 8, every 21 days, for a maximum of 6 cycles (total dosage/cycle = 40 mg/m^2), *followed by:*
Gemcitabine 1000 mg/m^2 per dose; administer intravenously, diluted in 0.9% NS to a concentration as low as 0.1 mg/mL over 30 minutes, for 2 doses on days 1 and 8, every 21 days, for a maximum of 6 cycles (total dosage/cycle = 2000 mg/m^2), *followed by:*
Doxorubicin HCl liposome injection 15 mg/m^2 per dose; administer intravenously in 250 mL D5W over 60 minutes, for 2 doses on days 1 and 8, every 21 days, for a maximum of 6 cycles (total dosage/cycle = 30 mg/m^2)

For patients who previously received an ASCT:
Vinorelbine 15 mg/m^2 per dose; administer intravenously, diluted in 0.9% sodium chloride injection (0.9% NS) or 5% dextrose injection (D5W) to a concentration between 1.5 and 3 mg/mL, over 6–10 minutes, for 2 doses on days 1 and 8, every 21 days, for a maximum of 6 cycles (total dosage/cycle = 30 mg/m^2), *followed by:*
Gemcitabine 800 mg/m^2 per dose; administer intravenously, diluted in 0.9% NS to a concentration as low as 0.1 mg/mL, over 30 minutes, for 2 doses on days 1 and 8, every 21 days, for a maximum of 6 cycles (total dosage/cycle = 1600 mg/m^2), *followed by:*
Doxorubicin HCl liposome injection 10 mg/m^2 per dose; administer intravenously in 250 mL D5W over 60 minutes, for 2 doses on days 1 and 8, every 21 days, for a maximum of 6 cycles (total dosage/cycle = 20 mg/m^2)

Supportive Care
Antiemetic prophylaxis
Emetogenic potential on Days 1 and 8 is **MODERATE**
See Chapter 39 for antiemetic recommendations

Hematopoietic growth factor (CSF) prophylaxis
Primary prophylaxis may be indicated. Administer in case of febrile neutropenia after dose reduction
See Chapter 43 for more information

Antimicrobial prophylaxis
Risk of fever and neutropenia is INTERMEDIATE
Antimicrobial primary prophylaxis to be considered:

- Antibacterial—consider a fluoroquinolone or no prophylaxis; *P. jirovecii* prophylaxis is recommended (eg, cotrimoxazole)
- Antifungal—consider use during neutropenia and for anticipated mucositis
- Antiviral—not indicated, unless patient previously had an episode of HSV

See Chapter 47 for more information

Treatment Modifications

Toxicity	Dose Modification
Episode of febrile neutropenia	Reduce each chemotherapy dose as follows during subsequent cycles: gemcitabine 800 mg/m^2, vinorelbine, 15 mg/m^2; liposomal doxorubicin 10 mg/m^2
Febrile neutropenia despite dose reduction	Reduce doses of gemcitabine and vinorelbine an additional 25% or add hematopoietic growth factor support
Febrile neutropenia despite a second dose reduction or after the addition of growth factor support	Discontinue chemotherapy
Platelet nadir <20,000/mm^3	Reduce gemcitabine and vinorelbine doses by 25% during subsequent cycles
Day 1 ANC <1200/mm^3 or platelet count <100,000/mm^3	Delay start of next cycle until ANC ≥1200/mm^3 and platelet count ≥100,000/mm^3
Day 8 ANC 500–1199/mm^3 or platelet count 75,000–99,000/mm^3	Reduce day 8 gemcitabine and vinorelbine doses by 25%
Day 8 ANC <500/mm^3 or platelet count <75,000/mm^3	Delay day 8 therapy until ANC ≥500/mm^3 and platelet count ≥75,000/mm^3, then administer day 8 gemcitabine and vinorelbine doses at doses decreased by 25%
Left ventricular ejection fraction <45%	Seek an alternative therapy that does not include liposomal doxorubicin

Patient Population Studied

Phases I/II multicenter trial of 91 patients with refractory or relapsed HL, ages 19–83 years. Both transplant-naïve and patients who had undergone ASCT were enrolled. Patients had not been previously treated with gemcitabine, vinorelbine, or liposomal doxorubicin. This therapy was not considered for patients *in lieu of* SCT

Of 91 patients, 40 had previously undergone ASCT and relapsed. Among transplant-naïve patients ($n = 51$), 79% had received 1 prior regimen, 17% 2 prior regimens, and 4% 3 or more prior regimens. Seventy percent of previously transplanted patients received 3 or more prior regimens. Most patients had chemosensitive disease, among whom 84% (61/73 with available data) had responded to their most recent treatment, including 89% of patients in whom the prior transplant had failed. Eighty-seven percent of patients (67/77 with available data) had previously received ABVD

Efficacy

	No Prior ASCT	Prior ASCT
Complete response	20	18
Partial response	45	59
Stable disease	31	13
Progressive disease	2	0
Indeterminate	2	10

Toxicity

Grade 3–4 Toxic Effects at Maximum Tolerated Dose

Toxicity	Transplant-Naïve (N = 43)		Prior Transplant (N = 37)	
	G3	G4	G3	G4
Blood and Bone Marrow				
ANC	28%	35%	27%	24%
Leucocytes	28%	5%	13%	3%
Hemoglobin	14%	2%	16%	0
Platelets	12%	2%	40%	3%
Constitutional Symptoms				
Fatigue	5%	0	11%	0
Gastrointestinal				
Anorexia	5%	0	0	0
Nausea/vomiting	2%	0	3%	0
Stomatitis/pharyngitis	21%	2%	0	0
Infection and Febrile Neutropenia				
Infection without neutropenia	5%	0	3%	0
Febrile neutropenia	7%	0	8%	3%
Infection (documented clinically)	5%	0	5%	0
Infection with unknown ANC	0	0	3%	0
Pulmonary				
Dyspnea	7%	2%	11%	0
Summary				
Maximum toxicity	44%	40%	54%	27%

Note: Of patients with prior autologous stem cell transplantation, 1 of 37 died

Therapy Monitoring

1. *Semiweekly and before each cycle:* CBC with differential
2. *Before each cycle:* Physical exam
3. *Response evaluation:* Every 2 cycles, CT of all initially involved sites. Bone marrow biopsy if BM involvement before start of therapy

Notes

1. Patients with prior stem cell transplantation received reduced doses of chemotherapy from the outset (**gemcitabine** 800 mg/m^2 per dose; **vinorelbine** 15 mg/m^2 per dose; and **liposomal doxorubicin** 10 mg/m^2 per dose)
2. Of transplant-naïve patients, 80% received high-dose chemotherapy and autologous stem cell transplantation after completion of GVD
3. EFS rate for patients with additional ASCT after GVD is 53%, compared to 50% for patients who did not have a transplant

SALVAGE/INDUCTION REGIMEN HODGKIN LYMPHOMA

DEXAMETHASONE, CARMUSTINE (BCNU), ETOPOSIDE, CYTARABINE (Ara-C), MELPHALAN (Alkeran) (Dexa-BEAM)

Pfreundschuh MG. J Clin Oncol 1994;12:580–586

Dexamethasone 8 mg; administer orally every 8 hours for 10 consecutive days (30 doses) on days 1–10, every 28 days (total dose/cycle = 240 mg)

Carmustine 60 mg/m^2; administer intravenously in 100–250 mL 5% dextrose injection (D5W) over at least 60 minutes on day 2, every 28 days (total dosage/cycle = 60 mg/m^2)

Melphalan 20 mg/m^2; administer intravenously, diluted in 0.9% sodium chloride injection (0.9% NS) to a concentration ≤0.45 mg/mL, over 15–20 minutes on day 3, every 28 days (total dosage/cycle = 20 mg/m^2)

Etoposide 75 mg/m^2 per day; administer intravenously, diluted in 0.9% NS or D5W to a concentration within the range 0.2–0.4 mg/mL, over 1 hour for 4 doses on days 4–7, every 28 days (total dosage/cycle = 300 mg/m^2)

Cytarabine 100 mg/m^2 per dose; administer intravenously in 25–500 mL 0.9% NS or D5W over 2 hours every 12 hours for 8 doses on days 4–7, every 28 days (total dosage/cycle = 800 mg/m^2)

Supportive Care

Antiemetic prophylaxis

Emetogenic potential on Day 2 is **HIGH**

Emetogenic potential on Day 3 is **MODERATE**

Emetogenic potential on Days 4–7 is **LOW**

See Chapter 39 for antiemetic recommendations

Hematopoietic growth factor (CSF) prophylaxis

Primary prophylaxis is indicated with one of the following:

Filgrastim (G-CSF) 5 mcg/kg per day, by subcutaneous injection, or

Pegfilgrastim (pegylated filgrastim) 6 mg/0.6 mL, by subcutaneous injection for one dose

• Begin use 24–72 h after myelosuppressive chemotherapy is completed

See Chapter 43 for more information

Antimicrobial prophylaxis

Risk of fever and neutropenia is INTERMEDIATE

Antimicrobial primary prophylaxis to be considered:

• Antibacterial—consider a fluoroquinolone or no prophylaxis; *P. jirovecii* prophylaxis is recommended (eg, cotrimoxazole)

• Antifungal—consider use during neutropenia and for anticipated mucositis

• Antiviral—antiherpes antivirals (eg, acyclovir)

See Chapter 47 for more information

Steroid-associated gastritis

Add a **proton pump inhibitor** concurrent with steroid use to prevent gastritis and duodenitis

Treatment Modifications

Adverse Event	Dose Modification
WBC <4000/mm^3 or platelet count <125,000/mm^3	Delay start of therapy 1 week, or reduce dosages of carmustine, melphalan, etoposide, and cytarabine by 20%

Toxicity (N = 54)*

Toxicity	% Patients/ Cycles
G3/4 granulocytopenia	92
G3/4 thrombocytopenia	87
Mucositis	21
G3/4 infection	10[†]
Nausea/vomiting	10
Cardiotoxicity	1.9
Psychosis	1.9
Death[‡]	7.5

*WHO Criteria
[†]Ten percent of cycles
[‡]Gram-negative sepsis during neutropenia

Therapy Monitoring

1. *Weekly:* CBC with differential
2. *Before each cycle:* History and physical exam, CBC with differential, chest x-ray
3. *Response evaluation:* Clinical examination, CT of chest, abdomen, and pelvis. FDG-PET scan at conclusion of therapy to document extent of remission. Bone marrow biopsy (if disease existed before therapy) performed 1 cycle after clinical complete response

Patient Population Studied

A study of 55 patients with HL who had received prior therapy with COPP + ABVD or COPP + ABVD + IMEP. Forty-two patients had received radiation as well; 28 patients were at first relapse, 22 were on second salvage, and 5 patients had previously received 3 chemotherapy regimens

Efficacy (N = 54)

Response to Prior Therapy	% Complete Response	% Partial Response
Complete response; relapse >12 months (n = 12)	58	25
Complete response; relapse <12 months (n = 15)	27	33
Progressive disease (n = 27)	22	30
Total (N = 54)	31.5	29.6

SALVAGE/INDUCTION REGIMEN HODGKIN LYMPHOMA

HIGH-DOSE IFOSFAMIDE, ETOPOSIDE AND EPIRUBICIN (IVE)

Proctor SJ et al. Ann Oncol 2003;14:i47–i50

Anticonvulsant prophylaxis:
Phenytoin 300 mg/day; administer orally for 6 consecutive days, from day −1 (1 day before chemotherapy begins) through day 5, every 21 days (total dose/cycle = 1800 mg)
Epirubicin 50 mg/m²; administer by intravenous injection over 3–5 minutes on day 1, every 21 days, for a maximum of 3 cycles (total dosage/cycle = 50 mg/m²)
Etoposide 200 mg/m² per day; administer intravenously, diluted in 0.9% sodium chloride injection (0.9% NS) to a concentration within the range of 0.2–0.4 mg/mL, over 60 minutes for 3 consecutive days, days 1–3, every 21 days, for a maximum of 3 cycles (total dosage/cycle = 600 mg/m²)
Ifosfamide 3000 mg/m² per day; administer intravenously, diluted in 0.9% NS or 5% dextrose injection (D5W) to a concentration within the range 0.6 to 20 mg/mL, over 22 hours on 3 consecutive days, days 1–3, every 21 days for a maximum of 3 cycles (total dosage/cycle = 9000 mg/m²)
Mesna 1800 mg/m²; administer intravenously in 10–50 mL 0.9% NS or D5W over 15 minutes on day 1 just before starting ifosfamide administration, every 21 days, then:
Mesna 3000 mg/m² per day; administer intravenously, diluted in 25–1000 mL 0.9% NS or D5W over 22 hours, for 3 consecutive days, days 1–3, every 21 days, for a maximum of 3 cycles (total dosage/cycle = 9000 mg/m²), *followed on day 3 by*
Mesna 1636 mg/m²; administer intravenously in 50–1000 mL 0.9% NS or D5W over 12 hours on day 3, after ifosfamide administration is completed, every 21 days (total mesna dosage/cycle = 12,436 mg/m²)
- Mesna administered by prolonged infusion over 22 hours at the same time as ifosfamide may be prepared conveniently as an admixture (in the same container) with ifosfamide
- Proctor et al. did not identify the amount of mesna they gave after ifosfamide administration was completed. The amount of mesna identified for administration on day 3 after ifosfamide administration is completed is calculated from the amount of mesna given within a 12-hour interval during continuous ifosfamide administration over 22 hours

Note: Hematopoietic growth factor support is not routinely given as primary prophylaxis

Supportive Care
Antiemetic prophylaxis
Emetogenic potential on day 1 is **HIGH**
Emetogenic potential on days 2 and 3 is **MODERATE**
See Chapter 39 for antiemetic recommendations

Hematopoietic growth factor (CSF) prophylaxis
Primary prophylaxis may be indicated
See Chapter 43 for more information

Antimicrobial prophylaxis
Risk of fever and neutropenia is INTERMEDIATE
Antimicrobial primary prophylaxis to be considered:
- Antibacterial—consider a fluoroquinolone or no prophylaxis; *P. jirovecii* prophylaxis is recommended (eg, cotrimoxazole)
- Antifungal—consider use during neutropenia
- Antiviral—antiherpes antivirals (eg, acyclovir)

See Chapter 47 for more information

Patient Population Studied

Phase II multicenter trial, 51 patients with refractory or relapsed HL, ages 16–53 years. The majority of patients were treated following a first relapse. Disease histologies included lymphocyte predominant (*n* = 4), mixed cellularity (*n* = 8), and nodular sclerosing subtypes (*n* = 39)

Treatment Modifications

None specified as part of this regimen. Often used as a preparative regimen for hematopoietic stem cell transplantation

Efficacy

Response	Percent of Patients
Complete response	61
Partial response	22
SD or progression	16

Overall Survival According to Response to Prior Therapy

<PR to primary therapy	8 months
PR to primary therapy	24 months
CR to primary therapy; first relapse	Not reached
CR to primary therapy; second relapse	46 months
CR to primary therapy; second relapse	18 months

Toxicity

Toxicity	Frequency
G4 hematologic toxicity	100% of patients
G3 infections	10% of all courses
Neurotoxicity	2% of patients
Treatment-related deaths	0

Therapy Monitoring

1. *Semi-weekly and before each cycle:* CBC with differential
2. *Before each cycle:* Physical exam
3. *Response evaluation after 3 cycles:* CT scan, and bone marrow biopsy if BM-involvement before start of therapy

Notes

Often used as a preparative regimen; 61% of the patients proceeded to high-dose chemotherapy and autologous stem cell transplantation

HIGH DOSE/CONDITIONING REGIMEN (PRETRANSPLANTATION)

CARMUSTINE (BCNU) + ETOPOSIDE + CYTARABINE (Ara-C) + MELPHALAN (BEAM)

Schmitz N et al. Lancet 2002;359:2065–2071

Carmustine 300 mg/m²; administer intravenously in 100–500 mL 5% dextrose injection (D5W) over at least 60 minutes on day −7 (total dosage = 300 mg/m²)
Etoposide 150 mg/m² per dose; administer intravenously, diluted in 0.9% sodium chloride injection (0.9% NS) to a concentration within the range of 0.2–0.4 mg/mL, over 60 minutes every 12 hours for 4 consecutive days (8 doses) on days −7 to −4 (total dosage = 1200 mg/m²)
Cytarabine 200 mg/m² per dose; administer intravenously in 25–1000 mL 0.9% NS or D5W over 30 minutes every 12 hours for 4 consecutive days (8 doses) on days −7 to −4 (total dosage = 1600 mg/m²)
Melphalan 140 mg/m²; administer intravenously, diluted in 0.9% NS to a concentration ≤0.45 mg/mL, over 15–20 minutes on day −3 (total dosage = 140 mg/m²)

Note: Hematopoietic stem cell transplantation (**HSCT**) occurs on **day 0**. See notes at end of this regimen

Supportive Care
Antiemetic prophylaxis
Emetogenic potential on day −7 is **HIGH**
Emetogenic potential on days −6, −5, and −4 is **LOW**
Emetogenic potential on day −3 is **MODERATE**
See Chapter 39 for antiemetic recommendations

Hematopoietic growth factor (CSF) prophylaxis
Primary prophylaxis is indicated with one of the following:
Filgrastim (G-CSF) 10 mcg/kg per day by subcutaneous injection, *or*
Sargramostim (GM-CSF) 250 mcg/m² per day by subcutaneous injection
- Begin use on day 0 (after cryopreserved hematopoietic progenitor cells are administered, and continue until leukocyte counts recover)
See Chapter 43 for more information

Antimicrobial prophylaxis
Risk of fever and neutropenia is HIGH
Antimicrobial primary prophylaxis is recommended:
- Antibacterial—consider fluoroquinolone prophylaxis; *P. jirovecii* prophylaxis is recommended (eg, cotrimoxazole)
- Antifungal—recommended
- Antiviral—antiherpes antivirals (eg, acyclovir)
See Chapter 47 for more information

Treatment Modifications

None specified as part of this preparative regimen

Patient Population Studied

Phase III multicenter trial in patients with relapsed Hodgkin disease. Comparison of high-dose chemotherapy followed by transplantation of autologous hemopoietic stem cells (BEAM-HSCT) with conventional aggressive chemotherapy without stem cell transplantation (Dexa-BEAM). Included 61 patients with chemosensitive relapse after treatment for advanced stage HL; age range: 21–57 years; treated with BEAM

Efficacy

3 Months After End of Treatment (N = 61)

Response	Percent
Unconfirmed complete response	85
Partial response	5
Failure	8
Died of complications	2 (1 patient)

3 Years After End of Treatment (N = 61)

	% FFTF	% OS
All patients (N = 61)	55	71
Early relapse (N = 21)	41	43
Late relapse (N = 29)	75	93
Multiple relapses (N = 11)	34	70

FFTF, Freedom from treatment failure; OS, overall survival

Therapy Monitoring

Intensive in-hospital monitoring

Notes

1. Preparative regimen for HSCT
2. Patients assigned **BEAM**-HSCT underwent high-dose chemotherapy (2 cycles of Dexa-BEAM) followed by transplantation of either autologous bone marrow or peripheral-blood-progenitor cells
3. **BEAM** was started 4 weeks after white blood cell count returned to normal after 2 cycles of Dexa-BEAM
4. Cryopreserved bone-marrow or peripheral-blood progenitor cells were infused on day 0 followed by granulocyte-colony-stimulating factor until leucocyte recovery
5. Bone-marrow or progenitor cells were harvested after the first or second course of Dexa-BEAM. Only patients who had complete or partial remission after 2 courses of Dexa-BEAM continued treatment. These patients were considered "chemosensitive"
6. Involved-field radiotherapy was recommended for all patients with residual lesions judged to represent active Hodgkin disease

Toxicity (N = 51)

Toxicity	% WHO G3/4
Infection	47
Oral (mucositis)	37
Gastrointestinal	14
Pulmonary or respiratory	4
Cardiac	2
Neurologic	2

HIGH DOSE/CONDITIONING REGIMEN (PRETRANSPLANTATION)

CYCLOPHOSPHAMIDE, CARMUSTINE (BCNU), ETOPOSIDE (VP-16) (CBV)

Jagannath S et al. J Clin Oncol 1989;7:179–185

Note: Treatment days are enumerated with respect to autologous hematopoietic stem cell transplantation (HSCT), in which the autologous graft is readministered on day zero
Carmustine 300 mg/m²; administer intravenously in 100–500 mL 5% dextrose injection (D5W) over at least 60 minutes on day −6 (total dosage = 300 mg/m²)
Cyclophosphamide 1500 mg/m² per day; administer intravenously in 100–1000 mL 0.9% sodium chloride injection (0.9% NS) or D5W over 30–60 minutes for 4 consecutive days on days −6, −5, −4, and −3 (total dosage = 6000 mg/m²)
Etoposide 125 mg/m² per dose; administer intravenously, diluted in 0.9% NS to a concentration within the range 0.2–0.4 mg/mL, over 1 hour every 12 hours for 6 doses on days −6, −5, and −4 (total dosage = 750 mg/m²)
Autologous BMT/HSCT is administered on day zero

Supportive Care
Antiemetic prophylaxis
Emetogenic potential on Days −6, −5, −4, and −3 is **HIGH**
See Chapter 39 for antiemetic recommendations

Hematopoietic growth factor (CSF) prophylaxis
Primary prophylaxis is indicated with one of the following:
  Filgrastim (G-CSF) 5 mcg/kg per day, by subcutaneous injection, or
  Sargramostim (GM-CSF) 250 mcg/m² per day, by subcutaneous injection
  • Begin use 24–72 h after myelosuppressive chemotherapy is completed (or transplant day 0)
See Chapter 43 for more information

Antimicrobial prophylaxis
Risk of fever and neutropenia is HIGH
Antimicrobial primary prophylaxis is recommended:
  • Antibacterial—consider fluoroquinolone prophylaxis; *P. jirovecii* prophylaxis is recommended (eg, cotrimoxazole)
  • Antifungal—recommended
  • Antiviral—Ganciclovir 5 mg/kg; administer intravenously every 12 hours for 10 consecutive days (adjust dose for renal insufficiency) on days 1–10 after transplantation
See Chapters 47 and 50 for more information

Treatment Modifications

None specified as part of this preparative regimen

Toxicity (N = 61)

	% of Patients
Nausea/vomiting	89
Severe mucositis	27
Hematuria	13.1
Seizures	3.3
Congestive heart failure	1.6
Febrile neutropenia	>90
Death*	6.6
Median time to ANC >500/mm³	22 days
Median time to platelets >50,000/mm³	26 days

*Candidemia in 2 patients; pulmonary fibrosis in 2 patients; all had received a cumulative etoposide dosage of 900 mg/m²

Therapy Monitoring

Intensive in-hospital monitoring. See Chapter 50, *Complications and Follow-up After Hematopoietic Stem Cell Transplantation*, for additional information

Patient Population Studied

A study of 61 patients with relapsed HL. Median age 28 years (range: 15–56 years). Median time from diagnosis to BMT 35 months (range: 6–11 months). Marrow stored an average of 1 month (range: 1–113 weeks) before transplantation. Zubrod performance status: 0 (n = 35), 1 (n = 18), 2 (n = 6), and 3 (n = 2). Disease staging: stage I (n = 5), stage II (n = 11), stage III (n = 6), and stage IV (n = 37), with 2 patients intensified in third complete response. Twenty-one patients had nodal disease only; 38 also had extranodal disease, including lung (n = 23), pleura (n = 7), bone (n = 5), and liver (n = 3)

Efficacy (N = 59)

	%	Median Survival
Complete response	46	>30 months
Partial response*	31	15 months
No response	23	2.7 months
All patients		30 months

*Six of 18 patients with partial response achieved complete response after radiation therapy to local sites

PALLIATIVE REGIMEN
RELAPSED OR REFRACTORY
HODGKIN LYMPHOMA
BRENTUXIMAB VEDOTIN

Younes A et al. J Clin Oncol 2012;30:2183–2189

Brentuximab vedotin 1.8 mg/kg (maximum dose = 180 mg); administer intravenously in a volume of 0.9% sodium chloride injection or 5% dextrose injection sufficient to produce a concentration with the range 0.4–1.8 mg/mL (minimum volume, 100 mL) over 30 minutes on day 1, every 3 weeks for up to 16 doses (total dosage/cycle = 1.8 mg/kg; maximum dose/cycle = 180 mg)

Notes:
- The dose for patients whose body weight is >100 kg should be calculated based on a weight of 100 kg (maximum single dose = 180 mg)
- The recommended starting dose in patients with severe renal impairment (creatinine clearance <30 mL/min [<0.5 mL/s]) is 1.2 mg/kg intravenously over 30 minutes every 3 weeks
- The recommended starting dose in patients with hepatic impairment is 1.2 mg/kg intravenously over 30 minutes every 3 weeks
- Do not administer brentuximab vedotin as an intravenous injection or more rapidly than over 30 minutes

Supportive Care
Antiemetic prophylaxis
Emetogenic potential is **LOW**
See Chapter 39 for antiemetic recommendations

Hematopoietic growth factor (CSF) prophylaxis
Primary prophylaxis is indicated with one of the following:
 Filgrastim (G-CSF) 5 mcg/kg per day, by subcutaneous injection, *or*
 Pegfilgrastim (pegylated filgrastim) 6 mg/0.6 mL, by subcutaneous injection for 1 dose
- Begin use from 24–72 hours after myelosuppressive chemotherapy is completed
- Continue daily filgrastim use until ANC ≥10,000/mm^3 on 2 measurements separated temporally by ≥12 hours
- Discontinue daily filgrastim use at least 24 hours before administering myelosuppressive treatment. Do not administer pegfilgrastim within 14 days before administering myelosuppressive treatment
See Chapter 43 for more information

Antimicrobial prophylaxis
Risk of fever and neutropenia is LOW
 Antimicrobial primary prophylaxis to be considered:
- Antibacterial—not indicated
- Antifungal—not indicated
- Antiviral—not indicated unless patient previously had an episode of HSV
See Chapter 47 for more information

Diarrhea management
 Loperamide 4 mg orally initially after the first loose or liquid stool, *then*
 Loperamide 2 mg orally every 2 hours during waking hours, *plus*
 Loperamide 4 mg orally every 4 hours during hours of sleep
- Continue for at least 12 hours after diarrhea resolves
- Recurrent diarrhea after a 12-hour diarrhea-free interval is treated as a new episode
- Rehydrate orally with fluids and electrolytes during a diarrheal episode
- If a patient develops blood or mucus in stool, dehydration, or hemodynamic instability, or if diarrhea persists >48 hours despite loperamide, stop loperamide and hospitalize the patient for IV hydration
Alternatively, a trial of **Diphenoxylate hydrochloride** 2.5 mg **with Atropine sulfate** 0.025 mg (eg, Lomotil)
- Initial adult dose is 2 tablets 4 times daily until control has been achieved, after which the dose may be reduced to meet individual requirements. Control may often be maintained with as little as 2 tablets daily
- Clinical improvement of acute diarrhea is usually observed within 48 hours. If improvement of chronic diarrhea after treatment with a maximum daily dose of 8 tablets is not observed within 10 days, control is unlikely with further administration

Treatment Modification

Adverse Event	Dose Modification
New or worsening G2/3 peripheral neuropathy	Hold brentuximab vedotin until neuropathy improves to G <1 or baseline, and then, restart at 1.2 mg/kg
G4 peripheral neuropathy	Discontinue brentuximab vedotin
G3/4 neutropenia	Hold brentuximab vedotin until neutropenia improves to G ≤2 or baseline. Consider filgrastim support
Recurrent G4 neutropenia despite the use of filgrastim (or another G-CSF)	Discontinue brentuximab vedotin or hold until neutropenia resolves, and then, restart at 1.2 mg/kg

Patient Population Studied

Patients with relapsed or refractory HL after high-dose chemotherapy and auto-SCT with histologically documented CD30-positive Hodgkin Reed-Sternberg cells. Patients could not have previously received allogeneic stem-cell transplantation (SCT)

Demographics and Baseline Clinical Characteristics

Demographic or Clinical Characteristic	Patients	
	Number	Percent
Age, median (range)	31 years (15–77 years)	
Sex, male-to-female ratio	48/54	47/53
Race		
Asian	7	7
Black or African American	5	5
White	89	87
Other	1	1
ECOG performance status		
0	42	41
1	60	59
Baseline "B" symptoms	35	34
Bone marrow involvement	8	8
Prior radiation	67	66
Prior chemotherapy regimens, median (range)	3.5 (1–13)	
Primary refractory disease*	72	71
Disease status relative to most recent prior therapy[†]		
Relapsed[†]	59	58
Refractory[†]	43	42
Best response with most recent systemic regimen		
Complete response	12	12
Partial response	35	34
Stable disease	23	23
Progressive disease	26	25
Unknown/other	6	6
Number of prior auto-SCT		
1	91	89
2	11	11
Months from auto-SCT to first posttransplantation relapse[‡]	6.7 (0–131)	
Months from initial diagnosis to first dose of study drug[‡]	39.9 (11.8–219.7)	

auto-SCT, autologous stem-cell transplantation; ECOG, Eastern Cooperative Oncology Group
*Primary refractory disease = failure to obtain a CR with front-line therapy or relapse within 3 months of front-line therapy
[†]Relapsed indicates best response of CR or PR to most recent prior therapy, and refractory indicates best response of SD or PD to most recent prior therapy
[‡]Median (range)

Efficacy (N = 102)

	Patients	
	Number	Percent
Objective response	76	75
Complete remission	35	34
Partial remission	41	40
Stable disease	22	22
Progressive disease	3	3
Not evaluable	1	1

	Median (95% CI)
Duration of objective response, months	6.7 (3.6–14.8)
Duration of response for patients with CR, months	20.5 (10.8–NE)
Progression-free survival, months	5.6 (5.0–9.0)
Overall survival, months	22.4 (21.7–NE)

NE, not estimable

Therapy Monitoring

1. *Every 3 weeks:* CBC with differential
2. *Every 3 weeks:* Physical exam, chest x-ray
3. *Response evaluation:* CT of chest, abdomen, and pelvis every 2 cycles starting after 6 weeks

Toxicity

Drug-Related Adverse Events Reported by >10% of Patients and G3/4 Incidence of These Events Regardless of Relationship to Brentuximab Vedotin

Adverse Event	Events Related to Brentuximab Vedotin (any G)		Any G3 Events		Any G4 Events	
	Patients					
	Number	Percent	Number	Percent	Number	Percent
Peripheral sensory neuropathy	43	42	8	8	0	0
Nausea	36	35	0	0	0	0
Fatigue	35	34	2	2	0	0
Neutropenia	19	19	14	14	6	6
Diarrhea	18	18	1	1	0	0
Pyrexia	14	14	2	2	0	0
Vomiting	13	13	0	0	0	0
Arthralgia	12	12	0	0	0	0
Pruritus	12	12	0	0	0	0
Myalgia	11	11	0	0	0	0
Peripheral motor neuropathy	11	11	1	1	0	0
Alopecia	10	10	0	0	0	0

PALLIATIVE REGIMEN HODGKIN LYMPHOMA

GEMCITABINE

Venkatesh H et al. Clin Lymphoma 2004;5:110–115

Gemcitabine 1000 mg/m^2 per dose; administer intravenously, diluted with 0.9% sodium chloride injection to a concentration as low as 0.1 mg/mL, over 30 minutes for 2 doses on days 1 and 8, every 3 weeks (total dosage/cycle = 2000 mg/m^2)

Supportive Care
Antiemetic prophylaxis
Emetogenic potential on Day 1 is **LOW**
See Chapter 39 for antiemetic recommendations

Hematopoietic growth factor (CSF) prophylaxis
Primary prophylaxis is NOT indicated
See Chapter 43 for more information

Antimicrobial prophylaxis
Risk of fever and neutropenia is LOW
  Antimicrobial primary prophylaxis to be considered:
  • Antibacterial—*P. jirovecii* prophylaxis is recommended (eg, cotrimoxazole)
  • Antifungal—not indicated
  • Antiviral—not indicated, unless patient previously had an episode of HSV
See Chapter 47 for more information

Efficacy (N = 27)

Complete response	0%
Partial response	22%
Median duration of partial response	5.1 months (range: 2.3–19.3 months)

Toxicity (N = 27)

Toxicity	% G3	% G4
Hematologic (1000 mg/m^2; N = 19)		
Anemia	5.3	—
Leukopenia	10.5	—
Neutropenia	21.1	—
Thrombocytopenia	—	10.5
Neutropenia and fever	5.3	—
Hematologic (1250 mg/m^2; N = 8)		
Anemia	12.5	—
Leukopenia	25	—
Neutropenia	37.5	12.5
Thrombocytopenia	75	12.5
Neutropenia and fever	—	—

Treatment Modifications

Adverse Event	Dose Modification
WBC <3500/mm^3, ANC <1500/mm^3, or platelet count <100,000/mm^3	Delay treatment until WBC >3500/mm^3, ANC >1500/mm^3, and platelet count >100,000/mm^3

Patient Population Studied

A study of 29 patients with relapsed HL. All patients had received at least 2 (range: 2–7) prior regimens for HL; 62% experienced a relapse after autologous BMT. Performance status among patients Eastern Cooperative Oncology Group (ECOG) was 0 (41.4%), 1 (48.3%), and 2 (10.3%)

Therapy Monitoring

1. *Weekly:* CBC with differential
2. *Every 2–3 cycles:* History and physical exam, chest x-ray
3. *Response evaluation:* Every 3 cycles, CT of chest, abdomen, and pelvis. FDG-PET scan at conclusion of therapy to document extent of remission

Notes

Gemcitabine has been increasingly used for the treatment of refractory or relapsed HL, either alone or in combination with other drugs such as cisplatin or dexamethasone. Gemcitabine doses usually range between 1000 and 1250 mg/m^2 given weekly 2 or 3 times per 21- or 28-day cycle

PALLIATIVE REGIMEN HODGKIN LYMPHOMA

VINORELBINE

Devizzi L et al. Ann Oncol 1994;5:817–820

Vinorelbine 30 mg/m^2 per dose; administer intravenously, diluted in a volume of 0.9% sodium chloride injection or 5% dextrose injection sufficient to produce a solution with a concentration within the range 1.5–3 mg/mL, over 6–10 minutes every week for 4 consecutive weeks (total dosage/cycle = 120 mg/m^2)

Supportive Care
Antiemetic prophylaxis
Emetogenic potential on Day 1 is **MINIMAL**
See Chapter 39 for antiemetic recommendations

Hematopoietic growth factor (CSF) prophylaxis
Primary prophylaxis is NOT indicated
See Chapter 43 for more information

Antimicrobial prophylaxis
Risk of fever and neutropenia is LOW
  Antimicrobial primary prophylaxis to be considered:
  • Antibacterial—*P. jirovecii* prophylaxis is recommended (eg, cotrimoxazole)
  • Antifungal—not indicated
  • Antiviral—not indicated, unless patient previously had an episode of HSV
See Chapter 47 for more information

Treatment Modifications

Adverse Event	Dose Modification
WBC <3500/mm^3, ANC <1500/mm^3, or platelet count <100,000/mm^3	Delay treatment until WBC >3500/mm^3, ANC >1500/mm^3, and platelet count >100,000/mm^3

Therapy Monitoring

1. *Weekly:* CBC with differential
2. *Every 4 weeks:* Physical exam, chest x-ray
3. *Response evaluation:* Every 4–8 courses, CT of chest, abdomen, and pelvis. FDG-PET scan at conclusion of therapy to document extent of remission. Bone marrow biopsy (if disease existed before therapy) performed 1 cycle after clinical complete response

Patient Population Studied

A study of 24 patients who had received at least 2 (range: 2–7) prior regimens for HL, consisting of MOPP and ABVD given sequentially or in alternation, followed by various salvage regimens, including autologous BMT in 4 cases. All patients had been previously treated with at least 2 vinca alkaloids. Fifteen patients had undergone extensive radiation therapy

Efficacy (N = 22)

No. of Prior Regimens	% Complete Response	% Partial Response
<3 (n = 4)	25	—
≥3 (n = 18)	11	44
Total (N = 22)	14	36

Toxicity (N = 23)*

	% G1	% G2	% G3	% G4
Leukopenia	9	26	52	9
Granulocytopenia	13	30	44	9
Thrombocytopenia	4	0	0	4
Anemia	39	22	4	4
Alopecia	—	—	4	—
Injection site reaction	—	—	22	—
Stomatitis	—	9	—	—
Infection	—	9	13	—
Fever	9	39	—	—
Constipation	—	9	4	—
Peripheral neuropathy	48	13	—	—

*NCI CTC, National Cancer Institute (USA) Common Toxicity Criteria, version 2.0. Available at: http://ctep.cancer.gov/protocolDevelopment/electronic_applications/ctc.htm [accessed December 7, 2013]

PALLIATIVE REGIMEN
RELAPSED OR REFRACTORY
HODGKIN LYMPHOMA

BENDAMUSTINE HCl

Moskowitz AJ et al. J Clin Oncol 2012;31:456–460

Bendamustine HCl 120 mg/m^2 per dose; administer intravenously in a volume of 0.9% sodium chloride injection sufficient to produce a concentration with the range 0.2–0.6 mg/mL over 60 minutes, on 2 consecutive days, days 1 and 2, every 28 days for a total of 6 cycles (total dosage/cycle = 240 mg/m^2)

Supportive Care
Antiemetic prophylaxis
Emetogenic potential is **MODERATE**
See Chapter 39 for antiemetic recommendations

Hematopoietic growth factor (CSF) prophylaxis
Primary prophylaxis may be indicated
Note: Growth factor support with pegfilgrastim or filgrastim was administered with each cycle of treatment
See Chapter 43 for more information

Antimicrobial prophylaxis
Risk of fever and neutropenia is LOW
  Antimicrobial primary prophylaxis to be considered:
  • Antibacterial—not indicated
  • Antifungal—not indicated
  • Antiviral—not indicated, unless patient previously had an episode of HSV
See Chapter 47 for more information

Diarrhea management
  Loperamide 4 mg orally initially after the first loose or liquid stool, *then*
  Loperamide 2 mg orally every 2 hours during waking hours, *plus*
  Loperamide 4 mg orally every 4 hours during hours of sleep
  • Continue for at least 12 hours after diarrhea resolves
  • Recurrent diarrhea after a 12-hour diarrhea-free interval is treated as a new episode
  • Rehydrate orally with fluids and electrolytes during a diarrheal episode
  • If a patient develops blood or mucus in stool, dehydration, or hemodynamic instability, or if diarrhea persists >48 hours despite loperamide, stop loperamide and hospitalize the patient for IV hydration
  Alternatively, a trial of **Diphenoxylate hydrochloride** 2.5 mg **with Atropine sulfate** 0.025 mg (eg, Lomotil)
  • Initial adult dose is 2 tablets 4 times daily until control has been achieved, after which the dose may be reduced to meet individual requirements. Control may often be maintained with as little as 2 tablets daily
  • Clinical improvement of acute diarrhea is usually observed within 48 hours. If improvement of chronic diarrhea after treatment with a maximum daily dose of 8 tablets is not observed within 10 days, control is unlikely with further administration

Patient Population Studied

Patients with biopsy-confirmed relapsed/refractory classical Hodgkin lymphoma (HL) were eligible. Failure of ASCT or ineligibility for ASCT was required. Previous alloSCT was allowed if relapse was >6 months after transplantation

Patient Demographic and Clinical Characteristics (N = 36)

Characteristic		
Age, median (range)	34 yrs (21–75 yrs)	
Sex, male (%)/ female (%)	13 (36)/23 (64)	
Number of prior therapies, median (range)	4 (1–17)	
Response to last chemotherapy, sensitive (%)/resistant (%)	18 (50)/18 (50)	

	Patients	
	Number	Percent
History of autologous transplantation	27	75
Relapse ≤3 months after autologous transplantation	5	—
Relapse >3 months after autologous transplantation	22	—
History of allogeneic transplantation	6	17
Disease extent at enrollment		
Nodal only	11	31
Extranodal	25	69
B symptoms at enrollment	7	19

Efficacy

Parameter	N	CR #	CR %	PR #	PR %	ORR #	ORR %	P*
Response by intention to treat	36	12	33	7	19	19	53	
Response for evaluable patients	34†	12	35	7	21	19	56	
Median number of prior therapies								
<4 prior therapies	16	6	38	3	19	9	56	1.0
≥4 prior therapies	18	6	33	4	22	10	55	
Response to last chemotherapy								
Sensitive	16	9	56	2	13	11	69	0.185
Resistant	18	3	17	5	28	8	45	
Previous ASCT	26	10	38	5	19	15	57	
Relapsed within 3 months after ASCT	5	0	0	0	0	0	0	0.011
Previous alloSCT	6	2	33	2	33	4	66	0.672

alloSCT, allogeneic stem-cell transplantation; ASCT, autologous stem-cell transplantation; CR, complete response; ORR, overall response rate (CR + PR); PR, partial response
*Fisher's exact test
†Two patients could not be evaluated: 1 died in a motor vehicle accident; 1 withdrew consent after 1 cycle. Both had clinical evidence of response to treatment

Toxicity

Adverse Events in ≥5% of Patients

Toxicity	Total (%)	% G1	% G2	% G3	% G4
Hematologic					
Thrombocytopenia	50	17	14	17	3
Anemia*	14			14	
Neutropenia	8			8	
Nonhematologic					
Fatigue	84	64	17	3	
Nausea	50	42	6	3	
Cough	22	22			
Vomiting	22	14	8		
Dyspnea	19	19			
Diarrhea	17	17			
Fever	11	8		3	
Pneumonia	11			8	3
Respiratory infection	9	6		3	
Constipation	8	8			
Mucositis	6	6			
Febrile neutropenia	6			6	
Hematuria	6	3		3	

*Only G3 and G4 reported

Treatment Modification

Adverse Event	Treatment Modification
ANC <1000/mm³ and/or platelet count <75,000/mm³ on day 1 of a cycle	Hold bendamustine until ANC ≥1000/mm³ and platelet count ≥75,000/mm³. If start is delayed by >5 days, reduce the bendamustine dosage to 90–100 mg/m²
ANC <1,000/mm³ and/or platelet count <75,000/mm³ on day 1 of a cycle after bendamustine 90–100 mg/m² in previous cycle	Hold bendamustine until ANC ≥1000/mm³ and platelet count ≥75,000/mm³. If start is delayed by >5 days reduce the bendamustine dose to 60–70 mg/m²
ANC <1000/mm³ and/or platelet count <75,000/mm³ on day 1 of a cycle that does not resolve within 21 days	Discontinue bendamustine
Clinically significant G ≥2 nonhematologic toxicity	Hold bendamustine until nonhematologic toxicity has recovered to G ≤1. If toxicity was G ≥3 reduce the bendamustine dose to 90–100 mg/m² in subsequent cycles
Clinically significant G ≥2 nonhematologic toxicity after bendamustine 90–100 mg/m² in previous cycle	Hold bendamustine until nonhematologic toxicity has recovered to G ≤1. If toxicity was G ≥3, reduce the bendamustine dose to 60–70 mg/m² in subsequent cycles

Treatment Monitoring

1. *Baseline assessment:* Computed tomography of the chest, abdomen, and pelvis, [18F] fluorodeoxyglucose–positron emission tomography (FDG-PET) scan, and bone marrow biopsy within 28 days before beginning treatment
2. *Twice weekly and before each cycle:* CBC with differential
3. *Before each cycle:* Physical exam, chest x-ray
4. *Response evaluation:* CT of chest, abdomen, and pelvis every 2 cycles starting after cycle 4. FDG-PET scan at conclusion of therapy to document extent of remission
5. Bone marrow biopsy to document response (if disease existed before therapy)

24. Lymphoma, Non-Hodgkin

Carla Casulo, MD, Julia Schaefer-Cutillo, MD, Jonathan W. Friedberg, MD, MMSc and Richard Fisher, MD

Epidemiology

Incidence: 70,800 (male: 38,270; female: 32,530. Estimated new cases for 2014 in the United States)
23.9 per 100,000 male, 16.4 per 100,000 female

Deaths: Estimated 18,990 in 2014
(male: 10,470; female: 8,520)

Median age: 66 years

Male to female ratio: 1.5 to 1.6 for all lymphoid neoplasms

Siegel R et al. CA Cancer J Clin 2013;63:11–30
Surveillance, Epidemiology and End Results (SEER) Program, available from http://seer.cancer.gov (accessed in 2013)

Pathology (WHO 2008)

AIDS-related lymphoma

Primary cutaneous CD30 positive T-cell lymphoproliferative disorders
• Lymphomatoid papulosis
• Primary cutaneous anaplastic large cell lymphoma
• Primary cutaneous peripheral T-cell lymphoma

Cutaneous B-cell lymphoma
• Primary marginal zone
• Follicular center
• Primary cutaneous diffuse large B-cell lymphoma of leg
• Primary cutaneous diffuse large B-cell lymphoma, other

2008 WHO Classification of Lymphomas

Precursor Lymphoid Neoplasms
• B lymphoblastic leukemia/lymphoma NOS
• B lymphoblastic leukemia/lymphoma with recurrent genetic abnormalities
• B lymphoblastic leukemia/lymphoma with t(9;22); bcr-abl1
• B lymphoblastic leukemia/lymphoma with t(v;11q23); MLL rearranged
• B lymphoblastic leukemia/lymphoma with t(12;21); TEL-AML1 and ETV6-RUNX1
• B lymphoblastic leukemia/lymphoma with hyperploidy
• B lymphoblastic leukemia/lymphoma with hypodiploidy
• B lymphoblastic leukemia/lymphoma with t(5;14); IL3-IGH
• B lymphoblastic leukemia/lymphoma with t(1;19); E2A-PBX1 and TCF3-PBX1
• T lymphoblastic leukemia/lymphoma

Mature B-Cell Neoplasms
• Chronic lymphocytic leukemia/small lymphocytic lymphoma
• B-cell prolymphocytic leukemia
• Splenic marginal zone lymphoma
• Hairy cell leukemia

(continued)

Work-up

1. Immunophenotyping
2. Cytogenetics for CLL/SLL and Burkitt lymphoma
3. PET scan
   Aggressive histology
   • PET scan recommended before and after treatment, mid cycle only appropriate in clinical trial setting
   • Also indicated for relapsed indolent disease when suspect aggressive transformation

Seam P et al. Blood 2007;110:3507–3516

CNS lymphomas (non–HIV-related; additional staging work-up recommended)

1. Slit-lamp exam by ophthalmologist
2. HIV testing
3. Lumbar puncture
4. Brain and spine MRI
5. Testicular exam in men

Staging

Ann Arbor Staging Classification for Hodgkin and Non-Hodgkin Lymphomas

Stage	Description
I	Involvement of a single lymph node region (I) or involvement of a single extralymphatic organ or site (IE)
II	Involvement of ≥2 lymph node regions or lymphatic structures on the same side of the diaphragm alone (II) or with involvement of limited, contiguous extralymphatic organ or tissue (IIE)
III	Involvement of lymph node regions on both sides of the diaphragm (III), which may include the spleen (IIIS) or limited, contiguous extralymphatic organ or site (IIIE) or both (IIIES)
IV	Diffuse or disseminated foci of involvement of one or more extralymphatic organs or tissues, with or without associated lymphatic involvement

(continued)

Pathology (WHO 2008) *(continued)*

- Lymphoplasmacytic lymphoma/Waldenström's macroglobulinemia
- Heavy-chain disease
- Plasma cell myeloma
- Solitary plasmacytoma of bone
- Extraosseous plasmacytoma
- Extranodal marginal zone B-cell lymphoma of mucosa-associated lymphoid tissue (MALT) type
- Nodal marginal zone lymphoma
- Follicular lymphoma
- Primary cutaneous follicular lymphoma
- Mantle cell lymphoma
- Diffuse large B-cell lymphoma, NOS
  - T-cell/histiocyte-rich large B-cell lymphoma
  - EBV+ DLBCL of the elderly
  - Diffuse large B-cell lymphoma associated with chronic inflammation
  - Lymphomatoid granulomatosis
- Primary CNS type
- Primary leg skin type
- Primary mediastinal large B-cell lymphoma
- Intravascular large B-cell lymphoma
- ALK+ large B-cell lymphoma
- Plasmablastic lymphoma
- Large B-cell lymphoma associated with HHV8+ Castleman disease
- Primary effusion lymphoma
- Burkitt lymphoma
- B-cell lymphoma, unclassifiable, Burkitt-like
- B-cell lymphoma, unclassifiable, Hodgkin lymphoma-like

Mature T-Cell and NK-Cell Neoplasms
- T-cell prolymphocytic leukemia
- T-cell large granular lymphocytic leukemia
- Chronic lymphoproliferative disorder of NK-cells
- Aggressive NK-cell leukemia
- Systemic EBV+ T-cell lymphoproliferative disorder of childhood
- Hydroa vacciniforme-like lymphoma
- Adult T-cell lymphoma/leukemia
- Extranodal T-cell/NK-cell lymphoma, nasal type
- Enteropathy-associated T-cell lymphoma
- Hepatosplenic T-cell lymphoma
- Subcutaneous panniculitis-like T-cell lymphoma
- Mycosis fungoides
- Sézary syndrome
- Primary cutaneous CD30+ T-cell lymphoproliferative disorder
- Primary cutaneous gamma-delta T-cell lymphoma
- Peripheral T-cell lymphoma, NOS
- Angioimmunoblastic T-cell lymphoma
- Anaplastic large cell lymphoma, ALK+ type
- Anaplastic large cell lymphoma, ALK− type

Swerdlow SH, Campo E, Harris NL, Jaffe ES, Pileri SA, Stein H, Thiele J, Vardiman JW, eds. World Health Organization Classification of Tumours of Haematopoietic and Lymphoid Tissues. Lyon, France: IARC Press, 2008

Staging *(continued)*

Stage	Description
	Abbreviations
A	Asymptomatic
B	Unexplained persistent or recurrent fever with temperature higher than 38°C (100.4°F), or recurrent drenching night sweats within 1 month, or unexplained loss of >10% body weight within 6 months
E	Limited direct extension into extralymphatic organ from adjacent lymph node
X	Bulky disease (mediastinal tumor width > one-third of the transthoracic diameter at T5/6, or a tumor diameter >10 cm)

Moormeier JA et al. Semin Oncol 1990;17:43–50

5-Year Survival Rate

NHL Subtype	5-Year Survival Rates
Diffuse large B-cell lymphoma	Varies according to IPI and treatment
Follicular lymphoma	Varies according to FLIPI
Mantle cell lymphoma	≈30%

IPI, International Prognostic Index; FLIPI, Follicular Lymphoma International Prognostic Index

Fisher RI et al. Blood 1995;85:1075–1082

Expert Opinion

The choice of therapy requires consideration of many factors, including age, comorbid pathologies, and future therapies (eg, stem cell transplantation). Therefore, treatment selection should be individualized

Diffuse Large B-cell Lymphoma

First-line therapy
- Rituximab-CHOP (rituximab, cyclophosphamide, doxorubicin, vincristine, prednisone)
- Dose-adjusted EPOCH-R (etoposide, prednisone, vincristine, cyclophosphamide, doxorubicin, rituximab)
- R-CHOP-14

For elderly (over 80):
- RminiCHOP (cyclophosphamide, doxorubicin, vincristine, prednisone)
- R-CEOP (cyclophosphamide, etoposide, vincristine, prednisone)

(continued)

Expert Opinion (continued)

Second-line therapy
- RICE (rituximab, ifosfamide, carboplatin, etoposide)
- ESHAP (etoposide, methylprednisolone, cytarabine, cisplatin)
- Dose-adjusted EPOCH + rituximab
- DHAP (dexamethasone/high dose cytarabine/cisplatin)
- GDP (gemcitabine/dexamethasone/cisplatin)
- Autologous or allogeneic (experimental) hematopoietic progenitor cell transplantation for sensitive diseases
- Clinical trials, if available

Follicular Lymphoma
First-line therapy
- CVP (cyclophosphamide, vincristine, prednisone) ± rituximab
- Rituximab + CHOP (cyclophosphamide, doxorubicin, vincristine, prednisone)
- Fludarabine ± rituximab
- Bendamustine + rituximab
- FND (fludarabine, mitoxantrone, dexamethasone) ± rituximab
- Alkylating agents (eg, chlorambucil or cyclophosphamide) ± prednisone ± rituximab
- Rituximab (selected circumstances)
- Maintenance/extended schedule rituximab

Second-line therapy
- Rituximab
- Treatments listed under *First-line therapy*
- Radioimmunotherapy
- Allogeneic hematopoietic progenitor cell transplantation (experimental)
- Clinical trials, if available

Small Lymphocytic Lymphoma
First-line therapy
- Fludarabine ± rituximab
- FC ± rituximab
- Alkylating agents (eg, chlorambucil or cyclophosphamide) ± prednisone ± rituximab
- CVP ± rituximab
- FCR (fludarabine, cyclophosphamide, and rituximab)
- Bendamustine + rituximab

Second-line therapy
- PC (pentostatin, cyclophosphamide) ± rituximab
- Treatments listed under *First-line therapy*
- Allogeneic hematopoietic progenitor cell transplantation (experimental)
- Ibrutinib

Prognostic Indices
International Prognostic Index (IPI)

A predictive model for aggressive non-Hodgkin's lymphoma. The International Non-Hodgkin's Lymphoma Prognostic Factors Project. N Engl J Med 1993;329:987–994

The **International Prognostic Index (IPI)** is a clinical tool to aid in predicting the prognosis of patients with aggressive non-Hodgkin lymphoma. First developed in 1993, it replaced the Ann Arbor stage as a prognosis tool. The original report was a retrospective analysis performed on 2031 patients with aggressive non-Hodgkin lymphoma treated between 1982 and 1987. Patients of all ages were included; all had been treated with doxorubicin-based regimens, most commonly CHOP (Shipp et al. A predictive model for aggressive non-Hodgkin's lymphoma. The International Non-Hodgkin's Lymphoma Prognostic Factors Project. N Engl J Med 1993;329:987–994). Five patient characteristics emerged as significant. Although the IPI has been shown to be a useful clinical tool, it should be kept in mind that the studies on which it was based did not include rituximab. How this omission may impact the IPI in the era of rituximab and newer agents targeting CD20 is uncertain

One point is assigned for each of the following risk factors:
- Age greater than 60 years
- Stage III or IV disease
- Elevated serum LDH
- ECOG/Zubrod performance status of 2, 3, or 4
- More than 1 extranodal site

The sum of the points allotted correlates with the following risk groups:

Points	Risk Category	5-Year Survival
0–1 points	Low risk	73%
2 points	Low-intermediate risk	51%
3 points	High-intermediate risk	43%
4–5 points	High risk	26%

Age-Adjusted IPI
A simplified index can be used when comparing patients within an age group (ie 60 or younger, or over 60) and includes only 3 of the above risk factors

One point is assigned for each of the following risk factors:
- Stage III or IV disease
- Elevated serum LDH
- ECOG/Zubrod performance status of 2, 3, or 4

The sum of the points allotted correlates with the following risk groups:

Points	Risk Category	5-Year Survival
0 point	Low risk	83%
1 point	Low-intermediate risk	69%
2 points	High-intermediate risk	46%
3 points	High risk	32%

(continued)

Expert Opinion (continued)

Mantle Cell Lymphoma

First-line therapy
- Rituximab + CHOP
- Hyper-CVAD (cyclophosphamide, vincristine, doxorubicin, and dexamethasone, alternating with high-dose methotrexate and cytarabine) + rituximab
- Bendamustine + rituximab
- Consolidation with autologous stem cell transplant

Second-line therapy
- Treatments listed under *First-line therapy*
- FC (fludarabine + cyclophosphamide) ± rituximab
- PCR (pentostatin, cyclophosphamide, rituximab)
- Bortezomib
- Lenalidomide
- Ibrutinib
- Older patients – R-FC or R-CHOP
- Autologous or allogeneic hematopoietic progenitor cell transplantation (experimental)
- Lenalidomide
- Ibrutinib

T-Cell Lymphomas

First-line therapy
- CHOP (cyclophosphamide, doxorubicin, vincristine, prednisone))
- CHEOP (cyclophosphamide, doxorubicin, etoposide, vincristine, prednisone)

Second-line therapy
- Romidepsin
- Pralatrexate

Burkitt's Lymphoma
- EPOCH-R
- Cyclophosphamide, vincristine (oncovin), doxorubicin, methotrexate (CODOX-M) + Ifosfamide, etoposide (VP-16), and cytarabine (ARA-C) (I-VAC)
- NHL-BFM 86 (Berlin-Frankfurt-Münster 86)
- Rituximab + hyperfractionated cyclophosphamide, vincristine, doxorubicin (adriamycin), and dexamethasone (R-hyper-CVAD)
- Methotrexate, cytarabine (ARA-C), cyclophosphamide, vincristine (oncovin), prednisone, and bleomycin (MACOP-B)

Prognostic Indices (continued)

Follicular Lymphoma International Prognostic Index (FLIPI)

Solal-Céligny et al. Blood 2004;104:1258–1265

Developed for the most common low-grade lymphoma, follicular lymphoma, following the success of the IPI. Five prognostic factors emerged

One point is assigned for each of the following adverse prognostic factors:
- Age greater than 60 years
- Stage III or IV disease
- Greater than 4 lymph node groups involved
- Serum hemoglobin less than 12 g/dL
- Elevated serum LDH

The sum of the points allotted correlates with the following risk groups:

Points	Risk Category	5-Year Survival	10-Year Survival
0–1 points	Low risk	91%	71%
2 points	Intermediate risk	78%	51%
3–5 points	High risk	53%	36%

Mantle Cell Lymphoma International Prognostic Index (MIPI)

Hoster et al. Blood 2008;11:558–565

A similar effort has led to a prognostic index predictive of outcome in advanced mantle cell lymphoma. Four prognostic factors emerged

The point values are assigned as follows:

Points	Factors
0 point	• Age less than 50 years • ECOG performance status of 0–1 • LDH less than 0.67 of the upper limit of normal • WBC of less than 6700 cells/mcl
1 point	• Age 50–59 • LDH 0.67–0.99 of the upper limit of normal • WBC 6700 to 9999 cells/mcl
2 points	• Age 60–69 • ECOG performance status of 2–4 • LDH 1–1.49 times the upper limit of normal • WBC 10,000–14,000 cells/mcl
3 points	• Age 70 or greater • LDH 1.5 times the upper limit of normal or greater • WBC of 15,000 cells/mcl or greater

The sum of the allotted points correlates with the following risk groups:

Points	Risk Category	Median Survival
0–3 points	Low risk	Not yet reached
4–5 points	Intermediate risk	51 months
6–11 points	High risk	29 months

REGIMEN

CYCLOPHOSPHAMIDE, DOXORUBICIN (HYDROXYLDAUNORUBICIN), VINCRISTINE (ONCOVIN), PREDNISONE (CHOP) + RITUXIMAB

Coiffier B et al. N Engl J Med 2002;346:235–242

Premedication for rituximab:
Acetaminophen 650–1000 mg; administer orally, *plus*
Diphenhydramine 25–50 mg; administer orally or intravenously, 30–60 minutes before starting rituximab
Rituximab 375 mg/m^2; administer intravenously in 0.9% sodium chloride injection (0.9% NS) or 5% dextrose injection (D5W), diluted to a concentration of 1–4 mg/mL, on day 1, every 21 days (total dosage/cycle = 375 mg/m^2)

Notes on rituximab administration:
• Infuse initially at 50 mg/hour. If hypersensitivity or infusion reactions do not occur during the first 30 minutes, increase the rate by 50 mg/hour every 30 minutes, as tolerated, to a maximum rate of 400 mg/hour. Subsequently, if previous administration was well tolerated, start at 100 mg/hour and increase by 100 mg/hour every 30 minutes, as tolerated, to a maximum rate of 400 mg/hour
• Interrupt rituximab administration for fever, chills, edema, congestion of the head and neck mucosa, hypotension, and other serious adverse events. Resume rituximab administration after adverse events abate

Intravenous hydration before and after cyclophosphamide administration:
500–1000 mL 0.9% NS

Cyclophosphamide 750 mg/m^2; administer intravenously in 25–250 mL 0.9% NS or D5W over 10–30 minutes, given on day 1, every 3 weeks (total dosage/cycle = 750 mg/m^2)
Doxorubicin 50 mg/m^2; administer by intravenous injection over 3–5 minutes, given on day 1, every 3 weeks (total dosage/cycle = 50 mg/m^2)
Vincristine 1.4 mg/m^2 (maximum dose = 2 mg); administer by intravenous injection over 1–2 minutes, given on day 1, every 3 weeks (total dosage/cycle = 1.4 mg/m^2; maximum dose/cycle = 2 mg)
Prednisone 40 mg/m^2 per day; administer orally for 5 consecutive days, days 1–5 every 3 weeks (total dosage/cycle = 200 mg/m^2)

Supportive Care
Antiemetic prophylaxis
Emetogenic potential on day 1 is **MODERATELY HIGH**
See Chapter 39 for antiemetic recommendations

Hematopoietic growth factor (CSF) prophylaxis
Primary prophylaxis is indicated with 1 of the following:
   Filgrastim (G-CSF) 5 mcg/kg per day; administer by subcutaneous injection, *or*
   Pegfilgrastim (pegylated filgrastim) 6 mg/0.6 mL; administer by subcutaneous injection for 1 dose
   • Begin use from 24–72 hours after myelosuppressive chemotherapy is completed
See Chapter 43 for more information

Antimicrobial prophylaxis
Risk of fever and neutropenia is INTERMEDIATE
   Antimicrobial primary prophylaxis to be considered:
   • Antibacterial—consider a fluoroquinolone or no prophylaxis; *Pneumocystis jirovecii* prophylaxis is recommended (eg, cotrimoxazole)
   • Antifungal—consider use during neutropenia and for anticipated mucositis
   • Antiviral—antiherpes antivirals (eg, acyclovir)
See Chapter 47 for more information

Steroid-associated gastritis
Add a **proton pump inhibitor** during prednisone use to prevent gastritis and duodenitis

Treatment Modifications

Adverse Event	Dose Modification
G4 ANC or febrile neutropenia after any cycle of chemotherapy	Filgrastim prophylaxis after chemotherapy during subsequent cycles*
G4 ANC during a cycle in which filgrastim was administered	Reduce cyclophosphamide and doxorubicin dosages 50% during subsequent cycles
G3/4 thrombocytopenia	
ANC <1500/mm^3 or platelet count <100,000/mm^3 on first day of a repeated cycle	Delay cycle for up to 2 weeks. Stop treatment if recovery has not occurred after a 2-week delay

*Filgrastim 5 mcg/kg per day; administer subcutaneously, starting on day 2 and continuing beyond ANC nadir until ANC exceeds 5000/mm^3 on 1 reading

Rituximab Infusion-Related Toxicities

Onset of infusion-related events (fevers, chills, rigors edema, congestion of the head and neck mucosa, hypotension):
1. Interrupt rituximab infusion
2. For fever, chills: Give additional dose of acetaminophen 650 mg orally and diphenhydramine 25–50 mg by intravenous injection
3. For rigors: Give meperidine 12.5–25 mg by intravenous injection ± promethazine 12.5–25 mg by intravenous infusion in at least 10 mL 0.9% NS or D5W over 5–15 minutes. If after 15–20 minutes the response to a single dose is considered inadequate, the dose may be repeated
4. After symptoms resolve, resume rituximab infusion at 50 mg/hour and increase by 50 mg/hour every 30 minutes, as tolerated, up to a maximum rate of 200 mg/hour

Dyspnea or wheezing, without allergic findings (urticaria, or tongue or laryngeal edema):
1. Interrupt rituximab infusion immediately
2. Give hydrocortisone 100 mg by intravenous injection (or glucocorticoid equivalent)
3. Give a histamine H$_2$-antagonist (ranitidine 150 mg, cimetidine 300 mg, or famotidine 20 mg) by intravenous injection
4. After symptoms resolve, resume rituximab infusion at 25 mg/hour with close monitoring. Do not increase rate

Note: Medications for the treatment of hypersensitivity reactions should be available for immediate use in the event of a reaction during administration (eg, intravenous fluids, epinephrine, antihistamines, glucocorticoids, and O$_2$)

Patient Population Studied

Previously untreated patients with diffuse large B-cell lymphoma 60–80 years of age were randomly assigned to receive 8 cycles of CHOP every 3 weeks (197 patients) or 8 cycles of CHOP plus rituximab given on the first day of each cycle (202 patients). Patients who were serologically positive for HIV and patients with active hepatitis B infection were excluded

Efficacy

	CHOP	RCHOP	
CR and CRu	63%	75%	
PR and SD	6%	8%	
PD during treatment	22%	9.5%	$p = 0.005$
Death during treatment	6%	6%	
Median OS	3.1 years	Not reached	
5-Year PFS	30%	54%	
5-Year PFS in low aaIPI* risk	34%	69%	$p = 0.00013$
5-Year PFS in high aaIPI* risk	29%	47%	$p = 0.00078$
5-Year DFS	45%	66%	
5-Year OS	45%	58%	
5-Year OS in low aaIPI* risk	62%	80%	$p = 0.023$
5-Year OS in high aaIPI* risk	39%	48%	$p = 0.062$

*Age-adjusted International Prognostic Index

Feugier P et al. J Clin Oncol 2005;23:4117–4126

Toxicity*,† (N = 202)

	% Any Grade	% G3/4
Fever	64	2
Infection	65	12
Mucositis	27	3
Liver toxicity	46	3
Cardiac toxicity	47	8
Neurologic toxicity	51	5
Renal toxicity	11	1
Lung toxicity	33	8
Nausea or vomiting	42	2
Constipation	38	2
Alopecia	97	39
Other toxicities	84	20

*NCI CTC
†Percentage of patients with event during at least 1 cycle

Coiffier B et al. N Engl J Med 2002;346:235–242

Therapy Monitoring

1. *Weekly:* CBC with differential
2. *Before each cycle:* LFTs, serum BUN, creatinine, PE

REGIMEN

DOSE-ADJUSTED ETOPOSIDE, PREDNISONE, VINCRISTINE (ONCOVIN), CYCLOPHOSPHAMIDE, AND DOXORUBICIN (HYDROXYLDAUNORUBICIN) WITH RITUXIMAB (DA-EPOCH WITH RITUXIMAB)

Wilson et al. Haematologica 2012;97(5):758–765

Premedication for rituximab:

Acetaminophen 650–1000 mg; administer orally, *plus*

Diphenhydramine 25–50 mg; administer orally or intravenously, 30–60 minutes before starting rituximab

Rituximab 375 mg/m²; administer intravenously diluted to a concentration of 1–4 mg/mL in 0.9% sodium chloride injection (0.9% NS) or 5% dextrose injection (D5W) on day 1, every 21 days (total dosage/cycle = 375 mg/m²)

Notes on rituximab administration:

- Infuse initially at 50 mg/hour. If hypersensitivity or infusion reactions do not occur during the first 30 minutes, increase the rate by 50 mg/hour every 30 minutes, as tolerated, to a maximum rate of 400 mg/hour. Subsequently, if previous administration was well tolerated, start at 100 mg/hour, and increase by 100 mg/hour every 30 minutes, as tolerated, to a maximum rate of 400 mg/hour

- Interrupt rituximab administration for fever, chills, edema, congestion of the head and neck mucosa, hypotension, and other serious adverse events. Resume rituximab administration after adverse events abate

Etoposide 50 mg/m² per day; administer by continuous intravenous infusion over 24 hours for 4 consecutive days on days 1–4, every 21 days (total dosage/cycle = 200 mg/m²)

Doxorubicin 10 mg/m² per day; administer by continuous intravenous infusion over 24 hours for 4 consecutive days on days 1–4, every 21 days (total dosage/cycle = 40 mg/m²)

Vincristine 0.4 mg/m² per day; administer by continuous intravenous infusion over 24 hours for 4 consecutive days on days 1–4, every 21 days (total dosage/cycle = 1.6 mg/m²)

Intravenous hydration before and after cyclophosphamide administration:

Cyclophosphamide Dosage	Volume of 0.9% NS Before and After Dosage
≤900 mg/m²	500 mL
1080–1555 mg/m²	1000 mL
≥1866 mg/m²	1250 mL

Cyclophosphamide 750 mg/m²; administer intravenously in 100 mL 0.9% NS or D5W over 15–30 minutes, given on day 5 after completing etoposide + doxorubicin + vincristine infusion, every 21 days (total dosage/cycle = 750 mg/m²)

Prednisone 60 mg/m² twice daily; administer orally for 5 consecutive days on days 1–5, every 21 days (total dosage/cycle = 600 mg/m²)

Filgrastim 5 mcg/kg per day; administer subcutaneously, starting on day 6 and continuing until ANC >5000/mm³

Notes:

- See instructions below for preparing a 3-in-1 admixture with etoposide, doxorubicin, and vincristine

- Etoposide + doxorubicin + vincristine admixtures are administered with an ambulatory (portable) infusion pump through a central venous access device

- Repeated cycles begin on day 22 if the ANC is ≥1000/mm³ and the platelet count is ≥100,000/mm³

Supportive Care

Antiemetic prophylaxis

Emetogenic potential on days 1–4 is **LOW**

Emetogenic potential on day 5 is **MODERATE**

See Chapter 39 for antiemetic recommendations

(continued)

Treatment Modifications

Events*	Dose Modification†
Previous cycle ANC nadir count ≥500/mm³	Increase etoposide, doxorubicin, and cyclophosphamide dosages by 20% greater than the dosages given during the previous cycle
Previous cycle ANC nadir <500/mm³ on 1 or 2 measurements	Give the same dosages as last cycle
Previous cycle ANC nadir <500/mm³ on at least 3 measurements	Reduce etoposide, doxorubicin, and cyclophosphamide dosages by 20% less than the dosages given during the previous cycle
Previous cycle platelet nadir <25,000/mm³ on 1 measurement	
Total bilirubin >4.0 mg/dL (>68.4 μmol/L)	Hold vincristine‡
Total bilirubin >3.0 mg/dL, but <4.0 mg/dL (>51.3 μmol/L but <68.4 μmol/L)	Reduce vincristine dosage by 75%‡
Total bilirubin >1.5 mg/dL but <3.0 mg/dL (>25.6 μmol/L but <51.3 μmol/L)	Reduce vincristine dosage by 50%‡
G2 neuropathy	Reduce vincristine dosage by 25%‡
G3 neuropathy	Reduce vincristine dosage by 50%‡

*ANC and platelet nadir measurements are based on *twice-weekly* CBC with differential only

†Dosage adjustments *greater than the starting dose level* apply to etoposide, doxorubicin, and cyclophosphamide only. Dose adjustments *less than the starting dose level* apply to cyclophosphamide only

‡Vincristine dosage is increased to 100% if neuropathy resolves to G ≤1 or total bilirubin to <1.5 mg/dL (<25.6 μmol/L)

(continued)

(*continued*)

Hematopoietic growth factor (CSF) prophylaxis
Primary prophylaxis is indicated with:

Filgrastim (G-CSF) 5 mcg/kg per day; administer by subcutaneous injection, starting on day 4, and continue use until the ANC >5000/mm³

See Chapter 43 for more information

Antimicrobial prophylaxis

Risk of fever and neutropenia is INTERMEDIATE

Antimicrobial primary prophylaxis to be considered:

- Antibacterial—consider a fluoroquinolone or no prophylaxis; *Pneumocystis jirovecii* prophylaxis is recommended (eg, cotrimoxazole)
- Antifungal—consider use during neutropenia and for anticipated mucositis
- Antiviral—antiherpes antivirals (eg, acyclovir)

See Chapter 47 for more information

Additional prophylaxis

Add a **proton pump inhibitor** during prednisone use to prevent gastritis and duodenitis
Give **stool softeners** and/or laxatives during and after infusional vincristine administration

Instructions for Preparing a 3-in-1 Admixture with Etoposide, Doxorubicin, and Vincristine

Dilute the 3 drugs in 0.9% NS as follows:

Total Dose of Etoposide	Volume of 0.9% NS
≤62 mg	250 mL
62.1–125 mg	500 mL
>125 mg	1000 mL

Etoposide (base) + doxorubicin + vincristine 3-in-1 admixtures:
Etoposide 50 mg/m², doxorubicin hydrochloride 10 mg/m², and vincristine sulfate 0.4 mg/m² admixtures diluted in 0.9% NS to produce a final etoposide concentration <250 mcg/mL in polyolefin-lined infusion bags were stable and compatible for 72 hours at 23°–25°C (73.4°–77°F), and at 31°–33°C (87.8°–91.4°F) when protected from exposure to light

Wolfe JL et al. Am J Health Syst Pharm 1999;56:985–989

Etoposide (PHOSphate) + doxorubicin + vincristine 3-in-1 admixtures:
Etoposide PHOSphate, doxorubicin hydrochloride, and vincristine sulfate admixtures diluted in 0.9% NS to produce a final etoposide concentration <250 mcg/mL in polyolefin-lined infusion bags were stable and compatible for up to 124 hours at 2°–6°C (35.6°–42.8°F) and 35°–40°C (95°–104°F) in the dark and in regular fluorescent light. In admixtures stored at 35°–40°C (95°–104°F) and exposed to light, the initial drug concentrations decreased slightly, but remained within acceptable concentrations

Yuan P et al. Am J Health Syst Pharm 2001;58:594–598

The 3-in-1 admixtures described above do not prevent microbial growth after exposure to bacterial and fungal contamination. With respect to product sterility, expiration dating should be determined by the aseptic techniques used in preparation and local and national guidelines

Efficacy*

CR/Cru	94%
CR/CRu; high-risk IPI (3–5 IPI factors)	82%
PFS	79% at 5 years
OS	80% at 5 years

*Five-year follow up of 72 patients with untreated de novo DLBCL who were at least 18 years of age and at stage II or higher. Radiation consolidation was not permitted

Wilson WH et al. J Clin Oncol 2008;26:2717–2724

Patient Population Studied

A study of 69 patients with newly diagnosed diffuse large B-cell lymphoma. All patients were serologically negative for HIV

Therapy Monitoring

1. *Twice weekly:* CBC with differential
2. *At the beginning of every cycle:* CBC with differential and LFTs

Treatment Modifications
(*continued*)

Rituximab Infusion-Related Toxicities

Onset of infusion-related events (fevers, chills, rigors edema, congestion of the head and neck mucosa, hypotension):

1. Interrupt rituximab infusion
2. For fever, chills: Give additional dose of acetaminophen 650 mg orally and diphenhydramine 25–50 mg by intravenous injection
3. For rigors: Give meperidine 12.5–25 mg by intravenous injection ± promethazine 12.5–25 mg by intravenous infusion in at least 10 mL 0.9% NS or D5W over 5–15 minutes. If after 15–20 minutes the response to a single dose is considered inadequate, the dose may be repeated
4. After symptoms resolve, resume rituximab infusion at 50 mg/hour and increase by 50 mg/hour every 30 minutes, as tolerated, up to a maximum rate of 200 mg/hour

Dyspnea or wheezing, without allergic findings (urticaria, or tongue or laryngeal edema):

1. Interrupt rituximab infusion immediately
2. Give hydrocortisone 100 mg by intravenous injection (or glucocorticoid equivalent)
3. Give a histamine H₂-antagonist (ranitidine 150 mg, cimetidine 300 mg, or famotidine 20 mg) by intravenous injection
4. After symptoms resolve, resume rituximab infusion at 25 mg/hour with close monitoring. Do not increase rate

Note: Medications for the treatment of hypersensitivity reactions should be available for immediate use in the event of a reaction during administration (eg, intravenous fluids, epinephrine, antihistamines, glucocorticoids, and O₂)

Toxicity*
72 Patients/414 Cycles

ANC nadir ≥100/mm³, ≤499/mm³	38% of cycles
ANC <100/mm³	24% of cycles
Platelet count <25,000/mm³	9% of cycles
Hospitalization for fever with neutropenia	19% of cycles
G 3 gastrointestinal toxicities	5% of cycles
G 3 neurologic toxicities	5% of cycles
Deaths†	4.2% (3/72)

*Five-year follow up of 72 patients with untreated de novo DLBCL who were at least 18 years of age and at stage II or higher. Radiation consolidation was not permitted
†*Aspergillus fumigatus* infection; subdural hematoma after anticoagulation for a pulmonary embolus; and presumed sepsis

Wilson WH et al. J Clin Oncol 2008;26:2717–2724

REGIMEN

CYCLOPHOSPHAMIDE, DOXORUBICIN (HYDROXYDAUNORUBICIN), VINCRISTINE (ONCOVIN), PREDNISONE (CHOP) + RITUXIMAB EVERY 14 DAYS (R-CHOP-14)

Pfreundschuh M et al. Lancet Oncol 2008;9:105–116

Premedication for rituximab:

Acetaminophen 650–1000 mg; administer orally, *plus*

Diphenhydramine 25–50 mg; administer orally or intravenously, 30–60 minutes before starting rituximab

Rituximab 375 mg/m^2; administer by intravenous infusion in 0.9% sodium chloride injection (0.9% NS) or 5% dextrose injection (D5W), diluted to a concentration of 1–4 mg/mL, once every 2 weeks (total dosage: 2250 mg/m^2 for 6 cycles; 3000 mg/m^2 for 8 cycles)

Notes on rituximab administration:

- Infuse initially at 50 mg/hour. If hypersensitivity or infusion reactions do not occur during the first 30 minutes, increase the rate by 50 mg/hour every 30 minutes, as tolerated, to a maximum rate of 400 mg/hour. Subsequently if previous administration was well tolerated, start at 100 mg/hour and increase by 100 mg/hour every 30 minutes, as tolerated, to a maximum rate of 400 mg/hour

- Interrupt rituximab administration for fever, chills, edema, congestion of the head and neck mucosa, hypertension, and other serious adverse events. Resume rituximab administration after adverse events abate

Hydration: 500–1000 mL 0.9% sodium chloride injection (0.9% NS); administer intravenously before and after cyclophosphamide administration

- May be administered concurrently or after completing rituximab

Cyclophosphamide 750 mg/m^2; administer intravenously in 25–250 mL 0.9% NS or 5% dextrose injection, over 10–30 minutes on day 1, every 14 days (total dosage/cycle = 750 mg/m^2)

Doxorubicin 50 mg/m^2; administer by intravenous injection over 3–5 minutes on day 1, every 14 days (total dosage/cycle = 50 mg/m^2)

Vincristine 2 mg; administer by intravenous injection over 1–2 minutes on day 1, every 14 days (total dosage/cycle = 2 mg)

Prednisone 100 mg/day; administer orally for 5 consecutive days, days 1–5, every 14 days (total dose/cycle = 500 mg)

Notes on administration of drug regimen:

- *R-CHOP is repeated every 2 weeks for 6 or 8 cycles after WBC count >2500/mm^3 and platelet count >80,000/mm^3 are achieved*

- Patients with poor performance status are given **Prephase Treatment** before starting R-CHOP-14

    Vincristine 1 mg; administer by intravenous injection over 1–2 minutes, *plus*

    Prednisone 100 mg/day; administer orally for 7 days before starting R-CHOP-14

Supportive Care

Antiemetic prophylaxis

Emetogenic potential on day *1* is **HIGH**

See Chapter 39 for antiemetic recommendations

Hematopoietic growth factor (CSF) prophylaxis

Primary prophylaxis is indicated with:

   Filgrastim (G-CSF) 5 mcg/kg per day; administer by subcutaneous injection, starting on day 4

   - Obtain a CBC before starting filgrastim therapy, and monitor twice weekly during filgrastim use until the ANC has reached 10,000/mm^3 following the expected chemotherapy-induced neutrophil nadir

See Chapter 43 for more information

Antimicrobial prophylaxis

Risk of fever and neutropenia is INTERMEDIATE

   Antimicrobial primary prophylaxis to be considered:

   - Antibacterial—consider a fluoroquinolone or no prophylaxis; *Pneumocystis jirovecii* prophylaxis is recommended (eg, cotrimoxazole)

   - Antifungal—consider use during neutropenia and for anticipated mucositis

   - Antiviral—antiherpes antivirals (eg, acyclovir)

See Chapter 47 for more information

(continued)

Treatment Modifications

Day 15 WBC count <2500/mm^3 or platelet count <80,000/mm^3	Hold start of next chemotherapy cycle until WBC count >2500/mm^3 and platelet count >80,000/mm^3

Patient Population Studied

A study of 1222 elderly patients (61–80 years of age) who had not received any prior therapy were randomly assigned to 6 or 8 cycles of CHOP-14 with or without rituximab. Median age was 68 years, approximately 50% had advanced stage disease, and 38% were classified as bulky. Excluded patients with HIV or other major comorbidities, WBC <2500/mm^3, platelet count <100,000/mm^3. Radiotherapy was planned to sites of initial bulky disease with or without extranodal involvement. The primary endpoint was event-free survival; secondary end points were response, progression during treatment, progression-free survival, overall survival, and frequency of toxic effects. Analyses were done by intention to treat

Therapy Monitoring

Prior to each cycle

1. CBC with differential
2. Serum chemistry with LFTs

(*continued*)

Steroid-associated gastritis

Add a **proton pump inhibitor** during prednisone use to prevent gastritis and duodenitis

Note: Patients with initial bulky disease (defined as lymphoma masses or conglomerates with a diameter ≥7.5 cm) or extranodal involvement received radiotherapy (36 Gy) to these areas irrespective of the result of chemotherapy. However, the role of additional radiotherapy to treat bulky disease and sites of extranodal involvement in patients assigned to radiotherapy (54% of patients) is unclear and was not studied in this trial. Comparison to 150 elderly patients with a very similar risk profile treated with 6 cycles of R-CHOP-14 without radiotherapy in a subsequent phase II study suggests the effect of radiotherapy in these patients is marginal, if existing at all

Efficacy

	6 × CHOP-14 (n = 307)	8 × CHOP-14 (n = 305)	6 × R-CHOP-14 (n = 306)	8 × R-CHOP-14 (n = 304)
CR	68%	72%	78%	76%
	—	$p = 0.3150$	$p = 0.0069$	$p = 0.0372$
3-Year PFS	56.9%	56.9%	73.4%	68.8%
	—	$p = 0.6155$	$p = 0.0001$	$p = 0.0001$
3-Year OS	67.7%	66%	78.1%	72.5%
	—	$p = 0.8358$	$p = 0.0181$	$p = 0.2602$

Toxicity

Grade 3 and 4 Common Toxicity Criteria Toxicities and Therapeutic Interventions

	6 × CHOP-14 (n = 307)	8 × CHOP-14 (n = 305)	6 × R-CHOP-14 (n = 306)	8 × R-CHOP-14 (n = 304)	*p*-Value
Leukocytopenia	48%	48%	52%	50%	0.8017
Infection	29%	31%	28%	35%	0.2784
Interventional antibiotics	45%	55%	53%	62%	0.0008
Anemia	16%	23%	16%	27%	0.0013
Red blood cell transfusions	41%	51%	47%	52%	0.0312
Thrombocytopenia	10%	17%	12%	16%	0.1242
Platelet transfusions	2%	4%	3%	4%	0.5840
Mucositis	3%	6%	5%	9%	0.0278
Neuropathy	7%	11%	7%	8%	0.3946
Arrhythmia	5%	3%	4%	6%	0.2437
Cardiac function	2%	2%	3%	3%	0.7917

REGIMEN

Elderly Patients (Age >80 Years)

R-miniCHOP (RITUXIMAB + CYCLOPHOSPHAMIDE + DOXORUBICIN + VINCRISTINE [ONCOVIN] + PREDNISONE)

Peyrade F et al. Lancet Oncol 2011;12:460–468

Premedication for rituximab:
Acetaminophen 650–1000 mg; administer orally, *plus*
Diphenhydramine 25–50 mg; administer orally or intravenously, 30–60 minutes before each dose of rituximab
Rituximab 375 mg/m²; administer intravenously in 0.9% sodium chloride injection (0.9% NS) or 5% dextrose injection (D5W) diluted to a concentration of 1–4 mg/mL on day 1 every 3 weeks for a total of 6 cycles (total dosage/cycle = 375 mg/m²)

Notes on rituximab administration:
• Infuse initially at 50 mg/h. If hypersensitivity or infusion reactions do not occur during the first 30 minutes, increase the rate by 50 mg/h every 30 minutes as tolerated to a maximum rate of 400 mg/h. Subsequently, if previous administration was well tolerated, start at 100 mg/h and increase by 100 mg/h every 30 minutes as tolerated to a maximum rate of 400 mg/h
• Interrupt rituximab administration for fever chills, edema, congestion of the head and neck mucosa, hypertension, and other serious adverse events. Resume rituximab administration after adverse events abate

Hydration: 500–1000 mL 0.9% sodium chloride injection (0.9% NS); administer intravenously before and after cyclophosphamide administration
• May be administered concurrently with rituximab or after completing administration
Cyclophosphamide 400 mg/m²; administer intravenously in 25–250 mL 0.9% NS or D5W over 10–30 minutes on day 1 every 3 weeks for a total of 6 cycles (total dosage/cycle = 400 mg/m²)
Doxorubicin 25 mg/m²; administer by intravenous injection over 3–5 minutes on day 1 every 3 weeks for a total of 6 cycles (total dosage/cycle = 25 mg/m²)
Vincristine 1 mg; administer by intravenous injection over 1–2 minutes on day 1 every 3 weeks for a total of 6 cycles (total dose/cycle = 1 mg)
Prednisone 40 mg/m² per dose; administer orally for 5 consecutive days on days 1–5 every 3 weeks for a total of 6 cycles (total dosage/cycle = 200 mg/m²)

Supportive Care
Antiemetic prophylaxis
Emetogenic potential on day 1 is **HIGH**. *Potential for delayed emetic symptoms*
See Chapter 39 for antiemetic recommendations

Hematopoietic growth factor (CSF) prophylaxis
Primary prophylaxis may be indicated
See Chapter 43 for more information

Antimicrobial prophylaxis
Risk of fever and neutropenia is INTERMEDIATE
Antimicrobial primary prophylaxis to be considered:
• Antibacterial—consider a fluoroquinolone or no prophylaxis; *Pneumocystis jirovecii* prophylaxis is recommended (eg, cotrimoxazole)
• Antifungal—consider use during neutropenia and for anticipated mucositis
• Antiviral—antiherpes antivirals (eg, acyclovir)
See Chapter 47 for more information

(continued)

Patient Characteristics (N = 149)

	Number of Patients (%)
Age, median (range)	83 years (80–95 years)
Men	51 (34%)
Performance status: 0/1/2	27 (18%)/72 (48%)/50 (34%)
Ann Arbor stage	
I	13 (9%)
II	24 (16%)
III	35 (23%)
IV	77 (52%)
Tumor mass ≥10 cm	30 (20%)
>1 extranodal sites	55 (37%)
LDH concentration >618 U/L	102 (68%)
B symptoms*	49 (33%)
β_2-Microglobulin ≥3 mg/L	82/112 (73%)
Serum albumin <35 g/L	69/137 (50%)
IPI	
0–1	13 (9%)
2	31 (21%)
3	46 (31%)
4–5	59 (40%)
Age-adjusted IPI	
0	15 (10%)
1	36 (24%)
2	66 (44%)
3	32 (21%)
IADL scale†	
Without limitation (score 4)	63 (47%)
With limitation (score <4)	72 (53%)

IADL, instrumental activities of daily living; IPI, International Prognostic Index; LDH, lactate dehydrogenase
*Fever, night sweats, and weight loss
†Completed by 135 patients
Note: Percentages do not add up to 100% in some cases because of rounding

(*continued*)

Infusion reactions associated with rituximab

Fevers, chills, and rigors

1. Interrupt rituximab administration for severe symptoms, and give:
   - **Acetaminophen** 650 mg orally for fever. For persistent or recurrent symptoms, repeat administration every 4–6 hours as needed during rituximab administration
   - **Diphenhydramine** 25–50 mg orally or by intravenous injection for pruritus, hypotension, or angioedema. For persistent or recurrent symptoms, repeat administration every 4–6 hours as needed during rituximab administration
   - **Meperidine** 12.5–25 mg by intravenous injection every 10–20 minutes as needed for shaking chills (generally, cumulative doses >100 mg are not needed; use repeated doses with caution in persons with moderate or more severely impaired renal function)
2. If rituximab administration was interrupted, resume infusion at a slower rate than the maximum rate previously attempted. Rate escalation may be reattempted at smaller incremental steps with close monitoring. Do not exceed the maximum recommended rate of 400 mg/h

Dyspnea or wheezing without allergic findings (urticaria, or tongue or laryngeal edema)

1. Interrupt rituximab administration immediately
2. Give **hydrocortisone** 100 mg by intravenous injection (or an alternative steroid with equivalent glucocorticoid potency)
3. Give a **histamine (H$_2$) receptor antagonist** (ranitidine 50 mg, cimetidine 300 mg, or famotidine 20 mg) intravenously over 15–30 minutes
4. After symptoms resolve, resume rituximab administration at 25 mg/h with close monitoring. Do not increase the administration rate

Steroid-associated gastritis

Add a **proton pump inhibitor** during prednisone use to prevent gastritis and duodenitis

Decreased bowel motility prophylaxis

Give **stool softeners** in a scheduled regimen, and **saline, osmotic, and lubricant laxatives**, as needed to prevent constipation associated with vincristine use. If needed, circumspectly add **stimulant (irritant) laxatives** in the least amounts and for the briefest durations needed cause defecation

Treatment Modifications

Adverse Event	Treatment Modifications
Severe neutropenia (G3 lasting ≥7 days or G4) or fever + neutropenia	Do not adjust dosages. Administer filgrastim during subsequent cycles from days 6–13 (8 doses) or until ANC is ≥1000/mm³
Any hematologic toxicity	Do not adjust dosages
On day 1 of a cycle, ANC <1000/mm³ or platelet count <100,000/mm³	Delay start of cycle until ANC ≥1000/mm³ and platelet count ≥100,000/mm³ with a maximum of 28 days between two consecutive cycles
ANC <1000/mm³ or platelet count <100,000/mm³ 1 week (day 28) after day 1 of a cycle despite withholding chemotherapy	Discontinue therapy
G2 neurologic vincristine-related toxicity including sensory or motor polyneuritis, constipation, or visual or auditory changes	Discontinue vincristine

Treatment Monitoring

1. *Within 1 month before the first treatment cycle:* full history, physical examination, instrumental activities of daily living (IADL) scale, thoracic and abdominal computerized scans, electrocardiogram, and assessment of resting left ventricular ejection fraction by echocardiography or an isotopic method
2. *Laboratory assessments within 1 week before first chemotherapy:* lactate dehydrogenase, β$_2$-microglobulin, serum creatinine, serum transaminases, bilirubin, alkaline phosphatase, and C-reactive protein concentrations
3. *Tumor response assessment:* after 3 cycles and at the end of treatment
4. *Follow-up:* every 3 months for the first 2 years after treatment and every 6 months thereafter

Efficacy

Response at End of Treatment (N = 149)

	Number of Patients (%)
Complete response	59 (40%)
Unconfirmed complete response	34 (23%)
Partial response	16 (11%)
Stable disease	2 (1%)
Progression during treatment	8 (5%)
Death	27 (18%)
Not assessed	3 (2%)

Prognostic Factors for Overall Survival: Univariate Analyses

	2-Year Overall Survival	Hazard Ratio (95% CI)	Log-Rank p Value
Performance status ≥2	40.4% vs. 68.4%	2.9 (1.8–4.9)	<0.0001
Ann Arbor stages III–IV	55.9% vs. 68.5%	1.6 (0.8–2.9)	0.17
LDH concentration >618 U/L	54.4% vs. 67.6%	1.6 (0.9–2.9)	0.12
Age-adjusted IPI 2–3	50.4% vs. 74.7%	2.6 (1.4–4.9)	0.0024
Number of extranodal sites >1	45.1% vs. 67%	2.1 (1.3–3.6)	0.0033
Serum albumin ≤3.5 g/dL	40.5% vs. 80.4%	3.6 (1.9–6.6)	<0.0001
β_2-Microglobulin ≥3 mg/L	59.6% vs. 58%	1.1 (0.6–2.2)	0.69
Tumor mass >10 cm	30.3% vs. 65.1%	2.2 (1.2–3.8)	0.0071
IADL score <4	52.7% vs. 65.6%	1.8 (1.0–3.1)	0.0394

CI, confidence interval; IADL, instrumental activities of daily living; IPI, International Prognostic Index; LDH, lactate dehydrogenase
Note: IADL consisted of a simple questionnaire that included the following items: ability to use a telephone, shopping, medication use, and ability to handle finance. The sum score of all 4 items was calculated and patients were classified as being without limitation in the event of a full sum score (4) and with limitation in the event of a sum score less than 4

Prognostic Factors for Overall Survival: Multivariate Analyses

	Hazard Ratio (95% CI)	p Value
Age-adjusted IPI 2–3	1.4 (0.6–3.5)	0.46
Number of extranodal sites >1	1.2 (0.6–2.4)	0.59
Serum albumin ≤3.5 g/dL	3.2 (1.4–7.1)	0.0053
β_2-Microglobulin ≥3 mg/L	0.9 (0.4–1.9)	0.75
Tumor mass >10 cm	1.4 (0.6–2.9)	0.43
IADL score <4	1.9 (1.0–3.9)	0.064

CI, confidence interval; IADL, instrumental activities of daily living; IPI, International Prognostic Index
Note: IADL consisted of a simple questionnaire that included the following items: ability to use a telephone, shopping, medication use, and ability to handle finance. The sum score of all 4 items was calculated and patients were classified as being without limitation in the event of a full sum score (4) and with limitation in the event of a sum score less than 4

Toxicity

Incidence of Nonhematologic Toxicity by Grade (N = 149)

	Number of Patients (%)				
	No Toxicity	G1/2	G3	G4	G5
Infection without neutropenia	113 (76%)	22 (15%)	12 (8%)	0 (0%)	2 (1%)
Febrile neutropenia	138 (93%)	1 (1%)	7 (5%)	0 (0%)	3 (2%)
Constitutional symptoms	69 (46%)	68 (46%)	7 (5%)	2 (1%)	3 (2%)
Neurologic toxicity	109 (73%)	30 (20%)	7 (5%)	3 (2%)	0 (0%)
Pulmonary toxicity	118 (79%)	25 (17%)	4 (3%)	1 (0%)	1 (1%)
Renal toxicity	137 (92%)	8 (5%)	2 (1%)	1 (0%)	1 (1%)
Cardiac arrhythmia	134 (90%)	11 (7%)	2 (1%)	2 (1%)	0 (0%)
Cardiac (other)	133 (89%)	13 (9%)	2 (1%)	0 (0%)	1 (1%)
Vascular toxicity	137 (92%)	8 (5%)	3 (2%)	1 (1%)	0 (0%)
Mucositis	138 (93%)	11 (7%)	0 (0%)	0 (0%)	0 (0%)
Creatinine	117 (79%)	31 (21%)	0 (0%)	1 (1%)	0 (0%)
Transaminases	128 (86%)	20 (13%)	0 (0%)	1 (1%)	0 (0%)

Note: Percentages do not add up to 100% in some cases because of rounding

Serious Adverse Events (N = 70)

	Number of Patients (%)
Infections and infestations	19 (27%)
General disorders	12 (17%)
Respiratory and mediastinal disorders	10 (14%)
Gastrointestinal disorders	7 (10%)
Nervous system disorders	7 (10%)
Renal and urinary disorders	4 (6%)
Cardiac and vascular disorders	4 (6%)
Injury and procedural complications	3 (4%)
Hepatobiliary disorders	2 (3%)
Skin disorders	1 (1%)
Musculoskeletal tissue disorders	1 (1%)

REGIMEN

Elderly Patients (Age >80 Years)

Mini-CEOP (CYCLOPHOSPHAMIDE + EPIRUBICIN + VINBLASTINE + PREDNISONE)

Merli et al. Leuk Lymphoma 2007;48:367–373

Hydration: 500–1000 mL 0.9% sodium chloride injection (0.9% NS); administer intravenously before and after cyclophosphamide administration

Cyclophosphamide 750 mg/m²; administer intravenously in 25–250 mL 0.9% NS or 5% dextrose injection over 10–30 minutes on day 1 every 3 or 4 weeks, according to hematologic toxicity (total dosage/cycle = 750 mg/m²)

Epirubicin 50 mg/m²; administer by intravenous injection over 3–5 minutes on day 1 every 3 or 4 weeks, according to hematologic toxicity (total dosage/cycle = 50 mg/m²)

Vinblastine 5 mg/m²; administer by intravenous injection over 1–2 minutes on day 1 every 3 or 4 weeks, according to hematologic toxicity (total dosage/cycle = 5 mg/m²)

Prednisone 50 mg/m² per dose; administer orally for 5 consecutive days on days 1–5 every 3 or 4 weeks, according to hematologic toxicity (total dosage/cycle = 250 mg/m²)

Supportive Care
Antiemetic prophylaxis
Emetogenic potential on day 1 is HIGH. Potential for delayed emetic symptoms
See Chapter 39 for antiemetic recommendations

Hematopoietic growth factor (CSF) prophylaxis
Primary prophylaxis is indicated with 1 of the following:
Filgrastim (G-CSF) 5 mcg/kg per day; administer by subcutaneous injection, *or*
Pegfilgrastim (pegylated filgrastim) 6 mg/0.6 mL; administer by subcutaneous injection for 1 dose
• Begin use from 24–72 hours after myelosuppressive chemotherapy is completed
• Continue daily filgrastim use until ANC ≥10,000/mm³ on 2 measurements separated temporally by ≥12 hours
• Discontinue daily filgrastim use at least 24 hours before administering myelosuppressive treatment. Do not administer pegfilgrastim within 14 days before administering myelosuppressive treatment
See Chapter 43 for more information

Antimicrobial prophylaxis
Risk of fever and neutropenia is INTERMEDIATE
Antimicrobial primary prophylaxis to be considered:
• Antibacterial—consider a fluoroquinolone or no prophylaxis; *Pneumocystis jirovecii* prophylaxis is recommended (eg, cotrimoxazole)
• Antifungal—recommended; consider use during periods of neutropenia
• Antiviral—antiherpes antivirals (eg, acyclovir, famciclovir, valacyclovir)
See Chapter 47 for more information

Steroid-associated gastritis
Add a **proton pump inhibitor** during steroid use to prevent gastritis and duodenitis

Treatment Modifications

Adverse Event	Treatment Modifications
ANC ≥1000/mm³	Administer full doses of epirubicin and cyclophosphamide
ANC 500–999/mm³	Administer 2/3 doses of epirubicin and cyclophosphamide
Anemia or thrombocytopenia	No reduction in treatment intensity
On day 1 of a cycle, ANC <500/mm³	Delay start of cycle until ANC ≥1000/mm³ with a maximum of 28 days between two consecutive cycles.
ANC <500/mm³ 1 week (day 35) after day 1 of a cycle despite withholding chemotherapy	Discontinue therapy
G2 neurologic vinblastine-related toxicity including sensory or motor polyneuritis, constipation, or visual or auditory changes	Discontinue vinblastine

Toxicity

Adverse Event	Percentage of Patients (Number)
Treatment program stopped for toxicity	2% (2)
Toxic deaths	7% (9)
Grades 3/4 neutropenia	27%
Cardiac events	6%
Nausea and vomiting	5%
Severe infections	10%
Neurologic problems	4%

Patient Population Studied

Patient Characteristics
Mini-CEOP (N = 125)

	Number of Patients (%)
Median age (range)	73 years (66–87 years)
Male gender	47 (38)
Performance Status 2–4	33 (27)
Ann Arbor stage III–IV	94 (75)
Bulky disease	29 (23)
Extranodal involvement ≥2 sites	38 (31)
Bone Marrow involvement	29 (24)
Elevated LDH	66 (55)
Age Adjusted IPI	
Low	17 (15)
Low-Intermediate	39 (33)
Intermediate-High	38 (32)
High	23 (20)
NA	8

IPI, International Prognostic Index;
LDH, lactate dehydrogenase; NA, not assessed

A study of 90 patients with recurrent or refractory NHL

Velasquez WS et al. Blood 1988;71:117–122

Treatment Monitoring

1. *Within 1 month before the first treatment cycle:* full history, physical examination, instrumental activities of daily living (IADL) scale, thoracic and abdominal computerized scans, electrocardiogram, and assessment of resting left ventricular ejection fraction by echocardiography or an isotopic method
2. *Laboratory assessments within 1 week before first chemotherapy:* lactate dehydrogenase, β_2-microglobulin, serum creatinine, serum transaminases, and bilirubin
3. *Tumor response assessment:* after 3 cycles and at the end of treatment
4. *Follow-up:* every 3 months for the first 2 years after treatment and every 6 months thereafter

Efficacy

Response to Treatment
(N = 104)

	Number of Patients (%)
Complete remission	69 (66)
Partial remission	12 (12)
Overall response	81 (78)
Stable disease/progressive disease	23 (22)

	Number of Patients and/or Percent
5-Year relapse-free survival*	48%
5-Year relapse-free survival†	21%
Number of deaths	93 (89.4%)
Death from lymphoma	73%
Treatment-related deaths	10 (8.8%)
5-Year overall survival	32%
Median overall survival	18 months

Variable	P Value
Univariate analysis of survival Correlations for entire group	
Age as a continuous variable and ↓ overall survival	<0.001
Bone marrow involvement and ↓ overall survival	0.04
Elevated lactate dehydrogenase (LDH) and ↓ overall survival	<0.001
Age Adjusted International Prognostic Index and ↓ overall survival	0.004
Bone marrow involvement and ↓ relapse-free survival	<0.001
Cox multivariate analysis Correlations for entire group	
Age as a continuous variable and ↓ overall survival	<0.001
Elevated lactate dehydrogenase (LDH) and ↓ overall survival	<0.001
Bone marrow involvement and ↓ relapse-free survival	<0.001
Quality of Life (Qol) Improvements—All Patients	
Pain	0.003
Appetite	0.006
Sleep	0.015
Global health	0.027
Quality of Life (Qol) Improvements—Patients with A Complete Response	
Emotional state	0.10
Role	0.05
Constipation	0.04
Global QoL	0.05

*After a median follow-up for living patients of 72 months (range: 9–104 months)
†Among eligible patients

REGIMEN

RITUXIMAB, IFOSFAMIDE, CARBOPLATIN, AND ETOPOSIDE (RICE)

Kewalramani T et al. Blood 2004;103:3684–3688

Premedication for rituximab:
Acetaminophen 650–1000 mg; administer orally, *plus*
Diphenhydramine 25–50 mg; administer orally or intravenously, 30–60 minutes before starting rituximab

Induction phase:
Rituximab 375 mg/m²; administer intravenously in 0.9% sodium chloride injection (0.9% NS) or 5% dextrose injection (D5W), diluted to a concentration of 1–4 mg/mL, 48 hours before initiation of the first cycle, then every 2 weeks on day 1 of each cycle (total dosage/3 cycles = 1500 mg/m²)

Notes on rituximab administration:
- An initiating dose was given 48 hours before the first cycle of RICE. Subsequently, rituximab was given on the first day of each cycle of RICE
- Infuse initially at 50 mg/hour. If hypersensitivity or infusion reactions do not occur during the first 30 minutes, increase the rate by 50 mg/hour every 30 minutes, as tolerated, to a maximum rate of 400 mg/hour. Subsequently, if previous administration was well tolerated, start at 100 mg/hour and increase by 100 mg/hour every 30 minutes, as tolerated, to a maximum rate of 400 mg/hour
- Interrupt rituximab administration for fever, chills, edema, congestion of the head and neck mucosa, hypertension, and other serious adverse events. Resume rituximab administration after adverse events abate

Note: ICE chemotherapy is administered on an inpatient basis beginning on day 3 of each cycle Cycles are administered at 2-week intervals such that the second and third cycles of RICE would begin on day 15 of the previous cycle

Etoposide 100 mg/m² per day; administer intravenously diluted in 0.9% NS to a concentration within the range of 0.2–0.4 mg/mL, over 1 hour for 3 consecutive days, days 3–5, every 2 weeks (total dosage/cycle = 300 mg/m²)
Carboplatin (calculated dose) AUC = 5 mg/mL · min* (maximum absolute dose/cycle = 800 mg); administer intravenously in 100–500 mL D5W or 0.9% NS over 15–30 minutes on day 4, every 2 weeks (total dosage/cycle calculated to produce an AUC = 5 mg/mL · min; maximum absolute dose/cycle = 800 mg)
Ifosfamide 5000 mg/m² with **mesna** 5000 mg/m²; administer by continuous intravenous infusion diluted in 0.9% NS or D5W to an ifosfamide concentration within the range of 0.6–20 mg/mL over 24 hours on day 4, every 2 weeks (total ifosfamide and mesna dosages/cycle = 5000 mg/m²)
- Ifosfamide and mesna may be combined in a single container, or may be administered separately

*Carboplatin dose is based on a formula developed by Calvert et al. to achieve a target area under the plasma concentration versus time curve (AUC; AUC units = mg/mL · min)

$$\text{Total Carboplatin Dose (mg)} = (\text{Target AUC}) \times (\text{GFR} + 25)$$

In practice, creatinine clearance (Clcr) is used in place of glomerular filtration rate (GFR). Clcr can be calculated from the equation of Cockcroft and Gault:

$$\text{For males, Clcr} = \frac{(140 \pm \text{age [years]}) \times (\text{body weight [kg]})}{72 \times (\text{serum creatinine [mg/dL]})}$$

$$\text{For females, Clcr} = \frac{(140 - \text{age [years]}) \times (\text{body weight [kg]})}{72 \times (\text{serum creatinine [mg/dL]})} \times 0.85$$

Calvert AH et al. J Clin Oncol 1989;7:1748–1756
Cockcroft DW, Gault MH. Nephron 1976;16:31–41
Jodrell DI et al. J Clin Oncol 1992;10:520–528
Sorensen BT et al. Cancer Chemother Pharmacol 1991;28:397–401

(continued)

Patient Population Studied

A study comparing 37 patients 18–72 years of age who had diffuse large B-cell lymphoma (DLBCL), according to the World Health Organization classification, that relapsed after, or was refractory to, a single standard anthracycline-based regimen, to historical control treated with ICE alone

Treatment Modifications

Adverse Event	Dose Modification
ANC <1000/mm³ and platelet count <50,000/mm³	Delay start of treatment until ANC is >1000/mm³ and platelet count is >50,000/mm³

Toxicity

G3/4 Toxicity	No. of Events
Neutropenia and fever	8
Infection	4
Cardiac ischemia	2
Venous thromboembolism	2
Hemorrhagic cystitis	2
Nausea/vomiting	2
Syncope	1
G3/4 neutropenia resulting in treatment delay	11
G3/4 thrombocytopenia resulting in treatment delay	14
G3/4 neutropenia and thrombocytopenia resulting in treatment delay	11

(continued)

Note: A carboplatin dose calculated with an IDMS-measured serum creatinine result using the Calvert formula could exceed an expected exposure (AUC) and result in increased drug-related toxicity. The FDA recommends capping an estimated GFR at 125 mL/min for any targeted AUC value. No greater estimated GFR values should be used [online] May 23, 2013. Available from: http://www.fda.gov/AboutFDA/CentersOffices/OfficeofMedicalProductsandTobacco/CDER/ucm228974.htm [accessed February 26, 2014]

Supportive Care
Antiemetic prophylaxis
Emetogenic potential on days 1, 3, and 5 is **LOW**
Emetogenic potential on day 4 is **MODERATE–HIGH. *Potential for delayed symptoms***
See Chapter 39 for antiemetic recommendations

Hematopoietic growth factor (CSF) prophylaxis
Primary prophylaxis is indicated with:
  Filgrastim (G-CSF) 5 mcg/kg per day; administer by subcutaneous injection for 8 consecutive days, on days 5–12
See Chapter 43 for more information

Antimicrobial prophylaxis
Risk of fever and neutropenia is LOW
  Antimicrobial primary prophylaxis to be considered:
  • Antibacterial—*Pneumocystis jirovecii* prophylaxis is recommended (eg, cotrimoxazole)
  • Antifungal—not indicated
  • Antiviral—not indicated unless patient previously had an episode of HSV
See Chapter 47 for more information

Therapy Monitoring

Before each cycle: CBC with differential, serum BUN, and creatinine

Notes

1. Used for cytoreduction and stem cell mobilization in transplant-eligible patients. There were no dose reductions. Of 381 cycles, 66 were delayed because of hematologic toxicity
2. Four patients developed confusion that resolved without intervention. These patients were not retreated

Efficacy

Response Rates to RICE Compared with ICE Historical Controls

Patient Subgroup	Overall Response Rate (%)			Complete Response Rate (%)		
	R-ICE	ICE*	*p*-Value	R-ICE	ICE*	*p*-Value
All patients	78	71	0.53	53	27	0.01
Relapsed	96	79	0.07	65	34	0.01
Refractory	46	63	0.36	31	19	0.46
sAAIPI L/LI	79	86	0.47	53	39	0.42
sAAIPI H/HI	76	61	0.28	53	19	0.01

sAAIP, Second-line age-adjusted international prognostic index; L, low risk; LI, low–intermediate risk; HI, high–intermediate risk; H, high risk
*ICE historical control

REGIMEN

ETOPOSIDE, METHYLPREDNISOLONE (SOLU-MEDROL), CYTARABINE (ARA-C), CISPLATIN (ESHAP)

Sweetenham JW, Johnson PWM. [Comment] J Clin Oncol 1994;12:2766
Velasquez WS et al. J Clin Oncol 1994;12:1169–1176

Hydration:
≥1000 mL 0.9% sodium chloride injection (0.9% NS) + 25–50 g mannitol daily; administer intravenously, continuously throughout chemotherapy administration or longer if medically appropriate, every 21–28 days, for 6–8 cycles. Monitor and replace magnesium/electrolytes as needed

Cisplatin 25 mg/m^2 per day; administer by continuous intravenous infusion in 100 mL to >1000 mL 0.9% NS over 24 hours for 4 consecutive days on days 1–4, every 21–28 days, for 6–8 cycles (total dosage/cycle = 100 mg/m^2)

Etoposide 40 mg/m^2 per day; administer intravenously, diluted in 0.9% NS to a concentration within the range 0.2–0.4 mg/mL over 1 hour for 4 consecutive days on days 1–4, every 21–28 days, for 6–8 cycles (total dosage/cycle = 160 mg/m^2)

Methylprednisolone 250–500 mg per day; administer intravenously in 25–500 mL 0.9% NS over 15 minutes for 5 consecutive days on days 1–5, every 21–28 days, for 6–8 cycles (total dose/cycle = 1250–2500 mg)

Cytarabine 2000 mg/m^2; administer intravenously in 25–1000 mL 0.9% NS or 5% dextrose injection over 2 hours on day 5, every 21–28 days, for 6–8 cycles (total dosage/cycle = 2000 mg/m^2)

Supportive Care
Antiemetic prophylaxis
Emetogenic potential on days 1–4 is **HIGH**
Emetogenic potential on day 5 is **MODERATE**
See Chapter 39 for antiemetic recommendations

Hematopoietic growth factor (CSF) prophylaxis
Primary prophylaxis is indicated with 1 of the following:
  Filgrastim (G-CSF) 5 mcg/kg per day; administer by subcutaneous injection, *or*
  Pegfilgrastim (pegylated filgrastim) 6 mg/0.6 mL; administer by subcutaneous injection for 1 dose
  • Begin use from 24–72 hours after myelosuppressive chemotherapy is completed
See Chapter 43 for more information

Antimicrobial prophylaxis
Risk of fever and neutropenia is INTERMEDIATE
  Antimicrobial primary prophylaxis to be considered:
  • Antibacterial—consider a fluoroquinolone or no prophylaxis; *Pneumocystis jirovecii* prophylaxis is recommended (eg, cotrimoxazole)
  • Antifungal—consider use during neutropenia and for anticipated mucositis
  • Antiviral—antiherpes antivirals (eg, acyclovir)
See Chapter 47 for more information

Steroid-associated gastritis
Add a **proton pump inhibitor** during methylprednisolone use to prevent gastritis and duodenitis

Patient Population Studied

A study of 122 patients with relapsed or refractory NHL

Efficacy (N = 122)

Complete response	37%
Partial response	27%
Overall response rate	64%

Treatment Modifications

Adverse Event*	Dose Modification
Previous cycle ANC nadir ≤200/mm^3	Reduce etoposide dosage by 20% and reduce cytarabine dosage by 50% during subsequent cycles
Previous cycle platelet count nadir ≤20,000/mm^3	
Documented sepsis during previous cycles	
Nonhematologic adverse events G3/4 in previous cycles	
Serum creatinine 1.5–2.0 mg/dL (133–177 μmol/L) immediately prior to a cycle	Reduce cisplatin dosage by 25% during subsequent cycles
Serum creatinine 2.1–3.0 mg/dL (186–265 μmol/L) immediately prior to a cycle	Reduce cisplatin dosage by 50% during subsequent cycles
Serum creatinine >3.0 mg/dL (>265 μmol/L) immediately before a cycle	Hold cisplatin

*For neutropenia consider Filgrastim 5 mcg/kg per day subcutaneously, starting on day 6 and continuing beyond ANC nadir until ANC exceeds 5000/mm^3 on 1 reading

Toxicity (N = 122)

Median ANC nadir	500/mm^3
Median platelet nadir	70,000/mm^3
G1/2 nausea/vomiting	49%
G3 nausea/vomiting	6%
>2-Fold increase in creatinine from baseline measurement	
Reversible	18%
Permanent	4%
Fever and neutropenia	30%
Treatment-related death	5%

Therapy Monitoring

1. *Before each cycle:* PE, CBC with differential, serum electrolytes, BUN, creatinine, and LFTs
2. *Daily on days of drug administration:* Serum electrolytes, magnesium, calcium, and phosphorus. Cardiac, pulmonary, and renal status should be carefully monitored during administration of fluids
3. *Weekly:* CBC with differential

REGIMEN

DEXAMETHASONE, CYTARABINE (HIGH-DOSE ARA-C), AND CISPLATIN (DHAP)

Gisselbrecht C et al. J Clin Oncol 2010;28:4184–4190

Hydration:
0.9% sodium chloride injection (0.9% NS) + at a rate of 250 mL/hour for 36 hours; administer intravenously beginning at least 6 hours before starting cisplatin administration, every 3–4 weeks, for 6–10 cycles. Monitor and replace magnesium/electrolytes as needed
Cisplatin 100 mg/m²; administer by continuous intravenous infusion over 24 hours in a volume equivalent to the dose, or diluted in 100 mL to ≥1000 mL 0.9% NS. Begin administration on day 1 after completing 6 hours of hydration, every 3–4 weeks, for 6–10 cycles (total dosage/cycle = 100 mg/m²)
Cytarabine
Patients ≤ 70 years: **Cytarabine** 2000 mg/m² per dose; administer intravenously over 3 hours in 50–500 mL 0.9% NS or 5% dextrose injection (D5W) every 12 hours for 2 doses, starting after the completion of cisplatin administration on day 2, every 3–4 weeks, for 6–10 cycles (total dosage/cycle = 4000 mg/m²)
Patients > 70 years: **Cytarabine** 1000 mg/m² per dose; administer intravenously over 3 hours in 50–500 mL 0.9% NS or D5W every 12 hours for 2 doses, starting after the completion of cisplatin administration on day 2, every 3–4 weeks, for 6–10 cycles (total dosage/cycle = 2000 mg/m²)
Dexamethasone 40 mg/day; administer orally or intravenously in 10–100 mL 0.9% NS or D5W over 10–30 minutes for 4 consecutive days on days 1–4, every 3–4 weeks, for 6–10 cycles (total dosage/cycle = 160 mg)

Supportive Care
Antiemetic prophylaxis
Emetogenic potential on day 1 is **HIGH.** *Potential for delayed symptoms*
Emetogenic potential on day 2 is **MODERATE–HIGH**
See Chapter 39 for antiemetic recommendations

Hematopoietic growth factor (CSF) prophylaxis
Primary prophylaxis is indicated with **1** *of the following:*
    Filgrastim (G-CSF) 5 mcg/kg per day; administer by subcutaneous injection, *or*
    Pegfilgrastim (pegylated filgrastim) 6 mg/0.6 mL; administer by subcutaneous injection for 1 dose
    • Begin use from 24–72 hours after myelosuppressive chemotherapy is completed
See Chapter 43 for more information

Antimicrobial prophylaxis
Risk of fever and neutropenia is INTERMEDIATE
    Antimicrobial primary prophylaxis to be considered:
    • Antibacterial—consider a fluoroquinolone or no prophylaxis; *Pneumocystis jirovecii* prophylaxis is recommended (eg, cotrimoxazole)
    • Antifungal—consider use during neutropenia and for anticipated mucositis
    • Antiviral—antiherpes antivirals (eg, acyclovir)
See Chapter 47 for more information

Steroid-associated gastritis
Add a **proton pump inhibitor** during dexamethasone use to prevent gastritis and duodenitis

Treatment Modifications

Adverse Event*	Dose Modification
ANC <200/mm³ during any cycle	Reduce cytarabine dosage to 1000 mg/m² per dose; maintain cisplatin dosage at 100 mg/m²
Platelet count <20,000/mm³ during any cycle	
Sepsis associated with neutropenia during any cycle	Reduce cytarabine dosage to 500 mg/m² per dose; maintain cisplatin dosage at 100 mg/m²
Serum creatinine increase to 1.5–2.0 mg/mL (133–177 µmol/L)	Reduce cisplatin dosage to 75 mg/m²
Serum creatinine increase to 2.1–3.0 mg/mL (186–265 µmol/L)	Reduce cisplatin dosage to 50 mg/m²

*For neutropenia consider Filgrastim 5 mcg/kg per day subcutaneously, starting on day 6 and continuing beyond ANC nadir until ANC exceeds 5000/mm³ on 1 reading

Patient Population Studied

A study of 90 patients with recurrent or refractory NHL

Efficacy (N = 90)

Complete response	31%
Partial response	24%
Overall response rate	55%
2-Year survival	25%

Toxicity (N = 90)

	% of Patients
ANC nadir <300/mm^3	53
Platelet count nadir <20,000/mm^3	39
Gastrointestinal (severe)	20
Acute cerebellar syndrome	1
Acute tumor lysis syndrome	6
Early deaths	
Because of tumor lysis syndrome	3
Because of sepsis	2
Because of thromboembolism	1
Because of subdural hemorrhage	1
Reversible ↑ serum creatinine to >2 × baseline	16
Permanent ↑ serum creatinine to >2 × baseline	4
Chronic polyneuritis	4
Tinnitus	4
Severe hearing loss	3
Respiratory failure	6
Hospitalization for IV antibiotics	48
Documented sepsis	31
Death from complications of sepsis	11

Therapy Monitoring

1. *Before each cycle:* PE, CBC with differential, serum electrolytes, BUN, creatinine, LFTs
2. *Daily on days of drug administration:* Serum electrolytes. Cardiac, pulmonary, and renal status are carefully monitored during administration of fluids
3. *Weekly:* CBC with differential

REGIMEN

GEMCITABINE + DEXAMETHASONE + CISPLATIN (GDP)

Crump et al. Cancer 2004;101:1835–1842
Crump et al. Clin Lymphoma 2005;6:56–60

Gemcitabine 1000 mg/m^2 per dose; administer intravenously in 0.9% sodium chloride injection (0.9% NS) to a concentration within the range 0.1–38 mg/mL over 30 minutes for 2 doses, on days 1 and 8, every 21 days (total dosage/cycle = 2000 mg/m^2)

Dexamethasone 40 mg/dose; administer orally in 2 or more divided doses for 4 consecutive days, on days 1–4, every 21 days (total dose/cycle = 160 mg)

Hydration before cisplatin: 1000 mL 0.9% NS; administer intravenously over a minimum of 1 hour before commencing cisplatin administration

(Optional) **Mannitol** 12.5–50 g; administer by intravenous injection or intravenous infusion over 5–60 minutes either before or concurrent with cisplatin administration

• Mannitol may be given to patients who have received adequate hydration. Continued hydration is essential to ensure diuresis

• Mannitol may be prepared as an admixture (in the same container) with cisplatin

Cisplatin 75 mg/m^2; administer intravenously in 50–500 mL 0.9% NS over 60 minutes on day 1 every 21 days (total dosage/cycle = 75 mg/m^2)

Hydration after cisplatin: ≥1000 mL 0.9% NS; administer intravenously over a minimum of 2 hours on day 1. Encourage patients to increase oral intake of nonalcoholic fluids, and provide electrolyte replacement as needed (potassium, magnesium, sodium)

Notes:
• The initial dexamethasone dose may be administered intravenously before chemotherapy commences as part of antiemetic primary prophylaxis

Supportive Care
Antiemetic prophylaxis
Emetogenic potential on day 1 is **HIGH**. *Potential for delayed emetic symptoms*
Emetogenic potential on day 8 is **LOW**
See Chapter 39 for antiemetic recommendations

Hematopoietic growth factor (CSF) prophylaxis
Primary prophylaxis may be indicated
See Chapter 43 for more information

Antimicrobial prophylaxis
Risk of fever and neutropenia is INTERMEDIATE
Antimicrobial primary prophylaxis to be considered:
• Antibacterial—consider a fluoroquinolone or no prophylaxis; *Pneumocystis jirovecii* prophylaxis is recommended (eg, cotrimoxazole)
• Antifungal—recommended; consider use during periods of neutropenia and in anticipation of mucositis
• Antiviral—antiherpes antivirals (eg, acyclovir, famciclovir, valacyclovir)
See Chapter 47 for more information

Steroid-associated gastritis
Add a **proton pump inhibitor** during steroid use to prevent gastritis and duodenitis

Oral care
Prophylaxis and treatment for mucositis/stomatitis
General advice:
• Encourage patients to maintain intake of nonalcoholic fluids
• Evaluate patients for oral pain and provide analgesic medications
• Consider histamine (H$_2$-subtype) receptor antagonists (eg, ranitidine, famotidine), or a proton pump inhibitor for epigastric pain
• *Lactobacillus* sp.-containing probiotics may be beneficial in preventing diarrhea

(continued)

Treatment Modifications

ANC <1000/mm^3 or platelet count <100,000/mm^3 on day 1 of a cycle	Delay start of next treatment cycle by 1 week or until ANC ≥1000/mm^3 and platelet count ≥100,000/mm^3
Day 8 ANC <500/mm^3 or platelet count <50,000/mm^3	Omit day 8 gemcitabine dose, or delay treatment 1 week and administer gemcitabine only if ANC ≥500/mm^3 and platelet count ≥50,000/mm^3
Day 8 ANC <500/mm^3 with platelet count >50,000/mm^3	Administer full dose of gemcitabine and begin therapy with filgrastim, or administer gemcitabine with a dose reduction of 25%
Day 8 platelet count 50,000–99,000/mm^3 with ANC >500/mm^3	Reduce day 8 gemcitabine dose by 25%
One dose delay or dosage attenuation for neutropenia	Administer filgrastim with subsequent treatment cycles to maintain dose intensity
One episode of febrile neutropenia	Administer filgrastim with subsequent treatment cycles

(continued)

Patients with intact oral mucosa:

- Clean the mouth, tongue, and gums by brushing after every meal and at bedtime with an ultrasoft toothbrush with fluoride toothpaste
- Floss teeth gently every day unless contraindicated. If gums bleed and hurt, avoid bleeding or sore areas, but floss other teeth
- Patients may use saline or commercial brand, nonalcoholic rinses
  - Do not use mouthwashes that contain alcohols

If mucositis or stomatitis is present:

- Keep the mouth moist utilizing water, ice chips, sugarless gum, sugar-free hard candies, or a saliva substitute
- Rinse mouth several times a day to remove debris
  - Use a solution of ¼ teaspoon (1.25 g) each of baking soda and table salt (sodium chloride) in 1 quart (~950 mL) of warm water. Follow with a plain water rinse
  - Do not use mouthwashes that contain alcohols
- Foam-tipped swabs (eg, Toothettes) are useful in moisturizing oral mucosa, but ineffective for cleansing teeth and removing plaque
- Advise patients who develop mucositis to:
  - Choose foods that are easy to chew and swallow
  - Take small bites of food, chew slowly, and sip liquids with meals
  - Encourage soft, moist foods such as cooked cereals, mashed potatoes, and scrambled eggs
  - For trouble swallowing, soften food with gravies, sauces, broths, yogurt, or other bland liquids
  - Avoid sharp, crunchy foods; hot, spicy, or highly acidic foods (eg, citrus fruits and juices); sugary foods; toothpicks; tobacco products; alcoholic drinks

Efficacy (N = 51)

All Patients

CR after 2 cycles of GDP	8 (16%)
PR after 2 cycles of GDP	17 (33%)
ORR after 2 cycles of GDP	25 (49%, 95% CI = 37–63%)
CR after completing all cycles of GDP	11 (22%)
PR after completing all cycles of GDP	16 (31%)
ORR after completing all cycles of GDP	27 (53%, 95% CI = 40–67%)

Patients >65 Years of Age not Usually Considered for High-dose Chemotherapy + ASCT

Median time to progression	3.1 months (95% CI = 2.3–9.2)
Median overall survival	8.9 months (95% CI = 5.2–18.5)

CI, confidence interval; CR, complete response; GDP, gemcitabine + dexamethasone + cisplatin; ORR, overall response rate (CR = PR); PR, partial response

Patient Population Studied

Patients with diffuse large B-cell, large-cell immunoblastic, anaplastic large-cell (B-cell or null-cell type), primary mediastinal large B-cell, or T-cell–rich B-cell lymphoma with disease recurrence after or refractory to 1 previous anthracycline-containing chemotherapy regimen. Patients with a diagnosis of transformed or composite lymphoma were excluded

Patient Characteristics (N = 51)

	Number
Median age–years (range)	57 (18–84)
Stage at study entry (Ann Arbor staging system)	
I/II	19
III/IV	32
B symptoms	11
Histology	
Diffuse large B cells	40
Immunoblastic cells	3
Anaplastic large cells	3
T-cell–rich B cells	3
Mediastinal large cells	2
Response to previous therapy	
CR/Cru	22
PR	25
No response	4
Months to disease recurrence/progression from end of initial therapy	
<3 mo	18
3–12 mo	19
>12 mo	14
Previous radiation	18
LDH at disease recurrence	
Elevated	32
Normal	19
IPI risk factors at disease recurrence	
0	4
1	15
2	13
3	16
4	2
5	1

Toxicities (Worst Ever by Patient; N = 51)[*]

	% G1	% G2	% G3	% G4
Hematologic Toxicities				
Hemoglobin	47	33	14	2
Granulocytes	6	18	33	31
Platelets	31	6	25	4
Febrile neutropenia[†]			14	
Infection[†]	4	6	6	2
Melena/GI bleeding	4		2	
Epistaxis	10		2	
Petechiae/purpura	2	6		
Nonhematologic Toxicities				
Fatigue	35	43	10	2
Nausea	39	20	8	
Emesis	18	12	10	
Constipation	18	27	2	
Stomatitis	16	10		
Diarrhea	22	10		
Cough	24	6		
Dyspnea	2	10	4	
Edema	12	12	2	
Thrombosis/embolism			8	6
Motor neuropathy	2	2	2	2
Sensory neuropathy	20	8	2	
Ototoxicity	2	24		
Elevated creatinine	14	6		
Elevated AST	8	2	2	2
Elevated ALT	10	4	4	

[*]National Cancer Institute (USA) Common Toxicity Criteria, version 2.0
[†]One grade 5 toxicity

Treatment Monitoring

1. Before treatment
   - History and physical examination
   - CBC with differential, serum creatinine, AST, ALT, alkaline phosphatase, and serum bilirubin
2. During treatment
   - History and physical examination before each cycle
   - CBC with differential, serum creatinine, AST, ALT, alkaline phosphatase, and serum bilirubin on day 1 of each treatment cycle
   - CBC with differential on day 8
3. Reassessment of efficacy: CT scan or sonographic examination after 2 and 4 cycles and at the end of treatment

REGIMEN

CYCLOPHOSPHAMIDE, VINCRISTINE, AND PREDNISONE (CVP)

Bagley CM Jr et al. Ann Intern Med 1972;76:227–234
Flinn IW et al. Ann Oncol 2000;11:691–695

Cyclophosphamide 400 mg/m^2 per day; administer orally for 5 consecutive days on days 1–5, every 3 weeks, for at least 4 cycles, +2 additional cycles after complete response (total dosage/cycle = 2000 mg/m^2)

or

Cyclophosphamide 1000 mg/m^2; administer intravenously, as either undiluted cyclophosphamide (20 mg/mL) or diluted in 100–1000 mL 0.9% sodium chloride injection (0.9% NS) or 5% dextrose injection (D5W), over 15–60 minutes, given on day 1, every 3 weeks, for at least 4 cycles, +2 additional cycles after complete response (total dosage/cycle = 1000 mg/m^2)
Vincristine 1.4 mg/m^2; administer by intravenous injection over 1–2 minutes, given on day 1, every 3 weeks, for at least 4 cycles, +2 additional cycles after complete response (total dosage/cycle = 1.4 mg/m^2)
Prednisone 100 mg/m^2 per day; administer orally for 5 consecutive days on days 1–5, every 3 weeks, for at least 4 cycles, +2 additional cycles after complete response (total dosage/cycle = 500 mg/m^2)

Supportive Care
Antiemetic prophylaxis
Emetogenic potential on days 1–5 is **MODERATE–HIGH**. *Potential for delayed emetic symptoms*
See Chapter 39 for antiemetic recommendations

Hematopoietic growth factor (CSF) prophylaxis
Primary prophylaxis may be indicated
See Chapter 43 for more information

Antimicrobial prophylaxis
Risk of fever and neutropenia is LOW
  Antimicrobial primary prophylaxis to be considered:
  • Antibacterial—*Pneumocystis jirovecii* prophylaxis is recommended (eg, cotrimoxazole)
  • Antifungal—not indicated
  • Antiviral—not indicated, unless patient previously had an episode of HSV
See Chapter 47 for more information

Steroid-associated gastritis
Add a **proton pump inhibitor** during steroid use to prevent gastritis and duodenitis

Decreased bowel motility prophylaxis
Give **stool softeners** in a scheduled regimen, and **saline, osmotic, and lubricant laxatives**, as needed to prevent constipation for as long as vincristine use continues. If needed, circumspectly add **stimulant (irritant) laxatives** in the least amounts and for the briefest durations needed to produce defecation

Toxicity (N = 35)

Severe infections	14%
Mild cystitis without bleeding	8.6%

Hematologic Nadirs During 6 Consecutive Cycles

Cycle	WBC Count	Platelet Count
1	2400/mm^3	220,000/mm^3
2	2300/mm^3	204,000/mm^3
3	3100/mm^3	192,000/mm^3
4	2000/mm^3	200,000/mm^3
5	3200/mm^3	224,000/mm^3
6	2800/mm^3	213,000/mm^3

Therapy Monitoring

1. *Prior to each cycle:* PE, CBC, differential, LFTs, serum BUN, and creatinine
2. *Weekly:* CBC with differential and LFTs

Patient Population Studied

A study of 35 patients with advanced NHL, among whom 32 previously had not received antineoplastic therapy

Efficacy (N = 35)

Complete response	57%
Partial response	34%
Overall response rate	91%

Treatment Modifications

At the start of a treatment cycle:

ANC	Platelet Count	% of Planned Dosages		
		C	V	P
>4000/mm^3	≥100,000/mm^3	100	100	100
3–4000/mm^3	50–100,000/mm^3	75	100	100
2–3000/mm^3	50–100,000/mm^3	50	100	100
1–2000/mm^3	<50,000/mm^3	25	50	100
0–1000/mm^3	<50,000/mm^3	0	0	0

C, cyclophosphamide; V, vincristine; P, prednisone
Note: Repeated cycles may be delayed for up to 1 week for incomplete hematologic recovery (ie, day 1 ANC must be >1000/mm^3 from prior treatment)

REGIMEN

RITUXIMAB + CYCLOPHOSPHAMIDE, VINCRISTINE, AND PREDNISONE (R-CVP)

Marcus R et al. Blood 2005;105:1417–1423

Premedication for rituximab:

Acetaminophen 650–1000 mg; administer orally, *plus*

Diphenhydramine 25–50 mg; administer orally or intravenously 30–60 minutes before starting rituximab

Rituximab 375 mg/m^2; administer intravenously in 0.9% sodium chloride injection (0.9% NS) or 5% dextrose injection (D5W), diluted to a concentration of 1–4 mg/mL, on day 1, every 3 weeks, for a maximum of 8 cycles (total dosage/cycle = 375 mg/m^2)

Notes on rituximab administration:

- Infuse initially at 50 mg/hour. If hypersensitivity or infusion reactions do not occur during the first 30 minutes, increase the rate by 50 mg/hour every 30 minutes, as tolerated, to a maximum rate of 400 mg/hour. Subsequently, if previous administration was well tolerated, start at 100 mg/hour and increase by 100 mg/hour every 30 minutes, as tolerated, to a maximum rate of 400 mg/hour

- Interrupt rituximab administration for fever, chills, edema, congestion of the head and neck mucosa, hypertension, and other serious adverse events. Resume rituximab administration after adverse events abate

Cyclophosphamide 750 mg/m^2; administer intravenously in 25–250 mL 0.9% NS or D5W, over 10–30 minutes on day 1, every 3 weeks, for a maximum of 8 cycles (total dosage/cycle = 750 mg/m^2)

Vincristine 1.4 mg/m^2 (maximum single dose = 2 mg); administer by intravenous injection over 1–2 minutes, on day 1, every 3 weeks, for a maximum of 8 cycles (total dosage/cycle = 1.4 mg/m^2, maximum dose/cycle = 2 mg)

Prednisone 40 mg/m^2 per day; administer orally for 5 consecutive days, days 1–5, every 3 weeks, for a maximum of 8 cycles (total dosage/cycle = 200 mg/m^2)

Supportive Care

Antiemetic prophylaxis

Emetogenic potential on day 1 is **MODERATE**

See Chapter 39 for antiemetic recommendations

Hematopoietic growth factor (CSF) prophylaxis

Primary prophylaxis is indicated with 1 of the following:

Filgrastim (G-CSF) 5 mcg/kg per day, by subcutaneous injection, *or*

Pegfilgrastim (pegylated filgrastim) 6 mg/0.6 mL, by subcutaneous injection for 1 dose

- Begin use from 24–72 hours after myelosuppressive chemotherapy is completed

See Chapter 43 for more information

Antimicrobial prophylaxis

Risk of fever and neutropenia is LOW

Antimicrobial primary prophylaxis to be considered:

- Antibacterial—*Pneumocystis jirovecii* prophylaxis is recommended (eg, cotrimoxazole)

- Antifungal—not indicated

- Antiviral—not indicated unless patient previously had an episode of HSV

See Chapter 47 for more information

Toxicity

Adverse Event	CVP	R-CVP
At least 1 adverse event	95%	97%
Life-threatening events	—	3.1%
Adverse event within 24 hours after an infusion	51%	71%
G 3/4, rituximab infusion-related reaction	N/A	9%
G 3/4 neutropenia	14%	24%
Overall infection rate or incidence of neutropenia and sepsis	No difference	

Patient Population Studied

A study of 321 patients age 18 years or older with advanced stage untreated CD20+ follicular lymphoma who were randomized to RCVP or CVP for 8 cycles. All patients had stage III or IV disease, an Eastern Clinical Oncology Group (ECOG) performance status of 0–2, and a need for therapy in the opinion of the participating clinician. Median age was 52–53 years. Majority were grade 1 or 2 follicular lymphoma

Treatment Modification

		Dose Modification		
	Adverse Event	Percent of Planned Dosages		
ANC	Platelet Count	C	V	P
>4000/mm^3	≥100,000/mm^3	100%	100%	100%
3000–4000/mm^3	50,000–100,000/mm^3	75%	100%	100%
2000–3000/mm^3	50,000–100,000/mm^3	50%	100%	100%
1000–2000/mm^3	<50,000/mm^3	25%	50%	100%
0–1000/mm^3	<50,000/mm^3	0	0	0
G2 neurotoxicity		Reduce vincristine dosage 50%		
G3/4 neurotoxicity		Discontinue vincristine		
Rituximab-induced infusion reaction		Interrupt therapy; resume rituximab and CVP once symptoms resolve		

C, cyclophosphamide; V, vincristine; P, prednisone
Note: Repeated cycles may be delayed for up to 1 week for incomplete hematologic recovery (ie, day 1 ANC must be >1000/mm^3 from prior treatment)

Efficacy
(Median Follow-up: 30 Months)

	CVP (N = 159)	R-CVP (N = 162)
Tumor Response*		
Complete response	8%	30%
Complete response, unconfirmed	3%	11%
Partial response	47%	40%
CR + CRu + PR	57%	81%
Stable disease	21%	7%
Progressive disease	20%	11%
Could not be assessed	3%	1%
Median time to progression*	15 months	32 months
Median time to treatment failure*	7 months	27 months
Median duration of response*	14 months	35 months
Median disease-free survival†	21 months	Not reached
Median time to new antilymphoma treatment or death	14 months	Not reached
KM estimates for overall survival at 30 months‡	85%	89%

CVP, Cyclophosphamide, vincristine, and prednisone; CR, complete response; CRu, complete response, unconfirmed; PR, partial response
*P <0.001
†P = 0.0009
‡Not significant

Therapy Monitoring

1. *Prior to each cycle:* PE, CBC with differential, LFTs, serum BUN, and creatinine
2. *Weekly:* CBC with differential and LFTs

REGIMEN

FLUDARABINE

Solal-Céligny P et al. J Clin Oncol 1996;14:514–519

Prophylaxis against tumor lysis:
See also Chapter 39

Allopurinol 300 mg per day; administer orally for 9 consecutive days, beginning the day before fludarabine treatment starts. Repeat a course of prophylaxis during at least the first 2 treatment cycles and for additional cycles if judged clinically appropriate

Fludarabine 25 mg/m² per day; administer intravenously in 100–125 mL 0.9% sodium chloride injection or 5% dextrose injection over 30 minutes for 5 consecutive days on days 1–5, every 4 weeks, for up to 9 cycles (total dosage/cycle = 125 mg/m²)
Note: The maximum planned treatment duration is 9 cycles. Treatment is discontinued in the event of disease progression or after 6 cycles for patients who achieve a CR after 3 cycles and for those whose disease does not respond during the first 6 cycles

Supportive Care
Antiemetic prophylaxis
Emetogenic potential on days 1–5 is **MINIMAL**
See Chapter 39 for antiemetic recommendations

Hematopoietic growth factor (CSF) prophylaxis
Primary prophylaxis is NOT indicated
See Chapter 43 for more information

Antimicrobial prophylaxis
Risk of fever and neutropenia is LOW
Antimicrobial primary prophylaxis to be considered:
• Antibacterial—*Pneumocystis jirovecii* prophylaxis is recommended (eg, cotrimoxazole)
• Antifungal—not indicated
• Antiviral—not indicated unless patient previously had an episode of HSV
See Chapter 47 for more information

Patient Population Studied

A study of 54 untreated patients with advanced follicular lymphoma. All patients were serologically negative for HIV

Efficacy (N = 49)

Overall response	65%
Complete response	37%
Partial response	28%

Treatment Modifications

Adverse Event	Dose Modification
ANC <1500/mm³ or platelet count <100,000/mm³	Delay treatment until ANC is ≥500/mm³ and platelet count ≥100,000/mm³, then resume treatment but reduce fludarabine dosage to 20 mg/m² per day for 5 days
Treatment delay >2 weeks	Discontinue fludarabine treatment

Therapy Monitoring

Before each cycle: CBC with differential, LFTs, serum BUN, and creatinine

Toxicity*
(N = 53 Patients; 336 Cycles)

Toxicity	% of Patients	% of Cycles
G ≥3 neutropenia	41	14.4
G ≥3 thrombocytopenia	5.7	1.2
	% of Patients	
G1 Infections	15	
G2 infections	9	
G ≥3 infections	0	
Neurologic toxicity	3.8	
Interstitial pneumonitis	1.9	
Hepatitis	1.9	

*WHO Criteria

REGIMEN

FLUDARABINE + RITUXIMAB

Czuczman MS et al. J Clin Oncol 2005;23:694–704

Cycle 1 (duration 35 days)
Premedication for rituximab:
Acetaminophen 650–1000 mg; administer orally *plus* **diphenhydramine** 25–50 mg; administer orally or intravenously 30–60 minutes before each dose of rituximab
Rituximab 375 mg/m² per dose; administer intravenously in 0.9% sodium chloride injection (0.9% NS) or 5% dextrose injection (D5W) diluted to a concentration of 1–4 mg/mL for 2 doses on days 1 and 5 (total dosage/cycle = 750 mg/m²)

Notes on rituximab administration:
- Infuse initially at 50 mg/h. If hypersensitivity or infusion reactions do not occur during the first 30 minutes, increase the rate by 50 mg/h every 30 minutes as tolerated to a maximum rate of 400 mg/h. Subsequently, if previous administration was well tolerated, start at 100 mg/h and increase by 100 mg/h every 30 minutes as tolerated to a maximum rate of 400 mg/h
- Interrupt rituximab administration for fever chills, edema, congestion of the head and neck mucosa, hypertension, and other serious adverse events. Resume rituximab administration after adverse events abate

Fludarabine 25 mg/m² per dose; administer intravenously in 100–125 mL 0.9% NS or D5W over 30 minutes for 5 consecutive days, on days 8–12 during a 35-day cycle (total dosage/cycle = 125 mg/m²)

Note: Fludarabine administration commences 72 hours after the second dose of rituximab given during cycle 1

Cycles 2, 4, and 6
Premedication for rituximab:
Acetaminophen 650–1000 mg; administer orally *plus* **diphenhydramine** 25–50 mg; administer orally or intravenously 30–60 minutes before each dose of rituximab
Rituximab 375 mg/m²; administer intravenously in 0.9% NS or D5W diluted to a concentration of 1–4 mg/mL, 3 days before commencing retreatment with fludarabine (total dosage/cycle = 375 mg/m²)

Cycles 2–6 (five 28-day cycles)
Fludarabine 25 mg/m² per dose; administer intravenously in 100–125 mL 0.9% NS or D5W over 30 minutes for 5 consecutive days, on days 1–5, every 28 days for 5 cycles (total dosage/cycle = 125 mg/m²)

Note: During cycles 2, 4, and 6, fludarabine administration begins 72 hours after rituximab doses are administered

Cycle 7 (after completing six 28-day cycles with fludarabine)
Premedication for rituximab:
Acetaminophen 650–1000 mg; administer orally *plus* **diphenhydramine** 25–50 mg; administer orally or intravenously 30–60 minutes before each dose of rituximab
Rituximab 375 mg/m² per dose; administer intravenously diluted to a concentration of 1–4 mg/mL with 0.9% NS or D5W diluted to a concentration of 1–4 mg/mL for 2 doses on days 1 and 5 (total dosage/cycle = 750 mg/m²)

Supportive Care
Treatment support included transfusion of blood and blood products, antibiotics, antiemetics, and colony-stimulating factors (filgrastim or granulocyte macrophage colony-stimulating factor)

Antiemetic prophylaxis
Emetogenic potential is **MINIMAL**
See Chapter 39 for antiemetic recommendations

(continued)

Treatment Modifications

Adverse Event	Treatment Modifications
G3/4 neutropenia, G3/4 thrombocytopenia, or G3/4 anemia	Observe without treatment until these hematologic parameters recover to within 20% of the baseline value. Thereafter, if toxicity = G3, administer 75% of the original fludarabine dosage for subsequent cycles. If toxicity = G4, administer 50% of the original fludarabine dosage for subsequent cycles. If G ≥3 persists ≥3 consecutive weeks, discontinue therapy
Nonhematologic toxicities, including nausea, vomiting, fatigue, diarrhea, and drug-related fever or chills	Administer symptomatic treatment but do not reduce dosages
G ≥2 nonhematologic toxicities other than nausea, vomiting, fatigue, diarrhea, and drug-related fever or chills attributed to fludarabine	Hold fludarabine therapy until toxicity G <2, then reduce the fludarabine dosage by 50% in subsequent cycles. If after 3 weeks toxicity has not resolved to G ≤1, discontinue treatment
G2 irreversible nonhematologic toxicity and G3/4 nonhematologic toxicities	Evaluate to determine appropriateness of continuing the fludarabine therapy
Infection in the absence of G3/4 neutropenia	Observe without further CLL treatment until the infection resolves, but do not alter chemotherapy dosages
Major infection	Reduce fludarabine dosage to 20 mg/m² · d × 5 days. If further dose reduction is needed, reduce the fludarabine dosage to 15 mg/m² · d × 5 days. Rituximab dosage is not reduced

(*continued*)

Hematopoietic growth factor (CSF) prophylaxis
Primary prophylaxis may be indicated
See Chapter 43 for more information

Antimicrobial prophylaxis
Risk of fever and neutropenia is INTERMEDIATE
Antimicrobial primary prophylaxis to be considered:

- Antibacterial—consider a fluoroquinolone or no prophylaxis; *Pneumocystis jirovecii* prophylaxis is recommended (eg, cotrimoxazole)

- Antifungal—recommended; consider use during periods of neutropenia, and in anticipation of mucositis

- Antiviral—antiherpes antivirals (eg, acyclovir, famciclovir, valacyclovir)

- *Note:* Antiviral prophylaxis was prescribed to patients for 6 to 12 months after completion of therapy because of the relatively high incidence of herpes infections (6 of 40 patients; 15%) believed to be secondary to T-cell depletion from fludarabine. No patient receiving acyclovir prophylaxis developed herpes infection

See Chapter 47 for more information

Infusion reactions associated with rituximab
Fevers, chills, and rigors
1. Interrupt rituximab administration for severe symptoms and give:

- **Acetaminophen** 650 mg orally for fever. For persistent or recurrent symptoms, repeat administration every 4–6 hours as needed during rituximab administration

- **Diphenhydramine** 25–50 mg orally or by intravenous injection for pruritus, hypotension, or angioedema. For persistent or recurrent symptoms, repeat administration every 4–6 hours as needed during rituximab administration

- **Meperidine** 12.5–25 mg by intravenous injection every 10–20 minutes as needed for shaking chills (generally, cumulative doses >100 mg are not needed; use repeated doses with caution in persons with moderate or more severely impaired renal function)

2. If rituximab administration was interrupted, resume infusion at a slower rate than the maximum rate previously attempted. Rate escalation may be reattempted at smaller incremental steps with close monitoring. Do not exceed the maximum recommended rate of 400 mg/h

Dyspnea or wheezing without allergic findings (urticaria, or tongue or laryngeal edema)
1. Interrupt rituximab administration immediately

2. Give **hydrocortisone** 100 mg by intravenous injection (or an alternative steroid with equivalent glucocorticoid potency)

3. Give a **histamine (H$_2$) receptor antagonist** (ranitidine 50 mg, cimetidine 300 mg, or famotidine 20 mg) intravenously over 15–30 minutes

4. After symptoms resolve, resume rituximab administration at 25 mg/hs with close monitoring. Do not increase the administration rate

Patient Population Studied

Baseline Clinical Characteristics	Number of Patients (%)
Age, median (range)	53 years (40–77)
Sex, female-to-male ratio	20 (50%)/ 20 (50%)
Disease type, new/relapsed	27 (67.5%)/ 13 (32.5%)
Disease stage	
III	14 (35%)
IV	26 (65%)
Histology*	
IWFA	7 (18%)
IWFB	26 (65%)
IWFC	6 (15%)
IWFD	1 (3%)
Extranodal sites of disease	
Marrow	26 (65%)
Splenomegaly	3 (8%)
Lung	1 (3%)
Liver	3 (8%)
IPI score	
0–1	20 (50%)
2	15 (38%)
3	4 (10%)
4–5	1 (3%)

IPI, International Prognostic Index; IWF, International Working Formulation
*Histology in WHO classification is as follows: CLL/SLL (n = 7; 18%); follicular, grade 1 (n = 13; 33%); follicular, grade 1 or 2, (n = 1; 3%); follicular, grade 2 (n = 7, 18%); follicular, grades 2 to 3A (n = 5; 13%); follicular, grade 3A (n = 4; 10%); follicular, grade 3B (n = 1; 3%); not available (n = 2; 5%)

Efficacy

Clinical Outcome (N = 40)

Outcome	Number of Patients (%)
Response	
Complete (CR/CRu)	32 (80%)
Partial (PR/PRu)	4 (10%)
Progressive disease*	4 (10%)
G-CSF, yes	14 (35%)

CR, complete response; CRu, unconfirmed complete response; G-CSF, granulocyte colony-stimulating factor; PR, partial response; PRu, unconfirmed partial response
*Includes 2 patients who demonstrated responsive disease (ie, equivalent to PR and a CRu) at mid-therapy, but in whom repeat scans at completion of therapy demonstrated disease progression

Association of Clinical Characteristics versus Time to Progression (N = 40)

Variable	Relative Risk (95% CI)	P Value
Age, >60 vs. ≤60 years	2.59 (1.02–6.55)	0.04
Disease type, relapsed vs. new	0.32 (0.09–1.11)	0.07
IPI score, ≥2 vs. ≤1	2.37 (0.89–6.32)	0.08
Histology, IWFA vs. others	0.82 (0.24–2.82)	0.75
Sex, female vs. male	0.89 (0.35–2.27)	0.81

IPI, International Prognostic Index; IWF, International Working Formulation

Toxicity

Clinical Outcome (N = 40)

Outcome	All Patients (N = 40)	Subgroup 1* (N = 10)	Subgroup 2* (N = 30)
	Number of Patients (Percent)		
Anemia grade			
0	26 (65%)	6 (60%)	20 (67%)
1	1 (2.5%)	1 (10%)	0
2	10 (25%)	2 (20%)	8 (27%)
3/4	3 (7.5%)	1 (10%)	2 (7%)
Neutropenia grade			
0	3 (7.5%)	1 (10%)	2 (7%)
1	6 (15%)	1 (10%)	5 (17%)
2	1 (2.5%)	0	1 (35)
3/4†	29 (72.5%)	8 (80%)	21 (72%)
Thrombocytopenia grade			
0	17 (42.5)	2 (20%)	15 (50%)
1	15 (37.5%)	4 (40%)	11 (37%)
2	4 (10%)	3 (30%)	1 (3%)
3/4	4 (10%)	1 (10%)	3 (10%)

CR, complete response; CRu, unconfirmed complete response; G-CSF, granulocyte colony-stimulating factor; PR, partial response; PRu, unconfirmed partial response
*"Unexpected" hematologic toxicities in the first 10 patients (subgroup 1), prompted treatment modifications instituted by protocol amendment. The subsequent 30 patients were designated subgroup 2. However, hematologic toxicities were very similar between both groups
†Overall, G3/4 neutropenia was transient and reversible in subgroup 2. Whereas 70% in subgroup 1 required G-CSF support, only 24% in subgroup 2 received G-CSF support including 2/7 who received G-CSF transiently only after completion of all scheduled study drugs. In subgroup 2 patients, transient therapy delay was required in 9 patients: starting with the third cycle of therapy in 4 patients, the fourth cycle in 2 patients, the fifth cycle in 1 patient, and the sixth cycle in 2 patients. Excluding a single patient removed from study at mid-therapy secondary to prolonged cytopenia in subgroup 2, 3 patients required a 40% fludarabine dose reduction: 1 patient starting at cycle 4 and 2 patients with cycle 6 only

(continued)

Toxicity (*continued*)

Association of Clinical Characteristics to Grade 3 or 4 Neutropenia (Subgroup 2 Patients) in Univariate Analysis

Variable	Odds Ratio (95% CI)	*P* Value
International Prognostic Index (IPI) score, ≥2 vs. ≤1	22.40 (2.19–2,228.70)	0.009
Marrow involvement, positive vs. negative	0.19 (0.02–1.84)	0.15

(N = 40 + Infectious Complications, Hospitalizations, and Nonhematologic Toxicities*)

Staphylococcal or culture-negative Mediport infections	3 (7.5%)
Fever + neutropenia requiring hospitalization	4 (10%)
Primary or secondary herpes simplex/zoster skin infections[†]	6 (15%)
Recurrent urinary tract infection	1 (2.5%)
Rituximab infusional toxicities	"Usual"
Intermittent G1/2 fludarabine-associated nausea/vomiting and liver function test abnormalities[‡]	1 (2.5%)
Interstitial pneumonitis believed secondary to fludarabine[§]	1 (2.5%)

*There were no differences in infectious complications noted between patients in subgroup 1 vs. subgroup 2
[†]Acyclovir prophylaxis was subsequently prescribed to all treated patients for 6–12 months after completion of therapy because of the relatively high incidence of herpes infections (6 of 40 patients; 15%) believed to be secondary to T-cell depletion from fludarabine. No patient receiving acyclovir prophylaxis developed herpes infection
[‡]Resolved after completion of therapy
[§]One case was seen in a single patient in subgroup 1 that necessitated taking the patient off of study after fludarabine cycle 5. This patient's symptoms resolved quickly with initiation of corticosteroids

Treatment Monitoring

1. *Pretreatment/screening period:* medical history and baseline laboratory and imaging studies, serum pregnancy test, bilateral bone marrow aspirates and core biopsies for assessment of the extent of disease
2. *Evaluations performed during and after treatment:* physical examination, CBC counts, serum chemistry, imaging studies for disease assessment

REGIMEN

Indolent (Follicular) Lymphoma
Small Lymphocytic Lymphoma
Mantle Cell Lymphoma

BENDAMUSTINE + RITUXIMAB

Rummel MJ et al. Lancet 2013;381:1203–1210

Bendamustine HCl 90 mg/m^2 per dose; administer intravenously in a volume of 0.9% sodium chloride injection (0.9% NS) sufficient to produce a concentration with the range 0.2–0.7 mg/mL over 30–60 minutes, on 2 consecutive days, days 1 and 2, every 4 weeks for up to 6 cycles (total dosage/cycle = 180 mg/m^2)

Premedication for rituximab:
Acetaminophen 650–1000 mg; administer orally *plus* **diphenhydramine** 25–50 mg; administer orally or intravenously 30–60 minutes before each dose of rituximab
Rituximab 375 mg/m^2; administer intravenously in 0.9% NS or 5% dextrose injection diluted to a concentration of 1–4 mg/mL on day 1, every 4 weeks for up to 6 cycles (total dosage/cycle = 375 mg/m^2)

Notes on rituximab administration:
• Infuse initially at 50 mg/h. If hypersensitivity or infusion reactions do not occur during the first 30 minutes, increase the rate by 50 mg/h every 30 minutes as tolerated to a maximum rate of 400 mg/h. Subsequently, if previous administration was well tolerated, start at 100 mg/h and increase by 100 mg/h every 30 minutes as tolerated to a maximum rate of 400 mg/h
• Interrupt rituximab administration for fever chills, edema, congestion of the head and neck mucosa, hypertension, and other serious adverse events. Resume rituximab administration after adverse events abate
• The regimen did not include maintenance or consolidation treatment with rituximab

Supportive Care
Antiemetic prophylaxis
Emetogenic potential is **MODERATE**
See Chapter 39 for antiemetic recommendations

Hematopoietic growth factor (CSF) prophylaxis
Primary prophylaxis may be indicated
See Chapter 43 for more information

Antimicrobial prophylaxis
Risk of fever and neutropenia is INTERMEDIATE
Antimicrobial primary prophylaxis to be considered:
  • Antibacterial—consider a fluoroquinolone or no prophylaxis; *Pneumocystis jirovecii* prophylaxis is recommended (eg, cotrimoxazole)
  • Antifungal—recommended; consider use during periods of neutropenia, and in anticipation of mucositis
  • Antiviral—antiherpes antivirals (eg, acyclovir, famciclovir, valacyclovir)
See Chapter 47 for more information

Infusion reactions associated with rituximab
Fevers, chills, and rigors
1. Interrupt rituximab administration for severe symptoms, and give:
  • **Acetaminophen** 650 mg orally for fever. For persistent or recurrent symptoms, repeat administration every 4–6 hours as needed during rituximab administration
  • **Diphenhydramine** 25–50 mg orally or by intravenous injection for pruritus, hypotension, or angioedema. For persistent or recurrent symptoms, repeat administration every 4–6 hours as needed during rituximab administration
  • **Meperidine** 12.5–25 mg by intravenous injection every 10–20 minutes as needed for shaking chills (generally, cumulative doses >100 mg are not needed; use repeated doses with caution in persons with moderate or more severely impaired renal function)
2. If rituximab administration was interrupted, resume infusion at a slower rate than the maximum rate previously attempted. Rate escalation may be reattempted at smaller incremental steps with close monitoring. Do not exceed the maximum recommended rate of 400 mg/h
Dyspnea or wheezing without allergic findings (urticaria, or tongue or laryngeal edema)
1. Interrupt rituximab administration immediately
2. Give **hydrocortisone** 100 mg by intravenous injection (or an alternative steroid with equivalent glucocorticoid potency)
3. Give a **histamine (H$_2$) receptor antagonist** (ranitidine 50 mg, cimetidine 300 mg, or famotidine 20 mg) intravenously over 15–30 minutes
4. After symptoms resolve, resume rituximab administration at 25 mg/hs with close monitoring. Do not increase the administration rate

Treatment Modifications

Adverse Effect	Treatment Modifications
WBC <2000/mm³, ANC <1000/mm³, or platelet count <100,000/mm³ at time of cycle start	Delay start of next treatment cycle for 1 week or until WBC ≥2000/mm³ (or ANC ≥1000/mm³) and platelet count ≥100,000/mm³. If restarting treatment is delayed by >5 days, reduce the bendamustine dosage to 70–80 mg/m² per day ×2 days
ANC <1000/mm³ and/or platelet count <75,000/mm³ on day 1 of a cycle with bendamustine dosage during the previous cycle = 70–80 mg/m²	Hold bendamustine until ANC ≥1000/mm³ and platelet count ≥75,00/mm³. If restarting treatment is delayed by >5 days, reduce the bendamustine dosage to 60–70 mg/m² per day ×2 days
ANC <1000/mm³ and/or platelet count <75,000/mm³ on day 1 of a cycle that does not resolve within 21 days	Discontinue bendamustine
WBC <1000/mm³ or platelet count <50,000/mm³ on 2 consecutive days between cycles	Reduce the bendamustine dosage to 70 mg/m² per day ×2 days during subsequent cycles
Clinically significant G ≥2 nonhematologic toxicity	Hold bendamustine until nonhematologic toxicity has recovered to G ≤1. If toxicity was G ≥3, reduce the bendamustine dosage to 70–80 mg/m² per day ×2 days during subsequent cycles
Clinically significant G ≥2 nonhematologic toxicity with bendamustine dosage during the previous cycle = 70–80 mg/m²	Hold bendamustine until nonhematologic toxicity has recovered to G ≤1. If toxicity was G ≥3, reduce the bendamustine dosage to 60–70 mg/m² per day ×2 days during subsequent cycles

Patient Population Studied

Patients with a histologically confirmed mantle cell or indolent non-Hodgkin lymphoma, including CD20-positive subtypes: grades 1/2 follicular, lymphoplasmacytic (Waldenström's macroglobulinemia), small lymphocytic, and marginal-zone lymphoma. All had previously untreated stages III/IV disease, and patients with indolent lymphoma subtypes had at least 1 of the following criteria: impaired hemopoiesis (Hgb <10 g/dL, ANC <1500/mm³, or platelet count <100,000/mm³); presence of B symptoms; large tumor burden (3 areas >5 cm or 1 area >7.5 cm); bulky disease with impingement on internal organs; progressive disease, defined as a more than 50% increase of tumor mass within 6 months; or a hyperviscosity syndrome. Patients younger than 65 years with mantle cell lymphoma were referred to clinical trials incorporating autologous stem cell transplantation

Patient Characteristics (N = 261 + 253 = 514)

Open-label, Multicenter, Randomized, Phase 3, Noninferiority Trial Comparing Bendamustine Plus Rituximab (B-R) versus Chop Plus Rituximab (Chop-R) as First-line Treatment for Patients with Indolent and Mantle Cell Lymphomas

	B-R (n = 261)	CHOP-R (n = 253)
Age (years)	64 (34–83)	63 (31–82)
<60	94 (36%)	90 (36%)
61–70	107 (41%)	105 (42%)
>70	60 (23%)	58 (23%)
Stage		
II	9 (3%)	9 (4%)
III	50 (19%)	47 (19%)
IV	202 (77%)	197 (78%)
Histology		
Follicular	139 (53%)	140 (55%)
Mantle cell	46 (18%)	48 (19%)
Marginal zone	37 (14%)	30 (12%)
Lymphoplasmacytic*	22 (8%)	19 (8%)
Small lymphocytic	10 (4%)	11 (4%)
Low grade, unclassifiable	7 (3%)	5 (2%)
B symptoms	100 (38%)	74 (29%)
Bone marrow involved	177 (68%)	170 (67%)
Extranodal involved sites ≥1	212 (81%)	193 (76%)
Lactate dehydrogenase >240 U/L	100 (38%)	84 (33%)
Median β₂-microglobulin (mg/L)	2.6 (0.7–17.8)	2.4 (1.1–23.2)
Prognostic groups for all patients (IPI)		
>2 risk factors	96 (37%)	89 (35%)
Prognostic groups according to FLIPI		
Low risk (0–1 risk factor)	16/139 (12%)	26/140 (19%)
Intermediate risk (2 risk factors)	57/139 (41%)	44/140 (31%)
Poor risk (3–5 risk factors)	63/136 (46%)	64/134 (48%)

FLIPI, Follicular Lymphoma International Prognostic Index

Efficacy (N = 514)

Open-label, Multicenter, Randomized, Phase 3, Noninferiority Trial Comparing Bendamustine Plus Rituximab versus CHOP Plus Rituximab as First-line Treatment for Patients with Indolent and Mantle Cell Lymphomas

	Bendamustine + R (N = 261)	CHOP + R (N = 253)	HR (95% CI) P Value
Median PFS*,†	69.5 months (26.1–NR)	31.2 months (15.2–65.7)	0.58 (0.44–0.74) <0.0001
Overall response rate	242 (93%)	231 (91%)	
Complete response	104 (40%)	76 (30)	0.021

Exploratory Subgroup Analysis to Assess the Progression-free Survival Benefit of Bendamustine Plus Rituximab versus CHOP Plus Rituximab

	HR (95% CI)	P Value
Age (years)		
≤60 (n = 199)	0.52 (0.33–0.79)	0.002
>60 (n = 315)	0.62 (0.45–0.84)	0.002
LDH concentration		
Normal (n = 319)	0.48 (0.34–0.67)	<0.0001
Elevated (n = 184)	0.74 (0.50–1.08)	0.118
FLIPI subgroup		
Favorable (0–2 risk factors; n = 143)	0.56 (0.31–0.98)	0.043
Unfavorable (3–5 risk factors; n = 127)	0.63 (0.38–1.04)	0.068

FLIPI, Follicular Lymphoma International Prognostic Index; HR, hazard ratio; LDH, lactate dehydrogenase; NR, not reached; PFS, progression-free survival; R, rituximab
*Progression-free survival at median follow-up of 45 months (IQR 25–57)
†A significant benefit for PFS was shown with bendamustine + R versus CHOP + R for all histologic subtypes, except for marginal-zone lymphoma

Toxicity

Hematologic Toxic Events in Patients Receiving ≥1 Dose of Study Treatment

Toxicity	G1		G2		G3		G4		G3/4	
	R-C	B-R	R-C	B-R	R-C	B-R	R-C	B-R	R-C	B-R
Leukocytopenia	13 (5%)	52 (19%)	39 (15%)	80 (30%)	110 (44%)	85 (32%)	71 (28%)	13 (5%)	181 (72%)*	98 (37%)*
Neutropenia	6 (2%)	30 (11%)	19 (8%)	61 (23%)	70 (28%)	53 (20%)	103 (41%)	24 (9%)	173 (69%)*	77 (29%)*
Lymphocytopenia	12 (5%)	14 (5%)	72 (29%)	38 (14%)	87 (35%)	122 (46%)	19 (8%)	74 (28%)	106 (43%)	196 (74%)
Anaemia	115 (46%)	102 (38%)	84 (33%)	44 (16%)	10 (4%)	6 (2%)	2 (<1%)	2 (<1%)	12 (5%)	8 (3%)
Thrombocytopenia	89 (35%)	104 (39%)	20 (8%)	19 (7%)	11 (4%)	15 (6%)	5 (2%)	2 (<1%)	16 (6%)	13 (5%)

B-R, bendamustine + rituximab; R-C, rituximab + cyclophosphamide + doxorubicin + vincristine + prednisone (R-CHOP)
*p <0.0001 between groups

(continued)

Toxicity (continued)

All Grades of Nonhematologic Toxic Events in Patients Receiving ≥1 Dose of Study Treatment

	Bendamustine + R (N = 261)	CHOP + R (N = 253)	*p* Value
Alopecia	0	245 (100%)*	<0.0001
Paresthesia	18 (7%)	73 (29%)	<0.0001
Stomatitis	16 (6%)	47 (19%)	<0.0001
Skin (erythema)	42 (16%)	23 (9%)	0.024
Skin (allergic reaction)	40 (15%)	15 (6%)	0.0006
Infectious episodes	96 (37%)	127 (50%)	0.0025
Sepsis	1 (<1%)	8 (3%)	0.019

CHOP + R, cyclophosphamide + doxorubicin + vincristine + prednisone + rituximab (R-CHOP); R, rituximab
*Includes only patients who received 3 or more cycles

Treatment Monitoring

1. *Before treatment:* physical examination; CBC with differential; assessment of serum chemistry; serum immunoelectrophoresis; measurement of immunoglobulin concentrations; CT scan of the chest, abdomen, and pelvis; sonography of the abdomen; and bone marrow aspiration and biopsy as indicated. If clinically relevant, endoscopy of the gastrointestinal tract is done
2. *Weekly:* CBC with differential once weekly
3. *Assessment of efficacy:* CT scan or sonographic examination after cycles 3 and 6, or at the end of treatment

REGIMEN

FLUDARABINE, MITOXANTRONE (NOVANTRONE), AND DEXAMETHASONE (FN-D)

McLaughlin P et al. J Clin Oncol 1996;14:1262–1268

Fludarabine 25 mg/m² per day; administer intravenously in 100–125 mL 0.9% sodium chloride injection (0.9% NS) or 5% dextrose injection (D5W) over 30 minutes for 3 consecutive days on days 1–3, every 4 weeks, for up to 8 cycles (total dosage/cycle = 75 mg/m²)

Mitoxantrone 10 mg/m²; administer intravenously in 50–150 mL 0.9% NS or D5W over 5–30 minutes, given on day 1, every 4 weeks, for up to 8 cycles (total dosage/cycle = 10 mg/m²)

Dexamethasone 20 mg/day; administer orally or by intravenous infusion in 10–100 mL 0.9% NS or D5W over 10–30 minutes for 5 consecutive days on days 1–5, every 4 weeks, for up to 8 cycles (total dose/cycle = 100 mg)

Supportive Care

Antiemetic prophylaxis
Emetogenic potential on day *1* is **MODERATE**
Emetogenic potential on days *2–5* is **MINIMAL**
See Chapter 39 for antiemetic recommendations

Hematopoietic growth factor (CSF) prophylaxis
Primary prophylaxis may be indicated
See Chapter 43 for more information

Antimicrobial prophylaxis
Risk of fever and neutropenia is INTERMEDIATE
  Antimicrobial primary prophylaxis to be considered:
  • Antibacterial—consider a fluoroquinolone or no prophylaxis; *Pneumocystis jirovecii* prophylaxis is recommended (eg, cotrimoxazole)
  • Antifungal—consider use during neutropenia and for anticipated mucositis
  • Antiviral—antiherpes antivirals (eg, acyclovir)
See Chapter 47 for more information

Additional prophylaxis
Add a **proton pump inhibitor** during prednisone use to prevent gastritis and duodenitis

Patient Population Studied

A study of 224 patients (median age: 58 years) with >10 million CD5+/19+/23+ cells. Patients with serum creatinine >2 mg/dL (176.8 μmol/L) or total bilirubin >2 mg/dL (34.2 μmol/L) were excluded

Efficacy

	FC	FCR
Complete response	35%	70%*
Nodular partial response	29%	10%
Overall response rate	88%	95%
Flow-negative complete response	12%	66%

FC, Fludarabine and cyclophosphamide; FCR, fludarabine, cyclophosphamide, and rituximab
*p <0.05

Treatment Modifications

Adverse Event	Dose Modification
Sepsis during any cycle ANC <100/mm³ or platelet count <20,000/mm³ during any cycle	Reduce fludarabine and mitoxantrone dosages by 20% during subsequent cycles

Therapy Monitoring

1. *On days of drug administration:* CBC with differential, LFTs, serum BUN, and creatinine
2. *Cardiac status:* Monitor every 2–3 cycles with a cardiac scan or echo cardiogram

Notes

In monitoring cardiac status and deciding whether to continue mitoxantrone, the authors used the following approach: Monitoring of cardiac status was performed after every 2–3 courses with cardiac scan or echocardiogram. For patients who had received prior anthracyclines, a potential cumulative cardiotoxic dose was estimated by assuming that a full cardiotoxic dose of mitoxantrone was 160 mg/m², and that of doxorubicin, by bolus, was 450 mg/m². (For doxorubicin by continuous infusion, the thresholds used were 675 mg/m² for 48-hour infusion and 800 mg/m² for 96-hour infusion.) The following calculation was used: if the total doses of mitoxantrone and doxorubicin per square meter are "m" and "d" respectively, then m/160 + d/450 must be less than 1. If this potential cardiotoxic threshold was exceeded, or if cardiac symptoms occurred, discontinuation of mitoxantrone was advised

Toxicity
(N = 51 Patients; 182 Cycles)

Adverse Event	% of Cycles
ANC <500/mm³	20
Platelet count <100,000/mm³	31
Platelet count <50,000/mm³	8
Infectious complications	12

Toxicity	% of Patients
Nausea	20
Vomiting	6
Stomatitis	12
Neurologic toxicities	8
Congestive heart failure	4
Diarrhea	4

REGIMEN

RITUXIMAB

Davis TA et al. J Clin Oncol 1999;17:1851–1857

Premedication for rituximab:

Acetaminophen 650–1000 mg; administer orally, *plus*

Diphenhydramine 25–50 mg; administer orally or intravenously 30–60 minutes before starting rituximab

Rituximab 375 mg/m²; administer intravenously diluted to a concentration of 1–4 mg/mL in 0.9% sodium chloride injection or 5% dextrose injection, weekly, for 4 consecutive weeks (days 1, 8, 15, and 22) (total dosage/course = 1500 mg/m²)

Notes on rituximab administration:

- Infuse initially at 50 mg/hour. If hypersensitivity or infusion reactions do not occur during the first 30 minutes, increase the rate by 50 mg/hour every 30 minutes, as tolerated, to a maximum rate of 400 mg/hour. Subsequently, if previous administration was well tolerated, start at 100 mg/hour, and increase by 100 mg/hour every 30 minutes, as tolerated, to a maximum rate of 400 mg/hour

- Interrupt rituximab administration for fever, chills, edema, congestion of the head and neck mucosa, hypotension, and other serious adverse events. Resume rituximab administration after adverse events abate

Supportive Care

Antiemetic prophylaxis

Emetogenic potential is **MINIMAL**

See Chapter 39 for antiemetic recommendations

Hematopoietic growth factor (CSF) prophylaxis

Primary prophylaxis is NOT indicated

See Chapter 43 for more information

Antimicrobial prophylaxis

Risk of fever and neutropenia is LOW

Antimicrobial primary prophylaxis to be considered:

- Antibacterial—*Pneumocystis jirovecii* prophylaxis is recommended (eg, cotrimoxazole)

- Antifungal—not indicated

- Antiviral—not indicated unless patient previously had an episode of HSV

See Chapter 47 for more information

Patient Population Studied

A study of 31 patients who had either low-grade or follicular B-cell NHL with either relapsed disease or primary therapy failure and progressive disease that required further treatment. Additional requirements included a demonstrable monoclonal CD20-positive B-cell population in a pathologic lymph node or bone marrow specimen and a WHO PS of 0, 1, or 2. Concurrent steroid use was not permitted

Efficacy (N = 28)

Complete response	4%
Partial response	39%
Overall response rate	43%

Toxicity*

	% of Patients
Transient fever	61
Leukopenia	23
Nausea	19
Dizziness	19
Throat irritation	19
G1/2 chills	36
G3/4 chills	3
G3/4 pulmonary disorders	6
G3/4 infusion-related hypotension	3

*NCI Adult Toxicity Criteria (February 1988 guidelines)

Treatment Modifications

Treatment prerequisites: Within 2 weeks before starting rituximab, study patients were required to have a hemoglobin ≥8.0 g/dL, ANC ≥1500/mm³, platelet count ≥75,000/mm³, serum creatinine concentration ≤2 mg/dL (≤177 μmol/L), total bilirubin level ≤2 mg/dL (≤34.2 μmol/L), and alkaline phosphatase and AST ≤2 times the upper limit of normal

Rituximab Infusion-Related Toxicities

Onset of infusion-related events (fevers, chills, rigors edema, congestion of the head and neck mucosa, hypotension):

1. Interrupt rituximab infusion

2. For fever, chills: Give additional dose of acetaminophen 650 mg orally and diphenhydramine 25–50 mg by intravenous injection

3. For rigors: Give meperidine 12.5–25 mg by intravenous injection ± promethazine 12.5–25 mg by intravenous infusion in at least 10 mL 0.9% NS or D5W over 5–15 minutes. If after 15–20 minutes the response to a single dose is considered inadequate, the dose may be repeated

4. After symptoms resolve, resume rituximab infusion at 50 mg/hour and increase by 50 mg/hour every 30 minutes, as tolerated, up to a maximum rate of 200 mg/hour

Dyspnea or wheezing, without allergic findings (urticaria, or tongue or laryngeal edema):

1. Interrupt rituximab infusion immediately

2. Give hydrocortisone 100 mg by intravenous injection (or glucocorticoid equivalent)

3. Give a histamine H₂-antagonist (ranitidine 150 mg, cimetidine 300 mg, or famotidine 20 mg) by intravenous injection

4. After symptoms resolve, resume rituximab infusion at 25 mg/hour with close monitoring. Do not increase rate

Note: Medications for the treatment of hypersensitivity reactions should be available for immediate use in the event of a reaction during administration (eg, intravenous fluids, epinephrine, antihistamines, glucocorticoids, and O₂)

Therapy Monitoring

Weekly: CBC with differential, LFTs, serum BUN, and creatinine

REGIMEN

EXTENDED-SCHEDULE RITUXIMAB

Ghielmini M et al. Blood 2004;103:4416–4423

Premedication for rituximab:
Acetaminophen 650–1000 mg; administer orally, *plus*
Diphenhydramine 25–50 mg; administer orally or intravenously, 30–60 minutes before starting rituximab

Induction phase:
Rituximab 375 mg/m^2; administer intravenously in 0.9% sodium chloride injection (0.9% NS) or 5% dextrose injection (D5W), diluted to a concentration of 1–4 mg/mL, once per week for 4 consecutive weeks (total dosage: 1500 mg/m^2), *followed by:*

Extended schedule phase:
Rituximab 375 mg/m^2; administer intravenously in 0.9% NS or D5W , diluted to a concentration of 1–4 mg/mL, at week 12 (8 weeks after the last *induction phase* dose), and again at months 5, 7, and 9, for a total of 4 doses (total dosage during maintenance phase = 1500 mg/m^2; total dosage during induction phase plus extended schedule phase = 3000 mg/m^2)

Notes on rituximab administration:
- Infuse initially at 50 mg/hour. If hypersensitivity or infusion reactions do not occur during the first 30 minutes, increase the rate by 50 mg/hour every 30 minutes, as tolerated, to a maximum rate of 400 mg/hour. Subsequently, if previous administration was well tolerated, start at 100 mg/hour and increase by 100 mg/hour every 30 minutes, as tolerated, to a maximum rate of 400 mg/hour
- Interrupt rituximab administration for fever, chills, edema, congestion of the head and neck mucosa, hypertension, and other serious adverse events. Resume rituximab administration after adverse events abate

Supportive Care

Antiemetic prophylaxis
Emetogenic potential is **MINIMAL**
See Chapter 39 for antiemetic recommendations

Hematopoietic growth factor (CSF) prophylaxis
Primary prophylaxis is NOT indicated
See Chapter 43 for more information

Antimicrobial prophylaxis
Risk of fever and neutropenia is LOW
  Antimicrobial primary prophylaxis to be considered:
  - Antibacterial—*Pneumocystis jirovecii* prophylaxis is recommended (eg, cotrimoxazole)
  - Antifungal—not indicated
  - Antiviral—not indicated unless patient previously had an episode of HSV
See Chapter 47 for more information

Toxicity

Toxicity After Randomized Phase

	No Maintenance	Maintenance
G3/4 nonhematologic	3%	10%
G3/4 hematologic	17%	18%

Toxicity During Induction Phase

Nonhematologic	
Overall	9.5%
Hypotension	2.5%
Asthenia	4%
Other	6.4%

Hematologic	
Anemia	2%
Leukocytopenia	3%
Neutropenia	9.4%
Thrombocytopenia	4%

Patient Population Studied

A study of 202 newly diagnosed (32%) or relapsed/refractory follicular lymphoma patients. Biopsy-proven CD20+ follicular lymphoma, grade I (34%), II (45%), or III (12%) according to the REAL classification. ECOG performance status 0 (73%), 1 (21%), or 2 (6%), and a cardiac ejection fraction (EF) of at least 50% as determined by echocardiography. Median age was 57 years

Therapy Monitoring

Before each rituximab administration: CBC before each rituximab and at months 2 and 12

Efficacy

(N = 185; Median follow-up time in 126 living patients = 36 months)

Randomization:
- Rituximab 375 mg/m² weekly for 4 weeks then no further treatment *versus*
- Rituximab 375 mg/m² weekly for 4 weeks followed by extended schedule with a single infusion of rituximab 375 mg/m² at week 12 (3 months) and again at months 5, 7, and 9

	All Evaluable (N = 185)	Chemotherapy-Naïve (N = 57)	Previously Treated (N = 128)
Month 3 RR	52%	67% with 9% CR	46% with 8% CR
	OR = 2.34; P = 0.0097		

	No Maintenance	Maintenance	p Value
Median EFS (151 randomized patients)	11.8 months	23.2 months	HR = 0.61; p = 0.024
Median EFS (chemotherapy-naïve patients)	19 months	36 months	p = 0.009
EFS by Response to Induction Phase			
Response at first restaging	16 months	36 months	p = 0.004
SD at first restaging	8 months	11 months	p = 0.35
Overall best response	77% (31% CR)	75% (38% CR)	NS
Overall best response (chemotherapy-naïve)	81% (31% CR)	92% (52% CR)	NS
Median remission duration among week-12 responders	16 months	36 months	p = 0.0039 (Marginally significant for chemotherapy-naïve vs. pretreated patients)
RR Over Time			
Month 3	67%	62%	NS at 3 and 7 months 7 but p = 0.046 >12 months
Month 12	44%	60%	
Month 24	28%	45%	
% in CR Over Time			
Month 3	8%	12%	NS at any time point
Month 24	19%	29%	

CR, complete response; EFS, event-free survival; OR, overall response; RR, Response rate; SD, stable disease

REGIMEN

MAINTENANCE RITUXIMAB

Salles G et al. Lancet 2011;377:42–51

Premedication for rituximab:
Acetaminophen 650–1000 mg; administer orally, *plus*
Diphenhydramine 25–50 mg; administer orally or intravenously, 30–60 minutes before starting rituximab

Induction phase:
Rituximab 375 mg/m²; administer intravenously in 0.9% sodium chloride injection (0.9% NS) or 5% dextrose injection (D5W), diluted to a concentration of 1–4 mg/mL, once per week, for 4 weeks (total dosage/4-week course = 1500 mg/m²), *followed by:*

Maintenance phase:
Rituximab 375 mg/m²; administer intravenously in 0.9% NS or D5W, diluted to a concentration of 1–4 mg/mL, once per week for 4 weeks, administered at 6-month intervals times 4 cycles (total dosage = 1500 mg/m² every 6 months; potential total dosage during maintenance phase [4 cycles] = 6000 mg/m²)

Notes on rituximab administration:
- Infuse initially at 50 mg/hour. If hypersensitivity or infusion reactions do not occur during the first 30 minutes, increase the rate by 50 mg/hour every 30 minutes, as tolerated, to a maximum rate of 400 mg/hour. Subsequently, if previous administration was well tolerated, start at 100 mg/hour and increase by 100 mg/hour every 30 minutes, as tolerated, to a maximum rate of 400 mg/hour
- Interrupt rituximab administration for fever, chills, edema, congestion of the head and neck mucosa, hypertension, and other serious adverse events. Resume rituximab administration after adverse events abate

Supportive Care
Antiemetic prophylaxis
Emetogenic potential is **MINIMAL**
See Chapter 39 for antiemetic recommendations

Hematopoietic growth factor (CSF) prophylaxis
Primary prophylaxis is NOT indicated
See Chapter 43 for more information

Antimicrobial prophylaxis
Risk of fever and neutropenia is LOW
  Antimicrobial primary prophylaxis to be considered:
  - Antibacterial—*Pneumocystis jirovecii* prophylaxis is recommended (eg, cotrimoxazole)
  - Antifungal—not indicated
  - Antiviral—not indicated unless patient previously had an episode of HSV
See Chapter 47 for more information

Patient Population Studied

A study of 114 patients who had received previous chemotherapy (previous rituximab not allowed) for indolent non-Hodgkin lymphoma (follicular and small lymphocytic), who were treated with a standard 4-week course of rituximab. Patients with objective response or stable disease were randomly assigned to receive either maintenance rituximab therapy (standard 4-week courses administered at 6-month intervals) or rituximab retreatment at the time of lymphoma progression. The duration of rituximab benefit was measured from the date of first rituximab treatment until the date other treatment was required

Toxicities

	Retreatment Group (No Maintenance; N = 46)	Maintenance Group (N = 44)
G3 infusion reactions	0%	4.5%
G3 hematologic toxicity	2.2%	2.3%
G3 nonhematologic toxicity	2.2%	2.3%

Therapy Monitoring

Every 3 months: CBC with differential and serum chemistries

Efficacy

	Retreatment Group (No Maintenance)	Maintenance Group	*p* Value
Response to initial rituximab			
CR	0	9	
ORR	15	39	
Response to subsequent treatment			
CR	4	27	0.007
ORR	35	52	—
Median PFS	7.4 months	31.3 months	0.007
Median duration rituximab benefit	27.4 months	31.3 months	0.94
3-year survival	68%	72%	NS

REGIMEN

FLUDARABINE + CYCLOPHOSPHAMIDE + RITUXIMAB (FCR)

Keating MJ et al. J Clin Oncol 2005;23:4079–4088

Prophylaxis against tumor lysis syndrome (cycle 1):
Allopurinol 300 mg/day; administer orally or intravenously, for 7 consecutive days, days 1–7

Premedication for rituximab (all cycles):
Acetaminophen 650 mg; administer orally, *plus*
Diphenhydramine 25 mg; administer intravenously, 30–60 minutes before starting rituximab

Cycle 1	Cycles 2–6
Rituximab 375 mg/m²; administer intravenously in 0.9% sodium chloride injection (0.9% NS) or 5% dextrose injection (D5W), diluted to a concentration within the range of 1–4 mg/mL, on day 1, every 28 days (total dosage/cycle = 375 mg/m²)	**Rituximab** 500 mg/m²; administer intravenously in 0.9% NS or D5W, diluted to a concentration within the range of 1–4 mg/mL, on day 1, every 28 days (total dosage/cycle = 500 mg/m²)

Notes on rituximab administration:
• Infuse initially at 50 mg/hour. If hypersensitivity or infusion reactions do not occur during the first 30 minutes, increase the rate by 50 mg/hour every 30 minutes, as tolerated, to a maximum rate of 400 mg/hour. Subsequently, if previous administration was well tolerated, start at 100 mg/hour, and increase by 100 mg/hour every 30 minutes, as tolerated, to a maximum rate of 400 mg/hour

Cycle 1	Cycles 2–6
Cyclophosphamide 250 mg/m² per day; administer intravenously in 25–250 mL 0.9% NS or D5W over 10–30 minutes, daily for 3 consecutive days, days 2–4, every 28 days (total dosage/cycle = 750 mg/m²)	**Cyclophosphamide** 250 mg/m² per day; administer intravenously in 25–250 mL 0.9% NS or D5W over 10–30 minutes, daily for 3 consecutive days, days 1–3, every 28 days (total dosage/cycle = 750 mg/m²)
Fludarabine 25 mg/m² per day; administer intravenously in 100–125 mL 0.9% NS or D5W over 20–30 minutes, daily for 3 consecutive days, days 2–4, every 28 days (total dosage/cycle = 75 mg/m²)	**Fludarabine** 25 mg/m² per day; administer intravenously in 100–125 mL 0.9% NS or D5W over 20–30 minutes, daily for 3 consecutive days, days 1–3, every 28 days (total dosage/cycle = 75 mg/m²)

Supportive Care
Antiemetic prophylaxis
Emetogenic potential on cycle 1, day 1 is **LOW**
Emetogenic potential on cycle 1, days 2–4 is **MODERATE**
Emetogenic potential on cycle 2 and subsequent cycles, days 1–3 is **MODERATE**
See Chapter 39 for antiemetic recommendations

Hematopoietic growth factor (CSF) prophylaxis
Primary prophylaxis is indicated with 1 of the following:
   Filgrastim (G-CSF) 5 mcg/kg per day; administer by subcutaneous injection, *or*
   Pegfilgrastim (pegylated filgrastim) 6 mg/0.6 mL; administer by subcutaneous injection for 1 dose
   • Begin use from 24–72 hours after myelosuppressive chemotherapy is completed
See Chapter 43 for more information

Hematopoietic growth factor (CSF) prophylaxis
Primary prophylaxis may be indicated
See Chapter 43 for more information

Antimicrobial prophylaxis
Risk of fever and neutropenia is INTERMEDIATE
   Antimicrobial primary prophylaxis to be considered:
   • Antibacterial—consider a fluoroquinolone or no prophylaxis; *Pneumocystis jirovecii* prophylaxis is recommended (eg, cotrimoxazole)
   • Antifungal—not indicated
   • Antiviral—antiherpes antivirals (eg, acyclovir)
See Chapter 47 for more information

Toxicity (N = 224)
First Infusion of Rituximab

	% G1/2	% G3/4
Fever and chills	42	1
Hypotension	10	1
Dyspnea	13	—
Nausea	11	—
Vomiting	5	—
Back pain	3	—
Urticaria	3	—
Headache	2	—

Fludarabine + Cyclophosphamide + Rituximab

	% G3	% G4
Neutropenia	24	28
Thrombocytopenia	4	<1
Infections Major	2.6%	
Minor	10%	

Efficacy (N = 224)

Complete response:	70%
Nodular partial remission:	10%
Partial response:	15%
No response:	5%

Treatment Modifications

ANC ≤1000/mm³ or platelet ≤80,000/mm³ after the first treatment cycle	Treatment postponed until ANC >1000/mm³ and platelets >80,000/mm³. If delay >1 week, restart treatment with reduction of the cyclophosphamide dosage to 200 mg/m² and fludarabine dosage to 20 mg/m². If further dose reduction is needed, reduce the cyclophosphamide dosage to 150 mg/m² and fludarabine dosage to 15 mg/m². The rituximab dose is not reduced
Major infection	Reduce cyclophosphamide dosage to 200 mg/m² and fludarabine dosage to 20 mg/m². If further dose reduction is needed, reduce the cyclophosphamide dosage to 150 mg/m² and fludarabine dosage to 15 mg/m². The rituximab dose is not reduced

Rituximab Infusion-Related Toxicities

Onset of infusion-related events (fevers, chills, rigors edema, congestion of the head and neck mucosa, hypotension):
1. Interrupt rituximab infusion
2. For fever, chills: Give additional dose of acetaminophen 650 mg orally and diphenhydramine 50 mg by intravenous injection
3. For rigors: Give meperidine 12.5–25 mg by intravenous injection ± promethazine 12.5–25 mg by intravenous infusion in at least 10 mL 0.9% NS or D5W over 5–15 minutes. If after 15–20 minutes the response to a single dose is considered inadequate, the dose may be repeated
4. After symptoms resolve, resume rituximab infusion at 50 mg/hour and increase by 50 mg/hour every 30 minutes, as tolerated, up to a maximum rate of 200 mg/hour

Dyspnea or wheezing, without allergic findings (urticaria, or tongue or laryngeal edema):
1. Interrupt rituximab infusion immediately
2. Give hydrocortisone 100 mg by intravenous injection (or glucocorticoid equivalent)
3. Give a histamine H_2-antagonist (ranitidine 150 mg, cimetidine 300 mg, or famotidine 20 mg) by intravenous injection
4. After symptoms resolve, resume rituximab infusion at 25 mg/hour with close monitoring. Do not increase rate

Patient Population Studied

A study of 224 patients (median age: 58 years) with CLL (Rai stages I–II, 67%; Rai stages III–IV, 33%)

Therapy Monitoring

1. *Prior to each cycle:* CBC with differential, serum electrolytes, BUN, creatinine, and LFTs
2. *Response evaluation:* Every 2–3 cycles

Notes

Keating MJ et al. [abstract 2118] Blood 2005;106:599a; reported at the 2005 American Society of Hematology meeting. Three hundred previously untreated patients with CLL who received FCR had 83% 4-year survival, and 77% (CR + PR) had a 4-year remission duration. Autoimmune hemolytic anemia or red cell aplasia occurred in 25 and 6 cases, respectively. Three cases of acute myelogenous leukemia and 3 additional cases of myelodysplastic syndrome occurred

REGIMEN

^{131}I TOSITUMOMAB

Kaminski MS et al. J Clin Oncol 2001;19:3918–3928

Note: The treatment regimen consists of 2 products: tositumomab, a murine IgG$_{2a}$ lambda monoclonal antibody that reacts specifically with the CD20 antigen, and ^{131}I-tositumomab, a radioiodinated derivative of tositumomab that has been covalently linked to iodine-131 (^{131}I)

Treatment requirements:
- *Within 2 weeks of therapy:* Bone marrow ≤25% involvement with lymphoma
- *Within 4 weeks of therapy:* ANC >1500/mm^3 and platelet count >100,000/mm^3
- Adequate liver and renal function

Premedication:
Saturated solution of potassium iodide (SSKI); administer 4 drops orally, 3 times daily, starting 24 hours prior to dosimetric dose and continuing for 14 days post therapy to prevent uptake of ^{131}I by the thyroid
Note: Patients should not receive the dosimetric dose of iodine ^{131}I-tositumomab unless they have received at least 3 doses of SSKI, 3 doses of Lugol solution, or 1 dose of potassium iodide 130 mg at least 24 hours prior to the dosimetric dose
Acetaminophen 650 mg; administer orally prior to dosimetric and therapeutic doses
Diphenhydramine 50 mg; administer orally prior to dosimetric and therapeutic doses

The administration of iodine ^{131}I-tositumomab follows a procedure in which a dosimetric dose precedes a subsequent therapeutic dose

	Dosimetric Step
Day 0	(Unlabeled) Tositumomab 450 mg; administer intravenously in 50 mL 0.9% sodium chloride injection (0.9% NS) over 60 minutes • Decrease the rate of infusion by 50% for mild-to-moderate infusional toxicity; interrupt administration for severe infusional toxicity • After complete resolution of severe infusional toxicity, administration may resume at a rate of infusion decreased by 50%
	Iodine ^{131}I-tositumomab (containing 5.0 mCi iodine ^{131}I + 35 mg tositumomab); administer intravenously in 30 mL 0.9% NS over 20 minutes • Decrease the rate of infusion by 50% for mild-to-moderate infusional toxicity; interrupt administration for severe infusional toxicity • After complete resolution of severe infusional toxicity, administration may resume at a rate of infusion decreased by 50%
Day 0; day 2, 3, or 4; and day 6 or 7	Measure whole-body gamma dosimetry and evaluate biodistribution using a gamma camera. Use the measurements to determine the patient-specific activity (in mCi) of radiolabeled tositumomab required to deliver a maximum tolerated therapeutic dose of 75 cGy total-body dose based on standard internal radiation dosimetry methods
Day 6 or 7	Calculate patient-specific activity of iodine ^{131}I-tositumomab to deliver 75 cGy total body dose (in mCi)

(continued)

Treatment Modifications

Platelet count between <150,000/mm^3	Attenuate therapeutic iodine ^{131}I dose to 65 Gy total-body dose
Obese patients (patients weighing more than 137% of their lean body weight)	Adjust dose in the dosimetry calculations based on 137% of their lean body weight

Patient Population Studied

Sixty patients with chemotherapy-refractory low-grade or transformed low-grade CD20+ B-cell non-Hodgkin lymphomas who had been treated with at least 2 protocol-specified qualifying chemotherapy regimens and had not responded or progressed within 6 months after their last qualifying chemotherapy lymphoma. Median age was 60 years; 98% had stage 3 or 4 disease. Patients who had >25% involvement of bone marrow, CNS lymphoma, HIV, or those with human antimouse antibodies (HAMA) were excluded

Efficacy

	^{131}I Tositumomab	Last Chemotherapy Received
CR	20%	2%
CR + PR	65%	28%
Median duration of response	6.5 months	3.4 months

(continued)

	Therapeutic Step
Days 7–14	(Unlabeled) Tositumomab 450 mg; administer intravenously in 50 mL 0.9% NS over 60 minutes • Decrease the rate of infusion by 50% for mild-to-moderate infusional toxicity; interrupt administration for severe infusional toxicity • After complete resolution of severe infusional toxicity, administration may resume at a rate of infusion decreased by 50%
	The activity of iodine ^{131}I calculated to deliver 75 cGy total-body irradiation (in mCi) conjugated with 35 mg tositumomab; administer intravenously in 30 mL 0.9% NS over 20 minutes • Decrease the rate of infusion by 50% for mild-to-moderate infusional toxicity; interrupt administration for severe infusional toxicity • After complete resolution of severe infusional toxicity, administration may resume at a rate of infusion decreased by 50%

Safety note
Radiation safety = minimal risk, but check with local and institutional policies regarding radiation safety

Supportive Care
Antiemetic prophylaxis
Emetogenic potential is **LOW**
See Chapter 39 for antiemetic recommendations

Hematopoietic growth factor (CSF) prophylaxis
Primary prophylaxis is NOT indicated
See Chapter 43 for more information

Antimicrobial prophylaxis
Risk of fever and neutropenia is LOW
Antimicrobial primary prophylaxis to be considered:
• Antibacterial—*Pneumocystis jirovecii* prophylaxis is recommended (eg, cotrimoxazole)
• Antifungal—not indicated
• Antiviral—not indicated unless patient previously had an episode of HSV
See Chapter 47 for more information

Toxicity
Common Adverse Events Related to Iodine ^{131}I-Tositumomab by NCI Toxicity Grade

Adverse Event	% G1/2	% G3/4	% All Grades
Asthenia	43%	0%	43%
Fever	28%	2%	30%
Nausea	25%	0%	25%
Chills	13%	2%	15%
Vomiting	13%	0%	13%
Pruritus	13%	0%	13%
Anorexia	10%	0%	10%
Hypotension	10%	0%	10%
Elevation in TSH	—	2%	—
Neutropenia*	—	18%	—
Thrombocytopenia	—	22%	—
Anemia	—	0%	—
MDS in expanded access studies	3%		

*One patient hospitalized for fever and neutropenia; time to count nadir is 4–7 weeks with recovery after 2–3 weeks

Subgroup Analyses of Response* (N = 60)

Characteristic	Number of Patients	Response Rate (%)	P Value†
Tumor burden			
>500 g	23	39	0.002
≤500 g	37	81	
Prior radiotherapy			
Yes	16	31	0.003
No	44	77	
Histology			
Low-grade	36	81	
Transformed low-grade	23	39	0.004
Mantle cell	1	100	
Bone marrow involvement			
Yes	33	82	0.004
No	26	42	
Number of prior therapies			
2–3	20	90	0.010
4	40	53	

*Investigator-assessed responses
†χ^2 Test

Therapy Monitoring

1. Baseline liver and renal function tests
2. Baseline TSH, then annual TSH
3. CBC 2 days prior to therapeutic dose, and weekly until at least week 10. Continue if cytopenias are prolonged. Patients with more severe cytopenias need more frequent monitoring. Monitoring should be more frequent in patients who develop moderate or severe cytopenia, or as clinically indicated
4. Vital signs and signs and symptoms of infusion-related or allergic reactions should be monitored during each of the infusions
5. *Note:* Patients who had prior exposure to murine proteins should be screened for HAMA prior to treatment as they may be at increased risk for hypersensitivity

REGIMEN

YTTRIUM ^{90}Y IBRITUMOMAB TIUXETAN (ZEVALIN) + RITUXIMAB

Witzig TE et al. J Clin Oncol 2002;20:2453–2463

Note: Zevalin is a radionuclide tagged immunoconjugate resulting from a stable covalent bond between the monoclonal antibody, ibritumomab, the murine IgG_1 kappa monoclonal anti-CD20 parent of the chimeric antibody rituximab, and the linker-chelator tiuxetan, which provides a high affinity, conformationally restricted chelation site for indium-111 (^{111}In) or yttrium-90 (^{90}Y)

Premedication for all rituximab doses:
Acetaminophen 650 mg; administer orally prior to dosimetric and therapeutic doses
Diphenhydramine 50 mg; administer orally prior to dosimetric and therapeutic doses

Day 1	Administer **rituximab** 250 mg/m²; administer intravenously
	Notes on rituximab administration:
	• Infuse initially at 50 mg/hour. If hypersensitivity or infusion reactions do not occur during the first 30 minutes, increase the rate by 50 mg/hour every 30 minutes, as tolerated, to a maximum rate of 400 mg/hour. If administration on day 1 was well tolerated, start subsequent treatments at 100 mg/hour and increase in increments of 100 mg/hour every 30 minutes, as tolerated, to a maximum rate of 400 mg/hour
	• Immediately stop rituximab administration for serious infusion reactions and discontinue the ibritumomab tiuxetan regimen
	• Interrupt rituximab administration for fever, chills, edema, congestion of the head and neck mucosa, hypertension, and other serious adverse events. Resume rituximab administration after adverse events abate
	• Temporarily slow or interrupt rituximab administration for less-severe infusion reactions. If symptoms improve, continue administration at 50% the previous rate
	• For signs or symptoms of extravasation, immediately stop rituximab administration and restart in another limb
	Within 4 hours after completing rituximab infusion, administer **indium ^{111}In ibritumomab tiuxetan** (containing 5.0 mCi [185 MBq] ^{111}In + up to 1.6 mg ibritumomab tiuxetan) by intravenous injection over 10 minutes
	• Use a 0.22-μm, low-protein-binding, inline filter between the syringe containing indium ^{111}In ibritumomab tiuxetan and the port into which it is injected
	• After injection, flush the line through which indium ^{111}In ibritumomab tiuxetan was given with at least 10 mL 0.9% NS
Days 2–7	Wiseman GA et al. Crit Rev Oncol Hematol 2001;39:181–194
	Assess for biodistribution (see below). Proceed only if biodistribution is normal. Dosimetry using indium ^{111}In ibritumomab tiuxetan should be conducted for all patients who are receive treatment with yttrium ^{90}Y ibritumomab. Eligibility for treatment with yttrium ^{90}Y ibritumomab tiuxetan is based on MIRDOSE3-estimated radiation-absorbed doses to normal organs and red marrow. Yttrium ^{90}Y ibritumomab tiuxetan should not be administered if the predicted delivered dose of radiation is more than 20 Gy to any nontumor organ or more than 3 Gy to the bone marrow

(continued)

Patient Population Studied

Phase 3 randomized trial comparing traditional weekly rituximab for 4 doses versus rituximab plus a single dose of ^{90}Y ibritumomab tiuxetan. One hundred forty-three patients with histologically confirmed, relapsed or refractory low-grade or follicular or transformed NHL requiring treatment as determined by an increase in overall tumor size, the presence of B symptoms, and/or the presence of masses that were causing ongoing clinical symptomatology. Prior therapy had to be completed at least 3 weeks prior to receiving ^{90}Y ibritumomab tiuxetan. Median age 59 years; 65% had stage 3 or 4 disease. Also required: hemoglobin ≥8 g/dL, absolute neutrophil count ≥1500 cells/mm³, platelet count ≥150,000 cells/mm³, total bilirubin <2.0 mg/dL (34.2 μmol/L), alkaline phosphatase and AST (aspartate aminotransferase) <4 times the upper limit of normal range, and serum creatinine level less than 2.0 mg/dL (176.8 μmol/L). Patients were excluded if their bone marrow biopsy or aspirate demonstrated ≥25% involvement with NHL, if their peripheral blood lymphocyte count was ≥5000 cells/mm³, if they had prior external beam radiation therapy to more than 25% of their bone marrow, or if they had a history of human antimurine antibodies (HAMA) or human antichimeric antibodies (HACA). Patients with CNS NHL, chronic lymphocytic leukemia, mantle-cell lymphoma, human immunodeficiency virus, prior radioimmunotherapy, hematopoietic growth factors within 2 weeks before treatment, or prior autologous or allogeneic stem cell transplant were not eligible

(continued)

Day 8	Administer **rituximab** 250 mg/m² by intravenous infusion as described above for day 1
	Within 4 hours after completing rituximab infusion, administer **yttrium ⁹⁰Y ibritumomab tiuxetan** by intravenous injection over 10 minutes

Platelet Count	Yttrium ⁹⁰Y Ibritumomab Tiuxetan Dose (per kg actual body weight)*
≥150,000/mm³	0.4 mCi (14.8 MBq)
100,000–149,000/mm³	0.3 mCi (11.1 MBq)

*DO NOT administer ⁹⁰Y doses >32 mCi (>1184 MBq) regardless of a patient's body weight
- Use a 0.22-µm, low-protein-binding, inline filter between the syringe containing yttrium ⁹⁰Y ibritumomab tiuxetan and the port into which it is injected
- After injection, flush the line through which yttrium ⁹⁰Y ibritumomab tiuxetan was given with at least 10 mL 0.9% NS

Safety note:
Radiation safety = minimal risk, but check with local and institutional policies regarding radiation safety

Expected biodistribution
- Activity in the blood pool areas (heart, abdomen, neck, and extremities) may be faintly visible
- Moderately high to high uptake in normal liver and spleen
- Moderately low or very-low uptake in normal kidneys, urinary bladder, and normal (uninvolved) bowel
- Nonfixed areas within the bowel lumen that change position with time; delayed imaging as described above may be necessary to confirm gastrointestinal clearance
- Focal fixed areas of uptake in the bowel wall (localization to lymphoid aggregates in bowel wall)

Tumor uptake may be visualized however tumor visualization on the ¹¹¹In scan is not required for treatment with yttrium ⁹⁰Y ibritumomab tiuxetan

Altered biodistribution
The criteria for altered biodistribution are met if any of the following is detected on visual inspection of the required gamma images:
- Intense localization of radiotracer in the liver and spleen and bone marrow indicative of reticuloendothelial system uptake
- Increased uptake in normal organs (not involved by tumor) such as:
  - Diffuse uptake in normal lung more intense than the liver
  - Kidneys have greater intensity than the liver on the posterior view
  - Fixed areas (unchanged with time) of uptake in the normal bowel greater than uptake in the liver
  - In less than 0.5% of patients receiving indium ¹¹¹In ibritumomab tiuxetan, prominent bone marrow uptake was observed, characterized by clear visualization of the long bones and ribs

Supportive Care
Antiemetic prophylaxis
Emetogenic potential is **LOW**
See Chapter 39 for antiemetic recommendations

Hematopoietic growth factor (CSF) prophylaxis
Primary prophylaxis is NOT indicated
See Chapter 43 for more information

Antimicrobial prophylaxis
Risk of fever and neutropenia is LOW
  Antimicrobial primary prophylaxis to be considered:
  - Antibacterial—*Pneumocystis jirovecii* prophylaxis is recommended (eg, cotrimoxazole)
  - Antifungal—not indicated
  - Antiviral—not indicated unless patient previously had an episode of HSV
See Chapter 47 for more information

Therapy Monitoring

1. Baseline liver and renal function tests
2. Baseline TSH, then annual TSH
3. CBC 2 days prior to therapeutic dose and weekly until at least week 10. Continue if cytopenias are prolonged. Patients with more severe cytopenias need more frequent monitoring. Monitoring should be more frequent in patients who develop moderate or severe cytopenia, or as clinically indicated
4. Vital signs and signs and symptoms of infusion-related or allergic reactions should be monitored during each of the infusions
5. *Note:* Patients who have had prior exposure to murine proteins should be screened for HAMA prior to treatment as they may be at increased risk for hypersensitivity

Efficacy

	Rituximab	^{90}Y Ibritumomab Tiuxetan	*p*-Value
ORR	56%	80%	0.002
CR	16%	30%	0.04
Median duration of response	12.1 months	14.2 months	
Durable response			
>6 months	53%	68%	0.046
>9 months	41%	53%	0.110
>12 months	31%	40%	0.231
Median time to next treatment	13.1 months	>32 months	

Toxicity

	% G1/2 (% G3/4)	
	Rituximab	^{90}Y Ibritumomab Tiuxetan
Asthenia	41%	44% (4%)
Chills	29%	25%
Headache	23%	16%
Nausea	19%	43%
Fever	17%	19%
Throat irritation	16%	18%
Pruritus	16% (1%)	11%
Angioedema	16%	8%
Pain	14% (1%)	19% (1%)
Abdominal pain	11% (1%)	19%
Vomiting	7%	19%
Cough	7%	15%
Dyspnea	7%	15%
Dizziness	7%	15%
Anorexia	3%	11%
Hematologic Toxicity		
Neutropenia		(57%)
Thrombocytopenia		(60%)
Anemia		(2%)
Time to count nadir: 4–7 weeks; recovery after 2–3 weeks		
MDS reported in 1.5% of expanded market follow-up		

REGIMEN

FLUDARABINE + RITUXIMAB

Byrd JC et al. Blood 2003;101:6–14
Byrd JC et al. Blood 2005;105:49–53

Induction (Concurrent) Regimen
Cycles 1–6
Fludarabine 25 mg/m² per dose; administer intravenously in 100–125 mL 0.9% sodium chloride injection (0.9% NS) or 5% dextrose injection (D5W) over 20–30 minutes for 5 consecutive days, on days 1–5, every 28 days for 6 cycles (total dosage/cycle = 125 mg/m²)
Cycle 1
Premedication for rituximab:
Acetaminophen 650–1000 mg; administer orally, *plus* **diphenhydramine** 25–50 mg; administer orally or intravenously 30–60 minutes before each dose of rituximab
Rituximab 375 mg/m² per dose; administer intravenously in 0.9% NS or D5W diluted to a concentration of 1–4 mg/mL for 2 doses on days 1 and 4 (total dosage/cycle = 750 mg/m²)

Notes on rituximab administration:
- Infuse initially at 50 mg/h. If hypersensitivity or infusion reactions do not occur during the first 30 minutes, increase the rate by 50 mg/h every 30 minutes as tolerated to a maximum rate of 400 mg/h. Subsequently, if previous administration was well tolerated, start at 100 mg/h and increase by 100 mg/h every 30 minutes as tolerated to a maximum rate of 400 mg/h
- The investigators altered the dosage-schedule for rituximab for the last 7 patients who received study treatment based on their observation that stepped-up dosing improved patients' tolerability for rituximab
- For those patients, rituximab was given as follows:

Cycle and Day of Treatment	Rituximab Dosage	Rituximab Rate
Cycle 1, Day 1	Rituximab 50 mg/m²	Dose given over 4 hours without rate escalation
Cycle 1, Day 3	Rituximab 325 mg/m²	1. Initial rate = 50 mg/h 2. If administration was tolerated during the first 30 min, the rate was escalated every 30 min as tolerated to a maximum rate of 400 mg/h
Cycle 1, Day 5	Rituximab 375 mg/m²	1. Initial rate = 100 mg/h for 15 min 2. If administration was tolerated during the first 15 min, the remainder of the dose was administered over 45 min to complete administration over a 1-hour period
Cycles 2–6, Day 1	Rituximab 375 mg/m²	

- Interrupt rituximab administration for fever chills, edema, congestion of the head and neck mucosa, hypertension, and other serious adverse events. Resume rituximab administration after adverse events abate

Cycles 2–6
Premedication for rituximab:
Acetaminophen 650–1000 mg; administer orally, *plus* **diphenhydramine** 25–50 mg; administer orally or intravenously 30–60 minutes before each dose of rituximab
Rituximab 375 mg/m²; administer intravenously in 0.9% NS or D5W diluted to a concentration of 1–4 mg/mL on day 1, every 28 days for 5 cycles (total dosage/cycle = 375 mg/m²)

Consolidation Regimen
Patients were observed for 2 months after completing 6 cycles of fludarabine + rituximab. Those judged to have achieved stable disease or a better response were treated with 4 additional weekly doses of rituximab, *thus:*
Rituximab 375 mg/m² per dose; administer intravenously in 0.9% NS or D5W diluted to a concentration of 1–4 mg/mL once weekly for 4 weeks (total dosage/4-week course = 1500 mg/m²)

Supportive Care
The investigators administered **allopurinol** 300 mg orally, once daily for 14 consecutive days, days 1–14 during cycle 1 only
Note: Persons who express a variant human leukocyte antigen allele, HLA-B*58:01, are at increased risk for severe cutaneous adverse reactions from allopurinol (Hershfield MS et al. Clin Pharmacol Ther 2013;93:153–158, Zineh I et al. Pharmacogenomics 2011;12:1741–1749)

Antiemetic prophylaxis
Emetogenic potential is **MINIMAL**
See Chapter 39 for antiemetic recommendations

Hematopoietic growth factor (CSF) prophylaxis
Primary prophylaxis may be indicated
See Chapter 43 for more information

(continued)

(*continued*)

Antimicrobial prophylaxis

Risk of fever and neutropenia is INTERMEDIATE

Antimicrobial primary prophylaxis to be considered:

- Antibacterial—consider a fluoroquinolone or no prophylaxis; *Pneumocystis jirovecii* prophylaxis is recommended (eg, cotrimoxazole)
- Antifungal—recommended; consider use during periods of neutropenia
- Antiviral—antiherpes antivirals (eg, acyclovir, famciclovir, valacyclovir)

See Chapter 47 for more information

Infusion reactions associated with rituximab

Fevers, chills, and rigors

1. Interrupt rituximab administration for severe symptoms, and give:

- **Acetaminophen** 650 mg orally for fever. For persistent or recurrent symptoms, repeat administration every 4–6 hours as needed during rituximab administration
- **Diphenhydramine** 25–50 mg orally or by intravenous injection for pruritus, hypotension, or angioedema. For persistent or recurrent symptoms, repeat administration every 4–6 hours as needed during rituximab administration
- **Meperidine** 12.5–25 mg by intravenous injection every 10–20 minutes as needed for shaking chills (generally, cumulative doses >100 mg are not needed; use repeated doses with caution in persons with moderate or more severely impaired renal function)

2. If rituximab administration was interrupted, resume infusion at a slower rate than the maximum rate previously attempted. Rate escalation may be reattempted at smaller incremental steps with close monitoring. Do not exceed the maximum recommended rate of 400 mg/h

Dyspnea or wheezing without allergic findings (urticaria, or tongue or laryngeal edema)

1. Interrupt rituximab administration immediately

2. Give **hydrocortisone** 100 mg by intravenous injection (or an alternative steroid with equivalent glucocorticoid potency)

3. Give a **histamine (H$_2$) receptor antagonist** (ranitidine 50 mg, cimetidine 300 mg, or famotidine 20 mg) intravenously over 15–30 minutes

4. After symptoms resolve, resume rituximab administration at 25 mg/h with close monitoring. Do not increase the administration rate

Treatment Modifications

Adverse Event	Treatment Modifications
G3/4 neutropenia, G3/4 thrombocytopenia, or G3/4 anemia	Observe without treatment until these hematologic parameters recover to within 20% of the baseline value. Thereafter, if toxicity = G3, administer 75% of the original fludarabine dosage during subsequent cycles. If toxicity = G4, administer 50% of the original fludarabine dosage during subsequent cycles
Nonhematologic toxicities, including nausea, vomiting, fatigue, diarrhea, and drug-related fever or chills	Administer symptomatic treatment but do not reduce chemotherapy dosages
G ≥2 nonhematologic toxicities other than nausea, vomiting, fatigue, diarrhea, and drug-related fever or chills attributed to fludarabine	Hold fludarabine therapy until toxicity G <2, then reduce the fludarabine dosage by 50% in subsequent cycles
G2 irreversible nonhematologic toxicity and G3/4 nonhematologic toxicities	Evaluate to determine appropriateness of continuing fludarabine therapy
Infection in the absence of G3/4 neutropenia	Observe without further CLL treatment until the infection resolves, but do not modify chemotherapy dosages
Major infection	Reduce fludarabine dosage to 20 mg/m². If further dose reduction is needed, reduce the fludarabine dosage to 15 mg/m². Rituximab dosage is not reduced

Notes:
Grade hematologic toxicity according to the modified NCI criteria for CLL
(Cheson BD et al. Blood 1996;87:4990–4997)
Grade nonhematologic toxicity according to National Cancer Institute (USA) Common Terminology Criteria for Adverse Events, version 4.0. At: http://ctep.cancer.gov/protocolDevelopment/electronic_applications/ctc.htm (accessed December 7, 2013)

Patient Population Studied

CALGB 9712, a randomized phase II trial open to accrual from 1997–1999, examined administration of rituximab either concurrently (n = 51) or sequentially (n = 53) with fludarabine therapy. At a median follow-up of 43 months among patients followed for progression, the PFS and overall survival (OS) of the concurrent and sequential arms were found to be similar. On the basis of this finding, all 104 patients enrolled on this trial were combined into 1 comparison group for the analyses reported here. CALGB 9011, open to accrual from 1990–1994, randomly assigned patients to either fludarabine, chlorambucil, or the combination. The fludarabine-only arm of that trial, with a sample size of 178, was used as the comparison group

Demographic and Clinical Characteristics of Patients According to Treatment

Characteristics	Fludarabine + Rituximab (CALGB 9712)	Fludarabine Alone (CALGB 9011)	P Value
No. of patients	104	178	
Median age, years (range)	63 (38–88)	64 (37–87)	0.75
Patients, ages <50 years	14%	14%	0.93
Patients, ages ≥70 years	23%	25%	0.88
Rai stage I	2%	2%	
Rai stage II	57%	55%	
Rai stage III	14%	41%	<0.0001
Rai stage IV	26%	2%	
Enlarged liver	15%	20%	0.43
Enlarged spleen	61%	68%	0.19
Median WBC, $\times 10^9$/L (range)	83 (9–436)	77 (9–709)	0.39
Median Hgb, g/dL (range)	12.3 (1.3–16.1)	12.0 (4.6–16.6)	0.26
Median platelets, $\times 10^9$/L (range)	158 (33–316)	155 (12–451)	0.57
Median, LDH, IU (range)	212 (92–950)	198 (39–1389)	0.20

Efficacy

Treatment Outcome

Response Evaluation	Percent (95% CI)
Induction CR	33 (20–46)
Induction CR + PR	90 (82–98)
Consolidation PR to CR[6–150]*	10 (2–18)
Overall CR	47 (33–61)
Overall PR + CR	90 (82–98)

CR, complete response; PR, partial response
*Includes patients with PR after induction except for those with residual cytopenias

(*continued*)

Efficacy (continued)

Retrospective comparative analysis of CALGB 9712 and CALGB 9011

	CALGB 9712 (Fludarabine + Rituximab)	CALGB 9011 Fludarabine alone	*P* Value
Complete response*	38%	20%	*P* = 0.002
Overall response*	84%	63%	*P* = 0.0003
PFS	Patients who received fludarabine + rituximab had significantly improved PFS as compared patients who received fludarabine alone		*P* <0.0001
2-Year PFS probability†	0.67 (CI, 0.58–0.76)	0.45 (CI, 0.37–0.52)	—
	Patients who received fludarabine + rituximab had significantly improved OS as compared patients who received fludarabine alone		*P* = 0.003
2-Year OS probability‡	0.93 (CI, 0.88–0.98)	0.81 (CI, 0.75–0.87)	—

*Multivariate analyses of the effect of treatment assignment on response, controlling for sex, age, WBC, LDH, and stage, showed that the treatment effect remained essentially unchanged after controlling for these covariates
†The treatment effect was unchanged in a multivariate analysis controlling for age, WBC, LDH, stage, and splenomegaly. Fludarabine-alone treatment assignment (P <0.0001), high WBC (P = 0.0003), and high LDH (P = 0.01) were significantly associated with early progression
‡The treatment effect was unchanged in a multivariate analysis controlling for age, WBC, LDH, stage, and splenomegaly. Fludarabine-alone treatment assignment (P = 0.0006), high WBC (P = 0.009), older age (P = 0.001), and high LDH (P = 0.02) were significantly associated with shortened survival

Hazard Ratios from Multivariate Analysis of Overall Survival*

Clinical Predictor (Hazard Ratio Comparison)	Hazard Ratio (95% CI)	*P* Value
Treatment, CALGB 9712 vs. CALGB 9011†	2.59 (1.50–4.46)	0.0006
WBC, 75th vs. 25th percentile	1.23 (1.05–1.44)	0.009
Age, 75th vs. 25th percentile	1.59 (1.18–1.93)	0.001
LDH, 75th vs. 25th percentile	1.18 (1.03–1.36)	0.02
Sex, male vs. female	1.25 (0.86–1.81)	0.24
Rai stage, high vs. intermediate	1.22 (0.88–1.69)	0.23
Splenomegaly, present vs. absent	1.20 (0.84–1.71)	0.33

*These comparative data are retrospective and could be confounded by differences in supportive care or dissimilar enrollment of genetic subsets on each trial
†CALGB 9712 = Fludarabine + Rituximab; CALGB 9011 = Fludarabine alone

Toxicity

Fludarabine + Rituximab: Maximum Toxicity During Induction

Toxicity	Toxicity Grade			
	G1	G2	G3	G4
Neutropenia	2%	6%	33%	43%
Thrombocytopenia	33%	14%	14%	6%
Anemia	47%	18%	4%	0
Infection	16%	27%	20%	0
Nausea	38%	10%	0	0
Vomiting	8%	8%	0	0
Dyspnea	6%	6%	10%	4%
Hypotension	2%	8%	6%	0
Fever	14%	18%	0	0
Chills	28%	8%	0	0
Myalgias	22%	6%	0	0
Fatigue/malaise	48%	14%	0	0

(continued)

Toxicity (continued)

Fludarabine + Rituximab: Maximum Toxicity During Consolidation

Toxicity	Toxicity Grade			
	G1	G2	G3	G4
Neutropenia	13%	18%	11%	8%
Thrombocytopenia	24%	8%	0	0
Anemia	14%	5%	0	3%
Infection	11%	27%	3%	3%
Nausea	6%	0	0	0
Vomiting	0	0	0	0
Dyspnea	0	9%	6%	0
Hypotension	6%	0	0	0
Fever	8%	0	0	0
Chills	3%	0	0	0
Myalgias	14%	3%	0	0
Fatigue/malaise	24%	6%	0	0

Grades 3 or 4 Toxicity

Toxicity	Fludarabine + Rituximab (CALGB 9712)	Fludarabine Alone (CALGB 9011)	*P* Value
Platelets	0.16	0.11	>0.2
Hemoglobin	0.07	0.10	>0.2
Granulocytes	0.61	0.21	<0.001
Infection	0.26	0.23	>0.2
Herpes virus	0.12	0.09	>0.2
Dyspnea	0.14	0.03	0.002
Hypotension	0.05	0.01	0.03

Treatment Monitoring

1. *Before each cycle:* CBC with manual differential

2. *After 6 cycles of fludarabine + rituximab:* clinical restaging (physical examination with lymph node, liver, and spleen measurement; and CBC with differential)

3. *Two months after completion of the initial 6 cycles of fludarabine + rituximab:* clinical restaging (physical examination, CBC with manual differential) and bone marrow aspirate and biopsy to determine response to induction therapy

4. *After completion of weekly rituximab × 4:* clinical staging (physical examination with lymph node, liver, and spleen measurement; and CBC with differential)

5. *Two months after completion of weekly rituximab × 4:* complete restaging (physical examination with lymph node, liver, and spleen measurement; and CBC with differential) and bone marrow aspirate and biopsy to determine overall response according to the NCI 1996 CLL criteria (Cheson BD et al. Blood 1996;87:4990–4997)

REGIMEN

FLUDARABINE + CYCLOPHOSPHAMIDE + RITUXIMAB

Hallek M et al. Lancet 2010;376:1164–1174

Premedication for rituximab:

Acetaminophen 650–1000 mg; administer orally *plus* **diphenhydramine** 25–50 mg; administer orally or intravenously 30–60 minutes before each dose of rituximab

Rituximab; administer intravenously in 0.9% sodium chloride injection (0.9% NS) or 5% dextrose injection (D5W) diluted to a concentration of 1–4 mg/mL, every 4 weeks for 6 cycles

	Cycle 1	Cycles 2–6
Dosage	375 mg/m^2	500 mg/m^2
Treatment day	0 (zero; the day before commencing treatment with fludarabine and cyclophosphamide	Day 1
Total dosage per cycle	375 mg/m^2	500 mg/m^2

Notes on rituximab administration:

Infuse initially at 50 mg/h. If hypersensitivity or infusion reactions do not occur during the first 30 minutes, increase the rate by 50 mg/h every 30 minutes as tolerated to a maximum rate of 400 mg/h. Subsequently, if previous administration was well tolerated, start at 100 mg/h and increase by 100 mg/h every 30 minutes as tolerated to a maximum rate of 400 mg/h

Fludarabine 25 mg/m^2 per day; administer intravenously in 100–125 mL 0.9% NS or D5W over 20–30 minutes for 3 consecutive days, on days 1–3, every 28 days for 6 cycles (total dosage/cycle = 75 mg/m^2)

Cyclophosphamide 250 mg/m^2 per day; administer intravenously in 25–250 mL 0.9% NS or D5W over 10–30 minutes for 3 consecutive days, on days 1–3, every 28 days for 6 cycles (total dosage/cycle = 750 mg/m^2)

Supportive Care

Antiemetic prophylaxis

Emetogenic potential on days 1–3 is **MODERATE**

See Chapter 39 for antiemetic recommendations

Hematopoietic growth factor (CSF) prophylaxis

Primary prophylaxis is indicated with 1 of the following:

　Filgrastim (G-CSF) 5 mcg/kg per day; administer by subcutaneous injection, *or*

　Pegfilgrastim (pegylated filgrastim) 6 mg/0.6 mL; administer by subcutaneous injection for 1 dose

- Begin use from 24–72 hours after myelosuppressive chemotherapy is completed
- Continue daily filgrastim use until ANC ≥10,000/mm^3 on 2 measurements separated temporally by ≥12 hours
- Discontinue daily filgrastim use at least 24 hours before administering myelosuppressive treatment. Do not administer pegfilgrastim within 14 days before administering myelosuppressive treatment

See Chapter 43 for more information

Antimicrobial prophylaxis

Risk of fever and neutropenia is INTERMEDIATE

Antimicrobial primary prophylaxis to be considered:

- Antibacterial—consider a fluoroquinolone or no prophylaxis; *Pneumocystis jirovecii* prophylaxis is recommended (eg, cotrimoxazole)
- Antifungal—recommended; consider use during periods of neutropenia
- Antiviral—antiherpes antivirals (eg, acyclovir, famciclovir, valacyclovir)

See Chapter 47 for more information

Infusion reactions associated with rituximab

Fevers, chills, and rigors

1. Interrupt rituximab administration for severe symptoms, and give:

- **Acetaminophen** 650 mg orally for fever. For persistent or recurrent symptoms, repeat administration every 4–6 hours as needed during rituximab administration
- **Diphenhydramine** 25–50 mg orally or by intravenous injection for pruritus, hypotension, or angioedema. For persistent or recurrent symptoms, repeat administration every 4–6 hours as needed during rituximab administration
- **Meperidine** 12.5–25 mg by intravenous injection every 10–20 minutes as needed for shaking chills (generally, cumulative doses >100 mg are not needed; use repeated doses with caution in persons with moderate or more severely impaired renal function)

2. If rituximab administration was interrupted, resume infusion at a slower rate than the maximum rate previously attempted. Rate escalation may be reattempted at smaller incremental steps with close monitoring. Do not exceed the maximum recommended rate of 400 mg/h

(continued)

(continued)

Dyspnea or wheezing without allergic findings (urticaria, or tongue or laryngeal edema)
1. Interrupt rituximab administration immediately
2. Give **hydrocortisone** 100 mg by intravenous injection (or an alternative steroid with equivalent glucocorticoid potency)
3. Give a **histamine (H$_2$) receptor antagonist** (ranitidine 50 mg, cimetidine 300 mg, or famotidine 20 mg) intravenously over 15–30 minutes
4. After symptoms resolve, resume rituximab administration at 25 mg/hs with close monitoring. Do not increase the administration rate

Patient Population Studied

Randomized phase II trial investigating whether the addition of rituximab to first-line chemotherapy with fludarabine and cyclophosphamide would improve the outcome of patients with chronic lymphocytic leukemia/small lymphocytic lymphoma

Patients' Demographics and Baseline Characteristics

Characteristics	Chemotherapy*,† (FC)	Chemoimmunotherapy*,‡ (FCR)
Age (years; median, range)	61 (36–81)	61 (30–80)
Age (years)		
≥65	119/409 (29%)	126/408 (31%)
≥70	37/409 (9%)	44/408 (11%)
Men	304/409 (74%)	303/408 (74%)
Binet stage		
A	22/409 (5%)	18/408 (4%)
B	259/409 (63%)	263/408 (64%)
C	126/409 (31%)	126/408 (31%)
ECOG 0	226/390 (58%)	221/395 (56%)
Presence of B symptoms	197/406 (49%)	167/407 (41%)
Cumulative illness rating scale§	1 (0–8)	1 (0–7)
CD20+ cells by flow cytometry§	81% (0–100)	79% (0–100)
Creatinine clearance <1.17 mL/s	88/392 (22%)	94/398 (24%)
IGHV unmutated	194/310 (63%)	196/309 (63%)
Cytogenetic abnormalities		
Del(13q)	182/305 (60%)	168/312 (54%)
Del(11q)	69/307 (22%)	84/314 (27%)
Trisomy 12	44/306 (14%)	30/312 (10%)
Del(17p)	29/306 (10%)	22/315 (7%)
β$_2$-Microglobulin (≥3.5 mg/L)	85/266 (32%)	91/277 (33%)
Serum thymidine kinase (≥10 U/L)	206/266 (77%)	202/277 (73%)
ZAP70 expression	55/147 (37%)	59/142 (42%)
Positive CD38	239/359 (67%)	237/360 (66%)

ECOG, Eastern Cooperative Oncology Group
*Data are n/N (%), unless otherwise indicated
†Chemotherapy = fludarabine + cyclophosphamide
‡Chemoimmunotherapy = fludarabine + cyclophosphamide + rituximab
§Data as median (range)

Treatment Modifications

Adverse Event	Treatment Modifications
ANC ≤1000/mm³ or platelet ≤80,000/mm³ after the first treatment cycle	Treatment postponed until ANC >1000/mm³ and platelet count is >80,000/mm³. If delayed >1 week, restart treatment with reduction of the cyclophosphamide dosage to 200 mg/m² per day and fludarabine dosage to 20 mg/m² per day. If further dosage reduction is needed, reduce the cyclophosphamide dosage to 150 mg/m² per day and fludarabine dosage to 15 mg/m² per day. Rituximab dosage is not reduced
Major infection	Reduce cyclophosphamide dosage to 200 mg/m² per day and fludarabine dosage to 20 mg/m² per day. If further dosage reduction is needed, reduce the cyclophosphamide dosage to 150 mg/m² per day and fludarabine dosage to 15 mg/m² per day. Rituximab dosage is not reduced

Treatment Monitoring

1. CBC with differential before each cycle
2. History and physical exam before each cycle
3. Response assessments every 3 cycles

Efficacy

Response to Treatment in Prognostic Subgroups

Groups	Chemotherapy*,† (FC)	Chemoimmunotherapy*,‡ (FCR)	*p* Value
All (n = 817)			
CR	88/409 (22%)	180/408 (44%)	**<0.0001**
ORR	328/409 (80%)	369/408 (90%)	**<0.0001**
Binet stage A (n = 40)			
CR	6/22 (27%)	13/18 (72%)	0.010
ORR	15/22 (68%)	18/18 (100%)	0.11
Binet stage B (n = 522)			
CR	66/259 (25%)	124/263 (47%)	<0.0001
ORR	220/259 (85%)	245/263 (93%)	0.003
Binet stage C (n = 252)			
CR	16/126 (13%)	43/126 (34%)	<0.0001
ORR	92/126 (73%)	106/126 (84%)	0.04
Patients with cytogenetic results and response assessment (n = 623)§			
CR	59/307 (19%)	138/316 (44%)	<0.0001
ORR	243/307 (79%)	290/316 (92%)	<0.0001
Age <65 years (n = 572)			
CR	59/290 (20%)	126/282 (45%)	<0.0001
ORR	229/290 (79%)	252/282 (89%)	0.001
Age ≥65 years (n = 245)			
CR	29/119 (24%)	54/126 (43%)	0.003
ORR	99/119 (83%)	117/126 (93%)	0.028
Del(17p) (n = 51)			
CR	0/29	1/22 (5%)	0.43
ORR	10/29 (34%)	15/22 (68%)	0.025
Del(11q) (n = 142)€			
CR	9/62 (15%)	41/80 (51%)	<0.0001
ORR	54/62 (87%)	74/80 (93%)	0.40
Trisomy 12 (n = 61)**			
CR	7/37 (19%)	17/24 (71%)	0.0001
ORR	31/37 (84%)	24/24 (100%)	0.07
Del(13q) (n = 224)††			
CR	27/119 (23%)	50/105 (48%)	0.0001
ORR	95/119 (80%)	101/105 (96%)	0.0002
No abnormalities according to the hierarchical model (n = 138)‡‡			
CR	16/58 (28%)	28/80 (35%)	0.5
ORR	53/58 (91%)	71/80 (89%)	0.78
IGHV mutated (n = 229)			
CR	24/116 (21%)	56/113 (50%)	<0.0001
ORR	98/116 (84%)	105/113 (93%)	0.06
IGHV unmutated (n = 390)			
CR	36/194 (19%)	79/196 (40%)	<0.0001
ORR	148/194 (76%)	179/196 (91%)	<0.0001

CR, complete remission; ORR, overall response rate
*Data are n/N (%), unless otherwise indicated
†Chemotherapy = fludarabine + cyclophosphamide
‡Chemoimmunotherapy = fludarabine + cyclophosphamide + rituximab
§Including 7 patients with cytogenetic results outside the hierarchical model
€Not including del(17p)
**Not including del(17p) or del(11q)
††Not including del(17p), del(11q), or trisomy 12
‡‡Not including del(17p), del(11q), trisomy 12, or del(13q) (ie, genetic classification according to the hierarchical model)

(*continued*)

Efficacy (*continued*)

Progression-free Survival 3 years After Randomization in Prognostic Subgroups

Groups	FC[*,†]	FCR[*,‡]	Hazard Rate (95% CI)	*p* Value
All (n = 817)	45%	65%	0.56 (0.46–0.69)	<0.0001
Binet stage				
A (n = 40)	42%	62%	0.42 (0.16–1.14)	0.08
B (n = 522)	45%	69%	0.50 (0.39–0.65)	<0.0001
C (n = 252)	45%	57%	0.73 (0.51–1.04)	0.08
Age				
<65 years (n = 572)	46%	64%	0.57 (0.45–0.73)	<0.0001
≥65 years (n = 245)	43%	68%	0.55 (0.38–0.79)	0.001
Del(17p) (n = 51)	0	18%	0.47 (0.24–0.90)	0.019
Del(11q) (n = 142)[§]	32%	64%	0.34 (0.24–0.61)	<0.0001
Trisomy 12 (n = 61)[ϵ]	48%	83%	0.32 (0.13–0.80)	0.01
Del(13q) (n = 224)[**]	52%	76%	0.43 (0.28–0.68)	0.0002
No abnormalities according to the hierarchical model (n = 138)[††]	48%	58%	0.78 (0.48–1.30)	0.3
IGHV mutated (n = 229)	55%	80%	0.43 (0.27–0.69)	0.0002
IGHV unmutated (n = 390)	35%	55%	0.62 (0.48–0.81)	0.0003

CI, confidence interval; IGHV, immunoglobulin heavy-chain variable gene region
*Data are percentages (Kaplan-Meier estimates), unless otherwise indicated
†FC = chemotherapy (fludarabine + cyclophosphamide)
‡FCR = chemoimmunotherapy (fludarabine + cyclophosphamide + rituximab)
§Not including del(17p)
ϵNot including del(17p) or del(11q)
**Not including del(17p), del(11q), or trisomy 12
††Not including del(17p), del(11q), trisomy 12, or del(13q) (ie, genetic classification according to the hierarchical model)

Overall Survival at 3 years After Randomization in Prognostic Subgroups

Groups	FC[*,†]	FCR[*,‡]	Hazard Rate (95% CI)	*p* Value
All (n = 817)	83%	87%	0.67 (0.48–0.92)	0.012
Binet stage				
A (n = 40)	84%	94%	0.19 (0.02–1.61)	0.091
B (n = 522)	81%	90%	0.45 (0.30–0.69)	0.0002
C (n = 252)	85%	81%	1.48 (0.84–2.62)	0.168
Age				
<65 years (n = 572)	85%	87%	0.68 (0.46–1.02)	0.059
≥65 years (n = 245)	78%	88%	0.63 (0.37–1.10)	0.103
Del(17p) (n = 51)	37%	38%	0.66 (0.32–1.36)	0.25
Del(11q) (n = 142)[§]	83%	94%	0.42 (0.18–0.97)	0.036
Trisomy 12 (n = 61)[ϵ]	86%	96%	0.23 (0.03–1.94)	0.142
Del(13q) (n = 224)[**]	89%	95%	0.30 (0.13–0.71)	0.004
No abnormalities according to the hierarchical model (n = 138)[††]	87%	83%	1.56 (0.67–3.64)	0.303
IGHV mutated (n = 229)	89%	91%	0.70 (0.33–1.49)	0.354
IGHV unmutated (n = 390)	79%	86%	0.62 (0.41–0.94)	0.023

CI, confidence interval; IGHV, immunoglobulin heavy-chain variable gene region
*Data are percentages (Kaplan-Meier estimates), unless otherwise indicated
†FC = chemotherapy (fludarabine + cyclophosphamide)
‡FCR = chemoimmunotherapy (fludarabine + cyclophosphamide + rituximab)
§Not including del(17p)
ϵNot including del(17p) or del(11q)
**Not including del(17p), del(11q), or trisomy 12
††Not including del(17p), del(11q), trisomy 12, or del(13q) (ie, genetic classification according to the hierarchical model)

(*continued*)

Efficacy (continued)

Multivariate Analysis of the Effects of Various Prognostic Variables on Progression-free Survival and Overall Survival in 524 Patients

Variable	Progression-Free Survival		Overall Survival	
	Hazard Ratio (95% CI)	*p* Value	Hazard Ratio (95% CI)	*p* Value
Chemoimmunotherapy*	0.48 (0.37–0.61)	<0.0001	0.6 (0.41–0.91)	0.017
Serum β_2-microglobulin ≥3.5 mg/L	1.40 (1.09–1.81)	0.009	1.82 (1.19–2.79)	0.006
ECOG performance status ≥1	—	—	1.85 (1.23–2.78)	0.003
Serum thymidine kinase ≥10 U/L	—	—	1.87 (1.02–3.41)	0.042
Del(17p)	7.49 (4.83–11.61)	<0.0001	9.32 (5.24–16.56)	<0.0001
IGHV unmutated	1.51 (1.11–2.05)	0.008	—	—
White blood cell count ≥50 × 10⁹/L	1.41 (1.08–1.86)	0.013	—	—

CI, confidence interval; ECOG, Eastern Cooperative Oncology Group; IGHV, immunoglobulin heavy-chain variable gene region
*Chemoimmunotherapy = fludarabine, cyclophosphamide, and rituximab

Toxicity

Incidence of G3/4 Adverse Events

	FC*,† (N = 396)	FCR*,‡ (N = 404)	*p* Value	<65 Years* (N = 560)	≥65 Years* (N = 240)	*p* Value
Total number of patients with more than 1 G3/4 event	249 (63%)	309 (76%)	<0.0001	375 (67%)	183 (76%)	0.009
Hematologic toxicity	157 (40%)	225 (56%)	<0.0001	254 (45%)	128 (53%)	0.04
Neutropenia	83 (21%)	136 (34%)	<0.0001	146 (26%)	73 (30%)	0.21
Leukocytopenia	48 (12%)	97 (24%)	<0.0001	106 (19%)	39 (16%)	0.37
Thrombocytopenia	44 (11%)	30 (7%)	0.07	50 (9%)	24 (10%)	0.63
Anaemia	27 (7%)	22 (5%)	0.42	35 (6%)	14 (6%)	0.82
Autoimmune hemolytic anemia	4 (1%)	3 (<1%)	0.69	4 (<1%)	3 (1%)	0.46
Tumor lysis syndrome	2 (<1%)	1 (<1%)	0.55	3 (<1%)	0	0.26
Cytokine release syndrome	0	1 (<1%)	0.32	1 (<1%)	0	0.51
Infections, total	85 (21%)	103 (25%)	0.18	127 (23%)	61 (25%)	0.4
Infections, not specified	68 (17%)	83 (21%)	0.19	104 (19%)	46 (19%)	0.84
Bacterial infection	5 (1%)	11 (3%)	0.14	6 (1%)	10 (4%)	0.004
Viral infection	17 (4%)	17 (4%)	0.95	26 (5%)	8 (3%)	0.4
Fungal infection	1 (<1%)	3 (<1%)	0.33	3 (<1%)	1 (<1%)	0.83
Parasitic infection	0	1 (<1%)	0.32	0	1 (<1%)	0.13

CI, confidence interval; G-CSF, granulocyte colony-stimulating factor (filgrastim); IGHV, immunoglobulin heavy-chain variable gene region
*Data are number (%), unless otherwise indicated
†FC = chemotherapy (fludarabine + cyclophosphamide)
‡FCR = chemoimmunotherapy (fludarabine + cyclophosphamide + rituximab)
Notes:
- Filgrastim was administered in 86 treatment cycles, for a median of 7 days in the FC group and 6 days in the FCR group. It was given more frequently in the FCR group (n = 75 vs. n = 11). In 40 treatment cycles, filgrastim was given as prophylaxis without any sign of neutropenia; in 46 cycles, it was administered to treat an adverse event (neutropenia or leukocytopenia)
- Ten (3%) deaths were related to treatment in the FC group, and 8 (2%) in the FCR group. Of these, 6 FC-treated patients and 5 FCR-treated patients died from infections (septicemia [n = 6], pneumonia [n = 3], hepatitis B [n = 1], and cryptosporidium gastroenteritis [n = 1]). In 7 patients (3 in the FC group and 4 in the FCR group), death occurred before the third treatment course (fatal septicemia [n = 6], sudden cardiac death [n = 1])

REGIMEN

CYCLOPHOSPHAMIDE + PENTOSTATIN + RITUXIMAB

Lamanna N et al. J Clin Oncol 2006;24:1575–1581

Cycle 1 (clinicians' discretion during subsequent cycles)
Premedication: prophylaxis against hyperuricemia with **allopurinol** 300 mg/day for 5–7 days, starting the day before chemotherapy commences
• Persons who express a variant human leukocyte antigen allele, HLA-B*58:01, are at increased risk for severe cutaneous adverse reactions from allopurinol (Hershfield MS et al. Clin Pharmacol Ther 2013;93:153–158; Zineh I et al. Pharmacogenomics 2011;12:1741–1749)

Cycles 1–6
Hydration on day 1: Administer intravenously at least 1500 mL 5% dextrose injection (D5W), 0.45% sodium chloride injection, or 0.9% sodium chloride injection (0.9% NS) on day 1 before starting chemotherapy
Cyclophosphamide 600 mg/m^2; administer intravenously in 50–250 mL 0.9% NS or 5% dextrose injection (D5W) over 15–60 minutes on day 1 every 3 weeks for 6 cycles (total dosage/cycle = 600 mg/m^2)
Pentostatin 4 mg/m^2; administer intravenously in 25–50 mL D5W or 0.9% NS over 20–30 minutes on day 1, every 3 weeks for 6 cycles (total dosage/cycle = 4 mg/m^2)
Filgrastim; administer by subcutaneous injection, daily, starting on cycle day 3 and continue until a patient achieves a single postnadir ANC >5000/mm^3 or an ANC >1500/mm^3 on 2 consecutive days
• Filgrastim doses are based on a patient's body weight as follows:

Body Weight	Filgrastim Dose
≤70 kg	300 mcg/day
>70 kg	480 mcg/day

Cycles 2–6
Premedication for rituximab:
Acetaminophen 650–1000 mg; administer orally *plus* **diphenhydramine** 25–50 mg; administer orally or intravenously 30–60 minutes before each dose of rituximab
Rituximab 375 mg/m^2; administer intravenously in D5W or 0.9% NS diluted to a concentration within the range of 1–4 mg/mL on day 1 after cyclophosphamide and pentostatin administration were completed, every 3 weeks for 5 cycles (total dosage/cycle = 375 mg/m^2)

Notes on rituximab administration:
• Infuse initially at 50 mg/h. If hypersensitivity or infusion reactions do not occur during the first 30 minutes, increase the rate by 50 mg/h every 30 minutes as tolerated to a maximum rate of 400 mg/h. Subsequently if previous administration was well tolerated, start at 100 mg/h and increase by 100 mg/h every 30 minutes as tolerated to a maximum rate of 400 mg/h

• Rituximab was not given during cycle 1. The investigators explained that infusion reactions to rituximab tend to be more severe in patients with hyperleukocytosis, which in a prior study had been shown to be alleviated by treatment with pentostatin and cyclophosphamide; therefore, rituximab was withheld until the second treatment cycle

Notes: Chemotherapy was administered in the following sequence: cyclophosphamide, then pentostatin, then rituximab
After 3 cycles, patients who did not achieve ≥PR were considered to have experienced treatment failure and were removed from study. Responding patients continued on treatment for a total of 6 cycles

Supportive Care
Antiemetic prophylaxis
Emetogenic potential with or without rituximab is **MODERATE**
See Chapter 39 for antiemetic recommendations

(continued)

Treatment Modifications

Adverse Event	Treatment Modification
Serum creatinine ≥2.0 mg/dL (≥177 μmol/L) or more than 20% higher than the baseline value measured at the start of treatment	Withhold pentostatin until serum creatinine <2.0 mg/dL (<177 μmol/L) or <120% the baseline measured at the start of treatment, or the creatinine clearance ≥50 mL/min (≥0.83 mL/s)
Severe rash	Withhold pentostatin therapy until rash resolves
Patients showing evidence of nervous system toxicity	Withhold therapy until toxicity resolves to baseline or consider discontinuing treatment with pentostatin
ANC ≤1000/mm^3 or platelet count ≤80,000/mm^3 after the first treatment cycle	Postponed treatment until ANC >1000/mm^3 and platelet count is >80,000/mm^3. If delay is >1 week, restart treatment cyclophosphamide dosage decreased to 500 mg/m^2. If further dosage reduction is needed, reduce the cyclophosphamide dosage to 400 mg/m^2. Pentostatin and rituximab dosages are not reduced
Major infection	Reduce cyclophosphamide dosage to 500 mg/m^2. If further dosage reduction is needed, reduce the cyclophosphamide dosage to 400 mg/m^2. Pentostatin and rituximab dosages are not reduced

Note: Reductions in pentostatin dosages are not recommended during treatment in patients with anemia and thrombocytopenia if patients can be otherwise supported hematologically. Pentostatin should be temporarily withheld if the absolute neutrophil count during treatment decreases to <200 cells/mm^3 in a patient whose initial ANC was >500 cells/mm^3. Pentostatin use may resume when ANC returns to pretreatment levels

(*continued*)

Hematopoietic growth factor (CSF) prophylaxis
Primary prophylaxis is indicated with 1 of the following:
Filgrastim (G-CSF) 5 mcg/kg per day; administer by subcutaneous injection, *or*
Pegfilgrastim (pegylated filgrastim) 6 mg/0.6 mL; administer by subcutaneous injection for 1 dose
- Discontinue daily filgrastim use at least 24 hours before administering myelosuppressive treatment. Do not administer pegfilgrastim within 14 days before administering myelosuppressive treatment

See Chapter 43 for more information

Antimicrobial prophylaxis
Risk of fever and neutropenia is INTERMEDIATE
Antimicrobial primary prophylaxis to be considered:
- Antibacterial—consider a fluoroquinolone or no prophylaxis; *Pneumocystis jirovecii* prophylaxis is recommended (eg, cotrimoxazole)
- Antifungal—recommended; consider use during periods of neutropenia, and in anticipation of mucositis
- Antiviral—antiherpes antivirals (eg, acyclovir, famciclovir, valacyclovir)

See Chapter 47 for more information

Infusion reactions associated with rituximab
Fevers, chills, and rigors
1. Interrupt rituximab administration for severe symptoms, and give:
   - **Acetaminophen** 650 mg orally for fever. For persistent or recurrent symptoms, repeat administration every 4–6 hours as needed during rituximab administration
   - **Diphenhydramine** 25–50 mg orally or by intravenous injection for pruritus, hypotension, or angioedema. For persistent or recurrent symptoms, repeat administration every 4–6 hours as needed during rituximab administration
   - **Meperidine** 12.5–25 mg by intravenous injection every 10–20 minutes as needed for shaking chills (generally, cumulative doses >100 mg are not needed; use repeated doses with caution in persons with moderate or more severely impaired renal function)
2. If rituximab administration was interrupted, resume infusion at a slower rate than the maximum rate previously attempted. Rate escalation may be reattempted at smaller incremental steps with close monitoring. Do not exceed the maximum recommended rate of 400 mg/h
Dyspnea or wheezing without allergic findings (urticaria, or tongue or laryngeal edema)
1. Interrupt rituximab administration immediately
2. Give **hydrocortisone** 100 mg by intravenous injection (or an alternative steroid with equivalent glucocorticoid potency)
3. Give a **histamine (H₂) receptor antagonist** (ranitidine 50 mg, cimetidine 300 mg, or famotidine 20 mg) intravenously over 15–30 minutes
4. After symptoms resolve, resume rituximab administration at 25 mg/h with close monitoring. Do not increase the administration rate

Patient Population Studied

Characteristic (N = 46)	Number (Percent)
Age, median (range)	62 years (30–80 years)
Sex, male-to-female ratio	30 (65%)/16 (35%)
Patient diagnosis	
SLL*	9 (20%)
Waldenström's macroglobulinemia	1 (2%)
Follicular lymphoma	4 (9%)
CLL intermediate risk	7 (15%)
CLL high risk	25 (54%)
Blood	
WBC, median (range)	49 cells/mm³ (2.6–256.9)
Hemoglobin, median (range)	10.8 g/dL (6.5–15.8)
PLT, median (range)	96 cells/mm³ (34–380)
CLL patients (N = 32)	
Anemia (hemoglobin <11 g/dL)	16 (50%)
Thrombocytopenia (<100,000 cells/mm³)	17 (53%)
β₂-microglobulin, mg/L median (range)	3.8 (0.8–12.1)
Patients with β₂-microglobulin >4	12 (38%)
CD38 expression >20%	28 (87%)

CLL, chronic lymphocytic leukemia; PLT, platelets; SLL, small lymphocytic lymphoma
*SLL, histologically (and immunophenotypically); most had the "CLL type" of SLL but did not meet the NCI Working Group definition of CLL because of the degree of blood and BM involvement

(*continued*)

Efficacy

Response	Number (%)
CLL Patients (N = 32)	
Total responses	24 (75%)
Complete responses	8 (25%)
Nodular responses	1 (3%)
Partial responses	15 (47%)
Median duration of response	25 months
Median time to treatment failure	40 months
Median time to treatment failure for patients with CR/NR	Not reached
Median time to treatment failure for patients with PR	17 months
Median overall survival	44 months
Median overall survival (patients with CR/NR)	Not reached
Median overall survival at 36 months (patients with CR/NR)	100%
Median overall survival (patients with PR/No Response)	32 months
Median overall survival at 36 months (patients with PR/No Response)	28%
Non-CLL Patients (N = 14)	
Total responses	7 (50%)
Complete responses	1 (7%)
Partial responses	6 (43%)

CLL, chronic lymphocytic leukemia

Toxicity

G3/4 neutropenia	53%
G3/4 anemia	9%
G3/4 thrombocytopenia	16%
G3/4 infections (including fever of unknown origin) in CLL patients	9/32 (28%)*
G3 nausea	1/32 (3%)
Asymptomatic tumor lysis in CLL	56%†
Number of CLL patients who did not receive the planned number of cycles	9/32 (28%)‡

*Eight of these patients had pneumonia. There was 1 death from progressive pneumonia
†The fraction may underestimate the true risk of tumor lysis syndrome because all patients received hydration and allopurinol before initiating therapy. Rapid cytoreduction was manifested as a prompt decline in the number of circulating lymphocytes, with a median reduction of 78% seen following the first cycle of chemotherapy
‡Therapy stopped in 5 because of infections and in 4 other patients for a variety of comorbid conditions (lung cancer, amegakaryocytic thrombocytopenia, chylous pleural effusion, and an acute confusional state of undetermined etiology)

Patient Population Studied
(continued)

Prior Therapy	Number of Patients (%)
CLL Patients (N = 32)	
Number prior regimens, median (range)	2 (1–7)
Prior fludarabine	25 (78%)
Refractory	8 (25%)
Prior alkylating agent	25 (78%)
Refractory	7 (22%)
Prior rituximab therapy	7 (22%)
Refractory	4 (13%)
Non-CLL Patients (N = 14)	
Number prior regimens, median (range)	2 (1–6)
Prior fludarabine	6
Refractory	1
Prior alkylating agents	13
Refractory	4
Prior rituximab	9
Refractory	5

CLL, chronic lymphocytic leukemia

Treatment Monitoring

1. *Baseline and response assessment (performed pretreatment, then after 3 and 6 cycles of therapy):* complete physical examination, CBC with differential, BM aspirate, and biopsy. Peripheral blood and/or BM samples analyzed by flow cytometry for CD5/CD19 (or CD5/CD20) dual staining and kappa/lambda clonal excess. Trisomy 12 also tested at the time of response assessment in patients shown to have trisomy 12. Patients who had abnormal computed tomography imaging pretreatment had repeat computed tomography imaging for response assessment

2. *Before each dose and at other appropriate intervals during therapy:* serum creatinine

3. *After completion of therapy:* follow patients at 2- to 3-month intervals for at least 1 year

REGIMEN

Small Lymphocytic Lymphoma
Mantle Cell Lymphoma
IBRUTINIB

Byrd JC et al. N Engl J Med 2013;369:32–42
Wang ML et al. N Engl J Med 2013;369:507–516

Ibrutinib 420–560 mg/day; administer orally, continually (total dose/week = 2940–3920 mg)
• Administration with food increases ibrutinib exposure approximately 2-fold compared with administration after overnight fasting (IMBRUVICA [ibrutinib] capsules, for oral use; November 2013 product label. Janssen Biotech, Inc. Horsham, PA-C, USA)

Supportive Care
Antiemetic prophylaxis
Emetogenic potential is **LOW**
See Chapter 39 for antiemetic recommendations

Hematopoietic growth factor (CSF) prophylaxis
Primary prophylaxis is NOT indicated
See Chapter 43 for more information

Antimicrobial prophylaxis
Risk of fever and neutropenia is LOW
 Antimicrobial primary prophylaxis to be considered:
 • Antibacterial—not indicated
 • Antifungal—not indicated
 • Antiviral—not indicated unless patient previously had an episode of HSV
See Chapter 47 for more information

Diarrhea management
 Loperamide 4 mg orally, initially after the first loose or liquid stool, *then*
 Loperamide 2 mg orally every 2 hours during waking hours, *plus*
 Loperamide 4 mg orally every 4 hours during hours of sleep
 • Continue for at least 12 hours after diarrhea resolves
 • Recurrent diarrhea after a 12-hour diarrhea-free interval is treated as a new episode
 • Rehydrate orally with fluids and electrolytes during a diarrheal episode
 • If a patient develops blood or mucus in stool, dehydration, or hemodynamic instability, or if diarrhea persists >48 hours despite loperamide, stop loperamide and hospitalize the patient for IV hydration
 Alternatively, a trial of **Diphenoxylate hydrochloride** 2.5 mg **with Atropine sulfate** 0.025 mg (eg, Lomotil)
 • Initial adult dose is 2 tablets 4 times daily until control has been achieved, after which the dose may be reduced to meet individual requirements. Control may often be maintained with as little as 2 tablets daily
 • Clinical improvement of acute diarrhea is usually observed within 48 hours. If improvement of chronic diarrhea after treatment with a maximum daily dose of 8 tablets is not observed within 10 days, control is unlikely with further administration

Oral care
Prophylaxis and treatment for mucositis/stomatitis
 General advice:
 • Encourage patients to maintain intake of nonalcoholic fluids
 • Evaluate patients for oral pain and provide analgesic medications
 • Consider histamine (H_2-subtype) receptor antagonists (eg, ranitidine, famotidine), or a proton pump inhibitor for epigastric pain
 • *Lactobacillus* sp.-containing probiotics may be beneficial in preventing diarrhea
 Patients with intact oral mucosa:
 • Clean the mouth, tongue, and gums by brushing after every meal and at bedtime with an ultra-soft toothbrush with fluoride toothpaste
 • Floss teeth gently every day unless contraindicated. If gums bleed and hurt, avoid bleeding or sore areas, but floss other teeth
 • Patients may use saline or commercial brand, nonalcoholic rinses
  ▪ Do not use mouthwashes that contain alcohols
 If mucositis or stomatitis is present:
 • Keep the mouth moist utilizing water, ice chips, sugarless gum, sugar-free hard candies, or a saliva substitute
 • Rinse mouth several times a day to remove debris
  ▪ Use a solution of ¼ teaspoon (1.25 g) each of baking soda and table salt (sodium chloride) in 1 quart (~950 mL) of warm water. Follow with a plain water rinse
  ▪ Do not use mouthwashes that contain alcohols

(continued)

(continued)

- Foam-tipped swabs (eg, Toothettes) are useful in moisturizing oral mucosa, but ineffective for cleansing teeth and removing plaque
- Advise patients who develop mucositis to:
  - Choose foods that are easy to chew and swallow
  - Take small bites of food, chew slowly, and sip liquids with meals
  - Encourage soft, moist foods such as cooked cereals, mashed potatoes, and scrambled eggs
  - For trouble swallowing, soften food with gravies, sauces, broths, yogurt, or other bland liquids
  - Avoid sharp, crunchy foods; hot, spicy, or highly acidic foods (eg, citrus fruits and juices); sugary foods; toothpicks; tobacco products; alcoholic drinks

Patient Population Studied

Byrd JC et al. N Engl J Med 2013;369:32–42

Patients with a diagnosis of relapsed or refractory CLL or small lymphocytic lymphoma, defined according to the International Workshop on Chronic Lymphocytic Leukemia and World Health Organization classifications. Those enrolled were deemed to be in need of treatment. The first and second cohorts were required to have received ≥2 previous therapies, including a purine analog. A third cohort included patients with high-risk disease that did not respond to a chemoimmunotherapy regimen or whose disease progressed within 24 months after completion of the regimen

Patient Characteristics (N = 85)

Age—median (range)	66 (37–82)
≥70 years	30 (35%)
Sex—male-to-female ratio	65 (76%)/20 (24%)
Diagnosis	
Chronic lymphocytic leukemia	82 (96%)
Small lymphocytic lymphoma	3 (4%)
Time since last systemic anticancer therapy—median (range)	3 months (1–98)
Rai stage at treatment initiation*—[Data missing = 1 (1%)]	
0, I, or II	29 (34%)
III or IV	55 (65%)
Number of previous therapies—median (range)	4 (1–12)
Previous therapy	
Nucleoside analog	81 (95%)
Rituximab	83 (98%)
Alkylator	76 (89%)
Alemtuzumab	18 (21%)
Bendamustine	33 (39%)
Ofatumumab	22 (26%)
Bulky nodes—[Data missing = 3 (4%)]	
≥5 cm in diameter	44 (52%)
≥10 cm in diameter 13 (15)	
Unmutated immunoglobulin variable-region heavy-chain gene	
Patients with data that could be evaluated	69 (81%)
Data missing	4 (5%)
Interphase cytogenetic abnormality—no. (%)	
17p13.1 deletion	28 (33%)
11q22.3 deletion	31 (36%)
β_2-Microglobulin level >3 mg/L [Data missing = 5 (6%)]	39 (46%)
Disease resistant to purine analogue[†]	41 (48%)

*Rai stage 0 = low-risk, stages I/II = intermediate-risk, and stages III/IV = high-risk
[†]Defined as treatment failure (stable disease or progressive disease) or disease progression within 12 months after receipt of a regimen containing a purine analogue

(continued)

Patient Population Studied (*continued*)

Wang ML et al. N Engl J Med 2013;369:507–516

Patients with a confirmed diagnosis of mantle cell lymphoma with cyclin D_1 overexpression or translocation breakpoints at t(11;14) and measurable disease (lymph-node diameter ≥2 cm). All had received at least 1 but no more than 5 previous lines of treatment, with no partial or better response to the most recent treatment

Patient Characteristics (N = 111)*

Age—median (range)	68 years (40–84 years)
Sex—male-to-female ratio	85 (77%)/26 (23%)
ECOG performance status	
0 or 1	99 (89%)
2	11 (10%)
>2	1 (1%)
Number of prior regimens—median (range)	3 (1–5)
≥3	61 (55%)
Previous therapy	
Hyper-CVAD†	33 (30%)
Stem cell transplantation	12 (11%)
Lenalidomide	27 (24%)
Rituximab or rituximab-containing regimen	99 (89%)
Simplified MIPI‡	
Low risk	15 (14%)
Intermediate risk	42 (38%)
High risk	54 (49%)
Bulky mass§	9 (8%)
At least 1 node ≥5 cm	43 (39%)
Refractory disease⁴	50 (45%)
Advanced disease**	80 (72%)

*Four patients enrolled but did not receive ibrutinib (investigator's decision)
†Hyperfractionated cyclophosphamide, vincristine, doxorubicin, and dexamethasone
‡The simplified Mantle-Cell Lymphoma International Prognostic Index (MIPI) score was derived with the use of the 4 prognostic factors of age, ECOG score, lactate dehydrogenase level, and white-cell count at baseline, and its range depends on the range of these characteristics. The index classifies patients as having low-risk (0–3), intermediate-risk (4 or 5), or high-risk (6–11) disease
§Bulky mass = tumor with a diameter ≥10 cm
⁴Refractory disease = lack of at least a partial response to the last therapy before study
**Advanced disease = involvement of bone marrow, extranodal sites, or both
Note: Percentages may not add up to 100% because of rounding

Efficacy (N = 85)

Byrd JC et al. N Engl J Med 2013;369:32–42

Subgroup	Number	ORR (95% CI)*
All patients	85	71% (60–80)
Dose		
420 mg	51	71% (56–82)
840 mg	34	71% (52–85)
Age		
<70 years	55	69% (55–81)
≥70 years	30	73% (54–88)
Rai stage at baseline		
0 (low-risk) I, or II (intermediate-risk)	29	69% (49–85)
III or IV (high risk)	55	71% (57–82)
Previous chemotherapy		
<3 Regimens	27	74% (54–89)
≥3 Regimens	58	69% (56–81)
17p13.1 deletion		
Positive	28	68% (48–84)
Negative	52	71% (57–83)
11q22.3 deletion		
Positive	31	77% (59–90)
Negative	49	65% (50–78)
IGHV (immunoglobulin variable-region heavy-chain gene)		
Mutated	12	33% (10–65)
Unmutated	69	77% (65–86)
β_2-Microglobulin		
≤3 mg/L	39	72% (55–85)
>3 mg/L	41	68% (52–82)

*Only patients who received ibrutinib and had at least one post-baseline assessment

Best Response to Therapy*

Wang ML et al. N Engl J Med 2013;369:507–516

Variable	Prior Bortezomib Treatment		All Patients (N = 111)
	No (N = 63)	Yes (N = 48)	
Response—no. (%)			
Overall	43 (68%)	32 (67%)	75 (68%)
Complete	12 (19%)	11 (23%)	23 (21%)
Partial	31 (49%)	21 (44%)	52 (47%)
None†	20 (32%)	15 (31%)	35 (32%)
Response duration	15.8 (5.6–NR)	NR (NR–NR)	17.5 (15.8–NR)
Progression-free survival	7.4 (5.3–19.2)	16.6 (8.3–NR)	13.9 (7.0–NR)
Overall survival	NR (10.0–NR)	NR (11.9–NR)	NR (13.2–NR)

*Only patients who received ibrutinib and had at least one post-baseline assessment
†Median values in months with 95% Confidence Intervals (95% CI)

Toxicity (N = 111)*

Wang ML et al. N Engl J Med 2013;369:507–516

Adverse Events	% G1	% G2	% G3	% G4	% All Grades
	Number of Patients with Event (%)				
Hematologic Event					
Neutropenia	1%	1%	6%	10%	18%
Thrombocytopenia	4%	4%	7%	4%	18%
Non-hematologic Event					
Diarrhea	32%	12%	6%	0	50%
Fatigue	20%	17%	5%	0	41%
Nausea	23%	7%	0	0	31%
Peripheral edema	19%	7%	1%	1%	28%
Dyspnea[†]	13%	10%	4%	0	27%
Constipation	18%	7%	0	0	25%
Upper respiratory tract infection	5%	18%	0	0	23%
Vomiting	17%	5%	0	0	23%
Decreased appetite	10%	9%	2%	0	21%
Cough	12%	6%	0	0	18%
Pyrexia	13%	5%	1%	0	18%
Abdominal pain	9%	3%	5%	0	17%
Contusion	15%	2%	0	0	17%
Rash	10%	4%	2%	0	15%

*Data = adverse events reported during treatment in the 111 patients included in the study. Listed events occurred in at least 15% of patients on or before the data-cutoff date. For 4 events (1 event each of diarrhea, depression, asthenia, and hypersomnia), the grade was not available; these 4 events are included as G3
[†]One grade 5 event

Treatment Monitoring

1. *Before treatment:* physical examination; CBC with differential; assessment of serum chemistry; serum immunoelectrophoresis; measurement of immunoglobulin concentrations; CT scan of the chest, abdomen, and pelvis; and bone marrow aspiration and biopsy as indicated. If clinically relevant, endoscopy of the gastrointestinal tract is done
2. *Weekly:* CBC with differential and platelet count once weekly
3. *Assessment of efficacy:* CT scan or sonographic examination at 2- or 3-cycle intervals after and at the end of treatment in MCL. Cycles 2, 5, 8, 12, 15, and 24 in SLL

REGIMEN

RITUXIMAB WITH HYPERFRACTIONATED CYCLOPHOSPHAMIDE + VINCRISTINE + DOXORUBICIN + DEXAMETHASONE (R-HYPER-CVAD) ALTERNATING WITH RITUXIMAB WITH METHOTREXATE + CYTARABINE (R-MC)

Romaguera JE et al. J Clin Oncol 2005;23:7013–7023
Wang M et al. Cancer 2008;113:2734–2741

If indicated: Prophylaxis against tumor lysis syndrome during the first cycle:
Hydration with 2500–3000 mL/day, as tolerated; administer intravenously at 100–125 mL/hour
Notes:
- Sodium bicarbonate is added to parenteral hydration solutions in the presence of plasma uric acid >9 mg/dL to maintain urine pH >7.0, but pH <8. The choice of hydration fluid and amount of sodium bicarbonate added to the fluid should NOT EXCEED the sodium concentration present in 0.9% sodium chloride injection (154 mEq/L); for example:
  - 5% Dextrose/0.45% sodium chloride injection with sodium bicarbonate 50–75 mEq/1000 mL, *or*
  - 5% Dextrose/0.2% sodium chloride injection with sodium bicarbonate 100–125 mEq/1000 mL, *or*
  - 5% Dextrose injection with sodium bicarbonate 125–150 mEq/1000 mL
- Potassium is NOT added to parenteral hydration solutions during the first few days of induction therapy unless serum potassium decreases to <3.0 mEq/dL
- Furosemide 20–40 mg; administer intravenously every 12–24 hours to maintain fluid balance
- Diuresis is maintained for at least the first 72 hours after starting chemotherapy in the absence of metabolic aberrations, or after metabolic complications normalize
- **Allopurinol** 300 mg/day; administer orally for 7 consecutive days on days 1–7 (longer treatment may be needed)
  - Persons who express a variant human leukocyte antigen allele, HLA-B*58:01, are at increased risk for severe cutaneous adverse reactions from allopurinol (Hershfield MS et al. Clin Pharmacol Ther 2013;93:153–158; Zineh I et al. Pharmacogenomics 2011;12:1741–1749)

R-Hyper-CVAD (odd-numbered cycles; ie, 1, 3, 5, ±7)
Premedication for rituximab:
Acetaminophen 650–1000 mg; administer orally, *plus*
Diphenhydramine 25–50 mg; administer orally or intravenously 30–60 minutes before starting rituximab
Rituximab 375 mg/m² per dose; administer intravenously in 0.9% sodium chloride injection (0.9% NS) or 5% dextrose injection (D5W), diluted to a concentration within the range of 1–4 mg/mL on day 1, for 3–4 cycles, cycles 1, 3, 5 (±7). Cycle duration is 21 days (total dosage/cycle = 375 mg/m²)

Notes on rituximab administration:
- Infuse initially at 50 mg/h. If hypersensitivity or infusion reactions do not occur during the first 30 minutes, increase the rate by 50 mg/h every 30 minutes, as tolerated, to a maximum rate of 400 mg/h. Subsequently, if previous administration was well tolerated, start at 100 mg/h and increase by 100 mg/h every 30 minutes, as tolerated, to a maximum rate of 400 mg/h
- Interrupt rituximab administration for fever, chills, edema, congestion of the head and neck mucosa, hypertension, and other serious adverse events. Resume rituximab administration after adverse events abate
- *Patients with evidence of peripheral blood involvement (as determined by flow cytometric analysis at the time of initial presentation) may have their first dose of rituximab delayed or omitted when they are believed to be at risk for tumor lysis syndrome or cytokine-release syndrome*

Cyclophosphamide 300 mg/m² per dose; administer intravenously in 500 mL 0.9% NS over 3 hours, every 12 hours for 6 doses, on days 2, 3, and 4, for 3–4 cycles, cycles 1, 3, 5 (±7). Cycle duration is 21 days (total dosage/cycle = 1800 mg/m²)
Mesna 600 mg/m² per day; administer by continuous intravenous infusion over 24 hours in 1000–2000 mL 0.9% NS on days 2, 3, and 4, starting 1 hour before cyclophosphamide and continuing until 12 hours after the last dose of cyclophosphamide, for 3–4 cycles, cycles 1, 3, 5 (±7). Cycle duration is 21 days (total duration of mesna administration per cycle is approximately 76 hours; total dosage/cycle is approximately 1900 mg/m²)
Vincristine 1.4 mg/m² per dose (maximum single dose = 2 mg); administer by intravenous injection over 1–2 minutes for 2 doses, 12 hours after the last dose of cyclophosphamide on day 5 and on day 12, for 3–4 cycles, cycles 1, 3, 5 (±7). Cycle duration is 21 days (total dosage/cycle = 2.8 mg/m²; maximum total dose/cycle = 4 mg)
Doxorubicin 16.6 mg/m² per day; administer by continuous intravenous infusion over 24 hours in 25–250 mL 0.9% NS or D5W for 3 consecutive days starting 12 hours after the last dose of cyclophosphamide, on days 5, 6, and 7, for 3–4 cycles, cycles 1, 3, 5 (±7). Cycle duration is 21 days (total dosage/cycle ~50 mg/m²)
Dexamethasone 40 mg/day; administer orally or intravenously in 25–150 mL 0.9% NS or D5W over 15–30 minutes for 8 doses, on days 2–5 and days 12–15 for 3–4 cycles, cycles 1, 3, 5 (±7). Cycle duration is 21 days (total dosage/cycle = 320 mg)

R-MC (even-numbered cycles; ie, 2, 4, 6, ±8)
Premedication for rituximab:
Acetaminophen 650–1000 mg; administer orally, *plus*
Diphenhydramine 25–50 mg; administer orally or intravenously, 30–60 minutes before starting rituximab

(continued)

(*continued*)

Rituximab 375 mg/m² per dose; administer intravenously in 0.9% NS or D5W diluted to a concentration within the range of 1–4 mg/mL on day 1 for 3–4 cycles, cycles 2, 4, 6 (±8). Cycle duration is 21 days (total dosage/cycle = 375 mg/m²)

Notes on rituximab administration:
- Infuse initially at 100 mg/h. If hypersensitivity or infusion reactions do not occur during the first 30 minutes, increase the rate by 100 mg/h every 30 minutes, as tolerated, to a maximum rate of 400 mg/h. Subsequently, if previous administration was well tolerated, start at 100 mg/h and increase by 100 mg/h every 30 minutes, as tolerated, to a maximum rate of 400 mg/h
- Interrupt rituximab administration for fever, chills, edema, congestion of the head and neck mucosa, hypertension, and other serious adverse events. Resume rituximab administration after adverse events abate

Hydration with 2500–3000 mL/day, as tolerated; administer intravenously at 100–125 mL/hour
Notes:
- Sodium bicarbonate is added to parenteral hydration solutions in the presence of plasma uric acid >9 mg/dL to maintain urine pH ≥7.0, but pH <8. The choice of hydration fluid and amount of sodium bicarbonate added to the fluid should NOT EXCEED the sodium concentration present in 0.9% sodium chloride injection (154 mEq/L); for example:
  - 5% Dextrose/0.45% sodium chloride injection with sodium bicarbonate 50–75 mEq/1000 mL, *or*
  - 5% Dextrose/0.2% sodium chloride injection with sodium bicarbonate 100–125 mEq/1000 mL, *or*
  - 5% dextrose injection with sodium bicarbonate 125–150 mEq/1000 mL

Methotrexate 200 mg/m²; administer intravenously in 250 mL to >1000 mL 0.9% NS or D5W (or saline and dextrose combinations) over 2 hours, *followed by:*
Methotrexate 800 mg/m²; administer intravenously in 250 mL to >1000 mL 0.9% NS or D5W (or saline and dextrose combinations) over 22 hours, on day 2, for 3–4 cycles, cycles 2, 4, 6 (±8). Cycle duration is 21 days (total dosage/cycle [not including intrathecal methotrexate] = 1000 mg/m²)

Notes on methotrexate administration:
- Patients with an initial serum creatinine level >1.5 mg/dL (>133 μmol/L), reduce the dose of methotrexate by 50%
- Patients with evidence of third spacing of fluids, remove the fluid as completely as possible or, if this is not possible, repeat rituximab plus hyper-CVAD until third spacing of fluid is resolved

Cytarabine 3000 mg/m² per dose; administer intravenously in 50–500 mL 0.9% NS or D5W over 2 hours, every 12 hours, for 4 doses, on days 3 and 4, for 3–4 cycles, cycles 2, 4, 6 (±8). Cycle duration is 21 days (total dosage/cycle [not including intrathecal cytarabine] = 12,000 mg/m²)

Notes on cytarabine administration:
- Reduce the cytarabine dose to 1000 mg/m² in patients whose age is ≥60 years and in those with a serum creatinine level >1.5 mg/dL (>133 μmol/L)
- Administer a **1% ophthalmic solution of**, at a rate of 2 drops in each eye 4 times daily, beginning on day 3 at the start of cytarabine infusion and continue for 7 days to prevent chemical conjunctivitis

Leucovorin calcium 50 mg; administer intravenously in 10–100 mL 0.9% NS or D5W over 10–20 minutes, on day 3, 36 hours after methotrexate administration began (12 hours after completing methotrexate), followed 6 hours later by:
Leucovorin calcium 15 mg; administer orally *or* intravenously in 10–100 mL 0.9% NS or D5W over 10–20 minutes, every 6 hours, for 8 doses or until blood methotrexate concentrations is <0.1 μmol/L
If methotrexate elimination is delayed or attenuated, both the dose and administration schedule for leucovorin calcium are escalated, thus:
leucovorin calcium 100 mg/dose intravenously every 3 hours, if serum methotrexate concentrations are:

Time After Methotrexate Administration Began	Serum Methotrexate Concentration
24 hours	>20 μmol/L (>20 × 10²⁶ mol/L)
48 hours	>1 μmol/L (>1 × 10²⁶ mol/L)
72 hours	>0.1 μmol/L (>1 × 10²⁷ mol/L)

If methotrexate elimination is delayed, measure serum methotrexate concentrations at daily intervals and continue leucovorin administration until serum methotrexate concentration is ≤0.05 μmol/L (≤5 × 10²⁸ mol/L) or undetectable

Treatment Duration:
- Patients who achieved a CR after the first 2 cycles (1 cycle with rituximab plus hyper-CVAD and 1 cycle with rituximab plus methotrexate and cytarabine) received 4 more cycles, for a total of 6 cycles
- Patients who achieved a partial response (PR) after 2 cycles and a complete remission after 6 cycles received 2 more cycles, for a total of 8 cycles
- Patients with evidence of disease after 6 cycles did not receive further therapy
- Patients whose disease was responding could be referred at any time during treatment for consolidation with stem cell transplantation

Supportive Care
Antiemetic prophylaxis for R-Hyper-CVAD (cycles 1, 3, 5, ± 7)
Emetogenic potential on day 1 is MINIMAL
Emetogenic potential on days 2, 3, and 4 is MODERATE

(*continued*)

(continued)

Emetogenic potential on days 5, 6, and 7 is **LOW–MODERATE**
Emetogenic potential on day 12 is **MINIMAL**
See Chapter 39 for antiemetic recommendations

Antiemetic prophylaxis for R-MC (cycles 2, 4, 6, ± 8)
Emetogenic potential on day 1 is **MINIMAL**
Emetogenic potential on day 2 is **MODERATE**
Emetogenic potential on days 3 and 4 is **MODERATE**
See Chapter 39 for antiemetic recommendations

Hematopoietic growth factor (CSF) prophylaxis (all cycles)
Primary prophylaxis is indicated with:

 Filgrastim (G-CSF) 5 mcg/kg per day; administer by subcutaneous injection for 10 days
 • Begin use from 24–36 hours after myelosuppressive chemotherapy is completed
 • Discontinue daily filgrastim use at least 24 hours before restarting myelosuppressive treatment
See Chapter 43 for more information

Antimicrobial prophylaxis
Risk of fever and neutropenia is HIGH
 Antimicrobial primary prophylaxis is recommended:

R-Hyper-CVAD (cycles 1, 3, 5, ±7)		
Antibacterial prophylaxis	Ciprofloxacin 500 mg orally, twice daily (or an alternative fluoroquinolone at an equivalent dose and schedule)	Days 8–17 (10 days)
	Cotrimoxazole (160 mg trimethoprim + 800 mg sulfamethoxazole), orally	One dose, 3 days per week, continually throughout all cycles
Antifungal prophylaxis	Fluconazole 100 mg/day, orally	Days 8–17 (10 days)
Antiviral prophylaxis	Valacyclovir 500 mg/day, orally (or acyclovir or famciclovir at an equivalent dose and schedule)	Days 8–17 (10 days)
R-MC (cycles 2, 4, 6, ±8)		
Antibacterial prophylaxis	Ciprofloxacin 500 mg, orally, twice daily (or an alternative fluoroquinolone at an equivalent dose and schedule)	Days 5–14 (10 days)
	Cotrimoxazole (160 mg trimethoprim + 800 mg sulfamethoxazole), orally	One dose, 3 days per week, continually throughout all cycles
Antifungal prophylaxis	Fluconazole 100 mg/day, orally	Days 5–14 (10 days)
Antiviral prophylaxis	Valacyclovir 500 mg/day, orally (or acyclovir or famciclovir at an equivalent dose and schedule)	Days 5–14 (10 days)

See Chapter 47 for more information

Infusion reactions associated with rituximab
 Fevers, chills, and rigors
 1. Interrupt rituximab administration for severe symptoms, and give:
  • **Acetaminophen** 650 mg orally for fever. For persistent or recurrent symptoms, repeat administration every 4–6 hours as needed during rituximab administration
  • **Diphenhydramine** 25–50 mg orally or by intravenous injection for pruritus, hypotension, or angioedema. For persistent or recurrent symptoms, repeat administration every 4–6 hours as needed during rituximab administration
  • **Meperidine** 12.5–25 mg; by intravenous injection every 10–20 minutes as needed for shaking chills (generally, cumulative doses >100 mg are not needed; use repeated doses with caution in persons with moderate or more severely impaired renal function)
 2. If rituximab administration was interrupted, resume infusion at a slower rate than the maximum rate previously attempted. Rate escalation may be reattempted at smaller incremental steps with close monitoring. Do not exceed the maximum recommended rate of 400 mg/h
 Dyspnea or wheezing without allergic findings (urticaria, or tongue or laryngeal edema)
 1. Interrupt rituximab administration immediately
 2. Give **hydrocortisone** 100 mg by intravenous injection (or an alternative steroid with equivalent glucocorticoid potency)
 3. Give a **histamine (H₂) receptor antagonist** (ranitidine 50 mg, cimetidine 300 mg, or famotidine 20 mg) intravenously over 15–30 minutes
 4. After symptoms resolve, resume rituximab administration at 25 mg/h with close monitoring. Do not increase the administration rate

Steroid-associated gastritis
Add a **proton pump inhibitor** during steroid use to prevent gastritis and duodenitis

Decreased bowel motility prophylaxis
Give **stool softeners** in a scheduled regimen, and **saline, osmotic, and lubricant laxatives**, as needed to prevent constipation for as long as vincristine use continues. If needed, circumspectly add **stimulant (irritant) laxatives** in the least amounts and for the briefest durations needed to produce defecation

Patient Population Studied

Prior Therapies and Responses to Prior Therapies in 29 Patients with Relapsed or Refractory Mantle Cell Lymphoma

Wang M et al. Cancer 2008;113:2734–2741

Prior Therapies

Therapy	Number of Patients
Median prior no. of regimens (range)	1 (1–5)
Doxorubicin-containing regimens	21
Fludarabine-containing regimens	5
Rituximab-containing regimens	18
Radiotherapy (excluding TBI)	9
Zevalin or Bexxar	2
Rituximab plus hyper-CVAD alternating with rituximab plus methotrexate-cytarabine	4
Autologous stem cell transplantation or TBI	5

Responses to Prior Therapies

	Number of Patients (%)
CR	10 (35)
PR	7 (24)
Less than PR	12 (41)

Bexxar, tositumomab and iodine (^{131}I) tositumomab; TBI indicates total body irradiation; Zevalin, ibritumomab tiuxetan

Patient Characteristics (N = 97)

Romaguera JE et al. J Clin Oncol 2005;23:7013–7023

Characteristic	Number of patients		
	All Ages	≤65 Years	>65 Years
Number of patients	97	65	32
Age, median (range)	61 years (41–80 years)		
Male-to-female ratio	3:1	3:1	3:1
Ann Arbor stage IV	99	98	100
Bone marrow involvement	91	89	94
GI involvement	88	85	94
Performance status, 0–1 (Zubrod)	98	98	97
Diffuse histologic pattern, n = 83*	89	88	88
Blastoid cytologic variant	14	14	16
Serum lactate dehydrogenase > normal	24	20	31
Serum/β_2-microglobulin ≥3 mg/L	55	46	72
Peripheral blood involvement	49	35	41
Large spleen	40	40	41
International Prognostic Index >2	57	34	91

*Fourteen patients had no lymph node to biopsy

Treatment Modifications

Adverse Event	Treatment Modifications
Platelet count 75,000–100,000/mm³, or an ANC 750–1000/mm³ on day 21 of a treatment cycle	Delay start of next cycle until platelets >100,000/mm³ and ANC >1000/mm³, reevaluating hematologic values every 3 days. Then resume therapy without a decrease in drug dosages
Platelet count was <75,000/mm³ or ANC was <750/mm³ on day 21 of a treatment cycle	Delay start of next cycle until platelet count >100,000/mm³ and ANC >1000/mm³ reevaluating hematologic values every 3 days. Then resume therapy with a decrease in the dose of cyclophosphamide and doxorubicin (cycles 1, 3, 5, ±7) or methotrexate and cytarabine (cycles 2, 4, 6, ± 8) by 25–50%
Patient age ≥60 years	Reduce cytarabine dosage to 1000 mg/m² per dose
Blood methotrexate concentration >20 µmol/L at the start of cytarabine treatment	Reduce cytarabine dosage to 2000 mg/m² per dose and reduce methotrexate dosage by 50% in subsequent cycles
Serum creatinine >2 mg/dL (>177 µmol/L)	
Serum creatinine >3 mg/dL (>265 µmol/L)	Reduce methotrexate dosage by 75%
Delayed methotrexate excretion or nephrotoxicity attributable to previous methotrexate treatment	Reduce methotrexate dosage by 50–75% (commensurate with the severity of nephrotoxicity)
Total bilirubin >2 g/dL (>34.2 µmol/L)	Reduce vincristine dose to 1 mg/dose
Total bilirubin 2–3 g/dL (34.2–51.3 µmol/L)	Reduce doxorubicin dosage by 25%
Total bilirubin 3–4 g/dL (51.3–68.4 µmol/L)	Reduce doxorubicin dosage by 50%

(continued)

Efficacy

Response Rates Among 29 Patients with Relapsed or Refractory Mantle Cell Lymphoma
Wang M et al. Cancer 2008;113:2734–2741

Response	Number (%)
Complete response/unconfirmed complete response	13 (45)
Partial response	14 (48)
Complete response/unconfirmed complete response + Partial response	27 (93)
No benefit	2 (7)

Failure-free and Overall Survival

Median failure-free survival (FFS)*	11 months
Median overall survival (OS)	19 months

*Note: No pretreatment variable (number of prior chemotherapy regimens, response to the previous regimen, pretreatment serum levels of β_2-microglobulin or LDH, and age) was associated with better FFS

Romaguera JE et al. J Clin Oncol 2005;23:7013–7023

CR/CRu Rates After 6 Courses

Variable	CR/CRu Response Rate (%) [95% CI (%)]			$X^2 P$
Overall	87 [79 to 93]			
High serum β_2M: No vs. Yes	98 [88 to 100]	vs.	79 [66 to 89]	0.01
High serum LDH: No vs. Yes	91 [81 to 96]	vs.	78 [56 to 93]	0.15
GI: Negative vs. Positive	91 [59 to 100]	vs.	89 [79 to 95]	0.16
IPI score: ≤2 vs. >2	93 [81 to 99]	vs.	84 [71 to 92]	0.10
BM involvement: No vs. Yes	78 [40 to 97]	vs.	89 [80 to 94]	0.31
Blastoid cytology: No vs. Yes	89 [80 to 95]	vs.	79 [49 to 95]	0.37
Age: ≤65 years vs. >65 years	89 [79 to 96]	vs.	84 [67 to 95]	0.52
Enlarged spleen: No vs. Yes	90 [75 to 95]	vs.	85 [69 to 94]	0.54
Age: <60 years vs. 61–65 years	90 [77 to 97]	vs.	88 [64 to 99]	—
Peripheral blood: No vs. Yes	89 [75 to 95]	vs.	86 [75 to 95]	0.76
IPI score: ≤1 vs. >1	89 [52 to 100]	vs.	88 [79 to 94]	0.99

3-Year FFS and OS Estimates

Overall	No Patients	% 3-Year FFS			P Value	% 3-Year OS			P Value
		65%				82%			
Serum β_2M ≥3 mg/L: No vs. Yes	44/53	79	vs.	51	.001	87	vs.	78	0.1
Serum LDH normal: No vs. Yes	74/23	74	vs.	39	.002	84	vs.	77	0.87
BM involvement: No vs. Yes	9/88	78	vs.	62	0.25	83	vs.	82	0.86
Blastoid cytology: No vs. Yes	83/14	66	vs.	50	0.33	86	vs.	61	0.06
Age: ≤65 years vs. >65 years	65/32	75	vs.	50	0.01	85	vs.	75	0.05
Enlarged spleen: No vs. Yes	58/39	68	vs.	66	0.36	81	vs.	83	0.52
Peripheral blood: No vs. Yes	61/36	69	vs.	58	0.22	86	vs.	76	0.51
IPI score: ≤2 vs. >2	42/55	78	vs.	54	0.03	87	vs.	78	0.41

β_2M, β_2-microglobulin; BM, bone marrow; CR, complete response; CRu, complete response unconfirmed; FFS, failure-free survival; LDH, lactate dehydrogenase; IPI, International Prognostic Index; OS, overall survival

Treatment Modifications
(continued)

Adverse Event	Treatment Modifications
Total bilirubin >4 g/dL (>68.4 µmol/L)	Reduce doxorubicin dosage by 75%
Disease involving the stomach or small bowel	Eliminate doxorubicin during the first hyper-CVAD cycle
If cytarabine is eliminated because of adverse effects	Omit the high-dose methotrexate + cytarabine regimen, replacing it with repeated cycles of hyper-CVAD
Peripheral neuropathy	Discontinue vincristine
Proximal myopathy	Discontinue dexamethasone
Cerebellar neurotoxicity	Reduce cytarabine dosage or omit cytarabine during subsequent treatments
G3 mucositis	Reduce methotrexate dosage

Cycles with Dose Reductions According to Age and Regimen
Romaguera JE et al. J Clin Oncol 2005;23:7013–7023

Age/Regimen	Number of Patients	Number of Cycles	Reduced Cycles Number	%	P Value
Patient age					
All ages	97	602	142	24	
≤65 years	65	410	70	17	.00001
>65 years	32	192	72	38	
Regimens					
R-hyper-CVAD		302	51	17	.0002
R-MC		300	91	30	

R-hyper-CVAD, rituximab with fractionated cyclophosphamide, vincristine, doxorubicin, and dexamethasone; R-MC, rituximab with methotrexate and cytarabine

Toxicity

Toxicity Rates in 104 Cycles of Rituximab Plus Hyper-CVAD Alternating with Rituximab Plus Methotrexate + Cytarabine Therapy

Wang M et al. Cancer 2008;113:2734–2741

Toxicity Grade	% G1	% G2	% G3	% G4
Fever and neutropenia	0	3	11	0
Fever without neutropenia	11	0	0	0
Neutropenia	6	6	14	60
Thrombocytopenia	21	15	9	54
Fatigue	36	6	0	0
Sensory loss	18	2	1	0
Nausea	17	21	0	0
Pruritus	15	3	2	0
Edema	13	18	0	0
Diarrhea	10	6	0	0
Muscle weakness	10	0	0	0
Stomatitis	5	6	0	0
Constipation	4	11	0	0
Vomiting	4	10	0	0

Hematologic Toxic Effects After 602 Courses

Romaguera JE et al. J Clin Oncol 2005; 23:7013–7023

Course Number	Neutropenia (%)		Thrombocytopenia (%)	
	G3	G4	G3	G4
1	10	51	12.5	2
2	7	64	9	28
3	7	28	23	14
4	5	64	9	42
5	7	31	17	12
6	3	68	5	46
7	14	37	15	17
8	4	55	7	50

Nonhematologic Toxic Effects After 602 Cycles

G3/4 Toxic Effect	Number of Events (%)
Neutropenic fever*	80 (13)
R-hyper-CVAD	20[†]
R-MC	60[†]
Infection*	35 (6)
Bacteremia	20 (3)
Pneumonia	6 (1)
Other	9 (1.5)
Fatigue	18 (3)
Stomatitis	6 (1)
Bleeding	3 (0.5)
Pancreatitis	1 (0.1)
Kidney failure	1 (0.1)
CNS	1 (0.1)

R-hyper-CVAD, rituximab plus fractionated cyclophosphamide, vincristine, doxorubicin, and dexamethasone; R-MC, rituximab plus methotrexate and cytarabine

*No difference for patients ≤65 years vs. patients >65 years

[†]$P = 0.00001$

Note: Lethal acute toxicity occurred in five patients: sepsis in 3 patients (*Staphylococcus aureus, Escherichia coli, Proteus mirabilis*); pulmonary hemorrhage in 1 patient; unknown cause in 1 patient

Therapy Monitoring

1. *Before each cycle:* PE, CBC with differential, LFTs, serum BUN, creatinine, and urinalysis
2. *Daily during treatment:* serum electrolytes, glucose, BUN, creatinine, total bilirubin, LFTs, LDH, uric acid, albumin, alkaline phosphatase, and CBC with differential
3. *Daily following high-dose systemic methotrexate administration:* methotrexate levels
4. *Response assessment every 2 cycles:* CT of the chest, abdomen, and pelvis; gallium scan or PET, and bilateral bone marrow biopsy with unilateral aspiration

   Note: To confirm CR, esophagogastroduodenoscopy and colonoscopy were performed, with biopsies performed randomly
5. *Response assessment upon completion of therapy:* CT of the chest, abdomen, and pelvis every 3 months during the first year, every 4 months during the second year, every 6 months during the third and fourth years, and yearly thereafter

REGIMEN

BORTEZOMIB

Fisher RI et al. J Clin Oncol 2006;24:4867–4874
Goy A et al. Ann Oncol 2009;20:520–525

Bortezomib 1.3 mg/m² per dose; administer by intravenous injection over 3–5 seconds for 4 doses on days 1, 4, 8, and 11, every 21 days for up to 17 cycles or four cycles beyond initial reporting of CR/CRu (total dosage/cycle = 5.2 mg/m²)

Supportive Care

Antiemetic prophylaxis
Emetogenic potential is **MINIMAL–LOW**
See Chapter 39 for antiemetic recommendations

Hematopoietic growth factor (CSF) prophylaxis
Primary prophylaxis is NOT indicated
See Chapter 43 for more information

Antimicrobial prophylaxis
Risk of fever and neutropenia is LOW
Antimicrobial primary prophylaxis to be considered:
- Antibacterial—not indicated
- Antifungal—not indicated
- Antiviral—not indicated, unless patient previously had an episode of HSV

See Chapter 47 for more information

Baseline Patient and Disease Characteristics

(N = 155, unless otherwise noted)

Characteristic	Patients Number (%)
Sex, Male	125 (81)
Race/ethnicity	
White	142 (92)
Black	6 (4)
Hispanic	4 (3)
Asian or Pacific Islander	3 (2)
Age, median (range)	65 years (42–89 y)
KPS, <90%	44/153 (29)
IPI, ≥3	65/147 (44)
LDH > ULN	54/149 (36)

(continued)

Dose Modifications

Bortezomib Dose Levels

Starting dose	1.3 mg/m² per dose on days 1, 4, 8, and 11
Level −1	1 mg/m² per dose on days 1, 4, 8, and 11
Level −2	0.7 mg/m² per dose on days 1, 4, 8, and 11
Level −3	1.3 mg/m² per dose on days 1 and 8

Adverse Event	Treatment Modifications
G3 thrombocytopenia (platelet count <50,000/mm³)	Reduce bortezomib dosage by 1 dose level
G ≥3 neutropenia with fever, or G4 neutropenia lasting longer than 7 days,	Hold treatment until toxicity resolves to G ≤1, then resume with bortezomib at 1 dose level lower
G3 nonhematologic toxicity or G4 hematologic toxicity	
Second occurrence of G3 nonhematologic toxicity or G4 hematologic toxicity	

Treatment Modification for Bortezomib-Induced Peripheral Neuropathy

Richardson PG et al. J Clin Oncol 2006;24:3113–3120

Severity of Peripheral Neuropathy	Modification of Dose and Schedule
G1 (paresthesias or loss of reflexes) without pain or loss of function	No action
G1 with pain or G2 (interferes with function but not with activities of daily living)	Reduce bortezomib dosage 1 dose level
G2 with pain or G3 (interferes with activities of daily living)	Withhold bortezomib treatment until toxicity resolves, then reinitiate reducing bortezomib dosage 1 dose level
G4 (permanent sensory loss that interferes with function)	Discontinue treatment

Efficacy

Median Efficacy Values in Months
(95% confidence interval)

	All Patients (N = 155)	CR/Cru + PR (N = 45)*	CR/Cru (N = 11)*	PR (N = 34)*	SD (N = 52)*	PD (N = 34)*
TTP	6.7 (4.0, 7.3)	12.4 (7.4, 16.3)	NE (14.6, NE)	9.1 (7.4, 12.5)	6.9 (4.2, 7.2)	1.2 (1.2, 1.3)
PFS	6.5 (4.0, 7.2)	12.4 (7.4, 17.3)	20.3 (14.6, NE)	9.7 (7.2, 15.2)	7.2 (6.4, 11.6)	1.2 (1.2, 1.3)
TTNT	7.4 (5.6, 9.3)	14.3 (11.1, 22.6)	23.9 (17.6, 33.9)	13.3 (9.0, 20.5)	7.0 (4.4, 8.7)	2.3 (1.9, 2.9)
OS	23.5 (20.3, 27.9)	35.4 (24.9, 37.5)	36.0 (NE, NE)	35.1 (23.4, 37.5)	27.8 (21.3, NE)	13.7 (6.7, 22.3)

CR, complete response; CRu, unconfirmed complete response; NE, not estimable; OS, overall survival; PD, progressive disease; PFS, progression-free survival; R, partial response; SD, stable disease; TTNT, time to next therapy; TTP, time to progression
*Of the 141 response-evaluable patients, 10 had no postbaseline assessment

(continued)

Baseline Patient and Disease Characteristics (continued)

Characteristic	Patients Number (%)
Stage IV MCL	119 (77)
Time from diagnosis, median (range)	2.3 years (0.2–11.2)
Diagnosed <3 years prior to first dose	103 (66)
Positive bone marrow evaluation	84/154 (55)
Number of prior lines of therapy for MCL 1/2/3*	84 (54)/65 (42)/6 (4)
Received prior regimen	
Anthracycline/mitoxantrone	152 (98)
Alkylating agents	150 (97)
Rituximab	149 (96)
At least 2 of 3 of the above	155 (100)
All 3 of the above	141 (91)
Prior high-intensity therapy[†]	58 (37)
Prior radioimmunotherapy	8 (5)
Prior radiation therapy (not including radioimmunotherapy)	29 (19)

IPI, International prognostic index; KPS, Karnofsky performance status; LDH, lactate dehydrogenase; MCL, mantle cell lymphoma; ULN, upper limit of normal
*Protocol deviation: eligibility violation exemption granted
[†]High-intensity regimens + (1) stem cell transplantation, (2) hyper-CVAD, (3) ICE, (4) ESHAP, or (5) DHAP, all with or without rituximab

Efficacy (continued)

Response Rate, DOR, TTP, PFS, TTNT, and OS in Patients with Refractory MCL and Patients with Prior High-intensity Therapy*

Parameter	Refractory MCL* (N = 58)	Prior High-Intensity Therapy* (N = 58)
Response rate (95% CI)	N = 51	N = 52
CR + PR	29% (17%, 44%)	25% (14%, 39%)
CR/CRu	6% (1%, 16%)	10% (3%, 21%)
Median DOR, months (95% CI)		
All responders	5.9 (4.7, NE)	Not reached (6.1, NE)
Patients achieving CR/CRu	Not reached (4.7, NE)	NE
Patients achieving PR	5.9 (4.9, 9.6)	NE
Median TTP, months (95% CI)	3.9 (1.7, 7.3)	4.2 (4.0, 7.4)
Median PFS, months (95% CI)	4.1 (1.7, 6.9)	4.5 (2.8, 7.4)
Median TTNT, months (95% CI)	4.6 (2.9, 8.0)	6.2 (3.4, 9.7)
Median OS, months (95% CI)	17.3 (7.7, 27.2)	20.3 (12.0, 28.8)

CI, confidence interval; CR, complete response; CRu, unconfirmed complete response; DOR, duration of response; MCL, mantle cell lymphoma; NE, not estimable; OS, overall survival; PFS, progression-free survival; PR, partial response; TTNT, time to next therapy; TTP, time to progression
*Note that patients with prior high-intensity therapy may also be included with patients refractory to their prior therapy

Baseline Characteristics of Patients Achieving CR/CRu to Bortezomib by Independent Radiology Review

Age*	Disease Duration[†]	Stage[‡]	IPI[§]	Prior Therapies	RD[ϵ]	Largest Mass**
52	4.6	III	1	CHOP Rituximab	Yes	11.0 × 7.7
73	2.3	IV	2	R-EPOCH	No	7.3 × 6.7
68	4.1	IV	2	R-CHOP Hyper-CVAD + ASCT	No	6.8 × 1.9
63	5.1	IV	2	Hyper-CVAD + ASCT R-CVP	Yes	5.9 × 4.4
72	2.7	IV	3	R-CHOP ^{90}Y-ibritumomab tiuxetan	Yes	5.5 × 3.0
58	5.2	IV	3	R-hyper-CVAD + ASCT ^{90}Y-ibritumomab tiuxetan	No	4.7 × 2.6
58	1.0	III	1	R-hyper-CVAD	No	3.9 × 2.8
78	2.0	IV	3	R-EPOCH CNOP	No	3.0 × 2.3
79	3.0	IV	3	CVP Rituximab R-pentostatin + mitoxantrone	No	3.0 × 2.7
74	0.9	III	2	R-CHOP + oblimersen	No	2.8 × 2.5
62	4.3	IV	2	R-CHOP Hyper-CVAD + ASCT	No	1.5 × 1.1

*Age in years
[†]Time since diagnosis in years
[‡]Disease stage
[§]IPI, International Prognostic Index
[ϵ]Refractory disease
**Largest tumor mass in centimeters

Toxicity

Adverse Events Reported in ≥20% Total Patients (N = 155)
Plus Incidences of Grade ≥3 and Drug-related Adverse Events

	Any Grade Number (%)	Grade ≥3 Number (%)	Drug Related Number (%)
Fatigue	95 (61)	19 (12)	81 (52)
Peripheral neuropathy	85 (55)	20 (13)	84 (54)
Constipation	77 (50)	4 (3)	52 (34)
Diarrhea	73 (47)	11 (7)	60 (39)
Nausea	68 (44)	4 (3)	56 (36)
Rash	43 (28)	4 (3)	36 (23)
Vomiting	42 (27)	4 (3)	35 (23)
Anorexia	36 (23)	5 (3)	22 (14)
Dizziness (excluding vertigo)	36 (23)	5 (3)	28 (18)
Dyspnea	35 (23)	7 (5)	10 (6)
Insomnia	33 (21)	1 (<1)	15 (10)
Thrombocytopenia	33 (21)	17 (11)	25 (16)
Musculoskeletal pain	31 (20)	3 (2)	15 (10)
Edema lower limb	31 (20)	1 (<1)	13 (8)

REGIMEN

LENALIDOMIDE

Goy A et al. J Clin Oncol 2013;31:3688–3695

Lenalidomide; administer orally for 21 consecutive days on days 1–21, every 28 days

Note: The investigators based lenalidomide dose on a patient's renal function, thus:

Creatinine Clearance	Lenalidomide Doses	
	Daily Dose	Total Weekly Dose
≥60 mL/min (≥1 mL/s)	25 mg/day	175 mg
≥30 to <60 mL/min (≥0.5 to <1 mL/s)	10 mg/day	70 mg

Supportive Care

Antiemetic prophylaxis
Emetogenic potential is **MINIMAL–LOW**
See Chapter 39 for antiemetic recommendations

Hematopoietic growth factor (CSF) prophylaxis
Primary prophylaxis may be indicated
See Chapter 43 for more information

Antimicrobial prophylaxis
Risk of fever and neutropenia is LOW
  Antimicrobial primary prophylaxis to be considered:
  • Antibacterial—not indicated
  • Antifungal—not indicated
  • Antiviral—not indicated unless patient previously had an episode of HSV
See Chapter 47 for more information

Thromboprophylaxis

Risk assessment and recommendations for VTE prophylaxis in patients with risk factors related to treatment

Geerts WH et al. Chest 2008;133(6 Suppl):381S–453S
Venous Thromboembolic Disease, V.2.2013. National Comprehensive Cancer Network, Inc., 2013 (Accessed October 8, 2013, at www.nccn.org)

Individual Risk Factors

• Obesity (BMI ≥30 kg/m²)
• H/O VTE
• CVAD or pacemaker
• Comorbid pathologies
  Cardiac disease
  Chronic renal disease
  Diabetes
  Acute infection
  Immobilization
• Surgery
  General surgery
  Any anesthesia
  Trauma
• Medications
  Erythropoietin (epoetin alfa, darbepoetin)
  Estrogenic compounds
  Bevacizumab
• Clotting disorders
  Thrombophilia
	For patients at low thromboembolic risk with ≤1 Individual risk factor present:
	• **Aspirin** 81–325 mg daily
	
	≥2 Individual risk factors present:
	• **LMWH,*** equivalent to enoxaparin sodium 40 mg/day *or* **dalteparin sodium** 5000 IU/day, subcutaneously, *or*
	• **Warfarin**, targeting an INR = 2–3

CVAD, central vascular access device; INR, international normalized ratio; LMWH, low-molecular-weight heparin; VTE, venous thromboembolic disease
*LMWHs should be used with caution in individuals with impaired renal function (creatinine clearance <30 mL/min). Refer to product labeling for information about doses and administration schedules in renally impaired patients, and guidance for monitoring anti-factor Xa concentrations

Lenalidomide Dose Levels

Starting dose	25 mg/day
Level −1	20 mg/day
Level −2	15 mg/day
Level −3	10 mg/day
Level −4	5 mg/day
Level −5	Discontinue

Adverse Event (AE)	Treatment Modifications
G ≥2 allergic reaction or hypersensitivity	Hold lenalidomide dosing for up to 21 days to allow toxicity to resolve, then restart at the same dose or reduce the lenalidomide dosage by 1 dose level
>3× upper limit of normal AST, ALT, or bilirubin	
G ≥1 tumor lysis syndrome	
G ≥3 neutropenia for ≥7 days or associated with fever (≥38.5°C [≥101.3°F])	
Platelets <50,000/mm³	
Constipation	
Venous thrombosis/embolism	
New peripheral neuropathy	
Lenalidomide-related nonhematologic AE	
Tumor flare reaction	
G3/4 neutropenia	Hold lenalidomide dosing for up to 21 days to allow toxicity to resolve to G ≤2, then restart at the same dose or reduce the lenalidomide daily dose by 1 dose level
Febrile neutropenia (ANC <1000/mm³ with fever ≥38°C [≥101.3°F])	
Desquamating (blistering) rash (or G4 non-desquamating rash)	
Any AE G ≥3 excluding nausea, vomiting, diarrhea, or lenalidomide-induced maculopapular rash	
G ≥3 nausea, vomiting, or diarrhea despite maximal therapy	
G4 fatigue lasting >7 days	

Patient Population Studied

Characteristic	Number of Patients	Percent
Age—median (range)	67 years (43–83 years)	
≥65 years	85	63
Male	108	81
Stage III to IV	124	93
ECOG PS		
0–1	116	87
2	18	13
Moderate-severe renal insufficiency*	29	22
Time from original MCL diagnosis to enrollment, years		
<3 years/≥3 years	52/82	39/61
MIPI score group at enrollment		
Intermediate/High	51/39	38/29
Positive bone marrow involvement†	55	41
High tumor burden‡	77	57
Bulky disease§	44	33
Number of prior treatment regimens—median (range)	4 (2–10)	
Number of prior systemic therapies: 2/3/≥4	29/34/71	22/25/53
Prior bortezomib: Received/Refractory	134/81	100/60
Refractory to last therapy	74	55
Prior high-dose or dose-intensive therapy‖	44	33
Prior ABMT or ASCT	39	29
Time from prior systemic therapy—median (range)	3.1 months (0.3–37.7 months)	
<6 months/≥6 months	96/38	72/28

ABMT, autologous bone marrow transplantation; ASCT, autologous stem cell transplantation; ECOG PS, Eastern Cooperative Oncology Group performance status; MCL, mantle cell lymphoma; MIPI, MCL International Prognostic Index

*Moderate renal insufficiency was defined as creatinine clearance (CrCl) ≥30 to <60 mL/min; severe renal insufficiency defined as CrCl <30 mL/min

†Bone marrow involvement was not required per protocol; prior data for bone marrow biopsy and aspirate were collected in 115 evaluable patients

‡Defined as at least 1 lesion ≥5 cm in diameter, or ≥3 lesions that were ≥3 cm in diameter by central radiology review

§Defined as at least 1 lesion ≥7 cm in diameter by central radiology review

‖Includes stem cell transplantation, hyper-CVAD (hyperfractionated cyclophosphamide, vincristine, doxorubicin, dexamethasone), or R-hyper-CVAD (rituximab plus hyper-CVAD)

Efficacy

(N = 134)

Efficacy Parameter	Central Review		Investigator Review	
	Number	Percent	Number	Percent
ORR	37	28	43	32
CR/CRu	10	7.5	22	16
PR	27	20	21	16
SD	39	29	36	27
PD	35	26	43	32
Missing response assessment*	23	17	12	9

Efficacy Parameter	Median	Range	Median	Range
TTR, months	2.2	1.7–13.1	2.0	1.7–15.9
TTCR/CRu, months	3.7	1.9–29.5	5.6	1.8–24.2
	Median	95% CI	Median	95% CI
DOR, months	16.6	7.7−26.7	18.5	12.8−26.7
Duration of CR/CRu, months	16.6	16.6−N/R	26.7	26.7−N/R
Duration of PR, months	9.2	5.7−20.5	7.7	3.7−21.4
PFS, months	4.0	3.6−5.6	3.8	3.5−6.8
TTP, months	5.4	3.7−7.5	4.0	3.6−7.5
TTF months	3.8	2.3−4.5	3.8	2.3−4.5
OS, months	19.0	12.5−23.9	19.0	12.5−23.9

CR, complete response; CRu, unconfirmed complete response; DOR, duration of response; MCL, mantle cell lymphoma; N/R, not reached; ORR, overall response rate; OS, overall survival; PD, progressive disease; PFS, progression-free survival; PR, partial response; SD, stable disease; TTCR/Cru, time to CR/Cru; TTF, time to treatment failure; TTP, time to progression; TTR, time to response

*Includes patients without or with incomplete postbaseline response assessment. For these 23 patients, the investigator's assessment for best ORR included 12 with progressive disease, 10 not assessable, and 1 CR (no identifiable target lesions by the central radiology reviewer who reported this patient as not evaluable, although a single GI [colon] lesion was reported by investigator readings). All 23 patients were included in the centrally reviewed response assessments as nonresponders

Summary of Subgroup Analyses of ORR and DOR by Baseline Demographics and Patient Characteristics with Lenalidomide in Evaluable Patients with Relapsed/Refractory MCL (Central Review)

Characteristic	Total Patients	ORR			DOR		
		No.	%	95% CI	No.	Median	95% CI
Median age							
<65 years	49	15	31	18−45	15	20.5	5.6−N/A
≥65 years	85	22	26	17−37	22	9.2	5.8−16.7
Sex							
Male	108	28	26	18−35	28	16.7	9.2−N/A
Female	26	9	35	17−56	9	7.7	2.1−20.5
ECOG PS							
0–1	116	31	27	19−36	31	16.7	14.8−N/A
2–4	18	6	33	13−59	6	7.7	1.7−9.2
Renal function							
Normal	99	28	28	20−38	28	20.5	5.7−N/A
Moderate insufficiency	28	7	25	11−45	7	9.2	7.7−16.6
Time from MCL diagnosis to first dose							
<3 years	52	12	23	13−37	12	16.6	5.1−N/A
≥3 years	82	25	31	21−42	25	14.8	5.8−20.5
MCL (Ann Arbor) stage							
I or II	10	1	10	0.3−45	1	7.7	N/A
III or IV	124	36	29	21−38	36	16.6	9.2−26.7

(*continued*)

Efficacy (*continued*)

Characteristic	Total Patients	ORR			DOR		
		No.	%	95% CI	No.	Median	95% CI
MIPI score at enrollment							
Low	39	14	36	21−53	14	20.5	5.6−N/A
Intermediate	51	12	23	13−38	12	16.7	5.7−26.7
High	39	10	26	13−42	10	7.7	3.6−N/A
LDH*							
Normal	84	32	38	28−49	32	16.7	14.8−N/A
High	47	5	11	4−23	5	5.8	1.7−7.7
WBC count							
$<6.7 \times 10^9$/L	67	22	33	22−45	22	14.8	5.6−20.5
6.7 to $<10 \times 10^9$/L	41	7	17	7−32	7	26.7	7.7−N/A
10 to $<15 \times 10^9$/L	9	6	67	30−93	6	N/A	3.6−N/A
$\geq15 \times 10^9$/L	12	1	8	0.2−39	1	N/A	N/A−N/A
Tumor burden							
High[†]	77	22	29	19−40	22	14.8	5.8−26.7
Low	54	15	28	17−42	15	16.6	5.6−16.6
Bulky disease							
Yes[‡]	44	13	30	17−45	13	14.8	5.7−N/A
No	87	24	28	19−38	24	16.6	5.8−N/A
Prior bone marrow involvement[§]							
Positive	55	13	24	13−37	13	9.2	3.6−N/A
Negative	52	13	25	14−39	13	16.7	5.1−N/A
Indeterminate	8	4	50	16−84	4	14.8	N/A−N/A
Number of prior systemic antilymphoma therapies							
<3	29	9	31	15−51	9	16.6	7.7−N/A
≥3	105	28	27	19−36	28	16.7	5.7−26.7
Received prior stem cell transplantation							
Yes	39	12	31	17−48	12	16.7	3.6−16.7
No	95	25	26	18−36	25	14.8	5.8−26.7
Received prior high-intensity therapy							
Yes	44	12	27	15−43	12	16.7	3.6−16.7
No	90	25	28	19−38	25	14.8	5.8−26.7
Time from last prior systemic anti-lymphoma therapy							
<6 months	96	23	24	16−34	23	7.7	3.6−26.7
≥6 months	38	14	37	22−54	14	16.7	14.8−N/A
Relapsed/refractory to prior bortezomib							
Refractory	81	22	27	18−38	22	20.5	7.7−N/A
Relapsed/progressed	51	15	29	18−44	15	16.6	5.0−16.7
Relapsed/refractory to last prior therapy							
Refractory	74	20	27	17−39	20	26.7	5.6−N/A
Relapsed/progressed	53	16	30	18−44	16	14.8	5.7−20.5
Starting dose of lenalidomide							
10 mg	29	6	21	8−40	6	9.2	7.7−14.8
25 mg	104	31	30	21−40	31	16.7	5.7−N/A

DOR, duration of response; ECOG PS, Eastern Cooperative Oncology Group performance status; LDH, lactate dehydrogenase; MCL, mantle-cell lymphoma; MIPI, MCL International Prognostic Index; N/A, not applicable; ORR, overall response rate

*The only factor that was significant in both the univariate and multivariate models was high lactate dehydrogenase at baseline

[†]Defined as at least 1 lesion ≥5 cm in diameter or ≥3 lesions that were ≥3 cm in diameter by central radiology review

[‡]Defined as at least 1 lesion ≥7 cm in diameter by central radiology review

[§]Bone marrow involvement was assessable in 115 evaluable patients

(*continued*)

Efficacy (*continued*)

All Treatment-Emergent Adverse Events After Lenalidomide (Regardless of Attribution) in ≥10% of Patients with Relapsed/Refractory MCL (N = 134)

Adverse Event (AE)	Any Grade Number (%)	G3 Number (%)	G4 Number (%)
Patients with ≥1 AEs	132 (99)	47 (35)	41 (31)
Hematologic			
Neutropenia	65 (49)	26 (19)	32 (24)
Thrombocytopenia	48 (36)	23 (17)	14 (10)
Anemia	41 (31)	11 (8)	4 (3)
Leukopenia	20 (15)	7 (5)	2 (1)
Nonhematologic			
Fatigue	45 (34)	9 (7)	0
Diarrhea	42 (31)	8 (6)	0
Nausea	40 (30)	0	1 (<1)
Cough	38 (28)	1 (<1)	0
Pyrexia*	31 (23)	1 (<1)	1 (<1)
Rash	30 (22)	2 (1)	0
Dyspnea*	24 (18)	6 (5)	1 (<1)
Pruritus	23 (17)	1 (<1)	0
Constipation	21 (16)	1 (<1)	0
Peripheral edema	21 (16)	0	0
Pneumonia†	19 (14)	10 ()	0
Asthenia*	19 (14)	2 (1)	1 (<1)
Decreased appetite	19 (14)	1 (<1)	0
Back pain	18 (13)	2 (1)	0
Hypokalemia	17 (13)	2 (1)	1 (<1)
Muscle spasms	17 (13)	1 (<1)	0
Upper respiratory tract infection	17 (13)	0	0
Decreased weight	17 (13)	0	0
Vomiting	16 (12)	0	1 (<1)

*One G5 event per AE
†Two G5 events

Treatment Monitoring

1. CBC with differential day 1
2. CT scans every 2 cycles
3. Confirmatory bone marrow aspirate and unilateral biopsy for patients achieving CR (by CT)

REGIMEN

(Older Patients)

RITUXIMAB + FLUDARABINE + CYCLOPHOSPHAMIDE (R-FC) *OR* RITUXIMAB + CYCLOPHOSPHAMIDE + DOXORUBICIN + VINCRISTINE + PREDNISONE (R-CHOP)

Kluin-Nelemans HC et al. N Engl J Med 2012;367:520–531

Notes:
- Induction therapy consisted of either R-FC or R-CHOP open-label chemoimmunotherapy
- Rituximab was added to the chemotherapy when the count of circulating lymphoma cells was $<10 \times 10^9$/L ($<$10,000/mm^3)

R-FC Regimen:
Premedication for rituximab:
Acetaminophen 650–1000 mg; administer orally *plus* **diphenhydramine** 25–50 mg; administer orally or intravenously 30–60 minutes before each dose of rituximab

Rituximab 375 mg/m^2 (maximum single dose, 750 mg); administer intravenously in 0.9% sodium chloride injection (0.9% NS) or 5% dextrose injection (D5W) diluted to a concentration of 1–4 mg/mL on day 1, every 28 days for 6 cycles (total dosage/cycle = 375 mg/m^2; maximum dose/cycle = 750 mg)

Notes on rituximab administration:
- Infuse initially at 50 mg/h. If hypersensitivity or infusion reactions do not occur during the first 30 minutes, increase the rate by 50 mg/h every 30 minutes as tolerated to a maximum rate of 400 mg/h. Subsequently, if previous administration was well tolerated, start at 100 mg/h and increase by 100 mg/h every 30 minutes as tolerated to a maximum rate of 400 mg/h
- Interrupt rituximab administration for fever chills, edema, congestion of the head and neck mucosa, hypertension, and other serious adverse events. Resume rituximab administration after adverse events abate

Fludarabine 30 mg/m^2; administer intravenously in 100–125 mL 0.9% NS or D5W over 30 minutes for 3 consecutive days, days 1–3, every 28 days for 6 cycles (total dosage/cycle = 90 mg/m^2)
Cyclophosphamide 250 mg/m^2; administer intravenously in 25–250 mL 0.9% NS or D5W over 30 minutes for 3 consecutive days, days 1–3, every 28 days for 6 cycles (total dosage/cycle = 750 mg/m^2)

R-CHOP Regimen:
Premedication for rituximab:
Acetaminophen 650–1000 mg; administer orally *plus* **diphenhydramine** 25–50 mg; administer orally or intravenously 30–60 minutes before each dose of rituximab
Rituximab 375 mg/m^2 (maximum single dose, 750 mg); administer intravenously on day 1, every 21 days for 8 cycles (total dosage/cycle = 375 mg/m^2; maximum dose/cycle = 750 mg)

Notes on rituximab administration:
- Infuse initially at 50 mg/h. If hypersensitivity or infusion reactions do not occur during the first 30 minutes, increase the rate by 50 mg/h every 30 minutes as tolerated to a maximum rate of 400 mg/h. Subsequently, if previous administration was well tolerated, start at 100 mg/h and increase by 100 mg/h every 30 minutes as tolerated to a maximum rate of 400 mg/h
- Interrupt rituximab administration for fever chills, edema, congestion of the head and neck mucosa, hypertension, and other serious adverse events. Resume rituximab administration after adverse events abate

Cyclophosphamide 750 mg/m^2; administer intravenously in 25–250 mL 0.9% NS or D5W over 30 minutes on day 1, every 21 days for 8 cycles (total dosage/cycle = 750 mg/m^2)
Doxorubicin 50 mg/m^2; administer by intravenous injection over 3–5 minutes on day 1, every 21 days for 8 cycles (total dosage/cycle = 50 mg/m^2)
Vincristine 1.4 mg/m^2 (maximum single dose, 2 mg); administer by intravenous injection over 1–2 minutes on day 1, every 21 days, for 8 cycles (total dosage/cycle = 1.4 mg/m^2; maximum dose/cycle = 2 mg)
Prednisone 100 mg; administer orally for 5 consecutive days, on days 1–5, every 21 days, for 8 cycles (total dose/cycle = 500 mg)

Supportive Care
Antiemetic prophylaxis: R-FC regimen
Emetogenic potential is **MODERATE** *on days 1–3*
Antiemetic prophylaxis: R-CHOP regimen
Emetogenic potential is **HIGH***. Potential for delayed emetic symptoms*
See Chapter 39 for antiemetic recommendations

Hematopoietic growth factor (CSF) prophylaxis
Primary prophylaxis is indicated with 1 of the following:
    Filgrastim (G-CSF) 5 mcg/kg per day; administer by subcutaneous injection, *or*
    Pegfilgrastim (pegylated filgrastim) 6 mg/0.6 mL; administer by subcutaneous injection for 1 dose
- Begin use from 24–72 hours after myelosuppressive chemotherapy is completed
- Continue daily filgrastim use until ANC $\geq$10,000/mm^3 on 2 measurements separated temporally by $\geq$12 hours

(continued)

(continued)

- Discontinue daily filgrastim use at least 24 hours before administering myelosuppressive treatment. Do not administer pegfilgrastim within 14 days before administering myelosuppressive treatment

See Chapter 43 for more information

Antimicrobial prophylaxis
Risk of fever and neutropenia is INTERMEDIATE
Antimicrobial primary prophylaxis to be considered:
- Antibacterial—consider a fluoroquinolone or no prophylaxis; *Pneumocystis jirovecii* prophylaxis is recommended (eg, cotrimoxazole)
- Antifungal—recommended; consider use during periods of neutropenia
- Antiviral—antiherpes antivirals (eg, acyclovir, famciclovir, valacyclovir)

See Chapter 47 for more information

Infusion reactions associated with rituximab
Fevers, chills, and rigors
1. Interrupt rituximab administration for severe symptoms, and give:
   - **Acetaminophen** 650 mg orally for fever. For persistent or recurrent symptoms, repeat administration every 4–6 hours as needed during rituximab administration
   - **Diphenhydramine** 25–50 mg orally or by intravenous injection for pruritus, hypotension, or angioedema. For persistent or recurrent symptoms, repeat administration every 4–6 hours as needed during rituximab administration
   - **Meperidine** 12.5–25 mg by intravenous injection every 10–20 minutes as needed for shaking chills (generally, cumulative doses >100 mg are not needed; use repeated doses with caution in persons with moderate or more severely impaired renal function)
2. If rituximab administration was interrupted, resume infusion at a slower rate than the maximum rate previously attempted. Rate escalation may be reattempted at smaller incremental steps with close monitoring. Do not exceed the maximum recommended rate of 400 mg/h

Dyspnea or wheezing without allergic findings (urticaria, or tongue or laryngeal edema)
1. Interrupt rituximab administration immediately
2. Give **hydrocortisone** 100 mg by intravenous injection (or an alternative steroid with equivalent glucocorticoid potency)
3. Give a **histamine (H₂) receptor antagonist** (ranitidine 50 mg, cimetidine 300 mg, or famotidine 20 mg) intravenously over 15–30 minutes
4. After symptoms resolve, resume rituximab administration at 25 mg/h with close monitoring. Do not increase the administration rate

Steroid-associated gastritis
Add a **proton pump inhibitor** during prednisone use to prevent gastritis and duodenitis

Decreased bowel motility prophylaxis
Give **stool softeners** in a scheduled regimen, and **saline, osmotic, and lubricant laxatives**, as needed to prevent constipation for as long as vincristine use continues. If needed, circumspectly add **stimulant (irritant) laxatives** in the least amounts and for the briefest durations needed to produce defecation

Treatment Modification

Adverse Event	Treatment Modifications
G2 neuropathy	Reduce the dose of vincristine by 25%
G3 neuropathy	Reduce the dose of vincristine by 50%
G4 neuropathy	Discontinue vincristine
WBC <4000/mm³ or platelet count <100,000/mm³ on day 1 of a cycle	Delay start of next cycle by 1 week. Then, if WBC >4000/mm³ and platelet count >100,000/mm³, resume therapy
Persistent cytopenias with WBC 2000–3000/mm³ and platelet count >100,000/mm³ after a 1-week treatment delay	Start the next cycle but reduce fludarabine, cyclophosphamide, and doxorubicin dosages by 75%
Persistent cytopenias WBC 1000–2000/mm³ and platelet count 50,000–100,000/mm³ after a 1-week treatment delay	Resume next cycle but reduce the doses of fludarabine, cyclophosphamide, and doxorubicin dosages by 50%
Persistent cytopenias with WBC <1000/mm³ and platelet count <50,000/mm³ after a 1-week treatment delay	Discontinue therapy
WBC nadir <1000/mm³ and/or platelet nadir <50,000/mm³	Decrease fludarabine, cyclophosphamide, and/or doxorubicin dosages by 25%

Baseline Characteristics

Characteristic	Total (N = 485)	R-FC (N = 246)	R-CHOP (N = 239)
Age—median (range)	70 years (60–87 years)	70 years (60–83 years)	70 years (61–87 years)
Male sex—no. (%)	340 (70)	178 (72)	162 (68)
Ann Arbor stage—no. (%)			
II	30 (6)	18 (7)	12 (5)
III	55 (11)	30 (12)	25 (10)
IV	400 (82)	198 (80)	202 (85)
Systemic symptom— no. (%)*	182 (38)	93 (38)	89 (37)
ECOG performance status of 2—no. (%)†	39 (8)	21 (9)	18 (8)
Bone-marrow involvement— no. (%)	364 (75)	182 (74)	182 (76)
LDH elevation—no. (%)	206 (42)	104 (42)	102 (43)
Median ratio of LDH activity to ULN	0.94	0.93	0.95
Median leukocyte count— $\times 10^{-9}$/L	7.8	7.7	7.9
MIPI‡			
Median score	6.20	6.20	6.18
Low risk—no. (%)	42 (9)	24 (10)	18 (8)
Intermediate risk— no. (%)	201 (41)	98 (40)	103 (43)
High risk—no. (%)	242 (50)	124 (50)	118 (49)

LDH denotes lactate dehydrogenase; R-CHOP rituximab, cyclophosphamide, doxorubicin, vincristine, and prednisone; R-FC rituximab, fludarabine, and cyclophosphamide; ULN upper limit of the normal range
*Systemic symptoms were defined as B symptoms in the Ann Arbor classification
†Scores on the Eastern Cooperative Oncology Group (ECOG) performance status range from 0 to 5, with 0 indicating asymptomatic, 1 symptomatic but ambulatory, and 2 symptomatic and in bed less than half the day; 5 indicates death
‡The Mantle-Cell Lymphoma International Prognostic Index (MIPI) score is calculated from the individual patient characteristics of age, ECOG performance status, LDH, and leukocyte count, and its range depends on the range of these characteristics. Scores range from 0 to 11, with higher scores indicating higher-risk disease. The index classifies patients as having low-, intermediate-, or high-risk disease

Toxicity*

Event	R-FC (N = 268)	R-CHOP (N = 249)
Anemia		
G1/2	59	68
G3/4	20	12†
Leukocytopenia		
G1/2	18	29
G3/4	73	59‡
Lymphocytopenia		
G1/2	9	19
G3/4	78	69‡
Neutropenia		
G1/2	18	20
G3/4	69	60
Thrombocytopenia		
G1/2	39	33
G3/4	41	18§
Elevated bilirubin		
G1/2	15	8
G3/4	1	1†
Nausea		
G1/2	36	26
G3/4	2	1†
Constipation		
G1/2	15	28
G3/4	2	3‡
Neuropathy		
G1/2	7	36
G3/4	1	4§

(continued)

Efficacy

	R-FC (N = 246)	R-CHOP (N = 239)	P Value
CR >induction therapy	98/246 (40%)	81/239 (34%)	0.10
ORR	192/246 (78%)	206/239 (86%)	0.06
CR + uCR	53%	49%	—
PD	14%	5%	—
TTF >37 months median follow-up	26 months	28 months	—
Duration of remission	37 months	36 months	—
Overall survival at 4 years	47%	62%	0.005 (HR for death, 1.50; 95% CI, 1.13–1.99)

	R-FC (N = 280)	R-CHOP (N = 280)
Deaths (N = 199)	115 (41.1%)[*,†]	84 (30%)[*,†]
Death from progression of lymphoma	64 (22.9%)	47 (16.8%)
Death from infection	19 (6.8%)	12 (4.3%)
Death from a secondary cancer	9 (3.2%)	3 (1%)
Death while in remission	29 (10.3%)	11 (3.9%)

CR, complete response; ORR, overall response rate; PD, progressive disease; R-CHOP rituximab, cyclophosphamide, doxorubicin, vincristine, and prednisone; R-FC rituximab, fludarabine, and cyclophosphamide; TTF, time to treatment failure; uCR, unconfirmed CR

*The remaining causes of death in the R-FC and R-CHOP groups, respectively, were related to cardiac causes (4 and 9 patients), pulmonary causes (3 and 2), central nervous system bleeding or ischemia (2 and 1), leukoencephalopathy (1 and 1), and unknown causes (13 and 9)

†Owing to the observed difference in overall survival, the independent data and safety monitoring committee recommended closing the R-FC group

Toxicity* (continued)

Fatigue		
G1/2	50	52
G3/4	4	6
Infection		
G1/2	18	31
G3/4	17	14[‡]
Myalgia or arthralgia		
G1/2	9	12
G3/4	0	3[†]
Febrile neutropenia[€]	11	17

*Adverse events were graded according to the National Cancer Institute (USA) Common Toxicity Criteria, version 2.0. At: http://ctep.cancer.gov/protocolDevelopment/electronic_applications/ctc.htm (accessed December 7, 2013). The maximal grade is the highest grade of adverse event that a patient had during the treatment period; patients were included only in the percentage for the highest grade of event they had. The following events were associated with no significant difference between the 2 induction regimens or between the 2 maintenance regimens and were grades 3 or 4 in none to 8% of patients: elevated creatinine, elevated aminotransferases, vomiting, diarrhea, mucositis, decreased cardiac function, decreased pulmonary function, depression, allergy, weight loss, and bleeding

†P <0.05 for adverse events of maximal grade 0 versus G1/2 versus G3/4 for R-FC versus R-CHOP

‡P <0.01 for adverse events of maximal grade 0 versus G1/2 versus G3/4 for R-FC versus R-CHOP

§P <0.001 for adverse events of maximal grade 0 versus G1/2 versus G3/4 for R-FC versus R-CHOP

€This adverse event was graded only within the G3 and G4 categories

Treatment Monitoring

1. *Before treatment:* physical examination; CBC with differential; assessment of serum chemistries; CT scan of the chest, abdomen, and pelvis; and bone marrow aspiration and biopsy as indicated. If clinically relevant, endoscopy of the gastrointestinal tract is done

2. *Weekly:* CBC with differential and platelet count once weekly

3. *Assessment of efficacy:* CT scan or sonographic examination at 2- or 3-cycle intervals after and at the end of treatment in MCL

REGIMEN

CYCLOPHOSPHAMIDE + DOXORUBICIN + VINCRISTINE + ETOPOSIDE + PREDNISOLONE (CHOEP)

Pfreundschuh M et al. Ann Oncol 2008;19:545–552
Schmitz et al. Blood 2010;116:3418–3425

Hydration with 500–1000 mL 0.9% sodium chloride injection (0.9% NS); administer intravenously before starting cyclophosphamide administration and 500–1000 mL 0.9% NS after completing cyclophosphamide

Cyclophosphamide 750 mg/m²; administer intravenously in 25–250 mL 0.9% NS or 5% dextrose injection (D5W) over 30 minutes on day 1, every 21 days (total dosage/cycle = 750 mg/m²)

Doxorubicin 50 mg/m²; administer by intravenous injection over 3–5 minutes on day 1, every 21 days (total dosage/cycle = 50 mg/m²)

Vincristine 2 mg; administer by intravenous injection over 1–2 minutes on day 1, every 21 days (total dose/cycle = 2 mg)

Etoposide 100 mg/m² per day; administer intravenously in a volume of 0.9% NS or D5W sufficient to produce a concentration within the range 0.2–0.4 mg/mL over 60 minutes for 3 consecutive days, on days 1–3, every 21 days (total dosage/cycle = 300 mg/m²)

Prednisolone *or* **prednisone** 100 mg/day; administer orally for 5 consecutive days, on days 1–5, every 21 days (total dose/cycle = 500 mg)

Notes:

- Prednisolone and prednisone may be used interchangeably at the same dose and administration schedule
- In the study reported by Pfreundschuh et al., patients were to receive radiotherapy (36 Gy) to sites of primary bulky and extranodal disease, and 85% of patients received radiotherapy according to protocol

Supportive Care

Antiemetic prophylaxis

Emetogenic potential on day 1 is **HIGH**. *Potential for delayed symptoms*
Emetogenic potential on days 2 and 3 is **LOW**
See Chapter 39 for antiemetic recommendations

Hematopoietic growth factor (CSF) prophylaxis

Primary prophylaxis may be indicated
See Chapter 43 for more information

Antimicrobial prophylaxis

Risk of fever and neutropenia is LOW

Antimicrobial primary prophylaxis to be considered:

- Antibacterial—*Pneumocystis jirovecii* prophylaxis is recommended (eg, cotrimoxazole)
- Antifungal—not indicated
- Antiviral—not indicated, unless patient previously had an episode of HSV

See Chapter 47 for more information

Steroid-associated gastritis

Add a **proton pump inhibitor** during steroid use to prevent gastritis and duodenitis

Patient Population Studied

A total of 343 patients with mature nodal or extranodal T-cell or NK-cell lymphoma who were enrolled on several protocols of the German High-Grade Non-Hodgkin Lymphoma Study Group between October 1993 and May 2007. Of 343 patients, 320 could be assigned to 1 of the following subtypes:

Anaplastic large cell lymphoma kinase-positive, ALK-positive (ALCL, ALK-positive)	78 (24.4%)
Anaplastic large cell lymphoma kinase-positive, ALK-negative (ALCL, ALK-negative)	113 (35.3%)
Peripheral T-cell lymphoma unspecified (PTCLU)	70 (21.9%)
Angioimmunoblastic T-cell lymphoma (AITL)	28 (8.8%)
NK/T-cell lymphoma	19 (5.9%)
Lymphoblastic lymphoma	7 (2.2%)
Enteropathy-type T-cell lymphoma	2 (0.6%)
Hepatosplenic gamma/delta (γ/δ) T-cell lymphoma	2 (0.6%)
Subcutaneous panniculitis-like T-cell lymphoma	1 (0.3%)

- All patients were treated on either phase II or phase III trials. The phase II studies were dose-finding studies using escalating doses of cyclophosphamide, doxorubicin, and etoposide compared with standard CHOP plus etoposide protocols. The phase III trials compared the standard CHOP regimen to 6 or 8 courses of CHOP given every 2 weeks (CHOP-14) or to CHOP plus etoposide (CHOEP-14 or -21), or compared CHOEP to a dose-escalated (Hi-CHOEP), or a mega-dose (Mega CHOEP) variant, the latter regimen necessitated repeated transplantation of hematopoietic stem cells
- Radiotherapy to sites of bulky disease (>7.5 cm) and to extranodal disease was part of all protocols except for the Mega CHOEP phase II trial where radiotherapy was optional
- Extranodal disease was common in all subtypes (41–56%)
- Highly significant (*P* <0.001) differences were seen for involvement of soft tissues (21% in ALK-positive ALCL, 8% in ALK-negative ALCL, 0–1% in other subtypes) and bone marrow (none in ALK-positive ALCL, 4% in ALK-negative ALCL, 11% in PTCLU, 27% in AITL, and 13% in other subtypes) when the 4 major subgroups were compared

Treatment Modification

Adverse Event	Treatment Modifications
G4 ANC or febrile neutropenia after any cycle	Administer filgrastim during subsequent cycles
G4 neutropenia during a cycle in which filgrastim was administered	Cyclophosphamide, doxorubicin, and etoposide dosages are reduced by 25–50% during subsequent cycles
G3/4 thrombocytopenia	Cyclophosphamide, doxorubicin, and etoposide dosages are reduced by 25–50% during subsequent cycles
ANC <1500/mm³ or platelets <100,000/mm³ on day 1 of a scheduled cycle	The cycle is delayed for up to 2 weeks. Treatment is stopped if recovery has not occurred after a 2-week delay

Efficacy (N = 289)

(Median Follow-up of 43.8 Months for the Whole Group)

	ALK-positive ALCL (N = 78)	ALK-negative ALCL (N = 113)	PTCLU (N = 70)	AITL (N = 28)	NK/T (N = 19)
3-Year EFS % (95% CI)	75.8% (65.8%–85.8%)	45.7% (36.3%–55.1%)	41.1% (29.5%–52.7%)	50.0% (31.6%–68.4%)	36.1% (14.1%–58.1%)
3-Year OS % (95% CI)	89.8% (82.5%–97.1%)	62.1% (52.9%–71.3%)	53.9% (41.7%–66.1%)	67.5% (50.1%–84.9%)	46.3% (23.4%–69.2%)

Younger Patients (<60 years) with Normal LDH NHLB1 Trial*

	CHOP (N = 41)	CHOEP (N = 42)	
3-Year EFS % (95% CI)	75.4% (62.1%–88.7%)	51.0% (35.7%–66.3%)	P = 0.003
3-Year OS % (95% CI)	—	—	P = 0.176

Younger Patients (<60 years) with Normal LDH NHLB1 Trial + Hi-CHOEP Phase II/II Trials*

	CHOP (N = 41)	CHOEP (N = 103)	
3-Year EFS % (95% CI)	51.0% (35.7%–66.3%)	70.5% (61.3%–79.7%)	P = 0.004
3-Year OS % (95% CI)	75.2% (61.9%–88.5%)	81.3% (73.5%–89.1%)	P = 0.285

ALK-positive ALCL

	CHOP (N = 12)	CHOEP (N = 34)	
3-Year EFS	57.1% (28.5%–85.7%)	91.2% (81.6%–100.0%)	P = 0.012

AITL, angioimmunoblastic T-cell lymphoma; ALK-negative ALCL, anaplastic large cell lymphoma kinase ALK-negative; ALK-positive, ALCL, anaplastic large cell lymphoma kinase ALK-positive; CI, confidence interval; EFS, event-free survival; NK/T, NK-/T-cell lymphoma; PTCLU, peripheral T-cell lymphoma, unspecified; OS, overall survival
*In patients >60 years of age, 6 courses of CHOP administered every 3 weeks remains the standard therapy

Toxicity

(N = 194)

Pfreundschuh M et al. Ann Oncol 2008;19:545–552

Leukocytopenia	87.2%
Thrombocytopenia	9.6%
Anemia	11.8%
Infection	10.8%
Polyneuropathy	3.3%
Mucositis	2.7%
Cardiac toxicity	0.5%
Renal toxicity	0
Lung toxicity	0
Nausea or vomiting	4.8%
Alopecia	69.8%

Therapeutic Interventions

Red blood cell transfusions (per patient/per cycle)	11.2/4.1
Platelet transfusion (per patient/per cycle)	2.1/0.4
Intravenous antibiotics (per patient/per cycle)	32.6/8.7

Treatment Monitoring

1. *Before treatment:* physical examination; CBC with differential; assessment of serum chemistries; CT scan of the chest, abdomen, and pelvis and bone marrow aspiration and biopsy as indicated
2. *Before each cycle:* CBC with differential and platelet count
3. *Assessment of efficacy:* Radiographic examination at 2- or 3-cycle intervals and at the end of treatment

REGIMEN
ROMIDEPSIN

Coiffier B et al. J Clin Oncol 2012;30:631–636

Romidepsin 14 mg/m^2 per dose; administer intravenously in 500 mL 0.9% sodium chloride injection over 4 hours for 3 doses, on days 1, 8, and 15, every 28 days for up to 6 cycles (total dosage/cycle = 43.2 mg/m^2)

Notes:
• Check serum magnesium and serum potassium before each dose to ensure serum magnesium ≥1.5 mg/dL and serum potassium ≥4 mEq/L. Supplement potassium and magnesium in all patients BEFORE administering romidepsin if laboratory results do not meet these criteria
• In the study, patients with stable disease (SD), partial response (PR), or CR/CRu could continue to receive romidepsin until they demonstrated disease progression (PD) or met another criterion for withdrawal

Supportive Care
Antiemetic prophylaxis
Emetogenic potential is **LOW–MODERATE**
See Chapter 39 for antiemetic recommendations

Hematopoietic growth factor (CSF) prophylaxis
Primary prophylaxis is NOT indicated
See Chapter 43 for more information

Antimicrobial prophylaxis
Risk of fever and neutropenia is LOW
   Antimicrobial primary prophylaxis to be considered:
    • Antibacterial—*Pneumocystis jirovecii* prophylaxis is recommended (eg, cotrimoxazole)
    • Antifungal—not indicated
    • Antiviral—not indicated unless patient previously had an episode of HSV
See Chapter 47 for more information

Decreased bowel motility prophylaxis
Give a bowel regimen to prevent constipation based initially on **stool softeners**, and **saline, osmotic, and lubricant laxatives**, as needed to prevent constipation for as long as romidepsin use continues. If needed, circumspectly add **stimulant (irritant) laxatives** in the least amounts and for the briefest durations needed to produce defecation

---

Treatment Modifications

Adverse Event	Treatment Modifications
G2/3 nonhematologic toxicities except alopecia	Withhold treatment with romidepsin until toxicity returns to G ≤1 or baseline. Resume romidepsin therapy at 14 mg/m^2 per dose
Recurrent G3 nonhematologic toxicities	Withhold treatment with romidepsin until toxicity returns to G ≤1 or baseline. Resume romidepsin therapy at 10 mg/m^2 per dose. Do not attempt to escalate the dose
G4 nonhematologic toxicity	Withhold treatment with romidepsin until toxicity returns to G ≤1 or baseline. Resume romidepsin therapy at 10 mg/m^2 per dose. Do not attempt to escalate the dose
Recurrent G3/4 nonhematologic toxicities after romidepsin 10 mg/m^2	Discontinue romidepsin
G3/4 neutropenia or thrombocytopenia	Withhold treatment with romidepsin until the specific cytopenia recovers to ANC ≥1500/mm^3 and/or platelet count ≥75,000/mm^3 or baseline. Resume romidepsin therapy at 14 mg/m per dose^2
Grade 4 febrile (≥38.5°C [101.3°F]) neutropenia	Withhold treatment with romidepsin until the specific cytopenia recovers to G ≤1 or baseline. Resume romidepsin therapy at 10 mg/m^2 per dose. Do not attempt to escalate the dose
Thrombocytopenia requiring platelet transfusion	

Note: In patients with congenital long QT syndrome, patients with a history of significant cardiovascular disease, and patients taking antiarrhythmic medicines or medicinal products that lead to significant QT prolongation, appropriate cardiovascular monitoring precautions should be considered, such as the monitoring of electrolytes and ECGs at baseline and periodically during treatment

Patient Population Studied

A prospective, single-arm, phase II trial that enrolled patients with PTCL. Patients had relapsed or had disease refractory to one or more systemic therapies. Concomitant use of any other anticancer therapy, drugs that could significantly prolong the QTc interval, moderate-to significant inhibitors of CYP3A4, or therapeutic warfarin were prohibited. Patients were excluded if they had nontransformed mycosis fungoides or Sézary syndrome, or any known significant cardiac abnormalities (eg, congenital long QT syndrome, QTc interval >480 msec, myocardial infarction within previous 6 months, other significant ECG abnormalities, symptomatic coronary artery disease, congestive heart failure, hypertrophic cardiomyopathy or restrictive cardiomyopathy, uncontrolled hypertension, cardiac arrhythmia requiring antiarrhythmic medications, known history of sustained ventricular tachycardia, ventricular fibrillation, torsades de pointes, or cardiac arrest)

Demographic Characteristics at Study Baseline (Histologically Confirmed Population, N = 130)

	Number (%)
Age, years—median (range)	61 (20–83)
Sex–male-to-female ratio	88 (68%)/42 (32%)
White race/ethnicity	116 (89%)
ECOG performance status*	
0	46 (35)
1	66 (51)
2	17 (13)
International Prognostic Index <2/≥2	31 (24%)/99 (76%)
Time since diagnosis, years—median (range)	1.3 (0.2–17.0)
PTCL subtype based on central diagnosis[†]	
PTCL NOS	69 (53%)
Angioimmunoblastic T-cell lymphoma	27 (21%)
ALK-1–negative ALCL	21 (16%)
Enteropathy-type T-cell lymphoma	6 (5%)
Subcutaneous panniculitis-like T-cell lymphoma	3 (2%)
ALK-1–positive ALCL[‡]	1 (1%)
Cutaneous gamma/delta T-cell lymphoma	1 (1%)
Extranodal NK/T-cell lymphoma, nasal type	1 (1%)
Transformed mycosis fungoides	1 (1%)
Type of prior systemic therapy	
Chemotherapy	129 (99%)
Monoclonal antibody therapy	20 (15%)
Other type of immunotherapy	14 (11%)
Number of prior systemic therapies—median (range)	2 (1–8)
1	38 (29%)
2	44 (34%)
3	19 (15%)
4	15 (12%)
>4	14 (11%)
Received prior autologous stem cell transplantation	21 (16%)
Refractory to most recent therapy	49 (38%)

ALCL, anaplastic large-cell lymphoma; ALK-1, anaplastic lymphoma kinase-1; NK, natural killer; NOS, not otherwise specified; PTCL, peripheral T-cell lymphoma

*One patient had missing ECOG performance status at baseline

[†]Also eligible but not enrolled: hepatosplenic TCL

[‡]Eligible because disease progressed after prior autologous bone marrow transplant

Efficacy (N = 130)

Response Rates*

Best Response Category

Objective disease response	
(CR/CRu + PR)	38 (29%)
CR/CRu	21 (16%)
CR	19 (15%)
CRu	2 (2%)
PR	17 (13%)
SD	22 (17%)
PD or N/E†	70 (54%)

Time to response, months	
All responders (CR/CRu + PR)—median (range)	1.8 (1.0–4.3)
CR/Cru—median (range)	2.4 (1.6–9.6)

Duration of response in months	
All responders (CR/CRu + PR)—median (range)	11.6 (0.5‡–34.0)‡
CR/Cru—median (range)	N/E (1.2–34.0)‡

CR, complete response; CRu, unconfirmed complete response; N/E, not evaluable; PD, progressive disease; PR, partial response; SD, stable disease
*Based on Investigator Assessment. Comparable to Independent Review Committee
†Insufficient efficacy data to determine response because of early termination (ie, includes patients determined to have PD by investigators prior to first postbaseline assessment and therefore assessed as N/E according to the IRC)
‡Denotes a censored value

CR/CRu Rate and ORR Based on Overall IRC Assessment in Patient Subgroups (Histopathologically confirmed population; N = 130)

Subgroup	Total Number of Patients	CR/CRu Rate	P Value	ORR	P Value
Sex					
Male	88	12 (14%)	0.79	22 (25%)	1.00
Female	42	7 (17%)		11 (26%)	
Age, years					
>65	81	12 (15%)	1.00	20 (25%)	0.84
≤65	49	7 (14%)		13 (27%)	
PTCL subtype					
PTCL NOS	69	10 (14%)	0.83*	20 (29%)	0.92*
AITL	27	5 (19%)		8 (30%)	
ALK-1–negative ALCL	21	4 (19%)		5 (24%)	
Other subgroups	13	0		0	
International Prognostic Index, baseline					
<2	31	3 (10%)	0.56	7 (23%)	0.81
≥2	99	16 (16%)		26 (26%)	
No. of prior systemic therapies					
≤2	82	11 (13%)	0.62	18 (22%)	0.30
>2	48	8 (17%)		15 (31%)	
Prior stem cell transplantation					
Yes	21	2 (10%)	0.74	5 (24%)	1.00
No	109	17 (16%)		28 (26%)	
Prior monoclonal antibody therapy†					
Yes	20	4 (20%)	1.00	5 (25%)	0.49
No	110	15 (14%)		28 (25%)	
Other immunotherapy‡					
Yes	14	2 (14%)	1.00	2 (14%)	0.52
No	116	17 (15%)		31 (27%)	
Refractory to last prior therapy					
Yes	49	9 (18%)	0.44	14 (29%)	0.54
No	81	10 (12%)		19 (23%)	

AITL, angioimmunoblastic T-cell lymphoma; ALCL, anaplastic large-cell lymphoma; ALK-1, anaplastic lymphoma kinase-1; CR, complete response; CRu, complete response, unconfirmed; IRC, Independent Review Committee; NOS, not otherwise specified; ORR, objective response rate; PTCL, peripheral T-cell lymphoma
*Based on PTCL NOS, AITL, and ALK-1-negative ALCL
†Including alemtuzumab and siplizumab
‡Including denileukin diftitox and interferon (type NOS)

Adverse Events Reported in at Least 10% of Patients: All Events and Drug-Related Events

(As treated population, N = 131)

Event	All Events		Drug-Related Events	
	All Grades	G ≥3	All Grades	G ≥3
Nausea	77 (59%)	3 (2%)	71 (54%)	2 (2%)
Infections SOC*	72 (55%)	25 (19%)	24 (18%)	8 (6%)
Asthenia/fatigue	72 (55%)	11 (8%)	68 (52%)	7 (5%)
Thrombocytopenia	53 (41%)	32 (24%)	52 (40%)	30 (23%)
Vomiting	51 (39%)	6 (5%)	44 (34%)	5 (4%)
Diarrhea	47 (36%)	3 (2%)	30 (23%)	2 (2%)
Pyrexia	46 (35%)	7 (5%)	22 (17%)	5 (4%)
Neutropenia	39 (30%)	26 (20%)	38 (29%)	24 (18%)
Constipation	39 (30%)	1 (1%)	19 (15%)	0
Anorexia	37 (28%)	2 (2%)	34 (26%)	2 (2%)
Anemia	32 (24%)	14 (11%)	27 (21%)	7 (5%)
Dysgeusia	27 (21%)	0	27 (21%)	0
Cough	23 (18%)	0	2 (2%)	0
Headache	19 (15%)	0	14 (11%)	0
Abdominal pain	18 (14%)	3 (2%)	8 (6%)	0
Dyspnea	17 (13%)	3 (2%)	7 (5%)	1 (1%)
Leukopenia	16 (12%)	8 (6%)	16 (12%)	8 (6%)
Chills	14 (11%))	1 (1%)	6 (5%)	0
Hypokalemia	14 (11%)	3 (2%)	7 (5%)	2 (2%)
Peripheral edema	13 (10%)	1 (1%)	3 (2%)	0
Decreased weight	13 (10%)	0	10 (8%)	0
Stomatitis	13 (10%)	0	9 (7%)	0
Tachycardia	13 (10%)	0	6 (5%)	0

SOC, system organ class (according to Medical Dictionary for Regulatory Activities)
*None of the individual preferred term events in the infections SOC were reported with an incidence ≥10%

Treatment Monitoring

1. *Before treatment:* physical examination; CBC with differential; assessment of serum chemistries; CT scan of the chest, abdomen, and pelvis and bone marrow aspiration and biopsy as indicated

2. *Before each romidepsin dose:* CBC with differential and platelet count; serum electrolytes, including potassium and magnesium

3. *Assessment of efficacy:* radiographic examination at 2- or 3-cycle intervals and at the end of treatment

REGIMEN
PRALATREXATE

O'Connor OA et al. J Clin Oncol 2011;29:1182–1189

Vitamin supplementation to ameliorate mucositis associated with pralatrexate use:

Cyanocobalamin (vitamin B_{12}) 1 mg; administer by intramuscular injection within **2 weeks** before the first dose of pralatrexate repeated every 8–10 weeks after previously administered doses

Folic acid 1–1.25 mg/day; administer orally, continually, starting at least 10 days before the first dose of pralatrexate, and continuing for 30 days after the last dose of pralatrexate

Notes:
• Increased methylmalonic acid (>200 nmol/L [>0.2 μmol/L]) or homocysteine (>10 μmol/L) at screening required initiating vitamin supplementation ≥10 days before the first dose of pralatrexate

• Vitamin B_{12} injections may be given on the same day as pralatrexate administration

Pralatrexate 30 mg/m² per dose; administer by intravenous injection over 3–5 minutes once weekly for 6 consecutive weeks followed by 1 week without treatment, every 7 weeks (total dosage/7-week cycle = 180 mg/m²)

Note: Continue treatment until progressive disease (PD) or unacceptable toxicity occurs or at patient/physician discretion

Supportive Care
Antiemetic prophylaxis
Emetogenic potential is **LOW**
See Chapter 39 for antiemetic recommendations

Hematopoietic growth factor (CSF) prophylaxis
Primary prophylaxis may be indicated
See Chapter 43 for more information

Antimicrobial prophylaxis
Risk of fever and neutropenia is LOW
   Antimicrobial primary prophylaxis to be considered:
   • Antibacterial—*Pneumocystis jirovecii* prophylaxis is recommended (eg, cotrimoxazole)

   • Antifungal—not indicated

   • Antiviral—not indicated unless patient previously had an episode of HSV
See Chapter 47 for more information

Oral care
Prophylaxis and treatment for mucositis/stomatitis
   General advice:
   • Encourage patients to maintain intake of nonalcoholic fluids

   • Evaluate patients for oral pain and provide analgesic medications

   • Consider histamine (H_2-subtype) receptor antagonists (eg, ranitidine, famotidine), or a proton pump inhibitor for epigastric pain

   • *Lactobacillus* sp.-containing probiotics may be beneficial in preventing diarrhea

   Patients with intact oral mucosa:
   • Clean the mouth, tongue, and gums by brushing after every meal and at bedtime with an ultrasoft toothbrush with fluoride toothpaste

   • Floss teeth gently every day unless contraindicated. If gums bleed and hurt, avoid bleeding or sore areas, but floss other teeth

   • Patients may use saline or commercial brand, nonalcoholic rinses
      ▪ Do not use mouthwashes that contain alcohols

   If mucositis or stomatitis is present:
   • Keep the mouth moist utilizing water, ice chips, sugarless gum, sugar-free hard candies, or a saliva substitute

   • Rinse mouth several times a day to remove debris
      ▪ Use a solution of ¼ teaspoon (1.25 g) each of baking soda and table salt (sodium chloride) in 1 quart (~950 mL) of warm water. Follow with a plain water rinse

      ▪ Do not use mouthwashes that contain alcohols

   • Foam-tipped swabs (eg, Toothettes) are useful in moisturizing oral mucosa, but ineffective for cleansing teeth and removing plaque

   • Advise patients who develop mucositis to:
      ▪ Choose foods that are easy to chew and swallow

      ▪ Take small bites of food, chew slowly, and sip liquids with meals

      ▪ Encourage soft, moist foods such as cooked cereals, mashed potatoes, and scrambled eggs

      ▪ For trouble swallowing, soften food with gravies, sauces, broths, yogurt, or other bland liquids

      ▪ Avoid sharp, crunchy foods; hot, spicy, or highly acidic foods (eg, citrus fruits and juices); sugary foods; toothpicks; tobacco products; alcoholic drinks

Patient Population Studied

Patients with PTCL according to the Revised European American Lymphoma WHO disease classification were eligible for study (Harris NL, Jaffe ES, Diebold J et al: Lymphoma classification-from controversy to consensus: The R.E.A.L. and WHO Classification of lymphoid neoplasms. Ann Oncol 2000;11[Suppl 1]:S3–S10). Patients were required to have documented disease progression after ≥1 prior treatment

Additional exclusion criteria included: prior allogeneic stem cell transplant (SCT); relapse <75 days after ASCT

Baseline Characteristics of Patients (N = 111)

Sex, male-to-female ratio	76 (68%)/35 (32%)
Ethnicity	
White	80 (72%)
African American	14 (13%)
Asian	6 (5%)
Hispanic	9 (8%)
Other/Unknown	1 (1%)/1 (1%)
Age, years—mean (range)	55.7 (21–85)
≥65 y	40 (36%)
Number of prior therapies for PTCL—median (range)	3 (1–13)
Number of prior systemic therapies for PTCL—median (range)	3 (1–12)
Type of prior therapy for PTCL	
Local therapy	
Radiation therapy	25 (23%)
Photopheresis	10 (9%)
Topical nitrogen mustard	4 (4%)
Systemic therapy	
CHOP	78 (70%)
Platinum-containing multiagent chemotherapy	45 (41%)
Non–platinum-containing multiagent chemotherapy	43 (39%)
Single-agent chemotherapy	36 (32%)
Autologous stem cell transplant	18 (16%)
Bexarotene	15 (14%)
Other	13 (12%)
Corticosteroids alone	8 (7%)
Hyper-CVAD	8 (7%)
Denileukin diftitox	7 (6%)
Systemic investigational agents	7 (6%)
Histopathology per central review	
PTCL unspecified	59 (53%)
Anaplastic large cell lymphoma, primary systemic type*	17 (15%)
Angioimmunoblastic T-cell lymphoma	13 (12%)
Transformed mycosis fungoides	12 (11%)
Blastic NK lymphoma (skin, lymph node, or visceral involved)	4 (4%)
Other	2 (2%)
T/NK-cell lymphoma nasal	2 (2%)
Extranodal peripheral T/NK-cell lymphoma unspecified	1 (<1%)
Adult T-cell leukemia/lymphoma (HTLV-1+)	1 (<1%)

CHOP, cyclophosphamide, doxorubicin, vincristine, and prednisone; HTLV, human T-lymphotropic virus; ALK, anaplastic lymphoma kinase; Hyper-CVAD, hyperfractionated cyclophosphamide with vincristine, doxorubicin, and corticosteroids; NK, natural killer; PTCL, peripheral T-cell lymphoma
*Eleven ALK-negative, 4 ALK-positive, 2 did not have ALK status determined
Note: Patients treated with corticosteroids alone received other systemic therapies

Dose Modification

Adverse Event	Treatment Modifications
G2 mucositis	Withhold pralatrexate therapy or omit dose. When toxicity recovers to G ≤1, resume pralatrexate therapy at previous dose
Recurrent G2 mucositis G3 mucositis	Withhold pralatrexate therapy or omit dose. When toxicity recovers to G ≤1, resume pralatrexate therapy at 20 mg/m² per week. Do not attempt to escalate dose
G4 mucositis	Discontinue pralatrexate therapy
G3 nonhematologic toxicity	Withhold pralatrexate therapy or omit dose. When toxicity recovers to G ≤1, resume pralatrexate therapy at 20 mg/m² per week. Do not attempt to escalate dose
G4 nonhematologic toxicity	Discontinue pralatrexate therapy
Platelet count <50,000/mm³ for 1 week	Withhold pralatrexate therapy or omit dose. When platelet count >50,000/mm³, resume pralatrexate therapy at previous dose
Platelet count <50,000/mm³ for 2 weeks	Withhold pralatrexate therapy or omit dose. When platelet count >50,000/mm³, resume pralatrexate therapy at 20 mg/m² per week. Do not attempt to escalate dose
Platelet count <50,000/mm³ for ≥3 weeks	Discontinue pralatrexate therapy
ANC 500–1000/mm³ without fever for 1 week	Withhold pralatrexate therapy or omit dose. When ANC >1000/mm³, resume pralatrexate therapy at previous dose

(*continued*)

Efficacy

Best Response to Treatment and Time-to-event Data (Total N = 109)

Response and Time to Event	Central Review IWC	Central Review IWC + PET	Local Investigator
Best response			
CR + CRu + PR	32 (29%)	28 (26%)	43 (39%)
CR	11 (10%)	15 (14%)	17 (16%)
CRu	1 (1%)	0	3 (3%)
PR	20 (18%)	13 (12%)	23 (21%)
SD	21 (19%)	18 (17%)	21 (19%)
PD	40 (37%)	31 (28%)	40 (37%)
UE	2 (2%)	18 (17%)	0
Missing, off treatment in cycle 1	14 (13%)	14 (13%)	5 (5%)
Time-to-event (number)	32	28	43
Median time to response, days			
First response (Range)	46 (37–349)	48 (37–248)	50 (38–358)
Best response (Range)	141 (37–726)	136 (37–542)	51 (38–542)
Median duration of response, months	10.1	12.7	8.1

CR, complete response; CRu, complete response unconfirmed; IWC, International Workshop Criteria;
PD, progressive disease; PET, positron emission tomography; PR, partial response; SD, stable disease; UE, unevaluable

Response Rate by Key Subsets

Parameter	Number (%)	IWC Response Rate Number (%) [95% CI]
Age, years		
<65	70 (64%)	19 (27%) [17 to 39]
≥65	39 (36%)	13 (33%) [19 to 50]
Prior systemic therapy		
1 regimen	23 (21%)	8 (35%) [16 to 57]
2 regimens	29 (27%)	7 (24%) [10 to 44]
>2 regimens	57 (52%)	17 (30%) [18 to 43]
Prior transplant		
Yes	18 (17%)	6 (33%) [13 to 59]
No	91 (83%)	26 (29%) [20 to 39]
Prior methotrexate		
Yes	21 (19%)	5 (24%) [8 to 47]
No	88 (81%)	27 (31%) [21 to 41]
Histology		
PTCL NOS	59 (54%)	19 (32%) [21 to 46]
Angioimmunoblastic	13 (12%)	1 (8%) [0 to 36]
Anaplastic LC	17 (16%)	6 (35%) [14 to 62]
Transformed MF	12 (11%)	3 (25%) [5 to 57]
Other	8 (7%)	3 (38%) [9 to 76]

CI, confidence interval; IWC, International Workshop Criteria; LC, large cell; MF, mycosis fungoides;
NOS, not otherwise specified; PTCL, peripheral T-cell lymphoma

Dose Modification (continued)

Adverse Event	Treatment Modifications
ANC 500–1000/mm^3 with fever or ANC <500/mm^3 for 1 week	Withhold pralatrexate therapy or omit dose. Administer growth factor support. When ANC >1000/mm^3, resume pralatrexate therapy at previous dose with growth factor support
ANC 500–1000/mm^3 with fever or ANC <500/mm^3 for 2 weeks Recurrent ANC 500–1000/mm^3 with fever or ANC <500/mm^3 that lasts 1 week	Withhold pralatrexate therapy or omit dose. Administer growth factor support. When ANC >1000/mm^3, resume pralatrexate therapy at 20 mg/m^2 per week with growth factor support. Do not attempt to escalate dose
ANC 500–1000/mm^3 with fever or ANC <500/mm^3 that lasts 3 weeks Second recurrence of ANC 500–1000/mm^3 with fever or ANC <500/mm^3 that lasts 1 week	Discontinue pralatrexate therapy

Toxicity

Adverse Events in ≥10% of Patients
(Safety Population, ≥1 Dose of Study Drug)

Event	Total	G3	G4
Any event*	111 (100%)	47 (42%)	35 (32%)
General events and administration site conditions			
Mucositis[†]	79 (71%)	20 (18%)	4 (4%)
Fatigue	40 (36%)	6 (5%)	2 (2%)
Pyrexia	38 (34%)	1 (1%)	1 (1%)
Edema[†]	34 (31%)	1 (1%)	0
Hematologic events			
Thrombocytopenia[†‡]	45 (41%)	15 (14%)	21 (19%)
Anemia[†]	38 (34%)	18 (16%)	2 (2%)
Neutropenia[†]	28 (25%)	15 (14%)	9 (8%)
Leukopenia[†]	12 (11%)	4 (4%)	4 (4%)
GI event			
Nausea	46 (41%)	4 (4%)	0
Constipation	38 (34%)	0	0
Vomiting	28 (25%)	2 (2%)	0
Diarrhea	25 (23%)	2 (2%)	0
Dyspepsia[†]	11 (10%)	0	0
Respiratory, thoracic, and mediastinal events			
Cough	32 (29%)	1 (1%)	0
Epistaxis	29 (26%)	0	0
Dyspnea	21 (19%)	8 (7%)	0
Skin and subcutaneous tissue events			
Rash	17 (15%)	0	0
Pruritus[†]	16 (14%)	2 (2%)	0
Night sweats	12 (11%)	0	0
Infections			
Upper respiratory tract infection	12 (11%)	1 (1%)	0
Sinusitis	11 (10%)	1 (1%)	0
Other conditions			
Hypokalemia[†]	18 (16%)	4 (4%)	1 (1%)
Anorexia[†]	18 (16%)	3 (3%)	0
Pharyngolaryngeal pain	15 (14%)	1 (1%)	0
Liver function test abnormal[†]	14 (13%)	6 (5%)	0
Back pain	14 (13%)	3 (3%)	0
Abdominal pain	13 (12%)	4 (4%)	0
Headache	13 (12%)	0	0
Pain in extremity	13 (12%)	0	0
Asthenia	12 (11%)	2 (2%)	0
Tachycardia	11 (10%)	0	0

*Twenty-three percent (n = 26) withdrew from treatment because of AEs, most frequently for mucositis (6%) or thrombocytopenia (5%)
[†]Included a grouping of similar preferred terms
[‡]Platelet count <10,000/mm^3 was seen in 5 patients
Note: Patients could have >1 adverse event

Treatment Monitoring

1. *Before treatment:* physical examination; CBC with differential; assessment of serum chemistries, as well as methylmalonic acid and homocysteine levels; CT scan of the chest, abdomen, and pelvis and bone marrow aspiration and biopsy as indicated
2. *Before each pralatrexate dose:* CBC with differential and platelet count
3. *Assessment of efficacy:* radiographic examination at 2- or 3-cycle intervals and at the end of treatment

REGIMEN

DOSE-ADJUSTED ETOPOSIDE + PREDNISONE + VINCRISTINE + CYCLOPHOSPHAMIDE + DOXORUBICIN + RITUXIMAB (DA-EPOCH-R)

Dunleavy K et al. New Engl J Med 2013;369:1915–1925

Prophylaxis against hyperuricemia during cycle 1: **Allopurinol** 600 mg; administer orally for 1 dose 24 hours before administering antineoplastic treatment, *and then:*

Allopurinol 300 mg/day; administer orally for 6 consecutive days, on days 2–7

Notes:

• Monitor chemistries (uric acid, potassium, phosphorus, calcium) for tumor lysis

• The initial 600-mg dose may be replaced by a 300-mg dose in patients who are already receiving allopurinol

• Additional measures, such as hospitalization with aggressive intravenous hydration, were used at investigators' discretion

• Persons who express a variant human leukocyte antigen allele, HLA-B*58:01, are at increased risk for severe cutaneous adverse reactions from allopurinol (Hershfield MS et al. Clin Pharmacol Ther 2013;93:153–158; Zineh I et al. Pharmacogenomics 2011;12:1741–1749)

   ▪ Consider alternative prophylaxis (rasburicase) in patients at high risk for hyperuricemia, and for treatment

Prednisone 60 mg/m²; administer orally, twice daily for 5 consecutive days, on days 1–5 (10 doses), every 21 days, for 6–8 cycles (total dosage/cycle = 600 mg/m²)

• The first prednisone dose should be given at least 1 hour before rituximab administration begins

• Patients who were unable to ingest oral medications may receive a parenterally administered steroid at a glucocorticoid equivalent dosage for the same number of doses on the same administration schedule (eg, methylprednisolone 48 mg/m² per dose)

Premedication for rituximab:

Acetaminophen 650–1000 mg; administer orally *plus* **diphenhydramine** 25–50 mg; administer orally or intravenously 30–60 minutes before each dose of rituximab

Rituximab 375 mg/m²; administer intravenously in 0.9% sodium chloride injection (0.9% NS) or 5% dextrose injection (D5W) diluted to a concentration within the range of 1–4 mg/mL, on day 1, every 21 days, for 6–8 cycles (total dosage/cycle = 375 mg/m²)

Notes on rituximab administration:

• Infuse initially at 50 mg/h. If hypersensitivity or infusion reactions do not occur during the first 30 minutes, increase the rate by 50 mg/h every 30 minutes as tolerated to a maximum rate of 400 mg/h. Subsequently, if previous administration was well tolerated, start at 100 mg/h and increase by 100 mg/h every 30 minutes as tolerated to a maximum rate of 400 mg/h

• Interrupt rituximab administration for fever chills, edema, congestion of the head and neck mucosa, hypertension, and other serious adverse events. Resume rituximab administration after adverse events abate

Etoposide + doxorubicin + vincristine "3-in-1" admixture (preparation instructions appear below*)

   Etoposide; administer by continuous intravenous infusion over 24 hours for 4 consecutive days, on days 1–4, every 21 days, for 6–8 cycles (see the table below for daily dosage and total dosage/cycle†)

   Doxorubicin; administer by continuous intravenous infusion over 24 hours for 4 consecutive days, on days 1–4, every 21 days, for 6–8 cycles (see the table below for daily dosage and total dosage/cycle†)

   Vincristine; administer by continuous intravenous infusion over 24 hours for 4 consecutive days, on days 1–4, every 21 days, for 6–8 cycles (total dosage/cycle = 1.6 mg/m²)

Hydration before and after cyclophosphamide administration: Give 0.9% NS (volumes specified below) at 300–500 mL/h

EPOCH Dose Level	Total Volume of Hydration Fluid‡
1 and 2	1000 mL
3, 4, and 5	2000 mL
≥6	2500 mL

Cyclophosphamide 750 mg/m²; administer intravenously in 100–150 mL 0.9% NS or D5W over 30 minutes on day 5 (after completing infusional etoposide + doxorubicin + vincristine), every 21 days for 6–8 cycles (see the table below for dosage specifications†)

Filgrastim 480 mcg/day; administer by subcutaneous injection, daily for 10 consecutive days, on days 6–15, *or* until postnadir ANC is >5000/mm³

*Etoposide + doxorubicin + vincristine "3-in-1" admixtures—preparation, storage, and stability

• To prepare a "3-in-1" admixture with etoposide + doxorubicin + vincristine, dilute all 3 drug products in 0.9% sodium chloride injection (0.9% NS) as follows:

Total Dose of Etoposide	0.9% NS Volume to Use
≤130 mg	500 mL
>130 mg	1000 mL

(continued)

(*continued*)

- Admixture with etoposide (base):
  - Etoposide 50 mg/m², doxorubicin hydrochloride 10 mg/m², and vincristine sulfate 0.4 mg/m² admixtures diluted in 0.9% NS to produce an etoposide concentration <250 mcg/mL, in polyolefin-lined infusion bags are stable and compatible for 72 hours at 23°–25°C (73.4°–77°F), and at 31°–33°C (87.8°–91.4°F) when protected from exposure to light (Wolfe JL et al. Am J Health Syst Pharm 1999;56:985–989)

- Admixture with etoposide PHOSphate:
  - Etoposide PHOSphate, doxorubicin hydrochloride, and vincristine sulfate admixtures diluted in 0.9% NS to produce an etoposide concentration <250 mcg/mL, in polyolefin-lined infusion bags are stable and compatible for up to 124 hours at 2°–6°C (35.6°–42.8°F) and 35°–40°C (95°–104°F) in the dark and in regular fluorescent light. In admixtures stored at 35°–40°C (95°–104°F) and exposed to light, the initial drug concentrations decreased slightly, but remained within acceptable concentrations (Yuan P et al. Am J Health Syst Pharm 2001;58:594–598)
- The "3-in-1" admixtures described above will not prevent microbial growth after exposure to bacterial and fungal contamination. With respect to product sterility, expiration dating should be determined by the aseptic techniques used in preparation and local and national guidelines

†EPOCH Dosage Levels:
- At dosage levels 1 through 6, adjustments apply *only* to etoposide, doxorubicin, and cyclophosphamide
- At dosage levels −1 or −2, adjustments apply *only* to cyclophosphamide (20% dosage reductions for each dosage decrement)

	Dosage Levels							
	−2	−1	1	2	3	4	5	6
Drugs	Daily Dosages (mg/m² · day)							
Doxorubicin	10	10	10	12	14.4	17.3	20.7	24.8
Etoposide	50	50	50	60	72	86.4	103.7	124.4
Cyclophosphamide	480	600	750	900	1080	1296	1555	1866

	Total Dosage per Cycle (mg/m² · 96 hours)							
Doxorubicin	40	40	40	48	57.6	69.2	82.8	99.2
Etoposide	200	200	200	240	288	345.6	414.8	497.6
Cyclophosphamide	480	600	750	900	1080	1296	1555	1866

‡Give half the total volume of fluid is before starting cyclophosphamide administration and give half the total volume after completing cyclophosphamide

Notes:
- Patients received 2 cycles after complete remission was established, for a total of 6–8 cycles
- HIV-positive patients did not receive antiretroviral therapy during chemotherapy
- DA-EPOCH-R was pharmacodynamically dose-adjusted on the basis of the ANC nadir
- Patients without evidence of cerebrospinal fluid (CSF) involvement received prophylactic intrathecal methotrexate 12 mg via lumbar puncture. Intrathecal treatment was administered on days 1 and 5, every 3 weeks (8 doses), during cycles 3, 4, 5, and 6 (total dose/cycle = 24 mg)
- Patients with evidence of CSF involvement received intrathecal treatment with methotrexate 12 mg via lumbar puncture *or* methotrexate 6 mg via an Ommaya reservoir, twice weekly until 2 weeks after CSF samples are cytologically negative for lymphoma *or* for a minimum duration of 4 weeks, then once weekly for 6 weeks, and then once monthly for 6 months

Antiemetic prophylaxis
*Emetogenic potential on Days 1–4 is **LOW***
*Emetogenic potential on Day 5 is **MODERATE***
See Chapter 39 for antiemetic recommendations

Hematopoietic growth factor (CSF) prophylaxis
Primary prophylaxis is indicated with:
Filgrastim (G-CSF) use is integral within the R-EPOCH regimen described above

Antimicrobial prophylaxis
Risk of fever and neutropenia is INTERMEDIATE
Antimicrobial primary prophylaxis to be considered:
- Antibacterial—consider a fluoroquinolone or no prophylaxis; *Pneumocystis jirovecii* prophylaxis is recommended (eg, cotrimoxazole)
- Antifungal—recommended; consider use during periods of neutropenia, and in anticipation of mucositis
- Antiviral—antiherpes antivirals (eg, acyclovir, famciclovir, valacyclovir)
See Chapter 47 for more information

(*continued*)

(continued)

Infusion reactions associated with rituximab
Fevers, chills, and rigors
1. Interrupt rituximab administration for severe symptoms, and give:
   - **Acetaminophen** 650 mg orally for fever. For persistent or recurrent symptoms, repeat administration every 4–6 hours as needed during rituximab administration
   - **Diphenhydramine** 25–50 mg orally or by intravenous injection for pruritus, hypotension, or angioedema. For persistent or recurrent symptoms, repeat administration every 4–6 hours as needed during rituximab administration
   - **Meperidine** 12.5–25 mg by intravenous injection every 10–20 minutes as needed for shaking chills (generally, cumulative doses >100 mg are not needed; use repeated doses with caution in persons with moderate or more severely impaired renal function)
2. If rituximab administration was interrupted, resume infusion at a slower rate than the maximum rate previously attempted. Rate escalation may be reattempted at smaller incremental steps with close monitoring. Do not exceed the maximum recommended rate of 400 mg/h

Dyspnea or wheezing without allergic findings (urticaria, or tongue or laryngeal edema)
1. Interrupt rituximab administration immediately
2. Give **hydrocortisone** 100 mg by intravenous injection (or an alternative steroid with equivalent glucocorticoid potency)
3. Give a **histamine (H$_2$) receptor antagonist** (ranitidine 50 mg, cimetidine 300 mg, or famotidine 20 mg) intravenously over 15–30 minutes
4. After symptoms resolve, resume rituximab administration at 25 mg/h with close monitoring. Do not increase the administration rate

Steroid-associated gastritis
Add a **proton pump inhibitor** during steroid use to prevent gastritis and duodenitis

Decreased bowel motility prophylaxis
Give **stool softeners** in a scheduled regimen, and **saline, osmotic, and lubricant laxatives**, as needed to prevent constipation for as long as vincristine use continues. If needed, circumspectly add **stimulant (irritant) laxatives** in the least amounts and for the briefest durations needed to produce defecation

Oral care
Prophylaxis and treatment for mucositis/stomatitis
General advice:
- Encourage patients to maintain intake of nonalcoholic fluids
- Evaluate patients for oral pain and provide analgesic medications
- Consider histamine (H$_2$-subtype) receptor antagonists (eg, ranitidine, famotidine), or a proton pump inhibitor for epigastric pain
- *Lactobacillus* sp.-containing probiotics may be beneficial in preventing diarrhea

Patients with intact oral mucosa:
- Clean the mouth, tongue, and gums by brushing after every meal and at bedtime with an ultrasoft toothbrush with fluoride toothpaste
- Floss teeth gently every day unless contraindicated. If gums bleed and hurt, avoid bleeding or sore areas, but floss other teeth
- Patients may use saline or commercial brand, nonalcoholic rinses
  - Do not use mouthwashes that contain alcohols

If mucositis or stomatitis is present:
- Keep the mouth moist utilizing water, ice chips, sugarless gum, sugar-free hard candies, or a saliva substitute
- Rinse mouth several times a day to remove debris
  - Use a solution of ¼ teaspoon (1.25 g) each of baking soda and table salt (sodium chloride) in 1 quart (~950 mL) of warm water. Follow with a plain water rinse
  - Do not use mouthwashes that contain alcohols
- Foam-tipped swabs (eg, Toothettes) are useful in moisturizing oral mucosa, but ineffective for cleansing teeth and removing plaque
- Advise patients who develop mucositis to:
  - Choose foods that are easy to chew and swallow
  - Take small bites of food, chew slowly, and sip liquids with meals
  - Encourage soft, moist foods such as cooked cereals, mashed potatoes, and scrambled eggs
  - For trouble swallowing, soften food with gravies, sauces, broths, yogurt, or other bland liquids
  - Avoid sharp, crunchy foods; hot, spicy, or highly acidic foods (eg, citrus fruits and juices); sugary foods; toothpicks; tobacco products; alcoholic drinks

Treatment Modifications

Adverse Events*	Treatment Modifications†
Creatinine clearance <50 mL/min (<0.83 mL/s)	At any dosage level, decrease etoposide dosage by 50%. If creatinine clearance recovers to >50 mL/min (>0.83 mL/s), etoposide should be given at 100% of planned dosage level
Previous cycle ANC nadir count ≥500/mm³	Increase etoposide, doxorubicin, and cyclophosphamide dosages by 20% greater than the dosages given during the previous cycle (increase by 1 dosage level)
Previous cycle ANC nadir count <500/mm³ on 1 or 2 measurements	Give the same dosages as last cycle
Previous cycle ANC nadir count <500/mm³ on at least 3 measurements	Reduce etoposide, doxorubicin, and cyclophosphamide dosages by 20% less than the dosages given during the previous cycle (decrease by 1 dosage level)
Previous cycle platelet nadir count <25,000/mm³ on 1 measurement	Continue treatment, but withhold vincristine‡
Total bilirubin >4.0 mg/dL (>68.4 μmol/L)	Reduce vincristine dosage by 75%‡
Total bilirubin >1.5 mg/dL but <3 mg/dL (>25.7 μmol/L but <51.3 μmol/L)	Reduce vincristine dosage by 50%‡
G2 neuropathy	Reduce vincristine dosage by 25%‡
G3 neuropathy	Reduce vincristine dosage by 50%‡

*ANC and platelet values based on twice weekly CBC with differential
†Dosage adjustment *greater than the starting dose levels* applies only to etoposide, doxorubicin, and cyclophosphamide. Dosage adjustment *less than the starting dose levels* applies only to cyclophosphamide
‡Vincristine dosage is increased to 100% if neuropathy resolves to G ≤1 or serum total bilirubin is <1.5 mg/dL (<25.7 μmol/L)

Characteristics of the Patients

Characteristic	All Patients (N = 30)	DA-EPOCH-R (N = 19)	SC-EPOCH-RR (N = 11)
Age in years—median (range)	33 (15–88)§	25 (15–88)§	44 (24–60)§
Age ≥40 years—number (%)	12 (40)	5 (26)	7 (64)
Male sex—number (%)	22 (73)	13 (68)	9 (82)
Ann Arbor stage III or IV—number (%)	20 (67)	11 (58)	9 (82)
ECOG-PS score ≥2—number (%)	9 (30)ᶜ	3 (16)ᶜ	6 (55)ᶜ
Serum LDH >ULN—number (%)	16 (53)**	7 (37)**	9 (82)**
Extranodal site—number (%)*	19 (63)	10 (53)	9 (82)
Bowel	15 (50)	9 (47)	6 (55)
Bone marrow or blood	4 (13)	3 (16)	1 (9)
Central nervous system	1 (3)	1 (5)	0
LMB risk group—number (%)†			
A	5 (17)	5 (26)	0
B	22 (73)	12 (63)	10 (91)
C	3 (10)	2 (10)	1 (9)
Burkitt lymphoma variant—number (%)**			
Sporadic	17 (57)	17 (89)	0
Immunodeficiency-associated‡	13 (43)	2 (11)	11 (100)
Secondary	11 (37)	0	11 (100)
Primary	2 (7)	2 (11)	0

(continued)

Treatment Modifications *(continued)*

Characteristics of the Patients

Characteristic	All Patients (N = 30)	DA-EPOCH-R (N = 19)	SC-EPOCH-RR (N = 11)
Molecular marker—number/total number (%)			
MYC rearrangement	22/22 (100)	14/14 (100)	8/8 (100)
BCL6 protein expression	24/24 (100)	15/15 (100)	9/9 (100)
BCL2 protein expression	0/26	0/16	0/10
EBER in situ hybridization	6/21 (29)	4/14 (29)	2/7 (29)

DA-EPOCH-R, dose-adjusted infusional therapy with etoposide, doxorubicin, vincristine, with cyclophosphamide, prednisone, and rituximab; ECOG-PS, Eastern Cooperative Oncology Group performance status; EBER, Epstein-Barr virus-encoded RNA; SC-EPOCH-RR short-course infusional therapy with etoposide, doxorubicin, and vincristine, with cyclophosphamide, prednisone, and 2 doses of rituximab; ULN upper limit of the normal range
*Patients may have had more than 1 extranodal site
†Lymphomes malins B (LMB) risk groups are defined as follows:
  • Group A includes patients with low-risk disease (resected stage I or abdominal stage II cancer)
  • Group B includes those with intermediate-risk disease (patients not in group A or C)
  • Group C includes those with high-risk disease (central nervous system involvement, at least 25% blasts in bone marrow, or both characteristics)
(Société Française d'Oncologie Pédiatrique lymphomes malins B (LMB) prognostic categories [Patte C et al. Blood 2007;109:2773–2780])
‡Patients with the immunodeficiency-associated variant may have had HIV infection, the autoimmune lymphoproliferative syndrome, or a deficiency of dedicator of cytokinesis 8
§P value = 0.03
¶P value = 0.04; P value = 0.03
**P value <0.001; all other P values >0.06

Efficacy

Clinical Outcome	Immunodeficiency-associated Burkitt Lymphoma	DA-EPOCH-R (N = 19)	SC-EPOCH-RR (N = 11)
Median duration of follow-up	—	86 months	73 months
Rate of freedom from progression	92%	100% (95% CI, 72–100)	95% (95% CI, 75–99)
Overall survival	92%	90% (95% CI, 60–98)	100% (95% CI, 82–100)

CI, confidence interval; DA-EPOCH-R, dose-adjusted infusional therapy with etoposide, doxorubicin, vincristine, with cyclophosphamide, prednisone, and rituximab; SC-EPOCH-RR short-course infusional therapy with etoposide, doxorubicin, and vincristine with cyclophosphamide, prednisone, and 2 doses of rituximab
None of the patients in either group had a recurrence of disease or died from Burkitt lymphoma. However, 1 patient with primary immunodeficiency-associated Burkitt lymphoma did not have a pathologic complete response and received localized radiotherapy. Acute myeloid leukemia developed in 1 HIV-positive patient 2.5 years after the completion of SC-EPOCH-RR, and the patient died 4 months later

Toxicity

Adverse Events

Event	All Cycles (N = 155)	DA-EPOCH-R Cycles (N = 116)	SC-EPOCH-RR Cycles (N = 39)
TLS—no. of cycles (%)	1 (1)	0	1 (3)
Absolute neutropenia—number of cycles (%)			
ANC nadir <500/mm³	72 (46)	60 (52)	12 (31)
ANC nadir <100/mm³	26 (17)	20 (17)	6 (15)
Thrombocytopenia—number of cycles (%)			
Platelets nadir <50,000/mm³	12 (8)	7 (6)	5 (13)
Platelets nadir <25,000/mm³	3 (2)	2 (2)	1 (3)
Fever and neutropenia necessitating hospital admission			
Any patient—no. of cycles (%)	30 (19)	26 (22)	4 (10)
Patients ≥40 years of age—number of cycles/total number (%)	4/54 (7)	2/30 (7)	2/24 (8)
Gastrointestinal event—number of cycles (%)*			
Mucositis	8 (5)	7 (6)	1 (9)
Constipation	2 (1)	0	2 (5)
Ileus	2 (1)	2 (2)	0
Neurologic event—number of patients/total number (%)†			
Sensory impairment	5/30 (17)	4/19 (21)	1/11 (9)
Motor impairment	2/30 (7)	2/19 (11)	0/11

NA, not applicable; TLS, Tumor lysis syndrome
*All the gastrointestinal events were G3
†All the sensory-impairment events were G3, and all the motor-impairment events were G2

Treatment Monitoring

1. *Twice weekly:* CBC with differential
2. *At the beginning of every cycle:* CBC with differential and LFTs

REGIMEN

CYCLOPHOSPHAMIDE, VINCRISTINE (ONCOVIN), DOXORUBICIN, METHOTREXATE (CODOX-M) + IFOSFAMIDE, ETOPOSIDE (VP-16), AND CYTARABINE (ARA-C) (I-VAC)

Magrath I et al. J Clin Oncol 1996;14:925–934

Patients are stratified into high-risk and low-risk groups according to extent of disease and LDH at presentation

Findings at Presentation	Treatment Regimen
Low Risk	
A single extraabdominal mass or completely resected abdominal disease, *and* serum LDH <350 units/L or a concentration within institutional normal range	3 Cycles A → A → A
High Risk	
All other patients	4 Cycles A → B → A → B

High- and Low-Risk Patients

Preparation for definitive therapy:

Allopurinol; administer orally or intravenously
- *Initial dosage:* **Allopurinol** 3.3 mg/kg per dose, 3 times daily (daily dosage = 10 mg/kg)
- *Three days after induction treatment commences:* Allopurinol dosage may be decreased to 1.7 mg/kg per dose, 3 times daily (daily dosage = 5 mg/kg)
- *Two weeks after beginning induction treatment:* Allopurinol may be discontinued

Hydration with allopurinol:
3000–4500 mL/m² per day, as tolerated; administer intravenously with a solution containing at least 75 mEq sodium/1000 mL
- **Sodium bicarbonate** is added to parenteral hydration solutions in the presence of plasma uric acid ≥9 mg/dL to maintain urine pH ≥7.0

Notes:
- Discontinue urinary alkalinization after serum uric acid decreases to <8 mg/dL and before starting chemotherapy
- **Potassium** is not added to parenteral hydration solutions during the first few days of induction therapy unless serum potassium decreases to <3.0 mEq/dL
- **Furosemide** 20–40 mg; administer orally or intravenously, is used to ensure that fluid output is consistent with intake
- Diuresis is maintained for at least the first 72 hours after starting chemotherapy in the absence of metabolic aberrations or after metabolic complications have normalized

High-Risk Patients

4 Cycles A → B → A → B

Regimen A: CODOX-M
Cyclophosphamide 800 mg/m²; administer intravenously in 50–100 mL 0.9% sodium chloride (0.9% NS) or 5% dextrose injection (D5W) over 30 minutes, given on day 1, *followed by:*
Cyclophosphamide 200 mg/m² per day; administer intravenously in 50–100 mL 0.9% NS D5W over 15 minutes for 4 consecutive days, on days 2–5 (total dosage/cycle = 1600 mg/m²)
Doxorubicin 40 mg/m²; administer by intravenous injection over 3–5 minutes, given on day 1 (total dosage/cycle = 40 mg/m²)
Vincristine 1.5 mg/m² per dose (maximum single dose is 2.5 mg); administer by intravenous injection over 1–2 minutes, as follows:
- During cycle 1, for 2 doses, on days 1 and 8 (total dosage/cycle = 3 mg/m²; maximum dose/cycle = 5 mg)
- During cycle 3, for 3 doses, on days 1, 8, and 15 (total dosage/cycle = 4.5 mg/m²; maximum dose/cycle = 7.5 mg)

Hydration with methotrexate:
3000 mL/m² per day with a solution containing at least 75 mEq sodium/1000 mL; administer intravenously during methotrexate administration (day 10) and for at least 24 hours afterward. **Sodium bicarbonate** 50–100 mEq/1000 mL is added to the parenteral solution to maintain urine pH ≥7.0
Methotrexate 1200 mg/m²; administer intravenously in 25–250 mL dextrose or saline fluids ± 50–100 mEq sodium bicarbonate over 1 hour on day 10, *followed immediately by:*
Methotrexate 240 mg/m² per hour; administer by continuous intravenous infusion in 250–6000 mL dextrose or saline fluids ± sodium bicarbonate 50–100 mEq/1000 mL over 23 hours on day 10 (total dosage/cycle [not including intrathecal methotrexate] = 6720 mg/m²)

Notes:
- For logistical practicality and efficiency, parenteral admixtures containing methotrexate may include a portion or all of the fluid and sodium bicarbonate needed to meet hydration and urinary alkalinization requirements during methotrexate administration
- Methotrexate administration is discontinued after a total duration of 24 hours without regard for any portion not administered

(continued)

(continued)

Calcium leucovorin 192 mg/m^2; administer intravenously in 25–250 mL 0.9% NS or D5W over 1 hour at 36 hours after methotrexate administration began, *followed 6 hours later by:*
Calcium leucovorin 12 mg/m^2 per dose; administer intravenously in 25–250 mL 0.9% NS or D5W over 15 minutes every 6 hours until serum methotrexate concentration is <0.05 μmol/L
Note:
• Calcium leucovorin may be administered orally after completing 1 day of parenteral administration if patients are compliant, not vomiting, and without other potentially mitigating complications

Regimen B: IVAC
Ifosfamide 1500 mg/m^2 + **mesna** 360 mg/m^2 per day; administer intravenously in 100–250 mL 0.9% NS or D5W over 1 hour, for 5 consecutive days, on days 1–5 (total ifosfamide dosage/cycle = 7500 mg/m^2)
Mesna 360 mg/m^2 per dose; administer intravenously in 25–150 mL 0.9% NS or D5W over 15 minutes every 3 hours, for 6 doses, starting 3 hours after each ifosfamide + mesna administration is completed (total mesna dosage/day [7 doses/24 hours] = 2520 mg/m^2; total mesna dosage/cycle = 12,600 mg/m^2)
Etoposide 60 mg/m^2 per day; administer intravenously in 150 mL 0.9% NS or D5W over 1 hour for 5 consecutive days, on days 1–5 (total dosage/cycle = 300 mg/m^2)
Cytarabine 2000 mg/m^2 per dose; administer intravenously in 150 mL D5W over 3 hours every 12 hours, for 4 doses, on days 1 and 2 (total dosage/cycle = 8000 mg/m^2)

Supportive Care
Antiemetic prophylaxis for Regimen A, CODOX-M
Emetogenic potential on days 1 and 10 is **HIGH**
Emetogenic potential on days 2–5 is **MODERATE**
Emetogenic potential on days 8 and 15 is **MINIMAL**
See Chapter 39 for antiemetic recommendations

Antiemetic prophylaxis for Regimen B, IVAC
Emetogenic potential on days 1–5 is **HIGH**
See Chapter 39 for antiemetic recommendations

Hematopoietic growth factor (CSF) prophylaxis after CODOX-M and IVAC
Primary prophylaxis is indicated with 1 of the following:
Filgrastim (G-CSF) 5 mcg/kg per day; administer by subcutaneous injection, starting on day 13 and continuing until the next treatment cycle (ie, when ANC recovers to ≥1000/mm^3)
See Chapter 43 for more information

Antimicrobial prophylaxis after CODOX-M and IVAC
Risk of fever and neutropenia is HIGH
Antimicrobial primary prophylaxis is recommended:
• Antibacterial—consider fluoroquinolone prophylaxis; *Pneumocystis jirovecii* prophylaxis is recommended (eg, cotrimoxazole)
• Antifungal—recommended
• Antiviral—antiherpes antivirals (eg, acyclovir)
See Chapter 47 for more information

Additional prophylaxis
Give **stool softeners** and/or laxatives during and after vincristine administration

Intrathecal Medications for Prophylaxis of High-Risk Patients and Treatment of Patients with CNS Disease

Dose in Milligrams Adjusted to Patient's Age in Years (y)			Days of Administration			
			Prophylaxis		Treatment	
≥3 y	2 y	1 y	A	B	A	B
Cytarabine by Lumbar Puncture						
70	50	35	1, 3	—	1, 3, 5	7, 9
Cytarabine by Intraventricular Route						
15	12	9	1, 3	—	1, 3, 5	7, 9
Methotrexate by Lumbar Puncture*						
12	10	8	15	5	15, 17	5
Methotrexate by Intraventricular Route*						
2	1.5	1	15	5	15, 17	5

A, CODOX-M Cycles 1 and 3; B, IVAC cycles 2 and 4
*Calcium leucovorin 12 mg/m^2 orally for 1 dose at 24 hours after each intrathecal dose of methotrexate

Low-Risk Patients

3 Cycles: A → A → A

Modified regimen A: (modified) CODOX-M
Cyclophosphamide 800 mg/m²; administer intravenously in 50–100 mL 0.9% NS or D5W over 30 minutes, given on day 1, *followed by:*
Cyclophosphamide 200 mg/m² per day; administer intravenously in 50–100 mL 0.9% NS D5W over 15 minutes, for 4 consecutive days, on days 2–5 (total dosage/cycle = 1600 mg/m²)
Doxorubicin 40 mg/m²; administer by intravenous injection over 3–5 minutes, given on day 1 (total dosage/cycle = 40 mg/m²)
Vincristine 1.5 mg/m² per dose (maximum single dose is 2.5 mg); administer by intravenous injection over 1–2 minutes, for 2 doses, on days 1 and 8 (total dosage/cycle = 3 mg/m²; maximum dose/cycle = 5 mg)

Hydration with methotrexate:
3000 mL/m² per day with a solution containing at least 75 mEq sodium/1000 mL; administer intravenously during methotrexate administration (day 10) and for at least 24 hours afterward. **Sodium bicarbonate** 50–100 mEq/1000 mL is added to the parenteral solution to maintain urine pH ≥7.0
Methotrexate 1200 mg/m²; administer intravenously in 25–250 mL dextrose or saline fluids ± 50–100 mEq sodium bicarbonate over 1 hour on day 10, *followed immediately by:*
Methotrexate 240 mg/m² per hour; administer by continuous intravenous infusion in 250–6000 mL dextrose or saline fluids ± sodium bicarbonate 50–100 mEq/1000 mL, over 23 hours on day 10 (total dosage/cycle [not including intrathecal methotrexate] = 6720 mg/m²)
Notes:
• For logistical practicality and efficiency, parenteral admixtures containing methotrexate may include a portion or all of the fluid and sodium bicarbonate needed to meet hydration and urinary alkalinization requirements during methotrexate administration
• Methotrexate administration is discontinued after a total duration of 24 hours without regard for any portion not administered

Calcium leucovorin 192 mg/m²; administer intravenously in 25–250 mL 0.9% NS or D5W over 1 hour at 36 hours after methotrexate administration began, *followed 6 hours later by:*
Calcium leucovorin 12 mg/m² per dose; administer intravenously in 25–250 mL 0.9% NS or D5W over 15 minutes every 6 hours until serum methotrexate concentration is <0.05 μmol/L
Note:
• Calcium leucovorin may be administered orally after completing 1 day of parenteral administration if patients are compliant, are not vomiting, and have no other potentially mitigating complications

Supportive Care
Antiemetic prophylaxis
Emetogenic potential on days 1 and 10 is **HIGH**
Emetogenic potential on days 2–5 is **MODERATE**
Emetogenic potential on days 8 and 15 is **MINIMAL**
See Chapter 39 for antiemetic recommendations

Hematopoietic growth factor (CSF) prophylaxis
Primary prophylaxis is indicated with
  Filgrastim (G-CSF) 5 mcg/kg per day; administer by subcutaneous injection, starting on day 13 and continuing until the next treatment cycle (ie, when ANC recovers to ≥1000/mm³)
See Chapter 43 for more information

Antimicrobial prophylaxis
Risk of fever and neutropenia is HIGH
  Antimicrobial primary prophylaxis is recommended:
  • Antibacterial—consider fluoroquinolone prophylaxis; *Pneumocystis jirovecii* prophylaxis is recommended (eg, cotrimoxazole)
  • Antifungal—recommended
  • Antiviral—antiherpes antivirals (eg, acyclovir)
See Chapter 47 for more information

Additional prophylaxis
Give **stool softeners** and/or laxatives during and after vincristine administration

CNS Prophylaxis*

Cytarabine on Day 1/Methotrexate on Day 3		
Patient's Age	Cytarabine	Methotrexate
1 year	35 mg	8 mg
2 years	50 mg	10 mg
≥3 years	70 mg	12 mg

*Administer intrathecally by lumbar puncture

Toxicity (N = 41)

	Regimen	Patient's Age (Years)	% of Cycles G3	% of Cycles G4
Neutropenia	A	<18	0	97.6
	A	≥18	2.2	97.8
	B	<18	0	100
	B	≥18	0	100
Leukopenia	A	<18	0	97.6
	A	≥18	4.4	95.6
	B	<18	0	100
	B	≥18	0	100
Thrombocytopenia	A	<18	17.1	53.7
	A	≥18	9.3	39.5
	B	<18	14.3	82.9
	B	≥18	3.7	96.3
Liver function abnormalities	A	<18	24.4	2.4
	A	≥18	24.4	2.4
	B	<18	5.9	0
	B	≥18	0	0
Stomatitis	A	<18	26.8	41.5
	A	≥18	28.9	20
	B	<18	5.7	2.9
	B	≥18	3.4	0
Documented infection	A	All ages	46.6	
	B	All ages	54.5	
Fever of unknown origin	A + B	<18	46.3	
	A + B	≥18	32.4	
Septicemia	A + B	<18	22.5	
	A + B	≥18	21.6	

Neurologic Adverse Events (N = 41 Patients)

Toxicity	% of Patients
Painful disabling neuropathy	26.8
Marked motor/severe sensory neuropathy	19.5
Severe motor weakness	7.3
Mild-moderate neuropathy	29.3

A, CODOX-M; B, IVAC

Magrath I et al. J Clin Oncol 1996;14:925–934
Weintraub M et al. J Clin Oncol 1996;14:935–940

Efficacy

Complete response	95%
Partial response	5%
Event-free survival	92% at 2 years

Patient Population Studied

A study of 41 previously untreated patients with small noncleaved (Burkitt or Burkitt-like) lymphoma. Thirty-four patients (15 adults + 19 children) were considered to be at high risk by the criteria stated above. Seven patients (5 adults + 2 children) were considered low risk

Therapy Monitoring

1. *Before each cycle:* PE, CBC with differential, LFTs, serum BUN, creatinine, creatinine clearance, urinalysis
2. *During the first 3–5 days of induction therapy:*
   - *Every 4–6 hours:* Serum creatinine and electrolytes, calcium, and phosphorus
   - *Daily until normal levels are achieved:* LDH
   - *On days of chemotherapy:* CBC with differential, serum creatinine, electrolytes, calcium, and phosphorus
3. *Weekly during the intervals between treatments:* CBC with differential, serum creatinine and electrolytes, calcium, and phosphorus
4. *After high-dose systemic methotrexate administration:* Daily methotrexate levels

Treatment Modifications

Treatment prerequisites:
• Cycles 2, 3, and 4 are started, when possible, on the day that the ANC recovers to $\geq 1000/mm^3$ after prior treatment
• A platelet count $\geq 50,000/mm^3$ without platelet transfusion support is required before starting repeated cycles. If a patient's ANC recovers to $\geq 1000/mm^3$, but the platelet count has not recovered to $\geq 50,000/mm^3$ without platelet transfusion, the patient should continue to receive daily filgrastim until the platelet count recovers to $\geq 50,000/mm^3$
• For CODOX-M, methotrexate is given without regard for blood counts
• Intravenously administered methotrexate is given only if creatinine clearance is > 50 mL/min (> 0.83 mL/s)

Adverse Event	Dose Modification
Motor weakness or unremitting obstipation	Continue treatment, but hold vincristine. When symptoms resolve, reintroduce vincristine at 50% dosage during subsequent treatments
Severe sensory symptoms	Reduce vincristine dosage by 50% during subsequent treatment
Serum sodium < 130 mmol/L	Hold cyclophosphamide. Resume cyclophosphamide after serum sodium recovers to ≥ 130 mmol/L and change hydration fluid and diluent fluids to 0.9% NS
Hemorrhagic cystitis	Hold cyclophosphamide
Total bilirubin > 2.5 mg/dL (42.8 μmol/L)	Reduce doxorubicin dosage by 50%
Total bilirubin > 3.0 mg/dL (51.3 μmol/L)	Hold doxorubicin
Cerebellar toxicity	Hold cytarabine
Acute renal failure	Hold ifosfamide

NCI CTC, National Cancer Institute (USA) Common Toxicity Criteria, version 2.0. Available at: http://ctep.cancer.gov/protocolDevelopment/electronic_applications/ctc.htm [accessed December 7, 2013]

BURKITT'S LYMPHOMA • *NHL-BFM 86* **789**

REGIMEN

NHL-BFM 86 (BERLIN-FRANKFURT-MÜNSTER 86)

Reiter A et al. J Clin Oncol 1995;13:359–372

Group B Regimen: Treatment was stratified by stage into 3 arms of different intensity. All patients received a cytoreductive prephase followed by 2 alternating courses of chemotherapy as follows:

B-SRG: Stage I and Completely Resected Stage II	
3 cycles	A → B → A

B-RG: Stage II Nonresected and Stage III	
6 cycles	A → B → A → B → A → B

B-IV/ALL: Stage IV and B-ALL	
6 cycles	AA → BB → AA → BB → AA → BB

Prophylaxis against tumor lysis syndrome during the first cycle:
Hydration with 2400–3000 mL/day, as tolerated, 5% dextrose/0.45% sodium chloride injection (D5W/0.45% NS) with sodium bicarbonate injection 100 mEq/1000 mL; administer intravenously at 100–125 mL/hour (2400–3000 mL/day)

Notes:

• **Sodium bicarbonate** is added to parenteral hydration solutions in the presence of plasma uric acid ≥9 mg/dL to maintain urine pH ≥7.0

• **Potassium** is not added to parenteral hydration solutions during the first few days of induction therapy unless serum potassium decreases to <3.0 mEq/L

• **Furosemide** 20–40 mg; administer intravenously every 12–24 hours to maintain fluid balance

Note: Diuresis is maintained for at least the first 72 hours after starting chemotherapy in the absence of metabolic aberrations or after metabolic complications normalize

Allopurinol; administer orally or intravenously

• *Initial dosage:* **Allopurinol** 3.3 mg/kg per dose 3 times daily (daily dosage = 10 mg/kg)

• *Three days after induction treatment commences:* Allopurinol dosage may be decreased to 1.7 mg/kg per dose 3 times daily (daily dosage = 5 mg/kg)

• *Two weeks after beginning induction treatment:* Allopurinol may be discontinued

Cytoreductive prephase:
Prednisone 30 mg/m² per day; administer orally for 5 consecutive days on days 1–5 (total dosage = 150 mg/m²)
Cyclophosphamide 200 mg/m² per day; administer intravenously in 50–1000 mL 0.9% sodium chloride injection (0.9% NS) or 5% dextrose injection (D5W) over 15–60 minutes for 5 consecutive days on days 1–5 (total dosage = 1000 mg/m²)

Supportive Care
Antiemetic prophylaxis
Emetogenic potential on days 1–5 is **MODERATE**
See Chapter 39 for antiemetic recommendations

Hematopoietic growth factor (CSF) prophylaxis
Primary prophylaxis may be indicated
See Chapter 43 for more information

Additional prophylaxis
Add a **proton pump inhibitor** during prednisone use to prevent gastritis and duodenitis

Course A:
Dexamethasone 10 mg/m² per day; administer orally for 5 consecutive days on days 1–5 (total dosage/course = 50 mg/m²)
Ifosfamide 800 mg/m² per day; administer intravenously in 100–250 mL 0.9% NS or D5W over 1 hour for 5 consecutive days on days 1–5 (total dosage/course = 4000 mg/m²)
Methotrexate 50 mg/m²; administer intravenously in 25–250 mL 0.9% NS or D5W over 30 minutes, given on day 1, *followed immediately by:*
Methotrexate 450 mg/m²; administer by continuous intravenous infusion in 250 mL to ≥1000 mL 0.9% NS or D5W (or saline and dextrose combinations) over 23.5 hours on day 1 (total dosage/course [not including intrathecal methotrexate] = 500 mg/m²)
Methotrexate 12 mg*; administer intrathecally on day 1, 2 hours after systemic methotrexate began (total dose/course [not including systemic methotrexate] = 12 mg)

(continued)

(continued)

Cytarabine 30 mg*; administer intrathecally on day 1, 2 hours after systemic methotrexate began (total dose/course [not including systemic cytarabine] = 30 mg)

Prednisolone 10 mg; administer intrathecally on day 1, 2 hours after systemic methotrexate began (total dose/course = 10 mg)

Leucovorin calcium 15 mg/m^2 per dose; administer intravenously in 10–250 mL 0.9% NS or D5W over 15–30 minutes for 3 doses at hours 48, 51, and 54 after systemic methotrexate began (total dosage/course = 45 mg/m^2)

Cytarabine 150 mg/m^2 per dose; administer intravenously in 25–500 mL 0.9% NS or D5W over 1 hour every 12 hours, for 4 doses, on days 4 and 5 (total dosage/course [not including intrathecal cytarabine] = 600 mg/m^2)

Teniposide 100 mg/m^2 per day; administer intravenously, diluted in 0.9% NS or D5W to a concentration of 0.1, 0.2, or 0.4 mg/mL, over 1 hour, for 2 consecutive days, on days 4 and 5 (total dosage/course = 200 mg/m^2)

Course B:

Dexamethasone 10 mg/m^2 per day; administer orally for 5 consecutive days on days 1–5 (total dosage/course = 50 mg/m^2)

Cyclophosphamide 200 mg/m^2 per day; administer intravenously in 50–1000 mL 0.9% NS or D5W over 1 hour for 5 consecutive days on days 1–5 (total dosage/course = 1000 mg/m^2)

Methotrexate 50 mg/m^2; administer intravenously in 25–250 mL 0.9% NS or D5W over 30 minutes, given on day 1, *followed immediately by*:

Methotrexate 450 mg/m^2; administer by continuous intravenous infusion in 250 mL to ≥1000 mL 0.9% NS or D5W (or saline and dextrose combinations) over 23.5 hours on day 1 (total dosage/course [not including intrathecal methotrexate] = 500 mg/m^2)

Methotrexate 12 mg*; administer intrathecally on day 1, 2 hours after systemic methotrexate began (total dose/course [not including systemic methotrexate] = 12 mg)

Cytarabine 30 mg*; administer intrathecally on day 1, 2 hours after systemic methotrexate began (total dose/course = 30 mg)

Prednisolone 10 mg; administer intrathecally on day 1, 2 hours after systemic methotrexate began (total dose/course = 10 mg)

Leucovorin calcium 15 mg/m^2 per dose; administer intravenously in 10–250 mL 0.9% NS or D5W over 15–30 minutes for 3 doses at hours 48, 51, and 54 after systemic methotrexate began (total dosage/course = 45 mg/m^2)

Doxorubicin 25 mg/m^2 per day; administer intravenously in 25–250 mL 0.9% NS or D5W over 1 hour, for 2 consecutive days, on days 4 and 5 (total dosage/course = 50 mg/m^2)

Course AA:

Dexamethasone 10 mg/m^2 per day; administer orally for 5 consecutive days on days 1–5 (total dosage/course = 50 mg/m^2)

Ifosfamide 800 mg/m^2 per day; administer intravenously in 100–250 mL 0.9% NS or D5W over 1 hour, for 5 consecutive days on days 1–5 (total dosage/course = 4000 mg/m^2)

Vincristine 1.5 mg/m^2 (maximum: 2 mg/dose); administer by intravenous injection over 1–2 minutes, given on day 1 (total dosage/course = 1.5 mg/m^2; maximum 2 mg/dose)

Methotrexate 500 mg/m^2; administer intravenously in 50–250 mL 0.9% NS or D5W over 30 minutes, given on day 1, *followed immediately by*:

Methotrexate 4500 mg/m^2; administer by continuous intravenous infusion in 250 mL to ≥1000 mL 0.9% NS or D5W over 23.5 hours on day 1 (total dosage/course [not including intrathecal methotrexate] = 5000 mg/m^2)

Methotrexate 6 mg/dose*; administer intrathecally for 2 doses on days 1 and 5, 2 hours after systemic methotrexate began on day 1 and then again on day 5 (total dose/course [not including systemic methotrexate] = 12 mg)

Cytarabine 15 mg/dose*; administer intrathecally for 2 doses on days 1 and 5, 2 hours after systemic methotrexate began on day 1, and then again on day 5 (total dose/course [not including systemic cytarabine] = 30 mg)

Prednisolone 5 mg/dose; administer intrathecally for 2 doses on days 1 and 5, 2 hours after systemic methotrexate began on day 1, and then again on day 5 (total dose/course = 10 mg)

Leucovorin calcium 15 mg/m^2 per dose; administer by intravenous infusion in 10–250 mL 0.9% NS or D5W over 15–30 minutes every 6 hours for 6 doses, starting 36 hours after systemic methotrexate began (total dosage/course = 90 mg/m^2)

Cytarabine 150 mg/m^2 per dose; administer intravenously in 25–500 mL 0.9% NS or D5W over 1 hour every 12 hours, for 4 doses, on days 4 and 5 (total dosage/course [not including intrathecal cytarabine] = 600 mg/m^2)

Teniposide 100 mg/m^2 per day; administer intravenously, diluted in 0.9% NS or D5W to a concentration of 0.1, 0.2, or 0.4 mg/mL, over 1 hour, for 2 consecutive days on days 4 and 5 (total dosage/course = 200 mg/m^2)

Course BB:

Dexamethasone 10 mg/m^2 per day; administer orally for 5 consecutive days on days 1–5 (total dosage/course = 50 mg/m^2)

Cyclophosphamide 200 mg/m^2 per day; administer intravenously in 50–1000 mL 0.9% NS or D5W over 1 hour, for 5 consecutive days, on days 1–5 (total dosage/course = 1000 mg/m^2)

Vincristine 1.5 mg/m^2 (maximum 2 mg/dose); administer by intravenous injection over 1–2 minutes, given on day 1 (total dosage/course = 1.5 mg/m^2; maximum 2 mg/dose)

Methotrexate 500 mg/m^2; administer intravenously in 50–250 mL 0.9% NS or D5W over 30 minutes, given on day 1, *followed immediately by*:

Methotrexate 4500 mg/m^2; administer by continuous intravenous infusion in 250 mL to ≥1000 mL 0.9% NS or D5W over 23.5 hours on day 1 (total dosage/course [not including intrathecal methotrexate] = 5000 mg/m^2)

Methotrexate 6 mg/dose*; administer intrathecally for 2 doses on days 1 and 5, 2 hours after systemic methotrexate began on day 1, and then again on day 5 (total dose/course [not including systemic methotrexate] = 12 mg)

Cytarabine 15 mg/dose*; administer intrathecally for 2 doses on days 1 and 5, 2 hours after systemic methotrexate began on day 1, and then again on day 5 (total dose/course = 30 mg)

Prednisolone 5 mg/dose; administer intrathecally for 2 doses on days 1 and 5, 2 hours after systemic methotrexate began on day 1, and then again on day 5 (total dose/course = 10 mg)

(continued)

(continued)

Leucovorin calcium 15 mg/m² per dose; administer intravenously in 10–250 mL 0.9% NS or D5W over 15–30 minutes every 6 hours for 6 doses, starting 36 hours after systemic methotrexate began (total dosage/course = 90 mg/m²)

Doxorubicin 25 mg/m² per day; administer intravenously in 25–250 mL 0.9% NS or D5W over 1 hour, for 2 consecutive days, on days 4 and 5 (total dosage/course = 50 mg/m²)

*Doses are adjusted for patients <3 years of age. See following table

CNS Prophylaxis (Intrathecal)

A and B: Cytarabine/Methotrexate on Day 1
(AA and BB: Cytarabine/Methotrexate on Days 1–5)

Patient's Age	Cytarabine (Dose/Day)	Methotrexate (Dose/Day)
1 year	18 mg (9 + 9)	8 mg (4 + 4)
2 years	24 mg (12 + 12)	10 mg (5 + 5)
≥3 years	30 mg (15 + 15)	12 mg (6 + 6)

Supportive Care
Antiemetic prophylaxis, courses A, B, AA, and BB
Emetogenic potential on days 1, 4, and 5 is **HIGH**
Emetogenic potential on days 2 and 3 is **MODERATE**
See Chapter 39 for antiemetic recommendations

Hematopoietic growth factor (CSF) prophylaxis
Primary prophylaxis may be indicated
See Chapter 43 for more information

Antimicrobial prophylaxis
Risk of fever and neutropenia is HIGH
Antimicrobial primary prophylaxis is recommended:
• Antibacterial—consider fluoroquinolone prophylaxis; *Pneumocystis jirovecii* prophylaxis is recommended (eg, cotrimoxazole)
• Antifungal—recommended
• Antiviral—antiherpes antivirals (eg, acyclovir)
See Chapter 47 for more information

Additional prophylaxis
Add a **proton pump inhibitor** during dexamethasone use to prevent gastritis and duodenitis
Give **stool softeners** and/or laxatives during and after vincristine administration

Therapy Monitoring

1. *After the first 2 treatment courses, and then before each subsequent treatment course:* Evaluation of tumor response
2. *Daily methotrexate levels:* Following high-dose systemic methotrexate administration
3. In patients with proven bone marrow or CNS involvement, bone marrow biopsies and CSF sampling, respectively, were repeated only until there was no more evidence of disease

Notes

1. Second-look surgery was projected for patients who had residual tumors by physical examination or imaging modalities after completing 2 treatment courses
2. Most patients were treated before the widespread use of filgrastim

Patient Population Studied

A study of 319 pediatric patients (ages ≤18 years), among whom 111 patients had a diagnosis of Burkitt lymphoma. Group B included Burkitt-type lymphomas, B-ALL, and most large cell lymphomas, including Ki-1 anaplastic large-cell lymphoma

Efficacy

For 152 patients with Burkitt lymphoma or B-ALL, the probability of event-free survival at 7 years was 79% ± 3%

Treatment Group	Probability of Event-Free Survival at 7 Years
SRG (N = 42)	98 ± 2%
RG (N = 117)	79 ± 4%
IV/B-ALL (N = 66)	75 ± 5%

Treatment Modifications

Treatment prerequisites
1. *Conditions for starting treatment courses 2, 3, and 4:* Platelet count >50,000/mm³; WBC count >1000/mm³; ANC >200/mm³
2. *Conditions for starting treatment courses 5 and 6:* WBC count >2000/mm³; ANC >500/mm³
3. Minimally, a 2-week interval must elapse between the first days of 2 courses in succession

Treatment notes
1. All treatments were completed within 2–3 months for the B-SRG arm, and within 4–5 months for the B-RG and B-IV/B-ALL arms
2. Cranial irradiation was optional for patients with overt CNS disease
3. Patients without CNS disease did not receive cranial radiation
4. Males with testicular involvement were to receive radiation to the testes
5. Local radiation therapy was limited to patients with residual unresectable active disease

Toxicity

Not described

REGIMEN

RITUXIMAB + HYPERFRACTIONATED CYCLOPHOSPHAMIDE, VINCRISTINE, DOXORUBICIN (ADRIAMYCIN), AND DEXAMETHASONE (R-HYPER-CVAD)

Thomas DA et al. J Clin Oncol 1999;17:2461–2470
Thomas DA et al. Cancer 2006;106:1569–1580

Prophylaxis against tumor lysis syndrome during the first cycle:
Hydration with 2500–3000 mL/day, as tolerated; administer intravenously
at 100–125 mL/hour (2500–3000 mL/day)

Notes:
- **Sodium bicarbonate** is added to parenteral hydration solutions in the presence of plasma uric acid ≥9 mg/dL to maintain urine pH ≥7.0, but pH <8. The choice of hydration fluid and amount of sodium bicarbonate added to the fluid should NOT EXCEED the sodium concentration present in 0.9% sodium chloride injection (154 mEq/L); for example:
  - 5% Dextrose/0.45% sodium chloride injection, USP, with sodium bicarbonate 50–75 mEq/1000 mL *or*
  - 5% Dextrose/0.2% sodium chloride injection, USP, with sodium bicarbonate 100–125 mEq/1000 mL *or*
  - 5% dextrose injection, USP, with sodium bicarbonate 125–150 mEq/1000 mL
- **Potassium** is NOT added to parenteral hydration solutions during the first few days of induction therapy unless serum potassium decreases to <3.0 mEq/dL

Furosemide 20–40 mg; administer intravenously every 12–24 hours to maintain fluid balance
Note: Diuresis is maintained for at least the first 72 hours after starting chemotherapy in the absence of metabolic aberrations, or after metabolic complications normalize
Allopurinol 300 mg/day; administer orally for 7 consecutive days, on days 1–7 (longer treatment may be needed)

Hyper-CVAD (cycles 1 and 3), premedication for rituximab:
Acetaminophen 650–1000 mg; administer orally, *plus*
Diphenhydramine 25–50 mg; administer orally or intravenously, 30–60 minutes before starting rituximab

Rituximab 375 mg/m² per dose; administer intravenously in 0.9% sodium chloride injection (0.9% NS) or 5% dextrose injection (D5W), diluted to a concentration of 1–4 mg/mL, for 2 doses during cycles 1 and 3, on days 1 and 11 of hyper-CVAD (total dosage/cycle = 750 mg/m²)

Notes on rituximab administration:
- Infuse initially at 50 mg/hour. If hypersensitivity or infusion reactions do not occur during the first 30 minutes, increase the rate by 50 mg/hour every 30 minutes, as tolerated, to a maximum rate of 400 mg/hour. Subsequently, if previous administration was well tolerated, start at 100 mg/hour and increase by 100 mg/hour every 30 minutes, as tolerated, to a maximum rate of 400 mg/hour
- Interrupt rituximab administration for fever, chills, edema, congestion of the head and neck mucosa, hypertension, and other serious adverse events. Resume rituximab administration after adverse events abate

Hyper-CVAD (cycles 1, 3, 5, and 7)
Cyclophosphamide 300 mg/m² per dose; administer intravenously over 2 hours in 500 mL 0.9% sodium chloride injection (0.9% NS) every 12 hours for 6 doses (days 1, 2, and 3), for 4 cycles, cycles 1, 3, 5, and 7 (total dosage/cycle = 1800 mg/m²)
Mesna 600 mg/m² per day; administer by continuous intravenous infusion over 24 hours in 1000–2000 mL 0.9% NS, starting 1 hour before cyclophosphamide and continuing until 12 hours after the last dose of cyclophosphamide (total duration approximately 76 hours/cycle), for 4 cycles, cycles 1, 3, 5, and 7 (total dosage/cycle = 1900 mg/m²)
Vincristine 2 mg/dose; administer by intravenous injection over 1–2 minutes for 2 doses, on days 4 and 11 (total dose/cycle = 4 mg)
Doxorubicin 50 mg/m²; administer intravenously via central venous access in 25–250 mL 0.9% NS or 5% dextrose injection (D5W) over 2 hours on day 4 (total dosage/cycle = 50 mg/m²)

(continued)

Treatment Modifications

Treatment prerequisites
- Second and subsequent cycles are implemented when WBC count ≥3000/mm³ and platelet count ≥60,000/mm³ at least 24 hours after a filgrastim dose was administered

- Subsequent cycles may be repeated at intervals less than every 21 days, but not more frequently than 14 days after the previous cycle

Adverse Event	Dose Modification
On day 21 of a treatment cycle, if WBC count ≥3000/mm³, but platelet count <60,000/mm³	Reevaluate hematologic laboratories every 3 days until platelet count ≥60,000/mm³
On day 21 of a treatment cycle, if WBC count ≥30,000/mm³, but platelet count <60,000/mm³	Hold filgrastim and reevaluate hematologic laboratories every 3 days until platelet count ≥60,000/mm³
Patient age ≥60 years	Reduce cytarabine dosage to 1000 mg/m² per dose
Blood methotrexate concentration >20 μmol/L at the start of treatment	Reduce cytarabine dosage to 2000 mg/m² per dose and reduce methotrexate dosage by 50%
Serum creatinine >2 mg/dL (>177 μmol/L)	
Serum creatinine >3 mg/dL (>265 μmol/L)	Reduce methotrexate dosage by 75%
Delayed methotrexate excretion or nephrotoxicity attributable to previous methotrexate treatment	Reduce methotrexate dosage by 50–75% (commensurate with the severity of nephrotoxicity)
Total bilirubin >2 g/dL (34.2 μmol/L)	Reduce vincristine dose to 1 mg
Total bilirubin 2–3g/dL (34.2–51.3 μmol/L)	Reduce doxorubicin dosage by 25%
Total bilirubin 3–4g/dL (51.3–68.4 μmol/L)	Reduce doxorubicin dosage by 50%
Total bilirubin >4g/dL (68.4 μmol/L)	Reduce doxorubicin dosage by 75%

(continued)

(continued)

Dexamethasone 40 mg/day; administer orally or by intravenous infusion in 25–150 mL 0.9% NS or D5W over 15–30 minutes for 8 doses, on days 1–4 and days 11–14 (total dosage/cycle = 320 mg)

High-dose methotrexate and cytarabine (cycles 2 and 4), premedication for rituximab:
Acetaminophen 650–1000 mg; administer orally, *plus*
Diphenhydramine 25–50 mg; administer orally or intravenously, 30–60 minutes before starting rituximab

Rituximab 375 mg/m² per dose; administer intravenously in 0.9% NS or D5W, diluted to a concentration of 1–4 mg/mL, for 2 doses during cycles 2 and 4, on days 2 and 8 of high-dose methotrexate and cytarabine (total dosage/cycle = 750 mg/m²)

Notes on rituximab administration:
• Infuse initially at 100 mg/hour. If hypersensitivity or infusion reactions do not occur during the first 30 minutes, increase the rate by 100 mg/hour every 30 minutes, as tolerated, to a maximum rate of 400 mg/hour. Subsequently if previous administration was well tolerated, start at 100 mg/hour and increase by 100 mg/hour every 30 minutes, as tolerated, to a maximum rate of 400 mg/hour

• Interrupt rituximab administration for fever, chills, edema, congestion of the head and neck mucosa, hypertension, and other serious adverse events. Resume rituximab administration after adverse events abate

High-dose methotrexate and cytarabine (cycles 2, 4, 6, and 8)
Hydration with 2500–3000 mL/day, as tolerated; administer intravenously at 100–125 mL/hour (2500–3000 mL/day)

Notes
• **Sodium bicarbonate** is added to parenteral hydration solutions in the presence of plasma uric acid ≥9 mg/dL to maintain urine pH ≥7.0, but pH <8. The choice of hydration fluid and amount of sodium bicarbonate added to the fluid should NOT EXCEED the sodium concentration present in 0.9% sodium chloride injection (154 mEq/L); for example:
  ▪ 5% Dextrose/0.45% sodium chloride injection, USP, with sodium bicarbonate 50–75 mEq/1000 mL *or*
  ▪ 5% Dextrose/0.2% sodium chloride injection, USP, with sodium bicarbonate 100–125 mEq/1000 mL *or*
  ▪ 5% dextrose injection, USP, with sodium bicarbonate 125–150 mEq/1000 mL

Methotrexate 1000 mg/m²; administer by continuous intravenous infusion in 250 mL to ≥1000 mL 0.9% NS or D5W (or saline and dextrose combinations) over 24 hours on day 1 (total dosage/cycle [not including intrathecal methotrexate] = 1000 mg/m²)
Cytarabine 3000 mg/m² per dose; administer intravenously in 50–500 mL 0.9% NS or D5W over 2 hours, every 12 hours, for 4 doses, on days 2 and 3 (total dosage/cycle [not including intrathecal cytarabine] = 12,000 mg/m²)
Calcium leucovorin 50 mg; administer intravenously in 10–100 mL 0.9% NS or D5W over 10–20 minutes for 1 dose, 12 hours after methotrexate administration is completed (36 hours after starting methotrexate), *followed 6 hours later by:*
Calcium leucovorin 15 mg; administer intravenously in 10–100 mL 0.9% NS or D5W over 10–20 minutes, every 6 hours, for 8 doses or until blood methotrexate concentrations is <0.1 μmol/L

• Calcium leucovorin doses are escalated to 50–100/dose intravenously every 4–6 hours if serum methotrexate concentrations are:
  ▪ >20 μmol/L at the end of methotrexate administration (hour 24)
  ▪ >1 μmol/L at 24 hours after the end of methotrexate administration (hour 48), *or*
  ▪ >0.1 μmol/L at 48 hours after the end of methotrexate administration (hour 72)

CNS prophylaxis (all patients)
Methotrexate; administer intrathecally on day 2 for 8 cycles (8 doses): 12 mg/dose via lumbar puncture or 6 mg/dose via intraventricular route (eg, Ommaya reservoir; total dose throughout 8 cycles [not including systemic methotrexate] = 96 mg via lumbar puncture or 48 mg intraventricularly)

(continued)

Treatment Modifications
(continued)

Adverse Event	Dose Modification
Disease involving the stomach or small bowel	Eliminate doxorubicin during the first hyper-CVAD cycle
If high-dose cytarabine is eliminated because of adverse effects	Omit the high-dose methotrexate + cytarabine regimen, replacing it with repeated cycles of hyper-CVAD
Peripheral neuropathy	Discontinue vincristine
Proximal myopathy	Discontinue dexamethasone
Cerebellar neurotoxicity	Reduce cytarabine dosage or omit cytarabine during subsequent treatments
Tumor lysis syndrome during induction with renal failure requiring hemodialysis	Reduce methotrexate dosage
G3 mucositis	

Patient Population Studied

A study of 26 consecutive adult patients with newly diagnosed, untreated Burkitt-type acute lymphoblastic leukemia (23 patients with FAB L3 subtype; 3 patients classified L1 or L2)

Therapy Monitoring

1. *Before each cycle:* PE, CBC with differential, LFTs, serum BUN, creatinine, and urinalysis
2. *Daily during treatment:* Serum electrolytes, glucose, BUN, creatinine, total bilirubin, LFTs, LDH, uric acid, albumin, alkaline phosphatase, and CBC with differential
3. *Daily following high-dose systemic methotrexate administration:* Methotrexate levels

(*continued*)

Cytarabine 100 mg; administer intrathecally via lumbar puncture or intraventricular routes, on day 7 for 8 cycles (total of dose 8 doses throughout 8 cycles [not including systemic cytarabine] = 800 mg)

CNS treatment
Methotrexate 12 mg/dose; administer intrathecally via lumbar puncture or 6 mg/dose via intraventricular route twice weekly until CSF cell count normalizes and cytology becomes negative for malignant disease, then administer intrathecally during subsequent cycles on day 2 per the regimen for CNS prophylaxis
Cytarabine 100 mg; administer intrathecally via lumbar puncture or intraventricular route, twice weekly until CSF cell count normalizes and cytology becomes negative for malignant disease, then administer intrathecally during subsequent cycles on day 7 per the regimen for CNS prophylaxis

Supportive Care
Antiemetic prophylaxis with Hyper-CVAD (cycles 1, 3, 5, and 7)
Emetogenic potential on days 1–4 is **MODERATE**

Antiemetic prophylaxis with high-dose methotrexate and cytarabine (cycles 2, 4, 6, and 8)
Emetogenic potential on days 1, 2, and 3 is **MODERATE**
See Chapter 39 for antiemetic recommendations

Hematopoietic growth factor (CSF) prophylaxis
Primary prophylaxis is indicated with hyper-CVAD (cycles 1, 3, 5, and 7) and with high-dose methotrexate and cytarabine (cycles 2, 4, 6, and 8):

Filgrastim (G-CSF) 10 mcg/kg per day; administer by subcutaneous injection starting 24 hours after the last dose of chemotherapy; and continuing until postnadir WBC count ≥3000/mm³
See Chapter 43 for more information

Antimicrobial prophylaxis
Risk of fever and neutropenia is HIGH
  Antimicrobial primary prophylaxis is recommended:
  • Antibacterial—consider fluoroquinolone prophylaxis; *Pneumocystis jirovecii* prophylaxis is recommended (eg, cotrimoxazole)
  • Antifungal—recommended
  • Antiviral—antiherpes antivirals (eg, acyclovir)
See Chapter 47 for more information

Additional prophylaxis
Add a **proton pump inhibitor** during dexamethasone use to prevent gastritis and duodenitis
Give **stool softeners** and/or laxatives during and after vincristine administration

Efficacy

Sequential comparison of hyper-CVAD plus rituximab versus hyper-CVAD alone

Parameter	Hyper-CVAD Plus Rituximab (N = 31)	Hyper-CVAD Alone (N = 48)	*p* Value
Percent CR	86%	85%	
Median follow-up	22 months	74 months	
Induction deaths	0%	13%	0.04
Percent relapse	7%	30%	0.008
Percent 3-year survival	89%	53%	<0.01
Percent 3-year EFS	80%	52%	0.02
Percent 3-year DFS	88%	60%	0.03
Percent 3-year CRD	91%	66%	0.024

EFS, Event-free survival; DFS, disease-free survival; CRD, complete response duration

Toxicity*

Toxicities in Patients with CR (N = 21)

	Age <60 Years (N = 13)	Age ≥60 Years (N = 8)
G3/4 neurotoxicity	15%	29%
Tumor lysis in first cycle	8%	25%
Creatinine increased more than 2-fold after methotrexate	23%	12%
Infection with cycle 2	54%	38%

Infectious Complications During First Cycle (N = 37)

Febrile neutropenia	86%
Fever of unknown origin	38%
Pneumonia	32%
Sepsis	11%
Bacterial meningitis	3%
Herpes simplex virus infections	3%

Infectious Complications in Cycles After First (N = 152)

Febrile neutropenia during high-dose methotrexate/cytarabine	47–55%
Febrile neutropenia during hyper-CVAD	30–39%
Herpes simplex virus infections	8%

Events Concurrent with Thrombocytopenia (N = 152)

Hemorrhage with thrombocytopenia (all)	12%
Severe epistaxis	4%
Retinal	2%
Gastrointestinal	2%
CNS	2%
Pulmonary	1%
Antecubital hematoma	1%

Other Toxicities

Deaths during induction	19%
Cerebellar neurotoxicity	3.8%

*NCI CTC

REGIMEN

METHOTREXATE, CYTARABINE (ARA-C), CYCLOPHOSPHAMIDE, VINCRISTINE (ONCOVIN), PREDNISONE, AND BLEOMYCIN (MACOP-B)

Klimo P, Connors JM. Ann Intern Med 1985;102:596–602

Odd-Numbered Weeks: 1, 3, 5, 7, 9, and 11

Doxorubicin 50 mg/m^2 per dose; administer by intravenous injection over 3–5 minutes for 6 doses on day 1 during weeks 1, 3, 5, 7, 9, and 11 (total dosage/12-week course = 300 mg/m^2)

Oral hydration before and after cyclophosphamide administration:
32–64 oz/day on the day cyclophosphamide is administered and for at least 1 day afterward

or

Intravenous hydration before and after cyclophosphamide administration:
500–1000 mL 0.9% sodium chloride injection (0.9% NS)
Cyclophosphamide 350 mg/m^2 per dose; administer intravenously in 25–250 mL 0.9% NS or 5% dextrose injection (D5W) over 10–30 minutes for 6 doses on day 1 during weeks 1, 3, 5, 7, 9, and 11 (total dosage/12-week course = 2100 mg/m^2)

Even-Numbered Weeks: 2, 4, 6, 8, 10, and 12

Oral hydration with methotrexate:
100–128 oz/day

or

Intravenous hydration with methotrexate:
100–150 mL/hour 0.9% NS, D5W or 5% dextrose/0.45% sodium chloride (D5W/0.95% NS) injection, before, during, and after intravenous methotrexate administration
Sodium bicarbonate 500–2000 mg (sufficient to increase urine pH to 7.0); administer orally every 6 hours for 48–60 hours, starting 8–12 hours before starting methotrexate administration

Notes:
• Sodium bicarbonate may be administered parenterally to patients who require intravenous hydration (50–100 mEq sodium bicarbonate/1000 mL of parenteral fluid)
• In patients with measurable serum or plasma methotrexate concentrations ≥48 hours after methotrexate administration is completed, continue sodium bicarbonate administration and vigorous oral or parenteral hydration until methotrexate is no longer detectable

Methotrexate 100 mg/m^2 per dose; administer intravenously in 10–50 mL 0.9% NS or D5W over 5–15 minutes or by intravenous injection over 0.5–2 minutes, on day 1, *followed by*
Methotrexate 300 mg/m^2 per dose; administer intravenously in 50–1000 mL 0.9% NS or D5W over 4 hours for 3 doses on day 1 during weeks 2, 6, and 10 (total intravenously administered dosage/12-week course = 1300 mg/m^2)

Leucovorin rescue:
Leucovorin calcium 15 mg/dose; administer orally every 6 hours for 6 doses, starting 28 hours after starting methotrexate during weeks 2, 6, and 10 (total dose during each week intravenous methotrexate is given = 90 mg)

Note: For patients with mucositis that precedes methotrexate administration and for those who develop mucositis during methotrexate or leucovorin administration, increase the total number of leucovorin doses from 6–12 doses

Vincristine 1.4 mg/m^2 per dose (maximum single dose = 2 mg); administer by intravenous injection over 1–2 minutes for 6 doses on day 1 during weeks 2, 4, 6, 8, 10, and 12 (total dosage/12-week course = 8.4 mg/m^2; maximum dose/12-week course = 12 mg)
Bleomycin 10 units/m^2 per dose; administer by slow intravenous injection over 10 minutes for 3 doses on day 1 during weeks 4, 8, and 12 (total dosage/12-week course = 30 units/m^2)
Prednisone 75 mg/day; administer orally for 69 consecutive days, then taper the daily dose during the last 15 days of treatment (days 70–84)

Treatment Modifications

Adverse Event	Dose Modification
ANC ≥1000/mm^3 on a day of treatment	Administer 100% of planned chemotherapy doses
ANC 100–999/mm^3 on a day of treatment	Administer 65% of planned chemotherapy doses
ANC <100/mm^3 on a day of treatment	Delay treatment for 1 week
Thrombocytopenia (any severity)	Do not modify treatment, but give platelet transfusions for platelet count <10,000/mm^3
Creatinine clearance <60 mL/min (<1 mL/s)	Give bleomycin 10 units/m^2 instead of methotrexate on weeks 2, 6, and 10*

*If low creatinine clearance is a result of lymphoma and improves during treatment, reintroduce methotrexate

Patient Population Studied

A study of 61 patients with advanced newly diagnosed diffuse large B-cell lymphoma

Efficacy (N = 61)

Complete response	84%
Partial response	16%

(*continued*)

CNS prophylaxis:
For all patients with lymphoma involving bone marrow, starting after documented remission in bone marrow
Methotrexate 12 mg; administer intrathecally via lumbar puncture twice weekly for 6 doses (total dose/week = 24 mg)
Cytarabine 30 mg/m²; administer intrathecally via lumbar puncture twice weekly for 6 doses (total dose/week = 60 mg/m²)

Supportive Care
Antiemetic prophylaxis
Odd-numbered weeks (1, 3, 5, 7, 9, and 11)
Emetogenic potential on day 1 is **HIGH**. *Potential for delayed emetic symptoms*
Even-numbered weeks (2, 6, and 10)
Emetogenic potential on day 1 is **MODERATE**
Emetogenic potential on day 1 is **MINIMAL**
See Chapter 39 for antiemetic recommendations

Hematopoietic growth factor (CSF) prophylaxis
Primary prophylaxis may be indicated
See Chapter 43 for more information

Antimicrobial prophylaxis
Risk of fever and neutropenia is HIGH
  Antimicrobial primary prophylaxis is recommended:
  • Antibacterial—consider fluoroquinolone prophylaxis; *Pneumocystis jirovecii* prophylaxis is recommended (eg, cotrimoxazole)
  • Antifungal—recommended
  • Antiviral—antiherpes antivirals (eg, acyclovir, famciclovir, valacyclovir)
See Chapter 47 for more information

Steroid-associated gastritis
Add a **proton pump inhibitor** during steroid use to prevent gastritis and duodenitis

Oral care
  • Encourage patients to maintain intake of non-alcoholic fluids
  If mucositis or stomatitis is present:
  • Rinse mouth several times a day with ¼ teaspoon (1.25 g) each of baking soda and table salt in one quart of warm water. Follow with a plain water rinse
    ▪ Do not use mouthwashes that contain alcohols

Toxicity (N = 61)

	% G1/2	% G3/4
Mucositis	56	26
Neurologic	92	8
Cutaneous	39	3

Hematologic

Granulocytopenia (<500/mm³)	21
Thrombocytopenia (<50,000/mm³)	2
Anemia requiring red cell transfusion	20
Infection requiring hospitalization	11
Infection not requiring hospitalization	11

Endocrinologic

Transient symptomatic hyperglycemia	3
Femoral osteonecrosis	2

Other Toxicities

Disabling weakness	8
Hand and feet dermal blistering	
Overall	39
Severe	3

Therapy Monitoring

1. *Weekly:* CBC with differential, LFTs, serum BUN, and creatinine
2. *Daily following systemic methotrexate administration:* Methotrexate levels

REGIMEN

THE BONN PROTOCOL

Pels H et al. J Clin Oncol 2003;21:4489–4495

Sequence of cycles (periods of drug administration are separated by a 2-week interval)

A1	→	B1	→	C1	→	A2	→	B2	→	C2
D1–5		D22–26		D43–49		D64–68		D85–89		D106–112

Cycle A:

Hydration with 5% dextrose/0.45% sodium chloride injection (D5W/0.45% NS) with sodium bicarbonate injection 100 mEq/1000 mL; administer intravenously at 100–125 mL/hour (2400–3000 mL/day). Monitor fluid status carefully

Patients ≤64 years:

Methotrexate loading dose 500 mg/m²; administer intravenously in 25–500 mL 0.9% sodium chloride injection (0.9% NS) or 5% dextrose injection (D5W) over 30 minutes, given on day 1, *followed immediately by:*

Methotrexate continuous infusion 4500 mg/m²; administer by continuous intravenous infusion in 250–3000 mL 0.9% NS or D5W over 23.5 hours on day 1 (total dosage/cycle [not including intrathecal methotrexate] = 5000 mg/m²)

Patients >64 years:

Methotrexate loading dose 500 mg/m²; administer intravenously in 25–500 mL 0.9% sodium chloride injection (0.9% NS) or 5% dextrose injection (D5W) over 30 minutes, given on day 1, *followed immediately by:*

Methotrexate continuous infusion 2500 mg/m²; administer by continuous intravenous infusion in 250–3000 mL 0.9% NS or D5W over 23.5 hours on day 1 (total dosage/cycle [not including intrathecal methotrexate] = 3000 mg/m²)

All patients:

Leucovorin calcium 30 mg/m²; administer intravenously in 5–50 mL D5W or 0.9% NS over 10–30 minutes

Leucovorin Administration Schedule

Normal Methotrexate Clearance Anticipated	Delayed Methotrexate Clearance
At 10, 18, 24, 30, and 42 hours after methotrexate administration concludes	Every 4 hours until serum methotrexate is <0.2 μmol/L

Vincristine 2 mg; administer by intravenous injection over 1–2 minutes, given on day 1 (total dose/cycle = 2 mg)

Ifosfamide 800 mg/m² per day; administer intravenously in 100–250 mL 0.9% NS or D5W over 1 hour, for 4 consecutive days, on days 2–5 (total dosage/cycle = 3200 mg/m²)

Mesna 800 mg/m² per day; administer by continuous intravenous infusion in 250–1000 mL 0.9% NS or D5W over 24 hours, for 4 consecutive days, on days 2–5 (total dosage/cycle = 3200 mg/m²)

Dexamethasone 10 mg/m² per day; administer orally for 4 consecutive days on days 2–5, *only during the A2 cycle* (total dosage/cycle = 40 mg/m²)

Prednisolone 2.5 mg per day; administer intrathecally for 3 consecutive days on days 1–4 (total dose/cycle = 10 mg)

Methotrexate 3 mg per day; administer intrathecally for 3 consecutive days on days 1–4 (total dose/cycle [not including systemic methotrexate] = 12 mg)

Cytarabine 30 mg; administer intrathecally on day = (total dose/cycle = 30 mg)

(continued)

Treatment Modifications

Adverse Event	Dose Modification
Creatinine clearance (Clcr) <100 mL/min	Decrease methotrexate dosage by a percentage equivalent to the percentage decrease from creatinine clearance of 100 mL/min (eg, for Clcr = 90 mL/min, decrease methotrexate dosage by 10%)
G ≥3 peripheral neuropathy	Omit vincristine and vindesine from subsequent cycles. Can reinstitute at reduced dosage (50%) if neuropathy improves to G ≤2

Patient Population Studied

A study of 65 consecutive patients with newly diagnosed primary central nervous system lymphoma. Radiation therapy was deferred

Efficacy (N = 61)

Complete response	61%
Partial response	10%
Progressive disease	20%
Not evaluated	9%
Estimated time to treatment failure*	21 months
Estimated median overall survival*	50 months
Estimated 2-year survival	69% (57–80%)
Estimated 5-year survival	43% (26–60%)

*Kaplan-Meser estimate

(continued)

Cycle B:
Hydration with D5W/0.45% NS with sodium bicarbonate injection 100 mEq/1000 mL; administer intravenously at 100–125 mL/hour (2400–3000 mL/day). Monitor fluid status carefully

Patient ≤64 years:
Methotrexate loading dose 500 mg/m^2; administer intravenously in 25–500 mL 0.9% sodium chloride injection (0.9% NS) or 5% dextrose injection (D5W) over 30 minutes, given on day 1, *followed immediately by:*
Methotrexate continuous infusion 4500 mg/m^2; administer by continuous intravenous infusion in 250–3000 mL 0.9% NS or D5W over 23.5 hours on day 1 (total dosage/cycle [not including intrathecal methotrexate] = 5000 mg/m^2)

Patient >64 years:
Methotrexate loading dose 500 mg/m^2; administer intravenously in 25–500 mL 0.9% sodium chloride injection (0.9% NS) or 5% dextrose injection (D5W) over 30 minutes, given on day 1, *followed immediately by:*
Methotrexate continuous infusion 2500 mg/m^2; administer by continuous intravenous infusion in 250–3000 mL 0.9% NS or D5W over 23.5 hours on day 1 (total dosage/cycle [not including intrathecal methotrexate] = 3000 mg/m^2)

All patients:
Leucovorin calcium 30 mg/m^2; administer intravenously in 5–50 mL D5W or 0.9% NS over 10–30 minutes

Leucovorin Administration Schedule

Normal Methotrexate Clearance Anticipated	Delayed Methotrexate Clearance
At 10, 18, 24, 30, and 42 hours after methotrexate administration concludes	Every 4 hours until serum methotrexate is <0.2 μmol/L

Vincristine 2 mg; administer by intravenous injection over 1–2 minutes, given on day 1 (total dose/cycle = 2 mg)
Cyclophosphamide 200 mg/m^2 per day; administer intravenously in 25–1000 mL 0.9% NS over 1 hour for 4 consecutive days on days 2–5 (total dosage/cycle = 800 mg/m^2)
Mesna 200 mg/m^2 per day; administer by continuous intravenous infusion in 250–1000 mL 0.9% NS or D5W over 24 hours, for 4 consecutive days, on days 2–5 (total dosage/cycle = 800 mg/m^2)
Dexamethasone 10 mg/m^2 per day; administer orally, for 4 consecutive days, on days 2–5, *only during the B2 cycle* (total dosage/cycle = 40 mg/m^2)
Prednisolone 2.5 mg per day; administer intrathecally, for 3 consecutive days, on days 1–4 (total dose/cycle = 10 mg)
Methotrexate 3 mg per day; administer intrathecally, for 3 consecutive days, on days 1–4 (total dose/cycle [not including systemic methotrexate] = 12 mg)
Cytarabine 30 mg; administer intrathecally on day 5 (total dose/cycle = 30 mg)

Cycle C:
Cytarabine 3000 mg/m^2 per day; administer intravenously in 50–500 mL 0.9% NS or D5W over 3 hours for 2 doses on days 1 and 2 (total dosage/cycle [not including intrathecal cytarabine] = 6000 mg/m^2)
Vindesine* 5 mg; administer by intravenous injection over 1–2 minutes, given on day 1 (total dose/cycle = 5 mg)
Dexamethasone 10 mg/m^2 per day; administer orally for 5 consecutive days on days 3–7 (total dosage/cycle = 50 mg/m^2)
Prednisolone 2.5 mg per day; administer intrathecally for 4 consecutive days on days 3–6 (total dose/cycle = 10 mg)
Methotrexate 3 mg per day; administer intrathecally for 4 consecutive days on days 3–6 (total dose/cycle = 12 mg)
Cytarabine 30 mg; administer intrathecally on day 7 (total dose/cycle [not including systemic cytarabine] = 30 mg)

*Although vindesine had once received FDA approval for commercial use, it is not currently marketed in the United States

(continued)

Toxicity* (N = 65)

Toxicity	% Patients
G3/4 leukopenia	94
G3/4 thrombocytopenia	89
Febrile neutropenia	17
G4 infection	9
G3 infection	9
Sepsis	8
Treatment-related death	9
Ommaya reservoir-associated infections	19
G2 nephrotoxicity (transient)	14
G ≥3 mucositis	12
Deep venous thrombosis	5
Transient vasculitis	3
Transient encephalopathy†	9
Clinical peripheral neuropathy	2
White matter changes on MRI	35‡

*WHO Toxicity Scale
†With methotrexate and ifosfamide
‡Twenty of 57 patients

Therapy Monitoring

1. *Daily on days of chemotherapy:* CBC with differential, serum electrolytes, BUN, creatinine, and LFTs
2. *Weekly:* CBC with differential, serum electrolytes, BUN, creatinine, and LFTs
3. *Following methotrexate administration:* Daily methotrexate levels

(continued)

Supportive Care
Antiemetic prophylaxis during A and B cycles
Emetogenic potential on day 1 is **HIGH**
Emetogenic potential on days 2–5 is **MODERATE**

Antiemetic prophylaxis during C cycles
Emetogenic potential on days 1 and 2 is **HIGH**
See Chapter 39 for antiemetic recommendations

Hematopoietic growth factor (CSF) prophylaxis
Primary prophylaxis may be indicated
See Chapter 43 for more information

Antimicrobial prophylaxis
Risk of fever and neutropenia is INTERMEDIATE
  Antimicrobial primary prophylaxis to be considered:
  • Antibacterial—consider a fluoroquinolone or no prophylaxis; *Pneumocystis jirovecii* prophylaxis
    is recommended (eg, cotrimoxazole)
  • Antifungal—consider use during neutropenia and for anticipated mucositis
  • Antiviral—antiherpes antivirals (eg, acyclovir)
See Chapter 47 for more information

Additional prophylaxis
Add a **proton pump inhibitor** during dexamethasone use to prevent gastritis and duodenitis
Give **stool softeners** and/or laxatives during and after vincristine administration

Oral care
Prophylaxis and treatment for mucositis/stomatitis
  General advice:
  • Encourage patients to maintain intake of non-alcoholic fluids
  • Evaluate patients for oral pain and provide analgesic medications
  • Consider histamine (H_2-subtype) receptor antagonists (eg, ranitidine, famotidine),
    or a proton pump inhibitor for epigastric pain
  • *Lactobacillus* sp.-containing probiotics may be beneficial in preventing diarrhea

  Patients with intact oral mucosa:
  • Clean the mouth, tongue, and gums by brushing after every meal and at bedtime with an
    ultra-soft toothbrush with fluoride toothpaste
  • Floss teeth gently every day unless contraindicated. If gums bleed and hurt, avoid bleeding
    or sore areas, but floss other teeth
  • Patients may use saline or commercial bland, non-alcoholic rinses
    ▪ Do not use mouthwashes that contain alcohols

  If mucositis or stomatitis is present:
  • Keep the mouth moist utilizing water, ice chips, sugarless gum, sugar-free hard candies,
    or a saliva substitute
  • Rinse mouth several times a day to remove debris
    ▪ Use a solution of ¼ teaspoon (1.25 g) each of baking soda and table salt (sodium
      chloride) in one quart (~950 mL) of warm water. Follow with a plain water rinse
    ▪ Do not use mouthwashes that contain alcohols
  • Foam-tipped swabs (eg, Toothettes®) are useful in moisturizing oral mucosa, but ineffective
    for cleansing teeth and removing plaque
  • Advise patients who develop mucositis to:
    ▪ Choose foods that are easy to chew and swallow
    ▪ Take small bites of food, chew slowly, and sip liquids with meals
    ▪ Encourage soft, moist foods such as cooked cereals, mashed potatoes, and scrambled eggs
    ▪ For trouble swallowing, soften food with gravies, sauces, broths, yogurt, or other bland
      liquids
    ▪ Avoid sharp, crunchy foods; hot, spicy, or highly acidic foods (eg, citrus fruits and juices);
      sugary foods; toothpicks; tobacco products; alcoholic drinks

REGIMEN

NEW APPROACHES TO BRAIN TUMOR THERAPY (NABTT) CNS CONSORTIUM 96-07

Batchelor T et al. J Clin Oncol 2003;21:1044–1049
Herrlinger U et al. Ann Neurol 2002;51:247–252

Hydration with each cycle:
5% Dextrose/0.45% sodium chloride injection with sodium bicarbonate 50–75 mEq/1000 mL, *or* 5% Dextrose/0.2% sodium chloride injection with sodium bicarbonate 100–125 mEq/1000 mL; administer intravenously at a rate sufficient to produce a urine output >100 mL/hour and urine pH ≥7.0. Continue until serum methotrexate concentration is <0.1 μmol/L. Begin methotrexate administration after urine output >100 mL/hour and urine pH ≥7.0 for ≥4 hours

Induction
Methotrexate 8000 mg/m²; administer by continuous intravenous infusion in 100 mL to ≥1000 mL 0.9% sodium chloride injection (0.9% NS) or 5% dextrose injection (D5W) over 4 hours, every 14 days until complete response or a maximum of 8 cycles (total dosage/cycle = 8000 mg/m²)
Calcium leucovorin 25 mg; administer intravenously in 25–250 mL 0.9% NS or D5W over 5–30 minutes every 6 hours, starting 24 hours after methotrexate began, continuing until serum methotrexate <0.10 μmol/L

Consolidation (after CR):
Methotrexate 8000 mg/m²; administer by continuous intravenous infusion in 100 mL to ≥1000 mL 0.9% NS or D5W over 4 hours, every 14 days, for 2 cycles (total dosage/cycle = 8000 mg/m²), *then:*
Calcium leucovorin 25 mg; administer intravenously in 25–250 mL 0.9% NS or D5W over 5–30 minutes every 6 hours, starting 24 hours after methotrexate began, continuing until serum methotrexate <0.10 μmol/L

Maintenance:
Methotrexate 8000 mg/m²; administer by continuous intravenous infusion in 100 mL to ≥1000 mL 0.9% NS or D5W over 4 hours, every 28 days, for 11 cycles (total dosage/cycle = 8000 mg/m²)
Calcium leucovorin 25 mg; administer intravenously in 25–250 mL 0.9% NS or D5W over 5–30 minutes every 6 hours, starting 24 hours after methotrexate begun, continuing until serum methotrexate <0.10 μmol/L

Supportive Care
Antiemetic prophylaxis
Emetogenic potential on day 1 is **MODERATE**
See Chapter 39 for antiemetic recommendations

Hematopoietic growth factor (CSF) prophylaxis
Primary prophylaxis is NOT indicated
See Chapter 43 for more information

Antimicrobial prophylaxis
Risk of fever and neutropenia is LOW
  Antimicrobial primary prophylaxis to be considered:
  • Antibacterial—*Pneumocystis jirovecii* prophylaxis is recommended (eg, cotrimoxazole)
  • Antifungal—not indicated
  • Antiviral—not indicated unless patient previously had an episode of HSV
See Chapter 47 for more information

Toxicity

1. After 287 cycles of high-dose methotrexate, 12 patients experienced 18 episodes of G3/4 adverse events (unspecified)
2. Mini-Mental State Evaluation score declined from 29 at baseline to 27 at follow-up in 1 of 19 patients

Therapy Monitoring

1. *Daily during hospital admission for high-dose methotrexate:* Serum BUN, creatinine, WBC, hemoglobin, platelet count, and methotrexate level
2. *Before each repeated cycle:* 24-hour urine collection for creatinine clearance, CBC with differential, ophthalmologic examination, and CSF cytopathology if it was originally positive before repeated cycles

Treatment Modification

Adverse Event	Dose Modification
Creatinine clearance (Clcr) <100 mL/min (<1.66 mL/s)	Decrease methotrexate dosage by a percentage equivalent to the percentage decrease from creatinine clearance of 100 mL/min (eg, for Clcr = 90 mL/min, decrease methotrexate dosage by 10%)

Patient Population Studied

A study of 25 patients with primary CNS lymphoma, among whom 5 patients had evidence of ocular lymphoma

Efficacy (N = 23)

Radiographic complete response	52%
Radiographic partial response	22%
Disease progression during treatment	22%
Among 5 Patients with Ocular Involvement	
Radiographic complete response in brain	80%
Radiographic partial response in brain	20%
Resolution of ocular signs	80%

REGIMEN

MEMORIAL SLOAN-KETTERING REGIMEN (RTOG 93-10)

DeAngelis LM et al. J Clin Oncol 2002;20:4643–4648

Induction (pre-irradiation) chemotherapy

Methotrexate 2500–3500 mg/m² per dose; administer intravenously in 250 mL to ≥1000 mL 0.9% sodium chloride injection (0.9% NS) or 5% dextrose injection (D5W) (or saline and dextrose combinations) over 2–3 hours, every second week, for 5 doses on day 1 during weeks 1, 3, 5, 7, and 9 (total dosage/10-week course [not including intrathecal methotrexate] = 12,500–17,500 mg/m²)

Hydration after methotrexate:
D5W , 5% dextrose/0.2% sodium chloride injection (D5W/0.2% NS), or 5% dextrose/0.45% sodium chloride injection (D5W/0.45% NS), with sodium bicarbonate injection 50–125 mEq/1000 mL; administer intravenously at 1500–1800 mL/m² for 24 hours, then 1000 mL/m² per day for the next 48 hours

Vincristine 1.4 mg/m² per dose (maximum single dose = 2.8 mg); administer by intravenous injection over 1–2 minutes every second week for 5 doses on day 1 during weeks 1, 3, 5, 7, and 9 (total dosage/10-week course = 7 mg/m²; maximum dose/10-week course = 14 mg)

Procarbazine 100 mg/m² per day; administer orally for 7 consecutive days every 28 days for 3 cycles on days 1–7 during weeks 1, 5, and 9 (total dosage/cycle = 700 mg/m²; total dosage/10 week course = 2100 mg/m²)

Methotrexate 12 mg/dose; administer intrathecally via intraventricular catheter or reservoir (eg, Ommaya) every second week for 5 doses, weeks 2, 4, 6, 8, and 10 (total dosage/10-week course [not including systemic methotrexate] = 60 mg)

Leucovorin calcium 10 mg/dose; administer orally every 6 hours for 8 doses, starting the evening after each intrathecal methotrexate administration

Dexamethasone; administer orally every day on a deescalating dose sequence during weeks 1–6, as follows:

Dexamethasone Dose*

Week	Daily	Total per week
1	16 mg	112 mg
2	12 mg	84 mg
3	8 mg	56 mg
4	6 mg	42 mg
5	4 mg	28 mg
6	2 mg	14 mg

*Dexamethasone dose can be adjusted based on a patient's neurologic condition; can discontinue after week 6

Supportive Care

Antiemetic prophylaxis during induction chemotherapy (weeks 1, 5, and 9)
Emetogenic potential on day 1 is **HIGH**
Emetogenic potential on days 2–7 is **MODERATE**

Antiemetic prophylaxis during induction chemotherapy (weeks 3 and 7)
Emetogenic potential on day 1 is **MODERATE**

Antiemetic prophylaxis during postirradiation chemotherapy (weeks 16 and 19)
Emetogenic potential on days 1 and 2 is **MODERATE**
See Chapter 39 for antiemetic recommendations

(continued)

Treatment Modifications

None described

Patient Population Studied

A study of 102 patients with primary CNS lymphoma

(*continued*)

Hematopoietic growth factor (CSF) prophylaxis
Primary prophylaxis is NOT indicated during induction (preradiation) chemotherapy
Primary prophylaxis is indicated after postirradiation chemotherapy (weeks 16 and 19) with 1 of the following:
Filgrastim (G-CSF) 5 mcg/kg per day; administer by subcutaneous injection, *or*
Pegfilgrastim (pegylated filgrastim) 6 mg/0.6 mL; administer by subcutaneous injection for 1 dose
  • Begin use from 24–72 hours after myelosuppressive chemotherapy is completed
See Chapter 43 for more information

Antimicrobial prophylaxis
Risk of fever and neutropenia is LOW
  Antimicrobial primary prophylaxis to be considered:
  • Antibacterial—*Pneumocystis jirovecii* prophylaxis is recommended (eg, cotrimoxazole)
  • Antifungal—consider use during neutropenia and for anticipated mucositis
  • Antiviral—not indicated unless patient previously had an episode of HSV
See Chapter 47 for more information

Additional prophylaxis
Add a **proton pump inhibitor** during dexamethasone use to prevent gastritis and duodenitis
Give **stool softeners** and/or laxatives during and after vincristine administration

Whole-brain radiation therapy
Consider delaying RT in patients >60 years of age because of concern for delayed neurotoxicity
1.8 Gy/fraction per day for 5 days/week for 5 weeks, weeks 11–15 (ie, "standard radiation therapy"; total dose/course = 45 Gy)

Notes:
• For ocular lymphoma, both eyes are included in the irradiated field at 1.8 Gy/fraction to a total dose of 36 Gy in 20 fractions
• Dose rate is modified for patients who achieve a CR at the end of the initial 10 weeks of chemotherapy to 1.2 Gy/fraction, 2 fractions/day separated by ≥6 hours, for 15 days (total dose/course = 36 Gy)

Postirradiation chemotherapy
Cytarabine 3000 mg/m² per day by intravenous infusion in 50–500 mL 0.9% NS over 3 hours for 2 consecutive days, weeks 16 and 19 (total dosage/course = 6000 mg/m²)

Efficacy (N = 50*)

Response after pre-irradiation chemotherapy	
Complete response	58%
Partial response	36%

*Patients in whom tumors had not been completely resected prior to study treatment

Toxicity*			
Adverse Event	All Ages	Age <60 Years	Age ≥60 Years
Induction Therapy (N = 98 Patients)			
Any G3/4 adverse event	53%	46%	63%
G3/4 myelosuppression	28%	—	—
G3/4 nephrotoxicity	3%	—	—
G3/4 acute CNS symptoms	9%	—	—
Radiation Therapy (N = 82 Patients)			
Any G3/4/5 adverse event	73%	—	—
G3/4 myelosuppression†	46%	—	—
Severe delayed neurologic toxicities‡	15%	—	—
Leukoencephalopathy	16%	14%	19%
Death as a result of neurologic toxicity	10%	6%	16%
Patients with a CR After Chemotherapy and Standard Radiation Therapy (N = 27)			
G3 neurotoxicity	3.7%	—	—
Patients with a CR After Chemotherapy and Hyperfractionated Radiation Therapy (N = 13)			
G4/5 neurotoxicity	23%	—	—

*NCI CTC, National Cancer Institute (USA) Common Toxicity Criteria, version 2.0. Available at: http://ctep.cancer.gov/protocolDevelopment/electronic_applications/ctc.htm [accessed December 7, 2013]
†The final chemotherapy cycle may have contributed to this toxicity
‡Median time of onset = 504 days (range: 80–1540 days) after start of cranial irradiation

Therapy Monitoring

1. *Before each cycle:* PE, CBC with differential, LFTs, BUN, and creatinine
2. *Daily during hospital admission for high-dose methotrexate:* Serum BUN, creatinine, WBC count, hemoglobin, platelet count, and methotrexate level
3. *Before each repeated cycle:* 24-hour urine collection for creatinine clearance, CBC with differential, ophthalmologic examination, and CSF cytopathology if it was originally positive before repeated cycles

25. Melanoma

Ahmad A. Tarhini, MD, PhD, Amanda L. Gillespie-Twardy, MD, and John M. Kirkwood, MD

Epidemiology

Incidence: 76,100 (male: 43,890; female: 32,210. Estimated new cases for 2014 in the United States)

21.1 per 100,000 male and female per year (27.4 per 100,000 male 16.7 per 100,000 female)

Deaths: Estimated 9,710 in 2014 (male: 6,470; female: 3,240)

Median age: 61 years

Male to female ratio: 1.5:1

Stage at Presentation

Stage 0:	49.3%
Stage I:	36.3%
Stage II:	7.3%
Stage III:	3.7%
Stage IV:	3.4%

Koh HK. N Engl J Med 1991;325:171–182
National Cancer Institute, Surveillance, Epidemiology and End Results (SEER) Program
Siegel R et al. CA Cancer J Clin 2014;64:9–29
Surveillance, Epidemiology and End Results (SEER) Program, available from http://seer.cancer.gov (accessed in 2013)

Work-up

Stage	Work-up
Stage IB Stage II	Chest x-ray (optional), LDH Further imaging as clinically indicated for stage IIB, IIC patients (CT scan ± PET/MRI)
Stage IIIA	Chest x-ray, LDH. Further imaging if clinically indicated (CT scan ± PET, and/or MRI)
Stage IIIB Stage IIIC	FNA preferred, if feasible, otherwise lymph node biopsy Chest x-ray, LDH, pelvic CT and if inguinofemoral nodes positive Further imaging if clinically indicated (CT scan ± PET, or MRI)
Stage IV	FNA preferred, if feasible, otherwise lymph node biopsy Chest x-ray and/or chest CT, LDH; consider abdomen/pelvic CT, head MRI and/or PET Further imaging if clinically indicated

Notes:
1. Consider sentinel lymph node biopsy (SLNB) for stage IA with adverse features (positive deep margins, lymphovascular invasion, mitotic rate ≥ 1 mm^2)
2. Encourage SLNB for stage IB and II
3. Discuss the impact of SLNB as an important staging tool and that the impact on survival is still unclear

Five-Year Relative Survival

Stage I:	91–99%
Stage II:	56–77%
Stage III:	27–59%*
Stage IV:	18%

*Rates are not available for stage IIIA patients (with microscopic lymph node involvement) because patients have at most 4 years of follow-up

Gimotty PA et al. A population-based validation of the American Joint Committee on Cancer melanoma staging system. J Clin Oncol 2005;23:8065–8075
NCI, Surveillance, Epidemiology and End Results (SEER) Program

Pathology

Melanoma types
1. Superficial spreading melanoma 60–70%
2. Nodular melanoma 15–30%
3. Lentigo maligna melanoma 5%
4. Acral lentiginous melanoma 2–8%

Lotze MT, Dollard RM, Kirkwood JM, Flickinger JC. Cutaneous melanoma. In: DeVita VT et al.: Cancer: Principles & Practice of Oncology, 6th ed. Lippincott Williams & Wilkins, 2001

Staging

Primary Tumor (T)

Classification	Thickness (mm)	Ulceration Status/Mitoses
Tis	NA	NA
T1	≤1.00	a. Without ulceration and mitosis <1/mm² b. With ulceration or mitoses ≥1/mm²
T2	1.01–2.00	a. Without ulceration b. With ulceration
T3	2.01–4.00	a. Without ulceration b. With ulceration
T4	>4.00	a. Without ulceration b. With ulceration

NA, Not applicable

Distant Metastases (M)

M	Site	Serum LDH
M0	No distant metastases	NA
M1a	Distant skin, subcutaneous, or nodal metastases	Normal
M1b	Lung metastases	Normal
M1c	All other visceral metastases Any distant metastasis	Normal Elevated

LDH, Lactate dehydrogenase; NA, not applicable

Balch CM et al. J Clin Oncol 2009;27:6199–6206
Edge SB, Byrd DR, Compton CC, Fritz AG, Greene FL, Trotti A, editors. AJCC Cancer Staging Manual. 7th ed. New York: Springer; 2010

Regional Lymph Nodes (N)

N	Number of Metastatic Nodes	Nodal Metastatic Burden
N0	0	NA
N1	1	a. Micrometastasis* b. Macrometastasis†
N2	2–3	a. Micrometastasis* b. Macrometastasis† c. In transit metastases/satellites without metastatic nodes
N3	≥4 metastatic nodes, or Matted nodes, or In transit metastases/satellites with metastatic nodes	

NA, Not applicable

*Micrometastases are diagnosed after sentinel lymph node biopsy
†Macrometastases are defined as clinically detectable nodal metastases confirmed pathologically

Anatomic Stage Grouping for Cutaneous Melanoma

Clinical Staging

	T	N	M
0	Tis	N0	M0
IA	T1a	N0	M0
IB	T1b	N0	M0
IB	T2a	N0	M0
IIA	T2b	N0	M0
IIA	T3a	N0	M0
IIB	T3b	N0	M0
IIB	T4a	N0	M0
IIC	T4b	N0	M0
III	Any T	N >N0	M0
IV	Any T	Any N	M1

Note: Clinical staging includes microstaging of the primary melanoma and clinical/radiologic evaluation for metastases. By convention, it should be used after complete excision of the primary melanoma with clinical assessment for regional and distant metastases

Anatomic Stage Grouping for Cutaneous Melanoma

Pathologic Staging

	T	N	M
0	Tis	N0	M0
IA	T1a	N0	M0
IB	T1b	N0	M0
	T2a	N0	M0
IIA	T2b	N0	M0
	T3a	N0	M0
IIB	T3b	N0	M0
	T4a	N0	M0
IIC	T4b	N0	M0
IIIA	T1–4a	N1a	M0
	T1–4a	N2a	M0
IIIB	T1–4b	N1a	M0
	T1–4b	N2a	M0
	T1–4a	N1b	M0
	T1–4a	N2b	M0
	T1–4a	N2c	M0
IIIC	T1–4b	N1b	M0
	T1–4b	N2b	M0
	T1–4b	N2c	M0
	Any T	N3	M0
IV	Any T	Any N	M1

Note: Pathologic staging includes microstaging of the primary melanoma and pathologic information about the regional lymph nodes after partial (ie, sentinel node biopsy) or complete lymphadenectomy. Pathologic stage 0 or stage IA patients are the exception; they do not require pathologic evaluation of their lymph nodes

Expert Opinion

Tumor Thickness	Recommended Margins*
In situ	0.5 cm
≤1.0 mm	1.0 cm
1.01–2.0 mm	1–2 cm
2.01–4.0 mm	2.0 cm
>4.0 mm	2.0 cm

*The recommended surgical margin in the treatment of melanoma depends on the tumor thickness

- **Prognosis according to stage:**
  - *Stage I:* Excellent prognosis with surgical treatment alone and a cure rate of more than 85%
  - *Stages IIA and IIB:* The 3–5-year postsurgical relapse rate in patients with stages IIA and IIB is 20–30% and 40–55%, respectively
  - *Stage III:* Patients with regional lymph node involvement have a 5-year relapse rate of 60–80%
  - *Stage IV:* Continues to be associated with a dismal prognosis with a median survival of 6–9 months
- Diagnosis and initial surgical management:
  - For patients with a suspicious pigmented lesion, an **excisional biopsy** is preferred
  - When an excisional biopsy is thought inappropriate because of location (eg, face, ear, palm, sole, digit, subungual), a full-thickness **incisional biopsy** or a punch biopsy rather than a shave is acceptable
  - Patients with initial presentation of melanoma T1–4 should be treated by wide excision of the primary. Definitive surgery should include **wide excision of the primary and lymphadenectomy**. For subungual melanoma, a distal interphalangeal amputation with histologically negative margins constitutes an adequate **wide excision**
  - Consider **sentinel lymph node biopsy (SLNB)** for stage IA with adverse features (positive deep margins, lymphovascular invasion, mitotic rate ≥1/mm^2). Encourage SLNB for stage IB and II. SLNB is an important staging tool, but its effect on survival is still unclear
- **Adjuvant therapy**
  - For the adjuvant treatment of malignant melanoma, the current U.S. Food and Drug Administration (FDA) approved regimens are high-dose interferon alfa-2b (HDI), which was approved in 1995, and pegylated interferon alfa-2b, which was recently approved for the treatment of stage III disease based on the EORTC 18991 study
  - HDI is the only form of adjuvant therapy that has ever shown a consistent, significant, and durable relapse-free survival benefit in multicenter randomized controlled trials from U.S. Cooperative Groups. Estimated relapse frequency reductions of 24–38% and mortality reductions of 22–32% based on the hazard ratios for patients treated with interferon alfa versus observation, or the GMK vaccine have been demonstrated
  - Based on the EORTC 18991 study, pegylated interferon alfa-2b has recurrence-free survival benefits that seem to be confined to the subpopulation of patients with microscopic nodal disease, and therefore, it can be offered to patients who cannot undertake high-dose interferon alfa-2b treatment
- **Metastatic melanoma**
  - For metastatic melanoma, survival is estimated at less than 2% at 5 or more years. However, major improvements in patient survival have been demonstrated with recently approved agents (ipilimumab, vemurafenib) and with several agents that are still in development (dabrafenib, PD1/PDL1 inhibitors)
  - Single-agent **dacarbazine** is the only *cytotoxic* chemotherapy agent approved by the FDA for metastatic melanoma. Response rates range from 20% in early trials to 6.7% in one of the largest recent phase III trials. Median response durations range from 4–6 months. Higher response rates have been achieved with strategies involving combination chemotherapy and autologous bone marrow transplant, but with higher toxicities and no benefit in terms of relapse or survival

  Bedikian AY et al. J Clin Oncol 2006;24:4738–4745
  Chapman PB et al. J Clin Oncol 1999;17:2745–2751
  Kirkwood JM. Cancer Principles and Practice of Oncology, 1993, pp 1–16

  - **Temozolomide (TMZ)** is transformed *in vivo* to monomethyltriazenoimidazole carboxamide (MTIC), the same active metabolite derived from hepatic metabolism of dacarbazine. Temozolomide crosses the blood–brain barrier and does not require metabolic activation; it undergoes spontaneous chemical degradation to MTIC at physiologic pH. A large randomized trial compared temozolomide with dacarbazine in patients with melanoma after the first presentation of metastatic disease. The median overall survival was 7.7 months with temozolomide and 6.4 months with dacarbazine (HR = 1.18; p = 0.2). The 6-month overall survival rate for temozolomide compared to dacarbazine was 61% versus 51%, respectively (HR = 1.36; p = 0.063). The difference between the treatment groups for overall survival did not reach statistical

(continued)

Expert Opinion (*continued*)

significance (p = 0.20), the 95% confidence interval for the HR (0.92–1.52) indicated temozolomide was at least equivalent to dacarbazine. Continuous prolonged daily administration of temozolomide has been found to more effectively deplete the activity of the DNA repair enzyme O_6-methylguanine-DNA-methyltransferase (MGMT) (73% after 21 days, with low levels persisting up to day 28). In phase I studies of daily temozolomide use, including a trial in which the drug was administered for 21 days during a 28-day cycle, temozolomide 75 mg/m² per day resulted in a 2.1-fold greater exposure to drug per 28-day period than a 5-day schedule. A recent Phase III trial described temozolomide use on an extended schedule (150 mg/m² per day orally on days 1–7, repeated every 14 days). There was no significant difference in overall survival (HR = 0.99, median 9.13 months [temozolomide] vs. 9.36 months [dacarbazine]), progression-free survival (HR = 0.92, median 2.30 months [temozolomide] vs. 2.17 months [dacarbazine]),or overall response rates (CR/PR) (14% temozolomide vs. 10 % dacarbazine)

Brock CS et al. Cancer Res 1998;58:4363–4367

Middleton MR et al. J Clin Oncol 2000;18:158–166

Patel PM et al. In: Proceedings of the 33rd ESMO Congress; 2008 Sept 12–16; Stockholm, Sweden. (EORTC 18032). Available from: www.esmo.org/fileadmin/media/presentations/977/2132/Media%20briefing%20PATEL.ppt.pdf

- **High-dose aldesleukin** (high-dose IL-2, HD IL-2) is approved by the U.S. Food and Drug Administration for metastatic melanoma based on a retrospective analysis of 8 phase II trials that demonstrated an objective response rate of 16% with durable responses in approximately 4% of patients. However, the major toxicities associated with this regimen, including a capillary leak syndrome leading to hypotension, renal insufficiency, and hypoxia, has precluded its widespread application. The use of high-dose aldesleukin is currently limited to specialized programs with experienced personnel, and it is generally offered to patients with good performance and excellent organ function

Atkins MB et al. J Clin Oncol 1999;17:2105–2116

- Promising results from a single-arm study of **paclitaxel and carboplatin plus sorafenib (PC + SOR)** in advanced melanoma has led to further investigation in a randomized phase III trial as second-line treatment. The addition of SOR to PC did not improve PFS or ORR, but overall, PC showed an improvement in the disease control rate (DCR) compared to historical data (DCR 62%; ORR 11%; SD 51%)
- Agarwala SS et al. J Clin Oncol 2007;25(June 20 Suppl) [abstract 8510]
- In 2011, the FDA approved ipilimumab for late-stage (metastatic) melanoma. Ipilimumab (Yervoy; Bristol-Myers Squibb Company, Princeton, NJ) is a monoclonal antibody to cytotoxic T-lymphocyte antigen-4 (CTLA4), which is also known as CD152 (cluster of differentiation 152). *CTLA4, a member of the immunoglobulin superfamily, is expressed on the surface of **T** cells and transmits an **inhibitory** signal*. CTLA4 is similar to **CD28**, a **costimulatory protein** that is also present on the surface of T-cells. Both CTLA4 and CD28 bind to CD80 (B7–1) and CD86 (B7–2) on antigen-presenting cells (APCs). Response to an antigen begins when an APC loads a peptide on its major histocompatibility complex (MHC) antigen and presents this to a resting T cell through its T-cell receptor (TCR). The outcome depends in part on the interaction of CD80 and CD86 on the APC with CTLA4 and CD28 on the T-cell surface. An interaction with CTLA4 transmits an inhibitory signal to T cells, whereas CD28 transmits a stimulatory signal. By targeting CTLA4, ipilimumab reduces inhibitory signals and may augment the immune response. Ipilimumab's safety and effectiveness were established in a single international study of 676 patients. All patients in the study had stopped responding to other FDA approved or commonly used treatments for melanoma. Because of the unusual and severe side effects associated with ipilimumab, it was approved with a Risk Evaluation and Mitigation Strategy to inform healthcare professionals about these serious risks. A medication guide is also provided to patients to inform them about potential side effects

Hodi FS et al. N Engl J Med 2010;363:711–723

- In 2011, the FDA also approved vemurafenib for the treatment of late-stage (metastatic) or unresectable melanoma with the BRAF V600E mutation. Vemurafenib is a potent inhibitor of oncogenic BRAF kinase activity. In the BRIM-3 study, vemurafenib produced improved rates of overall and progression-free survival in patients with previously untreated melanoma with the BRAF V600E mutation. Vemurafenib resulted in a 63% relative reduction in the risk of death and a 74% relative reduction in the risk of either death or disease progression when compared to dacarbazine

Chapman PB et al. N Engl J Med 2011;364:2507–2516

- In 2013 the FDA approved the MEK inhibitor trametinib in combination with the BRAF inhibitor dabrafenib to treat patients with advanced melanoma that is unresectable or metastatic. The FDA had approved both drugs as single agents to treat patients with unresectable or metastatic melanoma. They were approved as a combination therapy for patients with melanoma whose tumors express BRAF V600E and V600K. Trametinib in combination with dabrafenib was the first drug approved for combination treatment of melanoma. The safety and effectiveness of the combination were demonstrated in a clinical trial of 162 participants with unresectable or metastatic melanoma with the BRAF V600E or V600K mutation, most of whom had not received prior therapy. Participants received either the combination or dabrafenib as a single agent. Results showed that 76% of participants treated with the combination had an OR that lasted 10.5 months. In contrast, 54% of participants treated with dabrafenib as a single agent experienced an OR that lasted 5.6 months. One of the serious side effects of dabrafenib—the development of a new squamous cell carcinoma of the skin—was reduced with the combination, consistent with the biology of the effects of these two drugs on the targeted molecular pathway. The incidence of squamous cell carcinoma of the skin in this trial was 7% with the combination compared to 19% with single agent dabrafenib. The FDA approved the combination under the agency's accelerated approval program.

Flaherty et al. N Engl J Med 2012;367:1694–1703

Expert Opinion (continued)

- The programmed death-1 (PD-1) receptor is a T-cell co-inhibitory molecule that binds to PD-1 and PD-2 ligands (PD-L1 and PD-L2) on antigen-presenting cells and suppresses T-cell activation. These ligands are aberrantly expressed in several tumors, including melanoma. Inhibiting the interaction between PD-1 and PD-L1 has been shown to enhance T-cell responses in vitro and mediates preclinical anti-tumor activity. As a result, the anti-PD-1 monoclonal antibody BMS-936558 (also known as MDX-1106 and ONO-4538) and the anti-PD-L1 monoclonal antibody BMS-936559 were developed. In a phase I dose-escalation study, the anti-PD-1 antibody BMS-936558 was administered to 104 patients with advanced melanoma. Twenty-six objective responses were observed in 94 evaluable patients (28%) at doses ranging from 0.1 to 10 mg/kg. At a dose of 3 mg/kg, the response rate was 41% (in 7 of 17 patients). The response was also durable; in 13 of the 26 patients with an objective response, the response lasted for 1 year or more. Stable disease lasting at least 24 weeks was seen in 6 patients (6%). PFS at 24 weeks was 41%. The most common treatment-related adverse events were fatigue, rash, diarrhea, pruritis, decreased appetite, and nausea. Grade 3 or 4 treatment-related adverse events were seen in 14%, and there were 3 drug-related deaths (1%) due to pneumonitis. In a separate phase I study, the anti-PD-L1 antibody BMS-936559 was tested in 55 patients with advanced melanoma. Nine out of 52 patients with melanoma (17%) had an objective response at escalating dose ranges (1 to 10 mg/kg), with 3 patients achieving a complete response. All 9 patients started treatment at least 1 year before the data analysis, and of these patients, 5 had an objective response lasting for at least 1 year. In addition, 14 of 52 patients (27%) had stable disease lasting at least 24 weeks. PFS at 24 weeks was 42%. The most common treatment-related adverse events were fatigue, infusion reactions, diarrhea, arthralgia, rash, nausea, pruritis, and headache. Grade 3 or 4 treatment-related adverse events were seen in 9%

Batus M et al. Am J Clin Dermatol 2013
Brahmer JR et al. N Engl J Med 2012;366:2455–2465
Topalian SL et al. N Engl J Med 2012;366:2443–2454

REGIMEN

INTERFERON ALFA-2B

Kirkwood JM et al. J Clin Oncol 1996;14:7–17 [Trial E1684]

Interferon alfa-2b 20 million units/m² per dose; administer intravenously over 20 minutes in 0.9% sodium chloride injection (0.9% NS), sufficient to produce a solution with an interferon concentration ≥10 million units/100 mL, 5 consecutive days/week for 4 weeks (total dosage/week = 100 million units/m²), *then:*

Interferon alfa-2b 10 million units/m² per dose; administer subcutaneously 3 days/week for 48 weeks (total dosage/week = 30 million units/m²)

Supportive Care
Antiemetic prophylaxis
Emetogenic potential is **MINIMAL**
See Chapter 39 for antiemetic recommendations

Hematopoietic growth factor (CSF) prophylaxis
Primary prophylaxis is NOT indicated
See Chapter 43 for more information

Antimicrobial prophylaxis
Risk of fever and neutropenia is LOW
   Antimicrobial primary prophylaxis to be considered:
   • Antibacterial—not indicated
   • Antifungal—not indicated
   • Antiviral—not indicated unless patient previously had an episode of HSV
See Chapter 47 for more information

Patient Population Studied

ECOG 1684 was a study of 143 patients with deep primary (T4) or regionally metastatic (N1) cutaneous melanoma who had no evidence of distant metastatic disease or significant medical or psychiatric comorbidity and who had not previously received systemic adjuvant therapy

Efficacy (N = 143)

Median relapse-free survival	1.72 years
Overall median survival	3.8 years
5-Year relapse-free survival rate	37%

Treatment Modifications

Adverse Event	Dose Modification
First occurrence of a DLT*	Hold dose until resolution, then reduce interferon alfa dosage by 33%
Second occurrence of a DLT*	Hold dose until resolution, then decrease interferon alfa dosage by 66%
Third occurrence of a DLT*	Discontinue interferon alfa therapy

*Definitions of dose-limiting toxicities (DLTs): hematologic DLT, granulocyte count <500/mm³; hepatic DLT, SGPT (ALT) or SGOT (AST) >5 times ULN (upper limit of normal)

Notes:
1. Dose reductions or delays are usually required at least once for 50% of patients during the IV treatment phase and for 48% during the subcutaneous treatment phase
2. Of patients with appropriate dose reductions, 74–90% continue treatment on protocol for 1 year or until relapse
3. Dose delays and reductions as a result of adverse events occur in 28–44% of patients during the induction phase and in 36–52% of patients during the maintenance phase
4. A response to other adverse events is determined largely by the patient and treating physician. Side effects are rarely life-threatening and should not lead to discontinuation if appropriate and proactive supportive care is provided

Kirkwood JM et al. J Clin Oncol 2002;20:3703–3718

Three U.S. national cooperative group studies have evaluated the benefit of HDI as an adjuvant for high-risk melanoma. All demonstrate significant and durable reduction in the frequency of relapse, while the first and third trials demonstrated significant improvement in the fraction of patients surviving compared to observation (E1684) or to GMK that was a promising vaccine in 1994. E1684 showed a median relapse-free survival (RFS) of 1.72 years for HDI versus 0.98 year with observation (P1 = 0.0023), and a median OS of 3.82 versus 2.78 years (P1 = 0.0237), respectively. E1694 was closed early, based on analysis demonstrating significantly increased mortality and relapse risk for patients who did not receive HDI. E1690 was inconsistent in that mortality benefit did not track with RFS benefit as it did in the E1684 and E1694 trials, but was unique in that it began before FDA approval of HDI, but was completed after FDA approval of HDI for treatment of high-risk melanoma. Not surprisingly, patients who were assigned observation in this trial, where no nodal staging by either elective or sentinel lymph node surgery was required, were associated with systematic crossover from observation to posttrial treatment at nodal relapse with HDI. This may explain why this trial showed RFS, but not OS differences that were observed in the prior and subsequent U.S. Cooperative Group trials. The analysis of each of the foregoing studies has been updated to April 2001, representing a median follow-up of 12.6 years for E1684, where significant clinical benefit of HDI versus observation is evident with respect to RFS (HR = 1.38; P2 = 0.02). Improvement of OS with HDI over observation remains, with diminished magnitude, at this most recent update (HR = 1.22; P2 = 0.18). The changes observed with late reanalysis of this study do not detract from the meaning of the mature observation published at a median follow-up of 6.9 years—considerably longer than many other trial reports. It raises interesting questions regarding competing causes of mortality, because the differences in RFS for the HDI group remain stable out to more than 15 years—and may be a result of deaths from vascular or other events, among the treatment cohort now well into the eighth decade of life (median age now >70 years). In E1694, at a median follow-up of 2.1 years, HDI continued to demonstrate superiority to the GMK in terms of both RFS (HR = 1.33; P2 = 0.006) and OS (HR = 1.32; P2 = 0.04).

Toxicity (N = 143)

	% G1/2	% G3/4
Constitutional*	50	48
Myelosuppression	66	24
Neutropenia		26
Neurologic	55	28
Depression		10
Hepatotoxicity	48	14

*Fever, chills, fatigue, malaise, diaphoresis
Notes:
1. Other adverse effects of IFN alfa-2b: anorexia, weight loss, alopecia, transient mild rash-like erythema, exacerbation of psoriasis, erythema or induration at the site of injection, impaired cognitive function, alternating episodes of manic depression
2. Rare adverse effects of IFN alfa-2b: rhabdomyolysis, delirium, cutaneous necrosis at the site of injection
3. Thyroid dysfunction (hypothyroidism or hyperthyroidism) occurs in 8–20% of patients

Kirkwood JM et al. J Clin Oncol 1996;14:7–17
Kirkwood JM et al. J Clin Oncol 2002;20:3703–3718

Therapy Monitoring

1. *WBC, LFTs, electrolytes, and mineral panel:* Weekly during induction, monthly during maintenance therapy for at least 3 months, then no less frequently than every 3 months in patients who are stable with no new complaints
2. *Other standard tests (eg, serum electrolytes, thyroid-stimulating hormone [TSH] creatine kinase [CK] levels):* Recommended at baseline and at least every 3 months during treatment

Note

Developed as an adjuvant regimen

REGIMEN

PEGYLATED INTERFERON ALFA-2B

Eggermont AMM et al. J Clin Oncol 2012;30:3810–3818
Eggermont AMM et al. Lancet 2008;372:117–126

Premedication:

Acetaminophen 650–1000 mg; administer orally 30 minutes before the first dose and as needed prior to subsequent doses of peginterferon alfa-2b

Peginterferon alfa-2b 6 mcg/kg per dose; administer subcutaneously, once weekly for 8 consecutive weeks (induction phase; total dosage/week = 6 mcg/kg), *and then:*

Peginterferon alfa-2b 3 mcg/kg per dose; administer subcutaneously, once weekly for 5 years (maintenance phase; total dosage/week = 3 mcg/kg)

Supportive Care
Antiemetic prophylaxis
Emetogenic potential is LOW
See Chapter 39 for antiemetic recommendations

Hematopoietic growth factor (CSF) prophylaxis
Primary prophylaxis is NOT indicated
See Chapter 43 for more information

Antimicrobial prophylaxis
Risk of fever and neutropenia is LOW
Antimicrobial primary prophylaxis to be considered:
- Antibacterial—not indicated
- Antifungal—not indicated
- Antiviral—not indicated unless patient previously had an episode of HSV

See Chapter 47 for more information

Treatment Modifications

Adverse Event	Dose Modification
Absolute neutrophil count (ANC) <500/mm³, platelet count <50,000/mm³, ECOG PS ≥2, or nonhematologic toxicity G ≥3	Hold dose until ANC ≥500/mm³, platelet count ≥50,000/mm³, ECOG PS 0-1, and nonhematologic toxicity G ≤1. Then, resume at a reduced dose (see below)
Persistent or worsening severe neuropsychiatric disorders, G4 nonhematologic toxicity, inability to tolerate a dose of 1 mcg/kg per week, or new or worsening retinopathy	Permanently discontinue treatment

ECOG PS, Eastern Cooperative Oncology Group Performance Status

Starting Dose	Dose Modification
6 mcg/kg per week	**For doses 1 to 8** First modification: 3 mcg/kg per week Second modification: 2 mcg/kg per week Third modification: 1 mcg/kg per week Permanently discontinue peginterferon if patient is unable to tolerate 1 mcg/kg per week
3 mcg/kg per week	**For doses 9 to 260** First modification: 2 mcg/kg per week Second modification: 1 mcg/kg per week Permanently discontinue peginterferon if patient is unable to tolerate 1 mcg/kg per week

Toxicity (N = 608)

	% All Grades	% G3	% G4
Any	99	40	5
Fatigue	94	15	1
Liver abnormalities	79	10	<1
Pyrexia	75	4	<1
Headache	70	4	0
Myalgia	67	4	<1
Depression	59	6	<1

Patient Population Studied

Included in the study were 627 patients with histologically confirmed stage III melanoma (Tx N1-2 M0) whose primary cutaneous melanoma was completely excised with adequate surgical margins and complete regional lymphadenectomy. Patients with ocular or mucous membrane melanoma, evidence of distant metastasis or in-transit metastasis, prior malignancy within the past 5 years, autoimmune disease, uncontrolled infections, cardiovascular disease, liver or renal disease, use of systemic corticosteroids, and previous use of systemic therapy for melanoma were excluded

Efficacy

	Recurrence-Free Survival		Distant Metastasis-Free Survival		Overall Survival	
	3.8 Years	7.6 Years	3.8 Years	7.6 Years	3.8 Years	7.6 Years
Number of events	328	384	304	370	262	332
Rate of recurrence-free survival	45.6%	39.1%	48.2%	41.7%	56.8%	47.8%
Median time to event	months	years	months	years	NR	years
Hazard ratio	0.82	0.87	0.88	0.93	0.98	0.96
p Value	0.01	0.055	0.11	0.33	0.78	0.57

NR, Not reported

Therapy Monitoring

Every 3 months for 3 years and then every 6 months for 2 years: CBC with differential, LFTs, basic metabolic panel, LDH, physical examination, chest x-ray, and CT scans

REGIMEN

DACARBAZINE (DTIC)

Middleton MR et al. J Clin Oncol 2000;18:158–166

Dacarbazine 250 mg/m² (initial dosage) per day; administer intravenously in 50–250 mL of either 5% dextrose injection (D5W) or 0.9% sodium chloride injection (0.9% NS) over 30 minutes for 5 consecutive days on days 1–5, every 21 days (total dosage/cycle = 1250 mg/m²)

Alternative regimen:

Eggermont AMM, Kirkwood JM. Eur J Cancer 2004;40:1825–1836

Dacarbazine 1000 mg/m²; administer intravenously in 50–250 mL D5W or 0.9% NS over 30 minutes on day 1, every 28 days, for 2 cycles (total dosage/cycle = 1000 mg/m²)

Supportive Care
Antiemetic prophylaxis
Emetogenic potential on days of chemotherapy is **HIGH**
Potential for delayed symptoms
See Chapter 39 for antiemetic recommendations

Hematopoietic growth factor (CSF) prophylaxis
Primary prophylaxis is NOT indicated
See Chapter 43 for more information

Antimicrobial prophylaxis
Risk of fever and neutropenia is LOW
  Antimicrobial primary prophylaxis to be considered:
  • Antibacterial—not indicated
  • Antifungal—not indicated
  • Antiviral—not indicated unless patient previously had an episode of HSV
See Chapter 47 for more information

Treatment Modifications

Retreatment allowed if ANC ≥1500/mm³ and platelet count ≥100,000/mm³

Adverse Event	Dose Modification
Retreatment delayed by ≥2 weeks	Reduce dacarbazine dosage by 25%
G3/4 nonhematologic toxicity	Reduce dacarbazine dosage by 50%
>2 Dosage reductions	Discontinue therapy

Therapy Monitoring

1. *Before each cycle:* CBC with differential, LFTs, mineral panel, and electrolytes
2. *Response evaluation every 2 cycles:* PE, chest x-ray, and CT scans

Patient Population Studied

A study of 136 patients with histologically confirmed incurable or unresectable advanced metastatic melanoma. Patients with nonmeasurable disease, ocular melanoma, or CNS metastases were excluded

Efficacy (N = 136)

Complete response	2.9%
Partial response	10.3%
Stable disease	17.7%
Progressive disease	69.1%
Median overall survival	6.4 months

Toxicity (N = 136)

	% All Grades	% G3	% G4
Hematologic			
Anemia	11	0	1
Neutropenia	3	1	1
Thrombocytopenia	9	4	4
Nonhematologic			
Asthenia	14	1	0
Fatigue	18	2	0
Fever	18	2	0
Headache	12	1	0
Pain	39	13	0
Anorexia	20	2	0
Constipation	29	3	0
Nausea	38	4	0
Vomiting	24	4	0
Somnolence	13	1	0

REGIMEN

TEMOZOLOMIDE

Middleton MR et al. J Clin Oncol 2000;18:158–166

Temozolomide 200 mg/m² per day; administer orally for 5 consecutive days on days 1–5, every 28 days (total dosage/cycle = 1000 mg/m²)

Alternative regimens:

Brock CS et al. Cancer Res 1998;58:4363–4367

Temozolomide 75 mg/m² per day; administer orally for 21 consecutive days, every 28 days, for 2 cycles, followed by reevaluation of index measurable disease (total dosage/week = 525 mg/m²; total dosage/28-day cycle = 1575 mg/m²)

Patel PM et al. EORTC 18032 [poster]. In: 33rd Annual ESMO Congress. Stockholm, Sweden; 2008

Temozolomide 150 mg/m² per day; administer orally for 7 consecutive days, on days 1–7, every 14 days ("7 days on/7 days off"; total dosage/14-day cycle = 1050 mg/m²)

Supportive Care
Antiemetic prophylaxis
Emetogenic potential is **MODERATE**
See Chapter 39 for antiemetic recommendations

Hematopoietic growth factor (CSF) prophylaxis
Primary prophylaxis is NOT indicated
See Chapter 43 for more information

Antimicrobial prophylaxis
Risk of fever and neutropenia is LOW
   Antimicrobial primary prophylaxis to be considered:
   • Antibacterial—not indicated
   • Antifungal—not indicated
   • Antiviral—not indicated unless patient previously had an episode of HSV
See Chapter 47 for more information

Treatment Modifications

Retreatment allowed if ANC ≥1500/mm³ and platelet count ≥100,000/mm³

Adverse Event	Dose Modification
Retreatment delayed by ≥2 weeks	Reduce temozolomide dosage by 25%
G3/4 hematologic toxicity	Reduce temozolomide dosage by 25%
G3/4 nonhematologic toxicity	Reduce temozolomide dosage by 50%
>2 Dosage reductions	Discontinue therapy

Therapy Monitoring

1. *Before each cycle:* CBC with differential, LFTs, mineral panel, and electrolytes
2. *Response evaluation every 2 cycles:* PE, chest x-ray, and CT scans

Patient Population Studied

A study of 144 patients with histologically confirmed incurable or unresectable advanced metastatic melanoma. Patients with nonmeasurable disease, ocular melanoma, or CNS metastases were excluded

Efficacy (N = 144)

Complete response	2.8%
Partial response	11.8%
Stable disease	19.4%
Progressive disease	66%
Median overall survival	7.7 months

Toxicity (N = 144)

	% All Grades	% G3	% G4
Asthenia	12	3	0
Fatigue	20	3	0
Fever	11	1	1
Headache	22	5	1
Pain	34	7	0
Anorexia	15	0	0
Constipation	30	3	0
Nausea	52	4	0
Vomiting	34	4	1
Somnolence	12	0	0
Anemia	8	1	1
Neutropenia	5	1	2
Thrombocytopenia	9	2	5

ADVANCED DISEASE REGIMEN
CARBOPLATIN + PACLITAXEL

Hauschild A et al. J Clin Oncol 2009;27:2823–2830

Premedications:

Dexamethasone 20 mg per dose; administered orally or intravenously for 2 doses: the first dose between 12 and 14 hours before starting paclitaxel, and a second dose 6–7 hours before starting paclitaxel

Diphenhydramine 50 mg; administer intravenously per push 30 minutes before starting paclitaxel

Ranitidine 50 mg; administer intravenously in 25–100 mL of 0.9% sodium chloride injection (0.9% NS) or 5% dextrose injection (D5W) over 15–30 minutes, 30–60 minutes before starting paclitaxel

Cycles 1 through 4

Paclitaxel 225 mg/m^2; administer intravenously, diluted in 0.9% sodium chloride injection (0.9% NS) or 5% dextrose injection (D5W) to a concentration between 0.3 and 1.2 mg/mL, over 3 hours before carboplatin on day 1, every 21 days cycle (total dosage/cycle = 225 mg/m^2)

Carboplatin AUC = 6 mg/mL • min*; administer intravenously, diluted in 0.9% NS or D5W to a concentration >0.5 mg/mL, over 30 minutes on day 1 every 21 days (total dose/cycle calculated to produce an AUC = 6 mg/mL • min*)

Cycles 5 through 10

Paclitaxel 175 mg/m^2; administer intravenously, diluted in 0.9% NS or D5W to a concentration between 0.3 and 1.2 mg/mL, over 3 hours on day 1, every 21 days (total dosage/cycle = 175 mg/m^2)

Carboplatin AUC = 5 mg/mL • min*; administer intravenously, diluted in 0.9% NS or D5W to a concentration >0.5 mg/mL, over 30 minutes on day 1, every 21 days (total dose/cycle calculated to produce an AUC = 5 mg/mL • min*)

*Carboplatin dose is based on a formula described by Calvert et al. to achieve a target area under the plasma concentration versus time curve (AUC)

$$\text{Total Carboplatin Dose (mg)} = (\text{target AUC}) \times (\text{GFR} + 25)$$

In practice, creatinine clearance (Clcr) is used in place of glomerular filtration rate (GFR). Clcr can be estimated from the equation of Cockcroft and Gault, thus:

$$\text{For males, Clcr} = \frac{(140 - \text{age [years]}) \times \text{body weight (kg)}}{72 \times (\text{Serum creatinine [mg/dL]})}$$

$$\text{For females, Clcr} = \frac{(140 - \text{age [years]}) \times \text{body weight (kg)}}{72 \times (\text{Serum creatinine [mg/dL]})} \times 0.85$$

Note: A carboplatin dose calculated with an IDMS-measured serum creatinine result using the Calvert formula could exceed an expected exposure (AUC) and result in increased drug-related toxicity. The FDA recommends capping an estimated GFR at 125 mL/min for any targeted AUC value. No greater estimated GFR values should be used [online] May 23, 2013. Available from: http://www.fda.gov/AboutFDA/CentersOffices/OfficeofMedicalProductsandTobacco/CDER/ucm228974.htm [accessed February 26, 2014]

Notes:

1. If paclitaxel is discontinued because of hypersensitivity, carboplatin may be continued

2. If carboplatin is discontinued because of hypersensitivity, tinnitus, or hearing loss, paclitaxel may be continued

3. After 4 cycles of chemotherapy, the dose of both chemotherapy agents will be reduced to carboplatin AUC of = 5 mg/mL • min and paclitaxel 175 mg/m^2. Patients who had a dose reduction during the first 4 chemotherapy cycles will continue at reduced doses. There is no additional dose reduction at cycle 5; a second dose reduction would be triggered by an occurrence of toxicity

4. In the absence of unacceptable toxicity, patients may continue to receive chemotherapy until disease progression. After completing 10 cycles of chemotherapy, carboplatin and paclitaxel may be discontinued at the discretion of a treating physician

Supportive Care
Antiemetic prophylaxis
Emetogenic potential is **HIGH** *with potential for delayed symptoms*
See Chapter 39 for antiemetic recommendations

Hematopoietic growth factor (CSF) prophylaxis
Primary prophylaxis is indicated with one of the following:

Filgrastim (G-CSF) 5 mcg/kg per day by subcutaneous injection, *or*

Pegfilgrastim (pegylated filgrastim) 6 mg/0.6 mL by subcutaneous injection for 1 dose

• Begin use from 24–72 hours after myelosuppressive chemotherapy is completed

See Chapter 43 for more information

Antimicrobial prophylaxis
Risk of fever and neutropenia is LOW
See Chapter 47 for more information

Dose Modifications

Adverse Event	Dose Modification
If carboplatin target dose is an AUC = 6 mg/mL · min and paclitaxel dose is 225 mg/m² and one of the following occurs: • G4 neutropenia (ANC <500/mm³) lasting >7 days • G4 neutropenia (ANC <500/mm³) with fever (≥38°C [≥100.5°F]) • G4 thrombocytopenia (<25,000/mm³) • Lack of ANC or platelet count recovery to pretreatment levels by day 28 of each cycle • Any G3/4 nonhematologic toxicity (including neuropathy) attributed to carboplatin or paclitaxel, with the exception of G4 hypersensitivity reactions	Reduce carboplatin dose to AUC = 5 mg/mL · min and paclitaxel dose to 175 mg/m² on the same administration schedule *Note:* This dose reduction is permanent. Do not increase doses during subsequent cycles
If carboplatin target dose is an AUC = 5 mg/mL · min and paclitaxel dose is 175 mg/m² and one of the following occurs: • G4 neutropenia (ANC <500/mm³) lasting >7 days • G4 neutropenia (ANC <500/mm³) with fever (≥38°C [≥100.5°F]) • G4 thrombocytopenia (<25,000/mm³) • Lack of ANC or platelet count recovery to pretreatment levels by day 28 of each cycle • Any G3/4 nonhematologic toxicity (including neuropathy) attributed to carboplatin or paclitaxel, with the exception of G4 hypersensitivity reaction	Reduce carboplatin dose to AUC = 4 mg/mL · min and paclitaxel dose to 125 mg/m² on the same administration schedule *Note:* This dose reduction is permanent. Do not increase doses during subsequent cycles *Note:* If any of the criteria for dose reduction are met after this second dose reduction, discontinue carboplatin and paclitaxel
G4 hypersensitivity reactions to either paclitaxel or carboplatin	Discontinue the agent responsible for the hypersensitivity reaction *Note:* Continue the remaining chemotherapy agent at the same dose and administration schedule, in the absence of the discontinued agent

Toxicity (N = 134)

Adverse Event	% G3	% G4
Any event	31%	39%
Hematologic events	25%	34%
Neutrophils	13%	32%
Platelets	9%	3%
Hemoglobin	12%	2%
Infection	11%	4%
Febrile neutropenia	5%	2%
Constitutional symptoms	11%	2%
Fatigue	8%	2%
Gastrointestinal	12%	2%
Diarrhea	3%	0
Metabolic/laboratory	6%	5%
Lipase	1%	2%
Neurology	19%	2%
Neuropathy, sensory	13%	1%
Pain	16%	2%

Patient Population Studied

A study of 270 patients with unresectable stages III/IV melanoma with disease progression on a dacarbazine- or temozolomide-containing regimen. Prior adjuvant immunotherapy was allowed. Patients with active brain metastases were excluded

Efficacy (N = 135)

Response	N (%)
CR	0
PR	15 (11%)
SD	69 (51%)
PD	48 (36%)
Not evaluated	3 (2%)
Median PFS	17.9 weeks
Median OS	42.0 weeks

Therapy Monitoring

1. *Before each cycle:* CBC with differential, serum sodium, potassium, BUN, creatinine, glucose, SGOT (AST), SGPT (ALT), total bilirubin, alkaline phosphatase, LDH, albumin, amylase, lipase
2. *Response evaluation:* Every 2 cycles

ADVANCED/UNRESECTABLE MELANOMA REGIMEN

IPILIMUMAB

Hodi FS et al. N Engl J Med 2010;363:711–723

Ipilimumab 3 mg; administer intravenously, diluted in 0.9% sodium chloride injection or 5% dextrose injection to a concentration between 1 and 2 mg/mL, over 90 minutes, once every 3 weeks, for a total of 4 doses (total dosage/3-week cycle = 3 mg/kg)

Note: Adverse events associated with the administration of ipilimumab consist primarily of reactions that are immune in nature. Almost all immune-related adverse events can be managed with supportive care or corticosteroids. Corticosteroids do not appear to adversely affect patients who had an immune-related adverse event or alter objective antitumor responses. Glucocorticoids do not appear to alter the activity of activated CD8+ cells, and, therefore, may explain this unique characteristic of CTLA4 inhibition. Rash and colitis are reported most often during early use, whereas hypophysitis is reported with later doses. Ipilimumab immune-related adverse events are dose-dependent in incidence, and occurred more frequently after 10-mg/kg doses than with lower dosages

Patient Population Studied

Patients with a diagnosis of unresectable stage III or IV melanoma who had previously received therapy, including one or more of the following: dacarbazine, temozolomide, fotemustine, carboplatin, or aldesleukin. Other inclusion criteria were: Eastern Cooperative Oncology Group performance status of 0 or 1, and positive status for HLA-A*0201. Exclusion criteria included long-term use of systemic corticosteroids

Dose Modifications

Adverse Event	Dose Modification
Note: Among almost 3000 patients treated with ipilimumab, approximately 60% reported an adverse immune-related event; however, only 15% reported a serious adverse immune-related event	
Dermatologic Immune-Related Adverse Event	
Transient G1/2 skin rash	Continue therapy and treat symptoms with antihistamines or similar
G1/2 skin rash persisting >1–2 weeks	Administer topical or systemic corticosteroids
G3/4 skin rash	Administer intravenous corticosteroids until control is achieved
Stevens-Johnson syndrome, toxic epidermal necrolysis, or rash complicated by full-thickness dermal ulceration; or necrotic, bullous, or hemorrhagic manifestations; or erythema Multiforme	Permanently discontinue ipilimumab. Administer systemic glucocorticoid at a dose equivalent to 1–2 mg/kg per day of prednisone. When dermatitis is controlled, corticosteroid dose tapering toward discontinuation should occur over a period of at least 1 month
Nondermatologic Immune-Related Adverse Events	
Nondermatologic G1 toxicities	Continue therapy and treat symptoms
G2 enterocolitis	Withhold scheduled ipilimumab doses; administer antidiarrheal treatment and, if symptoms persist for >1 week, initiate systemic glucocorticoid at a dose equivalent to 0.5 mg/kg per day prednisone. If toxicities resolve to G ≤1, and if patient is receiving >7.5 mg prednisone per day or another glucocorticoid at an equivalent daily dose, resume ipilimumab at a dose of 3 mg/kg every 3 weeks until all 4 planned ipilimumab doses are administered, or 16 weeks after the first dose was given have elapsed, whichever occurs earlier. If toxicity does not improve to G ≤1, discontinue treatment permanently
G2 hepatotoxicity: aspartate aminotransferase (AST) or alanine aminotransferase (ALT) >3–5 times the ULN, or total bilirubin >1.5–3 times the ULN, or alkaline phosphatase >2.5–5 times the ULN	Withhold scheduled ipilimumab doses until toxicity improves to G ≤1. If toxicities resolve to G ≤1, and if patient is receiving >7.5 mg prednisone per day or another glucocorticoid at an equivalent daily dose, resume ipilimumab at a dose of 3 mg/kg every 3 weeks until all 4 planned ipilimumab doses are administered, or 16 weeks after the first dose was given have elapsed, whichever occurs earlier. If toxicity does not improve to G ≤1, discontinue treatment permanently
G2 neuropathy (not interfering with daily activities)	
G2 immune-mediated adverse reaction other than enterocolitis or symptomatic endocrinopathy	

(continued)

Dose Modifications (continued)

Adverse Event	Dose Modification
G2 immune-mediated endocrinopathies	Withhold scheduled dose of ipilimumab until toxicity improves to G ≤1. If toxicities resolve to G ≤1, and if patient is receiving less than 7.5 mg prednisone or equivalent per day, resume ipilimumab at a dose of 3 mg/kg every 3 weeks until administration of all 4 planned doses or 16 weeks from first dose have elapsed, whichever occurs earlier. If toxicity does not improve to G ≤1, discontinue treatment permanently. **Initiate appropriate hormone replacement therapy**
G2 immune-mediated ocular disease	Withhold scheduled dose of ipilimumab. If toxicities resolve to G ≤1, and if patient is receiving less than 7.5 mg prednisone or equivalent per day, resume ipilimumab at a dose of 3 mg/kg every 3 weeks until administration of all 4 planned doses or 16 weeks from first dose have elapsed, whichever occurs earlier. If toxicity does not improve to G≤1, discontinue treatment permanently. **Administer corticosteroid eye drops to patients who develop uveitis, iritis, or episcleritis**
Persistent G2 immune-mediated adverse reaction, or symptomatic endocrinopathy, or inability to reduce corticosteroid dose to 7.5 mg prednisone per day, or another glucocorticoid at an equivalent daily dose

Failure to complete full treatment course within 16 weeks after administration of first dose of ipilimumab | Permanently discontinue ipilimumab |
G3/4 immune-mediated colitis with abdominal pain, fever, ileus, or peritoneal signs; increase in stool frequency (≥7 over baseline); or stool incontinence, need for intravenous hydration for >24 hours, gastrointestinal hemorrhage, or gastrointestinal perforation	Permanently discontinue ipilimumab and initiate systemic corticosteroids at a dose of 1–2 mg/kg of prednisone per day or another glucocorticoid at an equivalent daily dose. Upon improvement to G ≤1, initiate corticosteroid taper and continue to taper over at least 1 month. In clinical trials, rapid corticosteroid tapering resulted in recurrence or worsening symptoms of enterocolitis in some patients
G3/4 hepatotoxicity: aspartate aminotransferase (AST) or alanine aminotransferase (ALT) >5 times the ULN, or total bilirubin >3 times the ULN, or alkaline phosphatase >5 times the ULN	Permanently discontinue ipilimumab and administer systemic corticosteroids at a dose of 1–2 mg/kg of prednisone per day or another glucocorticoid at an equivalent daily dose. When liver function tests show sustained improvement or return to baseline, initiate corticosteroid tapering and continue to taper over 1 month. During clinical development, **mycophenolate** treatment was administered to patients who had persistent severe hepatitis despite high-dose corticosteroids
G3/4 motor or sensory neuropathy (interfering with daily activities), Guillain-Barré syndrome, or myasthenia gravis	Permanently discontinue ipilimumab. Institute medical intervention as appropriate for management of severe neuropathy. Consider initiation of systemic corticosteroids at a dose of 1–2 mg/kg of prednisone per day or another glucocorticoid at an equivalent daily dose for severe neuropathies
G3/4 immune-mediated endocrinopathy	Permanently discontinue ipilimumab. Initiate systemic corticosteroids at a dose of 1–2 mg/kg of prednisone per day or another glucocorticoid at an equivalent daily dose, and **initiate appropriate hormone replacement therapy**
G3/4 immune-mediated ocular disease or disease that is unresponsive to topical immunosuppressive therapy (conjunctivitis, blepharitis, episcleritis, scleritis)

G3/4 immune-mediated reactions involving any organ system (eg, nephritis, pneumonitis, pancreatitis, noninfectious myocarditis, angiopathy, temporal arteritis, vasculitis, polymyalgia rheumatica, leukocytoclastic vasculitis, or arthritis) | Permanently discontinue ipilimumab |

ULN, Upper limit of normal

Efficacy (N = 137)

Median overall survival	10.1 months (95% CI, 8.0–13.8)
Rate of overall survival at 12 months	45.6%
Rate of overall survival at 18 months	33.2%
Rate of overall survival at 24 months	23.5%
Objective response[*,†]	10.9%
Complete response[†]	1.5%
Partial response[†]	9.5%
Stable disease[†]	17.5%

Reinduction (n = 8)

Complete response	12.5% (1/8)
Partial response	25% (2/8)
Stable disease	37.5% (3/8)

*Responses to ipilimumab continued to improve beyond week 24: 2 patients with SD improved to a PR, and 3 patients with a PR improved to a CR. Among 31 patients given reinduction therapy with ipilimumab, 21 patients achieved a CR, PR, or SD
†Duration of response: 60.0% maintained an objective response for at least 2 years (26.5–44 months, ongoing)

Toxicity (N = 131)

Adverse Event	Total % (All Grades)	% G3	% G4
Any event	96.9	37.4	8.4
Any drug-related event	80.2	19.1	3.8
Gastrointestinal disorders			
Diarrhea	32.8	5.3	0
Nausea	35.1	2.3	0
Constipation	20.6	2.3	0
Vomiting	23.7	2.3	0
Abdominal pain	15.3	1.5	0
Other			
Fatigue	42.0	6.9	0
Decrease appetite	26.7	1.5	0
Pyrexia	12.2	0	0
Headache	14.5	2.3	0
Cough	16.0	0	0
Dyspnea	14.5	3.1	0.8
Anemia	11.5	3.1	0
Any immune-related event			
Any immune-related event	61.1	12.2	2.3
Dermatologic	43.5	1.5	0
Pruritus	24.4	0	0
Rash	19.1	0.8	0
Vitiligo	2.3	0	0
Gastrointestinal	29.0	7.6	0
Diarrhea	27.5	4.6	0
Colitis	7.6	5.3	0
Endocrine	7.6	2.3	1.5
Hypothyroidism	1.5	0	0
Hypopituitarism	2.3	0.8	0.8
Hypophysitis	1.5	1.5	0
Adrenal insufficiency	1.5	0	0

Long-term adverse effects in survivors for >2 years (N = 94)

Injection-site reactions	17%
Vitiligo	12.8%
Proctocolitis with rectal pain	4.3%
Endocrine immune-related adverse event*	8.5%

*Required hormone-replacement therapy

Therapy Monitoring	Toxicity (N = 131) (*continued*)
1. Monitor liver function tests (LFTs), thyroid function tests (TFTs) and clinical chemistries at the start of treatment, before each dose, and as clinically indicated based on symptoms 2. Monitor patients for signs and symptoms of enterocolitis (diarrhea, abdominal pain, mucus or blood in stool, with or without fever) and bowel perforation 3. Monitor patients for signs and symptoms of dermatitis 4. Monitor for symptoms of motor or sensory neuropathy 5. Monitor patients for clinical signs and symptoms of hypophysitis, adrenal insufficiency, and hyper- or hypothyroidism. Patients may present with fatigue, headache, mental status changes, abdominal pain, unusual bowel habits, and hypotension, or nonspecific symptoms that may resemble other causes such as brain metastasis or underlying disease 6. Imaging studies (enlargement of the pituitary gland) may be considered in the diagnosis of hypophysitis 7. Endoscopy may be considered for persistent or severe gastrointestinal symptoms	*Toxicity—General Notes:* 1. All immune-related events occurred during the induction and reinduction periods 2. Median time to the resolution of immune-related adverse events of G2–4 was 4.9 weeks (95% CI, 3.1–6.4) 3. After administration of corticosteroids, median time to resolution of diarrhea G ≥2 was 2.3 weeks for 14 of 15 patients 4. In addition to corticosteroids, 4 patients received infliximab (antitumor necrosis factor-α antibody) for diarrhea G ≥3 or colitis 5. Ongoing events in 94 persons who survived ≥2 years included rash, pruritus, diarrhea, anorexia, and fatigue, generally G1/2 (5–15% of patients) and G3 leukocytosis (1 patient) 6. There were 14 deaths related to the study drugs (2.1%), of which 7 were associated with immune-related adverse events *Toxicity—Specific Notes:* *Skin:* 1. Rash is the most common immune related toxicity associated with ipilimumab (incidence ≈20%) 2. Median time to onset of moderate, severe, or life-threatening immune-mediated dermatitis was 3.1 weeks (range: days to 17.3 weeks after initiation) *Gastrointestinal:* 1. Most common serious adverse event affects the lower gastrointestinal tract and manifests as diarrhea and/or intestinal bleeding 2. Serious lower intestinal toxicity was reported in ≈13% of patients treated at 10 mg ipilimumab/kg of body weight 3. *Onset of diarrhea occurred within first 12 weeks after starting treatment, and was generally reversible* *Hepatic:* 1. Immune-related hepatotoxicity consists of elevated LFTs and immune hepatitis 2. Patients with right upper quadrant pain, nausea, or vomiting should have LFTs evaluated immediately, although hepatotoxicity can occur in the absence of symptoms 3. In patients with hepatotoxicity, rule out infectious or malignant causes and increase frequency of LFT monitoring until resolution *Endocrine:* 1. Most patients with hypophysitis/hypopituitarism present with headache; however, visual disturbances, fatigue, confusion, and impotency are common symptoms 2. Median time to onset of moderate-to-severe immune-mediated endocrinopathy was 11 weeks (range: days to 19.3 weeks after initiation) 3. Of 21 patients with moderate to life-threatening endocrinopathy, 17 required long-term hormone replacement therapy, most commonly adrenal (n = 10) and thyroid (n = 13) replacement *Neurologic:* 1. Myasthenia gravis and cases of Guillain-Barré syndrome have been reported in association with ipilimumab use 2. Monitor for symptoms of motor and sensory neuropathy

ADVANCED/UNRESECTABLE MELANOMA REGIMEN

VEMURAFENIB

Chapman PB et al. N Engl J Med 2011;364:2507–2516

Vemurafenib 960 mg/dose; administer orally, twice daily without regard to food, continually (total dose/week = 13,440 mg)

Supportive Care
Antiemetic prophylaxis
Emetogenic potential is **MINIMAL–LOW**
See Chapter 39 for antiemetic recommendations

Hematopoietic growth factor (CSF) prophylaxis
Primary prophylaxis is NOT indicated
See Chapter 43 for more information

Antimicrobial prophylaxis
Risk of fever and neutropenia is LOW
  Antimicrobial primary prophylaxis to be considered:
  • Antibacterial—not indicated
  • Antifungal—not indicated
  • Antiviral—not indicated unless patient previously had an episode of HSV
See Chapter 47 for more information

Toxicity

Adverse Event	Dose Modification
G1 or G2 (tolerable)	None; maintain dose at 960 mg twice daily
G2 (intolerable) or G3	Hold dose until G ≤1, then resume vemurafenib at 720 mg twice daily. If the adverse event recurs, hold dose until G ≤1, then further reduce the vemurafenib dose to 480 mg twice daily. If the adverse event occurs a third time, permanently discontinue vemurafenib
G4	Discontinue permanently or hold dose until G ≤1 and then resume vemurafenib at 480 mg twice daily. If the adverse event recurs, discontinue permanently
Cutaneous squamous cell carcinoma	None; maintain dose at 960 mg twice daily; resect lesion

Patient Population Studied

The study evaluated 337 patients with unresectable, previously untreated stage IIIC or stage IV melanoma that tested positive for the BRAF V600E mutation. Patients were excluded if they had a history of cancer within the past 5 years (except basal or squamous cell carcinoma of the skin or carcinoma of the cervix), metastases to the central nervous system (unless such metastases were definitively treated more than 3 months previously with no progression and no requirement for continued glucocorticoid therapy), or if they were on any other concomitant anticancer therapy

Therapy Monitoring

1. *At baseline:* Contrast CT or MRI of the brain, chest, abdomen, pelvis, and other anatomical regions as clinically indicated; physical and dermatologic examination; electrocardiography; CBC with differential; LFTs; basic metabolic panel; and LDH
2. *Every 3 weeks:* Physical examination, CBC with differential, LFTs, basic metabolic panel, and LDH
3. *Every 6 weeks:* Electrocardiography
4. Tumor assessments are performed at baseline, at weeks 6 and 12, and every 9 weeks thereafter

Therapy Modifications

Dose Levels	Vemurafenib Dose
Initial dose	960 mg twice daily
First dose reduction	720 mg twice daily
Second dose reduction	480 mg twice daily

Efficacy

Overall Survival (N = 336)

Hazard ratio	0.37
p Value	<0.001
6 months OS	84%

Progression-Free Survival (N = 275)

Hazard ratio	0.26
p Value	<0.001
Median PFS	5.3 months

Tumor Response (N = 219)

Complete response	2 (1%)
Partial response	104 (47%)
Median time to response	1.45 months

Toxicity (N = 336)

	% G2	% G3	% G4
Arthralgia	18	3	
Rash	10	8	
Fatigue	11	2	
Cutaneous squamous cell carcinoma		12	
Keratoacanthoma	2	6	
Nausea	7	1	
Alopecia	8		
Pruritis	6	1	
Hyperkeratosis	5	1	
Diarrhea	5	<1	
Headache	4	<1	
Vomiting	3	1	
Neutropenia	<1	0	<1

ADVANCED/UNRESECTABLE MELANOMA REGIMEN

DABRAFENIB + TRAMETINIB

Flaherty et al. N Engl J Med 2012;367:1694–1703

Dabrafenib 150 mg; administer orally twice daily at least 1 hour before or 2 hours after a meal
Trametinib 2 mg; administer orally once daily at least 1 hour before or 2 hours after a meal

Supportive Care
Antiemetic prophylaxis
Emetogenic potential is **MINIMAL–LOW**
See Chapter 39 for antiemetic recommendations

Hematopoietic growth factor (CSF) prophylaxis
Primary prophylaxis is NOT indicated
See Chapter 43 for more information

Antimicrobial prophylaxis
Risk of fever and neutropenia is LOW
   Antimicrobial primary prophylaxis to be considered:
   • Antibacterial—not indicated
   • Antifungal—not indicated
   • Antiviral—not indicated unless patient previously had an episode of HSV
See Chapter 47 for more information

Patient Population Studied

Patients with histologically confirmed metastatic melanoma with either BRAF V600E or BRAF V600K mutations were eligible for inclusion. Eligible patients had measurable disease, an ECOG PS of 0 or 1. Patients with treated brain metastases and at least a 3-month history of stable disease were allowed to enroll. Patients were randomly assigned to receive 150 mg of dabrafenib twice daily plus once-daily trametinib at a dose of either 1 mg (combination 150/1) or 2 mg (combination 150/2) or 150 mg of dabrafenib monotherapy twice daily. There were no significant differences among groups except that patients in the combination 150/2 group were older than those in the monotherapy group (P = 0.04).

Dabrafenib and Trametinib Dose Modifications

Dabrafenib Dose Levels

Dose Reductions	Dose and Schedule
First dose reduction	100 mg dabrafenib orally twice daily
Second dose reduction	75 mg dabrafenib orally twice daily
Third dose reduction	50 mg dabrafenib orally twice daily
If unable to tolerate 50 mg twice daily	Discontinue dabrafenib

Dabrafenib Dose Modification

Target Organ	Adverse Reactions*	Dose Modification
Febrile drug reaction	Fever of 101.3°F to 104°F	Withhold dabrafenib until AE resolves then resume dabrafenib at same dose or at a reduced dose
	• Fever higher than 104°F • Fever complicated by rigors, hypotension, dehydration or renal failure	• Permanently discontinue dabrafenib or • Withhold dabrafenib until AE resolves then resume dabrafenib at same dose or at a reduced dose
Other	• Intolerable G2 AE • Any G3 AE	Withhold dabrafenib until AE resolves to ≤G1 then resume dabrafenib at a reduced dose
	First occurrence of any G4 AE	Either: • Permanently discontinue dabrafenib or • Withhold dabrafenib until AE resolves to ≤G1 then resume dabrafenib at a reduced dose
	Recurrent G4 AE Intolerable G2 or any G3/4 AE on dabrafenib 50 mg twice daily	Permanently discontinue dabrafenib

(continued)

Dabrafenib and Trametinib Dose Modifications (*continued*)

Trametinib Dose Modification

Target Organ	Adverse Reactions*	Dose Modification
Cutaneous	G2 rash	Reduce dose of trametinib by 0.5 mg or discontinue trametinib in patients taking trametinib 1 mg daily
	Intolerable G2 rash that does not improve within 3 weeks following dose reduction G3/4 rash	Withhold trametinib for up to 3 weeks. If improved resume trametinib at a lower dose (reduced by 0.5 mg)
	Intolerable G2 or G3/4 rash that does not improve within 3 weeks despite interruption of trametinib dosing	Permanently discontinue trametinib
Cardiac	Asymptomatic, absolute decrease in LVEF of 10% **or** greater from baseline **and** is below institutional lower limits of normal (LLN) from pretreatment value	Withhold trametinib for up to 4 weeks
	Asymptomatic, absolute decrease in LVEF of ≥10% from baseline **and is** <LLN that improves to normal LVEF value within 4 weeks following interruption of trametinib	If improved within 4 weeks, resume trametinib at a lower dose (reduced by 0.5 mg) or discontinue trametinib in patients taking trametinib 1 mg daily
	• Symptomatic congestive heart failure • ≤Absolute decrease in LVEF of ≥20% from baseline that is <LLN • Absolute decrease in LVEF of ≥10% from baseline and is <LLN that does not improve to normal LVEF value within 4 weeks following interruption of trametinib	Permanently discontinue trametinib
Ocular	G2/3 retinal pigment epithelial detachments (RPED)	Withhold trametinib for up to 3 weeks
	G2/3 RPED that improves to Grade 0–1 within 3 weeks	If improved within 3 weeks, resume trametinib at a lower dose (reduced by 0.5 mg)
	• Retinal vein occlusion • G2/3 RPED that does not improve to at least G1 within 3 weeks	Permanently discontinue trametinib
Pulmonary	Interstitial lung disease/pneumonitis	Permanently discontinue trametinib
Other	G3 AE	Withhold trametinib for up to 3 weeks
	If G3 AE improves to G0/1 following interruption of trametinib within 3 weeks	Reduce dose of trametinib by 0.5 mg or discontinue trametinib in patients taking trametinib 1 mg daily
	• G4 AE • G3 AE that does not improve to G0/1 within 3 weeks	Permanently discontinue trametinib

AE, adverse event; RPED, retinal pigment epithelial detachments
*National Cancer Institute Common Terminology Criteria for Adverse Events (CTCAE) version 4.0

Efficacy End Points as Assessed by the Site Investigators (Intention-to-Treat Population)*			
End Point	Dabrafenib Monotherapy (N = 54)	Dabrafenib 150 mg + Trametinib 1 mg (N = 54)	Dabrafenib 150 mg + Trametinib 2 mg (N = 54)
Progression-free survival — mo			
Median (95% CI)	5.8 (4.6–7.4)	9.2 (6.4–11.0)	9.4 (8.6–16.7)
HR for death or progression (95% CI)	Reference	0.56 (0.37–0.87)	0.39 (0.25–0.62)
P value	Reference	0.006	<0.001
PFS at 12 mo (95% CI) — %	9 (3–20)	26 (15–39)	41 (27–54)
Best response — no. (%)			
Complete response	2 (4)	3 (6)	5 (9)
Partial response	27 (50)	24 (44)	36 (67)
Stable disease	22 (41)	24 (44)	13 (24)
Progressive disease	3 (6)	2 (4)	0
Could not be evaluated	0	1 (2)	0
Complete or partial response			
Number of patients	29	27	41
Percent of patients (95% CI)	54 (40–67)	50 (36–64)	76 (62–86)
P value	Reference	0.77	0.03
Duration of response — mo			
Median (95% CI)	5.6 (4.5–7.4)	9.5 (7.4–NA)	10.5 (7.4–14.9)

HR, hazard ratio; PFS, progression-free survival; NA, not achieved
*Hazard ratios and P values are for the comparison between each combination-therapy group and the monotherapy group

Adverse Events*

Adverse Event	Dabrafenib Monotherapy (N = 53)†		Dabrafenib 150 mg + Trametinib 1 mg (N = 54)		Dabrafenib 150 mg + Trametinib 2 mg (N = 55)†	
	G3/4	All Grades	G3/4	All Grades	G3/4	All Grades
	Number of Patients (percent)					
Any event	23 (43)	53 (100)	26 (48)	53 (98)	32 (58)	55 (100)
Pyrexia	0	14 (26)	5 (9)	37 (69)	3 (5)	39 (71)
Chills	0	9 (17)	1 (2)	27 (50)	1 (2)	32 (58)
Fatigue	3 (6)	21 (40)	1 (2)	31 (57)	2 (4)	29 (53)
Nausea	0	11 (21)	3 (6)	25 (46)	1 (2)	24 (44)
Vomiting	0	8 (15)	2 (4)	23 (43)	1 (2)	22 (40)
Diarrhea	0	15 (28)	0	14 (26)	1 (2)	20 (36)
Headache	0	15 (28)	1 (2)	20 (37)	0	16 (29)

(continued)

Adverse Events (continued)

Adverse Event	Dabrafenib Monotherapy (N = 53)[†]		Dabrafenib 150 mg + Trametinib 1 mg (N = 54)		Dabrafenib 150 mg + Trametinib 2 mg (N = 55)[†]	
	G3/4	All Grades	G3/4	All Grades	G3/4	All Grades
	Number of Patients (percent)					
Peripheral edema	0	9 (17)	0	13 (24	0	16 (29)
Cough	0	11 (21)	0	6 (11)	0	16 (29)
Arthralgia	0	18 (34)	0	24 (44)	0	15 (27)
Rash	0	19 (36)	0	11 (20)	0	15 (27)
Night sweats	0	3 (6)	0	8 (15)	0	13 (24)
↓ Appetite	0	10 (19)	0	16 (30)	0	12 (22)
Myalgia	1 (2)	12 (23)	0	13 (24)	1 (2)	12 (22)
Constipation	0	6 (11)	1 (2)	9 (17)	0	12 (22)
↑ alkaline phosphatase	0	1 (2)	3 (6)	12 (22)	0	5 (9)
Hyperkeratosis	0	16 (30)	0	3 (6)	0	5 (9)
Alopecia	0	18 (34)	0	5 (9)	0	3 (5)
	G3[‡]	All Grades	G3[‡]	All Grades	G3[‡]	All Grades
Cutaneous squamous-cell carcinoma[§]	9 (17)	10 (19)	1 (2)	1 (2)	3 (5)	4 (7)
Skin papilloma	0	8 (15)	0	4 (7)	0	2 (4)
Hyperkeratosis	0	16 (30)	0	3 (6)	0	5 (9)
↑ ejection fraction	0	0	1 (2)	2 (4)	0	5 (9)
Cardiac failure	0	0	1 (2)	1 (2)	0	0
Hypertension	0	2 (4)	0	2 (4)	1 (2)	5 (9)
Chorioretinopathy	0	0	0	0	1 (2)	1 (2)

*Adverse events reported in ≥20% of patients in any group, regardless of whether a causal relationship was likely. In addition to these events, there was one death from sepsis in 150/1 combination group and three deaths in the 150/2 combination group (two from brain hemorrhage and one from pulmonary embolism). None were considered related to study drug. Neutropenia (G3/4) occurred in 11% of patients in the 150/2 combination group, with one case of febrile neutropenia. Acneiform dermatitis occurred in 11% of patients in the 150/1 combination group, 16% in the combination group, and 4% in the 150/2 monotherapy group, with no G3/4 events reported

[†]One patient who was assigned to the monotherapy group received combination 150/2 and so was included in the combination 150/2 safety analyses

[‡]For these categories, no G4 events were reported

[§]Keratoacanthoma was classified as cutaneous squamous-cell carcinoma

Treatment Monitoring

1. At baseline: Contrast CT or MRI of the brain, chest, abdomen, pelvis, and other anatomical regions as clinically indicated; physical and dermatologic examination; electrocardiography; CBC with differential; LFTs; basic metabolic panel; and LDH

2. Every 3 weeks: Physical examination, CBC with differential, LFTs, basic metabolic panel, and LDH

3. Tumor assessments are performed at baseline, at weeks 6 and 12, and every 9 weeks thereafter

26. Mesothelioma

Verna Vanderpuye, MD, Anish Thomas, MD, and Nicholas J. Vogelzang, MD

Pleural Mesothelioma

Epidemiology

Incidence: 3000 new cases per year
Median age: 60 years
Male to female ratio: 3:1

Peto J et al. Lancet 1995;345:535–539
Vogelzang NJ et al. Cancer 1984;53:377–383

Pathology

H & E staining
1. Epithelioid: 60% of cases = tubopapillary, granular, solid (occasional 5-year survival)
2. Sarcomatoid/mixed: 40% of cases (0% 5-year survival)

Immunohistochemical staining: Keratin positive, CEA negative, Leu M negative, calretinin positive
Cytogenetics: Deletion of short arm of chromosome 1 and 3 and long arm of chromosome 22

Chaihinan AP et al. In: Holland JC, Frei E, eds. Cancer Medicine. 5th ed. Hamilton, ON: BC Decker; 2000:1293–1312
Corson JM. Semin Thorac Cardiovasc Surg 1997;9:347–355

Staging

No defined universal staging system

Rusch VW. Chest 1995;108:1122–1128

Additional information
1. *Thoracic lymph node involvement:* 20% at presentation/70% at autopsy
2. *Hematogenous metastases:* Liver, lung, and bone: usually late in disease course

Curran D et al. J Clin Oncol 1998;16:145–152
Herndon JE et al. Chest 1998;113:723–731
Symanowski JT et al. Proc Am Soc Clin Oncol 2003;22:647 [Abstract 2602]

Work-up

1. *Chest x-ray:* Initial tool in diagnosing pleural plaques and effusion
2. *CT scan or MRI:* CT scan or MRI can be used to assess extent of disease. Calcifications are not generally visible on CT scan. Furthermore, the CT scan is less sensitive than the MRI in depicting diaphragmatic, pericardial, and chest wall involvement
3. *PET scan:* Has shown benefit in assessing lymph node involvement but is useful in only 50–70% of cases
4. *Thoracentesis:* Used when there is a pleural effusion (30% diagnostic yield)
5. *CT-guided biopsy:* Depends on CT findings. If tumor is thick and easily biopsied, do a CT-directed biopsy
6. *Video-assisted thorascopic (VAT) surgery:* Do if on CT scan disease is thin or minimal or in a difficult location and thoracentesis is negative (90% diagnostic yield)

Flores RM et al. Proc Am Soc Clin Oncol 2003;22:620 [Abstract 2495]
Patz EF Jr et al. AJR Am J Roentgenol 1992;159: 961–966
Schneider DB et al. J Thorac Cardiovasc Surg 2000;120: 128–133
Steele JPC. Semin Oncol 2002;29:36–40

Survival

Overall survival: 6–18 months

Expert Opinion

Surgical management

Data regarding the choice of surgical procedure are derived mostly from observational studies involving selected patient populations treated with a variety of surgical techniques and adjuvant chemotherapies

- Pleurectomy and decortication (lung sparing surgery): Indicated for minimal bulky disease associated with massive or recurrent pleural effusions
- Extrapleural pneumonectomy (en bloc resection of ipsilateral lung, pleura [parietal and visceral], pericardium, and hemidiaphragm): Indicated for highly selected patients with early stage epithelioid type disease with extensive involvement of the diaphragm and visceral pleural surfaces, no nodal metastases, good performance status, and no comorbidities

Radiation therapy

Because of the large volume of lung in the radiation field, delivery of tumoricidal doses of radiation is difficult without causing serious toxicities. Hence, radiation is not usually recommended as single-modality treatment. It is, however, recommended for palliating pain and to prevent or treating chest wall masses that are the result of seeding from sites of invasive procedures, such as prior thoracocentesis or thorascopic surgery. It is also used as part of a combined modality approach in patients with surgically resectable disease

Chemotherapy

Chemotherapy is indicated in patients with malignant pleural mesothelioma whose disease is either unresectable or who are not otherwise candidates for curative surgery. Pemetrexed in combination with cisplatin is the standard first-line chemotherapy with vitamin B_{12} and folic acid given prophylactically to mitigate leukopenia and gastrointestinal adverse effects associated with pemetrexed

Boutin C et al. Chest 1995;108:754–758
Flores RM et al. J Thorac Cardiovasc Surg 2008;135:620–626
Flores RM. Semin Thorac Cardiovasc Surg 2009;2:149–153
Maasilta P et al. Int J Radiat Oncol Biol Phys 1991;20:433–438
Rice D. Ann Diagn Pathol 2009;13:65–72
Vogelzang NJ et al. J Clin Oncol 2003;21:2636–2644
Yanagawa J, Rusch V. Thorac Surg Clin 2013;23:73–78

REGIMEN

PEMETREXED + CISPLATIN

Vogelzang NJ et al. J Clin Oncol 2003;21:2636–2644

Folic acid 350–1000 mcg daily; administer orally, beginning 1–3 weeks before chemotherapy and continuing throughout treatment with pemetrexed + cisplatin, *and* **Cyanocobalamin (vitamin B$_{12}$)** 1000 mcg; administer intramuscularly every 9 weeks, beginning 1–3 weeks before chemotherapy and continuing throughout treatment with pemetrexed + cisplatin

Dexamethasone 4 mg; administer intravenously or orally twice daily for 3 consecutive days, starting the day before pemetrexed administration to decrease the risk of severe skin rash associated with pemetrexed (total dose/cycle = 24 mg)

Hydration: 0.9% Sodium chloride injection (0.9% NS), ≥1000 mL before and after cisplatin; administer intravenously over a minimum of 2–4 hours. Encourage patients to increase oral nonalcoholic fluid intake. Monitor and replace magnesium/electrolytes as needed

Pemetrexed 500 mg/m^2; administer intravenously in 100 mL 0.9% NS over 10 minutes, given before cisplatin on day 1, every 21 days (total dosage/cycle = 500 mg/m^2)

Cisplatin 75 mg/m^2; administer intravenously in 1000 mL 0.9% NS over 2 hours on day 1, beginning 30 minutes after pemetrexed has been administered, every 21 days (total dosage/cycle = 75 mg/m^2)

Supportive Care

Antiemetic prophylaxis

*Emetogenic potential is **HIGH**. Potential for delayed symptoms*

See Chapter 39 for antiemetic recommendations

Hematopoietic growth factor (CSF) prophylaxis

Primary prophylaxis is NOT indicated

See Chapter 43 for more information

Antimicrobial prophylaxis

Risk of fever and neutropenia is LOW

Antimicrobial primary prophylaxis to be considered:

- Antibacterial—not indicated
- Antifungal—not indicated
- Antiviral—not indicated unless patient previously had an episode of HSV

See Chapter 47 for more information

Additional supportive care

Add a **proton pump inhibitor** during dexamethasone use to prevent gastritis and duodenitis

Patient Population Studied

A study of 456 patients with advanced measurable pleural mesothelioma

Efficacy

Response rate	40–45%
Median time to progression	5–6 months
1-Year survival	50%
Median survival	12–13 months

Therapy Monitoring

1. *Before initial and repeated treatments:* H&P, CBC with differential, calculated creatinine clearance, serum electrolytes glucose, calcium, LFTs, and vitamin metabolites
2. *Treatment evaluation:* Every 2 cycles

Toxicity
(N = 168 Fully Supplemented with Vitamins)

	% CTC G3/4
Hematologic	
Hemoglobin	4.2
Leukocytes	14.9
Neutrophils	23.2
Platelets	5.4
Febrile neutropenia	0.6
Nonhematologic	
Nausea	11.9
Fatigue	10.1
Vomiting	10.7
Diarrhea	3.6
Dehydration	4.2
Stomatitis	3
Anorexia	1.2
Rash	0.6

Three deaths thought possibly related to pemetrexed + cisplatin occurred before folic acid and vitamin B$_{12}$ supplementation was added; none occurred thereafter

Treatment Modifications

Delay cycle until ANC is >1500/mm^3 and platelet >100,000/mm^3

Adverse Event	Dose Modification
G3 hematologic toxicities	Hold therapy until returns to baseline. Then decrease both drug dosages by 25%
G4 hematologic toxicities (thrombocytopenia)	Hold therapy until returns to baseline. Then decrease both drug dosages by 50%
Serum creatinine 1.6–2 mg/dL (141–177 μmol/L)	Decrease cisplatin dosage by 25%
Serum creatinine ≥2 mg/dL (≥177 μmol/L)	Hold therapy until serum creatinine <2 mg/dL (<177 μmol/L), then decrease cisplatin dosage by 25%
G ≥2 diarrhea	Hold chemotherapy until toxicity resolves to grade <2, then decrease both drug dosages by 25%
G3/4 mucositis	Decrease pemetrexed dosage 50%
Increased liver transaminases	Hold therapy until toxicity resolves, then decrease pemetrexed dosage by 25%
Other G ≥3 nonhematologic toxicities (except N/V, elevated transaminases and alopecia)	Delay treatment until toxicity resolves to baseline, then, decrease both drug dosages by 25% from previous dose levels

Delays of ≤42 days are permitted for recovery from pemetrexed- and cisplatin-related toxicities

Patients requiring 3 dose reductions: discontinue therapy

Notes

1. G2 neutropenia and anemia secondary to pemetrexed are brief and not cumulative
2. Anemia is cumulative with cisplatin. Consider using erythropoietin therapy if anemia G >1 occurs
3. Folate deficiency is best measured with homocysteine levels
4. Vitamin B$_{12}$ deficiency can be tested most readily with methylmalonic acid (MMA) levels

REGIMEN

PEMETREXED + CARBOPLATIN

Ceresoli GL et al. J Clin Oncol 2006;24:1443–1448

Folic acid 350–1000 mcg/day orally beginning at least 1 week before the first dose of pemetrexed and continued throughout the duration of treatment

Cyanocobalamin (vitamin B$_{12}$) 1000 mcg intramuscularly at least 1 week before the first dose of pemetrexed and repeated every 9 weeks (every 3 cycles) throughout treatment

Dexamethasone 4 mg/dose orally twice daily for 3 consecutive days (6 doses), starting the day before pemetrexed administration to decrease the risk of severe skin rash associated with pemetrexed (total dose/cycle = 24 mg)

Pemetrexed 500 mg/m^2; administer intravenously in 100 mL 0.9% sodium chloride injection over 10 minutes on day 1, every 21 days (total dosage/cycle = 500 mg/m^2), *followed 30 minutes later by:*

Carboplatin AUC 5 mg/mL per min; administer intravenously in 50–250 mL D5W over 30 minutes on day 1, every 21 days (total dosage/cycle calculated to produce an AUC = 5 mg/mL per min)

Notes:

Salicylates and nonsteroidal antiinflammatory agents (NSAIDs) were not allowed during the 2 days before (5 days for NSAIDs with a long half-life), the day of, and for 2 days after chemotherapy

Carboplatin dose calculation is based on formulas developed to achieve consistent drug exposure within and among patients. In the method that follows, area under the plasma concentration versus time curve (AUC) is the targeted pharmacokinetic endpoint used to obtain consistent exposure

Current product labeling for carboplatin approved by the U.S. Food and Drug Administration describes dose calculation based on a formula described by Calvert et al[*,†,‡]:

$$\text{Total Carboplatin Dose (mg)} = (\text{target AUC}) \times (\text{GFR} + 25)$$

In practice, creatinine clearance (Clcr) is used in place of glomerular filtration rate (GFR). Clcr can be measured from a 24-hour urine collection or estimated from 1 among several equations, such as the method of Cockcroft and Gault[§]:

$$\text{For males, Clcr} = \frac{(140 - \text{age [years]}) \times (\text{body weight [kg]})}{72 \times (\text{serum creatinine [mg/dL]})}$$

$$\text{For females, Clcr} = \frac{(140 - \text{age [years]}) \times (\text{body weight [kg]})}{72 \times (\text{serum creatinine [mg/dL]})} \times 0.85$$

Note: On October 8, 2010, the U.S. Food and Drug Administration (FDA) identified a potential safety issue with carboplatin dosing based on recent changes in the measurement of serum creatinine. Since the end of 2010, all clinical laboratories in the United States use the standardized Isotope Dilution Mass Spectrometry (IDMS) method to measure serum creatinine, which could result in an overestimation of the GFR in some patients with normal renal function. A carboplatin dose calculated with an IDMS-measured serum creatinine result using the Calvert formula could exceed an expected exposure (AUC) and result in increased drug-related toxicity

Provided actual GFR measurements are made to assess renal function, carboplatin can be safely dosed according to the Calvert formula described in product labeling

If GFR (or creatinine clearance) is estimated based on serum creatinine measurements by the IDMS method, the FDA recommends capping an estimated GFR at 125 mL/min for any targeted AUC value for patients with normal renal function. No greater estimated GFR values should be used

U.S. FDA. Carboplatin dosing. [online] October 8, 2010. Available from: http://www.fda.gov/aboutfda/centersoffices/officeofmedicalproductsandtobacco/cder/ucm228974.htm [last accessed September 4, 2013]

[*]Calvert AH, Newell DR, Gumbrell LA et al. Carboplatin dosage: prospective evaluation of a simple formula based on renal function. J Clin Oncol 1989;7:1748–1756
[†]Sørensen BT, Strömgren A, Jakobsen P, Jakobsen A. Dose-toxicity relationship of carboplatin in combination with cyclophosphamide in ovarian cancer patients. Cancer Chemother Pharmacol 1991;28:397–401
[‡]Jodrell DI, Egorin MJ, Canetta RM et al. Relationships between carboplatin exposure and tumor response and toxicity in patients with ovarian cancer. J Clin Oncol 1992;10:520–528
[§]Cockcroft DW, Gault MH. Prediction of creatinine clearance from serum creatinine. Nephron 1976;16:31–41

(*continued*)

(*continued*)

Supportive Care

Antiemetic prophylaxis

Emetogenic potential is at least **MODERATE**. *Potential for delayed emetic symptoms*

See Chapter 39 for antiemetic recommendations

Hematopoietic growth factor (CSF) prophylaxis

Primary prophylaxis may be indicated

See Chapter 43 for more information

Antimicrobial prophylaxis

Risk of fever and neutropenia is LOW

Antimicrobial primary prophylaxis to be considered:

- Antibacterial—not indicated
- Antifungal—not indicated
- Antiviral—not indicated unless patient previously had an episode of HSV

See Chapter 47 for more information

Oral care

Prophylaxis and treatment for mucositis / stomatitis

General advice:

- Encourage patients to maintain intake of nonalcoholic fluids
- Evaluate patients for oral pain and provide analgesic medications
- Consider histamine (H$_2$-subtype) receptor antagonists (eg, ranitidine, famotidine), or a proton pump inhibitor for epigastric pain
- *Lactobacillus* sp.-containing probiotics may be beneficial in preventing diarrhea

Patients with intact oral mucosa:

- Clean the mouth, tongue, and gums by brushing after every meal and at bedtime with an ultrasoft toothbrush with fluoride toothpaste
- Floss teeth gently every day unless contraindicated. If gums bleed and hurt, avoid bleeding or sore areas, but floss other teeth
- Patients may use saline or commercial brand, nonalcoholic rinses
  - Do not use mouthwashes that contain alcohols

If mucositis or stomatitis is present:

- Keep the mouth moist utilizing water, ice chips, sugarless gum, sugar-free hard candies, or a saliva substitute
- Rinse mouth several times a day to remove debris
  - Use a solution of ¼ teaspoon (1.25 g) each of baking soda and table salt (sodium chloride) in 1 quart (~950 mL) of warm water. Follow with a plain water rinse
  - Do not use mouthwashes that contain alcohols
- Foam-tipped swabs (eg, Toothettes) are useful in moisturizing oral mucosa, but ineffective for cleansing teeth and removing plaque
- Advise patients who develop mucositis to:
  - Choose foods that are easy to chew and swallow
  - Take small bites of food, chew slowly, and sip liquids with meals
  - Encourage soft, moist foods such as cooked cereals, mashed potatoes, and scrambled eggs
  - For trouble swallowing, soften food with gravies, sauces, broths, yogurt, or other bland liquids
  - Avoid sharp, crunchy foods; hot, spicy or highly acidic foods (eg, citrus fruits and juices); sugary foods; toothpicks; tobacco products; alcoholic drinks

Treatment Modifications

Adverse Event	Dose Modification
ANC <1500/mm^3 or platelet count <100,000/mm^3	Delay start of cycle up to 42 days until ANC ≥1500/mm^3 and platelet count ≥100,000/mm^3
ANC nadir <500/mm^3 *and* platelets ≥50,000/mm^3	Administer 75% of the previous pemetrexed dose, *or* carboplatin AUC = 4 mg/mL per min
Platelet nadir count <50,000/mm^3 *and* any ANC	Administer 50% of the previous pemetrexed dose, *or* carboplatin AUC = 3 mg/mL per min
Recurrence of G3/4 thrombocytopenia or neutropenia after 2 dose reductions	Discontinue therapy
G3/4 nonhematologic toxicities	Delay treatment until there is resolution to G ≤1 then proceed with pemetrexed reduced to 75% of the previous dose and carboplatin at AUC = 4 mg/mL per min
Creatinine clearance* <45 mL/min (<0.75 mL/s)	Delay the next cycle until creatinine clearance ≥45 mL/min (≥0.75 mL/s)

*Calculated by the Cockcroft and Gault formula before each dose

Efficacy (N = 102)

Response Rate*,†

Objective response rate	18.6% (95% CI, 11.6–27.5%)
Complete response	1.96% (2 patients) (10+ and 11 months)
Partial response	16.66% (17 patients)
Stable disease	47% (95% CI, 37.1–57.2%) (48 patients)
Progressive disease	34.3% (35 patients)

Response According to Histology

Epithelial MPM	15/80 (18.8%)
Mixed histotype MPM	4/8 (50%)
Sarcomatoid MPM	0/7

Effect on ECOG Performance Status‡

Patients with OR/baseline PS (N = 19)	0 (3)/1 (16)
Patients with OR/posttreatment PS	0 (10)/1 (9)
Patients with SD/baseline PS (N = 48)	0 (21)/1 (25)/2 (2)
Patients with SD/posttreatment PS	0 (23)/1 (22)/2 (3)

Median Follow-Up Time of 14.2 Months (95% CI, 12.2–15 Months) 26 without any Evidence of Disease Progression

Median TTP§	6.5 months
Median OS⁄	12.7 months
6-month survival estimates	70.0% (95% CI, 60.0–78.0%)
1-year survival estimates	51.6% (95% CI, 40.7–61.5%)

*Best tumor response was assessed according to an intent-to-treat analysis

†Response to treatment showed a trend that correlated with OS in univariate analysis (P = 0.069) and reached statistical significance in the multivariate model (P = 0.024). When SD patients were grouped with responders, the correlation with OS was much more significant (P <0.001)

‡Sixty-nine patients (68%) were symptomatic at the time of study enrollment. ECOG PS improved or was stable in the majority of patients who achieved response or SD

§TTP was significantly related to good PS (P = 0.047) and epithelial histology (P = 0.02) in both univariate and multivariate analyses

⁄Patients' PS was the only factor significantly related to OS in univariate and multivariate analyses (P = 0.04)

Patient Population Studied

Patients with histologically proven malignant pleural mesothelioma who were not candidates for curative surgery. Eligibility criteria included ages >18 years, Eastern Cooperative Oncology Group (ECOG) performance status (PS) ≤2, and an estimated life expectancy of ≥12 weeks. Creatinine clearance ≥45 mL/min. Patients were excluded if they were unable to discontinue administration of aspirin and/or other nonsteroidal antiinflammatory agents for 2 days before (5 days for long-acting agents), the day of, and 2 days after the dose of pemetrexed

Patient Characteristics

Characteristic	Number of Patients (N = 102)	Percent
Sex		
Male	76	74.5
Female	26	25.5
Age, years		
Median	65	
Range	38–79	
ECOG performance status		
0	33	32
1	61	60
2	8	8
Histologic subtype		
Mixed cell	8	8
Unspecified	7	7
Epithelial	80	78
Sarcomatoid	7	7
EORTC prognostic score		
Good	25	24.5
Poor	77	75.5
IMIG stage		
II	11	11
III	34	33
IV	49	48
Relapse after EPP	8	8

Toxicity

Hematologic Toxicity by Cycle (N = 482)

Toxicity	Toxicity Grade (Number of Patients)				% G3/4
	G1	G2	G3	G4	
Neutropenia	60	59	36	11	9.7
Thrombocytopenia	51	12	7*	3*	2
Anemia	166	79	16†	1†	3.5

Hematologic Toxicity by Patient (N = 102)

Neutropenia	17	25	9	11‡	19.6
Thrombocytopenia	17	3	6	2	7.8
Anemia	33	30	11	1	11.7

Nonhematologic Toxicity by Patient (N = 102)§

Nausea/vomiting	47	17	1	0	1
Fatigue	31	13	1	0	1
Stomatitis	3	7	0	0	0
Conjunctivitis	20	3	0	0	0
Diarrhea	2	0	3	0	3
Constipation	5	1	0	0	0

*G3/4 thrombocytopenia occurred after the second cycle in 7/10 (70%) patients
†G3/4 anemia occurred after the second cycle in 15 (88%) of 17 patients
‡Febrile neutropenia was reported in 2 patients
§Other toxicities reported as rare events included G4 rhabdomyolysis (1 patient), G2 hepatotoxicity (1 patient), G2 arthralgia-myalgia (2 patients), G2 genitourinary mucositis (2 patients), and G1 skin rash (2 patients)

Therapy Monitoring

1. *Before initial and repeated treatments:* H&P, CBC with differential, calculated or measured creatinine clearance, serum electrolytes, glucose, calcium, LFTs, and vitamin metabolites

2. *Treatment evaluation:* Every 2 cycles

REGIMEN

GEMCITABINE + CISPLATIN

Byrne MJ et al. J Clin Oncol 1999;17:25–30
van Haarst JW et al. Br J Cancer 2002;86(3):342–345

Hydration: 0.9% Sodium chloride injection (0.9% NS) ≥1000 mL before and after cisplatin; administer intravenously over a minimum of 2–4 hours. Monitor and replace magnesium/electrolytes as needed

Cisplatin 100 mg/m²; administer intravenously in 100–250 mL 0.9% NS over 60 minutes, given before gemcitabine on day 1, every 28 days for 6 cycles (total dosage/cycle = 100 mg/m²), *plus*

Gemcitabine 1000 mg/m² per dose; administer intravenously in 50–250 mL 0.9% NS over 30 minutes, given on days 1, 8, and 15, every 28 days for 6 cycles (total dosage/cycle = 3000 mg/m²)

or

Cisplatin 80 mg/m²; administer intravenously in 100–250 mL 0.9% NS over 60 minutes, on day 1, every 3 weeks for a maximum of 6 cycles (total dosage/cycle = 80 mg/m²), *plus*

Gemcitabine 1250 mg/m² per dose; administer intravenously in 50–250 mL 0.9% NS over 30 minutes, on days 1 and 8, every 3 weeks for a maximum of 6 cycles (total dosage/cycle = 2500 mg/m²)

Supportive Care

Antiemetic prophylaxis
*Emetogenic potential on day 1 is **HIGH**. Potential for delayed symptoms*
*Emetogenic potential with gemcitabine alone is **LOW***
See Chapter 39 for antiemetic recommendations

Hematopoietic growth factor (CSF) prophylaxis
Primary prophylaxis is NOT indicated
See Chapter 43 for more information

Antimicrobial prophylaxis
Risk of fever and neutropenia is LOW
  Antimicrobial primary prophylaxis to be considered:
  • Antibacterial—not indicated
  • Antifungal—not indicated
  • Antiviral—not indicated unless patient previously had an episode of HSV
See Chapter 47 for more information

Patient Population Studied

A study of 21 patients with advanced measurable pleural mesothelioma (Byrne MJ et al.)
A study of 25 patients with advanced measurable pleural mesothelioma (van Haarst JW et al.)

Therapy Monitoring

1. *Before chemotherapy on cycle days 1, 8, and 15:* CBC with differential, serum electrolytes, creatinine, bilirubin, ALT, and alkaline phosphatase
2. *Treatment evaluation:* Every 2 cycles

Byrne MJ et al. J Clin Oncol 1999;17:25–30

Efficacy (N = 46)

Response rate	18–47%
Duration of response	5–7 months
Estimated median survival	9.5–12 months
Estimated 1-year survival	41%

Nine of 10 responding patients achieved substantial or complete symptomatic improvement. Symptoms decreased significantly in 3 additional patients who achieved disease stabilization

From Byrne MJ et al. J Clin Oncol 1999;17:25–30
van Haarst JW et al. Br J Cancer 2002;86(3):342–345

Treatment Modifications

Serum creatinine >1.4 mg/dL (>124 µmol/L), but <1.7 mg/dL (<150 µmol/L)	Decrease cisplatin by 50% and gemcitabine by 25%
Serum creatinine >1.7 mg/dL (>150 µmol/L)	Withhold cisplatin and gemcitabine until serum creatinine <1.7 mg/dL (<150 µmol/L), then administer 50% of the previous cisplatin dosage and 75% of the previous gemcitabine dosage
WBC <3000/mm³ or platelet <100,000/mm³ on days 1 and 8 or days 1, 8, and 15 when gemcitabine treatment is planned	Decrease gemcitabine by 25%
WBC <2000/mm³ or platelet <75,000/mm³ when gemcitabine treatment is planned for day 8 or days 8 and 15	Omit gemcitabine

Byrne MJ et al. J Clin Oncol 1999;17:25–30

Toxicity (N = 21)

	Worst Toxicity Grade (%)				
	0	1	2	3	4
Hematologic					
Leukopenia	29	10	24	38	0
Thrombocytopenia*	24	14	29	14	19
Anemia	14	29	57	0	0
Nonhematologic					
Nausea/vomiting†	0	14	52	33	0
Stomatitis	62	38	0	0	0
Alopecia	71	24	5	0	0
Hearing loss	57	33	5	5	0
Neurologic	90	10	0	0	0

*Thrombocytopenia on days 8 and 15 was the major cause of dose modification
†One-third of patients had ≥1 episodes of severe nausea and vomiting, and symptoms were worse >24 hours after treatment

From Byrne MJ et al. J Clin Oncol 1999;17:25–30

Peritoneal Mesothelioma

Epidemiology

Incidence: 10% of all mesothelioma (200–400 new cases per year)
Median age: 53 years
Male to female ratio: 1:1

Survival

Median survival: 1 year

Expert Opinion

1. No standard treatment
2. Resectable disease
   a. *In women:* Treatment is the same as for ovarian cancer because these tumors behave and respond similarly to cytoreduction followed by cisplatin-based chemotherapy. Intraperitoneal (IP) chemotherapy has shown superiority over intravenous chemotherapy for advanced ovarian cancer
   b. *In men:* Treatment is the same as for pleural mesothelioma, or if disease is not related to asbestos exposure, it can be treated with IP chemotherapy
3. Locally advanced or recurrent disease: Give systemic chemotherapy as for pleural mesothelioma

Alberts DS et al. [Editorial]. J Clin Oncol 2002;20:3944–3949
Eltabbakh GH et al. J Surg Oncol 1999;70:6–12
Markman M, Kelsen D. J Cancer Res Clin Oncol 1992;118:547–550
Markman M et al. J Clin Oncol 2001;19:1001–1007

REGIMEN

INTRAPERITONEAL (IP) CISPLATIN + PACLITAXEL

Rothenberg ML et al. J Clin Oncol 2003;21:1313–1319

Dexamethasone 20 mg/dose; administer orally for 2 doses, 12 hours and 6 hours before paclitaxel on days 1 and 8, *plus*

Diphenhydramine 50 mg; administer by intravenous injection 30–60 minutes before paclitaxel on days 1 and 8, *plus*

Ranitidine 50 mg or **cimetidine** 300 mg; administer intravenously in 25–100 mL of a compatible solution; for example, 0.9% sodium chloride injection (0.9% NS) or 5% dextrose injection (D5W) over 5–30 minutes beginning 30–60 minutes before paclitaxel on days 1 and 8

Paclitaxel 135 mg/m^2; administer intravenously in a volume of 0.9% NS or D5W sufficient to produce a solution with concentration within the range 0.3–1.2 mg/mL over 24 hours on day 1, every 21 days for 6 cycles (total paclitaxel dosage/cycle given intravenously = 135 mg/m^2)

Cisplatin 100 mg/m^2; administer intraperitoneally in 2000 mL 0.9% NS warmed to body temperature on day 2, every 21 days for 6 cycles (total dosage/cycle = 100 mg/m^2)

Paclitaxel 60 mg/m^2; administer intraperitoneally in 2000 mL 0.9% NS, warmed to body temperature on day 8, every 21 days for 6 cycles (total paclitaxel dosage/cycle from IP route = 60 mg/m^2)

Additional information: Drug distribution is facilitated by sequentially placing patients R side down, L side down, in Trendelenburg and in reverse Trendelenburg position for 15 minutes each after drugs are instilled IP. Cisplatin- and paclitaxel-containing fluids are not drained after instillation

Supportive Care

Antiemetic prophylaxis

Emetogenic potential on days 1 and 8 is **LOW**

Emetogenic potential on day 2 is **HIGH**. *Potential for delayed symptoms*

See Chapter 39 for antiemetic recommendations

Hematopoietic growth factor (CSF) prophylaxis

Primary prophylaxis may be indicated

See Chapter 43 for more information

Antimicrobial prophylaxis

Risk of fever and neutropenia is LOW

Antimicrobial primary prophylaxis to be considered:

- Antibacterial—not indicated
- Antifungal—not indicated
- Antiviral—not indicated unless patient previously had an episode of HSV

See Chapter 47 for more information

Toxicity (N = 68)

	% G3	% G4
Hematologic		
Neutropenia	21	59
Anemia	15	4
Thrombocytopenia	9	0
Infection with neutropenia	12	0
Nonhematologic		
Nausea	50	0
Vomiting	29	4
Abdominal pain	12	1
Diarrhea	4	1
Fatigue/malaise/lethargy	24	0
Sensory neuropathy	3	0
Catheter-related infection	10	0
	% G1	**% G2**
Alopecia	10	66

96% of patients experienced ≥1 G3/4 toxicity

Therapy Monitoring

1. *Before each treatment cycle:* PE, CBC with differential, serum creatinine, and serum bilirubin
2. *Weekly:* CBC, serum electrolytes, serum creatinine, calcium, magnesium, and LFTs

Patient Population Studied

A study of 68 patients with FIGO stage III epithelial ovarian cancer (tumor extending outside the pelvis and/or positive retroperitoneal or inguinal lymph nodes) with residual peritoneal disease ≤1 cm in largest dimension after surgical staging by GOG standards

Efficacy (N = 68)

Median disease-free survival	33 months
Median survival	51 months
2-Year survival rate	91%

Treatment Modifications

ANC ≥3000/mm^3 and platelet ≥100,000/mm^3 required to start cycle. Delay therapy up to 2 weeks to allow hematologic recovery

Adverse Event	Dose Modification
Hematologic toxicity	No dose modifications. Day 8 paclitaxel given without regard for CBC
G >2 peripheral neuropathy	Delay therapy until toxicity grade ≤2, then decrease all drug dosages by 20%
G2 abdominal pain	Decrease IP drug dosages by 20%
G3/4 abdominal pain	Decrease IP drug dosages by 40%
CrCl <50 mL/min	Hold cisplatin until CrCl >50 mL/min (>0.83 mL/s), then decrease cisplatin dosage to 75 mg/m^2 during all subsequent cycles
Peritoneal catheter dysfunction or inability to administer therapy IP	Modify regimen schedule and route of administration for all remaining cycles: Paclitaxel 135 mg/m^2 intravenously over 24 hours on day 1, every 21 days; cisplatin 100 mg/m^2 intravenously over 60 minutes on day 2, every 21 days

27. Multiple Myeloma

Aldo Roccaro, MD, PhD, Giada Bianchi, MD, Irene M. Ghobrial, MD, and Kenneth C. Anderson, MD

Epidemiology

Incidence: 24,050 (male: 13,500; female: 10,550.
Estimated new cases for 2014 in the United States)
7.5 per 100,000 males, 4.8 per 100,000 females
Deaths: Estimated 11,090 in 2014 (male: 6,110; female: 4,980)
Median age: 69 years
Male to female ratio: 1.4:1

Durie-Salmon Stage at presentation
Stage I   6%
Stage II   21%
Stage III 73%

Durie BGM, Salmon SE. Cancer 1975;36:842–854
Siegel R et al. CA Cancer J Clin 2014;64:9–29
Surveillance, Epidemiology and End Results (SEER) Program, available from http://seer.cancer.gov (accessed in 2013)

Pathology

Monoclonal gammopathy of uncertain significance (MGUS)
- Stable serum M-protein level <3 g/dL and bone marrow clonal plasma cells <10%
- Urine Bence Jones protein absent or minimal
- No related organ/tissue impairment (ROTI)*
- No evidence of other B-lymphoproliferative disorders
- Progression to multiple myeloma (MM) in ~1% per year (median 10 years)

Smoldering (asymptomatic) myeloma
- M-protein in serum ≥30 g/L and/or bone marrow clonal plasma cells ≥10%
- No ROTI or symptoms

Active (symptomatic) myeloma[†]
- Requires one or more of the following (CRAB criteria):
- Calcium elevation (>11.5 mg/dL [>2.88 mmol/L])
- Renal insufficiency (creatinine >2 mg/dL [>177 μmol/L])
- Anemia (hemoglobin <10 g/dL or 2 g less than normal)
- Bone disease (lytic or osteopenic)

Extramedullary plasmacytoma
- Extramedullary tumor of clonal plasma cells
- Normal bone marrow
- Normal skeletal survey
- M-protein absent or disappears from blood/urine after excision or irradiation of solitary lesion
- Absence of ROTI*
- Progression to MM in ~15%

Solitary plasmacytoma of bone
- Three to 5% of plasma cell dyscrasias
- Isolated bone tumor consisting of monoclonal plasma cells
- Normal bone marrow
- M-protein absent or disappears from blood/urine after excision or irradiation of solitary lesion
- Absence of other myeloma ROTI*
- Multiple or recurrent in up to 5% of patients
- Progression to MM in ~50%

Work-up

All patients
1. H&P
2. CBC with differential; serum electrolytes, BUN, creatinine, calcium and albumin, LDH
3. Quantitative immunoglobulins, serum protein electrophoresis, and immunofixation
4. Twenty-four–hour urine protein electrophoresis, immunofixation, and Bence Jones quantitation
5. Serum free light-chain assay
6. Skeletal survey
7. Unilateral bone marrow aspirate and biopsy with flow and immunohistochemistry
8. Bone marrow cytogenetics and interphase FISH
9. Albumin and β_2-microglobulin (see staging system)

Selected patients
1. MRI of the spine (evaluate for solitary plasmacytoma of bone or suspected cord compression)
2. FDG-PET/CT scan in selected patients to evaluate for increased uptake
3. Tissue biopsy (evaluate for solitary plasmacytoma)
4. Serum viscosity (if M-protein level is markedly elevated or symptoms of hyperviscosity are present)
5. *Additional tests (prognostic markers):* plasma cell labeling index, C-reactive protein, and LDH

(continued)

Pathology (*continued*)

Plasma cell leukemia
- Five percent of newly presenting MM patients
- Peripheral blood absolute plasma cell count ≥2000/mm³
- More than 20% plasma cells in differential count of peripheral blood leukocytes

*ROTI: myeloma-related organ/tissue impairment:
1. Hypercalcemia
2. Renal insufficiency
3. Recurrent bacterial infections (>2 episodes in 12 months)
4. Bone lesions (lytic or osteoporotic with compression fractures)
5. Symptomatic hyperviscosity
6. Amyloidosis
7. Anemia

†Other examples of active disease include:
- Repeated infections
- Secondary amyloidosis
- Hyperviscosity
- Hypogammaglobulinemia

The International Myeloma Working Group. Br J Haematol 2003;121:749–757

Staging

Durie-Salmon Staging System

	Stage I	Stage II*	Stage III†
Myeloma cell mass	Low	Intermediate	High
Hemoglobin	>10 g/dL	8.5–10 g/dL	<8.5 g/dL
Serum calcium	≤12 mg/dL (≤3 mmol/L)	Fitting neither stage I nor stage II	>12 mg/dL (>3 mmol/L)
Skeletal survey	Normal‡		Advanced lytic bone lesions
Serum M-protein levels: IgG	<5 g/dL	5–7 g/dL	>7 g/dL
Serum M-protein levels: IgA	<3 g/dL	3–5 g/dL	>5 g/dL
24-hour urinary light chain excretion	<4 g/24 hours	4–12 g/24 hours	>12 g/24 hours

*Not meeting criteria for either stage I or stage III
†Need to meet 1 or more of the criteria listed
‡Or solitary plasmacytoma
Note: Subclassification: For each stage, "A" denotes serum creatinine <2 mg/dL (<177 μmol/L) and "B" denotes serum creatinine ≥2 mg/dL (≥177 μmol/L)

International Staging System

	Stage I	Stage II		Stage III
Serum β_2-microglobulin	<3.5 mg/L	<3.5 mg/L	3.5 to <5.5 mg/mL	≥5.5 mg/L
Serum albumin	≥3.5 g/dL (≥35 g/L)	<3.5 g/dL	—	—

Durie BGM, Salmon SE. Cancer 1975;36:842–854
Greipp PR et al. J Clin Oncol 2005;23:3412–3420

Response Criteria

International Myeloma Working Group Uniform Response Criteria CR and Other Response Categories

CR = Complete Response

- Negative immunofixation on the serum and urine
- Disappearance of any soft tissue plasmacytomas
- ≤5% plasma cells in bone marrow

sCR = Stringent Complete Response

CR as described above, **PLUS:**
- Normal free light chain (FLC) ratio **AND**
- Absence of clonal cells in bone marrow by immunohistochemistry or immunofluorescence

VGPR = Very Good Partial Response

- Serum and urine M-protein detectable by immunofluorescence but not on electrophoresis **OR**
- ≥90% reduction in serum M-protein + urine M-protein level <100 mg/24 hours

PR = Partial Response

- ≥50% reduction of serum M-protein + reduction in 24-hour urinary M-protein by ≥90% or to <200 mg/24 hours

If the serum and urine M-protein are unmeasurable:
- A ≥50% decrease in the difference between involved and uninvolved FLC levels is required in place of the M-protein criteria

If serum and urine M-protein are unmeasurable, and serum FLC assay is also unmeasurable:
- ≥50% reduction in plasma cells is required in place of M-protein, provided baseline bone marrow plasma cell percentage was ≥30%

Note: In addition to the above listed criteria, if present at baseline, a ≥50% reduction in the size of soft-tissue plasmacytomas is also required

SD = Stable Disease*

- Not meeting criteria for CR, VGPR, PR, or progressive disease

*Not recommended for use as an indicator of response; stability of disease is best described by providing the time-to-progression estimates

Median Survival

Treatments for myeloma have expanded in the last decade. A recent study[1] examined the survival trends over time of 2 groups of patients seen at Mayo Clinic, one from time of diagnosis and the other from the time of relapse:

- Among 387 patients who relapsed after stem cell transplantation, a clear improvement was seen in overall survival from the time of relapse. Patients whose disease relapsed after the year 2000 had a median overall survival of 23.9 months versus 11.8 months ($P < 0.001$) for those who relapsed prior to this date. This improvement was independent of other prognostic factors

- Patients treated with 1 or more of the newer drugs (thalidomide, lenalidomide, bortezomib) had longer survival from relapse (30.9 vs. 14.8 months; $P < 0.001$)

- In a larger group of 2981 patients with newly diagnosed myeloma, those diagnosed during the last decade had a 50% improvement in overall survival (44.8 vs. 29.9 months; $P < 0.001$)

A second study[2,3] estimated trends in age-specific 5- and 10-year relative survival of patients with multiple myeloma (MM) in the United States from 1990–1992 to 2002–2004 from the 1973–2004 database of the Surveillance, Epidemiology, and End Results (SEER) Program. Techniques of period analysis were used to show most recent developments:

Five- and 10-Year Estimates of Relative Survival of Patients with MM by Age Group and Calendar Period

	1990–1992		2002–2004		Increase[†]	P[‡]
	PE*	SE*	PE	SE		
5-Year Relative Survival						
All ages	28.8	0.9	34.7	0.9	5.9	<0.001
Younger than 50 years	44.8	3.5	56.7	3.0	11.9	0.001
50 to 59 years	38.8	2.5	48.2	2.1	9.4	0.001
60 to 69 years	30.6	1.8	36.3	1.8	5.7	0.09
70 to 79 years	27.1	1.7	28.7	1.6	1.6	0.21
80 years and older	13.8	2.0	15.2	1.9	1.4	0.96

International Myeloma Working Group Uniform Response Criteria

Disease Progression and Relapse

Progressive Disease*

Any one or more of the following:
- Increase of ≥25% from baseline in serum M-component (absolute increase must be ≥0.5 g/dL)
- Increase of ≥25% from baseline in urine M-component (absolute increase must be ≥200 mg/24 hours)
- Increase of ≥25% from baseline in the difference between involved and uninvolved FLC levels—only in patients without measurable serum and urine M-protein levels (absolute increase must be ≥10 mg/dL)
- Increase of ≥25% from baseline in bone marrow plasma cell percentage (absolute percentage must be ≥10%)
- Definite development of new bone lesions or soft-tissue plasmacytomas or definite increase in the size of existing bone lesions or soft-tissue plasmacytomas
- Development of hypercalcemia (corrected serum calcium >11.5 mg/dL or >2.88 mmol/L) that can be attributed solely to the plasma cell proliferative disorder

Clinical Relapse

One or more of the following:
- Development of new soft-tissue plasmacytomas or bone lesions
- Definite increase in the size of existing plasmacytomas or bone lesions. A definite increase is defined as a 50% (and at least 1 cm) increase as measured serially by the sum of the products of the cross-diameters of the measurable lesion
- Hypercalcemia >11.5 mg/dL (>2.88 mmol/L)
- Decrease in hemoglobin of ≥2 g/dL
- Rise in serum creatinine by ≥2 mg/dL (≥177 μmol/L)

Relapse from CR[†]

One or more of the following:
- Reappearance of serum or urine M-protein by immunofixation or electrophoresis
- Development of ≥5% plasma cells in the bone marrow
- Appearance of any other sign of progression (ie, new plasmacytoma, lytic bone lesion, or hypercalcemia)

*Used for calculation of time to progression and progression-free survival outcomes for all patients, including those in CR (includes primary progressive and disease progression on or off therapy)
†Used only if the outcome studied is disease-free survival (DFS)

Durie BGM et al. International uniform response criteria for multiple myeloma. Leukemia 2006;20:1467–1473

Median Survival (continued)

Five- and 10-Year Estimates of Relative Survival of Patients with MM by Age Group and Calendar Period

	1990–1992		2002–2004			
	PE*	SE*	PE	SE	Increase[†]	P[‡]
10-Year Relative Survival						
All ages	11.1	0.8	17.4	0.8	6.3	<0.001
Younger than 50 years	24.5	3.4	41.3	3.2	16.8	<0.001
50 to 59 years	17.2	2.1	28.6	2.2	11.4	<0.001
60 to 69 years	10.8	1.3	15.4	1.5	4.6	0.03
70 to 79 years	7.4	1.4	10.4	1.4	3.0	0.09
80 years and older	7.1	2.3	5.7	1.7	−1.4	0.94

*PE indicates point estimate; and SE, standard error
[†]Increase from 1990–1992 to 2002–2004 in percentage points
[‡]P for trend from 1990–1992 to the last period 2002–2004

1. Kumar SK et al. Improved survival in multiple myeloma and the impact of novel therapies. Blood 2008;111:2516–2520
2. Brenner H et al. Recent major improvement in long-term survival of younger patients with multiple myeloma. Blood 2008;111:2521–2526
3. Ghobrial IM, Anderson KC. The road to cure in multiple myeloma. Blood 2008;111:2503

A recent update (Pulte et al. Leuk Lymphoma 2013 Sep 3. [Epub ahead of print]) continues to demonstrate increased survival for patients with myeloma, but with a disparity in survival between non-Hispanic whites and minorities that has been persistent or slightly increasing over time, especially for younger patients. The reasons for these differences cannot be definitively ascertained from the SEER database, the source of the data since it lacks important information concerning several critical factors including cytogenetics, staging of myeloma, chemotherapeutic regimens employed and insurance data.

Number of Cases and Median Age at Presentation, Overall and by Ethnic Group*

Period	Case Numbers			Median Age		
	1998–2001	2002–2005	2006–2009	1998–2001	2002–2005	2006–2009
All	6443	6993	7120	69	68	67
NHW	4227	4378	4283	70	70	68
All nonwhite	2174	2551	2702	66	65	65
AA	1075	1245	1354	65	64	64
Hispanic	631	736	780	65	66	64
API	414	491	514	69	69	69

AA, African American; API, Asian and Pacific Islander; NWH, non-Hispanic white
*Note that number of NHW plus all nonwhites does not equal total case number because patients with missing information on ethnicity/race and more than 1 race or ethnic group were not included in analysis of individual racial groups

Adapted from Pulte et al. Leuk Lymphoma 2013; Early Online: 1–7

(continued)

Median Survival (continued)

Five- and 10-Year Relative Survival by Ethnic/Racial Group for All Age Groups

Period	Unadjusted Relative Survival (SE)			Adjusted Relative Survival (SE)*		
	1998–2001	2002–2005	2006–2009	1998–2001	2002–2005	2006–2009
5-Year Survival						
All	34.8 (0.6)	39.7 (0.4)	44.6 (0.6)	35.6 (0.6)	39.8 (0.4)	44 (0.6)
δ/p Value[†]	+9.8/<0.0001			+8.4/<0.0001		
NHW	34.2 (0.7)	39.6 (0.5)	44.9 (0.8)	36.4 (0.7)	40.9 (0.5)	45.3 (0.7)
δ/p Value[†]	+10.7/<0.0001			+8.9/<0.0001		
All nonwhite	35.4 (1)	39.5 (0.7)	43.5 (1)	33.8 (1)	37.6 (0.7)	41.4 (1)
δ/p Value[†]	+8.1/<0.0001			+7.6/<0.0001		
AA	35.1 (1.5)	39.7 (1)	44.3 (1.4)	33.4 (1.4)	37.4 (0.9)	41.5 (1.4)
δ/p Value[†]	+9.2/<0.0001			+8.1/<0.0001		
Hispanic	35.3 (1.9)	38.9 (1.2)	42.5 (1.8)	32.6 (1.8)	36.2 (1.2)	39.8 (1.8)
δ/p Value[†]	+7.2/0.01			+7.2/0.007		
API	37.3 (2.5)	39.8 (1.6)	42.4 (2.3)	37.5 (2.3)	40.4 (1.5)	43.3 (2.2)
δ/p Value[†]	+5.1/0.16			+5.8/0.09		
10-Year Survival						
All	16.1 (0.5)	20.4 (0.4)	25 (0.6)	16.6 (0.5)	20.2 (0.4)	24.1 (0.5)
δ/p Value[†]	+8.9/<0.0001			+7.7/<0.0001		
NHW	15.3 (0.6)	19.7 (0.5)	24.5 (0.7)	17 (0.6)	20.5 (0.5)	24.6 (0.7)
δ/p Value[†]	+9.2/<0.0001			+7.8/<0.0001		
All nonwhite	17.4 (1)	21.3 (0.8)	25.6 (1.2)	16.1 (0.8)	19.4 (0.6)	23 (0.9)
δ/p Value[†]	+8.2/<0.0001			+7.3/<0.0001		
AA	16.1 (1.2)	20.1 (1)	24.5 (1.4)	14.8 (1.1)	18.2 (0.9)	21.6 (1.2)
δ/p Value[†]	+8.4/<0.0001			+7.0/<0.0001		
Hispanic	17.4 (1.7)	21.1 (1.3)	25.2 (1.8)	15.3 (1.5)	18.6 (1.2)	22 (1.6)
δ/p Value[†]	+7.8/0.001			+6.9/0.0006		
API	22 (2.3)	24.9 (1.7)	27.8 (2.3)	21.4 (2.1)	24.4 (1.6)	28.1 (2.2)
δ/p Value[†]	+5.8/0.07			+7.0/0.03		

AA, African American; API, Asian and Pacific Islander; NHW, non-Hispanic white
*Age adjusted to International Cancer Survival Standard
[†]δ = Delta or difference between 1998–2001 and 2006–2009 periods and p value for trend

Adapted from Pulte et al. Leuk Lymphoma 2013; Early Online: 1–7

(continued)

Median Survival (continued)

Five- and 10-year Relative Survival by Ethnic and Age Groups

Period	15–49		50–69		70 and Older	
	5-Year Relative Survival (SE)		5-Year Relative Survival (SE)		5-Year Relative Survival (SE)	
	1998–2001	2006–2009	1998–2001	2006–2009	1998–2001	2006–2009
5-Year Survival						
All	52.9 (1.9)	66.1 (1.7)	39.9 (0.9)	52.2 (0.9)	26 (0.8)	30.8 (0.9)
δ/p Value*	**+13.2/<0.0001**		**+12.5/<0.0001**		**+4.8/<0.0001**	
NHW	54.4 (2.6)	71.2 (2.2)	40.8 (1.2)	53.7 (1.1)	25.6 (1)	31 (1.1)
δ/p Value*	**+16.8/<0.0001**		**+13.3/<0.0001**		**+5.4/<0.0001**	
All nonwhite	50.7 (2.9)	60.1 (2.6)	38.1 (1.5)	49 (1.4)	26.7 (1.9)	29.9 (1.8)
δ/p Value*	**+9.4/0.03**		**+11.7/<0.0001**		+3.2/0.23	
AA	46.1 (4)	60.5 (3.6)	39 (2.1)	48.9 (2)	25.9 (2.3)	30 (2.3)
δ/p Value*	**+14.4/0.01**		**+10.3/0.0007**		+4.1/0.21	
Hispanic	52.4 (5)	58.2 (4.5)	36.6 (2.7)	47.4 (2.6)	25.2 (3.1)	29.3 (2.9)
δ/p Value*	+5.8/0.42		**+9.2/0.02**		+4.1/0.34	
API	60.3 (7.3)	63.4 (8)	39 (3.8)	51.3 (3.4)	30.1 (3.5)	30.5 (3.2)
δ/p Value*	+3.1/0.79		**+14.2/0.01**		+0.4/0.93	
10-Year Survival						
All	34.6 (1.9)	47.3 (1.9)	17.6 (0.8)	30 (0.9)	9.8 (0.6)	13 (0.7)
δ/p Value*	**+12.7/<0.0001**		**+12.4/<0.0001**		**+3.2/<0.0001**	
NHW	36.6 (2.7)	53.7 (2.6)	17.7 (1)	30.1 (1.1)	9 (0.7)	12.4 (0.9)
δ/p Value*	**+17.1/<0.0001**		**+12.4/<0.0001**		**+3.4/<0.0001**	
All nonwhite	30 (3.3)	39.4 (3.4)	17.4 (1.5)	29.6 (1.7)	12.5 (1.6)	14.7 (1.7)
δ/p Value*	+9.4/0.06		**+12.2/<0.0001**		+2.2/0.25	
AA	27 (3.6)	38.9 (3.9)	16.6 (1.7)	27.5 (2)	10.5 (1.8)	12.7 (2)
δ/p Value*	**+11.9/0.03**		**+10.9/<0.0001**		+2.2/0.31	
Hispanic	36.6 (5.5)	41.3 (4.7)	16.4 (2.3)	28.2 (2.6)	8.5 (2.4)	11.8 (2.6)
δ/p Value*	+4.7/0.54		**+1.8/<0.0001**		+3.3/0.24	
API	37.8 (7.3)	39.3 (7.8)	21.6 (3.5)	35 (3.6)	18 (3.4)	19.2 (3.1)
δ/p Value*	+1.5/0.89		**+13.4/0.008**		+1.2/0.78	

AA, African American; API, Asian and Pacific Islander; NHW, non-Hispanic white

*δ = Delta or difference between 1998–2001 and 2006–2009 periods and p value for trend

Adapted from Pulte et al. Leuk Lymphoma 2013; Early Online: 1–7

Expert Opinion

1. *Treatment by stage:*

Asymptomatic MGUS, smoldering MM, and Stage I MM

These patients do not need primary therapy and should be ***monitored without therapy*** unless they have evidence of disease progression. Clinical trials are being conducted in these stages. Follow-up every 3 to 6 months is recommended. Progression of the disease to stage II or higher, is defined by:

- 25% increase in the monoclonal component (serum or urine)
- >25% increase in plasma cells bone marrow infiltration
- Increased size of bone lesions or development of new lytic lesions
- Hypercalcemia
- Increased plasmacytoma tumor volume

Symptomatic patients (Stages II and III MM)

These patients should be ***treated with combination therapy followed by consideration for stem cell transplantation*** if eligible. Determine whether a patient is a candidate for high-dose therapy with autologous peripheral blood stem cell (PBSC) transplantation before initiating chemotherapy. Avoid alkylating agents in such patients before autologous PBSCs are collected, because exposure to alkylating agents may prevent the collection of an adequate number of PBSCs for autologous transplantation

Regimens

Newly Diagnosed Multiple Myeloma—Transplantation Candidates

Lenalidomide + low-dose dexamethasone	Rajkumar SV et al. Lancet Oncol 2010;11:29–37
Bortezomib + dexamethasone	Harousseau J-L et al. J Clin Oncol 2010;28:4621–4629
Bortezomib + lenalidomide + dexamethasone	Richardson PG et al. Blood 2010;116:679–686
Bortezomib + thalidomide + dexamethasone	Cavo M et al. Lancet 2010;376:2075–2085 Kaufman JL et al. Cancer 2010;116:3143–3151
Bortezomib + doxorubicin + dexamethasone	Sonneveld P et al. J Clin Oncol 2012;30:2946–2955
Cyclophosphamide + bortezomib + dexamethasone	Reeder CB et al. Leukemia 2009;23:1337–1341
Carfilzomib + lenalidomide + dexamethasone	Jakubowlak AJ et al. Blood 2012;120:1801–1809
Thalidomide + dexamethasone	Rajkumar SV et al. J Clin Oncol 2006;24:431–436

Newly Diagnosed Multiple Myeloma—Those Not Transplantation Candidates

Melphalan + prednisone + thalidomide	Palumbo A et al. Lancet 2006;367:825–831 Palumbo A et al. Blood 2008;112:3107–3114
Bortezomib + melphalan + prednisone	San Miguel JFS et al. N Engl J Med 2008;359:906–917
Melphalan + prednisone + lenalidomide	Palumbo A et al. J Clin Oncol 2007;25:4459–4465

Relapsed/Refractory Multiple Myeloma

Bortezomib	Richardson PG et al. N Engl J Med 2003;348:2609–2617
Lenalidomide + dexamethasone	Dimopoulos M et al. N Engl J Med 2007;357:2123–2132 Weber DM et al. N Engl J Med 2007;357:2133–2142
Carfilzomib (bortezomib-naïve)	Vij R et al. Blood 2012;119:5661–5670
Carfilzomib (prior bortezomib)	Vij R et al. Br J Haematol 2012;158:739–748
Pomalidomide + dexamethasone	Lacy MQ et al. Leukemia 2010;24:1934–1939 Leleu X et al. Blood 2013;121:1968–1975
Pomalidomide + cyclophosphamide + prednisone	Larocca A et al. Blood 2013;122:2799–2806
Bortezomib + liposomal doxorubicin HCl	Orlowski RZ et al. J Clin Oncol 2007;25:3892–3901

(continued)

Expert Opinion (*continued*)

High-Dose Conditioning for Stem Cell Transplantation in Relapsed/Refractory Multiple Myeloma	
High-dose melphalan	Moreau P et al. Blood 2002;99:731–735
Maintenance Therapy Multiple Myeloma	
Bortezomib	Sonneveld P et al. J Clin Oncol 2012;30:2946–2955
Lenalidomide	Attal M et al. N Engl J Med 2012;366:1782–1791 Dimopoulos MA et al. Haematologica 2013;98:784–788 McCarthy PL et al. N Engl J Med 2012;366:1770–1781 Palumbo A et al. N Engl J Med 2012;366:1759–1769
Thalidomide	Morgan GJ et al. Blood 2012;119:7–15

2. *Indications for treatment:*
   - Monoclonal plasma cells in the bone marrow >10% and/or presence of a biopsy-proven plasmacytoma
   - Monoclonal protein present in the serum and/or urine*
   - Myeloma-related organ dysfunction (≥1)[†]

   [C] Calcium elevation in the blood (serum calcium >10.5 mg/dL [>2.63 mmol/L] or greater than the upper limit of normal range)
   [R] Renal insufficiency (serum creatinine >2 mg/dL [>177 μmol/L])
   [A] Anemia (hemoglobin <10 g/dL or 2 g less than the lower limit of normal range)
   [B] Lytic bone lesions or osteoporosis[‡]

*If no monoclonal protein is detected (nonsecretory disease), then >30% monoclonal bone marrow plasma cells and/or a biopsy-proven plasmacytoma required
[†]A variety of other types of end-organ dysfunctions can occasionally occur and lead to a need for therapy. Such dysfunction is sufficient to support classification of myeloma if proven to be myeloma related
[‡]If a solitary (biopsy-proven) plasmacytoma or osteoporosis alone (without fractures) is the sole defining criteria, then >30% plasma cells are required in the bone marrow

Note: THESE CRITERIA IDENTIFY STAGE IB and STAGES II and III A/B MYELOMA BY DURIE/SALMON STAGE. Stage IA becomes smoldering or indolent myeloma

3. *Solitary plasmacytoma:*
   - Primary radiation therapy (≥45 Gy) to the involved fields represents the initial treatment for patients diagnosed with osseous plasmacytoma
   - Same approach and/or surgery represent the initial treatment for patients with extraosseous plasmacytomas
   - Follow-up for either solitary or extraosseous plasmacytomas includes blood and urine tests every 4 weeks to monitor response to radiation treatment
   - If a complete disappearance of the monoclonal component is demonstrated, blood and urine tests will be performed every 3–6 months
   - If the monoclonal component persists, follow-up should continue every 4 weeks
   - If a progression in the disease is documented, a reevaluation for recurrent extraosseous plasmacytomas and/or myeloma should be considered

Dimopoulos MA et al. J Clin Oncol 1992;10:587–590
Hu K, Yahalom J. Oncology (Williston Park) 2000;14:101–108, 111; discussion 111–112, 115

(*continued*)

Expert Opinion (*continued*)

4. Treatment with a bisphosphonate is recommended to reduce skeletal complications for all myeloma patients with skeletal lesions. Alternatives that have demonstrated efficacy in this setting include:
   - Pamidronate, *or*
   - Zoledronic acid, *or*
   - Clodronate

Notes:
   - Because renal toxicity can result from bisphosphonate therapy, renal function should be monitored closely. Bisphosphonate doses may need to be modified or discontinued in renally impaired individuals
   - Myeloma patients with bone lesions should receive treatment with a bisphosphonate. Whether to administer bisphosphonates to myeloma patients without evidence of bone disease is unclear. Some research has shown bisphosphonates may have a clinical benefit even in patients without bone disease. Recommendations on how often bisphosphonates should be administered will likely evolve over time. Current recommendations are to administer standard doses of bisphosphonates every 3–4 weeks. The duration for which repeated doses should be administered is also unclear. Currently, there are no data from randomized studies to guide bisphosphonate use for more than 2 years. The risks and benefits of continuing bisphosphonate treatment after 2 years must be considered in each patient. To prevent osteonecrosis of the jaw, patients treated with bisphosphonates should maintain good dental hygiene and should stop bisphosphonate treatment for 90 days before and after invasive dental procedures. Caregivers must ensure that myeloma patients get enough vitamin D and calcium. This is a concern because 60% of myeloma patients are vitamin D and calcium deficient. U.S. Food and Drug Administration product labeling for both zoledronic acid and pamidronate disodium recommend vitamin D and calcium supplementation in conjunction with bisphosphonate treatment, but calcium supplementation should be used cautiously for patients with kidney problems

5. Anemia is present in most patients with multiple myeloma. Reversible causes of anemia should be evaluated and treated. Patients with symptomatic anemia may benefit from therapy with recombinant erythropoietin (see Chapter 43)

6. Waldenström macroglobulinemia presents with lymphoplasmacytic bone marrow infiltration and IgM paraproteinemia. Therapy usually consists of rituximab along with an alkylating agent such as cyclophosphamide, or bortezomib or nucleoside analogs such as fludarabine. Other management considerations focus on complications caused by macroglobulinemia, such as hyperviscosity, cryoglobulinemia, and hemolytic anemia

7. Primary amyloidosis is characterized by organ dysfunction resulting from monoclonal light-chain production and tissue deposition. Carefully selected patients may benefit from high-dose melphalan with autologous PBSC support, which can result in hematologic remission, regression of light-chain deposition, and improvement in organ function. Other options include the use of bortezomib- or lenalidomide-based regimens

8. The optimal prophylaxis strategy for thromboembolic complications of IMiD therapy (thalidomide and lenalidomide) is not clear. Therapy with low-molecular-weight heparins or full-dose warfarin anticoagulation are standard treatments for DVT and pulmonary embolism in the general population. However, in patients with multiple myeloma, data exist supporting the protective effect of aspirin against VTE, despite its mechanism of arterial anticoagulation. Until more is known about the nature and mechanism of thromboembolism induced by the IMiDs, it is difficult to say which agent is most appropriate. At this time, any of the agents may be considered reasonable; however, all patients receiving combination therapy with lenalidomide or thalidomide should have some form of thromboembolic prophylaxis incorporated into therapy

Palumbo A et al. Enoxaparin or aspirin for the prevention of recurrent thromboembolism in newly diagnosed myeloma patients treated with melphalan and prednisone plus thalidomide or lenalidomide. J Thromb Haemost 2006;4:1842–1845

Palumbo A et al. Prevention of thalidomide- and lenalidomide-associated thrombosis in myeloma. Leukemia 2008;22:414–423

REGIMEN
NEWLY DIAGNOSED MULTIPLE MYELOMA (TRANSPLANTATION CANDIDATES)

INDUCTION PRIOR TO AUTOLOGOUS STEM CELL TRANSPLANTATION (ASCT)
LENALIDOMIDE + LOW-DOSE DEXAMETHASONE

Rajkumar SV et al. Lancet Oncol 2010;11:29–37

Lenalidomide 25 mg/day; administer orally, continually, for 21 consecutive days on days 1–21, every 28 days (total dose/cycle = 525 mg)
Dexamethasone 40 mg/dose; administer orally for 4 doses on days 1, 8, 15, and 22, every 28 days (total dose/cycle = 160 mg)

Supportive Care
Antiemetic prophylaxis
*Emetogenic potential is **MINIMAL–LOW***
See Chapter 39 for antiemetic recommendations

Hematopoietic growth factor (CSF) prophylaxis
Primary prophylaxis is NOT indicated
See Chapter 43 for more information

Antimicrobial prophylaxis
Risk of fever and neutropenia is INTERMEDIATE
Antimicrobial primary prophylaxis to be considered:
- Antibacterial—consider a fluoroquinolone or no prophylaxis; *P. jirovecii* prophylaxis is recommended (eg, cotrimoxazole)
- Antifungal—consider concomitant use of clotrimazole during periods of neutropenia
- Antiviral—antiherpes antivirals (eg, acyclovir, famciclovir, valacyclovir)

Caution: Acyclovir and famciclovir accumulate in patients with impaired renal function and may exacerbate renal dysfunction (valacyclovir is a *prodrug* for acyclovir). Monitor kidney function serially during acyclovir, valacyclovir, and famciclovir use
- Acyclovir and famciclovir elimination is inversely related to renal function
- Acyclovir, famciclovir, and valacyclovir utilization is modified in renally impaired individuals (consult product labeling or Summary of Product Characteristics for guidance about dose/dosage and administration frequency modifications, and, when relevant, recommendations for drug dilution, administration rate, concurrent fluid administration, and fluid supplementation as a function of urine output)
- Impaired acyclovir elimination is associated with neurologic adverse effects, including agitation, ataxia, coma, confusion, dizziness, dysarthria, encephalopathy, hallucinations, paresthesia, seizure, somnolence, and tremors
See Chapter 47 for more information

(continued)

Treatment Modifications

Adverse Event	Treatment Modification
Platelet count <30,000/mm³	Interrupt lenalidomide treatment, follow CBC weekly. Resume lenalidomide at 15 mg/day after platelet count is ≥30,000/mm³
For each subsequent platelet count <30,000/mm³	Interrupt lenalidomide treatment, follow CBC weekly. After platelet count recovers to ≥30,000/mm³, resume lenalidomide at a dose decreased from the previous dose by 5 mg/day, but the daily dose should not be less than 5 mg/day
ANC <1000/mm³	Interrupt lenalidomide treatment, follow CBC weekly. Resume lenalidomide at 15 mg/day after ANC ≥1000/mm³
For each subsequent ANC <1000/mm³	Interrupt lenalidomide treatment, follow CBC weekly. After ANC recovers to ≥1000/mm³, resume lenalidomide at a dose decreased from the previous dose by 5 mg/day, but the daily dose should not be less than 5 mg/day
Febrile neutropenia	Interrupt lenalidomide treatment, follow closely, and resume lenalidomide at 15 mg/day after fever abates
G3/4 nonhematologic toxicity	Interrupt lenalidomide treatment, follow clinically. After toxicity abates to G ≤2, resume lenalidomide at a dose decreased from the previous dose by 5 mg/day, but the daily dose should not be less than 5 mg/day

(continued)

(*continued*)

Thromboprophylaxis

Risk assessment and recommendations for VTE prophylaxis in patients with multiple myeloma with individual or myeloma-related risk factors, or risk factors related to treatment

Individual risk factors	
• Obesity (BMI ≥30 kg/m²)	
• H/O VTE	
• CVC or pacemaker	
• Comorbid pathologies	
Cardiac disease	
Chronic renal disease	≤1 Individual or myeloma risk factor present:
Diabetes	• **Aspirin** 81–325 mg daily
Acute infection	
Immobilization	
• Surgery	≥2 Individual or myeloma risk factors present:
General surgery	• **LMWH*, equivalent to enoxaparin sodium** 40 mg/day *or* **dalteparin sodium** 5000 IU/day; administer subcutaneously, *or*
Any anesthesia	
Trauma	
• Medications	• **Warfarin**, targeting an INR = 2–3
Erythropoietin (epoetin alfa, darbepoetin)	
Estrogenic compounds	
Bevacizumab	
• Clotting disorders	
Thrombophilia	
Myeloma-related risk factors	
• Diagnosis of multiple myeloma	
• Hyperviscosity	
Concomitant treatment-related risk factors	**LMWH*, equivalent to enoxaparin sodium** 40 mg/day *or* **dalteparin sodium** 5000 IU/day; administer subcutaneously, *or*
Thalidomide or lenalidomide in combination with:	
• High-dose dexamethasone (≥480 mg/month)	**Warfarin**, targeting an INR = 2–3
• Doxorubicin	
• Multiagent chemotherapy	

CVC, central venous catheter; INR, international normalized ratio; LMWH, low-molecular-weight heparin; VTE, venous thromboembolic disease

*LMWHs should be used with caution in individuals with impaired renal function (creatinine clearance <30 mL/min). Refer to product labeling for information about doses and administration schedules in renally impaired patients, and guidance for monitoring anti-Factor Xa concentrations

Geerts WH et al. Chest 2008;133(6 Suppl):381S–453S
Multiple Myeloma, V.1.2014. National Comprehensive Cancer Network, Inc., 2013. (Accessed October 8, 2013, at http://www.nccn.org)
Palumbo A et al. Leukemia 2008;22:414–423
Venous Thromboembolic Disease, V.2.2013. National Comprehensive Cancer Network, Inc., 2013. (Accessed October 8, 2013, at http://www.nccn.org)

Bisphosphonates

All patients receiving primary therapy for symptomatic multiple myeloma should receive a bisphosphonate adjunctively; *for example*:

• **Pamidronate disodium** 90 mg; administer intravenously over 2–4 hours, every month, *or*

• **Zoledronic acid** 4 mg; administer intravenously over 15 minutes, every month

Consider baseline bone densitometry evaluation

See Chapter 43 for more information

Treatment Modifications
(continued)

Adverse Event	Treatment Modification
Toxicities ascribed to dexamethasone such as severe manifestations of hypercorticism, including hyperglycemia, irritability, insomnia, and oral candidiasis	Reduce dexamethasone dose to 20 mg per day

Lenalidomide starting dose adjustment for Renal Impairment in Multiple Myeloma (Days 1–21 of Each 28-day Cycle)

Moderate renal impairment CrCl 30–60 mL/min (0.5–1 mL/s)	10 mg lenalidomide every 24 hours
Severe renal impairment CrCl <30 mL/min (<0.5 mL/s), not requiring dialysis	15 mg lenalidomide every 48 hours
End-stage renal disease CrCl <30 mL/min (<0.5 mL/s), requiring dialysis	5 mg/day. On dialysis days, administer a daily dose following dialysis

CrCl, Creatinine clearance

Patient Population Studied

Randomized phase III trial of 445 patients with newly diagnosed multiple myeloma. Patients were eligible if they had previously untreated symptomatic multiple myeloma, bone marrow plasmacytosis (≥10% plasma cells or sheets of plasma cells), or a biopsy-proven plasmacytoma, and measurable disease defined as serum monoclonal protein >10 g/L or urine monoclonal protein ≥0.2 g/day or more. Study eligibility also required hemoglobin >7 g/dL, platelet count ≥75,000/mm³, ANC ≥1000/mm³, and an acceptable serum creatinine. Patients were excluded if they had G ≥2 peripheral neuropathy, active infection, current or prior deep vein thrombosis, or Eastern Cooperative Oncology Group performance status = 3/4

Efficacy (N = 208)

Best overall Response to Therapy	Percent of Patients
Overall response rate (partial response or better)	70%
Complete plus very good partial response	40%
Complete response	4%
Immunofixation-negative complete response	10%
Very good partial response	26%
Partial response	30%
Minimal response	13%
No response/stable disease	8%
Progressive disease	2%
Unevaluable	7%

1-year overall survival*	96% (95% CI, 94–99)
2-year overall survival*	87% (95% CI, 81–93)
1-year overall survival, ages <65 years old	98% (95% CI, 92–99)
1-year overall survival, ages ≥65 years old	94% (95% CI, 89–99)
Median time to partial response or better	1 month[†]
Median response duration	24.1 months (95% CI, 21.5–28.1)
Median progression-free survival	25.3 months (22.3–not reached)

*Overall survival was not a protocol-specified end point in this study. However, the study was stopped on recommendations of the independent data monitoring committee at a median follow-up of 12.5 months (95% CI, 11.5–14.6), because overall survival was significantly higher with low-dose dexamethasone than with high-dose dexamethasone ($p = 0.0002$). All patients in the high-dose group were instructed to crossover to receive low-dose dexamethasone
[†]Among patients who responded

Toxicity

G ≥3 Toxicities (N = 220)

Toxicity	Percent of patients
Hematologic	
Hemoglobin	7%
Platelets	5%
Neutrophils	20%
Nonhematologic	
Deep vein thrombosis or pulmonary embolism	12%
Infection or pneumonia	9%
Hyperglycemia	6%
Cardiac ischemia	<1%
Atrial fibrillation or flutter	<1%
Fatigue	9%
Neuropathy	2%
Nonneuropathic weakness	4%
Summary	
Any G ≥3 toxicity in first 4 months	35%
Any G ≥3 nonhematologic toxicity at any time during therapy	48%
Any G ≥4 nonhematologic toxicity at any time during therapy	14%
Early mortality (first 4 months)	<1%

Reason for Discontinuation (N = 222)

Treatment completed per protocol	25%
Disease progression	17%
Adverse events or complications	23%
Death on study	3%
Patient withdrawal or refusal	5%
Alternative therapy	17%
Other complicating disease	1%
Other	8%

Therapy Monitoring

1. *Before each cycle:* CBC with differential and blood chemistries (including BUN, creatinine, and calcium)
2. *Every 6 weeks to 3 months:* Measure serum and urine M-protein

REGIMEN
NEWLY DIAGNOSED MULTIPLE MYELOMA (TRANSPLANTATION CANDIDATES)

INDUCTION PRIOR TO AUTOLOGOUS STEM CELL TRANSPLANTATION (ASCT)
BORTEZOMIB + DEXAMETHASONE

Harousseau J-L et al. J Clin Oncol 2010;28:4621–4629

Bortezomib 1.3 mg/m^2 per dose; administer by intravenous injection over 3–5 seconds for 4 doses on days 1, 4, 8, and 11, every 3 weeks for 4 cycles (total dosage/cycle = 5.2 mg/m^2)

Dexamethasone 40 mg/dose; administer orally, as follows:
- *Cycles 1 and 2:* For 4 consecutive days on days 1–4, and for 4 consecutive days on days 9–12, every 3 weeks for 2 cycles (total dose/cycle = 320 mg)
- *Cycles 3 and 4:* For 4 consecutive days on days 1–4, every 3 weeks for 2 cycles (total dose/cycle = 160 mg)

Supportive Care
Antiemetic prophylaxis
Emetogenic potential is **MINIMAL**
See Chapter 39 for antiemetic recommendations

Hematopoietic growth factor (CSF) prophylaxis
Primary prophylaxis is NOT indicated
See Chapter 43 for more information

Antimicrobial prophylaxis
Risk of fever and neutropenia is HIGH
 Antimicrobial primary prophylaxis is recommended:
- Antibacterial—consider fluoroquinolone prophylaxis; *P. jirovecii* prophylaxis is recommended (eg, cotrimoxazole)
- Antifungal—recommended
- Antiviral—antiherpes antivirals (eg, acyclovir, famciclovir, valacyclovir)

Caution: Acyclovir and famciclovir accumulate in patients with impaired renal function and may exacerbate renal dysfunction (valacyclovir is a *prodrug* for acyclovir). Monitor kidney function serially during acyclovir, valacyclovir, and famciclovir use
- Acyclovir and famciclovir elimination is inversely related to renal function
- Acyclovir, famciclovir, and valacyclovir utilization is modified in renally impaired individuals (consult product labeling or Summary of Product Characteristics for guidance about dose/dosage and administration frequency modifications, and, when relevant, recommendations for drug dilution, administration rate, concurrent fluid administration, and fluid supplementation as a function of urine output)
- Impaired acyclovir elimination is associated with neurologic adverse effects, including agitation, ataxia, coma, confusion, dizziness, dysarthria, encephalopathy, hallucinations, paresthesia, seizure, somnolence, and tremors
See Chapter 47 for more information

(continued)

Treatment Modifications

Adverse Event	Treatment Modification
Febrile neutropenia	Withhold therapy until fever abates, then resume therapy at the same dosages and schedules
G4 hematologic toxicity	Withhold therapy until counts recover to ANC >750/mm^3 and platelets >50,000/mm^3, then resume therapy
G3/4 nonhematologic toxicity	Interrupt therapy, follow clinically and resume therapy when toxicity G ≤2
Toxicities ascribed to dexamethasone such as severe manifestations of hypercorticism, including hyperglycemia, irritability and insomnia, oral candidiasis	Reduce dexamethasone dose to 20 mg per dose

Treatment Modification for Bortezomib-Induced Peripheral Neuropathy*

Severity of Peripheral Neuropathy	Modification of Dose and Schedule
G1 (paresthesias or loss of reflexes) without pain or loss of function	No action
G1 with pain or G2 (interferes with function, but not with activities of daily living)	Reduce bortezomib dosage to 1 mg/m^2 per dose
G2 with pain or G3 (interferes with activities of daily living)	Withhold bortezomib treatment until toxicity resolves, then reinitiate at a dosage of 0.7 mg/m^2 per dose once weekly
G4 (permanent sensory loss that interferes with function)	Discontinue treatment

*Richardson PG et al. J Clin Oncol 2006;24:3113–3120

(*continued*)

Thromboprophylaxis

Risk assessment and recommendations for VTE prophylaxis in patients with multiple myeloma with individual or myeloma-related risk factors, or risk factors related to treatment

Individual risk factors
• Obesity (BMI $\geq$30 kg/m^2)
• H/O VTE
• CVC or pacemaker
• Comorbid pathologies
  Cardiac disease
  Chronic renal disease
  Diabetes
  Acute infection
  Immobilization
• Surgery
  General surgery
  Any anesthesia
  Trauma
• Medications
  Erythropoietin (epoetin alfa, darbepoetin)
  Estrogenic compounds
  Bevacizumab
• Clotting disorders
  Thrombophilia
Myeloma-related risk factors
• Diagnosis of multiple myeloma
• Hyperviscosity
	$\leq$1 Individual or myeloma risk factor present:
	• **Aspirin** 81–325 mg daily
	
	$\geq$2 Individual or myeloma risk factors present:
	• **LMWH***, **equivalent to enoxaparin sodium** 40 mg/day *or* **dalteparin sodium** 5000 IU/day; administer subcutaneously, *or*
	• **Warfarin**, targeting an INR = 2–3

Concomitant treatment-related risk factors Thalidomide or lenalidomide in combination with: • High-dose dexamethasone ($\geq$480 mg/month) • Doxorubicin • Multiagent chemotherapy	**LMWH***, **equivalent to enoxaparin sodium** 40 mg/day *or* **dalteparin sodium** 5000 IU/day; administer subcutaneously, *or* **Warfarin**, targeting an INR = 2–3

CVC, central venous catheter; INR, international normalized ratio; LMWH, low-molecular-weight heparin; VTE, venous thromboembolic disease

*LMWHs should be used with caution in individuals with impaired renal function (creatinine clearance <30 mL/min). Refer to product labeling for information about doses and administration schedules in renally impaired patients, and guidance for monitoring anti-Factor Xa concentrations

Geerts WH et al. Chest 2008;133(6 Suppl):381S–453S

Multiple Myeloma, V.1.2014. National Comprehensive Cancer Network, Inc., 2013. (Accessed October 8, 2013, at http://www.nccn.org)

Palumbo A et al. Leukemia 2008;22:414–423

Venous Thromboembolic Disease, V.2.2013. National Comprehensive Cancer Network, Inc., 2013. (Accessed October 8, 2013, at http://www.nccn.org)

Bisphosphonates

All patients receiving primary therapy for symptomatic multiple myeloma should receive a bisphosphonate adjunctively; *for example*:

• **Pamidronate disodium** 90 mg; administer intravenously over 2–4 hours, every month, *or*

• **Zoledronic acid** 4 mg; administer intravenously over 15 minutes, every month

Consider baseline bone densitometry evaluation

See Chapter 43 for more information

Patient Population Studied

Phase III study of 482 patients with multiple myeloma who were $\leq$65 years of age and eligible for autologous stem cell transplantation. All patients had untreated symptomatic MM with measurable paraprotein in serum (>10 g/L) or urine (>0.2 g/24 hours). Key eligibility criteria, included Eastern Cooperative Oncology Group PS $\leq$2, adequate renal function (no end-stage renal failure requiring dialysis), and hematologic (platelets $\geq$50,000/mm^3, neutrophils $\geq$750/mm^3), and hepatic (bilirubin $\leq$3 times the upper limit of normal range [ULN] and AST and ALT $\leq$4 times ULN) indices. Patients with confirmed diagnosis of amyloidosis and G $\geq$2 peripheral neuropathy were excluded

Efficacy

Response to Induction Therapy Overall and According to Baseline Disease Stage and Prognostic Factors

Evaluable Population (N = 223)

ORR (at least PR)	78.5%
At least VGPR	37.7%
CR/nCR	14.8%
CR	5.8%
MR + SD	12.6%
PD	4.5%
Death	0.5%
Not assessable	4%

ORR and at Least VGPR and CR/nCR Response Rates by Disease Stage

ISS 1

ORR	81.4%
At least VGPR	37.3%
CR/nCR	15.7%

ISS 2

ORR	71.6%
At least VGPR	35.8%
CR/nCR	14.8%

ISS 3

ORR	76.9%
At least VGPR	40.4%
CR/nCR	13.5%

Response to First Transplantation and Overall at Least VGPR and CR/nCR Rates, Including Second Transplantation, Among All Evaluable Patients

Response to First Transplantation

ORR (at least PR)	80.3%
At least VGPR	54.3%
CR/nCR	35%
CR	16.1%
MR + SD + PD	2.7%
Death	0.5%
No transplantation	11.7%

Overall, Including Second Transplantation

At least VGPR	67.7%
CR/nCR	39.5%

CR, complete response; CR/nCR, complete response/near complete response; ISS, International Staging System; MR, minimal response; ORR, overall response rate; PD, progressive disease; PR, partial response; SD, stable disease; VGPR, very good partial response

Toxicity (N = 239)

Toxicity	Percent of Patients
Any AE	96.7%
Any grade ≥3 AE	46.9%
Any grade ≥4 AE	11.3%
Any serious AE	27.2%
Toxicity leading to study drug discontinuation or delay	18.4%
Toxicity leading to bortezomib dose reduction	6.9% (64/931 cycles)
Death related to toxicity	0

Hematologic Toxicity	G1–4	G3/4
Anemia	15.9%	4.2%
Neutropenia	8%	5%
Thrombocytopenia	10.9%	2.9%
Infections	48.1%	8.8%
Herpes zoster*	9.2%	—
Thrombosis	4.6%	1.7%

Nonhematologic Toxicities	G1–4
Fatigue	28.5%
Rash	11.7%
GI symptoms	26.8%
Cardiac disorders	5.9%
Pneumopathy	3.4%
G1 Peripheral neuropathy†	21.3%
G2 Peripheral neuropathy†	15.5%
G3 Peripheral neuropathy†	7.1%

*No antiviral prophylaxis for *Herpes zoster* was specified in the protocol
†Medical Dictionary for Regulatory Activities (MedDRA) Preferred Terms used by investigators that were considered related to neurologic toxicity included accommodation disorder, anosmia, areflexia, difficulty in walking, dysesthesia, fall, formication, hypoesthesia, hyporeflexia, muscle spasms, pain in limb, paraparesis, paresthesia, peripheral motor neuropathy, peripheral neuropathy, sensory loss, vertigo, and vision blurred

Therapy Monitoring

1. *Before each cycle:* CBC with differential and blood chemistries (including BUN, creatinine, and calcium)
2. *Every 6 weeks to 3 months:* Measure serum and urine M-protein

REGIMEN
NEWLY DIAGNOSED MULTIPLE MYELOMA (TRANSPLANTATION CANDIDATES)

INDUCTION PRIOR TO AUTOLOGOUS STEM CELL TRANSPLANTATION (ASCT)
BORTEZOMIB + LENALIDOMIDE + DEXAMETHASONE

Richardson PG et al. Blood 2010;116:679–686

All Cycles:
Bortezomib 1–1.3 mg/m^2 per dose; administer by intravenous injection over 3–5 seconds for 4 doses on days 1, 4, 8, and 11, every 3 weeks for 8 cycles (total dosage/cycle for 1 mg/m^2 per dose = 4 mg/m^2; total dosage/cycle for 1.3 mg/m^2 per dose = 5.2 mg/m^2)
Lenalidomide 15–25 mg per day; administer orally for 14 consecutive days on days 1–14, every 3 weeks for 8 cycles (total dose/cycle for 15 mg/day = 210 mg; total dose/cycle for 25 mg/day = 350 mg)
Cycles 1–4:
Dexamethasone 40 mg per dose; administer orally for 8 doses on days 1, 2, 4, 5, 8, 9, 11, and 12, every 3 weeks for 4 cycles (total dose/cycle = 320 mg), *then*
Cycles 5–8:
Dexamethasone 20 mg per dose; administer orally for 8 doses on days 1, 2, 4, 5, 8, 9, 11, and 12, every 3 weeks for 4 cycles (total dose/cycle = 160 mg)

Supportive Care
Antiemetic prophylaxis
Emetogenic potential is **MINIMAL**
See Chapter 39 for antiemetic recommendations

Hematopoietic growth factor (CSF) prophylaxis
Primary prophylaxis is NOT indicated
See Chapter 43 for more information

Antimicrobial prophylaxis
Risk of fever and neutropenia is HIGH
Antimicrobial primary prophylaxis is recommended:
- Antibacterial—consider fluoroquinolone prophylaxis; *P. jirovecii* prophylaxis is recommended (eg, cotrimoxazole)
- Antifungal—recommended
- Antiviral—antiherpes antivirals (eg, acyclovir, famciclovir, valacyclovir)

Caution: Acyclovir and famciclovir accumulate in patients with impaired renal function and may exacerbate renal dysfunction (valacyclovir is a *prodrug* for acyclovir). Monitor kidney function serially during acyclovir, valacyclovir, and famciclovir use
- Acyclovir and famciclovir elimination is inversely related to renal function
- Acyclovir, famciclovir, and valacyclovir utilization is modified in renally impaired individuals (consult product labeling or Summary of Product Characteristics for guidance about dose/dosage and administration frequency modifications, and, when relevant, recommendations for drug dilution, administration rate, concurrent fluid administration, and fluid supplementation as a function of urine output)
- Impaired acyclovir elimination is associated with neurologic adverse effects, including agitation, ataxia, coma, confusion, dizziness, dysarthria, encephalopathy, hallucinations, paresthesia, seizure, somnolence, and tremors
See Chapter 47 for more information

Decreased bowel motility prophylaxis
Give a bowel regimen to prevent constipation based initially on **stool softeners**

(continued)

Treatment Modifications

Adverse Event	Treatment Modification
Platelet count <30,000/mm^3	Interrupt lenalidomide treatment, follow CBC weekly. Resume lenalidomide at 15 mg/day after platelet count is ≥30,000/mm^3
For each subsequent platelet count <30,000/mm^3	Interrupt lenalidomide treatment, follow CBC weekly. After platelet count recovers to ≥30,000/mm^3, resume lenalidomide at a dose decreased from the previous dose by 5 mg/day, but the daily dose should not be less than 5 mg/day
ANC <1000/mm^3	Interrupt lenalidomide treatment, follow CBC weekly. Resume lenalidomide at 15 mg/day after ANC ≥1000/mm^3
For each subsequent ANC <1000/mm^3	Interrupt lenalidomide treatment, follow CBC weekly. After ANC recovers to ≥1000/mm^3, resume lenalidomide at a dose decreased from the previous dose by 5 mg/day, but the daily dose should not be less than 5 mg/day
Febrile neutropenia	Interrupt lenalidomide treatment, follow closely, and resume lenalidomide at 15 mg/day after fever abates
G3/4 non-hematologic toxicity	Interrupt lenalidomide treatment and follow clinically. After toxicity abates to G ≤2, resume lenalidomide at a dose decreased from the previous dose by 5 mg/day, but the daily dose should not be less than 5 mg/day
Toxicities ascribed to dexamethasone such as severe manifestations of hypercorticism, including hyperglycemia, irritability, insomnia, and oral candidiasis	Reduce dexamethasone dose to 20 mg per day

(continued)

(*continued*)

Thromboprophylaxis
Risk assessment and recommendations for VTE prophylaxis in patients with multiple myeloma with individual or myeloma-related risk factors, or risk factors related to treatment

Individual risk factors
• Obesity (BMI ≥30 kg/m²)
• H/O VTE
• CVC or pacemaker
• Comorbid pathologies
  Cardiac disease
  Chronic renal disease
  Diabetes
  Acute infection
  Immobilization
• Surgery
  General surgery
  Any anesthesia
  Trauma
• Medications
  Erythropoietin (epoetin alfa, darbepoetin)
  Estrogenic compounds
  Bevacizumab
• Clotting disorders
  Thrombophilia
Myeloma-related risk factors
• Diagnosis of multiple myeloma
• Hyperviscosity
	≤1 Individual or myeloma risk factor present:
	• **Aspirin** 81–325 mg daily
	
	≥2 Individual or myeloma risk factors present:
	• **LMWH***, equivalent to enoxaparin sodium 40 mg/day *or* **dalteparin sodium** 5000 IU/day; administer subcutaneously, *or*
	• **Warfarin**, targeting an INR = 2–3

Concomitant treatment-related risk factors Thalidomide or lenalidomide in combination with: • High-dose dexamethasone (≥480 mg/month) • Doxorubicin • Multiagent chemotherapy	**LMWH***, equivalent to enoxaparin sodium 40 mg/day *or* **dalteparin sodium** 5000 IU/day; administer subcutaneously, *or* **Warfarin**, targeting an INR = 2–3

CVC, central venous catheter; INR, international normalized ratio; LMWH, low-molecular-weight heparin; VTE, venous thromboembolic disease
*LMWHs should be used with caution in individuals with impaired renal function (creatinine clearance <30 mL/min). Refer to product labeling for information about doses and administration schedules in renally impaired patients, and guidance for monitoring anti-Factor Xa concentrations

Geerts WH et al. Chest 2008;133(6 Suppl):381S–453S
Multiple Myeloma, V.1.2014. National Comprehensive Cancer Network, Inc., 2013. (Accessed October 8, 2013, at http://www.nccn.org)
Palumbo A et al. Leukemia 2008;22:414–423
Venous Thromboembolic Disease, V.2.2013. National Comprehensive Cancer Network, Inc., 2013. (Accessed October 8, 2013, at http://www.nccn.org)

Bisphosphonates
All patients receiving primary therapy for symptomatic multiple myeloma should receive a bisphosphonate adjunctively; *for example*:
• **Pamidronate sodium** 90 mg; administer intravenously over 2–4 hours, every month, *or*
• **Zoledronic acid** 4 mg; administer intravenously over 15 minutes, every month
Consider baseline bone densitometry evaluation
See Chapter 43 for more information

Treatment Modifications
(*continued*)

Treatment Modification for Bortezomib-Induced Peripheral Neuropathy*

Severity of Peripheral Neuropathy	Modifications of Dose and Schedule
G1 (paresthesias or loss of reflexes) without pain or loss of function	No action
G1 with pain or G2 (interferes with function but not with activities of daily living)	Reduce bortezomib dosage to 1 mg/m² per dose
G2 with pain or G3 (interferes with activities of daily living)	Withhold bortezomib treatment until toxicity resolves, then reinitiate at a dosage of 0.7 mg/m² per dose once weekly
G4 (permanent sensory loss that interferes with function)	Discontinue treatment

Lenalidomide Starting Dose Adjustment for Renal Impairment in Multiple Myeloma (Days 1–21 of Each 28-Day Cycle)

Moderate renal impairment CrCl 30–60 mL/min (0.5–1 mL/s)	10 mg lenalidomide every 24 hours
Severe renal impairment CrCl <30 mL/min (<0.5 mL/s), not requiring dialysis	15 mg lenalidomide every 48 hours
End-stage renal disease CrCl <30 mL/min (<0.5 mL/s), requiring dialysis	Lenalidomide 5 mg/day. On dialysis days, administer a daily dose following dialysis

CrCl, Creatinine clearance
*Richardson PG et al. J Clin Oncol 2006;24:3113–3120

Efficacy

Best Response to Treatment for Treated and Phase II Populations

Response	All Patients (N = 66)		Phase II Population (N = 35)	
	Percentage	90% CI	Percentage	90% CI
CR	29	20–39	37	24–52
nCR	11	5–19	20	10–34
VGPR	27	18–38	17	8–31
PR	33	24–44	26	14–41
CR + nCR	39	29–50	57	42–71
CR + nCR + VGPR	67	56–76	74	59–86
At least PR	100	96–100	100	92–100
Estimated 18-month duration of response			68% (95% CI, 55–79%)	

Percentages of Patients Achieving a Best Response of VGPR or Better, and Estimated 18-Month PFS Rates

Characteristic/Value	n	Response ≥VGPR n (%)	Estimated 18-Month PFS, % (95% CI)
Baseline Characteristic			
All patients	66	100 (96–100)	75 (63–84)
ISS disease stage I	29	21 (72)	89 (70–96)
ISS disease stage II/III	37	23 (62)	65 (47–78)
Durie-Salmon disease stage I	22	12 (55)	82 (59–93)
Durie-Salmon disease stage II/III	44	32 (73)	72 (56–83)
β_2-Microglobulin <3.5 mg/L	44	32 (73)	77 (61–87)
β_2-Microglobulin ≥3.5 mg/L	22	12 (55)	73 (49–87)
Albumin <3.5 g/dL	24	17 (71)	63 (40–78)
Albumin ≥3.5 g/dL	42	27 (64)	83 (67–91)
Cytogenetics Present			
Abnormal metaphase cytogenetics = Yes	6	5 (83)	(27–97)
Abnormal metaphase cytogenetics = No	60	39 (65)	75 (62–84)
Del 13/13q by FISH = Yes	24	79 (57–91)	18 (75)
Del 13/13q by FISH = No	27	16 (59)	65 (43–80)
Del 17p by FISH = Yes	5	3 (60)	100
Del 17p by FISH = No	45	30 (67)	68 (52–80)
t(4;14) by FISH = Yes	2	2 (100)	100
t(4;14) by FISH = No	39	24 (62)	63 (46–77)

(*continued*)

Patient Population Studied

A phase I/II study of 66 patients with newly diagnosed symptomatic multiple myeloma who had not previously received systemic antimyeloma therapy, and had a Karnofsky Performance Status ≥60%. Patients were excluded if they had G ≥2 peripheral neuropathy, serum creatinine >2.5 mg/dL (>221 μmol/L), platelets <50,000/mm³, ANC <1000/mm³, hemoglobin <8 g/dL, or transaminases ≥2 times the upper limit of normal range

Toxicity

Adverse Events in ≥15% of Patients and All G3/4 (N = 66)

Event	% Total	% G3	% G4
Neuropathy, sensory*	80	2	0
Fatigue	64	3	0
Constipation	61	0	0
Edema limb	45	0	0
Muscle pain	44	2	0
Rash/desquamation	36	2	0
Diarrhea	35	0	0
Nausea	32	0	0
Neuropathic pain	32	3	0
Extremity, limb pain	30	3	0
Insomnia	30	2	0
Hyperglycemia	27	2	0
Dizziness	26	3	0
Constitutional	18	0	0
Dyspnea	18	2	0
Neuropathy, motor	18	2	0
Platelets	18	2	5
Pruritus/itching	18	0	0
Neutrophils	15	8	2
Anxiety	14	2	0
Dry skin	14	2	0
Lymphopenia	14	11	3
Vision, blurred	12	2	0

(*continued*)

Efficacy (continued)

Characteristic/Value	n	Response ≥VGPR n (%)	Estimated 18-Month PFS, % (95% CI)
Cytogenetics Present			
t(11;14) by FISH = Yes	11	7 (64)	73 (37–90)
t(11;14) by FISH = No	40	28 (70)	72 (55–83)
Del 17p and/or t(4;14) by FISH = Yes	6	4 (67)	100
Del 17p and/or t(4;14) by = No	44	29 (66)	68 (51–79)
Estimated 18-month OS (with/without ASCT)		97% (95% CI, 88–99%)	

CI, confidence interval; CR, complete response; FISH, fluorescence in situ hybridization; ISS, International Staging System; nCR, near-complete response; OS, overall survival; PFS, progression-free survival; PR, partial response; VGPR, very good partial response
Note: Per European Group for Blood and Marrow Transplant criteria, all response categories required 2 confirmatory assessments at least 6 weeks apart

Toxicity (continued)

Event	% Total	% G3	% G4
Alanine transaminase	12	3	0
Hypokalemia	11	5	0
Mental status	11	2	0
Hyperkalemia	9	2	0
Hyponatremia	9	2	0
Hypophosphatemia	9	5	0
Pulmonary/upper respiratory, other	9	3	0
Agitation	6	2	0
Hearing	6	2	0
Hemoglobin	6	2	0
QTc interval	6	3	0
Thrombosis/ thrombus/embolism	6	3	2
Creatinine	3	2	0
Leukocytes	3	3	0
Atrial fibrillation	2	2	0
Infection, other	2	2	0
Stomach hemorrhage	2	2	0

*Including 34 (52%) = G1 and 18 (27%) = G2

Therapy Monitoring

1. *Before each cycle:* CBC with differential and blood chemistries (including BUN, creatinine, and calcium)
2. *Every 6 weeks to 3 months:* Measure serum and urine M-protein

REGIMEN
NEWLY DIAGNOSED MULTIPLE MYELOMA (TRANSPLANTATION CANDIDATES)

INDUCTION PRIOR TO AUTOLOGOUS STEM CELL TRANSPLANTATION (ASCT)
BORTEZOMIB + THALIDOMIDE + DEXAMETHASONE

Cavo M et al. Lancet 2010;376:2075–2085

Bortezomib 1.3 mg/m² per dose; administer by intravenous injection over 3–5 seconds for 4 doses on days 1, 4, 8, and 11, every 21 days for 3 cycles (total dosage/cycle = 5.2 mg/m²)

Thalidomide 200 mg/day; administer orally, continually, for 21 consecutive days on days 1–21, every 21 days for 3 cycles (total dose/cycle = 4200 mg)

Dexamethasone 40 mg per dose; administer orally for 8 doses on days 1, 2, 4, 5, 8, 9, 11, and 12, every 21 days for 3 cycles (total dose/cycle = 320 mg)

Supportive Care
Antiemetic prophylaxis
Emetogenic potential is **MINIMAL**
See Chapter 39 for antiemetic recommendations

Hematopoietic growth factor (CSF) prophylaxis
Primary prophylaxis is NOT indicated
See Chapter 43 for more information

Antimicrobial prophylaxis
Risk of fever and neutropenia is HIGH
Antimicrobial primary prophylaxis is recommended:
- Antibacterial—consider fluoroquinolone prophylaxis; *P. jirovecii* prophylaxis is recommended (eg, cotrimoxazole)
- Antifungal—recommended
- Antiviral—antiherpes antivirals (eg, acyclovir, famciclovir, valacyclovir)

Caution: Acyclovir and famciclovir accumulate in patients with impaired renal function and may exacerbate renal dysfunction (valacyclovir is a *prodrug* for acyclovir). Monitor kidney function serially during acyclovir, valacyclovir, and famciclovir use
- Acyclovir and famciclovir elimination is inversely related to renal function
- Acyclovir, famciclovir, and valacyclovir utilization is modified in renally impaired individuals (consult product labeling or Summary of Product Characteristics for guidance about dose/dosage and administration frequency modifications, and, when relevant, recommendations for drug dilution, administration rate, concurrent fluid administration, and fluid supplementation as a function of urine output)
- Impaired acyclovir elimination is associated with neurological adverse effects, including agitation, ataxia, coma, confusion, dizziness, dysarthria, encephalopathy, hallucinations, paresthesia, seizure, somnolence, and tremors

See Chapter 47 for more information

(continued)

Treatment Modifications

Bortezomib Dosage Levels

Dose Level 1	1.3 mg/m²
Dose Level −1	1 mg/m²
Dose Level −2	0.7 mg/m²

Thalidomide Dose Levels

Dose Level 1	200 mg daily
Dose Level −1	100 mg daily
Dose Level −2	50 mg daily

Adverse Event	Treatment Modification
Febrile neutropenia	Withhold therapy until fever abates then resume therapy
G4 hematologic toxicity	Withhold therapy until ANC >750/mm³ and platelets >50,000/mm³, then resume therapy at a dose decreased by 1 dose level
G3/4 nonhematologic toxicity	Interrupt therapy, follow clinically. After toxicity abates to G ≤2, resume therapy at a dose decreased by 1 dose level
G ≥3 thalidomide neuropathy	Interrupt therapy and follow clinically. After toxicity abates to G ≤2, resume therapy at a dose decreased by 1 dose level
Toxicities ascribed to dexamethasone such as severe manifestations of hypercorticism, including hyperglycemia, irritability, insomnia, and oral candidiasis	Reduce dexamethasone dose to 20 mg per dose

(continued)

(*continued*)

Thromboprophylaxis

Risk assessment and recommendations for VTE prophylaxis in patients with multiple myeloma with individual or myeloma-related risk factors, or risk factors related to treatment

Individual risk factors	
• Obesity (BMI ≥30 kg/m²)	
• H/O VTE	
• CVC or pacemaker	
• Comorbid pathologies	
• Cardiac disease	
Chronic renal disease	≤1 Individual or myeloma risk factor present:
Diabetes	• **Aspirin** 81–325 mg daily
Acute infection	
Immobilization	
• Surgery	
General surgery	≥2 Individual or myeloma risk factors present:
Any anesthesia	• **LMWH***, equivalent to enoxaparin sodium 40 mg/day *or* **dalteparin sodium** 5000 IU/day; administer subcutaneously, *or*
Trauma	
• Medications	
Erythropoietin (epoetin alfa, darbepoetin)	• **Warfarin**, targeting an INR = 2–3
Estrogenic compounds	
Bevacizumab	
• Clotting disorders	
Thrombophilia	
Myeloma-related risk factors	
• Diagnosis of multiple myeloma	
• Hyperviscosity	
Concomitant treatment-related risk factors Thalidomide or lenalidomide in combination with:	**LMWH***, equivalent to enoxaparin sodium 40 mg/day *or* **dalteparin sodium** 5000 IU/day; administer subcutaneously, *or*
• High-dose dexamethasone (≥480 mg/month)	
• Doxorubicin	**Warfarin**, targeting an INR = 2–3
• Multiagent chemotherapy	

CVC, central venous catheter; INR, international normalized ratio; LMWH, low-molecular-weight heparin; VTE, venous thromboembolic disease
*LMWHs should be used with caution in individuals with impaired renal function (creatinine clearance <30 mL/min). Refer to product labeling for information about doses and administration schedules in renally impaired patients, and guidance for monitoring anti-Factor Xa concentrations

Geerts WH et al. Chest 2008;133(6 Suppl):381S–453S
Multiple Myeloma, V.1.2014. National Comprehensive Cancer Network, Inc., 2013. (Accessed October 8, 2013, at http://www.nccn.org)
Palumbo A et al. Leukemia 2008;22:414–423
Venous Thromboembolic Disease, V.2.2013. National Comprehensive Cancer Network, Inc., 2013. (Accessed October 8, 2013, at http://www.nccn.org)

Bisphosphonates

All patients receiving primary therapy for symptomatic multiple myeloma should receive a bisphosphonate adjunctively; *for example*:

• **Pamidronate disodium** 90 mg; administer intravenously over 2–4 hours, every month, *or*

• **Zoledronic acid** 4 mg; administer intravenously over 15 minutes, every month

Consider baseline bone densitometry evaluation
See Chapter 43 for more information

Treatment Modifications
(*continued*)

Treatment Modification for Bortezomib-Induced Peripheral Neuropathy*

Severity of Peripheral Neuropathy	Modification of Dose and Schedule
G1 (paresthesias or loss of reflexes) without pain or loss of function	No action
G1 with pain or G2 (interferes with function, but not with activities of daily living)	Reduce bortezomib dosage to 1 mg/m² per dose
G2 with pain or G3 (interferes with activities of daily living)	Withhold bortezomib treatment until toxicity resolves, then reinitiate at a dosage of 0.7 mg/m² per dose once weekly
G4 (permanent sensory loss that interferes with function)	Discontinue treatment

*Richardson PG et al. J Clin Oncol 2006;24:3113–3120

Patient Population Studied

A phase III study of 480 patients, ages 18 to 65 years, with previously untreated, symptomatic newly diagnosed multiple myeloma who were eligible for stem cell transplantation

Eligible subjects demonstrated a Karnofsky performance status ≥60%, adequate hematologic function (ANC ≥1000/mm³ and platelet count ≥70,000/mm³), and serum creatinine ≤2 mg/dL (≤177 μmol/L). Patients with peripheral neuropathy G ≥2, a history of venous thromboembolism, or a previous diagnosis of thrombophilic alterations, were ineligible

Efficacy	

Response to Different Treatment Phases and Best Response

N = 236	% (95% CI)
After Induction Therapy	
Complete response	19% (13.7–23.6)
Complete or near complete response	31% (25–36.8)
Very good partial response or better	62% (55.7–68.1)
Partial response or better	93% (90–96.4)
Minimal response or stable disease	7% (3.6–10)
Progressive disease	5% (2.3–7.8)
After First Autologous Stem Cell Transplantation	
Complete response	38% (31.5–43.9)
Complete or near complete response	52% (45.7–58.5)
Very good partial response or better	79% (73.6–84)
Partial response or better	93% (90–96.4)
Minimal response or stable disease	6% (3.2–9.5)
Progressive disease	<1% (0–1.3)
After Second Autologous Stem Cell Transplantation	
Complete response	42% (35.2–47.8)
Complete or near complete response	55% (48.7–61.4)
Very good partial response or better	82% (76.9–86.7)
Partial response or better	93% (90–96.4)
Minimal response or stable disease	6% (2.9–8.9)
Progressive disease	8% (4.9–11.9)
After Consolidation Therapy	
Complete response	49% (42.8–55.5)
Complete or near complete response	62% (56.1–68.5)
Very good partial response or better	85% (80.6–89.7)
Partial response or better	92% (89–95.8)
Minimal response or stable disease	5% (2.3–7.9)
Progressive disease	9% (5.2–12.4)
Best Response to Overall Treatment Protocol	
Complete response	58% (51.3–63.9)
Complete or near complete response	71% (65.4–77)
Very good partial response or better	89% (85–93)
Partial response or better	96% (93.7–98.6)
Minimal response, stable disease, or progressive disease	4% (1.4–6.3)

Toxicity

Serious and G3/4 Adverse Events Reported in ≥2% of Patients During Induction Therapy

Any serious adverse event	13%
Any grade 3 or 4 adverse event	56%
Any grade 3 or 4 nonhematologic adverse event	51%
Skin rash	10%
Peripheral neuropathy	10%
Deep vein thrombosis	3%
Constipation	4%
Infections excluding herpes zoster	3%
Gastrointestinal events (excluding constipation)	2%
Cardiac toxicity	2%
Liver toxicity	2%
Discontinuation during or after induction therapy	6%
Toxic effects	4%
Disease progression	0
Other reasons	1%
Early death	<1%

Nonhematologic Adverse Events of Any Grade Reported in at Least 10% of Patients During Induction Therapy (N = 236)

	% G1–4	% G3/4
Constipation	42	4
Neuropathy	34	10
Skin rash	28	10
Fever	12	1
Infections	10	3
Edema	11	1
Gastrointestinal events (excluding constipation)	19	2

Therapy Monitoring

1. *Before each cycle:* CBC with differential and blood chemistries (including BUN, creatinine, and calcium)
2. *Every 6 weeks to 3 months:* Measure serum and urine M-protein

REGIMEN
NEWLY DIAGNOSED MULTIPLE MYELOMA (TRANSPLANTATION CANDIDATES)

INDUCTION PRIOR TO AUTOLOGOUS STEM CELL TRANSPLANTATION (ASCT)
BORTEZOMIB + DOXORUBICIN + DEXAMETHASONE

Sonneveld P et al. J Clin Oncol 2012;30:2946–2955

Induction:

Bortezomib 1.3 mg/m² per dose intravenously over 3–5 seconds for 4 doses on days 1, 4, 8, and 11, every 28 days for 3 cycles (total dosage/cycle = 5.2 mg/m²)

Doxorubicin 9 mg/m² per day by slow intravenous injection over 3–5 minutes for 4 consecutive days on days 1–4, every 28 days for 3 cycles (total dosage/cycle = 36 mg/m²)

Dexamethasone 40 mg/dose orally for 12 doses on days 1–4, days 9–12, and days 17–20 for 3 cycles (total dose/cycle = 480 mg)

Notes:

- Stem cell collection was performed 4–6 weeks after induction
- High-dose melphalan (HDM) 200 mg/m², and autologous stem cell transplantation (ASCT) were administered
- Starting 4 weeks after HDM, patients received maintenance with bortezomib 1.3 mg/m² intravenously every 2 weeks for 2 years
- Patients with an HLA-identical sibling could proceed to nonmyeloablative allogeneic stem cell transplantation (alloSCT) after HDM
- Maintenance therapy was not given after alloSCT

Supportive Care
Antiemetic prophylaxis
Emetogenic potential on days with doxorubicin is **LOW**
Emetogenic potential on days with bortezomib ± dexamethasone is **MINIMAL**
See Chapter 39 for antiemetic recommendations

Hematopoietic growth factor (CSF) prophylaxis
Primary prophylaxis is NOT indicated
See Chapter 43 for more information

Antimicrobial prophylaxis
Risk of fever and neutropenia is INTERMEDIATE
Antimicrobial primary prophylaxis to be considered:

- Antibacterial—consider a fluoroquinolone or no prophylaxis; *Pneumocystis jirovecii* prophylaxis is recommended (eg, cotrimoxazole)
- Antifungal—recommended; consider use during periods of neutropenia
- Antiviral—antiherpes antivirals (eg, acyclovir, famciclovir, valacyclovir) throughout bortezomib induction

See Chapter 47 for more information

Steroid-associated gastritis
Add a **proton pump inhibitor** during steroid use to prevent gastritis and duodenitis

(continued)

Treatment Modifications

Adverse Event	Treatment Modification
G3 nonhematologic toxicity or G4 hematologic toxicity	Hold treatment until toxicity resolves to G ≤1, then resume with bortezomib 1 mg/m² per dose and/or 25% reduction in doxorubicin dosage
G3 nonhematologic toxicity or G4 hematologic toxicity in a patient receiving bortezomib 1 mg/m²	Hold treatment until toxicity resolves to G ≤1, then resume with bortezomib 0.7 mg/m² per dose and/or 25% reduction in doxorubicin dosage
Severe manifestations of hypercorticism, including severe hyperglycemia, irritability, insomnia, or oral candidiasis	Reduce daily dexamethasone dose by 20% for G3 toxicity, and by 40% for G4 or recurrent G3 toxicity

Treatment Modification for Bortezomib-Induced Peripheral Neuropathy*

Severity of Peripheral Neuropathy	Modification of Dose and Schedule
G1 (paresthesias or loss of reflexes) without pain or loss of function	No action
G1 with pain or G2 (interferes with function but not with activities of daily living)	Reduce bortezomib dosage to 1 mg/m² per dose
G2 with pain or G3 (interferes with activities of daily living)	Withhold bortezomib treatment until toxicity resolves, then reinitiate with bortezomib 0.7 mg/m² per dose once weekly
G4 (permanent sensory loss that interferes with function)	Discontinue treatment

*Richardson PG et al. J Clin Oncol 2006;24:3113–3120

(continued)

Thromboprophylaxis
Risk assessment and recommendations for VTE prophylaxis in patients with multiple myeloma with individual or myeloma-related risk factors, or risk factors related to treatment

Individual risk factors
• Obesity (BMI ≥30 kg/m²)
• H/O VTE
• CVAD or pacemaker
• Comorbid pathologies
  Cardiac disease
  Chronic renal disease
  Diabetes
  Acute infection
  Immobilization
• Surgery
  General surgery
  Any anesthesia
  Trauma
• Medications
  Erythropoietin (epoetin alfa, darbepoetin)
  Estrogenic compounds
  Bevacizumab
• Clotting disorders
  Thrombophilia
Myeloma-related risk factors
• Diagnosis of multiple myeloma
• Hyperviscosity
	≤1 Individual or myeloma risk factor present:
	• **Aspirin** 81–325 mg daily
	
	≥2 Individual or myeloma risk factors present:
	• **LMWH***, equivalent to enoxaparin sodium 40 mg/day *or* **dalteparin sodium** 5000 IU/day; administer subcutaneously, *or*
	• **Warfarin**, targeting an INR = 2–3

Concomitant treatment-related risk factors Thalidomide or lenalidomide in combination with: • High-dose dexamethasone (≥480 mg/month) • Doxorubicin • Multiagent chemotherapy	**LMWH***, equivalent to enoxaparin sodium 40 mg/day *or* **dalteparin sodium** 5000 IU/day; administer subcutaneously, *or* **Warfarin**, targeting an INR = 2–3

CVAD, central vascular access device; INR, international normalized ratio; LMWH, low-molecular-weight heparin; VTE, venous thromboembolic disease

*LMWHs should be used with caution in individuals with impaired renal function (creatinine clearance <30 mL/min). Refer to product labeling for information about doses and administration schedules in renally impaired patients, and guidance for monitoring antifactor Xa concentrations

Geerts WH et al. Chest 2008;133(6 Suppl):381S–453S
Multiple Myeloma, V.1.2014. National Comprehensive Cancer Network, Inc., 2013. (Accessed October 8, 2013, at http://www.nccn.org)
Palumbo A et al. Leukemia 2008;22:414–423
Venous Thromboembolic Disease, V.2.2013. National Comprehensive Cancer Network, Inc., 2013. (Accessed October 8, 2013, at http://www.nccn.org)

Bisphosphonates
All patients receiving primary therapy for symptomatic multiple myeloma should receive a bisphosphonate adjunctively; *for example*:
• **Pamidronate disodium** 90 mg; administer intravenously over 2–4 hours, every month, *or*
• **Zoledronic acid** 4 mg; administer intravenously over at least 15 minutes, every month
Consider baseline bone densitometry evaluation
See Chapter 43 for more information

Patient Population Studied
Patients 18–65 years of age with newly diagnosed MM (Durie-Salmon stages II to III) WHO performance status 0 to 2, or WHO 3 when caused by MM. Exclusion criteria were systemic amyloid light chain amyloidosis, nonsecretory MM, neuropathy G ≥2, serum bilirubin ≥1.8 mg/dL (≥30 μmol/L) or aminotransferases ≥2.5 times the upper limit of normal range. Prior corticosteroids were allowed for a maximum of 5 days. Patients with renal impairment were not excluded. Local radiotherapy for painful MM lesions was allowed

Patient Characteristic (N = 413)	No (%)
ISIS Stage	
I	144 (35)
II	150 (36)
III	81 (20)
IV	38 (9)
M-Protein Isotype	
IgA	92 (22)
IgG	251 (61)
IgD	5 (1)
LCD	63 (15)
Other	2
M-Protein Light Chain [unknown = 1 (0%)]	
Kappa	277 (67)
Lambda	135 (33)
Creatinine, mg/dL [unknown = 1 (0%)]	
≤2	376 (91)
>2	36 (9)
Number of Skeletal Lesions [unknown = 12 (3%)]	
0	102 (25)
1–2	44 (11)
≥3	255 (62)

(continued)

Efficacy (N = 413)

Response	Number (%)
Response After Induction	
CR	29 (7)
≥nCR	46 (11)
≥VGPR	174 (42)
≥PR	322 (78)
Response After High-Dose Melphalan (HDM)	
CR	85 (21)
≥nCR	127 (31)
≥VGPR	254 (62)
≥PR	363 (88)
Response Overall	
CR	147 (36)
≥nCR	201 (49)
≥VGPR	312 (76)
≥PR	373 (90)
Response Upgrade During Maintenance	
Any response upgrade*	93 (23)
<CR → CR	48 (12)
<nCR → nCR	23 (6)
<VGPR → VGPR	20 (5)
<PR → PR	2*
ISS Stage I (*n* = 144)	
CR	59 (41)
≥nCR	78 (54)
≥VGPR	115 (80)
≥PR	132 (92)
ISS Stage II (*n* = 150)	
CR	51 (34)
≥nCR	70 (47)
≥VGPR	109 (73)
≥PR	134 (89)
ISS Stage III (*n* = 81)	
CR	26 (32)
≥nCR	35 (43)
≥VGPR	56 (69)
≥PR	70 (86)

Response	Number (%)
ISS Stage Unknown (*n* = 38)	
CR	11 (29)
≥nCR	18 (47)
≥VGPR	32 (84)
≥PR	37 (97)
β_2-Microglobulin >3 mg/L (*n* = 223)	
CR	77 (35)
≥nCR	103 (46)
≥VGPR	163 (73)
≥PR	189 (79)
Creatinine >2 mg/dL (*n* = 36)	
CR	13 (36)
≥nCR	19 (53)
≥VGPR	28 (78)
≥PR	31 (86)
Genetic Abnormalities	
del(13/13q14) (*n* = 148)	
≥nCR	76 (51)
≥VGPR	124 (84)
t(4;14) (*n* = 35)	
≥nCR	20 (57)
≥VGPR	30 (86)
del(17p13) (*n* = 25)	
≥nCR	13 (52)
≥VGPR	18 (72)

CR, complete response; ISS, International Staging System; nCR, near complete response; PR, partial response; VGPR, very good partial response
*Median time to any response upgrade after start of maintenance was 7 months (range: 1–57 months)

Median PFS	35 months
Median PFSA (ie, without censoring of alloSCT)	34 months
Median OS	Not reached at 66 months
5-year OS	61%
PFS calculated from the time of last HDM	31 months

Patient Population Studied
(*continued*)

Serum LDH [unknown = 12 (3%)]	
≤ULN	329 (80)
>ULN	72 (17)
Genetic Abnormalities	
del(13q) done in 361 (88%)	148/361 (41)
t(4;14) done in 250 (615)	35/250 (14)
del(17p13) done in 289 (70%)	25/289 (9)
Hematologic Abnormalities	
Median β_2-microglobulin, mg/L	3.40
Median hemoglobin, mmol/L	6.6
Median calcium, mmol/L	2.34
Median number of bone marrow plasma cells	40

| | Toxicity | | | | Therapy Monitoring |

Variable	Induction (*n* = 410)		Bortezomib Maintenance (*n* = 229)	
	No.	%	No.	%
Any AE	400	98	222	97
AE G3/4	258	63	110	48
AE classified as SAE	187	46	77	34
AE leading to discontinuation, dose reduction, or delay of bortezomib	112	27	81	35
Death from AE	7	2	0	0

	All Grades	G3/4	All Grades	G3/4
Hematologic Toxicities (%)				
Anemia	28	8	27	1
Neutropenia	4	3	2	0
Thrombocytopenia	39	10	37	4
Infections	56	26	75	24
Herpes zoster	2	0	2	0
Nonhematologic Toxicities (%)				
Wasting, fatigue	27	4	20	1
GI symptoms	67	11	48	5
Cardiac disorders	27	8	19	3
Thrombosis	6	4	1	1
Peripheral neuropathy	37	24	33	5

AE, adverse event (including infection); N/A, not applicable; SAE, serious adverse event

Therapy Monitoring

1. Blood counts and physical examinations on day 1 of each cycle
2. Serum and urinary protein electrophoresis studies on day 1 of each cycle as indicated and at the end of treatment

REGIMEN
NEWLY DIAGNOSED MULTIPLE MYELOMA (TRANSPLANTATION CANDIDATES)

INDUCTION PRIOR TO AUTOLOGOUS STEM CELL TRANSPLANTATION (ASCT)
CYCLOPHOSPHAMIDE + BORTEZOMIB + DEXAMETHASONE (CyBorD)

Reeder CB et al. Leukemia 2009;23:1337–1341

Bortezomib 1.3 mg/m^2 per dose intravenously over 3–5 seconds for 4 doses on days 1, 4, 8, and 11, every 28 days, for 4 cycles (total dosage/cycle = 5.2 mg/m^2)
Cyclophosphamide 300 mg/m^2 per dose orally for 4 doses on days 1, 8, 15, and 22, every 28 days, for 4 cycles (total dosage/cycle = 1200 mg/m^2)
Dexamethasone 40 mg/dose orally for 12 doses on days 1–4, days 9–12, and days 17–20 for 3 cycles (total dose/cycle = 480 mg)

Notes:
• Dose escalation was not allowed
• At the end of 4 cycles patients proceeded to stem cell mobilization and harvest

Supportive Care
Antiemetic prophylaxis
Emetogenic potential on days with cyclophosphamide is **MODERATE–HIGH**
Emetogenic potential on days with bortezomib $\pm$ dexamethasone is **MINIMAL**
See Chapter 39 for antiemetic recommendations

Hematopoietic growth factor (CSF) prophylaxis
Primary prophylaxis may be indicated
See Chapter 43 for more information

Antimicrobial prophylaxis
Risk of fever and neutropenia is INTERMEDIATE
Antimicrobial primary prophylaxis to be considered:
• Antibacterial—consider a fluoroquinolone or no prophylaxis; *Pneumocystis jirovecii* prophylaxis is recommended (eg, cotrimoxazole)
• Antifungal—recommended; consider use during periods of neutropenia
• Antiviral—antiherpes antivirals (eg, acyclovir, famciclovir, valacyclovir) throughout bortezomib induction
See Chapter 47 for more information

Steroid-associated gastritis
Add a **proton pump inhibitor** during steroid use to prevent gastritis and duodenitis

(continued)

Treatment Modifications

Note: Dose reduction was allowed after the first cycle, but cyclophosphamide and bortezomib can be held during cycle 1 for neutropenia or thrombocytopenia G $\geq$3

Cyclophosphamide Dose Levels

Starting dose	300 mg/m^2 per dose on days 1, 8, 15, and 22
Level −1	300 mg/m^2 per dose on days 1, 8, and 15
Level −2	300 mg/m^2 per dose on days 1 and 8
Level −3	300 mg/m^2 on day 1

Adverse Event	Treatment Modification
G3 hematologic toxicity	Reduce cyclophosphamide 1 dose level
G1/2 cystitis	Reduce cyclophosphamide 1 dose level
G3/4 cystitis	Discontinue cyclophosphamide

Bortezomib Dose Levels

Starting dose	1.3 mg/m^2 per dose on days 1, 4, 8, and 11
Level −1	1 mg/m^2 per dose on days 1, 4, 8, and 11
Level −2	0.7 mg/m^2 per dose on days 1, 4, 8, and 11
Level −3	1.3 mg/m^2 per dose on days 1 and 8

Adverse Event	Treatment Modification
G3 thrombocytopenia (platelet count <50,000/mm^3)	Reduce bortezomib dosage by 1 dose level

(continued)

(*continued*)

Thromboprophylaxis

Risk assessment and recommendations for VTE prophylaxis in patients with multiple myeloma with individual or myeloma-related risk factors, or risk factors related to treatment

Individual risk factors	

• Obesity (BMI $\geq$30 kg/m^2)
• H/O VTE
• CVAD or pacemaker
• Comorbid pathologies
  Cardiac disease
  Chronic renal disease
  Diabetes
  Acute infection
  Immobilization
• Surgery
  General surgery
  Any anesthesia
  Trauma
• Medications
  Erythropoietin (epoetin alfa, darbepoetin)
  Estrogenic compounds
  Bevacizumab
• Clotting disorders
  Thrombophilia
Myeloma-related risk factors
• Diagnosis of multiple myeloma
• Hyperviscosity
	$\leq$1 Individual or myeloma risk factor present:
	• **Aspirin** 81–325 mg daily
	
	$\geq$2 Individual or myeloma risk factors present:
	• **LMWH***, equivalent to enoxaparin sodium 40 mg/day *or* **dalteparin sodium** 5000 IU/day; administer subcutaneously, *or*
	• **Warfarin**, targeting an INR = 2–3

Concomitant treatment-related risk factors Thalidomide or lenalidomide in combination with: • High-dose dexamethasone ($\geq$480 mg/month) • Doxorubicin • Multiagent chemotherapy	**LMWH***, equivalent to enoxaparin sodium 40 mg/day *or* **dalteparin sodium** 5000 IU/day; administer subcutaneously, *or* **Warfarin**, targeting an INR = 2–3

CVAD, central vascular access device; INR, international normalized ratio; LMWH, low-molecular-weight heparin; VTE, venous thromboembolic disease

*LMWHs should be used with caution in individuals with impaired renal function (creatinine clearance <30 mL/min). Refer to product labeling for information about doses and administration schedules in renally impaired patients, and guidance for monitoring antifactor Xa concentrations

Geerts WH et al. Chest 2008;133(6 Suppl):381S–453S

Multiple Myeloma, V.1.2014. National Comprehensive Cancer Network, Inc., 2013. (Accessed October 8, 2013, at http://www.nccn.org)

Palumbo A et al. Leukemia 2008;22:414–423

Venous Thromboembolic Disease, V.2.2013. National Comprehensive Cancer Network, Inc., 2013. (Accessed October 8, 2013, at http://www.nccn.org)

Bisphosphonates

All patients receiving primary therapy for symptomatic multiple myeloma should receive a bisphosphonate adjunctively; *for example*:

• **Pamidronate disodium** 90 mg; administer intravenously over 2–4 hours, every month, *or*

• **Zoledronic acid** 4 mg; administer intravenously over at least 15 minutes, every month

Consider baseline bone densitometry evaluation

See Chapter 43 for more information

Treatment Modifications
(continued)

Treatment Modification for Bortezomib-Induced Peripheral Neuropathy*

Severity of Peripheral Neuropathy	Modification of Dose and Schedule
G1 (paresthesias or loss of reflexes) without pain or loss of function	No action
G1 with pain or G2 (interferes with function but not with activities of daily living)	Reduce bortezomib dosage 1 dose level
G2 with pain or G3 (interferes with activities of daily living)	Withhold bortezomib treatment until toxicity resolves, then reinitiate reducing bortezomib dosage 1 dose level
G4 (permanent sensory loss that interferes with function)	Discontinue treatment

Dexamethasone Dose Levels

Starting dose	40 mg per dose on days 1–4, 9–12, and 17–20
Level –1	20 mg per dose on days 1–4, 9–12, and 17–20
Level –2	20 mg per dose on days 1–4
Level –3	10 mg per dose on days 1–4

Adverse Event	Treatment Modification
G2 muscle weakness, G3 gastrointestinal tract, hyperglycemia, confusion or mood alteration	Reduce dexamethasone dose by 1 dose level

*Richardson PG et al. J Clin Oncol 2006;24:3113–3120

Efficacy

Responses	By ITT (N = 33)	By ITT if Completed 4 Cycles (N = 28)	After SCT (N = 23)
ORR (≥PR)	29 (88%)	27 (96%)	23 (100%)
≥VGPR	20 (61%)*	20 (71%)	17 (74%)
PR	9 (27%)	7 (25%)	6 (26%)

ITT, intention to treat; ORR, overall response (partial response or better); PR, partial response; SCT, stem cell transplantation; ≥VGPR, very good partial response or better
*One in CR, 12 in nCR, and 7 in VGPR

Risk Category as Assessed by Bone Marrow Plasma Cell Fish Analysis and ISS Stage, and Corresponding Response After 4 Cycles

Risk Category	Frequency	ORR	≥VGPR
Deletion 13	50% (16/32)	94% (15/16)	63% (10/16)
Deletion 17	13% (4/31)	75% (3/4)	50% (2/4)
t(4;14)	18% (6/33)	83% (5/6)	50% (3/6)
Hyperdiploid	21% (7/33)	100% (7/7)	71% (5/7)
ISS stage 3	30% (10/33)	80% (8/10)	60% (6/10)

FISH, fluorescent in situ hybridization; ISS, international staging system; ORR, overall response; VGPR, very good partial response

Therapy Monitoring

1. Blood counts and physical examinations on day 1 of each cycle
2. Serum and urinary protein electrophoresis studies on day 1 of each cycle as indicated and at the end of treatment

Patient Population Studied

Newly diagnosed, symptomatic MM of Durie–Salmon stage II or III, Eastern Cooperative Oncology Group performance status ≤2, creatinine ≤3.5 mg/dL (≤309 μmol/L), absolute neutrophil count ≥1000/mm³, platelets ≥100,000/mm³

Patient Characteristics

Mean age	60 (38–75) years
Gender: M/F	52%/48%
International Staging System, stages I/II/III,	33/36/30%
Durie–Salmon stage II or III; symptomatic disease	100%
del13 in 16/32	16/32 (50%)
del17*	4/31 (13%)
t(4;14)*	6/33 (18%)
Favorable hyperdiploid karyotype	7/33 (21%)

*Genetic high-risk categories

Toxicity

Adverse Events	G3/4*
Anemia	12%
Neutropenia	13%
Thrombocytopenia	25%
Hyperglycemia	13%
Diarrhea	6%
Hypokalemia	9%
Neuropathy	7%
Thrombosis	7%

*National Cancer Institute Common Terminology Criteria for Adverse Events (version 3.0) severity grades

REGIMEN
NEWLY DIAGNOSED MULTIPLE MYELOMA (TRANSPLANTATION CANDIDATES)

INDUCTION PRIOR TO AUTOLOGOUS STEM CELL TRANSPLANTATION (ASCT)
CARFILZOMIB + LENALIDOMIDE + DEXAMETHASONE (CRd)

Jakubowlak AJ et al. Blood 2012;120:1801–1809

Hydration with carfilzomib: During cycle 1, days 1 and 2, administer intravenously 250–500 mL 0.9% NS before each carfilzomib dose, *and* an additional 250–500 mL of fluid after carfilzomib. During repeated treatments, continue intravenous hydration as needed. Encourage oral hydration

Carfilzomib 36 mg/m^2 per dose intravenously in 50-mL 5% dextrose injection over 30 minutes
- *Cycles 1–8:* for 6 doses, on days 1, 2, 8, 9, 15, and 16, every 28 days (total dosage/cycle = 216 mg/m^2)
- *Cycle 9 and subsequent cycles:* for 4 doses, on days 1, 2, 15, and 16, every 28 days (total dosage/cycle = 144 mg/m^2)

Lenalidomide 25 mg/day orally, continually for 21 consecutive days on days 1–21, every 28 days (total dose/cycle = 525 mg)

Dexamethasone administer orally or intravenously for 4 doses on days 1, 8, 15, and 22, every 28 days
- *Cycles 1–4:* 40 mg/dose (total dose/cycle = 160 mg)
- Cycle 5 and subsequent cycles: 20 mg/dose (total dose/cycle = 80 mg)

Notes:
- After cycle 4, transplantation-eligible candidates underwent stem cell collection (SCC) then continued CRd with the option of transplantation
- Thirty-five patients underwent SCC, 7 proceeded to transplantation, and the remainder resumed CRd
- After 8 cycles, patients received maintenance CRd. Per initial design, CRd maintenance was planned for an indefinite period of time, but because progression events were limited and no maintenance treatments were discontinued because of toxicity, the study was amended to 24 total cycles of CRd. After completion of 24 cycles, single-agent lenalidomide off protocol was recommended

Supportive Care
Antiemetic prophylaxis
Emetogenic potential on days with lenalidomide ± carfilzomib is **LOW**
See Chapter 39 for antiemetic recommendations

Hematopoietic growth factor (CSF) prophylaxis
Primary prophylaxis may be indicated
See Chapter 43 for more information

Antimicrobial prophylaxis
Risk of fever and neutropenia is INTERMEDIATE
Antimicrobial primary prophylaxis to be considered:
- Antibacterial—consider a fluoroquinolone or no prophylaxis; *Pneumocystis jirovecii* prophylaxis is recommended (eg, cotrimoxazole)
- Antifungal—recommended; consider use during periods of neutropenia
- Antiviral—antiherpes antivirals (eg, acyclovir, famciclovir, valacyclovir)

See Chapter 47 for more information

Steroid-associated gastritis
Add a **proton pump inhibitor** during steroid use to prevent gastritis and duodenitis

(continued)

(continued)

Thromboprophylaxis

Risk assessment and recommendations for VTE prophylaxis in patients with multiple myeloma with individual or myeloma-related risk factors, or risk factors related to treatment

Individual risk factors
• Obesity (BMI $\geq$30 kg/m²)
• H/O VTE
• CVAD or pacemaker
• Comorbid pathologies
  Cardiac disease
  Chronic renal disease
  Diabetes
  Acute infection
  Immobilization
• Surgery
  General surgery
  Any anesthesia
  Trauma
• Medications
  Erythropoietin (epoetin alfa, darbepoetin)
  Estrogenic compounds
  Bevacizumab
• Clotting disorders
  Thrombophilia
Myeloma-related risk factors
• Diagnosis of multiple myeloma
• Hyperviscosity
	$\leq$1 Individual or myeloma risk factor present:
	• **Aspirin** 81–325 mg daily
	
	$\geq$2 Individual or myeloma risk factors present:
	• **LMWH*, equivalent to enoxaparin sodium** 40 mg/day *or* **dalteparin sodium** 5000 IU/day; administer subcutaneously, *or*
	• **Warfarin**, targeting an INR = 2–3

Concomitant treatment-related risk factors Thalidomide or lenalidomide in combination with: • High-dose dexamethasone ($\geq$480 mg/month) • Doxorubicin • Multiagent chemotherapy	**LMWH*, equivalent to enoxaparin sodium** 40 mg/day *or* **dalteparin sodium** 5000 IU/day; administer subcutaneously, *or* **Warfarin**, targeting an INR = 2–3

CVAD, central vascular access device; INR, international normalized ratio; LMWH, low-molecular-weight heparin; VTE, venous thromboembolic disease
*LMWHs should be used with caution in individuals with impaired renal function (creatinine clearance <30 mL/min). Refer to product labeling for information about doses and administration schedules in renally impaired patients, and guidance for monitoring antifactor Xa concentrations

Geerts WH et al. Chest 2008;133(6 Suppl):381S–453S
Multiple Myeloma, V.1.2014. National Comprehensive Cancer Network, Inc., 2013. (Accessed October 8, 2013, at http://www.nccn.org)
Palumbo A et al. Leukemia 2008;22:414–423
Venous Thromboembolic Disease, V.2.2013. National Comprehensive Cancer Network, Inc., 2013. (Accessed October 8, 2013, at http://www.nccn.org)

Bisphosphonates

All patients receiving primary therapy for symptomatic multiple myeloma should receive a bisphosphonate adjunctively; *for example*:

• **Pamidronate disodium** 90 mg; administer intravenously over 2–4 hours, every month, *or*

• **Zoledronic acid** 4 mg; administer intravenously over at least 15 minutes, every month

Consider baseline bone densitometry evaluation

See Chapter 43 for more information

(continued)

(*continued*)

Diarrhea management

Loperamide 4 mg orally initially after the first loose or liquid stool, *then*

Loperamide 2 mg orally every 2 hours during waking hours, *plus*

Loperamide 4 mg orally every 4 hours during hours of sleep

- Continue for at least 12 hours after diarrhea resolves
- Recurrent diarrhea after a 12-hour diarrhea-free interval is treated as a new episode
- Rehydrate orally with fluids and electrolytes during a diarrheal episode
- If a patient develops blood or mucus in stool, dehydration, or hemodynamic instability, or if diarrhea persists >48 hours despite loperamide, stop loperamide and hospitalize the patient for IV hydration

Alternatively, a trial of **Diphenoxylate hydrochloride** 2.5 mg **with Atropine sulfate** 0.025 mg (eg, Lomotil)

- Initial adult dose is 2 tablets 4 times daily until control has been achieved, after which the dose may be reduced to meet individual requirements. Control may often be maintained with as little as 2 tablets daily
- Clinical improvement of acute diarrhea is usually observed within 48 hours. If improvement of chronic diarrhea after treatment with a maximum daily dose of 8 tablets is not observed within 10 days, control is unlikely with further administration

Lenalidomide Starting Dose Adjustment for Renal Impairment in Multiple Myeloma (Days 1–21 of Each 28-Day Cycle)*

Moderate renal impairment: CrCl 30–60 mL/min (0.5–1 mL/s)	Lenalidomide 10 mg q24h
Severe renal impairment: CrCl <30 mL/min (<30 mL/s), not requiring dialysis	Lenalidomide 15 mg q48h
End-stage renal disease: requiring dialysis	Lenalidomide 5 mg/day. On dialysis days, administer the daily dose following dialysis

CrCl, creatinine clearance
*Richardson PG et al. J Clin Oncol 2006;24:3113–3120

Treatment Modifications

Carfilzomib Dose Levels

Starting dose	36 mg/m^2 per dose
Level −1	27 mg/m^2 per dose
Level −2	20 mg/m^2 per dose
Level −3	15 mg/m^2 per dose
Level −4	11 mg/m^2 per dose
Level −5	Discontinue

Adverse Event	**Treatment Modification**
Hematologic Toxicity	
G3/4 neutropenia	Hold carfilzomib dosing for up to 21 days to resolve toxicity and then restart at the same dosage, or reduce the carfilzomib dosage by 1 dose level. If counts recover to G2 neutropenia or G3 thrombocytopenia, reduce carfilzomib dosage by 1 dose level. If tolerated, the reduced dose may be escalated to the previous dose level
Febrile neutropenia (ANC <1000/mm^3 with fever ≥38°C)	
G4 thrombocytopenia	
G3/4 thrombocytopenia associated with bleeding	
Nonhematologic Toxicity	
G3/4 cardiac toxicity New onset or worsening: • Congestive heart failure • Decreased left ventricular function • Myocardial ischemia	Hold carfilzomib dosing for up to 21 days to resolve toxicity and then restart at the same dosage or reduce the carfilzomib dosage by 1 dose level. If tolerated, the reduced dosage may be escalated to the previous dose level
Pulmonary hypertension	
G3/4 pulmonary complications	
G3/4 elevation of transaminases, bilirubin, or other liver abnormalities	

(*continued*)

Treatment Modifications (*continued*)

Nonhematologic Toxicity

Serum creatinine ≥2× baseline	If attributable to carfilzomib, hold carfilzomib doses for up to 21 days to resolve toxicity to G1 or to baseline and then restart at the same dosage, or reduce the carfilzomib dosage by 1 dose level. If tolerated, the reduced dosage may be escalated to the previous dose level
G2 neuropathy with pain G3/4 peripheral neuropathy	Hold carfilzomib dosing for up to 21 days to resolve toxicity and then restart at the same dose, or reduce the carfilzomib dosage by 1 dose level. If tolerated, the reduced dosage may be escalated to the previous dose level
Other G3/4 nonhematologic toxicities	If attributable to carfilzomib, hold carfilzomib doses for up to 21 days to resolve toxicity to G1 or to baseline and then restart at the same dosage or reduce the carfilzomib dosage by 1 dose level. If tolerated, the reduced dosage may be escalated to the previous dose level

Lenalidomide Dose Levels

Starting dose	25 mg/day
Level −1	20 mg/day
Level −2	15 mg/day
Level −3	10 mg/day
Level −4	5 mg/day
Level −5	Discontinue

Adverse Event	**Treatment Modification**
G3/4 neutropenia Febrile neutropenia (ANC <1000/mm³ with fever ≥38°C)	Hold lenalidomide dosing for up to 21 days to resolve toxicity and then restart at the same dosage or reduce the lenalidomide dosage by 1 dose level
G3/4 nonhematologic toxicity	Hold lenalidomide dosing for up to 21 days to resolve toxicity to G ≤2 and then restart at the same dosage or reduce the lenalidomide dosage by 1 dose level
• Any adverse event G ≥3 (excluding nausea, vomiting, diarrhea, lenalidomide-induced maculopapular rash or dexamethasone-induced hyperglycemia) • G ≥3 nausea, vomiting, or diarrhea despite maximal therapy • G4 fatigue lasting >7 days	Hold carfilzomib and lenalidomide dosing for up to 21 days to resolve toxicity to G ≤2 and then, depending on presumed attribution of toxicity, restart at the same dosage or reduce the carfilzomib dosage and/or lenalidomide daily dose by 1 dose level
Toxicities ascribed to dexamethasone such as severe manifestations of hypercorticism, including hyperglycemia, irritability, insomnia, or oral candidiasis	Hold dexamethasone dosing for up to 21 days to resolve toxicity and then restart at the same dose, or reduce dexamethasone doses by 50%

Patient Population Studied

Enrolled both transplantation-eligible and -ineligible patients with newly diagnosed, symptomatic MM. Patients were required to have an Eastern Cooperative Oncology Group performance status of 0–2. Patients were ineligible if they had G3/4 neuropathy, and an estimated creatinine clearance <50 mL/min (<0.83 mL/s) or serum creatinine ≥2 g/dL (>177 μmol/L)

Baseline Characteristics

Characteristics	N = 53
Age	
Median, years (range)	59 (35–81)
≥65 years, *n* (%)	23 (43)
Sex	
Male, *n* (%)	39 (74)
Female	14 (26)
ISS Stage, *n* (%)	
I	21 (40)
II	18 (34)
III	14 (26)
Durie-Salmon Stage, *n* (%)	
I	7 (13)
II	12 (24)
III	34 (63)
Unfavorable cytogenetics, *n* (%)*	17/51 (33)
del 13†/hypodiploidy	10/50 (20)
t(4;14)	5/49 (10)
t(14;16)	0/48
del 17p	7/48 (15)

ISS, International Staging System
*One or more of the abnormalities listed
†del 13 by metaphase only

Efficacy

Best Response to Treatment in Evaluable Patients

	Responses, *n* (%)			
	≥PR	≥VGPR	≥nCR	sCR
All patients (N = 53)	52 (98)	43 (81)	33 (62)	22 (42)
Treatment Duration				
>4 cycles (*n* = 49)	49 (100)	43 (88)	33 (67)	22 (45)
>8 cycles (*n* = 36)	36 (100)	33 (92)	28 (78)	22 (61)
>12 cycles (*n* = 29)	29 (100)	25 (86)	21 (72)	18 (62)

nCR, near-complete response; PR, partial response; sCR, stringent complete response; VGPR, very good partial response

Best Response to Treatment by Carfilzomib Dose, ISS Stage, and Cytogenetics (N = 53)*

	Responses, *n* (%)			
	≥PR	≥VGPR	≥nCR	sCR
Carfilzomib Dose, mg/m²				
20 (*n* = 4)	4 (100)	4 (100)	3 (75)	1 (25)
27 (*n* = 13)	13 (100)	13 (100)	10 (77)	7 (54)
36 (*n* = 36)	35 (97)	26 (72)	20 (55)	14 (39)
ISS Stage				
I (*n* = 21)	21 (100)	16 (76)	12 (57)	7 (33)
II (*n* = 18)	18 (100)	15 (75)	10 (55)	8 (44)
III (*n* = 14)	13 (93)	12 (86)	11 (79)	7 (50)
Cytogenetics				
Normal/favorable (*n* = 34)[†]	34 (100)	26 (76)	20 (59)	13 (38)
Unfavorable (*n* = 17)[†]	16 (94)	13 (76)	11 (65)	9 (53)

ISS, International Staging System; nCR, near-complete response; PR, partial response; sCR, stringent complete response; VGPR, very good partial response
*Assessed by Modified International Myeloma Working Group (IMWG) Uniform Criteria with the addition of nCR
[†]Any of del 13 by metaphase or hypodiploidy or t(4;14) or t(14;16) or del 17p considered as unfavorable; all others considered normal/favorable

Toxicity

Treatment-Emergent Adverse Events During Induction (Cycles 1–8; N = 53)

	Any Grade, *n* (%)	G3/4, *n* (%)
Nonhematologic		
Hyperglycemia	38 (72)	12 (23)
Edema	25 (47)	2 (4)
Hypophosphatemia	24 (45)	13 (25)
Fatigue	20 (38)	1 (2)
Muscle cramping	17 (32)	0
Rash	15 (28)	4 (8)
Elevated liver function test	15 (28)	4 (8)
Diarrhea	14 (26)	0
Infection*	12 (23)	2 (4)
Phlebitis	12 (23)	0
Peripheral neuropathy	12 (23)[†]	0
Dyspnea	8 (15)	2 (4)
Deep vein thrombosis	6 (11)	2 (4)
Pulmonary embolism	3 (6)	3 (6)
Nausea	7 (13)	0
Renal	5 (9)	1 (2)
Constipation	5 (9)	0
Mood alterations	5 (9)	1 (2)
Hematologic		
Thrombocytopenia	36 (68)	9 (17)
Anemia	32 (60)	11 (21)
Neutropenia	16 (30)	9 (17)

*Grade 3/4 events were pneumonia, and grade 1/2 events were upper respiratory infections
[†]Three (6%) grade 2, remaining grade 1

Therapy Monitoring

1. Blood counts and physical examinations on day 1 of each cycle
2. Serum and urinary protein electrophoresis studies on day 1 of each cycle as indicated and at the end of treatment

REGIMEN
NEWLY DIAGNOSED MULTIPLE MYELOMA (TRANSPLANTATION CANDIDATES)

INDUCTION PRIOR TO AUTOLOGOUS STEM CELL TRANSPLANTATION (ASCT)
THALIDOMIDE + DEXAMETHASONE

Rajkumar SV et al. J Clin Oncol 2006;24:431–436

Four-week cycles:

Thalidomide 200 mg/day; administer orally, continually, for 4 weeks (total dose/4-week cycle = 5600 mg)

Dexamethasone 40 mg/dose; administer orally for three 4-day periods on days 1 to 4, 9 to 12, and 17 to 20, every 4 weeks (total dose/4-week cycle = 480 mg)

Supportive Care
Antiemetic prophylaxis
Emetogenic potential is **MINIMAL - LOW**
See Chapter 39 for antiemetic recommendations

Hematopoietic growth factor (CSF) prophylaxis
Primary prophylaxis is NOT indicated
See Chapter 43 for more information

Antimicrobial prophylaxis
Risk of fever and neutropenia is INTERMEDIATE
Antimicrobial primary prophylaxis to be considered:
- Antibacterial—consider a fluoroquinolone or no prophylaxis; *P. jirovecii* prophylaxis is recommended (eg, cotrimoxazole)
- Antifungal—consider concomitant use of clotrimazole during periods of neutropenia
- Antiviral—antiherpes antivirals (eg, acyclovir, famciclovir, valacyclovir)

Caution: Acyclovir and famciclovir accumulate in patients with impaired renal function and may exacerbate renal dysfunction (valacyclovir is a *prodrug* for acyclovir). Monitor kidney function serially during acyclovir, valacyclovir, and famciclovir use
  - Acyclovir and famciclovir elimination is inversely related to renal function
  - Acyclovir, famciclovir, and valacyclovir utilization is modified in renally impaired individuals (consult product labeling or Summary of Product Characteristics for guidance about dose/dosage and administration frequency modifications, and, when relevant, recommendations for drug dilution, administration rate, concurrent fluid administration, and fluid supplementation as a function of urine output)
  - Impaired acyclovir elimination is associated with neurologic adverse effects, including: agitation, ataxia, coma, confusion, dizziness, dysarthria, encephalopathy, hallucinations, paresthesia, seizure, somnolence, and tremors
See Chapter 47 for more information

Thromboprophylaxis
Risk assessment and recommendations for VTE prophylaxis in patients with multiple myeloma with individual or myeloma-related risk factors, or risk factors related to treatment

(continued)

Treatment Modifications

Thalidomide Dose Levels	
Dose Level 1	200 mg daily
Dose Level −1	100 mg daily
Dose Level −2	50 mg daily

Adverse Event	Treatment Modification
Febrile neutropenia	Withhold therapy until fever abates, then resume therapy
G4 hematologic toxicity	Withhold therapy until ANC >750/mm^3 and platelets >50,000/mm^3, then resume therapy with thalidomide dose decreased by 1 dose level
G3/4 nonhematologic toxicity	Interrupt therapy and follow clinically. After toxicity abates to G ≤2, resume therapy with thalidomide dose decreased by 1 dose level
G ≥3 thalidomide neuropathy	
Toxicities ascribed to dexamethasone such as severe manifestations of hypercorticism, including hyperglycemia, irritability, insomnia, and oral candidiasis	Reduce dexamethasone dose to 20 mg per dose

Efficacy

Best response within 4 cycles of therapy	63%
Complete response within 4 cycles of therapy	4%
Disease progression within 4 cycles of therapy	2%
Stem cell harvest efficiency	90%

(*continued*)

Individual risk factors
- Obesity (BMI ≥30 kg/m²)
- H/O VTE
- CVC or pacemaker
- Comorbid pathologies
  Cardiac disease
  Chronic renal disease
  Diabetes
  Acute infection
  Immobilization
- Surgery
  General surgery
  Any anesthesia
  Trauma
- Medications
  Erythropoietin (epoetin alfa, darbepoetin)
  Estrogenic compounds
  Bevacizumab
- Clotting disorders
  Thrombophilia

Myeloma-related risk factors
- Diagnosis of multiple myeloma
- Hyperviscosity

≤1 Individual or myeloma risk factor present:
- **Aspirin** 81–325 mg daily

≥2 Individual or myeloma risk factors present:
- **LMWH*, equivalent to enoxaparin sodium 40 mg/day** *or* **dalteparin sodium 5000 IU/day**; administer subcutaneously, *or*
- **Warfarin**, targeting an INR = 2–3

Concomitant treatment-related risk factors
Thalidomide or lenalidomide in combination with:
- High-dose dexamethasone (≥480 mg/month)
- Doxorubicin
- Multiagent chemotherapy

LMWH*, equivalent to enoxaparin sodium 40 mg/day *or* **dalteparin sodium 5000 IU/day**; administer subcutaneously, *or*
Warfarin, targeting an INR = 2–3

CVC, central venous catheter; INR, international normalized ratio; LMWH, low-molecular-weight heparin; VTE, venous thromboembolic disease
*LMWHs should be used with caution in individuals with impaired renal function (creatinine clearance <30 mL/min). Refer to product labeling for information about doses and administration schedules in renally impaired patients, and guidance for monitoring anti-Factor Xa concentrations

Geerts WH et al. Chest 2008;133(6 Suppl):381S–453S
Multiple Myeloma, V.1.2014. National Comprehensive Cancer Network, Inc., 2013. (Accessed October 8, 2013, at http://www.nccn.org)
Palumbo A et al. Leukemia 2008;22:414–423
Venous Thromboembolic Disease, V.2.2013. National Comprehensive Cancer Network, Inc., 2013. (Accessed October 8, 2013, at http://www.nccn.org)

Bisphosphonates
All patients receiving primary therapy for symptomatic multiple myeloma should receive a bisphosphonate adjunctively; *for example*:
- **Pamidronate disodium** 90 mg; administer intravenously over 2–4 hours, every month, *or*
- **Zoledronic acid** 4 mg; administer intravenously over 15 minutes, every month

Consider baseline bone densitometry evaluation
See Chapter 43 for more information

Patient Population Studied

Phase III trial of 207 patients with newly diagnosed, previously untreated, measurable myeloma. Patients were eligible to enter onto the study if they had previously untreated symptomatic multiple myeloma, bone marrow plasmacytosis (≥10% plasma cells or sheets of plasma cells), or a biopsy-proven plasmacytoma, and measurable disease defined as serum monoclonal protein >1 g/dL and/or urine monoclonal protein ≥200 mg/24 hours. Study eligibility criteria also included hemoglobin >7 g/dL, platelet count >50,000 cells/mm³, absolute neutrophil count >1000 cells/mm³, creatinine <3 mg/dL (<265 μmol/L), bilirubin ≤1.5 mg/dL (≤26 μmol/L), and ALT and AST ≤2.5-times the upper limit of normal. No prior systemic therapy was permitted with the exception of bisphosphonates

Toxicity (N = 102)

Grade 3/4 neutropenia	9%
Deep venous thrombosis (G ≥3)	17%
Skin rash (G ≥3)	4%
Sinus bradycardia (G ≥3)	1%
Peripheral neuropathy (G ≥3)	7%
Toxicity of any type (G ≥4)	34%
Treatment-related deaths	5%
G ≥3 Thrombosis/embolism	20%
G ≥3 Hyperglycemia	15%
G ≥3 Fatigue	15%
G ≥3 Dyspnea	11%
G ≥3 Hypocalcemia	8%
G ≥3 Confusion	8%
G ≥3 Constipation	8%
G ≥3 Neuropathy-motor	7%
G ≥3 Muscle weakness	6%
G ≥3 Edema	6%
G ≥3 Pneumonitis/pulmonary infiltrates	5%
G ≥3 Hyponatremia	4%
G ≥3 Hypotension	4%
G ≥3 Dehydration	4%
G ≥3 Neuropathy-sensory	4%
G ≥3 Rash/desquamation	4%
G ≥3 Nausea	4%
G ≥3 Hypoxia	3%
G ≥3 Depressed level of consciousness	3%
G ≥3 Anorexia	3%
G ≥3 Seizure	3%

Therapy Monitoring

1. *Before each cycle:* CBC with differential and blood chemistries (including BUN, creatinine, and calcium)
2. *Every 6 weeks to 3 months:* Measure serum and urine M-protein

REGIMEN
NEWLY DIAGNOSED MULTIPLE MYELOMA (ELDERLY AND THOSE *NOT* TRANSPLANTATION CANDIDATES)

MELPHALAN + PREDNISONE + THALIDOMIDE (MPT)

Palumbo A et al. Lancet 2006;367:825–831
Palumbo A et al. Blood 2008;112:3107–3114

Induction:

Melphalan 4 mg/m^2 per day; administer orally for 7 consecutive days on days 1–7, every 4 weeks, for 6 cycles (total dosage/cycle = 28 mg/m^2)

Prednisone 40 mg/m^2 per day; administer orally for 7 consecutive days on days 1–7, every 4 weeks, for 6 cycles (total dosage/cycle = 280 mg/m^2)

Thalidomide 100 mg/day; administer orally for 28 consecutive day on days 1–28, every 4 weeks for 6 cycles (total dose/cycle = 2800 mg)

Maintenance:

Thalidomide 100 mg/day; administer orally, continually, until confirmation of relapsed or refractory disease (total dose/week = 700 mg)

Supportive Care

Antiemetic prophylaxis
Emetogenic potential is **MINIMAL–LOW**
See Chapter 39 for antiemetic recommendations

Hematopoietic growth factor (CSF) prophylaxis
Primary prophylaxis is NOT indicated
See Chapter 43 for more information

Antimicrobial prophylaxis
Risk of fever and neutropenia is INTERMEDIATE
  Antimicrobial primary prophylaxis to be considered:
  • Antibacterial—consider a fluoroquinolone or no prophylaxis; *P. jirovecii* prophylaxis is recommended (eg, cotrimoxazole)
  • Antifungal—consider concomitant use of clotrimazole during periods of neutropenia
  • Antiviral—antiherpes antivirals (eg, acyclovir, famciclovir, valacyclovir)

Caution: Acyclovir and famciclovir accumulate in patients with impaired renal function and may exacerbate renal dysfunction (valacyclovir is a *prodrug* for acyclovir). Monitor kidney function serially during acyclovir, valacyclovir, and famciclovir use
  ▪ Acyclovir and famciclovir elimination is inversely related to renal function
  ▪ Acyclovir, famciclovir, and valacyclovir utilization is modified in renally impaired individuals (consult product labeling or Summary of Product Characteristics for guidance about dose/dosage and administration frequency modifications, and, when relevant, recommendations for drug dilution, administration rate, concurrent fluid administration, and fluid supplementation as a function of urine output)
  ▪ Impaired acyclovir elimination is associated with neurologic adverse effects, including agitation, ataxia, coma, confusion, dizziness, dysarthria, encephalopathy, hallucinations, paresthesia, seizure, somnolence, and tremors
See Chapter 47 for more information

(continued)

Treatment Modifications

Melphalan Dosage Levels

Dosage Level 1	4 mg/m^2
Dosage Level −1	3 mg/m^2
Dosage Level −2	2 mg/m^2

Adverse Event	Treatment Modification
Febrile neutropenia	Withhold therapy until fever abates, then resume therapy
G4 hematologic toxicity	Withhold therapy until ANC >750/mm^3 and platelets >50,000/mm^3, then resume therapy with the melphalan dose decreased by 1 dose level
G3/4 nonhematologic toxicity	Interrupt therapy and follow clinically. After toxicity abates to G ≤2, resume therapy with thalidomide dose decreased by 1 dose level
G ≥3 thalidomide neuropathy	
If ANC nadir is ≤1000/mm^3 or platelets nadir is ≤50,000/mm^3	Continue treatment, but reduce melphalan dosage by 1 level
G2 nonhematologic toxicity	Reduce thalidomide dose by 50% to 50 mg/day
G ≥3 nonhematologic toxicity	Discontinue thalidomide
G3 toxicities ascribed to prednisone such as severe manifestations of hypercorticism, including hyperglycemia, irritability, insomnia, and oral candidiasis	Reduce daily prednisone dosage by 20%
G4 or recurrent G3 toxicities ascribed to prednisone such as severe manifestations of hypercorticism, including hyperglycemia, irritability, insomnia, and oral candidiasis	Reduce daily prednisone dosage by 40%

(continued)

Thromboprophylaxis

Risk assessment and recommendations for VTE prophylaxis in patients with multiple myeloma with individual or myeloma-related risk factors, or risk factors related to treatment

Individual risk factors	
• Obesity (BMI ≥30 kg/m^2)	
• H/O VTE	
• CVC or pacemaker	
• Comorbid pathologies	
Cardiac disease	
Chronic renal disease	≤1 Individual or myeloma risk factor present:
Diabetes	• **Aspirin** 81–325 mg daily
Acute infection	
Immobilization	
• Surgery	
General surgery	≥2 Individual or myeloma risk factors present:
Any anesthesia	• **LMWH*, equivalent to enoxaparin sodium** 40 mg/day *or* **dalteparin sodium** 5000 IU/day; administer subcutaneously, *or*
Trauma	
• Medications	
Erythropoietin (epoetin alfa, darbepoetin)	
Estrogenic compounds	• **Warfarin**, targeting an INR = 2–3
Bevacizumab	
• Clotting disorders	
Thrombophilia	
Myeloma-related risk factors	
• Diagnosis of multiple myeloma	
• Hyperviscosity	
Concomitant treatment-related risk factors Thalidomide or lenalidomide in combination with: • High-dose dexamethasone (≥480 mg/month) • Doxorubicin • Multiagent chemotherapy	**LMWH*, equivalent to enoxaparin sodium** 40 mg/day *or* **dalteparin sodium** 5000 IU/day; administer subcutaneously, *or* **Warfarin**, targeting an INR = 2–3

CVC, central venous catheter; INR, international normalized ratio; LMWH, low-molecular-weight heparin; VTE, venous thromboembolic disease
*LMWHs should be used with caution in individuals with impaired renal function (creatinine clearance <30 mL/min). Refer to product labeling for information about doses and administration schedules in renally impaired patients, and guidance for monitoring anti-Factor Xa concentrations

Geerts WH et al. Chest 2008;133(6 Suppl):381S–453S
Multiple Myeloma, V.1.2014. National Comprehensive Cancer Network, Inc., 2013. (Accessed October 8, 2013, at http://www.nccn.org)
Palumbo A et al. Leukemia 2008;22:414–423
Venous Thromboembolic Disease, V.2.2013. National Comprehensive Cancer Network, Inc., 2013. (Accessed October 8, 2013, at http://www.nccn.org)

Bisphosphonates

All patients receiving primary therapy for symptomatic multiple myeloma should receive a bisphosphonate adjunctively; *for example*:

• **Pamidronate sodium** 90 mg; administer intravenously over 2–4 hours, every month, *or*

• **Zoledronic acid** 4 mg; administer intravenously over 15 minutes, every month

Consider baseline bone densitometry evaluation
See Chapter 43 for more information

Patient Population Studied

A multicenter randomized trial of 331 previously untreated patients with Durie and Salmon stage II or III multiple myeloma who were older than 65 years (or younger but unable to undergo transplantation), and had measurable disease. Exclusion criteria included any G2 peripheral neuropathy. Abnormal cardiac function, chronic respiratory disease, and abnormal liver or renal function were not criteria for exclusion

Efficacy
(N = 129)

Complete or partial response	76%
Complete response	15.5%
Partial response	60.4%
Near-complete response	12.4%
90% to 99% myeloma protein reduction	8.5%
50% to 89% myeloma protein reduction	39.5%
Minimal response	5.4%
No response	5.4%
Progressive disease	7.8%
Responses not available	5.4%
Progression free survival*	21.8 months
Median overall survival†	45 months

*After a median follow-up of 38.1 months. The magnitude of PFS benefit was consistent irrespective of age, serum concentrations of β_2-microglobulin, or high International Staging System
†The median OS of 45 months for melphalan + prednisone (MP) + thalidomide (T) compared to a median OS of 47.6 months for MP was not statistically significant ($P = 0.79$). New agents in the management of relapsed disease could explain this finding

Toxicity
(N = 129)

Adverse Event	G3/4 Adverse Events Percent of Patients
≥1 Event	48%
Hematologic	22%
Neutropenia	16%
Anemia	3%
Thrombocytopenia	3%
Thrombosis/embolism	12%
Deep venous thrombosis	9%
Pulmonary embolism	2%
Neurologic	10%
Peripheral neuropathy	8%
Somnolence or fatigue	3%
Infection	10%
Pneumonia	5%
Fever of unknown origin	2%
Herpes zoster	1%
Upper respiratory	2%
Cardiac	7%
Arrhythmia	2%
Myocardial infarction/ angina	2%
Cardiac failure	3%
Hypertension	1%
Gastrointestinal	6%
Constipation	6%
Mucositis	0
Dermatologic	3%
Rash	2%
Toxic epidermal necrolysis	1%
Renal	1%
Creatinine increase	1%
Edema	1%
Bleeding	0

Therapy Monitoring

1. *Before each cycle:* CBC with differential and blood chemistries (including BUN, creatinine, and calcium)
2. *Every 6 weeks to 3 months:* Measure serum and urine M-protein

REGIMEN
NEWLY DIAGNOSED MULTIPLE MYELOMA (*NOT* TRANSPLANTATION CANDIDATES)

BORTEZOMIB + MELPHALAN + PREDNISONE

San Miguel JF et al. N Engl J Med 2008;359:906–917

All Cycles:

Melphalan 9 mg/m² per day; administer orally for 4 consecutive days on days 1–4, every 6 weeks, for 9 cycles (total dosage/cycle = 36 mg/m²)

Prednisone 60 mg/m² per day; administer orally for 4 consecutive days on days 1–4, every 6 weeks, for 9 cycles (total dosage/cycle = 240 mg/m²), *plus*

Cycles 1–4:

Bortezomib 1.3 mg/m² per dose; administer by intravenous injection over 3–5 seconds for 8 doses, on days 1, 4, 8, 11, 22, 25, 29, and 32, every 6 weeks, for 4 cycles (total dosage/cycle = 10.4 mg/m²)

Cycles 5–9:

Bortezomib 1.3 mg/m² per dose; administer by intravenous injection over 3–5 seconds for 4 doses on days 1, 8, 22, and 29, every 6 weeks, for 5 cycles (total dosage/cycle = 5.2 mg/m²)

Supportive Care

Antiemetic prophylaxis
Emetogenic potential is **MINIMAL–LOW**
See Chapter 39 for antiemetic recommendations

Hematopoietic growth factor (CSF) prophylaxis
Primary prophylaxis is NOT indicated
See Chapter 43 for more information

Antimicrobial prophylaxis
Risk of fever and neutropenia is HIGH
Antimicrobial primary prophylaxis is recommended:

- Antibacterial—consider fluoroquinolone prophylaxis; *P. jirovecii* prophylaxis is recommended (eg, cotrimoxazole)
- Antifungal—recommended
- Antiviral—antiherpes antivirals (eg, acyclovir, famciclovir, valacyclovir)

Caution: Acyclovir and famciclovir accumulate in patients with impaired renal function and may exacerbate renal dysfunction (valacyclovir is a *prodrug* for acyclovir). Monitor kidney function serially during acyclovir, valacyclovir, and famciclovir use

- Acyclovir and famciclovir elimination is inversely related to renal function
- Acyclovir, famciclovir, and valacyclovir utilization is modified in renally impaired individuals (consult product labeling or Summary of Product Characteristics for guidance about dose/dosage and administration frequency modifications, and, when relevant, recommendations for drug dilution, administration rate, concurrent fluid administration, and fluid supplementation as a function of urine output)
- Impaired acyclovir elimination is associated with neurologic adverse effects, including agitation, ataxia, coma, confusion, dizziness, dysarthria, encephalopathy, hallucinations, paresthesia, seizure, somnolence, and tremors

See Chapter 47 for more information

Decreased bowel motility prophylaxis
Give a bowel regimen to prevent constipation based initially on **stool softeners**

(continued)

Treatment Modifications

Bortezomib Dosage Levels (per dose)	
Dosage Level 1	1.3 mg/m²
Dosage Level −1	1 mg/m²
Dosage Level −2	0.7 mg/m²

Melphalan Dose Levels (per day)	
Dosage Level 1	9 mg/m²
Dosage Level −1	6.75 mg/m²
Dosage Level −2	4.5 mg/m²

Adverse Event	Treatment Modification
Febrile neutropenia	Withhold therapy until fever abates then resume therapy
G4 hematologic toxicity	Withhold therapy until ANC >750/mm³ and platelets >50,000/mm³, then resume therapy with bortezomib and melphalan dosages decreased by 1 dose level
G3/4 nonhematologic toxicity	Withhold therapy. After toxicity abates to G ≤2, resume therapy with bortezomib and melphalan dosages decreased by 1 dose level
G≥3 thalidomide neuropathy	Continue treatment, but reduce thalidomide dose by 1 dose level
If ANC nadir is ≤1000/mm³ or platelets nadir is ≤50,000/mm³	Continue treatment, but reduce bortezomib and melphalan dosages by 1 level
G3 toxicities ascribed to prednisone such as severe manifestations of hypercorticism, including hyperglycemia, irritability, insomnia, or oral candidiasis	Reduce daily prednisone dosage by 20%
G4 or recurrent G3 toxicities ascribed to prednisone such as severe manifestations of hypercorticism, including hyperglycemia, irritability, insomnia, or oral candidiasis	Reduce daily prednisone dosage by 40%

(continued)

(*continued*)

Thromboprophylaxis
Risk assessment and recommendations for VTE prophylaxis in patients with multiple myeloma with individual or myeloma-related risk factors, or risk factors related to treatment

Individual risk factors
• Obesity (BMI ≥30 kg/m²)
• H/O VTE
• CVC or pacemaker
• Comorbid pathologies
  Cardiac disease
  Chronic renal disease
  Diabetes
  Acute infection
  Immobilization
• Surgery
  General surgery
  Any anesthesia
  Trauma
• Medications
  Erythropoietin (epoetin alfa, darbepoetin)
  Estrogenic compounds
  Bevacizumab
• Clotting disorders
  Thrombophilia
Myeloma-related risk factors
• Diagnosis of multiple myeloma
• Hyperviscosity
	≤1 Individual or myeloma risk factor present:
	• **Aspirin** 81–325 mg daily
	
	≥2 Individual or myeloma risk factors present:
	• **LMWH*, equivalent to enoxaparin sodium** 40 mg/day *or* **dalteparin sodium** 5000 IU/day; administer subcutaneously, *or*
	• **Warfarin**, targeting an INR = 2–3

Concomitant treatment-related risk factors Thalidomide or lenalidomide in combination with: • High-dose dexamethasone (≥480 mg/month) • Doxorubicin • Multiagent chemotherapy	**LMWH*, equivalent to enoxaparin sodium** 40 mg/day *or* **dalteparin sodium** 5000 IU/day; administer subcutaneously, *or* **Warfarin**, targeting an INR = 2–3

CVC, central venous catheter; INR, international normalized ratio; LMWH, low-molecular-weight heparin; VTE, venous thromboembolic disease

*LMWHs should be used with caution in individuals with impaired renal function (creatinine clearance <30 mL/min). Refer to product labeling for information about doses and administration schedules in renally impaired patients, and guidance for monitoring anti-Factor Xa concentrations

Geerts WH et al. Chest 2008;133(6 Suppl):381S–453S
Multiple Myeloma, V.1.2014. National Comprehensive Cancer Network, Inc., 2013. (Accessed October 8, 2013, at http://www.nccn.org)
Palumbo A et al. Leukemia 2008;22:414–423
Venous Thromboembolic Disease, V.2.2013. National Comprehensive Cancer Network, Inc., 2013. (Accessed October 8, 2013, at http://www.nccn.org)

Bisphosphonates
All patients receiving primary therapy for symptomatic multiple myeloma should receive a bisphosphonate adjunctively; *for example*:
• **Pamidronate sodium** 90 mg; administer intravenously over 2–4 hours, every month, *or*
• **Zoledronic acid** 4 mg; administer intravenously over 15 minutes, every month

Consider baseline bone densitometry evaluation
See Chapter 43 for more information

Treatment Modifications
(*continued*)

Treatment Modification for Bortezomib-Induced Peripheral Neuropathy*

Severity of Peripheral Neuropathy	Modification of Dose and Schedule
G1 (paresthesias or loss of reflexes) without pain or loss of function	No action
G1 with pain, or G2 (interferes with function but not with activities of daily living)	Reduce bortezomib dosage to 1 mg/m² per dose
G2 with pain, or G3 (interferes with activities of daily living)	Withhold bortezomib treatment until toxicity resolves, then reinitiate at a dosage of 0.7 mg/m² per dose once weekly
G4 (permanent sensory loss that interferes with function)	Discontinue treatment

*Richardson PG et al. J Clin Oncol 2006;24:3113–3120

Patient Population Studied

A randomized, open-label, phase III trial of 682 patients with newly diagnosed, untreated, symptomatic, measurable myeloma who, because of age (≥65 years), were not candidates for high-dose therapy plus stem cell transplantation

Efficacy
(N = 337)*

European Group for Blood and Marrow Transplantation (EBMT) Criteria

Complete or partial response	71%
Complete response	30%
Partial response	40%
Minimal response	9%
Stable disease	18%
Progressive disease	1%

Time to Event

Median time to response[†]	
First response (months)	1.4
Complete response	4.2
Median duration of response[†]	
Complete or partial response	19.9
Complete response	24
Time to subsequent myeloma therapy[‡]	Not reached
Treatment-free interval[‡]	Not reached

International Uniform Response Criteria[§]

Complete, very good partial, or partial response	74%
Complete response	33%
Very good partial response	8%
Partial response	33%
Stable disease	23%
Progressive disease	1%

*Seven patients could not be evaluated for a response. Among patients evaluated, responses were not determined for 4. Percentages may not total 100 because of rounding
[†]Data determined by computer algorithm, applying EBMT criteria
[‡]Data based on 344 patients
[§]Of 79 patients considered to have stable disease on the basis of International Uniform Response Criteria who could be evaluated, 4 patients (1%) had negative results on immunofixation (complete response) and 19 (6%) had a reduction of at least 50% in M-protein (partial response). These patients were not recorded as having a complete or partial response because confirmatory results were missing. If these patients are included, the response rate is 81% and the complete-response rate is 34%. Patients could not be assessed for the category of stringent complete response because immunohistochemical, immunofluorescence, and free light-chain assays were not performed. International Uniform Response Criteria do not require changes in M-protein be confirmed a minimum of 6 weeks after the initial assessment

Toxicity (N = 340)*

	G1/2	G3	G4
Any Event	18	53	28
Hematologic Events[†]			
Thrombocytopenia	15	20	17
Neutropenia	9	30	10
Anemia	24	16	3
Leukopenia	10	20	3
Lymphopenia	5	14	5
Gastrointestinal Events			
Nausea	44	4	0
Diarrhea	38	7	1
Constipation	36	1	0
Vomiting	29	4	0
Infections			
Pneumonia	9	5	2
Herpes zoster	10	3	0
Nervous System Disorders			
Peripheral sensory neuropathy	31	13	<1
Neuralgia	27	8	1
Dizziness	14	2	0
Other Conditions			
Pyrexia	26	2	1
Fatigue	21	7	1
Asthenia	20	3	<1
Cough	21	0	0
Insomnia	20	<1	0
Peripheral edema	19	1	0
Rash	18	1	0
Back pain	14	3	<1
Dyspnea	11	3	1
Hypokalemia	6	6	1
Arthralgia	10	1	0
Deep venous thrombosis	1	1	0

*Listed adverse events were reported in ≥15% of patients, and G3 or G4 events were reported in ≥5% of patients. Patients may have more than 1 adverse event. Included are all patients who received at least 1 dose of a study drug
[†]Rates of red cell transfusions were 26%; erythropoiesis-stimulating agents for treatment-related anemia were used in 30% of patients

Therapy Monitoring

1. *Before each cycle:* CBC with differential and blood chemistries (including BUN, creatinine, and calcium)
2. *Every 6 weeks to 3 months:* Measure serum and urine M-protein

REGIMEN
NEWLY DIAGNOSED MULTIPLE MYELOMA
NOT TRANSPLANTATION CANDIDATES
MELPHALAN + PREDNISONE + LENALIDOMIDE

Palumbo A et al. J Clin Oncol 2007;25:4459–4465

Induction:
Melphalan 0.18 mg/kg per day; administer orally for 4 consecutive days on days 1–4, every 4 weeks, for 9 cycles (total dosage/cycle = 0.72 mg/kg)
Prednisone 2 mg/kg per day; administer orally for 4 consecutive days on days 1–4, every 4 weeks, for 9 cycles (total dosage/cycle = 8 mg/kg)
Lenalidomide 10 mg per day; administer orally for 21 consecutive days on days 1–21, every 4 weeks, for 9 cycles (total dose/cycle = 210 mg)
Maintenance:
Lenalidomide 10 mg/day; administer orally for 21 consecutive days on days 1–21, every 4 weeks until signs of relapse or disease progression (total dose/cycle = 210 mg)

Supportive Care
Antiemetic prophylaxis
Emetogenic potential is **MINIMAL–LOW**
See Chapter 39 for antiemetic recommendations

Hematopoietic growth factor (CSF) prophylaxis
Primary prophylaxis is NOT indicated
See Chapter 43 for more information

Antimicrobial prophylaxis
Risk of fever and neutropenia is INTERMEDIATE
Antimicrobial primary prophylaxis to be considered:
- Antibacterial—consider a fluoroquinolone or no prophylaxis; *P. jirovecii* prophylaxis is recommended (eg, cotrimoxazole)
- Antifungal—consider concomitant use of clotrimazole during periods of neutropenia
- Antiviral—antiherpes antivirals (eg, acyclovir, famciclovir, valacyclovir)

Caution: Acyclovir and famciclovir accumulate in patients with impaired renal function and may exacerbate renal dysfunction (valacyclovir is a *prodrug* for acyclovir). Monitor kidney function serially during acyclovir, valacyclovir, and famciclovir use
- Acyclovir and famciclovir elimination is inversely related to renal function
- Acyclovir, famciclovir, and valacyclovir utilization is modified in renally impaired individuals (consult product labeling or Summary of Product Characteristics for guidance about dose/dosage and administration frequency modifications, and, when relevant, recommendations for drug dilution, administration rate, concurrent fluid administration, and fluid supplementation as a function of urine output)
- Impaired acyclovir elimination is associated with neurological adverse effects, including agitation, ataxia, coma, confusion, dizziness, dysarthria, encephalopathy, hallucinations, paresthesia, seizure, somnolence, and tremors
See Chapter 47 for more information

Decreased bowel motility prophylaxis
Give a bowel regimen to prevent constipation based initially on **stool softeners**

(continued)

Treatment Modifications

Lenalidomide Dose Levels	
Dose Level 1	10 mg/day
Dose Level −1	5 mg/day

Melphalan Dose Levels	
Dosage Level 1	0.18 mg/kg
Dosage Level −1	0.135 mg/kg

Adverse Event	Treatment Modification
Febrile neutropenia	Withhold therapy until fever abates, then resume therapy
G4 neutropenia for ≥7 days despite filgrastim administration, any other G4 hematologic toxicities, or any G ≥3 nonhematologic toxicities	Withhold therapy until toxicities resolve to G ≤2 then resume therapy with a subsequent dose/dosage reduction in lenalidomide and melphalan at the start of the following cycle
G ≥3 neuropathy	Interrupt therapy and follow clinically. After toxicity abates to G ≤2, resume lenalidomide with a dose decreased by 1 dose level
G3/4 non-hematologic toxicity	Interrupt lenalidomide treatment and follow clinically. Resume lenalidomide at 5 mg/day after toxicity abates to G ≤2
ANC <1000/mm³, platelet count <50,000/mm³, or nonhematologic adverse events G ≥2	Withhold therapy as long as 2 weeks until ANC ≥1000/mm³, platelet count is ≥50,000/mm³, and nonhematologic toxicities are G ≤1, then resume therapy. A delay of 2 weeks is allowed without any dose modification. A new cycle delay beyond a maximum of 2 weeks requires a dose/dosage reduction in lenalidomide and melphalan by 1 dose level
Toxicities ascribed to prednisone such as severe manifestations of hypercorticism, including: hyperglycemia, irritability, insomnia, or oral candidiasis	Reduce prednisone dose to 20 mg/day

(continued)

(continued)

Thromboprophylaxis

Risk assessment and recommendations for VTE prophylaxis in patients with multiple myeloma with individual or myeloma-related risk factors, or risk factors related to treatment

Individual risk factors
• Obesity (BMI ≥30 kg/m²)
• H/O VTE
• CVC or pacemaker
• Comorbid pathologies
  Cardiac disease
  Chronic renal disease
  Diabetes
  Acute infection
  Immobilization
• Surgery
  General surgery
  Any anesthesia
  Trauma
• Medications
  Erythropoietin (epoetin alfa, darbepoetin)
  Estrogenic compounds
  Bevacizumab
• Clotting disorders
  Thrombophilia
Myeloma-related risk factors
• Diagnosis of multiple myeloma
• Hyperviscosity
	≤1 Individual or myeloma risk factor present:
	• **Aspirin** 81–325 mg daily
	
	≥2 Individual or myeloma risk factors present:
	• **LMWH***, equivalent to enoxaparin sodium 40 mg/day *or* **dalteparin sodium** 5000 IU/day; administer subcutaneously, *or*
	• **Warfarin**, targeting an INR = 2–3

Concomitant treatment-related risk factors Thalidomide or lenalidomide in combination with: • High-dose dexamethasone (≥480 mg/month) • Doxorubicin • Multiagent chemotherapy	**LMWH***, equivalent to enoxaparin sodium 40 mg/day *or* **dalteparin sodium** 5000 IU/day; administer subcutaneously, *or* **Warfarin**, targeting an INR = 2–3

CVC, central venous catheter; INR, international normalized ratio; LMWH, low-molecular-weight heparin; VTE, venous thromboembolic disease

*LMWHs should be used with caution in individuals with impaired renal function (creatinine clearance <30 mL/min). Refer to product labeling for information about doses and administration schedules in renally impaired patients, and guidance for monitoring anti-Factor Xa concentrations

Geerts WH et al. Chest 2008;133(6 Suppl):381S–453S
Multiple Myeloma, V.1.2014. National Comprehensive Cancer Network, Inc., 2013. (Accessed October 8, 2013, at http://www.nccn.org)
Palumbo A et al. Leukemia 2008;22:414–423
Venous Thromboembolic Disease, V.2.2013. National Comprehensive Cancer Network, Inc., 2013. (Accessed October 8, 2013, at http://www.nccn.org)

Bisphosphonates

All patients receiving primary therapy for symptomatic multiple myeloma should receive a bisphosphonate adjunctively; *for example*:

• **Pamidronate sodium** 90 mg; administer intravenously over 2–4 hours, every month, *or*

• **Zoledronic acid** 4 mg; administer intravenously over 15 minutes, every month

Consider baseline bone densitometry evaluation
See Chapter 43 for more information

Treatment Modifications
(continued)

Lenalidomide Starting Dose Adjustment for Renal Impairment in Multiple Myeloma (Days 1–21 of Each 28-Day Cycle)*

Moderate renal impairment CrCl 30–60 mL/min (0.5–1 mL/s)	10 mg lenalidomide every 24 hours
Severe renal impairment CrCl <30 mL/min, not requiring dialysis	15 mg lenalidomide every 48 hours
End-stage renal disease CrCl <30 mL/min, requiring dialysis	Lenalidomide 5 mg/day. On dialysis days, administer a daily dose following dialysis

CrCl, Creatinine clearance
*Richardson PG et al. J Clin Oncol 2006;24:3113–3120

Patient Population Studied

Phase I/II trial of 54 patients ages ≥65 years or younger if ineligible for high-dose therapy for newly diagnosed multiple myeloma. Karnofsky performance status ≥60%; platelet count ≥75,000/mm³; absolute neutrophil count ≥1500/mm³; corrected serum calcium ≤3.5 mmol/L (≤14 mg/dL)

Therapy Monitoring

1. *Before each cycle:* CBC with differential and blood chemistries (including BUN, creatinine, and calcium)
2. *Every 6 weeks to 3 months:* Measure serum and urine M-protein

Efficacy

	1	2	3 (MTD)	4
	\multicolumn{4}{c}{Dose Levels Evaluated}			
Lenalidomide (mg)	5	5	10	10
Melphalan (mg/kg)	0.18	0.25	0.18	0.25
Number of patients	6	6	21	20
Complete or partial response	66.7	83.3	81	85
CR, immunofixation negative	—	—	23.8	10
VGPR	—	33.3	23.8	30
Partial response	66.7	50	33.3	45
Minimal response	33.3	16.7	19	15
No response	—	—	—	—
Progressive Disease	—	—	—	—

Median time to best response	4 months
PR > first cycle	52.9%
PR > third cycle	66%
PR > sixth cycle	79.2%
1-year event-free survival	92.3% (95% CI, 85.1 to 99.5)
1-year event-free survival at MTD	95.2% (95% CI, 93.2 to 97.3).
1-year overall survival in all patients	100% (95% CI, 91.8% to 100%)

CR, complete response; MTD, Maximum tolerated doses; PR, partial response; VGPR, very good partial response

Toxicity

	Total G3/4 Events	Total G1/2 Events
Hematologic Events		
Neutropenia	67.9%	ND
Thrombocytopenia	32.1%	ND
Anemia	17%	ND
Nonhematologic Events		
Infective		
Febrile neutropenia	9.4%	—
Pneumonia	1.9%	5.7%
Upper respiratory	—	13.2%
Dermatologic events		
Rash	3.8%	35.8%
Vasculitis	3.8%	1.9%
Thromboembolism		
Deep venous thrombosis	3.8%	—
Pulmonary embolism	1.9%	—
Constitutional events		
Fatigue	3.8%	43.4%
Fever	—	18.9%
Gastrointestinal events		
Constipation	—	24.5%
Diarrhea	1.9%	22.6%
Nausea	—	18.9%
Anorexia	—	17%
Neurologic events		
Mood alterations	1.9%	9.4%
Dizziness	—	3.8%

ND, Not determined
Note: G1/2 adverse events reported by ≥10% of patients or G3/4 adverse events reported by ≥3% of patients

REGIMEN
RELAPSED/REFRACTORY MULTIPLE MYELOMA
BORTEZOMIB ± DEXAMETHASONE

Richardson PG et al. N Engl J Med 2003;348:2609–2617

Bortezomib 1.3 mg/m^2 per dose; administer by intravenous injection over 3–5 seconds for 4 doses on days 1, 4, 8, and 11, every 21 days (total dosage/cycle = 5.2 mg/m^2)

In patients with disease progression after 2 cycles, or stable disease after 4 cycles, add:
Dexamethasone 20 mg per dose; administer orally for 8 doses on days 1, 2, 4, 5, 8, 9, 11, and 12, every 21 days (total dose/cycle = 160 mg)

Supportive Care
Antiemetic prophylaxis
Emetogenic potential is **MINIMAL**
See Chapter 39 for antiemetic recommendations

Hematopoietic growth factor (CSF) prophylaxis
Primary prophylaxis is NOT indicated
See Chapter 43 for more information

Antimicrobial prophylaxis
Risk of fever and neutropenia is HIGH
Antimicrobial primary prophylaxis is recommended:
- Antibacterial—consider fluoroquinolone prophylaxis; *P. jirovecii* prophylaxis is recommended (eg, cotrimoxazole)
- Antifungal—recommended
- Antiviral—antiherpes antivirals (eg, acyclovir, famciclovir, valacyclovir)

Caution: Acyclovir and famciclovir accumulate in patients with impaired renal function and may exacerbate renal dysfunction (valacyclovir is a *prodrug* for acyclovir). Monitor kidney function serially during acyclovir, valacyclovir, and famciclovir use
  - Acyclovir and famciclovir elimination is inversely related to renal function
  - Acyclovir, famciclovir, and valacyclovir utilization is modified in renally impaired individuals (consult product labeling or Summary of Product Characteristics for guidance about dose/dosage and administration frequency modifications, and, when relevant, recommendations for drug dilution, administration rate, concurrent fluid administration, and fluid supplementation as a function of urine output)
  - Impaired acyclovir elimination is associated with neurological adverse effects, including agitation, ataxia, coma, confusion, dizziness, dysarthria, encephalopathy, hallucinations, paresthesia, seizure, somnolence, and tremors
See Chapter 47 for more information

Decreased bowel motility prophylaxis
Give a bowel regimen to prevent constipation based initially on **stool softeners**

(continued)

Treatment Modifications

Adverse Event	Treatment Modification
G3 nonhematologic toxicity or G4 hematologic toxicity	Hold treatment until toxicity resolves to G ≤1, then resume with bortezomib 1 mg/m^2
G3 nonhematologic toxicity or G4 hematologic toxicity in a patient receiving bortezomib 1 mg/m^2	Hold treatment until toxicity resolves to G ≤1, then resume with bortezomib 0.7 mg/m^2
Severe manifestations of hypercorticism, including severe hyperglycemia, irritability, insomnia, or oral candidiasis	Reduce daily dexamethasone dosage by 20% for G3 toxicity, and by 40% for G4 or recurrent G3 toxicity

Patient Population Studied

Study of 202 patients with relapsed multiple myeloma, refractory to the therapy subjects had most recently received. A multicenter, open-label, nonrandomized, phase II trial

Efficacy (N = 193)

European Group for Blood and Marrow Transplantation Criteria	
Complete response	10%
Partial response	18%
Minimal response	7%
No change	24%
Progressive disease	41%
Median time to first response	1.3 months
Median response duration*	12 months

*In the 67 patients with a complete, partial, or minimal response to bortezomib alone

(*continued*)

Thromboprophylaxis

Risk assessment and recommendations for VTE prophylaxis in patients with multiple myeloma with individual or myeloma-related risk factors, or risk factors related to treatment

Individual risk factors	
• Obesity (BMI $\geq$30 kg/m^2)	
• H/O VTE	
• CVC or pacemaker	
• Comorbid pathologies	
Cardiac disease	
Chronic renal disease	$\leq$1 Individual or myeloma risk factor present:
Diabetes	• **Aspirin** 81–325 mg daily
Acute infection	
Immobilization	
• Surgery	
General surgery	$\geq$2 Individual or myeloma risk factors present:
Any anesthesia	• **LMWH***, equivalent to enoxaparin sodium 40 mg/day *or* **dalteparin sodium** 5000 IU/day; administer subcutaneously, *or*
Trauma	
• Medications	
Erythropoietin (epoetin alfa, darbepoetin)	• **Warfarin**, targeting an INR = 2–3
Estrogenic compounds	
Bevacizumab	
• Clotting disorders	
Thrombophilia	
Myeloma-related risk factors	
• Diagnosis of multiple myeloma	
• Hyperviscosity	
Concomitant treatment-related risk factors	**LMWH***, equivalent to enoxaparin sodium 40 mg/day *or* **dalteparin sodium** 5000 IU/day; administer subcutaneously, *or*
Thalidomide or lenalidomide in combination with:	
• High-dose dexamethasone ($\geq$480 mg/month)	
• Doxorubicin	**Warfarin**, targeting an INR = 2–3
• Multiagent chemotherapy	

CVC, central venous catheter; INR, international normalized ratio; LMWH, low-molecular-weight heparin; VTE, venous thromboembolic disease

*LMWHs should be used with caution in individuals with impaired renal function (creatinine clearance <30 mL/min). Refer to product labeling for information about doses and administration schedules in renally impaired patients, and guidance for monitoring anti-Factor Xa concentrations

Geerts WH et al. Chest 2008;133(6 Suppl):381S–453S
Multiple Myeloma, V.1.2014. National Comprehensive Cancer Network, Inc., 2013. (Accessed October 8, 2013, at http://www.nccn.org)
Palumbo A et al. Leukemia 2008;22:414–423
Venous Thromboembolic Disease, V.2.2013. National Comprehensive Cancer Network, Inc., 2013. (Accessed October 8, 2013, at http://www.nccn.org)

Bisphosphonates

All patients receiving primary therapy for symptomatic multiple myeloma should receive a bisphosphonate adjunctively; *for example*:

• **Pamidronate disodium** 90 mg; administer intravenously over 2–4 hours, every month, *or*

• **Zoledronic acid** 4 mg; administer intravenously over 15 minutes, every month

Consider baseline bone densitometry evaluation
See Chapter 43 for more information

Toxicity (N = 202)

NCI Common Toxicity Criteria, version 2.0

Toxicity	Percentage of Patients	
	Bortezomib-Related	G3/4
Nonhematologic Toxicity		
Nausea	55	6
Diarrhea	44	8
Fatigue	41	12
Peripheral neuropathy	31	12
Vomiting	27	9
Anorexia	25	2
Fever	22	4
Headache	19	3
Constipation	16	2
Rash	15	<1
Limb pain	13	7
Dizziness, not vertigo	12	1
Weakness	11	6
Dehydration	10	7
Hematologic Toxicity		
Thrombocytopenia	40	31
Anemia	21	8
Neutropenia	19	14

Note: Ten deaths occurred within 20 days after the last bortezomib dose. Most deaths were attributed to progressive disease; 2 deaths were possibly related to treatment

Therapy Monitoring

1. *Weekly:* CBC with differential
2. *Every 2 cycles:* Serum BUN, creatinine, and LFTs. Serum and urine M-protein

REGIMEN
RELAPSED/REFRACTORY MULTIPLE MYELOMA
LENALIDOMIDE + DEXAMETHASONE

Weber DM et al. N Engl J Med 2007;357:2133–2142
Dimopoulos M et al. N Engl J Med 2007;357:2123–2132

Lenalidomide 25 mg per day; administer orally for 21 consecutive days on days 1–21, every 28 days (total dose/cycle = 525 mg)
Cycles 1–4:
Dexamethasone 40 mg per dose; administer orally for 12 doses on days 1–4, 9–12, and 17–20, every 28 days for 4 cycles (total dose/cycle = 480 mg)
Cycle 5 and subsequently:
Dexamethasone 40 mg per dose; administer orally for 4 doses on days 1–4, every 28 days, until the occurrence of disease progression or unacceptable toxic effects (total dose/cycle = 160 mg)

Supportive Care
Antiemetic prophylaxis
Emetogenic potential is **MINIMAL–LOW**
See Chapter 39 for antiemetic recommendations

Hematopoietic growth factor (CSF) prophylaxis
Primary prophylaxis is NOT indicated
See Chapter 43 for more information

Antimicrobial prophylaxis
Risk of fever and neutropenia is INTERMEDIATE
Antimicrobial primary prophylaxis to be considered:
- Antibacterial—consider a fluoroquinolone or no prophylaxis; *P. jirovecii* prophylaxis is recommended (eg, cotrimoxazole)
- Antifungal—consider concomitant use of clotrimazole during periods of neutropenia
- Antiviral—antiherpes antivirals (eg, acyclovir, famciclovir, valacyclovir)

Caution: Acyclovir and famciclovir accumulate in patients with impaired renal function and may exacerbate renal dysfunction (valacyclovir is a *prodrug* for acyclovir). Monitor kidney function serially during acyclovir, valacyclovir, and famciclovir use
- Acyclovir and famciclovir elimination is inversely related to renal function
- Acyclovir, famciclovir, and valacyclovir utilization is modified in renally impaired individuals (consult product labeling or Summary of Product Characteristics for guidance about dose/dosage and administration frequency modifications, and, when relevant, recommendations for drug dilution, administration rate, concurrent fluid administration, and fluid supplementation as a function of urine output)
- Impaired acyclovir elimination is associated with neurologic adverse effects, including agitation, ataxia, coma, confusion, dizziness, dysarthria, encephalopathy, hallucinations, paresthesia, seizure, somnolence, and tremors
See Chapter 47 for more information

(continued)

Treatment Modifications

Lenalidomide Dose Levels

Dose Level 1	25 mg
Dose Level −1	15 mg
Dose Level −2	10 mg
Dose Level −3	5 mg

Dexamethasone Dose Levels

Dose Level 1	40 mg/dose for 12 doses on days 1 to 4, 9 to 12, and 17 to 20
Dose Level −1	40 mg daily for 4 days every 2 weeks (days 1–4 and 15–18)
Dose Level −2	40 mg daily for 4 days every 4 weeks (days 1–4)
Dose Level −3	20 mg daily for 4 days every 4 weeks (days 1–4)

Adverse Event	Treatment Modification
G3/4 neutropenia	Interrupt lenalidomide treatment and follow clinically. After ANC recovers to ≥1000/mm³, resume lenalidomide at a dose decreased from the previous dose by 5 mg/day, but the daily dose should not be less than 5 mg/day
Febrile neutropenia	Interrupt lenalidomide treatment and follow closely. After fever abates, resume lenalidomide at a dose decreased from the previous dose by 5 mg/day, but the daily dose should not be less than 5 mg/day
G3/4 nonhematologic toxicity	Interrupt lenalidomide treatment and follow clinically. After toxicity abates to G ≤2, resume lenalidomide at a dose decreased from the previous dose by 5 mg/day, but the daily dose should not be less than 5 mg/day
Toxicities ascribed to dexamethasone such as severe manifestations of hypercorticism, including hyperglycemia, irritability, insomnia, or oral candidiasis	Reduce dexamethasone dose to the next lowest dose level

(continued)

(continued)

Thromboprophylaxis

Risk assessment and recommendations for VTE prophylaxis in patients with multiple myeloma with individual or myeloma-related risk factors, or risk factors related to treatment

Individual risk factors	

• Obesity (BMI ≥30 kg/m²)
• H/O VTE
• CVC or pacemaker
• Comorbid pathologies
  Cardiac disease
  Chronic renal disease
  Diabetes
  Acute infection
  Immobilization
• Surgery
  General surgery
  Any anesthesia
  Trauma
• Medications
  Erythropoietin (epoetin alfa, darbepoetin)
  Estrogenic compounds
  Bevacizumab
• Clotting disorders
  Thrombophilia
Myeloma-related risk factors
• Diagnosis of multiple myeloma
• Hyperviscosity
	≤1 Individual or myeloma risk factor present:
	• **Aspirin** 81–325 mg daily
	
	≥2 Individual or myeloma risk factors present:
	• **LMWH***, equivalent to enoxaparin sodium 40 mg/day *or* **dalteparin sodium** 5000 IU/day; administer subcutaneously, *or*
	• **Warfarin**, targeting an INR = 2–3

Concomitant treatment-related risk factors Thalidomide or lenalidomide in combination with: • High-dose dexamethasone (≥480 mg/month) • Doxorubicin • Multiagent chemotherapy	**LMWH***, equivalent to enoxaparin sodium 40 mg/day *or* **dalteparin sodium** 5000 IU/day; administer subcutaneously, *or* **Warfarin**, targeting an INR = 2–3

CVC, central venous catheter; INR, international normalized ratio; LMWH, low-molecular-weight heparin; VTE, venous thromboembolic disease
*LMWHs should be used with caution in individuals with impaired renal function (creatinine clearance <30 mL/min). Refer to product labeling for information about doses and administration schedules in renally impaired patients, and guidance for monitoring anti-Factor Xa concentrations

Geerts WH et al. Chest 2008;133(6 Suppl):381S–453S
Multiple Myeloma, V.1.2014. National Comprehensive Cancer Network, Inc., 2013. (Accessed October 8, 2013, at http://www.nccn.org)
Palumbo A et al. Leukemia 2008;22:414–423
Venous Thromboembolic Disease, V.2.2013. National Comprehensive Cancer Network, Inc., 2013. (Accessed October 8, 2013, at http://www.nccn.org)

Bisphosphonates

All patients receiving primary therapy for symptomatic multiple myeloma should receive a bisphosphonate adjunctively; *for example*:

• **Pamidronate disodium** 90 mg; administer intravenously over 2–4 hours, every month, *or*

• **Zoledronic acid** 4 mg; administer intravenously over 15 minutes, every month

Consider baseline bone densitometry evaluation
See Chapter 43 for more information

Treatment Modifications
(continued)

Lenalidomide Starting Dose Adjustment for Renal Impairment in Multiple Myeloma (Days 1–21 of Each 28-Day Cycle)*

Moderate renal impairment CrCl 30–60 mL/min (0.5–1 mL/s)	10 mg lenalidomide every 24 hours
Severe renal impairment CrCl <30 mL/min, not requiring dialysis	15 mg lenalidomide every 48 hours
End-stage renal disease CrCl <30 mL/min, requiring dialysis	Lenalidomide 5 mg/day. On dialysis days, administer a daily dose following dialysis

CrCl, Creatinine clearance
*Richardson PG et al. J Clin Oncol 2006;24:3113–3120

Patient Population Studied

Two multicenter, randomized, phase III studies that enrolled patients with progressive multiple myeloma not resistant to dexamethasone who had received at least 1 previous treatment. Patients were considered to have disease that was resistant to dexamethasone if they had had progression during previous therapy containing high-dose dexamethasone (total monthly dose >200 mg). Measurable disease was defined as a serum monoclonal protein (M-protein) level of ≥0.5 g/dL or a urinary Bence Jones protein level ≥0.2 g/day. Additional eligibility criteria included an Eastern Cooperative Oncology Group performance status ≤2

European Study
(Dimopoulos M et al. N Engl J Med 2007;357:2123–2132)

(351 patients: N = 176 lenalidomide group; N = 175 placebo group)

North America Study
(Weber DM et al. N Engl J Med 2007;357:2133–2142)

(353 patients: N = 177 lenalidomide group; N = 176 placebo group)

Efficacy

	North American Study (Weber et al.)		European Study (Dimopoulos et al.)	
	Lenalidomide N = 177	Placebo N = 176	Lenalidomide N = 176	Placebo N = 175
Overall response	61	19.9	60.2	24
Complete response	14.1	0.6	15.9	3.4
Near-complete response	10.2	1.1	8.5	1.7
Partial response	36.7	18.2	35.8	18.9
Stable disease	30.5	58	30.1	55.4
Progressive disease	2.8	14.2	1.7	14.3
Response not evaluable	5.6	8	8	6.3
Previous Thalidomide, Response Rate, and Time to Progression (TTP)				
Yes	56.8	12.5	49.1	16.4
Median TTP (months)	8.5	4.1	8.4	4.6
No	64.1	26	65	28.7
Median TTP (months)	—	—	13.5	4.7
Beta$_2$-Microglobulin Level, Response Rate				
<2.5 mg/L	75	27.5	70.6	37.5
≥2.5 mg/L	55.2	16.8	56	18.9
Previous Therapies (Number), Response Rate, and Time to Progression (TTP)				
1	64.7	22.4	66.1	29.8
Median TTP (months)	NR	5.1	—	—
≥2	58.7	18.3	57.5	21.2
Median TTP (months)	10.2	4.6	—	—
Previous Stem Cell Transplant, Response Rate				
Yes	66.1	19.4	61.9	28.4
No	52.9	20.6	58.2	18.8
Previous Use of Bortezomib, Response Rate, and Time to Progression (TTP)				
Yes	68.4	10	—	—
No	60.1	21.2	—	—
Median TTP (months)	10.3	3.3	—	—
Median TTP, All Patients (Months)	11.1	4.7	11.3	4.7
Median Overall Survival (Months)	26.2	12.9	NR	20.6

NR, not reached; TTP, Time to progression

Toxicity	North America Study (Weber et al.) G3/4 (N = 177)	European Study (Dimopoulos et al.) G3/4 (N = 176)
Hematologic Events		
Neutropenia	41.2	29.5
Anemia	13	8.6
Thrombocytopenia	14.7	11.4
Febrile neutropenia	3.4	3.4
Gastrointestinal Events		
Constipation	2.8	1.7
Diarrhea	3.4	2.8
Nausea	2.8	1.1
General Disorders		
Asthenia	3.4	6.2
Fatigue	6.2	6.8
Pyrexia	2.3	0.6
Peripheral edema	2.3	1.1
Infections		
Upper respiratory	1.1	1.7
Any infection	21.4	9.6
Pneumonia	12.4	Not reported
Neurologic Disorders		
Headache	Not reported	0.6
Tremor	Not reported	1.1
Dizziness	Not reported	0.6
Paresthesia	Not reported	0.6
Insomnia	Not reported	1.1
Musculoskeletal or Connective Tissue Disorder		
Muscle cramp	Not reported	0.6
Back pain	Not reported	2.3
Bone pain	Not reported	2.8
Muscle weakness	Not reported	7.4
Arthralgia	Not reported	0.6
Vascular Disorders		
Deep vein thrombosis	Not reported	4
Pulmonary embolism	Not reported	4.5
Venous thromboembolism	Not reported	11.4

Therapy Monitoring

1. Blood counts and physical examinations
   - Cycle 1: days 1, 8, and 15
   - Cycles 2 and 3: days 1 and 15
   - Cycle 4, and subsequently: day 1
2. Serum and urinary protein electrophoresis studies on day 1 of each cycle and at the end of treatment
3. Serum electrolytes and creatinine before beginning each treatment cycle

REGIMEN
RELAPSED/REFRACTORY MULTIPLE MYELOMA (PRIOR BORTEZOMIB AND BORTEZOMIB NAÏVE)

CARFILZOMIB

Vij R et al. Blood 2012;119:5661–5670 (Bortezomib-naïve)
Vij R et al. Br J Haematol 2012;158:739–748 (Prior bortezomib)

Hydration with carfilzomib: During cycle 1, days 1 and 2, administer intravenously 250–500 mL 0.9% NS before each carfilzomib dose, *and* an additional 250–500 mL of fluid intravenously after carfilzomib. During repeated treatments, continue intravenous hydration as needed. Encourage oral hydration

Carfilzomib 36 mg/m² per dose intravenously in 50-mL 5% dextrose injection over 30 minutes for 6 doses, on days 1, 2, 8, 9, 15, and 16, every 28 days for a maximum of 12 cycles (total dosage/cycle = 216 mg/m²)

Supportive Care
Antiemetic prophylaxis
Emetogenic potential is **LOW**
See Chapter 39 for antiemetic recommendations

Hematopoietic growth factor (CSF) prophylaxis
Primary prophylaxis may be indicated
See Chapter 43 for more information

Antimicrobial prophylaxis
Risk of fever and neutropenia is INTERMEDIATE
Antimicrobial primary prophylaxis to be considered:
- Antibacterial—consider a fluoroquinolone or no prophylaxis; *Pneumocystis jirovecii* prophylaxis is recommended (eg, cotrimoxazole)
- Antifungal—recommended; consider use during periods of neutropenia
- Antiviral—antiherpes antivirals (eg, acyclovir, famciclovir, valacyclovir)

See Chapter 47 for more information

Thromboprophylaxis
Risk assessment and recommendations for VTE prophylaxis in patients with multiple myeloma with individual or myeloma-related risk factors, or risk factors related to treatment

Individual risk factors	
• Obesity (BMI ≥30 kg/m²)	
• H/O VTE	
• CVAD or pacemaker	
• Comorbid pathologies	
Cardiac disease	**≤1 Individual or myeloma risk factor present:**
Chronic renal disease	• **Aspirin** 81–325 mg daily
Diabetes	
Acute infection	
Immobilization	
• Surgery	
General surgery	**≥2 Individual or myeloma risk factors present:**
Any anesthesia	• **LMWH***, equivalent to enoxaparin
Trauma	**sodium** 40 mg/day *or* **dalteparin sodium**
• Medications	**5000 IU/day**; administer subcutaneously,
Erythropoietin (epoetin alfa, darbepoetin)	*or*
Estrogenic compounds	• **Warfarin**, targeting an INR = 2–3
Bevacizumab	
• Clotting disorders	
Thrombophilia	
Myeloma-related risk factors	
• Diagnosis of multiple myeloma	
• Hyperviscosity	

Patient Population Studied

Characteristic	Bortezomib-Naïve* (N = 129)	Prior Bortezomib† (N = 35)
General		
Median age, years (range)	65 (38–85)	63 (40–77)
Male, *n* (%)	76 (58.9)	18 (51.4)
Median time from diagnosis, years (range)	3.6 (0.7–24.4)	3.6 (1.2–13.2)
Immunoglobulin Subtype, *n* (%)		
IgG	86 (66.7)	24 (68.6)
IgA	33 (25.6)	5 (14.3)
IgD	—	1 (2.9)
Not reported/ missing	10 (7.8)	5 (14.3)
Light Chain Subtype, *n* (%)		
Kappa	94 (72.9)	23 (65.7)
Lambda	35 (27.1)	12 (34.3)
ECOG PS, *n* (%)		
0	52 (40.3)	15 (42.9)
1 or 2	77 (59.7)	19 (54.3)
ISS Stage, *n* (%)		
I or II	94 (72.9)	27 (77.1%)
III	22 (17.1)	7 (20%)
Not reported/ missing	13 (10.1)	1 (2.9%)
Others Clinical History		
Neuropathy history‡	90 (69.8)	19 (54.3)§
CrCl <50 mL/min (<0.83 mL/s)	20 (15.5)	4 (11.4)
Cytogenetic/FISH Prognostic Markers, *n* (%)		
Normal/ favorable	103 (79.8)	25 (71.4)
Poor	19 (14.7)	9 (25.7)
Unknown or not done	7 (5.4)	1 (2.9%)

CrCl, creatinine clearance; FISH, fluorescence in situ hybridization
*Includes 2 patient cohorts: (a) cohort 1 (*n* = 59) was treated with 20 mg/m² carfilzomib; (b) cohort 2 (*n* = 70) was treated with 20/27 mg/m² carfilzomib
†Patients treated with 20 mg/m² carfilzomib
‡Baseline peripheral neuropathy (PN): 68 (52.7)
§Peripheral neuropathy G ≥1

(continued)

(continued)

(continued)

Concomitant treatment-related risk factors Thalidomide or lenalidomide in combination with: • High-dose dexamethasone (≥480 mg/month) • Doxorubicin • Multiagent chemotherapy	**LMWH*, equivalent to enoxaparin sodium** 40 mg/day *or* **dalteparin sodium** 5000 IU/day; administer subcutaneously, *or* **Warfarin**, targeting an INR = 2–3

CVAD, central vascular access device; INR, international normalized ratio; LMWH, low-molecular-weight heparin; VTE, venous thromboembolic disease

*LMWHs should be used with caution in individuals with impaired renal function (creatinine clearance <30 mL/min). Refer to product labeling for information about doses and administration schedules in renally impaired patients, and guidance for monitoring antifactor Xa concentrations

Geerts WH et al. Chest 2008;133(6 Suppl):381S–453S
Multiple Myeloma, V.1.2014. National Comprehensive Cancer Network, Inc., 2013. (Accessed October 8, 2013, at http://www.nccn.org)
Palumbo A et al. Leukemia 2008;22:414–423
Venous Thromboembolic Disease, V.2.2013. National Comprehensive Cancer Network, Inc., 2013. (Accessed October 8, 2013, at http://www.nccn.org)

Bisphosphonates

All patients receiving primary therapy for symptomatic multiple myeloma should receive a bisphosphonate adjunctively; *for example*:

• **Pamidronate disodium** 90 mg; administer intravenously over 2–4 hours, every month, *or*

• **Zoledronic acid** 4 mg; administer intravenously over at least 15 minutes, every month

Consider baseline bone densitometry evaluation
See Chapter 43 for more information

Diarrhea management

Loperamide 4 mg orally initially after the first loose or liquid stool, *then*
Loperamide 2 mg orally every 2 hours during waking hours, *plus*
Loperamide 4 mg orally every 4 hours during hours of sleep

• Continue for at least 12 hours after diarrhea resolves

• Recurrent diarrhea after a 12-hour diarrhea-free interval is treated as a new episode

• Rehydrate orally with fluids and electrolytes during a diarrheal episode

• If a patient develops blood or mucus in stool, dehydration, or hemodynamic instability, or if diarrhea persists >48 hours despite loperamide, stop loperamide and hospitalize the patient for IV hydration

Alternatively, a trial of **Diphenoxylate hydrochloride** 2.5 mg **with Atropine sulfate** 0.025 mg (eg, Lomotil)

• Initial adult dose is 2 tablets 4 times daily until control has been achieved, after which the dose may be reduced to meet individual requirements. Control may often be maintained with as little as 2 tablets daily

• Clinical improvement of acute diarrhea is usually observed within 48 hours. If improvement of chronic diarrhea after treatment with a maximum daily dose of 8 tablets is not observed within 10 days, control is unlikely with further administration

Patient Population Studied
(continued)

Prior Therapies	Bortezomib-Naïve* (N = 129) n (%)	Prior Bortezomib[†] (N = 35) n (%)
Median number of prior regimens (range)	2 (1–4)	3.0 (1–13)
Bortezomib	3 (2.3)[‡]	35 (100.0)[§]
Thalidomide	76 (58.9)	24 (68.6)
Lenalidomide	76 (58.9)	13 (37.1)
Thalidomide or lenalidomide	119 (92.2)	27 (77.1)
Corticosteroid	125 (96.9)	34 (97.1)
Alkylating agent	105 (81.4)	31 (88.6)
Anthracycline	30 (23.3)	11 (31.4)
Stem cell transplantation	94 (72.9)	28 (80.0)
Refractory to bortezomib in any prior regimen n (%)		7 (20.0)
Refractory to last therapy, n (%)		22 (62.9)

*Includes 2 patient cohorts: (a) cohort 1 (n = 59) was treated with 20 mg/m^2 carfilzomib; (b) cohort 2 (n = 70) was treated with 20/27 mg/m^2 carfilzomib
[†]Patients treated with 20 mg/m^2 carfilzomib
[‡]Bortezomib exposure not considered therapeutic
[§]20/35 (57.1%) had bortezomib in last regimen

Treatment Modifications

Carfilzomib Dose Levels

Starting dose	36 mg/m² per dose
Level −1	27 mg/m² per dose
Level −2	20 mg/m² per dose
Level −3	15 mg/m² per dose
Level −4	11 mg/m² per dose
Level −5	Discontinue

Adverse Event	Treatment Modification
Hematologic Toxicity	
G3/4 neutropenia	Hold carfilzomib dosing for up to 21 days to resolve toxicity and then restart at the same dosage, or reduce the carfilzomib dosage by 1 dose level. If counts recover to G2 neutropenia or G3 thrombocytopenia, reduce carfilzomib dosage by 1 dose level. If tolerated, the reduced dose may be escalated to the previous dose level
Febrile neutropenia (ANC <1.0 × 10⁹/L with fever ≥38°C)	
G4 thrombocytopenia	
G3/4 thrombocytopenia associated with bleeding	
Nonhematologic Toxicity	
G3/4 cardiac toxicity New onset or worsening of: • Congestive heart failure • Decreased left ventricular function • Myocardial ischemia	Hold carfilzomib dosing for up to 21 days to resolve toxicity and then restart at the same dosage or reduce the carfilzomib dosage by 1 dose level. If tolerated, the reduced dosage may be escalated to the previous dose level
Pulmonary hypertension	
G3/4 pulmonary complications	
G3/4 elevation of transaminases, bilirubin or other liver abnormalities	
Serum creatinine equal to or greater than 2× baseline	Hold carfilzomib dosing for up to 21 days to resolve toxicity to G1 or to baseline and then restart at the same dosage, or reduce the carfilzomib dosage by 1 dose level. If tolerated, the reduced dose may be escalated to the previous dose level
G2 neuropathy with pain	Hold carfilzomib dosing for up to 21 days to resolve toxicity and then restart at the same dose or reduce the carfilzomib dose by 1 level. If tolerated, the reduced dosage, or reduce the carfilzomib dosage by 1 dose may be escalated to the previous dose level
G3/4 peripheral neuropathy	
Other G3/4 nonhematologic toxicities	Hold carfilzomib dosing for up to 21 days to resolve toxicity to G1 or to baseline and then restart at the same dosage, or reduce the carfilzomib dosage by 1 dose level. If tolerated, the reduced dosage may be escalated to the previous dose level

Efficacy

Response	Bortezomib-Naïve* (N = 129) *n* (%)	Prior Bortezomib† (N = 35) *n* (%)
CR	3 (2.4)	1 (2.9)
VGPR	26 (20.6)	1 (2.9)
PR	31 (24.6)	4 (11.4)
MR	18 (14.3)	5 (14.3)
SD	23 (18.3)	13 (37.1)
PD	18 (14.3)	10 (28.6)
ORR (CR + VGPR + PR)	60 (47.6)	6 (17.1)
95% CI	38.7–56.7	
CBR (ORR + MR)	78 (61.9)	11 (31.4)
95% CI	52.8–70.4	

CBR, clinical benefit response; CR, complete response; MR, minimal response; ORR, overall response rate; PD, progressive disease; PR, partial response; SD, stable disease; VGPR, very good partial response
*Includes 2 patient cohorts: (a) cohort 1 (*n* = 59) was treated with 20 mg/m² carfilzomib; (b) cohort 2 (*n* = 70) was treated with 20/27 mg/m² carfilzomib. *Response is response rate after 6 cycles of treatment in response-evaluable population*
†Patients treated with 20 mg/m² carfilzomib. *Response is best overall response in response-evaluable population*

		Bortezomib-Naïve* (N = 129)		Prior Bortezomib† (N = 35)
	n	ORR % (95% CI)	*n*	ORR % (95% CI)
Overall	126‡	47.6 (38.7–56.7)	35	17.1 (6.6–33.7)
Baseline Characteristics				
Age, Years				
<65	58	58.6 (44.9–71.4)	21	9.5 (1.2–30.4)
≥65	68	38.2 (26.7–50.8)	14	28.6 (8.4–58.1)
ECOG Performance Status				
0	51	52.9 (38.5–67.1)	15	26.7 (7.8–55.1)
≥1	75	44.0 (32.5–55.9)	19	10.5 (1.3–33.1)
ISS Stage				
I	52	57.7 (43.2–71.3)	19	15.8 (3.4–39.6)
II	41	34.1 (20.1–50.6)	8	25.0 (3.2–65.1)
III	20	45.0 (23.1–68.5)	7	14.3 (0.4–57.9)
Baseline Neuropathy				
Grade 0	59	39.0 (26.5–52.6)	—	—
Grade ≥1	66	56.1 (43.3–68.3)	—	—

(continued)

Efficacy (continued)

Cytogenetic/FISH Prognostic Markers

Normal/favorable	100	51.0 (40.8–61.1)	25	16.0 (4.5–36.1)
Poor	19	36.8 (16.3–61.6)	9	11.1 (0.3–48.2)

Serum β_2-Microglobulin, mg/L

<5.5	93	47.3 (36.9–57.9)	—	—
≥5.5	20	45.0 (23.1–68.5)	—	—

Received Prior Lenalidomide

Yes	74	41.9 (30.5–53.9)	—	—
No	52	55.8 (41.3–69.5)	—	—

Received Prior Thalidomide

Yes	75	56.0 (44.1–67.5)	—	—
No	51	35.3 (22.4–49.9)	—	—

*Includes 2 patient cohorts: (a) cohort 1 ($n = 59$) was treated with 20 mg/m² carfilzomib; (b) cohort 2 ($n = 67$) was treated with 20/27 mg/m² carfilzomib. *Response is response rate after 6 cycles of treatment in response-evaluable population*
†Patients treated with 20 mg/m² carfilzomib. *Response is best overall response in response-evaluable population*
‡Reponse rate for the 2 cohorts as follows: cohort 1 (42.4%, 95% CI, 29.6–55.9); cohort 2 (52.2%, 95% CI, 39.7–64.6)

Response	Bortezomib-Naïve* (N = 126)		Prior Bortezomib† (N = 35)	
	n		*n*	

Duration of Response (DOR), Months

Median, mo (95% CI)	60	NR (13.1–NR)	17	
≥PR (ORR)			6	NE (10.6–NE)
≥MR (CBR)			11	10.6 (7.2–NE)

Duration of Clinical Benefit Response, Months

Median, (95% CI)	78	NR (11.5–NR)	11	

Time to Progression (TTP), Months

Median (95% CI)	126	12.0 (8.2–NR)		4.6 (1.9–11.1)

Time to Response, Months

Median, (min, max)	60	1.7 (0.5–3.7)	17	
≥PR (ORR)			6	1.4 (0.5–1.9)
≥MR (CBR)			11	1.0 (0.5–6.7)

Time to Clinical Benefit Response, Months

Median, (min, max)	78	0.5 (0.5–6.5)	11	

CBR, clinical benefit response; DOR, duration of response; NE, not estimable; NR, not reached; ORR, overall response rate
*Includes 2 patient cohorts: (a) cohort 1 ($n = 59$) was treated with 20 mg/m² carfilzomib; (b) cohort 2 ($n = 70$) was treated with 20/27 mg/m² carfilzomib. *Response is response rate after 6 cycles of treatment in response-evaluable population*
†Patients treated with 20 mg/m² carfilzomib. *Response is best overall response in response-evaluable population*

Toxicity					Therapy Monitoring

Treatment-Emergent Adverse Event, *n* (%)	Bortezomib-Naïve* (N = 129)		Prior Bortezomib† (N = 35)	
	All Grades‡	G ≥3§	All Grades‡	G ≥3§
Hematologic				
Anemia	54 (41.9)	19 (14.7)	12 (34.3)	5 (14.3)
Neutropenia	39 (30.2)	17 (13.2)	9 (25.7)	4 (11.4)
Thrombocytopenia	39 (30.2)	17 (13.2)	11 (31.4)	7 (20.0)
Lymphopenia	33 (25.6)	21 (16.3)	6 (17.1)	2 (5.7)
Nonhematologic				
Fatigue	80 (62.0)	8 (6.2)	22 (62.9)	1 (2.9)
Nausea	63 (48.8)	—	21 (60.0)	1 (2.9)
Dyspnea	50 (38.8)	7 (5.4)	13 (37.1)	2 (5.7)
Cough	44 (34.1)	—	8 (22.9)	0
Pyrexia	44 (34.1)	—	9 (25.7)	0
Headache	42 (32.6)	—	9 (25.7)	1 (2.9)
Diarrhea	40 (31.0)	—	13 (37.1)	0
Upper respiratory infection	40 (31.0)	—	12 (34.3)	2 (5.7)
Epiglottitis	—	—	2 (5.7)	2 (5.7)
Pneumonia	—	—	3 (8.6)	3 (8.6)
Peripheral edema	35 (27.1)	—	—	—
Congestive heart failure	—	6 (4.7)	—	—
Hypertension	—	—	8 (22.9)	1 (2.9)
Chills	29 (22.5)	—	—	—
Insomnia	29 (22.5)	—	—	—
Vomiting	29 (22.5)	—	15 (42.9)	1 (2.9)
Constipation	25 (19.4)	—	8 (22.9)	0
Asthenia	—	—	8 (22.9)	1 (2.9)
Muscle spasms	24 (18.6)	—	—	—
Arthralgia	22 (17.1)	—	—	—
Back pain	22 (17.1)	—	—	—
Pain	—	—	7 (20.0)	0
Hypoesthesia	—	—	9 (25.7)	0
Dizziness	22 (17.1)	—	7 (20.0)	0

(continued)

Therapy Monitoring

1. Blood counts and physical examinations on day 1 of each cycle
2. Serum and urinary protein electrophoresis studies on day 1 of each cycle as indicated and at the end of treatment

Toxicity *(continued)*				
Treatment-Emergent Adverse Event, n (%)	Bortezomib-Naïve* (N = 129)		Prior Bortezomib† (N = 35)	
	All Grades‡	G ≥3§	All Grades‡	G ≥3§
Laboratory				
Acute renal failure	—	6 (4.7)	—	—
Increased serum creatinine	24 (18.6)	—	12 (34.3)	1 (2.9)
Hypercalcemia	—	—	5 (14.3)	2 (5.7)
Hyperglycemia	—	6 (4.7)	—	—
Hypophosphatemia	—	6 (4.7)	—	—
Hypokalemia	—	5 (3.9)	—	—
Hyponatremia	—	5 (3.9)	—	—
Increased AST	—	3 (2.3)	7 (20.0)	0
Increased ALT	—	–	10 (28.6)	0

*Includes 2 patient cohorts: (a) cohort 1 (*n* = 59) was treated with 20 mg/m² carfilzomib; (b) cohort 2 (*n* = 70) was treated with 20/27 mg/m² carfilzomib

†Patients treated with 20 mg/m² carfilzomib

‡Treatment-emergent adverse events of all grades in ≥20% of the safety population

§Treatment-emergent adverse events G ≥3 in ≥5% of the safety population

REGIMEN
RELAPSED/REFRACTORY MULTIPLE MYELOMA

POMALIDOMIDE + DEXAMETHASONE

Leleu X et al. Blood 2013;121:1968–1975
Lacy MQ et al. Leukemia 2010;24:1934–1939

Pomalidomide 4 mg/day orally, continually, for 21 consecutive days, on days 1–21, every 28 days (total dose/cycle = 84 mg)
Dexamethasone 40 mg/dose; orally for 4 doses on days 1, 8, 15, and 22, every 28 days (total dose/cycle = 160 mg)

or

Pomalidomide 2 mg/day; orally, continually, for 28 consecutive days, on days 1–28, every 28 days (total dose/cycle = 56 mg)
Dexamethasone 40 mg daily orally on days 1, 8, 15, and 22, every 28 days (total dose/cycle = 160 mg)

Supportive Care
Antiemetic prophylaxis
Emetogenic potential is **MINIMAL–LOW**
See Chapter 39 for antiemetic recommendations

Hematopoietic growth factor (CSF) prophylaxis
Primary prophylaxis may be indicated
See Chapter 43 for more information

Antimicrobial prophylaxis
Risk of fever and neutropenia is INTERMEDIATE
  Antimicrobial primary prophylaxis to be considered:
  • Antibacterial—consider a fluoroquinolone or no prophylaxis; *Pneumocystis jirovecii* prophylaxis is recommended (eg, cotrimoxazole)
  • Antifungal—recommended; consider use during periods of neutropenia
  • Antiviral—antiherpes antivirals (eg, acyclovir, famciclovir, valacyclovir)
See Chapter 47 for more information

Thromboprophylaxis
Risk assessment and recommendations for VTE prophylaxis in patients with multiple myeloma with individual or myeloma-related risk factors, or risk factors related to treatment

Individual risk factors
• Obesity (BMI ≥30 kg/m²)
• H/O VTE
• CVAD or pacemaker
• Comorbid pathologies
  Cardiac disease
  Chronic renal disease
  Diabetes
  Acute infection
  Immobilization
• Surgery
  General surgery
  Any anesthesia
  Trauma
• Medications
  Erythropoietin (epoetin alfa, darbepoetin)
  Estrogenic compounds
  Bevacizumab
• Clotting disorders
  Thrombophilia
Myeloma-related risk factors
• Diagnosis of multiple myeloma
• Hyperviscosity
	≤1 Individual or myeloma risk factor present:
	• **Aspirin** 81–325 mg daily
	
	≥2 Individual or myeloma risk factors present:
	• **LMWH***, equivalent to enoxaparin sodium 40 mg/day *or* **dalteparin sodium** 5000 IU/day; administer subcutaneously, *or*
	• **Warfarin**, targeting an INR = 2–3

Treatment Modifications

Pomalidomide Dose Levels

Starting dose	4 mg/day
Level –1	3 mg/day
Level –2	2 mg/day
Level –3	1 mg/day
Level –4	Discontinue

Dexamethasone Dose Levels

Starting dose	40 mg/dose
Level –1	20 mg/dose
Level –2	12 mg/dose
Level –3	8 mg/dose
Level –4	4 mg/dose
Level –5	Discontinue

Adverse Event	Treatment Modification
ANC <500/mm³ Febrile neutropenia (fever ≥38.5°C + ANC <1000/mm³) Platelets <25,000/mm³	Interrupt pomalidomide treatment, and follow CBC weekly. When ANC ≥500/mm³ and platelet count 50,000/mm³, resume pomalidomide 1 dose level lower
Nonhematologic G3/4 toxicity	Interrupt pomalidomide treatment, and follow weekly or more frequently. Restart treatment 1 dose level lower than the previous dose when toxicity has resolved G ≤2
G4 rash, neuropathy, hypersensitivity, or G ≥3 bradycardia or cardiac arrhythmia	Permanently discontinue pomalidomide
G3/4 adverse events occurring on or after day 15 during a single cycle	Withhold pomalidomide for the remainder of the cycle and reduce by 1 dose level beginning with the next cycle
Toxicities ascribed to dexamethasone such as severe manifestations of hypercorticism, including hyperglycemia, irritability, insomnia, or oral candidiasis	Hold dexamethasone dosing for up to 21 days to resolve toxicity and then restart at the same dose or reduce the dexamethasone dose by 50%

(continued)

(continued)

Concomitant treatment-related risk factors Thalidomide or lenalidomide in combination with: • High-dose dexamethasone (≥480 mg/month) • Doxorubicin • Multiagent chemotherapy	**LMWH*, equivalent to enoxaparin sodium** 40 mg/day *or* **dalteparin sodium** 5000 IU/day; administer subcutaneously, *or* **Warfarin**, targeting an INR = 2–3

CVAD, central vascular access device; INR, international normalized ratio; LMWH, low-molecular-weight heparin; VTE, venous thromboembolic disease

*LMWHs should be used with caution in individuals with impaired renal function (creatinine clearance <30 mL/min). Refer to product labeling for information about doses and administration schedules in renally impaired patients, and guidance for monitoring antifactor Xa concentrations

Geerts WH et al. Chest 2008;133(6 Suppl):381S–453S
Multiple Myeloma, V.1.2014. National Comprehensive Cancer Network, Inc., 2013. (Accessed October 8, 2013, at http://www.nccn.org)
Palumbo A et al. Leukemia 2008;22:414–423
Venous Thromboembolic Disease, V.2.2013. National Comprehensive Cancer Network, Inc., 2013. (Accessed October 8, 2013, at http://www.nccn.org)

Bisphosphonates

All patients receiving primary therapy for symptomatic multiple myeloma should receive a bisphosphonate adjunctively; *for example*:
• **Pamidronate disodium** 90 mg; administer intravenously over 2–4 hours, every month, *or*
• **Zoledronic acid** 4 mg; administer intravenously over at least 15 minutes, every month
Consider baseline bone densitometry evaluation
See Chapter 43 for more information

Patient Population Studied

Patients were eligible if they had relapsed MM after at least 1 prior regimen. Patients were considered to be "nonresponders" to the last line of lenalidomide or bortezomib after having received ≥2 cycles of either drug if they did not achieve a response defined by International Myeloma Working Group (IMWG) criteria (stable disease [stable disease and minor response]) within 2 cycles of treatment

Characteristic	21/28 (N = 43)*	28/28 (N = 41)*
Median time from diagnosis to randomization, years (range)	5.1 (0.9–8.7)	6.5 (0.8–23.1)
≤3 years, *n* (%)	13 (30)	4 (10)
Median age, years (range)	60 (45–81)	60 (42–83)
Age ≥65 years, *n* (%)	11 (26)	15 (37)
ISS stage II/III [%][†]	32/24	42/17
Myeloma type, *n* (%)		
Intact Ig	36 (84)	34 (83)
Light chain	4 (9)	5 (12)
Freelite measurable only[‡]	3 (7)	2 (5)
Lytic bone lesions, *n* (%)	37 (86)	37 (90)
Number of lytic lesions: [3–6]	9 (25)	8 (22)
Number of lytic lesions: >6	11 (31)	17 (46)
Osseous Fracture	10 (29)	11 (32)
Medullary compression	0	3 (9)
Plasmacytoma	9 (21)	5 (12)

(continued)

Patient Population Studied (continued)

Characteristic	21/28 (N = 43)*	28/28 (N = 41)*
Median β_2-microglobulin, mg/L (range)	3.9 (1.0–13.2)	3.7 (1.6–12.0)
(3.5–5.5) mg/L, n (%)	19 (44)	11 (27.5)
>5.5 mg/L, n (%)	10 (23)	11 (27.5)
Median serum creatinine, (μmol/L) (range)	80.0 (0.9 mg/dL) (44.0–193.0)	87.0 (0.98 mg/dL) (42.0–196)
>115 μmol/L (1.3 mg/dL), n (%)	6 (14)	4 (10)
Median hemoglobin, g/dL (range)	10.5 (7.2–14.1)	10.5 (6.4–14.1)
<10 g/dL, n (%)	18 (42)	15 (37.5)
Median neutrophils, $\times 10^9$/L (range)	2.6 (0.04–10.4)	2.3 (0.9–8.3)
Median platelets, $\times 10^9$/L (range)	161 (51–366)	147 (33–269)
<100 $\times$ 10^9/L, n (%)	8 (19)	10 (25)
Median number of lines (min-max)	5 (1–13)	5 (2–10)

*Pomalidomide was given orally either daily on days 1 to 21 of each 28-day cycle (arm 21/28 days) or continuously of each 28-day cycle (arm 28/28 days)
†ISS classification at diagnosis
‡Patients whose disease was considered "not measurable" based on intact serum immunoglobulin and urine light-chain excretion but had serum immunoglobulin free light chain >100 mg/L and an abnormal free light chain ratio

Leleu X et al. Blood 2013;121:1968–1975

Incidence Rate (Number and Percentage) of Patients with Various Adverse Prognostic Factors by Arm (N = 84)

Prognostic Factor	21/28 (N = 43)	28/28 (N = 41)	Total (N = 84)
Patients >6 lines of therapy, n (%)	12 (28)	7 (17)	19 (23)
Refractory* to, n (%)			
Lenalidomide	36 (84)	39 (95)	75 (89)
Lenalidomide last prior therapy	15 (35)	11 (27)	26 (31)
Bortezomib	34 (79)	34 (83)	68 (81)
Both lenalidomide and bortezomib	32 (74)	32 (78)	64 (76)
Last prior therapy	36 (70)	35 (68)	71 (84.5)
FISH cytogenetics, n (%)†	N = 33	N = 32	
Deletion 17p	6 (21)	9 (33)	—
Translocation (4;14)	2 (7)	4 (17)	—

*Refractory by International Myeloma Working Group (IMWG) criteria
†High-risk cytogenetics by FISH consisted of deletion 17p or t(4;14) at diagnosis and/or at entry in the trial

Leleu X et al. Blood 2013;121:1968–1975

Efficacy

Response to Treatment and Survival End Points by Arm Based on Independent Review Committee Assessment

	21/28	28/28	Total
ITT (N = 84)			
	N = 43	N = 41	N = 84
ORR (≥PR), n (%)	15 (35)	14 (34)	29 (34.5)
CR*, n (%)	1 (2)	2 (5)	3 (4)
VGPR, n (%)	1 (2)	1 (2)	2 (2)
PR, n (%)	13 (30)	11 (27)	24 (27)
Stable disease, n (%)	19 (44)	21 (51)	40 (48)
Progressive disease, n (%)	5 (12)	3 (7)	8 (9.5)
Not evaluable, n (%)	4 (9)	3 (7)	7 (8)
Median time to first response (95% CI), months	2.7 (0.8, 9.5)	1.1 (0.6, 8)	1.8 (0.6, 9.5)
Median duration of response (95% CI), months	6.4 (4, —)	8.3 (6.5, 16)	7.3 (5, 15)
1 Year free of relapse	42%	47%	44%
Efficacy-Evaluable Population (N = 66)			
	N = 34	N = 32	N = 66
ORR (CR + PR), n (%)	15 (44)	12 (37.5)	27 (41)
≥VGPR, n (%)	2 (6)	3 (9)	5 (7.5)
Median survival (95% CI), months	21/28 (N = 43)	28/28 (N = 41)	Total
Time to progression	5.8 (3, 10)	4.8 (3, 7)	5.4 (4, 8)
At 1 year, %	31	25	28
Progression-free survival	5.4 (3, 9)	3.7 (2, 7)	4.6 (4, 7)
At 1 year, %	29	22	25.5
Overall survival	14.9 (9, —)	14.8 (9, 20)	14.9 (11, 20)
At 12 months, %	58	56	57
At 18 months, %	49	39	44

CR, complete response; ORR, overall response rate; PR, partial response; VGPR, very good partial response
*CR confirmed by bone marrow assessment

Leleu X et al. Blood 2013;121:1968–1975

Patient Outcomes

Confirmed response rate*,†	32% (95% CI: 19–53)
*Confirmed response rate**	32% (95% CI: 17–51)
Number of responders*	11
VGPR	2
PR	9
MR	4
Best response	
VGPR	3 (9%)
PR	8 (23%)
MR	5 (15%)
SD	12 (35%)
PD	6 (18%)
Median time to response*	2.0 months (range: 0.7–3.9)
Duration of response*,‡	9.1 months (95% CI: 6.5–NA)
Overall survival‡	13.9 months (95% CI: NA)
Progression free survival‡	4.8 months (95% CI: 2.7–10.1)

CI, confidence interval; MR, best response; NA, not attained; PD, progressive disease; PR, partial response; SD, stable disease; VGPR, very good partial response
*Does not include MR per study design
†Study design uses the first 32 patients
‡Kaplan–Meier method

Lacy MQ et al. Leukemia 2010;24:1934–1939

Toxicity
Summary of G3/4 (NCI-CTC*) Adverse Events that Occurred in >5% of Cases

Adverse Events, *n* (%)	21/28 (N = 43)	28/28 (N = 41)	Total (N = 84)
SAEs	32 (74)	33 (80)	65 (77)
Study drug-related SAEs	14 (33)	18 (44)	32 (38)
Any G3 or G4 AE	40 (93)	35 (85)	75 (89)
Hematologic			
Blood and lymphatic system	32 (74)	30 (73)	62 (74)
Anemia	16 (37)	14 (34)	30 (36)
Neutropenia	28 (65)	24 (58.5)	52 (62)
Thrombocytopenia	12 (28)	11 (27)	23 (27)
Nonhematologic			
General disorders	10 (23)	10 (24)	20 (24)
Asthenia	6 (14)	2 (5)	8 (9.5)
Infections and infestations	8 (19)	11 (27)	19 (23)
Pneumonia	3 (7)	8 (19.5)	11 (13)
Musculoskeletal/connective tissue	9 (21)	8 (19.5)	17 (20)
Bone pain	6 (14)	3 (7)	9 (11)
Renal and urinary disorders	7 (16)	2 (5)	9 (11)
Renal failure	7 (16)	2 (5)	9 (11)
Respiratory disorders	8 (19)	2 (5)	10 (12)
Dyspnea	5 (12)	0	5 (6)

*National Cancer Institute Common Terminology Criteria for Adverse Events, version 3.0

Leleu X et al. Blood 2013;121:1968–1975

Maximum Severity of Toxicities* (N = 34)

Toxicity[†]	G1	G2	G3	G4	All Grades
Hematologic					
Anemia	15	9	4	0	28
Lymphocyte count decreased	0	3	0	0	3
Neutrophil count decreased	5	7	6	4	22
Platelet count decreased	8	4	3	0	15
Leukopenia	9	5	7	1	22

(continued)

Toxicity (continued)

Toxicity[†]	G1	G2	G3	G4	All Grades
Nonhematologic					
Edema limbs	0	2	0	0	2
Musculoskeletal	0	1	0	0	1
Muscle weakness lower limb	0	1	0	0	1
Agitation	0	2	0	0	2
Anxiety	0	1	0	0	1
Confusion	0	1	0	0	1
Peripheral sensory neuropathy	6	3	0	0	9
Tremor	0	1	0	0	1
Myalgia	0	1	0	0	1
Dyspnea	0	1	0	0	1
Pneumonitis	0	0	1	0	1
Edema	0	0	1	0	1
Fatigue	8	9	3	0	20
Dermatology	0	0	1	0	1
Anorexia	5	1	0	0	6
Constipation	0	1	0	0	1
Diarrhea	4	0	0	0	4
Gastritis	0	1	0	0	1
Nausea	2	2	0	0	4
Metabolic/Laboratory					
Hyperglycemia	0	3	0	1	4
Infection/Febrile Neutropenia					
Infection—no ANC	0	1	0	0	1
Upper airway infection	0	1	0	0	1
Bladder infection	0	1	0	0	1
Pneumonia G0 to G2 ANC	0	0	1	0	1
Respiratory tract infection	0	2	0	0	2
Skin infection	0	1	0	0	1

*Possibly, probably, or definitely related
[†]National Cancer Institute Common Terminology Criteria for Adverse Events, version 3.0

Lacy MQ et al. Leukemia 2010;24:1934–1939

Therapy Monitoring

1. Blood counts and physical examinations on day 1 of each cycle
2. Serum and urinary protein electrophoresis studies on day 1 of each cycle as indicated and at the end of treatment

REGIMEN
RELAPSED/REFRACTORY MULTIPLE MYELOMA

POMALIDOMIDE + CYCLOPHOSPHAMIDE + PREDNISONE

Larocca A et al. Blood 2013;122:2799–2806

Induction:

Cyclophosphamide 50 mg/dose orally, every other day (eg, days 1, 3, 5..., etc. *or* days 2, 4, 6..., etc.) continually, for 14 doses every 28 days (total dose/cycle = 700 mg)

Prednisone 50 mg/dose orally, every other day (eg, days 1, 3, 5..., etc. *or* days 2, 4, 6..., etc.) continually, for 14 doses every 28 days (total dose/cycle = 700 mg)

plus

Pomalidomide 2–3 mg/day orally, continually, for 28 consecutive days, on days 1–28, every 28 days (total dose/cycle = 56–84 mg), *or*

Pomalidomide 4 mg/day orally, continually, for 21 consecutive days, on days 1–21, every 28 days (total dose/cycle = 84 mg)

Maintenance:

Pomalidomide 1 mg/day orally, continually, until disease relapse or progression (total dose/week = 7 mg)

Prednisone 25 mg/dose orally, every other day (eg, days 1, 3, 5..., etc. *or* days 2, 4, 6..., etc.) continually, until disease relapse or progression

Supportive Care

Antiemetic prophylaxis

*Emetogenic potential is **MINIMAL–LOW***

See Chapter 39 for antiemetic recommendations

Hematopoietic growth factor (CSF) prophylaxis

Primary prophylaxis may be indicated

See Chapter 43 for more information

Antimicrobial prophylaxis

Risk of fever and neutropenia is INTERMEDIATE

  Antimicrobial primary prophylaxis to be considered:

  • Antibacterial—consider a fluoroquinolone or no prophylaxis; *Pneumocystis jirovecii* prophylaxis is recommended (eg, cotrimoxazole)

  • Antifungal—recommended; consider use during periods of neutropenia, and in anticipation of mucositis

  • Antiviral—antiherpes antivirals (eg, acyclovir, famciclovir, valacyclovir)

See Chapter 47 for more information

(continued)

Treatment Modifications

Pomalidomide Dose Levels

Starting dose	2.5 mg/day
Level −1	2 mg/day
Level −2	1.5 mg/day
Level −3	1 mg/day
Level −4	0.5 mg/day
Level −5	Discontinue

Prednisone Dose Levels

Starting dose	50 mg/dose
Level −1	25 mg/dose
Level −2	20 mg/dose
Level −3	10 mg/dose
Level −4	5 mg/dose
Level −5	Discontinue

Adverse Event	Treatment Modification
ANC <500/mm³ Febrile neutropenia (fever ≥38.5°C + ANC <1000/mm³) Platelets <25,000/mm³	Interrupt pomalidomide and cyclophosphamide treatment, and follow CBC weekly. When ANC ≥500/mm³ and platelet count ≥50,000/mm³, resume pomalidomide 1 dose level lower and cyclophosphamide at a dose of 25 mg every other day
Nonhematologic G3/4 toxicity	Interrupt pomalidomide treatment, and follow weekly or more frequently. Restart treatment 1 dose level lower than the previous dose when toxicity has resolved G ≤2
ANC <1000/mm³, platelet count <50,000/mm³, hemoglobin <8 g/dL, and/or nonhematologic adverse events G ≥3	Delay the start of a new cycle. If delayed by ≥2 weeks, reduce the dose of pomalidomide by 1 dose level

(continued)

(*continued*)

Thromboprophylaxis

Risk assessment and recommendations for VTE prophylaxis in patients with multiple myeloma with individual or myeloma-related risk factors, or risk factors related to treatment

Individual risk factors
• Obesity (BMI $\geq$30 kg/m^2)
• H/O VTE
• CVAD or pacemaker
• Comorbid pathologies
  Cardiac disease
  Chronic renal disease
  Diabetes
  Acute infection
  Immobilization
• Surgery
  General surgery
  Any anesthesia
  Trauma
• Medications
  Erythropoietin (epoetin alfa, darbepoetin)
  Estrogenic compounds
  Bevacizumab
• Clotting disorders
  Thrombophilia
Myeloma-related risk factors
• Diagnosis of multiple myeloma
• Hyperviscosity
	$\leq$1 Individual or myeloma risk factor present:
	• **Aspirin** 81–325 mg daily
	
	$\geq$2 Individual or myeloma risk factors present:
	• **LMWH*, equivalent to enoxaparin sodium** 40 mg/day *or* **dalteparin sodium** 5000 IU/day; administer subcutaneously, *or*
	• **Warfarin**, targeting an INR = 2–3

Concomitant treatment-related risk factors Thalidomide or lenalidomide in combination with: • High-dose dexamethasone ($\geq$480 mg/month) • Doxorubicin • Multiagent chemotherapy	**LMWH*, equivalent to enoxaparin sodium** 40 mg/day *or* **dalteparin sodium** 5000 IU/day; administer subcutaneously, *or* **Warfarin**, targeting an INR = 2–3

CVAD, central vascular access device; INR, international normalized ratio; LMWH, low-molecular-weight heparin; VTE, venous thromboembolic disease
*LMWHs should be used with caution in individuals with impaired renal function (creatinine clearance <30 mL/min). Refer to product labeling for information about doses and administration schedules in renally impaired patients, and guidance for monitoring antifactor Xa concentrations

Geerts WH et al. Chest 2008;133(6 Suppl):381S–453S
Multiple Myeloma, V.1.2014. National Comprehensive Cancer Network, Inc., 2013. (Accessed October 8, 2013, at http://www.nccn.org)
Palumbo A et al. Leukemia 2008;22:414–423
Venous Thromboembolic Disease, V.2.2013. National Comprehensive Cancer Network, Inc., 2013. (Accessed October 8, 2013, at http://www.nccn.org)

Bisphosphonates

All patients receiving primary therapy for symptomatic multiple myeloma should receive a bisphosphonate adjunctively; *for example*:

• **Pamidronate disodium** 90 mg; administer intravenously over 2–4 hours, every month, *or*

• **Zoledronic acid** 4 mg; administer intravenously over at least 15 minutes, every month

Consider baseline bone densitometry evaluation
See Chapter 43 for more information

Treatment Modifications
(continued)

Adverse Event	Treatment Modification
G4 rash, neuropathy or hypersensitivity, or G $\geq$3 bradycardia or cardiac arrhythmia	Permanently discontinue pomalidomide
G3/4 adverse events occurring on or after day 15 during a single cycle	Withhold pomalidomide for the remainder of the cycle, and reduce pomalidomide dose by 1 dose level beginning with the next cycle
Toxicities ascribed to prednisone such as severe manifestations of hypercorticism, including: hyperglycemia, irritability, insomnia, or oral candidiasis	Hold prednisone doses for up to 21 days to resolve toxicity and then restart at the same dose level or reduce the prednisone dose by 50%

Efficacy

Best Responses to Pomalidomide + Cyclophosphamide + Prednisone

| | | | | | Relapsed | Refractory to | |
| | | | | | >LEN | LEN | LEN/BOR |
POL Dose	1 mg (N = 4)	1.5 mg (N = 4)	2 mg (N = 4)	2.5 mg (N = 55)	2.5 mg (N = 18)	2.5 mg (N = 37)	2.5 mg (N = 16)
Response							
CR/PR	1 (25%)	2 (50%)	2 (50%)	28 (51%)	11 (61%)	17 (46%)	8 (50%)
CR	—	—	—	3	1	2	2
VGPR	—	—	—	10	6	4	1
PR	1	2	2	15	4	11	5
MR	1	-	1	11	2	9	5
SD	1	1	1	15	5	10	3
PD	1	1	—	1	0	1	—

BOR, bortezomib; CR, complete response; LEN, lenalidomide; MR, minimal response; PD, progressive disease; POL, pomalidomide; PR, partial response; SD, stable disease; VGPR, very good partial response

Time to Event Analysis

	N	Median Follow-Up	Median PFS	Median OS	12-Month OS
		Months (Range)	Months (95% CI)		
All patients	67	15.0 (3.7–26.4)	8.6 (7.5–13.9)	NR	65% (51–76%)
LEN 1–2 mg	12	24.1 (3.7–26.4)	4.6 (3.3–8.0)	9 (5.2–NR)	44% (15–70%)
LEN 2.5 mg	55	14.8 (6.1–21.4)	10.4 (7.8–15.8)	NR	69% (54–81%)
Relapsed > LEN	18	12.7 (7.2–21.4)	15.7 (12.8–20.7)	NR	88% (60–97%)
Refractory to LEN	37	15.3 (6.1–21.4)	8.6 (7.5–13.9)	NR	60% (41–75%)
Refractory to LEN/BOR	16	15.8 (6.6–21.4)	8.6 (4.8–NR)	NR	67% (37–85%)

BOR, bortezomib; LEN, lenalidomide; NR, not reached; OS, overall survival; PFS, progression-free survival

Toxicity

Treatment—Related Adverse Events During Salvage Therapy Phase 2 (N = 55)

Event	G1	G2	G3	G4	G5	All Grades
Hematologic						
Neutropenia	6	10	14	9	—	33
Thrombocytopenia	15	5	3	3	—	26
Anemia	10	22	5	—	—	37
Nonhematologic						
Ischemia	—	—	—	1	—	1
Arrhythmia	—	3	—	—	—	3
Sensory neuropathy	6	2	—	—	—	8
Neuralgia	2	1	1	—	—	4
Motor neuropathy	—	—	1	—	—	1
Tremor	—	1	—	—	—	1
Confusion	—	1	—	1	—	2
Mood depression	—	1	—	—	—	1
Other neurologic	3	—	1	—	—	4
Upper respiratory	2	5	—	—	—	7
Pneumonia	2	5	3	—	1	11
Sepsis	—	—	—	—	1	1
Other infective	1	4	—	—	—	5
Diarrhea	1	—	—	—	—	1
Constipation	—	5	—	—	—	5
Nausea/vomiting	1	—	—	—	—	1
Other gastrointestinal	1	2	1	—	—	4
Increased transaminase	2	1	—	—	—	3
Liver failure	—	—	1	—	—	1
Pancreatitis	—	1	—	—	—	1
Deep vein thrombosis	—	1	—	1	—	2
Phlebitis	1	—	—	—	—	1

(continued)

Patient Population Studied

Patients with MM who had received 1–3 prior lines of therapy and whose disease had relapsed after lenalidomide or was refractory. Relapse was defined as reoccurrence of disease requiring the initiation of a salvage therapy. Refractory disease was defined as relapse while on salvage therapy or progression within 60 days after the most recent therapy. Patients were required to have Karnofsky performance status ≥60%, platelet count ≥50,000/mm³, neutrophil count ≥1000/mm³, corrected serum calcium ≤3.5 mmol/L (≤14 mg/dL), and serum creatinine ≤2 mg/dL (≤177 μmol/L)

Baseline Patients Characteristics (N = 66)

Median age, years (range)	69 (41–84)
Gender (F/M)	33 (48%)/36 (52%)
International Staging System stage I/II/III	34 (49%)/27 (39%)/8 (12%)
Myeloma protein class	
IgG	42 (61%)
IgA 4	16 (23%)
Bence-Jones protein	10 (15%)
Non-secretory	1 (1%)
Karnofsky performance status 60–70/80/90–100	10 (14%)/13 (19%)/46 (67%)
Serum β_2-microglobulin level: median (mg/L)	3 (1.6–12)
Months from diagnosis to on study: median (range)	53 (11–203)
Prior lines of therapy: median (range)	3 (1–3)
Prior therapies	
Lenalidomide	69 (100%)
Bortezomib	58 (84%)
Thalidomide	14 (20%)
Autologous transplant	23 (33%)
Allogeneic transplant	10 (15%)

(continued)

Toxicity (*continued*)

Event	G1	G2	G3	G4	G5	All Grades
Nonhematologic						
Fatigue	5	7	2	—	—	14
Fever	2	—	—	—	—	2
Drowsiness	1	—	—	—	—	1
Weight gain	—	1	—	—	—	1
Rash	—	2	4	—	—	6
Other dermatologic	—	1	—	—	—	1
Other	7	6	3	—	—	16

Therapy Monitoring

1. Blood counts and physical examinations on day 1 of each cycle
2. Serum and urinary protein electrophoresis studies on day 1 of each cycle as indicated and at the end of treatment

Patient Population Studied
(*continued*)

Baseline Patients Characteristics (N = 66)

Previous lenalidomide	
Relapsed	23 (33%)
Refractory	46 (67%)
Previous bortezomib [data not available for 14 (20%)]	
Relapsed	17 (25%)
Refractory	27 (39%)
FISH*	
High risk	18 (26%)
Standard risk	35 (51%)
Not available	16 (23%)
Chromosome abnormalities	
Del 13	24 (35%)
(4;14)	8 (12%)
t(11;14)	12 (17%)
t(14;16)	3 (4%)
Del17	8 (12%)

*High risk FISH = presence of at least 1 of the following: t(4;14), t(14;16), or del17

REGIMEN
RELAPSED/REFRACTORY MULTIPLE MYELOMA
LIPOSOMAL DOXORUBICIN + BORTEZOMIB

Orlowski RZ et al. J Clin Oncol 2007;25:3892–3901

Bortezomib 1.3 mg/m² per dose; administer by intravenous injection over 3–5 seconds for 4 doses on days 1, 4, 8, and 11, every 3 weeks (total dosage/cycle = 5.2 mg/m²)

Doxorubicin HCl Liposome Injection ([pegylated] liposomal doxorubicin) 30 mg/m²; administer intravenously in 250 mL (doses ≤90 mg) or 500 mL (doses >90 mg) 5% dextrose injection over 60 minutes after bortezomib on day 4, every 3 weeks (total dosage/cycle = 30 mg/m²)

Notes:

1. Liposomal doxorubicin doses >60 mg are administered at an initial rate of 1 mg/min to minimize the risk of infusion reactions. If no infusion-related adverse reactions are observed within 15 minutes after starting administration, the infusion rate may be increased to complete administration over 1 hour

2. Treatment on study continued until disease progression, unacceptable treatment-related toxicities, or for 8 cycles. Patients still responding after 8 cycles were permitted to continue, provided treatment was well tolerated

Supportive Care
Antiemetic prophylaxis
Emetogenic potential on days with bortezomib alone is **MINIMAL–LOW**
Emetogenic potential on days with liposomal doxorubicin is **LOW**
See Chapter 39 for antiemetic recommendations

Hematopoietic growth factor (CSF) prophylaxis
Primary prophylaxis may be indicated
See Chapter 43 for more information

Antimicrobial prophylaxis
Risk of fever and neutropenia is HIGH
Antimicrobial primary prophylaxis is recommended:
- Antibacterial—consider fluoroquinolone prophylaxis; *P. jirovecii* prophylaxis is recommended (eg, cotrimoxazole)
- Antifungal—recommended
- Antiviral—antiherpes antivirals (eg, acyclovir, famciclovir, valacyclovir)

Caution: Acyclovir and famciclovir accumulate in patients with impaired renal function and may exacerbate renal dysfunction (valacyclovir is a *prodrug* for acyclovir). Monitor kidney function serially during acyclovir, valacyclovir, and famciclovir use
- Acyclovir and famciclovir elimination is inversely related to renal function
- Acyclovir, famciclovir, and valacyclovir utilization is modified in renally impaired individuals (consult product labeling or Summary of Product Characteristics for guidance about dose/dosage and administration frequency modifications, and, when relevant, recommendations for drug dilution, administration rate, concurrent fluid administration, and fluid supplementation as a function of urine output)
- Impaired acyclovir elimination is associated with neurologic adverse effects, including agitation, ataxia, coma, confusion, dizziness, dysarthria, encephalopathy, hallucinations, paresthesia, seizure, somnolence, and tremors

See Chapter 47 for more information

(continued)

Toxicity (N = 318)

Overview of Treatment-Emergent Adverse Events	Percent of Patients
Any adverse event	98
Drug-related adverse events	94
Serious adverse events	36
Drug-related serious adverse events	22
G3/4 adverse events	80
Drug-related G3/4 adverse events	68
Adverse event leading to bortezomib discontinuation	30
Adverse event leading to liposomal doxorubicin discontinuation	36
Adverse event with fatal outcome	4
Drug-related adverse event with fatal outcome	2

Adverse Events During Treatment Reported by at Least 15% of Patients

	% Total	% G3/4
Hematologic Events		
Thrombocytopenia	30	23
Anemia	23	9
Neutropenia	35	29
Febrile neutropenia	3	3
Gastrointestinal Events		
Nausea	46	2
Diarrhea	43	7
Constipation	28	1
Vomiting	31	4
Constitutional Symptoms		
Fatigue	31	6
Pyrexia	29	1
Asthenia	19	6
Anorexia	18	2

(continued)

(continued)

Thromboprophylaxis

Risk assessment and recommendations for VTE prophylaxis in patients with multiple myeloma with individual or myeloma-related risk factors, or risk factors related to treatment

Individual risk factors	
• Obesity (BMI ≥30 kg/m²)	
• H/O VTE	
• CVC or pacemaker	
• Comorbid pathologies	
Cardiac disease	
Chronic renal disease	≤1 Individual or myeloma risk factor present:
Diabetes	• **Aspirin** 81–325 mg daily
Acute infection	
Immobilization	
• Surgery	≥2 Individual or myeloma risk factors present:
General surgery	• **LMWH***, equivalent to enoxaparin sodium 40 mg/day *or* **dalteparin sodium** 5000 IU/day; administer subcutaneously, *or*
Any anesthesia	
Trauma	
• Medications	• **Warfarin**, targeting an INR = 2–3
Erythropoietin (epoetin alfa, darbepoetin)	
Estrogenic compounds	
Bevacizumab	
• Clotting disorders	
Thrombophilia	
Myeloma-related risk factors	
• Diagnosis of multiple myeloma	
• Hyperviscosity	
Concomitant treatment-related risk factors Thalidomide or lenalidomide in combination with:	**LMWH***, equivalent to enoxaparin sodium 40 mg/day *or* **dalteparin sodium** 5000 IU/day; administer subcutaneously, *or*
• High-dose dexamethasone (≥480 mg/month)	
• Doxorubicin	**Warfarin**, targeting an INR = 2–3
• Multiagent chemotherapy	

CVC, central venous catheter; INR, international normalized ratio; LMWH, low-molecular-weight heparin; VTE, venous thromboembolic disease

*LMWHs should be used with caution in individuals with impaired renal function (creatinine clearance <30 mL/min). Refer to product labeling for information about doses and administration schedules in renally impaired patients, and guidance for monitoring anti-Factor Xa concentrations

Geerts WH et al. Chest 2008;133(6 Suppl):381S–453S

Multiple Myeloma, V.1.2014. National Comprehensive Cancer Network, Inc., 2013. (Accessed October 8, 2013, at http://www.nccn.org)

Palumbo A et al. Leukemia 2008;22:414–423

Venous Thromboembolic Disease, V.2.2013. National Comprehensive Cancer Network, Inc., 2013. (Accessed October 8, 2013, at http://www.nccn.org)

Hand-foot reaction (palmar-plantar erythrodysesthesia)

For patients who develop a hand-foot reaction, use topical emollients (eg, Aquaphor), topical or orally administered steroids, antihistamine agents (H_1-receptor antagonists), or pyridoxine Pyridoxine may provide relief for discomfort/pain associated with PPE, although the mechanism through which this occurs remains unclear

• The suggested pyridoxine starting dose is 50 mg/day, which may be increased to a maximum of 200 mg/day

Patients who have developed G1/2 PPE while receiving doxorubicin HCl liposome injection may receive a fixed daily dose of pyridoxine 200 mg. This may allow for treatment to be completed without dosage reduction, treatment delay, or recurrence of PPE

(continued)

Toxicity (N = 318) *(continued)*

Other		
Thromboembolic event	1	1
Bleeding/hemorrhage	14	4
Cough	16	0
Stomatitis	18	2
Hand-foot syndrome	16	5
Cardiac events	10	2
Neuralgia	14	3
Headache	18	1
Peripheral neuropathy	35	4
Alopecia	2	N/A

Efficacy (N = 324)

Total response (CR + PR)	44%
CR	4%
PR	40%
nCR	9%
CR + VGPR	27%

Median time to first response	43 days
Median number of cycles administered	5 cycles
Median treatment duration	105 days
Median duration of response	10.2 months
Median time to progression	9.3 months
Median progression-free survival	9 months
Median duration of overall survival	311 days
15-month survival rate	76%

CR, complete response; nCR, near-complete response; PR, partial response; VGPR, very good partial response

(*continued*)

Diarrhea management

Latent or delayed-onset diarrhea*:

Loperamide 4 mg; administer orally initially after the first loose or liquid stool, *then*
Loperamide 2 mg; administer orally every 2 hours during waking hours, *plus*
Loperamide 4 mg; administer orally every 4 hours during hours of sleep

- Continue for at least 12 hours after diarrhea resolves
- Recurrent diarrhea after a 12-hour diarrhea-free interval is treated as a new episode
- Rehydrate orally with fluids and electrolytes during a diarrheal episode
- If a patient develops blood or mucus in stool, dehydration, or hemodynamic instability, or if diarrhea persists >48 hours despite loperamide, stop loperamide and hospitalize the patient for IV hydration

Alternatively, a trial of **Diphenoxylate hydrochloride** 2.5 mg **with Atropine sulfate** 0.025 mg (eg, Lomotil)

- Initial adult dose is two tablets four times daily until control has been achieved, after which the dose may be reduced to meet individual requirements. Control may often be maintained with as little as two tablets daily
- Clinical improvement of acute diarrhea is usually observed within 48 hours. If improvement of chronic diarrhea after treatment with a maximum daily dose of 8 tablets is not observed within 10 days, control is unlikely with further administration

*Rothenberg ML et al. J Clin Oncol 2001;19:3801–3807
Wadler S et al. J Clin Oncol 1998;16:3169–3178

Oral care

Prophylaxis and treatment for mucositis/stomatitis

General advice:

- Encourage patients to maintain intake of non-alcoholic fluids
- Evaluate patients for oral pain and provide analgesic medications
- Consider histamine H_2-receptor antagonists (eg, ranitidine, famotidine), or a proton pump inhibitor for epigastric pain
- *Lactobacillus* sp.-containing probiotics may be beneficial in preventing diarrhea

Patients with intact oral mucosa:

- Clean the mouth, tongue, and gums by brushing after every meal and at bedtime with an ultra-soft toothbrush with fluoride toothpaste
- Floss teeth gently every day unless contraindicated. If gums bleed and hurt, avoid bleeding or sore areas, but floss other teeth
- Patients may use saline or commercial bland, non-alcoholic rinses
  - Do not use mouthwashes that contain alcohols

If mucositis or stomatitis is present:

- Keep the mouth moist utilizing water, ice chips, sugarless gum, sugar-free hard candies, or a saliva substitute
- Rinse mouth several times a day to remove debris
  - Use a solution of ¼ teaspoon (1.25 g) each of baking soda and table salt (sodium chloride) in one quart (~950 mL) of warm water. Follow with a plain water rinse
  - Do not use mouthwashes that contain alcohols
- Foam-tipped swabs (eg, Toothettes) are useful in moisturizing oral mucosa, but ineffective for cleansing teeth and removing plaque
- Advise patients who develop mucositis to:
  - Choose foods that are easy to chew and swallow
  - Take small bites of food, chew slowly, and sip liquids with meals
  - Encourage soft, moist foods such as cooked cereals, mashed potatoes, and scrambled eggs
  - For trouble swallowing, soften food with gravies, sauces, broths, yogurt, or other bland liquids
  - Avoid sharp, crunchy foods; hot, spicy or highly acidic foods (eg, citrus fruits and juices); sugary foods; toothpicks; tobacco products; alcoholic drinks

Bisphosphonates

All patients receiving primary therapy for symptomatic multiple myeloma should receive a bisphosphonate adjunctively; *for example*:

- **Pamidronate disodium** 90 mg; administer intravenously over 2–4 hours, every month, *or*
- **Zoledronic acid** 4 mg; administer intravenously over 15 minutes, every month

Consider baseline bone densitometry evaluation
See Chapter 43 for more information

Patient Population Studied

A randomized phase III study of 646 patients with relapsed refractory multiple myeloma. Eligible subjects had an Eastern Cooperative Oncology Group performance status ≤1, must have experienced disease progression after a response to 1 or more lines of therapy or were refractory to initial treatment, but were bortezomib naïve. Subjects were excluded if their disease progressed while receiving anthracycline-containing therapy, and if they had already received >240 mg/m² doxorubicin, clinically significant cardiac disease, a left ventricular ejection fraction less than institutional normal limits, or peripheral neuropathy G ≥2

Therapy Monitoring

1. Blood counts with differential leukocyte count and physical examinations on day 1 of each cycle
2. Serum and urinary protein electrophoresis studies on day 1 of each cycle and at the end of treatment

Treatment Modifications

Bortezomib Dosage Levels

Dosage Level 1	1.3 mg/m²
Dosage Level −1	1 mg/m²
Dosage Level −2	0.7 mg/m²

Modification Guidelines for Hematologic Toxicity on Day 1 of Planned Therapy

Toxicity	Treatment Modification
ANC 1000–1500/mm³ or platelets 75,000–100,000/mm³	Resume treatment with no dosage reduction
ANC 500–999/mm³ or platelets 50,000–75,000/mm³	Hold treatment until toxicity resolves to G ≤1 or 75% of the counts measured at the start of the previous cycle, then resume without dosage reduction
ANC <500/mm³ or platelets <25,000/mm³	First episode: Hold treatment until toxicity resolves to G ≤1, then resume with a 25% dosage reduction of both liposomal doxorubicin and bortezomib or continue full dose with hematopoietic growth factor support (filgrastim, sargramostim) Reduce dose by 25% if neutropenia occurs despite growth factor use
Febrile neutropenia	Withhold therapy until fever abates then resume therapy

Treatment Modification for Bortezomib-Induced Peripheral Neuropathy*

Severity of Peripheral Neuropathy	Modification of Dose and Schedule
G1 (paresthesias or loss of reflexes) without pain or loss of function	No action
G1 with pain or G2 (interferes with function but not with activities of daily living)	Reduce bortezomib dosage to 1 mg/m² per dose
G2 with pain or G3 (interferes with activities of daily living)	Withhold bortezomib treatment until toxicity resolves, then reinitiate at a dosage of 0.7 mg/m² per dose once weekly
G4 (permanent sensory loss that interferes with function)	Discontinue treatment

*Richardson PG et al. J Clin Oncol 2006;24:3113–3120

Liposomal Doxorubicin

Treatment Modification Guidelines for Cardiac Toxicity

Toxicity	Treatment Modification
LVEF decreases by ≥15% from baseline, or to <45%	Discontinue liposomal doxorubicin

LVEF, left ventricular ejection fraction

(continued)

Treatment Modifications (*continued*)

Treatment Modification Guidelines for Palmar-Plantar Erythrodysesthesia (PPE, Hand-Foot Syndrome)

Grade of Toxicity	Liposomal Doxorubicin Dosing Interval		
	4 Weeks	5 Weeks	6 Weeks
G1: Mild erythema, swelling, or desquamation not interfering with daily activities	Resume unless patient has previous G3/4 skin toxicity. If so, delay an additional week	Resume unless patient has previous G3/4 skin toxicity. If so, delay an additional week	Resume liposomal doxorubicin at a 25% dose reduction; return to a 4-week dosing interval or discontinue therapy
G2: Erythema, desquamation, or swelling interfering with, but not precluding, normal physical activities; small blisters or ulcerations <2 cm in diameter	Delay treatment 1 week	Delay treatment 1 week	Resume liposomal doxorubicin at a 25% dose reduction; return to 4-week dosing interval or discontinue therapy
G3: Blistering, ulceration, or swelling interfering with walking or normal daily activities; cannot wear regular clothing	Delay treatment 1 week	Delay treatment 1 week	Discontinue therapy
G4: Diffuse or local process causing infectious complications, or a bedridden state, or hospitalization	Delay treatment 1 week	Delay treatment 1 week	Discontinue therapy

REGIMEN
RELAPSED/REFRACTORY MULTIPLE MYELOMA
CONDITIONING REGIMEN BEFORE AUTOLOGOUS PERIPHERAL BLOOD STEM CELL TRANSPLANTATION
HIGH-DOSE MELPHALAN

Moreau P et al. Blood 2002;99:731–735

Conditioning for autologous PBSC transplant:

Melphalan 200 mg/m²; administer intravenously, diluted in sufficient 0.9% sodium chloride injection (0.9% NS) to produce a concentration ≤0.45 mg/mL over 30 minutes, 2 days before PBSC reinfusion (on day −2) (total dosage = 200 mg/m²). PBSC reinfusion on day 0 (zero), *or*

Melphalan 100 mg/m² per day; administer intravenously, diluted in sufficient 0.9% NS to produce a concentration ≤0.45 mg/mL over 30 minutes, for 2 consecutive days, starting 3 days before PBSC reinfusion (on days −3 and −2) (total dosage = 200 mg/m²). PBSC reinfusion on day 0 (zero)

Supportive Care
Antiemetic prophylaxis
Emetogenic potential is **HIGH** *on days melphalan is administered. Potential for delayed symptoms*
See Chapter 39 for antiemetic recommendations

Hematopoietic growth factor (CSF) prophylaxis
  Filgrastim (G-CSF), 5–10 mcg/kg per day; administer by subcutaneous injection starting on day +7 after PBSC reinfusion, and continue until granulocyte counts recover, *or*
  Sargramostim (GM-CSF) 5–10 mcg/kg per day; administer by subcutaneous injection starting on day +7 after PBSC reinfusion, and continue until granulocyte counts recover

Antimicrobial prophylaxis
Antibacterial prophylaxis (*P. jirovecii* pneumonia prophylaxis):
  Trimethoprim + Sulfamethoxazole (TMP + SMZ) 160 mg/800 mg; administer orally, daily, continually for 3 months, *or*
  TMP + SMZ 80 mg/400 mg; administer orally daily, continually for 3 months, *or*
  TMP + SMZ 160 mg/800 mg; administer orally 3 days per week, continually for 3 months
Antifungal prophylaxis
  Fluconazole 200–400 mg/day; administer orally or intravenously daily for 30 days after PBSC reinfusion or until neutrophil engraftment occurs (ANC >500/mm³)
Antiviral prophylaxis for HSV-seropositive recipients to prevent reactivation of HSV during the early posttransplant period
  Acyclovir 200 mg; administer orally every 8 hours for 30 days, *or*
  Acyclovir 250 mg/m² per dose; administer intravenously every 12 hours for 30 days, *or*
  Valacyclovir 500 mg; administer orally daily for 30 days

Note: Routine acyclovir prophylaxis for >30 days after HSCT is not recommended

Caution: Acyclovir and famciclovir accumulate in patients with impaired renal function and may exacerbate renal dysfunction (valacyclovir is a *prodrug* for acyclovir). Monitor kidney function serially during acyclovir, valacyclovir, and famciclovir use

• Acyclovir and famciclovir elimination is inversely related to renal function

• Acyclovir, famciclovir, and valacyclovir utilization is modified in renally impaired individuals (consult product labeling or Summary of Product Characteristics for guidance about dose/dosage and administration frequency modifications, and, when relevant, recommendations for drug dilution, administration rate, concurrent fluid administration, and fluid supplementation as a function of urine output)

• Impaired acyclovir elimination is associated with neurologic adverse effects, including agitation, ataxia, coma, confusion, dizziness, dysarthria, encephalopathy, hallucinations, paresthesia, seizure, somnolence, and tremors

See Chapter 47 for more information

(continued)

Patient Population Studied

A study of 142 patients ≤65 years of age with symptomatic multiple myeloma responding to primary chemotherapy with VAD

Exclusions:
1. Stable stage 1 MM deemed not to require therapy (Durie-Salmon classification)
2. Previous cytotoxic chemotherapy other than VAD in preparation for transplantation*
3. Previous radiation therapy
4. Severe abnormalities of cardiac, pulmonary, and hepatic function (not characterized)
5. Serum creatinine concentration >5.7 mg/dL (>504 μmol/L)

*VAD was chosen as the regimen because of its "speedy tumor cell reduction without induction of hematopoietic stem cell compromise"

Efficacy (N = 142)

Response to HDT	
Complete response	35%
Very good partial response*	20%
Partial response	39%
Stable or progressive disease	6%
Toxic death	0
Median event-free survival	20.5 months

*Ninety percent decrease in serum paraprotein level

(*continued*)

Oral care

Prophylaxis and treatment for mucositis/stomatitis

General advice:
- Encourage patients to maintain intake of non-alcoholic fluids
- Evaluate patients for oral pain and provide analgesic medications
- Consider histamine H_2-receptor antagonists (eg, ranitidine, famotidine), or a proton pump inhibitor for epigastric pain
- *Lactobacillus* sp.-containing probiotics may be beneficial in preventing diarrhea

Patients with intact oral mucosa:
- Clean the mouth, tongue, and gums by brushing after every meal and at bedtime with an ultra-soft toothbrush with fluoride toothpaste
- Floss teeth gently every day unless contraindicated. If gums bleed and hurt, avoid bleeding or sore areas, but floss other teeth
- Patients may use saline or commercial bland, non-alcoholic rinses
  - Do not use mouthwashes that contain alcohols

If mucositis or stomatitis is present:
- Keep the mouth moist utilizing water, ice chips, sugarless gum, sugar-free hard candies, or a saliva substitute
- Rinse mouth several times a day to remove debris
  - Use a solution of ¼ teaspoon (1.25 g) each of baking soda and table salt (sodium chloride) in one quart (~950 mL) of warm water. Follow with a plain water rinse
  - Do not use mouthwashes that contain alcohols
- Foam-tipped swabs (eg, Toothettes) are useful in moisturizing oral mucosa, but ineffective for cleansing teeth and removing plaque
- Advise patients who develop mucositis to:
  - Choose foods that are easy to chew and swallow
  - Take small bites of food, chew slowly, and sip liquids with meals
  - Encourage soft, moist foods such as cooked cereals, mashed potatoes, and scrambled eggs
  - For trouble swallowing, soften food with gravies, sauces, broths, yogurt, or other bland liquids
  - Avoid sharp, crunchy foods; hot, spicy or highly acidic foods (eg, citrus fruits and juices); sugary foods; toothpicks; tobacco products; alcoholic drinks

Notes:

This conditioning regimen was part of a more comprehensive therapy for multiple myeloma that included the following:

1. Before PBSC harvest, patients received 3 cycles of vincristine + doxorubicin + dexamethasone (VAD)

2. In the absence of tumor progression (>25% increase in tumor mass), and if cardiopulmonary, hepatic, and renal function (serum creatinine <1.7 mg/dL [<150 μmol/L]) remained adequate after a third course of VAD, peripheral blood stem cells (PBSCs) were collected

3. After PBSC collection, patients received a fourth course of VAD

(*continued*)

Adverse Events (N = 142)

Event	Duration in Days Median (Range)
Hematopoietic growth factor	7 (0–23)
Neutropenia	8 (4–34)
Thrombocytopenia	7 (0–30)
Intravenous antibiotics	8 (0–30)
Length of hospital stay	19 (11–47)

Supportive Measure	Number Median (Range)
Platelet transfusions	1 (0–18)
RBC transfusions	2 (0–9)

G3/4 Toxicity	WHO Criteria
Cardiac	0.7%
Mucositis	30%
Pulmonary	1.4%
Renal	2.1%
Liver	0.7%
Toxic death	0

Therapy Monitoring

CBC with differential, daily to every third day as hematological recovery occurs

(continued)

Response to VAD Regimen and Stem Cell Collection

Complete response	5%
Very good partial response*	12%
Partial response	61%
Stable disease	22%

Stem Cell Collection

G-CSF priming	75%
Stem cell factor + G-CSF	4%
Cyclophosphamide + G-CSF	21%
Median number of CD34 infused	5 (range: 1.2–132) $\times 10^6$/kg

G-CSF, granulocyte-colony stimulating factor
*Ninety percent decrease in serum paraprotein level

4. After completion of high-dose chemotherapy (HDT) and PBSCT, treatment with **recombinant interferon alfa** 3 million International Units was given by subcutaneous injection 3 times weekly after granulocytes exceeded 1500/mm^3 and platelets exceeded 100,000/mm^3 during the first year after transplantation. Interferon was continued at participating physicians' discretion in case of disease progression or when it induced severe and persistent adverse effects. The value of maintenance interferon in this or any setting is uncertain

REGIMEN
MAINTENANCE THERAPY—MULTIPLE MYELOMA
BORTEZOMIB

Sonneveld P et al. J Clin Oncol 2012;30:2946–2955

Induction:
Bortezomib 1.3 mg/m^2 per dose by intravenous injection over 3–5 seconds for 4 doses on days 1, 4, 8, and 11, every 28 days for 3 cycles (total dosage/cycle = 5.2 mg/m^2)
Doxorubicin 9 mg/m^2 per day by slow intravenous injection over 3–5 minutes for 4 consecutive days on days 1–4, every 28 days for 3 cycles (total dosage/cycle = 36 mg/m^2)
Dexamethasone 40 mg/dose orally for 12 doses on days 1–4, days 9–12, and days 17–20 for 3 cycles (total dose/cycle = 480 mg)

Notes:
• Stem cell collection was performed 4–6 weeks after induction
• One or 2 cycles of high-dose melphalan (HDM) 200 mg/m^2, and autologous stem cell transplantation (ASCT) were administered
• Starting 4 weeks after HDM, patients received maintenance with bortezomib 1.3 mg/m^2 intravenously every 2 weeks for 2 years
• Patients with an HLA-identical sibling could proceed to nonmyeloablative allogeneic stem cell transplantation (alloSCT) after HDM
• Maintenance therapy was not given after alloSCT

Maintenance therapy (starting 4 weeks after HDM):
Bortezomib 1.3 mg/m^2 per dose by intravenous injection over 3–5 seconds, continually, every 2 weeks for 2 years (total dosage/2-week course = 1.3 mg/m^2)

Supportive Care
Antiemetic prophylaxis
Emetogenic potential with bortezomib is **MINIMAL**
See Chapter 39 for antiemetic recommendations

Hematopoietic growth factor (CSF) prophylaxis
Primary prophylaxis is NOT indicated
See Chapter 43 for more information

Antimicrobial prophylaxis
Risk of fever and neutropenia is INTERMEDIATE
  Antimicrobial primary prophylaxis to be considered:
  • Antibacterial—consider a fluoroquinolone or no prophylaxis; *Pneumocystis jirovecii* prophylaxis is recommended (eg, cotrimoxazole)
  • Antifungal—recommended; consider use during periods of neutropenia
  • Antiviral—antiherpes antivirals (eg, acyclovir, famciclovir, valacyclovir) throughout bortezomib induction
See Chapter 47 for more information

(continued)

(*continued*)

Thromboprophylaxis

Risk assessment and recommendations for VTE prophylaxis in patients with multiple myeloma with individual or myeloma-related risk factors, or risk factors related to treatment

Individual risk factors	

• Obesity (BMI ≥30 kg/m²)
• H/O VTE
• CVAD or pacemaker
• Comorbid pathologies
  Cardiac disease
  Chronic renal disease
  Diabetes
  Acute infection
  Immobilization
• Surgery
  General surgery
  Any anesthesia
  Trauma
• Medications
  Erythropoietin (epoetin alfa, darbepoetin)
  Estrogenic compounds
  Bevacizumab
• Clotting disorders
  Thrombophilia
 	
Myeloma-related risk factors
• Diagnosis of multiple myeloma
• Hyperviscosity
	≤1 Individual or myeloma risk factor present:
	• **Aspirin** 81–325 mg daily
	
	≥2 Individual or myeloma risk factors present:
	• **LMWH***, equivalent to enoxaparin sodium 40 mg/day *or* **dalteparin sodium** 5000 IU/day; administer subcutaneously, *or*
	• **Warfarin**, targeting an INR = 2–3

Concomitant treatment-related risk factors Thalidomide or lenalidomide in combination with: • High-dose dexamethasone (≥480 mg/month) • Doxorubicin • Multiagent chemotherapy	**LMWH***, equivalent to enoxaparin sodium 40 mg/day *or* **dalteparin sodium** 5000 IU/day; administer subcutaneously, *or* **Warfarin**, targeting an INR = 2–3

CVAD, central vascular access device; INR, international normalized ratio; LMWH, low-molecular-weight heparin; VTE, venous thromboembolic disease

*LMWHs should be used with caution in individuals with impaired renal function (creatinine clearance <30 mL/min). Refer to product labeling for information about doses and administration schedules in renally impaired patients, and guidance for monitoring antifactor Xa concentrations

Geerts WH et al. Chest 2008;133(6 Suppl):381S–453S
Multiple Myeloma, V.1.2014. National Comprehensive Cancer Network, Inc., 2013. (Accessed October 8, 2013, at http://www.nccn.org)
Palumbo A et al. Leukemia 2008;22:414–423
Venous Thromboembolic Disease, V.2.2013. National Comprehensive Cancer Network, Inc., 2013. (Accessed October 8, 2013, at http://www.nccn.org)

Bisphosphonates

All patients receiving primary therapy for symptomatic multiple myeloma should receive a bisphosphonate adjunctively; *for example*:

• **Pamidronate disodium** 90 mg; administer intravenously over 2–4 hours, every month, *or*

• **Zoledronic acid** 4 mg; administer intravenously over at least 15 minutes, every month

Consider baseline bone densitometry evaluation
See Chapter 43 for more information

Treatment Modifications

Bortezomib Dose Level

Starting dose	1.3 mg/m² per dose on days 1, 4, 8, and 11
Level −1	1.0 mg/m² per dose on days 1, 4, 8, and 11
Level −2	0.7 mg/m² per dose on days 1, 4, 8, and 11
Level −3	1.3 mg/m² per dose on days 1 and 8

Adverse Event	Treatment Modification
G3 thrombocytopenia (<50,000/mm³)	Reduce bortezomib dosage by 1 dose level

Treatment Modification for Bortezomib-Induced Peripheral Neuropathy*

Severity of Peripheral Neuropathy	Modification of Dose and Schedule
G1 (paresthesias or loss of reflexes) without pain or loss of function	No action
G1 with pain or G2 (interferes with function but not with activities of daily living)	Reduce bortezomib dosage by 1 dose level
G2 with pain or G3 (interferes with activities of daily living)	Withhold bortezomib treatment until toxicity resolves, then reinitiate reducing bortezomib dosage by 1 dose level
G4 (permanent sensory loss that interferes with function)	Discontinue treatment

*Richardson PG et al. J Clin Oncol 2006;24:3113–3120

Patient Population Studied

Patients were newly diagnosed with MM Durie-Salmon stages II to III, WHO PS 0 to 2, or WHO 3 when caused by MM. Exclusion criteria included systemic amyloid light chain amyloidosis, nonsecretory MM, and neuropathy G ≥2. Local RT was allowed for painful MM lesions

Baseline Patient and Disease Characteristics (N = 413)

	No.	%
Age, years: median (range)	57 (31–65)	
Male sex	253	61
WHO performance stage		
0	193	47
1	170	41
2	31	8
3	15	4
ISS stage		
I	144	35
II	150	36
III	81	20
M-protein isotype		
IgA	92	22
IgG	251	61
IgD	5	1
LCD	63	15
M-protein light chain		
Kappa	277	67
Lambda	135	33
Number of skeletal lesions		
0	102	25
1–2	44	11
≥3	255	62
Genetic abnormalities (positive/# assessed, %)		
del(13q)	148/361	41%
t(4;14)	35/250	14%
del(17p13)	25/289	9%
Creatinine >2 mg/dL	36	9
Median β_2-microglobulin, mg/L	3.40	
Median hemoglobin, mmol/L (g/dL)	6.6 (10.6)	
Median calcium, mmol/L (mg/dL)	2.34 (9.4)	
Median number of bone marrow plasma cells	40	

Ig, immunoglobulin; ISS, International Staging System
*WHO performance stage, 4 = 1% unknown; ISS stage, 38 = 9% unknown; M-protein isotype, 2 = 0% other; M-protein light chain, 1 = 0% unknown; number of skeletal lesions, 12 = 3% unknown

Efficacy

An analysis of PFS calculated in 645 patients from the time of last high-dose melphalan (HDM) indicated that posttransplantation bortezomib contributed to improvement of PFS

Toxicity

- Bortezomib-emergent peripheral neuropathy (BiPN) was the prevalent toxicity during induction, preventing a substantial number of patients from starting maintenance therapy
- In those who started maintenance, 5% experienced G3/4 BiPN
- Prolonged administration of bortezomib on the once every-2-weeks schedule was deemed feasible; therefore, it is important to prevent BiPN during induction, which enables patients to continue into maintenance
- The tolerability of bortezomib given every-2-weeks is similar to the weekly schedule
- Subcutaneous bortezomib administration may further improve tolerability

Bortezomib Maintenance After Bortezomib + Doxorubicin + Dexamethasone Induction (N = 229)

Still on treatment after 6 months	90%
Still on treatment after 12 months	76%
Still on treatment after 18 months	64%
Still on treatment after 24 months	47%

Safety Profile and Toxicities

Variable	Bortezomib + Doxorubicin + Dexamethasone Induction (*n* = 410)		Bortezomib Maintenance (*n* = 229)	
	No.	%	No.	%
Any AE	400	98	222	97
AE grades 3 to 4	258	63	110	48
AE classified as SAE	187	46	77	34
AE leading to discontinuation, dose reduction, or delay of bortezomib	112	27	81	35
Death from AE	7	2	0	0

	All G	G3/4	All G	G3/4
Hematologic Toxicities				
Anemia	28	8	27	1
Neutropenia	4	3	2	0
Thrombocytopenia	39	10	37	4
Infections	56	26	75	24
Herpes zoster	2	0	2	0
Nonhematologic Toxicities				
Wasting, fatigue	27	4	20	1
GI symptoms	67	11	48	5
Cardiac disorders	27	8	19	3
Thrombosis	6	4	1	1
Peripheral neuropathy	37	24	33	5

AE, adverse event (including infection); N/A, not applicable; SAE, serious adverse event

Therapy Monitoring

1. Blood counts and physical examinations at regular intervals (1 to 3 months)
2. Serum and urinary protein electrophoresis studies as indicated at regular intervals (1 to 3 months)

REGIMEN
MAINTENANCE THERAPY—MULTIPLE MYELOMA
LENALIDOMIDE

Attal M et al. N Engl J Med 2012;366:1782–1791
Dimopoulos MA et al. Haematologica 2013;98:784–788
McCarthy PL et al. N Engl J Med 2012;366:1770–1781
Palumbo A et al. N Engl J Med 2012;366:1759–1769

Lenalidomide 10 mg/day orally, continually, for 21 consecutive days, on days 1–21, every 28 days (total dose/cycle = 210 mg)

or

Lenalidomide 15 mg/day orally, continually, for 21 consecutive days, on days 1–21, every 28 days (total dose/cycle = 315 mg)

Notes:

- Maintenance treatment may begin with lenalidomide 10 mg/day for 21 consecutive days every 28 days, and if tolerated, escalated to lenalidomide 15 mg/day for 21 consecutive days every 28 days

- Maintenance therapy is continued until disease progression or the development of unacceptable rates of adverse effects

Supportive Care

Antiemetic prophylaxis
Emetogenic potential is **MINIMAL–LOW**
See Chapter 39 for antiemetic recommendations

Hematopoietic growth factor (CSF) prophylaxis
Primary prophylaxis is NOT indicated
See Chapter 43 for more information

Antimicrobial prophylaxis
Risk of fever and neutropenia is INTERMEDIATE
Antimicrobial primary prophylaxis to be considered:

- Antibacterial—consider a fluoroquinolone or no prophylaxis; *Pneumocystis jirovecii* prophylaxis is recommended (eg, cotrimoxazole)

- Antifungal—recommended; consider use during periods of neutropenia

- Antiviral—antiherpes antivirals (eg, acyclovir, famciclovir, valacyclovir)

See Chapter 47 for more information

(continued)

Treatment Modifications

Lenalidomide Dose Levels	
Starting dose	25 mg/dose
Level –1	20 mg/dose
Level –2	15 mg/dose
Level –3	10 mg/dose
Level –4	5 mg/dose
Level –5	Discontinue

Adverse Event	Treatment Modification
G3/4 neutropenia Febrile neutropenia (ANC <1000/mm^3 with fever ≥38°C)	Hold lenalidomide dosing for up to 21 days to resolve toxicity and then restart at the same dose or reduce the lenalidomide dose by 1 dose level
G3/4 nonhematologic toxicity	Hold lenalidomide dosing for up to 21 days to resolve toxicity to G ≤2 and then restart at the same dose or reduce the lenalidomide dose by 1 dose level

(*continued*)

Thromboprophylaxis

Risk assessment and recommendations for VTE prophylaxis in patients with multiple myeloma with individual or myeloma-related risk factors, or risk factors related to treatment

Individual risk factors
• Obesity (BMI ≥30 kg/m²)
• H/O VTE
• CVAD or pacemaker
• Comorbid pathologies
  Cardiac disease
  Chronic renal disease
  Diabetes
  Acute infection
  Immobilization
• Surgery
  General surgery
  Any anesthesia
  Trauma
• Medications
  Erythropoietin (epoetin alfa, darbepoetin)
  Estrogenic compounds
  Bevacizumab
• Clotting disorders
  Thrombophilia
	≤1 Individual or myeloma risk factor present:
	• **Aspirin** 81–325 mg daily
	
	≥2 Individual or myeloma risk factors present:
	• **LMWH***, equivalent to enoxaparin sodium 40 mg/day *or* **dalteparin sodium** 5000 IU/day; administer subcutaneously, *or*
	• **Warfarin**, targeting an INR = 2–3

Myeloma-related risk factors • Diagnosis of multiple myeloma • Hyperviscosity	
Concomitant treatment-related risk factors Thalidomide or lenalidomide in combination with: • High-dose dexamethasone (≥480 mg/month) • Doxorubicin • Multiagent chemotherapy	**LMWH***, equivalent to enoxaparin sodium 40 mg/day *or* **dalteparin sodium** 5000 IU/day; administer subcutaneously, *or* **Warfarin**, targeting an INR = 2–3

CVAD, central vascular access device; INR, international normalized ratio; LMWH, low-molecular-weight heparin; VTE, venous thromboembolic disease

*LMWHs should be used with caution in individuals with impaired renal function (creatinine clearance <30 mL/min). Refer to product labeling for information about doses and administration schedules in renally impaired patients, and guidance for monitoring antifactor Xa concentrations

Geerts WH et al. Chest 2008;133(6 Suppl):381S–453S

Multiple Myeloma, V.1.2014. National Comprehensive Cancer Network, Inc., 2013. (Accessed October 8, 2013, at http://www.nccn.org)

Palumbo A et al. Leukemia 2008;22:414–423

Venous Thromboembolic Disease, V.2.2013. National Comprehensive Cancer Network, Inc., 2013. (Accessed October 8, 2013, at http://www.nccn.org)

Diarrhea management

  Loperamide 4 mg orally initially after the first loose or liquid stool, *then*

  Loperamide 2 mg orally every 2 hours during waking hours, *plus*

  Loperamide 4 mg orally every 4 hours during hours of sleep

  • Continue for at least 12 hours after diarrhea resolves

  • Recurrent diarrhea after a 12-hour diarrhea-free interval is treated as a new episode

  • Rehydrate orally with fluids and electrolytes during a diarrheal episode

  • If a patient develops blood or mucus in stool, dehydration, or hemodynamic instability, or if diarrhea persists >48 hours despite loperamide, stop loperamide and hospitalize the patient for IV hydration

(*continued*)

Patient Population Studied

Patients with symptomatic, measurable, newly diagnosed MM who were not candidates for transplantation (≥65 years of age) were eligible for this trial. Exclusion criteria were an ANC <1500/mm³, platelet count <75,000/mm³, a hemoglobin level <8.0 g/dL, a serum creatinine level of >2.5 mg/dL [>221 μmol/L], and peripheral neuropathy of G ≥2. A total of 459 patients were randomly assigned to receive nine 4-week cycles of melphalan-prednisone-lenalidomide induction (MPR) followed by lenalidomide maintenance therapy until a relapse or disease progression occurred (152 patients) or to receive MPR (153 patients) or melphalan-prednisone (MP) (154 patients) without maintenance therapy. Maintenance consisted of lenalidomide 10 mg daily for the first 21 days of 28-day cycles until disease progression or the development of unacceptable toxicity. The primary end point was progression-free survival

Palumbo A et al. N Engl J Med 2012;366:1759–1769

Patients with MM between 18 and 70 years of age, an Eastern Cooperative Oncology Group performance status of 0 or 1, symptomatic disease requiring treatment (Durie–Salmon stage ≥1) and any induction regimen of 2 to 12 months' duration, who had received ≤2 induction regimens (excluding dexamethasone alone). Patients with stable disease or a marginal, partial, or complete response during the first 100 days after stem cell transplantation were eligible. After disease restaging, patients were randomly assigned in a blinded manner to lenalidomide or placebo between days 100 and 110 after transplantation. A total of 460 patients <71 years of age with stable disease or a marginal, partial, or complete response 100 days after undergoing stem cell transplantation were randomly assigned to lenalidomide or placebo, which was administered until disease progression. The starting dose of lenalidomide was 10 mg/day (range: 5–15 mg/day). The time to disease progression was the primary end point

McCarthy PL et al. N Engl J Med 2012;366:1770–1781

(*continued*)

(*continued*)

Alternatively, a trial of **Diphenoxylate hydrochloride** 2.5 mg **with Atropine sulfate** 0.025 mg (eg, Lomotil)

- Initial adult dose is 2 tablets 4 times daily until control has been achieved, after which the dose may be reduced to meet individual requirements. Control may often be maintained with as little as 2 tablets daily
- Clinical improvement of acute diarrhea is usually observed within 48 hours. If improvement of chronic diarrhea after treatment with a maximum daily dose of 8 tablets is not observed within 10 days, control is unlikely with further administration

Bisphosphonates

All patients receiving primary therapy for symptomatic multiple myeloma should receive a bisphosphonate adjunctively; *for example*:

- **Pamidronate disodium** 90 mg; administer intravenously over 2–4 hours, every month, *or*
- **Zoledronic acid** 4 mg; administer intravenously over at least 15 minutes, every month

Consider baseline bone densitometry evaluation
See Chapter 43 for more information

Efficacy

Variable	MPR-R (N = 152)	MPR (N = 153)	MP (N = 154)
Best Response			
Complete or partial response—no. (%)	117 (77.0)*	104 (68.0)†	77 (50.0)
Complete response	15 (9.9)	5 (3.3)	5 (3.2)
Partial response‡	102 (67.1)	99 (64.7)	72 (46.8)
Very good partial response§	35 (23.0)	45 (29.4)	14 (9.1)
Stable disease—no. (%)	28 (18.4)	40 (26.1)	70 (45.5)
Progressive disease—no. (%)	0	2 (1.3)	0
Response could not be evaluated—no. (%)	7 (4.6)	7 (4.6)	7 (4.5)
Time to Event			
Median time to first evidence of response: months (range)	2*(1–9)	2*(1–6)	3 (1–15)
Duration of response—months			
Median complete or partial response (95% CI)	29ᶜ (22–NR)	13 (12–15)	13 (10–18)
Median complete response (95% CI)	NRᶜ (36–NR)	31 (23–33)	22 (10–24)
Median partial response‡ (95% CI)	19 (11–NR)	11 (9–13)	10 (9–15)
Median very good partial response§ (95% CI)	28* (22–NR)	15 (13–22)	18 (10–22)

MP, melphalan–prednisone induction without lenalidomide maintenance; MPR, melphalan–prednisone–lenalidomide induction without lenalidomide maintenance; MPR-R, melphalan–prednisone–lenalidomide induction followed by lenalidomide maintenance; NR, not reached
*P <0.001 for the comparison with the MP group
†P = 0.002 for the comparison with the MP group
‡Partial response defined as 50–99% reduction in serum/urinary levels of myeloma protein
§Very good partial response defined as 90–99% reduction in serum/urinary levels of myeloma protein
ᶜP <0.001 for the comparison with the MPR group and the comparison with the MP group

Palumbo A et al. N Engl J Med 2012;366:1759–1769

(*continued*)

Patient Population Studied
(*continued*)

Study patients were <65 years of age with MM that had not progressed during the interval between first-line autologous stem cell transplantation (1 or 2 procedures) within the previous 6 months, serum creatinine <1.8 mg/dL (<160 μmol/L), an ANC ≥1000/mm³, and platelet count >75,000/mm³. After undergoing transplantation, patients received consolidation treatment with 2 cycles of lenalidomide 25 mg daily for the first 21 days of 28-day cycles, and then, based on prior random assignment, received maintenance therapy with either placebo or lenalidomide 10 mg daily for the first 3 months, which, if tolerated, could be increased to 15 mg daily on the same administration schedule. Treatment was continued until the patient withdrew consent, disease progressed, or toxicity was unacceptable. Randomization was stratified according to baseline levels of serum β_2-microglobulin (≤3 mg/L or >3 mg/L), the presence or absence of a 13q deletion by FISH and treatment response after transplantation (a complete or very good partial response vs. a partial response or stable disease). The primary end point was progression-free survival

Attal M et al. N Engl J Med 2012;366:1782–1791

Efficacy (continued)

	Lenalidomide	Placebo	HR	*p* Value
At a Median of 18 Months				
Progression/death	47/231 (20%)	101/229 (44%)	0.37; 95% CI, 0.26–0.53	P <0.001
Median time to progression	39 months	21 months		P <0.001
Deaths	13/231	24/229	0.52; 95% CI, 0.26–1.02	P = 0.05
Median overall survival	NR	NR	—	—
At a Median of 34 Months				
Progression/death	86/231 (37%)	132/229 (58%)	0.48; 95% CI, 0.36–0.63	—
Median time to progression	46 months	27 months	—	P <0.001
Deaths	35 (15%)	53 (23%)	—	P = 0.03
3-Year rate freedom from progression/death	66%; 95% CI, 59–73	39%; 95% CI, 33–48	—	—
Overall survival at 3 years	88%; 95% CI, 84–93	80%; 95% CI, 74–86	0.62; 95% CI, 0.40–0.95	P = 0.03

McCarthy PL et al. N Engl J Med 2012;366:1770–1781

Response to Treatment as Assessed by the Independent Review Committee*

Variable	Lenalidomide (N = 307)	Placebo (N = 307)	*p* Value
Response at randomization			
Evaluable for response-# (%) of patients	266 (87)	274 (89)	0.18
Percent complete response	5	8	
Percent VGPR[†]	56	51	
Percent partial response	38	39	
Percent stable disease	1	2	
Percent complete response or VGPR	61	59	0.55
Best response during maintenance			
Evaluable for response-# (%) of patients	300 (98)	293 (95)	0.07
Percent complete response	29	27	
Percent VGPR[‡]	55	49	
Percent partial response	15	23	
Percent stable disease	1	1	
Percent complete response or VGPR	84	76	0.009

VGPR, very good partial response
*Responses assessed according to International Uniform Response Criteria for MM
[†]Includes 4 patients (2%) in lenalidomide group and 5 (2%) in placebo group with disappearance of M protein on immunofixation but no BM marrow evaluation
[‡]Includes 6 patients (2%) in lenalidomide group and 9 (3%) in placebo group with disappearance of M protein on immunofixation but no BM marrow evaluation

Attal M et al. N Engl J Med 2012;366:1782–1791

(continued)

Efficacy (continued)

Survival Endpoints

	Lenalidomide (N = 307)	Placebo (N = 307)	HR *p* value
Progressive disease	104	160	HR 1.25 *P* = 0.29
Median progression-free survival	41 months	23 months	*P* <0.001
Overall survival 3 years after randomization	80%	84%	

Rate of Progression-Free Survival 3 Years After Randomization*

Probability 3 year progression-free survival	59%	35%	
With VGPR at randomization	64%	49%	*P* = 0.006
Without VGPR at randomization	51%	18%	*P* <0.001
Baseline serum β_2-microglobulin ≤3 mg/L	71%	41%,	*P* <0.001
Baseline serum β_2-microglobulin >3 mg/L	50%	29%	*P* <0.001
With 13q deletion	53%	24%	*P* <0.001
Without 13q deletion	67%	44%	*P* <0.001

VGPR, very good partial response. Median follow-up = 30 months
*Age, sex, isotype of the monoclonal component, International Staging System stage, induction regimen, or number of transplantations did not modify the progression-free survival benefit with lenalidomide

Attal M et al. N Engl J Med 2012;366:1782–1791

Toxicity

Maintenance Therapy

	G3	G4
Hematologic Adverse Events—Number/Total (%)		
Neutropenia	4/88 (5)	2/88 (2)
Thrombocytopenia	0/88	5/88 (6)
Anemia	2/88 (2)	2/88 (2)
Nonhematologic Adverse Events—Number/Total (%)		
Infection*	3/88 (3)	2/88 (2)
Fatigue	2/88 (2)	1/88 (1)
Deep vein thrombosis	2/88 (2)	0/88
Diarrhea	3/88 (3)	1/88 (1)
Bone pain	4/88 (5)	0/88
Diabetes mellitus	2/88 (2)	0/88

*Infection was described in the following terms: pneumonia, lower respiratory tract infection, upper respiratory tract infection, bronchitis, sepsis, urinary tract infection, diverticulitis, herpes zoster, infective arthritis, bacteriuria, cellulitis, gastrointestinal tract infection, oral infection, tooth infection, septic shock, appendicitis, sinusitis, postprocedural infection, streptococcal bacteremia, *Escherichia coli* infection, and meningitis

Palumbo A et al. N Engl J Med 2012;366:1759–1769

(continued)

Toxicity (*continued*)

Hematologic Adverse Events Following Randomization to Placebo or Maintenance Lenalidomide

	Lenalidomide (N = 231)		Placebo (N = 229)		
	G3	G4	G3	G4	
Event	Number of Patients (%)				*p* Value
Neutropenia	74 (32)	30 (13)	27 (12)	7 (3)	<0.001
Thrombocytopenia	21 (9)	11 (5)	3 (1)	8 (3)	0.001
Lymphopenia	15 (6)	1 (<1)	3 (1)	1 (<1)	0.01
Anemia	9 (4)	2 (1)	1 (<1)	0	0.006
Leukopenia	24 (10)	3 (1)	7 (3)	1 (<1)	0.001
Any event	74 (32)	36 (16)	27 (12)	12 (5)	<0.001

McCarthy PL et al. N Engl J Med 2012;366:1770–1781

Adverse Events After Randomization in the Treated Population

	Lenalidomide Group (N = 306)		Placebo Group (N = 302)	
	All Events	G3/4	All Events	G3/4
Event	Number of Patients (%)			
Any event	305 (>99)	225 (74)	297 (98)	130 (43)
Hematologic Events				
Hematologic events	210 (69)	179 (58)	107 (35)	68 (22)
Neutropenia	180 (59)	157 (51)	78 (26)	53 (18)
Febrile neutropenia	6 (2)	4 (1)	1 (<1)	1 (<1)
Anemia	31 (10)	10 (3)	28 (9)	7 (2)
Thrombocytopenia	74 (24)	44 (14)	45 (15)	20 (7)
Nonhematologic Events				
Nausea and vomiting	48 (16)	1 (<1)	54 (18)	0
Constipation	61 (20)	2 (1)	58 (19)	0
Diarrhea	123 (40)	5 (2)	61 (20)	1 (<1)
Fatigue	145 (47)	15 (5)	122 (40)	6 (2)
Pyrexia	62 (20)	1 (<1)	33 (11)	0
Peripheral edema	20 (7)	0	19 (6)	0
Upper respiratory infection	215 (70)	7 (2)	194 (64)	2 (1)
Pneumonia	35 (11)	11 (4)	14 (5)	5 (2)
Herpes zoster	51 (17)	7 (2)	53 (18)	4 (1)

(*continued*)

Toxicity (continued)

Event	Lenalidomide Group (N = 306)		Placebo Group (N = 302)	
	All Events	G3/4	All Events	G3/4
	Number of Patients (%)			
Nonhematologic Events				
Deep vein thrombosis	14 (5)	7 (2)	6 (2)	3 (1)
Pulmonary embolism	5 (2)	4 (1)	0	0
Ischemic stroke	2 (1)	2 (1)	0	0
Peripheral neuropathy	71 (23)	4 (1)	49 (16)	3 (1)
Rash	61 (20)	10 (3)	51 (17)	6 (2)
Decreased appetite	18 (6)	0	12 (4)	1 (<1)
Dyspnea	20 (6)	1 (<1)	13 (4)	0
Muscle spasms	119 (39)	2 (1)	70 (23)	1 (<1)

Attal M et al. N Engl J Med 2012;366:1782–1791

Reasons for Discontinuing Treatment

Number in Lenalidomide Group Who Discontinued	Event (Disorder)	Number in Placebo Group Who Discontinued
10	Blood disorders	7
13	Gastrointestinal disorders	3
13	General disorders	3
8	Neoplasms	2
11	Nervous system disorders	6
12	Skin/subcutaneous tissue	8
6	Vascular disorders	3
4	Infections	4
17	Other events	17
83 (27.1%)	TOTAL (%)	44 (14.6%)

Second Primary Cancers

Second Cancer	McCarthy et al		Attal et al*	
	Lenalidomide (N = 231)	Placebo (N = 229)	Lenalidomide (N = 306)	Placebo (N = 302)
	Number of Patients		Number of Patients (Percent)	
Hematologic Cancers[†]				
Acute lymphoblastic leukemia	1	0	3	0
Acute myeloid leukemia	5	0	5[†]	4[‡]
Hodgkin lymphoma	1	0	4	0
Myelodysplastic syndrome	1	0	1	1
Non-Hodgkin lymphoma	0	1	—	—
Total	8	1	13 (4)	5 (2)

(continued)

Toxicity (continued)				Therapy Monitoring

Solid Tumor Cancers

Breast cancer	3	0	2	0
Carcinoid tumor	0	1	—	—
Central nervous system cancer	1	0	—	—
Colorectal cancer	—	—	3	0
Esophageal cancer	—	—	1	0
Gastrointestinal cancer	2	1	—	—
Gynecologic cancer	1	1	—	—
Lung cancer	—	—	0	1
Malignant melanoma	1	2	0	1
Prostate cancer	1	0	2	1
Renal cell carcinoma	—	—	1	1
Sinus cancer	—	—	1	0
Thyroid cancer	1	0	—	—
Total	10	5	10 (3)	4 (1)

Nonmelanoma Skin Cancers

Basal-cell carcinoma	2	1	5 (2)	3 (1)
Squamous-cell carcinoma	2	2		

*Thirty-two second primary cancers in 26 patients were reported in the lenalidomide group versus 12 second primary cancers in 11 patients in the placebo group. The incidence of second primary cancers was 3.1 per 100 patient-years in the lenalidomide group versus 1.2 per 100 patient-years in the placebo group ($P = 0.002$). In the multivariate analysis, the incidence of second primary cancers was significantly related to study-group assignment, age, sex, and International Staging System stage
†Median time to diagnosis of a hematologic cancer after randomization was 28 months (range: 12–46 months) in patients in the lenalidomide group, and 30 months in the 1 hematologic cancer in the placebo group. The median time to the diagnosis of a solid tumor cancer after randomization was 15 months (range: 3–51 months) in the lenalidomide group and 21 months (range: 6–34 months) in the placebo group
‡AML or MDS

Therapy Monitoring

1. Blood counts and physical examinations at regular intervals (1–3 months)
2. Serum and urinary protein electrophoresis studies as indicated at regular intervals (1–3 months)

REGIMEN
MAINTENANCE THERAPY—MULTIPLE MYELOMA
THALIDOMIDE

Morgan GJ et al. Blood 2012;119:7–15

Thalidomide 50 mg/day orally, continually (total dose/week = 350 mg). If tolerated for 4 weeks, dose was increased to:
Thalidomide 100 mg/day orally, continually until disease progression (total dose/week = 700 mg)

Supportive Care
Antiemetic prophylaxis
Emetogenic potential is **MINIMAL–LOW**
See Chapter 39 for antiemetic recommendations

Hematopoietic growth factor (CSF) prophylaxis
Primary prophylaxis is NOT indicated
See Chapter 43 for more information

Antimicrobial prophylaxis
Risk of fever and neutropenia is INTERMEDIATE
Antimicrobial primary prophylaxis to be considered:
- Antibacterial—consider a fluoroquinolone or no prophylaxis; *Pneumocystis jirovecii* prophylaxis is recommended (eg, cotrimoxazole)
- Antifungal—recommended; consider use during periods of neutropenia
- Antiviral—antiherpes antivirals (eg, acyclovir, famciclovir, valacyclovir)

See Chapter 47 for more information

Thromboprophylaxis
Risk assessment and recommendations for VTE prophylaxis in patients with multiple myeloma with individual or myeloma-related risk factors, or risk factors related to treatment

Individual risk factors
• Obesity (BMI ≥30 kg/m^2)
• H/O VTE
• CVAD or pacemaker
• Comorbid pathologies
  Cardiac disease
  Chronic renal disease
  Diabetes
  Acute infection
  Immobilization
• Surgery
  General surgery
  Any anesthesia
  Trauma
• Medications
  Erythropoietin (epoetin alfa, darbepoetin)
  Estrogenic compounds
  Bevacizumab
• Clotting disorders
  Thrombophilia
Myeloma-related risk factors
• Diagnosis of multiple myeloma
• Hyperviscosity
	≤1 Individual or myeloma risk factor present:
	• **Aspirin** 81–325 mg daily
	
	≥2 Individual or myeloma risk factors present:
	• **LMWH*, equivalent to enoxaparin sodium 40 mg/day** *or* **dalteparin sodium 5000 IU/day**; administer subcutaneously, *or*
	• **Warfarin**, targeting an INR = 2–3

(continued)

Treatment Modifications

Thalidomide Dose Levels

Dose Level 1	200 mg daily
Dose Level –1	100 mg daily
Dose Level –2	50 mg daily

Adverse Event	Treatment Modification
Febrile neutropenia	Withhold therapy until fever abates, then resume therapy
G4 hematologic toxicity	Withhold therapy until ANC >750/mm^3 and platelets >50,000/mm^3, then resume therapy with thalidomide dose decreased by 1 dose level
G3/4 nonhematologic toxicity G ≥3 thalidomide neuropathy	Interrupt therapy and follow clinically. After toxicity abates to G ≤2, resume therapy with thalidomide dose decreased by 1 dose level

Patient Population Studied

Patients ≥18 years of age with newly diagnosed MM. Exclusion criteria included asymptomatic myeloma, solitary bone plasmacytoma, and extramedullary plasmacytoma. Patients were assigned to induction treatment via either an "intensive" or a "nonintensive" treatment pathway, as determined by performance status, informed discussion, and patient preference. There was no rigid age cutoff. Patients who completed induction therapy were randomly assigned (1:1) to maintenance therapy with open-label thalidomide (*n* = 408) or no maintenance (*n* = 410). Maintenance randomization was not allowed for those who developed progressive disease or relapse. The target dose of thalidomide was 50 mg/day, which, if tolerated, was increased to 100 mg/day after 4 weeks at the lower dose and continued until disease progression

Standard iFISH (interphase FISH) analysis was used for cytogenetic profiling. "Adverse" iFISH was defined as the cytogenetic abnormalities gain(1q), t(4;14), t(14;16), t(14;20), and del(17p); del(1p32) was an adverse prognostic factor only in younger patients. "Favorable" iFISH was defined by the absence of these cytogenetic abnormalities and predominantly included hyperdiploidy, t(6;14), and t(11;14)

(continued)

Concomitant treatment-related risk factors Thalidomide or lenalidomide in combination with: • High-dose dexamethasone (≥480 mg/month) • Doxorubicin • Multiagent chemotherapy	**LMWH*, equivalent to enoxaparin sodium** 40 mg/day *or* **dalteparin sodium** 5000 IU/day; administer subcutaneously, *or* **Warfarin**, targeting an INR = 2–3

CVAD, central vascular access device; INR, international normalized ratio; LMWH, low-molecular-weight heparin; VTE, venous thromboembolic disease
*LMWHs should be used with caution in individuals with impaired renal function (creatinine clearance <30 mL/min). Refer to product labeling for information about doses and administration schedules in renally impaired patients, and guidance for monitoring antifactor Xa concentrations

Geerts WH et al. Chest 2008;133(6 Suppl):381S–453S
Multiple Myeloma, V.1.2014. National Comprehensive Cancer Network, Inc., 2013. (Accessed October 8, 2013, at http://www.nccn.org)
Palumbo A et al. Leukemia 2008;22:414–423
Venous Thromboembolic Disease, V.2.2013. National Comprehensive Cancer Network, Inc., 2013. (Accessed October 8, 2013, at http://www.nccn.org)

Bisphosphonates
All patients receiving primary therapy for symptomatic multiple myeloma should receive a bisphosphonate adjunctively; *for example*:
• **Pamidronate disodium** 90 mg; administer intravenously over 2–4 hours, every month, *or*
• **Zoledronic acid** 4 mg; administer intravenously over at least 15 minutes, every month
Consider baseline bone densitometry evaluation
See Chapter 43 for more information

Therapy Monitoring
1. Blood counts and physical examinations at regular intervals (1–3 months)
2. Serum and urinary protein electrophoresis studies as indicated at regular intervals (1–3 months)

Efficacy

Summary of Key Trials Evaluating Thalidomide Maintenance Therapy in Multiple Myeloma*

Trial	N	Primary Treatment	Maintenance	Cytogenetic Testing	EFS or PFS	OS
Brinker	112	BU/CY/VP-16 or HDM + ABMT or ASCT	THAL vs observation	—	—	Median OS 65 vs 54 months $P = 0.05$[†]
IFM-9902	597	Double ASCT	THAL/PAM vs no maintenance	del(13) only[‡]	3-year EFS 52% vs 37% $P <0.009$	4-year OS 87% vs 74% $P <0.04$
Total Therapy 2	668	Double ASCT	THAL vs no maintenance until disease progression	Any abnormality vs none	5-year EFS 56% vs 45% $P = 0.0005$	5-year OS 67% vs 65% $P = 0.09$
Spencer et al	243	Single ASCT	THAL (12 months) + PRED vs PRED	None	3-year PFS 42% vs 23% $P <0.001$	3-year OS 86% vs 75% $P = 0.004$
Ludwig et al	128	THAL/DEX vs MP	THAL/IFN vs IFN until disease progression	None	Median PFS 27.7 vs 13.2 months $P <0.0068$	Median OS 52.6 vs 51.4 months $P = NS$

(continued)

Efficacy (continued)

Summary of Key Trials Evaluating Thalidomide Maintenance Therapy in Multiple Myeloma*

Trial	N	Primary Treatment	Maintenance	Cytogenetic Testing	EFS or PFS	OS
MRC Myeloma IX	820	Single ASCT or nonintensive therapy (MP vs CTDa)	THAL vs no maintenance, until disease progression	Extensive§	Median PFS 23 vs 15 months P = 0.0003	Median OS 60 vs 58 months P = NS
Stewart	322	Various + HDM + ASCT	THAL/PRED vs observation	FISH on BM > ASCT€	4-year MS-PFS and PFS 32% vs 14% P <0.0001	4-year OS 68% vs 60% P = 0.18

ABMT, autologous bone marrow transplantation; ASCT, autologous stem cell transplantation; BU/CY/VP-16, busulfan, cyclophosphamide, and etoposide; CTDa, attenuated regimen of cyclophosphamide, thalidomide, and dexamethasone; DEX, dexamethasone; EFS, event-free survival; HDM, high-dose melphalan; IFN, interferon; MP, melphalan and prednisone; MS-PFS, myeloma-specific PFS; N, number of patients; NS, not significant; OS, overall survival; PAM, pamidronate; PFS, progression-free survival; PRED, prednisone; THAL, thalidomide
*Adapted from Morgan GJ et al. Blood 2012;119:7–15
†Comparing thalidomide maintenance vs thalidomide salvage
‡EFS benefit was seen in patients without del(13)
§PFS benefit was seen in patients with a favorable cytogenetic profile; thalidomide maintenance therapy was associated with worse OS than no maintenance therapy in patients with an unfavorable cytogenetic profile
€Both OS (multivariate HR = 2.24; 95% CI, 1.11–4.54; P = 0.02) and PFS (multivariate HR = 2.23; 95% CI, 1.34–3.69; P = 0.002) were worse in high-genetic-risk patients

Attal M et al. Blood 2006;108:3289–3294
Barlogie B et al. Blood 2008;112:3115–3121
Brinker BT et al. Cancer 2006;106:2171–2180
Ludwig H et al. Haematologica 2010;95:1548–1554
Morgan GJ et al. Blood 2012;119:7–15
Spencer A et al. J Clin Oncol 2009;27:1788–1793
Stewart AK et al. Blood 2013;121:1517–1523

Toxicity

Adverse Events (Safety Population)

Event	Intensive Induction Maintenance Yes (N = 246)	No (N = 247)	P	Nonintensive Induction Maintenance Yes (N = 164)*	No (N = 163)	P	Overall P*
Any SAE†	60 (24.4)	51 (20.6)	0.33	56 (34.1)	33 (20.2)	0.0061	0.012
Suspect unrelated to study drugs	48 (19.5)	46 (18.6)	0.82	43 (26.2)	31 (19.0)	0.15	0.26
Any serious adverse reaction‡	21 (8.5)	7 (2.8)	0.0064	16 (9.8)	4 (2.5)	0.0095	0.00014
Thromboembolic events	4 (1.6)	4 (1.6)	1.0	3 (1.8)	5 (3.1)	0.50	0.80
Hematologic disorders	0	2 (0.8)	0.50	0	0	NA	0.50
Cardiovascular disorders	2 (0.8)	1 (0.4)	0.62	4 (2.4)	0	0.12	0.12
Gastrointestinal disorders	2 (0.8)	0	0.25	0	1 (0.6)	0.50	1.0
Infection	6 (2.4)	0	0.015	1 (0.6)	1 (0.6)	1.0	0.069
Nervous system disorders	6 (2.4)	1 (0.4)	0.068	3 (1.8)	2 (1.2)	1.0	0.14
Renal and urinary disorders	3 (1.2)	0	0.12	1 (0.6)	0	1.0	0.12
Skin/subcutaneous disorders	3 (1.2)	0	0.12	2 (1.1)	0	0.50	0.062

NA, not applicable; SAE, serious adverse event
*P value for comparison of maintenance (n = 246 + 164 = 410) versus no maintenance (n = 247 + 163 = 410)
†Irrespective of suspected association with study drugs; patients who had >1 type of adverse event have been listed against all relevant types of events, but patients who had >1 occurrence of the same type of event are recorded only once
‡Suspected association with study drugs

28. Ovarian Cancer

Eddie Reed, MD

Epidemiology

Incidence: 21,980 (Estimated new cases for 2014 in the United States)
Deaths: Estimated 14,270 in 2014
Median age: 63 years

Stage at presentation
Limited (Stage I-II):   25–30%
Advanced (Stage III-IV):   70–75%

Siegel R et al. CA Cancer J Clin 2014;64:9–29
Surveillance, Epidemiology and End Results (SEER) Program, available from http://seer.cancer.gov (accessed in 2014)

Pathology

WHO classification of malignant ovarian tumors

1. Common epithelial tumors (60% of all neoplasms of ovary; 90% of all malignant neoplasms of ovary)
2. Sex cord–stromal tumor (5% of malignant neoplasms of ovary)
3. Lipid (lipoid) cell tumors (rare)
4. Gonadoblastoma (rare)

Tumor Grade
• Grade 1—Well differentiated
• Grade 2—Moderately differentiated
• Grade 3—Poorly differentiated

Note: Serous carcinoma can be classified into either low grade or high grade

Ozols RF, Schwartz PE, Eifel PJ. In: DeVita VT Jr, Hellman S, Rosenberg SA, eds. Cancer: Principles & Practice of Oncology, 6th ed. Philadelphia, PA: Lippincott Williams & Wilkins; 2001:1596–1632

Work-up

1. Personal and family history, physical examination
2. Liver function tests, BUN, creatinine, LDH
3. CBC with platelets, PT, PTT, INR
4. Tumor markers (CA-125, α-fetoprotein (AFP), HCG)
5. CT scan of abdomen and pelvis, and chest x-ray. CT of chest if chest x-ray is abnormal
6. Radiographic tests of unclear utility: MRI of abdomen and pelvis, PET scan

5-year Relative Survival by Stage at Diagnosis

Stage at Diagnosis	5-year Relative Survival (%)
Localized (confined to primary site)	91.9
Regional (spread to regional lymph nodes)	72.0
Distant (cancer has metastasized)	27.3

Surveillance, Epidemiology and End Results (SEER) Program, available from http://seer.cancer.gov (accessed in 2013)

Treatment and survival by stage cannot be summarized simply for ovarian cancer. Each stage is strongly influenced by whether the disease is amenable to surgery, by the histologic type and grade, by the bulk of residual disease after the completion of surgery, and by other factors
Differences in survival among patients with the same stage of disease may indicate incomplete staging. When comprehensive staging is performed, a substantial number of patients initially believed to have disease confined to the pelvis will be staged upward

Staging

Primary Tumor (T)

TNM Category	FIGO Stage	
TX		Primary tumor cannot be assessed
T0		No evidence of primary tumor
T1	I	Tumor limited to ovaries (one or both)
T1a	IA	Tumor limited to one ovary; capsule intact, no tumor on ovarian surface. No malignant cells in ascites or peritoneal washings
T1b	IB	Tumor limited to both ovaries; capsules intact, no tumor on ovarian surface. No malignant cells in ascites or peritoneal washings
T1c	IC	Tumor limited to one or both ovaries with any of the following: capsule ruptured, tumor on ovarian surface, malignant cells in ascites or peritoneal washings
T2	II	Tumor involves 1 or both ovaries with pelvic extension and/or implants
T2a	IIA	Extension and/or implants on uterus and/or tube(s). No malignant cells in ascites or peritoneal washings
T2b	IIB	Extension to and/or implants on other pelvic tissues. No malignant cells in ascites or peritoneal washings
T2c	IIC	Pelvic extension and/or implants (T2a or T2b) with malignant cells in ascites or peritoneal washings
T3	III	Tumor involves one or both ovaries with microscopically confirmed peritoneal metastasis outside the pelvis
T3a	IIIA	Microscopic peritoneal metastasis beyond pelvis (no macroscopic tumor)
T3b	IIIB	Macroscopic peritoneal metastasis beyond pelvis 2 cm or less in greatest dimension
T3c	IIIC	Peritoneal metastasis beyond pelvis more than 2 cm in greatest dimension and/or regional lymph node metastasis

Note: Liver capsule metastasis T3/Stage III; liver parenchymal metastasis M1/Stage IV
Pleural effusion must have positive cytology for M1/Stage IV

Regional Lymph Nodes (N)

TNM Category	FIGO Stage	
NX		Regional lymph nodes cannot be assessed
N0		No regional lymph node metastasis
N1	IIIC	Regional lymph node metastasis

Distant Metastasis (M)

TNM Category	FIGO Stage	
M0		No distant metastasis (no pathologic M0; use clinical M to complete stage group)
M1	IV	Distant metastasis (excludes peritoneal metastasis)

Staging

Group	T	N	M
I	T1	N0	M0
IA	T1a	N0	M0
IB	T1b	N0	M0
IC	T1c	N0	M0
II	T2	N0	M0
IIA	T2a	N0	M0
IIB	T2b	N0	M0
IIC	T2c	N0	M0
III	T3	N0	M0
IIIA	T3a	N0	M0
IIIB	T3b	N0	M0
IIIC	T3c	N0	M0
	Any T	N1	M0
IV	Any T	Any N	M1

Edge SB, Byrd DR, Compton CC, Fritz AG, Greene FL, Trotti A, eds. AJCC Cancer Staging Manual. 7th ed. New York, NY: Springer; 2010

Expert Opinion
Chemotherapy

Early Stage Disease

1. In good-prognosis, early stage disease, surgery alone is adequate therapy: there is a 95% 10-year survival rate (Ia or Ib)
2. In early stage patients who have an increased risk for recurrence (poorly differentiated histologies):
   - Three cycles of cisplatin + cyclophosphamide, reduced the risk of recurrence and improve survival
   - A comparable European study gives similar data for cisplatin alone versus ^{32}P
   - Three cycles of paclitaxel and carboplatin may offer as much benefit, but the data are not yet conclusive

Bolis G et al. Ann Oncol 1995;6:887–893
Young RC et al. J Clin Oncol 2003;21:4350–4355
Young RC. Semin Oncol 2000;27(3 Suppl 7):8–10

Advanced-Stage Disease (≥IIc)

1. Standard of care for advanced-stage disease: depends in part on the amount of residual disease
   - Patients with stage III disease that is optimally debulked with no residual mass greater than 1 cm in diameter after surgery should be treated, if possible, with intraperitoneal cisplatin and paclitaxel
   - Six cycles of paclitaxel + carboplatin are used if debulking surgery was not optimal
2. Benefit of 3-drug combinations in this setting is uncertain:
   - Paclitaxel + carboplatin, + topotecan
   - Paclitaxel + carboplatin + gemcitabine
   - Paclitaxel + cisplatin + cyclophosphamide (most effective 3-drug regimen)
3. Generally, dose-intense approaches requiring stem cell support are ill advised
4. Benefit of "consolidation" therapy, after an initial 6 cycles of systemic treatment is uncertain
   - Consolidation regimens: Several additional cycles of single-agent paclitaxel or a paclitaxel combination

Kohn EC et al. Gynecol Oncol 1996;62:181–191
McGuire WP et al. N Engl J Med 1996;334:1–6
Ozols RF et al. J Clin Oncol 2003;21:3194–200
Sarosy GA, Reed E. [Editorial] Ann Intern Med 2000;133:555–556

Recurrent Disease

1. Treatment of recurrent disease is complex. Decisions should be based on:
   - Likelihood of sensitivity/resistance to agents given in the past: platinum-sensitive or platinum-resistant disease
   - Residual toxicity from prior treatments
   - Comorbid illnesses, including renal, hepatic, and cardiac function
   - Desires of the patient
2. *Platinum-sensitive disease*
   - Epithelial ovarian cancer that recurs ≥1–2 years after platinum-based chemotherapy
   - Response rate to retreatment with another platinum agent-based regimen tends to be high (<70%)
3. *Platinum-resistant disease*
   - Disease progression in the face of appropriate initial platinum-based treatment
   - Disease recurrence within the first 6 months after an initial response to platinum-based therapy
   - Poor prognosis, especially if disease progresses during their initial 6 cycles of therapy with platinum agents
   - Use of non–cross-resistant agents in the second-line and third-line setting is critically important

Leitao MM Jr et al. Gynecol Oncol 2003;91:123–129
Markman M et al. J Cancer Res Clin Oncol 2004;130:25–28
Markman M et al. Gynecol Oncol 2004;93:699–701
Reed E et al. Gynecol Oncol 1992;46:326–329

Platinum Hypersensitivity

1. Platinum hypersensitivity can develop in patients who have received ≥6 cycles of cisplatin or carboplatin
2. A desensitization regimen should be used
3. Rarely, desensitization is unsuccessful. In this situation, consider doxorubicin with cyclophosphamide

Surgery

1. Ideally, a gynecologic oncologist should perform all surgical procedures for ovarian cancer, including:
   - Initial staging and debulking surgery
   - Second-look procedure (if done)
   - Any interval surgical debulking procedure
2. Goals of initial surgical procedure:
   - Stage disease
   - Remove all visible disease from the abdominopelvic cavity; or, if surgeon cannot remove all visible disease, remove all disease possible (debulking surgery)
3. Debulking important because subsequent survival and response to chemotherapy are linked to:
   - Dimension of the largest remaining tumor lesion after completion of surgery
   - Possibly, the overall volume of residual disease
4. Surgery alone is the preferred approach to patients with good-prognosis, early stage epithelial ovarian cancer:
   - Stage: Ia or Ib
   - Any epithelial histology other than clear cell
   - Well-differentiated or moderately well-differentiated histologic grade (low grade). (Any early stage patient other than the latter should have postsurgery chemotherapy.)
5. Neoadjuvant chemotherapy (has not received widespread acceptance):
   - Two to 3 cycles of chemotherapy before an initial staging and debulking procedure
   - Data suggest a less-morbid operation with reduced blood loss and a shorter operative procedure

Hoskins WJ et al. Am J Obstet Gynecol 1994;170:974–979; discussion 979–980
Schwartz PE, Zheng W. Gynecol Oncol 2003;90:644–650
Schwartz PE et al. Gynecol Oncol 1999;72:93–99

Germ Cell Tumors

The recommended laboratory evaluation for germ cell tumors should include:
1. A comprehensive metabolic panel, CBC with platelets, magnesium level, LDH, AFP, and HCG levels
2. Pulmonary function studies may be obtained
3. Complete surgical staging is recommended as initial surgery, with fertility-sparing surgery considered in those desiring fertility

Stage I dysgerminoma or immature teratoma

1. Patients who have had complete surgical staging and no evidence of disease is found outside the ovary should be observed
2. Patients who have had incomplete surgical staging for whom observation without chemotherapy is being considered, should undergo a complete staging procedure. If no evidence of disease is found outside the ovary these patients may be observed. If, at the time of a complete surgical staging, tumor is found outside the ovary, patients should receive bleomycin + etoposide + cisplatin (BEP) in the postoperative period

Stages II–IV dysgerminoma or stage I, grades 2–3 immature teratoma or embryonal tumors or endodermal sinus tumors

1. These patients should receive chemotherapy for 3–4 cycles with bleomycin + etoposide + cisplatin (BEP)
2. Patients achieving a complete clinical response should be observed clinically every 2–4 months with AFP and HCG levels (if initially elevated) for 2 years
3. Patients with radiographic evidence of residual tumor but with normal AFP and HCG levels should be considered for surgical resection of the tumor; observation can be considered
4. Patients with persistently elevated AFP and/or HCG after chemotherapy, or with clinically or radiographically evident disease, should receive chemotherapy or radiation or supportive care. Acceptable regimens for recurrent disease include:
   - Cisplatin + etoposide
   - VIP (etoposide + ifosfamide + cisplatin)
   - VeIP (vinblastine + ifosfamide + cisplatin)
   - VAC (vincristine + dactinomycin + cyclophosphamide)

Radiation

1. External beam radiation therapy:
   - Very useful in the treatment of some subsets of patients with early stage disease
   - Has fallen out of favor in the United States
   - Commonly used in some academic centers in Canada and Europe
   - Major drawback is the reduction in reserve function of organs within the radiation field, such as the bone marrow
   - Useful in the management of tumor masses that might cause extreme pain, bleeding, or other medical problems and in cases in which surgery is not a good option
   - On occasion, large lesions in the pelvis or metastases to bone (unusual) respond readily to radiation
2. Intraperitoneal colloidal ^{32}P:
   - Useful in the treatment of early stage disease
   - Can be of palliative value in other settings
   - Has fallen out of favor in the United States
3. Gamma-knife, intensity-modulated radiation therapy (IMRT), and standard whole-brain radiation:
   - Metastases to the brain occur uncommonly but are no longer considered rare
   - Several approaches are effective in controlling CNS disease
   - Use of these approaches depends on the clinical setting and the technology available

Ovarian Stromal Tumors

1. Patients with stages IA–C ovarian stromal tumors desiring fertility should be treated with fertility-sparing surgery. Otherwise, complete staging is recommended to all other patients
2. Those with surgical findings of stage I tumor should be observed
3. Patients having high-risk stage I (tumor rupture, poorly differentiated tumor, tumor size >10–15 cm) or stages II–IV tumors can be observed, or can receive radiation therapy or undergo cisplatin-based chemotherapy with germ cell regimens preferred
4. Patients subsequently having a clinical relapse may consider secondary cytoreductive surgery, enter a clinical trial, or be offered supportive care

Toxicities: Ovarian Cancer Chemotherapy

1. **Myelosuppression**

   Associated with all the agents listed in this chapter except tamoxifen. All 3 lineages are affected. Persistent thrombocytopenia is associated with the platinum compounds

2. **Nausea and vomiting**

   Preventive treatment is very important. Delayed nausea and vomiting is very common. Steroids, serotonin (HT_3)-receptor antagonists, and neurokinin (NK_1)-receptor antagonists are recommended for routine use with platinum-containing regimens

3. **Renal dysfunction**

   Seen with cisplatin and with carboplatin, but usually more clinically significant with cisplatin. Serum creatinine may be normal in the face of a markedly reduced creatinine clearance. This is important because other drugs that are eliminated by the kidney may be needed (eg, antibiotics). Platinum-related renal insufficiency is nonoliguric: be vigilant

4. **Neurotoxicity**

   Clinically occurs before detectable changes on EMG/NCTs. Bilateral paresthesias in stocking-and-glove distribution usually are progressive with repeated platinum doses and can become severe. Cisplatin is more likely to cause this problem than carboplatin

5. **Fatigue/weakness**

   May be related to anemia, but is a common side effect of several newer agents, including gemcitabine and topotecan

6. **Altered sexual function**

   A common side effect, but is seldom discussed spontaneously by a patient. It can be an underlying contributing factor to family disruption and clinical reactive depression; usually is a combined function of surgery and effect of neuroactive anticancer agent (platinum agents)

7. **Clinical depression**

   A common side effect. Many patients request medication for this. Sometimes may be a severe problem

8. **Rare toxicities**

   Acute hypersensitivity to paclitaxel. Acute hypersensitivity to cisplatin/carboplatin (usually occurs after 6–8 cycles of therapy). Desensitization is occasionally appropriate and can be successful. On most occasions, switch to another agent right away

Epithelial Ovarian Cancer (EOC), Primary Peritoneal Cancer (PPC), Fallopian Tube Cancer Chemotherapy: Expert Opinion

Early stage disease [IA, IB, IC]

1. IA, grades 1/2 and IB, grades 1/2 (good prognosis, early stage disease):
   - Surgery alone is adequate therapy with a 95% 10-year survival rate

2. IA, grade 3, IB, grade 3, IC, grades 1/2/3, and some IA/IB grade 2 (early stage patients who are at increased risk for recurrence):
   - Three cycles of cisplatin + cyclophosphamide: reduced risk of recurrence, and improved survival
   - A comparable European study gives similar data for cisplatin alone versus ^{32}P
   - Three to 6 cycles of paclitaxel and carboplatin may offer as much benefit, but the data are not yet conclusive

Bolis G et al. Ann Oncol 1995;6:887–893
Young RC et al. J Clin Oncol 2003;21:4350–4355
Young RC. Semin Oncol 2000;27(3 Suppl 7):8–10

Advanced stage disease (Stage II, III or IV)

1. **Standard of care** for advanced stage disease:
   - Six to 8 cycles of paclitaxel + carboplatin, after debulking surgery

2. Additional standard option in <1 cm, optimally debulked, Stages II/II patients:
   - **Intraperitoneal (IP) chemotherapy** every 3 weeks for 6 cycles
     - (Day 1) Paclitaxel 135 mg/m² by continuous intravenous infusion over 24 hours
     - (Day 2) Cisplatin 75–100 mg/m² intraperitoneally
     - (Day 8) Paclitaxel 60 mg/m² intraperitoneally

3. **Three-drug combinations** in this setting provide no added benefit
   - GOG 182/ICON5: Five-arm randomized trial, to determine if adding either topotecan, gemcitabine, or pegylated liposomal doxorubicin in the frontline setting would extend PFS or OS. Control arm = paclitaxel and carboplatin IV every 3 weeks × 8 cycles. Accrual >1200 patients/year; 4312 women enrolled. None of the 3-drug regimens demonstrated an improvement in either PFS or OS. Survival analyses of groups defined by size of residual disease (optimal or suboptimal cytoreduction) also failed to show experimental benefit in any subgroup (Bookman et al. J Clin Oncol 2009)

(continued)

Epithelial Ovarian Cancer (EOC), Primary Peritoneal Cancer (PPC), Fallopian Tube Cancer
Chemotherapy: Expert Opinion (*continued*)

4. **Dose-dense weekly paclitaxel**
   - A randomized phase III trial comparing a dose-dense regimen of weekly paclitaxel (days 1, 8, and 15) in combination with carboplatin every 3 weeks versus both agents administered once every 3 weeks, showed statistically significant improvement with the dose-dense paclitaxel regimen in: (a) PFS (28.0 vs. 17.2) and (b) OS at 3 years (72.1% vs. 65.1% [hazard ratio = 0.75; confidence interval, 0.57–0.98]). However, patient dropout was higher in the dose-dense group, primarily related to hematologic toxicity (Katsumata et al. Lancet 2009)

5. Generally, **dose-intense approaches requiring stem cell support** are ill advised

6. Benefit of **"consolidation" therapy** is uncertain (ie, several additional cycles of single-agent paclitaxel or a paclitaxel combination, after an initial 6 cycles of systemic treatment)

7. Whether **maintenance therapy** can increase PFS and, most importantly, increase OS is under evaluation. Most maintenance therapy strategies continue a regimen with lower toxicity and often include agents used in the primary treatment regimen
   - SWOG and GOG randomized women who achieved a CR with primary therapy to either 3 or 12 cycles of maintenance IV paclitaxel. Twelve cycles resulted in a 7-month PFS advantage but an uncertain OS advantage because of early termination
   - In Europe, Pecorelli et al. reported no gains in PFS or OS in patients given an additional 6 cycles of paclitaxel *after a complete response* from initial therapy
   - GOG 212 is ongoing (Paclitaxel or Polyglutamate Paclitaxel or Observation in Treating Patients With Stage III or Stage IV Ovarian Epithelial or Peritoneal Cancer or Fallopian Tube Cancer)

8. The benefit of adding **bevacizumab** to a standard frontline IV paclitaxel/carboplatin regimen administered every 3 weeks is under debate. Evidence suggests that in standard-risk patients, it does not confer any benefit. It remains to be determined whether it may be beneficial in high-risk patients. The GOG-218 and ICON7 trials suggest a role for maintenance bevacizumab in ovarian cancer; however, the absolute benefit in PFS is very modest, and neither trial showed an OS benefit. There is no level I evidence for (a) *the use of bevacizumab in patients receiving intraperitoneal (IP) chemotherapy*, or (b) *the use of bevacizumab as neoadjuvant chemotherapy prior to surgical cytoreduction*. In addition to resolving whether this therapy is indicated, future trials will need to address (a) an optimal bevacizumab dosage (7.5 mg/kg or 15 mg/kg every 3 weeks); (b) the optimal duration of bevacizumab maintenance (1 year, until progression, or beyond progression); and (c) any biologic predictors given bevacizumab's modest activity and substantial toxicity and cost
   - GOG 218 (3 arms): (a) cyclophosphamide + paclitaxel (CP); (b) CP + concomitant bevacizumab only, and (c) CP + concomitant and maintenance bevacizumab. After a median follow-up of 17.4 months, PFS was significantly prolonged with CP + concomitant and maintenance bevacizumab compared with CP alone (14.1 vs. 10.3 months; hazard ratio [HR] = 0.717; p <0.0001). Importantly there was no PFS advantage for CP + *concomitant bevacizumab only* over the CP-alone control arm (11.2 vs. 10.3 months; HR = 0.908; p = 0.080)
   - ICON7: Median PFS 19.8 months for women receiving concurrent and maintenance bevacizumab compared with 17.4 months for those in the control arm (*P* = 0.039). Overall survival, among all participants was not improved (HR for death of 0.85, 95% CI, 0.69–1.04). But in the high risk subgroup—stage III with ≥1 cm residual tumor after surgery and all stage IV patients—the HR was 0.64, 95% CI, 0.48–0.85, *P* = 0.002

Bookman MA et al. J Clin Oncol 2009;27:1419–1425. Erratum in: J Clin Oncol 2009;27:2305
Burger RA et al. Proc Am Soc Clin Oncol 2010;28(15S, Part I of II):5s [abstract LBA1]
du Bois A et al. Ann Oncol 2005;16(Suppl 8):viii7–viii12
Katsumata N et al. Lancet 2009;374:1331–1338
Kristensen G. Proc Am Soc Clin Oncol 2011;29(18S, Part II of II):781s [abstract LBA5006]
McGuire WP et al. N Engl J Med 1996;334:1–6
Ozols RF et al. J Clin Oncol 2003;21:3194–3200
Papadimitriou C et al. Bone Marrow Transplant 2008;41:547–554

Recurrent disease

1. Treatment of recurrent disease is complex. Decisions should be based on:
   - Likelihood of sensitivity/resistance to agents given in the past: platinum-sensitive or -resistant disease
   - Residual toxicity from prior treatments
   - Comorbid illnesses including renal, hepatic, and cardiac function
   - Desires of the patient

Definitions:

Platinum-refractory disease
- Disease that grows through initial platinum-containing therapy

Platinum-sensitive disease
- Epithelial ovarian cancer that recurs, ≥1–2 years after platinum-based chemotherapy
- Response rate to retreatment with another platinum agent-based regimen tends to be high (<70%)

Platinum-resistant disease
- *Definition:* Disease progression in the face of appropriate initial platinum-based treatment or disease recurrence within the first 6 months after an initial response to platinum-based therapy
- *Prognosis:* Poor, especially if disease progresses during the initial 6 cycles of therapy with platinum agents
- *Chemotherapy recommendations:* Use of non–cross-resistant agents in the second-line and third-line settings is critically important

(continued)

Epithelial Ovarian Cancer (EOC), Primary Peritoneal Cancer (PPC), Fallopian Tube Cancer

Chemotherapy: Expert Opinion (continued)

2. Patients with disease progression without evidence of benefit after the initial 2 therapies should either be enrolled on a clinical trial or enroll in hospice

3. Patients who have not received chemotherapy should be approached as discussed above under **Advanced stage disease (Stage II, III, or IV)**

4. Patients with "platinum-sensitive disease" can receive platinum doublets including:
   - Carboplatin + paclitaxel
   - Cisplatin + paclitaxel
   - Cisplatin + cyclophosphamide
   - Carboplatin + weekly paclitaxel
   - Carboplatin + docetaxel
   - Carboplatin + gemcitabine
   - Carboplatin + liposomal doxorubicin
   - Cisplatin + gemcitabine
   - Single-agent cisplatin
   - Single-agent carboplatin
   - Bevacizumab

5. Agents with activity in both platinum-sensitive and platinum-refractory disease include:
   - Docetaxel
   - Pemetrexed
   - Oral etoposide
   - Gemcitabine
   - Liposomal doxorubicin
   - Weekly paclitaxel
   - Topotecan
   - Fluorouracil
   - Altretamine (hexamethylmelamine)

6. **Bevacizumab** seems to be well tolerated and active in second-line and third-line treatments of patients with EOC/PPC. However, there is no evidence indicating that this is better tolerated or more active than myriad other agents previously examined in similar patients. Evidence must yet be developed to support its use in the second-line (or later) setting as a single agent or in combination with a cytotoxic drug (Burger RA et al. J Clin Oncol 2007; Cannistra SA et al. J Clin Oncol 2007)
   - OCEANS: A phase III trial comparing carboplatin and gemcitabine ± bevacizumab in women with platinum-sensitive recurrent ovarian cancer. A 3.7-month PFS advantage for women using bevacizumab, with an interim analysis of OS demonstrating a 5.6-month advantage for the bevacizumab arm

Burger RA et al. J Clin Oncol 2007;25:5165–5171
Cannistra SA et al. J Clin Oncol 2007;25:5180–5186
Leitao MM, Jr et al. Gynecol Oncol 2003;91:123–129
Markman M et al. Gynecol Oncol 2004;93:699–701
Markman M et al. J Cancer Res Clin Oncol 2004;130:25–28
Reed E et al. Gynecol Oncol 1992;46:326–329

Epithelial Ovarian Cancer (EOC), Primary Peritoneal Cancer (PPC), Fallopian Tube Cancer
Surgery: Expert Opinion

1. Ideally, a gynecologic oncologist should perform all surgical procedures for ovarian cancer, including:
   - Initial staging and debulking surgery
   - "Second look" procedures (if done)
   - Any interval surgical debulking procedure
2. Goals of initial surgical procedure:
   - Stage the disease
   - Remove all visible disease from the abdominopelvic cavity, or
   - If surgeon cannot remove all visible disease, remove all disease possible (debulking surgery)
3. Debulking is important because subsequent survival and response to chemotherapy are linked to:
   - Dimension of the largest remaining tumor lesions after the completion of surgery
   - Possibly the overall volume of residual disease
4. Surgery alone, is the preferred approach to patients with good prognosis early stage epithelial ovarian cancer:
   - *Stages:* IA or IB
   - *Histology:* Any epithelial histology other than clear cell
   - *Histologic grade:* Well-differentiated or moderately well-differentiated (any early stage patient other than these should have chemotherapy after surgery)
5. Neoadjuvant chemotherapy:
   - Two to 3 cycles of chemotherapy before an initial staging and debulking procedure
   - Data suggest a less-morbid operation, with reduced blood loss and a shorter operative procedure
   - Has not received widespread acceptance

Hoskins WJ et al. Am J Obstet Gynecol 1994;170:974–979; discussion 979–980
Schwartz PE et al. Gynecol Oncol 1999;72:93–99
Schwartz PE, Zheng W. Gynecol Oncol 2003;90:644–650

PLATINUM-SENSITIVE REGIMEN
CARBOPLATIN + PACLITAXEL

Ozols RF et al. J Clin Oncol 2003;21:3194–3200

Note: Regimen for optimally debulked ovarian cancer and suboptimally debulked disease as well

Premedication for paclitaxel:

Dexamethasone 10 mg/dose; administer orally for 2 doses 12 hours and 6 hours before paclitaxel, *or*

Dexamethasone 20 mg/dose; administer intravenously over 10–15 minutes, 30–60 minutes before paclitaxel (total dose/cycle = 20 mg)

Diphenhydramine 50 mg; administer by intravenous injection 30 minutes before paclitaxel

Cimetidine 300 mg (or **ranitidine** 50 mg, **famotidine** 20 mg, or an equivalent histamine receptor [H_2]-subtype antagonist); administer intravenously over 15–30 minutes, 30–60 minutes before paclitaxel

Paclitaxel 175 mg/m²; administer intravenously in a volume of 0.9% sodium chloride injection (0.9% NS) or 5% dextrose injection (D5W) sufficient to produce a concentration within the range 0.3–1.2 mg/mL, over 3 hours, on day 1, every 3 weeks (total dosage/cycle = 175 mg/m²)

Carboplatin (calculated dose) AUC = 7.5*; administer intravenously in 0.9% NS or D5W 100–500 mL over 60 minutes, on day 1 after completing paclitaxel, every 3 weeks for 6 cycles (total dosage/cycle calculated to produce a target AUC = 7.5 mg/mL · min)

*Carboplatin dose is based on a formula described by Calvert et al. to achieve a target area under the plasma concentration versus time curve (AUC)

$$\text{Total carboplatin dose (mg)} = (\text{target AUC}) \times (\text{GFR} + 25)$$

In practice, creatinine clearance (Clcr) is used in place of glomerular filtration rate (GFR). Clcr can be calculated from the equation of Cockcroft and Gault:

$$\text{For males, Clcr} = \frac{(140 - \text{age [years]}) \times (\text{body weight [kg]})}{72 \times (\text{serum creatinine [mg/dL]})}$$

$$\text{For females, Clcr} = \frac{(140 - \text{age [years]}) \times (\text{body weight [kg]})}{72 \times (\text{serum creatinine [mg/dL]})} \times 0.85$$

Calvert AH et al. J Clin Oncol 1989;7:1748–1756
Cockcroft DW, Gault MH. Nephron 1976;16:31–41
Jodrell DI et al. J Clin Oncol 1992;10:520–528
Sorensen BT et al. Cancer Chemother Pharmacol 1991;28:397–401

Note: On October 8, 2010, the U.S. Food and Drug Administration (FDA) identified a potential safety issue with carboplatin dosing based on recent changes in the measurement of serum creatinine. By the end of 2010, all clinical laboratories in the United States began using the standardized isotope dilution mass spectrometry (IDMS) method to measure serum creatinine, which could result in an overestimation of the GFR in some patients with normal renal function. A carboplatin dose calculated with an IDMS-measured serum creatinine result using the Calvert formula could exceed an expected exposure (AUC) and result in increased drug-related toxicity

Provided actual GFR measurements are made to assess renal function, carboplatin can be safely dosed according to the Calvert formula described in product labeling

If GFR (or creatinine clearance) is estimated based on serum creatinine measurements by the IDMS method, the FDA recommends capping an estimated GFR at 125 mL/min for any targeted AUC value for patients with normal renal function. No greater estimated GFR values should be used

U.S. FDA. Carboplatin dosing. [online] October 8, 2010. Available from: http://www.fda.gov/AboutFDA/CentersOffices/CDER/ucm228974.htm

Supportive Care
Antiemetic prophylaxis
Emetogenic potential is **HIGH**. *Potential for delayed symptoms*
See Chapter 39 for antiemetic recommendations

(continued)

Treatment Modifications

Adverse Event	Dose Modification
At start of a cycle, ANC ≤1000/mm³ or platelets ≤100,000/mm³	Delay start of cycle up to 2 weeks until ANC >1000/mm³ and platelets >100,000/mm³
ANC ≤1000/mm³ or platelets ≤100,000/mm³ for more than 2 but less than 3 weeks after scheduled start of next cycle	Reduce paclitaxel and carboplatin dosages by 20% (140 mg/m² and AUC = 6, respectively)
At start of a cycle, ANC ≤1000/mm³ and platelets ≤100,000/mm³ despite dose reduction	Delay start of cycle until ANC >1000/mm³ and platelets >1000/mm³; then administer filgrastim 5 mcg/kg per day subcutaneously for 14 days with same chemotherapy dosages
Serum creatinine >2 mg/dL (>177 μmol/L) or G ≥3 peripheral neuropathy	Delay start of cycle up to 2 weeks; if serum creatinine is not ≤2 mg/dL (≤177 μmol/L) or G <3 peripheral neuropathy, discontinue therapy

Toxicity* (Carboplatin: N = 392)

	% G3	% G4
Hematologic		
Leukopenia	53	6
Granulocytopenia	17	72
Thrombocytopenia	19	20
Nonhematologic		
Gastrointestinal	5	5
Neurologic†	7	0
Alopecia	0	0
Metabolic	2	1
Genitourinary	1	0
Pain	1	0

*GOG toxicity criteria
†Primarily peripheral neuropathy

(*continued*)

Hematopoietic growth factor (CSF) prophylaxis
Primary prophylaxis is NOT indicated
See Chapter 43 for more information

Antimicrobial prophylaxis
Risk of fever and neutropenia is LOW
   Antimicrobial primary prophylaxis to be considered:
   • Antibacterial—not indicated
   • Antifungal—not indicated
   • Antiviral—not indicated unless patient previously had an episode of HSV
See Chapter 47 for more information

Efficacy (Carboplatin: N = 392)

Median progression-free survival	20.7 months
Median overall survival	57.4 months

Therapy Monitoring

Before repeated cycles: PE, CBC with differential, and serum electrolytes, magnesium, calcium, BUN, and creatinine

Patient Population Studied

A randomized study of 792 women with pathologically verified Stage III epithelial ovarian cancer who were left with no residual disease >1 cm in diameter; 400 cisplatin arm and 392 carboplatin arm. McGuire et al. (N Engl J Med 1996;334:1–6) had shown that cisplatin plus paclitaxel was superior to cisplatin plus cyclophosphamide in advanced-stage epithelial ovarian cancer. This study was a **noninferiority trial** of cisplatin and paclitaxel versus carboplatin and paclitaxel to show equivalence of the 2 regimens

PLATINUM-SENSITIVE REGIMEN

CISPLATIN + PACLITAXEL

Ozols RF et al. J Clin Oncol 2003;21:3194–3200

Premedication with **Dexamethasone** 10 mg/dose; administer orally for 2 doses 12 hours and 6 hours before paclitaxel, *or*
Dexamethasone 20 mg; administer intravenously over 10–15 minutes, 30–60 minutes before paclitaxel (total dose/cycle = 20 mg)
Diphenhydramine 50 mg; administer by intravenous injection 30–60 minutes before paclitaxel
Cimetidine 300 mg (or **Ranitidine** 50 mg, **Famotidine** 20 mg, or an equivalent histamine receptor [H_2]-subtype antagonist); administer intravenously over 15–30 minutes, 30–60 minutes before paclitaxel

Paclitaxel 135 mg/m²; administer intravenously in a volume of 0.9% sodium chloride injection (0.9% NS) or 5% dextrose injection sufficient to produce a concentration within the range 0.3–1.2 mg/mL, over 24 hours on day 1, every 3 weeks, for 6 cycles (total dosage/cycle = 135 mg/m²)
Cisplatin 75 mg/m²; administer intravenously in 0.9% NS 100–250 mL over 1 hour, on day 2 after completing paclitaxel, every 3 weeks, for 6 cycles (total dosage/cycle = 75 mg/m²)
Note: Encourage patients to increase oral intake of nonalcoholic fluids, and provide electrolyte replacement as needed (potassium, magnesium, sodium)

Supportive Care
Antiemetic prophylaxis
*Emetogenic potential during paclitaxel administration is **LOW***
*Emetogenic potential during and after cisplatin administration is **HIGH**. Potential for delayed symptoms*
See Chapter 39 for antiemetic recommendations

Hematopoietic growth factor (CSF) prophylaxis
Primary prophylaxis is NOT indicated
See Chapter 43 for more information

Antimicrobial prophylaxis
Risk of fever and neutropenia is LOW
 Antimicrobial primary prophylaxis to be considered:
 • Antibacterial—not indicated
 • Antifungal—not indicated
 • Antiviral—not indicated unless patient previously had an episode of HSV
See Chapter 47 for more information

Efficacy (Comparison of Regimens)

	Cisplatin (N = 400)	Carboplatin (N = 392)
Median progression-free survival (months)	19.4	20.7
Median overall survival (months)	48.7	57.4

Toxicity

	Cisplatin (N = 400)		Carboplatin (N = 392)	
	% G3	% G4	% G3	% G4
Hematologic				
Leukopenia*	51	12	53	6
Granulo-cytopenia	15	78	17	72
Thrombo-cytopenia*	3	2	19	20
Nonhematologic				
Gastro-intestinal*	14	9	5	5
Neurologic	8	0	7	0
Alopecia	0	0	0	0
Metabolic*	6	2	2	1
Genitourinary*	3	0	1	0
Pain	1	0	1	0
	% G1/2		% G1/2	
Pain	15		26	

*Statistically significant difference at the 0.05 level

Treatment Modifications

Adverse Event	Dose Modification
Delay in achieving ANC ≥1000/mm³ and platelets ≥100,000/mm³ <2 weeks	No dose adjustment; no filgrastim
Delay in achieving ANC ≥1000/mm³ and platelets ≥100,000/mm³ ≥2 weeks but ≤3 weeks	Reduce cisplatin dosage by 20%
Recurrent delays in achieving ANC ≥1000/mm³ and platelets ≥100,000/mm³ ≥2 weeks but ≤3 weeks	Add filgrastim 5 mcg/kg per day subcutaneously. Start 24 hours after completing chemotherapy, and continue for 14 days without further dosage modification
Episode of febrile neutropenia after earlier delay in achieving ANC and platelets led to a reduction in cisplatin dosage	Add filgrastim 5 mcg/kg per day subcutaneously. Start 24 hours after completing chemotherapy, and continue for 14 days without further dosage modification
G3/4 Neurologic toxicity that has not resolved even after a 3-week delay	Discontinue therapy
Creatinine clearance* <30 mL/min (<0.5 mL/s)	Discontinue therapy

*Creatinine clearance used as a measure of glomerular filtration rate (GFR)

Notes

There were no differences in efficacy between the cisplatin + paclitaxel and the carboplatin + paclitaxel treatment regimens. However, there were differences with respect to toxicities. The authors interpreted the data as showing that the carboplatin + paclitaxel regimen was equally efficacious and significantly less toxic than the cisplatin + paclitaxel regimen

PLATINUM-SENSITIVE REGIMEN

INTRAPERITONEAL CISPLATIN AND PACLITAXEL

Armstrong DK et al. N Engl J Med 2006;354:34–43
Walker JL et al. Gynecol Oncol 2006;100:27–32
GOG Protocol #0172

Note: Regimen for Stage III epithelial ovarian or peritoneal carcinoma optimally debulked with no residual mass greater than 1 cm in diameter after surgery. Suboptimally debulked disease should not be treated with this regimen

Premedication for paclitaxel:
Dexamethasone 10 mg/dose; administer orally for 2 doses 12 hours and 6 hours before paclitaxel, *or*
Dexamethasone 20 mg/dose; administer intravenously over 10–15 minutes, 30–60 minutes before paclitaxel (total dose/cycle = 20 mg)
Diphenhydramine 50 mg; administer by intravenous injection 30 minutes before paclitaxel
Cimetidine 300 mg (or **ranitidine** 50 mg, **famotidine** 20 mg, or an equivalent histamine receptor [H_2]-subtype antagonist); administer intravenously over 15–30 minutes, 30–60 minutes before paclitaxel

Paclitaxel 135 mg/m²; administer intravenously in a volume of 0.9% sodium chloride injection (0.9% NS) or 5% dextrose injection (D5W) sufficient to produce a concentration within the range 0.3–1.2 mg/mL, over 24 hours on day 1, every 21 days, for 6 cycles (total dosage of paclitaxel intravenously/cycle = 135 mg/m²)

Intraperitoneal cisplatin
Hydration before cisplatin: ≥1000 mL 0.9% NS; administer by intravenous infusion over a minimum of 2–4 hours
Note: If a large amount of ascites is present, it should be drained prior to the instillation of cisplatin
Cisplatin 100 mg/m²; administer intraperitoneally as rapidly as possible in warmed (37°C [98.6°F]) 0.9% NS 2000 mL through an implanted peritoneal catheter on day 2, every 21 days, for 6 cycles (total dosage/21-day cycle = 100 mg/m²). Following the infusion, patients alternate position from prone, supine, and left and right lateral decubitus every 15 minutes over 2 hours to maximize drug distribution throughout the peritoneal cavity
Note: Do not attempt to retrieve the infusate
Hydration after cisplatin: ≥1000 mL 0.9% NS; administer by intravenous infusion over a minimum of 3–4 hours. Also encourage high oral fluid intake. Goal is to achieve a urine output of ≥100 mL/hour

Intraperitoneal paclitaxel
Note: If a large amount of ascites is present, it should be drained prior to the instillation of paclitaxel
Paclitaxel 60 mg/m²; administer intraperitoneally as rapidly as possible in warmed (37°C [98.6°F]) 0.9% NS or D5W 1000 mL through an implanted peritoneal catheter, followed by an additional 1000 mL of 0.9% NS or D5W on day 8, every 21 days, for 6 cycles (total dosage of paclitaxel administered intraperitoneally/21-day cycle = 60 mg/m²)
Note: Do not attempt to retrieve the infusate

Systemic cisplatin
If intraperitoneal therapy is discontinued, substitute:
Cisplatin 75 mg/m²; administer intravenously in 250 mL 0.9% NS over 30–60 minutes on day 2, every 21 days, for 3 cycles (total dosage/cycle = 75 mg/m²)

Supportive Care
Antiemetic prophylaxis
Emetogenic potential on days 1 and 8 is **LOW**
Emetogenic potential on day 2 is **HIGH**. *Potential for delayed symptoms*
See Chapter 39 for antiemetic recommendations

Hematopoietic growth factor (CSF) prophylaxis
Primary prophylaxis is NOT indicated
See Chapter 43 for more information

(continued)

Treatment Modifications

Dose Modification Levels for Treatment

	IV Paclitaxel	IP Cisplatin	IP Paclitaxel
Starting dose	135 mg/m²	100 mg/m²	60 mg/m²
Level −1	110 mg/m²	75 mg/m²	45 mg/m²

Note: No dose escalations performed

Dose Escalations for Hematologic Toxicity

Adverse Event	Treatment Modification
ANC <1500/mm³ or platelet count <100,000/mm³ on day 1 of a cycle	Delay start of next cycle until ANC ≥1500/mm³ and platelet count ≥100,000/mm³. Do not adjust dosages or add filgrastim if the delay is less than 2 weeks
>2 weeks, but ≤3 weeks delay to start next cycle because ANC <1500/mm³ or platelet count <100,000/mm³ on day 1	Reduce intravenous paclitaxel dosage 1 level
>2 weeks delay in start of a cycle because ANC <1500/mm³ or platelet count <100,000/mm³ on day 1 despite 1 dose reduction	Add filgrastim 5 mcg/kg per day beginning 24 hours after completion of intravenous chemotherapy and continue use for 14 days
>3 weeks delay to start next cycle because ANC <1500/mm³ or platelet count <100,000/mm³ on day 1 regardless of whether filgrastim was or was not used	Discontinue therapy
ANC <1500/mm³ or platelet count <100,000/mm³ on day 8 of a cycle	Do not delay nor adjust intraperitoneal paclitaxel dosage
Uncomplicated WBC or ANC nadirs	Do not modify dosages

(continued)

(continued)

Antimicrobial prophylaxis

Risk of fever and neutropenia is LOW

Antimicrobial primary prophylaxis to be considered:

• Antibacterial—not indicated

• Antifungal—not indicated

• Antiviral—not indicated unless patient previously had an episode of HSV

See Chapter 47 for more information

Arthralgia and myalgia G $\leqq$ 2 associated with chemotherapy

Dexamethasone 4–8 mg/dose orally twice daily for 6 doses after chemotherapy

Toxicity (N = 201)

Toxicity	% G3/4
Hematologic Toxicities	
WBC <1000/mm^3	76
Platelet count <25,000/mm^3	12
Other hematologic event	94
Nonhematologic Toxicities	
Gastrointestinal event	46
Metabolic event	27
Neurologic event	19
Fatigue	18
Infection	16
Pain	11
Cardiovascular event	9
Fever	9
Renal or genitourinary event	7
Pulmonary event	3
Hepatic event	3
Other	3
Cutaneous change	1
Event involving lymphatic system	1
Complications of IP Access Devices	
Port complications	19.5%
Inflow obstruction	8.8%
Infection	10.2%
Bowel Injury	2%

Armstrong DK et al. N Engl J Med 2006;354:34–43
Walker JL et al. Gynecol Oncol 2006;100:27–32

(continued)

Patient Population Studied

A study of 205 women with Stage III epithelial ovarian or peritoneal carcinoma optimally debulked with no residual mass greater than 1 cm in diameter after surgery. All patients had a Gynecologic Oncology Group (GOG) performance status of 0–2

Efficacy (N = 205)

Variable	Months
Median progression-free survival (PFS)	23.8
PFS in patients with gross residual disease	18.3
PFS in patients without visible residual disease	37.6
Median overall survival	65.6

Treatment Modifications
(continued)

Adverse Event	Treatment Modification
ANC <500/mm^3 on day 8	Add filgrastim 5 mcg/kg per day until ANC >5000–10,000/mm^3
Nadir platelet count <25,000/mm^3	Reduce intravenous paclitaxel dosage 1 dose level
First episode of febrile neutropenia or sepsis requiring intravenous antibiotics	Reduce intravenous paclitaxel dosage 1 dose level. Do not add filgrastim
Febrile neutropenia or sepsis requiring intravenous antibiotics despite reduction of paclitaxel 1 dosage level	Add filgrastim beginning 24 hours after completion of IV chemotherapy and continuing for 14 days without additional dosage modification

Abdominal Pain Score

G0	No pain
G1	Mild pain. Opioid analgesia not required; pain causes minimal interference with daily activities and lasts for less than 72 hours
G2	Moderate pain. Opioid analgesia required; pain causes moderate interference with daily activities and lasts longer than 72 hours
G3	Severe pain. Opioid analgesia required; pain confines patient to bed and causes severe interference with daily activities

(continued)

Toxicity (N = 201)
(continued)

Discontinuation of IP Therapy (N = 119)

Reason	Primary	Contributing
Catheter related	**40**	**10**
IP catheter infection	21	4
IP catheter blocked	10	0
IP catheter leak	3	2
Access problem	5	3
Fluid leak from vagina	1	1
Not IP catheter related	**34**	**28**
Nausea/Vomiting/Dehydration	16	16
Renal/Metabolic	15	12
Disease Progression	3	0
Possibly IP treatment related	**45**	**42**
Other infection (not catheter)	7	5
Abdominal pain	4	16
Patient refusal	19	8
Bowel complication	4	4
Other	11	9

Walker JL et al. Gynecol Oncol 2006;100:27–32

Notes

1. Among all randomized phase III trials conducted by the GOG among patients with advanced ovarian cancer, this therapy yielded the longest median survival (65.6 months)
2. Only 42% of patients received all 6 cycles of intraperitoneal therapy
3. The primary reason for discontinuation of intraperitoneal therapy was catheter-related complications
4. Among 205 patients randomly allocated to the intraperitoneal arm, 58% (119) did not complete all 6 cycles of intraperitoneal therapy. Of these 119 patients, 34% (40/119 = 34%) discontinued intraperitoneal therapy primarily as a result of catheter complications, whereas 29% (34/119 = 29%) discontinued for unrelated reasons. Additionally, 37% (45/119 = 37%) discontinued for reasons that were possibly related to the intraperitoneal treatment (see table under toxicities)
5. Hysterectomy, appendectomy, small bowel resection, and ileocecal resection were not associated with failure to complete 6 cycles
6. There appears to be an association between rectosigmoid colon resection and the ability to initiate intraperitoneal therapy. Intraperitoneal therapy was not initiated 16% of patients who had a left colon or rectosigmoid colon resection versus 5% of those who did not have such a resection (p = 0.015)
7. Intraperitoneal therapy should begin as soon as possible after surgery. A delay of intraperitoneal therapy allows opportunity for adhesions to develop and may limit intraperitoneal distribution of the IP fluid
8. The 2 L of intraperitoneal fluid administered with the intraperitoneal therapy does not replace the need for intravascular hydration administration and adequate urine output. Administration of at least 1 L of 0.9% sodium chloride injection both prior to and after cisplatin is essential

Armstrong DK et al. N Engl J Med 2006;354:34–43
Walker JL et al. Gynecol Oncol 2006;100:27–32

Therapy Monitoring

1. *Prior to start of therapy:* PE, CBC with differential, electrolytes, serum creatinine, BUN, mineral panel, LFTs, CA-125, audiogram only in patients with a history of hearing loss, and chest x-ray
2. *Weekly:* CBC with differential
3. *Prior to each cycle:* PE, CBC with differential, electrolytes, serum creatinine, BUN, mineral panel, LFTs

Treatment Modifications
(continued)

Adverse Event	Treatment Modification
G2 abdominal pain	Reduce intraperitoneal cisplatin or paclitaxel, whichever is causing symptoms, by 1 dose level
Recurrent G2 abdominal pain after a dose reduction or G3 abdominal pain or complications involving the intraperitoneal catheter prohibiting further intraperitoneal therapy	Discontinue intraperitoneal therapy and administer intravenous cisplatin instead
Any grade gastrointestinal toxicity	Hospitalize patient if necessary but do not adjust chemotherapy dosages
G2 peripheral neuropathy	Reduce cisplatin dosage by 1 dose level
G3/4 peripheral neuropathy	Hold therapy until peripheral neuropathy G ≤1 then restart therapy with cisplatin dosage reduced by 1 dose level. Consider discontinuing therapy if not recovered to baseline by 2–3 weeks
Increase in serum creatinine >0.7–1.0 mg/dL (>62–88 μmol/L) above baseline	Hold therapy until serum creatinine returns to baseline and reduce intraperitoneal cisplatin 1 dosage level. Consider discontinuing therapy if not recovered to baseline by 2–3 weeks

PLATINUM-SENSITIVE REGIMEN
CISPLATIN AND CYCLOPHOSPHAMIDE

Young RC et al. J Clin Oncol 2003;23:4350–4355

Cyclophosphamide 1000 mg/m²; administer intravenously in 1000 mL 0.9% sodium chloride injection (0.9% NS) over 30–60 minutes, on day 1, every 21 days, for 3 cycles (total dosage/cycle = 1000 mg/m²)
Cisplatin 100 mg/m²; administer intravenously in 250 mL 0.9% NS over 30–60 minutes, on day 1, after cyclophosphamide, every 21 days, for 3 cycles (total dosage/cycle = 100 mg/m²)
Note: Encourage patients to increase oral intake of nonalcoholic fluids, and provide electrolyte replacement as needed (potassium, magnesium, sodium)

Supportive Care
Antiemetic prophylaxis
Emetogenic potential is **HIGH**. *Potential for delayed symptoms*
See Chapter 39 for antiemetic recommendations

Hematopoietic growth factor (CSF) prophylaxis
Primary prophylaxis may be indicated
See Chapter 43 for more information

Antimicrobial prophylaxis
Risk of fever and neutropenia is LOW
   Antimicrobial primary prophylaxis to be considered:
   • Antibacterial—not indicated
   • Antifungal—not indicated
   • Antiviral—not indicated unless patient previously had an episode of HSV
See Chapter 47 for more information

Patient Population Studied

Prospective randomized clinical trial conducted by the GOG of 251 patients: 124 patients randomized to ³²P and 127 randomized to chemotherapy. Eligible patients were either FIGO Stage Ia or Ib (grade 3), or Stage Ic or II (any grade). In addition, all Stages I and II patients with clear cell histology (any grade) were eligible

Efficacy

10-Year Cumulative Incidence of Recurrence	
All patients	28%
Stage I	24%
Stage II	39%

Toxicity

	% G3/4
Hematologic	
Leukopenia	69.5
Granulocytopenia	68
Thrombocytopenia	8.5
Nonhematologic	
Gastrointestinal	11.9
Renal	1.7
Ototoxicity	0.8
Bowel perforation	0

Therapy Monitoring

Before repeated cycles: PE, CBC with differential, and serum electrolytes, magnesium, calcium, BUN, and creatinine

Notes

Although compared with intraperitoneal ³²P, there were no statistically significant differences in survival, the authors concluded: "The lower cumulative recurrence seen with CP (cisplatin + cyclophosphamide) and complications of ³²P administration make platinum-based combinations the preferred adjuvant therapy for early ovarian cancer patients at high-risk for recurrence"

Treatment Modifications

(Specific Recommendations Not Provided by Authors)

Adverse Event	Dose Modification
Creatinine clearance* 30–60 mL/min (0.5–1 mL/s)	Reduce cisplatin so that dose in milligrams equals the creatinine clearance value in mL/min†
Creatinine clearance* <30 mL/min (<0.5 mL/s)	Hold cisplatin
If on day 1 of a cycle, leukocyte count <3000/mm³, ANC <1000/mm³, or platelets <100,000/mm³	Hold chemotherapy for 1 week, then resume treatment if leukocytes ≥3000/mm³, ANC ≥1000/mm³, and platelets >100,000/mm³
If on day 1 of a cycle, G ≥2 nonhematologic adverse event or serum creatinine ≥1.8 mg/dL (≥159 μmol/L)	Hold chemotherapy for 1 week, then resume with chemotherapy dose reduced by 20–30% if nonhematologic toxicity resolved to G ≤1 and creatinine ≤1.5 mg/dL (≤133 μmol/L)
G4 neutropenia (with or without fever)	Add prophylaxis with filgrastim 5 mcg/kg per day subcutaneously for 14 days with same chemotherapy doses during all subsequent cycles
Febrile neutropenia despite filgrastim support	Hold treatment until adverse event resolves, then resume chemotherapy with chemotherapy dosage reduced by 20–30%

*Creatinine clearance used as a measure of glomerular filtration rate (GFR)
†Also applies to patients with creatinine clearance (GFR) of 30–60 mL/min (0.5–1 mL/s) at outset of treatment

PLATINUM-SENSITIVE REGIMEN

PLATINUM RETREATMENT (CISPLATIN OR CARBOPLATIN)

Leitao M et al. Gynecol Oncol 2003;91:123–129

Hydration before cisplatin: ≥1000 mL 0.9% sodium chloride injection (0.9% NS); administer intravenously over a minimum of 3–4 hours. Monitor and replace magnesium/electrolytes as needed

Cisplatin 80–100 mg/m²; administer intravenously in 100–500 mL 0.9% NS over 30–60 minutes on day 1, every 3 weeks, for a maximum of 8 cycles (total dosage/3-week cycle = 80–100 mg/m²)

Hydration after cisplatin: ≥1000 mL 0.9% NS; administer intravenously over a minimum of 3–4 hours. Also encourage high oral fluid intake. Goal is to achieve a urine output of ≥100 mL/hour

or

Carboplatin (calculated dose) AUC = 6; administer by intravenous infusion in 50–150 mL D5W over 15–30 minutes on day 1, every 3 weeks (total dosage/cycle calculated to produce an AUC = 6 mg/mL · min)

*Carboplatin dose is based on a formula described by Calvert et al. to achieve a target area under the plasma concentration versus time curve (AUC)

$$\text{Total carboplatin dose (mg)} = (\text{target AUC}) \times (\text{GFR} + 25)$$

In practice, creatinine clearance (Clcr) is used in place of glomerular filtration rate (GFR). Clcr can be estimated from the equation of Cockcroft and Gault, thus:

$$\text{For males, Clcr} = \frac{(140 - \text{age [years]}) \times (\text{body weight [kg]})}{72 \times (\text{serum creatinine [mg/dL]})}$$

$$\text{For females, Clcr} = \frac{(140 - \text{age [years]}) \times (\text{body weight [kg]})}{72 \times (\text{serum creatinine [mg/dL]})} \times 0.85$$

Calvert AH et al. J Clin Oncol 1989;7:1748–1756
Cockcroft DW, Gault MH. Nephron 1976;16:31–41
Jodrell DI et al. J Clin Oncol 1992;10:520–528
Sorensen BT et al. Cancer Chemother Pharmacol 1991;28:397–401

Note: On October 8, 2010, the U.S. Food and Drug Administration (FDA) identified a potential safety issue with carboplatin dosing based on recent changes in the measurement of serum creatinine. By the end of 2010, all clinical laboratories in the United States began using the standardized isotope dilution mass spectrometry (IDMS) method to measure serum creatinine, which could result in an overestimation of the GFR in some patients with normal renal function. A carboplatin dose calculated with an IDMS-measured serum creatinine result using the Calvert formula could exceed an expected exposure (AUC) and result in increased drug-related toxicity

Provided actual GFR measurements are made to assess renal function, carboplatin can be safely dosed according to the Calvert formula described in product labeling

If GFR (or creatinine clearance) is estimated based on serum creatinine measurements by the IDMS method, the FDA recommends capping an estimated GFR at 125 mL/min for any targeted AUC value for patients with normal renal function. No greater estimated GFR values should be used

U.S. FDA. Carboplatin dosing. [online] October 8, 2010. Available from: http://www.fda.gov/AboutFDA/CentersOffices/CDER/ucm228974.htm

Supportive Care
Antiemetic prophylaxis
Emetogenic potential is **MODERATE–HIGH** *(carboplatin) or* **HIGH** *(cisplatin). Potential for delayed symptoms with either carboplatin or cisplatin*
See Chapter 39 for antiemetic recommendations

(continued)

Treatment Modifications

Adverse Event	Dose Modification
Cisplatin	
Creatinine clearance 40–60 mL/min (0.66–1 mL/s)	Reduce cisplatin so that dose in milligrams equals the creatinine clearance* value in mL/min†
Creatinine clearance <40 mL/min (<0.66 mL/s)	Hold cisplatin
On treatment day 1, serum creatinine 1.6–2 mg/dL (141–177 μmol/L)	Reduce cisplatin dosage by 25%
On treatment day 1, serum creatinine >2 mg/dL (>177 μmol/L)	Hold cisplatin until serum creatinine ≤2.0 mg/dL (≤177 μmol/L)
Day 1 WBC <2000/mm³ or platelet count <100,000/mm³	Delay cisplatin for 1 week or until myelosuppression resolves, whichever occurs later
Second treatment delay because of myelosuppression / Sepsis during an episode of neutropenia	Delay cisplatin for 1 week, or until myelosuppression resolves, then decrease cisplatin dosage to 60–80 mg/m² during subsequent treatments
Bleeding associated with thrombocytopenia	Reduce cisplatin dosage to 60–80 mg/m²
Carboplatin	
ANC nadir <500/mm³, platelet nadir <50,000/mm³ or febrile neutropenia	Reduce carboplatin dosage to AUC = 5 mg/mL · min if previous cycle dose was AUC = 6; or to AUC = 4 if previous cycle dose was AUC = 5
ANC nadir <500/mm³, platelet nadir <50,000/mm³, or febrile neutropenia after 2 carboplatin dose reductions (AUC in previous cycle = 4 mg/mL · min)	Decrease carboplatin dosage to AUC = 3 mg/mL · min

(continued)

(*continued*)

Hematopoietic growth factor (CSF) prophylaxis
Primary prophylaxis is indicated with 1 of the following:

Filgrastim (G-CSF) 5 mcg/kg per day by subcutaneous injection, *or*
Pegfilgrastim (pegylated filgrastim) 6 mg/0.6 mL, by subcutaneous injection for 1 dose
- Begin use from 24–72 hours after myelosuppressive chemotherapy is completed
- Continue daily filgrastim use until ANC ≥10,000/mm³ on 2 measurements separated temporally by ≥12 hours
- Discontinue daily filgrastim use at least 24 hours before repeating myelosuppressive treatment. Do not administer pegfilgrastim within 14 days before administering myelosuppressive treatment

See Chapter 43 for more information

Antimicrobial prophylaxis
Risk of fever and neutropenia is LOW–INTERMEDIATE
  Antimicrobial primary prophylaxis to be considered:
- Antibacterial—consider a fluoroquinolone or no prophylaxis
- Antifungal—not indicated
- Antiviral—not indicated unless patient previously had an episode of HSV

See Chapter 47 for more information

Arthralgia and myalgia G ≥2 associated with chemotherapy
Dexamethasone 4–8 mg/dose orally twice daily for 6 doses after chemotherapy

Treatment Modifications
(continued)

Adverse Event	Dose Modification
Day 1 ANC <1500/mm³ or platelets <100,000/mm³	Delay chemotherapy until ANC >1500/mm³ and platelets >100,000/mm³, for maximum delay of 2 weeks
Delay of >2 weeks in reaching ANC >1500/mm³ or platelets >100,000/mm³	Discontinue therapy
Bleeding associated with thrombocytopenia	Reduce carboplatin dosages to AUC 4–5 mg/mL · min

*Creatinine clearance used as a measure of glomerular filtration rate
†This also applies to patients with creatinine clearance (GFR) of 40–60 mL/min (0.66–1 mL/s) at the outset of treatment

Efficacy (N = 30)

Variable	No. of Patients	% PR
Best Response to Last Platinum Regimen		
Complete or partial response	14	43
Stable or progressive disease	16	6
Platinum-Free Interval		
≤6 months	2	0
6–12 months	8	63
>12 months	20	10
Number of Intervening Nonplatinum Agents		
≤3	20	35
>3	10	0
Time to Progression After Last Platinum Regimen		
≤6 months	23	17
>6 months	6	50
Number of Prior Platinum Regimens		
1 prior regimen	9	33
2 or 3 prior regimens	21	19

Patient Population Studied

A study of 30 patients with platinum-resistant ovarian cancer, who received nonplatinum chemotherapy for recurrent epithelial ovarian cancer before additional platinum therapy. Platinum resistance was defined as less than a partial response to platinum therapy or progression within 6 months of the last platinum therapy

Therapy Monitoring

1. *Before repeated cycles:* PE, CBC with differential, serum electrolytes, magnesium, calcium, BUN, and creatinine
2. *Every month:* Serum CA-125 level
3. *Every 2–3 months:* Restaging radiographic studies

Toxicity

Cisplatin
(PLATINOL-AQ [cisplatin injection] product label, November 2002. Bristol-Myers Squibb)

Individual and cumulative dose-related renal toxicity: Increased serum creatinine, uric acid, and BUN *Renal tubular damage with electrolyte wasting:* Hypomagnesemia, hypocalcemia, hyponatremia, hypokalemia, and hypophosphatemia	28–36%*
Dose-related, cumulative peripheral neuropathies: Bilateral paresthesias, areflexia, loss of proprioception and vibratory sensation, motor neuropathies	30–100% depending on cumulative doses
Optic neuritis, papilledema, and cerebral blindness	Rare
Cumulative ototoxicity: With tinnitus or high frequency hearing loss. Vestibular toxicity	31%*
Nausea and vomiting at any dose: Severe and delayed emesis at dosages ≥50 mg/m²	Varies (moderate to severe in virtually all patients without effective antiemetic prophylaxis)
Transiently increased liver transaminases	Rare
Hypersensitivity reactions: Anaphylactoid reactions, facial edema, wheezing, tachycardia, and hypotension	1–20%
Coombs-positive hemolytic anemia	Rare
Dose-related leukopenia, thrombocytopenia, anemia	25–30%*

Carboplatin
(PARAPLATIN [carboplatin aqueous solution] Injection product label, January 2004. Bristol-Myers Squibb)

Nausea and vomiting	92%†
Diarrhea, constipation, other GI side effects	21%
Thrombocytopenia: <100,000/mm³ <50,000/mm³	62% 35%
Neutropenia: <1000/mm³	21%
Anemia: <11 g/dL <8 g/dL	90% 21%
Nephrotoxicity: Increased serum creatinine Increased BUN	10% 22%
Hyponatremia, hypomagnesemia, hypocalcemia, hypokalemia	47%, 43%, 31%, 28%
Peripheral neuropathies: Paresthesia, ataxia, distal motor deficits; decreased vibratory sense, light touch, pinprick, and joint position; areflexia	
Cumulative ototoxicity: Tinnitus, high-frequencies hearing loss, audiogram deficits	1.1%
Increased alkaline phosphatase, AST, total bilirubin	37%
Alopecia	19%
Hypersensitivity reactions: Facial flushing, generalized urticaria, hypotension, rash, pruritus, bronchospasm, shortness of breath	5%

*Incidence after a single treatment with cisplatin 50 mg/m²
†All data are based on the experience of 553 patients with previously treated ovarian carcinoma who received single-agent carboplatin, without regard for their baseline status

EPITHELIAL OVARIAN CANCER REGIMEN

GEMCITABINE + CARBOPLATIN

Pfisterer J et al. J Clin Oncol 2006;24:4699–4707

Gemcitabine 1000 mg/m² per dose; administer intravenously in 50–250 mL 0.9% sodium chloride injection (0.9% NS) over 30–60 minutes for 2 doses, on days 1 and 8, every 21 days (total dosage/cycle = 2000 mg/m²)
Note: On day 1, administer after hydration for carboplatin, then follow with carboplatin

Carboplatin (calculated dose) AUC = 4 mg/mL · min*; administer intravenously in 0.9% NS or 5% dextrose injection 100–500 mL over 1 hour, on day 1 after completing gemcitabine, every 3 weeks (total dosage/cycle calculated to produce a target AUC = 4 mg/mL · min)

*Carboplatin dose is based on a formula described by Calvert et al. to achieve a target area under the plasma concentration versus time curve (AUC)

$$\text{Total carboplatin dose (mg)} = (\text{target AUC}) \times (\text{GFR} + 25)$$

In practice, creatinine clearance (Clcr) is used in place of glomerular filtration rate (GFR). Clcr can be estimated from the equation of Cockcroft and Gault, thus:

$$\text{For males, Clcr} = \frac{(140 - \text{age [years]}) \times (\text{body weight [kg]})}{72 \times (\text{serum creatinine [mg/dL]})}$$

$$\text{For females, Clcr} = \frac{(140 - \text{age [years]}) \times (\text{body weight [kg]})}{72 \times (\text{Serum creatinine [mg/dL]})} \times 0.85$$

Calvert AH et al. J Clin Oncol 1989;7:1748–1756
Cockcroft DW , Gault MH. Nephron 1976;16:31–41
Jodrell DI et al. J Clin Oncol 1992;10:520–528
Sorensen BT et al. Cancer Chemother Pharmacol 1991;28:397–401

Note: On October 8, 2010, the U.S. Food and Drug Administration (FDA) identified a potential safety issue with carboplatin dosing based on recent changes in the measurement of serum creatinine. By the end of 2010, all clinical laboratories in the United States began using the standardized isotope dilution mass spectrometry (IDMS) method to measure serum creatinine, which could result in an overestimation of the GFR in some patients with normal renal function. A carboplatin dose calculated with an IDMS-measured serum creatinine result using the Calvert formula could exceed an expected exposure (AUC) and result in increased drug-related toxicity

Provided actual GFR measurements are made to assess renal function, carboplatin can be safely dosed according to the Calvert formula described in product labeling

If GFR (or creatinine clearance) is estimated based on serum creatinine measurements by the IDMS method, the FDA recommends capping an estimated GFR at 125 mL/min for any targeted AUC value for patients with normal renal function. No greater estimated GFR values should be used

U.S. FDA. Carboplatin dosing. [online] October 8, 2010. Available from: http://www.fda.gov/AboutFDA/CentersOffices/CDER/ucm228974.htm

Supportive Care
Antiemetic prophylaxis
Emetogenic potential on days with gemcitabine alone is **LOW**
Emetogenic potential on days with carboplatin is **MODERATE**. *Potential for delayed symptoms*
See Chapter 39 for antiemetic recommendations

Hematopoietic growth factor (CSF) prophylaxis
Primary prophylaxis is NOT indicated
See Chapter 43 for more information

Antimicrobial prophylaxis
Risk of fever and neutropenia is LOW
   Antimicrobial primary prophylaxis to be considered:
   • Antibacterial—not indicated
   • Antifungal—not indicated
   • Antiviral—not indicated unless patient previously had an episode of HSV
See Chapter 47 for more information

Patient Population Studied

Patients with platinum-sensitive recurrent ovarian cancer were randomly assigned to receive either gemcitabine plus carboplatin or carboplatin alone. The primary objective was to compare progression-free survival (PFS)

Dose Modifications

Adverse Event	Dose Modifications
ANC <1500/mm³ or platelet count <100,000/mm³	Hold day 1 chemotherapy until ANC ≥1500/mm³ and platelet count ≥100,000/mm³
ANC <1500/mm³ or platelet count <100,000/mm³ ≥2 weeks	Discontinue therapy
Intracycle: G1/2 nonhematologic toxicity or G1–3 nausea or vomiting	100% gemcitabine dosage on day 8
Intracycle: G3 nonhematologic toxicity, except nausea, vomiting, and alopecia	Reduce gemcitabine dosage by 50% on day 8, or hold treatment at clinician's discretion
Intracycle: G4 nonhematologic toxicity	Hold gemcitabine
Day 8 ANC ≥1000–1400/mm³ and/or platelet count ≥75,000–99,000/mm³	Reduce gemcitabine dosage by 50%
Day 8 ANC <1000/mm³ and platelet count <75,000/mm³	Hold gemcitabine

(continued)

Toxicity

Selected Toxicities* and Associated Supportive Care

	% G1	% G2	% G3	% G4
Hematologic				
Anemia	18.3	41.7	22.3	5.1
Neutropenia	5.1	15.4	41.7	28.6
Thrombocytopenia	23.4	20.6	30.3	4.6
Nonhematologic				
Allergic reaction/hypersensitivity	0.6	2.3	1.7	0.6
Alopecia	34.9	14.3	NA†	NA†
Diarrhea	9.1	4	1.7	0
Dyspnea	0.6	6.9	1.1	0
Fatigue	16.6	20	1.7	0.6
Febrile neutropenia	0	0	1.1	0
Infection without neutropenia	0.6	0.6	0	0.6
Infection with neutropenia	0.6	0	0	0
Neuropathy, motor	5.1	0.6	0.6	0
Neuropathy, sensory	24.6	4	1.1	0
Vomiting	23.4	16	2.9	0

Treatment

Parenteral Antibiotics	8.4%
G-CSF or GM-CSF‡	23.6%
RBCs	27%
EPO§	7.3%

*NCI-CTC, National Cancer Institute Common Toxicity Criteria
†NA, not applicable. Grade 3/4 alopecia are not recognized by NCI-CTC (version 2.0 and later)
‡G-CSF, granulocyte colony-stimulating factor; GM-CSF, granulocyte macrophage colony-stimulating factor
§Erythropoietin or epoetin alfa

Dose Modifications (continued)

Adverse Event	Dose Modifications
Febrile neutropenia, or ANC <500/mm³ for >5 days, or ANC <100/mm³ for >3 days, or Platelet count <25,000/mm³, or Platelet count <50,000/mm³ with bleeding, or G3/4 nonhematologic toxicity (except nausea/vomiting), or treatment delay for toxicity ≥1 week	Reduce gemcitabine dosage to 800 mg/m² per dose *Note:* If gemcitabine dosage is 800 mg/m² then discontinue gemcitabine
Significant hypersensitivity reaction to carboplatin (hypotension, dyspnea, and angioedema requiring therapy)*	Discontinue therapy

*Patients who experience G1/2 carboplatin hypersensitivity reactions may continue treatment if there is evidence of tumor response and appropriate preventive measures are instituted

Efficacy

Efficacy (N = 178)

Not assessable/not done	6.7
Progressive disease	7.9
Stable disease	38.2
Partial response (PR)	32.6
Complete response (CR)	14.6
Overall response rate: CR + PR (95% CI)	47.2 (39.9–54.5)

Therapy Monitoring

1. *Baseline:* LFTs, serum chemistry, CBC with differential and platelet count, and CA-125. Complete history and physical examination including a gynecologic examination
2. *Follow-up:* CBC with differential and platelet count on days 1, 8, and 15 of each cycle

EPITHELIAL OVARIAN CANCER REGIMEN

LIPOSOMAL DOXORUBICIN + CARBOPLATIN

Pujade-Lauraine E et al. J Clin Oncol 2010;28:3323–3329

Doxorubicin HCl liposome injection (liposomal doxorubicin) 30 mg/m^2; administer intravenously in 250 mL (doses ≤90 mg) 5% dextrose injection over 60 minutes, on day 1 before carboplatin, every 4 weeks (total dosage/cycle = 30 mg/m^2)

Note: Doxorubicin HCl liposome injection should be administered at an initial rate of 1 mg/min to minimize the risk of infusion reactions. If no infusion-related adverse events are observed, the rate of infusion can be increased to complete administration of the drug over 1 hour

Note: Experience with doxorubicin HCl liposome injection at high cumulative doses is too limited to have established its effects on the myocardium. Therefore, it should be assumed that it will have myocardial toxicity similar to conventional formulations of doxorubicin HCl. Irreversible myocardial toxicity leading to congestive heart failure often unresponsive to cardiac supportive therapy may be encountered as the total cumulative lifetime dosage of doxorubicin HCl approaches **450–550 mg/m^2**. Prior anthracyclines or anthracenediones will reduce the total dose of doxorubicin HCl that can be given without associated cardiac toxicity. Cardiac toxicity also may occur at lower cumulative doses in patients receiving concurrent cyclophosphamide therapy

Carboplatin (calculated dose) AUC = 5*; administer intravenously in 0.9% sodium chloride injection or D5W 100–500 mL over 60 minutes, on day 1 after completing liposomal doxorubicin administration, every 4 weeks (total dosage/cycle calculated to produce a target AUC = 5 mg/mL · min)

*Carboplatin dose is based on a formula described by Calvert et al. to achieve a target area under the plasma concentration versus time curve (AUC)

$$\text{Total carboplatin dose (mg)} = (\text{target AUC}) \times (\text{GFR} + 25)$$

In practice, creatinine clearance (Clcr) is used in place of glomerular filtration rate (GFR). Clcr can be estimated from the equation of Cockcroft and Gault, thus:

$$\text{For males, Clcr} = \frac{(140 - \text{age [years]}) \times (\text{body weight [kg]})}{72 \times (\text{serum creatinine [mg/dL]})}$$

$$\text{For females, Clcr} = \frac{(140 - \text{age [years]}) \times (\text{body weight [kg]})}{72 \times (\text{serum creatinine [mg/dL]})} \times 0.85$$

Calvert AH et al. J Clin Oncol 1989;7:1748–1756
Cockcroft DW , Gault MH. Nephron 1976;16:31–41
Jodrell DI et al. J Clin Oncol 1992;10:520–528
Sorensen BT et al. Cancer Chemother Pharmacol 1991;28:397–401

Note: On October 8, 2010, the U.S. Food and Drug Administration (FDA) identified a potential safety issue with carboplatin dosing based on recent changes in the measurement of serum creatinine. By the end of 2010, all clinical laboratories in the United States began using the standardized Isotope Dilution Mass Spectrometry (IDMS) method to measure serum creatinine, which could result in an overestimation of the GFR in some patients with normal renal function. A carboplatin dose calculated with an IDMS-measured serum creatinine result using the Calvert formula could exceed an expected exposure (AUC) and result in increased drug-related toxicity

Provided actual GFR measurements are made to assess renal function, carboplatin can be safely dosed according to the Calvert formula described in product labeling

If GFR (or creatinine clearance) is estimated based on serum creatinine measurements by the IDMS method, the FDA recommends capping an estimated GFR at 125 mL/min for any targeted AUC value for patients with normal renal function. No greater estimated GFR values should be used

U.S. FDA. Carboplatin dosing. [online] October 8, 2010. Available from: URL: http://www.fda.gov/AboutFDA/CentersOffices/CDER/ucm228974.htm

Supportive Care

Antiemetic prophylaxis

Emetogenic potential is **MODERATE**. *Potential for delayed symptoms*

See Chapter 39 for antiemetic recommendations

(continued)

Patient Population Studied

Patients with histologically proven ovarian cancer with recurrence ≥6 months after first- or second-line platinum and taxane-based therapies. Randomization against paclitaxel + carboplatin. Primary end point was progression-free survival (PFS); secondary end points were toxicity, quality of life, and overall survival

Efficacy

Efficacy (> Median Follow-up of 22 Months)*

PFS (intent-to-treat population)	11.3 months
Progression according to RECIST	79%
Progression according to CA-125 GCIG criteria	21%

*In the absence of unacceptable toxicity or disease progression, patients were treated for a total of 6 courses of therapy. In the event disease stabilization or partial response was achieved after 6 courses of therapy, patients were allowed to remain on therapy until progression

(continued)

Hematopoietic growth factor (CSF) prophylaxis
Primary prophylaxis is NOT indicated
See Chapter 43 for more information

Antimicrobial prophylaxis
Risk of fever and neutropenia is LOW
Antimicrobial primary prophylaxis to be considered:
- Antibacterial—not indicated
- Antifungal—not indicated
- Antiviral—not indicated unless patient previously had an episode of HSV

See Chapter 47 for more information

Hand-foot reaction (palmar-plantar erythrodysesthesia, PPE)
For patients who develop a hand-foot reaction, use topical emollients (eg, Aquaphor), topical or orally administered steroids, antihistamine agents (H_1-receptor antagonists), or pyridoxine
- Pyridoxine may provide relief for discomfort/pain associated with PPE although the mechanism through which this occurs remains unclear
- The suggested pyridoxine starting dose is 50 mg/day, which may be increased to a maximum of 200 mg/day

Patients who have developed G1/2 PPE while receiving doxorubicin HCl liposome injection may receive a fixed daily dose of pyridoxine 200 mg. This may allow for treatment to be completed without dosage reduction, treatment delay, or recurrence of PPE

Therapy Monitoring

1. Baseline: LFTs, serum chemistry, CBC with differential and platelet count, and CA-125. Complete history and physical examination including a gynecologic examination
2. Baseline ECG and left ventricular ejection fraction measurement by echocardiogram or multigated angiography. A left ventricular ejection fraction measurement before each course of therapy if cumulative anthracycline dose exceeds 450 mg/m²
3. Follow-up: CBC with differential and platelet count on days 1, 8, and 15 of each cycle, and LFTs prior to commencing repeated cycles

Toxicity

Adverse Event	% Any Grade	%G ≥2	%G 3–4
Toxicity (N = 466)*			
Hematologic Toxicity			
Neutropenia	79.6		35.2
Febrile neutropenia			2.6
Infection	20.4		2.6
Thrombo-cytopenia	38.4		15.9
Anemia	66.3		7.9
Bleeding			0.6
Nonhematologic Toxicity			
Alopecia	34.7		
Nausea	78.3	35.2‡	
Vomiting	48.9	22.5‡	
Constipation	55.4	21.5	
Diarrhea	23.2	5.4‡	
Fatigue	77.9	36.9‡	
Mucositis	39.1	13.9‡	
Neuropathy, Sensory	39.9	4.9‡	
Neuropathy, Motor	7.3	1.5	
Cardiovascular	10.5	2.1‡	
Allergic reaction	15.5	5.6‡	
Hand-foot syndrome	38.6	12‡	
Arthralgia/myalgia	22.3	4‡	

*NCI Common Terminology Criteria for Adverse Events, version 3.0
†Graded as 1, partial hair loss, or 2, complete hair loss
‡Grades 2 and 3 only (no reported grade 4 toxicities)

Note: Because of rounding, percentages may not total 100

Dose Modifications

Adverse Event	Dose Modifications
ANC <1000/mm³ or platelet count <75,000/mm³	Hold day 1 chemotherapy until ANC ≥1000/mm³ and platelet count ≥75,000/mm³
ANC <1000/mm³ or platelet count <75,000/mm³ ≥3 weeks	Discontinue therapy
G3/4 nonhematologic toxicity	Reduce carboplatin dosage to AUC = 4 mg/mL · min. If toxicity occurred at carboplatin dosage of AUC = 4 consider discontinuing therapy. Reduce liposomal doxorubicin dosage by 25% or add filgrastim support
Febrile neutropenia, *or* ANC <500/mm³ for ≥7 days, *or* Platelet count <10,000/mm³, *or* Platelet count 10,000–50,000/mm³ with bleeding, or treatment delay for hematological toxicity >1 week	
Total cumulative lifetime doxorubicin dosage ≥450 mg/m²	Obtain a left ventricular ejection fraction measurement before each course of therapy
Acute liposomal doxorubicin-associated infusion reactions, including: flushing, shortness of breath, facial swelling, headache, chills, back pain, tightness in the chest or throat, and/or hypotension	Decrease liposomal doxorubicin administration rate or terminate the infusion depending on the severity. Mild infusion reactions can be managed conservatively with a slowing of the rate of infusion*
G1 Palmar plantar erythrodysesthesia (PPE) = Mild erythema, swelling, or desquamation not interfering with daily activities†	Continue next cycle at the same liposomal doxorubicin dosage, unless patient has experienced previous G3/4 toxicity. If so, delay up to 2 weeks and decrease dosage by 25%. Return to original dose interval
G2 PPE = Erythema, desquamation, or swelling interfering with, but not precluding normal physical activities; small blisters or ulcerations <2 cm in diameter†	Delay liposomal doxorubicin dosing up to 2 weeks or until resolved to G0/1. If after 2 weeks there is no resolution discontinue liposomal doxorubicin
G3 PPE = Blistering, ulceration, or swelling interfering with walking or normal daily activities; cannot wear regular clothing†	Delay liposomal doxorubicin administration up to 2 weeks or until resolved to G0/1. Decrease liposomal doxorubicin dosage by 25% and return to original dose interval. If after 2 weeks there is no resolution, discontinue liposomal doxorubicin
G4 Palmar plantar erythrodysesthesia (PPE) = Diffuse or local process causing infectious complications, or a bed ridden state or hospitalization†	
G1 stomatitis = Painless ulcers, erythema, or mild soreness	Continue next cycle at the same liposomal doxorubicin dosage, unless patient has experienced previous G 3/4 toxicity. If so, delay up to 2 weeks and decrease liposomal doxorubicin dosage by 25%. Return to original dose interval
G2 stomatitis = Painful erythema, edema, or ulcers, but can eat	Delay liposomal doxorubicin administration up to 2 weeks or until resolved to G0/1. If at >2 weeks there is no resolution, discontinue liposomal doxorubicin
G3 stomatitis = Painful erythema, edema, or ulcers, but cannot eat	Delay liposomal doxorubicin administration up to 2 weeks or until resolved to G0/1. Decrease liposomal doxorubicin dosage by 25% and return to original dose interval. If at >2 weeks there is no resolution, discontinue liposomal doxorubicin
G4 stomatitis = Requires parenteral or enteral support	
Serum bilirubin 1.2–3 mg/dL (20.5–51.3 μmol/L)	Reduce dosage of liposomal doxorubicin by 50%
Serum bilirubin >3 mg/dL (>51.3 μmol/L)	Reduce dosage of liposomal doxorubicin by 75%
Significant hypersensitivity reaction to carboplatin (hypotension, dyspnea and angioedema requiring therapy)‡	Discontinue therapy

*For patients with a history of asthma or allergic reactions to drugs consider parenteral pre-medication with 100 mg hydrocortisone with or without 25–50 mg diphenhydramine
†Preventive measures for PPE include wearing loose-fitting clothes, avoiding activities that can lead to trauma to the vasculature of palms or soles, and use of ice packs to promote vasoconstriction and reduce inflammation. Patients should be advised to avoid hot baths and showers (jacuzzis and steam baths included) for 24 hours before and 72 hours after liposomal doxorubicin. Cool baths are recommended. Topical steroid creams provide no benefit. Topical antihistamine and anesthetic preparations may aggravate skin toxicity. Emollients and petroleum-based balms may provide some relief
‡Patients who experience G1/2 carboplatin hypersensitivity reactions may continue treatment if there is evidence of tumor response and appropriate preventive measures are instituted

EPITHELIAL OVARIAN CANCER REGIMEN

CARBOPLATIN + DOCETAXEL

Strauss HG et al. Gynecol Oncol 2007;104:612–616

Premedication with **Dexamethasone** 8 mg/dose; administer orally twice daily for 3 days (6 doses), starting on the day before docetaxel administration (total dose/cycle = 48 mg) *or* Dexamethasone 4 mg/dose; administer orally for 3 doses during the evening before, morning of, and evening after docetaxel administration (total dose/cycle = 12 mg)

Docetaxel 75 mg/m²; administer intravenously in a volume of 0.9% sodium chloride injection (0.9% NS) or 5% dextrose injection (D5W) sufficient to produce a docetaxel concentration within the range 0.3–0.74 mg/mL over 30 minutes on day 1 before carboplatin, every 3 weeks for 6 cycles (total dosage/cycle = 75 mg/m²), *followed by:*

Carboplatin [calculated dose] AUC = 5*; administer intravenously in 0.9% NS or D5W 100–500 mL over 60 minutes, on day 1 after completing docetaxel, every 3 weeks for 6 cycles (total dosage/cycle calculated to produce a target AUC = 5 mg/mL · min)

*Carboplatin dose is based on a formula described by Calvert et al. to achieve a target Area Under the plasma concentration versus time Curve (AUC)

$$\text{Total carboplatin dose (mg)} = (\text{target AUC}) \times (\text{GFR} + 25)$$

In practice, creatinine clearance (Clcr) is used in place of glomerular filtration rate (GFR). Clcr can be estimated from the equation of Cockcroft and Gault, thus:

$$\text{For males, Clcr} = \frac{(140 - \text{age [years]}) \times (\text{body weight [kg]})}{72 \times (\text{serum creatinine [mg/dL]})}$$

$$\text{For females, Clcr} = \frac{(140 - \text{age [years]}) \times (\text{body weight [kg]})}{72 \times (\text{serum creatinine [mg/dL]})} \times 0.85$$

Calvert AH et al. J Clin Oncol 1989;7:1748–1756
Cockcroft DW , Gault MH. Nephron 1976;16:31–41
Jodrell DI et al. J Clin Oncol 1992;10:520–528
Sorensen BT et al. Cancer Chemother Pharmacol 1991;28:397–401

Note: On October 8, 2010, the U.S. Food and Drug Administration (FDA) identified a potential safety issue with carboplatin dosing based on recent changes in the measurement of serum creatinine. By the end of 2010, all clinical laboratories in the United States began using the standardized isotope dilution mass spectrometry (IDMS) method to measure serum creatinine, which could result in an overestimation of the GFR in some patients with normal renal function. A carboplatin dose calculated with an IDMS-measured serum creatinine result using the Calvert formula could exceed an expected exposure (AUC) and result in increased drug-related toxicity

Provided actual GFR measurements are made to assess renal function, carboplatin can be safely dosed according to the Calvert formula described in product labeling

If GFR (or creatinine clearance) is estimated based on serum creatinine measurements by the IDMS method, the FDA recommends capping an estimated GFR at 125 mL/min for any targeted AUC value for patients with normal renal function. No greater estimated GFR values should be used

U.S. FDA. Carboplatin dosing. [online] October 8, 2010. Available from: http://www.fda.gov/AboutFDA/CentersOffices/CDER/ucm228974.htm

Supportive Care

Antiemetic prophylaxis

Emetogenic potential is **MODERATE**. *Potential for delayed symptoms*
See Chapter 39 for antiemetic recommendations

Hematopoietic growth factor (CSF) prophylaxis

Primary prophylaxis is NOT indicated
See Chapter 43 for more information

Antimicrobial prophylaxis

Risk of fever and neutropenia is LOW

Antimicrobial primary prophylaxis to be considered:

- Antibacterial—not indicated
- Antifungal—not indicated
- Antiviral—not indicated unless patient previously had an episode of HSV

See Chapter 47 for more information

Patient Population Studied

Eligible patients had recurrent ovarian, peritoneal or tubal cancer (platinum-free interval >6 months), performance status 0–2. Patients with had undergone surgical debulking for recurrent disease were excluded from the study. First-line chemotherapy in 25 patients included carboplatin/paclitaxel (21), carboplatin/docetaxel (1), carboplatin/cyclophosphamide (1), and carboplatin alone (2). Patients with preexisting peripheral neuropathy G ≥2 (NCI Common Toxicity Criteria, version 2.0; 1998) were excluded

Efficacy

Efficacy (N = 25)*

Strauss et al. Gynecol Oncol 2007;104:612–616

Intent-to-Treat Population (N = 25)	
Overall response rate*,†	72% [95% CI, 60%–84%]
Median progression-free survival	19 months [95% CI, 4–40 months]
Overall survival‡	26 months [95% CI, 11–44 months]

Efficacy-Evaluable Patients (N = 23)	
Overall response rate*,†	78.3% [95% CI, 64%–86%]
Complete response*	69.6% (16/23)
Partial response†	8.7 % (2/23)
Remission duration	50% (8/16 CR) at a median follow-up of 40.4 months

Complete response: Disappearance of all measurable disease assessed by imaging, disappearance of clinical signs and symptoms and normalization of CA-125 serum values without clinical evidence of progression for ≥4 weeks
†*Partial response:* Reduction of ≥50% in the sum of the greatest perpendicular diameters of all measurable lesions without appearance of new lesions for ≥4 weeks, no enlargement of any existing lesion, and decrease of elevated CA-125 values ≥50% from the pretherapeutic level
‡In an unplanned retrospective analysis, patients with a platinum-free interval ≥12 months showed significantly better OS than those with a platinum-free interval <12 months (p = 0.003/HR 8.6 [95% CI, 5.4–10.8])

Dose Modifications

Adverse Event	Dose Modifications
ANC <1000/mm^3 or platelet count <75,000/mm^{3*}	Hold day 1 chemotherapy until ANC ≥1000/mm^3 and platelet count ≥75,000/mm^3
ANC <1000/mm^3 or platelet count <75,000/mm^3 ≥3 weeks	Discontinue therapy
G3/4 nonhematologic toxicity	Reduce carboplatin dosage to AUC 4 mg/mL · min. If toxicity occurred at carboplatin dosage of AUC = 4 mg/mL · min, consider discontinuing therapy. Reduce docetaxel dosage to 60 mg/m^2
ANC <1500/mm^3 or platelet count <100,000/mm^3 on day 1 of a cycle, *or* Febrile neutropenia, *or* ANC <500/mm^3 despite filgrastim prophylaxis, *or* ANC <500/mm^3 for ≥7 days, *or* Platelet count <25,000/mm^3	Reduce carboplatin dosage to AUC = 4 mg/mL · min. Reduce docetaxel dosage to 60 mg/m^2
Second episode of febrile neutropenia	Continue docetaxel 60 mg/m^2, carboplatin AUC = 4 mg/mL · min, and give filgrastim* during subsequent cycles
ANC <1500/mm^3 or platelet count <100,000/mm^3 on despite 2-week delay, *or* febrile neutropenic despite filgrastim support, *or* Febrile neutropenia at docetaxel dosage of 60 mg/m^2 and carboplatin AUC 4 mg/mL · min, *or* Nonhematologic toxicity G >2 except mucositis, nausea or alopecia, *or* Significant hypersensitivity reaction to docetaxel or carboplatin (hypotension, dyspnea and angioedema requiring therapy)[†]	Discontinue therapy
G ≥3 peripheral neuropathy	Hold therapy for a maximum of 2 weeks, until toxicity G ≤2. Reinstitute therapy reducing docetaxel dosage to 30 mg/m^2. If toxicity recurs at docetaxel dosage = 30 mg/m^2, reduce carboplatin dosage to AUC = 4 mg/mL · min

*Filgrastim 5 mcg/kg per day subcutaneously for 8 consecutive days, days 3–10
[†]Patients who experience G1/2 carboplatin hypersensitivity reactions may continue treatment if there is evidence of tumor response and appropriate preventive measures are instituted

Toxicity

Acute Toxicity (N = 25)*

Strauss HG et al. Gynecol Oncol 2007;104:612–616

Toxicity	% G1	% G2	% G3	% G4
Neutropenia	12	16	28	32
Thrombo-cytopenia	4	12	20	4
Anemia	28	44	4	0
Infection	16	8	4	0
Nausea	48	32	4	4
Vomiting	32	16	4	0
Diarrhea	12	32	12	0
Stomatitis	16	20	0	0
Sensory neuropathy	20	20	0	0
Mood alteration (depression)	0	8	4	0
Alopecia	12	88	—	—
Epiphora	0	8	0	0
Skin	12	12	0	0
Peripheral edema	0	12	0	0
Joint pain	8	4	0	0

*NCI Clinical Trials Group Common Toxicity Criteria, version 2.0 (1998)

Therapy Monitoring

1. *Baseline:* LFTs, serum chemistry, CBC with differential and platelet count, and CA-125. Complete history and physical examination, including a gynecologic examination
2. *Follow-up:* CBC with differential and platelet count at least weekly through leukocyte and platelet count nadirs, and prior to beginning repeated cycles, and LFTs before commencing repeated cycles

EPITHELIAL OVARIAN CANCER REGIMEN

CARBOPLATIN + DOCETAXEL

Kushner DM et al. Gynecol Oncol 2007;105:358–364

Premedication:

Dexamethasone 4 mg/dose; administer orally for 3 doses during the evening before, morning of, and evening after docetaxel administration (total dose/cycle = 12 mg)

Docetaxel 35 mg/m² per dose (maximum single dose limited to 70 mg)*; administer intravenously in a volume of 0.9% sodium chloride injection (0.9% NS) or 5% dextrose injection (D5W) sufficient to produce a final docetaxel concentration within the range 0.3–0.74 mg/mL, over 60 minutes for 3 doses, before carboplatin on days 1, 8, and 15, every 28 days (total dosage/cycle = 105 mg/m²; maximum dose/cycle = 210 mg), *followed by:*

Carboplatin (calculated dose) AUC = 2[†]; administer intravenously in 0.9% NS or D5W 100–500 mL over 30 minutes for 3 doses, after completing docetaxel on days 1, 8, and 15, every 28 days (total dosage/cycle calculated to produce a cumulative target AUC = 6 mg/mL · min)

Notes: Carboplatin hypersensitivity led to 11 subjects coming off trial (31%). Diphenhydramine premedication produced a nonsignificant decrease in reaction rate

In the clinical trial, treatment was continued until evidence of disease progression, intolerable toxicity, patient refusal of further treatment, or physician decision that it was in the best interest of a patient to discontinue therapy. Patients who achieved a complete response (CR) continued therapy for 2 cycles following documentation of CR

*Patients with G2 neurotoxicity were treated at an initial docetaxel dosage of 30 mg/m²

[†]Carboplatin dose is based on a formula described by Calvert et al. to achieve a target area under the plasma concentration versus time curve (AUC)

$$\text{Total carboplatin dose (mg)} = (\text{target AUC}) \times (\text{GFR} + 25)$$

In practice, creatinine clearance (Clcr) is used in place of glomerular filtration rate (GFR). Clcr can be estimated from the equation of Cockcroft and Gault, thus:

$$\text{For males, Clcr} = \frac{(140 - \text{age [years]}) \times (\text{body weight [kg]})}{72 \times (\text{serum creatinine [mg/dL]})}$$

$$\text{For females, Clcr} = \frac{(140 - \text{age [years]}) \times (\text{body weight [kg]})}{72 \times (\text{serum creatinine [mg/dL]})} \times 0.85$$

Calvert AH et al. J Clin Oncol 1989;7:1748–1756
Cockcroft DW, Gault MH. Nephron 1976;16:31–41
Jodrell DI et al. J Clin Oncol 1992;10:520–528
Sorensen BT et al. Cancer Chemother Pharmacol 1991;28:397–401

Note: On October 8, 2010, the U.S. Food and Drug Administration (FDA) identified a potential safety issue with carboplatin dosing based on recent changes in the measurement of serum creatinine. By the end of 2010, all clinical laboratories in the United States began using the standardized isotope dilution mass spectrometry (IDMS) method to measure serum creatinine, which could result in an overestimation of the GFR in some patients with normal renal function. A carboplatin dose calculated with an IDMS-measured serum creatinine result using the Calvert formula could exceed an expected exposure (AUC) and result in increased drug-related toxicity

Provided actual GFR measurements are made to assess renal function, carboplatin can be safely dosed according to the Calvert formula described in product labeling

If GFR (or creatinine clearance) is estimated based on serum creatinine measurements by the IDMS method, the FDA recommends capping an estimated GFR at 125 mL/min for any targeted AUC value for patients with normal renal function. No greater estimated GFR values should be used

U.S. FDA. Carboplatin dosing. [online] October 8, 2010. Available from: http://www.fda.gov/AboutFDA/CentersOffices/CDER/ucm228974.htm

Supportive Care

Antiemetic prophylaxis

Emetogenic potential is **MODERATE**

See Chapter 39 for antiemetic recommendations

Hematopoietic growth factor (CSF) prophylaxis

Primary prophylaxis is NOT indicated

See Chapter 43 for more information

(continued)

Patient Population Studied

Thirty-six patients were enrolled in a prospective phase II study of a weekly docetaxel and carboplatin regimen. Patients eligible for the trial had an initial diagnosis of ovarian or primary peritoneal carcinoma. Initial treatment with a platinum-based regimen was required, with a treatment-free interval of at least 3 months. Patients could have received 1 prior regimen for recurrence. At the time of enrollment, patients were required to have a Gynecologic Oncology Group performance status of <2, neuropathy (sensory and motor) grade ≤2 (NCI Common Toxicity Criteria), and recovered from effects of recent surgery, radiotherapy, or chemotherapy. Biologically evaluable disease (CA-125) could be followed only if measurable disease was not present. The majority of patients had ovarian cancer (89%) and Stages III/IV (97%) disease, with a median initial disease-free interval of 12 months. Most subjects were treated for first recurrence (81%) and had measurable disease (58%)

Toxicity

Hematologic and Nonhematologic Toxicity*

Toxicity	% No Toxicity	% G1	% G2	% G3	% G4
Leukopenia	17	23	29	31	0
Neutropenia	26	9	17	34	14
Anemia	31	46	17	6	0
Thrombo-cytopenia	69	23	6	3	0
Gastro-intestinal	14	43	34	3	6
Neurologic	63	20	17	0	0
Carboplatin reaction[†]	63	11	11	14	0

*There was no detectable difference in quality of life as a consequence of therapy
[†]Carboplatin hypersensitivity reactions led to 11 subjects coming off trial (31%)

(continued)

Antimicrobial prophylaxis

Risk of fever and neutropenia is LOW

Antimicrobial primary prophylaxis to be considered:

- Antibacterial—not indicated
- Antifungal—not indicated
- Antiviral—not indicated unless patient previously had an episode of HSV

See Chapter 47 for more information

Dose Modifications

Adverse Event	Dose Modifications
ANC <1000/mm^3 or platelet count <75,000/mm^{3*}	Hold day 1 chemotherapy until ANC ≥1000/mm^3 and platelet count ≥75,000/mm^3
ANC <1500/mm^3 or platelet count <100,000/mm^3 on day 1 of a cycle	Reduce docetaxel dosage to 30 mg/m^2. If adverse effect occurred with docetaxel 30 mg/m^2, reduce each carboplatin dosage to AUC = 1 mg/mL · min per dose on the same administration schedule
ANC <1000/mm^3 or platelet count <75,000/mm^3 ≥3 weeks	Discontinue therapy
ANC <1000/mm^3, or Platelet count <100,000/mm^3, or G ≥3 renal toxicity, or G ≥2 toxicities with an adverse effect on organ function	Omit the scheduled weekly dose
ANC <500/mm^3 or platelet count <25,000/mm^3 for ≥7 days, or ANC <500/mm^3 despite filgrastim prophylaxis, or G4 neutropenia associated with fever, or G ≥3 anemia, or G ≥3 renal toxicity, or G ≥3 hepatic toxicity (bilirubin > ULN or transaminases >5 × ULN), or Uncontrolled G ≥3 nausea/vomiting, or G ≥2 stomatitis, or Other G ≥2 nonhematologic toxicities with an adverse effect on organ function, or Omission of 2 consecutive weekly doses	Reduce docetaxel dosage to 30 mg/m^2 per dose. If adverse effect occurred with docetaxel 30 mg/m^2, reduce carboplatin dosage to AUC = 1 mg/mL · min per dose on the same administration schedule
ANC <1500/mm^3 or platelet count <100,000/mm^3 despite 2-week delay, or Febrile neutropenia despite filgrastim support, or Febrile neutropenia at docetaxel dosages of 30 mg/m^2 and carboplatin AUC = 1 mg/mL · min, or Significant hypersensitivity reaction to docetaxel or carboplatin (hypotension, dyspnea and angioedema requiring therapy)*	Discontinue therapy
G ≥3 peripheral neuropathy	Hold therapy for a maximum of 2 weeks until toxicity G ≤2. Reinstitute therapy but reduce docetaxel dosage to 30 mg/m^2 per dose. If adverse effect occurred with docetaxel 30 mg/m^2, reduce carboplatin dosage to AUC = 1 mg/mL · min per dose on the same administration schedule

ULN, upper limit of normal range

*Patients who experience G1/2 carboplatin hypersensitivity reactions may continue treatment if there is evidence of tumor response and appropriate preventive measures are instituted

Efficacy*

Intention to Treat (N = 36)[†]

Overall response rate (ORR)	50% (18/36)
Complete response	11% (4/36)
Partial response	39% (14/36)

Evaluable for Response (N = 27)[†]

Overall response rate (ORR)	67% (18/27)
Complete response	15% (4/27)
Partial response	52% (14/27)
ORR biologically evaluable	65% (11/17)
ORR measurable disease	70% (7/10)
ORR platinum-resistant (treatment-free interval <6 months)	60% (3/5)
ORR platinum-sensitive disease (treatment-free interval >6 months)	68% (15/22)

Note: Data were not available concerning time to progression or survival

*RECIST (Response Evaluation Criteria in Solid Tumors) criteria were used to define response. If CA-125 was increased at baseline, normalization was required for a complete response (CR). Patients without measurable disease were evaluated by CA-125 values as described by Rustin et al. (J Clin Oncol 1996;14:1545–1551). Complete response = normalization of CA-125 lasting ≥4 weeks, documented with at least 3 normal values. Partial response (PR) = 50–75% improvement in the CA-125 level, lasting ≥ weeks. This could be documented in 1 of 2 ways: (a) 4 CA-125 levels, 2 initial elevated and 1 showing a 50% decrease requiring confirmation by a fourth sample, or (b) 3 CA-125 levels with a serial decrease of at least 75%. Progressive disease = a rise ≥50% documented on 2 separate occasions 1 week apart. Stable disease = any condition not meeting the above parameters

[†]Patients who received 1 or more cycles of drug and lived at least 3 weeks were evaluable for response. Twenty-seven patients were evaluable for response. Nine subjects were removed from study prior to the first response evaluation. Eight of these were removed because of toxicity and 1 subject withdrew consent for reasons other than toxicity

Therapy Monitoring

1. *Baseline:* LFTs, serum chemistry, CBC with differential and platelet count, and CA-125. Complete history and physical examination, including a gynecologic examination
2. *Follow-up:* CBC with differential and platelet count on days 1, 8, and 15, and LFTs before commencing repeated cycles

EPITHELIAL OVARIAN CANCER REGIMEN
CISPLATIN + GEMCITABINE

Rose PG et al. Gynecol Oncol 2003;88:17–21

Gemcitabine 750 mg/m^2 per dose; administer intravenously in 50–250 mL sodium chloride injection (0.9% NS) over 30–60 minutes for 2 doses, on days 1 and 8, every 21 days (total dosage/cycle = 1500 mg/m^2), *followed by:*

Hydration before cisplatin with ≥1000 mL 0.9% NS; administer intravenously over a minimum of 3–4 hours

Cisplatin 30 mg/m^2 per dose; administer intravenously in 100–500 mL 0.9% NS over 30–60 minutes for 2 doses, on days 1and 8, every 21 days (total dosage/cycle = 60 mg/m^2)

Hydration after cisplatin with ≥1000 mL 0.9% NS; administer intravenously over a minimum of 3–4 hours

Notes: Encourage increased oral intake of nonalcoholic fluids. Goal is to achieve a urine output ≥100 mL/hour. Monitor and replace electrolytes as needed (potassium, magnesium, sodium)

Supportive Care
Antiemetic prophylaxis
Emetogenic potential is **MODERATE–HIGH**. *Potential for delayed symptoms*
See Chapter 39 for antiemetic recommendations

Hematopoietic growth factor (CSF) prophylaxis
Primary prophylaxis is NOT indicated
See Chapter 43 for more information

Antimicrobial prophylaxis
Risk of fever and neutropenia is LOW
Antimicrobial primary prophylaxis to be considered:
- Antibacterial—not indicated
- Antifungal—not indicated
- Antiviral—not indicated unless patient previously had an episode of HSV

See Chapter 47 for more information

Patient Population Studied

Thirty-six patients with ovarian or peritoneal cancers whose disease was platinum- and paclitaxel-refractory, and who had failed to benefit from multiple second-line agents, were treated with a combination of gemcitabine and cisplatin. Tumors were defined as platinum-resistant if disease had progressed on or within 6 months after patients had completed their most recent platinum regimen. Patients had received a median of 2 (range: 1–5) prior platinum- or paclitaxel-based regimens, were heavily pretreated, and had received a median of 3 nonplatinum/nonpaclitaxel regimens (range: 0–6 regimens). Despite this, the majority of patients had an excellent performance status: ECOG = 0

Efficacy

Intention to Treat (N = 36)	
Overall response rate	41.6% (15/36)
Complete response	11.1% (4/36)
Partial response	30.5% (11/36)

Duration of Benefit (N = 35)	
Progression-free survival	6 months (range: 1–14 months)
Overall survival	12 months
Median response duration, responding patients	11 months (range: 4–14 months)

Intention to Treat/Evaluable Disease (N = 5)*,†	
Overall response rate	40% (2/5)

Intention to Treat/Measurable Disease (N = 31)†	
Overall response rate	42% (13/31)

Response According to Platinum-Free Interval	
<6 months	16.6% (1/6)
6–12 months	37.5% (3/8)
>12 months	50% (11/22)

Progression on Prior Gemcitabine (N = 6)	
Partial response	66% (4/6)

*In patients with "nonmeasurable" disease with only increased CA-125, a partial response was defined as a reduction in CA-125 value by ≥50%
†Neither maximum disease diameter nor a pretreatment CA-125 level correlated with response

Toxicity

Adverse Effects (First Cycle)

Adverse Effect	Grade				
	% G0	% G1	% G2	% G3	% G4
Leukopenia	27.8	11.1	36.1	22.2	2.8
Thrombocytopenia	8.3	22.2	50	16.7	2.8
Neutropenia	25	8.3	30.5	30.5	5.6
Anemia	5.6	38.9	47.2	8.8	—
Nausea/vomiting	86.1	—	5.6	—	8.3
Dermatologic	100	—	—	—	—
Renal	100	—	—	—	—
Peripheral neurotoxicity	100	—	—	—	—
Fever	100	—	—	—	—
Fatigue	100	—	—	—	—
Tinnitus	100	—	—	—	—
Hypomagnesemia	100	—	—	—	—
Pulmonary	100	—	—	—	—

Adverse Effects (All Cycles)

Adverse Effect	% G0	% G1	% G2	% G3	% G4
Leukopenia	25	13.9	16.7	41.7	2.8
Thrombocytopenia	8.8	19.4	38.9	30.6	5.6
Neutropenia	22.2	8.8	16.7	38.9	13.9
Anemia	—	22.2	58.3	19.4	—
Nausea/vomiting	86.1	—	5.6	—	8.8
Dermatologic	100	—	—	—	—
Renal	100	—	—	—	—
Peripheral neurotoxicity*	94.4	2.8	2.8	—	—
Fever	97.2	—	2.8	—	—
Fatigue	—	100	—	—	—
Tinnitus†	97.2	—	—	2.8†	—
Hypomagnesemia	100	—	—	—	—
Pulmonary	100	—	—	—	—

(continued)

Dose Modifications

Adverse Event	Dose Modifications
ANC <1500/mm³ or platelet count <100,000/mm³	Hold day 1 chemotherapy until ANC ≥1500/mm³ and platelet count ≥100,000/mm³
ANC <1500/mm³ or platelet count <100,000/mm³ ≥2 weeks	Discontinue therapy
Intracycle: G1/2 nonhematologic toxicity or G1–3 nausea or vomiting	100% gemcitabine dosage on day 8
Intracycle: G3 nonhematologic toxicity, except nausea, vomiting, and alopecia	Reduce gemcitabine dosage by 50% on day 8, or hold treatment at clinician's discretion
Intracycle: G4 nonhematologic toxicity	Hold gemcitabine
Intracycle: Day 8 ANC <1000/mm³ or platelet count <75,000/mm³	Do not administer day 8 therapy. In subsequent cycles, administer gemcitabine 600 mg/m² per dose on days 1 and 8. If adverse event occurred with gemcitabine 600 mg/m², administer gemcitabine 400 mg/m² per dose on days 1 and 8. If adverse event occurred with gemcitabine 400 mg/m², administer gemcitabine 300 mg/m² per dose on days 1 and 8.
Intracycle: Day 8 ANC 1000–1400/mm³ and/or platelet count 75,000–100,000/mm³	Reduce gemcitabine dosage to 600 mg/m². If adverse event occurred with gemcitabine 600 mg/m², administer gemcitabine 400 mg/m² per dose on days 1 and 8. If adverse event occurred with gemcitabine 400 mg/m², administer gemcitabine 300 mg/m² per dose on days 1 and 8

(continued)

Toxicity (continued)

Dose Reductions with Repeated Administrations

Toxicity Responsible for Reduction	Number of Dose Reductions			
	0	1	2	3
Thrombocytopenia and/or neutropenia	47.2	36.1	5.6	11.1

*Grade 1 peripheral neurotoxicity developed in all patients who received more than 8 cycles
†After 6 courses of therapy

Therapy Monitoring

1. *Baseline:* LFTs, serum chemistry (including potassium, magnesium, and sodium), CBC with differential and platelet count, and CA-125. Complete history and physical examination, including a gynecologic examination
2. *Follow-up:* CBC with differential and platelet count at least weekly through leukocyte and platelet count nadirs, and serum potassium, magnesium, and sodium before repeated treatment
3. Repeat LFTs before commencing repeated cycles

Dose Modifications (continued)

Adverse Event	Dose Modifications
Neutropenia and sepsis, *or* severe thrombocytopenia (platelets <20,000/mm³)	Administer gemcitabine 600 mg/m². If adverse event occurred with gemcitabine 600 mg/m², administer gemcitabine 400 mg/m² per dose on days 1 and 8. If adverse event occurred with gemcitabine 400 mg/m², administer gemcitabine 300 mg/m² per dose on days 1 and 8
G2 peripheral neuropathy	Reduce cisplatin dosage to 25 mg/m² per dose on days 1 and 8
G3/4 peripheral neuropathy	Hold therapy until peripheral neuropathy G ≤1, then restart therapy with cisplatin dosage reduced to cisplatin 20–25 mg/m² per dose on days 1 and 8. Consider discontinuing therapy if not recovered to baseline by 2–3 weeks
Creatinine clearance 40–60 mL/min (0.66–1 mL/s)	Reduce cisplatin so that dose in milligrams equals the creatinine clearance* value in mL/min†
Creatinine clearance <40 mL/min (<0.66 mL/s)	Hold cisplatin
On treatment day, serum creatinine 1.6–2 mg/dL (141–177 μmol/L)	Reduce cisplatin dosage by 25%
On treatment day 1, serum creatinine >2 mg/dL (>177 μmol/L)	Hold cisplatin until serum creatinine ≤2 mg/dL (≤177 μmol/L)

*Creatinine clearance is used as a measure of glomerular filtration rate
†This also applies to patients with creatinine clearance of 40–60 mL/min (0.66–1 mL/s) at the outset of treatment

EPITHELIAL OVARIAN CANCER REGIMEN

CARBOPLATIN + WEEKLY (DOSE-DENSE) PACLITAXEL

Katsumata N et al. Lancet 2009;374:1331–1338

Note: Regimen for optimally debulked ovarian cancer. Suboptimally debulked disease can be treated with this regimen as well

Premedication:

Dexamethasone 10 mg/dose; administer orally for 2 doses 12 hours and 6 hours before paclitaxel, *or*

Dexamethasone 20 mg/dose; administer intravenously over 10–15 minutes, 30–60 minutes before paclitaxel on days 1, 8, and 15 (total dose/cycle = 60 mg)

Diphenhydramine 50 mg; administer by intravenous injection 30–60 minutes before paclitaxel

Cimetidine 300 mg (or **ranitidine** 50 mg, **famotidine** 20 mg, or an equivalent histamine receptor [H_2]-subtype antagonist); administer intravenously over 15–30 minutes, 30–60 minutes before paclitaxel

Paclitaxel 80 mg/m^2 per dose; administer intravenously in a volume of 0.9% sodium chloride injection (0.9% NS) or 5% dextrose injection (D5W) sufficient to produce a concentration within the range 0.3–1.2 mg/mL, over 60 minutes for 3 doses, on days 1, 8, and 15, every 3 weeks (total dosage/cycle = 240 mg/m^2)

Carboplatin (calculated dose) AUC = 6*; administer intravenously in 0.9% NS or D5W 100–500 mL over 60 minutes, on day 1 after completing paclitaxel, every 3 weeks (total dosage/cycle calculated to produce a target AUC = 6 mg/mL · min)

*Carboplatin dose is based on a formula described by Calvert et al. to achieve a target area under the plasma concentration versus time curve (AUC)

$$\text{Total carboplatin dose (mg)} = (\text{target AUC}) \times (\text{GFR} + 25)$$

In practice, creatinine clearance (Clcr) is used in place of glomerular filtration rate (GFR). Clcr can be estimated from the equation of Cockcroft and Gault, thus:

$$\text{For males, Clcr} = \frac{(140 \pm \text{age [years]}) \times \text{body weight [kg]}}{72 \times (\text{serum creatinine [mg/dL]})}$$

$$\text{For females, Clcr} = \frac{(140 - \text{age [years]}) \times \text{body weight [kg]}}{72 \times (\text{serum creatinine [mg/dL]})} \times 0.85$$

Calvert AH et al. J Clin Oncol 1989;7:1748–1756
Cockcroft DW, Gault MH. Nephron 1976;16:31–41
Jodrell DI et al. J Clin Oncol 1992;10:520–528
Sorensen BT et al. Cancer Chemother Pharmacol 1991;28:397–401

Note: On October 8, 2010, the U.S. Food and Drug Administration (FDA) identified a potential safety issue with carboplatin dosing based on recent changes in the measurement of serum creatinine. By the end of 2010, all clinical laboratories in the United States began using the standardized isotope dilution mass spectrometry (IDMS) method to measure serum creatinine, which could result in an overestimation of the GFR in some patients with normal renal function. A carboplatin dose calculated with an IDMS-measured serum creatinine result using the Calvert formula could exceed an expected exposure (AUC) and result in increased drug-related toxicity

Provided actual GFR measurements are made to assess renal function, carboplatin can be safely dosed according to the Calvert formula described in product labeling

If GFR (or creatinine clearance) is estimated based on serum creatinine measurements by the IDMS method, the FDA recommends capping an estimated GFR at 125 mL/min for any targeted AUC value for patients with normal renal function. No greater estimated GFR values should be used U.S. FDA. Carboplatin dosing. [online] October 8, 2010. Available from: http://www.fda.gov/AboutFDA/CentersOffices/CDER/ucm228974.htm

Supportive Care

Antiemetic prophylaxis

Emetogenic potential on days with carboplatin is **HIGH**. *Potential for delayed symptoms*

Emetogenic potential on days with paclitaxel alone is **LOW**

See Chapter 39 for antiemetic recommendations

Hematopoietic growth factor (CSF) prophylaxis

Primary prophylaxis is NOT indicated

See Chapter 43 for more information

(continued)

Patient Population Studied

Phase III, open-label, randomized trial conducted in 95 centers in Japan. Patients had a histologically or cytologically proven diagnosis of Stages II to IV epithelial ovarian cancer, fallopian tube cancer, or primary peritoneal cancer. Eastern Cooperative Oncology Group (ECOG) performance status of 0–3, and adequate organ function. Patients were excluded if they had an ovarian tumor with a low malignant potential. Previous chemotherapy was not allowed

Dose Modifications

Adverse Event	Dose Modifications
ANC <1000/mm^3 or platelet count <75,000/mm^3	Hold day 1 chemotherapy until ANC ≥1000/mm^3 and platelet count ≥75,000/mm^3
ANC <1000/mm^3 or platelet count <75,000/mm^3 ≥3 weeks	Discontinue therapy
If on days 8 or 15, ANC <500/mm^3 or platelet count <50,000/mm^3	Hold chemotherapy until ANC ≥500/mm^3 and platelet count ≥50,000/mm^3
G3/4 nonhematologic toxicity	Reduce paclitaxel dosage to 70 mg/m^2
G3/4 nonhematologic toxicity with paclitaxel 70 mg/m^2	Reduce paclitaxel dosage to 60 mg/m^2
With carboplatin target AUC = 6 mg/mL · min: Febrile neutropenia, *or* ANC <500/mm^3 for ≥7 days, *or* Platelet count <10,000/mm^3, *or* Platelet count 10,000–50,000/mm^3 with bleeding, *or* Treatment delay for hematologic toxicity >1 week	Reduce carboplatin dosage to target an AUC = 5 mg/mL · min

(continued)

(*continued*)

Antimicrobial prophylaxis
Risk of fever and neutropenia is LOW
  Antimicrobial primary prophylaxis to be considered:
- Antibacterial—not indicated
- Antifungal—not indicated
- Antiviral—not indicated unless patient previously had an episode of HSV

See Chapter 47 for more information

Efficacy*

	Dose-Dense Paclitaxel[†] (N = 147)	Conventional Paclitaxel[‡] (N = 135)	p-Value
Complete response[§]	20%	16%	0.44
Partial response[§]	36%	38%	0.81
Stable disease[§]	29%	31%	0.8
Progressive disease[§]	3%	7%	0.16
Not evaluable[§]	12%	9%	0.44
Median progression-free survival	28 months	17.2 months	0.0015
Overall survival at 2 years	83.6%	77.7%	0.049
Overall survival at 3 years	72.1%	65.1%	0.03

*Katsumata N et al. Lancet 2009;374:1331–1338
[†]Carboplatin AUC = 6 mg/mL · min + paclitaxel 80 mg/m^2 per dose, on days 1, 8, and 15, every 21 days
[‡]Carboplatin AUC = 6 mg/mL · min + paclitaxel 180 mg/m^2 on day 1, every 21 days
[§]Clinical response in patients with measurable lesions

Toxicity*,†

	Dose-Dense Paclitaxel[‡] (N = 312)	Conventional Paclitaxel[§] (N = 314)	p-Value
Hematologic Toxicity			
Neutropenia	92%	88%	0.15
Thrombocytopenia	44%	38%	0.19
Anemia	69%	44%	<0.0001
Febrile neutropenia	9%	9%	1
Nonhematologic Toxicity			
Nausea	10%	11%	0.7
Vomiting	3%	4%	0.82
Diarrhea	3%	3%	0.64
Fatigue	5%	3%	0.14
Arthralgia	1%	2%	0.72
Myalgia	1%	1%	0.69
Motor neuropathy	5%	4%	0.56
Sensory neuropathy	7%	6%	0.87

*Katsumata N et al. Lancet 2009;374:1331–1338
[†]According to NCI Common Toxicity Criteria, version 2.0
[‡]Carboplatin AUC = 6 mg/mL · min + paclitaxel 80 mg/m^2 per dose, on days 1, 8, and 15, every 21 days
[§]Carboplatin AUC = 6 mg/mL · min + paclitaxel 180 mg/m^2 on day 1, every 21 days

Dose Modifications (*continued*)

Adverse Event	Dose Modifications
With carboplatin target AUC = 5 mg/mL · min: Febrile neutropenia, *or* ANC <500/mm^3 for ≥7 days, *or* Platelet count <10,000/mm^3, *or* Platelet count 10,000–50,000/mm^3 with bleeding, *or* Treatment delay for hematologic toxicity >1 week	Reduce carboplatin dosage to target an AUC = 4 mg/mL · min
G ≥2 peripheral neuropathy	Reduce paclitaxel dosage to 70 mg/m^2
G ≥2 peripheral neuropathy with paclitaxel 70 mg/m^2	Reduce paclitaxel dosage to 60 mg/m^2
Significant hypersensitivity reaction to carboplatin (hypotension, dyspnea, and angioedema requiring therapy)*	Discontinue therapy

*Patients who experience G1/2 carboplatin hypersensitivity reactions may continue treatment if there is evidence of tumor response and appropriate preventive measures are instituted

Therapy Monitoring

1. *Baseline:* LFTs, serum chemistry, CBC with differential and platelet count, and CA-125. Complete history and physical examination, including a gynecologic examination
2. *Follow-up:* CBC with differential and platelet count at least weekly through leukocyte and platelet count nadirs, and before beginning *repeated* cycles
3. *Before beginning repeated cycles:* Repeat LFTs

EPITHELIAL OVARIAN CANCER REGIMEN
PEMETREXED

Miller DS et al. J Clin Oncol 2009;27:2686–2691
Vergote I et al. Eur J Cancer 2009;45:1415–1423

Ancillary medications:
Folic acid 350–1000 mcg; administer daily beginning 1–2 weeks before the first dose of pemetrexed and continue until 3 weeks after the last pemetrexed dose
Cyanocobalamin (vitamin B_{12}) 1000 mcg; administer by intramuscular injection every 9 weeks, beginning 1–2 weeks before the first dose of pemetrexed, and continue until 3 weeks after the last pemetrexed dose
Dexamethasone 4 mg; administer orally twice daily for 3 days (6 doses) starting the day before each pemetrexed dose (total dose/cycle = 24 mg)
Notes: Nonsteroidal antiinflammatory drugs should be held for 2 days before and 2 days after pemetrexed administration
Pemetrexed 500 mg/m²; administer intravenously in 10 mL 0.9% sodium chloride injection (0.9% NS) over 10 minutes on day 1, every 21 days, for a maximum of 6 cycles (unless there was earlier evidence of disease progression or intolerance of the study treatment) (total dosage/cycle = 500 mg/m²)
Note: In a randomized double blind phase II study, pemetrexed 500 mg/m² had comparable activity with a more favorable toxicity profile than a dosage of 900 mg/m²

Supportive Care
Antiemetic prophylaxis
Emetogenic potential is **LOW**
See Chapter 39 for antiemetic recommendations

Hematopoietic growth factor (CSF) prophylaxis
Primary prophylaxis is NOT indicated
See Chapter 43 for more information

Antimicrobial prophylaxis
Risk of fever and neutropenia is LOW
  Antimicrobial primary prophylaxis to be considered:
  • Antibacterial—not indicated
  • Antifungal—not indicated
  • Antiviral—not indicated unless patient previously had an episode of HSV
See Chapter 47 for more information

Therapy Monitoring
1. *Baseline:* LFTs, serum chemistry, CBC with differential and platelet count, and CA-125. Complete history and physical examination including a gynecologic examination
2. *Follow-up:* CBC with differential and platelet count at least weekly through leukocyte and platelet count nadirs, and before beginning *repeated* cycles
3. *Before beginning repeated cycles:* Repeat LFTs

Dose Modifications

Adverse Event	Dose Modifications
ANC <1500/mm³ *or* Platelet count <100,000/mm³, or G ≥2 nonhematologic toxicity	Hold day 1 chemotherapy until: ANC ≥1500/mm³, platelet count ≥100,000/mm³, and nonhematologic toxicity is G ≤1
ANC <1500/mm³ ≥2 weeks, *or* Platelet count <100,000/mm³ ≥2 weeks, *or* G ≥2 nonhematologic toxicity ≥2 weeks	Discontinue therapy
Febrile neutropenia and/or G4 neutropenia persisting for >7 days, or G4 thrombocytopenia, or G2 bleeding	Reduce pemetrexed dosage by 100 mg/m² or discontinue therapy
G3/4 nonhematologic toxicity	Reduce pemetrexed dosage by 100 mg/m² or discontinue therapy
G>2 peripheral neuropathy	Reduce pemetrexed dosage by 100 mg/m² or discontinue therapy

Efficacy*

	Pemetrexed Dose		
	500 mg/m² (N = 43†)	900 mg/m² (N = 48†)	P Value‡
Best Study Response			
Overall response rate (95% CI)	9.3% (92.6–22.10)	10.4% (3.5–22.7)	1.000
Partial response rate	9.3%	10.4%	—
Stable disease	32.6%	29.2%	—
Progressive disease	48.8%	50%	—
Unknown	9.3%	10.4%	—
Time to Event Parameters (95% CI)			
Median time to response	2.1 (1.4–3.4)	1.5 (1.1–2.3)	0.270
Median duration of response	4 (3.1–6)	4.3 (3.2–6.1)	0.799
Median progression-free survival	2.8 (2.6–4.2)	2.8 (2.1–4.2)	0.786
Median overall survival	11.9 (7.9–14.8)	10.3 (7.7–14.8)	0.974

*Tumor response assessed according to RECIST. Elevated CA-125 levels were followed as target lesions if no other target lesions were present as defined in the Gynaecologic Cancer InterGroup (GCIG) criteria
†Reasons not evaluable for efficacy: pemetrexed 500 mg/m² per dose: One patient did not meet the CA-125 inclusion criterion, 1 did not have ovarian or primary peritoneal cancer, and 2 patients did not have platinum-resistant disease; pemetrexed 900 mg/m² per dose: 3 patients did not have platinum-resistant disease
‡Fisher's exact

Toxicity*

Toxicity†	Pemetrexed 500 mg/m² (N = 47)				Pemetrexed 900 mg/m² (N = 51)			
	% G1	% G2	% G3	% G4	% G1	% G2	% G3	% G4
Hematologic								
Anemia	2.1	14.9	6.4	4.3	5.9	23.5	11.8	2
Leukopenia	0	6.4	4.3	2.1	2	0	5.9	3.9
Neutropenia	2.1	2.1	2.1	10.6	2	3.9	7.8	5.9
Febrile neutropenia	0	0	2.1	4.3	0	2	3.9	0
Thrombocytopenia	2.1	2.1	2.1	2.1	3.9	0	5.9	5.9
Nonhematologic								
ALT, SGPT	0	2.1	2.1	0	2	0	5.9	0
Ascites	2.1	2.1	6.4	0	2	7.8	3.9	0
Fatigue (asthenia, lethargy, malaise)	31.9	38.3	6.4	0	33.3	25.5	13.7	0
Ileus	0	0	6.4	0	3.9	2	3.9	0
Vomiting	17	27.7	4.3	0	23.5	19.6	5.9	0

ALT, Alanine transaminase; SGPT, serum glutamic pyruvic transaminase
*NCI, Common Toxicity Criteria
†Toxicities reported are those for which ≥5% of patients experienced a G3/4 toxicity in at least 1 treatment arm, except for febrile neutropenia for which all patients are included

EPITHELIAL OVARIAN CANCER REGIMEN

DOCETAXEL

Kaye SB et al. Eur J Cancer 1995;31A(Suppl 4):S14–S17

Premedication:
Dexamethasone 8 mg/dose; administer orally twice daily for 3 days (6 doses) starting on the day before docetaxel administration (total dose/cycle = 48 mg) *or*
Dexamethasone 4 mg/dose; administer orally for 3 doses during the evening before, morning of, and evening after docetaxel administration (total dose/cycle = 12 mg)
Docetaxel 75–100 mg/m²; administer intravenously in a volume of 0.9% sodium chloride injection or 5% dextrose injection sufficient to produce a docetaxel concentration within the range of 0.3–0.74 mg/mL over 60 minutes on day 1, every 21 days, for 4 cycles (total dosage per cycle = 75–100 mg/m²)

Supportive Care
Antiemetic prophylaxis
*Emetogenic potential is **LOW–MODERATE***
See Chapter 39 for antiemetic recommendations

Hematopoietic growth factor (CSF) prophylaxis
Primary prophylaxis is NOT indicated
See Chapter 43 for more information

Antimicrobial prophylaxis
Risk of fever and neutropenia is LOW
  Antimicrobial primary prophylaxis to be considered:
  • Antibacterial—not indicated
  • Antifungal—not indicated
  • Antiviral—not indicated unless patient previously had an episode of HSV
See Chapter 47 for more information

Patient Population Studied

Evaluation of docetaxel administration in 293 patients with advanced ovarian cancer in 3 phase II trials. All patients had previously received cisplatin and/or carboplatin as first-line treatment. In all 3 studies, docetaxel 100 mg/m² was administered every 3 weeks, without premedication for hypersensitivity reactions or emesis. At the time of the analysis, 200 patients were evaluable for response

Therapy Monitoring

1. *Baseline:* LFTs, serum chemistry, CBC with differential and platelet count, and CA-125. Complete history and physical examination including a gynecologic examination
2. *Follow-up:* CBC with differential and platelet count at least weekly through leukocyte and platelet count nadirs, and prior to beginning *repeated cycles*
3. *Before beginning repeated cycles:* Repeat LFTs

Toxicity

Incidence and Severity of Major Adverse Effects of 100 mg/m² Docetaxel

Adverse Effect	Incidence
Neutropenia (grade 3 or 4)	83/99 patients (84%)
Acute hypersensitivity (grades 2–4)	13/207 patients (6%)
Skin reactions (grades 2–4)	98/188 patients (52%)
Fluid retention or effusions	102/181 patients (56%)*
Neuropathy (grades 2–3)	11/95 patients (12%)

*Incidence was 66% in patients who received 6 courses of docetaxel

Treatment Modifications

Adverse Events	Treatment Modifications
ANC <1500/mm³ on day of planned treatment*	Delay treatment until ANC ≥1500/mm³; administer filgrastim during subsequent cycles†
ANC <500/mm³ ≥7 days	Reduce docetaxel dosage by 20% during subsequent cycles (or add filgrastim†)
First episode of febrile neutropenia	Reduce docetaxel dosage by 20% during subsequent cycles (or add filgrastim†)
Second episode of febrile neutropenia	Continue docetaxel and give filgrastim† during subsequent cycles
Third episode of febrile neutropenia	Add ciprofloxacin‡
First episode of G4 documented infection	Reduce docetaxel dosage by 20% during subsequent cycles
Second episode of G4 documented infection	Continue docetaxel and give filgrastim† and ciprofloxacin‡ during subsequent cycles
Third episode of G4 documented infection	Discontinue docetaxel

*Although an ANC of 1500/mm³ is often identified as a minimum acceptable ANC to safely proceed with treatment, recent data show that an ANC ≥1000/mm³ is acceptable if filgrastim is given after chemotherapy
†Filgrastim 5 mcg/kg per day subcutaneously for 8 consecutive days, days 3–10
‡Ciprofloxacin 500 mg orally twice daily for 7 consecutive days starting on day 5

Efficacy*

Results of Phase II Trials of 100 mg/m² Docetaxel by Study and Type of Response

Response	Study (Number of Patients)				Percent of Evaluable Patients E = 200	Percent of Enrolled Patients N = 293
	ECTG N = 123 E = 85	CSG N = 126 E = 75	MDACC N = 44 E = 40	All Studies N = 293 E = 200		
Complete response	3	6	1	10	5	3.4
Partial response	23	17	13	53	26.5	18.1
Progressive disease	21	22	3	46	23	15.7
Evaluable, ORR	31	31	35	31.5	—	—
Enrolled ORR	21	18	32	21.5	—	—

ECTG, Early Clinical Trials Group of the European Organisation for Research and Treatment of Cancer; CSG, Clinical Screening Group of the EORTC; MDACC, The University of Texas MD Anderson Cancer Center, Houston, Texas, USA; N, number of patients enrolled; E, number of patients evaluable; ORR, overall response rate
*Response criteria were those accepted by UICC. Although CA-125 measurements were made with every course of treatment, the results were not used in the response assessment

PLATINUM-REFRACTORY OR PLATINUM-RESISTANT REGIMEN

FLUOROURACIL + LEUCOVORIN

Reed E et al. Gynecol Oncol 1992;46:326–329

Leucovorin 500 mg/m^2 per dose; administer intravenously in 25–100 mL 0.9% sodium chloride injection or 5% dextrose injection over 30 minutes, daily for 5 consecutive days, on days 1–5, every 21 days (total dosage/cycle = 2500 mg/m^2), *followed after 1 hour by:*
Fluorouracil 375 mg/m^2 per dose; administer by intravenous injection over 3–5 minutes, daily, 1 hour after the completion of leucovorin, for 5 consecutive days, days 1–5, every 21 days (total dosage/cycle = 1875 mg/m^2)

Supportive Care
Antiemetic prophylaxis
Emetogenic potential is **LOW**
See Chapter 39 for antiemetic recommendations

Hematopoietic growth factor (CSF) prophylaxis
Primary prophylaxis is NOT indicated
See Chapter 43 for more information

Antimicrobial prophylaxis
Risk of fever and neutropenia is LOW
Antimicrobial primary prophylaxis to be considered:
- Antibacterial—not indicated
- Antifungal—not indicated
- Antiviral—not indicated unless patient previously had an episode of HSV

See Chapter 47 for more information

Patient Population Studied

A study of 29 patients with recurrent advanced-stage ovarian cancer of epithelial histology who had progressive disease while receiving or had suffered relapse after high-dose cisplatin therapy

Efficacy (N = 29)

	Relapsed After Response to Platinum-Based Therapy (n = 8)	Progressive Disease on Platinum-Based Therapy (n = 21)
CR	13%	5%
PR	—	5%
SD*	38%	38%
PD	50%	52%

*SD: 5, 5, 7, 8, 8, 8, 10, 13, 14, 21, and 27 months

Toxicity* (N = 29/204 Cycles)

	Number of Cycles			
	G1	G2	G3	G4
Hematologic				
Neutropenia	1	5	7	4
Thrombocytopenia	7	2	4	4
Anemia	4	6	5	1
Nonhematologic				
Nausea/vomiting	9	3	2	0
Stomatitis	9	5	4	2
Diarrhea	11	3	3	0

*National Cancer Institute Common Toxicity Criteria, version 2

Treatment Modifications

Adverse Event	Dose Modification
G2 nonhematologic toxicity	Reduce fluorouracil daily dosage by 25% on the same administration schedule
WBC <3000/mm^3 or platelet count <75,000/mm^3 on treatment day	Delay cycle 1 week until WBC >3000/mm^3 and platelet count >75,000/mm^3

If no toxicity G >1 is documented in a cycle, then increase fluorouracil daily dosage by 25% on the same administration schedule

Therapy Monitoring

Before repeated cycles: PE, CBC with differential, and serum electrolytes

Notes

Because this regimen is well tolerated, it represents an option for patients when more attractive options have been exhausted

PLATINUM-REFRACTORY OR PLATINUM-RESISTANT REGIMEN

GEMCITABINE

Markman M et al. Gynecol Oncol 2003;90:593–596

Gemcitabine 1000 mg/m² per dose; administer intravenously diluted to a concentration ≥0.1 mg/mL in 0.9% sodium chloride injection over 30 minutes for 3 doses, on days 1, 8, and 15, every 28 days (total dosage/cycle = 3000 mg/m²)

Supportive Care
Antiemetic prophylaxis
Emetogenic potential is **LOW**
See Chapter 39 for antiemetic recommendations

Hematopoietic growth factor (CSF) prophylaxis
Primary prophylaxis is NOT indicated
See Chapter 43 for more information

Antimicrobial prophylaxis
Risk of fever and neutropenia is LOW
Antimicrobial primary prophylaxis to be considered:
- Antibacterial—not indicated
- Antifungal—not indicated
- Antiviral—not indicated unless patient previously had an episode of HSV

See Chapter 47 for more information

Patient Population Studied

A study of 51 patients with ovarian (41), fallopian tube (1), and primary peritoneal cancer (9) and prior chemotherapy with a platinum agent (cisplatin or carboplatin) and a taxane (paclitaxel or docetaxel). If a patient had previously responded to such therapy, and the treatment-free interval had been 3 months, the patient had to be retreated with a platinum agent or a taxane to confirm clinical resistance

Efficacy (N = 51)

Partial response	8%
≥75% decrease in CA-125	8%
Median duration of response	4 months
Survival (all patients)	7 months
Survival (patients with response)	15 months

Toxicity (N = 51)

	% Patients
Hematologic	
G4 neutropenia	24
G3 thrombocytopenia	7
Nonhematologic	
G3 fatigue	10
Fever/chills (no neutropenia)	15
Rash	4
Conjunctivitis	4

Treatment Modifications

Adverse Event	Dose Modification
ANC nadir <1000/mm³ or platelet count nadir ≤100,000/mm³	Hold treatment until ANC recovers to ≥ 1000/mm³ and platelets to >100,000/mm³, then resume with gemcitabine dosage decreased by 200 mg/m² per dose
Second occurrence of ANC nadir ≤1000/mm³ or platelet count nadir ≤100,000/mm³	Hold treatment until ANC recovers to >1000/mm³ and platelets to >100,000/mm³, then resume with gemcitabine dosage decreased by an additional 200 mg/m² per dose
Third occurrence of ANC nadir ≤1000/mm³ or platelet count nadir ≤100,000/mm³	Discontinue gemcitabine therapy
G3 nonhematologic toxicity	Hold treatment until toxicities resolve to G <1, then resume with gemcitabine dosage decreased by 200 mg/m² per dose
Second occurrence of G3 nonhematologic toxicity	Hold treatment until toxicities resolve to G ≤1, then resume with gemcitabine dosage decreased by an additional 200 mg/m² per dose

Therapy Monitoring

Before repeated cycles: PE, CBC with differential, and serum electrolytes, magnesium, calcium, BUN, creatinine, and LFTs

Notes

Gemcitabine dosages of 1250 mg/m² resulted in excessive toxicity

PLATINUM-REFRACTORY OR PLATINUM-RESISTANT REGIMEN

ORAL ALTRETAMINE (HEXAMETHYLMELAMINE)

Chan JK et al. Gynecol Oncol 2004;92:368–371

Altretamine 65 mg/m² per dose; administer orally 4 times daily, after meals and at bedtime, for 14 consecutive days, on days 1–14, every 28 days (total dosage/cycle = 3640 mg/m²) *or*
Altretamine 65 mg/m² per dose; administer orally 4 times daily, after meals and at bedtime, for 21 consecutive days, on days 1–21, every 28 days (total dosage/cycle = 5460 mg/m²)

Supportive Care
Antiemetic prophylaxis
Emetogenic potential is **MODERATE–HIGH**
See Chapter 39 for antiemetic recommendations

Hematopoietic growth factor (CSF) prophylaxis
Primary prophylaxis is NOT indicated
See Chapter 43 for more information

Antimicrobial prophylaxis
Risk of fever and neutropenia is LOW
   Antimicrobial primary prophylaxis to be considered:
   • Antibacterial—not indicated
   • Antifungal—not indicated
   • Antiviral—not indicated unless patient previously had an episode of HSV
See Chapter 47 for more information

Patient Population Studied

A report of 2 women with recurrent ovarian cancer. Includes review of the literature

Efficacy

Response to altretamine appears to be:
1. Correlated with response to initial platinum therapy: Higher in patients whose disease responded to initial therapy
2. Correlated with treatment-free interval after an initial response to platinum therapy: The longer the interval, the higher the response
3. Higher in platinum-sensitive (PS) disease than in platinum-resistant (PR) disease: Response rates for PS disease in several studies range from 17–50%, whereas response for PR disease range from 0–35%

Treatment Modifications

Adverse Event	Dose Modification
GI intolerance unresponsive to symptomatic measures	Discontinue altretamine for ≥14 days, then resume at 50 mg/m² per dose 4 times daily for the same planned treatment duration
WBC <2000/mm³ or ANC <1000/mm³	
Platelet count <75,000/mm³	
Progressive neurotoxicity	
Progressive neurotoxicity that does not stabilize on a reduced altretamine dosage	Discontinue altretamine indefinitely

Therapy Monitoring

Before repeated cycles: PE, CBC with differential, and serum electrolytes, magnesium, calcium, BUN, and creatinine

Toxicity

Hematologic

Moderate-to-severe anemia	13%
Platelet counts <50,000/mm³	≤10%
WBC counts <2000/mm³	≤1%

Nonhematologic

Nausea and vomiting	33%*
Severe nausea and vomiting	1%*
Moderate-to-severe peripheral sensory neuropathy	9%*
Mild sensory neuropathy	22%
Increased alkaline phosphatase	9%
Mood disorders*: depression, insomnia, confusion, personality changes, anxiety	≤1%
Movement and coordination disorders*	1%
Fatigue, malaise, lethargy	1%

*Symptoms are more likely to occur in patients who receive continuous daily treatment with high doses of altretamine than with moderate doses administered on an intermittent schedule

PLATINUM-REFRACTORY OR PLATINUM-RESISTANT REGIMEN

DOXORUBICIN HCL LIPOSOME INJECTION (LIPOSOMAL DOXORUBICIN)

Lorusso D et al. Oncology 2004;67:243–249
Thigpen JT et al. Gynecol Oncol 2005;96:10–18

Doxorubicin HCl liposome injection 40–50 mg/m^2; administer intravenously diluted in 250 mL 5% dextrose injection (D5W) for doses ≤90 mg and in 500 mL D5W for doses >90 mg every 3–4 weeks (total dosage/cycle = 40–50 mg/m^2)
Note: Administer at an initial rate of 1 mg/min for 10–15 minutes. If infusion reactions are not observed, the rate may be increased to complete drug administration over 60 minutes

Supportive Care
Antiemetic prophylaxis
Emetogenic potential is **LOW**
See Chapter 39 for antiemetic recommendations

Hematopoietic growth factor (CSF) prophylaxis
Primary prophylaxis is NOT indicated
See Chapter 43 for more information

Antimicrobial prophylaxis
Risk of fever and neutropenia is LOW
Antimicrobial Primary Prophylaxis to be Considered:
- Antibacterial—not indicated
- Antifungal—not indicated
- Antiviral—not indicated, unless patient previously had an episode of HSV

See Chapter 47 for more information

Hand-foot reaction (palmar-plantar erythrodysesthesia)
For patients who develop a hand-foot reaction, use topical emollients (eg, Aquaphor), topical or orally administered steroids, antihistamine agents (H$_1$-receptor antagonists), or pyridoxine Pyridoxine may provide relief for discomfort/pain associated with PPE although the mechanism through which this occurs remains unclear
- The suggested pyridoxine starting dose is 50 mg/day, which may be increased to a maximum of 200 mg/day

Patients who have developed G1/2 PPE while receiving doxorubicin HCl liposome injection may receive a fixed daily dose of pyridoxine, 200 mg. This may allow for treatment to be completed without dosage reduction, treatment delay, or recurrence of PPE.

Patient Population Studied

A study of 37 patients with advanced ovarian cancer in whom first-line therapy had failed to provide benefit

Efficacy

Response rates of 7.7–26% have been reported in several studies with a median progression-free survival of 4–6 months

Treatment Modifications

Adverse Event	Dose Modification
Hand-foot syndrome	Reduce dosage to 40 mg/m^2
G3/4 nonhematologic toxicity	
Stomatitis G ≥2	
Persistent (>3 weeks) G1/2 toxicity	Increase dosing interval to 4 weeks
Persistent (>4 weeks) G3/4 toxicity	Discontinue therapy

Therapy Monitoring

Before repeated cycles: PE, CBC with differential, and serum electrolytes, magnesium, calcium, BUN, and creatinine

Notes

The consensus of experts in the management of ovarian carcinoma:
1. Based on survival and toxicity advantages and a once-monthly administration schedule, liposomal doxorubicin is considered by some to be the first-choice nonplatinum agent for relapsed ovarian cancer
2. Tolerability is improved with the use of liposomal doxorubicin 40 mg/m^2 on an every-4-week schedule. Hand-foot syndrome (PPE) is the most commonly reported adverse event associated with liposomal doxorubicin. Avoid this toxicity by using lower dosages of liposomal doxorubicin (40 mg/m^2 every 4 weeks, or 10 mg/m^2 weekly), rather than omitting or decreasing doses as a consequence of adverse events

Thigpen JT et al. Gynecol Oncol 2005;96:10–18

Toxicity (N = 37)

	% G1	% G2	% G3	% G4
Hematologic				
Neutropenia	—	—	—	—
Thrombocytopenia	3	—	—	—
Anemia	24	—	—	—
Febrile neutropenia	—	—	—	—
Nonhematologic				
PPE	11	8	3	—
Stomatitis/mucositis	8	—	—	—
Nausea/vomiting	14	—	—	—
Asthenia	24	—	—	—
Hair loss	16	—	—	—
Anaphylactic reactions	5	—	—	—
Liver toxicity	—	—	—	—
Cardiac toxicity	—	—	—	—

Note: Toxicity grades for palmar plantar erythrodysesthesia (PPE):
G1 Mild erythema, swelling or desquamation not interfering with daily activities
G2 Erythema, swelling, or desquamation interfering with daily activities; small blisters or ulcerations <2 cm
G3 Blistering, ulcerations, or swelling interfering with daily activities; patient cannot wear regular clothing
G4 Diffuse or local process causing infectious complications, a bedridden state, or hospitalization

Lorusso D et al. Oncology 2004;67:243–249

REGIMEN
VINORELBINE

Rothenberg ML et al. Gynecol Oncol 2004;95: 506–512

Vinorelbine 30 mg/m² per dose; administer by intravenous injection over 1–2 minutes for 2 doses, on days 1 and 8, every 21 days (total dosage/cycle = 60 mg/m²)

Supportive Care
Antiemetic prophylaxis
Emetogenic potential is **MINIMAL**
See Chapter 39 for antiemetic recommendations

Hematopoietic growth factor (CSF) prophylaxis
Primary prophylaxis is NOT indicated
See Chapter 43 for more information

Antimicrobial prophylaxis
Risk of fever and neutropenia is LOW
   Antimicrobial primary prophylaxis to be considered:
   • Antibacterial—not indicated
   • Antifungal—not indicated
   • Antiviral—not indicated unless patient previously had an episode of HSV

See Chapter 47 for more information

Decreased bowel motility
Give a bowel regimen to prevent constipation based initially on stool softeners

Treatment Modifications

Adverse Event	Dose Modification
ANC <1000/mm³ or platelet count <75,000/mm³ on the day before or the day of vinorelbine administration	Hold vinorelbine dose on this day
ANC 1000–1499/mm³ or platelet count 75,000–99,999/mm³ on the day before or the day of vinorelbine administration	Administer vinorelbine, but reduce vinorelbine dosage by 7.5 mg/m²
On the day before or the day of repeated vinorelbine administration, ANC 1000–1499/mm³ or platelet count 75,000–99,999/mm³ after vinorelbine 15 mg/m²	Discontinue therapy

Toxicity* (N = 79)

	% G0	% G1	% G2	% G3	% G4
Hematologic					
Anemia	27	23	38	13	0
Granulocytopenia	24	4	16	28	28
Leukopenia	11	19	23	39	8
Thrombocytopenia	78	19	3	0	0
Nonhematologic					
Abdominal pain	72	10	13	5	0
Alopecia	71	16	13	0	0
Anorexia	76	24	0	0	0
Constipation	51	28	15	6	0
Dyspnea	78	0	18	3	1
Fever without infection	79	13	8	0	0
Insomnia	89	11	0	0	0
Malaise/fatigue/lethargy	34	27	28	11	0
Nausea	42	39	11	8	0
Numbness/other symptoms of peripheral neuropathy	75	0	25	0	0
Pain	69	15	11	5	0
Paresthesia	89	5	6	0	0
Vomiting	71	14	13	1	0
Weakness	86	8	3	3	0

*National Cancer Institute Common Toxicity Criteria, version 2

Patient Population Studied
A study of 79 patients with recurrent or resistant epithelial ovarian cancer after treatment with platinum and paclitaxel

Efficacy (N = 79)

Partial response (n = 71)	3%
Median time to progression	3 months
6-month survival rate	65%
Median Survival	
All patients (N = 79)	10.1 months
Chemotherapy-resistant (n = 52)	8 months
Chemotherapy-sensitive (n = 27)	16 months

Therapy Monitoring
Before repeated cycles: CBC with differential

Notes
During the initial 10 weeks of treatment, vinorelbine did not appear to be effective in relieving the symptom-related distress or progressive impairment of physical functioning associated with refractory ovarian cancer

PLATINUM-REFRACTORY OR PLATINUM-RESISTANT REGIMEN

PACLITAXEL (24-HOUR PACLITAXEL INFUSION EVERY 3 WEEKS; WEEKLY PACLITAXEL)

For both treatment strategies, give premedication for paclitaxel with:
Dexamethasone 10 mg/dose; administer orally for 2 doses 12 hours and 6 hours before paclitaxel, *or*
Dexamethasone 20 mg/dose; administer intravenously over 10–15 minutes, 30–60 minutes before paclitaxel (total dose/cycle = 20 mg)
Diphenhydramine 50 mg; administer by intravenous injection 30 minutes before paclitaxel
Cimetidine 300 mg (or **ranitidine** 50 mg, **famotidine** 20 mg, or an equivalent histamine receptor [H_2]-subtype antagonist); administer intravenously over 15–30 minutes, 30–60 minutes before paclitaxel

24-Hour Paclitaxel
Omura GA et al. J Clin Oncol 2003;21:2843–2848
Paclitaxel 175 mg/m²; administer intravenously in a volume of 0.9% sodium chloride injection (0.9% NS) or 5% dextrose injection (D5W) sufficient to produce a concentration within the range 0.3–1.2 mg/mL, over 3 hours, on day 1, every 3 weeks (total dosage/cycle = 175 mg/m²)

or

Weekly Paclitaxel Regimens
Ghamande S et al. Int J Gynecol Cancer 2003;13:142–147
Paclitaxel 70–80 mg/m² per dose; administer intravenously in a volume of 0.9% NS or D5W sufficient to produce a concentration within the range 0.3–1.2 mg/mL, over 60 minutes, weekly for a minimum of 6 consecutive weeks (total dosage/6-week cycle = 420–480 mg/m²), *or*
Paclitaxel 70–80 mg/m² per dose; administer intravenously in a volume of 0.9% NS or D5W sufficient to produce a concentration within the range 0.3–1.2 mg/mL, over 60 minutes for 3 doses, on days 1, 8, and 15, every 28 days (total dosage/28-day cycle = 210–240 mg/m²)

Supportive Care
Antiemetic prophylaxis for 24-hour (every-3-weeks) and weekly paclitaxel regimens
*Emetogenic potential is **LOW***
See Chapter 39 for antiemetic recommendations

Hematopoietic growth factor (CSF) prophylaxis for the 24-hour regimen
Primary prophylaxis is indicated with 1 of the following:
  Filgrastim (G-CSF) 5 mcg/kg per day, by subcutaneous injection, *or*
  Pegfilgrastim (pegylated filgrastim) 6 mg/0.6 mL, by subcutaneous injection for 1 dose
• Begin use from 24–72 hours after myelosuppressive chemotherapy is completed
• Continue daily filgrastim use until ANC ≥10,000/mm³ on 2 measurements temporally separated by ≥12 hours
• Discontinue daily filgrastim use at least 24 hours before administering another dose of paclitaxel. Do not administer pegfilgrastim within 14 days before a dose of paclitaxel
See Chapter 43 for more information

Hematopoietic growth factor (CSF) prophylaxis for the weekly regimen
Primary prophylaxis is indicated with:
  Filgrastim (G-CSF) 5 mcg/kg per day by subcutaneous injection
• Begin use approximately 24 hours after myelosuppressive chemotherapy is completed
• Discontinue use at least 24 hours before administering subsequent paclitaxel doses
See Chapter 43 for more information

Antimicrobial prophylaxis
Risk of fever and neutropenia is LOW–INTERMEDIATE
Antimicrobial primary prophylaxis to be considered:
• Antibacterial—consider a fluoroquinolone or no prophylaxis
• Antifungal—not indicated
• Antiviral—not indicated unless patient previously had an episode of HSV
See Chapter 47 for more information

Treatment Modifications

Adverse Event	Dose Modification
24-Hour Paclitaxel Infusion Every 3 Weeks	
G ≥3 Nonhematologic toxicity	Reduce paclitaxel dose to 135 mg/m²
Delay in achieving ANC ≥1000/mm³ and platelets ≥100,000/mm³ <2 weeks	No dose adjustment
Recurrent delays in achieving ANC ≥1000/mm³ and platelets ≥100,000/mm³ ≥2 weeks but ≤3 weeks	Add filgrastim 5 mcg/kg per day without further dosage modification If already using filgrastim, reduce paclitaxel dose to 135 mg/m²
G3/4 neurologic toxicity that has not resolved even after a 3-week delay	Discontinue therapy
Weekly Paclitaxel Regimen	
WBC <2500/mm³	Hold chemotherapy until WBC >2500/mm³
ANC <1500/mm³	Hold chemotherapy until ANC >1500/mm³
Platelets <75,000/mm³	Hold chemotherapy until Platelets >75,000/mm³
G3/4 neurologic toxicity that has not resolved even after a 3-week delay	Discontinue therapy

Patient Population Studied

A study of 164 patients with epithelial ovarian cancer who had been treated with not more than 1 platinum-based regimen and no prior taxane

Omura GA et al. J Clin Oncol 2003;21:2843–2848

A study of 23 patients with advanced recurrent ovarian cancer with disease deemed resistant to platinum agents and paclitaxel (defined as either progression of disease while on therapy or progression within 12 months of prior paclitaxel therapy)

Ghamande S et al. Int J Gynecol Cancer 2003;13:142–147

Efficacy

24-Hour Paclitaxel Infusion Every 3 Weeks (N = 164)

Median time to death	13.1 months

Platinum-Resistant Disease	
Complete response	5%
Partial response	17%
No response	78%

Platinum-Sensitive Disease	
Complete response	15%
Partial response	33%
No response	52%

Omura GA et al. J Clin Oncol 2003;21:2843–2848

Weekly Paclitaxel (N = 23)

	Paclitaxel-Free Interval	
	<12 Months (n = 10)	>12 Months (n = 13)
Partial response*	0	70%
Stable disease	30%	15%
Progressive disease	70%	15%

*Partial response based on Rustin's criteria with more than 50% reduction in CA-125 levels

Ghamande S et al. Int J Gynecol Cancer 2003;13:142–147

Toxicity (N = 164)

24-Hour Paclitaxel Infusion Every 3 Weeks

	% G3/4
Anemia	7
Thrombocytopenia	5
Nausea/vomiting	5
Neuropathy	7
Myalgia/arthralgia	3
G4 neutropenia	22 (first cycle without filgrastim)

Omura GA et al. J Clin Oncol 2003;21:2843–2848

Weekly Paclitaxel (N = 28)

	% Patients
G2 neutropenia	10.7
G3 neutropenia	21.4
G1 thrombocytopenia	3.6
G2 anemia	32.1
G2 neuropathy	7.1
G >2 neuropathy	3.6

Ghamande S et al. Int J Gynecol Cancer 2003;13:142–147

Therapy Monitoring

1. *Before repeated cycles:* CBC with differential
2. *Twice per week:* Obtain CBC with differential in patients treated with the weekly regimen

PLATINUM-REFRACTORY OR PLATINUM-RESISTANT REGIMEN

TOPOTECAN HCL

Bhoola SM et al. Gynecol Oncol 2004;95:564–569

Topotecan HCl 2.25–4 mg/m^2 (median: 3.7 mg/m^2) per dose; administer intravenously in 50–250 mL 0.9% sodium chloride injection or 5% dextrose injection over 30 minutes, weekly, continually (total dosage/week = 2.25–4 mg/m^2)

or

Topotecan HCl 1.5 mg/m^2 per dose; administer intravenously in 50–250 mL 0.9% NS or D5W over 30 minutes for 5 consecutive days, on days 1–5, every 21 days (total dosage/cycle = 7.5 mg/m^2)

Supportive Care for Both Weekly and Every-3-Weeks Regimens

Antiemetic prophylaxis
Emetogenic potential is LOW
See Chapter 39 for antiemetic recommendations

Hematopoietic growth factor (CSF) prophylaxis
Primary prophylaxis may be indicated
See Chapter 43 for more information

Antimicrobial prophylaxis
Risk of fever and neutropenia is LOW
  Antimicrobial primary prophylaxis to be considered:
  • Antibacterial—not indicated
  • Antifungal—not indicated
  • Antiviral—not indicated unless patient previously had an episode of HSV
See Chapter 47 for more information

Treatment Modifications

Adverse Event	Dose Modification
G3/4 neutropenia on treatment day 1 (every 21 day regimen)	Hold topotecan until ANC ≥1000/mm^3 ± Reduce topotecan dose 10–20% ± Administer filgrastim in subsequent cycles*
G3/4 neutropenia on treatment day 1 (weekly regimen)	Hold topotecan until ANC ≥1000/mm^3 ± reduce topotecan dose 10–20% ± administer filgrastim in subsequent cycles* ± change schedule to 2 weeks on/1 week off
G ≥2 anemia	Administer erythropoietin
G ≥2 fatigue	Administer erythropoietin

*With every 21-day administration schedule administer filgrastim 5 mcg/kg per day subcutaneously beginning 24 hours after the day 5 dose and continuing until ANC >10,000/mm^3 on 2 consecutive measurements

Toxicity: Weekly Regimen (N = 50)

	% G2	% G3	% G4
Hematologic			
Anemia	42	24	0
Leukopenia	38	2	2
Neutropenia	24	14	4
Thrombocytopenia	4	10	0

	% G1/2	% G3/4
Nonhematologic		
Fatigue	14	4
Neuropathy	6	0
Nausea	2	0
Dehydration	2	0
Diarrhea	2	0
Alopecia	2	0

Patient Population Studied

A study of 50 patients with ovarian cancer who had received multiple prior regimens

Efficacy: Weekly Regimen (N = 42*)

Measurable Disease (n = 35)	
Partial response	31%
Stable disease	43%
Progressive disease	26%

↑CA-125[†]		
	All with↑ CA-125 (n = 41)	↑CA-125[†] Only (n = 7)
Partial response	27	29
Stable disease	24	29
Progressive disease	49	42

Platinum-Sensitive Disease	
Partial response	39
Stable disease	43
Progressive disease	18

Platinum-Resistant or Platinum-Refractory Disease	
Partial response	21
Stable disease	37
Progressive disease	42

*Includes only patients who received ≥2 cycles
†Partial response defined as a 50% reduction in CA-125 levels maintained for ≥1 month. Progressive disease defined as a 25% increase in CA-125 levels

Therapy Monitoring

Before repeated cycles: CBC with differential

Notes

A retrospective chart review of patients with rapidly progressive disease or clinical deterioration excluded from analysis. Efficacy of both regimens are comparable; toxicity of weekly regimen tolerable

PLATINUM-REFRACTORY OR PLATINUM-RESISTANT REGIMEN

ORAL ETOPOSIDE

Moosavi AS et al. J Obstet Gynaecol 2004;24:292–293

Etoposide 50 mg/day; administer orally once daily for 21 consecutive days, days 1–21, every 4 weeks (total dose/cycle = 1050 mg)

Supportive Care
Antiemetic prophylaxis
Emetogenic potential is **LOW**
See Chapter 39 for antiemetic recommendations

Hematopoietic growth factor (CSF) prophylaxis
Primary prophylaxis is NOT indicated
See Chapter 43 for more information

Antimicrobial prophylaxis
Risk of fever and neutropenia is LOW
  Antimicrobial primary prophylaxis to be considered:
  • Antibacterial—not indicated
  • Antifungal—not indicated
  • Antiviral—not indicated unless patient previously had an episode of HSV
See Chapter 47 for more information

Treatment Modifications

Adverse Event	Dose Modification
Nausea and vomiting*	Ingest doses with food
G3/4 ANC	Hold therapy. Resume treatment when ANC ≥1500/mm³ using an alternative schedule† (every other day, MWF, 2 of every 3 days, M–F)

*Nausea and vomiting are more common after oral etoposide administration than after parenteral administration with bioequivalent doses. Food ingestion does not affect absorption of etoposide doses <200 mg
†The 50-mg etoposide capsules cannot be opened or broken because they contain a liquid product

Therapy Monitoring

Every week: CBC with differential and platelet count

Patient Population Studied

Ten patients with epithelial ovarian cancer and evidence of disease progression; GOG performance status ≤2

Efficacy (N = 10)

Partial response rate	20%*
Response duration	3.5 and 6 months
Median progression-free interval	7.5 months
Median survival time	8.5 months

*Both patients who responded were deemed to have platinum-sensitive disease

Toxicity (N = 10)

	% Patients
Hematologic	
G1 ANC	50%
G2 ANC	30%
Nonhematologic	
Nausea/vomiting	40%
Mild mucositis	10%
Alopecia	100%

Notes

Although oral etoposide has activity in recurrent ovarian cancer, response and survival durations are short with a high rate of complications

REGIMEN

TAMOXIFEN

Markman M et al. Gynecol Oncol 2004;93:390–393

Tamoxifen 10 mg/dose; administer orally twice daily, continually (total dose/week = 140 mg)

Supportive Care
Antiemetic prophylaxis
Emetogenic potential is **MINIMAL**
See Chapter 39 for antiemetic recommendations

Hematopoietic growth factor (CSF) prophylaxis
Primary prophylaxis is NOT indicated
See Chapter 43 for more information

Antimicrobial prophylaxis
Risk of fever and neutropenia is LOW
  Antimicrobial primary prophylaxis to be considered:
  • Antibacterial—not indicated
  • Antifungal—not indicated
  • Antiviral—not indicated unless patient previously had an episode of HSV
See Chapter 47 for more information

Patient Population Studied

A study of 56 patients with recurrent ovarian (n = 44), fallopian tube (n = 3), or primary peritoneal carcinoma (n = 9). All patients had a prior response to primary platinum/taxane–based therapy or a platinum therapy used in the second-line setting and a treatment-free interval of ≥3 months. *Patients had no symptoms believed to be caused by recurrent cancer*

Efficacy (N = 57)

Duration of tamoxifen therapy in asymptomatic patients with recurrent ovarian cancer (n = 57 episodes; one patient received tamoxifen after both primary and secondary-treatments)

Median duration of treatment	3 mo
Patients remaining on therapy ≥6 mo	42%
Patients remaining on treatment ≥12 mo	19%
Patients with recurrence after primary therapy remaining on treatment ≥12 mo (n = 45)	18%
Patients with recurrence after second-line therapy remaining on treatment ≥12 mo (n = 12)	25%

Treatment Modifications

Grade 3 toxicities with this dose of tamoxifen are very uncommon and usually do not require dose reductions

Toxicity

No patient discontinued tamoxifen because of unacceptable side effects. This is a very well-tolerated dose schedule. The most common toxicities in females are hot flashes and some degree of vaginal discharge and, in premenopausal females, menstrual irregularities, such as irregular menses or amenorrhea. The risk for thromboembolic events increases with tamoxifen treatment, but is very low at this dose and usually administered for a short period of time. Neuropsychiatric (depression and other mood disorders) toxicities are uncommon. Liver and dermatologic toxicities can be very serious, but are rare

Therapy Monitoring

1. *Every month:* Serum CA-125 level
2. *Every 2–3 months*: Restaging radiographic studies

Notes

Best used in asymptomatic cases with a rising CA-125, or in cases in which comorbid illnesses argue against more aggressive therapy

29. Pancreatic Cancer

Ramesh K. Ramanathan, MD, PhD, Sc and Daniel D. Von Hoff, MD, FACP

Epidemiology

Incidence: 46,420 (male: 23,530; female: 22,890. Estimated new cases for 2014 in the United States) (13.9 per 100,000 males; 10.9 per 100,000 females)

Deaths: Estimated 39,590 in 2014 (male: 20,170; female: 19,420)

Median age: 71 years

Male to female ratio: ~1:1

Stage at presentation:	
Stage I:	20%
Stage II:	40%
Stage III–IV:	40%

Siegel R et al. CA Cancer J Clin 2014;64:9–29

Surveillance, Epidemiology, and End Results (SEER) Program, available from http://seer.cancer.gov (accessed in 2013)

Takhar AS et al. BMJ 2004;329:668–673

Pathology

Most cancers of the pancreas arise in the head of the pancreas (60–70%), 15% in the body, and 5% in the tail; in 20%, the neoplasm diffusely involves the entire gland

Malignant Tumors of Pancreatic Origin

Ductal adenocarcinoma	85–90%
Acinar cell carcinoma	1–2%
Undifferentiated carcinoma (anaplastic giant cell, osteoclastic giant cell)	<1%
Sarcomatoid carcinoma/ carcinosarcoma	<1%

de Braud F et al. Crit Rev Oncol Hematol 2004;50: 147–155

Solcia E et al. Tumors of the pancreas. In: Atlas of Tumor Pathology, 3rd series. Washington, DC: Armed Forces Institute; 1997

Work-up

The diagnosis of pancreatic cancer is based on imaging studies and histologic confirmation performed by fine-needle aspiration by endoscopic ultrasonography (EUS), biopsy under CT or US guidance, or during laparotomy

- History and physical examination
- CBC and differential, serum electrolytes, creatinine, LFTs, PT, PTT, CA19-9
- Imaging:
  - Spiral CT: Spiral or a helical CT of the abdomen according to a defined pancreatic protocol is essential. CT provides localization, size of the primary tumor, and evidence of metastasis and evaluates major vessels adjacent to the pancreas for neoplastic invasion or thrombosis. CT is almost 100% accurate in predicting unresectable disease. However, the positive predictive value of the test is low and approximately 25–50% of patients predicted to have resectable disease on CT turn out to have unresectable lesions at laparotomy
  - Endoscopic retrograde cholangiopancreatography (ERCP) can also be useful in patients whom a CT scan is equivocal, because fewer than 3% of patients with pancreatic carcinoma have normal pancreatograms
  - EUS is a relatively new technique and provides useful information. However, EUS needs to be performed in centers with experience in this procedure. EUS is useful for characterizing cystic lesions and assessment of vascular invasion by tumor. In addition, an aspirate can be done for histologic diagnosis. A celiac plexus block can be done via EUS for relief of abdominal pain

Agawam B. Am J Gastroenterol 2004;99:844–850

Tamm EP et al. Radiographic Imaging: Daniel D. Von Hoff, Douglas B. Evans, Ralph H. Hruban, eds. Pancreatic Cancer, 1st ed. Jones & Bartlett Publishers, 2005:165–180

Staging

	Primary Tumor (T)
TX	Primary tumor cannot be assessed
T0	No evidence of primary tumor
Tis	Carcinoma in situ
T1	Tumor limited to the pancreas, 2 cm or less in greatest dimension
T2	Tumor limited to the pancreas, more than 2 cm in greatest dimension
T3	Tumor extends beyond the pancreas but without involvement of the celiac axis or the superior mesenteric artery
T4	Tumor involves the celiac axis or the superior mesenteric artery (unresectable primary tumor)

	Regional Lymph Nodes (N)
NX	Regional lymph nodes cannot be assessed
N0	No regional lymph node metastasis
N1	Regional lymph node metastasis

	Distant Metastasis (M)
M0	No distant metastasis (no pathologic M0; use clinical M to complete stage group)
M1	Distant metastasis

Stage	T	N	M
0	Tis	N0	M0
IA	T1	N0	M0
IB	T2	N0	M0
IIA	T3	N0	M0
IIB	T1	N1	M0
IIB	T2	N1	M0
IIB	T3	N1	M0
III	T4	Any N	M0
IV	Any T	Any N	M1

Edge SB, Byrd DR, Compton CC, Fritz AG, Greene FL, Trotti A, editors. AJCC Cancer Staging Manual. 7th ed. New York: Springer; 2010

Expert Opinion

Pancreatic cancer can be broadly divided into 2 groups: *surgically resectable* or *unresectable/advanced cancer*. Patients should be enrolled to suitable clinical trials for all stages of pancreatic cancer if possible

Surgery
- The only curative therapy for pancreatic cancer is resection of the tumor and the surrounding tissues. Patients with resectable disease comprise the smallest group (~15%)
- Criteria for unresectable tumors include:
  - Distant metastases
  - SMA, celiac encasement
  - SMV, portal vein occlusion
  - Aortic or IVC invasion, or encasement
  - Invasion of SMV below the transverse mesocolon
- Borderline resectable pancreatic cancer
  - Patients who present with localized pancreatic cancer but who have a high likelihood of a positive surgical margin (R1) are classified as borderline resectable. A commonly used criteria is as follows:
    - Severe unilateral SMV/Portal impingement
    - Tumor abutment on SMA
    - GDA encasement up to origin of hepatic artery
    - SMV occlusion, if of a short segment with open vein both proximally and distally
    - Adrenal, colon or kidney invasion

Key: GDA, Gastroduodenal artery; IVC, inferior vena cava; SMA, superior mesenteric artery; SMV, superior mesenteric vein

Preoperative Therapy
Treatment regimens include chemoradiation with fluorouracil similar to the regimen used in RTOG 97-04 (Regine et al.). Concurrent involved field radiation with gemcitabine is an alternate regimen. The E4201 study (Loehrer et al.) administered concurrent gemcitabine with RT to patients with locally advanced cancer. RT (50.4 GY in 28 fractions) plus gemcitabine (600 mg/m^2 per week for 6 weeks)

Loehrer P et al. Proc Am Soc Clin Oncol 2008;26(15S, Part I of II):214s [abstract 4506]
Regine WF et al. JAMA 2008;299:1019–1026

(continued)

Survival

1-Year survival for all stages	19%
5-Year survival for all stages	4%
5-Year survival in resected patients	25%

Jemal A et al. CA Cancer J Clin 2009;59:225–249
Katz MH. CA Cancer J Clin 2008;58:111–125
Li D et al. Lancet 2004;363:1049–1057

Expert Opinion (*continued*)

Adjuvant Therapy

- Following surgery, adjuvant therapy should be considered for patients who have recovered from surgery. Approximately 20–25% of patients will have a prolonged convalescence and/or a suboptimal performance status following surgery and will not be candidates for adjuvant therapy

- Evaluate all patients for adjuvant therapy. Gemcitabine 1000 mg/m^2 administered intravenously, may be given weekly for 3 consecutive weeks every 4 weeks for 6 cycles

- Administer radiation with chemosensitizing fluorouracil or capecitabine in addition to gemcitabine as a component of adjuvant therapy for patients at high risk of recurrence. These are patients with a microscopic positive margin (R1 resection), extracapsular lymph node extension, and multiple involved regional nodes ($\geq$4) at resection

- Adjuvant therapy with gemcitabine with or without concurrent chemoradiation with fluorouracil should be considered in most patients

- The efficacy of combined radiation and fluorouracil as adjuvant therapy for pancreatic cancer was first demonstrated by a small prospective randomized study conducted by the Gastrointestinal Tumor Study Group (GITSG). Twenty-two patients were randomized to no adjuvant treatment and 21 patients were assigned to receive combined modality therapy

Radiation Therapy

- Two courses of 2000 cGy, each given for 5 days separated by an interval of 2 weeks +

- Fluorouracil 500 mg/m^2 per day, administered intravenously in 25–250 mL 0.9% sodium chloride (0.9% NS) or 5% dextrose injection (D5W), USP, over 10–30 minutes for 3 consecutive days for the first 3 days of each 2000-cGy segment of radiation therapy (total dosage/3-day course = 1500 mg/m^2). Subsequently, treatment resumed 1 month after completion of radiation with fluorouracil 500 mg/m^2 per dose administered intravenously for 3 consecutive days, on days 1–3 of each week for 2 years of therapy

- The median survival for the treatment group was 20 months vs. 11 months for the control group, and the median disease-free survival was 11 months for the treated group vs. 9 months for the control group

This study and data from a subsequent confirmatory study of an additional 30 patients treated with the similar regimen of fluorouracil and RT provided evidence for the role of adjuvant therapy in resected pancreatic cancer

Gastrointestinal Tumor Study Group. Cancer 1987;59:2006–2010
Kalser MH et al. Arch Surg 1985;120:899–903

- The benefit of gemcitabine monotherapy was demonstrated by Oettle et al. This multicenter study randomized 368 patients following surgery to observation or adjuvant therapy starting 6 weeks after surgical resection:

  Gemcitabine 1000 mg/m^2 per dose administered intravenously in 0.9% NS, over 30 minutes for 3 doses on days 1, 8, and 15 every 4 weeks for 6 months (total dosage/4-week cycle = 3000 mg/m^2)

- Therapy with gemcitabine was well tolerated. The primary endpoint of disease-free survival was significantly improved in the treatment group (13.4 months vs. 6.9 months, P <0.001); the median survival (22.1 vs. 20.2 months) was similar in both groups

Oettle H et al. JAMA 2007;297:267–277

- The European Study Group for Pancreatic Cancer (ESPAC 1, 2, and 3) evaluated the role of fluorouracil, gemcitabine, and RT as adjuvant therapy and support the role of chemotherapy alone as adjuvant therapy. The role of RT and the detrimental effect of RT seen in these studies have been controversial as a result of the lack of quality control and central review. ESPAC-3 (n = 1088) compared gemcitabine to fluorouracil as adjuvant therapy. The median survival for both groups was approximately 23 months. However, the safety profile favors gemcitabine as the preferred regimen for adjuvant therapy

Neoptolemos JP et al. N Engl J Med 2004;350:1200–1210. Erratum in: N Engl J Med 2004;351:726
Neoptolemos JP et al. Br J Cancer 2009;100:246–250
Neoptolemos JP et al. Proc Am Soc Clin Oncol 2009;27(Suppl):18s [abstract LBA-4505]

(*continued*)

Expert Opinion (*continued*)

Therapy of Patients with Metastatic Pancreatic Cancer and "Good"
Performance Status—*First line regimen*
In this group are patients with an ECOG performance status of 0 or 1 and with minimal cancer-related symptoms. Meta-analyses have indicated that patients with a good performance status can benefit from combination therapy with gemcitabine regimens. Two regimens are considered to have activity and *are recommended in first line*:

- *nab*-Paclitaxel **+** gemcitabine: MPACT was a large, international study performed at community and academic centers. *nab*-Paclitaxel **+** gemcitabine was superior to gemcitabine monotherapy across all efficacy endpoints, had an acceptable toxicity profile. *nab*-Paclitaxel **+** gemcitabine is a new option for the treatment of metastatic pancreatic cancer that will now be studied in the adjuvant and locally advanced setting

- FOLFIRINOX: As compared with gemcitabine, FOLFIRINOX [oxaliplatin **+** irinotecan **+** fluorouracil **+** leucovorin] was associated with a survival advantage and had increased toxicity. FOLFIRINOX is an option for the treatment of patients with metastatic pancreatic cancer and a good performance status [younger than 76 years and who have a good performance status (ECOG 0 or 1), no cardiac ischemia, and normal or nearly normal bilirubin levels]

Therapy of Patients with Metastatic Pancreatic Cancer and "Good"
Performance Status—*Second line regimen*
In second line one can consider the alternate regimen of the two above or the **OFF regimen**

Conroy T et al. N Engl J Med 2011;364:1817–1825
Pelzer et al. European J Cancer 2011;47:1676–1681
Von Hoff DD et al. J Clin Oncol 2011;29:4548–4554
Von Hoff et al. J Clin Oncol 31, 2013(Suppl; abstr 4005)

- An intergroup study (RTOG 97-04) provides support for concurrent chemoradiation as adjuvant therapy. This study provided central review and quality assurance for RT. Regine et al., randomly assigned patients (n = 451) to 1 of 2 chemotherapy regimens following a pancreatectomy for 3 weeks prior to chemoradiation therapy, and then for an additional 12 weeks, starting 3–5 weeks after completing chemoradiation:

Pre-chemoradiation regimens
- Group 1:
  Fluorouracil 250 mg/m^2 per day in 25–500 mL 0.9% NS or D5W administered intravenously over 10–30 minutes, daily for 3 weeks (total dosage/3-week course = 5250 mg/m^2)
- Group 2:
  Gemcitabine 1000 mg/m^2 per dose diluted with 0.9% NS to concentrations as low as 0.1 mg/mL administered intravenously over 30 minutes once weekly for 3 weeks (total dosage/3-week course = 3000 mg/m^2)

During chemoradiation
- Groups 1 and 2:
  Fluorouracil 250 mg/m^2 per day in 25–1000 mL 0.9% NS or D5W administered by continuous intravenous infusion over 24 hours, daily throughout radiation therapy

Post-chemoradiation regimens:
- Group 1:
  Fluorouracil 250 mg/m^2 per day in 25–500 mL 0.9% NS or D5W administered intravenously over 10–30 minutes, daily for 4 consecutive weeks (28 days) every 6 weeks for two 6-week cycles (total dosage/6-week cycle = 7000 mg/m^2)
- Group 2:
  Gemcitabine 1000 mg/m^2 per dose diluted with 0.9% NS to concentrations as low as 0.1 mg/mL, administered intravenously over 30 minutes once weekly for 3 consecutive weeks every 4 weeks for three 4-week cycles (total dosage/4-week cycle = 3000 mg/m^2)

- Chemoradiation was given for a total dose of 50.4 Gy with fluorouracil. On multivariate analysis, patients with pancreatic head tumors (n = 388) had a survival advantage when treated in the gemcitabine arm with median survival of 20.5 months and 3-year survival of 31% compared to 16.9 months and 22%, respectively, in the fluorouracil arm (P = 0.5). There were no differences in survival for the overall study population

Regine WF et al. JAMA 2008;299:1019–1026

(*continued*)

Expert Opinion (continued)

Patients who have positive margins following surgery have a poor outcome. In this group of patients who have "borderline resectable" cancer, preoperative chemoradiation could be administered with or without 2–4 months of systemic chemotherapy followed by pancreatic resection

Treatment for Metastatic Disease

Chemotherapy similar to treatment of patients with metastatic disease is preferred. Concurrent chemoradiation is also an option. Evaluate patients after 4–6 cycles of systemic therapy. Patients who continue to have disease confined to the pancreas may be considered for concurrent chemoradiation therapy. Continuous infusion fluorouracil or capecitabine administration with radiation to the pancreas is preferred. There is limited experience with concurrent radiation and gemcitabine and these regimens should be administered with caution

We evaluate patients for therapy based on either a "good" or "poor" performance status

Therapy of Patients with "Poor" Performance Status

Outcome and survival are poor for a patient with an ECOG performance status ≥ 2 with severe fatigue, rapid weight loss, and/or biliary obstruction. This group of patients may be considered for treatment with gemcitabine alone or gemcitabine and erlotinib. Palliative care with symptom management should also be discussed with the patient and family

- Gemcitabine may be administered over 30 minutes or at a fixed dose rate (10 mg/m^2 per minute)
- The addition of erlotinib to gemcitabine was demonstrated in a randomized phase III trial to improve survival and progression-free survival in advanced pancreatic cancer. In this phase III trial, a total of 569 patients were randomly assigned to receive gemcitabine with erlotinib or placebo:

Gemcitabine 1000 mg/m^2 per dose diluted with 0.9% NS to concentrations as low as 0.1 mg/mL, administered intravenously over 30 minutes once weekly
  - *Cycle 1:* Gemcitabine was given on days 1, 8, 15, 22, 29, 36, and 43 during the initial 8-week cycle (total dosage = 7000 mg/m^2)
  - *Subsequent cycles:* Gemcitabine was given on days 1, 8, and 15 every 4 weeks (total dosage/4-week cycle = 3000 mg/m^2)
  - **Erlotinib** 100 mg/day or 150 mg/day orally, continually *or* placebo orally, continually
  - Most patients received erlotinib 100 mg/day, orally
- In the control arm of gemcitabine, the median survival was 5.91 months and 1-year overall survival was 17%. One-year survival was also greater with erlotinib plus gemcitabine (23% vs. 17%; P = 0.023). Patients who developed a skin rash following therapy with erlotinib had the best outcome and longest survival. The median survival for patients without a rash was 5.3 months (1-year survival = 16%) compared to 10.5 months (1-year survival 43%) for those who had a grade 2 + rash with treatment

Therapy of Patients with "Good" Performance Status

In this group are patients with an ECOG performance status of 0 or 1 and with minimal cancer-related symptoms. Meta-analyses have indicated that patients with a good performance status can benefit from combination therapy with gemcitabine regimens. Two new regimens are considered to have activity:

- *nab*-Paclitaxel + gemcitabine: MPACT was a large, international study performed at community and academic centers. *nab*-Paclitaxel + gemcitabine was superior to gemcitabine monotherapy across all efficacy endpoints, had an acceptable toxicity profile. *nab*-Paclitaxel + gemcitabine is a new option for the treatment of metastatic pancreatic cancer that will now be studied in the adjuvant and locally advanced setting
- FOLFIRINOX: As compared with gemcitabine, **FOLFIRINOX [oxaliplatin + irinotecan + fluorouracil + leucovorin]** was associated with a survival advantage and had increased toxicity. FOLFIRINOX is an option for the treatment of patients with metastatic pancreatic cancer and a good performance status [younger than 76 years and who have a good performance status (ECOG 0 or 1), no cardiac ischemia, and normal or nearly normal bilirubin levels]

Abbruzzese J. JAMA 2008;299:1066–1067
Conroy T et al. N Engl J Med 2011;364:1817–1825
Moore MJ et al. J Clin Oncol 2007;25:1960–1966
Philip PA. Lancet Oncol 2008;9:7–8
Russo S et al. Semin Oncol 2007;34:327–334
Sultana A et al. J Clin Oncol 2007;25:2607–2615
Ujiki MB, Talamonti MS. Semin Oncol 2007;34:311–320
Von Hoff DD et al. J Clin Oncol 2011;29:4548–4554
Von Hoff et al. J Clin Oncol 31, 2013(Suppl; abstr 4005)

ADJUVANT THERAPY REGIMEN

GEMCITABINE + RADIATION THERAPY (RTOG 97-04)

Regine WF et al. JAMA 2008;299:1019–1026

Pre-chemoradiation:
Gemcitabine 1000 mg/m² per dose diluted with 0.9% sodium chloride injection (0.9% NS) to concentrations as low as 0.1 mg/mL administer intravenously over 30 minutes once weekly for 3 consecutive weeks (total dosage/3-week course = 3000 mg/m²), *followed 1–2 weeks later by*
Chemoradiation therapy:
Radiation therapy for a total dose of 5040 cGy (28 fractions 5 days/week with a boost of 540 cGy) with
Fluorouracil 250 mg/m² per day in 25–1000 mL 0.9% NS or D5W administer by continuous intravenous infusion over 24 hours throughout radiation therapy, *followed 3–5 weeks later by*
Post-chemoradiation:
Gemcitabine 1000 mg/m² per dose diluted with 0.9% NS to concentrations as low as 0.1 mg/mL administer intravenously over 30 minutes once weekly for 3 consecutive weeks every 4 weeks for a total of 12 weeks (total dosage/4-week cycle = 3000 mg/m²)

Supportive Care
Emetogenic potential: **LOW**
See Chapter 39 for antiemetic recommendations

Hematopoietic growth factor (CSF) prophylaxis
Primary prophylaxis is NOT indicated
See Chapter 43 for more information

Antimicrobial prophylaxis
Risk of fever and neutropenia is LOW
Antimicrobial primary prophylaxis to be considered:
- Antibacterial—not indicated
- Antifungal—not indicated
- Antiviral—not indicated unless patient previously had an episode of HSV

See Chapter 47 for more information

Patient Population Studied

Study of 451 patients (388 with pancreatic head tumors) with resected pancreatic adenocarcinoma who were randomized and 221 who received the study arm of gemcitabine and fluorouracil/RT. The control group received fluorouracil and fluorouracil/RT. The margin positive rate following surgery (R1) was 34%. In patients with pancreatic head tumors there was an increase in survival, but this did not reach statistical significance (P = 0.5)

Toxicity (N = 221 Treated with Gemcitabine and Concurrent Chemoradiation)

Grade 3/4 Toxicity	Percentage (%)
Grade 3/4 hematologic	58
Grade 4 hematologic	14
Diarrhea	15
Stomatitis/mucositis	10
Nausea/vomiting	10

Comment: Grade 3/4 hematologic toxicity was higher in the gemcitabine arm than in the fluorouracil arm (58% vs. 9%, respectively). However, there was no difference in the incidence of febrile neutropenia or infection There was no difference in the ability to deliver chemotherapy (90% vs. 87%) or radiation therapy between the gemcitabine and fluorouracil groups (88% vs. 86%, respectively)

Treatment Modifications

Modifications for gemcitabine: see single-agent gemcitabine dosing

Burris HA et al. J Clin Oncol 1997;15:2403–2413

Concurrent chemoradiation dose modifications:
The following guidelines may be considered as Regine et al. did not specify modifications (Talamonti MS et al. J Clin Oncol 2000;18:3384–3389)
- Hold radiation therapy for grade 3/4 GI or grade 4 hematologic toxicity, and resume after toxicity resolves
- Dose reduce fluorouracil by 25% for grade 3 hematologic toxicity
- Hold fluorouracil in the case of grade 4 hematologic toxicity, grade 3/4 GI tract and other nonhematologic toxicity. Resume fluorouracil at a 25% reduced dose after toxicity resolves
- Hold fluorouracil for grade 2/3 hand-foot syndrome until symptoms resolve and resume with a 25% dose reduction

Efficacy

Pancreatic Head Tumors (N = 388)	Gemcitabine + Fluorouracil Arm	Fluorouracil Arm
Median survival	20.5 months	16.9 months
3-Year survival	31%	22%

Therapy Monitoring

1. *Every week:* CBC with differential
2. During the period of RT, monitor patients for toxicity every week
3. *Before each cycle of chemotherapy:* H&P, CBC, complete chemistry panel including electrolytes, liver function tests, and magnesium; CA19-9 level if initially elevated

Surveillance
1. H&P every 3–6 months for 2–3 years and then annually
2. At every visit, H&P, CBC, complete chemistry panel including electrolytes, liver function tests, and magnesium; CA19-9 level if initially elevated
3. CT scans for surveillance every 6 months for 2–3 years then annually

METASTATIC DISEASE REGIMEN
GEMCITABINE

Burris HA et al. J Clin Oncol 1997;15:2403–2413

Gemcitabine 1000 mg/m² per dose; administer by intravenous infusion in 50–250 mL 0.9% sodium chloride injection over 30 minutes on days 1, 8, and 15, every 28 days (total dosage/cycle = 3000 mg/m²)
- In the referenced trial, for the first cycle, patients received gemcitabine 1000 mg/m² once weekly for up to 7 weeks. Thereafter, gemcitabine was administered once weekly for 3 consecutive weeks out of every 4 weeks
- Single-agent gemcitabine given at the dose of 1500 mg/m² at the rate of 10 mg/min over 150 minutes is an alternative regimen

Tempero M et al. J Clin Oncol 2003;15:3402–3408

Supportive Care
Antiemetic prophylaxis
Emetogenic potential with gemcitabine: **LOW**
See Chapter 39 for antiemetic recommendations

Hematopoietic growth factor (CSF) prophylaxis
Primary prophylaxis is NOT indicated
See Chapter 43 for more information

Antimicrobial prophylaxis
Risk of fever and neutropenia is LOW
Antimicrobial primary prophylaxis to be considered:
- Antibacterial—not indicated
- Antifungal—not indicated
- Antiviral—not indicated unless patient previously had an episode of HSV

See Chapter 47 for more information

Persistent rash or flulike symptoms after gemcitabine:
Consider Dexamethasone 10 mg orally or intravenously before starting gemcitabine

Treatment Modifications

Adverse Events	Treatment Modifications
WBC <1000/mm³ to 500/mm³ or platelets <99,000/mm³ to 50,000/mm³ on day of treatment	Reduce gemcitabine dosages by 25%
G ≥3 nonhematologic adverse event during the previous treatment cycle	
WBC <500/mm³ or platelet <50,000/mm³ on day of treatment	Delay chemotherapy for up to 2 weeks
Treatment delay >2 weeks for recovery from hematologic adverse event	Discontinue treatment

Adverse Events (N = 63)

WHO Grade (%)	Grade I	Grade II	Grade III	Grade IV
WBC	26	36	10	0
Platelets	16	21	10	0
Hemoglobin	31	24	7	3
Bilirubin	3	10	2	2
Alkaline phosphatase	33	22	16	0
Aspartate transaminase	41	20	10	1.6
BUN	8	0	0	0
Creatinine	2	0	0	0
Diarrhea	18	5	2	0
Constipation	5	2	3	0
Pain	2	6	2	0
Fever	22	8	0	0
Infection	5	3	0	0
Pulmonary	3	3	0	0
Hair	16	2	0	0
Proteinuria	10	0	0	0
Hematuria	12.7	0	0	0
Nausea/vomiting	29	22	10	3

Patient Population Studied

Study of 63 patients with locally advanced or metastatic pancreatic cancer not amenable to curative surgical resection treated with single-agent gemcitabine. Patients who had received previous chemotherapy were not eligible

Therapy Monitoring

1. *Every week:* CBC with differential
2. *Before each cycle:* CBC with differential, serum electrolytes, creatinine, mineral panel, and LFT
3. *Response assessment:* CT scans every 2 months and CA19-9 monthly

Efficacy (N = 63)

Median survival	5.65 months
Survival rate at 12 months	18%
Clinical benefit response*	23.8%

*Clinical benefit response (CBR) is a composite measurement of pain, performance status, and weight that was sustained more than 4 weeks in at least 1 parameter without the worsening in any other parameter. The median time to achieve CBR in gemcitabine-treated patients was 7 weeks and duration of benefit was 18 weeks
Note: In this pivotal phase III clinical trial, gemcitabine was compared in a randomized fashion with fluorouracil (600 mg/m² per week). The median survival in the fluorouracil arm was 4.41 months, survival rate at 12 months was 2%, and clinical benefit response was 4.8%

METASTATIC DISEASE REGIMEN
GEMCITABINE + ERLOTINIB

Moore MJ et al. J Clin Oncol 2007;25:1960–1966

Gemcitabine 1000 mg/m^2 per dose; administer by intravenous infusion in 50–250 mL 0.9% sodium chloride injection over 30 minutes on days 1, 8, and 15, every 28 days (total dosage/cycle = 3000 mg/m^2)
- In the referenced trial, for the first cycle, patients received gemcitabine 1000 mg/m^2 once weekly for 7 consecutive weeks during an 8-week cycle. Thereafter, gemcitabine was administered once weekly for 3 consecutive weeks out of every 4 weeks

Erlotinib was administered orally 100 mg/day (n = 262) or 150 mg/day (n = 23), continually, until progression or intolerable toxicity

Supportive Care
Antiemetic prophylaxis
Emetogenic potential is: **LOW**
See Chapter 39 for antiemetic recommendations

Hematopoietic growth factor (CSF) prophylaxis
Primary prophylaxis is NOT indicated
See Chapter 43 for more information

Antimicrobial prophylaxis
Risk of fever and neutropenia is LOW
   Antimicrobial primary prophylaxis to be considered:
   - Antibacterial—not indicated
   - Antifungal—not indicated
   - Antiviral—not indicated unless patient previously had an episode of HSV
See Chapter 47 for more information

Diarrhea management
Latent or delayed onset diarrhea*:
   Loperamide 4 mg orally initially, then 2 mg orally every 2 hours during waking hours, plus **Loperamide** 4 mg orally every 4 hours during hours of sleep
   - Continue for at least 12 hours after diarrhea resolves
   - Recurrent diarrhea after a 12-hour diarrhea free interval is treated as a new episode
   - If diarrhea persists >48 hours despite loperamide, stop loperamide and hospitalize patient for IV hydration
Persistent or severe diarrhea (G ≥3):
   - Interrupt erlotinib treatment until symptoms resolve, then consider resuming at a decreased dose

*Rothenberg ML et al. J Clin Oncol 2001;19:3801–3807
Wadler S et al. J Clin Oncol 1998;16:3169–178

Adverse Events for Gemcitabine and Erlotinib

Grade 3/4 Toxicity	Percentage (%)
Diarrhea	6
Fatigue	15
Any infection	17
Rash	6

Consider regimen for patients with ECOG performance status 0–2 and total bilirubin ≤ ULN or ≤1.8 mg/dL (≤30.8 μmol/L); ALT and AST ≤5× ULN

Therapy Monitoring

1. *Every week:* CBC with differential
2. *Before each cycle:* CBC, complete chemistry panel including electrolytes, liver function tests, and magnesium; CA19-9 level if initially elevated
3. *Response assessment:* Every 8 weeks with CT scans or earlier if clinically indicated; CA19-9 monthly

Treatment Modifications

Adverse Events	Treatment Modifications
WBC <1000/mm^3 to 500/mm^3 or platelets <99,000/mm^3 to 50,000/mm^3 on day of treatment	Reduce gemcitabine dosages by 50%
WBC <500/mm^3 or platelet <50,000/mm^3 on day of treatment	Delay gemcitabine for up to 2 weeks
Patients with grade 4 granulocytopenia, thrombocytopenia, or nonhematologic toxicity during the previous treatment cycle	Reduce gemcitabine dosages by 25%

Erlotinib dose modifications
- Dose reductions should be made in 50-mg decrements
- Pulmonary symptoms: If acute onset (or worsening) of pulmonary symptoms (eg, dyspnea, cough, fever), interrupt treatment and evaluate for drug-induced interstitial lung disease; discontinue permanently with development of interstitial lung disease
- Severe skin reaction: Reduce dose or temporarily interrupt treatment

Patient Population Studied

A total of 569 patients were randomly assigned to receive erlotinib/placebo with gemcitabine. Locally advanced unresectable patients comprised 24% of the population. The majority received erlotinib at the dose of 100 mg/day

Efficacy (N = 569)

Variable	Gemcitabine + Erlotinib N = 285	Gemcitabine + Placebo N = 284
Median survival	6.24 months	5.91 months
1-Year survival	23%	17%

Of patients receiving gemcitabine + erlotinib, 16% had at least 1 dose reduction compared to 5% in the control group

ADVANCED OR METASTATIC PANCREATIC CANCER REGIMEN

GEMCITABINE + *nab*-PACLITAXEL

Von Hoff DD et al. J Clin Oncol 2011;29:4548–4554
Von Hoff DD et al. J Clin Oncol 2013;31(Suppl; abstr 4005)

Paclitaxel protein-bound particles for injectable suspension (*nab*-paclitaxel) 125 mg/m^2 per dose intravenously once weekly for 3 doses on days 1, 8, and 15 every 28 days (total dosage/ cycle = 375 mg/m^2), followed by

Gemcitabine HCl 1000 mg/m^2 per dose intravenously in 50–250 mL 0.9% sodium chloride injection for 3 doses on days 1, 8, and 15 every 28 days (total dosage/cycle = 3000 mg/m^2), *followed by:*

Supportive Care

Antiemetic prophylaxis

Emetogenic potential is **MODERATE**

See Chapter 39 for antiemetic recommendations

Hematopoietic growth factor (CSF) prophylaxis

Primary prophylaxis may be indicated

See Chapter 43 for more information

(Filgrastim may be given according to institutional guidelines for the treatment of neutropenic fever or infections associated with neutropenia and for the prevention of febrile neutropenia in patients with an ANC <500/mm^3. Patients not experiencing resolution of neutropenia within 21 days, despite uninterrupted filgrastim should discontinue therapy)

Antimicrobial prophylaxis

Risk of fever and neutropenia is LOW

Antimicrobial primary prophylaxis to be considered:

- Antibacterial—not indicated

- Antifungal—not indicated

- Antiviral—not indicated unless patient previously had an episode of HSV

See Chapter 47 for more information

(*Prophylaxis Against Sepsis:* At the first occurrence of fever ≥38.5°C [101.3°F] [regardless of ANC], institution of ciprofloxacin (500 mg orally, twice daily)—or amoxicillin/clavulanate [Augmentin, 500 mg orally, 2–3 times daily] in patients with allergy to fluoroquinolones—should be initiated. On their first visit, patients should be provided with enough ciprofloxacin [or the alternative antibiotic] for use at home, and they should be instructed to begin taking it when they first record a temperature of ≥38.5°C [101.3°F] [or if they feel they are developing a fever and a thermometer is not available]. They should also immediately contact their physician for guidance on where to go for blood counts to be evaluated for sepsis as soon as possible. Hospitalization or evaluation in the emergency room may be required depending on the clinical presentation)

Diarrhea management

Latent or delayed onset diarrhea*:

Loperamide 4 mg orally initially after the first loose or liquid stool, *then*
Loperamide 2 mg orally every 2 hours during waking hours, *plus*
Loperamide 4 mg orally every 4 hours during hours of sleep

- Continue for at least 12 hours after diarrhea resolves

- Recurrent diarrhea after a 12-hour diarrhea-free interval is treated as a new episode

- Rehydrate orally with fluids and electrolytes during a diarrheal episode

- If a patient develops blood or mucus in stool, dehydration, or hemodynamic instability, or if diarrhea persists >48 hours despite loperamide, stop loperamide and hospitalize the patient for IV hydration

Alternatively, a trial of **Diphenoxylate hydrochloride** 2.5 mg with **Atropine sulfate** 0.025 mg (eg, Lomotil)

- Initial adult dose is 2 tablets 4 times daily until control has been achieved, after which the dose may be reduced to meet individual requirements. Control may often be maintained with as little as 2 tablets daily

- Clinical improvement of acute diarrhea is usually observed within 48 hours. If improvement of chronic diarrhea after treatment with a maximum daily dose of 8 tablets is not observed within 10 days, control is unlikely with further administration

(continued)

(continued)

Persistent diarrhea:
  Octreotide 100–150 mcg subcutaneously 3 times daily. Maximum total daily dose is 1500 mcg
Antibiotic therapy during latent or delayed onset diarrhea:
  A fluoroquinolone (eg, **Ciprofloxacin** 500 mg orally every 12 hours) if absolute neutrophil
  count <500/mm³ with or without accompanying fever in association with diarrhea
    • Antibiotics should also be administered if patient is hospitalized with prolonged diarrhea
    and should be continued until diarrhea resolves

*Abigerges D et al. J Natl Cancer Inst 1994;86:446–449
Rothenberg ML et al. J Clin Oncol 2001;19:3801–3807
Wadler S et al. J Clin Oncol 1998;16:3169–3178

Note

Interstitial Pneumonitis
Monitor patients carefully for signs and symptoms of pneumonitis (ie, episodes of transient or repeated dyspnea with unproductive persistent cough or fever) and, if observed, perform immediate clinical evaluation and timely institution of appropriate management (emphasizing the need for corticosteroids if an infectious process has been ruled out, as well as appropriate ventilation and oxygen support when required)

Treatment Modifications

Dose Adjustments on Day 1 of Each Treatment Cycle for Hematologic Toxicity

ANC		Platelets	Timing
≥1500/mm³	AND	≥100,000/mm³	Treat on time
<1500/mm³	OR	<100,000/mm³	Delay by 1 week intervals until recovery

Dose Levels

	nab-Paclitaxel (mg/m²)	Gemcitabine HCl (mg/m²)
Starting dose	125	1000
Dose level −1	100	800
Dose level −2	75	600

Dose Adjustments within a Treatment Cycle for Hematologic Toxicity

Day 8			Day 15		
Blood Counts	*nab*-Paclitaxel	Gemcitabine	**Blood Counts**	*nab*-Paclitaxel	Gemcitabine
ANC >1000/mm³ *and* platelets ≥75,000/mm³	100%		ANC >1000/mm³ *and* platelets ≥75,000/mm³	100%	
			ANC 500–1000/mm³ *or* platelets 50,000–74,999/mm³	Full dose (treat on time) and administer filgrastim*	
			ANC <500/mm³ *or* platelets <50,000/mm³	Hold and administer filgrastim*	
ANC 500–1000/mm³ *or* platelets 50,000–74,999/mm³	Decrease dose by 1 level (treat on time)		ANC >1000/mm³ *and* platelets ≥75,000/mm³	Return to previous dose level (treat on time) and administer filgrastim*	
			ANC 500–1000/mm³ *or* platelets 50,000–74,999/mm³	Same dose as day 8 (treat on time) and administer filgrastim*	
			ANC <500/mm³ *or* platelets <50,000/mm³	Hold and administer filgrastim*	
ANC <500/mm³ *or* platelets <50,000/mm³	Hold		ANC >1000/mm³ *and* platelets ≥75,000/mm³	Decrease day 8 dose by 1 level (treat on time) and administer filgrastim*	
			ANC 500–1000/mm³ *or* platelets 50,000–74,999/mm³	Decrease day 8 dose by 1 level (treat on time) and administer filgrastim*	
			ANC <500/mm³ *or* platelets <50,000/mm³	Hold and administer filgrastim*	

*Febrile patients (regardless of ANC) should have chemotherapy treatment interrupted. A full sepsis diagnostic work-up should be performed while continuing broad-spectrum antibiotics. If cultures are positive, guide antibiotic therapy by the sensitivity profile of the isolated organism. Patients with persisting fever after 3 weeks, despite uninterrupted antibiotic treatment, should discontinue therapy. Febrile neutropenic patients can also receive filgrastim, in addition to antibiotic treatment, to hasten resolution of their febrile neutropenia

(continued)

Treatment Modifications (continued)

Dose Adjustments on Day 1 of Each Treatment Cycle for Nonhematologic Toxicity and/or Dose Hold with Previous Cycle

Toxicity/Dose Held	*nab*-Paclitaxel + Gemcitabine Dose This Cycle
G0/1/2 toxicity	Same as day 1 previous cycle (except for G2 cutaneous toxicity where doses of gemcitabine and *nab*-paclitaxel should be reduced to next lower dose level)
G3 toxicity*	Decrease *nab*-paclitaxel and gemcitabine to next lower dose level*
G ≥3 peripheral neuropathy	Hold *nab*-paclitaxel treatment but continue gemcitabine administration if indicated. Resume *nab*-paclitaxel treatment at next lower dose level after the peripheral neuropathy improves to G ≤1
G4 toxicity	Hold therapy†
Dose held in 2 previous consecutive cycles	Decrease gemcitabine to next lower dose level and continue throughout the rest of treatment

*Except for cutaneous toxicity: If the toxicity only affects neuropathy, then only *nab*-paclitaxel should be reduced
†The decision as to which drug should be modified depends upon the type of nonhematologic toxicity seen and which course is medically most sound in the judgment of the physician

Dose Adjustments within a Treatment Cycle for Nonhematologic Toxicity

CTC Grade	Percent of Day 1 *nab*-Paclitaxel + Gemcitabine Dose
G1/2, G3 nausea/vomiting and alopecia	100%*
G3 (except G3 nausea/vomiting and alopecia)	Hold either 1 or both drugs until resolution to G ≤1. Then resume treatment at the next lower dose level
G ≥3 peripheral neuropathy	Hold *nab*-paclitaxel treatment but continue gemcitabine administration if indicated. Resume *nab*-paclitaxel treatment at next lower dose level after the peripheral neuropathy improves to G ≤1
G4	Hold therapy†

*Except for cutaneous toxicity: If the toxicity only affects neuropathy, then only *nab*-paclitaxel should be reduced
†The decision as to which drug should be modified depends upon the type of nonhematologic toxicity seen and which course is medically most sound in the judgment of the physician

Patient Population Studied

Patients with histologically or cytologically confirmed metastatic pancreatic ductal adenocarcinoma (PDA) who had not previously received treatment for metastatic disease. Prior adjuvant treatment with fluorouracil or gemcitabine administered as a radiation sensitizer during and up to 4 weeks after radiation therapy was allowed. If a patient received adjuvant therapy, tumor recurrence must have occurred >6 months after the last treatment. Patients had an ECOG PS of 0 or 1. Twenty, 44, and 3 patients received 100, 125, and 150 mg/m² *nab*-paclitaxel, respectively

	nab-Paclitaxel (mg/m²)					
	100 (n = 20)		125 (n = 44)		150 (n = 3)	
Characteristic	No.	%	No.	%	No.	%
Age, years						
Median	62		61		69	
Range	30–86		28–78		53–72	
Female sex	9	45	25	57	1	33

(continued)

Patient Population Studied (continued)

Characteristic	nab-Paclitaxel mg/m²					
	100 (n = 20)		125 (n = 44)		150 (n = 3)	
	No.	%	No.	%	No.	%
ECOG						
0	9	45	22	50	2	67
1	11	55	22	50	1	33
Site of metastatic disease						
Abdomen/peritoneal	16	80	38	86	2	67
Liver	11	55	34	77	2	67
Liver only	1	5	2	5	1	33
Lung	5	25	18	41	1	33
Lung only	1	5	5	11	1	33
Other	10	50	12	27	1	33
Number of metastatic sites						
1	6	30	8	18	1	33
2	8	40	18	41	2	67
≥3	6	30	18	41	0	—
CA19-9 baseline levels, number	15		37		2	—
Normal*	2	13	6	16	1	50
Elevated	13	87	31	84	1	50
CA19-9 baseline, units/mL						
Median	1,148		881		181	
Range	14–180,062		1–96,990		23–339	
Previous treatment						
Prior chemotherapy (no prior adjuvant)	3	15	10	23	1	33
Prior adjuvant therapy	3	15	10	23	1	33
With gemcitabine	1	5	5	11	0	—
With capecitabine	1	5	4	9	0	—
With fluorouracil	2	10	1	2	0	—
With docetaxel	0		2	5	0	—
With erlotinib	0		0		1	33
Time since last dose adjuvant therapy, months						
Median	64		12		5	
Range	9–81		1–23			

ECOG, Eastern Cooperative Oncology Group; *nab*-paclitaxel, paclitaxel protein-bound particles for injectable suspension (albumin bound)

*Upper limit for normal range was <37 units/mL. Approximately 10–15% of patients with pancreatic cancer lack Lewis antigens and thus lack the ability to secrete CA19-9

MPACT Trial

A total of 861 patients with metastatic pancreatic ductal adenocarcinoma (PDA) and a Karnofsky performance status (KPS) ≥70 were randomized at 151 community and academic centers 1:1 to receive *nab*-paclitaxel 125 mg/m² + gemcitabine 1000 mg/m² days 1, 8, and 15 every 4 weeks or gemcitabine alone 1000 mg/m² weekly for 7 weeks followed by 1 week of rest (cycle 1) and then days 1, 8, and 15 every 4 weeks (cycle ≥2). The median age was 63 years (range: 27–88 years). KPS was 100 (16%), 90 (44%), 80 (32%), and 70 (7%). Patients had advanced disease with liver metastases (84%), ≥3 metastatic sites (46%), and CA19-9 ≥59 × upper limit of normal (46%)

Efficacy

Response Result	Gemcitabine 1000 mg/m² + *nab*-Paclitaxel 125 mg/m² (n = 44)		Gemcitabine 1000 mg/m² + *nab*-Paclitaxel 100, 125, or 150 mg/m² (n = 67)	
	Number	%	Number	%
Complete response	0		3	4
Partial response	21	48	28	42
Stable disease*	9	20	12	18
Progressive disease	7	16	15	22
Disease control rate†	30	68	43	64

Median OS of patients who received *nab*-paclitaxel 125 mg/m² + gemcitabine 1000 mg/m² (n = 44)	12.2 months	

Median OS according to metabolic response compared to baseline (EORTC criteria for absence of [¹⁸F]fluorodeoxyglucose uptake) (cohorts 1 + 2‡)	Metabolic Response		p Value
	Incomplete	Complete	
	10.2 months	20.1 months	0.01

Median OS correlated with SPARC (all cohorts§)	Average z-Score		p Value
	≥0, High SPARC	<0, Low SPARC	
	17.8 months	8.1 months	0.0431

EORTC, European Organization for Research and Treatment of Cancer; OS, overall survival; SPARC, secreted protein acidic and rich in cysteine

*Stable disease was defined as ≥16 weeks

†Disease control rate defined as percentage of patients with complete and partial response and stable disease ≥16 weeks

‡Cohort 1 = gemcitabine 1000 mg/m² + *nab*-paclitaxel 100 mg/m²; Cohort 2 = gemcitabine 1000 mg/m² + *nab*-paclitaxel 125 mg/m²

§Three cohorts. All received gemcitabine 1000 mg/m². The *nab*-paclitaxel dosages were 100, 125, or 150 mg/m²

Efficacy: MPACT

	nab-Paclitaxel + Gemcitabine	Gemcitabine Monotherapy	Hazard Ratios/ p Values
Median overall survival (OS)	8.5 months	6.7 months	HR 0.72; 95% CI, 0.617–0.835 p = 0.000015
Overall survival, 6 months	67%	55%	
Overall survival, 12 months	35%	22%	
Overall survival, 24 months	9%	4%	
Median progression-free survival (PFS)	5.5 months	3.7 months	HR 0.69; 95% CI, 0.581–0.821 p = 0.000024
ORR (RECIST v1.0 criteria)	23%	7%	p = 1.1 × 10⁻¹⁰
Metabolic response by PET (N = 257/861 patients)	63%	38%	p = 0.000051
ORR by CT scans in PET-evaluable patients	31%	11%	p = 0.0001
CA19-9 response (≥90% decrease)	31%	14%	p <0.0001
CA19-9 response (≥20% decrease)	61%	44%	p <0.0001
Median duration of treatment	3.9 months	2.8 months	—

Von Hoff et al. J Clin Oncol 2013;31(Suppl; abstr 4005)

Toxicity

Adverse Events	Gemcitabine 1000 mg/m² + *nab*-Paclitaxel 100 mg/m² (n = 20)		Gemcitabine 1000 mg/m² + *nab*-Paclitaxel 125 mg/m² (n = 44)	
	No.	%	No.	%
Nonhematologic Events				
Diarrhea				
G1	1	5	7	16
G2	1	5	6	14
G3	3	15	1	2
G4	0		0	
Fatigue				
G1	4	20	10	23
G2	9	45	13	30
G3	1	5	12	27
G4	0		0	
Nausea				
G1	7	35	11	25
G2	2	10	9	20
G3	0		1	2
G4	0		0	
Sensory neuropathy				
G1	5	25	15	34
G2	1	5	9	20
G3	1	5	9	20
G4	0		0	
Vomiting				
G1	1	5	10	23
G2	2	10	3	7
G3	0		3	7
G4	0		0	

(continued)

Toxicity (continued)

Adverse Events	Gemcitabine 1000 mg/m² + nab-Paclitaxel 100 mg/m² (n = 20)		Gemcitabine 1000 mg/m² + nab-Paclitaxel 125 mg/m² (n = 44)	
	No.	%	No.	%
Hematologic Events				
Anemia				
G1	7	35	10	23
G2	11	55	27	63
G3	1	5	6	14
G4	0		0	
Leukopenia				
G1	2	10	6	14
G2	12	60	9	21
G3	4	20	16	37
G4	0		8	19
Neutropenia				
G1	4	20	6	14
G2	3	15	1	2
G3	8	40	11	26
G4	2	10	21	49
Febrile Neutropenia				
G1	0		0	
G2	0		0	
G3	1	5	1	2
G4	1	5	0	
Thrombocytopenia				
G1	5	25	18	42
G2	5	25	9	21
G3	2	10	8	19
G4	1	5	4	9

National Cancer Institute Common Terminology Criteria for Adverse Events, version 3.0

Toxicity: MPACT

G ≥3 neutropenia	38%	27%
Febrile neutropenia	3%	1%
G ≥3 fatigue	17%	7%
G ≥3 diarrhea	6%	1%
G ≥3 peripheral neuropathy*	17%	1%

*Improved to grade ≤1 in median 29 days, and 44% of patients resumed nab-Paclitaxel treatment

Von Hoff et al. J Clin Oncol 2013;31(Suppl; abstr 4005)

Treatment Monitoring

1. *Days 1, 8, and 15:* CBC with differential

ADVANCED OR METASTATIC PANCREATIC CANCER REGIMEN

OXALIPLATIN + IRINOTECAN + FLUOROURACIL + LEUCOVORIN (FOLFIRINOX)

Conroy T et al. N Engl J Med 2011;364:1817–1825

Oxaliplatin 85 mg/m² intravenously in 250 mL 5% dextrose injection (D5W) over 2 hours on day 1, every 2 weeks (total dosage/cycle = 85 mg/m²)

Note: Oxaliplatin must not be mixed with sodium chloride injection

Either: **(racemic) Leucovorin calcium** 400 mg/m² *or* **levoleucovorin calcium** 200 mg/m² intravenously in 25–500 mL D5W or 0.9% sodium chloride injection over 2 hours on day 1, every 2 weeks (total dosage/cycle for racemic leucovorin = 400 mg/m², for levoleucovorin = 200 mg/m²), *followed 30 minutes after administration begins by:*

Irinotecan 180 mg/m² intravenously over 90 minutes in 500 mL D5W on day 1, 30 minutes after leucovorin (or levoleucovorin) administration begins, every 2 weeks (total dosage/cycle = 180 mg/m²), *followed by:*

(bolus) **Fluorouracil** 400 mg/m² by intravenous injection over 1–2 minutes after leucovorin (or levoleucovorin) and irinotecan administration are completed on day 1, every 2 weeks, *followed by:*

Fluorouracil 2400 mg/m² by continuous intravenous infusion over 46 hours in 100–1000 mL 0.9% NS or D5W, starting on day 1 every 2 weeks (total dosage/cycle = 2800 mg/m²)

Important note: This regimen is difficult for patients. Thus, FOLFIRINOX is a first-line option for patients with metastatic pancreatic cancer who are younger than 76 years and who have a good performance status (ECOG 0 or 1), no cardiac ischemia, and normal or nearly normal bilirubin levels

Notes:
- Patients must be instructed in the use of loperamide as treatment for diarrhea, and must have a supply of this drug upon starting FOLFIRINOX
- Filgrastim is not recommended as primary prophylaxis, but it could be considered for high-risk patients
- The dose of leucovorin is not modified for toxicity, but is omitted if fluorouracil is omitted. Once a fluorouracil dose is decreased, it is not re-escalated

Supportive Care
Antiemetic prophylaxis
Emetogenic potential is **MODERATE**
See Chapter 39 for antiemetic recommendations

Hematopoietic growth factor (CSF) prophylaxis
Primary prophylaxis may be indicated
See Chapter 43 for more information

Antimicrobial prophylaxis
Risk of fever and neutropenia is LOW
   Antimicrobial primary prophylaxis to be considered:
   - Antibacterial—not indicated
   - Antifungal—not indicated
   - Antiviral—not indicated unless patient previously had an episode of HSV
See Chapter 47 for more information

Acute cholinergic syndrome
Atropine sulfate 0.25–1 mg subcutaneously or intravenously if abdominal cramping or diarrhea develop during or within 1 hour after irinotecan administration
- If symptoms are severe, add as primary prophylaxis at least 30 minutes before irinotecan during subsequent cycles
- For irinotecan, acute cholinergic syndrome may be characterized by: abdominal cramping, diarrhea, diaphoresis, hypotension, flushing, bradycardia, rhinitis, increased salivation, meiosis, and lacrimation

(continued)

(*continued*)

Diarrhea management

Latent or delayed onset diarrhea*:

Loperamide 4 mg orally initially after the first loose or liquid stool, *then*

Loperamide 2 mg orally every 2 hours during waking hours, *plus*

Loperamide 4 mg orally every 4 hours during hours of sleep

- Continue for at least 12 hours after diarrhea resolves
- Recurrent diarrhea after a 12-hour diarrhea-free interval is treated as a new episode
- Rehydrate orally with fluids and electrolytes during a diarrheal episode
- If a patient develops blood or mucus in stool, dehydration, or hemodynamic instability, or if diarrhea persists >48 hours despite loperamide, stop loperamide and hospitalize the patient for IV hydration

   Alternatively, a trial of **Diphenoxylate hydrochloride** 2.5 mg **with Atropine sulfate** 0.025 mg (eg, Lomotil)
- Initial adult dose is 2 tablets 4 times daily until control has been achieved, after which the dose may be reduced to meet individual requirements. Control may often be maintained with as little as 2 tablets daily
- Clinical improvement of acute diarrhea is usually observed within 48 hours. If improvement of chronic diarrhea after treatment with a maximum daily dose of 8 tablets is not observed within 10 days, control is unlikely with further administration

Persistent diarrhea:

Octreotide 100–150 mcg subcutaneously 3 times daily. Maximum total daily dose is 1500 mcg

Antibiotic therapy during latent or delayed onset diarrhea:

A fluoroquinolone (eg, **Ciprofloxacin** 500 mg orally every 12 hours) if absolute neutrophil count <500/mm^3 with or without accompanying fever in association with diarrhea
- Antibiotics should also be administered if patient is hospitalized with prolonged diarrhea and should be continued until diarrhea resolves

*Abigerges D et al. J Natl Cancer Inst 1994;86:446–449
Rothenberg ML et al. J Clin Oncol 2001;19:3801–3807
Wadler S et al. J Clin Oncol 1998;16:3169–3178

Treatment Modifications

Event	Delay of Cycle	Dosage Reductions		
		Irinotecan	Oxaliplatin	Fluorouracil
First occurrence of ANC <1500/mm^3 on day 1	Hold treatment up to 2 weeks until granulocytes ≥1500/mm^3	Reduce dosage to 150 mg/m^2	Do not reduce dosage	Delete bolus fluorouracil
Second occurrence of ANC <1500/mm^3 on day 1	In case of nonrecovery >2 weeks delay, stop treatment	Maintain the dosage at 150 mg/m^2	Reduce the dosage to 60 mg/m^2	Continue without bolus fluorouracil
Third occurrence of ANC <1500/mm^3 on day 1	Discontinue treatment			
First occurrence of platelets <75,000/mm^3 on day 1	Hold treatment up to 2 weeks until platelets ≥75,000/mm^3. In case of nonrecovery >2 weeks delay, stop treatment	Do not reduce dosage	Reduce the dosage to 60 mg/m^2	Reduce both bolus and CI by 25% of original dosages
Second occurrence of platelets <75,000/mm^3 on day 1		Reduce the dosage to 150 mg/m^2	Maintain the dosage at 60 mg/m^2	Continue both bolus and CI at 75% of original dosages
Third occurrence of platelets <75,000/mm^3 on day 1	Discontinue treatment			
First occurrence febrile neutropenia or G4 neutropenia >7 days or infection with concomitant G3/4 neutropenia		Reduce the dosage to 150 mg/m^2	Do not reduce dosage	Delete bolus fluorouracil
Second occurrence febrile neutropenia or G4 neutropenia >7 days or infection with concomitant G3/4 neutropenia		Maintain the dosage at 150 mg/m^2	Reduce the dosage to 60 mg/m^2	Continue without bolus fluorouracil
		Note: Consider the use of filgrastim for recurrent G3/4 neutropenia despite a first-dose reduction or after febrile neutropenia		

(*continued*)

Treatment Modifications (continued)

Event	Delay of Cycle	Dosage Reductions		
		Irinotecan	Oxaliplatin	Fluorouracil
Third occurrence febrile neutropenia or G4 neutropenia >7 days or infection with concomitant G3/4 neutropenia	Discontinue treatment			
First occurrence G3/4 thrombocytopenia		Do not reduce dosage	Reduce the dosage to 60 mg/m²	Reduce both bolus and CI fluorouracil by 25% of the original dosages
Second occurrence G3/4 thrombocytopenia		Reduce the dosage to 150 mg/m²	Maintain the dosage at 60 mg/m²	Continue with bolus fluorouracil at 75% of the original dosage and reduce CI by an additional 25–50% of the original dosage
Third occurrence G3/4 thrombocytopenia	Discontinue treatment			
First occurrence G3/4 diarrhea, or diarrhea + fever and/or diarrhea + G3/4 neutropenia		Reduce the dosage to 150 mg/m². Do not retreat with irinotecan until recovered from diarrhea without loperamide for at least 24 hours	Do not reduce dosage	Delete bolus fluorouracil
Second occurrence G3/4 diarrhea, or diarrhea + fever and/or diarrhea + G3/4 neutropenia		Maintain the dosage at 150 mg/m². Do not retreat with irinotecan until recovered from diarrhea without loperamide for at least 24 hours	Reduce the dosage to 60 mg/m²	Continue without bolus fluorouracil and reduce the CI by 25% of the original dosage
Third occurrence G3/4 diarrhea or diarrhea + fever and/or diarrhea + G3/4 neutropenia	Discontinue treatment			
Diarrhea ≥48 hours despite high doses of loperamide	No systematic reduction of the irinotecan, oxaliplatin, or fluorouracil doses after complete recovery, unless G3/4 diarrhea, or diarrhea + fever, and/or concomitant neutropenia G3/4			
G3/4 mucositis or "hand-foot" syndrome		Do not reduce dosage	Do not reduce dosage	Reduce both bolus and CI fluorouracil by 25% of the original dosages
Angina pectoris or of myocardial infarction		Do not reduce dosage	Do not reduce dosage	Discontinue fluorouracil
Any toxicity G ≥2, except anemia and alopecia		Consider reducing the dosage to 150 mg/m²	Consider reducing the dosage to 60 mg/m²	Consider reducing both bolus and CI fluorouracil by 25% of the original dosages
Total bilirubin ≥1.5× ULN		Do not administer	Do not reduce dosage	Do not reduce dosage

CI, continuous infusion; ULN, upper limit of normal of laboratory value

Efficacy

Objective Responses in the Intention-to-Treat Population

Variable	FOLFIRINOX* (N = 171)	Gemcitabine (N = 171)	P Value
	Response—Number (%)		
Complete response	1 (0.6)	0	
Partial response	53 (31.0)	16 (9.4)	
Stable disease	66 (38.6)	71 (41.5)	
Progressive disease	26 (15.2)	59 (34.5)	
Could not be evaluated	25 (14.6)	25 (14.6)	
Rate of objective response†			<0.001
No. (%)	54 (31.6)	16 (9.4)	
95% CI	24.7–39.1	5.4–14.7	
Rate of disease control‡			<0.001
No. (%)	120 (70.2)	87 (50.9)	
95% CI	62.7–76.9	43.1–58.6	
Response duration—months			0.57
Median	5.9	3.9	
95% CI	4.9–7.1	3.1–7.1	

Variable	FOLFIRINOX* (N = 171)	Gemcitabine (N = 171)	HR [95% CI] P Value
Progression-free survival	6.4 months 95% CI, 5.5–7.2	3.3 months 95% CI, 2.2–3.6	0.47 [0.37–0.59] p <0.001
6-Month PFS rate	52.8%	17.2%	—
12-Month PFS rate	12.1%	3.5%	—
18-Month PFS rate	3.3%	0%	—
Overall survival§	11.1 months	6.8 months	0.57 [0.45–0.73] p <0.001
6-Month OS rate	75.9%	57.6%	—
12-Month OS rate	48.4%	20.6%	—
18-Month OS rate	18.6%	6.0%	—

95% CI, 95% confidence interval; HR, hazard ratio; OS, overall survival; PFS, progression-free survival
*FOLFIRINOX = oxaliplatin + irinotecan + fluorouracil + leucovorin
†Defined as percentage of patients who had a complete response or partial response
‡Defined as the percentage of patients who had a complete response, partial response, or stable disease
§Synchronous metastases, albumin level <3.5 g/dL (<35 g/L), hepatic metastases, and age >65 years were identified as independent adverse prognostic factors for overall survival

Patient Population Studied

Patients with histologically and cytologically confirmed metastatic pancreatic adenocarcinoma not previously treated with chemotherapy. Other inclusion criteria were an Eastern Cooperative Oncology Group (ECOG) performance status score of 0 or 1 and adequate bone marrow, liver function (total bilirubin ≤1.5 times the upper limit of normal range), and renal function. Exclusion criteria included an age ≥76 years and previous radiotherapy for measurable lesions

Patient Characteristics

Age (years)	
Median	61
Range	25–76

Sex—number (%)	
Male	106 (62.0)
Female	65 (38.0)

ECOG performance status score—number (%)	
0	64 (37.4)
1	106 (61.9)
2	(0.6)

Pancreatic tumor location—number (%)	
Head	67 (39.2)
Body	53 (31.0)
Tail	45 (26.3)
Multicentric	6 (3.5)

Biliary stent—number (%)	
Yes	27 (15.8)
No	144 (84.2)

Number of metastatic sites involved	
Median	2
Range	1–6

Number of measurable metastatic sites—number of patients/total number (%)	
Liver	149/170 (87.6)
Pancreas	90/170 (52.9)
Lymph node	49/170 (28.8)
Lung	33/170 (19.4)
Peritoneal	33/170 (19.4)
Other	18/170 (10.6)

	Toxicity			Treatment Monitoring

Toxicity

Most Common G3/4 Adverse Events*

Event	FOLFIRINOX (N = 171)	Gemcitabine (N = 171)	P Value
	Number of Patients/Total Number (%)		
Hematologic			
Neutropenia	75/164 (45.7)	35/167 (21.0)	<0.001
Febrile neutropenia	9/166 (5.4)	2/169 (1.2)	0.03
Thrombocytopenia	15/165 (9.1)	6/168 (3.6)	0.04
Anemia	13/166 (7.8)	10/168 (6.0)	NS†
Nonhematologic			
Fatigue	39/165 (23.6)	30/169 (17.8)	NS†
Vomiting	24/166 (14.5)	14/169 (8.3)	NS†
Diarrhea	21/165 (12.7)	3/169 (1.8)	<0.001
Sensory neuropathy	15/166 (9.0)	0/169	<0.001
↑ Alanine aminotransferase	12/165 (7.3)	35/168 (20.8)	<0.001
Thromboembolism	11/166 (6.6)	7/169 (4.1)	NS†

*Events listed are those that occurred in more than 5% of patients in either group
†NS denotes not significant

Note: Despite the higher incidence of adverse events associated with the FOLFIRINOX regimen, a significant increase in the time to definitive deterioration of the quality of life was observed in the FOLFIRINOX group as compared with the gemcitabine group

Treatment Monitoring

1. *At start of every cycle:* medical history, complete physical examination, CBC with differential and serum electrolytes and LFTs
2. *Weekly:* CBC with differential

ADVANCED OR METASTATIC PANCREATIC CANCER REGIMEN—SECOND LINE

OXALIPLATIN + FOLINIC ACID (Leucovorin) + FLUOROURACIL (OFF) + BSC (Best Supportive Care)

Pelzer U et al. Eur J Cancer 2011;47:1676–1681

Days 1, 8, 15, and 22 during 6-week cycles:
Leucovorin calcium 200 mg/m² per dose intravenously in 25–100 mL 0.9% sodium chloride injection (0.9% NS) or 5% dextrose injection (D5W) over 30 minutes for 4 doses on days 1, 8, 15, and 22, every 6 weeks (total dosage/6-week cycle = 800 mg/m²), *followed by:*
Fluorouracil 2000 mg/m² per dose by continuous intravenous infusion in 100–1000 mL 0.9% NS or D5W over 24 hours for 4 doses on days 1, 8, 15, and 22, every 6 weeks (total dosage/6-week cycle = 8000 mg/m²)

Days 8 and 22 during 6-week cycles:
Oxaliplatin 85 mg/m² per dose administer intravenously in 250 mL D5W over 2–4 hours for 2 doses prior to leucovorin and fluorouracil on days 8 and 22 (total dosage/6-week cycle = 170 mg/m²)

Note: Oxaliplatin must not be mixed with sodium chloride injection. If leucovorin or fluorouracil are diluted in solutions containing sodium chloride injection and administered through the same tubing or vascular access device as oxaliplatin, the fluid pathway should be flushed with D5W before administering oxaliplatin

Best supportive care (BSC) according to current palliative care guidelines includes:
• Adequate pain management
• Therapy of infection
• Biliary stent intervention if needed
• Social support and on-demand psychooncologic intervention
• Nutrition consultation/intervention

Supportive Care
Antiemetic prophylaxis
Emetogenic potential on days with fluorouracil and leucovorin is **LOW**
Emetogenic potential on days with oxaliplatin is **MODERATE**
See Chapter 39 for antiemetic recommendations

Hematopoietic growth factor (CSF) prophylaxis
Primary prophylaxis may be indicated
See Chapter 43 for more information

Antimicrobial prophylaxis
Risk of fever and neutropenia is LOW
  Antimicrobial primary prophylaxis to be considered:
  • Antibacterial—not indicated
  • Antifungal—not indicated
  • Antiviral—not indicated unless patient previously had an episode of HSV
See Chapter 47 for more information

Diarrhea management
Latent or delayed onset diarrhea*:
  Loperamide 4 mg orally initially after the first loose or liquid stool, *then*
  Loperamide 2 mg orally every 2 hours during waking hours, *plus*
  Loperamide 4 mg orally every 4 hours during hours of sleep
  • Continue for at least 12 hours after diarrhea resolves
  • Recurrent diarrhea after a 12-hour diarrhea-free interval is treated as a new episode
  • Rehydrate orally with fluids and electrolytes during a diarrheal episode
  • If a patient develops blood or mucus in stool, dehydration, or hemodynamic instability, or if diarrhea persists >48 hours despite loperamide, stop loperamide and hospitalize the patient for IV hydration

(continued)

(continued)

Alternatively, a trial of **Diphenoxylate hydrochloride** 2.5 mg **with Atropine sulfate** 0.025 mg (eg, Lomotil)

- Initial adult dose is 2 tablets 4 times daily until control has been achieved, after which the dose may be reduced to meet individual requirements. Control may often be maintained with as little as 2 tablets daily
- Clinical improvement of acute diarrhea is usually observed within 48 hours. If improvement of chronic diarrhea after treatment with a maximum daily dose of 8 tablets is not observed within 10 days, control is unlikely with further administration

Persistent diarrhea:

Octreotide 100–150 mcg subcutaneously 3 times daily. Maximum total daily dose is 1500 mcg

Antibiotic therapy during latent or delayed onset diarrhea:

A fluoroquinolone (eg, **Ciprofloxacin** 500 mg orally every 12 hours) if absolute neutrophil count <500/mm^3 with or without accompanying fever in association with diarrhea

- Antibiotics should also be administered if patient is hospitalized with prolonged diarrhea and should be continued until diarrhea resolves

*Abigerges D et al. J Natl Cancer Inst 1994;86:446–449
Rothenberg ML et al. J Clin Oncol 2001;19:3801–3807
Wadler S et al. J Clin Oncol 1998;16:3169–3178

Dose Modifications

Fluorouracil and Oxaliplatin

Any G2/3/4 nonhematologic toxicity	Delay start of next cycle until the severity of all toxicities are G ≤1
ANC ≤1500/mm^3 or platelet count ≤100,000/mm^3	Delay start of next cycle until ANC >1500/mm^3 and platelet count >100,000/mm^3
G3/4 Nonneurologic	Reduce fluorouracil and oxaliplatin dosages by 20%
G3/4 ANC	Reduce oxaliplatin dosage by 20%
Persistent (≥14 days) paresthesias	Reduce oxaliplatin dosage by 20%
Temporary (7–14 days) painful paresthesias	
Temporary (7–14 days) functional impairment	
Persistent (≥14 days) painful paresthesias	Discontinue oxaliplatin
Persistent (≥14 days) functional impairment	

Adapted in part from de Gramont A et al. J Clin Oncol 2000;18:2938–2947

Efficacy

	OFF	Best Supportive Care	Statistics
Median survival with therapy	4.82 months (95% CI: 4.29–5.35)	2.30 months (95% CI: 1.76–2.83)	HR 0.45 (95% CI: 0.24–0.83) p = 0.008
Median survival since diagnosis	9.09 months (95% CI: 6.97–11.21)	7.90 months (95% CI: 4.95–10.84)	HR 0.50 (95% CI: 0.27–0.95) p = 0.031

Treatment Monitoring

1. *At start of every cycle:* Medical history, complete physical examination, CBC with differential and serum electrolytes and LFTs
2. *Weekly:* CBC with differential

Patient Population Studied

Patients with histologically confirmed advanced pancreatic cancer whose disease had progressed during first-line gemcitabine therapy. Patients had a Karnofsky performance status (KPS) >60% and good hepatic function, defined as AST (aspartate aminotransferase) and ALT (alanine aminotransferase) <2.5× the upper normal limit (UNL), or, in case of liver metastasis <5× UNL

Total number of patients	23
Sex, male-to-female ratio	14/9
Median age (range)	60 (38–76)
Karnofsky Performance Status 70–80%	12
Karnofsky Performance Status 90–100%	11
Gemcitabine first-line therapy	23/23
PFS on gemcitabine <3 months	6
PFS on gemcitabine 3–6 months	10
PFS on gemcitabine >6 months	7
M0/M1 disease	6/17

Toxicity

Toxicity (NCI CTC 2.0)

	G1	G2	G3	G4
	(Number of Patients)			
Hemoglobin	5	1	1	0
Leucopenia	4	0	0	0
Thrombocytopenia	2	2	0	0
Diarrhea	5	1	2	0
Nausea/emesis	6	4	1	0
Paresthesia	10	1	0	0

Mean (range) cumulative doses administered:
Oxaliplatin 281 mg (0–850 mg)
Folinic acid 1591 mg (200–8000 mg)
Fluorouracil 15, 630 mg (2000–20,000 mg)

30. Pancreatic Endocrine Tumors

Sara Ekeblad, MD, PhD and Britt Skogseid, MD, PhD

Epidemiology

Incidence: 1/100,000

~85% sporadic; ~15% hereditary, for example, multiple endocrine neoplasia (MEN1), von Hippel-Lindau disease

Median age: 53–57 years

Male to female ratio: 0.8–1.3:1

Ekeblad SB et al. Clin Cancer Res 2008;14:7798–7803
Fischer L et al. Br J Surg 2008;95:627–635
Hochwald SN et al. J Clin Oncol 2002;20:2633–2642
Öberg K, Eriksson B. Best Pract Res Clin Gastroenterol 2005;19:753–781
Tomassetti PD et al. Ann Oncol 2005;16:1806–1810

Pathology

WHO classification: Pancreatic endocrine tumors

1. Well-differentiated *neuroendocrine tumor* (20–35%): no gross invasion
   - *Benign:* no angio- or perineural invasion, size <2 cm, <2 mitoses/10 high-power fields (HPF), <2% of cells Ki67-positive
   - *Of uncertain behavior:* angio- and/or perineural invasion and/or >2 cm and/or 2–10 mitoses/10 HPF and/or >2% of cells Ki67-positive
2. Well-differentiated *neuroendocrine carcinoma* (51–71%): gross local invasion and/or metastases
3. Poorly differentiated *neuroendocrine carcinoma* (9–21%): >10 mitoses/10 HPF

Functional status:

Nonfunctioning: 59–76%

Insulinoma: 8–17%

Gastrinoma: 10–14%

Glucagonoma: 1–6%

VIPoma: 2–5%

Ekeblad SB et al. Clin Cancer Res 2008;14:7798–7803
Fischer L et al. Br J Surg 2008;95:627–635
Pape U-F et al. Cancer 2008;113:256–265
Rindi G, Klöppel G. Neuroendocrinology 2004;80 (Suppl 1):12–15

Work-up

Radiology

1. Body CT or MRI
2. Somatostatin receptor scintigraphy: Uses *radioactive octreotide*, a drug similar to somatostatin that attaches to tumor cells that have somatostatin receptors
3. Positron emission tomography (PET) scan (in selected cases)
   - [^{11}C]5-hydroxy-L-tryptophan (5-HTP) PET for well-differentiated tumors
   - Fluorodeoxyglucose (FDG) PET for poorly differentiated tumors
4. Endoscopic ultrasound
5. Intraoperative ultrasound
   - To localize small tumors not visualized by other modalities but suspected because of biochemical findings
   - To localize multiple tumors in MEN1 patients

Biochemistry

1. In all patients with suspected pancreatic endocrine tumor
   - Fasting levels of:
     - insulin, proinsulin, blood glucose
     - gastrin
     - glucagon
     - pancreatic polypeptide
     - vasoactive intestinal peptide (VIP)
     - chromogranin A
2. If insulinoma is suspected (high fasting insulin or symptoms of hypoglycemia):
   - 72-hour fast with measurements of insulin, proinsulin, and plasma glucose
   - Consider differential diagnoses, for example, measurement of sulfonylurea in blood to exclude abuse of oral hypoglycemic drugs

(continued)

Work-up (continued)

3. If gastrinoma is suspected (high fasting gastrin in the absence of treatment with proton pump inhibitors, multiple ulcers, and/or steatorrhea):
   - Measure gastrin after *secretin stimulation test* (after withdrawal of proton pump inhibitors, ideally for 1 week)
   - Measure gastric pH together with fasting gastrin
4. If ectopic Cushing syndrome is suspected to be caused by a pancreatic tumor:
   - Measure 24-hour urine free cortisol excretion, *or* free cortisol to creatinine ratio
     A ratio of cortisol >95 mcg per gram of creatinine helps confirm hypercortisolism
   - Measure adrenocorticotropic hormone (ACTH) and corticotropin-releasing factor (CRF)

Biopsies
1. If possible, radiologically verified tumors should be biopsied under ultrasound guidance
2. Ideally, biopsy specimens should be evaluated by pathologists knowledgeable in endocrine pathology and stained for:
   - *General markers for pancreatic endocrine tumors:* Chromogranin A, synaptophysin
   - *Specific hormones:* Insulin, gastrin, glucagon, VIP, pancreatic polypeptide
   - *Markers of proliferation:* Ki67

MEN1 investigation
1. If MEN1 is suspected (family history, hyperparathyroidism)
   - Measure serum calcium, PTH, prolactin
   - Perform genetic testing

Survival

5-Year: 55–64%
10-Year: 44%
Median survival: 90–99 months

Stage	Mean Survival
I	231 months (≈19 years)
IIa	222 months (≈18.5 years)
IIb	153 months (≈13 years)
IIIa	94 months (≈8 years)
IIIb	133 months (≈11 years)
IV	76 months (≈6 years)

Staging

Stage	Location/Size/Extension	Percent of Cases
I	Limited to pancreas, <2 cm	5–31
IIa	Limited to pancreas, 2–4 cm	8–9
IIb	Limited to pancreas, >4 cm, *or* Invading duodenum or bile duct	5–7
IIIa	Invading adjacent organs (stomach, spleen, colon, adrenal gland), *or* Invading the wall of large vessels (celiac axis or superior mesenteric artery)	3–8
IIIb	Regional lymph node metastasis	14–15
IV	Distant metastasis	29–60

Ekeblad SB et al. Clin Cancer Res 2008;14:7798–7803
Fischer L et al. Br J Surg 2008;95:627–635
Pape U-F et al. Cancer 2008;113:256–265
Rindi G, Klöppel G. Virchows Arch 2006;449:395–401

Expert Opinion

Pancreatic endocrine tumors are rare, and there is a lack of solid evidence on treatment and outcomes. The following is our view of their management, based on available evidence and many years of clinical experience

Diagnosis and work-up

1. Always measure hormone levels if symptoms of a functioning tumor occur or a pancreatic mass is demonstrated

2. Obtain a CT scan if hormone levels are elevated

3. Obtain somatostatin receptor scintigraphy (radioactive octreotide scan) or 5-HTP PET if unclear

4. Patient history: always probe for family history, history of kidney stones, and history of hyperparathyroidism (MEN1)

5. If MEN1 is suspected, discuss performing genetic testing

6. For known MEN1 carriers, perform annual biochemical screening beginning in adolescence. CT and/or 5-HTP PET if hormone levels are elevated

7. Radiologically visualized tumor: biopsy if radical surgery seems impossible

Surgery

1. Preferably performed by experienced endocrine surgeon at a high-volume center

2. Radical surgery of tumors that can be demonstrated by imaging

3. For tumors that can only be detected biochemically, if fully confident of the analyses, perform a surgical exploration. If a tumor is identified, proceed to resection if possible

4. Aim for pancreas-preserving surgery. If MEN1, distal pancreatectomy in combination with enucleation of lesions in the head of the pancreas are preferable. In addition, consider duodenotomy in case of MEN1 gastrinoma

5. Use intraoperative ultrasound to localize possible additional tumors or very small functioning tumors (especially important for MEN1 tumors)

6. If there is evidence of disease dissemination, consider:
   - Radiofrequency ablation of liver metastases
     - Useful for limited numbers of liver metastases
     - One study showed 45% of patients rendered tumor-free with relatively few complications (Eriksson J et al. World J Surg 2008;32:930–938)
     - Metastases usually recur, but radiofrequency ablation can be performed repeatedly
     - Can alleviate hormonal symptoms
   - Liver embolization
     - Useful if there are a larger number of liver metastases than can be treated with radiofrequency ablation
     - Lessens tumor burden in many patients
     - Can alleviate hormonal symptoms

Systemic treatment

Treat inoperable tumors at once; do not wait for tumor progression to initiate treatment

1. Streptozocin + fluorouracil or streptozocin + doxorubicin have long been considered is the first choice for patients with *well-differentiated tumors*

2. Carboplatin + etoposide is effective, and, generally, the first choice in patients with *poorly differentiated carcinomas*

3. Temozolomide used as second-line treatment after the combinations mentioned above, or for patients who cannot tolerate more intensive chemotherapy
   - Easy to use for the patient as it is taken orally; thus, it can easily be taken in an outpatient setting
   - Test tumor material for O_6-methylguanine-methyltranferase, low levels of which might predict a favorable response to temozolomide

4. Two additional options for patients with well and moderately differentiated tumors include sunitinib malate and everolimus. There is no consensus on whether these agents should be used before or after cytotoxic chemotherapy regimens such as streptozocin + fluorouracil

5. Somatostatin analogs should be used to alleviate hormonal symptoms, and might possibly also have antitumor effects, although this is still unclear. Somatostatin analogs can be used in combination with chemotherapy

6. Radionuclide-tagged somatostatin analogs (^{177}Lu-DOTA^0, Tyr^3) are increasingly used although only in a trial setting
   - A recent study showed a 42% response rate with an acceptable safety profile

(continued)

Expert Opinion (*continued*)

Supportive care:

Regardless of the therapy used, attention should be given to symptom management as many patients present with debilitating symptoms for which amelioration can significantly improve the quality of their lives:

- *Gastric hyperacidity (patients with a diagnosis of gastrinoma):*

  Omeprazole 40–60 mg per day orally, or an equivalent **proton pump inhibitor** or **histamine (H_2) receptor antagonist** may be used

- *Steatorrhea:*

  Consider supplementation with **pancreatic enzymes** whenever steatorrhea or changes in bowel habits suggest malabsorption

- *Diarrhea*:*

  Loperamide 4 mg; administer orally initially after the first loose or liquid stool, *then*

  Loperamide 2 mg; administer orally every 2 hours during waking hours, *plus*

  Loperamide 4 mg; administer orally every 4 hours during hours of sleep

  - Continue for at least 12 hours after diarrhea resolves

  - Recurrent diarrhea after a 12-hour diarrhea-free interval is treated as a new episode

  - Rehydrate orally with fluids and electrolytes during a diarrheal episode

  - If a patient develops blood or mucus in stool, dehydration, or hemodynamic instability, or if diarrhea persists >48 hours despite loperamide, stop loperamide and hospitalize the patient for IV hydration

Persistent diarrhea:

  Tincture of opium: Doses are individually titrated. Begin with 2–4 drops mixed in water; administer orally 2–3 times per day, and titrate by decreasing or increasing the number of drops per dose as needed

  Octreotide 50–200 mcg; administer subcutaneously 3 times daily. Maximum total daily dose is 1500 mcg

Diarrhea in patients who have undergone ileocecal resection:

  Cholestyramine 4 g/dose; administer orally for 2–6 doses per day (up to 24 g/day)

Antibiotic therapy during latent or delayed onset diarrhea:

  A fluoroquinolone (eg, **Ciprofloxacin** 500 mg; administer orally every 12 hours) if absolute neutrophil count is <500/mm^3 with or without accompanying fever in association with diarrhea

  - Antibiotics should also be administered if patient is hospitalized with prolonged diarrhea and should be continued until diarrhea resolves

*Abigerges D et al. J Natl Cancer Inst 1994;86:446–449
Kulke MH et al. J Clin Oncol 2008;26:3403–3410
Rothenberg ML et al. J Clin Oncol 2001;19:3801–3807
Wadler S et al. J Clin Oncol 1998;16:3169–3178

Arnold R et al. Gut 1996;38:430–438
de Keizer B et al. Eur J Nucl Med Mol Imaging 2008;35:749–755
Ekeblad S et al. Clin Cancer Res 2007;13:2986–2991
Ekeblad SB et al. Clin Cancer Res 2008;14:7798–7803
Eriksson B et al. Cancer 1990;65:1883–1890
Eriksson J et al. World J Surg 2008;32:930–938
Fischer L et al. Br J Surg 2008;95:627–635
Fjällskog M–LH et al. Cancer 2001;92:1101–1107
Hochwald SN et al. J Clin Oncol 2002;20:2633–2642
Kwekkeboom DJ et al. J Clin Oncol 2008;26:2124–2130
Moertel CG et al. Cancer 1991;68:227–232
Moertel CG et al. N Engl J Med 1980;303:1189–1194
Moertel CG et al. N Engl J Med 1992;326:519–523
Öberg K, Eriksson B. Best Pract Res Clin Gastroenterol 2005;19:753–781
Pape U-F et al. Cancer 2008;113:256–265
Rindi G, Klöppel G. Neuroendocrinology 2004;80(Suppl 1):12–15
Rindi G, Klöppel G. Virchows Arch 2006;449:395–401
Tomassetti PD et al. Ann Oncol 2005;16:1806–1810

REGIMEN

SOMATOSTATIN ANALOGS
OCTREOTIDE ACETATE

Arnold R et al. Gut 1996;38:430–438

Starting dose: **Octreotide acetate** 50 mcg; administer by subcutaneous injection 3 times daily for 3 days

Followed by: **Octreotide acetate** 100 mcg; administer by subcutaneous injection 3 times daily for 3 days

Followed by: **Octreotide acetate** 200 mcg; administer by subcutaneous injection 3 times daily continually, starting on day 7

Duration of treatment: Treatment is continued indefinitely
Supportive Care
Supplemental therapy for all somatostatin analogs: Pancreatic enzymes to avoid steatorrhea. Individualize dosage by giving the number of tablets or capsules that optimally minimize steatorrhea

Antiemetic prophylaxis
Emetogenic potential is **MINIMAL**
See Chapter 39 for antiemetic recommendations

Hematopoietic growth factor (CSF) prophylaxis
Primary prophylaxis is NOT indicated
See Chapter 43 for more information

Antimicrobial prophylaxis
Risk of fever and neutropenia is LOW
Antimicrobial primary prophylaxis to be considered:
- Antibacterial—not indicated
- Antifungal—not indicated
- Antiviral—not indicated unless patient previously had an episode of HSV

See Chapter 47 for more information

Treatment Modifications

Adverse Event	Treatment Modification
Steatorrhea	Increase dose of pancreatic enzyme supplement to 3 capsules with every meal

Toxicity

	All Grades
Diarrhea	34%
Flatulence	27%
Pain at injection site	27%
Vomiting	11%
Steatorrhea	8%
Hyperglycemia	3%
Gall stones	2%
Septicemia	1%

Patient Population Studied

- One-hundred three patients with gastroenteropancreatic neuroendocrine tumors given somatostatin analogs in a multicenter phase II trial
- Patients with functional or nonfunctional, poorly differentiated, intermediate or small cell carcinoma with high-grade malignant behavior were not included

Efficacy (N = 52)

- No objective tumor regression was seen
- Of patients with progressive pancreatic endocrine tumor, 28% had stabilization of tumor growth for ≥3 months

Tumor Growth in 52 Patients with Confirmed Progression Before Treatment

Responses at Month 3	Responses Reassessed During Months 6–12			
	Death	Progression	Stable Disease	Regression
Death (8)	8			
Progression (30)	11	14	5	0
Stable disease (14)	3	4	7	0
Regression (0)	0	0	0	0
Total (52)	22	18	12	0

Response to octreotide occurred in 19 patients according to the study protocol. WHO criteria used. However, tumors growing slowly but continuously with progression of ≤25% within 3 months were also judged as "progression" if progression ≥25% occurred within 12 months
Response = stable disease or decrease in tumor growth after confirmed progression before treatment, or decrease in tumor growth after stable disease within the pretreatment period, if lasting for at least 3 months

(continued)

Efficacy (N = 52) *(continued)*

Effect of Octreotide on Flushing, Diarrhea, and Hormone Secretion in Patients with Functional Endocrine GEP Tumors

Symptoms	Normalization	Improvement >50%	No Change	Worse
Diarrhea*				
Month 3 (n = 28)	32.1%	32.1%	21.5%	14.3%
Month 12 (n = 20)	45%	40%	5%	10%
Flushing*				
Month 3 (n = 40)	35%	40%	22.5%	2.5%
Month 12 (n = 27)	44.4%	40.8%	11.1%	3.7%
Hormone secretion				
Month 3 (n = 61)	11.5%	29.5%	34.4%	24.6%
Month 12 (n = 39)	5.1%	28.2%	38.5%	28.2%

GEP tumors, gastroenteropancreatic neuroendocrine tumors
*Patients with carcinoid syndrome, patients with functional tumors

Therapy Monitoring

1. *Every 3 months:* Complete history and physical examination
2. *Every 3–6 months:* Conventional imaging (CT, MRI, or ultrasound), serum electrolytes and serum glucose
3. *Every year:* Somatostatin receptor scintigraphy (OctreoScan Kit for the Preparation of Indium In-111 Pentetreotide; Mallinckrodt Inc., St. Louis, MO) is controversial
4. *New symptoms:* Somatostatin receptor scintigraphy (OctreoScan)

REGIMEN

LONG-ACTING SOMATOSTATIN ANALOGS

Kvols LK et al. N Engl J Med 1986;315:663–666
Öberg K et al. Ann Oncol 2004;15:966–973

Octreotide acetate injection 100–500 mcg per dose subcutaneously 2 or 3 times daily, doubling the dose at 3- to 4-day intervals until maximum control of symptoms is achieved

or

Octreotide acetate for injectable suspension 10–30 mg per dose intragluteally every 4 weeks (avoid intramuscular injection into the deltoids)

or

Lanreotide acetate (powder for suspension for injection) 30 mg per dose intramuscularly every 10–14 days (not available in the United States)

Supportive Care
Supplemental therapy for all somatostatin analogs: Pancreatic enzymes to avoid steatorrhea. Individualize dosage by giving the number of tablets or capsules that optimally minimize steatorrhea

Antiemetic prophylaxis
Emetogenic potential is **MINIMAL**
See Chapter 39 for antiemetic recommendations

Hematopoietic growth factor (CSF) prophylaxis
Primary prophylaxis is NOT indicated
See Chapter 43 for more information

Antimicrobial prophylaxis
Risk of fever and neutropenia is LOW
Antimicrobial primary prophylaxis to be considered:
- Antibacterial—not indicated
- Antifungal—not indicated
- Antiviral—not indicated unless patient previously had an episode of HSV

See Chapter 47 for more information

Patient Population Studied

Primary symptomatic treatment in 25 patients with hormonally active tumors

Efficacy (N = 25)

(Octreotide 150 mcg/dose 3 times daily; 18 months' follow-up)

Biochemical response*	72%
Biochemical stable disease	28%
Tumor size stable (n = 13)	100%
Symptomatic relief†	76%

*>50% decrease in 24-hour urinary 5-HIAA
†>50% decrease in flushing and diarrhea

Kvols LK et al. N Engl J Med 1986;315:663–666

Treatment Modifications

(Patients Receiving Octreotide Acetate for Injectable Suspension or Lanreotide Acetate)

Escape from antisecretory response	Administer octreotide acetate injection 100–500 mcg per dose subcutaneously 2 or 3 times daily. Increase dose or reduce interval between doses of the long-acting preparation as needed
Steatorrhea	Increase dose of pancreatic enzyme supplement to 3 capsules with every meal

Therapy Monitoring

1. *Every 3 months:* Complete history and physical examination
2. *Every 3–6 months:* Conventional imaging (CT, MRI, or ultrasound), serum electrolytes, and serum glucose
3. *Every year:* Somatostatin receptor scintigraphy (OctreoScan Kit for the Preparation of Indium In-111 Pentetreotide; Mallinckrodt Inc., St. Louis, MO) is controversial
4. *New symptoms:* Somatostatin receptor scintigraphy (OctreoScan)

Toxicity (N = 25)

Steatorrhea*,†	Frequent (~66%)
Loose stools†	Common
Nausea†	Common
Abdominal cramps†	Common
Flatulence†	Common
Hyperglycemia‡/hypoglycemia	<10%
Gallbladder stone/sludge	50%
Bradycardia	<2%
Pain/erythema at injection site	Occasional
Gastric atony	Very rare

*Occurs frequently unless pancreatic enzyme supplements are administered. Etiology is presumed to be transient inhibition of pancreatic exocrine function and malabsorption of fat
†Starts within hours of the first subcutaneous injection and usually subsides spontaneously within the first few weeks of treatment
‡From transient inhibition of insulin secretion

Kvols LK et al. N Engl J Med 1986;315:663–666
Öberg K et al. Ann Oncol 2004;15:966–973

Notes

1. Performing an OctreoScan provides information about the somatostatin receptor status of the patient's tumor and should be performed before treatment with a somatostatin analog is initiated. Patients with receptor-positive tumors more frequently respond to such treatment than those with receptor-negative tumors

2. Because of adverse events, administration of the immediate-release formulation is recommended before administration of the intramuscular depot formulation

3. Patients should begin therapy with octreotide acetate injection subcutaneously for 3–7 days to test for tolerability before receiving a long-acting formulation (octreotide acetate for injectable suspension or lanreotide acetate) intramuscularly

4. Increase the dosage of the short-acting octreotide acetate injection until control of symptoms is achieved by doubling the dosage at 3- to 4-day intervals

5. Patients who are considered to be "responders" to the drug and who tolerate the short-acting formulation can then receive octreotide acetate for injectable suspension or lanreotide acetate

6. The subcutaneous injections should be continued for **at least 14 days after the start of the** long-acting formulation to allow time for therapeutic levels to be achieved

7. Conversion to the long-acting formulation provides greater patient convenience. If the dose of the short-acting formulation was 200–600 mcg per day, begin with a 20-mg dose of the long-acting formulation. If the dose of the short-acting formulation was 750–1500 mcg per day, begin with a 30-mg dose of the long-acting formulation

8. Supplementary ("rescue") administration of the short-acting octreotide acetate injection should be given to patients escaping the antisecretory effects of the long-acting octreotide acetate for injectable suspension. If the rescue therapy is required during the week before the next dose of the long-acting formulation, a reduction in the dosing interval by 1 week is recommended. If the rescue medication is administered sporadically throughout the month, then increasing the dose of octreotide acetate for injectable suspension stepwise in increments of 10 mg per month, up to 60 mg per month

Supplemental therapy for all somatostatin analogs: Pancreatic enzymes to avoid steatorrhea
Individualize dosage by giving the number of tablets or capsules that optimally minimize steatorrhea
Select Pancrelipase products with a high lipase content to avoid steatorrhea. In some patients, enteric-coated enzyme tablets may not dissociate as intended and may pass through the bowel intact
Administer Pancrelipase with meals or snacks
Adjust doses slowly; monitor symptoms and response

• Do not crush or chew enteric-coated products or the enteric-coated contents of opened capsules

• Capsules may be opened and shaken onto a small quantity of soft food that is not hot and does not require chewing

• Pancrelipase should be immediately swallowed without chewing to prevent mucosal irritation

• Ingested doses should be followed with a glass of juice or water to ensure complete ingestion

• Avoid mixing pancrelipase with foods that have a pH >5.5, which can dissolve enteric coatings

REGIMEN

STREPTOZOCIN + FLUOROURACIL

Eriksson B et al. Cancer 1990;65:1883–1890
Moertel CG et al. N Engl J Med 1980;303:1189–1194
Moertel CG et al. N Engl J Med 1992;326:519–523

Premedications and hydration:
≥1000 mL 0.9% sodium chloride injection (0.9% NS); administer intravenously, starting 1.5 hours before administration of chemotherapy, continuing during administration, and for approximately 1.5 hours afterward

Induction course:
Streptozocin 1000 mg/day; administer intravenously in 100–1000 mL 0.9% NS or 5% dextrose injection (D5W) over 30–120 minutes for 5 consecutive days, on days 1–5 (total dose/cycle = 5000 mg)
Fluorouracil 400 mg/m² per day; administer by intravenous injection over 1–2 minutes for 3 consecutive days, days 1–3 (total dosage/cycle = 1200 mg/m²)

Subsequent courses: (beginning 3 weeks after the induction cycle)
Streptozocin 2000 mg intravenously in 100–1000 mL 0.9% NS or D5W over 30–120 minutes on day 1, every 3 weeks (total dose/cycle = 2000 mg)
Fluorouracil 400 mg/m² by intravenous injection over 1–2 minutes on day 1, every 3 weeks (total dosage/cycle = 400 mg/m²)

Supportive Care
Antiemetic prophylaxis
Emetogenic potential on days with streptozocin is **HIGH**
See Chapter 39 for antiemetic recommendations

Hematopoietic growth factor (CSF) prophylaxis
Primary prophylaxis is NOT indicated
See Chapter 43 for more information

Antimicrobial prophylaxis
Risk of fever and neutropenia is LOW
  Antimicrobial primary prophylaxis to be considered:
  • Antibacterial—not indicated
  • Antifungal—not indicated
  • Antiviral—not indicated unless patient previously had an episode of HSV
See Chapter 47 for more information

Patient Populations Studied

• One-hundred eighteen patients with metastatic carcinoid tumor were randomly assigned to receive treatment with streptozocin combined with cyclophosphamide or with fluorouracil (Moertel CG et al. N Engl J Med 1980;303:1189–1194)

• A prospective, nonrandomized trial. Of 84 patients with advanced pancreatic endocrine tumor, 19 received streptozocin + fluorouracil (Eriksson B et al. Cancer 1990;65:1883–1890)

• A multicenter randomized trial in which responses to streptozocin + fluorouracil, streptozocin + doxorubicin, or chlorozotocin monotherapy were compared. One-hundred five patients with advanced pancreatic endocrine tumors (Moertel CG et al. N Engl J Med 1992;326:519–523)

Treatment Modifications

Adverse Event	Treatment Modification
Creatinine clearance on day 1 of a second and subsequent cycles = 60–75 mL/min (1–1.25 mL/s)	Give streptozocin 1000 mg/day for 2 consecutive days, on days 1 and 2 (total dose/cycle = 2000 mg)
Creatinine clearance on day 1 of a second and subsequent cycles = 50–60 mL/min (0.83–1 mL/s)	Give streptozocin 1000 mg on day 1 only (total dose/ cycle = 1000 mg)
Creatinine clearance on day 1 of a second and subsequent cycles <50 mL/min (<0.83 mL/s)	Discontinue streptozocin. Resume treatment after creatinine clearance >50 mL/min
Altered LFTs	No streptozocin adjustments recommended since hepatic metabolism does not appear to be important. Hold fluorouracil if total bilirubin >5 mg/dL (>85.5 μmol/L). In individual patients, titrate fluorouracil dosage to keep hematologic toxicities no greater than mild-to-moderate
Hematologic toxicities	Streptozocin and fluorouracil doses are titrated to produce no greater than mild-to-moderate hematologic toxicities

Efficacy

Study	Objective Response Rate	Median Duration of Response
Moertel et al, 1980	63% (CR 33%)	17 months
Eriksson et al, 1990*	45%	27.5 months
Moertel et al, 1992	45%	6.9 months

*Combined results of streptozocin in combination with fluorouracil or doxorubicin as first-line treatment

Toxicity

	All Grades	Grades 1/2	Grades 3/4
Nausea	54–85%	—	22–41% (severe)
Anemia	9%	N/A	N/A
Leukopenia	2–56%	—	25% G3; 4% G4
Thrombocytopenia	15–25%	4%	6–11%
Elevated creatinine	30–36%	N/A	N/A
Renal failure	—	—	7% (G4)
Diarrhea	—	33% (mild)	2% (severe)
Stomatitis	—	5–19% (mild)	5% (severe)
Urinary albumin >30 mg/day	65%	—	—
>1.25-times increase in LFTs	34%	—	—

Therapy Monitoring

Before each cycle of treatment: WBC with differential and platelet count, liver function tests, renal function tests

REGIMEN

STREPTOZOCIN + DOXORUBICIN

Moertel CG et al. N Engl J Med 1992;326:519–523

Premedications and hydration:
1000 mL 0.9% sodium chloride injection (0.9% NS); administer intravenously, starting 1.5 hours before administration of chemotherapy, continuing during administration and for approximately 1.5 hours afterward

Induction course:
Streptozocin 1000 mg/day; administer intravenously in 100–1000 mL 0.9% NS or 5% dextrose injection (D5W) over 30–120 minutes for 5 consecutive days, on days 1–5 (total dose/cycle = 5000 mg)
Doxorubicin 40 mg/m²; administer by intravenous injection over 3–5 minutes on day 1 (total dosage/cycle = 40 mg/m²)

Subsequent courses: (beginning 3 weeks after the induction cycle)
Streptozocin 2000 mg; administer intravenously in 100–1000 mL 0.9% NS or D5W over 30–120 minutes on day 1, every 3 weeks (total dose/cycle = 2000 mg)
Doxorubicin 40 mg/m²; administer by intravenous injection over 3–5 minutes on day 1 (total dosage/cycle = 40 mg/m²)

Supportive Care
Antiemetic prophylaxis
Emetogenic potential on days with streptozocin is **HIGH**
See Chapter 39 for antiemetic recommendations

Hematopoietic growth factor (CSF) prophylaxis
Primary prophylaxis is NOT indicated
See Chapter 43 for more information

Antimicrobial prophylaxis
Risk of fever and neutropenia is LOW
Antimicrobial primary prophylaxis to be considered:
• Antibacterial—not indicated
• Antifungal—not indicated
• Antiviral—not indicated unless patient previously had an episode of HSV
See Chapter 47 for more information

Patient Populations Studied

• A prospective study of 84 patients with neuroendocrine pancreatic tumors. Fifty-nine (70%) had malignant tumors and received 1 or more types of medical treatment (Eriksson B et al. Cancer 1990;65:1883–1890)

• A multicenter randomized trial comparing streptozocin + fluorouracil, streptozocin + doxorubicin, and chlorozotocin alone. One-hundred five patients with advanced islet-cell carcinoma (Moertel CG et al. N Engl J Med 1992;326:519–523)

Therapy Monitoring

1. *Before each cycle of treatment:* WBC with differential and platelet count, liver function tests, renal function tests

2. *Before initiation of treatment with doxorubicin, and before every third cycle:* Myocardial scintigraphy to assess cardiac function

Toxicity

	All Grades	Grades 1/2	Grades 3/4
Nausea	80%	—	20% (severe)
Anemia	9%	N/A	N/A
Leukopenia	57%	—	5%
Elevated creatinine	46%	N/A	N/A
Renal failure	—	—	4% (G4)
Diarrhea	—	5% (mild)	—
Stomatitis	—	5% (mild)	—

Treatment Modifications

Adverse Event	Treatment Modification
Creatinine clearance on day 1 of a second and subsequent cycles = 60–75 mL/min (1–1.25 mL/s)	Give streptozocin 1000 mg/day for 2 consecutive days, on days 1 and 2 (total dose/cycle = 2000 mg)
Creatinine clearance on day 1 of a second and subsequent cycles = 50–60 mL/min (0.83–1 mL/s)	Give streptozocin 1000 mg on day 1 only (total dose/cycle = 1000 mg)
Creatinine clearance on day 1 of a second and subsequent cycles <50 mL/min (<0.83 mL/s)	Discontinue streptozocin. Resume treatment after creatinine clearance >50 mL/min
Cumulative dose of doxorubicin ≥550 mg/m² (450 mg/m² in patients >70 years of age)	Monitor cardiac ejection fraction at baseline and reevaluate before repeating a treatment cycle or every other cycle
Altered LFTs	No streptozocin adjustments recommended since hepatic metabolism does not appear to be important Hold doxorubicin if total bilirubin >5 mg/dL (>85.5 μmol/L)
Hematologic toxicities	Streptozocin and doxorubicin doses are titrated to produce no greater than mild-to-moderate hematologic toxicities

Efficacy

Study	Objective Response Rate	Median Duration of Response
Eriksson et al, 1990*	45%	27.5 months
Moertel et al, 1992	69%	20 months

*Combined results of streptozocin in combination with fluorouracil or doxorubicin as first-line treatment

REGIMEN
SUNITINIB MALATE

Raymond E et al. N Engl J Med 2011;364:501–513

Sunitinib malate 37.5 mg per day orally, continually (total dose/week = 262.5 mg)

Notes:
In patients without an objective tumor response who had grade ≤1 nonhematologic or grade ≤2 hematologic treatment-related adverse events during the first 8 weeks, the dose may be increased to 50 mg per day
Patients can receive somatostatin analogs as needed

Supportive Care
Antiemetic prophylaxis
Emetogenic potential is **MINIMAL–LOW**
See Chapter 39 for antiemetic recommendations

Hematopoietic growth factor (CSF) prophylaxis
Primary prophylaxis is NOT indicated
See Chapter 43 for more information

Antimicrobial prophylaxis
Risk of fever and neutropenia is LOW
  Antimicrobial primary prophylaxis to be considered:
  • Antibacterial—not indicated
  • Antifungal—not indicated
  • Antiviral—not indicated unless patient previously had an episode of HSV
See Chapter 47 for more information

Diarrhea management
Latent or delayed onset diarrhea*:
  Loperamide 4 mg orally initially after the first loose or liquid stool, *then*
  Loperamide 2 mg orally every 2 hours during waking hours, *plus*
  Loperamide 4 mg orally every 4 hours during hours of sleep
  • Continue for at least 12 hours after diarrhea resolves
  • Recurrent diarrhea after a 12-hour diarrhea-free interval is treated as a new episode
  • Rehydrate orally with fluids and electrolytes during a diarrheal episode
  • If a patient develops blood or mucus in stool, dehydration, or hemodynamic instability, or if diarrhea persists >48 hours despite loperamide, stop loperamide and hospitalize the patient for IV hydration
  Alternatively, a trial of **Diphenoxylate hydrochloride** 2.5 mg **with Atropine sulfate** 0.025 mg (eg, Lomotil)
  • Initial adult dose is 2 tablets 4 times daily until control has been achieved, after which the dose may be reduced to meet individual requirements. Control may often be maintained with as little as 2 tablets daily
  • Clinical improvement of acute diarrhea is usually observed within 48 hours. If improvement of chronic diarrhea after treatment with a maximum daily dose of 8 tablets is not observed within 10 days, control is unlikely with further administration
Persistent diarrhea:
  Octreotide acetate (solution) 100–150 mcg; subcutaneously 3 times daily. Maximum total daily dose is 1500 mcg
Antibiotic therapy during latent or delayed onset diarrhea:
  A fluoroquinolone (eg, **Ciprofloxacin** 500 mg orally every 12 hours) if absolute neutrophil count <500/mm³ with or without accompanying fever in association with diarrhea
  • Antibiotics should also be administered if patient is hospitalized with prolonged diarrhea and should be continued until diarrhea resolves

*Abigerges D et al. J Natl Cancer Inst 1994;86:446–449
Rothenberg ML et al. J Clin Oncol 2001;19:3801–3807
Wadler S et al. J Clin Oncol 1998;16:3169–3178

Oral care
Prophylaxis and treatment for mucositis/stomatitis
  General advice:
  • Encourage patients to maintain intake of nonalcoholic fluids
  • Evaluate patients for oral pain and provide analgesic medications
  • Consider histamine (H₂-subtype) receptor antagonists (eg, ranitidine, famotidine), or a proton pump inhibitor for epigastric pain
  • *Lactobacillus* sp.-containing probiotics may be beneficial in preventing diarrhea

(continued)

(continued)

Patients with intact oral mucosa:
- Clean the mouth, tongue, and gums by brushing after every meal and at bedtime with an ultrasoft toothbrush with fluoride toothpaste
- Floss teeth gently every day unless contraindicated. If gums bleed and hurt, avoid bleeding or sore areas, but floss other teeth
- Patients may use saline or commercial bland, nonalcoholic rinses
  - Do not use mouthwashes that contain alcohols

If mucositis or stomatitis is present:
- Keep the mouth moist using water, ice chips, sugarless gum, sugar-free hard candies, or a saliva substitute
- Rinse mouth several times a day to remove debris
  - Use a solution of ¼ teaspoon (1.25 g) each of baking soda and table salt (sodium chloride) in 1 quart (~950 mL) of warm water. Follow with a plain water rinse
  - Do not use mouthwashes that contain alcohols
- Foam-tipped swabs (eg, Toothettes) are useful in moisturizing oral mucosa, but ineffective for cleansing teeth and removing plaque
- Advise patients who develop mucositis to:
  - Choose foods that are easy to chew and swallow
  - Take small bites of food, chew slowly, and sip liquids with meals
  - Encourage soft, moist foods such as cooked cereals, mashed potatoes, and scrambled eggs
  - For trouble swallowing, soften food with gravies, sauces, broths, yogurt, or other bland liquids
  - Avoid sharp, crunchy foods; hot, spicy or highly acidic foods (eg, citrus fruits and juices); sugary foods; toothpicks; tobacco products; alcoholic drinks

Hand–foot reaction (palmar–plantar erythrodysesthesia, PPE)
For patients who develop a hand–foot reaction, use topical emollients (eg, Aquaphor), topical or orally administered steroids, antihistamine agents (H_1-receptor antagonists), or pyridoxine
Pyridoxine may provide relief for discomfort/pain associated with PPE although the mechanism through which this occurs remains unclear
- The suggested pyridoxine starting dose is 50 mg/day, which may be increased to a maximum of 200 mg/day

Treatment Modifications

Adverse Event	Treatment Modification
Sunitinib Dose Levels	
Starting dose: Level 1	37.5 mg once daily
Level −1	25 mg once daily
Level +1	50 mg once daily
Cutaneous Toxicities	
Rash G ≥2	Hold sunitinib and provide immediate symptomatic treatment
If treatment is withheld for more than 3 weeks because of cutaneous toxicity	Discontinue therapy
When cutaneous toxicity resolves to G ≤1	Restart sunitinib at 1 dose level lower than the dose level administered at the time toxicity developed. Treatment for symptoms may continue indefinitely as a preventive measure
If cutaneous toxicity G3/4 recurs at reduced sunitinib doses	Again, hold sunitinib until the toxicity resolves to G ≤1, at which time sunitinib should be restarted at 1 dose level lower than the dose level administered at the time toxicity developed. Treatment for symptoms may continue indefinitely as a preventive measure
If cutaneous toxicity G3/4 recurs at dose level −1	Discontinue therapy
If cutaneous toxicity does not recur at reduced sunitinib doses with or without continued treatment for symptoms	The dose of sunitinib may be increased 1 dose level to the dose level administered at the time the cutaneous toxicity developed. Interrupt treatment by withholding sunitinib if toxicity recurs following the increase. When toxicity again resolves to G ≤1, resume sunitinib at the reduced dose previously tolerated

(continued)

Treatment Modifications (continued)

Diarrhea

G1/2 diarrhea	Focus on treatment for symptoms designed to resolve the diarrhea. No dose modifications will be made for G1/2 diarrhea unless G2 diarrhea persists for >2 weeks
If G2 diarrhea persists for more than 2 weeks	Follow the guidelines below for G3/4 diarrhea
If the diarrhea cannot be controlled with the preventive measures outlined, and is G3/4 or worsens by 1 grade level (G3 to G4) while on sunitinib and is not alleviated within 48 hours by antidiarrheal treatment	Hold sunitinib. Also withhold sunitinib if persistent G2 diarrhea (lasting >2 weeks) is not alleviated by antidiarrheal treatment while sunitinib use continues
If sunitinib is held for more than 3 weeks and the diarrhea does not resolve to G ≤1	Discontinue therapy
If within 3 weeks of holding sunitinib, diarrhea resolves to G ≤1	Restart sunitinib at 1 dose level less than the dose level administered at the time toxicity developed
If G3/4 diarrhea or persistent G2 diarrhea recurs at reduced sunitinib doses and the dose level at which persistent G2 diarrhea occurs is greater than dose level −1 (persistent is defined as lasting for >2 weeks)	Again, withhold sunitinib until the toxicity resolves to CTCAE (Common Terminology Criteria for Adverse Events) G ≤1, at which time sunitinib should be restarted at 1 dose level less than the dose level administered at the time toxicity developed. Treatment for symptoms may continue indefinitely as a preventive measure
If G3/4 diarrhea or persistent G2 diarrhea recurs at dose level −1 (persistent defined as lasting for more >2 weeks)	Discontinue therapy
If diarrhea does not recur at the reduced sunitinib doses with or without continued treatment for symptoms	The dose of sunitinib may be increased 1 dose level to the dose level administered at the time diarrhea developed. Interrupt treatment by withholding sunitinib if toxicity recurs following the increase. When toxicity again resolves to G ≤1, resume sunitinib at the reduced dose previously tolerated

Hypertension

Note: Patients should have their blood pressure checked once weekly during their first 24 weeks of therapy and for an 8-week period after an adjustment in their sunitinib dose

G1 Hypertension	Continue sunitinib at same dose and schedule
G2 Asymptomatic	Treat with antihypertensive medications and continue sunitinib at same dose and schedule
G2 Symptomatic, or persistent G2 despite antihypertensive medications, or diastolic BP >110 mm Hg, or G3 hypertension	Treat with antihypertensive medications. Hold sunitinib (maximum 3 weeks until symptoms resolve and diastolic BP <100 mm Hg); then continue sunitinib at 1 dose level lower. *Note:* Discontinue therapy if sunitinib is withheld >3 weeks
G4 Hypertension	Discontinue therapy

Other Adverse Events

Any other adverse event	Interrupt treatment. Resume at 25 mg/day when toxicity resolves to G ≤1. If symptoms do not recur, try increasing dose to the starting dose level, 37.5 mg daily
Recurrence of adverse event once dose increased to 37.5 mg/day	Interrupt treatment. Resume at 25 mg/day when toxicity resolves to G ≤1 but do not increase dose to the starting dose level, 37.5 mg daily
Coadministration of potent CYP3A4 inhibitors (eg, atazanavir, clarithromycin, itraconazole, ketoconazole, ritonavir, telithromycin, voriconazole)	Reduce sunitinib dose
Coadministration of potent CYP3A4 inducers (eg, carbamazepine, dexamethasone, phenytoin, phenobarbital, rifampin, St. John's wort)	Increase sunitinib dose (to a maximum of 87.5 mg daily)

Efficacy

Summary of Efficacy Measures in the Intention-to-Treat Population*

Outcome	Sunitinib (N = 86)	Placebo (N = 85)	p Value
Progression-Free Survival*			
Patients with events—no. (%)	30 (35)	51 (60)	
Progression	27 (31)	48 (56)	
Death without progression	3 (3)	3 (4)	
Patients with data censored—no. (%)	56 (65)	34 (40)	
Probability event-free at 6 months—% (95% CI)	71.3 (60.0–82.5)	43.2 (30.3–56.1)	
Estimated median progression-free survival, months	11.4 (7.4–19.8)	5.5 (3.6–7.4)	
Hazard ratio for progression or death (95% CI)	0.42 (0.26–0.66)		<0.001
Overall Survival			
Deaths—no. (%)	9 (10)	21 (25)	
Patients with data censored—no. (%)	77 (90)	64 (75)	
Survival probability at 6 months—% (95% CI)	92.6 (86.3–98.9)	85.2 (77.1–93.3)	
Estimated median overall survival	Not reached	Not reached	
Hazard ratio for death (95% CI)	0.41 (0.19–0.89)		0.02
Objective Tumor Response			
Best observed RECIST response—no. (%)			
Complete response	2 (2)	0	
Partial response	6 (7)	0	
Stable disease	54 (63)	51 (60)	
Progressive disease	12 (14)	23 (27)	
Could not be evaluated	12 (14)	11 (13)	
Objective response rate—%	9.3	0	0.007

CI, confidence interval; RECIST, Response Evaluation Criteria in Solid Tumors (Therasse P et al. J Natl Cancer Inst 2000;92:205–216)

*Data for a total of 3 patients (1 in the sunitinib group and 2 in the placebo group) were censored at day 1 in the analysis of PFS because of inadequate baseline tumor assessment

Patient Population Studied

A multinational, double-blind, placebo-controlled, phase III trial that randomly assigned patients in a 1:1 ratio to receive orally once daily placebo or sunitinib 37.5 mg. Patient characteristics included the following:

Demographic and Baseline Characteristics of the Patients	Sunitinib (N = 86)	Placebo (N = 85)
Variable		
Age		
Median—years	56	57
Range—years	25–84	26–78
≥65 y—no. (%)	22 (26)	23 (27)
Sex—no. (%)		
Male	42 (49)	40 (47)
Female	44 (51)	45 (53)
ECOG performance status—no. (%)		
0	53 (62)	41 (48)
1	33 (38)	43 (51)
2	0	1 (1)
Inherited genetic conditions—no. (%)		
Multiple endocrine neoplasia type 1	0	2 (2)
von Hippel–Lindau disease	2 (2)	0
Time since diagnosis—years		
Median	2.4	3.2
Range	0.1–25.6	0.1–21.3
Tumor functionality—no. (%)*		
Nonfunctioning	42 (49)	44 (52)
Functioning	25 (29)	21 (24)
Not specified	19 (22)	20 (24)
Ki-67 index		
Number of patients with data that could be evaluated	36	36

(*continued*)

Toxicity
Common Adverse Events in the Safety Population*

Event	Sunitinib (N = 83)			Placebo (N = 82)		
	All Grades	G1/2	G3/4	All Grades	G1/2	G3/4
	Number of Patients (%)					
Diarrhea	49 (59)	45 (54)	4 (5)	32 (39)	30 (37)	2 (2)
Nausea	37 (45)	36 (43)	1 (1)	24 (29)	23 (28)	1 (1)
Asthenia	28 (34)	24 (29)	4 (5)	22 (27)	19 (23)	3 (4)
Vomiting	28 (34)	28 (34)	0	25 (30)	23 (28)	2 (2)
Fatigue	27 (32)	23 (28)	4 (5)	22 (27)	15 (18)	7 (8)
Hair-color changes	24 (29)	23 (28)	1 (1)	1 (1)	1 (1)	0
Neutropenia	24 (29)	14 (17)	10 (12)	3 (4)	3 (4)	0
Abdominal pain	23 (28)	19 (23)	4 (5)	26 (32)	18 (22)	8 (10)
Hypertension	22 (26)	14 (17)	8 (10)	4 (5)	3 (4)	1 (1)
Palmar–plantar erythrodysesthesia	19 (23)	14 (17)	5 (6)	2 (2)	2 (2)	0
Anorexia	18 (22)	16 (19)	2 (2)	17 (21)	16 (20)	1 (1)
Stomatitis	18 (22)	15 (18)	3 (4)	2 (2)	2 (2)	0
Dysgeusia	17 (20)	17 (20)	0	4 (5)	4 (5)	0
Epistaxis	17 (20)	16 (19)	1 (1)	4 (5)	4 (5)	0
Headache	15 (18)	15 (18)	0	11 (13)	10 (12)	1 (1)
Insomnia	15 (18)	15 (18)	0	10 (12)	10 (12)	0
Rash	15 (18)	15 (18)	0	4 (5)	4 (5)	0
Thrombocytopenia	14 (17)	11 (13)	3 (4)	4 (5)	4 (5)	0
Mucosal inflammation	13 (16)	12 (14)	1 (1)	6 (7)	6 (7)	0
Weight loss	13 (16)	12 (14)	1 (1)	9 (11)	9 (11)	0
Constipation	12 (14)	12 (14)	0	16 (20)	15 (18)	1 (1)
Back pain	10 (12)	10 (12)	0	14 (17)	10 (12)	4 (5)

*Adverse events were defined on the basis of the National Cancer Institute, Common Terminology Criteria for Adverse Events, version 3.0. Events listed are those of any grade that occurred in more than 15% of patients in either group.

Therapy Monitoring

1. *Every 6 weeks to 3 months:* Physical examination and routine laboratory tests including thyroid function tests
2. *Response assessment:* Every 2–3 cycles. A cycle is defined as a 6-week period

Patient Population Studied
(continued)

Demographic and Baseline Characteristics of the Patients	Sunitinib (N = 86)	Placebo (N = 85)
Index—no. (%)		
≤2%	7 (19)	6 (17)
>2%–5%	16 (44)	14 (39)
>5%–10%	5 (14)	10 (28)
>10%	8 (22)	6 (17)
No. of sites of disease—no. (%)°		
1	30 (35)	23 (27)
2	31 (36)	26 (31)
≥3	24 (28)	35 (41)
Not reported	1 (1)	1 (1)
Presence of distant metastases—no. (%)		
Any, including hepatic	82 (95)	80 (94)
Extrahepatic	21 (24)	34 (40)
Previous treatment—no. (%)		
Surgery	76 (88)	77 (91)
Radiation therapy	9 (10)	12 (14)
Chemoembolization	7 (8)	14 (16)
Radiofrequency ablation	3 (3)	6 (7)
Percutaneous ethanol injection	1 (1)	2 (2)
Somatostatin analogs†	30 (35)	32 (38)
Previous systemic chemotherapy—no. (%)		
Any	57 (66)	61 (72)
Streptozocin	24 (28)	28 (33)
Anthracyclines	27 (31)	35 (41)
Fluoropyrimidines	20 (23)	25 (29)

*Tumor functionality was reported by investigators. On the basis of the investigators' assessment, patients included in the "unknown" category had clinical symptoms but no identified corresponding neuropeptide secretion
†This category includes patients who received somatostatin analogs (predominantly octreotide acetate and lanreotide acetate) before the first dose of study drug, regardless of whether they continued receiving somatostatin analogs concomitantly with the study drug

REGIMEN

EVEROLIMUS

Yao JC et al. N Engl J Med 2011;364:514–523

Everolimus 10 mg/day orally, continually (total dose/week = 70 mg)

Notes:
- Everolimus tablets should be swallowed whole (without breaking, crushing, or chewing) with water
- Everolimus tablets and tablets for oral suspension may be taken with or without food, but should be taken consistently either with or without food
- Commercially available formulations (a) tablets and (b) tablets for oral suspension should not be used in combination to administer a dose

Supportive Care
Antiemetic prophylaxis
Emetogenic potential is **MINIMAL–LOW**
See Chapter 39 for antiemetic recommendations

Hematopoietic growth factor (CSF) prophylaxis
Primary prophylaxis is NOT indicated
See Chapter 43 for more information

Antimicrobial prophylaxis
Risk of fever and neutropenia is LOW
  Antimicrobial primary prophylaxis to be considered:
  - Antibacterial—not indicated
  - Antifungal—not indicated
  - Antiviral—not indicated unless patient previously had an episode of HSV
See Chapter 47 for more information

Oral care
Prophylaxis and treatment for mucositis/stomatitis
  General advice:
  - Encourage patients to maintain intake of nonalcoholic fluids
  - Evaluate patients for oral pain and provide analgesic medications
  - Consider histamine (H_2-subtype) receptor antagonists (eg, ranitidine, famotidine), or a proton pump inhibitor for epigastric pain
  - *Lactobacillus* sp.-containing probiotics may be beneficial in preventing diarrhea
  Patients with intact oral mucosa:
  - Clean the mouth, tongue, and gums by brushing after every meal and at bedtime with an ultrasoft toothbrush with fluoride toothpaste
  - Floss teeth gently every day unless contraindicated. If gums bleed and hurt, avoid bleeding or sore areas, but floss other teeth
  - Patients may use saline or commercial bland, nonalcoholic rinses
    - Do not use mouthwashes that contain alcohols
  If mucositis or stomatitis is present:
  - Keep the mouth moist using water, ice chips, sugarless gum, sugar-free hard candies, or a saliva substitute
  - Rinse mouth several times a day to remove debris
    - Use a solution of ¼ teaspoon (1.25 g) each of baking soda and table salt (sodium chloride) in 1 quart (~950 mL) of warm water. Follow with a plain water rinse
    - Do not use mouthwashes that contain alcohols
  - Foam-tipped swabs (eg, Toothettes) are useful in moisturizing oral mucosa, but ineffective for cleansing teeth and removing plaque

(continued)

Treatment Modifications

Adverse Event	Treatment Modification
Invasive systemic fungal infection	Discontinue everolimus and treat with appropriate antifungal therapy
Noninfectious pneumonitis without symptoms with only radiologic changes	Observe carefully. Specific therapies or drug interruption may not be necessary
Noninfectious pneumonitis with mild-to-moderate symptoms	Withhold therapy. Glucocorticoids may be initiated. Resume everolimus at a reduced dose depending on the individual clinical circumstances
Noninfectious pneumonitis with severe symptoms (including a decrease in DL_{CO} on pulmonary function tests)	Discontinue therapy and consider administering high doses of glucocorticoids
ANC <1000/mm^3 or platelet count <75,000/mm^3	Withhold therapy. Resume everolimus when symptoms improve to G ≤2 with everolimus dose reduced to 5 mg/day or 5 mg every other day but not <15 mg/week
Any nonhematologic G3/4 toxicity	Withhold therapy. Restart everolimus when symptoms improve to G ≤2 with everolimus dose reduced to 5 mg/day or 5 mg every-other-day but not <15 mg/week
G1/2 oral ulcerations	Topical treatments are recommended, but alcohol- or peroxide-containing mouthwashes should be avoided. Focus on pain control, oral hygiene, and IV fluid replacement or parenteral nutrition if severe
Hyperglycemia	Monitor blood sugar levels and institute oral hypoglycemic agent or insulin as needed
Hypertriglyceridemia	Monitor triglycerides, instituting dietary interventions for minor elevations and lipid-lowering agents for levels >500 mg/dL (>5.65 mmol/L)

(*continued*)

- Advise patients who develop mucositis to:
  - Choose foods that are easy to chew and swallow
  - Take small bites of food, chew slowly, and sip liquids with meals
  - Encourage soft, moist foods such as cooked cereals, mashed potatoes, and scrambled eggs
  - For trouble swallowing, soften food with gravies, sauces, broths, yogurt, or other bland liquids
  - Avoid sharp, crunchy foods; hot, spicy, or highly acidic foods (eg, citrus fruits and juices); sugary foods; toothpicks; tobacco products; alcoholic drinks

Diarrhea management

Latent or delayed onset diarrhea*:

Loperamide 4 mg orally initially after the first loose or liquid stool, *then*
Loperamide 2 mg orally every 2 hours during waking hours, *plus*
Loperamide 4 mg orally every 4 hours during hours of sleep

- Continue for at least 12 hours after diarrhea resolves
- Recurrent diarrhea after a 12-hour diarrhea-free interval is treated as a new episode
- Rehydrate orally with fluids and electrolytes during a diarrheal episode
- If a patient develops blood or mucus in stool, dehydration, or hemodynamic instability, or if diarrhea persists >48 hours despite loperamide, stop loperamide and hospitalize the patient for IV hydration

Alternatively, a trial of **Diphenoxylate hydrochloride 2.5 mg with Atropine sulfate 0.025 mg** (eg, Lomotil)

- Initial adult dose is 2 tablets 4 times daily until control has been achieved, after which the dose may be reduced to meet individual requirements. Control may often be maintained with as little as 2 tablets daily
- Clinical improvement of acute diarrhea is usually observed within 48 hours. If improvement of chronic diarrhea after treatment with a maximum daily dose of 8 tablets is not observed within 10 days, control is unlikely with further administration

Persistent diarrhea:

Octreotide acetate (solution) 100–150 mcg subcutaneously 3 times daily. Maximum total daily dose is 1500 mcg

Antibiotic therapy during latent or delayed onset diarrhea:

A fluoroquinolone (eg, **Ciprofloxacin** 500 mg orally every 12 hours) if absolute neutrophil count <500/mm³ with or without accompanying fever in association with diarrhea

- Antibiotics should also be administered if patient is hospitalized with prolonged diarrhea and should be continued until diarrhea resolves

*Abigerges D et al. J Natl Cancer Inst 1994;86:446–449
Rothenberg ML et al. J Clin Oncol 2001;19:3801–3807
Wadler S et al. J Clin Oncol 1998;16:3169–3178

Patient Population Studied

International, multicenter, double-blind, phase III study. Patients were randomly assigned to treatment with oral everolimus 10 mg or matching placebo, both administered once daily in conjunction with best supportive care. Patients initially assigned to placebo who met criteria for disease progression could switch to open-label everolimus. Of the 203 patients initially assigned to receive placebo, 148 (73%) crossed over to open-label everolimus

Demographic and Baseline Clinical Characteristics of the Patients

Characteristic	Everolimus (N = 207)	Placebo (N = 203)
Age—years		
Median	58	57
Range	23–87	20–82
Sex—no. (%)		
Male	110 (53)	117 (58)
Female	97 (47)	86 (42)
WHO performance status—no. (%)		
0	139 (67)	133 (66)
1	62 (30)	64 (32)
2	6 (3)	6 (3)
Histologic status of tumor—no. (%)		
Well differentiated	170 (82)	171 (84)
Moderately differentiated	35 (17)	30 (15)
Unknown	2 (1)	2 (1)
Time from initial diagnosis—no. (%)		
≤6 months	24 (12)	33 (16)
>6 months to ≤2 years	65 (31)	43 (21)
>2 years to ≤5 years	54 (26)	81 (40)
>5 years	64 (31)	46 (23)

(*continued*)

Efficacy

Variable	Everolimus (N = 207)	Placebo (N = 203)
Progression-Free Survival (PFS)		
Assessment by local investigator		
Progression-free survival events—no. (%)	109 (53)	165 (81)
Censored data—no. (%)	98 (47)	38 (19)
Median progression-free survival—months	11.0	4.6
Hazard ratio for PFS with everolimus (95% CI); *p* value	0.35 (0.27–0.45); <0.001	
Review by central adjudication committee		
Progression-free survival events—no. (%)	95 (46)	142 (70)
Censored data—no. (%)	112 (54)	61 (30)
Median progression-free survival—months	11.4	5.4
Hazard ratio for PFS with everolimus (95% CI); *p* value	0.34 (0.26–0.44); <0.001	
Estimated proportion of patients alive and progression-free at 18 months—% (95% CI)	34% (26–43)	9% (4–16)

Response According to RECIST Criteria

	Everolimus (N = 207)	Placebo (N = 203)
Partial response—no. (%)	10 (5)	4 (2)
Percent with stable disease	73%	51%
Percent with some tumor shrinkage	64%	21%

Overall Survival*

Hazard ratio for death with everolimus	1.05; 95% CI, 0.71–1.55; *p* = 0.59

*Median overall survival not reached. Of the 203 patients initially assigned to receive placebo, 148 (73%) crossed over to receive open-label everolimus

Patient Population Studied
(continued)

Characteristic	Everolimus (N = 207)	Placebo (N = 203)
Time from disease progression to randomization—no. (%)		
≤1 months	73 (35)	61 (30)
>1 months to ≤2 months	43 (21)	53 (26)
>2 months to ≤3 months	30 (14)	29 (14)
>3 months to ≤12 months	58 (28)	54 (27)
>12 months	3 (1)	1 (<1)
No. of disease sites—no. of patients (%)		
1	51 (25)	62 (31)
2	85 (41)	64 (32)
≥3	70 (34)	77 (38)
Organ involved—no. (%)		
Liver	190 (92)	187 (92)
Pancreas	92 (44)	84 (41)
Lymph nodes	68 (33)	73 (36)
Lung	28 (14)	30 (15)
Bone	13 (6)	29 (14)

Toxicity[*][†]				
	Everolimus (N = 204)		Placebo (N = 203)	
Median treatment duration, months (range)	8.79 (0.25–27.47)		3.74 (0.01–37.79)	
Treatment a minimum of 12 months	31%		11%	
Mean relative dose intensity[‡]	0.86		0.97	
Percentage requiring dose adjustments[§]	59%		28%	
	All Grades	G3/4	All G	G3/4
Adverse Event	Number of Patients (%)			
Stomatitis[ϵ]	131 (64)	14 (7)	34 (17)	0
	Everolimus (N = 204)		Placebo (N = 203)	
Rash	99 (49)	1 (<1)	21 (10)	0
Diarrhea	69 (34)	7 (3)	20 (10)	0
Fatigue	64 (31)	5 (2)	29 (14)	1 (<1)
Infections[**]	46 (23)	5 (2)	12 (6)	1 (<1)
Nausea	41 (20)	5 (2)	37 (18)	0
Peripheral edema	41 (20)	1 (<1)	7 (3)	0
Decreased appetite	40 (20)	0	14 (7)	2 (1)
Headache	39 (19)	0	13 (6)	0
Dysgeusia	35 (17)	0	8 (4)	0
Anemia	35 (17)	12 (6)	6 (3)	0
Epistaxis	35 (17)	0	0	0
Pneumonitis[††]	35 (17)	5 (2)	0	0
Weight loss	32 (16)	0	9 (4)	0
Vomiting	31 (15)	0	13 (6)	0
Pruritus	30 (15)	0	18 (9)	0
Hyperglycemia	27 (13)	11 (5)	9 (4)	4 (2)
Thrombocytopenia	27 (13)	8 (4)	1 (<1)	0
Asthenia	26 (13)	2 (1)	17 (8)	2 (1)
Nail disorder	24 (12)	1 (<1)	2 (1)	0
Cough	22 (11)	0	4 (2)	0
Pyrexia	22 (11)	0	0	0
Dry skin	21 (10)	0	9 (4)	0

[*]Drug-related adverse events occurring in ≥10% of patients
[†]Median follow-up period of 17 months
[‡]Ratio of administered doses to planned doses
[§]Reductions or temporary interruptions
[ϵ]Includes stomatitis, aphthous stomatitis, mouth ulceration, and tongue ulceration
[**]Includes all types of infections
[††]Includes pneumonitis, interstitial lung disease, lung infiltration, and pulmonary fibrosis

Therapy Monitoring

1. *Prior to starting treatment and periodically thereafter:* Renal function, CBC with differential, blood glucose, and serum lipid profiles
2. *ECG:* A 12-lead ECG should be performed before the start of treatment, weekly for at least the first 2 weeks. Additional ECGs may be performed depending on the QTc. If the dose is increased, then at least 1 additional ECG should be obtained
3. *Safety assessment:* Every 2–4 weeks for the first 3 cycles; every 4–8 weeks, thereafter
4. *Response assessment:* Every 8–12 weeks

REGIMEN

CISPLATIN + ETOPOSIDE

Fjällskog M-LH et al. Cancer 2001;92:1101–1107
Moertel CG et al. Cancer 1991;68:227–232

Hydration days 2 and 3:
$\geq$1000 mL 0.9% sodium chloride injection
(0.9% NS); administer intravenously at a
rate that produces a diuresis $\geq$100 mL/h,
starting at least 2 hours before chemotherapy
administration. Continue hydration
during chemotherapy administration and
for at least 2 hours afterward. Mannitol
or furosemide may be given as needed
to enhance diuresis and prevent excessive
fluid retention. Encourage increased oral
intake of nonalcoholic fluids. Monitor and
replace electrolytes as needed (potassium,
magnesium, sodium)
Etoposide 100 mg/m^2 per day; administer
intravenously, diluted in a volume of
0.9% NS to a concentration within the range
of 0.2–0.4 mg/mL, over 60 minutes on
3 consecutive days, on days 1–3, every
4 weeks (total dosage/cycle = 300 mg/m^2)
Cisplatin 45 mg/m^2 per day; administer
intravenously in 100–250 mL 0.9% NS
over 1 hour on 2 consecutive days, on days 2
and 3, every 4 weeks (total dosage/cycle =
90 mg/m^2)

Supportive Care
Antiemetic prophylaxis
*Emetogenic potential on day 1 is **LOW***
*Emetogenic potential on days 2 and 3 is **HIGH**,
with a potential for delayed symptoms*
See Chapter 39 for antiemetic
recommendations

Hematopoietic growth factor (CSF) prophylaxis
Primary prophylaxis may be indicated
See Chapter 43 for more information

Antimicrobial prophylaxis
Risk of fever and neutropenia is LOW
Antimicrobial primary prophylaxis to be considered:
• Antibacterial—not indicated
• Antifungal—not indicated
• Antiviral—not indicated unless patient
previously had an episode of HSV
See Chapter 47 for more information

Toxicity

	All Grades	Grades 1/2	Grades 3/4
Nephrotoxicity	53–66%	—	2% (severe)
Anemia	89%	Decreased Hb: 1–3 g/dL (38%); 3–4 g/dL (29%); >4 g/dL (22%)	
Leukopenia	100%	35%	65%
Thrombocytopenia	—	49%	35%
Peripheral neuropathy	—	17%	75%
Ototoxicity	—	2–8%	—
Diarrhea	16%	—	—
Stomatitis	13%	11%	2%
Nausea	96%	83%	13%
Alopecia	100%	—	—
Dermatitis	—	4%,	—
Fever	—	—	2%

Patient Populations Studied

• Nonrandomized study of 15 patients with
malignant pancreatic endocrine tumors
(4 were poorly differentiated endocrine
carcinomas) treated with cisplatin +
etoposide as second- or third-line
treatment (Fjällskog M-LH et al. Cancer
2001;92:1101–1107)
• Prospective, nonrandomized study of
45 patients with neuroendocrine tumors
among whom 14 had well-differentiated
pancreatic endocrine tumors (Moertel CG
et al. Cancer 1991;68:227–232)

Efficacy

Study	Objective Response Rate	Median Duration of Response
Moertel et al, 1991*	67%	8 months
Fjällskog et al, 2001†	53%	9 months

*Tumor response was unrelated to primary site,
endocrine hyperfunction, or prior therapy experience.
The median survival of all patients with anaplastic
tumors was 19 months
†Includes foregut carcinoids and endocrine pancreatic
tumors. No difference in response between patients
with well-differentiated or poorly differentiated
endocrine pancreatic carcinoma

Treatment Modifications

Adverse Event	Treatment Modification
Day 1 ANC <1500/mm^3 or platelets <100,000/mm^3	Delay treatment 1 week or until ANC >1500/mm^3 and platelets >100,000/mm^3, then administer full doses
ANC at nadir <500/mm^3	Administer filgrastim during subsequent cycles: • Administer filgrastim on days 4–11, *or* • Administer pegfilgrastim at least 24 hours after completing chemotherapy, *and/or* • Decrease etoposide dosage by 25%
Albumin <3.2 g/dL (<32 g/L)	Reduce etoposide dosage by 50%
Albumin <2.5 g/dL (<25 g/L)	Discontinue etoposide until albumin $\geq$2.5 g/dL ($\geq$25 g/L)

Therapy Monitoring

1. *Before and during each cycle of treatment:* Body
weight to detect excessive fluid retention
2. *Days 7, 10, and 14 of each cycle:* WBC with
differential count
3. *Every cycle:* Liver and renal function tests

SECOND-LINE REGIMEN FOR INOPERABLE WELL- AND POORLY-DIFFERENTIATED NEUROENDOCRINE TUMORS AND FOR PATIENTS WHO CANNOT TOLERATE MORE INTENSIVE THERAPIES

TEMOZOLOMIDE

Ekeblad S et al. Clin Cancer Res 2007;13:2986–2991

Induction course:
Temozolomide 150 mg/m^2 per day; administer orally for 5 consecutive days, days 1–5 (total dosage during cycle 1 = 750 mg/m^2)

Subsequent courses:
Temozolomide 200 mg/m^2 per day; administer orally for 5 consecutive days, days 1–5, every 4 weeks (total dosage/cycle = 1000 mg/m^2)

Supportive Care
Antiemetic prophylaxis
Emetogenic potential is **MODERATE**
See Chapter 39 for antiemetic recommendations

Hematopoietic growth factor (CSF) prophylaxis
Primary prophylaxis is NOT indicated
See Chapter 43 for more information

Antimicrobial prophylaxis
Risk of fever and neutropenia is LOW
  Antimicrobial primary prophylaxis to be considered:
  • Antibacterial—not indicated
  • Antifungal—not indicated
  • Antiviral—not indicated unless patient previously had an episode of HSV
See Chapter 47 for more information

Patient Populations Studied

Retrospective study of 36 patients with advanced neuroendocrine tumors, among whom 12 had a diagnosis of pancreatic endocrine tumor

Treatment Modifications

Adverse Event	Treatment Modification
Leukopenia G ≥2 on day 1 of a new cycle	Delay starting the cycle for 1 week. Then, decrease temozolomide dosage by 50 mg/m^2 each day it is given; eg, from 200 mg/m^2 per day to 150 mg/m^2 per day, from 150 mg/m^2 per day to 100 mg/m^2 per day

Therapy Monitoring

Before each treatment cycle: WBC including differential and platelet count

Efficacy (N = 12)

Ekeblad S et al. Clin Cancer Res 2007;13:2986–2991

Complete response	0
Partial response	8%
Stable disease	67%
Progressive disease	25%
Median time to progression for whole group	7 months

Toxicity

Ekeblad S et al. Clin Cancer Res 2007;13:2986–2991

	Grade 1	Grade 2	Grade 3	Grade 4
Anemia	9 (26%)	1 (3%)	1 (3%)	0
Thrombocytopenia	8 (23%)	0	5 (14%)	0
Leukopenia	3 (9%)	1 (3%)	1 (3%)	0
Neutropenia	0	1 (3%)	0	1 (3%)
Fatigue	8 (23%)	3 (9%)	2 (6%)	1 (3%)
Nausea (with premedication)	10 (29%)	0	0	0

SECOND-LINE REGIMEN FOR INOPERABLE WELL- AND POORLY DIFFERENTIATED NEUROENDOCRINE TUMORS

^{177}Lu-OCTREOTATE ([^{177}Lu-DOTA^0, Tyr^3] OCTREOTATE) SOMATOSTATIN ANALOGS LABELED WITH RADIOACTIVE [^{177}Lu-DOTA^0, Tyr^3]

de Keizer B et al. Eur J Nucl Med Mol Imaging 2008;35:749–755

Pretreatment:
Long-acting somatostatin analogs were discontinued 1 month before starting ^{177}Lu-octreotate therapy, and replaced with octreotide acetate solution. Octreotide acetate solution was discontinued 1 day before starting ^{177}Lu-octreotate

Preparation of ^{177}Lu-octreotate ([^{177}Lu-DOTA^0,Tyr^3]octreotate)
[DOTA^0,Tyr^3]octreotate is obtained from Mallinckrodt Inc., St. Louis, MO
^{177}LuCl$_3$ is obtained from a facility with a nuclear reactor
^{177}Lu-octreotate is prepared locally

Premedication:
Granisetron 1–3 mg *or* **ondansetron** 8 mg acetate solution intravenously
An admixture of amino acids (lysine 2.5% and arginine 2.5%) in 1000 mL 0.9% sodium chloride injection) acetate solution intravenously over 4 hours starting 30 minutes before ^{177}Lu-octreotate administration

Administration of ^{177}Lu-octreotate ([^{177}Lu-DOTA^0,Tyr^3]octreotate)
^{177}**Lu-octreotate** is administered intravenously over 30 minutes
Cycle dosages: 100 mCi (3.7 GBq), 150 mCi (5.6 GBq) or 200 mCi (7.4 GBq) with 200 mCi (7.4 GBq) used most frequently
Interval between treatments: 6–10 weeks
Treatment duration: Treatment is continued up to a cumulative dose of 750–800 mCi (27.8–29.6 GBq; corresponding with a radiation dose to the bone marrow of 2 Gy)

Supportive Care
Antiemetic prophylaxis
Emetogenic potential is LOW
See Chapter 39 for antiemetic recommendations

Hematopoietic growth factor (CSF) prophylaxis
Primary prophylaxis is NOT indicated
See Chapter 43 for more information

Antimicrobial prophylaxis
Risk of fever and neutropenia is LOW
Antimicrobial primary prophylaxis to be considered:
- Antibacterial—not indicated
- Antifungal—not indicated
- Antiviral—not indicated unless patient previously had an episode of HSV

See Chapter 47 for more information

Treatment Modifications

Adverse Event	Treatment Modification
If dosimetric calculations indicate radiation dose to the kidneys will exceed 23 Gy	Reduce the cumulative dose to 500–700 mCi

Toxicity

de Keizer B et al. Eur J Nucl Med Mol Imaging 2008;35:749–755
Kwekkeboom DJ et al. J Clin Oncol 2008;26:2124–2130

Toxicity	All Grades
Nausea	25%
Vomiting	10%
Abdominal discomfort	10%
G3/4 hematologic toxicity	9.5% of patients (3.6% of administrations)
WHO G1 reversible hair loss	62%
Serious liver toxicity	<1%
Myelodysplastic syndrome*	<1%
Hormonal crisis	1.3%[†,‡]

*Two to 3 years after the last treatment with ^{177}Lu-octreotate
[†]Two of 3 patients with VIPoma
[‡]Hormone-release crisis occurred immediately or within 48 hours after ^{177}Lu-octreotate administration during 10 of 1691 (0.6%) treatments. The crisis was characterized by flushing and severe diarrhea in all patients ± nausea, hypotension, and metabolic abnormalities

Patient Populations Studied

- Nonrandomized prospective study of 310 patients with gastroenteropancreatic neuroendocrine tumors, among whom 91 had a diagnosis of pancreatic endocrine tumor. Of the whole group, 89% had liver metastases (Kwekkeboom DJ et al. J Clin Oncol 2008;26:2124–2130)
- Retrospective analysis of 479 patients with gastroenteropancreatic neuroendocrine tumors, among whom 159 had a diagnosis of pancreatic endocrine tumor. Of the group, 88% had liver metastases and 26% had bone metastases (de Keizer B et al. Eur J Nucl Med Mol Imaging 2008;35:749–755)

Efficacy (N = 91)

- A 43% objective radiologic response
- Median time to progression 40 months in patients who did not have progressive disease

Tumor Responses 3 Months After the Last Administration of ¹⁷⁷Lu-Octreotate

Tumor Type	Response: Number of Patients (%)				
	CR	PR	MR	SD	PD
Nonfunctioning pancreatic	4 (6%)	26 (36%)	13 (18%)	19 (26%)	10 (14%)
Gastrinoma	—	5 (42%)	4 (33%)	2 (17%)	1 (8%)
Insulinoma	—	3 (60%)	—	1 (20%)	1 (20%)
VIPoma	—	1 (50%)	—	—	1 (50%)
Total	4 (5%)	35 (38%)	17 (19%)	22 (24%)	13 (14%)

CR, Complete response; PR, partial response; MR, minimal response; SD, stable disease; PD, progressive disease; VIPoma, vasoactive intestinal peptide-secreting tumor

Therapy Monitoring

Before each therapy: CBC with differential, and renal and liver function tests

31. Pheochromocytoma

Karel Pacak, MD, PhD, DSc and Tito Fojo, MD, PhD

Epidemiology

Incidence*: 3–8 cases per one
million population
Median age: 42 years
Male to female ratio: 1:1

*The annual incidence of pheochromocytoma in the United States is not precisely known, but the high prevalence (0.05%) of pheochromocytomas found in autopsy series indicates that the tumor is underdiagnosed and that the annual incidence is likely to be higher than indicated

Eisenhofer G et al. Endocr Relat Cancer 2004;11:
423–436
Neumann HPH et al. N Engl J Med 2002;346:
1459–1466
Pacak K et al. Nat Clin Pract Endocrinol Metab
2007;3:91–102

Pathology

• Approximately 80–85% of pheochromocytomas are located in the adrenal gland. The remaining 15–20% are located along the paraaortic sympathetic chain, aortic bifurcation, and urinary bladder
• Bilateral tumors occur in ~10% of patients and are much more common in familial pheochromocytomas
• 5–36% of pheochromocytomas are malignant, but no widely accepted pathologic criteria exist for differentiating between benign and malignant pheochromocytoma
• A diagnosis of malignancy requires evidence of metastases at nonchromaffin sites distant from that of the primary tumor
• Although most cases of pheochromocytomas are sporadic, a significant proportion occur secondary to several hereditary syndromes. Hereditary contribution is approximately 30%. The propensity of malignancy in hereditary pheochromocytoma syndromes is highly variable

Pheochromocytoma in Hereditary Syndromes

Hereditary Syndrome	Gene	Frequency*	Predisposition to Malignancy	Adrenal Disease	Extraadrenal Disease
Von Hippel-Lindau disease (VHL)	*VHL*	6–20%	3%	++	+
Multiple endocrine neoplasia types IIA and IIB (MEN IIA, MEN IIB)	*RET*	30–50%	<3%	++	–
Neurofibromatosis type 1 (NF1)	*NF*	1–5%	<3%	++	+
Familial paraganglioma and/ or pheochromocytoma caused by mutation of succinate dehydrogenase gene family members	SDHB	4–9%	66–83%	+	++
	SDHD	2–8%	<2%	+	++
	SDHC	<1%	Not described	–	+ (head and neck)
	SDHA	<5%	Not described	+	+
	SDHAF2	Rare	Not described	–	+ (head and neck)
None described	TMEM127	3%	Not described	+	Unknown

++, very common; +, common; –, rare
*Frequency in sporadic tumors

Burnichon N et al. Hum Mol Genet 2010;19:3011–3020
Eisenhofer G et al. Endocr Relat Cancer 2004;11:423–436
Hao H-X et al. Science 2009;325:1139–1142
John H et al. Urology 1999;53:679–683
Mannelli M et al. J Med Genet 2007;44:586–587
O'Riordain DS et al. World J Surg 1996;20:916–921; discussion 922
Pacak K et al. Ann Intern Med 2001;134:315–329
Qin Y et al. Nat Genet 2010;42:229–233

Evaluation

The diagnosis of pheochromocytoma is confirmed by biochemical evidence of elevated catecholamine production (preferably with measurement of plasma metanephrines) and by radiologic studies (Figure 31–1)

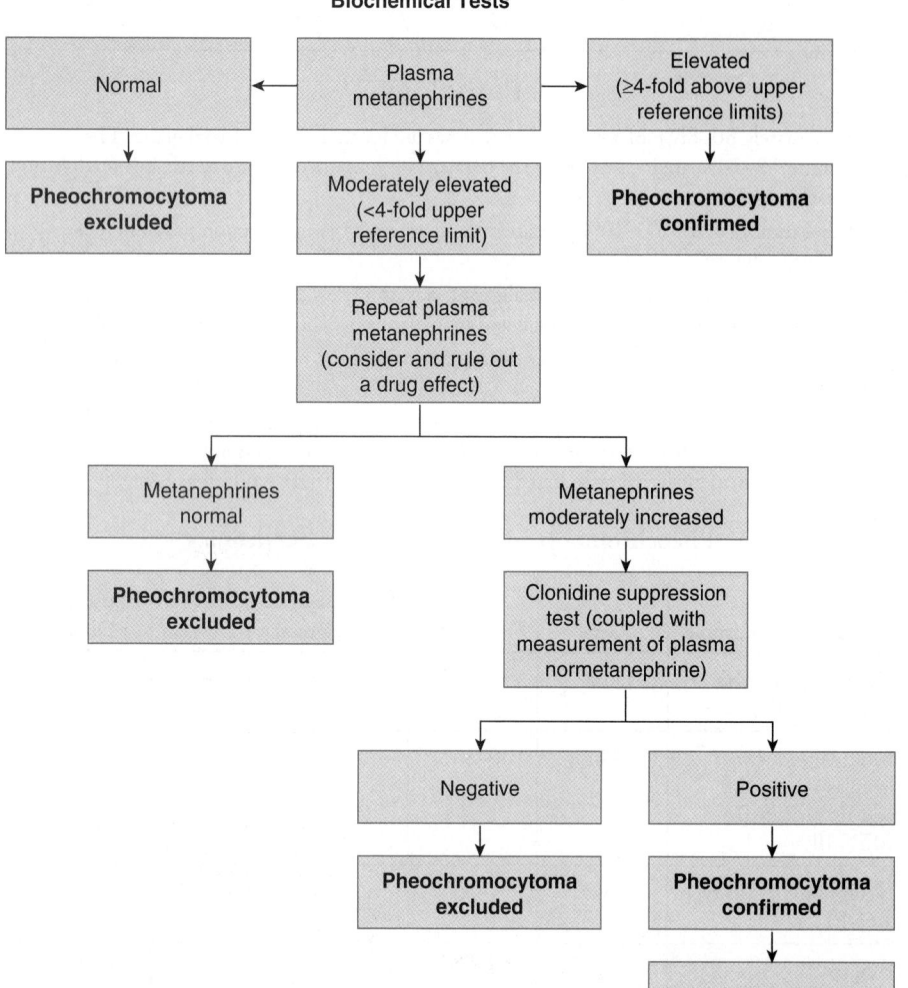

Figure 31–1. Biochemical tests.

Acetaminophen may interfere with measurement of plasma metanephrines. Other drugs, including benzodiazepines, buspirone, diuretics, levodopa, tricyclic antidepressants, and α- and β-adrenergic blockers, may cause false-positive elevations of plasma or urine catecholamines or metanephrines. Currently, there is no drug interference using the new liquid chromatography tandem mass spectrometry method

de Jong WHA et al. Clin Chem 2007;53:1684–1693

Survival

For patients with resectable pheochromocytoma, the overall survival is equal to that of the age-matched normal population. Although the 5-year survival of malignant pheochromocytomas is less than 50%, malignant pheochromocytomas can be slow-growing, and patients may have minimal morbidity and survive as long as 20 years

Bravo EL, Tagle R. Endocr Rev 2003;24:539–553
John H et al. Urology 1999;53:679–683
Remine WH et al. Ann Surg 1974;179:740–748
van Heerden JA et al. Surgery 1982;91:367–373

Imaging Studies

- *CT or MRI of abdomen (90–100% sensitivity):* Because of inadequate specificity, detection of a mass by these tests does not justify a diagnosis. [123]I metaiodobenzylguanidine (MIBG) scintigraphy is needed for confirmation

- *MIBG scan:* Used to confirm diagnosis when CT or MRI detects a tumor mass. In addition, if abdominal imaging is negative, whole-body evaluation by CT or MRI and MIBG scan are indicated to investigate for extraadrenal pheochromocytoma. Drugs that may interfere with MIBG study include labetalol, calcium channel blockers, guanethidine, reserpine, sympathomimetics, tricyclic antidepressants

- *6-[18F] Fluorodopamine positron emission tomography:* This is used when the biochemical tests are positive, but conventional studies cannot locate the tumor

- *6-[18F]-Fluorodeoxyglucose positron emission tomography:* This is used in patients with *SDHB*-related metastatic pheochromocytoma as the first-line imaging study

- *6-[18F]-Fluorodopa positron emission tomography:* This is recommended to be used in *SDHx*-related head and neck paraganglioma as the first-line imaging study (unpublished observations)

Eisenhofer G et al. J Clin Endocrinol Metab 2003;88:2656–2666
Ilias I, Pacak K. J Clin Endocrinol Metab 2004;89:479–491
King KS et al. J Clin Endocrinol Metab 2010;95:481–482
Pacak K et al. Ann Intern Med 2001;134:315–329
Timmers HJLM et al. J Clin Oncol 2007;25:2262–2269

Staging

There is no accepted staging system for pheochromocytoma

Treatment Notes

Surgery

- The definitive treatment for pheochromocytoma is surgical excision of the tumor. Surgical removal can cure pheochromocytoma in up to 90% of cases, whereas, if left untreated, the tumor can prove fatal. Laparoscopic adrenalectomy is now considered the standard approach for excision of most pheochromocytomas with the exception of very large (>10 cm) tumors. The survival rates after surgery are 97.7–100%
- Surgery for **malignant** pheochromocytoma is rarely curative, but resection of the primary mass or metastases can reduce exposure of the cardiovascular system and organs to toxic levels of circulating catecholamines. Consequently, aggressive surgical resection of accessible primary or recurrent disease or metastases should be attempted if the surgery renders the patient free of gross disease with the potential for normal biochemical determinations
- Surgery for **malignant** pheochromocytoma may be indicated for lesions in life-threatening or debilitating anatomic locations
- The value of surgical debulking for **malignant** pheochromocytoma before chemotherapy or radiation therapy is not proved
- The median time for recurrence of pheochromocytoma after initial resection is approximately 6 years and may be as long as 20 years
- Alternatives to surgical resection include external beam radiation, cryoablation, radiofrequency ablation, transcatheter arterial embolization, chemotherapy, and radiopharmaceutical therapy
- Biochemical testing should always be repeated after recovery from surgical resection of a primary mass to exclude any remaining disease or metastasis
- Postoperative follow-up of patients includes evaluation of plasma metanephrine levels 6 weeks and 6 and 12 months after surgery, then yearly. Imaging studies should be performed on the basis of follow-up test results. Exceptions: (a) Patients with SDHB because they have a higher risk of malignancy and (b) those with an extraadrenal tumor or a primary >5 cm who should be followed up more frequently (every 6 months for the first 5 years)
- Before surgery, patients with pheochromocytoma must undergo pharmacologic blockage of catecholamine synthesis and activity as well as volume expansion because they have reduced intravascular volume as a result of a persistent vasoconstricted state. The combination of phenoxybenzamine (an irreversible, nonselective α-adrenergic receptor antagonist) or doxazosin, terazosin, or prazosin (selective α_1-adrenergic receptor antagonists), with atenolol (a selective β_1-adrenergic receptor antagonist) and metyrosine (a tyrosine hydroxylase inhibitor), and liberal salt intake starting 2–3 weeks before surgery leads to better control of blood pressure and decreases surgical risks
- Routine preoperative use of phenoxybenzamine opposes catecholamine-induced vasoconstriction. A β-adrenoceptor blocker (atenolol) is added to prevent the reflex tachycardia associated with α-blockade. The pressor effects of a pheochromocytoma must be controlled by α-blockade before β-blockers are initiated

  Note: β-Blockade **alone** can be dangerous in patients with pheochromocytoma and is contraindicated because it does not prevent and can actually augment effects of catecholamines at α-adrenoceptors
- Metyrosine is used to reduce the synthesis of new catecholamines by the tumor

Drug	Mechanism	Oral Dose	Side Effects
Phenoxybenzamine hydrochloride	Long-acting nonselective α-adrenergic antagonist	Initial dose: 10 mg twice daily, gradually increased to 20 and 40 mg 2 or 3 times daily (approximately 1–2 mg/kg per day). Final dose is determined by the patient's blood pressure	Tachycardia, orthostatic hypotension, nausea, abdominal pain, nasal congestion, fatigue, and retrograde or difficulty in ejaculation
Atenolol	Long-acting β_1-selective (cardioselective) β-adrenergic antagonist	Initial dose: 25 mg once a day. This can be increased to 25 mg twice daily and 50 mg twice daily if needed. Dose should be decreased in renal impairment	Hypotension, bradycardia, postural hypotension, cardiac failure, dizziness, tiredness, fatigue, and depression
Metyrosine	Competitively inhibits tyrosine hydroxylase, the rate-limiting enzyme in catecholamine synthesis	Initially, 250 mg 4 times daily. This may be increased by 250–500 mg daily to a maximum dose of 66.7 mg/kg per day or 4000 mg/day (whichever is less); eg, 1000 mg 4 times daily. Doses should be decreased in renal failure and given as divided doses	Extrapyramidal neurologic symptoms, crystalluria, diarrhea, anxiety, depression, headache, fatigue, and xerostomia
Doxazosin mesylate	Short-acting α_1-antagonist	Initial dose: 1–2 mg daily. This can be gradually increased to 10–16 mg/day Recommended maximum daily dose is 16 mg as a single daily dose with either immediate- or extended-release formulations	Postural dizziness and vertigo, postural hypotension, syncope
Terazosin hydrochloride	Short-acting α_1-antagonist	Initial dose: 1–2 mg daily. This can be gradually increased to 5 mg/day Recommended maximum daily dose is 20 mg, either as a single daily dose, or 10 mg every 12 hours	
Prazosin hydrochloride	Short-acting α_1-antagonist	Initial dose: 1 mg 2 or 3 times daily. This can be gradually increased to 2–5 mg/dose, 2 or 3 times daily Recommended maximum daily dose is 20 mg given in 2 or 3 divided doses	

(continued)

Treatment Notes *(continued)*

Important note:

Several drugs (including some commonly used by oncologists) may lead to a hypertensive crisis in a patient with a diagnosis of pheochromocytoma and should be avoided. These include:

- ACTH
- Amphetamines
- Antibiotics such as linezolid
- Cocaine
- Droperidol*
- Glucagon*
- Histamine*
- **Morphine**
- **Metoclopramide*, chlorpromazine, prochlorperazine**
- Saralasin
- **Tricyclic and other antidepressants**
- Tyramine
- Weight-loss medications

*Has been used as a provocative test for pheochromocytoma

Eigelberger MS, Duh Q-Y. Curr Treat Options Oncol 2001;2:321–329
Eisenhofer G et al. Endocr Relat Cancer 2004;11:423–436
Pacak K et al. Ann Intern Med 2001;134:315–329
Pacak K. J Clin Endocrinol Metab 2007;92:4069–4079

U.S. Food and Drug Administration Maximum Recommended Therapeutic Dose (MRTD) Database http://www.fda.gov/AboutFDA/CentersOffices/OfficeofMedicalProductsandTobacco/CDER/ucm092199.htm [last accessed July 17, 2013]

Westphal SA. Am J Med Sci 2005;329:18–21

REGIMEN

CYCLOPHOSPHAMIDE, VINCRISTINE, DACARBAZINE (CVD)

Averbuch SD et al. Ann Intern Med 1988;109:267–273

Recommendation: Hospitalization while first cycle is administered given that a rare patient may have worsening of their hypertension or even a hypertensive crisis during administration or shortly thereafter

Cyclophosphamide 750 mg/m²; administer intravenously in 100–250 mL 0.9% sodium chloride injection (0.9% NS) or 5% dextrose injection (D5W) over 15–30 minutes on day 1, every 21 days (total dosage/cycle = 750 mg/m²)

Vincristine 1.4 mg/m²; administer by intravenous injection over 1–2 minutes on day 1, every 21 days (total dosage/cycle = 1.4 mg/m²)

Dacarbazine 600 mg/m² per dose; administer intravenously in 100–250 mL 0.9% NS or D5W over 15–30 minutes for 2 doses on days 1 and 2, every 21 days (total dosage/cycle = 1200 mg/m²)

Supportive Care
Antiemetic prophylaxis
Emetogenic potential on days 1 and 2 is **HIGH**. *Potential for delayed symptoms*
See Chapter 39 for antiemetic recommendations

Hematopoietic growth factor (CSF) prophylaxis
Primary prophylaxis is NOT indicated
See Chapter 43 for more information

Antimicrobial prophylaxis
Risk of fever and neutropenia is LOW
Antimicrobial primary prophylaxis to be considered:
- Antibacterial—not indicated
- Antifungal—not indicated
- Antiviral—not indicated unless patient previously had an episode of HSV

See Chapter 47 for more information

Efficacy (N = 14)

Tumor Response

Complete response	2 (14%)
Partial response	6 (43%)
Overall response	57%
Median duration	21 months

Biochemical Response

Complete response	3 (21%)
Partial response	8 (57%)
Overall response	78%
Median duration	22 months

Toxicity (N = 14)

Hematologic

WBC nadir <1000/mm³	21% (3/14)
Mean nadir WBC	2100/mm³
Platelet count nadir <50,000/mm³	29% (4/14)
Mean nadir platelet count	144,000/mm³

Nonhematologic

Mild sensory impairment	Mean grade 0.9/4
Paresthesias	Mean grade 0.9/4
Nausea and vomiting	Mean grade 1.6/4
Hypotension	4 episodes

Treatment Modifications

Counts on Day 1 of Repeated Cycles

WBC 3000–3999/mm³ or platelets 75,000–100,000/mm³	Vincristine 100%. Reduce cyclophosphamide and dacarbazine dosages by 25%
WBC 2000–2999/mm³ or platelets 50,000–75,000/mm³	Vincristine 100%. Reduce cyclophosphamide and dacarbazine dosages by 50%
WBC 1000–1999/mm³ or platelets 25,000–50,000/mm³	Vincristine 100%. Hold cyclophosphamide and dacarbazine
Total bilirubin 1.5–2 mg/dL (25.7–34.2 μmol/L) or serum AST 75–150 units/L	Reduce vincristine dosage by 50%
Total bilirubin 3–5.9 mg/dL (51.3–100.9 μmol/L) or serum AST 151–300 units/L	Reduce vincristine dosage by 75%
Total bilirubin >6 mg/dL (>102.6 μmol/L) or serum AST >300 units/L	Hold vincristine
G1/2 neuropathy	Decrease vincristine dosage by 50%
G3/4 neuropathy	Hold vincristine

Nadir Counts During the Previous Cycle

WBC 1000–1999/mm³ or platelets 50,000–75,000/mm³	Vincristine 100%. Reduce cyclophosphamide and dacarbazine dosages by 50%
WBC <1000/mm³ or platelets <50,000/mm³	Vincristine 100%. Reduce cyclophosphamide and dacarbazine dosages by 75%

Notes

Several drugs (including some commonly used by oncologists) may lead to a hypertensive crisis in a patient with a diagnosis of pheochromocytoma and should be avoided:

1. ACTH
2. Amphetamines
3. Antibiotics such as linezolid
4. Cocaine
5. Droperidol
6. Glucagon*
7. Histamine*
8. **Morphine**
9. **Metoclopramide***, chlorpromazine, prochlorperazine
10. Saralasin
11. **Tricyclic and other antidepressants**
12. Tyramine
13. Weight-loss medications

*Used as a provocative test for pheochromocytoma

Patient Population

A study of 14 patients with advanced malignant pheochromocytoma

Therapy Monitoring

1. *During initial treatment cycles:* Careful hemodynamic monitoring
2. *Before each cycle:* Plasma/serum metanephrines and catecholamines, CBC with differential, LFTs, and neurologic exam

32. Prostate Cancer

Avni Shah, MD, Wenhui Zhu, MD, PhD, and William L. Dahut, MD

Epidemiology

Incidence: 233,000 (Estimated new cases for 2014 in the United States) 152 per 100,000 males per year
Deaths: Estimated 29,480 in 2014
Median age: 66 years

Siegel R et al. CA Cancer J Clin 2014;64:9–29
Surveillance, Epidemiology and End Results (SEER) Program, available from http://seer.cancer.gov (accessed in 2013)

Stage at Presentation
Stage I: 50%
Stage II: 20%
Stage III: 17%
Stage IV: 13%

Pathology

Adenocarcinoma (acinar): >95%
Ductal adenocarcinoma*: <1%
Mucinous*: <1%
Small cell*: <1%
Transitional cell*: <1%
Small cell*: <1%

Gleason Score at Presentation
(Radical prostatectomy specimens)
2–4: 6%
5–6: 54%
7: 30%
8–9: 10%

*Poor prognosis
Kantoff PW et al. Prostate Cancer: Principles & Practice. Philadelphia: Lippincott

Work-up

Bone scan if:
T1 and PSA >20
T2 and PSA >10
Gleason > or >8
T3/T4 disease
Symptomatic

Pelvic CT/MRI if:
T3/T4
T1/2 and normogram indicates probability of LN invasion >10%

Staging

Primary Tumor (T)

Tx	Primary tumor cannot be assessed
T0	No evidence of primary tumor
T1	Clinically inapparent tumor neither palpable nor visible by imaging
T1a	Tumor incidental histologic finding in 5% or less of tissue resected
T1b	Tumor incidental histologic finding in more than 5% of tissue resected
T1c	Tumor identified by needle biopsy (eg, because of elevated PSA)
T2	Tumor confined within prostate*
pT2	Organ confined
T2a	Tumor involves one-half of 1 lobe or less
pT2a	Unilateral, one-half of 1 side or less
T2b	Tumor involves more than one-half of 1 lobe but not both lobes
pT2b	Unilateral, involving more than one-half of side but not both sides
T2c	Tumor involves both lobes
pT2c	Bilateral disease
T3	Tumor extends through the prostate capsule†
pT3	Extraprostatic extension
T3a	Extracapsular extension (unilateral or bilateral)
pT3a	Extraprostatic extension or microscopic invasion of bladder neck‡
T3b	Tumor invades seminal vesicle(s)
pT3b	Seminal vesicle invasion
T4	Tumor is fixed or invades adjacent structures other than seminal vesicles: such as external sphincter, rectum, bladder, levator muscles, and/or pelvic wall
pT4	Invasion of rectum, levator muscles, and/or pelvic wall

Note: There is no pathologic T1 classification
*Tumor found in one or both lobes by needle biopsy, but not palpable or reliably visible by imaging, is classified as T1c
†Invasion into the prostatic apex or into (but not beyond) the prostatic capsule is classified not as T3 but as T2
‡Positive surgical margin should be indicated by an R1 descriptor (residual microscopic disease)

Staging Groups

Group	T	N	M	PSA	Gleason
I	T1a–c	N0	M0	PSA <10	Gleason ≤6
	T2a	N0	M0	PSA <10	Gleason ≤6
	T1–2a	N0	M0	PSA X	Gleason X
IIA	T1a–c	N0	M0	PSA <20	Gleason 7
	T1a–c	N0	M0	PSA ≥10 <20	Gleason ≤6
	T2a	N0	M0	PSA <20	Gleason ≤7
	T2b	N0	M0	PSA <20	Gleason ≤7
	T2b	N0	M0	PSA X	Gleason X
IIB	T2c	N0	M0	Any PSA	Any Gleason
	T1–2	N0	M0	PSA ≥20	Any Gleason
	T1–2	N0	M0	Any PSA	Gleason ≥8
III	T3a–b	N0	M0	Any PSA	Any Gleason
IV	T4	N0	M0	Any PSA	Any Gleason
	Any T	N1	M0	Any PSA	Any Gleason
	Any T	Any N	M1	Any PSA	Any Gleason

When either PSA or Gleason is not available, grouping should be determined by T stage and/or either PSA or Gleason as available

Edge SB, Byrd DR, Compton CC, Fritz AG, Greene FL, Trotti A, editors. AJCC Cancer Staging Manual. 7th ed. New York: Springer; 2010

Regional Lymph Nodes (N)

NX	Regional lymph nodes were not assessed
pNX	Regional nodes not sampled
N0	No regional lymph node metastasis
pN0	No positive regional nodes
N1	Metastasis in regional lymph node(s)
pN1	Metastases in regional node(s)

Distant Metastasis (M)

M0	No distant metastasis
M1	Distant metastasis
M1a	Nonregional lymph node(s)
M1b	Bone(s)
M1c	Other site(s) with or without bone disease

Note: When more than 1 site of metastasis is present, the most advanced category is used. pM1c is most advanced

15-Year Relative Survival

Stages I–II	81%
Stage III	57%
Stage IV	6%

Predicting 15-year Prostate Cancer Specific Mortality After Radical Prostatectomy

Gleason Score	Mortality (from PrCa)
<6	0.2%–1.2%
3+4/4+3	4.2%–6.5%/6.6%–11%
8–10	26%–37%

Eggener et al. J Urol 2011;185:869–875

10-Year Free Disease Survival

(After radical prostatectomy for localized disease)

Gleason score 2–4	96%
Gleason score 5–6	82%
Gleason score 7	52%
Gleason score 8–9	35%

Expert Opinion

Screening for prostate cancer:
The optimal use of PSA in the diagnosis of prostate cancer remains a subject of continued controversy. In 2012 the USPSTF recommended against the use of PSA-based screening for prostate cancer to the general population, regardless of age. The American Urological Association has also revised their guidelines in response, advising against routine PSA based screening. However, in high-risk men ages 40–54 or all men between 55–69 the AUA advises the test to be a man's decision after a discussion of the full understanding of the risks and benefits of testing. Both groups agree that men above the age of 70 or under the age of 40 do not undergo screening

http://annals.org/article.aspx?articleID=1216568 (The Annals of Internal Medicine article for the USPSTF by Virginia A Moyer, 17 July 2012)
http://www.auanet.org/education/guidelines/prostate-cancer-detection.cfm (AUA guidelines)

The traditionally employed PSA threshold of 4 ng/mL has only a 70–80% sensitivity and 60–70% specificity. The positive predictive value of a PSA between 4 and 10 ng/mL is only 25%, and approximately 20% of patients with PSA between 2 and 4 ng/mL will have prostate cancer on biopsy. Free PSA percentage (<10%) has been shown to improve the positive predictive value in patients with total PSA between 4 and 10 ng/mL. In the Prostate Cancer Prevention Trial, 21.1% of prostate cancers were diagnosed in men with a PSA level between 2.6 and 3.9 ng/mL and 15.4% of the prostate cancers had a Gleason score of 7–10 when PSA was ≤2.5 ng/mL

Initial assessment and staging evaluation:
Patients are stratified at diagnosis for an initial treatment plan based on anticipated life expectancy and clinical symptoms
- For asymptomatic patients with life expectancy <10 years, treatment may be delayed until symptoms appear
- Once an abnormal digital rectal exam and/or an elevated PSA suggest prostate cancer is present, an ultrasound-guided prostate core biopsy with 10–12 cores is performed to help establish the diagnosis, and the 2 most common cellular patterns of the tumor are graded pathologically using the Gleason scale
- Pelvic CT or MRI is recommended for patients with T3/T4 tumor or T1/T2 tumor with a predicted probability of lymph node involvement >20%
- Bone scan is recommended for patients with T3/T4 tumor, symptomatic disease, or a T1/T2 tumor with PSA >20 ng/mL or a Gleason score ≥8

Localized prostate cancer:
Patients with newly diagnosed clinically localized prostate cancer are divided into 3 risk groups of occult metastasis and relapse after local initial therapy
- *Low risk:* PSA <10 ng/mL, Gleason score ≤6, T1/T2a tumor
- *Intermediate risk:* PSA 10–20 ng/mL, Gleason score 7, T2b/T2c tumor
- *High risk:* PSA >20 ng/mL, Gleason score 8–10, T3/T4 tumor

Treatment options for localized prostate cancer include active surveillance, radical prostatectomy (RP; including open surgery, laparoscopic, and robot-assisted procedures), and radiation therapy (RT; including high-dose external beam radiation therapy with 3D conformal or intensity-modulated radiation therapy, and brachytherapy with or without external beam therapy)
- The treatment decision is based on the probability of organ-confined disease, patient's life expectancy, and risk of relapse and metastasis
- Active surveillance is an option for patients with low-risk prostate cancer. Serial biopsy and close PSA monitoring are used to attempt to identify patients who may benefit from definitive local treatment. Some have suggested intervention if PSA doubling time is less than 3 years or Gleason grade progression to a predominant Gleason 4 pattern
- For patients with organ-confined disease, both RT and RP remain the standard of care, although surgery is not commonly performed in patients >70 years of age
- In nonrandomized patient cohort studies RP and RT appear to provide equivalent PSA-free relapse, but differ in the type and frequency of side effects. At 5 years, the rate of event-free survival was 81% for RP, 81% for high-dose external beam radiation therapy, and 83% for brachytherapy in 2991 patients with clinical stage T1-T2 localized prostate cancer treated between 1990 and 1998
- Patients undergoing RP should have extended pelvic lymph node dissection (PLND), except those with a low predicted probability of nodal metastasis by nomograms
- For T3/T4 disease, RP may be considered for selected patients with well-differentiated tumors. Most high-risk patients will receive XRT plus hormonal ablation
- For RP, nerve-sparing procedures with radical retropubic and robotic-assisted laparoscopic prostatectomy are the most common techniques. The main determinants of outcome are PSA level, Gleason score, and the TNM clinical stage. Adverse effects from surgery include incontinence, erectile dysfunction, bladder neck stricture, and bowel incontinence
- The biochemical control rate after RT depends largely upon the risk features associated with individual tumors. The probability of biochemical control 5 years after RT without hormonal ablation is 84% for low-risk disease, 62% for intermediate-risk disease, and 43% for high-risk disease

Adjuvant therapies after initial definitive therapies
- Adjuvant RT after RP should be considered for patients with positive surgical margins, seminal vesicle involvement, or pathological evidence of T3/T4 disease
- Immediate postoperative RT for patients with pathologic T3 disease improves PSA progression-free survival significantly (74% vs. 53% for placebo after 5 years of follow up), although there is no overall survival benefit
- Due to exclusion of patients with node positive disease in most clinical trials, it remains unclear whether adjuvant RT after RP should be considered in this subset of patients

(continued)

Expert Opinion (continued)

- Immediate androgen-deprivation therapy (ADT) provides significant overall survival benefit in patients with microscopically positive lymph nodes treated with RP, compared to hormonal therapy started at the time of symptomatic local recurrence or metastasis
- Neoadjuvant/adjuvant ADT of 2–3 years in combination with RT is the standard for high-risk patients. Neoadjuvant/adjuvant ADT (for 6 months) in combination with RT may improve progression-free disease and prostate cancer-specific and overall survival for patients with PSA >10 ng/mL, a Gleason score ≥7, or radiographic evidence of extraprostatic disease. This needs confirmation in a larger study limited only to intermediate-risk patients

Androgen-deprivation therapy
- Optimal ADT includes medical castration with a GnRH antagonist, an LHRH agonist, or surgical castration with bilateral orchiectomy. The addition of an antiandrogen can reduce the initial disease flare that may follow introduction of a LHRH agonist, but does not appear to add significantly to survival
- Side effects of ADT include osteoporosis, hot flashes, loss of libido, erectile dysfunction, fatigue, gynecomastia, cognitive dysfunction, depression, anemia, loss of muscle mass, glucose intolerance, and changes in lipids profile and increased risk of cardiovascular disease
- Hot flashes from hormonal therapy can be treated with clonidine (0.1 mg daily, orally), low-dose estrogens, or antidepressants
- Prophylactic breast XRT can reduce the incidence of painful gynecomastia
- Patients receiving long-term ADT should have a baseline bone density scan and supplemental vitamin D and calcium. Consider bisphosphonates if an evaluation demonstrates evidence of either osteopenia or osteoporosis

PSA Failure
PSA failure after RP:
- Following RP, it is expected that PSA will be undetectable. Biochemical recurrence following RP is defined as either failure to achieve an undetectable PSA level or a PSA rise after surgery on 2 or more laboratory determinations. The American Urological Association Prostate Guideline Update Panel has chosen a PSA level ≥0.2 ng/mL as the threshold
- Patients with biochemical recurrence because of local failure and without distant metastasis (clinical features include PSA <2 ng/mL, slow PSA doubling time, a long interval to failure after surgery) should be evaluated for salvage RT. Salvage RT provides durable disease-free survival in 60–70% of patients, but no confirmed overall survival benefits. Predictors of progression after salvage RT include a Gleason score of 8–10, pre-RT PSA >2 ng/mL, negative surgical margins, and a PSA doubling time <10 months

PSA failure after RT:
- PSA failure after RT is defined as a PSA rise ≥2 ng/mL above the nadir (the Phoenix definition)
- Patients with original clinical stage T1–T2, a life expectancy >10 years, and a current PSA <10 ng/mL may be candidates for local therapy such as salvage RP, cryotherapy, or brachytherapy. However, morbidity is high and there are no randomized trials that demonstrate improved survival. Further work-up is indicated to rule out distant metastasis before local therapy

For patients with PSA failure, timing of ADT is affected by PSA velocity, patient preference, and other medical comorbidities. Early implementation of ADT may delay the appearance of metastases; however, there are no data indicating early ADT provides any overall survival benefit

Advanced prostate cancer
- In patients with metastatic prostate cancer, local therapies are used primarily for symptom management. There are no conclusive data that local therapies improve survival
- ADT should begin immediately in the presence of tumor-related symptoms or overt metastasis
- **Combined androgen blockage** (castration combined with an antiandrogen) provides no definite survival improvement over castration alone in patients with metastatic disease
- Initiation of treatment with LHRH agonists is associated with a transient increase in testosterone production with initial use (tumor flare). For patients with overt metastases who are at risk of developing symptoms (such as spinal cord compression, worsening pain, or urinary outlet obstruction) an antiandrogen should be given concurrently with a LHRH agonist for at least 7 days after initiating treatment with the latter to competitively block testosterone at androgen receptors, and prevent potential exacerbation of disease. **Ketoconazole** may also be used in patients who are at high risk for complications associated with tumor flare
- Intermittent ADT can be used to reduce side effects and cost of ADT, but its long-term efficacy remains unproven
- **Abiraterone acetate** has been approved in patients pre-chemotherapy based on improved progression-free survival. The study was stopped before an overall-survival benefit could be seen, but there was a trend towards OS improvement as well [Ryan et al. N Engl J Med 2013;368:138–148]. **Enzalutamide** may be shown to be beneficial in this setting as well
- Second-line hormonal management includes antiandrogens, antiandrogen withdrawal, adrenal androgen inhibitors (**aminoglutethimide or ketoconazole with hydrocortisone replacement**), and estrogens. **Abiraterone acetate** targets cytochrome P450 17A1 (CYP17A1), leading to a decrease in the production of testosterone. It received FDA approval based on a study that demonstrated improved survival in patients who received it after docetaxel chemotherapy. **Abiraterone acetate** is administered daily in combination with prednisone. **Enzalutamide**, a potent anti-androgen, has also been approved for use post-chemotherapy based on an OS benefit. One advantage of enzalutamide over abiraterone acetate is that it does not require concomitant prednisone which can have side-effects in patients with prostate cancer. Selected patients may respond to sequential hormonal manipulations

(continued)

Expert Opinion (*continued*)

- **Sipuleucel-T** is a cellular immunotherapy consisting of peripheral blood mononuclear cells obtained by leukapheresis and cultured (activated) with a recombinant human protein consisting of prostatic acid phosphatase linked to granulocyte-macrophage colony-stimulating factor (PAP-GM-CSF). In a randomized trial this product had no effect on time to progression, but lead to an improvement in overall survival.

- Chemotherapy with **docetaxel** every 3 weeks plus prednisone is the preferred first-line chemotherapy for advanced prostate cancer, providing improved survival. **Cabazitaxel** is a semisynthetic derivative of a natural taxoid, which, when combined with prednisone, improved survival in patients who had progressed on docetaxel and prednisone. Alternative regimens include **every 3-week docetaxel and estramustine, weekly docetaxel and prednisone**, and **every 3-week mitoxantrone and prednisone**

- **Cabazitaxel** is approved as a second-line chemotherapeutic agent

- *Metastatic small cell carcinoma of the prostate* should be treated with a platinum-containing regimen, but mixed tumors (adenocarcinoma and small cell) may have some initial response to hormonal ablation

- **Zoledronic acid** prevents skeletal-related events in patients with castrate resistant prostate cancer and bone metastases

- **Radium-223** has been approved by the FDA-for prostate cancer and selectively targets bone metastases with alpha particles. It has been shown to improve overall survival but it remains to be seen where exactly it will be used in patients and whether or not it will be combined with other approved agents

American Cancer Society Guidelines for the Early Detection of Cancer. Prostate Cancer Early Detection. Available from: http://www.cancer.org/Cancer/ProstateCancer/MoreInformation/ProstateCancerEarlyDetection/prostate-cancer-early-detection-toc
Gulley JL, Dahut WL. Prostate cancer. In: Abraham J et al. eds. Bethesda Handbook of Clinical Oncology 2nd ed. Philadelphia, PA: Lippincott Williams & Wilkins; 2005:185–201
Parker et al. N Engl J Med. 2013;369:213–223
Pazdur R et al. Cancer Management: A Multidisciplinary Approach. 13th ed. Manhasset, NY: CMP Healthcare Media, Inc; 2010
The Partin Tables. Available from: http://urology.jhu.edu/prostate/partintables.php [last accessed July 8, 2011]
U.S. Preventive Services Task Force. Screening for prostate cancer: U.S. Preventive Services Task Force recommendation statement. Ann Intern Med 2008;149:185–191, W–42

REGIMEN

ABIRATERONE ACETATE
METASTATIC CASTRATION-RESISTANT PROSTATE CANCER—NO PRIOR CHEMOTHERAPY

Ryan CJ et al. N Engl J Med 2013;368:138–148

Abiraterone acetate 1000 mg orally once daily, continually for 28 consecutive days (total dose/28-day cycle = 28,000 mg)
Note: No food should be consumed for at least 2 hours before a dose of abiraterone acetate is taken and for at least 1 hour after a dose of abiraterone acetate is taken. Exposure (area under the curve) of abiraterone acetate increases up to 10-fold when abiraterone acetate is taken with meals

Prednisone 5 mg orally twice daily, continually for 28 consecutive days (total dose/28-day cycle = 280 mg)

Notes:
- For patients with baseline moderate hepatic impairment (Child-Pugh Class B), reduce the dose of abiraterone acetate to 250 mg once daily
- Avoid abiraterone acetate in patients with baseline severe hepatic impairment (Child-Pugh Class C), as abiraterone acetate has not been studied in this population, and no dose adjustment can be predicted
- Abiraterone acetate is an inhibitor of the polymorphically expressed cytochrome P450 (CYP) enzyme, CYP2D6
  - **Avoid coadministration** of abiraterone acetate with CYP2D6 substrates that have a low therapeutic index. If an alternative treatment cannot be used, exercise caution and consider a dose reduction of concomitantly used CYP2D6 substrates
- Monitor for symptoms and signs of adrenocortical insufficiency. Increased dosage of corticosteroids may be indicated before, during, and after stressful situations
- Monitor for signs and symptoms of mineralocorticoid excess, including hypokalemia, fluid retention, and hypertension. Prednisone dose may have to be supplemented in some patients or augmented with an aldosterone antagonist such as eplerenone
- Use abiraterone acetate with caution in patients with a history of cardiovascular disease. Control hypertension and correct hypokalemia before initiating treatment
- Abiraterone acetate is a substrate of CYP3A4. Avoid or use with caution strong CYP3A4 inhibitors (eg, atazanavir, clarithromycin, indinavir, itraconazole, ketoconazole, nefazodone, nelfinavir, ritonavir, saquinavir, telithromycin, voriconazole) or inducers (eg, carbamazepine, phenobarbital, phenytoin, rifabutin, rifapentine, rifampin) during abiraterone acetate treatment
- Abiraterone acetate was a strong inhibitor of CYP1A2 and CYP2D6, and a moderate inhibitor of CYP2C9, CYP2C19, and CYP3A4/5 in experimental systems. It is not yet known whether its effects on CYP1A2, CYP2C subfamily, or CYP3A subfamily enzymes in in vitro systems are representative of a potential for clinically important drug interactions
- Use abiraterone acetate with caution in patients with a history of cardiovascular disease. The safety of abiraterone acetate in patients with LVEF <50% or NYHA Class III or IV heart failure is not established. Control hypertension and correct hypokalemia before treatment

Supportive Care
Antiemetic prophylaxis
Emetogenic potential is **MINIMAL–LOW**
See Chapter 39 for antiemetic recommendations

Hematopoietic growth factor (CSF) prophylaxis
Primary prophylaxis is NOT indicated
See Chapter 43 for more information

Antimicrobial prophylaxis
Risk of fever and neutropenia is LOW
Antimicrobial primary prophylaxis to be considered:
- Antibacterial—not indicated
- Antifungal—not indicated
- Antiviral—not indicated unless patient previously had an episode of HSV

See Chapter 47 for more information

Treatment Modification

Adverse Event	Dose Modification
G2 hepatotoxicity	Hold abiraterone acetate until toxicity remits to G ≤1, then resume treatment at a dose of 750 mg once daily
G3 hepatotoxicity (elevations in ALT and/or AST >5 × upper limit of normal [ULN] or total bilirubin >3 × ULN) in a patient with baseline normal hepatic function	Withhold abiraterone acetate. Treatment may be restarted at a dose of 750 mg once daily following return of liver function tests to a patient's baseline or to AST and ALT G ≤1 (2.5 × ULN) and total bilirubin G ≤1 (≤1.5 × ULN). For patients who resume treatment, monitor serum transaminases
G3 hepatotoxicity (elevations in ALT and/or AST >5 × upper limit of normal [ULN] or total bilirubin >3 × ULN) in a patient with baseline normal hepatic impairment on a reduced dose of 750 mg/day because of prior hepatotoxicity at 1000 mg/day	Withhold abiraterone acetate. Treatment may be restarted at a dose of 500 mg once daily following return of liver function tests to a patient's baseline or to AST and ALT G ≤1 (2.5 × ULN) and total bilirubin G ≤1 (≤1.5 × ULN). For patients who resume treatment, monitor serum transaminases
G3 hepatotoxicity (elevations in ALT and/or AST >5 × upper limit of normal or total bilirubin >3 × ULN) in a patient with baseline normal hepatic impairment on a reduced dose of 500 mg/day because of prior hepatotoxicity at 750 mg/day	Discontinue abiraterone acetate

(continued)

Efficacy

Prespecified Secondary and Exploratory Efficacy End Points*

	Abiraterone + Prednisone (N = 546)	Prednisone Alone (N = 542)	Value (95% CI)†	P Value
End Point				
Secondary End Points				
Median Times in Months to:				
Opioid use for cancer-related pain	Not Reached	23.7	0.69 (0.57–0.83)	<0.001
Starting cytotoxic chemotherapy	25.2	16.8	0.58 (0.49–0.69)	<0.001
Decline in ECOG PS by ≥1 point	12.3	10.9	0.82 (0.71–0.94)	0.005
PSA progression‡	11.1	5.6	0.49 (0.42–0.57)	<0.001
Exploratory End Points§				
Median Times in Months to:				
Increase in pain⁋	26.7	18.4	0.82 (0.67–1.00)	0.049
Functional status decline**	12.7	8.3	0.78 (0.66–0.92)	0.003
Decline of ≥50% in PSA level (%)††	62	24	2.59 (2.19–3.05)‡‡	<0.001

Patients with Measurable Disease at Baseline and a RECIST Response (%)

	N = 220	N = 218		
Defined objective response	36	16	2.27 (1.59–3.25)‡‡	<0.001
Stable disease	61	69		
Progressive disease	2	15		

CI, Confidence interval; FACT-P, Functional Assessment of Cancer Therapy–Prostate; HR, hazard ratio; PS, performance score; PSA, prostate-specific antigen; RECIST, Response Evaluation Criteria in Solid Tumors
*Percentages may not sum to 100 because of rounding
†Values are hazard ratios unless otherwise specified
‡Based on Prostate Cancer Clinical Trials Working Group 2 (PCWG2) criteria
§The exploratory analyses are reported with no adjustment for multiplicity
⁋Increase in pain is defined as an increase in the baseline pain level by 30% or more, as measured by the average of the pain scores on the Brief Pain Inventory–Short Form (range: 0–10, with higher scores indicating worse average pain) at 2 consecutive visits, without a decrease in analgesic use
**Defined as months from randomization to the first date a patient has a decrease of 10 points or more on the FACT-P instrument (range: 0–156, with higher scores indicating better overall quality of life)
††A decline ≥50% in the PSA level was based on modified PCWG2 criteria
‡‡Values are relative risks

Treatment Modification
(continued)

Adverse Event	Dose Modification
G3 hepatotoxicity (elevations in ALT and/or AST >5 × ULN or total bilirubin >3 × ULN) in a patient with baseline moderate hepatic impairment on a reduced dose of 750 mg abiraterone acetate daily	Discontinue abiraterone acetate
G4 hepatotoxicity (elevations in ALT and/or AST >20 × ULN or total bilirubin >10 × ULN) in a patient with baseline moderate hepatic impairment	Discontinue abiraterone acetate
Hypertension, hypokalemia, and fluid retention caused by mineralocorticoid excess	Withhold abiraterone acetate. Ensure corticosteroids are being administered appropriately. Manage hypokalemia and hypertension
Suspicion of adrenocortical insufficiency	Perform appropriate tests to confirm the diagnosis of adrenocortical insufficiency. Consider administering increased corticosteroid doses during and after stressful situations

Toxicity
Adverse Events

Adverse Event	Abiraterone + Prednisone (N = 542)	Prednisone Alone (N = 540)
	Number of Patients (%)	
Any adverse event	537 (99)	524 (97)
G3/4 adverse event	258 (48)	225 (42)
Any serious adverse event	178 (33)	142 (26)
Adverse event leading to treatment discontinuation	55 (10)	49 (9)
Adverse event leading to death*	20 (4)	12 (2)
G1-4 adverse event ≥15% of patients in either group		
Fatigue	212 (39)	185 (34)
Back pain	173 (32)	173 (32)
Arthralgia	154 (28)	129 (24)
Nausea	120 (22)	118 (22)
Constipation	125 (23)	103 (19)
Hot flush	121 (22)	98 (18)
Diarrhea	117 (22)	96 (18)
Bone pain	106 (20)	103 (19)
Muscle spasm	75 (14)	110 (20)
Pain in extremity	90 (17)	85 (16)
Cough	94 (17)	73 (14)

Adverse Events of Special Interest[†]

Adverse Event	Abiraterone + Prednisone (N = 542)		Prednisone Alone (N = 540)	
	G 1–4	G 3 or 4	G 1–4	G 3 or 4
Fluid retention or edema	150 (28)	4 (<1)	127 (24)	9 (2)
Hypokalemia	91 (17)	13 (2)	68 (13)	10 (2)
Hypertension	118 (22)	21 (4)	71 (13)	16 (3)
Cardiac disorder[‡]	102 (19)	31 (6)	84 (16)	18 (3)
Atrial fibrillation	22 (4)	7 (1)	26 (5)	5 (<1)
ALT increased	63 (12)	29 (5)	27 (5)	4 (<1)
AST increased	58 (11)	16 (3)	26 (5)	5 (<1)

ALT, Alanine aminotransferase; AST, aspartate aminotransferase
*Most common adverse events leading to death were general disorders, including disease progression, decline in physical health, and infections including pneumonia and respiratory tract infection
[†]Adverse events of special interest were selected on the basis of the safety profile of phase 2 and phase 3 studies of abiraterone
[‡]Cardiac disorders included ischemic heart disease, myocardial infarction, supraventricular tachyarrhythmia, ventricular tachyarrhythmia, cardiac failure, and possible arrhythmia-related investigations, signs, and symptoms

Patient Population Studied

Inclusion criteria: (a) metastatic, histologically or cytologically confirmed adenocarcinoma of the prostate; (b) PSA progression according to Prostate Cancer Clinical Trials Working Group 2 (PCWG2) criteria or radiographic progression in soft tissue or bone ± PSA progression; (c) ongoing androgen deprivation with a serum testosterone level <50 ng/dL (<1.7 nmol/L); (d) ECOG performance status grade of 0 or 1; (e) no symptoms or mild symptoms, as defined according to the Brief Pain Inventory–Short Form (BPI-SF; scores of 0 to 1 [asymptomatic] or 2 to 3 [mildly symptomatic], respectively). Exclusion criteria: (a) No previous therapy with an antiandrogen; (b) visceral metastases; (c) previous ketoconazole >7 days

Treatment Monitoring

1. CBC every 8 weeks for the first 24 weeks, and then, every 12 weeks
2. *Evaluation including PSA:* Every 8 weeks for the first 24 weeks, and then, every 12 weeks
3. Monitor blood pressure, serum potassium, and symptoms of fluid retention at least every 8 weeks
4. Measure serum transaminases (ALT and AST) and bilirubin levels prior to starting treatment with abiraterone acetate, every 2 weeks for the first 3 months of treatment, and monthly thereafter. Modify, interrupt, or discontinue abiraterone acetate dosing as recommended
5. In patients with baseline moderate hepatic impairment receiving a reduced abiraterone acetate dose of 250 mg/day, measure ALT, AST, and bilirubin prior to the start of treatment, every week for the first month, every 2 weeks for the following 2 months of treatment, and monthly, thereafter. Promptly measure serum total bilirubin, AST, and ALT if clinical symptoms or signs suggestive of hepatotoxicity develop
6. For patients who resume treatment after LFTs return to G ≤1 from a G2/3/4 toxicity, monitor serum transaminases and bilirubin at a minimum of every 2 weeks for 3 months and monthly thereafter
7. Monitor for symptoms and signs of adrenocortical insufficiency. Increased dosage of corticosteroids may be indicated before, during, and after stressful situations

REGIMEN
DOCETAXEL + PREDNISONE

Tannock IF et al. N Engl J Med 2004;351:1502–1512

Dexamethasone 8 mg/dose orally for 3 doses at 12 hours, 3 hours, and 1 hour before docetaxel treatment commences (total dose/cycle = 24 mg)
Docetaxel 75 mg/m² intravenously over 1 hour, in a volume of 0.9% sodium chloride injection or 5% dextrose injection sufficient to produce a solution with concentration within the range 0.3–0.74 mg/mL, on day 1, every 21 days (total dosage/cycle = 75 mg/m²)
Prednisone 5 mg/dose orally twice daily, continually, for 21 consecutive days, on days 1–21, every 3 weeks (total dose/cycle = 210 mg)

Supportive Care
Antiemetic prophylaxis
Emetogenic potential on day 1 is LOW
See Chapter 39 for antiemetic recommendations

Hematopoietic growth factor (CSF) prophylaxis
Primary prophylaxis is NOT indicated
See Chapter 43 for more information

Antimicrobial prophylaxis
Risk of fever and neutropenia is LOW
  Antimicrobial primary prophylaxis to be considered:
  • Antibacterial—not indicated
  • Antifungal—not indicated
  • Antiviral—not indicated unless patient previously had an episode of HSV
See Chapter 47 for more information

Patient Population Studied

A study of 335 patients with castration-refractory metastatic prostate cancer and no prior chemotherapy other than estramustine

Efficacy

	Docetaxel + Prednisone	Mitoxantrone + Prednisone
Median survival	18.9 months (n = 335)	16.5 months (n = 357)
Pain response	35% (n = 153)	22% (n = 157)
50% ↓ PSA	45% (n = 291)	32% (n = 300)

Treatment Modifications

Adverse Event	Dose Modification
G4 Neutropenia ≥7 days duration, febrile neutropenia, infection, or ANC <1500/mm³ on day of therapy	Delay therapy until ANC >1500/mm³ *or* reduce dose of docetaxel by 25%
G3/4 thrombocytopenia	Delay therapy until thrombocytopenia G ≤2, or reduce dosage of docetaxel by 25%
G3/4 toxicities other than those listed above	Wait for toxicity to recover to G ≤1, then reduce docetaxel dosage to 60 mg/m²
G3/4 neurotoxicity	
G4 nonhematologic toxicity that occurs with 60 mg/m² docetaxel	Stop therapy
Aspartate/alanine aminotransferase (AST/ALT) >1.5 × upper limits of normal (ULN) and alkaline phosphatase >2.5 × ULN Bilirubin > ULN	Hold docetaxel until resolved

Therapy Monitoring

Before each cycle: CBC with differential, liver function tests, PSA if indicated

Toxicity (N = 332)

	% All Grades	% G3/4
Hematologic		
Neutropenia	—	32
Anemia	—	5
Thrombocytopenia	—	1
Febrile neutropenia	3	—
Infection	—	6
Nonhematologic		
Fatigue	53	5
Nausea/vomiting	42	—
Diarrhea	32	2
Sensory neuropathy	30	—
Stomatitis	20	—
Dyspnea	15	—
Peripheral edema	15	—
Myalgia	14	—

REGIMEN

MITOXANTRONE + PREDNISONE (M + P)

Hussain M et al. Semin Oncol 1999;26(5 Suppl 17):55–60
Tannock IF et al. J Clin Oncol 1996;14:1756–1764

Mitoxantrone 12 mg/m² intravenously in 50 mL 0.9% sodium chloride injection or 5% dextrose injection over 5–30 minutes, on day 1, every 21 days (total dosage/cycle = 12 mg/m²)
Prednisone 5 mg/dose orally twice daily continually, for 21 consecutive days, on days 1–21, every 3 weeks (total dose/cycle = 210 mg)
Usually administered for a total of 6 cycles

Supportive Care
Antiemetic prophylaxis
*Emetogenic potential on day 1 is **LOW***
See Chapter 39 for antiemetic recommendations

Hematopoietic growth factor (CSF) prophylaxis
Primary prophylaxis is NOT indicated
See Chapter 43 for more information

Antimicrobial prophylaxis
Risk of fever and neutropenia is LOW
  Antimicrobial primary prophylaxis to be considered:
  • Antibacterial—not indicated
  • Antifungal—not indicated
  • Antiviral—not indicated unless patient previously had an episode of HSV
See Chapter 47 for more information

Patient Population Studied

Patients with metastatic castration-refractory prostate cancer with symptoms (including pain) and disease progression despite standard hormonal therapy. Randomized comparison with prednisone alone

Efficacy (N = 80)

Palliative response*	29–38%
Palliative response duration	43 weeks

*Defined as a decrease in pain parameters

Efficacy: PSA Response (N = 57)

≥50% decrease	33%
≥75% decrease	23%

Toxicity* (N = 654 and 796 cycles)

	% Cycles	
	% G1/2	% G3/4
Hematologic (N = 796 cycles)		
Neutropenia	NA	45
Febrile neutropenia	NA	7
Thrombocytopenia	4.2	0.6
Nonhematologic (N = 654 cycles)		
Nausea/vomiting	29	0.5
Alopecia	24	—
Cardiac dysfunction	2.5	1.7

*WHO criteria

Treatment Modifications

Adverse Event	Dose Modification
WBC <3000/mm³, ANC <1500/mm³, or platelet <100,000/mm³	Delay therapy until WBC >3000/mm³, ANC >1500/mm³, platelet >100,000/mm³
Nadir ANC <500/mm³, or nadir platelet <50,000/mm³	Reduce mitoxantrone dosage by 2 mg/m² per dose
Nadir ANC >1000/mm³, and nadir platelet >100,000/mm³, and minimal nonhematologic toxicity	May increase mitoxantrone dosage to 14 mg/m² per dose
Patients who received a total cumulative lifetime mitoxantrone dosage of 140 mg/m²	Stop mitoxantrone, but continue prednisone

Therapy Monitoring

1. *Before starting therapy:* Echocardiogram
2. *Before each cycle:* CBC with differential, LFTs, PSA if indicated

ADVANCED DISEASE REGIMEN

ABIRATERONE ACETATE
METASTATIC CASTRATION-RESISTANT PROSTATE CANCER—PRIOR CHEMOTHERAPY

Fizazi K et al. Lancet Oncol 2012;13:983–992

Abiraterone acetate 1000 mg orally once daily on an empty stomach, continually for 28 consecutive days (total dose/28-day cycle = 28,000 mg)

Note: No food should be consumed for at least 2 hours before a dose of abiraterone acetate is taken and for at least 1 hour after a dose of abiraterone acetate is taken. Exposure (area under the curve) of abiraterone increases up to 10-fold when abiraterone acetate is taken with meals

Prednisone 5 mg orally, twice daily, continually for 28 consecutive days (total dose/28-day cycle = 280 mg)

Notes:
- For patients with baseline moderate hepatic impairment (Child-Pugh Class B), reduce the dose of abiraterone acetate to 250 mg once daily
- Avoid abiraterone acetate in patients with baseline severe hepatic impairment (Child-Pugh Class C), as abiraterone acetate has not been studied in this population, and no dose adjustment can be predicted
- Abiraterone acetate is an inhibitor of the polymorphically expressed cytochrome P450 (CYP) enzyme, CYP2D6
  - **Avoid coadministration** of abiraterone acetate with CYP2D6 substrates that have a low therapeutic index. If an alternative treatment cannot be used, exercise caution and consider a dose reduction of concomitantly used CYP2D6 substrates
- Monitor for symptoms and signs of adrenocortical insufficiency. Increased dosage of corticosteroids may be indicated before, during, and after stressful situations
- Monitor for signs and symptoms of mineralocorticoid excess, including hypokalemia, fluid retention, and hypertension. Prednisone dose may have to be supplemented in some patients or augmented with an aldosterone antagonist such as eplerenone
- Use abiraterone acetate with caution in patients with a history of cardiovascular disease. Control hypertension and correct hypokalemia before initiating treatment
- Abiraterone acetate is a substrate of CYP3A4. Avoid or use with caution strong CYP3A4 inhibitors (eg, atazanavir, clarithromycin, indinavir, itraconazole, ketoconazole, nefazodone, nelfinavir, ritonavir, saquinavir, telithromycin, voriconazole) or inducers (eg, carbamazepine, phenobarbital, phenytoin, rifabutin, rifapentine, rifampin) during abiraterone acetate treatment
- Abiraterone acetate was a strong inhibitor of CYP1A2 and CYP2D6, and a moderate inhibitor of CYP2C9, CYP2C19, and CYP3A4/5 in experimental systems. It is not yet known whether its effects on CYP1A2, CYP2C subfamily, or CYP3A subfamily enzymes in in vitro systems are representative of a potential for clinically important drug interactions
- Use abiraterone acetate with caution in patients with a history of cardiovascular disease. The safety of abiraterone acetate in patients with LVEF <50% or NYHA Class III or IV heart failure is not established. Control hypertension and correct hypokalemia before treatment

Supportive Care
Antiemetic prophylaxis
Emetogenic potential is **MINIMAL–LOW**
See Chapter 39 for antiemetic recommendations

Hematopoietic growth factor (CSF) prophylaxis
Primary prophylaxis is NOT indicated
See Chapter 43 for more information

Antimicrobial prophylaxis
Risk of fever and neutropenia is LOW
   Antimicrobial primary prophylaxis to be considered:
   - Antibacterial—not indicated
   - Antifungal—not indicated
   - Antiviral—not indicated unless patient previously had an episode of HSV
See Chapter 47 for more information

Treatment Modification

Adverse Event	Dose Modification
G2 hepatotoxicity	Hold abiraterone acetate until toxicity remits to G ≤1, then resume treatment at a dose of 750 mg once daily
G3 hepatotoxicity (elevations in ALT and/or AST >5 × upper limit of normal [ULN] or total bilirubin >3 × ULN) in a patient with baseline normal hepatic function	Withhold abiraterone acetate. Treatment may be restarted at a dose of 750 mg once daily following return of liver function tests to a patient's baseline or to AST and ALT G ≤1 (2.5 × ULN) and total bilirubin G ≤1 (≤1.5 × ULN). For patients who resume treatment, monitor serum transaminases
G3 hepatotoxicity (elevations in ALT and/or AST >5 × upper limit of normal [ULN] or total bilirubin >3 × ULN) in a patient with baseline normal hepatic impairment on a reduced dose of 750 mg/day because of prior hepatotoxicity at 1000 mg/day	Withhold abiraterone acetate. Treatment may be restarted at a dose of 500 mg once daily following return of liver function tests to a patient's baseline or to AST and ALT G ≤1 (2.5 × ULN) and total bilirubin G ≤1 (≤1.5 × ULN). For patients who resume treatment, monitor serum transaminases
G3 hepatotoxicity (elevations in ALT and/or AST >5 × upper limit of normal [ULN] or total bilirubin >3 × ULN) in a patient with baseline normal hepatic impairment on a reduced dose of 500 mg/day because of prior hepatotoxicity at 750 mg/day	Discontinue abiraterone acetate

(continued)

Treatment Modification
(*continued*)

Adverse Event	Dose Modification
G3 hepatotoxicity (elevations in ALT and/or AST >5 × ULN or total bilirubin >3 × ULN) in a patient with baseline moderate hepatic impairment on a reduced dose of 750 mg abiraterone acetate daily	Discontinue abiraterone acetate
G4 hepatotoxicity (elevations in ALT and/or AST >20 × ULN or total bilirubin >10 × ULN) in a patient with baseline moderate hepatic impairment	Discontinue abiraterone acetate
Hypertension, hypokalemia, and fluid retention caused by mineralocorticoid excess	Withhold abiraterone acetate. Ensure corticosteroids are being administered appropriately. Manage hypokalemia and hypertension
Suspicion of adrenocortical insufficiency	Perform appropriate tests to confirm the diagnosis of adrenocortical insufficiency. Consider administering increased corticosteroid doses during and after stressful situations

Patient Population Studied

A phase-3, double-blind, randomized placebo-controlled trial, in which men with histologically or cytologically confirmed metastatic castration-resistant prostate cancer were enrolled if they had (a) previous treatment with docetaxel and a maximum of 2 previous chemotherapies; (b) PSA progression according to Prostate Cancer Working Group criteria, or radiographic progression in soft tissue or bone ± PSA progression; (c) ongoing androgen deprivation to maintain serum testosterone concentration lower <50 ng/dL (<2.0 nmol/L by radioimmunoassay); and (d) ECOG performance status ≤2

	Abiraterone Acetate + Prednisone	Placebo + Prednisone
Age (years)		
Median (range)	69 (42–95)	69 (39–90)
≥75 years	220/797 (28%)	111/397 (28%)
Disease location		
Bone	709/797 (89%)	357/397 (90%)
Node	361/797 (45%)	164/397 (41%)
Liver	90/797 (11%)	30/397 (8%)
BPI-SF score for pain*		
Number of patients	792	394
Median score (range)	3.0 (0–10)	3.0 (0–10)
Number of previous cytotoxic chemotherapy regimens		
1	558/797 (70%)	275/398 (69%)
2	239/797 (30%)	123/398 (31%)
ECOG performance status		
0 or 1	715/797 (90%)	353/398 (89%)
2	82/797 (10%)	45/398 (11%)
Prostate-specific antigen		
Number of patients	788	393
Median (range), ng/mL	128.8 (0.4–9253.0)	137.7 (0.6–10114.0)
Gleason score at initial diagnosis		
≤7	341/697 (49%)	161/350 (46%)
≥8	356/697 (51%)	189/350 (54%)
PSA at initial diagnosis (ng/mL)		
Number of patients	619	311
Median (range)	27.0 (0.1–16065.9)	35.5 (1.1–7378.0)
Previous cancer therapy		
Surgery	429/797 (54%)	193/398 (49%)
Radiotherapy	570/797 (72%)	285/398 (72%)
Hormonal	796/797 (100%)	396/398 (100%)
Other†	797/797 (100%)	398/398 (100%)
Extent of disease‡		
Viscera, not otherwise specified	1 (0%)	0 (0%)
Lungs	103 (13%)	45 (11%)
Prostate mass	60 (8%)	23 (6%)
Other viscera	46 (6%)	21 (5%)
Other tissue	40 (5%)	20 (5%)

BPI-SF, Brief Pain Inventory-Short Form
*The BPI-SF rates pain on a scale of 0–10: 0–3 = clinically significant pain is absent; 4–10 = clinically significant pain is present; the scores shown are for the worst pain over the previous 24 hours
†Including chemotherapy
‡Data are for the extent of disease in specific/relevant organs; therefore, numbers ≠ 797 and 398

Efficacy
Progression-Free Survival (PFS) and Objective Response OR

	Abiraterone Acetate + Prednisone N = 797 (95% CI)	Placebo + Prednisone N = 398 (95% CI)	Hazard Ratio (95% CI)	p Value
Time to PSA progression (months)*	8.5 (8.3–11.1)	6.6 (5.6–8.3)	0.63 (0.52–0.78)	<0.0001
Radiographic PFS (months)*	5.6 (5.6–6.5)	3.6 (2.9–5.5)	0.66 (0.58–0.76)	<0.0001
PSA response (%)†	235 (29.5%)	22 (5.5%)	—	<0.0001
OR by RECIST (%)‡	118 (14.8%)	13 (3.3%)	—	<0.0001

RECIST, Response Evaluation Criteria in Solid Tumors
Data are median (95% CI) or number (%)
*Calculated from date of randomization to date of PSA progression (per Prostate Specific Antigen Working Group criteria) or date of radiographically documented disease progression or death
†Proportion of patients with a PSA decline of 50% or higher according to Prostate Specific Antigen Working Group criteria; unstratified analysis
‡Additional (not secondary) end point

Overall Survival by Subgroup (Univariate Analysis)

	Abiraterone Acetate + Prednisone		Placebo + Prednisone		
	Events (N)	Median OS (Months; 95% CI)	Events (N)	Median OS (Months; 95% CI)	HR (95% CI)
Baseline ECOG status					
0–1	432/715	17.0 (15.6–17.7)	237/353	12.3 (10.8–14.5)	0.74 (0.63–0.87)
2	69/82	7.3 (6.4–8.6)	37/45	7.0 (4.0–8.1)	0.77 (0.50–1.17)
Pain at study entry					
Pain absent (0–3)	244/440	18.4 (17.2–19.9)	137/219	13.9 (11.7–15.9)	0.69 (0.56–0.85)
Pain present (4–10)	257/357	13.3 (11.1–14.7)	137/179	9.3 (7.9–10.7)	0.78 (0.63–0.96)
Previous lines of chemotherapy					
1	329/557	17.1 (15.6–18.2)	185/275	11.7 (10.4–13.9)	0.71 (0.59–0.85)
2	172/240	14.2 (11.8–15.3)	89/123	10.4 (8.8–13.5)	0.80 (0.61–1.02)
Type of progression before study entry					
PSA progression	126/238	18.3 (16.7–20.8)	79/125	13.6 (10.8–16.8)	0.63 (0.47–0.84)
Radiographic progression ± PSA progression	375/559	14.8 (14.0–16.1)	195/273	10.5 (8.9–12.5)	0.78 (0.65–0.93)
Previous docetaxel usage					
From first docetaxel dose	494/787	32.6 (30.7–35.0)	274/397	27.6 (25.9–30.3)	0.75 (0.65–0.88)
From last docetaxel dose	494/787	23.2 (22.4–24.5)	274/397	19.4 (17.5–20.8)	0.74 (0.64–0.86)
Reason for discontinuation of docetaxel					
Progressive disease	241/362	14.2 (12.0–15.8)	129/182	10.5 (9.3–11.8)	0.77 (0.62–0.97)
All other reasons	258/431	17.0 (15.6–18.2)	145/215	12.6 (10.4–14.9)	0.73 (0.59–0.89)
Treatment of abiraterone acetate plus prednisone started					
≤3 Months after last docetaxel dose	144/227	15.0 (13.7–17.4)	82/112	10.7 (8.9–13.0)	0.62 (0.47–0.83)
>3 Months after last docetaxel dose	346/554	16.1 (14.9–17.3)	190/282	11.8 (10.3–14.6)	0.77 (0.64–0.92)
Docetaxel exposure time					
≤3 Months	98/140	14.6 (11.9–16.7)	51/69	10.8 (8.4–14.9)	0.76 (0.53–1.08)
>3 Months	252/401	16.2 (14.9–17.3)	223/328	11.2 (10.3–13.6)	0.74 (0.63–0.87)

Patients who were not deceased at the time of analysis were censored on the last date the patient was known to be alive or lost to follow-up
Every test was done at a significance level of 0.05
Patient numbers are not consistent across subgroups because of missing data

Toxicity

	Abiraterone Acetate + Prednisone (n = 791)			Placebo + Prednisone (n = 394)		
	All Grades N (%)	G3 N (%)	G4 N (%)	All Grades N (%)	G3 N (%)	G4 N (%)
Hematologic						
Anemia	198 (25%)	53 (7%)	9 (1%)	110 (28%)	26 (7%)	6 (2%)
Thrombocytopenia	30 (4%)	8 (1%)	3 (<1%)	15 (4%)	1 (<1%)	1 (<1%)
Neutropenia	8 (1%)	1 (<1%)	0	2 (<1%)	1 (<1%)	0
Febrile neutropenia	3 (<1%)	0	3 (<1%)	0	0	0
Nonhematologic						
Diarrhea	156 (20%)	8 (1%)	1 (<1%)	58 (15%)	5 (1%)	0
Fatigue	372 (47%)	70 (9%)	2 (<1%)	174 (44%)	38 (10%)	3 (<1%)
Asthenia	122 (15%)	26 (3%)	0	54 (14%)	7 (2%)	1 (<1%)
Back pain	262 (33%)	53 (7%)	3 (<1%)	141 (36%)	39 (10%)	1 (<1%)
Nausea	258 (33%)	16 (2%)	1 (<1%)	130 (33%)	11 (3%)	0
Vomiting	191 (24%)	20 (3%)	1 (<1%)	101 (26%)	12 (3%)	0
Hematuria	73 (9%)	12 (2%)	0	34 (9%)	9 (2%)	0
Abdominal pain	102 (13%)	18 (2%)	0	47 (12%)	8 (2%)	0
Pain in extremity	156 (20%)	23 (3%)	1 (<1%)	82 (21%)	20 (5%)	0
Dyspnea	116 (15%)	12 (2%)	2 (<1%)	49 (12%)	7 (2%)	2 (<1%)
Constipation	223 (28%)	10 (1%)	0	126 (32%)	4 (1%)	0
Pyrexia	80 (10%)	3 (<1%)	0	36 (9%)	5 (1%)	0
Arthralgia	239 (30%)	40 (5%)	0	95 (24%)	17 (4%)	0
Urinary tract infection	105 (13%)	12 (2%)	0	29 (7%)	3 (<1%)	0
Pain	38 (5%)	7 (<1%)	0	21 (5%)	7 (2%)	1 (<1%)
Bone pain	216 (27%)	49 (6%)	2 (<1%)	117 (30%)	27 (7%)	4 (1%)
Adverse Events of Special Interest						
Fluid retention or edema	261 (33%)	18 (2%)	2 (<1%)	94 (24%)	4 (1%)	0
Hypokalemia	143 (18%)	31 (4%)	4 (<1%)	36 (9%)	3 (<1%)	0
Cardiac disorders*	126 (16%)	32 (4%)	9 (1%)	46 (12%)	7 (2%)	2 (<1%)
Abnormalities in LFTs	89 (11%)	28 (4%)	2 (<1%)	35 (9%)	11 (3%)	3 (<1%)
Hypertension	88 (11%)	10 (1%)	0	32 (8%)	1 (<1%)	0

LFTs, Liver function tests
*Cardiac disorders associated with abiraterone acetate treatment as defined by the standardized *Medical Dictionary for Regulatory Activities Queries* included ischemic heart disease, myocardial infarction, supraventricular tachyarrhythmias, ventricular tachyarrhythmias, cardiac failure, and possible arrhythmia-related investigations, signs, and symptoms

Treatment Monitoring

1. CBC before each cycle
2. *Evaluation including PSA:* Every 6 weeks
3. Monitor blood pressure, serum potassium, and symptoms of fluid retention at least monthly
4. Measure serum transaminases (ALT and AST) and bilirubin levels prior to starting treatment with abiraterone acetate, every 2 weeks for the first 3 months of treatment, and monthly thereafter. Modify, interrupt, or discontinue abiraterone acetate dosing as recommended
5. In patients with baseline moderate hepatic impairment receiving a reduced abiraterone acetate dose of 250 mg/day, measure ALT, AST, and bilirubin prior to the start of treatment, every week for the first month, every 2 weeks for the following 2 months of treatment, and monthly, thereafter. Promptly measure serum total bilirubin, AST, and ALT if clinical symptoms or signs suggestive of hepatotoxicity develop
6. For patients who resume treatment after LFTs return to G ≤1 from a G2/3/4 toxicity, monitor serum transaminases and bilirubin at a minimum of every 2 weeks for 3 months and monthly thereafter
7. Monitor for symptoms and signs of adrenocortical insufficiency. Increased dosage of corticosteroids may be indicated before, during, and after stressful situations

ADVANCED DISEASE REGIMEN

ENZALUTAMIDE
METASTATIC CASTRATION-RESISTANT PROSTATE CANCER—PRIOR CHEMOTHERAPY

Scher HI et al. N Engl J Med 2012;367:1187–1197

Enzalutamide 160 mg orally, once daily, continually

Notes:
• Can be taken with or without food
• Swallow capsules whole. Do not chew, dissolve, or open the capsules

Notes:
• If possible, avoid concomitant use of strong CYP2C8 inhibitors. If patients must receive a strong CYP2C8 inhibitor concomitantly, reduce the enzalutamide dose to 80 mg once daily. If coadministration of the strong inhibitor is discontinued, the enzalutamide dose should be returned to the dose used prior to initiation of a strong CYP2C8 inhibitor
• Coadministration of a strong CYP3A4 inhibitor (eg, itraconazole) increased the composite AUC of enzalutamide plus *N*-desmethyl enzalutamide by 1.3-fold in healthy volunteers
• The effects of CYP3A4 inducers on the pharmacokinetics of enzalutamide have not been evaluated in vivo
• Coadministration of enzalutamide with strong CYP3A4 inducers may decrease the plasma exposure of enzalutamide and should be avoided if possible
• Moderate CYP3A4 inducers and St. John's wort may also reduce the plasma exposure of enzalutamide and should be avoided if possible
• Enzalutamide is a strong CYP3A4 inducer and a moderate CYP2C9 and CYP2C19 inducer in humans. At steady state, enzalutamide reduced the plasma exposure to midazolam (CYP3A4 substrate), warfarin (CYP2C9 substrate), and omeprazole (CYP2C19 substrate). Concomitant use of enzalutamide with narrow therapeutic index drugs that are metabolized by CYP3A4, CYP2C9 (eg, phenytoin, warfarin) and CYP2C19 should be avoided, as enzalutamide may decrease their exposure. If coadministration with warfarin cannot be avoided, conduct additional INR monitoring

Treatment Modification

Adverse Event	Treatment Modification
G ≥3 adverse event or an intolerable side effect	Withhold dosing for 1 week or until symptoms improve to G ≤2, then resume at the same or a reduced dose (120 mg or 80 mg daily), if warranted
Occurrence of a seizure	Discontinue enzalutamide

Patient Population Studied

Patients had (a) a histologically or cytologically confirmed diagnosis of prostate cancer; (b) castrate levels of testosterone (<50 ng/dL; [<1.7 nmol/L]); (c) previous treatment with docetaxel; and (d) progressive disease defined according to Prostate Cancer Working Group 2 criteria (including 3 increasing values for PSA or radiographically confirmed progression with or without a rise in the PSA level)

Efficacy

Multivariate Analysis of Hazard Ratios for Death*

Variable	Measurement Estimates		Hazard Ratio for Death (95% CI)[†]
	Coefficient	P Value	
Study treatment (enzalutamide vs. placebo)	−0.54 ± 0.09	<0.001	0.58 (0.49–0.70)
ECOG performance score (0 or 1 vs. 2)	−0.33 ± 0.14	0.02	0.72 (0.55–0.95)
BPI-SF mean pain score (question no. 3) (<4 vs. ≥4)[‡]	−0.23 ± 0.10	0.02	0.79 (0.65–0.97)
Progression at study entry (PSA only vs. radiographic)	−0.29 ± 0.09	0.002	0.75 (0.62–0.90)
Visceral disease at screening (no vs. yes)	−0.47 ± 0.10	<0.001	0.63 (0.52–0.76)

(*continued*)

Efficacy (*continued*)

Secondary End Points Related to Response and Disease Progression§

End Point	Enzalutamide (N = 800)	Placebo (N = 399)	Hazard Ratio (95% CI)	P Value
Confirmed PSA decline§				
≥1 Postbaseline PSA assessment—no. (%)	731 (91)	330 (83)		
PSA response—no./total no. (%)				
Decline ≥50% from baseline	395/731 (54)	5/330 (2)		<0.001
Decline ≥90% from baseline	181/731 (25)	3/330 (1)		<0.001
Soft-tissue objective response				
Patients with measurable disease—no. (%)	446 (56)	208 (52)		
CR or PR—no./total no. (%)	129/446 (29)	8/208 (4)		<0.001
FACT-P quality-of-life response§				
No (%) with ≥1 postbaseline assessment	651 (81)	257 (64)		
Quality-of-life response—no./total no. (%)€	281/651 (43)	47/257 (18)		<0.001
Progression indicators				
Time to PSA progression			0.25 (0.20–0.30)	<0.001
Median, months	8.3	3.0		
95% CI	5.8–8.3	2.9–3.7		
Radiographic progression-free survival			0.40 (0.35–0.47)	<0.001
Median, months	8.3	2.9		
95% CI	8.2–9.4	2.8–3.4		
Time to first skeletal-related event			0.69 (0.57–0.84)	<0.001
Median, months	16.7	13.3		
95% CI	14.6–19.1	9.9–NYR		

BPI-SF, Brief Pain Inventory–Short Form; CI, confidence interval; CR, complete response; ECOG, Eastern Cooperative Oncology Group; FACT-P, Functional Assessment of Cancer Therapy–Prostate; LDH, lactate dehydrogenase; NYR, not yet reached; PR, partial response

*Patients alive at the time of analysis were censored at the date patient was last known to be alive

†Hazard ratios for death were calculated after adjustment for prognostic factors. These included age (<65 years vs. ≥65 years), region (North America vs. other), number of previous chemotherapy regimens (1 vs. 2), and baseline serum PSA level (per increase of 1 ng/mL). The Gleason score for prostate tumors was excluded owing to a large number of missing values

‡On the Brief Pain Inventory–Short Form (BPI-SF) scores of 0–3 indicate clinically significant pain is absent and scores of 4–10 indicate clinically significant pain is present. Higher scores indicate greater pain

§Only patients with both baseline and postbaseline assessments are included

€Defined as 10-point improvement in the global score on the FACT-P questionnaire, as compared with baseline, on 2 consecutive measurements obtained at least 3 weeks apart

Toxicity

Adverse Events, According to Grade

Adverse Event	Enzalutamide (N = 800)		Placebo (N = 399)	
	Any Grade	G ≥3	Any Grade	G ≥3
	Number of Patients (Percent)			
≥1 Adverse event	785 (98)	362 (45)	390 (98)	212 (53)
Any serious adverse event	268 (34)	227 (28)	154 (39)	134 (34)
Discontinuation owing to adverse event	61 (8)	37 (5)	39 (10)	28 (7)
Adverse event leading to death	23 (3)	23 (3)	14 (4)	14 (4)
Frequent adverse events more common with enzalutamide*				
Fatigue	269 (34)	50 (6)	116 (29)	29 (7)
Diarrhea	171 (21)	9 (1)	70 (18)	1 (<1)
Hot flash	162 (20)	0	41 (10)	0
Musculoskeletal pain	109 (14)	8 (1)	40 (10)	1 (<1)
Headache	93 (12)	6 (<1)	22 (6)	0
Clinically significant adverse events				
Cardiac disorder				
Any	49 (6)	7 (1)	30 (8)	8 (2)
Myocardial infarction	2 (<1)	2 (<1)	2 (<1)	2 (<1)
Abnormality on liver-function testing†	8 (1)	3 (<1)	6 (2)	3 (<1)
Seizure	5 (<1)	5 (<1)	0	0

*Includes adverse events that occurred in >10% of patients in the enzalutamide group and those that occurred in the enzalutamide group at a rate ≥2% higher than in the placebo group
†Includes hyperbilirubinemia and increased levels of aspartate or alanine aminotransferases

Treatment Monitoring

Evaluation including PSA: Every 6 weeks

ADVANCED DISEASE REGIMEN
CABAZITAXEL + PREDNISONE

de Bono JS et al. Lancet 2010;376:1147–1154

Note: Severe hypersensitivity reactions can occur with cabazitaxel administration. These may include generalized rash/erythema, hypotension, and bronchospasm. Severe hypersensitivity reactions require immediate discontinuation of cabazitaxel infusion and administration of appropriate therapy. Patients should receive primary prophylaxis against hypersensitivity reactions as described below. Cabazitaxel must not be given to patients who have a history of severe hypersensitivity reactions to other drugs formulated with polysorbate 80, such as fosaprepitant dimeglumine (the parenteral formulation of aprepitant [Emend]), darbepoetin alfa, docetaxel, etoposide, recombinant human papillomavirus quadrivalent vaccine (Gardasil), and various vaccines. Patients should be observed closely for hypersensitivity reactions, especially during the first and second infusions. Hypersensitivity reactions may occur within a few minutes following the initiation of the cabazitaxel infusion, thus facilities and equipment for the treatment of hypotension and bronchospasm should be available

Premedication:
At least 30 minutes prior to each cabazitaxel dose, administer the following medications to reduce the risk and/or severity of hypersensitivity:

- **Diphenhydramine** 25 mg, or an equivalent H_1-receptor antihistamine, orally or intravenously
- **Dexamethasone** 8 mg or an equipotent glucocorticoid
- **Ranitidine** 50 mg intravenously or 150 mg orally, or an equivalent histamine (H_2)-receptor antagonist

Cabazitaxel 25 mg/m² intravenously over 60 minutes, diluted in a volume of 0.9% sodium chloride injection or 5% dextrose injection sufficient to produce a solution with concentration within the range 0.1–0.26 mg/mL, on day 1, every 3 weeks (total dosage/cycle = 25 mg/m²)

Prednisone 10 mg/day orally, continually for 21 consecutive days (total dose/21-day cycle = 210 mg)

Note:
- Cabazitaxel is extensively metabolized in the liver (>95%), primarily by cytochrome P450 (CYP) CYP3A4/5 enzymes (80–90%), and, to a lesser extent, by the polymorphically expressed enzyme, CYP2C8. Consequently hepatic impairment is likely to increase cabazitaxel concentrations
- Although no formal drug interaction trials with cabazitaxel have been conducted, clinicians should use caution with respect to the following:
  - *CYP3A4 inhibitors:* Concomitant administration of strong CYP3A subfamily inhibitors (eg, atazanavir, clarithromycin, indinavir, itraconazole, ketoconazole, nefazodone, nelfinavir, ritonavir, saquinavir, telithromycin, voriconazole) is expected to increase concentrations of cabazitaxel. Therefore, coadministration with strong CYP3A inhibitors should be avoided. Caution should be exercised with concomitant use of moderate CYP3A subfamily inhibitors
  - *CYP3A4 inducers:* The concomitant administration of strong CYP3A subfamily inducers (eg, carbamazepine, phenobarbital, phenytoin, rifabutin, rifapentine, rifampin) is expected to decrease cabazitaxel concentrations. Therefore, coadministration with strong CYP3A inducers should be avoided. In addition, patients should also refrain from taking St. John's wort

Supportive Care
Antiemetic prophylaxis
Emetogenic potential is **LOW**
See Chapter 39 for antiemetic recommendations

Hematopoietic growth factor (CSF) prophylaxis
Primary prophylaxis is NOT indicated
See Chapter 43 for more information

Antimicrobial prophylaxis
Risk of fever and neutropenia is LOW
Antimicrobial primary prophylaxis to be considered:
- Antibacterial—not indicated
- Antifungal—not indicated
- Antiviral—not indicated unless patient previously had an episode of HSV

See Chapter 47 for more information

Treatment Modifications

Adverse Event	Dose Modification
Prolonged grade ≥3 neutropenia (>1 week) despite appropriate medication including filgrastim	Delay treatment until neutrophil count is >1500 cells/mm³, then reduce cabazitaxel dosage to 20 mg/m². Use filgrastim for secondary prophylaxis
Prolonged grade ≥3 neutropenia (>1 week) despite appropriate medication including filgrastim at a cabazitaxel dosage of 20 mg/m²	Discontinue cabazitaxel
Febrile neutropenia	Delay treatment until improvement or resolution, and until neutrophil count is >1500 cells/mm³, then resume treatment with cabazitaxel dosage decreased to 20 mg/m². Use filgrastim for secondary prophylaxis
Febrile neutropenia at a cabazitaxel dosage of 20 mg/m²	Discontinue cabazitaxel
Grade ≥3 diarrhea or diarrhea that persists despite appropriate medication, fluid, and electrolytes replacement	Delay treatment until improvement or resolution, then resume treatment with cabazitaxel dosage decreased to 20 mg/m²
Grade ≥3 diarrhea or diarrhea that persists despite appropriate medication, fluid, and electrolytes replacement at a cabazitaxel dosage of 20 mg/m²	Discontinue cabazitaxel
Total bilirubin ≥ ULN, or AST and/or ALT ≥1.5 times ULN)	Discontinue cabazitaxel

Toxicity* (N = 371)

	% All Grades	% G ≥3
Hematologic		
Neutropenia	94	82
Febrile neutropenia	—	8
Leukopenia	96	68
Anemia	97	11
Thrombocytopenia	47	4
Nonhematologic		
Diarrhea	47	6
Fatigue	37	5
Asthenia	20	5
Back pain	16	4
Nausea	34	2
Vomiting	23	2
Hematuria	17	2
Abdominal pain	12	2
Pain in extremity	8	2
Dyspnea	12	1
Constipation	20	1
Pyrexia	12	1
Arthralgia	11	1
Urinary tract infection	7	1
Pain	5	1
Bone pain	5	1

*NCI Common Terminology Criteria for Adverse Events, version 3

Efficacy

	Mitoxantrone	Cabazitaxel	p-Value
Tumor Response Rate*			
Number of evaluable patients	204	201	
Response rate (%)	4.4%	14.4%	0.0005
PSA Response Rate†			
Number of evaluable patients	325	329	
Response rate (%)	17.8%	39.2%	0.0002
Pain Response Rate‡			
Number of evaluable patients	168	174	
Response rate (%)	7.7%	9.2%	0.63
Progression			
Number pts in intention-to-treat analysis	377	378	
Median time to tumor progression (months)	5.4	8.8	<0.0001
Median time to PSA progression (months)	3.1	6.4	0.001
Median time to pain progression (months)§	NR	11.1 (2.9-NR)	0.52

NR, Not reached
*Tumor response was evaluated only for patients with measurable disease according to RECIST
†PSA response was defined as ≥50% reduction in serum PSA concentrations, established only for patients with a serum PSA concentration of 20 mcg/L or more at baseline, confirmed by a repeat PSA measurement after at least 3 weeks
‡Pain response was established only for patients with a median present pain intensity (PPI) score ≥2, a mean analgesic score (AS) ≥10 points at baseline, or both, and was defined as a reduction from baseline median PPI score ≥2 points without an increased AS or a decrease ≥50% in the AS without an increase in the PPI score, maintained for at least 3 weeks
§Data for 265 patients in the cabazitaxel group and 279 patients in the mitoxantrone group were censored as a result of ≥2 PPI or AS assessments or both, being missed during the same week (unless a complete evaluation of ≥5 values showed pain progression)

Patient Population Studied

A study of 755 patients with pathologically proven castration-refractory prostate cancer with documented disease progression during or after completion of docetaxel treatment. Eligible patients had an Eastern Cooperative Oncology Group performance status of 0–2. Patients with measurable disease were required to have documented disease progression by Response Evaluation Criteria in Solid Tumors (RECIST) criteria with at least 1 metastatic visceral or soft-tissue lesion. Patients with nonmeasurable disease were required to have rising serum prostate-specific antigen (PSA) concentrations (at least 2 consecutive increases relative to a reference value measured at least a week apart) or the appearance of at least 1 new demonstrable radiographic lesion. Additional inclusion criteria were: previous and ongoing castration by orchiectomy, LHRH agonists, or both interventions

Therapy Monitoring

1. *Before each cycle:* Physical exam, CBC and LFTs
2. *Evaluation including PSA:* Every 6 weeks to every 3 months

ADVANCED DISEASE REGIMEN

KETOCONAZOLE + HYDROCORTISONE

Bok RA, Small EJ. Drug Saf 1999;20:451–458
Small EJ et al. J Urol 1997;157:1204–1207

Ketoconazole 400 mg orally every 8 hours, continually
Hydrocortisone 20 mg orally every morning, continually
Hydrocortisone 10 mg orally every evening, continually

Notes:

1. Ketoconazole absorption can be decreased with concurrent use of antacids, H_2-antagonist antihistamines, and proton pump inhibitors (PPIs). Avoid H_2-antagonists and PPIs. If antacid treatment is needed, ketoconazole should be taken at least 2 hours before antacids

2. To avoid nausea, start ketoconazole at a low dose (eg, 200 mg 3 times daily) and gradually increase to full doses after several days

Supportive Care

Antiemetic prophylaxis
The regimen is not emetogenic. Primary prophylaxis is not indicated
See Chapter 39 for antiemetic recommendations

Hematopoietic growth factor (CSF) prophylaxis
Primary prophylaxis is NOT indicated
See Chapter 43 for more information

Antimicrobial prophylaxis
Risk of fever and neutropenia is LOW
Antimicrobial primary prophylaxis to be considered:
• Antibacterial—not indicated
• Antifungal—not indicated
• Antiviral—not indicated unless patient previously had an episode of HSV
See Chapter 47 for more information

Patient Population Studied

A study of 48 patients with castration-refractory metastatic prostate cancer with progression after antiandrogen withdrawal

Efficacy

>50% PSA decline (≥8 weeks)	62.5%
Median change in PSA	79.5% decline
Mean duration of response	3.5 months

Small EJ et al. J Urol 1997;157:1204–1207

Treatment Modifications

Adverse Event	Dose Modification
Toxicity G ≥2	Hold ketoconazole until adverse events have resolved

Note: Ketoconazole is a potent inhibitor of the cytochrome P450 enzyme, CYP3A4. It has been reported to inhibit the metabolism of many drugs and drug metabolites that are metabolized by CYP3A-subfamily enzymes, resulting in elevated concentrations of the drugs. Affected drugs include (but are not limited to):

1. Warfarin (enhances anticoagulant effect)
2. Dihydropyridine calcium channel antagonists (eg, amlodipine, felodipine, nifedipine)
3. Loratadine
4. Some HIV protease inhibitors (saquinavir, indinavir and nelfinavir)
5. Statin hypolipidemic drugs (HMG-CoA reductase inhibitors)
6. Many other drugs and natural products

Drugs that are susceptible to pharmacokinetic interactions because of concomitant use with ketoconazole may require dose or schedule adjustments. It may be prudent to consider alternative treatment options, or if clinically appropriate, discontinue drugs that are known to interact with ketoconazole

Therapy Monitoring

Monthly: LFTs including AST, ALT, bilirubin, alkaline phosphatase, PSA if indicated

Notes

1. Liver transaminases may be transiently increased. Therapy can be continued in a setting of a grade 1 increase in transaminases with close monitoring, but there is a small risk (0.1–1%) of idiosyncratic hepatitis, which can be fatal
2. Some clinicians administer higher doses of hydrocortisone (30 mg in the morning and 20 mg in the evening)
3. In addition to glucocorticoid replacement, some patients require mineralocorticoid supplementation with fludrocortisone 100–200 mcg daily orally in the morning

Toxicity (N = Varies)

	% Patients	
	Mild (G1/2)	Moderate/ Severe
Nausea/vomiting	10	—
LFT abnormalities*	4–20	—
Fulminant hepatitis	—	0.1–1
Fatigue	6	—
Edema	6	—
"Sticky skin"[†,‡]	10	—
Rash[‡]	4	—
Nail dystrophy[‡]	Common	—
Dry mouth[‡]	Often	—
Gynecomastia[§]	10–15	—
Adrenal insufficiency[¶]	Varies	
Impotence	Anticipated	

*Asymptomatic increases; usually resolve with discontinuation of treatment
[†]Subjective sensation of stickiness to the skin, usually noted in axillary area
[‡]Cutaneous and mucosal effects probably related to inhibitory effect on retinoic acid metabolism
[§]Not observed with ketoconazole 200–400 mg/day, but may occur with higher doses
[¶]Steroid replacement recommended

From Bok RA, Small EJ. Drug Saf 1999;20:451–458

ADVANCED DISEASE REGIMEN

RADIUM-223
METASTATIC CASTRATION-RESISTANT PROSTATE CANCER WITH BONE METASTASES

Parker et al. N Engl J Med 2013;369:213–223
XOFIGO (radium 223) Package Insert (http://labeling.bayerhealthcare.com/html/products/pi/Xofigo_PI.pdf)

Radium (Ra)-223 dichloride 50 kBq (^{223}Ra 1.35 μCi) per kilogram of body weight by slow intravenous injection over 1 minute every 4 weeks for 6 injections

Note:

• Flush the intravenous access line or cannula with 0.9% sodium chloride injection before and after injection of radium-223

• Safety and efficacy beyond 6 injections with radium-223 have not been studied

Calculate volume to be administered to a given patient using the:

• Patient's body weight (kg)

• Dosage level 50 kBq/kg body weight or 1.35 μCi/kg body weight

• Radioactivity concentration of the product (1000 kBq/mL; 27 μCi/mL) at the reference date

• Decay correction factor to correct for physical decay of radium-223

Calculate total volume to be administered as follows:

$$\text{Volume to be administered (mL)} = \frac{\text{Body weight in kg} \times 50 \text{ kBq/kg body weight}}{\text{Decay factor} \times 1000 \text{ kBq/mL}}$$

OR

$$\text{Volume to be administered (mL)} = \frac{\text{Body weight in kg} \times 1.35 \text{ μCi/kg body weight}}{\text{Decay factor} \times 27 \text{ μCi/mL}}$$

Decay Correction Factor Table

Days from Reference Date	Decay Factor	Days from Reference Date	Decay Factor
−14	2.296	0	0.982
−13	2.161	1	0.925
−12	2.034	2	0.870
−11	1.914	3	0.819
−10	1.802	4	0.771
−9	1.696	5	0.725
−8	1.596	6	0.683
−7	1.502	7	0.643
−6	1.414	8	0.605
−5	1.330	9	0.569
−4	1.252	10	0.536
−3	1.178	11	0.504
−2	1.109	12	0.475
−1	1.044	13	0.447
		14	0.420

The Decay Correction Factor Table is corrected to 12 noon Central Standard Time (CST). To determine the decay correction factor, count the number before or after the reference date. The Decay Correction Factor Table includes a correction to account for the 7-hour time difference between 12 noon European Time (CET) at the site of manufacture and 12 noon U.S. CST, which is 7 hours earlier than CET

(continued)

(continued)

Note: Immediately before and after administration, the net patient dose of administered radium-223 should be determined by measurement in an appropriate radioisotope dose calibrator that has been calibrated with a National Institute of Standards and Technology (NIST) traceable radium-223 standard and corrected for decay using the date and time of calibration

Safety Information: Radium-223 is primarily an alpha emitter, with 95.3% of energy emitted as alpha particles. Only 3.6% is emitted as beta particles and 1.1% as gamma radiation. Thus the external radiation exposure associated with handling of patient doses is expected to be low, because the typical treatment activity will be <8000 kBq (<216 µCi). Nevertheless care should be used as follows:

Precautions:
- The administration of radium-223 is associated with potential risks to other persons from radiation or contamination from spills of bodily fluids such as urine, feces, or vomit. Therefore, radiation protection precautions must be taken in accordance with national and local regulations
- Whenever possible, patients should use a toilet (commode) and the toilet should be flushed several times after each use. When handling bodily fluids, simply wearing gloves and hand washing will protect caregivers. Clothing soiled with radium-223 or patient fecal matter or urine should be washed promptly and separately from other clothing

Instructions to Patients:
- Stay well hydrated and monitor oral intake, fluid status, and urine output. Report signs of dehydration
- There are no restrictions regarding contact with other people after receiving radium-223. Follow good hygiene practices for at least 1 week after the last injection so as to minimize radiation exposure from bodily fluids to household members and caregivers
- Flush toilets several times after each use
- Promptly wash clothing soiled with fecal matter or urine separately from other clothing
- Caregivers should use universal precautions when handling body fluids to avoid contamination. When handling bodily fluids, wearing gloves and hand washing will protect caregivers
- Patients who are sexually active should use condoms and their female partners of reproductive potential should use a highly effective method of birth control during treatment and for 6 months following completion of radium-223 treatment

Toxicity

Adverse Events That Occurred in at Least 5% of Patients in Either Study Group in the Safety Population*

Adverse Event	Radium-223 (N = 600)				Placebo (N = 301)			
	% All Grades	% G3	% G4	% G5	% All Grades	% G3	% G4	% G5
Hematologic								
Anemia	31	11	2	0	31	12	1	<1
Thrombocytopenia	12	3	3	<1	6	2	<1	0
Neutropenia	5	2	1	0	1	1	0	0
Nonhematologic								
Constipation	18	1	0	0	15	2	0	0
Diarrhea	25	2	0	0	15	2	0	0
Nausea	36	2	0	0	35	2	0	0
Vomiting	18	2	0	0	14	2	0	0
Asthenia	6	1	0	0	6	1	0	0
Fatigue	26	4	1	0	26	5	1	0
Deterioration general physical health	4	2	<1	1	7	3	1	1
Peripheral edema	13	2	0	0	10	1	<1	0
Pyrexia	6	1	0	0	6	1	0	0
Pneumonia	3	2	0	1	5	2	1	0
Urinary tract infection	8	1	0	0	9	1	<1	<1

(continued)

Toxicity (continued)

Adverse Event	Radium-223 (N = 600)				Placebo (N = 301)			
	% All Grades	% G3	% G4	% G5	% All Grades	% G3	% G4	% G5
Weight loss	12	1	0	0	15	2	0	0
Anorexia	17	2	0	0	18	1	0	0
Decreased appetite	6	<1	0	0	4	0	0	0
Bone pain	50	20	1	0	62	25	1	0
Muscular weakness	2	<1	<1	0	6	2	0	0
Pathologic fracture	4	2	0	0	5	3	<1	0
Progression malignant neoplasm	13	2	1	9	15	1	<1	11
Dizziness	7	<1	0	0	9	1	0	0
Spinal cord compression	4	2	1	<1	8	5	<1	0
Insomnia	4	0	0	0	7	<1	0	0
Hematuria	5	1	0	0	5	1	0	0
Urinary retention	4	2	0	0	6	2	0	0
Dyspnea	8	2	<1	<1	9	2	0	1

*Only 1 G5 hematologic adverse event was considered possibly related to study drug: thrombocytopenia in 1 patient in the radium-223 group

Patient Population Studied

Inclusion criteria: (a) histologically confirmed, progressive castration-resistant prostate cancer (b) 2 or more bone metastases detected on skeletal scintigraphy and no known visceral metastases; (c) received docetaxel, or were not healthy enough or declined to receive it, or it was not available; (d) symptomatic disease with regular use of analgesic medication or treatment with external beam radiation therapy required for cancer-related bone pain within the previous 12 weeks; (e) a baseline PSA ≥5 ng/mL or with evidence of progressively increasing PSA values (2 consecutive increases over the previous reference value); (f) an ECOG performance-status score of 0–2; and (g) a life expectancy ≥6 months. Exclusion criteria: (a) chemotherapy within the previous 4 weeks; (b) previous hemibody external radiotherapy; (c) systemic radiotherapy with radioisotopes within the previous 24 weeks; (d) a blood transfusion or use of erythropoietin-stimulating agents within the previous 4 weeks; (e) malignant lymphadenopathy ≥3 cm in the short-axis diameter; (f) history of or the presence of visceral metastases; and (g) imminent or established spinal cord compression

Castration-resistant disease was defined as a serum testosterone level ≤50 ng/dL (≤1.7 nmol/L) after bilateral orchiectomy or during maintenance treatment consisting of androgen-ablation therapy with a luteinizing hormone-releasing hormone agonist or polyestradiol phosphate. Patients with castration-resistant disease during maintenance treatment were required to continue that treatment throughout the study

Baseline Characteristics of the Patients*

Characteristic	Radium-223 (N = 614)	Placebo (N = 307)
Age		
Median (range)—years	71 (49–90)	71 (44–94)
>75 years—no. (%)	171 (28)	90 (29)
Total alkaline phosphatase—no. (%)		
<220 U/L	348 (57)	169 (55)
≥220 U/L	266 (43)	138 (45)

Treatment Modifications

None

Treatment Monitoring

1. Weekly CBC with differential and platelet count
2. Monitor oral intake, fluid status, and urine output during treatment with radium-223
   - Instruct patients to report signs of dehydration, hypovolemia, urinary retention, or renal failure or insufficiency

(continued)

Patient Population Studied (*continued*)

Characteristic	Radium-223 (N = 614)	Placebo (N = 307)
Current use of bisphosphonates—no. (%)		
Yes	250 (41)	124 (40)
No	364 (59)	183 (60)
Any previous use of docetaxel—no. (%)		
Yes	352 (57)	174 (57)
No	262 (43)	133 (43)
ECOG performance-status score—no. (%)		
0	165 (27)	78 (25)
1	371 (60)	187 (61)
≥2	77 (13)	41 (13)
WHO ladder for cancer pain—no. (%)[†]		
1 (mild pain/no opioid use)	257 (42)	137 (45)
2 (moderate pain/occasional opioid use)	151 (25)	78 (25)
3 (severe pain/regular daily opioid use)	194 (32)	90 (29)
Extent of disease—no. (%)		
<6 metastases	100 (16)	38 (12)
6–20 metastases	262 (43)	147 (48)
>20 metastases	195 (32)	91 (30)
Superscan[‡]	54 (9)	30 (10)
External beam radiation therapy within 12 weeks after screening—no. (%)		
Yes	99 (16)	48 (16)
No	515 (84)	259 (84)
Median biochemical values (Range)		
Hemoglobin (normal range = 13.4–17.0 g/dL)	12.2 (8.5–15.7)	12.1 (8.5–16.4)
Albumin (normal range: 36–45 g/L)	40 (24–53)	40 (23–50)
Total alkaline phosphatase >105 U/L	211 (32–6431)	223 (29–4805)
Lactate dehydrogenase >255 U/L	315 (76–2171)	336 (132–3856)
PSA >3.999 ng/mL	146 (3.8–6026)	173 (1.5–14500)

ECOG, Eastern Cooperative Oncology Group
*Percentages may not sum to 100 due to rounding
[†]A total of 12 patients in the radium-223 group (2%) and 2 patients in the placebo group (1%) had no pain or analgesic use at baseline
[‡]Superscan refers to a bone scan showing diffuse, intense skeletal uptake of the tracer without renal and background activity

Efficacy

Overall Survival and Subgroup Analyses of Hazard Ratios for Death

End Point	Radium-223 (N = 614)	Placebo (N = 307)	Hazard Ratio (95% CI)	P Value
Median overall survival, months	14.9	11.3	0.70 (0.58–0.83)	<0.001
Total AP at baseline				
<220 U/L	—	—	0.82 (0.64–1.07)	—
≥220 U/L	—	—	0.62 (0.49–0.79)	—
Current bisphosphonate use				
Yes	—	—	0.70 (0.52–0.93)	—
No	—	—	0.74 (0.59–0.92)	—
Previous docetaxel use				
Yes	—	—	0.71 (0.56–0.89)	—
No	—	—	0.74 (0.56–0.99)	—
ECOG performance-status score				
0 or 1	—	—	0.68 (0.56–0.82)	—
≥2	—	—	0.82 (0.50–1.35)	—
Extent of disease				
<6 metastases	—	—	0.95 (0.46–1.95)	—
6–20 metastases	—	—	0.71 (0.54–0.92)	—
>20 metastases	—	—	0.64 (0.47–0.88)	—
Superscan*	—	—	0.71 (0.40–1.27)	—
Opioid use				
Yes	—	—	0.68 (0.54–0.86)	—
No	—	—	0.70 (0.52–0.93)	—

Main Secondary Efficacy End Points in the Intention-to-Treat Population

End Point	Radium-223 (N = 614)	Placebo (N = 307)	Hazard Ratio (95% CI)	P Value
Median time to first symptomatic skeletal event	15.6 mo	9.8 mo	0.66 (0.52–0.83)	<0.001
Median time to increase in total alkaline phosphatase	7.4 mo	3.8 mo	0.17 (0.13–0.22)	<0.001
Median time to increase in PSA level	3.6 mo	3.4 mo	0.64 (0.54–0.77)	<0.001
≥30% reduction in total alkaline phosphatase	233/497 (47)	7/211 (3)	—	<0.001
Normalization of total alkaline phosphatase	109/321 (34)	2/140 (1)	—	<0.001

*Superscan refers to a bone scan showing diffuse, intense skeletal uptake of the tracer without renal and background activity

REGIMENS

HORMONAL AGENTS

Bolla M et al. Lancet 2002;360:103–108
Delaere KPJ, Van Thillo EL. Semin Oncol 1991;18(5 Suppl 6):13–18
Iversen P et al. J Urol 2000;164:1579–1582
Janknegt RA. Cancer 1993;72(12 Suppl 17):3874–3877
Janknegt RA et al. J Urol 1993;149:77–83
Periti P et al. Clin Pharmacokinet 2002;41:485–504
Tyrrell CJ. Eur Urol 1994;26(Suppl 1):15–19

Treatment options:
1. Surgical castration: Orchiectomy
2. Medical castration: LHRH agonists
3. Nonsteroidal antiandrogens
4. Androgen-deprivation therapy (ADT)
   • GnRH antagonist
   • Orchiectomy + antiandrogen
   • LHRH agonist + antiandrogen

LHRH agonists:
1. **Leuprolide depot** 7.5 mg intramuscularly every month
2. **Leuprolide depot** 22.5 mg intramuscularly every 3 months
3. **Leuprolide depot** 30 mg intramuscularly every 4 months
4. **Leuprolide depot** 45 mg intramuscularly every 6 months
5. **Goserelin implant** 3.6 mg subcutaneously every 4 weeks
6. **Goserelin implant** 10.8 mg subcutaneously every 3 months

Nonsteroidal antiandrogens:
1. **Flutamide** 250 mg/dose orally 3 times per day, continually
2. **Bicalutamide** 50 mg or 150 mg/day if given as monotherapy orally, continually
3. **Nilutamide** 300 mg/day orally for 1 month with castration, followed by nilutamide 150 mg/day orally, continually

GnRH antagonist
Degarelix, starting dose, 240 mg given as two subcutaneous injections of 120 mg in the first month followed by maintenance dose of 80 mg given as one subcutaneous injection monthly thereafter

Supportive Care
Antiemetic prophylaxis
The regimens are not emetogenic. Primary prophylaxis is not indicated
See Chapter 39 for antiemetic recommendations

Hematopoietic growth factor (CSF) prophylaxis
Primary prophylaxis is NOT indicated
See Chapter 43 for more information

Antimicrobial prophylaxis
Risk of fever and neutropenia is LOW
Antimicrobial primary prophylaxis to be considered:
• Antibacterial—not indicated
• Antifungal—not indicated
• Antiviral—not indicated unless patient previously had an episode of HSV
See Chapter 47 for more information

Efficacy

Metastatic disease
1. LHRH agonists >85% response rate
2. No significant differences among LHRH agonists
3. Single-agent antiandrogen therapy may be inferior to medical (LHRH agonist) or surgical castration
4. Use of combined androgen blockade (CAB) as frontline therapy is controversial with limited evidence of clinical benefit

Locally advanced disease
Concurrent radiation and hormonal therapy in locally advanced disease appears to have a survival benefit. LHRH agonist + an antiandrogen are used for up to 3 months before, during, and for 3 years after radiation treatment

Bolla M et al. Lancet 2002;360:103–108
Laverdière J et al. Int J Radiat Oncol Biol Phys 1997;37:247–252
Prostate Cancer Trialists' Collaborative Group. Lancet 2000;355:1491–1498
Seidenfeld J et al. Ann Intern Med 2000;132:566–577. Erratum in: Ann Intern Med 2005;143:764–765; comment in: Ann Intern Med 2000;132:584–585

Patient Population Studied

Patients with metastatic and locally advanced prostate cancer treated with hormonal therapy

Therapy Monitoring

All antiandrogens
1. *Monthly for the first 4 months:* LFTs
2. *Every 2–3 months after the first 4 months:* LFTs

Nilutamide
1. Baseline chest x-ray before therapy
2. *For respiratory symptoms:* Discontinue therapy pending evaluation

Wysowski DK, Fourcroy JL. J Urol 1996;155:209–212

Toxicity

Common Toxicities of Androgen Deprivation

Hot flashes	LHRH Ag > AA
Loss of libido, impotence	LHRH Ag >> AA
Bone and muscle loss	LHRH Ag >> AA
Breast tenderness	AA >> LHRH Ag
Gynecomastia	AA >> LHRH Ag
Skin and hair changes	N/A
Weight gain	N/A
Asthenia	N/A

AA, antiandrogens; LHRH Ag, LHRH agonists

Toxicities of Individual Androgen Therapies

	% Patients
LHRH Agonists	
Tumor flare	Variable
Injection-site reactions	Variable
Flutamide	
Gynecomastia	45–50
Diarrhea	20
Nausea/vomiting	5
Hepatitis	2.5
Vertigo	2.5
Hot flashes	2.5
Bicalutamide	
Gynecomastia	49
Breast tenderness	40
Constipation	14
Aggravation reaction	13
Hot flashes	13
Asthenia	12
Urinary retention	10
Diarrhea	6
Nausea/vomiting	5
Nilutamide	
Hot flashes	28
Visual disturbance*	27–50
Nausea	10 (7–20)
Dyspnea	6
Interstitial pneumonitis	1–2
Gynecomastia	4
Alcohol intolerance	5–19
Increased LFTs†	4–8
Anemia	4

*Includes decreased adaptation to darkness, blurred vision
†Transient in a majority of patients

Notes

1. For patients with metastatic prostate cancer being treated with an LHRH agonist alone, a testosterone level should be checked at 1 month. If it is >20 ng/dL, consider orchiectomy or adding antiandrogen

2. Concurrent antiandrogen therapy can be used with LHRH agonist for the first 2–4 weeks of treatment to avoid tumor flare

3. Antiandrogen withdrawal should be considered the first therapeutic maneuver in men whose disease has progressed after treatment with combined androgen blockade. Approximately 20% of patients have a significant decrease in serum PSA when antiandrogen is withdrawn

4. Degarelix binds to the GnRH receptor in the pituitary gland and blocks LH/FSH release from the pituitary. Patients typically achieve castrate levels of testosterone by day 3 of treatment without a testosterone surge. A Phase 3, one year multicenter, randomized, open-label trial compared the efficacy and safety of degarelix with leuprolide. Six-hundred and ten patients with all stages of histologically confirmed prostate cancer for whom androgen deprivation therapy was indicated were enrolled. Patients receiving degarelix showed a significantly lower risk of PSA progression or death compared with leuprolide (p = 0.05). PSA recurrences occurred primarily in patients with advanced disease and exclusively in those with baseline PSA >20 ng/mL. The latter had a significantly longer time to PSA recurrence with degarelix. The results suggest degarelix offers improved PSA control compared with leuprolide. However, further studies are warranted to confirm these findings

5. With acute cord compression or other oncologic emergency caused by a growing prostate tumor, Degarelix is the preferred treatment

Kelly WK, Scher HI. J Urol 1993;149:607–609
Pont A. J Urol 1987;137:902–904
Tombal et al. Eur Urol 2010;57:836–842

IMMUNOTHERAPY REGIMEN
SIPULEUCEL-T

Kantoff PW et al. N Engl J Med 2010;363:411–422

General notes:
- Patients are scheduled for 3 leukapheresis procedures (at weeks 0, 2, and 4), each followed approximately 3 days later by infusion of sipuleucel-T
- Infusions are prepared from PBMCs collected by means of a single standard leukapheresis processing 1.5 to 2 times a patient's estimated blood volume
- Sipuleucel-T is prepared at a designated manufacturing facility by culturing APCs for 36–44 hours at 37°C (98.6°F) with media containing PA2024. The cells are washed before final formulation

Premedication:
Acetaminophen 650 mg orally approximately 30 minutes prior to the administration of sipuleucel-T, *and*
Diphenhydramine 25–50 mg, or an equivalent H_1-receptor antihistamine orally approximately 30 minutes prior to the administration of sipuleucel-T

Sipuleucel-T suspension for intravenous infusion containing a minimum of 50 million autologous CD54+ cells activated with PAP-GM-CSF/dose in 250 mL lactated Ringer injection, intravenously over a period of approximately 60 minutes. Administer a total of 3 doses at approximately 2-week intervals (total dose/single treatment is at least 50 million autologous CD54+ cells activated with PAP-GM-CSF)

Notes for acute infusion reactions: Interrupt or slow infusion depending on the severity of the reaction. Administer appropriate medical therapy including:
- **Diphenhydramine** 25–50 mg, or an equivalent H_1-receptor antihistamine, intravenously
- **Ranitidine** 50 mg, **cimetidine** 300 mg, **famotidine** 20 mg, or an equivalent histamine receptor [H_2]-subtype antagonist, intravenously over 15–30 minutes
- *Note:* In healthy subjects, cimetidine reduces the clearance and volume of distribution of meperidine; thus, use caution when these drugs are used concomitantly
- **Meperidine** 10–25 mg intravenously as needed for chills

Important:
- Sipuleucel-T is for *autologous use only*. Before infusion, confirm that a patient's identity matches patient identifiers on the infusion containers
- Do not initiate infusion of expired sipuleucel-T. If, for any reason, a patient is unable to receive a scheduled infusion of sipuleucel-T, the patient will need to undergo an additional leukapheresis procedure if the course of treatment is to be continued. Patients should be advised of this possibility prior to initiating treatment
- The sipuleucel-T infusion bag must remain within its insulated polyurethane container until the time of administration. Do not remove the insulated polyurethane container from its outer cardboard shipping box
- DO NOT USE a cell filter to administer sipuleucel-T

Supportive Care
Antiemetic prophylaxis
Emetogenic potential is **MINIMAL**
See Chapter 39 for antiemetic recommendations

Hematopoietic growth factor (CSF) prophylaxis
Primary prophylaxis is NOT indicated
See Chapter 43 for more information

Antimicrobial prophylaxis
Risk of fever and neutropenia is LOW
 Antimicrobial primary prophylaxis to be considered:
 - Antibacterial—not indicated
 - Antifungal—not indicated
 - Antiviral—not indicated unless patient previously had an episode of HSV
See Chapter 47 for more information

Treatment Modifications

Adverse Event	Dose Modification
Acute infusion reactions	Interrupt or slow infusion depending on the severity of the reaction and administer appropriate medical therapy including intravenous H_1/H_2 antagonists ± low-dose meperidine

Patient Population Studied

A study of 512 patients with metastatic castration-resistant prostate cancer and an expected survival ≥6 months (341 randomized to sipuleucel-T and 171 to placebo). Initially, only men without disease-related symptoms and a Gleason score ≤7 were enrolled. Eligibility criteria were later amended to include men with any Gleason score, as well as those with minimal disease-related symptoms. Additional eligibility criteria were a serum PSA ≥5 mcg/L, a serum testosterone level <50 ng/dL (<1.7 nmol/L), and progressive disease on the basis of imaging studies or PSA measurements. Exclusion criteria included an Eastern Cooperative Oncology Group (ECOG) performance status ≥2, visceral metastases, pathologic long-bone fractures, spinal cord compression, and treatment within the previous 28 days with systemic glucocorticoids, external beam radiation, surgery, or systemic therapy for prostate cancer (except medical or surgical castration). Patients were also excluded if they had undergone chemotherapy within the previous 3 months. Continuation of medical castration or bisphosphonate therapy was required at least until the time of disease progression

Efficacy*

Median time to objective disease progression	14.6 weeks[†]
Adjusted HR for death, sipuleucel-T *vs.* placebo	0.78 (95% CI, 0.61–0.98)
Median overall survival	25.8 months[‡]
Estimated probability of survival at 36 months	31.7%[§]
Reductions of PSA ≥50% on two visits ≥4 weeks apart	2.6%[ϵ]
Antibody titers against the immunizing antigen, PA2024 >400 at any time after baseline	66.2%[**,‡‡]
Antibodies titers against prostatic acid phosphatase >400 at any time after baseline	28.5%[†,‡,‡‡]

*Median follow up time: 34.1 months
[†]Placebo group: 14.4 weeks
[‡]Placebo group: 21.7 months
[§]Placebo group: 23%
[ϵ]Placebo group: 1.3%
[**]Placebo group: 2.9%
[††]Placebo group: 1.4%
[‡‡]In prespecified analyses, patients in the sipuleucel-T group who had an antibody titer >400 against PA2024 or prostatic acid phosphatase at any time after baseline lived longer than those who had an antibody titer ≤400 (P <0.001 and P = 0.08, respectively, by the log-rank test)

Therapy Monitoring

1. *Before each cycle:* CBC with LFTs
2. *Evaluation including PSA:* Every 6 weeks

Toxicity*

Toxicity	Sipuleucel-T (N = 338)		Placebo (N = 168)	
	% All Grades	% G3/4/5	% All Grades	% G3/4/5
Any	98.8	31.7	96.4	35.1
Chills	54.1	1.2	12.5	0
Fatigue	39.1	1.1	38.1	1.8
Back pain	34.3	3.6	36.3	4.8
Pyrexia	29.3	0.3	13.7	1.8
Nausea	28.1	0.6	20.8	0
Arthralgia	20.7	2.1	23.8	3.0
Citrate toxicity[†]	20.1	0	20.2	0
Vomiting	17.8	0	11.9	0
Headache	16.0	0.3	4.8	0
Dizziness	14.5	0	9.5	0
Pain	13.0	1.8	7.1	1.2
Influenza-like illness	9.8	0	3.6	0
Bone pain	9.5	0.9	10.7	1.2
Hypertension	7.4	0.6	3.0	0
Anorexia	7.1	0.3	16.1	1.8
Weight loss	5.9	0.6	10.7	0.6
Hyperhidrosis	5.3	0	0.6	0
Groin pain	5.0	0	2.4	0
Anxiety	3.8	0	8.3	0
Flank pain	2.7	0	6.0	0
Depression	2.4	0.3	6.5	0
	% Mild/Moderate (G1/2)		% Severe (G3)[§]	
Acute infusion reactions[‡]	67.7		3.5	

*NCI Common Terminology Criteria for Adverse Events, version 3
[†]Citrate toxicity has been associated with leukapheresis; paresthesia and oral paresthesia are likely symptoms of citrate toxicity
[‡]Acute infusion reactions (*reported within 1 day after infusion*) included chills, fever, fatigue, asthenia, dyspnea, hypoxia, bronchospasm, dizziness, headache, hypertension, tachycardia, muscle ache, nausea, and vomiting. The most common events (≥20%) were chills, fever, and fatigue. Fevers and chills generally resolved within 2 days (71.9% and 89.0%, respectively)
[§]The incidence of severe events was greater following the second sipuleucel-T infusion in comparison with the first infusion (2.1% vs. 0.8%, respectively), and decreased to 1.3% following the third infusion. Some (1.2%) patients in the sipuleucel-T group were hospitalized within 1 day after infusion for management of acute infusion reactions. No G4/5 acute infusion reactions were reported with sipuleucel-T

33. Renal Cell Cancer

Susan Bates, MD and Olivier Rixe, MD, PhD

Epidemiology

Incidence: 63,920 (male: 39,140; female: 24,780. Estimated new cases for 2014 in the United States) 21 per 100,000 men, 10.6 per 100,000 women

Deaths: Estimated 13,860 in 2014 (male: 8,900; female: 4,960)

Median age: 64 years

Male to female ratio: 1.6:1

Stage at Presentation:

Stage	Percentage
Stage I:	50.4%
Stage II:	14.6%
Stage III:	20.7%
Stage IV:	14.3%

Siegel R et al. CA Cancer J Clin 2014;64:9–29
Surveillance, Epidemiology and End Results (SEER) Program, available from http://seer.cancer.gov (accessed in 2013)

Pathology

Clear cell	70–80%
Papillary	10–15%
Chromophobe	5%
Collecting duct	0.4–2.6%

Zambrano NR et al. J Urol 1999;162:1246–1258

Work-up
(For Suspicious Renal Mass)

1. H&P
2. CBC, chemistry profile
3. Urinalysis
4. Chest x-ray
5. Abdominal and pelvic CT with contrast
6. Chest CT if abnormal chest x-ray or advanced lesion
7. MRI if CT suggests caval thrombosis or renal insufficiency
8. Bone scan or brain MRI if clinically indicated

Staging

Primary Tumor (T)

TX	Primary tumor cannot be assessed
T0	No evidence of primary tumor
T1	Tumor 7 cm or less in greatest dimension, limited to the kidney
T1a	Tumor 4 cm or less in greatest dimension, limited to the kidney
T1b	Tumor more than 4 cm but not more than 7 cm in greatest dimension, limited to the kidney
T2	Tumor more than 7 cm in greatest dimension, limited to the kidney
T2a	Tumor more than 7 cm but less than or equal to 10 cm in greatest dimension, limited to the kidney
T2b	Tumor more than 10 cm, limited to the kidney
T3	Tumor extends into major veins or perinephric tissues but not into the ipsilateral adrenal gland and not beyond Gerota's fascia
T3a	Tumor grossly extends into the renal vein or its segmental (muscle containing) branches, or tumor invades perirenal and/or renal sinus fat but not beyond Gerota's fascia
T3b	Tumor grossly extends into the vena cava below the diaphragm
T3c	Tumor grossly extends into the vena cava above the diaphragm or invades the wall of the vena cava
T4	Tumor invades beyond Gerota's fascia (including contiguous extension into the ipsilateral adrenal gland)

Regional Lymph Nodes (N)

NX	Regional lymph nodes cannot be assessed
N0	No regional lymph node metastasis
N1	Regional lymph node metastasis

Distant Metastasis (M)

M0	No distant metastasis
M1	Distant metastasis

Staging Groups

	T	N	M
I	T1	N0	M0
II	T2	N0	M0
III	T1 or T2	N1	M0
	T3	N0 or N1	M0
IV	T4	Any N	M0
	Any T	Any N	M1

Edge SB, Byrd DR, Compton CC, Fritz AG, Greene FL, Trotti A, editors. AJCC Cancer Staging Manual. 7th ed. New York: Springer; 2010

Relative 5-Year Survival

Stage I	91%
Stage II	86%
Stage III	67%
Stage IV	17%

National Cancer Institute, Surveillance, Epidemiology, and End Results (SEER) Program

Risk Group Criteria

Memorial Sloan-Kettering Cancer Center (MSKCC) Criteria

(Motzer RJ et al. J Clin Oncol 2002;20:289–296)

1. <12 Months from initial RCC diagnosis to start of therapy
2. Lactate dehydrogenase >1.5 × ULN
3. Hemoglobin < lower limit of normal range
4. Corrected serum calcium >10 mg/dL (>2.5 mmol/L)
5. Karnofsky performance score <80
6. ≥2 Metastatic sites

Favorable: 0 risk factors
Intermediate: 1 or 2 risk factors
Poor: ≥3 risk factors

Cleveland Clinic Foundation Criteria

(Mekhail TM et al. J Clin Oncol 2005;23:832–841)

1. <12 Months from initial RCC diagnosis to start of therapy
2. Lactate dehydrogenase >1.5 × ULN
3. Hemoglobin < lower limit of normal range
4. Corrected serum calcium >10 mg/dL (>2.5 mmol/L)
5. Prior radiotherapy
6. ≥2 Metastatic sites

Favorable: 0–1 risk factors
Intermediate: 2 risk factors
Poor: ≥3 risk factors

Expert Opinion

Primary Treatment:
Surgical candidates: Treatment-naïve patients. Important factors include:
1. MSKCC risk group
2. Histologic subtype
3. Patient-specific factors

Stage 1A:
1. Partial nephrectomy (preferred)
2. Radical nephrectomy (in patients with centrally located tumors, or when other reasons make partial nephrectomy impossible)
3. Thermal ablation or cryoablation (in nonsurgical candidates), although must be prepared to proceed to open resection if needed
4. Active surveillance (AS) in selected patients: Although the standard of care for treatment of renal masses has been surgical removal, many elderly patients are at high risk for perioperative morbidity and mortality. AS has emerged as a management option for these patients and for those who choose not to have surgery. Many studies show that most renal masses grow slowly and do not display aggressive behavior. The risk of AS is progression to metastatic disease, but, fortunately, the rate of metastases for renal masses during AS appears to be low

Stage 1B:
1. Partial nephrectomy (preferred)
2. Radical nephrectomy (in patients with centrally located tumors, or when other reasons make partial nephrectomy impossible)

Stages II, III:
1. Radical nephrectomy

Stage IV:
1. Partial or radical nephrectomy for cytoreduction prior to systemic therapy
2. Partial or radical nephrectomy plus metastasectomy if oligometastases are surgically resectable

Primary treatment references:
Flanigan RC et al. J Urol 2004;171:1071–1076
Mason RJ et al. Eur Urol 2011;59:863–867

(continued)

Expert Opinion (continued)

Systemic Therapy, Clear Cell Histology:
First-line therapy for treatment-naïve patients, MSKCC intermediate or favorable risk group, clear cell histology:
1. Sunitinib

2. Bevacizumab plus interferon alfa

3. Pazopanib

4. Sorafenib

5. High-dose aldesleukin (interleukin-2) for selected patients; only therapy with the potential to give long-term disease-free survival that can be assumed to be curative

First-line therapy for treatment-naïve patients, MSKCC poor risk group, clear cell histology:
1. Temsirolimus: There is level 1 evidence for a survival advantage compared with interferon alfa alone in the first-line setting

Second-line therapy, clear cell histology patients, after disease progression on first-line therapy:
1. Everolimus

2. Axitinib

3. Temsirolimus

4. Interferon alfa

5. Aldesleukin

6. Sunitinib

7. Pazopanib

8. Sorafenib

9. Bevacizumab

FDA Approved Indications:
- **Axitinib (Inlyta):** Advanced renal cell carcinoma after failure of one prior systemic therapy
- **Bevacizumab (Avastin):** Metastatic renal cell carcinoma in combination with interferon alfa
- **Everolimus (Afinitor):** Advanced renal cell carcinoma after failure of treatment with sunitinib or sorafenib
- **Pazopanib (Votrient):** Advanced renal cell carcinoma
- **Sorafenib (Nexavar):** Advanced renal cell carcinoma
- **Sunitinib (Sutent):** Advanced renal cell carcinoma
- **Temsirolimus (Torisel):** Advanced renal cell carcinoma

Systemic Therapy, Non–Clear Cell Histologies
First-line therapy for treatment-naïve patients, non–clear cell histologies:
1. Temsirolimus

2. Sorafenib

3. Sunitinib

4. Pazopanib

5. Erlotinib

6. Gemcitabine + doxorubicin (*Note:* sarcomatoid histology only)

Considerations in Selecting First- and Second-Line Therapies Clear Cell and Non–Clear Cell Histologies
1. Patients' comorbidities that could be exacerbated by agent-specific toxicities such as hypertension with VEGF-targeting agents (sunitinib, sorafenib, pazopanib, axitinib, bevacizumab)

2. Convenience of oral agents

Managing Hypertension Associated with Inhibitors of the VEGF Signaling Pathway Inhibitors (VEGFi)[1,2]

Graded Severity	Antihypertensive Therapy	Blood Pressure Monitoring	VEGFi Dose Modification
CTCAE G1 *Pre-hypertension* [SBP 120–139 mm Hg or DBP 80–89 mm Hg]	None	At least weekly initially and after changes in dose and administration schedule of the *VEGFi*. After stable BP is achieved increase monitoring intervals to every 2–3 wks or schedule to coincide with clinical evaluations	No change
CTCAE G2 *Stage 1 HTN* [SBP 140–159 mm Hg or DBP 90–99 mm Hg]; Recurrent or persistent (≥24 h) HTN; medical intervention indicated; Symptomatic increase by >20 mm Hg (diastolic) or to >140/90 mm Hg if previously WNL; monotherapy indicated	*Step 1:* Initiate DHP-CCB treatment, and, if needed, after 24–48h, increase the dose in incremental steps every 24–48h until BP is controlled or a maximum antihypertensive dose is reached *Step 2:* If BP still is not controlled, add another antihypertensive, a BB, ACEI, ARB, or ABB. Increase dose of 2nd drug as described in Step 1 (above) *Step 3:* If BP still is not controlled, add 3rd drug from categories listed in Step 2; increase dose of 3rd drug as described in Step 1 (above) *Step 4:* If BP is still not controlled, consider either decreasing *VEGFi* dose one dose level or discontinuing *VEGFi* *Note:* If the dose of the *VEGFi* is reduced or the *VEGFi* is stopped, BP is expected to decrease. Monitor patient for hypotension and adjust number and doses of antihypertensive medications accordingly	Monitor BP as recommended by treating clinician	No changes except as described for Step 4 [If BP is still not controlled, consider either decreasing *VEGFi* dose one dose level or discontinuing *VEGFi*]
CTCAE G3 *Stage 2 HTN* [SBP ≥160 mm Hg or DBP ≥100 mm Hg]; medical intervention indicated; more than one drug or more intensive therapy than previously used indicated	Withhold *VEGFi* until systolic BP <159 mm Hg and diastolic BP <99 mm Hg. BP management identical to that for **G2** *(Stage 1) HTN (see Steps 1–4 above)* with two exceptions: 1. If SBP >180 mm Hg or DBP >110 mm Hg *and patient is symptomatic,* optimal management should include intensive IV support in an ICU setting. Discontinue *VEGFi* and notify other medically responsible health care providers that stopping *VEGFi* may result in a decrease in BP 2. If SBP >180 mm Hg or DBP >110 mm Hg *and the patient is asymptomatic,* two new antihypertensives must be given together in Step 1, and dose escalated as in Step 1 *Note:* If the dose of the *VEGFi* is reduced or the *VEGFi* is stopped, BP is expected to decrease. Monitor patient for hypotension and adjust number and doses of antihypertensive medications accordingly	BP should be monitored as recommended by the treating clinician unless the patient is symptomatic with SBP >180 mm Hg or DBP >110 mm Hg in which cases, monitoring should be intensive	1. Withhold the *VEGFi* until SBP <159 mm Hg and DBP <99 mm Hg 2. If BP cannot be controlled after an optimal trial of antihypertensive medications, consider either reducing the dose of the *VEGFi* or discontinuing its use 3. If a patient requires hospitalization for symptomatic SBP >180 mm Hg or DBP >110 mm Hg, permanently discontinue the *VEGFi*, or if BP is controlled, resume the *VEGFi* at a reduced dose

(continued)

Managing Hypertension Associated with Inhibitors of the VEGF Signaling Pathway Inhibitors (*VEGFi*)[1,2] (continued)

Graded Severity	Antihypertensive Therapy	Blood Pressure Monitoring	*VEGFi* Dose Modification
CTCAE G4 Life-threatening consequences (eg, malignant hypertension, transient or permanent neurologic deficit, hypertensive crisis)	1. Optimal management with intensive parenteral support in an ICU setting 2. Discontinue the *VEGFi* and notify other medically responsible health care providers that stopping a *VEGFi* may result in a decrease in BP	Intensive	Permanently discontinue the *VEGFi*, or if BP is controlled, resume the *VEGFi* at a reduced dose

ABB, α/β-adrenergic blockers; ACEI, angiotensin converting enzyme inhibitors; ARB, angiotensin II receptor blockers; BB, selective β-adrenergic blockers; CTCAE, National Cancer Institute (USA), Common Terminology Criteria for Adverse Events; DBP, diastolic blood pressure; DHP-CCB, dihydropyridine calcium-channel blockers; HTN, hypertension; ICU, intensive (*or* critical) care unit; SBP, systolic blood pressure; VEGF, vascular endothelial growth factor; *VEGFi*, **VEGF** signaling pathway inhibitor

Notes:
- Hypertension grading is based on CTCAE, version 4.0 criteria
- When SBP and DBP fall into different categories, the higher category should be selected in classifying blood pressure status
- Discontinue the *VEGFi* if patients require delaying treatment >2 weeks for management of hypertension
- Discontinue the *VEGFi* if patients require >2 *VEGFi* dose reductions
- Patients may receive up to two drugs for managing hypertension prior to decreasing *VEGFi* doses
- Allow an interval of at least 24 hours between modifications of antihypertensive therapy
- Treatment with a *VEGFi*, including aflibercept, axitinib, bevacizumab, cediranib, pazopanib, sunitinib, sorafenib, and vandetanib has rarely been associated with developing reversible posterior leukoencephalopathy syndrome (RPLS). Presenting symptoms associated with RPLS have included mild to severe hypertension, headache, lethargy, decreased alertness, confusion, altered mental functioning, and visual loss, seizure, and other neurologic disturbances
  - Discontinue the *VEGFi* in patients experiencing signs and symptoms referable to RPLS
  - MRI is the most sensitive imaging modality for detecting RPLS, and is recommended in suspected cases to confirm the diagnosis
  - RPLS usually is reversible upon removal of precipitating factors and application of measures to alleviate symptoms and control blood pressure; however, some patients have experienced ongoing neurological effects and death

Commercially Available Orally Administered Antihypertensives

Pharmacological Categories	Drug Name[†] (formulation)	Doses and Administration Schedules*			Metabolism
		Initial	Intermediate	Maximum Recommended	
Dihydropyridine calcium-channel blockers (DHP-CCB)	Nifedipine (extended release)	30 mg daily	60 mg daily	90 mg daily	CYP3A4 substrate
	Amlodipine besylate[3]	2.5 mg daily	5 mg daily	10 mg daily	CYP3A4 substrate
	Felodipine (extended release)	2.5 mg daily	5 mg daily	10 mg daily	CYP3A4 substrate and inhibitor[4]
Selective β-adrenergic blockers (BB)	Metoprolol tartrate[3]	25 mg twice daily	50 mg twice daily	100 mg twice daily	CYP2D6 substrate
	Atenolol	25 mg daily	50 mg daily	100 mg daily	Eliminated unchanged in urine and feces
	Acebutolol HCl	100 mg twice daily	200–300 mg twice daily	400 mg twice daily	Yes (CYP450 unknown)
	Bisoprolol fumarate	2.5 mg daily	5–10 mg daily	20 mg daily	Substrate for CYP2D6 and CYP3A4; ~50% renally eliminated as intact bisoprolol
	Nebivolol HCl[5,6]	5 mg daily	—	40 mg daily	Substrate for CYP2D6 and UGT enzymes
		Caution: Consider use for BP maintenance rather than titration. Product labeling recommends dose adjustments not more frequently than every 2 weeks			

(continued)

Commercially Available Orally Administered Antihypertensives (continued)

Pharmacological Categories	Drug Name[†] (formulation)	Doses and Administration Schedules[*]			Metabolism
		Initial	Intermediate	Maximum Recommended	
Angiotensin converting enzyme inhibitors (ACEIs)	Captopril	12.5 mg three times daily	25 mg three times daily	50 mg three times daily	CYP2D6 substrate
	Enalapril maleate[7]	5 mg daily	10–20 mg daily	40 mg daily	CYP3A4 substrate
	Ramipril	2.5 mg daily	5 mg daily	10 mg daily	Metabolism by liver esterases and phase II metabolism; ie, not CYP450
	Lisinopril	5 mg daily	10–20 mg daily	40 mg daily	Minimally, not CYP450
	Fosinopril sodium	10 mg daily	20 mg daily	40 mg daily	Hydrolyzed by intestinal and hepatic esterases; ie, not CYP450
	Perindopril erbumine	4 mg daily	none	8 mg daily	Hydrolysis and phase II metabolism; ie, not CYP450
	Quinapril	10 mg daily	20 mg daily	40 mg daily	Hydrolysis to quinaprilat, which is renally eliminated
Angiotensin II receptor blockers (ARBs)	Losartan	25 mg daily	50 mg daily	100 mg daily	CYP3A4 substrate
	Candesartan	4 mg daily	8–16 mg daily	32 mg daily	CYP2C9 substrate
	Irbesartan[7]	75 mg daily	150 mg daily	300 mg daily	CYP2C9 substrate
	Telmisartan	40 mg daily	none	80 mg daily	Phase II metabolism; ie, not CYP450
	Valsartan	80 mg daily	none	160 mg daily	Minimally, not CYP450
α-/β-adrenergic blocker	Labetolol HCl	100 mg twice daily	200 mg twice daily	400 mg twice daily	CYP2D6 substrate and inhibitor

ABC, ATP binding cassette proteins; CYP450, cytochrome P450 superfamily microsomal enzymes; FMO, flavin-containing monooxygenase family microsomal enzymes; UGT, uridine diphosphate-glucuronosyltransferase

[*]Recommendations for use are for adult patients without renal or hepatic impairment. Consult complete prescribing information for use in persons with impaired renal and/or hepatic function and other special populations

[†]Drugs in emboldened characters are suggested as optimal choices to avoid or minimize potential drug interactions with *VEGFi* through unilateral or mutual effects on CYP3A4

Notes:
Axitinib
- A substrate for metabolism by CYP3A4/5 (primary catalyst) and, to a lesser extent, CYP1A2, CYP2C19, and UGT1A1 in an *in vitro* system
- In an *in vitro* system is an inhibitor of ABCB1 (P-glycoprotein, MDR1); however, it is not expected to inhibit ABCB1-mediated transport at therapeutic plasma concentrations
Pazopanib
- A substrate for metabolism by CYP3A4 (primary catalyst) with minor contributions from CYP1A2 and CYP2C8
- Drug interaction trials conducted in patients with cancer suggest that pazopanib is a weak inhibitor of CYP3A4, CYP2C8, and CYP2D6 *in vivo*, but had no effect on CYP1A2, CYP2C9, or CYP2C19. Consequently, concomitant use of pazopanib with CYP3A4, CYP2D6, or CYP2C8 substrates that have with low therapeutic indices or narrow ranges of therapeutic concentrations is not recommended
- Pazopanib has been shown to inhibit UGT1A1 and OATP1B1 in an *in vitro* system with IC_{50} of 1.2 μmol/L and 0.79 μmol/L, respectively, ie, systemically achievable concentrations. Thus, drugs eliminated by UGT1A1 and OATP1B1 may be increased during concomitant use with pazopanib
Sorafenib
- A substrate for phase I and II metabolism by CYP3A4 and UGT1A9, respectively
- Sorafenib inhibits UGT1A1[8] and UGT1A9, and ABCB1 (P-glycoprotein, MDR1) *in vitro*, and may increase the systemic exposure of concomitantly administered drug substrates for metabolism and/or transport by these proteins
Sunitinib and its primary active (N-deethylated) metabolite, SU12662
- Substrates for metabolism by CYP3A4. Consequently, concomitant administration of sunitinib with strong CYP3A4 inhibitors or inducers should be avoided

References

1. Maitland ML, Bakris GL, Black HR et al. Initial assessment, surveillance, and management of blood pressure in patients receiving vascular endothelial growth factor signaling pathway inhibitors. J Natl Cancer Inst 2010;102:596–604
2. de Jesus-Gonzalez N, Robinson E, Moslehi J, Humphreys BD. Management of antiangiogenic therapy-induced hypertension. Hypertension 2012;60:607–615
3. Szmit S, Nurzynski P, Szalus N, Opolski G, Szczylik C. Reversible myocardial dysfunction in a young woman with metastatic renal cell carcinoma treated with sunitinib. Acta Oncol 2009;48:921–925
4. Gomo C, Coriat R, Faivre L et al. Pharmacokinetic interaction involving sorafenib and the calcium-channel blocker felodipine in a patient with hepatocellular carcinoma. Invest New Drugs 2011;29:1511–1514
5. Bamias A, Manios E, Karadimou A et al. The use of 24-h ambulatory blood pressure monitoring (ABPM) during the first cycle of sunitinib improves the diagnostic accuracy and management of hypertension in patients with advanced renal cancer. Eur J Cancer 2011;47:1660–1668
6. Bamias A, Lainakis G, Manios E et al. Diagnosis and management of hypertension in advanced renal cell carcinoma: prospective evaluation of an algorithm in patients treated with sunitinib. J Chemother 2009;21:347–350
7. Costero O, Picazo ML, Zamora P, Romero S, Martinez-Ara J, Selgas R. Inhibition of tyrosine kinases by sunitinib associated with focal segmental glomerulosclerosis lesion in addition to thrombotic microangiopathy. Nephrol Dial Transplant 2010;25:1001–1003
8. Liu Y, Ramírez J, Ratain MJ. Inhibition of paracetamol glucuronidation by tyrosine kinase inhibitors. Br J Clin Pharmacol 2011;71:917–920

REGIMEN

SORAFENIB TOSYLATE

Escudier B et al. N Engl J Med 2007;356:125–134
Escudier B et al. J Clin Oncol 2009;27:3312–3318

Sorafenib tosylate 400 mg; administer orally every 12 hours (eg, morning and evening) continually in 28-day cycles (total dose/day = 800 mg; total dose/cycle = 22,400 mg)

Notes:

- Patients should swallow tablets whole with approximately 250 mL (8 oz) of water. Tablets may be taken with or without food

- *Special precautions:* Sorafenib is metabolized by cytochrome P450 (CYP) CYP3A subfamily enzymes and has been shown in preclinical studies to inhibit multiple CYP isoforms. Therefore, all patients who are taking concomitant medications metabolized by CYP enzymes should be closely observed for side effects associated with concomitantly administered medications. Special caution should be used with any of the following medications: ketoconazole, itraconazole, voriconazole, ritonavir, clarithromycin, cyclosporine, carbamazepine, phenytoin, and phenobarbital. Furthermore, patients taking medications with a low therapeutic index (eg, warfarin, quinidine, digoxin) should be monitored proactively. *Patients using sorafenib should be advised to avoid consuming grapefruit products for as long as they continue to use sorafenib*

Supportive Care: Hand-foot reaction
For patients who develop a hand-foot reaction, use topical emollients (eg, Aquaphor®), topical and/or oral steroids, antihistamine agents (H_1-receptor antagonists), or pyridoxine 50–150 mg/day orally

Antiemetic prophylaxis
Emetogenic potential is **MINIMAL**
See Chapter 39 for antiemetic recommendations

Hematopoietic growth factor (CSF) prophylaxis
Primary prophylaxis is NOT indicated
See Chapter 43 for more information

Antimicrobial prophylaxis
Risk of fever and neutropenia is LOW
  Antimicrobial primary prophylaxis to be considered:
  - Antibacterial—not indicated
  - Antifungal—not indicated
  - Antiviral—not indicated unless patient previously had an episode of HSV
See Chapter 47 for more information

Diarrhea management
Latent or delayed onset diarrhea*:
  Loperamide 4 mg orally initially after the first loose or liquid stool, *then*
  Loperamide 2 mg orally every 2 hours during waking hours, *plus*
  Loperamide 4 mg orally every 4 hours during hours of sleep
  - Continue for at least 12 hours after diarrhea resolves
  - Recurrent diarrhea after a 12-hour diarrhea-free interval is treated as a new episode
  - Rehydrate orally with fluids and electrolytes during a diarrheal episode
  - If a patient develops blood or mucus in stool, dehydration, or hemodynamic instability, or if diarrhea persists >48 hours despite loperamide, stop loperamide and hospitalize the patient for IV hydration

(continued)

Patient Population Studied

A study of 903 patients (451 randomly assigned to sorafenib tosylate, 452 to placebo) with histologically confirmed metastatic clear cell renal cell carcinoma, which had progressed after 1 systemic treatment within the previous 8 months. Additional eligibility criteria included performance status of 0 or 1 on the basis of Eastern Cooperative Oncology Group (ECOG) criteria and an intermediate-risk or low-risk status, according to the Memorial Sloan-Kettering Cancer Center (MSKCC) prognostic score. Most patients (99%) had clear cell renal cell carcinoma. Of those patients, 51% had low-risk disease, and 49% had intermediate-risk disease according to MSKCC criteria. Most patients had undergone previous nephrectomy and had received cytokine-based treatment

Median age	59 years (range: 19–86 years)
Median time from diagnosis	2 years (range: <1–19 years)

Characteristic	
Clear cell	100%
ECOG PS 0/1/2	48%/49%/2%
Low Motzer criteria	52%
Intermediate Motzer criteria	48%
Prior nephrectomy	93%
Prior radiation	28%
Prior cytokine-based therapy	83%
Metastatic sites: 1/2/≥2	15%/27%/57%
Lung metastases	75%
Liver metastases	26%

(continued)

Persistent diarrhea:
> **Octreotide** 100–150 mcg subcutaneously 3 times daily. Maximum total daily dose is 1500 mcg

Antibiotic therapy during latent or delayed onset diarrhea:
> A fluoroquinolone (eg, **Ciprofloxacin** 500 mg orally every 12 hours) if absolute neutrophil count <500/mm³ with or without accompanying fever in association with diarrhea
> • Antibiotics should also be administered if patient is hospitalized with prolonged diarrhea and should be continued until diarrhea resolves

*Abigerges D et al. J Natl Cancer Inst 1994;86:446–449
Rothenberg ML et al. J Clin Oncol 2001;19:3801–3807
Wadler S et al. J Clin Oncol 1998;16:3169–3178

Treatment Modifications

Sorafenib Dose Levels

Starting dose: Level 1	400 mg every morning; 400 mg every evening
Level −1	200 mg every morning; 400 mg every evening
Level −2	200 mg every morning; 200 mg every evening
Level −3	200 mg once daily

Adverse Event	Dose Modification
Cutaneous Toxicities	
Rash G ≥2	Hold sorafenib and provide *immediate* symptomatic treatment
If treatment is withheld for more than 3 weeks because of cutaneous toxicity	Discontinue therapy
When toxicity resolves to G ≤1	Restart sorafenib at 1 dose level less than the dose level administered at the time toxicity developed. Treatment for symptoms may continue indefinitely as a preventive measure
If cutaneous toxicity G3/4 recurs at reduced sorafenib doses	Again, hold sorafenib until the toxicity resolves to G ≤1, at which time sorafenib should be restarted at 1 dose level lower than the dose level administered at the time toxicity developed. Treatment for symptoms may continue indefinitely as a preventive measure
If cutaneous toxicity G3/4 recurs at dose levels −2 or lower	Discontinue therapy
If cutaneous toxicity does not recur at reduced sorafenib doses with or without continued treatment for symptoms	The dose of sorafenib may be increased 1 dose level to the dose level administered at the time cutaneous toxicity developed. If toxicity recurs following the increase, then follow the guidelines above, with the exception that when drug is restarted the sorafenib dose should be reduced 1 dose level

(continued)

Efficacy (N = 903)*

	Sorafenib (N = 451)	Placebo (N = 452)
Complete response	1 (<1%)	0
Partial response	43 (9.5%)	8 (1.7%)
Median progression-free survival (PFS)†	5.5 months	2.8 months
Median time to response	80 days (range: 35–275 days)	
Median duration of response	18 days (range: 36–378 days)	
Median overall survival‡	19.3 months	15.9 months
Median overall survival§	17.8 months	15.2 months
Median overall survivalᶜ	17.8 months	14.3 months

*RECIST (Response Evaluation Criteria in Solid Tumors) (Therasse P et al. J Natl Cancer Inst 2000;92:205–216)
†Benefit in PFS was independent of age, MSKCC score, previous use of cytokine therapy, presence of lung or liver metastases, and the time since diagnosis (<1.5 years or ≥1.5 years)
‡Differences in OS: Hazard ratio = 0.77 (95% CI, 0.63–0.95), P = 0.02. The analyses did not reach prespecified O'Brien-Fleming boundaries for statistical significance. Reference: Escudier B et al. N Engl J Med 2007;356:125–134
§HR = 0.88; P = 0.146. Reference: Escudier B et al. J Clin Oncol 2009;27:3312–3318
ᶜHR = 0.78; P = 0.029 if survival data for placebo patients who crossed over to sorafenib is censored. Reference: Escudier B et al. J Clin Oncol 2009;27:3312–3318

Treatment Modifications (*continued*)	
Adverse Event	**Dose Modification**
Diarrhea	
G1/2 diarrhea	Focus on treatment for symptoms designed to resolve the diarrhea. No dose modifications will be made for G1/2 diarrhea unless G2 diarrhea persists for more than 2 weeks
If G2 diarrhea persists for more than 2 weeks	Follow the guidelines below for G3/4 diarrhea
If diarrhea cannot be controlled with the preventive measures outlined, and is G3/4 or worsens by 1 grade level (G3 to G4) while on sorafenib and is not alleviated within 48 hours by antidiarrheal treatment	Hold sorafenib. Also, withhold sorafenib if persistent G2 diarrhea is not alleviated by antidiarrheal treatment while sorafenib use continues (persistent is defined as lasting for >2 weeks)
If sorafenib is held for more than 3 weeks and diarrhea does not resolve to G ≤1	Discontinue therapy
If within 3 weeks of withholding sorafenib, diarrhea resolves to G ≤1	Restart sorafenib at 1 dose level less than the dose level administered at the time toxicity developed
If G3/4 diarrhea or persistent G2 diarrhea recurs at reduced doses of sorafenib (persistent is defined as lasting >2 weeks)	Again, withhold sorafenib until the toxicity resolves to CTCAE G ≤1, at which time sorafenib should be restarted at one dose level lower than the dose level administered at the time toxicity developed. Treatment for symptoms may continue indefinitely as a preventive measure
If G3/4 diarrhea or persistent G2 diarrhea recurs at dose level −2 (persistent defined as lasting for >2 weeks)	Discontinue therapy
If diarrhea does not recur at reduced sorafenib doses with or without continued treatment for symptoms	The dose of sorafenib may be increased 1 dose level to the dose level administered at the time the diarrhea developed. If toxicity recurs following the increase, then follow the guidelines above, with the exception that when drug is restarted the sorafenib dose should be reduced 1 dose level
Hypertension	
Note: Patients should have their blood pressure checked once weekly during their first 24 weeks of therapy and for an 8-week period after an adjustment in their sorafenib dose	
G1 hypertension	Continue sorafenib at same dose and schedule
G2 asymptomatic	Treat with antihypertensive medications and continue sorafenib at same dose and schedule
G2 symptomatic, or persistent G2 despite antihypertensive medications, or diastolic BP >110 mm Hg, or G3 hypertension	Treat with antihypertensive medications. Hold sorafenib (maximum 3 weeks until symptoms resolve and diastolic BP <100 mm Hg); then continue sorafenib at 1 dose level lower *Note:* Discontinue therapy if sorafenib is withheld >3 weeks
G4 hypertension	Discontinue therapy

Therapy Monitoring

1. *Every 6 weeks to 3 months:* Physical examination and routine laboratory tests
2. *Response assessment:* Every 2–3 cycles. A cycle defined as 28 days of oral therapy

Toxicity (N = 902)*						
	Sorafenib (N = 451)			Placebo (N = 451)		
	% Any Grade	% G2	% G3/4	% Any Grade	% G2	% G3/4	P Value[†]
Cardiac							
Hypertension	17	10	4	2	<1	<1	<0.001
Hematologic							
Decreased Hemoglobin	8	3	3	7	2	4	0.28
Constitutional							
Fatigue	37	12	5	28	9	4	0.12
Other symptoms	10	2	1	6	2	1	1
Weight loss	10	5	<1	6	2	0	0.009
Gastrointestinal							
Diarrhea	43	12	2	13	3	1	<0.001
Nausea	23	6	<1	19	5	1	0.46
Anorexia	16	5	<1	13	4	1	0.26
Vomiting	16	6	1	12	4	1	0.54
Constipation	15	5	1	11	4	1	0.75
Neurologic							
Sensory Neuropathy	13	3	<1	6	1	1	0.05
Pain							
Abdominal	11	5	2	9	4	2	0.41
Headache	10	4	<1	6	2	<1	0.04
Joint[‡]	10	3	2	6	3	<1	1
Bone[§]	8	4	1	8	3	3	0.35
Tumor	6	2	3	5	2	2	0.82
Dermatologic							
Rash or desquamation	40	13	1	16	2	<1	<0.001
Hand-foot skin reaction	30	12	6	7	1	0	<0.001
Alopecia	27	4	<1	3	<1	0	<0.001
Pruritus	19	5	<1	6	<1	0	<0.001
Pulmonary							
Cough	13	5	<1	14	4	<1	0.87
Dyspnea	14	6	4	12	4	2	0.35

*NCI Common Terminology Criteria for Adverse Events v3.0
[†]p Values for the comparison between sorafenib and placebo groups with respect to G2 adverse events
[‡]p-Value for grades 3/4 = 0.07
[§]p-Value for grades 3/4 = 0.007

REGIMEN

SUNITINIB MALATE

Motzer RJ et al. N Engl J Med 2007;356:115–124
Motzer RJ et al. J Clin Oncol 2009;27:3584–3590

Sunitinib malate 50 mg; administer orally once daily, continually, without regard for meals, in 6-week cycles consisting of 4 consecutive weeks of daily treatment followed by 2 weeks without treatment (total dose/6-week cycle = 1400 mg)

Supportive Care: Hand-foot reaction
For patients who develop a hand-foot reaction, use topical emollients (eg, Aquaphor), topical and/or oral steroids, antihistamine agents (H_1-receptor antagonists), or pyridoxine 50–150 mg/day orally

Antiemetic prophylaxis
Emetogenic potential is **MINIMAL**
See Chapter 39 for antiemetic recommendations

Hematopoietic growth factor (CSF) prophylaxis
Primary prophylaxis is NOT indicated
See Chapter 43 for more information

Antimicrobial prophylaxis
Risk of fever and neutropenia is LOW
  Antimicrobial primary prophylaxis to be considered:
  • Antibacterial—not indicated
  • Antifungal—not indicated
  • Antiviral—not indicated unless patient previously had an episode of HSV
See Chapter 47 for more information

Diarrhea management
Latent or delayed onset diarrhea*:
  Loperamide 4 mg orally initially after the first loose or liquid stool, *then*
  Loperamide 2 mg orally every 2 hours during waking hours, *plus*
  Loperamide 4 mg orally every 4 hours during hours of sleep
  • Continue for at least 12 hours after diarrhea resolves
  • Recurrent diarrhea after a 12-hour diarrhea-free interval is treated as a new episode
  • Rehydrate orally with fluids and electrolytes during a diarrheal episode
  • If a patient develops blood or mucus in stool, dehydration, or hemodynamic instability, or if diarrhea persists >48 hours despite loperamide, stop loperamide and hospitalize the patient for IV hydration
Persistent diarrhea:
  Octreotide 100–150 mcg subcutaneously 3 times daily. Maximum total daily dose is 1500 mcg
Antibiotic therapy during latent or delayed onset diarrhea:
  A fluoroquinolone (eg, **Ciprofloxacin** 500 mg orally every 12 hours) if absolute neutrophil count <500/mm³ with or without accompanying fever in association with diarrhea
  • Antibiotics should also be administered if patient is hospitalized with prolonged diarrhea and should be continued until diarrhea resolves

*Abigerges D et al. J Natl Cancer Inst 1994;86:446–449
Rothenberg ML et al. J Clin Oncol 2001;19:3801–3807
Wadler S et al. J Clin Oncol 1998;16:3169–3178

Patient Population Studied

A study of 375 patients with metastatic renal cell carcinoma with a clear cell histologic component, who had not previously received treatment with systemic therapy for renal cell carcinoma. Other key eligibility criteria included an Eastern Cooperative Oncology Group (ECOG) performance status of 0 or 1, and adequate hematologic, coagulation, hepatic, renal, and cardiac functions

Efficacy (N = 375)*

Confirmed PR[†]	31% (95% CI, 26–36%)
Median progression-free survival (PFS)[‡]	11 months (95% CI, 10–12 months)
Median overall survival[§]	26.4 months (95% CI, 23.0–32.9 months)

*RECIST (Therasse P et al. J Natl Cancer Inst 2000;92:205–216)
[†]Central review; reference: Motzer RJ et al. N Engl J Med 2007;356:115–124
[‡]Central review and investigator assessment; reference: Motzer RJ et al. N Engl J Med 2007;356:115–124
[§]Motzer RJ et al. J Clin Oncol 2009;27:3584–3590: Median overall survival time was greater in the sunitinib group than in the interferon alfa group (HR = 0.821; 95% CI, 0.673–1.001; P = 0.051) based on the primary analysis of the unstratified log-rank test (P = 0.013 using the unstratified Wilcoxon test). By stratified log-rank test, the HR was 0.818 (95% CI, 0.669–0.999; P = 0.049)

Treatment Modifications

Sunitinib Dose Levels

Starting dose: Level 1	50 mg once daily, 4 weeks on/2 weeks off
Level −1	37.5 mg once daily, 4 weeks on/2 weeks off
Level −2	25 mg once daily, 4 weeks on/2 weeks off

Adverse Event	Dose Modification
Cutaneous Toxicities	
Rash G ≥2	Hold sunitinib and provide *immediate* symptomatic treatment
If treatment is withheld for more than 3 weeks because of cutaneous toxicity	Discontinue therapy
When toxicity resolves to G ≤1	Restart sunitinib at 1 dose level lower than the dose level administered at the time toxicity developed. Treatment for symptoms may continue indefinitely as a preventive measure
If cutaneous toxicity G3/4 recurs at reduced sunitinib doses	Again, hold sunitinib until the toxicity resolves to G ≤1, at which time sunitinib should be restarted at 1 dose level lower than the dose level administered at the time toxicity developed. Treatment for symptoms may continue indefinitely as a preventive measure
If cutaneous toxicity G3/4 recurs at dose levels −2 or lower	Discontinue therapy
If cutaneous toxicity does not recur at reduced sunitinib doses with or without continued treatment for symptoms	The dose of sunitinib may be increased 1 dose level to the dose level administered at the time the cutaneous toxicity developed. If toxicity recurs following the increase, then follow the guidelines above, with the exception that when drug is restarted the sunitinib dose should be reduced 1 dose level
Diarrhea	
G1/2 diarrhea	Focus on treatment for symptoms designed to resolve the diarrhea. No dose modifications will be made for G1/2 diarrhea unless G2 diarrhea persists for more than 2 weeks
If G2 diarrhea persists for more than 2 weeks	Follow the guidelines below for G3/4 diarrhea
If the diarrhea cannot be controlled with the preventive measures outlined, and is G3/4 or worsens by 1 grade level (G3 to G4) while on sunitinib and is not alleviated within 48 hours by antidiarrheal treatment	Hold sunitinib. Also withhold sunitinib if persistent G2 diarrhea is not alleviated by antidiarrheal treatment while sunitinib use continues (persistent defined as lasting for >2 weeks)
If sunitinib is held for more than 3 weeks and the diarrhea does not resolve to G ≤1	Discontinue therapy

(continued)

Therapy Monitoring

1. Every 6 weeks to 3 months: Physical examination and routine laboratory tests including thyroid function tests
2. *Response assessment:* Every 2–3 cycles. A cycle is defined as a 6-week period (4 consecutive weeks of daily sunitinib use, followed by 2 consecutive weeks without sunitinib)

Treatment Modifications (*continued*)

Adverse Event	Dose Modification
If within 3 weeks of holding sunitinib, diarrhea resolves to G ≤1	Restart sunitinib at 1 dose level less than the dose level administered at the time toxicity developed
If G3/4 diarrhea or persistent G2 diarrhea recurs at reduced sunitinib doses and the dose level at which persistent G2 diarrhea occurs is greater than dose level −1 (persistent is defined as lasting for >2 weeks)	Again, withhold sunitinib until the toxicity resolves to CTCAE G ≤1, at which time sunitinib should be restarted at 1 dose level less than the dose level administered at the time toxicity developed. Treatment for symptoms may continue indefinitely as a preventive measure
If G3/4 diarrhea or persistent G2 diarrhea recurs at dose level −2 (persistent defined as lasting for more >2 weeks)	Discontinue therapy
If diarrhea does not recur at the reduced sunitinib doses with or without continued treatment for symptoms	The dose of sunitinib may be increased 1 dose level to the dose level administered at the time diarrhea developed. If toxicity recurs following the increase, then follow the guidelines above, with the exception that when drug is restarted, the sunitinib dose should be reduced 1 dose level

Hypertension

Note: Patients should have their blood pressure checked once weekly during their first 24 weeks of therapy and for an 8-week period after an adjustment in their sunitinib dose

G1 hypertension	Continue sunitinib at same dose and schedule
G2 asymptomatic	Treat with antihypertensive medications and continue sunitinib at same dose and schedule
G2 symptomatic, or persistent G2 despite antihypertensive medications, or diastolic BP >110 mm Hg, or G3 hypertension	Treat with antihypertensive medications. Hold sunitinib (maximum 3 weeks until symptoms resolve and diastolic BP <100 mm Hg); then continue sunitinib at 1 dose level lower *Note:* Discontinue therapy if sunitinib is withheld >3 weeks
G4 hypertension	Discontinue therapy
Coadministration of potent CYP3A4 inhibitors (eg, ketoconazole, itraconazole, voriconazole, clarithromycin, atazanavir, ritonavir, telithromycin)	Reduce sunitinib dose
Coadministration of potent CYP3A4 inducers (eg, rifampin, phenytoin, phenobarbital, dexamethasone, carbamazepine, St. John's wort)	Increase sunitinib dose (to a maximum of 87.5 mg daily)

Toxicity (N = 375)*

Adverse Event	% Any Grade	% G3	% G4
Diarrhea	53	5	0
Fatigue	51	7	0
Nausea	44	3	0
Stomatitis	25	1	0
Vomiting	24	4	0
Hypertension	24	8	0
Hand-foot syndrome	20	5	0
Mucosal inflammation	20	2	0
Rash	19	1	1
Asthenia	17	4	0
Dry skin	16	1	0
Skin discoloration	16	0	0
Changes in hair color	14	0	0
Epistaxis	12	1	0
Pain in limb	11	1	0
Headache	11	1	0
Dry mouth	11	0	0
Decline in ejection fraction†	10	2	0
Pyrexia	7	1	0
Chills	6	1	0
Myalgia	5	1	0

Laboratory Abnormalities

	% Any Grade	% G3	% G4
Leukopenia	78	5	0
Neutropenia	72	11	1
Anemia	71	3	1
Increased creatinine	66	1	0
Thrombocytopenia	65	8	0
Lymphopenia	60	12	0
Increased lipase	52	13	3
Increased aspartate aminotransferase	52	2	0
Increased alanine aminotransferase	46	2	1
Increased alkaline phosphatase	42	2	0
Increased uric acid	41	0	12
Hypophosphatemia	36	4	1
Increased amylase	32	4	1
Increased total bilirubin	19	1	0

*NCI Common Terminology Criteria for Adverse Events v3.0. Listed are all treatment-related adverse events of interest and those occurring in at least 10% of patients in the sunitinib group

†The incidence of a G3 decline in the LVEF was 2% with sunitinib. This was not associated with clinical sequelae and was reversible after dose modification or discontinuation of treatment. No G4 events were reported in this category

REGIMEN

PAZOPANIB HYDROCHLORIDE

Sternberg CN et al. J Clin Oncol 2010;28:1061–1068

Pazopanib HCl 800 mg; administer orally once daily at least 1 hour before or 2 hours after a meal

Note: Tablets are swallowed whole (without breaking, chewing, or crushing). Oral bioavailability was increased after crushing tablets and when ingested concurrently with a high-fat or low-fat meal, resulting in increased systemic exposure ($AUC_{[0-72 \text{ hour}]}$) and maximum concentration achieved

Note: Caution in patients with hepatic dysfunction
- In patients with baseline moderate hepatic impairment administer **pazopanib** 200 mg orally once daily
- The safety of pazopanib in patients with pr-existing severe hepatic impairment, defined as total bilirubin $>3 \times$ ULN with any level of ALT, is unknown. Treatment with pazopanib is not recommended in patients with severe hepatic impairment

Note: When using pazopanib, monitor patients electrocardiographically at baseline and periodically thereafter. Evaluate serum electrolytes (calcium, magnesium, potassium) at baseline and periodically thereafter, supplementing as needed to maintain electrolytes within normal ranges

Supportive Care
Antiemetic prophylaxis
Emetogenic potential is **MINIMAL**
See Chapter 39 for antiemetic recommendations

Hematopoietic growth factor (CSF) prophylaxis
Primary prophylaxis is NOT indicated
See Chapter 43 for more information

Antimicrobial prophylaxis
Risk of fever and neutropenia is LOW
  Antimicrobial primary prophylaxis to be considered:
  - Antibacterial—not indicated
  - Antifungal—not indicated
  - Antiviral—not indicated unless patient previously had an episode of HSV
See Chapter 47 for more information

Diarrhea management
Latent or delayed onset diarrhea*:
  Loperamide 4 mg orally initially after the first loose or liquid stool, *then*
  Loperamide 2 mg orally every 2 hours during waking hours, *plus*
  Loperamide 4 mg orally every 4 hours during hours of sleep
  - Continue for at least 12 hours after diarrhea resolves
  - Recurrent diarrhea after a 12-hour diarrhea-free interval is treated as a new episode
  - Rehydrate orally with fluids and electrolytes during a diarrheal episode
  - If a patient develops blood or mucus in stool, dehydration, or hemodynamic instability, or if diarrhea persists >48 hours despite loperamide, stop loperamide and hospitalize the patient for IV hydration
Persistent diarrhea:
  Octreotide 100–150 mcg subcutaneously 3 times daily. Maximum total daily dose is 1500 mcg
Antibiotic therapy during latent or delayed onset diarrhea:
  A fluoroquinolone (eg, **Ciprofloxacin** 500 mg orally every 12 hours) if absolute neutrophil count $<500/mm^3$ with or without accompanying fever in association with diarrhea
  - Antibiotics should also be administered if patient is hospitalized with prolonged diarrhea and should be continued until diarrhea resolves

*Abigerges D et al. J Natl Cancer Inst 1994;86:446–449
Rothenberg ML et al. J Clin Oncol 2001;19:3801–3807
Wadler S et al. J Clin Oncol 1998;16:3169–3178

Patient Population Studied

A study of 435 patients enrolled in a placebo-controlled, randomized, double-blind, global, multicenter, phase III study. Randomization was stratified on the basis of ECOG PS (0 vs. 1), prior nephrectomy (yes vs. no), and prior systemic treatment for advanced RCC (treatment naïve vs. cytokine pretreated). Patients were centrally randomly assigned in a 2:1 ratio (290 vs. 145) to receive either 800 mg pazopanib HCl once daily or matching placebo. The study initially enrolled patients with advanced and/or metastatic RCC who had progressed on 1 prior cytokine-based systemic therapy but was subsequently amended to include treatment-naïve patients. Additional eligibility criteria included a diagnosis of clear cell or predominantly clear cell histology. Patients were excluded if they had poorly controlled hypertension (systolic blood pressure of ≥140 mm Hg or diastolic blood pressure of ≥90 mm Hg, despite antihypertensive therapy). The experimental and control arms were well balanced with regards to MSKCC risk category (94% vs. 92% with favorable/intermediate group, respectively) and prior nephrectomy (89% vs. 88%, respectively). Patients who experienced disease progression after treatment with placebo, had the option of receiving pazopanib via an open-label study provided they met predefined eligibility criteria. Seventy (48%) of 145 placebo-arm patients enrolled in the open-label study

Treatment Modifications

Pazopanib Dose Levels

Starting dose: Level 1	800 mg once daily
Level −1	600 mg once daily
Level −2	400 mg once daily
Level −3	200 mg once daily

Adverse Event	Dose Modification

Hepatotoxicity

Adverse Event	Dose Modification
Isolated ALT elevations between 3 × ULN and 8 × ULN	Continue pazopanib with weekly monitoring of LFTs until ALT returns to G1 or baseline
Isolated ALT elevations of >8 × ULN	Discontinue pazopanib administration until ALT decreases to G ≤1 or baseline. If the potential benefit for reinitiating treatment with pazopanib is considered to outweigh the risk for hepatotoxicity, then restart pazopanib at a reduced dose of not more than 400 mg once daily and measure serum liver tests weekly for 8 weeks
ALT >3 × ULN recurs after restarting pazopanib at a dose of 400 mg once daily	Discontinue pazopanib permanently
ALT >3 × ULN concurrently with bilirubin elevations >2 × ULN	Discontinue pazopanib permanently. Monitor patients until resolution *Note:* Pazopanib is a UGT1A1 inhibitor. Mild, indirect (unconjugated) hyperbilirubinemia may occur in patients with Gilbert syndrome. In these patients, an elevation in ALT >3 × ULN should be managed as per the recommendations outlined for isolated ALT elevations

Proteinuria

Adverse Event	Dose Modification
G4 proteinuria	Discontinue pazopanib permanently

Diarrhea

Adverse Event	Dose Modification
G1/2 diarrhea	Focus on treatment for symptoms designed to resolve the diarrhea. No dose modifications for G1/2 diarrhea unless G2 diarrhea persists for >2 weeks
G2 diarrhea that persists ≥2 weeks	Follow guidelines for G3/4 diarrhea (below)
If diarrhea cannot be controlled with preventive measures outlined, and is G3/4 or worsens by one grade level (G3 to G4) while on pazopanib, and is not alleviated by symptomatic treatment within 48 hours	Hold pazopanib. Also, withhold pazopanib if persistent G2 diarrhea while on pazopanib is not alleviated by treatment for symptoms (persistent defined as lasting for >2 weeks)
If pazopanib is held for >3 weeks and diarrhea does not resolve to G ≤1	Discontinue therapy
If within 3 weeks of withholding pazopanib diarrhea resolves to G ≤1	Restart pazopanib at 1 dose level less than the dose level administered at the time toxicity developed

(*continued*)

Toxicity (N = 290 Pazopanib; 145 Placebo)*

Adverse Event[†]	Placebo % Any Grade	Pazopanib % Any Grade	% G3	% G4
Diarrhea	13	52	3	<1
Hypertension	15	40	4	—
Hair color changes	4	38	<1	—
Nausea	13	26	<1	—
Anorexia	14	22	2	—
Vomiting	11	21	2	<1
Fatigue	11	19	2	—
Asthenia	12	14	3	—
Abdominal pain	2	11	2	—
Headache	7	10	—	—

Clinical Chemistry[‡]

	Placebo % Any Grade	Pazopanib % Any Grade	% G3	% G4
ALT increase	32	53	10	2
AST increase	27	53	7	<1
Hyperglycemia	47	41	<1	—
Total bilirubin increase	15	36	3	<1
Hypophosphatemia	16	34	4	—
Hypocalcemia	35	33	1	1
Hyponatremia	35	31	4	1
Hypomagnesemia	13	11	3	—
Hypoglycemia	4	17	—	<1

Hematologic[‡]

	Placebo % Any Grade	Pazopanib % Any Grade	% G3	% G4
Leukopenia	9	37	—	—
Neutropenia	9	34	1	<1
Thrombocytopenia	7	32	<1	<1
Lymphocytopenia	34	31	4	<1

*NCI Common Terminology Criteria for Adverse Events v3.0
[†]Adverse events with an incidence of ≥10% in the pazopanib arm are displayed
[‡]Clinical laboratory abnormalities with an incidence of ≥30% in the pazopanib arm or with a 5% increase in incidence in the pazopanib arm compared with the placebo arm are displayed

Treatment Modifications (*continued*)

Adverse Event	Dose Modification
Diarrhea	
If G3/4 diarrhea or persistent G2 diarrhea recurs at reduced pazopanib doses (persistent defined as lasting for >2 weeks)	Again, withhold pazopanib until the toxicity resolves to CTCAE G ≤1, at which time pazopanib should be restarted at 1 dose level less than the dose level administered at the time toxicity developed. Treatment for symptoms may continue indefinitely as a preventive measure
If G3/4 diarrhea or persistent G2 diarrhea recurs at a dose of 200 mg once daily (persistent defined as lasting for >2 weeks)	Discontinue therapy
If diarrhea does not recur at reduced pazopanib doses with or without continued treatment for symptoms	The dose of pazopanib may be increased 1 dose level to the dose level that was being administered at the time diarrhea developed. If toxicity recurs following the increase, then follow the guidelines above, with the exception that when drug is restarted the pazopanib dose should be reduced 1 dose level
Hypertension	
Note: Patients should have their blood pressure checked once per week during their first 24 weeks of therapy and for an 8-week period after an adjustment is made in their pazopanib dose	
G1 hypertension	Continue pazopanib at same dose and schedule
G2 asymptomatic	Treat with antihypertensive medications and continue pazopanib at same dose and schedule
G2 symptomatic or persistent G2 despite anti-hypertensive medications or diastolic BP >110 mm Hg or G3 hypertension	Treat with antihypertensive medications. Hold pazopanib (maximum 3 weeks until symptoms resolve and diastolic BP <100 mm Hg); then continue pazopanib at 1 dose level lower *Note:* Discontinue therapy if pazopanib is withheld >3 weeks
G4 hypertension	Discontinue therapy
QTc Abnormalities	
ECGs and electrolytes should be checked 3 times per week if any QTc abnormalities are noted	
QTc prolongation defined as: • A single measurement of ≥550 msec • An increase of ≥100 msec from baseline • Two consecutive measurements (within 48 hours of each other) that were ≥500 msec but ≤550 msec • An increase of ≥60 msec, but <100 msec from baseline to a value ≥480 msec	Hold pazopanib until QTc <480 msec, then resume pazopanib at 1 dose level lower

Therapy Monitoring

1. *At baseline, day 8, every 3 weeks until week 24, and every 4 weeks thereafter:* Physical examinations, vital signs, with blood pressure monitoring and clinical laboratory evaluations. Serum chemistries, particularly: calcium, magnesium, and potassium. 12-Lead ECG should be performed before the start of treatment (additional ECGs only if clinically indicated)

2. *Thyroid function tests:* Monitor every 12 weeks. If thyroid-stimulating hormone levels are abnormal, evaluations of free triiodothyronine and thyroxine should be obtained

3. *LFTs:* Monitor at baseline, once every 4 weeks for the first 4 months, then periodically thereafter

4. *Response assessment:* Every 2–3 cycles

Efficacy (N = 290)*

Pazopanib Response Rate, Overall Study Population		95% CI
Complete response	<1%	
Partial response	30%[†]	25.1–35.6
Median duration of response, weeks	58.7	52.1–68.1
Median time to response, weeks	11.9	9.4–12.3
Pazopanib Response Rate, Subsets		
Treatment-naïve population	32%	24.3–38.9
Cytokine pre-treated subpopulation	29%	21.2–36.5

Progression-Free Survival[‡]		HR vs. Placebo
Pazopanib, overall study population	9.2 months	0.46 (0.34–0.62)
Pazopanib, treatment-naïve population	11.1 months	0.40 (0.27–0.60)
Pazopanib, cytokine pre-treated subpopulation	7.4 months	0.54 (0.35–0.84)
Placebo	2.8–4.2 months	

*RECIST (Therasse P et al. J Natl Cancer Inst 2000;92:205–216)
[†]Median duration = 58.7 weeks
[‡]Prespecified subgroup analyses showed that PFS was improved for patients treated with pazopanib compared with placebo regardless of MSKCC risk category, sex, age, or ECOG PS (HR range: 0.40–0.52; $P < 0.001$ by log-rank test for all)

Mixed-Model Repeated-Measures Analyses for QoL Change from Baseline

Model	Number of Patients		Difference[†]	95% CI	P Value
	Pazopanib	Placebo*			
EORTC Quality of Life Questionnaire-C30: Global Health Status/QoL by Week					
6	243	110	−1.90	−5.84–2.04	0.34
12	219	81	−2.82	−7.17–1.53	0.20
18	191	61	−2.05	−6.95–2.86	0.41
24	164	49	0.39	−4.47–5.25	0.88
48	96	24	−0.67	−6.48–5.14	0.82
EuroQuol Questionaire-5D Index by Week					
6	253	125	0.01	−0.04–0.05	0.84
12	219	86	−0.04	−0.09–0.01	0.08
18	196	62	−0.02	−0.08–0.04	0.50
24	166	51	−0.03	−0.09–0.04	0.44
48	98	24	0.03	−0.03–0.10	0.33
EQ-5D Visual Analog Scale by Week					
6	239	111	1.85	−2.41–6.12	0.39
12	212	80	0.06	−4.79–4.91	0.98
18	189	60	−0.08	−5.04–4.89	0.98
24	161	49	−0.15	−4.83–4.53	0.95
48	95	23	−1.97	−9.02–5.09	0.58

*More patients in the placebo arm discontinued study treatment because of disease progression compared with patients in the pazopanib arm
[†]The minimal important differences for the questionnaires have been previously established as 5–10 for the EORTC-QLQ-C30, 0.08 for the EQ-5D Index, and 7 for the EQ-5D VAS. Values greater than 0 indicate a trend in favor of pazopanib, and values less than 0 indicate a trend in favor of placebo

REGIMEN

BEVACIZUMAB + INTERFERON ALFA-2A OR -2B

Escudier B et al. Lancet 2007;370:2103–2111
Escudier B et al. J Clin Oncol 2010;28:2144–2150
Rini BI et al. J Clin Oncol 2008;26:5422–5428
Rini BI et al. J Clin Oncol 2010;28:2137–2143

Bevacizumab 10 mg/kg per dose; administer intravenously in 100 mL 0.9% sodium chloride injection every 2 weeks until disease progression, unacceptable toxicity, or withdrawal of consent. No dose reduction permitted

Interferon alfa-2a *or* **interferon alfa-2b** 9 million IU/dose; administer by subcutaneous injection 3 times weekly for a maximum of 52 weeks, or until disease progression, unacceptable toxicity, or withdrawal of consent (total weekly dose = 27 million IU)

Note: If needed, the starting dose may be less than 9 million IU but every effort should be made to reach the recommended dose within the first 2 weeks of treatment

Supportive Care

Antiemetic prophylaxis
Emetogenic potential is **MINIMAL**
See Chapter 39 for antiemetic recommendations

Hematopoietic growth factor (CSF) prophylaxis
Primary prophylaxis is NOT indicated
See Chapter 43 for more information

Antimicrobial prophylaxis
Risk of fever and neutropenia is LOW
　Antimicrobial primary prophylaxis to be considered:
　• Antibacterial—not indicated

　• Antifungal—not indicated

　• Antiviral—not indicated unless patient previously had an episode of HSV
See Chapter 47 for more information

Treatment Modifications

Dose Levels

Starting dose: Level 1	Interferon alfa-2a *or* -2b 9 million IU + bevacizumab 10 mg/kg
Level −1	Interferon alfa-2a *or* -2b 6 million IU + bevacizumab 10 mg/kg
Level −2	Interferon alfa-2a *or* -2b 3 million IU + bevacizumab 10 mg/kg

Note: Across all NSCLC studies, for example, bevacizumab was discontinued in 8.4–21% of patients because of adverse reactions

Adverse Event	Dose Modification
G3/4 nonhematologic toxicity attributable to interferon alfa at a dose of 9 million IU	Reduce dose of interferon alfa to 6 million IU
G3/4 nonhematologic toxicity attributable to interferon alfa at a dose of 6 million IU	Reduce dose of interferon alfa to 3 million IU
Gastrointestinal (GI) perforations, fistula formation in the GI tract, intraabdominal abscess, fistula formation involving an internal organ, serious hemorrhage (ie, requiring medical intervention)	Discontinue bevacizumab

(continued)

Patient Population Studied

A study of 649 patients with metastatic RCC who were randomly assigned to receive either interferon alfa-2 alone or interferon alfa-2 plus bevacizumab. The RCC had to have predominantly (>50%) clear cell renal cell carcinoma and patients had to have undergone a prior nephrectomy or partial nephrectomy (if resection margins were clearly negative of disease). Patients had to have a Karnofsky performance status ≥70%. The primary end point of the trial was OS. The study was designed to have 80% power to detect an improvement in OS with an HR of 0.76, assuming an improvement of median survival from 13 months to 17 months, at a two-sided alpha level of 0.05 (Escudier B et al. Lancet 2007;370:2103–2111)

A study of 732 patients with metastatic RCC who were randomly assigned to receive either interferon alfa-2 alone or interferon alfa-2 plus bevacizumab. The RCC had to have predominantly a clear cell histologic component. Prior systemic therapy for RCC was not allowed. Patients were required to have a Karnofsky performance status ≥70%. The primary end point was OS (Rini BI et al. J Clin Oncol 2008;26:5422–5428)

Treatment Modifications (*continued*)

Hypertensive crisis or hypertensive encephalopathy	Discontinue bevacizumab
Reversible posterior leukoencephalopathy syndrome (RPLS)*	Discontinue bevacizumab
Severe arterial thromboembolic event (ATE)—cerebral infarction, transient ischemic attacks, myocardial infarction, angina*	Discontinue bevacizumab *Note:* The safety of resumption of bevacizumab therapy after resolution of an ATE has not been studied
Nephrotic syndrome (proteinuria [>3.5 g/day], hypoalbuminemia, hyperlipidemia, and edema)*	Discontinue bevacizumab
Moderate-to-severe proteinuria	Suspend bevacizumab administration for proteinuria ≥2 g/24 hours and resume when proteinuria is <2 g/24 hours. Patients with moderate-to-severe proteinuria based on 24-hour urine collections should be monitored regularly until improvement or resolution is observed. The safety of continued treatment in patients with moderate to severe proteinuria has not been evaluated *Note:* Data from a postmarketing safety study showed poor correlation between urine protein-to-creatinine ratio and 24-hour urine protein
Protein in urine ≥2+ per dipstick measurement	Perform further assessment with a 24-hour urine collection
Wound dehiscence or wound healing complications requiring medical intervention	Discontinue bevacizumab
Prior surgery	Do not initiate bevacizumab for at least 28 days after surgery, and not before the surgical wound is fully healed
Serious hemorrhage or recent hemoptysis (≥2.5 mL red blood)	Do not administer bevacizumab
Planned elective surgery	Temporarily suspend bevacizumab for at least 4 weeks
Severe infusion reactions	Temporarily suspend bevacizumab and administer appropriate medical therapy

*The safety of resuming bevacizumab therapy in patients who experience RPLS, ATE, and moderate-to-severe proteinuria (nephrotic syndrome) is unknown

Hypertension

Note: Patients should have their blood pressure checked once weekly during their first 24 weeks of therapy and during an 8-week period after any adjustment is made in their bevacizumab dose

G1 hypertension	Continue bevacizumab at same dose and schedule
G2 asymptomatic hypertension	Treat with antihypertensive medications and continue bevacizumab at same dose and schedule
G2 symptomatic hypertension or persistent G2 hypertension despite antihypertensive medications, or diastolic BP >110 mm Hg, or G3 hypertension	Treat with antihypertensive medications. Hold bevacizumab (maximum 3 weeks until symptoms resolve and diastolic BP <100 mm Hg); then, continue bevacizumab at 1 dose level lower *Note:* Discontinue therapy if bevacizumab is withheld >3 weeks
G4 hypertension	Discontinue therapy

Therapy Monitoring

1. *ECG:* Unless additional ECGs are clinically indicated, 12-lead ECGs are performed before the start of treatment, weekly for the first 8 weeks, and then every 12 weeks thereafter. If the dose is increased, then weekly monitoring is indicated for approximately 6 weeks

2. *Response assessment:* Every 2–3 cycles

3. *BP monitoring:* Should be conducted every 2–3 weeks during treatment. Patients who develop hypertension may require BP monitoring at more frequent intervals (even if they have discontinued therapy)

4. *Proteinuria monitoring:* Patients should also be monitored for the development or worsening of proteinuria with serial urinalyses. Patients with a urine dipstick reading >2+ should undergo further assessment (24-hour urine collection) and should be monitored regularly until improvement or resolution is observed

Efficacy[*]

	Escudier et al. 2007	Rini et al. 2008
Complete response, percent	1%	—
Partial response, percent	30%	25.5%
ORR (patients with G ≥2 hypertension)	—	13.1%[†]
ORR (patients without G ≥2 hypertension)	—	9.0%[†]
Time to response, median	2.2 months	—
Time to response, range	2–14 months	—
Duration of response, median	13.5 months	8.7 months
Duration of response, range	1.8–20.3 months	—
PFS		
PFS (patients with G ≥2 hypertension)	—	13.2 months[‡]
PFS (patients without G ≥2 hypertension)	—	8.0 months[‡]
OS	23.3 months	18.3
OS, MSKCC favorable risk	35.1 months	—
OS, MSKCC intermediate risk	22.6 months	—
OS, MSKCC poor risk	6 months	—
OS (patients with G ≥2 hypertension)	—	41.6 months[‡]
OS (patients without G ≥2 hypertension)	—	16.2 months[‡]

[*]RECIST (Therasse P et al. J Natl Cancer Inst 2000;92:205–216)
[†]$p = 0.95$
[‡]$p < 0.001$

Toxicity (N = Various)[*]

	Escudier et al. 2007 N = 337 (304)[†]		Rini et al. 2008 N = 366 (349)[†]	
	% All Grades	% G3/4	% G3	% G4
Nonhematologic				
Fatigue	33 (27)[†]	12 (8)[†]	35 (28)[†]	2 (2)[†]
Asthenia/weight loss	32 (28)	10 (7)	15 (5)	0
Proteinuria	18 (3)	7 (0)	13 (0)	2 (0)
Hypertension	26 (9)	3 (<1)	9 (0)	1 (0)
Bleeding	33 (9)	3 (<1)	—	—
Influenza-like illness	24 (25)	3 (2)	—	—
Anorexia	36 (30)	3 (3)	17 (8)	0
Nausea	—	—	7 (4)	0
Depression	12 (10)	3 (1)	—	—

(continued)

Toxicity (N = Various)* (continued)

	Escudier et al. 2007 N = 337 (304)†		Rini et al. 2008 N = 366 (349)†	
	% All Grades	% G3/4	% G3	% G4
Nonhematologic				
Pyrexia	45 (43)	2 (<1)	0	1 (0)
Headache	23 (16)	2 (1)	—	—
Diarrhea	20 (15)	2 (<1)	—	—
Venous thromboembolic event	3 (<1)	2 (<1)	1 (0)	1 (1)
Dyspnea	30 (30)	<1 (2)	5 (3)	1 (0)
Arterial thromboembolic event	1 (<1)	1 (<1)	—	—
Cerebrovascular ischemia	—	—	1 (0)	1 (0)
Gastrointestinal perforation	1 (0)	1 (0)	>1 (0)	>1 (0)
Wound healing complications	1 (1)	<1 (0)	—	—
Congestive heart failure	<1 (<1)	<1 (0)	<1 (<1)	<1 (0)
Hematologic				
Neutropenia	7 (7)	4 (2)	8 (8)	1 (0)
Anemia	10 (13)	3 (6)	3 (3)	1 (0)
Thrombocytopenia	6 (4)	2 (<1)	2 (1)	0

Adverse Events Leading to Study Discontinuation

	Escudier et al. 2007 N = 337 (304)†	Rini et al. 2008 N = 366 (349)†
Any study drug	28 (12)	24 (19)
Bevacizumab/placebo	19 (6)	—
Interferon alfa-2	23 (12)	—
Death not from disease progression	2 (2)	—
Disease progression or death	—	56 (61)
Refused further treatment	—	11 (9)

*NCI Common Terminology Criteria for Adverse Events v3.0
†Numbers in parentheses are those for the control arm treated with interferon alfa-2 plus placebo

Bevacizumab Toxicities

http://www.accessdata.fda.gov/drugsatfda_docs/label/2009/125085s0169lbl.pdf

Hypertension:
- Across clinical studies, the incidence of grade 3 or 4 hypertension ranged from 5–18%

Proteinuria and nephrotic syndrome:
- Across clinical studies, the incidence of grades 3–4 proteinuria (characterized as >3.5 g/24 hours) ranged up to 3% in bevacizumab-treated patients
- Nephrotic syndrome (proteinuria [>3.5 g/day], hypoalbuminemia, hyperlipidemia, and edema) occurred in <1% of patients who received bevacizumab in clinical trials, in some instances with fatal outcomes

Arterial thromboembolic events (ATEs):
- Across indications, the incidence of grade ≥3 ATEs (cerebral infarction, transient ischemic attacks, myocardial infarction, angina, and a variety of other ATEs) in the bevacizumab-containing arms was 2.4%
- Among patients who received bevacizumab in combination with chemotherapy, the risk of developing ATEs during therapy was increased in patients with a history of arterial thromboembolism, or age >65 years

Gastrointestinal (GI) perforation:
- The incidence of GI perforation ranged from 0.3–2.4% across clinical studies
- The typical presentation may include abdominal pain, nausea, emesis, constipation, and fever
- Perforation can be complicated by intraabdominal abscess and fistula formation
- The majority of cases occurred within the first 50 days after initiation of bevacizumab

Surgery and wound healing complications:
- The incidence of wound healing complications, including serious and fatal complications, in patients with metastatic colorectal cancer who underwent surgery during the course of bevacizumab treatment was 15%

Hemorrhage:
- Bevacizumab can result in 2 distinct patterns of bleeding: minor hemorrhage, most commonly grade 1 epistaxis, and serious, and, in some cases fatal, hemorrhagic events
- Severe or fatal hemorrhage, including hemoptysis, gastrointestinal bleeding, hematemesis, CNS hemorrhage, epistaxis, and vaginal bleeding occurred up to 5-fold more frequently in patients who received bevacizumab compared to patients who received only chemotherapy
- Across indications, the incidence of grade ≥3 hemorrhagic events among patients receiving bevacizumab ranged from 1.2–4.6%

REGIMEN

TEMSIROLIMUS

Hudes G et al. N Engl J Med 2007;356:2271–2281

Premedication:

Diphenhydramine 25–50 mg; administer intravenously approximately 30 minutes before each dose of temsirolimus as prophylaxis against hypersensitivity reactions (other histamine H$_1$-receptor antagonists may be substituted)

Temsirolimus 25 mg diluted in 250 mL 0.9% sodium chloride injection; administer intravenously over 30–60 minutes once weekly (total dose/week = 25 mg)

Notes:
- The concomitant use of strong cytochrome P450 (CYP) **CYP3A4 inhibitors** should be avoided. Ingestion of grapefruit products (fruit, juice) may also increase plasma concentrations of sirolimus (a major metabolite of temsirolimus) and should be avoided. If a strong **CYP3A4 inhibitor** must be administered, a temsirolimus dose reduction to 12.5 mg/week should be considered. However, there are no clinical data with this dose adjustment in patients receiving strong CYP3A4 inhibitors

- If a concomitantly administered strong **CYP3A4 inhibitor** is discontinued, a washout period of approximately 1 week should be allowed before the temsirolimus dose is adjusted back to the dose used prior to initiation of the strong CYP3A4 inhibitor

- The use of concomitant strong **CYP3A4 inducers** should be avoided. If a strong **CYP3A4 inducer** must be administered, a temsirolimus dose increase from 25 mg/week up to 50 mg/week should be considered. However, there are no clinical data with this dose adjustment in patients receiving strong CYP3A4 inducers

- If a concomitantly administered strong **CYP3A4 inducer** is discontinued, the temsirolimus dose should be returned to the dose used prior to initiation of the strong CYP3A4 inducer

- Temsirolimus has immunosuppressive properties and may predispose patients to infections. Localized and systemic infections (bacterial and invasive fungal infections) have occurred. Some of these infections have been severe or fatal. Complete the treatment for preexisting invasive fungal infections prior to starting treatment with temsirolimus

- Elevations in serum glucose can occur with temsirolimus. When possible, optimal glucose and lipid control should be achieved before starting a patient on temsirolimus

Supportive Care

Antiemetic prophylaxis
Emetogenic potential is **MINIMAL**
See Chapter 39 for antiemetic recommendations

Hematopoietic growth factor (CSF) prophylaxis
Primary prophylaxis is NOT indicated
See Chapter 43 for more information

Antimicrobial prophylaxis
Risk of fever and neutropenia is LOW
   Antimicrobial primary prophylaxis to be considered:
- Antibacterial—not indicated
- Antifungal—not indicated
- Antiviral—not indicated unless patient previously had an episode of HSV
See Chapter 47 for more information

Patient Population Studied

A study of 626 patients were randomly assigned to receive interferon (207), temsirolimus (209), or a combination of interferon and temsirolimus (210). Eligibility criteria included patients with histologically confirmed advanced renal cell carcinoma (stage IV or recurrent disease) and a Karnofsky performance score of ≥60 (on a scale of 0–100, with higher scores indicating better performance) who had not previously received systemic therapy for renal cancer. A fasting level of total cholesterol of no more than 350 mg/dL (≤9.1 mmol/L) and a triglyceride level of no more than 400 mg/dL (≤4.5 mmol/L) were required. At least 3 of the following 6 predictors of short survival were required: (a) a serum lactate dehydrogenase level ≥1.5-times the upper limit of normal range; (b) a hemoglobin level less than the lower limit of normal range; (c) a corrected serum calcium level >10 mg/dL (>2.5 mmol/L); (d) <1 year from initial diagnosis of renal cell carcinoma to randomization; (e) a Karnofsky performance score of 60 or 70; or (f) metastases in multiple organs

Treatment Modifications

Temsirolimus Dose Levels

Starting dose: Level 1	25 mg once daily
Level −1	20 mg once daily
Level −2	15 mg once daily

Adverse Event	Dose Modification
Invasive systemic fungal infection	Discontinue temsirolimus and treat with appropriate antifungal therapy
Noninfectious pneumonitis without symptoms with only radiologic changes	Observe carefully. Specific therapies or drug interruption may not be necessary
Noninfectious pneumonitis with mild-to-moderate symptoms	Withhold therapy. Glucocorticoids may be initiated. Resume temsirolimus at a reduced dose depending on the individual clinical circumstances
Noninfectious pneumonitis with severe symptoms (including a decrease in DL_{CO} on pulmonary function tests)	Discontinue therapy and consider administering high doses of glucocorticoids
ANC <1000/mm³ or platelet count <75,000/mm³	Withhold therapy. Resume temsirolimus when symptoms improve to G ≤2 with temsirolimus dose reduced by 5 mg/week to a dose not less than 15 mg/week
Any nonhematologic G3/4 toxicity	Withhold therapy. Resume temsirolimus when symptoms improve to G ≤2 with temsirolimus dose reduced by 5 mg/week to a dose not less than 15 mg/week
G1/2 oral ulcerations	Topical treatments are recommended, but alcohol- or peroxide-containing mouthwashes should be avoided. Focus on pain control, oral hygiene, and IV fluid replacement, or total parenteral nutrition if severe
Hyperglycemia	Monitor blood sugar levels and institute oral hypoglycemic agent or insulin as needed
Hypertriglyceridemia	Monitor triglycerides, instituting dietary interventions for minor elevations and lipid-lowering agents for levels exceeding 500 mg/dL

Efficacy (N = 209)*

Percent objective response rate	8.6 (range: 4.8–12.4)
Median overall survival (95% CI), months	10.9 (range: 8.6–12.7)
Median progression-free survival (95% CI), months	5.5 (range: 3.9–7.0)
Median time to treatment failure (95% CI), months	3.8 (range: 3.5–3.9)

*RECIST (Therasse P et al. J Natl Cancer Inst 2000;92:205–216)

Therapy Monitoring

1. *Prior to starting treatment and periodically thereafter:* Renal function, CBC with differential, blood glucose, and serum lipid profile
2. *ECG:* A 12-lead ECG should be performed before the start of treatment, weekly for at least the first 2 weeks. Additional ECGs may be performed depending on the QTc. If the dose is increased then at least 1 additional ECG should be obtained
3. *Response assessment:* Every 8–12 weeks

Toxicity (N = 208)*

Adverse Event	% All Grades	% G3/4
Asthenia	51	11
Rash	47	4
Nausea	37	2
Anorexia	32	3
Pain	28	5
Dyspnea	28	9
Infection	27	5
Diarrhea	27	1
Peripheral edema	27	2
Fever	24	1
Abdominal pain	21	4
Stomatitis	20	1
Constipation	20	0
Back pain	20	3
Vomiting	19	2
Weight loss	19	1
Headache	15	1
Chills	8	1

Laboratory Abnormalities

Anemia	45	20
Hyperlipidemia	27	3
Hyperglycemia	26	11
Hypercholesterolemia	24	1
Increased creatinine level	14	3
Thrombocytopenia	14	1
Increased aspartate aminotransferase level (AST)	8	1
Neutropenia	7	3
Leukopenia	6	1

*NCI Common Terminology Criteria for Adverse Events v3.0

SECOND-LINE REGIMEN
EVEROLIMUS

Motzer RJ et al. Lancet 2008;372:449–456
Motzer RJ et al. Cancer 2010;116:4256–4265

Everolimus 10 mg/day; administer orally in a fasting state or with a light, fat-free meal, continually. Treatment cycles are 28 days in duration (total dose/28-day cycle = 280 mg)

Notes:
- For patients with mild-to-moderate hepatic impairment (Child-Pugh Class B), reduce the dose to 5 mg daily
- Everolimus has not been evaluated in patients with severe hepatic impairment (Child-Pugh Class C) and should not be used in this population
- A missed dose may be taken up to 6 hours after the regular scheduled time; otherwise, it should be skipped. After missing a dose, take everolimus at the usual time the following day. Doubling doses on subsequent days to compensate for missed doses should not be attempted
- Everolimus has immunosuppressive properties and may predispose patients to infections. Localized and systemic infections (bacterial and invasive fungal infections) have occurred. Some of these infections have been severe or fatal. Complete treatment for preexisting invasive fungal infections prior to starting treatment with everolimus
- Elevations in serum glucose can occur with everolimus. When possible, optimal glucose and lipid control should be achieved before starting a patient on everolimus
- Avoid concomitant use with strong inhibitors of CYP3A4 or PgP (MDR1, ABCB1 transport protein). If coadministration with moderate CYP3A4 or PgP inhibitors is required, use caution and reduce the everolimus dose to 2.5 mg daily
- Increase the everolimus dose if coadministered with a strong CYP3A4 inducer

Supportive Care
Antiemetic prophylaxis
Emetogenic potential is **MINIMAL**
See Chapter 39 for antiemetic recommendations

Hematopoietic growth factor (CSF) prophylaxis
Primary prophylaxis is NOT indicated
See Chapter 43 for more information

Antimicrobial prophylaxis
Risk of fever and neutropenia is LOW
Antimicrobial primary prophylaxis to be considered:
- Antibacterial—not indicated
- Antifungal—not indicated
- Antiviral—not indicated unless patient previously had an episode of HSV

See Chapter 47 for more information

Treatment Modifications

Everolimus Dose Levels	
Starting dose: Level 1	10 mg once daily
Level −1	5 mg once daily
Level −2	2.5 mg once daily

(continued)

Patient Population Studied

A study of 410 patients with metastatic renal cell carcinoma that showed a clear cell component that had progressed either during or within 6 months after stopping treatment with sunitinib, sorafenib, or both drugs. Previous therapy with bevacizumab, aldesleukin (interleukin-2), or interferon alfa, was also permitted. Key eligibility criteria included a Karnofsky performance status score ≥70%. Patients were randomly assigned in a 2:1 ratio to receive everolimus 10 mg once daily (n = 272) or placebo (n = 138) in conjunction with best supportive care. Randomization was stratified by Memorial Sloan-Kettering Cancer Center prognostic score and previous anticancer therapy. The primary endpoint was progression-free survival

Treatment Modifications (*continued*)

Adverse Event	Dose Modification
Invasive systemic fungal infection	Discontinue everolimus and treat with appropriate antifungal therapy
Noninfectious pneumonitis without symptoms with only radiologic changes	Observe carefully. Specific therapies or drug interruption may not be necessary
Noninfectious pneumonitis with mild-to-moderate symptoms	Withhold therapy. Glucocorticoids may be initiated. Resume everolimus at a reduced dose depending on the individual clinical circumstances
Noninfectious pneumonitis with severe symptoms (including a decrease in DL_{CO} on pulmonary function tests)	Discontinue therapy and consider administering high doses of glucocorticoids
ANC <1000/mm^3 or platelet count <75,000/mm^3	Withhold therapy. Resume everolimus when symptoms improve to G ≤2 with everolimus dose reduced to 5 mg/day, or 5 mg every other day but not less than 15 mg/week
Any nonhematologic G3/4 toxicity	Withhold therapy. Restart everolimus when symptoms improve to G ≤2 with everolimus dose reduced to 5 mg/day, or 5 mg every other day but not less than 15 mg/week
G1/2 oral ulcerations	Topical treatments are recommended, but alcohol- or peroxide-containing mouthwashes should be avoided. Focus on pain control, oral hygiene, and IV fluid replacement, or total parenteral nutrition if severe
Hyperglycemia	Monitor blood sugar levels and institute oral hypoglycemic agent or insulin as needed
Hypertriglyceridemia	Monitor triglycerides, instituting dietary interventions for minor elevations and lipid-lowering agents for levels exceeding 500 mg/dL

Therapy Monitoring

1. *Prior to starting treatment and periodically thereafter:* Renal function, CBC with differential, blood glucose, and serum lipid profiles
2. *ECG:* A 12-lead ECG should be performed before the start of treatment, weekly for at least the first 2 weeks. Additional ECGs may be performed depending on the QTc. If the dose is increased, then at least 1 additional ECG should be obtained
3. *Safety assessment:* Every 2–4 weeks for the first 3 cycles; every 4–8 weeks thereafter
4. *Response assessment:* Every 8–12 weeks

Efficacy (Everolimus N = 272; Placebo N = 138)*

Partial response	1%
Median progression-free survival	4 months[†]
Probability of being progression-free at 6 months	26%[‡]
Median duration of treatment	95 days
Median overall survival[§]	Hazard ratio consistent with placebo: 14.8 months (everolimus) vs. 14.4 months (placebo) (HR: 0.87; P = 0.162)

*RECIST (Therasse P et al. J Natl Cancer Inst 2000;92:205–216)
[†]1.9 months in the placebo group. Predefined subset analyses (MSKCC risk classification) plus a series of exploratory analyses across relevant patient subgroups (number of previous VEGF receptor tyrosine kinase inhibitors, age, sex, and geographic region) indicated benefit was maintained across subgroups
[‡]2% in placebo group
[§]Confounded by crossover: Of the 98 patients in the placebo group whose disease progressed per investigator assessment, 79 crossed over to open-label everolimus after disease progression. Of these 79 patients, 60 developed progressive disease within 8 weeks after enrollment. By the rank-preserving structural failure time model, the survival corrected for crossover was 1.9-fold longer (95% CI, 0.5–8.5) with everolimus compared with placebo only. Independent prognostic factors for shorter OS in the study included low performance status, high corrected serum calcium, low hemoglobin, and prior sunitinib use (P <0.01) (Motzer RJ et al. Cancer 2010;116:4256–4265)

Toxicity (Placebo N = 135; Everolimus N = 269)*

Adverse Event	Placebo % All Grades	Everolimus % All Grades	% G3	% G4
Stomatitis†	8	40	3	0
Rash	4	25	<1	0
Fatigue	16	20	3	0
Asthenia	8	18	1	0
Diarrhea	3	17	1	0
Anorexia	6	16	<1	0
Nausea	8	15	0	0
Mucosal inflammation	2	14	1	0
Vomiting	4	12	0	0
Cough	4	12	0	0
Dry skin	4	11	<1	0
Infections‡	2	10	2	1
Pneumonitis§		8	3	0
Dyspnea	2	8	1	0

Laboratory Abnormality				
Anemia	76	91	9	<1
Hypercholesterolemia	32	76	3	0
Hypertriglyceridemia	30	71	<1	0
Hyperglycemia	23	50	12	0
Increased creatinine	33	46	<1	0
Lymphopenia	29	42	14	1
Increased alkaline phosphatase	30	37	<1	0
Hypophosphatemia	7	32	4	0
Leukopenia	8	26	0	0
Increased aspartate aminotransferase (AST)	7	21	<1	0
Thrombocytopenia	2	20	<1	0
Increased alanine aminotransferase (ALT)	4	18	<1	0
Hypocalcemia	6	17	0	0
Neutropenia	3	11	0	0

Adjustment in Therapy	Placebo	Everolimus
Treatment discontinuation for toxicity	10%	4%
Dose interruption required	34%	15%
Dose reduction with no previous interruption	5%	<1%

*NCI Common Terminology Criteria for Adverse Events v3.0
†Includes aphthous stomatitis, mouth ulceration, and stomatitis
‡Includes all infections
§Includes interstitial lung disease, lung infiltration, pneumonitis, pulmonary alveolar haemorrhage, and pulmonary toxicity

SECOND-LINE REGIMEN
AXITINIB

Rini BI et al. Lancet 2011;378:1931–1939

Axitinib 5 mg; administer orally twice daily (approximately every 12 hours), continually (total dose/week = 35 mg)

- Axitinib should be swallowed whole (no breaking, crushing, or chewing) with water
- Axitinib may be administered without respect to food ingestion

Notes:

1. Patients who tolerate axitinib for at least two consecutive weeks with no adverse reactions G >2, who remain normotensive, and are not receiving anti-hypertension medications may have their dose increased to 7 mg twice daily, and further to 10 mg twice daily using the same criteria

2. *Strong CYP3A4/5 Inhibitors:* The concomitant use of strong CYP3A4/5 inhibitors should be avoided (eg, atazanavir, clarithromycin, indinavir, itraconazole, ketoconazole, nefazodone, nelfinavir, ritonavir, saquinavir, telithromycin, and voriconazole). Selection of an alternate concomitant medication with no or minimal CYP3A4/5 inhibition potential is recommended. Although axitinib dose adjustment has not been studied in patients receiving strong CYP3A4/5 inhibitors, if a strong CYP3A4/5 inhibitor must be co-administered, a dose decrease of axitinib by approximately half is recommended, as this dose reduction is predicted to adjust the axitinib area under the plasma concentration vs time curve (AUC) to the AUC range observed without inhibitors. Subsequent doses can be increased or decreased based on individual safety and tolerability. If co-administration of a strong inhibitor is discontinued, the axitinib dose should be returned (after 3–5 elimination half-lives of the inhibitor) to that used prior to initiation of the strong CYP3A4/5 inhibitor

3. The axitinib starting dose should be reduced by approximately half in patients with baseline moderate hepatic impairment (Child-Pugh class B)

4. If axitinib is interrupted, patients receiving antihypertensive medications should be monitored for hypotension

Supportive Care
Antiemetic prophylaxis
Emetogenic potential is **MINIMAL–LOW**
See Chapter 39 for antiemetic recommendations

Hematopoietic growth factor (CSF) prophylaxis
Primary prophylaxis is NOT indicated
See Chapter 43 for more information

Antimicrobial prophylaxis
Risk of fever and neutropenia is LOW
  Antimicrobial primary prophylaxis to be considered:
  - Antibacterial—not indicated
  - Antifungal—not indicated
  - Antiviral—not indicated, unless patient previously had an episode of HSV
See Chapter 47 for more information

Diarrhea management
Latent or delayed-onset diarrhea*:
  Loperamide 4 mg orally initially after the first loose or liquid stool, *then*
  Loperamide 2 mg orally every 2 hours during waking hours, *plus*
  Loperamide 4 mg orally every 4 hours during hours of sleep
  - Continue for at least 12 hours after diarrhea resolves
  - Recurrent diarrhea after a 12-hour diarrhea-free interval is treated as a new episode
  - Rehydrate orally with fluids and electrolytes during a diarrheal episode
  - If a patient develops blood or mucus in stool, dehydration, or hemodynamic instability, or if diarrhea persists >48 hours despite loperamide, stop loperamide and hospitalize the patient for IV hydration

(continued)

(continued)

Alternatively, a trial of **Diphenoxylate hydrochloride** 2.5 mg **with Atropine sulfate** 0.025 mg (eg, Lomotil®)
- Initial adult dose is two tablets four times daily until control has been achieved, after which the dose may be reduced to meet individual requirements. Control may often be maintained with as little as two tablets daily
- Clinical improvement of acute diarrhea is usually observed within 48 hours. If improvement of chronic diarrhea after treatment with a maximum daily dose of 8 tablets is not observed within 10 days, control is unlikely with further administration

Persistent diarrhea:

Octreotide 100–150 mcg subcutaneously 3 times daily. Maximum total daily dose is 1500 mcg

Antibiotic therapy during latent or delayed-onset diarrhea:

A fluoroquinolone (eg, **Ciprofloxacin** 500 mg orally every 12 hours) if absolute neutrophil count $<500/mm^3$ with or without accompanying fever in association with diarrhea
- Antibiotics should also be administered if patient is hospitalized with prolonged diarrhea and should be continued until diarrhea resolves

*Abigerges D et al. J Natl Cancer Inst 1994;86:446–449
Rothenberg ML et al. J Clin Oncol 2001;19:3801–3807
Wadler S et al. J Clin Oncol 1998;16:3169–3178

Treatment Modifications

Adverse Event	Treatment Discontinuation
Any hypertension	Treat as needed with standard anti-hypertensive therapy
Persistent hypertension despite use of anti-hypertensive medications	Reduce the dose of axitinib ($10 \rightarrow 7 \rightarrow 5 \rightarrow 3 \rightarrow 2$ mg twice daily)
Evidence of hypertensive crisis	Discontinue axitinib
Moderate to severe proteinuria	Reduce the dose of axitinib ($10 \rightarrow 7 \rightarrow 5 \rightarrow 3 \rightarrow 2$ mg twice daily), or withhold axitinib treatment until protein returns to baseline values

Patient Population Studied

Multicenter, phase 3, randomized, controlled trial that included patients with histologically or cytologically confirmed RCC with a clear cell component. All patients had RECIST-defined progressive disease after one previous systemic first-line regimen with a sunitinib-based, bevacizumab plus interferon alfa-based, temsirolimus-based, or cytokine-based regimen. Eligibility criteria included 2 weeks or more since the end of previous systemic treatment (4 weeks or more for bevacizumab plus interferon alfa) and an ECOG PS of 0 or 1. Exclusion criteria included present use or anticipated need for cytochrome P450 (CYP)3A4-inhibiting, CYP3A4-inducing, or CYP1A2-inducing drugs

Baseline Demographics and Clinical Characteristics

	Axitinib (n = 361)	Sorafenib (n = 362)
Age (Years)		
Median (range)	61 (20–82)	61 (22–80)
Sex		
Male	265 (73%)	258 (71%)
Female	96 (27%)	104 (29%)
ECOG Performance Status		
0	195 (54%)	200 (55%)
1	162 (45%)	160 (44%)
MSKCC Risk Subgroup*		
Favorable	100 (28%)	101 (28%)
Intermediate	134 (37%)	130 (36%)
Poor	118 (33%)	120 (33%)
NA	9 (2%)	11 (3%)
Heng et al. Risk Factors†		
Favorable	66 (18%)	79 (22%)
Intermediate	236 (65%)	225 (62%)
Poor	37 (10%)	34 (9%)
NA	22 (6%)	24 (7%)

(continued)

Efficacy

[Independent Review Committee Assessment]

	Axitinib (n = 361)	Sorafenib (n = 362)	HR for Progression or Death (95% CI)	p Value
Progression-Free Survival (PFS) in Months				
Estimated median PFS	6.7 (6.3–8.6)	4.7 (4.6–5.6)	0.665 (0.544–0.812)*	<0.0001
Stratified Estimated Median PFS (Months) Depending on Previous Regimens				
Previous cytokine	12.1 (10.1–3.9)	6.5 (6.3–8.3)	0.464 (0.318–0.676)†	<0.0001
Previous sunitinib	4.8 (4.5–6.4)	3.4 (2.8–4.7)	0.741 (0.573–0.958)†	0.0107
Previous bevacizumab	4.2 (2.8–6.5)	4.7 (2.8–6.7)	1.147 (0.568–2.317)†	0.6366
Previous temsirolimus	10.1 (1.5–10.2)	5.3 (1.5–10.1)	0.511 (0.140–1.865)†	0.1425

Objective Tumor Response

Best RECIST Response Observed, n (%)

	Axitinib	Sorafenib		
Complete response	0	0	—	—
Partial response	70 (19%)	34 (9%)	—	—
Stable disease ≥20 weeks	96 (27%)	77 (21%)	—	—
Stable disease <20 weeks	84 (23%)	120 (33%)	—	—
Progressive disease	78 (22%)	76 (21%)	—	—
Not assessed	0	0	—	—
Indeterminate‡	22 (6%)	42 (12%)	—	—
Objective response rate§	70 (19%)	34 (9%)	—	<0.001
95% CI	15.4–23.9	6.6–12.9	—	—

HR, Hazard ratio; RECIST, Response Evaluation Criteria In Solid Tumors; ECOG, Eastern Cooperative Oncology Group
*One-sided log-rank test stratified by ECOG performance status and previous treatment
†One-sided log-rank test stratified by ECOG performance status
‡Includes patients with no post-baseline scans, target lesions that were indeterminate at subsequent timepoints, or patients randomized and not treated
§One-sided Cochran-Mantel-Haenszel test of treatment stratified by ECOG performance status and previous treatment

Patient Population Studied
(continued)

	Axitinib (n = 361)	Sorafenib (n = 362)
Previous Systemic Therapy		
Sunitinib	194 (54%)	195 (54%)
Cytokines	126 (35%)	125 (35%)
Bevacizumab	29 (8%)	30 (8%)
Temsirolimus	12 (3%)	12 (3%)

ECOG, Eastern Cooperative Oncology Group; MSKCC, Memorial Sloan-Kettering Cancer Center; NA, not available
*MSKCC risk groups were derived with three risk factors: (1) hemoglobin (≤13 g/dL [≤130 g/L] vs >13 g/dL [>130 g/L] for men, and ≤11.5 g/dL [≤115 g/L] vs >11.5 g/dL [>115 g/L] for women), (2) corrected calcium (<10 mg/dL [<2.5 mmol/L] vs ≥10 mg/dL [≥2.5 mmol/L]), and (3) ECOG performance status (0 vs 1) MSKCC risk groups were defined as favorable (0 factors), intermediate (1 factor), or poor (2–3 factors)
†Heng risk groups were defined as favorable (0 factors), intermediate (1–2 factors), or poor (≥3 factors)

Toxicity

Common Treatment-Emergent All-Causality Adverse Events

Adverse Events	Axitinib (n = 359)		Sorafenib (n = 355)	
	All Grades	G ≥3	All Grades	G ≥3
Diarrhea	197 (55%)	38 (11%)	189 (53%)	26 (7%)
Hypertension	145 (40%)	56 (16%)	103 (29%)	39 (11%)
Fatigue	140 (39%)	41 (11%)	112 (32%)	18 (5%)
Decreased appetite	123 (34%)	18 (5%)	101 (29%)	13 (4%)
Nausea	116 (32%)	9 (3%)	77 (22%)	4 (1%)
Dysphonia	111 (31%)	0	48 (14%)	0
PPE	98 (27%)	18 (5%)	181 (51%)	57 (16%)
Weight decreased	89 (25%)	8 (2%)	74 (21%)	5 (1%)
Vomiting	85 (24%)	12 (3%)	61 (17%)	3 (1%)
Asthenia	74 (21%)	19 (5%)	50 (14%)	9 (3%)
Constipation	73 (20%)	4 (1%)	72 (20%)	3 (1%)
Hypothyroidism	69 (19%)	1 (<1%)	29 (8%)	0
Cough	55 (15%)	3 (1%)	59 (17%)	2 (1%)
Mucosal inflammation	55 (15%)	5 (1%)	44 (12%)	2 (1%)
Arthralgia	54 (15%)	5 (1%)	39 (11%)	5 (1%)
Stomatitis	54 (15%)	5 (1%)	44 (12%)	1 (<1%)
Rash	45 (13%)	1 (<1%)	112 (32%)	14 (4%)
Alopecia	14 (4%)	0	115 (32%)	0

Laboratory Abnormalities*

Anemia	113/320 (35%)	1/320 (<1%)	165/316 (52%)	12/316 (4%)
Hemoglobin elevation	31/320 (10%)	NA	3/316 (1%)	NA
Neutropenia	19/316 (6%)	2/316 (1%)	26/308 (8%)	2/308 (1%)
Thrombocytopenia	48/312 (15%)	1/312 (<1%)	44/310 (14%)	0
Lymphopenia	106/317 (33%)	10/317 (3%)	111/309 (36%)	11/309 (4%)
Creatinine elevation	185/336 (55%)	0	131/318 (41%)	1/318 (<1%)
Hypophosphatemia	43/336 (13%)	6/336 (2%)	158/318 (50%)	51/318 (16%)
Hypercalcemia	19/336 (6%)	0	5/319 (2%)	0
Hypocalcemia	132/336 (39%)	4/336 (1%)	188/319 (59%)	5/319 (2%)
Lipase elevation	91/338 (27%)	16/338 (5%)	148/319 (46%)	47/319 (15%)

PPE, Palmar-plantar erythrodysesthesia; NA, not available
*Denominator for each laboratory abnormality differed depending on the availability of baseline and at least one on-study test result

Treatment Monitoring

1. *At baseline, week 2, week 4, and every 4 weeks thereafter:* Clinical assessments including medical history and physical examination, vital signs, and CBC with differential

2. *At screening, after 6 and 12 weeks of therapy, and every 8 weeks thereafter:* Tumor assessments, including CT and MRI. Thyroid function tests. 24-hour or spot urine for protein measurement

REGIMEN

HIGH-DOSE ALDESLEUKIN (INTERLEUKIN-2 [IL-2])

Yang JC et al. J Clin Oncol 2003;21:3127–3132

Aldesleukin 720,000 units/kg per dose; administer intravenously in 50 mL of albumin (human) 5% over 15 minutes every 8 hours for a maximum of 15 doses/cycle, if tolerated, for 2 cycles (after treatment commences the administration schedule is preserved; treatment is not extended to replace doses that were omitted owing to adverse events). Each cycle is separated by 7–10 days of rest. Treatment is repeated every 2 months

Supportive Care
Antiemetic prophylaxis
Emetogenic potential is **MODERATE**
See Chapter 39 for antiemetic recommendations

Hematopoietic growth factor (CSF) prophylaxis
Primary prophylaxis is NOT indicated
See Chapter 43 for more information

Antimicrobial prophylaxis
Risk of fever and neutropenia is LOW
Antimicrobial primary prophylaxis to be considered:
• Antibacterial—not indicated
• Antifungal—not indicated
• Antiviral—not indicated unless patient previously had an episode of HSV
See Chapter 47 for more information

Ancillary medications: See special section below

Patient Population Studied

A study of 156 patients with metastatic RCC without prior IL-2 therapy. Patients with brain metastases, coronary artery disease, active autoimmune disorder, or significant renal, pulmonary, or hepatic insufficiency were excluded

Efficacy (N = 155)

Complete response	6%
Partial response	15%

Treatment Modifications: Guidelines for Delay or Discontinuation of Aldesleukin and for Treatment of Adverse Events

Relative Criteria	Absolute Criteria
Cardiac	
Sinus tachycardia (120–130 beats/min)	Sustained sinus tachycardia (>130 beats/min) despite correcting hypotension, fever, and tachycardia, and stopping dopamine) *ECG changes:* Atrial fibrillation Supraventricular tachycardia Ventricular arrhythmias (frequent PVCs, bigeminy tachycardia) Changes suggestive of ischemia *Laboratory:* Elevated CPK isoenzymes or troponin
Dermatologic	
	Moist desquamation
Gastrointestinal	
Diarrhea, 1000 mL/8 hours Ileus/abdominal distention *Laboratory:* Bilirubin >7 mg/dL (120 µmol/L)	Diarrhea, 1000 mL/8 hours × 2 Vomiting not responsive to medication Severe abdominal distention affecting breathing Severe abdominal pain, unrelenting
Hemodynamic	
Maximum phenylephrine 1–1.5 mg/kg per minute	Maximum phenylephrine 1.5–2 µg/kg per minute
Minimum phenylephrine >0.5 mg/kg per minute	Minimum phenylephrine >0.8 µg/kg per minute

(continued)

Treatment Modifications: Guidelines for Delay or Discontinuation of Aldesleukin and for Treatment of Adverse Events (continued)

Relative Criteria	Absolute Criteria
Hemorrhagic	
Guaiac-positive sputum, emesis, or stool *Laboratory:* Platelets 30,000–50,000/mm³	Frank blood in sputum, emesis, or stool *Laboratory:* Platelets <30,000/mm³
Infectious	
	Strong clinical suspicion or documented infection
Musculoskeletal	
Weight gain >15%	
Extremity tightness	Extremity paresthesias
Neurologic	
Vivid dreams	Hallucinations
Emotional lability	Persistent crying Mental status changes not reversible in 2 hours Inability to subtract serial 7s or spell words backwards Disorientation
Pulmonary	
Resting shortness of breath	
3–4 L O_2 by nasal cannula for saturation ≥95%	>4 L O_2 by nasal cannula for saturation ≥95% *or* 40% O_2 mask for saturation ≥95%
Rales one-third up lower chest	Endotracheal intubation Moist rales halfway up chest Pleural effusion requiring thoracentesis or chest tube while on therapy
Renal	
Urine 80–160 mL/shift Urine 10–20 mL/hour *Laboratory:* Creatinine 2.5–2.9 mg/dL (221–256 µmol/L)	Urine <80 mL/shift Urine <10 mL/hour *Laboratory:* Creatinine >3 mg/dL (>265 µmol/L)

When to Delay or Discontinue Aldesleukin

Observation	Action
Any relative criteria	Initiate corrective measure ± delay aldesleukin
>3 Relative criteria	Initiate corrective measure, delay aldesleukin Stop aldesleukin if not easily reversible
Any absolute criteria	Initiate corrective measures, delay aldesleukin Stop aldesleukin if not easily reversible

Adapted from Schwartzentruber DJ. J Immunother 2001;24:287–293

(continued)

Toxicity* (N = 156)

Adverse Event	% G3/4
Hypotension	36
Malaise	21
Nausea or vomiting	13
Oliguria (<80 mL/8 hours)	12
CNS: Orientation	10
Thrombocytopenia	9
Diarrhea	9
Arrhythmia, atrial	4
Hyperbilirubinemia	3
Elevated ALT	3
CNS: level of consciousness	3
Infection	3
Peripheral edema	0.4

*All toxicities were reversible and no deaths occurred

Treatment Modifications: Guidelines for Delay or Discontinuation of Aldesleukin and for Treatment of Adverse Events *(continued)*

Corrective Measures for Aldesleukin Symptoms/Findings

Symptom	Corrective Measure
Cardiac	
Tachycardia (sinus)	Correct fever, hypotension, hypoxia, anemia; consider discontinuation of dopamine if used
Arrhythmia (other than sinus tachycardia)	Stop aldesleukin (most arrhythmias); correct electrolytes, minerals, anemia, hypoxia; use medications as indicated
Creatine kinase elevation	Measure isoenzymes or troponin, and obtain ECG; if evidence of myocarditis, stop aldesleukin; will need exercise ECHO before next cycle of aldesleukin to rule out myocardial dysfunction; future aldesleukin may be considered if ECHO is normal
Troponin elevation	Must stop aldesleukin; will need exercise ECHO before next cycle of aldesleukin to rule out myocardial dysfunction; future aldesleukin may be considered if the ECHO is normal
Constitutional	
Chills (generally after first or second aldesleukin dose)	Warm blankets as first measure; intravenous meperidine if chills persist
Fever breakthrough	Increase indomethacin to every 6 hours; consider septic work-up if happens after first 24 hours of therapy (ie, high spike above baseline during therapy)
Nasal congestion	Room humidifier, decongestant (no aerosolized steroids)
Dermatologic	
Moist desquamation	Oatmeal baths, lotions (no steroid- or alcohol-containing lotions)
Pruritus	Oatmeal baths, lotions, antipruritics
Gastrointestinal	
Diarrhea	Antidiarrheals (alternate medications); avoid overuse because of complicating ileus and distention
Nausea/vomiting	Antiemetics (alternate medications and routes if any medication is not effective)
Abdominal pain	Evaluate cause; give indomethacin rectally; consider antacids
Mucositis/stomatitis	Frequent oral care, mouthwashes, topical anesthetics, room humidifier
Hemodynamic	
Hypotension	Initially fluids; add phenylephrine after 1–1.5 L of fluid boluses
Acidosis: CO_2 <20 mmol/L	Give 50 mEq sodium bicarbonate intravenously
Acidosis: CO_2 <18 mmol/L	Give 100 mEq sodium bicarbonate intravenously
Hemorrhagic	
Anemia	Transfuse packed red blood cells to maintain hematocrit above 28% during aldesleukin dosing
Thrombocytopenia	Consider transfusion if platelet count <20,000/mm^3

(continued)

Notes

1. Patients are retreated with another course of aldesleukin if disease is stable or regressing
2. Therapy is stopped and patients observed if they have 2 consecutive posttreatment evaluations that are unchanged
3. In a 2-arm comparison with low-dose aldesleukin (72,000 units/kg), there was no overall survival difference

Treatment Modifications: Guidelines for Delay or Discontinuation of Aldesleukin and for Treatment of Adverse Events (continued)

Corrective Measures for Aldesleukin Symptoms/Findings

Symptom	Corrective Measure
Infectious	
Infection	Stop aldesleukin and treat infection as indicated
Laboratory	
Hypoalbuminemia	Observe
Hypocalcemia	Maintain above lowest normal value
Hypokalemia	Maintain potassium above 3.6 mmol/L
Hypomagnesemia	Maintain above lowest normal value
Musculoskeletal	
Weight gain >15%	Use fluids judiciously
Pulmonary	
Shortness of breath	Check transcutaneous O_2 saturation; if <95%, use O_2; use fluids judiciously; do not use aerosolized steroids
Renal	
Edema	Elevate symptomatic extremity; use fluids judiciously
Oliguria	Initially fluids; add dopamine after 1–1.5 L of fluid boluses

Adapted from Schwartzentruber DJ. J Immunother 2001;24:287–293

Ancillary Medications for Adverse Events Associated with High-Dose Aldesleukin Therapies

Adverse Event	Medication	Dose, Schedule, and Route of Administration
Scheduled Medications		
Fever/myalgia	Acetaminophen	650 mg/4 hours PO/PR
	Indomethacin	50–75 mg/6–8 hours PO/PR
Gastritis	Ranitidine HCl	50 mg/8 hours IV
Nausea	Granisetron HCl	0.01 mg/kg daily
Prevent central line sepsis	Cefazolin sodium Clindamycin phosphate	1000–2000 mg/6 hours, IV or 900 mg every 8 hours, IV
As Needed (PRN) Medications		
Agitation/ combativeness	Haloperidol lactate	1–5 mg/1 hour IV/IM
Anxiety	Lorazepam	0.5–1 mg/6 hours PO/IV
Chills	Meperidine HCl	25–50 mg/1 hour IV
Diarrhea	Loperamide HCl	2 mg/3 hours PO
	Diphenoxylate HCl/atropine sulfate	2.5 mg/0.025 mg every 3 hours PO
	Codeine sulfate	30–60 mg/4 hours PO

(continued)

Ancillary Medications for Adverse Events Associated with High-Dose Aldesleukin Therapies (continued)

Adverse Event	Medication	Dose, Schedule, and Route of Administration
As Needed (PRN) Medications		
Gastric upset	Al(OH)$_3$/Mg(OH)$_2$ simethicone	200 mg/200 mg/20 mg every 3 hours PO
Hypocalcemia	Calcium gluconate 10%	1000 mg over 1 hour IV
Hypokalemia	Potassium chloride	10 mEq over 1 hour IV
Hypomagnesemia	Magnesium sulfate	1000 mg (8.12 mEq) over 1 hour IV
Hypophosphatemia	Potassium phosphate	10–15 mmol over 6 hours IV
Hypotension	0.9% sodium chloride injection	250–500 mL IV
	Phenylephrine HCl	0.1–2 mcg/kg/min IV
Insomnia	Temazepam	15–30 mg at bedtime PO
	Zolpidem tartrate	5–10 mg at bedtime PO
Mucositis	Sodium bicarbonate	30 g (~6 tsp)/1500 mL, swish and swallow
Nausea	Prochlorperazine	25 mg/4 hours PR; or 10 mg/6 hours IV
	Ondansetron HCl	10 mg/8 hours IV
	Lorazepam	0.5–1 mg/6 hours PO/IV
Oliguria	0.9% sodium chloride injection	250–500 mL IV
	Dopamine HCl	2–5 mcg/kg per minute IV
Perianal discomfort	Tucks® (hamamelis water pads)	Apply locally
Pruritus	Hydroxyzine HCl	10–25 mg/6 hours PO
	Diphenhydramine HCl	25–50 mg/4 hours PO/IV
	Oatmeal powder/baths	Apply locally
	Lubriderm® (topical emollient)/camphor/menthol	Apply locally
Sinus congestion	Pseudoephedrine HCl	30 mg/6 hours PO

Adapted from Schwartzentruber DJ. J Immunother 2001;24:287–293

Therapy Monitoring (In-Patient Aldesleukin Administration)

Parameter to Monitor	Not Requiring Vasopressors	Requiring ICU/ Vasopressors
1. Monitoring during therapy		
Vital signs	Every 4 hours	Every 1 hour
Intake and output	Every 8 hours	Every 1 hour
Weight	Daily	Daily
Mental status	Every 8 hours	Every 8 hours
IV site/injection site*	Every 8 hours	Every 8 hours
CBC and leukocyte differential count	Daily	Twice daily
Electrolytes, glucose, BUN, creatinine	Daily	Twice daily
AST, ALT, alkaline phosphatase, total bilirubin	Daily	Daily
Albumin, calcium, magnesium, phosphorus	Daily	Daily
Creatine phosphokinase	Daily	Daily
PTT, PT	Every 3 days	Every 3 days
Thyroid-stimulating hormone and free T_4	Each cycle	Each cycle
Urinalysis	Each cycle	Each cycle
ECG	Each cycle	Each cycle
Chest x-ray	Each cycle	Each cycle
2. Response evaluation		
Radiologic evaluation or physical measurement of all sites of disease	Every 2 months	

*Monitor for extravasation or irritation. Change peripheral IV site every 3 days

Rosenberg SA. Principles and Practice of the Biologic Therapy of Cancer, 3rd ed. Philadelphia, PA: Lippincott Williams & Wilkins; 2000

REGIMEN

SUBCUTANEOUS LOW-DOSE ALDESLEUKIN (INTERLEUKIN-2 [IL-2])

Yang JC et al. J Clin Oncol 2003;21:3127–3132

Aldesleukin 250,000 units/kg; administer subcutaneously 5 days per week during the first week, *followed by:*

Aldesleukin 125,000 units/kg; administer subcutaneously 5 days per week during the next 5 weeks, followed by 2 weeks without aldesleukin (total dosage/cycle = 4,375,000 units/kg) Eight-week treatment cycle = 6 consecutive weeks of treatment followed by 2 weeks without aldesleukin

Supportive Care
Antiemetic prophylaxis
Emetogenic potential is **MINIMAL**
See Chapter 39 for antiemetic recommendations

Hematopoietic growth factor (CSF) prophylaxis
Primary prophylaxis is NOT indicated
See Chapter 43 for more information

Antimicrobial prophylaxis
Risk of fever and neutropenia is LOW
  Antimicrobial primary prophylaxis to be considered:
  • Antibacterial—not indicated
  • Antifungal—not indicated
  • Antiviral—not indicated unless patient previously had an episode of HSV
See Chapter 47 for more information

Therapy Monitoring (Outpatient IL-2 Administration)

Parameter to Monitor Outpatient	Frequency
1. *Monitoring during therapy*	
Vital signs	As needed
Intake and output	Not strictly measured
Weight	Daily
Mental status	Daily
IV site/injection site*	Daily
CBC and leukocyte differential counts	Weekly
Electrolytes, glucose, BUN, creatinine	Weekly
AST, ALT, alkaline phosphatase, bilirubin	Weekly
Albumin, calcium, magnesium, phosphorus	Each course
Creatine phosphokinase	Weekly
PTT, PT	Weekly
Thyroid-stimulating hormone and free T$_4$	Each course
Urinalysis	Each course
ECG	Each course
Chest x-ray	Each course
2. *Response evaluation*	
Radiologic evaluation or physical measurements of all sites of disease	Every 2 months

*Monitor for extravasation or irritation. Change peripheral IV site every 3 days

Rosenberg SA. Principles and Practice of the Biologic Therapy of Cancer, 3rd ed. Philadelphia, PA: Lippincott Williams & Wilkins; 2000

Patient Population Studied

A study of 94 patients with metastatic RCC who had not previously received aldesleukin. Patients with brain metastases, coronary artery disease, active autoimmune disorder, or significant renal, pulmonary, or hepatic insufficiency were excluded

Efficacy (N = 93)

Complete response	2%
Partial response	8%

Toxicity (N = 94)

	% G3/4
Malaise	9*
Nausea or vomiting	4*
Diarrhea	2*
CNS: orientation	2
Oliguria (<80 mL/8 hours)	1
Infection	1*
Increased ALT	0.6
Hyperbilirubinemia	0
Peripheral edema	0
Thrombocytopenia	0
Hypotension	0
CNS: Level of consciousness	0

*All toxicities were reversible and no deaths occurred

Treatment Modifications

Adverse Event	Dose Modification
G3/4 toxicities except reversible G3 toxicities commonly seen with low-dose aldesleukin (see *Toxicity*)	Skip doses until toxicity resolves
G3/4 toxicities easily reversed by supportive measures	No dose adjustment or delay
Local inflammation at the injection site with or without nodular induration	No dose adjustment or delay. Apply local measures

Notes

1. Doses may be skipped, depending on patient tolerance
2. Patients are retreated with another course of aldesleukin if disease is stable or regressing
3. Therapy is stopped and patients observed if they have 2 consecutive posttreatment evaluations that are unchanged
4. Patients without evidence of disease receive 1 additional consolidation cycle
5. Comparison of objective responses achieved with high-dose intravenous aldesleukin and subcutaneous aldesleukin demonstrated a small, but statistically significant, difference that favored high-dose treatment

REGIMEN

INTERFERON ALFA-2A

Negrier S et al. N Engl J Med 1998;338:1272–1278

Induction:
Interferon alfa-2a 18 million units; administer subcutaneously, 3 doses per week for 10 weeks (total dose/10-week induction = 540 million units)

Maintenance:
Interferon alfa-2a 18 million units; administer subcutaneously, 3 doses per week for 13 weeks (total dose/13-week maintenance = 702 million units)
Note: Patients should take interferon doses around bedtime, allowing them to sleep through a period of the most severe symptoms

Supportive Care
Antiemetic prophylaxis
Emetogenic potential is **MINIMAL**
See Chapter 39 for antiemetic recommendations

Hematopoietic growth factor (CSF) prophylaxis
Primary prophylaxis is NOT indicated
See Chapter 43 for more information

Antimicrobial prophylaxis
Risk of fever and neutropenia is LOW
  Antimicrobial primary prophylaxis to be considered:
  • Antibacterial—not indicated
  • Antifungal—not indicated
  • Antiviral—not indicated unless patient previously had an episode of HSV
See Chapter 47 for more information

Primary antipyretic prophylaxis
Acetaminophen 650–1000 mg orally *or* **ibuprofen** 400–600 mg orally, administer 1 hour before interferon, then every 4 hours as needed

Efficacy (N = 147)

Week 10
Complete response	0%
Partial response	7%
Disease stabilization	31%
Disease progression	Not evaluated

Week 25
Complete response	1%
Partial response	5%
Disease stabilization	13%
Disease progression	Not evaluated

Patient Population Studied

A study of 147 patients with RCC and progressive metastasis. Patients were excluded if they had brain metastases, cardiac dysfunction, any contraindications to the use of vasopressor agents, active infection, previous aldesleukin or interferon alfa treatment, chemotherapy, or radiation therapy within 6 weeks before enrollment, or current treatment with steroids

Therapy Monitoring

1. *Before each cycle:* CBC with differential, serum electrolytes, BUN, creatinine, LFTs, and mineral panel
2. *Response evaluation:* After each maintenance cycle

Toxicity* (N = 147)

	% G3/4
Impaired performance status	16
Anemia	6
Nausea or vomiting	5
Fever	5
Weight loss	4
Increased ALT or AST	3
Pulmonary symptoms	3
Diarrhea	1
Hypotension resistant to pressors	1
Neurologic symptom	1
Cardiac signs	1
Leukopenia	1
Infection	1
Cutaneous signs	0
Thrombocytopenia	0
Increased creatinine	0
Renal symptoms	0
Hyperbilirubinemia	0

*WHO criteria

Treatment Modifications

Adverse Event	Dose Modification
Hypotension resistant to intravenous vasopressors	Stop treatment. Resume cautiously if blood pressure recovers
Life-threatening or persistent, severe toxic reactions	Discontinue therapy
WHO G ≥3 toxicity	Stop treatment. Resume when toxicity G ≤1 at original dose
Recurrent WHO G ≥3 toxicity	Stop treatment. Resume when toxicity G ≤1, with interferon alfa-2a dose decreased by 50%

Notes

Interferon alfa-2a has been used in the treatment of metastatic RCC at different doses (3–18 million units) and modes of administration with a median overall survival of 13 months

Motzer RJ et al. JCO 2002;20:289–296

34. Sarcomas

Brigitte Widemann, MD, Tito Fojo, MD, PhD, and Jean-Yves Blay, MD

Primary Malignant Bone Tumors

Epidemiology

Incidence: 3,020 (male: 1,680; female: 1,340. Estimated new cases for 2014 in the United States) 1.1 per 100,000 males, 0.8 per 100,000 females

Deaths: Estimated 1,460 in 2014 (male: 830; female: 630)

Median age: 42 years

Male to female ratio: 1.5:1

Siegel R et al. CA Cancer J Clin 2014;64:9–29
Surveillance, Epidemiology and End Results (SEER) Program, available from http://seer.cancer.gov (accessed in 2013)

Classification
WHO Classification of Malignant Bone Tumors

Osteogenic tumors
Osteosarcoma
  a. Conventional
   • Chondroblastic
   • Fibroblastic
   • Osteoblastic
  b. Telangiectatic
  c. Small cell
  d. Low-grade central
  e. Secondary
  f. Parosteal
  g. Periosteal
  h. High-grade surface

Ewing sarcoma/primitive neuroectodermal tumor
Ewing sarcoma

Cartilage tumors
Chondrosarcoma
  a. Central, primary, and secondary
  b. Peripheral
  c. Dedifferentiated
  d. Mesenchymal
  e. Clear cell

Fibrogenic tumors
Fibrosarcoma

Fibrohistiocytic tumors
Malignant fibrous histiocytoma

Giant cell tumor
Malignancy in giant cell tumor

Notochordal tumors
Chordoma

Vascular tumors
Angiosarcoma

Smooth muscle tumors
Leiomyosarcoma

Lipogenic tumors
Liposarcoma

Miscellaneous tumors
Adamantinoma

Hematopoietic tumors (see respective sections)
1. Plasma cell myeloma
2. Malignant lymphoma, NOS

Work-up

1. History and physical examination
2. *Laboratory tests:* CBC with differential; electrolytes; liver function tests; mineral panel, including alkaline phosphatase; lactate dehydrogenase
3. Plain films of affected bone
4. Chest x-ray (PA and lateral)
5. CT scan of chest, abdomen, and pelvis (particularly chest because 80% of metastatic lesions occur here)
6. MRI to ascertain extent of the tumor, involvement of surrounding neurovascular structures, invasion of the adjacent joint, and the presence of skip metastases
7. Bone scan to identify skip lesions within affected bones or distant metastatic disease
8. Bone marrow aspirate for light microscopy examination in the case of Ewing sarcoma
9. No radiologic studies are pathognomonic, so bone biopsy remains essential to diagnosis
10. Echocardiogram or MUGA scan to determine cardiac ejection fraction as clinically indicated
11. Audiogram before cisplatin chemotherapy

Surgical Staging

The surgical system as described by Enneking et al. is based on the GTM classification. Stage is determined by 3 different subcategories: grade (G), location or site (T), and lymph node involvement and metastases (M)

Grade [G]

G1	Low grade, uniform cell type without atypia, few mitoses
G2	High grade, atypical nuclei, mitoses pronounced

Site [T]

T1	Intracompartmental = Confined within limits of periosteum
T2	Extracompartmental = Breach in an adjacent joint cartilage, bone cortex (or periosteum) fascia lata, quadriceps, and joint capsule

Lymph Node Involvement and Metastases [M]

M0	No identifiable skip lesions or distant metastases
M1	Any skip lesions, regional lymph nodes, or distant metastases

Enneking Staging System of Malignant Bone Tumors

Stage		G	T	M
IA	Low grade, intracompartmental	G1	T1	M0
IB	Low grade, extracompartmental	G1	T2	M0
IIA	High grade, intracompartmental	G2	T1	M0
IIB	High grade, extracompartmental	G2	T2	M0
IIIA	Low or high grade, intracompartmental with metastases	G1/2	T1	M1
IIIB	Low or high grade, extracompartmental with metastases	G1/2	T2	M1

Enneking WF et al. Clin Orthop 1980;153:106–120

Clinical Staging
IUCC and TNM Staging

Primary Tumor

TX	Primary tumor cannot be assessed
T0	No evidence of primary tumor
T1	Tumor ≤8 cm in greatest dimension
T2	Tumor >8 cm in greatest dimension
T3	Discontinuous tumors in the primary bone site

Nodal Status

NX	Regional lymph nodes cannot be assessed
N0	No regional metastasis
N1	Regional lymph nodes metastasis

Metastases

MX	Distant metastasis cannot be assessed
M0	No distant metastases
M1	Distant metastases
	M1a Lung
	M1b Other distant sites, including lymph nodes

Grade

GX	Grade cannot be assessed
G1	Well differentiated–low grade
G2	Moderately differentiated–low grade
G3	Poorly differentiated–high grade
G4	Undifferentiated–high grade

Stage Grouping

IA	G1,2	T1	N0	M0
IB	G1,2	T2	N0	M0
IIA	G3,4	T1	N0	M0
IIB	G3,4	T2	N0	M0
III	Any G	T3	N0	M0
IVA	Any G	Any T	N0	M1a
IVB	Any G	Any T	N1	Any M
IVB	Any G	Any T	Any N	M1b

International Union Against Cancer (IUCC) and American Joint Committee on Cancer (AJCC) TNM Staging, 6th ed. System for Bone Sarcomas
Reproduced by permission of the American Joint Committee on Cancer (AJCC), Chicago, Illinois. The original source for this material is the AJCC Cancer Staging Manual, 7th ed. (2009) published by Springer-Verlag, New York, NY, http://www.springeronline.com

Histologic Grading Systems for Assessing Response to Induction Chemotherapy in Osteosarcoma

Salzer-Kuntschik

I:	No viable cells
II:	Single viable tumor cells or cluster <0.5 cm
III:	Viable tumor <10%
IV:	Viable tumor 10–50%
V:	Viable tumor >50%
VI:	No effect on chemotherapy

Picci

Total response:	No viable tumor
Good response:	90–99% necrosis
Fair response:	60–89% necrosis
Poor response:	<60% necrosis

Huvos (Wunder et al)

IV:	No histologic evidence of viable tumor
III:	Only scattered foci of viable tumor cells
II:	Areas of necrosis with areas of viable tumor
I:	Little or no chemotherapy effect

Picci P et al. Cancer 1985;56:1515–1521
Salzer-Kuntschik M et al. Pathologe 1983;4:135–141
Wunder JS et al. J Bone Joint Surg Am 1998;80:1020–1033

5-Year Survival

Nonmetastatic (80% of Patients at Diagnosis)	
Good histologic response (>90% necrosis)	75%
Poor histologic response (<90% necrosis)	55%
Metastatic (20% of patients at diagnosis)	20%

Expert Opinion

Primary Bone Tumors
General
1. Rare, account for <0.2% of malignant tumors
2. *Relatively high incidence in children and adolescents,* although even in the young, benign bone tumors are more common
3. Considerably outnumbered by metastases to the bone in older patients
4. Presentations:
   - Nonmechanical pain or night pain around the knee are cause for concern
   - Swelling only if tumor extends through the cortex distending periosteum
5. Referral to reference center is strongly encouraged
6. Frequently difficult to recognize as malignant by clinicians, radiologists as well as pathologists → major diagnostic difficulties in nonspecialized centers
7. Ideally, all cases of suspected bone tumor should be discussed at a multidisciplinary team meeting

Diagnosis and Local Staging
1. Conventional radiographs in 2 planes should be the first investigation
2. CT in the case of a diagnostic problem or doubt, to visualize calcification, periosteal bone formation, cortical destruction, or soft-tissue involvement
3. When malignancy is uncertain on radiographs, the next step is MRI, in particular for limbs
4. General staging to assess the extent of distant disease includes
   - Bone scintigraphy
   - Chest radiographs and chest CT
5. Whole-body MRI and PET under evaluation for staging and treatment assessment

Biopsy
1. Experienced physician(s) should biopsy suspicious sites, as exact staging of disease has impact on treatment and outcome (III, B)
2. Principles of biopsy:
   - Determine stage before the biopsy → may guide location of biopsy
   - Minimal contamination of normal tissues
   - Core needle biopsy often more than adequate often guided by ultrasound, X-ray, or CT
   - Samples for microbiologic culture as well as histology
   - Samples should be snap-frozen for future studies
   - An experienced pathologist should evaluate samples
   - Excision biopsy is contraindicated because it may contaminate tissue compartments
   - Open biopsy requires a longitudinal incision
   - In aggressive and malignant tumors of bone, consider biopsy tract contaminated with tumor and removed together with the resection specimen to avoid local recurrences
3. Spinal column involvement, avoid laminectomy or decompression resulting in incomplete resection unless necessary to relieve spinal cord compression

Prevention and Management of Pathologic Fracture
1. Pathologic fractures may disseminate tumor cells into surrounding tissues and increase the risk of local recurrence
2. Patients with weakened bone → immobilize following biopsy with an external splint. In cases of fracture, internal fixation is contraindicated as it disseminates tumor further into both bone and soft tissues increasing the risk of local recurrence. Neoadjuvant chemotherapy used with expectation of a good response will allow fracture hematoma to contract and allow subsequent resection
3. If response to chemotherapy is poor or in tumors unlikely to respond → consider early surgery obtaining wide margins including amputation
4. Consider postoperative radiotherapy to decrease the risk of local recurrence

Systemic Therapy
(Also see individual histologies)
1. Strongly consider treatment in reference centers or networks (IV, A)
2. High-grade osteosarcoma, Ewing sarcoma, and spindle cell sarcoma should receive primary chemotherapy

Surgery
(Also see individual histologies)
1. Surgery should be performed only after adequate preoperative staging, and, depending on the tumor, primary chemotherapy
2. Striving to obtain adequate surgical margins → narrower margins are associated with an increased risk of local recurrence

(continued)

Expert Opinion (continued)

3. If possible perform a wide en-bloc resection
   - General *intracompartmental* resection
   - Occasionally *extracompartmental* resection if entire bone/muscle compartment can be removed easily (III, B)
4. If postoperative radiotherapy is likely, risk areas and close margins should be identified with clips
5. Surgical reconstruction varies; discuss with patient

Follow-up
1. To detect local recurrence or metastatic disease when early treatment is still possible and might be effective
2. Recommended intervals for follow-up after completion of chemotherapy:
   - Every 6 weeks to 3 months for the first 2 years
   - Every 2–4 months for years 3–4
   - Every 6 months for years 5–10
   - Every 6–12 months thereafter
   Note: These suggested intervals of follow-up can be balanced against evidence that excessive exposure to radiation may increase the risk of developing leukemia, especially in children
3. Recommended intervals for follow-up for low-grade bone sarcoma
   - Every 6 months for 2 years, and then, annually
4. Late metastases as well as local recurrences and functional deficits may occur >10 years after diagnosis, and there is no universally accepted stopping point for tumor surveillance
5. It is important to evaluate long-term toxicity of therapy for >10 years. Secondary cancers and leukemia, particularly acute myeloid leukemia, may occur (III, B)

Note: Levels of Evidence (I–V) and Grades of Recommendation (A–D) are as used by the American Society of Clinical Oncology

Hogendoorn PCW et al. ESMO/EUROBONET Working Group Bone sarcomas: ESMO Clinical Practice Guidelines for diagnosis, treatment and follow-up. Ann Oncol 2010;21 Suppl 5:v204–v213

Osteosarcoma
Background:
1. Most frequent primary cancer of bone (incidence: 0.2–0.03/100,000/year)
2. Higher incidence in adolescents (0.8–1.1/100,000/year at ages 15–19 years); accounts for >10% of all solid cancers
3. Male to female ratio: 1.4:1
4. Usually arises in the metaphysis of a long bone, most commonly around the knee, axial skeleton, and craniofacial bones, primarily in adults
5. Risk factors:
   - Previous radiation therapy
   - Paget disease of bone
   - Germ-line abnormalities (Rb mutations, p53 mutations)

Staging and risk assessment:
1. 75% arise around the knee
2. Typically there is pain that begins insidiously, gradually becomes constant, may be present at night and is often nonmechanical in nature
3. Localized swelling and limitation of joint movement are later findings
4. Adverse prognostic or predictive factors:
   - Detectable metastases
   - Poor histologic response to preoperative chemotherapy
   - Axial or proximal extremity site
   - Large tumor volume
   - Elevated serum AP or LDH
   - Older age, >40 years (III, B)
   - Paget disease

Treatment: General
1. Changes in the size and ossification of tumor are not reliable indicators of response to neoadjuvant chemotherapy
2. Sequential dynamic MRI that evaluate changes in vascularity are reliable
3. Assessment of response usually is apparent only after several cycles of chemotherapy → do not discontinue and change chemotherapy regimen early

(continued)

Expert Opinion (continued)

Treatment: Radiation therapy
1. Limited role but may be appropriate in highly selected cases or for palliation (IV, C)
2. Consider boost techniques to increase local dose including intensity modulated radiotherapy (IMRT), proton therapy or samarium

Treatment: Multimodality
Localized disease
1. High-grade tumors should receive primary chemotherapy
2. Curative treatment for high-grade osteosarcoma = surgery + chemotherapy (I, A)
   Compared with surgery alone, multimodal treatment of high-grade osteosarcoma increases DFS probabilities from 10–20% to >60%
3. Goal of surgery is to safely remove the tumor and preserve as much function as possible → consider limb salvage
4. Whenever possible, patients should receive chemotherapy in the context of prospective trials
5. Agents with activity (I, A)
   • Doxorubicin
   • Cisplatin
   • High-dose methotrexate
   • Ifosfamide
6. Combinations:
   • Doxorubicin and cisplatin frequently are the basis of treatment
   • Evidence exists that combinations with methotrexate and/or ifosfamide might provide additional benefit over 2-drug schedules (II, A)
   • Ideal combination and optimal treatment durations (commonly given over periods of 6–12 months) are yet to be defined
7. Most current protocols include a period of preoperative chemotherapy → although not proven to add survival benefit over postoperative chemotherapy alone (I, B)
8. Extent of histologic response to preoperative chemotherapy offers important prognostic information (I, A)
9. The multimodal treatment principles were generated in children, adolescents and young adults with high-grade central osteosarcoma, but also relate to adults at least up to the age of 60 years (III, B)
10. Chemotherapy also is recommended for older patients with osteosarcoma using protocols extrapolated from those designed for pediatric/adolescent patients
11. Extraosseous osteosarcoma: Use high-grade soft-tissue sarcoma or osteosarcoma regimens. No consensus amongst experts as to best approach

Metastatic disease
1. Some have very similar or even identical prognosis to the prognosis of patients with localized disease, with surgical removal of all known metastatic lesions (III, B)
2. ≈30% of all patients with primary metastatic osteosarcoma and >40% of those who achieve a complete surgical remission become long-term survivors

Recurrent disease
1. Treatment is primarily surgical. Complete removal of all metastases must be attempted (III, B)
2. Prognosis is poor, with long-term post-relapse survival <20%. However, >1/3 with second surgical remission survive for >5 years
3. Multiple recurrences curable as long as they are resectable, and repeated thoracotomies are often warranted (III, B)
4. Role of second-line chemotherapy is less well-defined than that of surgery and there is no accepted standard regimen
5. Choice may take into account the prior disease-free interval, and often includes: ifosfamide, with or without etoposide, with or without carboplatin

Ewing Sarcoma
Background:
1. Second most common primary malignant bone cancer
2. Occurs most frequently in children and adolescents (median age: 15 years)
3. Male to female ratio: 1.5:1
4. ≈25% pelvic bones/≈50% extremity tumors
5. Occasionally arises in soft tissue

Staging and risk assessment:
1. All are high-grade tumors
2. All share common gene rearrangement involving the EWS gene on chromosome 22. Most involve reciprocal translocation
3. 20–25% of patients are diagnosed with metastatic disease (10% lung, 10% bones/bone marrow, 5% combinations or others)

(continued)

Expert Opinion (*continued*)

4. Work-up and staging
   - Scan to detect lung and bone metastases
   - Perform bone marrow biopsy and aspirate
   - Light microscopic analysis of bone marrow aspirates and biopsies from sites distal to the lesion (metastases) are mandatory
   - Most are recognized with classical hematoxylin and eosin (H&E) stain and immunohistochemistry, but translocation detection by FISH and RT-PCR is mandatory when diagnosis by light microscopy techniques are in doubt (II, B)
     - RT-PCR with frozen tissue
     - FISH with formalin-fixed paraffin-embedded tissue or touch preps (imprints)
5. Adverse prognostic or predictive factors:
   - Tumor size or volume
   - Serum LDH levels
   - Axial localization
   - Older age (>15 years)
   - Poor histologic response to preoperative chemotherapy
   - Incomplete or no surgery is possible (II, B)
   - The presence of bone metastases is associated with a poorer outcome than lung/pleura metastases (<20% compared with 20–40% 5-year survival)

Treatment: General
1. Change in the size of lesions on MRI is a rather reliable indicator of response
2. Dynamic MRI is not as reliable in evaluating response to treatment as in osteosarcoma
3. Sequential FDG-PET might be of value

Treatment: Radiation therapy
1. Radiation-responsive tumor
2. Radiotherapy, in combination with chemotherapy achieves local control
3. Incomplete surgery, even when combined with postoperative radiotherapy, is not superior to radiotherapy alone and should be avoided
4. If surgery is incomplete follow with postoperative radiotherapy
5. Give radiotherapy alone only if complete surgery is not possible
6. Consider postoperative RT if surgical margins are inadequate and consider RT after chemotherapy for patients who do not achieve a good response to chemotherapy (ie, >10% viable tumor cells) (IV, C)

Treatment: Multimodality
Localized disease
1. Should receive primary chemotherapy
2. Complete surgery, where feasible, best modality for local control
3. With surgery or radiotherapy alone, the 5-year survival is <10%
4. Current multimodality approaches include chemotherapy. Survival is ≈60–70% in localized and ≈20–40% in metastatic disease
5. Agents considered most active
   - Doxorubicin
   - Cyclophosphamide
   - Ifosfamide
   - Vincristine
   - Dactinomycin
   - Etoposide
6. Most protocols are based on 4- to 6-drug combinations (I, A). Current trials initially employ 3–6 cycles of chemotherapy after biopsy, followed by local therapy, then 6–10 cycles of chemotherapy (treatment duration ≈10–12 months)
7. Chemotherapy intensity is positively associated with outcome. However, high-dose chemotherapy with stem cell transplantation is still investigational in high-risk localized Ewing sarcoma
8. Treatment of adult patients follows the same principles as for younger patients, but be aware of tolerability of treatment
9. Extra-skeletal Ewing sarcoma same approach as for bone Ewing sarcoma

Metastatic disease
1. Patients with metastases at diagnosis have a worse prognosis; bone or bone marrow metastases are associated with a 5-year survival <20%
2. Experience with intensive, time-compressed, or high-dose chemotherapy approaches, followed by autologous stem cell transplantation are promising but evidence of benefit is pending (III, B)

(*continued*)

Expert Opinion (continued)

3. With lung metastases, whole-lung irradiation may confer a survival advantage (III, B)

4. Surgical resection of residual metastases is less well defined

Recurrent disease

1. With recurrent disease, 5-year survival is <20%, although relapse >2 years from initial diagnosis is associated with a better outcome (III, B)

2. Doxorubicin often cannot be used because of the cumulative lifetime dosages already administered

3. The choice of chemotherapy in relapse is not standardized (III, B):
   - Alkylating agents (cyclophosphamide, high-dose ifosfamide) in combination with topoisomerase inhibitors (etoposide, topotecan), *or*
   - Irinotecan with temozolomide

Chondrosarcoma

Background:

1. Most frequent bone sarcoma of adults (≈0.1/100,000 per year)

2. Male to female ratio: ~1:1

3. The majority are staged as low grade (grade I) rather than high-grade (grades II–III)

4. Most arise centrally in the diametaphyseal region of long bones

5. Most present as a painless mass → pain at the site of a cartilaginous lesion suggest malignancy

Staging and risk assessment:

1. Differentiation is difficult between benign enchondroma or osteochondroma and malignant grade I chondrosarcoma

2. Although they are extremely rare in hands and feet, lesions found in long bones and central cartilaginous lesions should be considered potential low-grade chondrosarcoma until proved otherwise

3. Inoperable, locally advanced, and metastatic lesions have poor prognosis because of resistance to radiotherapy and chemotherapy

4. Prognosis depends on histologic grade; however, assessing grade is difficult

Treatment: Radiation therapy

1. Role of radiotherapy is limited but may be appropriate in highly selected cases or for palliation (IV, C)

Treatment: Multimodality

1. Low-grade cartilage tumors are unlikely to metastasize, but may recur locally

2. Higher-grade chondrosarcomas and all chondrosarcomas of the pelvis or axial skeleton should be surgically excised with wide margins

3. Recent evidence suggests mesenchymal chondrosarcoma may be chemotherapy sensitive → consider for adjuvant or neoadjuvant therapy

4. Dedifferentiated chondrosarcoma
   - Uncertainty about chemotherapy sensitivity; often treated like osteosarcoma, but with a poorer outcome
   - There is a high risk of local recurrence following excision, particularly in the presence of a pathologic fracture

Spindle Cell Sarcomas of Bone (Malignant Fibrous Histiocytoma/Fibrosarcoma of Bone [MFH/FS])

Background:

1. Heterogeneous group of tumors including
   - Fibrosarcoma (FS)
   - Malignant fibrous histiocytoma (MFH)
   - Leiomyosarcoma
   - Undifferentiated sarcoma

2. 2–5% of primary bone malignancies

3. Similar age group as chondrosarcoma

4. Similar skeletal distribution as osteosarcoma

5. Typically present with pain and have a high incidence of fracture at presentation

Staging and risk assessment:

1. Typically present in an older patient with a lytic lesion in bone

2. Differential diagnosis includes a metastasis

3. Pathologic fractures are common

Treatment:

1. Treatment strategies are similar to those used for osteosarcoma, with chemotherapy and complete en-bloc resection including any soft-tissue component

REGIMEN

HIGH-DOSE METHOTREXATE, CISPLATIN, AND DOXORUBICIN

Meyers PA et al. J Clin Oncol 2005;23:2004–2011

The regimen consists of 10 weeks of induction chemotherapy followed by limb-sparing surgery or amputation, which is followed by adjuvant maintenance chemotherapy beginning in week 12 and continuing until week 31

Note: Adjuvant maintenance chemotherapy should begin at week 12 provided wound healing is adequate

Hydration before and after cisplatin: ≥1000 mL 0.45% sodium chloride injection (0.45% NS); administer intravenously over a minimum of 2–4 hours

Cisplatin 120 mg/m²; administer intravenously in 150–1000 mL 0.9% sodium chloride injection (0.9% NS) over 4 hours, for 4 cycles, during weeks 0 and 5 in the induction phase and weeks 12 and 17 in the maintenance phase (total dosage/cycle = 120 mg/m²)

Note: Encourage patients to increase oral intake of nonalcoholic fluids, and monitor serum electrolytes and replace as needed (potassium, magnesium, sodium)

Doxorubicin 25 mg/m² per day; administer intravenously in 50–1000 mL 0.9% NS or 5% dextrose injection (D5W) over 24 hours for 3 consecutive days, on days 1–3, for 6 cycles, during weeks 0 and 5 in the induction phase, and weeks 12, 17, 22, and 27 in the maintenance phase (total dosage/cycle = 75 mg/m²)

Hydration: 1500–3000 mL/m² per day; administer intravenously. Use a solution containing a total amount of sodium not >0.9% NS (ie, ≤154 mEq sodium/1000 mL) by intravenous infusion during methotrexate administration and for at least 24 hours afterward

• Fluid administration may commence 2–12 hours before starting methotrexate, depending on a patient's fluid status
• Urine output should be at least 100 mL/hour before starting methotrexate infusion
• Maintain hydration at a rate that maintains urine output ≥100 mL/hour until the serum methotrexate concentration is <0.1 µmol/L
• Urine pH should be increased within the range ≥7.0 to ≤8.0 to enhance methotrexate solubility and ensure elimination
  ▪ Adverse effects attributable to methotrexate are related to systemic methotrexate concentrations *and* the duration for which concentrations are maintained

Sodium bicarbonate 50–150 mEq/1000 mL is added to the parenteral solution to maintain urine pH ≥7.0 to ≤8.0

Base Solution Sodium Content	Sodium Bicarbonate Additive	Total Sodium Content
0.45% Sodium Chloride Injection (0.45% NS)		
77 mEq/L	50–75 mEq	127–152 mEq/L
0.2% Sodium Chloride Injection (0.2% NS)		
34 mEq/L	100–125 mEq	134–159 mEq/L
5% Dextrose Injection (D5W)		
0 mEq/L	125–150 mEq	125–150 mEq/L
D5W/0.45% NS		
77 mEq/L	50–75 mEq	127–152 mEq/L
D5W/0.2% NS		
34 mEq/L	100–125 mEq	134–159 mEq/L

(continued)

Treatment Modifications

Adverse Event	Dose Modification
Delayed methotrexate clearance during weeks 3, 15, 20, and 25	Do not administer the scheduled course of methotrexate during the ensuing weeks (4, 16, 21, and 26) to ensure that doxorubicin is administered on schedule

Patient Population Studied

A prospective randomized intergroup phase III study of newly diagnosed patients with histologically confirmed high-grade, intramedullary osteosarcoma who were 30 years of age or younger. There were 677 patients enrolled without clinically detectable metastases; 340 received this regimen, including 168 who also received liposomal muramyl tripeptide

(*continued*)

Methotrexate 12,000 mg/m² (maximum dose = 20,000 mg); administer intravenously in
500–2000 mL 0.9% NS or D5W (or saline and dextrose combinations) over 4 hours for
12 cycles during weeks 3, 4, 8, and 9 in the induction phase, and weeks 15, 16, 20, 21, 25, 26,
30, and 31 in the maintenance phase (total dosage/cycle = 12,000 mg/m²; maximum dose/
cycle = 20,000 mg)
Note: For logistical practicality and efficiency, parenteral admixtures containing methotrexate
may include a portion, or all of the fluid and sodium bicarbonate needed to meet hydration
and urinary alkalinization requirements during methotrexate administration

Leucovorin 10 mg (a fixed dose); administer intravenously in 25–250 mL 0.9% NS or D5W
over 15 minutes every 6 hours, starting 24 hours after methotrexate administration *began* and
continuing until the serum methotrexate concentration is <0.1 μmol/L (ie, <1 × 10⁻⁷ mol/L,
or <100 nmol/L)
Note: Leucovorin may be administered orally after completing 1 day of parenteral
administration if patients are compliant, are not vomiting, and have no other potentially
mitigating complications
Leucovorin 10 mg (fixed dose); administer orally every 6 hours until the serum methotrexate
concentration is <0.1 μmol/L (ie, <1 × 10⁻⁷ mol/L, or <100 nmol/L)

Leucovorin rescue for delayed methotrexate excretion:
• Hydration, urinary alkalinization, and a more intensive leucovorin regimen are required if
  methotrexate excretion is delayed (eg, worsening renal function, effusions present)
• If 24 hours after the completion of methotrexate administration a patient's serum creatinine
  is increased by ≥50% above the baseline value, or if serum methotrexate concentration is
  ≥5 μmol/L (≥5 × 10⁻⁶ mol/L), increase the leucovorin dosage and schedule to 100 mg/
  m² per dose intravenously (*not* orally) every 3 hours until serum methotrexate level is <0.1
  μmol/L (<1 × 10⁻⁷ mol/L, <100 nmol/L); then resume leucovorin 10 mg/dose orally or
  intravenously every 6 hours until serum methotrexate concentration is <0.05 μmol/L (<5 ×
  10⁻⁸ mol/L, or <50 nmol/L), or until undetectable (if the lower limit of assay sensitivity is
  ≥0.05 μmol/L [≥5 × 10⁻⁸ mol/L, or ≥50 nmol/L])

Supportive Care
Antiemetic prophylaxis
Emetogenic potential during cycles with cisplatin + doxorubicin is **HIGH**. *Potential for delayed symptoms*
Emetogenic potential with doxorubicin alone is **MODERATE**
Emetogenic potential with methotrexate is **MODERATE**
See Chapter 39 for antiemetic recommendations

Hematopoietic growth factor (CSF) prophylaxis
Primary prophylaxis is indicated with 1 of the following:
  Filgrastim (G-CSF) 5 mcg/kg per day by subcutaneous injection, *or*
  Sargramostim (GM-CSF) 250 mcg/m² per day by subcutaneous injection
  • Begin use from 24–72 hours after doxorubicin is completed
  • Discontinue use at least 24 hours before resuming chemotherapy
See Chapter 43 for more information

Antimicrobial prophylaxis
Risk of fever and neutropenia is HIGH
  Antimicrobial primary prophylaxis is recommended:
  • Antibacterial—consider fluoroquinolone prophylaxis; *P. jirovecii* prophylaxis is
    recommended (eg, cotrimoxazole)
  • Antifungal—recommended
  • Antiviral—antiherpes antivirals (eg, acyclovir, famciclovir, valacyclovir)
See Chapter 47 for more information

Oral care
Prophylaxis and treatment for mucositis/stomatitis
  General advice:
  • Encourage patients to maintain intake of non-alcoholic fluids
  • Evaluate patients for oral pain and provide analgesic medications
  • Consider histamine (H₂-subtype) receptor antagonists (eg, ranitidine, famotidine), or a
    proton pump inhibitor for epigastric pain
  • *Lactobacillus* sp.-containing probiotics may be beneficial in preventing diarrhea

(*continued*)

Efficacy (N = 172)

Event free-survival at 3 years	71%
Event free-survival at 5 years	64%
Second malignant neoplasm	3 occurrences
Favorable necrosis (Huvos III/IV)	43%

Toxicity (N = 172)

	Frequency
Elevations in ALT after methotrexate	Common
Stomatitis	Common
Infections	Common
Objective hearing loss	11%
Renal dysfunction	Rare

(continued)

Patients with intact oral mucosa:

- Clean the mouth, tongue, and gums by brushing after every meal and at bedtime with an ultra-soft toothbrush with fluoride toothpaste
- Floss teeth gently every day unless contraindicated. If gums bleed and hurt, avoid bleeding or sore areas, but floss other teeth
- Patients may use saline or commercial bland, non-alcoholic rinses
  - Do not use mouthwashes that contain alcohols

If mucositis or stomatitis is present:

- Keep the mouth moist utilizing water, ice chips, sugarless gum, sugar-free hard candies, or a saliva substitute
- Rinse mouth several times a day to remove debris
  - Use a solution of ¼ teaspoon (1.25 g) each of baking soda and table salt (sodium chloride) in one quart (~950 mL) of warm water. Follow with a plain water rinse
  - Do not use mouthwashes that contain alcohols
- Foam-tipped swabs (eg, Toothettes®) are useful in moisturizing oral mucosa, but ineffective for cleansing teeth and removing plaque
- Advise patients who develop mucositis to:
  - Choose foods that are easy to chew and swallow
  - Take small bites of food, chew slowly, and sip liquids with meals
  - Encourage soft, moist foods such as cooked cereals, mashed potatoes, and scrambled eggs
  - For trouble swallowing, soften food with gravies, sauces, broths, yogurt, or other bland liquids
  - Avoid sharp, crunchy foods; hot, spicy or highly acidic foods (eg, citrus fruits and juices); sugary foods; toothpicks; tobacco products; alcoholic drinks

Therapy Monitoring

1. *During treatment cycles:* Daily renal function
2. *After high-dose systemic methotrexate administration:* Daily methotrexate levels
3. *Before each cycle:* CBC with differential, serum electrolytes, BUN, and creatinine

REGIMEN
ETOPOSIDE + HIGH-DOSE IFOSFAMIDE + MESNA

Goorin AM et al. J Clin Oncol 2002;20:426–433

This regimen was initially developed for newly diagnosed osteosarcoma and included high-dose methotrexate, cisplatin, and doxorubicin as part of the continuation therapy. The protocol summarized here assumes that patients previously received high-dose methotrexate, cisplatin, and doxorubicin as part of their upfront therapy

	Induction Chemotherapy
Start: Hour 0 End: Hour 1	**Etoposide** 100 mg/m^2 per day; administer intravenously in 250 mL/m^2 5% dextrose and 0.2% sodium chloride injection (D5W/0.2% NS) over 1 hour for 5 consecutive days, on days 1–5, every 21 days (total dosage/cycle = 500 mg/m^2)
Start: Hour 1 End: Hour 5	An admixture containing **ifosfamide** 3500 mg/m^2 + **mesna** 700 mg/m^2 per day; administer intravenously in 800 mL/m^2 D5W/0.2% NS over 4 hours, starting immediately after etoposide administration is completed, for 5 consecutive days, on days 1–5, every 21 days (total ifosfamide dosage/cycle = 17,500 mg/m^2)
Start: Hour 5 End: Hour 8	**Mesna** 700 mg/m^2 per day; administer by continuous intravenous infusion in 600 mL/m^2 D5W/0.2% NS over 3 hours, starting after ifosfamide administration is completed, for 5 consecutive days, on days 1–5, every 21 days
Start: Hour 8 End: Hour 14	**Hydration** with D5W/0.2% NS; administer intravenously at 150 mL/m^2 per hour for 6 hours for 5 consecutive days on days 1–5, every 21 days
Start: Hours 8, 11, and 14 End: 8:15, 11:15, and 14:15	**Mesna** 700 mg/m^2 per dose; administer intravenously diluted with 0.9% sodium chloride injection (0.9% NS) or 5% dextrose injection (D5W) to a concentration of 1–20 mg/mL, over 15 minutes, every 3 hours for 3 doses/day, starting 3 hours after ifosfamide administration is completed, for 5 consecutive days, on days 1–5, every 21 days (total mesna dosage/cycle = 17,500 mg/m^2; this total also includes Hour 1 and Hour 5 doses)
Start: Hour 14 End: Hour 24	**Hydration** with D5W/0.2% NS; administer intravenously at 100 mL/m^2 per hour for 10 hours for 5 consecutive days on days 1–5, every 21 days

Note: After 2 cycles of treatment, radiologic evaluation is completed and patients should have surgery for any metastatic sites of disease. Surgical removal of all metastatic sites is recommended when feasible

	Continuation Chemotherapy
Start: Hour 0 End: Hour 1	**Etoposide** 100 mg/m^2 per day; administer intravenously in 250 mL/m^2 D5W/0.2% NS over 1 hour for 5 consecutive days, on days 1–5, every 21 days (total dosage/cycle = 500 mg/m^2)
Start: Hour 1 End: Hour 5	An admixture containing **ifosfamide** 2400 mg/m^2 + **mesna** 480 mg/m^2 per day; administer intravenously in 800 mL/m^2 D5W/0.2% NS over 4 hours, starting immediately after etoposide administration is completed, for 5 consecutive days, on days 1–5, every 21 days (total ifosfamide dosage/cycle = 12,000 mg/m^2)
Start: Hour 5 End: Hour 8	**Mesna** 480 mg/m^2 per day; administer intravenously in 600 mL/m^2 D5W/0.2% NS over 3 hours, starting after ifosfamide administration is completed, for 5 consecutive days, on days 1–5, every 21 days
Start: Hour 8 End: Hour 14	**Hydration** with D5W/0.2% NS; administer intravenously at 150 mL/m^2 per hour for 6 hours, for 5 consecutive days, on days 1–5, every 21 days
Start: Hours 8, 11, and 14 End: 8:15, 11:15, and 14:15	**Mesna** 480 mg/m^2 per dose; administer intravenously diluted with 0.9% NS or D5W to a concentration of 1–20 mg/mL, over 15 minutes, every 3 hours for 3 doses/day, starting 3 hours after ifosfamide administration is completed, for 5 consecutive days, on days 1–5, every 21 days (total mesna dosage/cycle = 12,000 mg/m^2; this total also includes Hour 1 and Hour 5 doses)
Start: Hour 14 End: Hour 24	**Hydration** with D5W/0.2% NS; administer intravenously at 100 mL/m^2 per hour for 10 hours for 5 consecutive days, on days 1–5, every 21 days

Supportive Care
Antiemetic prophylaxis
Emetogenic potential is **MODERATE**. *Potential for delayed symptoms*
See Chapter 39 for antiemetic recommendations

Hematopoietic growth factor (CSF) prophylaxis
Primary prophylaxis is indicated with 1 of the following:
  Filgrastim (G-CSF) 5 mcg/kg per day by subcutaneous injection, *or*

(continued)

(continued)

Pegfilgrastim (pegylated filgrastim) 6 mg/0.6 mL by subcutaneous injection for 1 dose
- Begin use on day 6, at least 24 hours after myelosuppressive chemotherapy is completed
- Continue daily filgrastim use after the neutrophil nadir until ANC ≥5000/mm³ on 2 measurements separated temporally by ≥12 hours
- Discontinue daily filgrastim use at least 24 hours before administering myelosuppressive treatment. Do not administer pegfilgrastim within 14 days before administering myelosuppressive treatment

See Chapter 43 for more information

Antimicrobial prophylaxis
Risk of fever and neutropenia is INTERMEDIATE
Antimicrobial primary prophylaxis to be considered:
- Antibacterial—consider a fluoroquinolone or no prophylaxis; *P. jirovecii* prophylaxis is recommended (eg, cotrimoxazole)
- Antifungal—consider concomitant use of clotrimazole during periods of neutropenia
- Antiviral—antiherpes antivirals (eg, acyclovir, famciclovir, valacyclovir)

See Chapter 47 for more information

Oral care
Prophylaxis and treatment for mucositis / stomatitis
General advice:
- Encourage patients to maintain intake of non-alcoholic fluids
- Evaluate patients for oral pain and provide analgesic medications
- Consider histamine (H_2-subtype) receptor antagonists (eg, ranitidine, famotidine), or a proton pump inhibitor for epigastric pain
- *Lactobacillus* sp.-containing probiotics may be beneficial in preventing diarrhea
Patients with intact oral mucosa:
- Clean the mouth, tongue, and gums by brushing after every meal and at bedtime with an ultra-soft toothbrush with fluoride toothpaste
- Floss teeth gently every day unless contraindicated. If gums bleed and hurt, avoid bleeding or sore areas, but floss other teeth
- Patients may use saline or commercial bland, non-alcoholic rinses
  - Do not use mouthwashes that contain alcohols
If mucositis or stomatitis is present:
- Keep the mouth moist utilizing water, ice chips, sugarless gum, sugar-free hard candies, or a saliva substitute
- Rinse mouth several times a day to remove debris
  - Use a solution of ¼ teaspoon (1.25 g) each of baking soda and table salt (sodium chloride) in one quart (~950 mL) of warm water. Follow with a plain water rinse
  - Do not use mouthwashes that contain alcohols
- Foam-tipped swabs (eg, Toothettes®) are useful in moisturizing oral mucosa, but ineffective for cleansing teeth and removing plaque
- Advise patients who develop mucositis to:
  - Choose foods that are easy to chew and swallow
  - Take small bites of food, chew slowly, and sip liquids with meals
  - Encourage soft, moist foods such as cooked cereals, mashed potatoes, and scrambled eggs
  - For trouble swallowing, soften food with gravies, sauces, broths, yogurt, or other bland liquids
  - Avoid sharp, crunchy foods; hot, spicy or highly acidic foods (eg, citrus fruits and juices); sugary foods; toothpicks; tobacco products; alcoholic drinks

Patient Population Studied

A prospective phases II/III trial in 41 evaluable patients ≤30 years of age with measurable, newly diagnosed, biopsy-proven, high-grade, metastatic osteosarcoma with normal renal, hepatic, and bone marrow profile and ECOG performance status ≤2

Efficacy (N = 23–41)

Response Rate*	
Combined pathologic + radiologic response (n = 39)	59% ± 8%
Pathologic response alone† (n = 23)	65% ± 10%
Radiologic response alone (n = 27)	52% ± 9%

*Assessed after 2 cycles of etoposide + ifosfamide with mesna
†As measured by necrosis of the primary tumor

Toxicity* (N = 41)

	% G3	% G4
Hematopoietic		
WBC count	2	83
ANC	2	29
Platelets	17	27
Hemoglobin	5	5
Nonhematopoietic		
Sepsis	10	—
Bacterial infection	7	—
Viral infection	2	—
Fanconi syndrome	7	—
Stomatitis	7	—
Sodium	2	—
Creatinine	2	—
Hematuria	2	—
Poor Karnofsky score	2	—
Vomiting	2	—
Potassium	2	—

*Toxicities listed are those pertaining only to the 2 cycles of induction chemotherapy using ifosfamide and etoposide

Treatment Modifications

Repeat chemotherapy 3 weeks after the initiation of treatment if ANC >1,000/μL and the platelet count >120,000/μL

Therapy Monitoring

1. *Before each cycle:* CBC with differential, serum electrolytes, BUN, and creatinine
2. *During treatment cycles:* Daily serum electrolytes, BUN, and creatinine; CBC with differential at least twice weekly

Notes

1. Although few patients were treated, the response to ifosfamide and etoposide seemed to be dose dependent
2. This combination may be more active against bony metastases than other regimens

REGIMEN

Recurrent or Refractory Bone [or Soft-Tissue Sarcoma] (Children and Young Adults)

GEMCITABINE + DOCETAXEL

Navid F et al. Cancer 2008;113:419–425

Gemcitabine 675 mg/m^2 per dose; administer intravenously, diluted in 0.9% sodium chloride injection (0.9% NS) to a concentration as low as 0.1 mg/mL, over 90 minutes for 2 doses, on days 1 and 8, every 21 days (total dosage/cycle = 1350 mg/m^2)

Premedication for docetaxel:
Dexamethasone 8 mg/dose; administer orally twice daily for 3 days, starting 1 day before docetaxel administration (total dose/cycle = 48 mg)

Optional premedication for docetaxel:
• **Diphenhydramine HCl** 25 mg; administer orally 30–60 minutes *or* intravenously 5–30 minutes prior to docetaxel administration

• **Ranitidine** 150 mg; administer orally 30–60 minutes prior to docetaxel administration, *or*

• **Ranitidine** 50 mg; administer intravenously 5–30 minutes prior to docetaxel administration

Docetaxel 75–100 mg/m^2; administer intravenously, in a volume of 0.9% NS or D5W sufficient to produce a docetaxel concentration within the range 0.3–0.74 mg/mL, over 60 minutes, on day 8 after completing gemcitabine administration, every 21 days (total dosage/cycle = 75–100 mg/m^2)

Supportive Care
Antiemetic prophylaxis
Emetogenic potential is LOW
See Chapter 39 for antiemetic recommendations

Hematopoietic growth factor (CSF) prophylaxis
Primary prophylaxis is indicated with 1 of the following:
Filgrastim (G-CSF) 5 mcg/kg per day by subcutaneous injection, *or*
Pegfilgrastim (pegylated filgrastim) 6 mg/0.6 mL by subcutaneous injection for one dose
• Begin use on cycle day 9; that is, 24 hours after myelosuppressive chemotherapy is completed

• Continue daily filgrastim use until ANC ≥10,000/mm^3 on 2 measurements separated temporally by ≥12 hours

• Discontinue daily filgrastim use at least 24 hours before administering myelosuppressive treatment. Do not administer pegfilgrastim within 14 days before administering myelosuppressive treatment

See Chapter 43 for more information

Antimicrobial prophylaxis
Risk of fever and neutropenia is LOW
Antimicrobial primary prophylaxis to be considered:
• Antibacterial—not indicated

• Antifungal—not indicated

• Antiviral—not indicated unless patient previously had an episode of HSV

See Chapter 47 for more information

Patient Population Studied

A retrospective analysis of 22 patients with recurrent or progressive bone or soft-tissue sarcoma

Therapy Monitoring

1. *At start of therapy:* Clinical examination and laboratory testing

2. *Day 1 of each treatment cycle:* Physical examination, ECOG PS, complete blood count with leukocyte differential count, and serum chemistries

3. *Weekly CBC with leukocyte differential count:* At least the first 6 cycles of therapy

4. *After every 2 cycles of therapy:* Tumor measurements

Treatment Modifications

Adverse Event	Dose Modification
Febrile neutropenia or platelet count of less than 25,000/mm^3 lasting >5 days	Reduce gemcitabine and docetaxel dosages by 25% in all subsequent cycles
ANC <1000/mm^3 at start of next cycle	Withhold treatment until ANC ≥1000/mm^3, then reduce gemcitabine and docetaxel dosages by 25%
Platelet count <100,000/mm^3 at start of next cycle	Withhold treatment until platelet count ≥100,000/mm^3, then reduce gemcitabine and docetaxel dosages by 25%
ANC <1000/mm^3 or platelet count <100,000/mm^3 despite 2-week delay	Discontinue therapy
Day 8 ANC 500–999/mm^3, or day 8 platelet count 50,000–99,000/mm^3	Reduce day 8 gemcitabine and docetaxel dosages by 25%
Day 8 ANC <500/mm^3, or day 8 platelet count <50,000/mm^3	Do not administer day 8 gemcitabine and docetaxel
G3/4 nonhematologic toxicity other than alopecia, fatigue, malaise, and nail changes	Hold chemotherapy up to 2 weeks until toxicity resolves to G ≤1. If toxicity does not resolve to G ≤1 within 2 weeks, discontinue therapy. Resume treatment if toxicity resolves to G ≤1 within 2 weeks, but reduce gemcitabine and docetaxel dosages by 25%
G3/4 nonhematologic toxicity other than alopecia, fatigue, malaise, and nail changes, despite a 25% reduction in initial gemcitabine and docetaxel dosages	Hold chemotherapy up to 2 weeks until toxicity resolves to G ≤1. If toxicity does not resolve to G ≤1 within 2 weeks, discontinue therapy. Resume treatment if toxicity resolves to G ≤1 within 2 weeks, but reduce gemcitabine and docetaxel dosages by an additional 25%

(continued)

Efficacy (N = 14)

Tumor Response Categorization Using RECIST in 14 Patients by Disease Type*

Disease Type	Number of Patients	RECIST Category			
		CR	PR	SD	PD
Osteosarcoma[†]	10	0	3	1	6
Ewing sarcoma family of tumors[‡]	2	0	0	1	1
Malignant fibrous histiocytoma	1	1	0	0	0
Undifferentiated sarcoma	1	0	0	0	1
Total	14	1	3	2	8

Median number of cycles	4 (range: 1–13)
Median duration of PR/CR	3.8 months (range: 1.6–9.7+ months)
Median time to progressive disease	2.3 months (range: 0.8–14 months)
Number of patients dead and cause of death	19 (18 from PD and 1 from unknown cause)
Patients alive	3 with osteosarcoma (alive with disease at 7, 52, and 69 months after recurrence)

RECIST, Response Evaluation Criteria in Solid Tumors; CR, complete response; PR, partial response; SD, stable disease; PD, progressive disease (Therasse P et al. J Natl Cancer Inst 2000;92:205–216)
*Eight of the 22 patients were not evaluable for objective tumor response: 5 patients had tumors that did not qualify as target lesions as defined by RECIST, 3 patients had no evidence of disease by imaging studies at the initiation of gemcitabine and docetaxel treatment, and 1 patient died before undergoing imaging for response evaluation. Of the 5 patients with no target lesions, 4 had tumors measuring <1 cm and 1 had pleural-based lung disease. Lesions decreased in size in 2 of these patients, were stable in 2 patients, and progressed in 1 patient during therapy
[†]Duration of SD: 13 months
[‡]Duration of SD: 3.5 months

Treatment Modifications
(continued)

G ≥3 liver function test abnormalities	Hold chemotherapy up to 2 weeks until toxicity resolves to G ≤1. If toxicity does not resolve to G ≤1 within 2 weeks, discontinue therapy. Resume treatment if toxicity resolves to G ≤1 within 2 weeks, but reduce gemcitabine and docetaxel dosages by 25%
G ≥3 liver function test abnormalities despite a 25% reduction in initial gemcitabine and docetaxel dosages	Hold chemotherapy up to 2 weeks until toxicity resolves to G ≤1. If toxicity does not resolve to G ≤1 within 2 weeks, discontinue therapy. Resume treatment if toxicity resolves to G ≤1 within 2 weeks, but reduce gemcitabine and docetaxel dosages by an additional 25%
G4 mucositis and diarrhea	Discontinue therapy
G2 neuropathy	Delay therapy 1 week. If symptoms do not resolve to G ≤1, reduce docetaxel dosage by 25%
G3 neuropathy	Discontinue therapy
Febrile neutropenia (T >38°C [>100.4°F] with ANC <1000/mm³)	Reduce gemcitabine and docetaxel doses by 25%
G3/4 hematologic toxicity	Hold chemotherapy up to 2 weeks until toxicity resolves to G ≤1. If toxicity does not resolve to G ≤1 within 2 weeks, discontinue therapy

Toxicity (N = 22)

Grade 3/4 Toxicities in 22 Patients (109 Courses of Gemcitabine + Docetaxel)*

Toxicity	Grade 3		Grade 4	
	Number of Events (%)	Number of Patients (%)	Number of Events (%)	Number of Patients (%)
Myelosuppression				
Anemia	14 (13)	7 (32)	2 (2)	2 (9)
Neutropenia	18 (17)	11 (50)	15 (14)	8 (36)
Thrombocytopenia	14 (13)	9 (41)	24 (22)	9 (41)
Gastrointestinal				
Diarrhea	2 (2)	2 (9)	—	—
Nausea	1 (1)	1 (5)	—	—
Vomiting	1 (1)	1 (5)	—	—
Colitis	1 (1)	1 (5)	—	—
Hepatic				
Elevated ALT/AST	5 (5)	3 (14)	—	—
Metabolic				
Hypokalemia	4 (4)	4 (18)	1 (1)	1 (5)
Hypophosphatemia	8 (7)	5 (23)	—	—
Hyperglycemia	1 (1)	1 (5)	—	—
Infection				
Without neutropenia	3 (3)	3 (14)	—	—
With neutropenia	1 (1)	1 (5)	—	—
Febrile neutropenia	3 (3)	2 (9)	—	—
Neurology				
Sensory neuropathy	1 (1)	1 (5)	—	—
Other				
Fluid retention	2 (2)	2 (9)	—	—

ALT, alanine aminotransferase; AST, aspartate aminotransferase
*Toxicities were graded according to National Cancer Institute Common Terminology Criteria for Adverse Events (v. 3.0)

Primary Malignant Bone Tumors: Ewing Sarcoma

Epidemiology

Incidence: Estimated annual incidence from birth to age 20 years is 2.9/million population. Approximately 10% of patients are 20–30 years of age. Cases in patients >30 years of age are infrequent

Median age: 14 years; 90% of patients, <20 years of age

Mortality rate: 0.05/100,000 population

Male to female ratio: Slightly more prevalent in males

American Cancer Society: Cancer Facts and Figures 2005 http://cancer.org
Gurney JG et al. Malignant bone tumors. In: Reis LAG, Smith MA, Gurney JG et al., eds. Cancer incidence and survival among children and adolescents: United States SEER program, 1975–1995. NIH Pub. No. 99-4649. Bethesda, MD: National Cancer Institute SEER Program; 1999:99–110

Stage at Diagnosis	
Nonmetastatic	80%
Metastatic	20%

5-Year Survival	
Localized	60–70%
Metastatic	20%

Expert Opinion

Treatment of Ewing sarcoma is similar to that of osteosarcoma because it involves the use of neoadjuvant chemotherapy followed by local therapy (surgery or radiation), which is then followed by adjuvant chemotherapy

Chemotherapy
1. The most commonly used drugs are doxorubicin, vincristine, ifosfamide, etoposide, dactinomycin, and cyclophosphamide
2. The use of combination chemotherapy as part of a multidisciplinary approach has increased 5-year survival rates from <10% to approximately 60%

Local therapy
1. Local therapy in the treatment of Ewing sarcoma varies from surgery alone, to radiation alone, to a combination of both modalities, depending on where disease is located
2. Surgery remains the preferred route of local control. A wide surgical margin should be attempted
3. In contrast to osteosarcoma and the soft-tissue sarcomas, Ewing tumors are radiosensitive. Therefore, in patients in whom surgery is not possible or for those patients with marginal and intralesional surgery, radiation is an effective therapeutic option
4. The behavior of Ewing sarcoma and PNET (Primitive neuroectodermal tumors) in adults is no different from its behavior in children

Adverse prognostic factors
1. Metastatic disease
2. Pelvic localization
3. Tumor diameter >8–10 cm
4. Age >15 years
5. Elevated LDH
6. Poor histologic response to preoperative chemotherapy
7. Radiation therapy as the only local treatment

Grier HE et al. N Engl J Med 2003;348:694–701
Verrill MW et al. J Clin Oncol 1997;15:2611–2621

Pathology

Ewing sarcoma family of tumors (includes primitive neuroectodermal tumors):
1. Rare tumors arising in the bone marrow from primitive neural crest elements
2. Constitute approximately 10% of bone sarcomas
3. Subtypes include:
   - Classic Ewing sarcoma (most commonly associated with bone)
   - Primitive neuroectodermal tumor (generally not associated with bones)
4. Distinguished immunohistochemically from other pediatric tumors by expression of the MIC2 gene
5. Most commonly detected translocation is **t(11;22)(q24;q12)**, one of a series of related translocations that occur in >95% of the Ewing sarcoma family of tumors (including primitive neuroectodermal tumors)
6. The t(11;22) translocation joins the Ewing sarcoma gene *EWS* on chromosome 22 to friend leukemia insertion (*FLI1*) on chromosome 11 (ie, t[11;22])
   Note: FLI1 is a member of the ETS (E-twenty six) family
7. The *EWS-FLI1* fusion transcript encodes a 68-kDa protein with 2 primary domains
   - *EWS* domain = a potent transcriptional activator
   - *FLI1* domain = a highly conserved *ETS* DNA-binding domain

   The EWS-FLI1 fusion protein thus acts as an aberrant transcription factor
8. In an individual patient, t(11;22) fuses one of many observed combinations of exons from *EWS* and *FLI1* to form the fused message. Most common combination = *EWS* exon 7 fused to *FLI1* exon 6 ("7/6") in ≈50–64% of tumors of the Ewing sarcoma family

REGIMEN

Newly Diagnosed—Ewing Sarcoma, Primitive Neuroectodermal Tumor of Bone, Primitive Sarcoma of Bone

VINCRISTINE, CYCLOPHOSPHAMIDE, AND DOXORUBICIN OR DACTINOMYCIN ALTERNATING WITH IFOSFAMIDE AND ETOPOSIDE

Grier HE et al. N Engl J Med 2003;348:694–701

Patients receive 2 complete courses of alternating induction chemotherapy (1 course includes 1 cycle with vincristine, doxorubicin, and cyclophosphamide followed by 1 cycle with ifosfamide and etoposide). Local therapy (surgery or radiation) occurs at week 12 and, after recovery, adjuvant chemotherapy with the same chemotherapy regimens ensues for a further 7 cycles of vincristine, doxorubicin, and cyclophosphamide, in alternation with 6 cycles of ifosfamide and etoposide (total: 17 cycles of chemotherapy)

Cycles of vincristine, doxorubicin (or dactinomycin), and cyclophosphamide + mesna:
Vincristine 2 mg/m^2 (maximum single dose "capped" at 2 mg); administer by intravenous injection over 1–3 minutes on day 1, every 42 days (total dosage/cycle = 2 mg/m^2; maximum dose/cycle = 2 mg)
Doxorubicin 75 mg/m^2; administer by intravenous injection over 3–5 minutes on day 1, every 42 days (total dosage/cycle = 75 mg/m^2; total cumulative dosage permitted = 375 mg/m^2)
• When a total doxorubicin dosage of 375 mg/m^2 has been administered, no additional doxorubicin is given. Instead, doxorubicin is *replaced by:*
Dactinomycin 1.25 mg/m^2; administer by intravenous injection over 3–5 minutes on day 1, every 42 days (total dosage/cycle = 1.25 mg/m^2)
• Dactinomycin is used only after doxorubicin is discontinued from the regimen
An admixture containing **cyclophosphamide** 1200 mg/m^2 + **mesna** 240 mg/m^2; administer intravenously in 100–250 mL 0.9% sodium chloride injection (0.9% NS) or 5% dextrose injection (D5W) over 15–30 minutes on day 1 every 42 days (total cyclophosphamide dosage/cycle = 1200 mg/m^2)
Then, either:
Mesna 240 mg/m^2 per dose; administer intravenously diluted with 0.9% NS or D5W to a concentration of 1–20 mg/mL, over 15 minutes for 2 doses at 4 hours and 8 hours after cyclophosphamide administration is completed, on day 1, every 42 days (total mesna dosage/cycle = 720 mg/m^2; includes 240 mg dose given with cyclophosphamide), *or*
Mesna 480 mg/m^2 per dose; administer orally for 2 doses at 2 hours and 6 hours after cyclophosphamide administration is completed on day 1, every 42 days (total mesna dosage/cycle = 1200 mg/m^2; includes 240 mg dose given with cyclophosphamide)

Cycles of ifosfamide + mesna and etoposide:
An admixture containing **ifosfamide** 1800 mg/m^2 + **mesna** 360 mg/m^2 per day; administer intravenously in a volume of 0.9% NS or D5W sufficient to produce ifosfamide concentrations between 0.6 and 20 mg/mL, over 60 minutes for 5 consecutive days, on days 22–26, every 42 days (total ifosfamide dosage/cycle = 9000 mg/m^2)
Then, either:
Mesna 360 mg/m^2 per dose; administer intravenously diluted with 0.9% NS or D5W to a concentration of 1–20 mg/mL, over 15 minutes for 2 doses per day at 4 hours and 8 hours after ifosfamide administration is completed, for 5 consecutive days, on days 22–26, every 42 days (total mesna dosage/cycle = 5400 mg/m^2; includes 360 mg doses given daily with cyclophosphamide), *or*
Mesna 720 mg/m^2 per dose; administer orally for 2 doses per day at 2 hours and 6 hours after ifosfamide administration is completed, for 5 consecutive days, on days 22–26, every 42 days (total mesna dosage/cycle = 9000 mg/m^2; includes 360 mg doses given daily with cyclophosphamide)
Etoposide 100 mg/m^2 per day; administer intravenously diluted with 0.9% NS to a concentration of 0.2–0.4 mg/mL over 60 minutes for 5 consecutive days, on days 22–26, every 42 days (total dosage/cycle = 500 mg/m^2)

After the first 4 cycles of chemotherapy (2 complete courses, 12 weeks), local control is planned to consist of radiation therapy, surgery, or both

(continued)

Treatment Modifications

None specified

Patient Population Studied

This was a prospective randomized intergroup phase III study in newly diagnosed patients with primary bone tumors who were 30 years of age or younger. Patients had adequate renal, liver, and cardiac function; 300 patients were enrolled and 198 received this regimen

Efficacy (N = 198)

5-year event-free survival	69%
5-year overall survival	72%
Pattern of Treatment Failure	
Local progression	4.5%
Systemic progression	22.2%
Local and systemic progression	2%
Progression at unknown site	0.5%
Death	3.5%
Infection	3%
Hemorrhage	0.5%
Second malignant neoplasms	2%

(continued)

Radiation alone:
- Treat the extent of the initial soft tissue and osseous involvement with a 3-cm margin to a dose 4500 cGy
- Then treat with an additional 1080 cGy to the postchemotherapy, preradiation therapy tumor volume

Surgery without residual disease:
- No radiation therapy is administered

Gross residual tumor after surgery
- Treat as if treating with radiation alone

Microscopic residual disease after surgery
- Treat the extent of the initial soft tissue and osseous involvement with a 1-cm margin to a dose 4500 cGy

Supportive Care
Antiemetic prophylaxis
Emetogenic potential during cycles with vincristine, doxorubicin or dactinomycin, and cyclophosphamide is **HIGH**. *Potential for delayed symptoms*
Emetogenic potential during cycles with ifosfamide and etoposide is **MODERATE**
See Chapter 39 for antiemetic recommendations

Hematopoietic growth factor (CSF) prophylaxis
Primary prophylaxis is indicated with 1 of the following:
    Filgrastim (G-CSF) 5 mcg/kg per day by subcutaneous injection, *or*
    Pegfilgrastim (pegylated filgrastim) 6 mg/0.6 mL by subcutaneous injection for 1 dose
- Begin use at least 24 hours after myelosuppressive chemotherapy is completed (days 6 and 27)
- Continue daily filgrastim use after the neutrophil nadir until ANC $\geq 5000/mm^3$ on 2 measurements separated temporally by ≥ 12 hours
- Discontinue daily filgrastim use at least 24 hours before administering myelosuppressive treatment. Do not administer pegfilgrastim within 14 days before administering myelosuppressive treatment

See Chapter 43 for more information

Antimicrobial prophylaxis
Risk of fever and neutropenia is INTERMEDIATE
    Antimicrobial primary prophylaxis to be considered:
- Antibacterial—consider a fluoroquinolone or no prophylaxis; *P. jirovecii* prophylaxis is recommended (eg, cotrimoxazole)
- Antifungal—consider concomitant use of clotrimazole during periods of neutropenia
- Antiviral—antiherpes antivirals (eg, acyclovir, famciclovir, valacyclovir)

See Chapter 47 for more information

Therapy Monitoring

1. *Weekly:* CBC with differential
2. *Before each cycle:* CBC with differential, serum creatinine, liver function tests, and urinalysis
3. *Response evaluation:* At conclusion of first 4 cycles of chemotherapy

REGIMEN

CYCLOPHOSPHAMIDE + TOPOTECAN

Saylors RL, III et al. J Clin Oncol 2001;19:3463–3469

Pretreatment hydration: 500 mL/m^2 0.9% sodium chloride injection (0.9% NS), *or* 0.45% sodium chloride injection, *or* 5% dextrose injection/0.45% sodium chloride injection; administer intravenously over 2–4 hours before starting chemotherapy

Cyclophosphamide 250 mg/m^2 per day; administer intravenously in 25–250 mL 0.9% NS or 5% dextrose injection (D5W) over 30 minutes for 5 consecutive days, on days 1–5, every 21 days (total dosage/cycle = 1250 mg/m^2)

Topotecan HCl 0.75 mg/m^2 per day; administer intravenously in 50–250 mL 0.9% NS or D5W over 30 minutes for 5 consecutive days, after cyclophosphamide on days 1–5, every 21 days (total dosage/cycle = 3.75 mg/m^2)

Posttreatment hydration: Hydration continues orally or intravenously at a rate of 3000 mL/m^2 per 24 hours until 24 hours after the last dose of chemotherapy is completed

Supportive Care
Antiemetic prophylaxis
Emetogenic potential is **MODERATE**
See Chapter 39 for antiemetic recommendations

Hematopoietic growth factor (CSF) prophylaxis
Primary prophylaxis is indicated with 1 of the following:
 Filgrastim (G-CSF) 5 mcg/kg per day by subcutaneous injection, *or*
 Pegfilgrastim (pegylated filgrastim) 6 mg/0.6 mL by subcutaneous injection for 1 dose
 • Begin use at least 24 hours after myelosuppressive chemotherapy is completed (day 6)
 • Continue daily filgrastim use after the neutrophil nadir until ANC ≥5000/mm^3 on 2 measurements separated temporally by ≥12 hours
 • Discontinue daily filgrastim use at least 24 hours before administering myelosuppressive treatment. Do not administer pegfilgrastim within 14 days before administering myelosuppressive treatment
See Chapter 43 for more information

Antimicrobial prophylaxis
Risk of fever and neutropenia is INTERMEDIATE
 Antimicrobial primary prophylaxis to be considered:
 • Antibacterial—consider a fluoroquinolone or no prophylaxis; *P. jirovecii* prophylaxis is recommended (eg, cotrimoxazole)
 • Antifungal—consider concomitant use of clotrimazole during periods of neutropenia
 • Antiviral—antiherpes antivirals (eg, acyclovir, famciclovir, valacyclovir)
See Chapter 47 for more information

Toxicity* (N = 307 Cycles)

	% of Cycles with G3/4
Neutropenia	53
Thrombocytopenia	44
Anemia	27
Infection†	11
Nausea/vomiting	0.65
Hematuria‡	0.65
Perirectal mucositis	0.33
Transaminase elevation	0.33

*National Cancer Institute (USA) Common Toxicity Criteria, version 2.0
†Includes admissions for fever/neutropenia: 5 bacteremia or fungemia, 1 herpes zoster, 1 infectious cystitis
‡In 2 patients with history of hematuria on ifosfamide

Therapy Monitoring

1. *Daily during therapy:* Urinalysis
2. *Twice weekly:* CBC with differential until recovery from hematopoietic toxicity
3. *Weekly:* Physical examination
4. *Before each cycle:* Serum creatinine, LFTs with bilirubin, serum electrolytes, including calcium, magnesium, and phosphorus
5. *Response evaluation:* After the first and second cycles, then after every 2 cycles

Treatment Modifications

None specified

Patient Population Studied

A study of 91 pediatric patients with recurrent or refractory solid tumors, including Ewing sarcoma (n = 17), rhabdomyosarcoma (n = 15), and neuroblastoma (n = 13)

Efficacy

Ewing Sarcoma (n = 17)	
Complete response	12%
Partial response	24%
Rhabdomyosarcoma (n = 15)	
Complete response	0
Partial response	67%

Notes

Responses were observed in patients who had received >1 year of intensive alkylating agent therapy and/or ablative therapy with autologous stem cell rescue

REGIMEN

Relapsed/Refractory Ewing Sarcoma or Peripheral Neuroectodermal Tumor (PNET)

TEMOZOLOMIDE + IRINOTECAN

Casey DA et al. Pediatr Blood Cancer 2009;53:1029–1034
Wagner LM et al. Pediatr Blood Cancer 2007;48:132–139

Temozolomide 100 mg/m² per day; administer orally for 5 consecutive days, on days 1–5, 1 hour before irinotecan, every 21–28 days (total dosage/cycle = 500 mg/m²)
Note: Temozolomide doses are rounded to the nearest 5 mg by using commercially available products
Irinotecan 10–20 mg/m² per dose; administer intravenously, diluted with 5% dextrose injection to a concentration within the range of 0.12–2.8 mg/mL, over 90 minutes for 10 doses, on days 1–5 and days 8–12, every 21–28 days (total dosage/cycle = 100–200 mg/m²)

Supportive Care

Antiemetic prophylaxis
Emetogenic potential is **MODERATE**
See Chapter 39 for antiemetic recommendations

Hematopoietic growth factor (CSF) prophylaxis
Primary prophylaxis is NOT indicated
See Chapter 43 for more information

Antimicrobial prophylaxis
Risk of fever and neutropenia is LOW
   Antimicrobial primary prophylaxis to be considered:
   • Antibacterial—not indicated
   • Antifungal—not indicated
   • Antiviral—not indicated unless patient previously had an episode of HSV
See Chapter 47 for more information

Acute cholinergic syndrome

Atropine sulfate 0.25–1 mg subcutaneously or intravenously if abdominal cramping or diarrhea develop during or within 1 hour after irinotecan administration
• If symptoms are severe, add as primary prophylaxis at least 30 minutes before irinotecan during subsequent cycles
• For irinotecan, acute cholinergic syndrome may be characterized by abdominal cramping, diarrhea, diaphoresis, hypotension, flushing, bradycardia, rhinitis, increased salivation, meiosis, and lacrimation

Diarrhea management

• The potential for developing diarrhea and abdominal pain should be discussed with all patients and their caretakers, and instructions given to start loperamide immediately if these symptoms occur and to ensure adequate hydration is maintained. See "Dose Modifications" (below) for instructions
Latent or delayed onset diarrhea*:
   Loperamide 4 mg orally initially after the first loose or liquid stool, *then*
   Loperamide 2 mg orally every 2 hours during waking hours, *plus*
   Loperamide 4 mg orally every 4 hours during hours of sleep
   • Continue for at least 12 hours after diarrhea resolves
   • Recurrent diarrhea after a 12-hour diarrhea-free interval is treated as a new episode
   • Rehydrate orally with fluids and electrolytes during a diarrheal episode
   • If a patient develops blood or mucus in stool, dehydration, or hemodynamic instability, or if diarrhea persists >48 hours despite loperamide, stop loperamide and hospitalize the patient for IV hydration

(continued)

Dose Modifications

Irinotecan Dose Levels*

Level 1 starting dosage	10–20 mg/m² per day
Level −1	7.5–15 mg/m² per day
Level −2	5–10 mg/m² per day

Temozolomide Dose Levels

Level 1 starting dosage	100 mg/m² per day orally on days 1–5
Level −1	75 mg/m² per day orally on days 1–5
Level −2	50 mg/m² per day orally on days 1–5

Adverse Event	Dose Modification
G1 ANC 1500–1999/mm³, or G1 thrombocytopenia during a cycle	Maintain dose and schedule
G2 ANC 1000–1499/mm³, or G2 thrombocytopenia during a cycle	Reduce dosage of both agents by 1 dosage level
G4 neutropenia >7 days duration	Reduce dosage of both agents for the following cycle by 1 dose level
G3/4 infection	
Day 21 ANC <1000/mm³, or platelet count <75,000/mm³	Delay start of next cycle by 1 week and reduce dosage of both agents 1 level
Day 28 ANC still <1000/mm³, or platelet count still <75,000/mm³	Delay start of next cycle by 1 additional week and reduce dosage of both agents 1 level
Day 35 ANC still <1000/mm³, or platelet count still <75,000/mm³	Discontinue therapy

Diarrhea in Children 2–15 Years of Age

Children 2–15 years, with first liquid stools	Begin oral loperamide liquid immediately with the first liquid stool at a dosage of 0.18 mg/kg per day (0.03 mg/kg administered orally every 4 hours)

(continued)

(continued)

Alternatively, a trial of **Diphenoxylate hydrochloride** 2.5 mg **with Atropine sulfate** 0.025 mg (eg, Lomotil)

- Initial adult dose is 2 tablets 4 times daily until control has been achieved, after which the dose may be reduced to meet individual requirements. Control may often be maintained with as little as 2 tablets daily
- Clinical improvement of acute diarrhea is usually observed within 48 hours. If improvement of chronic diarrhea after treatment with a maximum daily dose of 8 tablets is not observed within 10 days, control is unlikely with further administration

Persistent diarrhea:

Octreotide 100–150 mcg subcutaneously 3 times daily. Maximum total daily dose is 1500 mcg

Antibiotic primary prophylaxis and treatment during latent or delayed onset diarrhea:

Consider the following to prevent or lessen irinotecan-associated diarrhea:

- Prophylactic oral **cefixime** 8 mg/kg (maximum dose of 400 mg) orally once daily, beginning 1–2 days prior to the start of irinotecan therapy and continuing continue until completion of the cycle, *alternatively:*
- **Cefpodoxime proxetil** 5 mg/kg/day per day orally twice daily (maximum dose of 200 mg twice daily)
  - Previous studies suggest prophylaxis with cephalosporin antibiotics can ameliorate irinotecan-associated diarrhea by reducing the enteric bacteria responsible for producing β-glucuronidase, which regenerates in the gut irinotecan's toxic metabolite, SN-38, by cleaving the glucuronide moiety from SN-38 (Wagner LM et al. Pediatr Blood Cancer 2008;50:201–207)
- Alternatively, **activated charcoal** at a dose equal to 5 times the irinotecan dose up to a maximum dose of 260 mg orally 3 times daily during irinotecan therapy (Michael M et al. J Clin Oncol 2004;22:4410–4417)

Antibiotic treatment during latent or delayed onset diarrhea

- A fluoroquinolone (eg, **Ciprofloxacin** 500 mg orally every 12 hours) if absolute neutrophil count <500/mm³ with or without accompanying fever in association with diarrhea

Antibiotics should also be administered if a patient is hospitalized with prolonged diarrhea, and should be continued until diarrhea resolves

*Abigerges D et al. J Natl Cancer Inst 1994;86:446–449
Rothenberg ML et al. J Clin Oncol 2001;19:3801–3807
Wadler S et al. J Clin Oncol 1998;16:3169–3178

Efficacy (N = 14)*

Wagner LM et al. Pediatr Blood Cancer 2007;48:132–139

Complete response	1 (7%)
Partial response	3 (21%)
Minor response	3 (21%)
Median duration of response	30 (range: 12–64) weeks
Median time to progression	20 weeks
Marked symptomatic pain relief with reduction in medication usage[†]	7 (50%)

*WHO criteria; 2 patients started treatment with no measurable disease following other salvage therapies. Consequently, only 14 patients were fully evaluable for response
[†]In first course of therapy, irrespective of ultimate imaging response

Dose Modifications
(continued)

G3/4 diarrhea within the first 24 hours	Hospitalize for optimal managements. Begin loperamide 0.06 mg/kg every 4 hours. Reduce irinotecan dosage for the following cycle by 1 dose level

Delayed Diarrhea in Patients >15 Years of Age

G1 (2–3 stools/day > baseline)	Maintain dose and schedule
G2 (4–6 stools/day > baseline)	Delay until diarrhea resolves to baseline, then reduce irinotecan dosage by 1 dosage level
G3 (7–9 stools/day > baseline)	Delay until diarrhea resolves to baseline, then reduce dosage of irinotecan by 1 dosage level
G4 (≥10 stools/day > baseline)	Delay until diarrhea resolves to baseline, then reduce dosage of irinotecan by 2 dosage levels

Other Nonhematologic Toxicities

Any G1 toxicity	Maintain dose and schedule
Any G2 toxicity	Hold treatment until toxicity resolves to G ≤1, then reduce dosage of both agents by 1 dosage level
Any G3 toxicity	Hold treatment until toxicity resolves to G ≤1, then reduce dosage of both agents by 1 dosage level
Any G4 toxicity	Hold treatment until toxicity resolves to G ≤1, then reduce dosage of both agents by 2 dosage levels

*Treatment should be stopped in case of recurrent toxicity at dose level −2, unless there is perceived clinical benefit from irinotecan that justifies continuation

André T et al. Eur J Cancer 1999;35:1343–1347
Camptosar irinotecan hydrochloride injection, product label, August 2010. Pharmacia & Upjohn Company, Division of Pfizer, Inc., New York, NY
Douillard JY et al. Lancet 2000;355:1041–1047
Tournigand C et al. J Clin Oncol 2004;22:229–237

Efficacy (N = 20)*

Casey DA et al. Pediatr Blood Cancer 2009;53:1029–1034

Best response achieved (n = 19)	
Complete response[†]	5 patients[‡]
Partial response	7 patients
Progressive disease	7 patients
Stable disease	0
Overall objective response	63%
Overall survival (n = 20)[§]	55%[§]
Median TTP	
All evaluable patients (n = 20)	8.3 months
Patients with recurrent ES (n = 14)	16.2 months
>2-year remission after primary diagnosis (n = 6)[ϵ]	22.8 months
<2-year remission after primary diagnosis (n = 14)	3.7 months
Localized disease at initial diagnosis (n = 9)	16.4 months
Metastatic disease at initial diagnosis (n = 11)	2.4 months
Single-site disease recurrence	24.3 months
Multiple-site recurrence	2.4 months

*WHO criteria
[†]Each of the 5 completed 12 planned cycles of irinotecan/temozolomide; all were in remission with a median follow-up time of 28.3 months
[‡]Two patients disease free > additional radiation or chemotherapy. Five patients experienced PD > a median of 6 months and 9 cycles of therapy
[§]Eleven patients (55%) alive with median follow up 25.7 months at conclusion of cohort analysis
[ϵ]Four of 6 achieved a CR and were in remission >12 cycles of therapy with a median follow-up time of 26.4 months

Patient Population Studied

All patients had either progressive disease (PD) during initial therapy (n = 5) or relapse within 2 years of diagnosis (n = 1). Twelve patients had metastatic disease at diagnosis, including 5 with bone and/or marrow metastases

Therapy Monitoring

1. *Prior to enrollment:* Complete medical history, clinical examination, performance status, hematologic and serum chemistries cardiac evaluation in case of prior treatment with anthracyclines or mediastinal irradiation, and tumor target assessment
2. *Day 1 of each treatment cycle:* Physical examination, ECOG PS, complete blood count with leukocyte differential count, and serum chemistries
3. *Weekly CBC with leukocyte differential count:* At least the first 6 cycles of therapy
4. *After every 2 cycles of therapy:* Tumor measurements

Toxicity

(N = 154 cycles of irinotecan + temozolomide)*

Casey DA et al. Pediatr Blood Cancer 2009;53:1029–1034

Toxicity	No. G3	No. G4	Percent G3/4
Diarrhea	7	0	7 (4.5%)
Colitis	1	0	1 (0.6%)
Neutropenia	12	7	19 (12.3%)
Thrombocytopenia[†]	13	3	16 (10.4%)
Pneumonitis	1	0	1 (0.6%)
Hospitalizations			
Febrile neutropenia	—	2	1 (1.2%)
Diarrhea/dehydration	—	3	1 (1.9%)
Colitis	—	1	1 (0.6%)
Pneumonitis	—	1	1 (0.6%)

*National Cancer Institute (USA) Common Toxicity Criteria, version 2.0 (NCI-CTC v2.0)
[†]150 cycles/19 patients. One patient had thrombocytopenia prior to enrollment

Toxicity (*continued*)

Wagner LM et al. Pediatr Blood Cancer 2007;48:132–139*

Toxicity	21-Day Schedule	28-Day Schedule	Cumulative
Total number of patients	9	7	16
Total number of courses	67	28	95
Median courses per patient (range)	6 (2–17)	3 (1–7)	5 (1–17)
Courses with grade 3–4 neutropenia	1 (2%) of 59[†]	1 (4%) of 28	2 (2%)[‡]
10 mg/m² per day	0 of 24	1 (5%) of 21	—
15 mg/m² per day	0 of 12	0 of 7	—
20 mg/m² per day	1 (4%) of 23	—	—
Courses with G3/4 thrombocytopenia	1(2%) of 59[†]	2 (7%) of 28	3 (3%)[‡]
10 mg/m² per day	0 of 24	2 (10%) of 21	—
15 mg/m² per day	0 of 12	0 of 7	—
20 mg/m² per day	1(4%) of 23	—	—
Courses with G3/4 vomiting	5 (7%) of 67	3 (11%) of 28	8 (8%)
10 mg/m² per day	0 of 32	0 of 21	—
15 mg/m² per day	4 (33%) of 12	3 (43%) of 7	—
20 mg/m² per day	1 (4%) of 23	—	—
Courses with G3/4 diarrhea	6 (9%)	4 (14%)	10 (11%)
10 mg/m² per day	0 of 32	0 of 21	—
15 mg/m² per day	4 (33%) of 12	4 (57%) of 7	—
20 mg/m² per day	2 (9%) of 23	—	—

*NCI-CTC, v.2.0
[†]Of 59 courses assessable for hematologic toxicity
[‡]Of 87 total courses assessable for hematologic toxicity

Sarcomas: Soft-Tissue Sarcomas
(Including Rhabdomyosarcoma, But Not Including GIST)
Epidemiology

Incidence: 12,020 (male: 6,550; female: 5,470. Estimated new cases for 2014 in the United States)
Deaths: Estimated 4,740 in 2014 (male: 2,550; female: 2,190)
Male to female ratio: 1.2:1

Siegel R et al. CA Cancer J Clin 2014;64:9–29

Cellular Classification of Adult Soft-Tissue Sarcoma
Soft-tissue sarcomas are classified histologically according to the soft-tissue cell of origin. The histologic grade reflects the metastatic potential of these tumors more accurately than the classic cellular classification listed below. Pathologists assign grade based on the number of mitoses per high-powered field, presence of necrosis, cellular and nuclear morphology, and the degree of cellularity. Discordance among expert pathologists can reach 40%

Alphabetical Listing (Percent of All Soft-Tissue Sarcomas)
(Note, however, that the frequency of histologic type is site dependent)
- Alveolar soft-part sarcoma (≤3%)
- Angiosarcoma (≤3%)
- Dermatofibrosarcoma protuberans (≤3%)
- Epithelioid sarcoma (≤3%)
- Extraskeletal chondrosarcoma (≤3%)
- Extraskeletal osteosarcoma (≤3%)
- Fibrosarcoma (≤3%)
- Gastrointestinal stromal tumor (GIST) (≤3%) (see separate section on GIST)
- **Leiomyosarcoma (≈12%)**
- **Liposarcoma (≈15–25%)**
- **Malignant fibrous histiocytoma (≈28–40%)**
- Malignant hemangiopericytoma (≤3%)
- Malignant mesenchymoma (≤3%)
- Malignant schwannoma (≤3%)
- **Malignant peripheral nerve sheath tumor (≈6%)**
- Peripheral neuroectodermal tumors (≤3%)
- **Rhabdomyosarcoma (≈5%)** (see separate section on rhabdomyosarcoma)
- **Synovial sarcoma (≈10%)**
- Sarcoma, NOS (not otherwise specified) (≤3%)

Abraham JA et al. Ann Surg Oncol 2007;14:1953–1967
Alvegård TA, Berg NO. J Clin Oncol 1989;7:1845–1851
Fayette J et al. Ann Oncol 2007;18:2030–2036
Fury MG et al. Cancer J 2005;11:241–247
Gaynor JJ et al. J Clin Oncol 1992;10:1317–1329
Marcus SG et al. Arch Surg 1993;128:1336–1343
Mendenhall WM et al. Cancer 2004;101:2503–2508
van Ruth S et al. Eur J Cancer 2002;38:1324–1328

Work-up
1. History and physical examination
2. *Laboratory tests:* CBC with differential, electrolytes, liver function tests, and mineral panel, including alkaline phosphatase and lactate dehydrogenase
3. Radiologic imaging modality is variable and dictated by the site of disease. This involves a combination of plain x-rays, CT, MRI, and PET imaging. Although CT remains the imaging modality of choice in the staging of retroperitoneal soft-tissue sarcoma, MRI is used more frequently to stage soft-tissue sarcoma of the extremity
4. Bone marrow aspirate for light microscopy examination in Ewing sarcoma
5. No radiologic studies are pathognomonic, so biopsy remains essential to diagnosis. Carefully plan biopsy to establish grade and histologic subtype and if needed molecular and cytogenetic studies
6. Echocardiogram or MUGA scan to determine cardiac ejection fraction as clinically indicated

Disease Distribution

Extremity	43%
Lower	30%
Upper	13%
Intraabdominal	34%
Visceral	19%
Retroperitoneal	15%
Trunk	10%
Other	13%

Soft tissue sarcoma. In: DeVita V, Lawrence T, Rosenberg S, eds. DeVita, Hellman, and Rosenberg's Cancer Principles & Practice of Oncology. 9th ed. (2011) published by Lippincott Williams & Wilkins: Philadelphia, 1533–1577
American Cancer Society: Cancer Facts and Figures 2011. http://cancer.org
http://www.cancer.gov/aboutnci/servingpeople/snapshots/sarcoma.pdf

Soft-Tissue Sarcomas: Adult Soft-Tissue Sarcomas, Other Than GIST

Classification of Malignant Adult Soft-Tissue Sarcomas

1. Fibrous tumors
   a. Fibrosarcoma:
      (1) Adult fibrosarcoma
      (2) Inflammatory fibrosarcoma
2. Fibrohistiocytic tumors
   a. Malignant fibrous histiocytoma
      (1) Storiform-pleomorphic
      (2) Myxoid (myxofibrosarcoma)
      (3) Giant cell (malignant giant cell tumor of the soft parts)
      (4) Inflammatory
3. Lipomatous
   a. Liposarcoma
      (1) Well-differentiated liposarcoma
         (a) Lipoma-like liposarcomas
         (b) Sclerosing liposarcoma
         (c) Inflammatory liposarcoma
      (2) Dedifferentiated liposarcoma
      (3) Myxoid or round cell liposarcoma
      (4) Pleomorphic liposarcoma
4. Smooth muscle tumors
   a. Leiomyosarcoma
   b. Epithelioid leiomyosarcoma
5. Skeletal muscle tumors
   a. Rhabdomyosarcoma
      (1) Embryonal rhabdomyosarcoma
      (2) Botryoid rhabdomyosarcoma
      (3) Spindle cell rhabdomyosarcoma
      (4) Alveolar rhabdomyosarcoma
      (5) Pleomorphic rhabdomyosarcoma
   b. Rhabdomyosarcoma with ganglionic differentiation (ectomesenchymoma)
6. Tumors of the blood and lymph nodes
   a. Epithelioid hemangioendothelioma
   b. Angiosarcoma and lymphangiosarcoma
   c. Kaposi sarcoma
7. Perivascular tumors
   a. Malignant glomus tumor (glomangiosarcoma)
   b. Malignant hemangiopericytoma

8. Synovial tumors
   a. Malignant giant cell tumor of tendon sheath
9. Neural tumors
   a. Malignant peripheral nerve sheath tumor (MPNST)
      (1) Malignant triton tumor (MPSNT with rhabdomyosarcoma)
      (2) Glandular MPNST
      (3) Epithelioid MPNST
   b. Malignant granular cell tumor
   c. Primitive neuroectodermal tumor
      (1) Neuroblastoma
      (2) Ganglioneuroblastoma
      (3) Neuroepithelioma (peripheral neuroectodermal tumor)
10. Paraganglionic tumors
    a. Malignant paraganglioma
11. Extraskeletal cartilaginous and osseous tumors
    a. Extraskeletal chondrosarcoma
       (1) Myxoid chondrosarcoma
       (2) Mesenchymal chondrosarcoma
    b. Extraskeletal osteosarcoma
12. Pluripotential mesenchymal tumors
    a. Malignant mesenchyma
13. Miscellaneous tumors
    a. Alveolar soft-part sarcoma
    b. Epithelioid sarcoma
    c. Malignant extrarenal rhabdoid tumor
    d. Desmoplastic small cell tumor
    e. Ewing sarcoma—extraskeletal
    f. Clear cell sarcoma
    g. Gastrointestinal stromal tumors
    h. Synovial sarcoma
    i. Dermatofibrosarcoma protuberans

Brennan MF et al. Sarcomas of the soft tissues and bone. In: DeVita VT Jr, Hellman S, Rosenberg SA, eds. Cancer: Principles & Practice of Oncology, 7th ed. Philadelphia, PA: Lippincott Williams & Wilkins; 2005:1581–1637

Expert Opinion

Adult-Type Soft-Tissue Sarcomas Arising from Limbs and Superficial Trunk

Note: Levels of Evidence (I–V) and Grades of Recommendation (A–D) are as used by the American Society of Clinical Oncology

Casali PG, Blay JY. Soft tissue sarcomas: ESMO clinical practice guidelines for diagnosis, treatment and follow-up. ESMO/CONTICANET/EUROBONET Consensus Panel of experts. Ann Oncol 2010;21 Suppl 5:v198–v203

Incidence

Adult soft-tissue sarcomas are rare tumors, with an estimated incidence averaging 5/100,000 population per year in Europe

Diagnosis and General Guidelines

- Multidisciplinary approach is mandatory in all cases; ideally in referral centers
- Enrollment in clinical trials is highly encouraged
- Biopsy options:
  - Standard approach: multiple core needle biopsies (using needles >16G)
  - Excisional biopsy may be the most practical option for superficial lesions <5 cm
  - Open biopsy is another option
- Frozen-section technique for immediate diagnosis is not encouraged
- Biopsy should be performed in such a way that the biopsy pathway and the scar can be safely removed on definitive surgery. The biopsy entrance point is preferably tattooed
- Tumor samples should be fixed in formalin (Bouin fixation should be banned because it prevents molecular analysis)
- Recommend using a grading system that distinguishes 3 malignancy grades based on differentiation, necrosis, and mitotic rate (The Federation Nationale des Centres de Lutte Contre le Cancer [FNCLCC] grading system, also used by the WHO)
- If preoperative treatment was carried out, the pathology report should include a tumor response assessment. However, in contrast to osteosarcoma and Ewing sarcoma, no validated system is available at present, and no percentage of residual "viable cells" is considered to have a specific prognostic significance
- Collection of fresh-frozen tissue and tumor imprints (touch preps) with appropriate consent is encouraged, because new molecular pathology assessments could become available

Stage Classification and Risk Assessment

- The American Joint Committee on Cancer (AJCC)/International Union against Cancer (UICC) stage classification system stresses the importance of the malignancy grade in sarcoma. However, its use in routine practice is limited
- Prognostic factors:
  1. Tumor grade
  2. Tumor size
  3. Tumor depth
  4. Tumor resectability

Staging Procedures

A chest spiral CT scan is mandatory for staging purposes
Depending on the histologic type and other clinical features, further staging assessments may be recommended (ie, regional lymph node clinical assessment for synovial sarcoma, epithelioid sarcoma, alveolar soft-part sarcoma, clear cell sarcoma; abdominal CT scan for myxoid liposarcoma, etc)

Treatment

Limited Disease
- Surgery is the standard treatment for all patients with adult type, localized soft-tissue sarcomas
- Standard surgical procedure is a wide excision with negative margins (R0). This implies removing the tumor with a rim of normal tissue around
- An excision with small margins may be acceptable in highly selected cases, in particular for extracompartmental atypical lipomatous tumors

(continued)

Staging

UICC and TNM Staging (AJCC) TNM

Primary Tumor

TX	Primary tumor cannot be assessed
T0	No evidence of primary tumor
T1	Tumor ≤5 cm in greatest dimension
T1a	Tumor above superficial fascia
T1b	Deep tumor*
T2	Tumor >5 cm in greatest dimension
T2a	Tumor above superficial fascia
T2b	Deep tumor

Nodal Status

NX	Regional lymph nodes cannot be assessed
N0	No regional lymph node metastasis
N1	Regional lymph nodes metastasis

Metastases

MX	Distant metastasis cannot be assessed
M0	No distant metastases
M1	Distant metastases
M1a	Lung
M1b	Other distant sites, including lymph nodes

GX	Grade cannot be assessed
G1	Well-differentiated—low-grade
G2	Moderately differentiated—low-grade
G3	Poorly differentiated—high-grade
G4	Undifferentiated—high-grade

Stage Groupings

Stage IA	T1a	N0	M0	G1, GX
	T1b	N0	M0	G1, GX
Stage IB	T2a	N0	M0	G1, GX
	T2b	N0	M0	G1, GX
Stage IIA	T1a	N0	M0	G2, G3
	T1b	N0	M0	G2, G3
Stage IIB	T2a	N0	M0	G2
	T2b	N0	M0	G2
Stage III	T2a, T2b	N0	M0	G3
	Any T	N1	M0	Any G
Stage IV	Any T	Any N	M1	Any G

*Deep tumors are tumors deep to the superficial fascia or those that have invaded through the fascia

Reprinted with permission from AJCC: Soft tissue sarcoma. In: Edge SB, Byrd DR, Compton CC et al., eds: AJCC Cancer Staging Manual. 7th ed. New York, NY: Springer; 2010:291–298

Expert Opinion (continued)

Radiation Therapy (RT):

1. *High-grade, deep lesions, >5 cm:* Wide excision followed by RT

2. *High-grade, deep, <5 cm:* Surgery followed by RT

3. *Low-grade, superficial, >5 cm, and low-grade, deep, <5 cm STS:* RT occasionally used

4. *Low-grade, deep, >5 cm STS:* Discuss RT in a multidisciplinary fashion

Notes:

- RT is not given in the case of a truly compartmental resection of a tumor entirely contained within the compartment

- Overall, RT has been shown to improve local control, but not overall survival

5. *Postoperative RT:* Follows marginal or R1 (microscopic residual disease) or R2 (gross residual disease) excisions, if these cannot be rescued through reexcision; 50–60 Gy, 1.8–2 Gy fractions, possibly with boosts up to 66 Gy

6. *Preoperative RT:* 50 Gy

7. *Intraoperative radiation therapy (IORT) and brachytherapy:* In selected cases

8. *Local relapse:* Approach parallels approach to primary local disease, except for a wider resort to preoperative or postoperative radiation therapy, if not previously performed

Surgery:

- Definitions:

  - R0 resection—No residual microscopic disease

  - R1 resection—Microscopic residual disease (presence of tumor cells on resection margins)

  - R2 resection—Gross residual disease

- R1 resections: Consider reoperation if adequate margins can be achieved without major morbidity, taking into account tumor extent and tumor biology

- R2 surgery: Reoperation is mandatory, possibly with preoperative treatments if adequate margins cannot be achieved, or surgery is mutilating. In the latter case, the use of multimodal therapy with less-radical surgery requires shared decision making with the patient under conditions of uncertainty

- In nonresectable tumors, or those amenable only to mutilating surgery, options that can be considered include:

  - Chemotherapy and/or radiotherapy

  - Isolated hyperthermic limb perfusion with tumor necrosis factor-α (TNFα) + melphalan, if the tumor is confined to an extremity

  - Regional hyperthermia combined with chemotherapy

Note:

- These treatment modalities added to surgery should not be viewed as truly "adjuvant," the context being in fact that of a likely systemic disease

- In 1 large randomized phase III study (in patients with G2–3, deep, >5-cm soft-tissue sarcomas), regional hyperthermia in addition to systemic chemotherapy was associated with a local and disease-free survival advantage

Adjuvant chemotherapy

- Might improve, or at least delay, distant and local recurrence in high-risk patients

- A metaanalysis found a statistically significant, limited benefit in terms of both survival and relapse-free survival. However, studies are conflicting, and a final demonstration of efficacy is lacking

- Therefore, adjuvant chemotherapy is not standard treatment in adult-type soft-tissue sarcomas, but can be considered as an option in high-risk patients (having a G >1, deep, >5-cm tumor) (II, C)

- Adjuvant chemotherapy is not used in histologies known to be insensitive to chemotherapy

- If the decision is made to use chemotherapy as upfront treatment, it may well be used preoperatively, at least in part

- If used, adjuvant chemotherapy should consist of the combination chemotherapy regimens proven to be most active in advanced disease

- A local benefit may be gained, facilitating surgery. In one large randomized phase III study (patients with G2–3, deep, >5-cm soft-tissue sarcomas), regional hyperthermia + systemic chemotherapy was associated with a local and disease-free survival advantage (no survival benefit demonstrated)

Follow-up

- There are no published data to indicate the optimal routine follow-up policy of surgically treated patients with localized disease

- Malignancy grade affects the likelihood and speed at which relapses may take place. Risk assessment is based on:

  - Tumor grade

  - Tumor size

  - Tumor site

- High-risk patients generally relapse within 2–3 years

- Low-risk patients may relapse later, although it is less likely

- Relapses most often occur to the lungs

- Early detection of local or metastatic recurrence to the lungs may have prognostic implications. Lung metastases typically are asymptomatic at a stage in which they are suitable for surgery

(continued)

Expert Opinion (*continued*)	5-Year Survival

Extensive Disease

General guidelines:

- Metachronous resectable lung metastases without extrapulmonary disease are managed with complete excision of all lesions as standard treatment (IV, B). There is a lack of formal evidence that chemotherapy improves results

- Chemotherapy is preferably given before surgery, in order to assess tumor response and thus modulate the length of treatment

- In the case of lung metastases being synchronous, in the absence of extrapulmonary disease, standard treatment is chemotherapy (IV, B). Especially when patient benefit is achieved, surgery of lung metastases is an option

- Extrapulmonary disease is treated with chemotherapy as standard treatment (I, A)

- In highly selected cases, surgery of responding metastases may be offered as an option following a multidisciplinary evaluation

Chemotherapy:

- Standard chemotherapy is based on **anthracyclines** as first-line treatment (I, A)

- No formal demonstration multiagent chemotherapy is superior to single-agent chemotherapy with doxorubicin alone in terms of overall survival. However, a higher response rate may be expected in a number of sensitive histologic types according to several, although not all, randomized clinical trials

- Multiagent chemotherapy with **anthracyclines plus ifosfamide** may be the treatment of choice, especially when a tumor response is felt to give an advantage and patient performance status is good

- In angiosarcoma, **taxanes** are an alternative option (III, B)

- **Imatinib** is standard medical therapy for rare patients with dermatofibrosarcoma protuberans whose disease is not amenable to nonmutilating surgery or with metastases requiring medical therapy (III, B)

- After failure of **anthracycline-based chemotherapy** or if an anthracycline cannot be used, the following criteria may apply (although it lacks high-level evidence):

  - Patients who have already received chemotherapy may be treated with **ifosfamide**, if they did not receive it previously

  - **High-dose ifosfamide** (≈ 14 g/m^2) may be an option for patients who have already received standard-dose ifosfamide (IV, C)

  - **Trabectedin** is a second-line option (II, B). It has proved effective in leiomyosarcoma and liposarcoma. Responses have also been observed in synovial sarcoma and other histotypes; however, it is not currently approved for use in the USA outside the context of a clinical trial

  - Single agent **gemcitabine** was also shown to have antitumor activity in leiomyosarcoma as a single agent

  - **Dacarbazine** has some activity as second-line therapy (mostly in leiomyosarcoma). It could also be combined **with gemcitabine**. One randomized trial has demonstrated a survival advantage with the combination of gemcitabine and dacarbazine (DTIC) over DTIC alone

  - **Best supportive care** is an option for pretreated patients with advanced soft-tissue sarcoma, particularly when secondary and later treatment options have already been used

- *Pretreated patients with advanced disease are candidates for clinical studies*

5-Year Survival

Nonmetastatic (80% of Patients at Diagnosis)	
Stage II	70%
Stage III	25%
Metastatic (20% of Patients at Diagnosis)	20%

SOFT-TISSUE SARCOMAS: RHABDOMYOSARCOMA

Epidemiology

Incidence: 350 estimated new cases in the United States per year; rhabdomyosarcoma represents 50% of all diagnosed soft-tissue sarcomas

Staging

For protocol purposes, patients are classified according to their risk of recurrence as low risk, intermediate risk, or high risk. The assignment proceeds as follows:
1. Determine the group (I, II, III, or IV)
2. Determine the stage (1, 2, 3, or 4)
3. Use the group and stage assignment together with histology to assign a risk category

Group classification system: A surgicopathologic grouping system with groups defined by the extent of disease and by the extent of initial surgical resection after pathologic review of the tumor specimens
Staging classification system: Classifies tumors based on primary site and size
Risk classification system: Used to assess the risk of recurrence as low, intermediate, and high risk; combines the clinical group and stage information

Group Classification System

Group	Extent of Disease and Initial Surgical Resection After Pathologic Review of Specimen	%*
I	Localized disease that is completely resected with no regional nodal involvement	14
IIA	Localized, grossly resected tumor with microscopic residual disease but no regional node involvement	20
IIB	Locoregional disease with tumor-involved lymph nodes with complete resection and no residual disease	
IIC	Locoregional disease with tumor-involved lymph nodes, grossly resected, but with evidence of microscopic residual tumor at the primary site and/or histologic involvement of the regional node (from the primary site)	
III	Localized, gross residual disease including incomplete resection or biopsy of the primary site	48
IV	Distant metastatic disease present at the time of diagnosis	18

*Percentage of all rhabdomyosarcomas

Staging Classification System

Stage	Description
1	Localized disease involving the orbit or head and neck (excluding parameningeal sites) or genitourinary region (excluding bladder/prostate sites) or biliary tract **(favorable sites)**
2	Localized disease of any other primary site not included in Stage 1 **(unfavorable sites)**. Primary tumor must be ≤5 cm in diameter with no clinical regional lymph node involvement by tumor
3	Localized disease of any other primary site not included in Stage 1 **(unfavorable sites)**. These patients differ from Stage 2 patients by having primary tumors >5 cm in diameter and/or regional node involvement
4	Metastatic disease at diagnosis

Lawrence W Jr et al. J Clin Oncol 1987;5:46–54

(continued)

Pathology

Embryonal Embryonal Botryoid* Spindle*	60–70%	Higher incidence in the 0–4 years age group
Alveolar	20%	Similar incidence throughout childhood
Pleomorphic	10–20%	

*These subtypes are associated with more favorable outcomes

Disease Sites at Diagnosis

Site	%
Parameningeal*	23
Nonparameningeal	8
Bladder and prostate	11
Non–bladder and prostate†	16
Limbs	16
Orbit	9
Other	17

*Sites in anatomic proximity to the base of the skull and adjacent meninges; eg, nasopharynx and middle ear
†Genitourinary other than bladder and prostate that include paratesticular, vagina, and uterus

Stevens MCG. Lancet Oncol 2005;6:77–84

5-Year Survival

Low risk	>90%
Intermediate risk	55–70%
High risk	20–25%

Staging (continued)

Risk Classification System

Risk	Histology	Stage	Group
Low	All	1	I, II, III
	Embryonal	2, 3	I, II
Intermediate	Embryonal	2, 3	III
	Embryonal*	4	IV
	Alveolar	1, 2, 3	I, II, III
	Undifferentiated	1, 2, 3	I, II, III
High	All†	4	IV
	Undifferentiated	4	IV

*Age <10 years
†Exception: Embryonal in children <10 years of age

Raney RB et al. J Pediatr Hematol Oncol 2001;23:215–220

Expert Opinion

1. Disease prognosis is related to the age of the adolescent, site of origin, resectability, presence of metastases, number of metastatic sites, and the unique biologic characteristics of the rhabdomyosarcoma tumor cells[1,2]

2. Distinctive molecular characteristics can be used to confirm alveolar and embryonal subtypes:

   Alveolar rhabdomyosarcoma: Unique translocation between the *FKHR* gene on chromosome 13 and either the *PAX3* gene on chromosome 2 (59% cases) or the *PAX7* gene on chromosome 1 (19% cases)
   Embryonal tumors: Often show loss of specific genomic material from the short arm of chromosome 11. The consistent loss of genomic material from the chromosome 11p15 region in embryonal tumors suggests the presence of a tumor suppressor gene. No such gene has yet been identified[3]

3. The variability with which rhabdomyosarcoma presents at different anatomic sites has a strong effect on treatment strategies

Barr FG. J Pediatr Hematol Oncol 1997;19:483–491
Breneman JC et al. J Clin Oncol 2003;21:78–84
Breneman J et al. [abstract 210] Int J Radiat Oncol Biol Phys 2001;51(3 Suppl 1):118

REGIMEN

VINCRISTINE + DACTINOMYCIN + CYCLOPHOSPHAMIDE (VAC)

Crist WM et al. J Clin Oncol 2001;19:3091–3102

Treatment Schedule

Drugs	Induction (Weeks 0–16)																
	0	1	2	3	4	5	6	7	8	9	10	11	12	13	14	15	16
Vincristine (V)	V	V	V	V	V	V	V	V	V	V	V	V	V				V
Dactinomycin (A)	A			A			A										A
Cyclophosphamide (C)	C			C			C			C			C				C
										Radiation therapy							

Drugs	Continuation (Weeks 20–28)											
	17	18	19	20	21	22	23	24	25	26	27	28
Vincristine (V)				V	V	V	V	V	V			
Dactinomycin (A)				A			A					
Cyclophosphamide (C)				C			C					

Vincristine 1.5 mg/m² per dose (maximum single dose = 2 mg); administer by intravenous injection over 1–2 minutes on day 1 (total dosage during the weeks in which vincristine is administered = 1.5 mg/m²; maximum dose/treatment = 2 mg)

Dactinomycin 0.015 mg/kg per day (maximum single dose = 0.5 mg); administer by intravenous injection over 1–2 minutes for 5 consecutive days, on days 1–5 (total dosage during the weeks in which dactinomycin is administered = 0.075 mg/kg; maximum dose/cycle = 2.5 mg)

An admixture containing **cyclophosphamide** 2200 mg/m² + **mesna** 120 mg/m²; administer intravenously in 100–1000 mL 0.9% sodium chloride injection (0.9% NS) or 5% dextrose injection (D5W) over 10–30 minutes, on day 1 (total dosage during the weeks in which cyclophosphamide is administered = 2200 mg/m²), *followed by*

Mesna 1200 mg/m²; administer intravenously in 250–1000 mL of 0.9% NS or D5W over 24 hours (rate of 50 mg/m² per hour), starting immediately after each dose of cyclophosphamide (total dosage during the weeks in which cyclophosphamide is administered = 1320 mg/m²; includes 120 mg administered with cyclophosphamide)

• The administration schedules for vincristine, dactinomycin, and cyclophosphamide appears in the table (above)

Supportive Care: Antiemetic prophylaxis
*Emetogenic potential during weeks with vincristine, dactinomycin, and cyclophosphamide is **HIGH**. Potential for delayed symptoms*
*Emetogenic potential on days with vincristine and cyclophosphamide is **HIGH***
*Emetogenic potential on days with vincristine alone is **MINIMAL***
See Chapter 39 for antiemetic recommendations

Hematopoietic growth factor (CSF) prophylaxis
Primary prophylaxis is indicated with:
  Filgrastim (G-CSF) 5 mcg/kg per day by subcutaneous injection
  • Begin use from 24 hours after myelosuppressive chemotherapy is completed; that is, day 6 during VAC cycles and day 2 during vincristine and cyclophosphamide (VC) cycles
  • Filgrastim may be given on days when vincristine is administered alone
  • Continue daily filgrastim use until ANC ≥15,000/mm³
  • Discontinue daily filgrastim use at least 24 hours before administering resuming myelosuppressive treatment (containing dactinomycin or cyclophosphamide)
See Chapter 43 for more information

Antimicrobial prophylaxis
Risk of fever and neutropenia is HIGH
  Antimicrobial primary prophylaxis is recommended:
  • Antibacterial—consider fluoroquinolone prophylaxis; *P. jirovecii* prophylaxis is recommended (eg, cotrimoxazole)
  • Antifungal—recommended
  • Antiviral—antiherpes antivirals (eg, acyclovir, famciclovir, valacyclovir)
See Chapter 47 for more information

Treatment Modifications

Percentage of Courses in Which ≥75% of Protocol-Specified Drugs Were Delivered

Vincristine	81%
Dactinomycin	81%
Cyclophosphamide	86%

Patients with severe toxicity attributed to VAC (eg, venoocclusive disease of the liver) were switched to VIE (vincristine, ifosfamide and etoposide) therapy

Toxicity* (N = 884†)

	% of Patients
Myelosuppression	>90
Severe infections	55
Severe renal toxicity	2
Second cancer‡	1.1
Death§	0.9

*National Cancer Institute (USA) Common Toxicity Criteria, version 2.0
†Combined data for patients receiving either VA (vincristine + dactinomycin, n = 134) ,VAC (n = 291), VAI (vincristine + dactinomycin + ifosfamide, n = 223), or VIE (vincristine, ifosfamide, and etoposide, n = 236). There were no statistically significant differences in toxicities among the different regimens
‡Among 10 patients who developed a secondary malignancy, 6 were treated with VAC; 3-year estimated cumulative incidence of secondary malignancy was 2%
§Fatality rate (5%) was highest in patients with preexisting renal abnormalities who were treated with VAC

Patient Population Studied

A study of 884 patients with previously untreated nonmetastatic rhabdomyosarcoma who had undergone surgery. Randomization to 1 of 4 study arms: VA (vincristine + dactinomycin, n = 134), VAC (n = 291), VAI (vincristine + dactinomycin + ifosfamide, n = 223), and VIE (vincristine, ifosfamide, and etoposide, n = 236). Patients with preexisting renal abnormalities predisposing to nephrotoxicity were assigned to VAC

Therapy Monitoring

1. *Daily during therapy:* Urinalysis
2. *Twice per week:* CBC with differential until recovery from hematopoietic toxicity
3. *Weekly:* Physical examination
4. *Before each cycle:* Serum creatinine, LFTs with bilirubin, serum electrolytes, including calcium, magnesium, and phosphorus
5. *Response evaluation:* After the third, sixth, and eighth cycles

Efficacy (N = 134)

	Failure-Free Survival (3-Year)	Overall Survival (3-Year)
Patients with preexisting renal abnormalities (n = 56)	75%*	80%*
All VAC patients (n = 134)	75%	84%

*Estimated

REGIMEN

IRINOTECAN

Cosetti M et al. J Pediatr Hematol Oncol 2002;24:101–105

Irinotecan 20 mg/m² per dose; administer intravenously in a volume of 5% dextrose injection (preferred) or 0.9% sodium chloride injection sufficient to produce a concentration within a range of 0.12–2.8 mg/mL over 60 minutes for 10 doses, on days 1–5 and days 8–12, every 21–28 days (total dosage/cycle = 200 mg/m²)

Supportive Care
Antiemetic prophylaxis
Emetogenic potential is **MODERATE**
See Chapter 39 for antiemetic recommendations

Hematopoietic growth factor (CSF) prophylaxis
Primary prophylaxis may be indicated
See Chapter 43 for more information

Antimicrobial prophylaxis
Risk of fever and neutropenia is LOW
  Antimicrobial primary prophylaxis to be considered:
- Antibacterial—not indicated
- Antifungal—not indicated
- Antiviral—not indicated unless patient previously had an episode of HSV

See Chapter 47 for more information

Acute cholinergic syndrome
Atropine sulfate 0.25–1 mg subcutaneously or intravenously if abdominal cramping or diarrhea develop during or within 1 hour after irinotecan administration
- If symptoms are severe, add as primary prophylaxis at least 30 minutes before irinotecan during subsequent cycles
- For irinotecan, acute cholinergic syndrome may be characterized by abdominal cramping, diarrhea, diaphoresis, hypotension, flushing, bradycardia, rhinitis, increased salivation, meiosis, and lacrimation

Diarrhea management
Latent or delayed onset diarrhea*:
  Loperamide 4 mg orally initially after the first loose or liquid stool, *then*
  Loperamide 2 mg orally every 2 hours during waking hours, *plus*
  Loperamide 4 mg orally every 4 hours during hours of sleep
- Continue for at least 12 hours after diarrhea resolves
- Recurrent diarrhea after a 12-hour diarrhea-free interval is treated as a new episode
- Rehydrate orally with fluids and electrolytes during a diarrheal episode
- If a patient develops blood or mucus in stool, dehydration, or hemodynamic instability, or if diarrhea persists >48 hours despite loperamide, stop loperamide and hospitalize the patient for IV hydration

Alternatively, a trial of **Diphenoxylate hydrochloride** 2.5 mg **with Atropine sulfate** 0.025 mg (eg, Lomotil)
- Initial adult dose is 2 tablets 4 times daily until control has been achieved, after which the dose may be reduced to meet individual requirements. Control may often be maintained with as little as 2 tablets daily
- Clinical improvement of acute diarrhea is usually observed within 48 hours. If improvement of chronic diarrhea after treatment with a maximum daily dose of 8 tablets is not observed within 10 days, control is unlikely with further administration

Persistent diarrhea:
  Octreotide 100–150 mcg subcutaneously 3 times daily. Maximum total daily dose is 1500 mcg

Antibiotic therapy during latent or delayed onset diarrhea:
  A fluoroquinolone (eg, **Ciprofloxacin** 500 mg orally every 12 hours) if absolute neutrophil count <500/mm³ with or without accompanying fever in association with diarrhea
- Antibiotics should also be administered if patient is hospitalized with prolonged diarrhea and should be continued until diarrhea resolves

*Abigerges D et al. J Natl Cancer Inst 1994;86:446–449
Rothenberg ML et al. J Clin Oncol 2001;19:3801–3807
Wadler S et al. J Clin Oncol 1998;16:3169–3178

Patient Population Studied

A study of 22 heavily pretreated children with multiply relapsed tumors. Four patients with rhabdomyosarcoma; the rest had other diagnoses, but clinically very similar

Efficacy (N = 4)

Complete response	50%
Partial response	25%

Four patients with rhabdomyosarcoma; the rest had other diagnoses, but clinically very similar

Toxicity* (N = 22)

	% G1	% G2	% G3	% G4
Hematologic				
Anemia	9.1	13.6	0	0
Leukopenia	18.2	22.7	18.2	0
Neutropenia	4.5	13.6	9.1	18.2
Thrombocytopenia	18.2	9.1	13.6	13.6
Nonhematologic				
SGOT	13.6	0	0	0
SGPT	4.5	4.5	0	0
Diarrhea	40.9	13.6	13.6	4.5
Pneumonitis/pulmonary infiltrates				4.5

SGOT, serum glutamic oxaloacetic transaminase (AST); SGPT, serum glutamic pyruvic transaminase (ALT)
*National Cancer Institute (USA) Common Toxicity Criteria, version 2.0

Treatment Modifications

None specified; the following are suggested

Adverse Event	Dose Modification
WBC <4000/mm³, platelet count <100,000/mm³, or diarrhea	Delay start of cycle by 1 week until WBC >4000/mm³, platelet count >100,000/mm³, and no diarrhea
Day 8 or 15 WBC <3000/mm³ or platelet count <100,000/mm³	Hold irinotecan
G >1 diarrhea	Hold irinotecan
If WBC <1000/mm³, platelet count <50,000/mm³, or diarrhea G >2 at any time in cycle	Reduce subsequent irinotecan dosage by 50%

Therapy Monitoring

1. *Weekly:* CBC with differential
2. *Before each cycle:* CBC with differential, LFTs with bilirubin
3. *Response evaluation:* After every 2 cycles

INTERMEDIATE RISK RHABDOMYOSARCOMA

VINCRISTINE, DOXORUBICIN, CYCLOPHOSPHAMIDE, AND ETOPOSIDE/IFOSFAMIDE (VDC/IE)

Arndt CAS et al. Eur J Cancer 1998;34:1224–1229
Arndt CAS et al. Pediatr Blood Cancer 2008;50:33–36

Schema for Chemotherapy Administration

Induction

Weeks	0	1	2	3	6	7	8	9	12*
	V	V	V	E	V	V	V	E	Evaluation
	D			I	D			I	
	C				C				

Consolidation

Weeks	12	15	18	21‡
	V	E	V	Evaluation
	D	I	D†	
	C		C	

Maintenance

Weeks	21	24	27	30	33	36§	39
	E	V	E	V	E	VDC or EI	E
	I	D†	I	D	I		I
		C		C			

V, Vincristine 1.5 mg/m² (maximum dose = 2 mg); D, doxorubicin 37.5 mg/m² per day for 2 days; C, cyclophosphamide 600 mg/m² per day for 2 days with mesna 360 mg/m² for 5 doses; E, etoposide 100 mg/m² per day for 5 days; I, ifosfamide 1800 mg/m² per day for 5 days with mesna 360 mg/m² for 5 doses per day
*If primary RT is given, it is given at week 12. Primary surgery also occurs at week 12
†Doxorubicin omitted if radiation therapy (RT) being given concomitantly
‡If surgery follows primary RT, surgery is performed here. If RT follows surgery, RT begins here
§VDC given if D previously omitted at week 18 or 24, otherwise EI given

VINCRISTINE + DOXORUBICIN + CYCLOPHOSPHAMIDE (VDC)

Vincristine 1.5 mg/m² (maximum dose 2 mg); administer by intravenous injection over 1–2 minutes on day 1, during weeks 0, 1, 2, 6, 7, 8, 12, 18, 24, 30, and 36 (week 36, if VDC is given) (total dosage/week = 1.5 mg/m²; maximum dose/week = 2 mg)

Doxorubicin 37.5 mg/m² per day; administer by intravenous infusion in 25–1000 mL 0.9% sodium chloride injection (0.9% NS) or 5% dextrose injection (D5W) over 18 hours for 2 consecutive days, on days 1 and 2, during weeks 0, 6, 12, 18, 24, 30, and 36 (if VDC is given) (total dosage/week = 75 mg/m²)

An admixture of **cyclophosphamide** 600 mg/m² plus **mesna** 360 mg/m² per dose; administer by intravenous infusion, in a volume of 0.9% NS or D5W sufficient to produce a mesna concentration within the range of 1–20 mg/mL, over 15–60 minutes for 2 consecutive days, on days 1 and 2, during weeks 0, 6, 12, 18, 24, 30, and 36 (week 36, if VDC is given) (total cyclophosphamide dosage/week = 1200 mg/m²), *followed each day by:*

Mesna 360 mg/m² per dose; administer by intravenous infusion, in a volume of 0.9% NS or D5W sufficient to produce a mesna concentration within the range of 1–20 mg/mL, over 15–60 minutes every 3 hours for 4 doses per day, starting 3 hours after commencing administration of cyclophosphamide + mesna (a total of 5 mesna doses/day), for 2 consecutive days, days 1 and 2, during weeks 0, 6, 12, 18, 24, 30, and 36 (if VDC is given) (total dosage/week = 3600 mg/m²; includes 360 mg doses given with cyclophosphamide)

(continued)

Dose Modifications

Adverse Event	Treatment Modification
G1 ANC 1500–1999/mm³, or G1 thrombocytopenia during a cycle	Maintain dosages and schedules. Administer filgrastim if not previously administered
Day 21 ANC <1000/mm³, or platelet count <75,000/mm³	Delay start of next cycle by 1 week. Reduce dosages in ensuing cycle or administer filgrastim if not previously administered
Day 28 ANC still <1000/mm³, or platelet count still <75,000/mm³	Delay start of next cycle by 1 additional week. Reduce dosages in ensuing cycle or administer filgrastim if not previously administered
Day 35 ANC still <1000/mm³, or platelet count still <75,000/mm³	Discontinue therapy
Postradiation mucositis	Reduce doxorubicin dosage
Decrease of cardiac ejection fraction from baseline	Reduce doxorubicin dosage
G2 neurotoxicity	Reduce vincristine dosage 50%
Foot drop	Reduce vincristine dosage 50%
G3/4 neurotoxicity	Discontinue vincristine
Any G1 nonhematologic toxicity	Maintain doses and schedules
Any G2/3 nonhematologic toxicity	Hold treatment until toxicity resolves to G ≤1, then reduce dosage of drug(s) felt responsible for the toxicity in subsequent cycles by 25%
Any G4 toxicity	Hold treatment until toxicity resolves to G ≤1, then reduce dosage of drug(s) felt responsible for the toxicity in subsequent cycles by 50%

(*continued*)

IFOSFAMIDE + ETOPOSIDE (IE)

An admixture of **ifosfamide** 1800 mg/m² plus **mesna** 360 mg/m² per dose; administer by intravenous infusion, in a volume of 0.9% NS or D5W sufficient to produce an ifosfamide concentration within the range of 0.6–20 mg/mL, and a mesna concentration within the range of 1–20 mg/mL over 15–60 minutes for 5 consecutive days, on days 1–5, during weeks 3, 9, 15, 21, 27, 33, 36 (week 36, if EI is given instead of VDC), and 39 (total ifosfamide dosage/week = 9000 mg/m²), *followed each day by:*

Mesna 360 mg/m² per dose; administer by intravenous infusion, in a volume of 0.9% NS or D5W sufficient to produce a mesna concentration within the range of 1–20 mg/mL, over 15–60 minutes, every 3 hours, for 4 doses per day, starting 3 hours after commencing administration of ifosfamide + mesna (a total of 5 mesna doses/day), for 5 consecutive days, on days 1–5, during weeks 3, 9, 15, 21, 27, 33, 36 (week 36, if EI is given instead of VDC), and 39 (total dosage/week = 9000 mg/m²; includes 360 mg doses given with cyclophosphamide)

Etoposide 100 mg/m² per day; administer intravenously, diluted in 0.9% NS to a concentration within the range of 0.2–0.4 mg/mL, over 60 minutes for 5 consecutive days, on days 1–5, during weeks 3, 9, 15, 21, 27, 33, 36 (week 36, if EI is given instead of VDC), and 39 (total dosage/week = 500 mg/m²)

Notes:
- Patients with positive cerebrospinal fluid cytology: Administer triple **intrathecal** chemotherapy with **methotrexate, cytarabine, and hydrocortisone**

CNS treatment (confirmed CNS disease)—possible regimen*:
Methotrexate 6 mg per dose +
Cytarabine 30 mg per dose +
Hydrocortisone 15 mg per dose

Induction: All 3 drugs are given together, twice weekly for at least 4 consecutive weeks, or for 2 weeks after CSF specimens are without evidence of lymphoma, whichever is greater

Administer intrathecally in a volume of **preservative-free** 0.9% NS equivalent to the amount of CSF removed via lumbar puncture, intraventricular catheter or reservoir. Total doses/week:

- **Methotrexate** = 12 mg
- **Cytarabine** = 60 mg
- **Hydrocortisone** = 30 mg

Consolidation: All 3 drugs are given together, once weekly for 6 weeks. Administer intrathecally in a volume of **preservative-free** 0.9% NS equivalent to the amount of CSF removed via intraventricular catheter or reservoir. Total doses/week:

- **Methotrexate** = 6 mg
- **Cytarabine** = 30 mg
- **Hydrocortisone** = 15 mg

Maintenance: All 3 drugs are given together, once monthly for 6 months. Administer intrathecally in a volume of preservative-free 0.9% NS equivalent to the amount of CSF removed. Total doses/month:

- **Methotrexate** = 6 mg
- **Cytarabine** = 30 mg
- **Hydrocortisone** = 15 mg

*Note: Monotherapy with methotrexate or cytarabine may be feasible in patients with sensitive disease

(*continued*)

Patient Population Studied

Patients with intermediate risk rhabdomyosarcoma defined as having Stage 2 or 3 (unfavorable site) Group III disease, or any nonmetastatic alveolar disease. Patients with metastatic disease were not eligible for the pilot study

Efficacy (N = 46)

Arndt CAS et al. Pediatr Blood Cancer 2008;50:33–36

Patients with parameningeal primaries

5-year FFS*	82% (95% CI, 59%–93%)
5-year overall survival	82% (95% CI, 59%–93%)

Patients with nonparameningeal primaries

Estimated 5-year FFS*	75%
Estimated 5-year FFS* for Stage 2 (n = 8)	63%
Estimated 5-year FFS* for Stage 3 (n = 12)	83%

*Failure-free survival (FFS) is defined as the time to the first occurrence of recurrence of rhabdomyosarcoma or death as a first event

(continued)

- Perform echocardiograms to monitor cardiac function at baseline and prior to weeks 12, 24, 30, at the end of therapy, 1 year after completion of therapy, and then, every 2 ± 5 years, depending on the result
- After week 12 (following 4 cycles of chemotherapy), patients undergo therapy for local control of the tumor. Either surgery or irradiation is used for local control. Patients receiving irradiation as primary local therapy should begin treatment at week 12, as soon as possible after completing doxorubicin. (*Example:* 5040 cGy in 28 fractions to the tumor followed by a boost of an additional 540 cGy in 3 fractions to the tumor plus a 2-cm margin.) If the patient undergoes surgery, postoperative irradiation is given for patients with gross or microscopic residual disease, or if the surgical margin is ≤1 cm. Postoperative irradiation then begins at week 21. (*Example:* Tumor bed plus a 3-cm margin for the initial 5040 cGy in 28 fractions, followed by a boost of an additional 540 cGy in three fractions to the tumor bed with a 2-cm margin.) Doxorubicin is not given during radiation therapy

Supportive Care

Antiemetic prophylaxis for the vincristine + doxorubicin + cyclophosphamide regimen
Emetogenic potential on days 1 and 2 is **HIGH**. *Potential for delayed symptoms*

Antiemetic prophylaxis for the ifosfamide + etoposide regimen
Emetogenic potential is **MODERATE–HIGH**
See Chapter 39 for antiemetic recommendations

Hematopoietic growth factor (CSF) prophylaxis
Primary prophylaxis is indicated with the following:

Filgrastim (G-CSF) 5 mcg/kg per day by subcutaneous injection
- Begin use 24 hours after myelosuppressive chemotherapy is completed
- Discontinue filgrastim use at least 24 hours before administering myelosuppressive treatment
- Do not give filgrastim during radiation therapy

See Chapter 43 for more information

Antimicrobial prophylaxis
Risk of fever and neutropenia is INTERMEDIATE
Antimicrobial primary prophylaxis to be considered:
- Antibacterial—consider a fluoroquinolone or no prophylaxis; *P. jirovecii* prophylaxis is recommended (eg, cotrimoxazole)
- Antifungal—consider concomitant use of clotrimazole during periods of neutropenia, and in anticipation of mucositis
- Antiviral—antiherpes antivirals (eg, acyclovir, famciclovir, valacyclovir)

See Chapter 47 for more information

Oral care
Prophylaxis and treatment for mucositis/stomatitis
General advice:
- Encourage patients to maintain intake of non-alcoholic fluids
- Evaluate patients for oral pain and provide analgesic medications
- Consider histamine (H_2-subtype) receptor antagonists (eg, ranitidine, famotidine), or a proton pump inhibitor for epigastric pain
- *Lactobacillus* sp.-containing probiotics may be beneficial in preventing diarrhea

Patients with intact oral mucosa:
- Clean the mouth, tongue, and gums by brushing after every meal and at bedtime with an ultra-soft toothbrush with fluoride toothpaste
- Floss teeth gently every day unless contraindicated. If gums bleed and hurt, avoid bleeding or sore areas, but floss other teeth
- Patients may use saline or commercial bland, non-alcoholic rinses
  - Do not use mouthwashes that contain alcohols

(continued)

Toxicity (Feasibility)

Arndt CAS et al. Eur J Cancer 1998;34:1224–1229

VDC cycles delivered at full dose	169/191 (88%)
EI cycles delivered at full dose	196/212 (92%)

Reasons for reductions in doxorubicin dose

Postradiation mucositis (all during maintenance)	10 cycles
Decrease of cardiac ejection fraction from baseline	2 cycles (1 patient)*
Decrease in doxorubicin and cyclophosphamide dosage (all during maintenance) as a result of delay in recovery of the neutrophil and platelet count	6 cycles
Vincristine dosage decreased because of foot drop	4 cycles (1 patient)

Reasons for decrease in etoposide and ifosfamide

Delay in recovery of neutrophil and platelet count	13 maintenance cycles
Mucositis	2 maintenance cycles
EI cycles omitted because of prolonged cytopenias	3 patients

Mean duration of induction chemotherapy (start of treatment to start of week 12; scheduled time = 84 days)

Patients without surgery prior to week 12	97 days (range: 82 ± 144)
Patients with surgery following first 4 cycles of chemotherapy (recovery from week 9)	106 days (range: 84 ± 126)
Mean duration of consolidation therapy (start of week 12 to start of week 21 therapy; scheduled time = 63 days)	80 days (range: 61 ± 154)
Mean duration of maintenance therapy (scheduled time = 144 days)	168 days (range: 90 ± 215)

*Although cardiac function still in the normal range

(continued)

(continued)

If mucositis or stomatitis is present:

- Keep the mouth moist utilizing water, ice chips, sugarless gum, sugar-free hard candies, or a saliva substitute
- Rinse mouth several times a day to remove debris
  - Use a solution of ¼ teaspoon (1.25 g) each of baking soda and table salt (sodium chloride) in one quart (~950 mL) of warm water. Follow with a plain water rinse
  - Do not use mouthwashes that contain alcohols
- Foam-tipped swabs (eg, Toothettes®) are useful in moisturizing oral mucosa, but ineffective for cleansing teeth and removing plaque
- Advise patients who develop mucositis to:
  - Choose foods that are easy to chew and swallow
  - Take small bites of food, chew slowly, and sip liquids with meals
  - Encourage soft, moist foods such as cooked cereals, mashed potatoes, and scrambled eggs
  - For trouble swallowing, soften food with gravies, sauces, broths, yogurt, or other bland liquids
  - Avoid sharp, crunchy foods; hot, spicy or highly acidic foods (eg, citrus fruits and juices); sugary foods; toothpicks; tobacco products; alcoholic drinks

Therapy Monitoring

1. *Prior to enrollment:* Complete medical history, clinical examination, performance status, hematologic and serum chemistries, and tumor target assessment
2. *Day 1 of each treatment cycle:* Physical examination, ECOG PS, complete blood count with leukocyte differential count, and serum chemistries
3. *Weekly CBC with leukocyte differential count:* At least the first 6 cycles of therapy
4. *After every 2 cycles of therapy:* Tumor measurements

REGIMEN

DOXORUBICIN

O'Bryan RM et al. Cancer 1973;32:1–8
O'Bryan RM et al. Cancer 1977;39:1940–1948

Doxorubicin 60 mg/m²; administer by intravenous injection over 3–5 minutes on day 1, every 21 days (total dosage/cycle = 60 mg/m²)

Supportive Care
Antiemetic prophylaxis
Emetogenic potential is **MODERATE**
See Chapter 39 for antiemetic recommendations

Hematopoietic growth factor (CSF) prophylaxis
Primary prophylaxis may be indicated
See Chapter 43 for more information

Antimicrobial prophylaxis
Risk of fever and neutropenia is LOW
   Antimicrobial primary prophylaxis to be considered:
   • Antibacterial—not indicated
   • Antifungal—not indicated
   • Antiviral—not indicated unless patient previously had an episode of HSV
See Chapter 47 for more information

Hand-foot reaction (palmar-plantar erythrodysesthesia)
For patients who develop a hand-foot reaction, use topical emollients (eg, Aquaphor), topical or orally administered steroids, antihistamine agents (H₁-receptor antagonists), or pyridoxine
   Pyridoxine may provide relief for discomfort/pain associated with PPE, although the mechanism through which this occurs remains unclear
• The suggested pyridoxine starting dose is 50 mg/day, which may be increased to a maximum of 200 mg/day

Oral care
Prophylaxis and treatment for mucositis/stomatitis
   General advice:
   • Encourage patients to maintain intake of non-alcoholic fluids
   • Evaluate patients for oral pain and provide analgesic medications
   • Consider histamine (H₂-subtype) receptor antagonists (eg, ranitidine, famotidine), or a proton pump inhibitor for epigastric pain
   • *Lactobacillus* sp.-containing probiotics may be beneficial in preventing diarrhea
   Patients with intact oral mucosa:
   • Clean the mouth, tongue, and gums by brushing after every meal and at bedtime with an ultra-soft toothbrush with fluoride toothpaste
   • Floss teeth gently every day unless contraindicated. If gums bleed and hurt, avoid bleeding or sore areas, but floss other teeth
   • Patients may use saline or commercial bland, non-alcoholic rinses
      ▪ Do not use mouthwashes that contain alcohols
   If mucositis or stomatitis is present:
   • Keep the mouth moist utilizing water, ice chips, sugarless gum, sugar-free hard candies, or a saliva substitute
   • Rinse mouth several times a day to remove debris
      ▪ Use a solution of ¼ teaspoon (1.25 g) each of baking soda and table salt (sodium chloride) in one quart (~950 mL) of warm water. Follow with a plain water rinse
      ▪ Do not use mouthwashes that contain alcohols
   • Foam-tipped swabs (eg, Toothettes®) are useful in moisturizing oral mucosa, but ineffective for cleansing teeth and removing plaque

(continued)

Patient Population Studied

Patients with metastatic or unresectable locoregional recurrent soft-tissue sarcoma

Efficacy (N = 64; N = 98)

	Partial Response*
All histologies (N = 64)	21 (32.8%)
Fibrosarcomas (n = 14)	2 (14.3%)
Leiomyosarcoma (n = 8)	3 (37.5%)
Hemangiosarcoma (n = 3)	2 (66.7%)
Other (n = 12)	4 (33.3%)
Rhabdomyosarcomas (n = 11)	3 (27.3%)
Osteogenic sarcoma (n = 9)	5 (55.5%)
Ewing sarcoma (n = 7)	2 (28.6%)

*Includes only patients who received 2 courses of doxorubicin

O'Bryan RM et al. Cancer 1973;32:1–8 (N = 64)

Risk Category and Dose (N = 98)*	Partial Response
Good risk; 75 mg/m² (n = 41)	15 (37%)
Good risk; 60 mg/m² (n = 10)	2 (20%)
Good risk; 45 mg/m² (n = 28)	5 (18%)
Poor risk; 50 mg/m² (n = 9)	1 (11%)
Poor risk; 25 mg/m² (n = 10)	0

*Patients were classified as "good risk" if in the opinion of the investigator they were able to tolerate 75 mg/m² for 3 doses. Poor-risk patients were expected to tolerate 50 mg/m² for 3 doses. The latter included those older than 65 years of age, those with prior radiation therapy or chemotherapy, and those with poor tolerance of myelosuppressive therapy

O'Bryan RM et al. Cancer 1977;39:1940–1948 (N = 98)

(*continued*)

- Advise patients who develop mucositis to:
  - Choose foods that are easy to chew and swallow
  - Take small bites of food, chew slowly, and sip liquids with meals
  - Encourage soft, moist foods such as cooked cereals, mashed potatoes, and scrambled eggs
  - For trouble swallowing, soften food with gravies, sauces, broths, yogurt, or other bland liquids
  - Avoid sharp, crunchy foods; hot, spicy or highly acidic foods (eg, citrus fruits and juices); sugary foods; toothpicks; tobacco products; alcoholic drinks

Treatment Modifications

Adverse Event	Dose Modification
WBC <3000/mm^3 or platelets <100,000/mm^3	Delay treatment 1 week until WBC ≥3000/mm^3 and platelets ≥100,000/mm^3
>2-Week delay in start of cycle	Reduce doxorubicin dose by 15 mg/m^2
WBC nadir <1000/mm^3 or platelet nadir <29,500/mm^3	Reduce doxorubicin dosage by 15 mg/m^2
WBC nadir 1000–1499/mm^3 or platelet nadir 30,000–49,500/mm^3	Reduce doxorubicin dosage by 30 mg/m^2
G ≥3 mucositis	Reduce doxorubicin dosage by 10–15 mg/m^2
Doxorubicin total cumulative lifetime dosage ≥400–450 mg/m^2	Obtain frequent MUGA scans to monitor cardiac function
A fall in ejection fraction (possible guidelines: resting cardiac ejection fraction decreased ≥10–15% below baseline or to <35–40%)	Discontinue therapy

Toxicity (N = 472; N = 818)

Toxicity			No. of Patients (%)
Hematologic			
WBC/mm^3	or	Platelets/mm^3	
3000–4000	or	75,000–100,000	91 (19.3)
2000–2999	or	50,000–74,500	113 (23.9)
1000–1999	or	25,000–49,500	91 (19.3)
<1000	or	<25,000	52 (11)
Nonhematologic			
Mild gastrointestinal toxicity			40 (8.5)
Moderate gastrointestinal toxicity			152 (32.2)
Severe gastrointestinal toxicity			10 (2.1)

O'Bryan RM et al. Cancer 1973;32:1–8 (N = 472)

(*continued*)

Toxicity (N = 472; N = 818) (continued)

Hematologic Toxicity			% of Patients		
Dosage (mg/m²)			75	60	45
WBC/mm³	or	Platelets/mm³			
3000–4000	or	75,000–100,000	3	13	19
2000–2999	or	50,000–74,500	28	31	6
1000–1999	or	25,000–49,500	27	23	31
<1000	or	<25,000	14	15	13

O'Bryan RM et al. Cancer 1977;39:1940–1948 (N = 818)

Congestive Heart Failure: According to Cumulative Dosage

Cumulative Dosage	No. of Patients (%)
<200 mg/m² (n = 491)	1 (0.2)
201–300 mg/m² (n = 145)	2 (1.4)
301–400 mg/m² (n = 84)	5 (5.9)
401–550 mg/m² (n = 98)	5 (5.1)
Total (N = 818)	13 (1.6)

O'Bryan RM et al. Cancer 1977;39:1940–1948 (N = 818)

General Summary of Toxicities

Myelosuppression	Dose-limiting toxicity. Leukopenia more common than thrombocytopenia or anemia; nadir usually on days 10–14 with recovery by day 21 after treatment
Nausea and vomiting	Moderate severity on the day of treatment; delayed symptoms (>24 hours after treatment) uncommon
Mucositis and diarrhea	Common, but not dose limiting
Cardiotoxicity (acute)	Incidence not related to dosage. Presents within 3 days after treatment as arrhythmias, conduction abnormalities, ECG changes, pericarditis, and/or myocarditis. Usually transient and asymptomatic
Cardiotoxicity (chronic)	Dosage-dependent dilated cardiomyopathy associated with congestive heart failure. Risk increases with increasing cumulative doses
Strong vesicant	Avoid extravasation
Skin	Hand-foot syndrome, with skin rash, swelling, erythema, pain, and desquamation. Onset at 5–6 weeks after starting treatment. Hyperpigmentation of nails, rarely skin rash, urticaria. Potential for radiation recall
Alopecia	Common, but generally reversible within 3 months after discontinuing doxorubicin
Infusion reactions	Signs and symptoms include flushing, dyspnea, facial swelling, headache, back pain, chest and/or throat tightness, and hypotension May occur with a first treatment. Symptoms resolve within several hours to a day after discontinuing doxorubicin
Urine discoloration	Red-orange discoloration usually within 1–2 days after drug administration

Therapy Monitoring

1. *During treatment cycles:* CBC with differential weekly
2. *Before each cycle after a cumulative doxorubicin dosage of 400–450 mg/m²:* Cardiac ejection fraction

Notes

1. Single-agent doxorubicin remains the standard therapy for palliation of metastatic disease
2. Although some advocate higher dosages up to 70–75 mg/m² per dose, the accumulated evidence does not convincingly support the use of these higher doses

REGIMEN

IFOSFAMIDE

van Oosterom AT et al. Eur J Cancer 2002;38:2397–2406

Hydration and mannitol diuresis:
1000 mL 5% Dextrose and 0.9% sodium chloride injection (D5W/0.9% NS); administer intravenously over 2 hours, beginning 2 hours before the start of chemotherapy
Mannitol is given to patients who have received adequate hydration. **Mannitol** 20% 200 mL; administer intravenously over 30 minutes, starting 1 hour before the start of chemotherapy. It is *essential* to continue hydration after mannitol administration

Mesna 600 mg/m^2; administer intravenously, diluted with 0.9% sodium chloride injection (0.9% NS) or 5% dextrose injection (D5W) to a concentration within the range of 1–20 mg/mL, over 15 minutes just before the start of the ifosfamide + mesna admixture (see "Note" below), *followed by:*
An admixture containing **ifosfamide** 5000 mg/m^2 + **mesna** 2500 mg/m^2; administer intravenously, diluted in a volume of D5W/0.9% NS sufficient to produce an ifosfamide concentration within the range of 0.6–20 mg/mL, over 24 hours, on day 1, every 21 days (total ifosfamide dosage/cycle = 5000 mg/m^2), *followed by:*
Mesna 1250 mg/m^2; administer intravenously in 2000 mL D5W/0.9% NS over 12 hours, on day 2 after completing ifosfamide administration, every 21 days (total mesna dosage per cycle = 4350 mg/m^2; includes mesna administered before and with ifosfamide)

or

Mesna 600 mg/m^2; administer intravenously, diluted with 0.9% NS or D5W to a concentration within the range of 1–20 mg/mL, over 15 minutes for 3 consecutive days, on days 1–3, just before the start of the ifosfamide + mesna admixture (see "Note" below), *followed by:*
An admixture containing **ifosfamide** 3000 mg/m^2 + **mesna** 1500 mg/m^2 per day; administer intravenously, diluted in a volume of D5W/0.9% NS sufficient to produce an ifosfamide concentration within the range of 0.6–20 mg/mL, over 4 hours, daily for 3 consecutive days, on days 1–3, every 21 days (total ifosfamide dosage/cycle = 9000 mg/m^2), *followed by:*
Mesna 500 mg/m^2 per dose; administer orally or intravenously diluted with 0.9% NS or D5W to a concentration within the range of 1–20 mg/mL, over 15 minutes, for 2 doses per day at 4 and 8 hours after completing ifosfamide administration, daily for 3 consecutive days, on days 1–3, every 21 days (total mesna dosage/cycle = 9300 mg/m^2; includes mesna administered before and with ifosfamide)

Note: Although the use of mesna before ifosfamide administration was reported with both regimens, ifosfamide, like cyclophosphamide, has to be metabolized to active (and toxic) metabolites *before* there is a need to protect the uroepithelium. Consequently, pretreating with mesna may be of little value

Supportive Care
Antiemetic prophylaxis
Emetogenic potential is **MODERATE** *each day of ifosfamide administration*
See Chapter 39 for antiemetic recommendations

Hematopoietic growth factor (CSF) prophylaxis
Primary prophylaxis may be indicated
See Chapter 43 for more information

Antimicrobial prophylaxis
Risk of fever and neutropenia is LOW
  Antimicrobial primary prophylaxis to be considered:
  • Antibacterial—not indicated
  • Antifungal—not indicated
  • Antiviral—not indicated unless patient previously had an episode of HSV
See Chapter 47 for more information

Patient Population Studied

A study of 182 adult patients with metastatic or unresectable locoregional recurrent soft-tissue sarcoma

Treatment Modifications

Adverse Event	Dose Modification
WHO G1 WBC or platelets	Reduce ifosfamide and mesna dosages by 10%
WHO G2 WBC or platelets	Delay start of therapy until WBC or platelets are G ≤1, then reduce ifosfamide and mesna dosages by 10%
3-Week delay in start of cycle because WBC or platelets have not increased to WHO toxicity G ≤1	Discontinue therapy
WBC nadir <500/mm^3 or platelet nadir <50,000/mm^3	Reduce ifosfamide and mesna dosages by 20%, regardless of WBC or platelet count on day 1
Resting cardiac ejection fraction <40%	Discontinue therapy

Efficacy* (N = 174)

	5000 mg/m^2	3000 mg/m^2 per day × 3 days
First-Line Therapy		
	n = 49	n = 49
Partial response	10%	24.5%
Median[†]	52 weeks	44 weeks
2-year survival	25%	25%
Second-Line Therapy		
	n = 36	n = 40
Complete response	3%	3%
Partial response	3%	5%
Median survival[†]	45 weeks	36 weeks

*WHO criteria
[†]Estimated median survival

Toxicity (N = 182)

Toxicity[*,†]	5000 mg/m²	3000 mg/m² per day × 3 days
First-Line Therapy: Hematologic		
	n = ≤48	n = ≤47
WBC G3/4	4%/15%	23%/34%
Nadir median	3050/mm³	1500/mm³
Nadir range	100–10,600/mm³	200–8900/mm³
ANC G3/4	7%/13%	12%/44%
Nadir median	1990/mm³	600/mm³
Nadir range	10–14,600/mm³	0.0–6520/mm³
Platelets G3/4	2%/2%	2%/2%
Nadir median	218,000/mm³	203,000/mm³
Nadir range	12,000–571,000/mm³	16,000–415,000/mm³
Hgb G3/4	6%/0	13%/2%
Nadir median	6.8 mmol/L (11 g/dL)	6.5 mmol/L (10.5 g/dL)
Nadir range	4.3–12.2 mmol/L (6.9–19.6 g/dL)	0.7–8.3 mmol/L (1.1–13.4 g/dL)
First-Line Therapy: Nonhematologic		
Alopecia	13%	30%
G3/G4 nausea/vomiting	10%/0	10%/0
G3/4 neurotoxicity	6%/0	11%/0
G3/4 infection	2%/2%	4%/6%
Second-Line Therapy: Hematologic		
	n = ≤37	n = ≤41
WBC G3/4	27%/5%	24%/39%
Nadir median	3200/mm³	1500/mm³
Nadir range	200–7700/mm³	0.0–10,000/mm³
ANC G3/4	19%/12%	31%/46%
Nadir median	1780/mm³	520/mm³
Nadir range	50–7810/mm³	0.0–5250/mm³
Platelets G3/4	3%/0	7%/7%
Nadir median	212,000/mm³	175,000/mm³
Nadir range	38,000–439,000/mm³	14,000–482,000/mm³

(*continued*)

Toxicity (N = 182) *(continued)*

Hgb G3/4	3%/3%	15%/5%
Nadir median	6.5 mmol/L (10.5 g/dL)	6 mmol/L (9.6 g/dL)
Nadir range	2.8–9.2 mmol/L (4.5–14.8 g/dL)	2.8–8.2 mmol/L (4.5–13.2 g/dL)

Second-Line Therapy: Nonhematologic

Alopecia	50%	65%
G3/G4 nausea/vomiting	9%/0	15%/2%
G3/4 neurotoxicity	3%/0	2%/2%
G3/4 infection	0/0	10%/0

*WHO criteria
†Worst WHO grade per patient

Therapy Monitoring

During treatment cycles: CBC with differential twice weekly

Notes

Despite differences in response rates in first-line therapy, there were no differences in survival between the 2 regimens

REGIMEN

DOXORUBICIN + IFOSFAMIDE

Le Cesne A et al. J Clin Oncol 2000;18:2676–2684

Hydration and mannitol diuresis:
1000 mL 5% Dextrose and 0.9% sodium chloride injection (D5W/0.9% NS); administer intravenously over 2 hours, starting 2 hours before the start of chemotherapy
Mannitol may be given to patients who have received adequate hydration
Mannitol 20% 200 mL; administer intravenously over 30 minutes, starting 1 hour before the start of chemotherapy. It is *essential* to continue hydration after mannitol administration

Doxorubicin 50 mg/m^2; administer by intravenous injection over 3–5 minutes, on day 1, every 21 days (total dosage/cycle = 50 mg/m^2), *followed by:*
Mesna 600 mg/m^2; administer intravenously, diluted with 0.9% sodium chloride injection (0.9% NS) or 5% dextrose injection (D5W) to a concentration within the range of 1–20 mg/mL, over 15 minutes just before the start of the ifosfamide + mesna admixture (see "Note" below), *followed by:*
An admixture containing **ifosfamide** 5000 mg/m^2 + **mesna** 2500 mg/m^2; administer intravenously, diluted in a volume of D5W/0.9% NS sufficient to produce an ifosfamide concentration within the range of 0.6–20 mg/mL, over 24 hours, on day 1, every 21 days (total ifosfamide dosage/cycle = 5000 mg/m^2), *followed by:*
Mesna 1250 mg/m^2; administer intravenously in 2000 mL D5W/0.9% NS over 12 hours, on day 2 after completing administration of the ifosfamide + mesna admixture, every 21 days (total mesna dosage/cycle = 4350 mg/m^2; includes mesna administered before and with ifosfamide)

Note: Although the use of mesna before ifosfamide administration was reported by the investigators, ifosfamide must be metabolized to active (and toxic) metabolites *before* there is a need to protect the uroepithelium. Consequently, pretreating with mesna may be of little value

Supportive Care
Antiemetic prophylaxis
Emetogenic potential is **HIGH**
See Chapter 39 for antiemetic recommendations

Hematopoietic growth factor (CSF) prophylaxis
Primary prophylaxis is indicated with 1 of the following:
  Filgrastim (G-CSF) 5 mcg/kg per day by subcutaneous injection, *or*
  Pegfilgrastim (pegylated filgrastim) 6 mg/0.6 mL by subcutaneous injection for 1 dose
- Begin use from 24–72 hours after myelosuppressive chemotherapy is completed
- Continue daily filgrastim use until ANC ≥10,000/mm^3 on 2 measurements separated temporally by ≥12 hours
- Discontinue daily filgrastim use at least 24 hours before administering myelosuppressive treatment. Do not administer pegfilgrastim within 14 days before administering myelosuppressive treatment

See Chapter 43 for more information

Antimicrobial prophylaxis
Risk of fever and neutropenia is LOW
Antimicrobial primary prophylaxis to be considered:
- Antibacterial—not indicated
- Antifungal—not indicated
- Antiviral—not indicated unless patient previously had an episode of HSV

See Chapter 47 for more information

(continued)

Patient Population Studied

A study of 294 adult patients with metastatic or unresectable locoregional recurrent soft-tissue sarcoma randomly assigned to receive ifosfamide with either standard-dose doxorubicin (50 mg/m^2; n = 147) or intensified doxorubicin (75 mg/m^2; n = 133) with sargramostim support

Treatment Modifications

Adverse Event	Dose Modification
WBC <3000/mm^3 or platelets <100,000/mm^3	Delay treatment 1 week until WBC ≥3000/mm^3 and platelets ≥100,000/mm^3
Treatment delay 3 times (3 weeks) without achieving a WBC ≥3000/mm^3 and platelets ≥100,000/mm^3	Discontinue therapy
Serum creatinine >1.7 mg/dL (>150 mmol/L) or creatinine clearance <50 mL/min (<0.83 mL/s)	Delay treatment until serum creatinine <1.7 mg/dL (<150 mmol/L) or creatinine clearance >50 mL/min (>0.83 mL/s)
Nonhematologic life-threatening toxicity	Discontinue therapy
Resting cardiac ejection fraction below 40%	Discontinue therapy

Efficacy (N = 147)

Complete response	3.4%
Partial response	17.7%
Early death from toxicity	1 patient
Median duration of response	47 weeks

(*continued*)

Hand-foot reaction (palmar-plantar erythrodysesthesia, PPE)
For patients who develop a hand-foot reaction, use topical emollients (eg, Aquaphor), topical or orally administered steroids, antihistamine agents (H$_1$-receptor antagonists), or pyridoxine
   Pyridoxine may provide relief for discomfort/pain associated with PPE, although the mechanism through which this occurs remains unclear
- The suggested pyridoxine starting dose is 50 mg/day, which may be increased to a maximum of 200 mg/day

Oral care
Prophylaxis and treatment for mucositis/stomatitis
  General advice:
- Encourage patients to maintain intake of non-alcoholic fluids
- Evaluate patients for oral pain and provide analgesic medications
- Consider histamine (H$_2$-subtype) receptor antagonists (eg, ranitidine, famotidine), or a proton pump inhibitor for epigastric pain
- *Lactobacillus* sp.-containing probiotics may be beneficial in preventing diarrhea
  Patients with intact oral mucosa:
- Clean the mouth, tongue, and gums by brushing after every meal and at bedtime with an ultra-soft toothbrush with fluoride toothpaste
- Floss teeth gently every day unless contraindicated. If gums bleed and hurt, avoid bleeding or sore areas, but floss other teeth
- Patients may use saline or commercial bland, non-alcoholic rinses
  - Do not use mouthwashes that contain alcohols
  If mucositis or stomatitis is present:
- Keep the mouth moist utilizing water, ice chips, sugarless gum, sugar-free hard candies, or a saliva substitute
- Rinse mouth several times a day to remove debris
  - Use a solution of ¼ teaspoon (1.25 g) each of baking soda and table salt (sodium chloride) in one quart (~950 mL) of warm water. Follow with a plain water rinse
  - Do not use mouthwashes that contain alcohols
- Foam-tipped swabs (eg, Toothettes®) are useful in moisturizing oral mucosa, but ineffective for cleansing teeth and removing plaque
- Advise patients who develop mucositis to:
  - Choose foods that are easy to chew and swallow
  - Take small bites of food, chew slowly, and sip liquids with meals
  - Encourage soft, moist foods such as cooked cereals, mashed potatoes, and scrambled eggs
  - For trouble swallowing, soften food with gravies, sauces, broths, yogurt, or other bland liquids
  - Avoid sharp, crunchy foods; hot, spicy or highly acidic foods (eg, citrus fruits and juices); sugary foods; toothpicks; tobacco products; alcoholic drinks

Toxicity* (N = 147)

Toxicity	% of Patients or Levels
Hematologic	
G3/4 WBC	86
G3/4 ANC	92
Median ANC nadir (all cycles)	200/mm^3
Range of ANC nadir (all cycles)	0–5500/mm^3
Infection	4.6
G3/4 platelets	8
Median platelet nadir (all cycles)	141,000/mm^3
Range of platelet nadir (all cycles)	5–323,000/mm^3
Nonhematologic	
G3/4 asthenia	4.5
G3/4 stomatitis	3.9
G3/4 vomiting	10
G2/3 myocardial insufficiency	1.3
G ≥2 diarrhea	6.5
G3/4 fever	2.6
G ≥2 flu-like syndrome	1
G ≥2 bone pain/myalgia	6

*National Cancer Institute (USA) Common Toxicity Criteria, version 2.0

Therapy Monitoring

1. *During treatment cycles:* CBC with differential twice weekly
2. *Before each cycle:* CBC with differential, serum electrolytes, BUN, and creatinine (creatinine clearance if serum creatinine >1.7 mg/dL (>150 mmol/L))
3. *Before each cycle after a cumulative doxorubicin dosage of 400–450 mg/m²:* Cardiac ejection fraction

Notes

Combination chemotherapy may produce a higher response rate than single-agent therapy, but toxicity is greater and survival advantages for the more aggressive regimens have not been reproducibly reported

METASTATIC SOFT-TISSUE SARCOMA (PATIENTS ≥10 YEARS OF AGE)

GEMCITABINE + DOCETAXEL
GEMCITABINE ALONE

Maki RG et al. J Clin Oncol 2007;25:2755–2763

Gemcitabine 900 mg/m^2 per dose; administer intravenously, diluted in 0.9% sodium chloride injection (0.9% NS) to a concentration as low as 0.1 mg/mL, over 90 minutes for 2 doses, on days 1 and 8, every 21 days (total dosage/cycle = 1800 mg/m^2)

Premedication for docetaxel:
Dexamethasone 8 mg/dose; administer orally twice daily for 3 days, starting 1 day before docetaxel administration (total dose/cycle = 48 mg)
Optional premedication for docetaxel:
• **Diphenhydramine HCl** 25 mg; administer orally 30–60 minutes *or* intravenously 5–30 minutes prior to docetaxel administration

• **Ranitidine** 150 mg; administer orally 30–60 minutes prior to docetaxel administration, *or*

• **Ranitidine** 50 mg; administer intravenously 5–30 minutes prior to docetaxel administration

Docetaxel 100 mg/m^2; administer intravenously, in a volume of 0.9% NS or 5% dextrose injection (D5W) sufficient to produce a docetaxel concentration within the range 0.3–0.74 mg/mL, over 60 minutes, on day 8 after completing gemcitabine administration, every 21 days (total dosage/cycle = 100 mg/m^2)

or

Gemcitabine 1200 mg/m^2 per dose; administer intravenously, diluted in 0.9% NS to a concentration as low as 0.1 mg/mL, over 2 hours for 2 doses, on days 1 and 8, every 21 days (total dosage/cycle = 2400 mg/m^2)

Notes:
• Patients with prior pelvic irradiation should begin therapy with gemcitabine or gemcitabine and docetaxel dosages decreased by 25%

• The investigators concluded that gemcitabine + docetaxel yielded superior progression-free and overall survival in comparison with gemcitabine alone, but with increased toxicity for the combination

Supportive Care
Antiemetic prophylaxis
*Emetogenic potential is **LOW–MODERATE***
See Chapter 39 for antiemetic recommendations

Hematopoietic growth factor (CSF) prophylaxis
Primary prophylaxis is indicated with 1 of the following:
    Filgrastim (G-CSF) 5 mcg/kg per day by subcutaneous injection, *or*
    Pegfilgrastim (pegylated filgrastim) 6 mg/0.6 mL by subcutaneous injection for 1 dose
• Begin use on cycle day 9; that is, 24 hours after myelosuppressive chemotherapy is completed

• Continue daily filgrastim use until ANC ≥10,000/mm^3 on 2 measurements separated temporally by ≥12 hours

• Discontinue daily filgrastim use at least 24 hours before administering myelosuppressive treatment. Do not administer pegfilgrastim within 14 days before administering myelosuppressive treatment

See Chapter 43 for more information

Antimicrobial prophylaxis
Risk of fever and neutropenia is LOW
Antimicrobial primary prophylaxis to be considered:
• Antibacterial—not indicated

• Antifungal—not indicated

• Antiviral—not indicated unless patient previously had an episode of HSV

See Chapter 47 for more information

Patient Population Studied

Patients with a diagnosis of recurrent or progressive soft-tissue sarcoma (excluding GI stromal tumor and Kaposi sarcoma); age >10 years; zero to 3 prior chemotherapy regimens; ECOG PS ≤2; peripheral neuropathy grade ≤1 by National Cancer Institute (USA) Common Terminology Criteria for Adverse Events, version 3.0

Efficacy (N = 73)

Outcome	Percent of Patients (Number of Patients)	
	Gemcitabine + Docetaxel	Gemcitabine Alone
Complete response	3% (2)	0
Partial response	14% (10)	8% (4)
SD ≥24 weeks	15% (11)	18% (9)
SD <24 weeks	38% (28)	35% (17)
Disease progression	25% (18)	37% (18)
Not assessable	4% (3)	2% (1)
Median progression-free survival	6.2 months	3 months
Median overall survival	17.9 months	11.5 months

Treatment Modifications

Adverse Event	Dose Modification
Febrile neutropenia or platelet count of <25,000/mm³ lasting more than 5 days	Reduce gemcitabine and docetaxel dosages by 25% in all subsequent cycles
ANC <1000/mm³ at start of next cycle	Withhold treatment until ANC ≥1000/mm³, then reduce gemcitabine and docetaxel dosages by 25%
Platelet count <100,000/mm³ at start of next cycle	Withhold treatment until platelet count ≥100,000/mm³, then reduce gemcitabine and docetaxel dosages by 25%
ANC <1000/mm³ or Platelet count <100,000/mm³ despite 2-week delay	Discontinue therapy
Day 8 ANC 500–999/mm³ or day 8 platelet count 50,000–99,000/mm³	Reduce day 8 gemcitabine and docetaxel dosages by 25%
Day 8 ANC <500/mm³ or day 8 platelet count <50,000/mm³	Do not administer day 8 gemcitabine and docetaxel
G3/4 nonhematologic toxicity other than alopecia, fatigue, malaise, and nail changes	Hold chemotherapy up to 2 weeks until toxicity resolves to G ≤1. If toxicity does not resolve to G ≤1 within 2 weeks, discontinue therapy. Resume treatment if toxicity resolves to G ≤1 within 2 weeks, but reduce gemcitabine and docetaxel dosages by 25%
G3/4 nonhematologic toxicity other than alopecia, fatigue, malaise, and nail changes despite a 25% reduction in initial gemcitabine and docetaxel dosages	Hold chemotherapy up to 2 weeks until toxicity resolves to G ≤1. If toxicity does not resolve to G ≤1 within 2 weeks, discontinue therapy. Resume treatment if toxicity resolves to G ≤1 within 2 weeks, but reduce gemcitabine and docetaxel dosages by an additional 25%
G ≥3 liver function test abnormalities	Hold chemotherapy up to 2 weeks until toxicity resolves to G ≤1. If toxicity does not resolve to G ≤1 within 2 weeks, discontinue therapy. Resume treatment if toxicity resolves to G ≤1 within 2 weeks, but reduce gemcitabine and docetaxel dosages by 25%
G ≥3 liver function test abnormalities despite a 25% reduction in initial gemcitabine and docetaxel dosages	Hold chemotherapy up to 2 weeks until toxicity resolves to G ≤1. If toxicity does not resolve to G ≤1 within 2 weeks, discontinue therapy. Resume treatment if toxicity resolves to G ≤1 within 2 weeks, but reduce gemcitabine and docetaxel dosages by an additional 25%
G4 mucositis and diarrhea	Discontinue therapy
G2 neuropathy	Delay therapy 1 week. If symptoms do not resolve to G ≤1, reduce docetaxel dosage by 25%
G3 neuropathy	Discontinue therapy
Febrile neutropenia (T >38°C [>100.4°F] with ANC <1000/mm³)	Reduce gemcitabine and docetaxel dosages by 25%
G3/4 hematologic toxicity	Hold chemotherapy up to 2 weeks until toxicity resolves to G ≤1. If toxicity does not resolve to G ≤1 within 2 weeks, discontinue therapy

Toxicity

Toxicity	Percent of Patients	
	Gemcitabine + Docetaxel (N = 49)	Gemcitabine Alone (N = 73)
G3/4 neutrophils*	16%	28%
G3 hemoglobin	7%	13%
Blood transfusion	16%	20%
G3/4 platelets	40%	35%
Platelet transfusion	15%	11%
Febrile neutropenia	5%	7%
G3/4 pulmonary	7%	6%
G3/4 fatigue	16%	8%
G3 myalgias or muscle weakness	8%	2%
All other G3†	23%	2%

*National Cancer Institute Common Terminology Criteria for Adverse Events, version 3.0
†Includes (1 each except as noted): deep venous thrombosis/pulmonary embolus (n = 5), nausea/vomiting or anorexia (n = 4), lymphopenia (n = 4), edema (n = 3), GI bleeding (n = 2), high serum glucose, abdominal pain, diarrhea, mucositis, cough, pleural effusion, hiccups, bone pain, back spasm/pain, rash, nail changes, hypokalemia

Best Response by Histology*

Histology (Number of Patients with the Histology)	Number of Patients in Each Category					
	CR	PR	SD ≥24 Weeks	SD <24 Weeks	PD	NA
Gemcitabine + Docetaxel (N = 73)						
Leiomyosarcoma (29)	—	5	3	13	8	—
MFH/HGUPS (11)	1	3	3	2	1	1
Liposarcoma (8)						
Well differentiated/ dedifferentiated	—	—	—	4	—	1
Myxoid-round cell	—	—	—	—	—	—
Pleomorphic	—	2	—	1	—	—
Synovial sarcoma (5)	—	—	1	1	2	1
Malignant peripheral nerve sheath tumor (4)	—	—	1	—	3	—
Unclassified sarcoma (1)	—	—	—	1	—	—
Fibrosarcoma (3)	—	—	1	2	—	—
Rhabdomyosarcoma (2)	1	—	—	—	1	—
Other sarcoma histology (10)	—	—	2	4	4	—
Gemcitabine Alone (N = 49)						
Leiomyosarcoma (9)	—	1	2	5	1	—
MFH/HGUPS (8)	—	2	2	1	3	—
Liposarcoma (11)						
Well differentiated/ dedifferentiated	—	—	2	3	3	—
Myxoid-round cell	—	—	—	2	1	—
Pleomorphic	—	—	—	—	—	—
Synovial sarcoma (4)	—	—	1	1	2	—
Malignant peripheral nerve sheath tumor (2)	—	—	—	1	1	—
Unclassified sarcoma (4)	—	—	1	2	1	—
Fibrosarcoma (3)	—	—	1	—	2	—
Rhabdomyosarcoma (0)	—	—	—	—	—	—
Other sarcoma histology (7)	1	—	—	2	4	—

CR, complete response; PR, partial response; PD, progressive disease; SD, stable disease; NA, not assessable; MFH/HGUPS, malignant fibrous histiocytoma/high-grade undifferentiated pleomorphic sarcoma
*Includes one Response Evaluation Criteria in Solid Tumors Group (RECIST; Therasse P et al. J Natl Cancer Inst 2000;92:205–216) unconfirmed PR on each arm: gemcitabine (MFH/HGUPS); gemcitabine-docetaxel (uterine leiomyosarcoma)

Therapy Monitoring

1. *At start of therapy:* Clinical examination and laboratory testing
2. *Day 1 of each treatment cycle:* Physical examination, ECOG PS, complete blood count with leukocyte differential count, and serum chemistries
3. *Weekly CBC with leukocyte differential count:* At least the first 6 cycles of therapy
4. *After every 2 cycles of therapy:* Tumor measurements

UNRESECTABLE/METASTATIC/ PROGRESSIVE SOFT-TISSUE SARCOMA

GEMCITABINE + DACARBAZINE

García-del-Muro X et al. J Clin Oncol 2011;29:2528–2533

Gemcitabine 1800 mg/m²; administer intravenously, diluted in 0.9% sodium chloride injection (0.9% NS) to a concentration as low as 0.1 mg/mL, over 3 hours, on day 1, every 2 weeks, for a total of 12 cycles (24 weeks) (total dosage/cycle = 1800 mg/m²), *followed by:*
Dacarbazine 500 mg/m²; administer intravenously in 50–250 mL 0.9% NS or 5% dextrose injection over 20 minutes, on day 1, every 2 weeks, for a total of 12 cycles (24 weeks) (total dosage/cycle = 500 mg/m²)

Notes:
• Treatment after 24 weeks may be continued if it is thought the treatment is providing benefit

Supportive Care
Antiemetic prophylaxis
Emetogenic potential is **HIGH**. *Potential for delayed symptoms*
See Chapter 39 for antiemetic recommendations

Hematopoietic growth factor (CSF) prophylaxis
Primary prophylaxis is NOT indicated
See Chapter 43 for more information

Antimicrobial prophylaxis
Risk of fever and neutropenia is LOW
   Antimicrobial primary prophylaxis to be considered:
    • Antibacterial—not indicated
    • Antifungal—not indicated
    • Antiviral—not indicated unless patient previously had an episode of HSV
See Chapter 47 for more information

Oral care
Prophylaxis and treatment for mucositis/stomatitis
   General advice:
• Encourage patients to maintain intake of non-alcoholic fluids
• Evaluate patients for oral pain and provide analgesic medications
• Consider histamine (H₂-subtype) receptor antagonists (eg, ranitidine, famotidine), or a proton pump inhibitor for epigastric pain
• *Lactobacillus* sp.-containing probiotics may be beneficial in preventing diarrhea

Patients with intact oral mucosa:
• Clean the mouth, tongue, and gums by brushing after every meal and at bedtime with an ultra-soft toothbrush with fluoride toothpaste
• Floss teeth gently every day unless contraindicated. If gums bleed and hurt, avoid bleeding or sore areas, but floss other teeth
• Patients may use saline or commercial bland, non-alcoholic rinses
   ■ Do not use mouthwashes that contain alcohols

If mucositis or stomatitis is present:
• Keep the mouth moist utilizing water, ice chips, sugarless gum, sugar-free hard candies, or a saliva substitute
• Rinse mouth several times a day to remove debris
   ■ Use a solution of ¼ teaspoon (1.25 g) each of baking soda and table salt (sodium chloride) in one quart (~950 mL) of warm water. Follow with a plain water rinse
   ■ Do not use mouthwashes that contain alcohols
• Foam-tipped swabs (eg, Toothettes®) are useful in moisturizing oral mucosa, but ineffective for cleansing teeth and removing plaque
• Advise patients who develop mucositis to:
   ■ Choose foods that are easy to chew and swallow
   ■ Take small bites of food, chew slowly, and sip liquids with meals
   ■ Encourage soft, moist foods such as cooked cereals, mashed potatoes, and scrambled eggs
   ■ For trouble swallowing, soften food with gravies, sauces, broths, yogurt, or other bland liquids
   ■ Avoid sharp, crunchy foods; hot, spicy or highly acidic foods (eg, citrus fruits and juices); sugary foods; toothpicks; tobacco products; alcoholic drinks

Patient Population Studied

Patients 18 years or older with a histologic diagnosis of soft-tissue sarcoma with unresectable or metastatic progressive disease after prior treatment with anthracyclines and ifosfamide, or with contraindication for their use. Patients with rhabdomyosarcoma, chondrosarcoma, osteosarcoma, Ewing sarcoma, and gastrointestinal stromal tumor were excluded

Therapy Monitoring

1. *Pretreatment Evaluations:* History and physical examination; complete blood count with differential and platelet count; serum chemistries; electrocardiogram; chest X-ray; computed tomography (CT) scan of the chest, abdomen, and pelvis; and documentation of tumor measurements
2. *Weekly during treatment:* Complete blood cell counts with leukocyte differential count
3. *Before each cycle:* History and physical examinations and assessment of toxicities. Serum chemistries
4. *Every 3–4 cycles:* CT scans to assess response

Treatment Modifications

Dosage Levels

	Gemcitabine	Dacarbazine
Starting dosage level	1800 mg/m²	500 mg/m²
Dosage level −1	1500 mg/m²	400 mg/m²
Dosage level −2	1200 mg/m²	400 mg/m²

Adverse Event	Dose Modification
G3/4 thrombocytopenia, G4 granulocytopenia, or febrile neutropenia	Reduce gemcitabine and dacarbazine dosages by 1 dosage level
ANC <1000/mm³ at start of next cycle	Withhold treatment until ANC ≥1000/mm³, then reduce gemcitabine and dacarbazine dosages by 1 level
Platelet count <100,000/mm³ at start of next cycle	Withhold treatment until platelet count ≥100,000/mm³, then reduce gemcitabine and dacarbazine dosages by 1 level
ANC <1000/mm³ or platelet count <100,000/mm³ despite a 2-week delay	Withhold treatment until ANC ≥1000/mm³, then reduce gemcitabine and dacarbazine dosages by 1 level. If needed, administer cycles at 3-week intervals instead of 2-week intervals
G4 hepatotoxicity or G3/4 nonhematologic toxicity other than alopecia, fatigue, malaise, and nail changes	Hold chemotherapy up to 2 weeks until toxicity resolves to G ≤1. Resume treatment if toxicity resolves to G ≤1, but reduce gemcitabine and dacarbazine dosages by 1 dosage level
G2/3 skin rash	Reduce gemcitabine dosage to 1500 mg/m². If G2/3 rash recurs, reduce gemcitabine dosage to 1200 mg/m²
G ≥3 emesis	Discontinue dacarbazine

Toxicity (N = 57)

Worst Toxicity by Patient (NCI CTCAE v3.0*)

Adverse Events	% Patients All Grades	% Patients G3	% Patients G4
Hematologic Toxicity			
Leukopenia	76	26	0
Neutropenia	76	32	16
Thrombocytopenia	40	2	4
Anemia	82	4	0
Febrile neutropenia	9	7	2
Nonhematologic Toxicity			
Nausea	40	0	—
Vomiting	35	2	—
Diarrhea	18	0	0
Stomatitis	18	2	0
Asthenia	76	7	—
Rash	15	0	0
Alopecia	7	0	0

*National Cancer Institute (USA) Common Terminology Criteria for Adverse Events, version 3.0

Efficacy* (N = 57)

Progression-free rate at 3 months	56%
Median progression-free survival	4.2 months
Median overall survival	16.8 months
Overall response rate†	12%
Median duration of response	10.2 months (range: 2.7–12.3 months)
Median progression-free survival, leiomyosarcoma	4.9 months
Median overall survival, leiomyosarcoma	18.3 months
Median progression-free survival, nonleiomyosarcoma	2.1 months
Median overall survival, nonleiomyosarcoma	7.8 months

*RECIST 1.0 (Response Evaluation Criteria in Solid Tumors; Therasse P et al. J Natl Cancer Inst 2000;92:205–216)
†Responses were seen in leiomyosarcoma (3 patients), undifferentiated pleomorphic sarcoma (1 patient), uterine sarcoma (1 patient), and nonclassifiable sarcoma (1 patient)

ADVANCED SOFT-TISSUE SARCOMA
TRABECTEDIN (ECTEINASCIDIN 743; ET-743)

Demetri GD et al. J Clin Oncol 2009;27:4188–4196
Garcia-Carbonero R et al. J Clin Oncol 2004;22:1480–1490
Grosso F et al. Lancet Oncol 2007;8:595–602

Trabectedin 1.5 mg/m^2; administer intravenously over 24 hours on day 1, every 3 weeks (total dosage/cycle = 1.5 mg/m^2)

Administration via:

- *Central venous access:* dilute trabectedin with a volume of 0.9% sodium chloride injection (0.9% NS) or 5% dextrose injection (D5W) sufficient to produce a concentration ≤0.03 mg/mL

- *Peripheral venous access:* dilute trabectedin with ≥1000 mL 0.9% NS or D5W

Note: Trabectedin has not received U.S. Food and Drug Administration approval for use in human subjects outside clinical trials

Supportive Care
Antiemetic prophylaxis
Emetogenic potential is **MODERATE**
See Chapter 39 for antiemetic recommendations

Hematopoietic growth factor (CSF) prophylaxis
Primary prophylaxis is indicated with 1 of the following:

Filgrastim (G-CSF) 5 mcg/kg per day by subcutaneous injection, *or*
Pegfilgrastim (pegylated filgrastim) 6 mg/0.6 mL by subcutaneous injection for 1 dose
- Begin use from 24–72 hours after myelosuppressive chemotherapy is completed
- Continue daily filgrastim use until ANC ≥10,000/mm^3 on 2 measurements separated temporally by ≥12 hours
- Discontinue daily filgrastim use at least 24 hours before administering myelosuppressive treatment. Do not administer pegfilgrastim within 14 days before administering myelosuppressive treatment

See Chapter 43 for more information

Antimicrobial prophylaxis
Risk of fever and neutropenia is LOW
Antimicrobial primary prophylaxis to be considered:
- Antibacterial—not indicated
- Antifungal—not indicated
- Antiviral—not indicated unless patient previously had an episode of HSV

See Chapter 47 for more information

Treatment Modifications

Starting dosage level	1.5 mg/m^2
Dosage level −1	1.2 mg/m^2
Dosage level −2	1 mg/m^2

Adverse Event	Dose Modification
Febrile neutropenia: T >38°C [>100.4°F] with ANC <1000/mm^3	Reduce trabectedin dosage by 1 dose level
Platelet count <25,000/mm^3 lasting more than 5 days	Reduce trabectedin dosage by 1 dose level
G4 neutropenia >5 days	
ANC <1000/mm^3 at start of next cycle	Withhold treatment until ANC ≥1000/mm^3, then reduce trabectedin dosage by 1 dose level

(continued)

Treatment Modifications (*continued*)

Platelet count <100,000/mm³ at start of next cycle	Withhold treatment until platelet count ≥100,000/mm³, then reduce trabectedin dosage by 1 dose level
ANC <1000/mm³, or platelet count <100,000/mm³ despite a 3-week delay	Discontinue trabectedin therapy
G2/3/4 nonhematologic toxicity other than alopecia, fatigue, malaise, and nail changes	Hold trabectedin up to 3 weeks until toxicity resolves to G ≤1. If toxicity does not resolve to G ≤1 within 3 weeks then discontinue trabectedin therapy. Resume treatment if toxicity resolves to G ≤1 within 3 weeks, but reduce trabectedin dosage by 1 dose level
G2/3/4 nonhematologic toxicity other than alopecia, fatigue, malaise, and nail changes despite a reduction in trabectedin by 1 dosage level	Hold trabectedin up to 3 weeks until toxicity resolves to G ≤1. If toxicity does not resolve to G ≤1 within 3 weeks, discontinue trabectedin therapy. Resume treatment if toxicity resolves to G ≤1 within 3 weeks, but reduce trabectedin dosage by an additional dose level
G ≥3 liver function test abnormalities	Hold trabectedin up to 3 weeks until toxicity resolves to G ≤1. If toxicity does not resolve to G ≤1 within 3 weeks, discontinue trabectedin therapy. Resume treatment if toxicity resolves to G ≤1 within 3 weeks, but reduce trabectedin dosage by 1 dose level
G ≥3 liver function test abnormalities despite a reduction in trabectedin 1 dosage level	Hold trabectedin up to 3 weeks until toxicity resolves to G ≤1. If toxicity does not resolve to G ≤1 within 3 weeks, discontinue trabectedin therapy. Resume treatment if toxicity resolves to G ≤1 within 3 weeks, but reduce trabectedin dosage by an additional dose level

Patient Populations Studied

Progressive Soft-Tissue Sarcoma

Garcia-Carbonero R et al. J Clin Oncol 2004;22: 1480–1490

Patients with histologically confirmed recurrent or metastatic soft-tissue sarcoma with disease progression despite prior chemotherapy with 2 or fewer prior regimens for advanced disease were eligible for the trial

Myxoid Liposarcoma

Grosso F et al. Lancet Oncol 2007;8:595–602

Retrospective analysis of 51 patients with advanced pretreated myxoid liposarcoma in a compassionate-use program

Metastatic Liposarcoma/Leiomyosarcoma

Demetri GD et al. J Clin Oncol 2009;27:4188–4196

Patients >18 years old with histologic confirmation of liposarcoma or leiomyosarcoma; unresectable and/or metastatic relapse or progressive disease after prior treatment with a regimen containing at least an anthracycline and ifosfamide (combined or sequential)

Efficacy*

Progressive Soft-Tissue Sarcoma

Garcia-Carbonero R et al. J Clin Oncol 2004;22:1480–1490

Response to Trabectedin According to Histologic Subtype

Histology	Complete Response	Partial Response	Minor Response	Overall Response
Leiomyosarcoma (n = 13)	0	8% (1)	0	8% (1)
Liposarcoma (n = 10)	10% (1)	10% (1)	10% (1)	20% (2)
Synovial sarcoma (n = 6)	0	0	0	0
Other (n = 7)	0	0	14% (1)	0
All histologies (n = 36)	3% (1)	6% 92)	6% (2)	8% (3)

Median time to progression (TTP)	1.7 months (95% CI, 1.3–4.4 months)
Estimated 1-year TTP rate	9.4% (95% CI, 3.2–27.4%)
Median overall survival (OS)	12.1 months (95% CI, 8.1–26.5 months)
Estimated 1-year OS rate	53.1% (95% CI, 38.7–72.8%)

(*continued*)

Efficacy* (continued)

Myxoid Liposarcoma

Grosso F et al. Lancet Oncol 2007;8:595–602

Overall (N = 51)	Percent (Number)	95% CI
Complete response	4% (2)	
Partial response	47% (24)	
Overall response rate (ORR)	51% (26)	36–65%
Minimal response	12% (6)	
Median follow-up	14 months	8.7–20 months
Median time to reach a response[†]	3.6 months	IQR 2.4–4.6 months
Median PFS	14 months	95% CI 13.1–21 months
PFS at 3 months	92%	85–99%
PFS at 6 months	88%	79–95%
Median PFS of patients with PR/CR[‡]	20.3 months	14–30.6 months
Median PFS of patients with SD/MR[‡]	12.5 months	8.1–21.4 months

*RECIST (Response Evaluation Criteria in Solid Tumors; Therasse P et al. J Natl Cancer Inst 2000;92:205–216)
[†]In a subgroup of 40 patients only 6 of 23 with confirmed CR/PR achieved responses by first assessment; of the other 17 patients, 8 had MR and 9 SD at first assessment; median time to reach objective response was 3.6 months. In patients without confirmed CR/PR by first assessment, early alterations in tumor appearance were detected by CT/MRI—the hallmark feature was a decrease in tumor density without substantial changes in tumor dimensions. Same early signs were seen in 12 of the 15 patients with SD as their best response confirmed during central review
[‡]PFS during previous chemotherapy (ie, before starting trabectedin treatment) for 34 patients for whom data were available was 8.4 months (3.1–11.1 months)

Metastatic Liposarcoma/Leiomyosarcoma

Demetri GD et al. J Clin Oncol 2009;27:4188–4196

	Time/Percent	95% CI
Time to Progression, Months (Independent Review)		
Number of events	104 (76/5%)	
Median	3.7 months	2.1–5.4 months
Number PD at 3 months	53.4%	44.6–66.2%
Number PD at 6 months	37.2%	28.4–46%
Ratio: TTP with Trabectedin-to-TTP with Last Prior Therapy		
Last prior therapy		
Number	119	
Ratio >1.33	33.6% (40)	
Last prior therapy for advanced/metastatic disease		
Number	109	
Ratio >1.33	36.7% (40)	
Median progression-free survival	3.3 months	
Median overall survival	13.9 months	

Toxicity

Progressive Soft-Tissue Sarcoma

Garcia-Carbonero R et al. J Clin Oncol 2004;22:1480–1490

Worst Nonhematologic Toxicity Per Patient and Per Cycle

CTC Grade*	0		1		2		3		4	
Toxicity	Pt†	Cy†	Pt†	Cy†	Pt†	Cy†	Pt†	Cy†	Pt†	Cy†
Creatinine	74	83	23	16	3	0.8	0	0	0	0
Alkaline phosphatase	66	70	31	29	3	0.8	0	0	0	0
Aspartate aminotransferase‡	17	20	29	46	29	24	23	10	3	0.8
Alanine aminotransferase§	14	16	26	43	40	30	14	10	6	1.6
Bilirubin	86	94	11	5	0	0	3	0.8	0	0
Creatine phosphokinase€	74	87	20	12	0	0	0	0	3	0.8
Nausea	43	65	43	31	9	3	6	1.6	0	0
Vomiting	77	90	17	7	3	1.6	3	0.8	0	0
Fatigue	31	55	40	33	29	12	0	0	0	0

Worst Hematologic Toxicity Per Patient and Per Cycle

Hemoglobin	3	8	43	60	46	29	6	1.6	3	0.8
White blood cell count	20	24	17	37	20	22	29	11	14	4
Absolute neutrophil count	29	44	20	26	17	15	23	11	11	3
Platelet count	63	74	14	15	6	6	11	3	6	1.6

*CTC, National Cancer Institute (USA), Common Toxicity Criteria, version 2.0
†Toxicities expressed as percent and per patient (Pt) or per cycle (Cy)
‡AST (SGOT)
§ALT (SGPT)
€CPK

Metastatic Liposarcoma/Leiomyosarcoma

Demetri GD et al. J Clin Oncol 2009;27:4188–4196

Worst Grade Trabectedin-Related Adverse Events

	Per patient (N = 130)				Per cycle (N = 950)			
	Grade 1/2		Grade 3/4		Grade 1/2		Grade 3/4	
Adverse Event	No.	%	No.	%	No.	%	No.	%
Abdominal pain	21	16	6	5	N/A	N/A	N/A	N/A
Anorexia	28	22	1	<1	N/A	N/A	N/A	N/A
Back pain	15	12	4	3	N/A	N/A	N/A	N/A
Constipation	45	35	—	—	260	27	—	—
Cough	23	18	—	—	114	12	—	—
Diarrhea	30	23	1	<1	112	12	1	<1
Dizziness	17	13	1	<1	N/A	N/A	N/A	N/A
Dyspnea	17	13	5	4	N/A	N/A	N/A	N/A

(continued)

Toxicity (continued)

Adverse Event	No.	%	No.	%	No.	%	No.	%
Fatigue	87	67	10	8	564	59	19	2
Headache	36	28	1	<1	142	15	1	<1
Nausea	90	69	7	5	509	53	8	<1
Pyrexia	32	25	1	<1	N/A	N/A	N/A	N/A
Vomiting	50	38	7	5	169	17	7	<1

Metastatic Liposarcoma/Leiomyosarcoma

Demetri GD et al. J Clin Oncol 2009;27:4188–4196

Worst On-Treatment Laboratory Abnormalities

	Per Patient (N = 130)						Per Cycle (N = 950)					
	G1/2		G3		G4		G1/2		G3		G4	
Abnormality	No.	%	No.	%	No.	%	No.	%	No.	%	No.	%
Hematologic												
Anemia	116	89	5	4	5	4	758	80	5	<1	5	<1
Neutropenia	35	27	34	26	27	21	357	38	151	16	28	5
Febrile Neutropenia	1		<1				1		<1			
Thrombocytopenia	55	42	12	9	3	2	316	33	20	2	3	<1
Biochemical												
ALT	64	49	59	45	3	2	574	60	122	13	3	<1
AST	81	62	41	32	—	—	590	62	57	6	—	—
AP	70	54	2	2	—	—	341	36	4	<1	—	—
Bilirubin	27	21	1	<1	—	—	52	5	1	<1	—	—
CPK	32	25	4	3	3	2	139	15	4	<1	3	<1
Creatinine	46	35	—	—	3	2	302	32	—	—	3	<1

ALT, alanine aminotransferase; AP, alkaline phosphatase; AST, aspartate aminotransferase; CPK, creatine phosphokinase

Therapy Monitoring

1. *Pretreatment evaluations:* History and physical examination; complete blood count with differential and platelet count; serum chemistries; electrocardiogram; chest x-ray; computed tomography (CT) scan of the chest, abdomen, and pelvis; and documentation of tumor measurements

2. *Weekly during treatment:* Complete blood cell counts with leukocyte differential count

3. *Before each cycle:* History and physical examinations and assessment of toxicities. Serum chemistries

4. *Every 2–3 cycles:* CT scans to assess response

UNRESECTABLE LEIOMYOSARCOMA
GEMCITABINE + DOCETAXEL

Hensley ML et al. J Clin Oncol 2002;20:2824–2831

Gemcitabine 900 mg/m² per dose; administer intravenously, diluted in 0.9% sodium chloride injection (0.9% NS) to a concentration as low as 0.1 mg/mL, over 90 minutes for 2 doses, on days 1 and 8, every 21 days (total dosage/cycle = 1800 mg/m²)

Premedication for docetaxel:
Dexamethasone 8 mg/dose; administer orally twice daily for 3 days, starting 1 day before docetaxel administration (total dose/cycle = 48 mg)
Optional premedication for docetaxel:
   Diphenhydramine HCl 25 mg; administer orally 30–60 minutes *or* intravenously 5–30 minutes prior to docetaxel administration
   Ranitidine 150 mg; administer orally 30–60 minutes prior to docetaxel administration, *or*
   Ranitidine 50 mg; administer intravenously 5–30 minutes prior to docetaxel administration

Docetaxel 100 mg/m²; administer intravenously, in a volume of 0.9% NS or 5% dextrose injection (D5W) sufficient to produce a docetaxel concentration within the range 0.3–0.74 mg/mL, over 60 minutes on day 8 after gemcitabine, every 21 days (total dosage/cycle = 100 mg/m²)

Notes:
• Patients previously treated with radiation therapy should receive *reduced* dosages as follows:
  Gemcitabine 675 mg/m² per dose; administer intravenously, diluted in 0.9% NS to a concentration as low as 0.1 mg/mL, over 90 minutes for 2 doses, on days 1 and 8, every 21 days (total dosage/cycle = 1350 mg/m²)

Premedication for docetaxel:
Dexamethasone 8 mg/dose; administer orally twice daily for 3 days, starting 1 day before docetaxel administration (total dose/cycle = 48 mg)
Optional premedication for docetaxel:
   Diphenhydramine HCl 25 mg; administer orally 30–60 minutes *or* intravenously 5–30 minutes prior to docetaxel administration
   Ranitidine 150 mg; administer orally 30–60 minutes prior to docetaxel administration, *or*
   Ranitidine 50 mg; administer intravenously 5–30 minutes prior to docetaxel administration
Docetaxel 75 mg/m²; administer intravenously in a volume of 0.9% NS or D5W sufficient to produce a docetaxel concentration within the range 0.3–0.74 mg/mL over 60 minutes on day 8 after gemcitabine, every 21 days (total dosage/cycle = 75 mg/m²)
• Patients who continue to respond after receiving 6 cycles may receive 2 additional cycles of therapy

Supportive Care
Antiemetic prophylaxis
Emetogenic potential is **LOW–MODERATE**
See Chapter 39 for antiemetic recommendations

Hematopoietic growth factor (CSF) prophylaxis
Primary prophylaxis is NOT indicated
See Chapter 43 for more information

Antimicrobial prophylaxis
Risk of fever and neutropenia is LOW
  Antimicrobial primary prophylaxis to be considered:
  • Antibacterial—not indicated
  • Antifungal—not indicated
  • Antiviral—not indicated unless patient previously had an episode of HSV
See Chapter 47 for more information

Treatment Modifications

Adverse Event	Dose Modification
Febrile neutropenia or platelet count <25,000/mm³ lasting more than 5 days	Reduce gemcitabine and docetaxel dosages by 25% in all subsequent cycles
ANC <1000/mm³ at start of next cycle	Withhold treatment until ANC ≥1000/mm³, then reduce gemcitabine and docetaxel dosages by 25%
Platelet count <100,000/mm³ at start of next cycle	Withhold treatment until platelet count ≥100,000/mm³, then reduce gemcitabine and docetaxel dosages by 25%
ANC <1000/mm³ or platelet count <100,000/mm³ despite 2-week delay	Discontinue therapy
Day 8 ANC 500–999/mm³ or day 8 platelet count 50,000–99,000/mm³	Reduce day 8 gemcitabine and docetaxel dosages by 25%
Day 8 ANC <500/mm³ or day 8 platelet count <50,000/mm³	Do not administer day 8 gemcitabine and docetaxel
G3/4 nonhematologic toxicity other than alopecia, fatigue, malaise, and nail changes	Hold chemotherapy up to 2 weeks until toxicity resolves to G ≤1. If toxicity does not resolve to G ≤1 within 2 weeks then discontinue therapy. Resume treatment if toxicity resolves to G ≤1 within 2 weeks but reduce gemcitabine and docetaxel dosages by 25%
G3/4 nonhematologic toxicity other than alopecia, fatigue, malaise, and nail changes despite a 25% reduction in initial gemcitabine and docetaxel dosages	Hold chemotherapy up to 2 weeks until toxicity resolves to G ≤1. If toxicity does not resolve to G ≤1 within 2 weeks, discontinue therapy. Resume treatment if toxicity resolves to G ≤1 within 2 weeks, but reduce gemcitabine and docetaxel dosages by an additional 25%
G ≥3 liver function test abnormalities	Hold chemotherapy up to 2 weeks until toxicity resolves to G ≤1. If toxicity does not resolve to G ≤1 within 2 weeks, discontinue therapy. Resume treatment if toxicity resolves to G ≤1 within 2 weeks, but reduce gemcitabine and docetaxel dosages by 25%
G ≥3 liver function test abnormalities despite a 25% reduction in initial gemcitabine and docetaxel dosages	Hold chemotherapy up to 2 weeks until toxicity resolves to G ≤1. If toxicity does not resolve to G ≤1 within 2 weeks then discontinue therapy. Resume treatment if toxicity resolves to G ≤1 within 2 weeks, but reduce gemcitabine and docetaxel dosages by an additional 25%
G4 mucositis and diarrhea	Discontinue therapy
G2 neuropathy	Delay therapy 1 week. If symptoms do not resolve to G ≤1, reduce docetaxel dosage by 25%
G3 neuropathy	Discontinue therapy
Febrile neutropenia (T >38°C [>100.4°F] with ANC <1000/mm³)	Reduce gemcitabine and docetaxel doses by 25%
G3/4 hematologic toxicity	Hold chemotherapy up to 2 weeks until toxicity resolves to G ≤1. If toxicity does not resolve to G ≤1 within 2 weeks, discontinue therapy

Efficacy
Leiomyosarcoma (LMS) (N = 34)*

Best Response	Percent (Number of Patients)	95% CI
Complete response	8.8 % (3)	
Partial response	44% (15)	
Minor response/stable disease	23.5% (8)	
Progression of disease	26.5% (9)	
Overall objective response†	53% (18)	35–70%
Median duration of response	4 months	3 months–NR‡
Median progression-free survival	5.6 months	4.3–9.9 months
Progression-free at 6 months	47%	32–68%
Median overall survival	17.9 months	11.6 months—NR
Alive at 6 months	66%	49–88%

Patients Previously Treated with Doxorubicin ± Ifosfamide (N = 16)

Overall objective response	50% (8)	

NR, Not reached
*RECIST criteria (Response Evaluation Criteria in Solid Tumors; Therasse P et al. J Natl Cancer Inst 2000;92:205–216)
†Among 5 patients with non-uterine primary LMS, 2 (40%) had PRs

Toxicity*
(N = 34 patients/160 cycles)

	Grade 3		Grade 4	
	Number of Patients	%	Number of Patients	%
Neutropenia	5	15	2	6
Thrombocytopenia	9	26	1	3
Neutropenia and fever	—	—	2	6
Anemia	4	12	1	3
Dyspnea	5	15	2	6
Diarrhea	3	9	1	3
Fatigue	7	21	—	—
Sensory neuropathy	2	6	—	—
Allergic reaction	1	3	—	—
Venous thrombosis	—	—	1	3

*National Cancer Institute (USA), Common Toxicity Criteria, version 2.0

Patient Population Studied

Patients with histologically confirmed LMS of the uterus or of other primary site that was considered unresectable for cure and who had received zero to 2 previous chemotherapy regimens for treatment of LMS

Therapy Monitoring

1. *Pretreatment evaluations:* History and physical examination; complete blood count with differential and platelet count; serum chemistries; electrocardiogram; chest X-ray, computed tomography (CT) scan of the chest, abdomen, and pelvis; and documentation of tumor measurements
2. *Weekly during treatment:* Complete blood cell counts with leukocyte differential count
3. *Before each cycle:* History and physical examinations and assessment of toxicities. Serum chemistries
4. *Every 2–3 cycles:* CT scans to assess response

RELAPSED/REFRACTORY SOFT-TISSUE AND BONE SARCOMA

VINCRISTINE, ORAL IRINOTECAN, AND TEMOZOLOMIDE (VOIT)

Wagner LM et al. Pediatr Blood Cancer 2010;54:538–545

Temozolomide 150 mg/m^2 per day; administer orally for 5 consecutive days at least 1 hour before vincristine and irinotecan, on days 1–5, every 21 days (total dosage/cycle = 750 mg/m^2)
• Temozolomide doses are rounded to the nearest 5 mg to utilize commercially available products

Vincristine 1.5 mg/m^2 (maximum dose = 2 mg); administer by intravenous injection over 1–2 minutes on day 1, every 21 days (total dosage/cycle = 1.5 mg/m^2; maximum dose/cycle = 2 mg)
Irinotecan 90 mg/m^2 per day; administer orally for 5 consecutive days, on days 1–5, every 21 days (total dosage/cycle = 450 mg/m^2)
• Doses were prepared from an injectable formulation of irinotecan
• Five doses were prepared in individual oral syringes and dispensed with instructions to store under refrigeration until they were used
• Irinotecan solution was mixed with cranberry-grape juice immediately before administration to mask its bitter flavor

Supportive Care
Antiemetic prophylaxis
Emetogenic potential on days 1–5 is **MODERATE–HIGH**
See Chapter 39 for antiemetic recommendations

Hematopoietic growth factor (CSF) prophylaxis
Primary prophylaxis is NOT indicated
See Chapter 43 for more information

Antimicrobial prophylaxis
Risk of fever and neutropenia is LOW
  Antimicrobial primary prophylaxis to be considered:
  • Antibacterial—not indicated
  • Antifungal—not indicated
  • Antiviral—not indicated unless patient previously had an episode of HSV
See Chapter 47 for more information

Acute cholinergic syndrome
Atropine sulfate 0.25–1 mg subcutaneously or intravenously if abdominal cramping or diarrhea develop during or within 1 hour after irinotecan administration
• If symptoms are severe, add as primary prophylaxis at least 30 minutes before irinotecan during subsequent cycles
• For irinotecan, acute cholinergic syndrome may be characterized by abdominal cramping, diarrhea, diaphoresis, hypotension, flushing, bradycardia, rhinitis, increased salivation, meiosis, and lacrimation

Diarrhea management
• The potential for developing diarrhea and abdominal pain should be discussed with all patients and their caretakers, and instructions given to start loperamide immediately if these symptoms occur and to ensure adequate hydration is maintained. See "Dose Modifications" below for instructions

Latent or delayed onset diarrhea*:
  Loperamide 4 mg orally initially after the first loose or liquid stool, *then*
  Loperamide 2 mg orally every 2 hours during waking hours, *plus*
  Loperamide 4 mg orally every 4 hours during hours of sleep
  • Continue for at least 12 hours after diarrhea resolves
  • Recurrent diarrhea after a 12-hour diarrhea-free interval is treated as a new episode
  • Rehydrate orally with fluids and electrolytes during a diarrheal episode
  • If a patient develops blood or mucus in stool, dehydration, or hemodynamic instability, or if diarrhea persists >48 hours despite loperamide, stop loperamide and hospitalize the patient for IV hydration

(continued)

(continued)

Alternatively, a trial of **Diphenoxylate hydrochloride** 2.5 mg **with Atropine sulfate** 0.025 mg (eg, Lomotil)
- Initial adult dose is 2 tablets 4 times daily until control has been achieved, after which the dose may be reduced to meet individual requirements. Control may often be maintained with as little as 2 tablets daily
- Clinical improvement of acute diarrhea is usually observed within 48 hours. If improvement of chronic diarrhea after treatment with a maximum daily dose of 8 tablets is not observed within 10 days, control is unlikely with further administration

Persistent diarrhea:
Octreotide 100–150 mcg subcutaneously 3 times daily. Maximum total daily dose is 1500 mcg

Antibiotic primary prophylaxis and treatment during latent or delayed onset diarrhea:
Consider the following to prevent or lessen irinotecan-associated diarrhea:
- Prophylactic oral **cefixime** 8 mg/kg (maximum dose of 400 mg) orally once daily, beginning 1–2 days prior to the start of irinotecan therapy and continuing until completion of the cycle, *alternatively:*
- **Cefpodoxime proxetil** 5 mg/kg orally, twice daily (maximum dose of 200 mg twice daily)
  - Previous studies suggest prophylaxis with cephalosporin antibiotics can ameliorate irinotecan-associated diarrhea by reducing the enteric bacteria responsible for producing β-glucuronidase, which regenerates in the gut irinotecan's toxic metabolite, SN-38, by cleaving the glucuronide moiety from SN-38 (Wagner LM et al. Pediatr Blood Cancer 2008;50:201–207)
- Alternatively, **activated charcoal** at a dose equal to 5-times the irinotecan dose up to a maximum dose of 260 mg orally 3 times daily during irinotecan therapy (Michael M et al. J Clin Oncol 2004;22:4410–4417)

Antibiotic treatment during latent or delayed onset diarrhea
- A fluoroquinolone (eg, **Ciprofloxacin** 500 mg orally every 12 hours) if absolute neutrophil count <500/mm^3 with or without accompanying fever in association with diarrhea

Antibiotics should also be administered if a patient is hospitalized with prolonged diarrhea, and should be continued until diarrhea resolves

*Abigerges D et al. J Natl Cancer Inst 1994;86:446–449
Rothenberg ML et al. J Clin Oncol 2001;19:3801–3807
Wadler S et al. J Clin Oncol 1998;16:3169–3178

Dose Modifications

Irinotecan Dosage Levels*

Level 1 starting dosage	90 mg/m^2 per day orally on days 1–5
Level −1	70 mg/m^2 per day orally on days 1–5
Level −2	50 mg/m^2 per day orally on days 1–5

Temozolomide Dosage Levels

Level 1 starting dosage	150 mg/m^2 per day orally on days 1–5
Level −1	125 mg/m^2 per day orally on days 1–5
Level −2	100 mg/m^2 per day orally on days 1–5

Vincristine Dosage Levels

Level 1 starting dosage	1.5 mg/m^2 (maximum single dose = 2 mg) by intravenous injection
Level −1	0.75 mg/m^2 (maximum single dose = 2 mg) by intravenous injection

(continued)

Patient Population Studied

Patients older than 12 months and younger than 21 years with solid tumors refractory to standard therapy and no other curative option. Patients were excluded if they had received treatment with agents known to affect irinotecan metabolism (eg, enzyme-inducing anticonvulsants), or if they had previously received treatment with temozolomide or irinotecan or had experienced prior progression of their tumor with either agent

Dose Modifications (*continued*)

Adverse Event	Dose Modification
G1 ANC (1500–1999/mm³) or G1 thrombocytopenia during a given cycle	Maintain dose and schedule
G2 ANC (1000–1499/mm³) or G2 thrombocytopenia during a given cycle	Reduce dosage of irinotecan and temozolomide by 1 dosage level
G4 neutropenia >7 days duration	Reduce dosage of irinotecan and temozolomide for the following cycle by 1 dose level
G3/4 infection	
Day 21 ANC <1000/mm³ or platelet count <75,000/mm³	Delay start of next cycle by 1 week and reduce dosage of irinotecan and temozolomide by 1 level
Day 28 ANC still <1000/mm³ or platelet count still <75,000/mm³	Delay start of next cycle by 1 additional week and reduce dosage of irinotecan and temozolomide by 1 level
Day 35 ANC still <1000/mm³ or platelet count still <75,000/mm³	Discontinue therapy

Diarrhea in Children 2–15 Years of Age

Children 2–15 years, with first liquid stools	Begin loperamide immediately with the first liquid stool at a dosage of loperamide 0.03 mg/kg administered orally every 4 hours (0.18 mg/kg/24h)
G3/4 diarrhea within the first 24 hours	Hospitalize for optimal management. Begin **loperamide** 0.06 mg/kg, orally, every 4 hours. Reduce irinotecan dosage for the following cycle by 1 dose level

Delayed Diarrhea in Patients >15 Years of Age

G1 (2–3 stools/day > baseline)	Maintain dose and schedule
G2 (4–6 stools/day > baseline)	Delay until diarrhea resolves to baseline, then reduce irinotecan dosage by 1 dosage level
G3 (7–9 stools/day > baseline)	Delay until diarrhea resolves to baseline, then reduce irinotecan dosage by 1 dosage level
G4 (≥10 stools/day > baseline)	Delay until diarrhea resolves to baseline, then reduce irinotecan dosage by 2 dosage levels

Other Nonhematologic Toxicities

Any G1 toxicity	Maintain dose and schedule
Any G2 toxicity	Hold treatment until toxicity resolves to G ≤1, then reduce dosage of 1 or all agents by 1 dosage level
Any G3 toxicity	Hold treatment until toxicity resolves to G ≤1, then reduce dosage of 1 or all agents by 1 dosage level
Any G4 toxicity	Hold treatment until toxicity resolves to G ≤1, then reduce dosage of 1 or all agents by 2 dosage levels
G 2 neurotoxicity	Reduce vincristine dosage by 50% (if receiving 2 mg maximum, reduce to 1 mg)
G 3/4 neurotoxicity	Discontinue vincristine

*Treatment should be stopped in case of recurrent toxicity at dose level −2, unless there is perceived clinical benefit from irinotecan that justifies continuation

André T et al. Eur J Cancer 1999;35:1343–1347
Camptosar irinotecan hydrochloride injection, product label, August 2010. Pharmacia & Upjohn Company, Division of Pfizer, Inc., New York, NY
Douillard JY et al. Lancet 2000;355:1041–1047
Tournigand C et al. J Clin Oncol 2004;22:229–237

Efficacy

Details for Patients With Response or Prolonged Stable Disease

Tumor Type	Dosages (mg/m²)		No. of Courses	Response/ Confirmed	Reason for Stopping
	Irino	Tem			
Osteosarcoma	35	100	3	PR/Yes	Weight loss, N/V
Ewing sarcoma	50	100	2	CR/No	Transaminitis
Ewing sarcoma	35	100	2	PR/No	New lesions
Ewing sarcoma	35	100	8	SD/Yes	PD
Medulloblastoma	35	100	7	SD/Yes	Infection
Neuroblastoma	50	100	6	SD/Yes	Weight loss
Hepatoblastoma	50	100	4	SD/Yes	PD
Alveolar soft parts sarcoma	70	100	6	SD/Yes	PD
Synovial sarcoma	90	100	4	SD/Yes	PD
Pleuropulmonary blastoma	90	125	16	SD/Yes	Other therapy
Neuroblastoma	90	125	8	SD/Yes	PD
Medulloblastoma	90	150	12	SD/Yes	PD
Brainstem glioma	90	150	8	SD/Yes	PD

Irino, Irinotecan; Tem, temozolomide

Therapy Monitoring

1. *Prior to enrollment:* Complete medical history, clinical examination, performance status, hematologic and serum chemistries, cardiac evaluation in case of prior treatment with anthracyclines or mediastinal irradiation, and tumor target assessment
2. *Day 1 of each treatment cycle:* Physical examination, ECOG PS, complete blood count with leukocyte differential count, and serum chemistries
3. *Weekly CBC:* At least during the first 6 cycles of therapy
4. *After every 2 cycles of therapy:* Tumor measurements

Toxicity

Non–Dose-Limiting Toxicities Observed in Evaluable Patients[*,†]

Toxicity Type	Course 1 (18 Courses) Maximum Toxicity Grade			Courses 2–8 (54 Courses) Maximum Toxicity Grade		
	No. G1 (%)	No. G2 (%)	No. G3 (%)	No. G1 (%)	No. G2 (%)	No. G3 (%)
Hemoglobin	7 (39%)	2(11%)	—	3(5.6%)	3(5.6%)	—
Leukocytes (total WBC)	9 (50%)	3(17%)	—	4(7.4%)	2(3.7%)	—
Lymphopenia	3 (17%)	6(33%)	—	3(5.6%)	1(1.8%)	2(3.7%)
Neutrophils/granulocytes	1 (5.6%)	2(11%)	3(17%)	—	2(3.7%)	2(3.7%)
Platelets	5 (28%)	—	—	5	1(1.8%)	—
Fatigue	3 (17%)	1(5.6%)	—	2(4%)	—	—
Anorexia	—	2(11%)	—	—	—	—
Constipation	3 (17%)	1(5.6%)	—	1(1.8%)	—	—
Diarrhea	3 (17%)	4(22%)	1(5.6%)	1(1.8%)	4	—
Nausea	3 (17%)	—	—	2(3.7%)	2(3.7%)	—
Vomiting	1 (5.6%)	2(11%)	2(11%)	3(5.6%)	2(3.7%)	2(4%)
Alkaline phosphatase	1(5.6%)	1(5.6%)	—	2(4%)	—	—
ALT (SGPT)	3 (17%)	1(5.6%)	1(5.6%)	2(4%)	1(1.8%)	—
AST (SGOT)	3 (17%)	1(5.6%)	—	4	—	—
Hyperbilirubinemia	3 (17%)	—	—	—	—	—
Hypophosphatemia	2 (11%)	—	—	—	1(1.8%)	—
Hypokalemia	2 (11%)	—	—	3(5.6%)	—	—
Hyponatremia	1 (5.6%)	—	1(5.6%)	4	—	—
Abdominal pain	3 (17%)	1(5.6%)	—	1(1.8%)	—	—
Jaw pain	1(5.6%)	1(5.6%)	—	—	—	—

*National Cancer Institute (USA) Common Terminology Criteria for Adverse Events, version 3
†No G4 toxicities reported

ADVANCED SOFT-TISSUE AND BONE SARCOMA
DOXORUBICIN + DACARBAZINE (AD)

Antman K et al. J Clin Oncol 1993;11:1276–1285

Doxorubicin 15 mg/m² per day; administer intravenously in 25–1000 mL 5% dextrose injection (D5W) or 0.9% sodium chloride injection (0.9% NS) over 24 hours, for 4 consecutive days (96 hours), every 21 days (total dosage/cycle = 60 mg/m²)

Dacarbazine 250 mg/m² per day; administer intravenously, in 100–250 mL 0.9% NS or D5W over 24 hours for 4 consecutive days (96 hours), every 21 days (total dosage/cycle = 1000 mg/m²)

Important:
- Doxorubicin and dacarbazine are sensitive to photodegradation
  - Doxorubicin product containers should be protected from light
  - Prevent dacarbazine exposure to sunlight. Cover dacarbazine product containers with opaque material or foil and use light opaque or light resistant administration sets, or wrap tubing with opaque material or foil during drug administration

Notes:
Treatment courses were repeated at 21 days or when the WBC count reached 3000/mm³ and the platelet count reached 100,000/mm³

Supportive Care
Antiemetic prophylaxis
Emetogenic potential is **HIGH**
See Chapter 39 for antiemetic recommendations

Hematopoietic growth factor (CSF) prophylaxis
Primary prophylaxis is indicated with 1 of the following:
    Filgrastim (G-CSF) 5 mcg/kg per day by subcutaneous injection, *or*
    Pegfilgrastim (pegylated filgrastim) 6 mg/0.6 mL by subcutaneous injection for 1 dose
- Begin use from 24–72 hours after myelosuppressive chemotherapy is completed
- Continue daily filgrastim use until ANC ≥10,000/mm³ on 2 measurements separated temporally by ≥12 hours
- Discontinue daily filgrastim use at least 24 hours before administering myelosuppressive treatment. Do not administer pegfilgrastim within 14 days before administering myelosuppressive treatment
See Chapter 43 for more information

Antimicrobial prophylaxis
Risk of fever and neutropenia is LOW
    Antimicrobial primary prophylaxis to be considered:
- Antibacterial—not indicated
- Antifungal—not indicated
- Antiviral—not indicated unless patient previously had an episode of HSV
See Chapter 47 for more information

Oral care
Prophylaxis and treatment for mucositis/stomatitis
    General advice:
- Encourage patients to maintain intake of non-alcoholic fluids
- Evaluate patients for oral pain and provide analgesic medications
- Consider histamine (H₂-subtype) receptor antagonists (eg, ranitidine, famotidine), or a proton pump inhibitor for epigastric pain
- *Lactobacillus* sp.-containing probiotics may be beneficial in preventing diarrhea
    Patients with intact oral mucosa:
- Clean the mouth, tongue, and gums by brushing after every meal and at bedtime with an ultra-soft toothbrush with fluoride toothpaste
- Floss teeth gently every day unless contraindicated. If gums bleed and hurt, avoid bleeding or sore areas, but floss other teeth
- Patients may use saline or commercial bland, non-alcoholic rinses
  - Do not use mouthwashes that contain alcohols

(continued)

(continued)

If mucositis or stomatitis is present:

- Keep the mouth moist utilizing water, ice chips, sugarless gum, sugar-free hard candies, or a saliva substitute
- Rinse mouth several times a day to remove debris
  - Use a solution of ¼ teaspoon (1.25 g) each of baking soda and table salt (sodium chloride) in one quart (~950 mL) of warm water. Follow with a plain water rinse
  - Do not use mouthwashes that contain alcohols
- Foam-tipped swabs (eg, Toothettes®) are useful in moisturizing oral mucosa, but ineffective for cleansing teeth and removing plaque
- Advise patients who develop mucositis to:
  - Choose foods that are easy to chew and swallow
  - Take small bites of food, chew slowly, and sip liquids with meals
  - Encourage soft, moist foods such as cooked cereals, mashed potatoes, and scrambled eggs
  - For trouble swallowing, soften food with gravies, sauces, broths, yogurt, or other bland liquids
  - Avoid sharp, crunchy foods; hot, spicy or highly acidic foods (eg, citrus fruits and juices); sugary foods; toothpicks; tobacco products; alcoholic drinks

Treatment Modifications

Adverse Event	Dose Modification
WBC <3000/mm³ or platelets <100,000/mm³	Delay treatment 1 week until WBC ≥3000/mm³ and platelets ≥100,000/mm³
>2-week delay in start of cycle	Reduce doxorubicin and dacarbazine dosages by 25%
WBC nadir <1000/mm³ or platelet nadir <30,000/mm³	Reduce doxorubicin and dacarbazine dosages by 50%
WBC nadir 1000–1499/mm³ or platelet nadir 30,000–49,500/mm³	Reduce doxorubicin and dacarbazine dosages by 25%
G ≥3 mucositis	Reduce doxorubicin dosage 10–15 mg/m²
Doxorubicin total cumulative lifetime dosage >400–450 mg/m²	Obtain frequent MUGA scans to monitor cardiac function
Decreased cardiac ejection fraction (suggested guidelines): resting cardiac ejection fraction decreased ≥10–15% from baseline, or to absolute values <35–40%	Discontinue therapy

Patient Population Studied

At the time the study was designed, doxorubicin alone or with dacarbazine (AD) was considered the best available therapy for metastatic adult sarcomas. Ifosfamide was thought to be active in sarcomas that did not respond to a doxorubicin-based regimen. The study was designed to determine if ifosfamide added to doxorubicin and dacarbazine (ADI) significantly affected toxicity, response rate, and survival. Patients with measurable metastatic or unresectable sarcoma were randomly assigned to receive AD or ADI. Patients with chondrosarcomas, fibrosarcomas, and other sarcomas of bone were eligible, although those with osteosarcoma, rhabdomyosarcoma, Ewing sarcoma, Kaposi sarcoma, and mesothelioma were excluded, as were patients with prior chemotherapy for sarcoma or prior doxorubicin

Efficacy

Response Rates and Duration (N = 169)

Complete response	2% (4)
Partial response	15% (25)

Responses by Measurements

No further x-rays	2% (3)
Stable	41% (69)
Increasing disease	35% (59)
Early death, assumed no response	2% (4)
No evaluation, assumed no response	3% (5)
Total	100 (169)
Time to progression, median	4 months
Duration of response, median	8 months

Responses for Radiation-Associated Sarcomas (N = 13)

Complete response	0
Partial response	8% (1)

Responses by Tumor Grade	Grade I or II	Grade III
Complete response	0% (0)	4% (4)
Partial response	12% (9)	17% (16)

Response by Measurements

No further x-rays	1% (1)	2% (2)
Stable	43% (32)	39% (37)
Increasing disease	40% (30)	31% (29)
Early death, assumed no response	1% (1)	3% (3)
No evaluation, assumed no response	3% (2)	3% (3)
Total	100% (75)	100% (94)

Responses by Histology	% CR	% ORR
Leiomyosarcoma (N = 59)	2	16
Other common histologies (N = 7)	0	71
All other histologies (N = 44)	5	14

Toxicity

Number of Cases of Severe, Life-Threatening, and Lethal Toxicities (N = 170)

	Severe/Life-Threatening	Lethal
Anemia	11	0
Leukopenia	55	0
Granulocytopenia	64	0
Infections	0	0
Thrombocytopenia	7	0
Bladder, hematuria	0	0
Renal, other	0	0
Cardiac	2	0
Pulmonary embolism	0	1
CNS, somnolence/coma	0	0
Nausea/vomiting	15	0
Mucositis/ulcers/stomatitis	12	0
Diarrhea	1	0
Weight loss	0	0
Hepatic	0	0
Maximum grade of any toxicity	94 (55%)	1 (0.6%)

Therapy Monitoring

1. *Pretreatment evaluations:* History and physical examination; complete blood count with differential and platelet count; serum chemistries; electrocardiogram; chest x-ray, computed tomography (CT) scan of the chest, abdomen, and pelvis; and documentation of tumor measurements

2. *Weekly during treatment:* Complete blood cell counts with leukocyte differential count

3. *Before each cycle:* History and physical examinations and assessment of toxicities. Serum chemistries

4. *Every 2–3 cycles:* CT scans to assess response

DERMATOFIBROSARCOMA PROTUBERANS
IMATINIB MESYLATE

Rutkowski P et al. J Clin Oncol 2010;28:1772–1779

Note: Dermatofibrosarcoma protuberans (DFSP) is a dermal sarcoma typically carrying a translocation between chromosomes 17 and 22 that generates functional platelet-derived growth factor B (PDGFB)

Starting dose: **Imatinib mesylate** 400 mg/day; administer orally with food and a large glass of water (total dose/week = 2800 mg)

Dose escalation: **Imatinib mesylate** 600–800 mg/day; administer orally with food and a large glass of water (total dose/week = 4200–5600 mg)

Notes:
- 400- and 600-mg doses may be given once daily, or, alternatively, may be split into 2 equal doses, one given during morning hours and a second dose during the evening
- 800-mg daily doses should be given as two 400-mg doses, one during morning hours and a second dose during the evening
- For patients unable to swallow the film-coated tablets, imatinib mesylate may be dispersed in a glass of water or apple juice. The required number of tablets should be placed in an appropriate volume of beverage (approximately 50 mL for a 100-mg tablet, and 200 mL for a 400-mg tablet) and stirred with a spoon. The suspension should be administered immediately after the tablets have completely disintegrated

Note: Response rates and TTP did not differ between patients taking 400 mg daily versus 400 mg twice a day

Supportive Care
Antiemetic prophylaxis
Emetogenic potential is **LOW**
See Chapter 39 for antiemetic recommendations

Hematopoietic growth factor (CSF) prophylaxis
Primary prophylaxis is NOT indicated
See Chapter 43 for more information

Antimicrobial prophylaxis
Risk of fever and neutropenia is LOW
  Antimicrobial primary prophylaxis to be considered:
  - Antibacterial—not indicated
  - Antifungal—not indicated
  - Antiviral—not indicated unless patient previously had an episode of HSV
See Chapter 47 for more information

Diarrhea management
Latent or delayed onset diarrhea*:
  Loperamide 4 mg orally initially after the first loose or liquid stool, *then*
  Loperamide 2 mg orally every 2 hours during waking hours, *plus*
  Loperamide 4 mg orally every 4 hours during hours of sleep
- Continue for at least 12 hours after diarrhea resolves
- Recurrent diarrhea after a 12-hour diarrhea-free interval is treated as a new episode
- Rehydrate orally with fluids and electrolytes during a diarrheal episode
- If a patient develops blood or mucus in stool, dehydration, or hemodynamic instability, or if diarrhea persists >48 hours despite loperamide, stop loperamide and hospitalize the patient for IV hydration

Alternatively, a trial of **Diphenoxylate hydrochloride** 2.5 mg **with Atropine sulfate** 0.025 mg (eg, Lomotil)
- Initial adult dose is 2 tablets 4 times daily until control has been achieved, after which the dose may be reduced to meet individual requirements. Control may often be maintained with as little as 2 tablets daily
- Clinical improvement of acute diarrhea is usually observed within 48 hours. If improvement of chronic diarrhea after treatment with a maximum daily dose of 8 tablets is not observed within 10 days, control is unlikely with further administration

*Abigerges D et al. J Natl Cancer Inst 1994;86:446–449
Rothenberg ML et al. J Clin Oncol 2001;19:3801–3807
Wadler S et al. J Clin Oncol 1998;16:3169–3178

Dose Modifications

Dosage Levels*

800 mg
600 mg
400 mg
300 mg
200 mg

Adverse Event	Treatment Modification
Hematologic*	
G1/2	No modifications
Recurrence of a G2 toxicity	Hold imatinib until toxicity resolves to G ≤1; then restart at 1 lower dose level
First episode of a G3/4 toxicity	Hold imatinib until toxicity resolves to G ≤1; then restart at the same dose
Second episode of a G3/4 toxicity	Hold imatinib until toxicity resolves to G ≤1; then restart at 1 lower dose level
Recurrent G2/3/4 at a reduced dose	Hold imatinib until toxicity resolves to G ≤1; then restart at 1 dose level lower, or for recurrent G4, consider discontinuing imatinib
Nonhematologic	
G1	No dose modifications
First episode of a G2 toxicity	Hold imatinib until toxicity resolves to G ≤1; then restart at the same dose
Recurrence of a G2 toxicity (second G2)	Hold imatinib until toxicity resolves to G ≤1; then restart at 1 lower dose level
G3/4	Hold imatinib until toxicity resolves to G ≤1; then restart at 1 lower dose level
Recurrent G2/3/4 at a reduced dose	Hold imatinib until toxicity resolves to G ≤1; then restart at 1 dose level lower, or for recurrent G4, consider discontinuing imatinib

*No dose modifications for anemia. Growth factors were allowed but not recommended

Patient Population Studied

Patients from 2 distinct phase II trials of imatinib (400–800 mg daily) in patients with locally advanced or metastatic DFSP were conducted and closed prematurely, one in Europe (European Organization for Research and Treatment of Cancer [EORTC]) with 14-week progression-free rate as the primary end point and the other in North America (Southwest Oncology Group [SWOG]) with confirmed objective response rate as the primary end point. In the EORTC trial, confirmation of *PDGFB* rearrangement was required, and surgery was undertaken after 14 weeks if feasible. The SWOG study confirmed t(17;22) after enrollment

Efficacy

Dermatofibrosarcoma Protuberans (DFSP) Best Response by Subtype (N = 24)

	Number of Patients					
	Partial Response*		Stable Disease		Progressive Disease	
	Imatinib (mg/day)					
	400	800	400	800	400	800
DFSP classic	2	4	3	2	—	—
DFSP fibrosarcomatous	2	3		1	—	2
DFSP pigmented	—	—	—	—	—	1
Not DFSP	—	—	—	—	1	—
All patients (N = 24)	45.9% (11/24)					
Primary tumors	71% (5/7)					
Locally recurrent tumors N =12)	33% (4/12)					

Response, Progression, and Survival Status of Patients with Dermatofibrosarcoma Protuberans After Imatinib Therapy in the EORTC and SWOG Trials

| Response, Progression, and Survival Status | EORTC (N = 16) | | SWOG (N = 8) | | Total (N = 24) | |
	No.	%	No.	%	No.	%
Response at 14–16 Weeks						
Partial response	5	31.3	4	50	9	37.5
Stable disease	6	37.5	2	25	8	33.3
Progressive disease	3	18.8	1	12.5	4	16.7
Not evaluable	2	12.4	1	12.5	3	12.5
Best Overall Response						
Partial response (confirmed)	3	18.8	4	50	7	29.2
Partial response (resected)	4	25	0	0	4	16.7
Stable disease	4	25	2	25	6	25
Progressive disease	3	18.8	1	12.5	4	16.6
Not evaluable	2	12.5	1	12.5	3	12.5
Progression Status						
Progression-free	8	50	4	50	12	50
Progression	8	50	4	50	12	50
Survival Status						
Alive	10	62.5	8	100	18	75
Dead	6	37.5	0	0	6	25
Cause of Death						
Progression	5	31.3	0	0	5	20.8

EORTC, European Organization for Research and Treatment of Cancer; SWOG, Southwest Oncology Group
*Four PRs not confirmed—resection of residual disease after >14 weeks of therapy

Toxicity
Adverse Events from Imatinib Reported in Patients with DFSP*

Adverse Event	EORTC (N = 16)						SWOG (N = 8)						Total (N = 24)					
	No.	%	No.	%	No.	%	No.	%	No.	%	No.	%	No.	%	No.	%	No.	%
Leukopenia	4	25	2	12.5	1	6.3	2	25	0	0	0	0	6	25	2	8.3	1	4.2
Neutropenia	2	12.5	1	6.3	2	12.5	0	0	0	0	2	25	2	8.3	1	4.2	4	16.7
Thrombocytopenia	1	6.3	0	0	1	6.3	0	0	0	0	0	0	1	4.2	0	0	1‡	4.2
Anemia	11	68.8	4	25	0	0	1	12.5	0	0	1	12.5	12	50	4	16.7	1	4.2
Bilirubin	4	25	1	6.3	1	6.3	0	0	0	0	0	0	4	16.7	1	4.2	1	4.2
AST increase	4	25	1	6.3	1	6.3	2	25	0	0	0	0	6	25	1	4.2	1‡	4.2
Hypertension†	1	6.3	1	6.3	0	0	0	0	0	0	0	0	1	4.2	1	4.2	0	0
Fatigue	3	18.8	2	12.5	2	12.5	5	62.5	0	0	2	25	8	33.3	2	8.3	4	16.7
Rash	4	25	1	6.3	1	6.3	3	37.5	0	0	0	0	7	29.2	1	4.2	1	4.2
Anorexia	2	12.5	0	0	0	0	2	25	0	0	0	0	4	16.7	0	0	0	0
Diarrhea	3	18.8	3	18.8	0	0	1	12.5	0	0	1	12.5	4	16.7	3	12.5	1	4.2
Nausea	3	18.8	2	12.5	1	6.3	4	50	0	0	0	0	7	29.2	2	8.3	1	4.2
Vomiting	1	6.3	0	0	2	12.5	1	12.5	0	0	0	0	2	8.3	0	0	2	8.3
H&N edema†	6	37.5	0	0	0	0	5	62.5	0	0	0	0	11	45.8	0	0	0	0
L/T/V edema†	6	37.5	1	6.3	1	6.3	5	62.5	0	0	0	0	11	45.8	1	4.2	1	4.2
Pain	3	18.8	0	0	0	0	0	0	0	0	1	12.5	3	12.5	0	0	1	4.2

DFSP, Dermatofibrosarcoma protuberans; EORTC, European Organization for Research and Treatment of Cancer; SWOG, Southwest Oncology Group; No., number of patients; %, percentage of patients
*National Cancer Institute (USA), Common Terminology Criteria for Adverse Events, version 3.0
†Hypertension, arterial hypertension; H&N edema, head and neck edema; L/T/V edema: limbs/truncal/visceral edema
‡Grade 4; 2 toxic grade 4 events were noted in 1 patient with preexisting liver disturbances and alcohol abuse history: thrombocytopenia and increased serum AST

Therapy Monitoring

1. *Day 7 and at least monthly for 6 months, then every 3 months:* History and physical examination
2. *Weekly:* Complete blood count with leukocyte differential count
3. *Twice monthly first 2 months, then monthly for 6, then every 3 months:* Liver function tests
4. *At end of month 2 and every 3 months thereafter:* Radiographic assessments were using the same modality as had been performed at baseline

SOFT-TISSUE SARCOMAS: GI STROMAL TUMORS (GIST)

Epidemiology

Incidence: 2000–5000 estimated cases in the United States annually
Male to female ratio: 1:1

Gastrointestinal stromal tumors (GIST) account for <1% of all primary tumors of the gastrointestinal tract

Site of Disease	% of Patients
Stomach	60–70
Small bowel	20–30
Other*	10

*Large bowel, esophagus, rectum, mesentery, and omentum

Work-up

1. History and physical examination
2. *Laboratory tests:* CBC with differential, electrolytes, LFTs
3. PA and lateral chest x-ray
4. Contrast-enhanced CT scan of chest, abdomen, and pelvis
5. PET scan can complement conventional CT helping to differentiate benign from malignant tissue (Van den Abbeele A, Badawi R. Eur J Cancer 2002;38(Suppl 5):S60–S65)
6. Upper endoscopy or endoscopic ultrasound-guided (EUS) fine-needle biopsy to obtain a tissue diagnosis. EUS can usually accurately differentiate leiomyoma and leiomyosarcoma

Histologic Classification

Cell Type	% of Tumors
Spindle	70
Epithelioid	20
Mixed	10

KIT Mutations

Mutation	Site	% Incidence
Exon 11	Juxtamembrane domain	67
Exon 9	External domain	17
Exon 13	TK1	2
Exon 17	TK2	2
None*		13

*Wild-type *KIT*, although some have mutant *PDGFRA*
Heinrich MC et al. J Clin Oncol 2002;21:4342–4349

Expert Opinion

1. GIST consist of mesenchymal tumors that arise from the interstitial cells of Cajal (ICC) in the myenteric plexus
2. The true incidence of these tumors remains unknown, because until relatively recently, they were classified as tumors either of smooth muscle (eg, leiomyosarcomas) or of neural crest origin (eg, schwannomas)
3. Because nearly all GIST express the cell surface tyrosine kinase receptor, c-*KIT*, immunohistochemical staining facilitates the diagnosis
4. More than 90% of patients with GIST have activating *KIT* or *PDGFR-α* mutations (platelet-derived growth factor receptor-α)
5. Oncogenic mutations result in activation of *KIT* and its downstream pathways leading to uncontrolled cell division and resistance to apoptosis
6. Complete surgical resection remains the gold standard in the treatment of localized GIST. The goal of surgery is to remove all disease with negative resection margins. This is accomplished in up to 60% of GIST. Because nodal metastases are rare, lymphadenectomy is unnecessary. However, peritoneal surfaces and liver should be closely examined at laparotomy for evidence of metastatic spread
7. Despite curative resection, most patients subsequently have recurrence; the median time to recurrence is 1.5–2 years. The most acceptable and easily applied morphologic criteria for predicting tumor behavior are tumor size and mitotic rate
8. GIST is considered resistant to standard chemotherapy regimens for sarcomas such as doxorubicin and ifosfamide
9. Imatinib (STI571/Glivec/Gleevec) is an orally administered small-molecule selective tyrosine kinase inhibitor that is active in GIST (Demetri et al). Imatinib inhibits the activity of tyrosine kinases such as Bcr-Abl, PDGFR-α and the stem cell factor receptor c-*KIT*. As a competitive antagonist of ATP binding, imatinib blocks the ability of the kinases to transfer phosphate groups from ATP to tyrosine residues on substrate proteins, interrupting signal transduction
10. Clinical response to imatinib and survival rates seem to correlate with the presence or absence of certain *KIT* mutations: Mutations in exon 11 that encodes the intracellular juxtamembrane domain account for ≈70% of cases and are associated with an 85% response rate to imatinib
11. Imatinib is less effective in tumors without *KIT* mutations and in those with *KIT* mutations other than exon 11
12. The mutational status of *KIT* also seems to influence the progression-free survival, with longer survival in patients who harbor exon 11 mutations compared with those lacking an exon 11 mutation (Singer et al, J Clin Oncol 2002;20:3898–3905)
13. Because PDGFR-α is also an imatinib substrate, some tumors without *KIT* mutations respond to imatinib. However, unlike *KIT* mutations, most *PDGFR-α* mutations occur in the kinase domain and are unresponsive to imatinib
14. Over time, acquired resistance to imatinib is seen in approximately 20% of patients. In view of the high likelihood of tumor recurrence in these patients, imatinib is now recommended in the adjuvant setting. It is possible that it will have its maximal effect in the setting of minimal disease
15. The ACOSOG Z9001 trial demonstrated that the risk of recurrence in patients with resected GIST could be reduced by 1 year of adjuvant imatinib. Subsequently, the SSGXVIII/AIO trial demonstrated that 3 years of adjuvant imatinib was superior to 1 year of therapy in patients at high risk of recurrence after surgery by prolonging both recurrence-free survival and overall survival

Demetri GD et al. N Engl J Med 2002;347:472–480
Singer S et al. J Clin Oncol 2002;20:3898–3905

ADJUVANT REGIMEN

IMATINIB MESYLATE FOR 1 YEAR
(ACOSOG Z9001)

DeMatteo RP et al. Lancet 2009;373:1097–1104

Starting dose: **Imatinib mesylate** 400 mg/day; administer orally with food and a large glass of water (total dose/week = 2800 mg)

Dose escalation: **Imatinib mesylate** 600–800 mg/day; administer orally with food and a large glass of water (total dose/week = 4200–5600 mg)

Notes:

• 400- and 600-mg doses may be given once daily, or, alternatively, may be split into 2 equal doses, one given during morning hours and a second dose during the evening

• 800-mg daily doses should be given as two 400-mg doses, one during morning hours and a second dose during the evening

• For patients unable to swallow the film-coated tablets, imatinib mesylate may be dispersed in a glass of water or apple juice. The required number of tablets should be placed in an appropriate volume of beverage (approximately 50 mL for a 100-mg tablet, and 200 mL for a 400-mg tablet) and stirred with a spoon. The suspension should be administered immediately after the tablets have completely disintegrated

Supportive Care

Antiemetic prophylaxis

Emetogenic potential is **LOW**

See Chapter 39 for antiemetic recommendations

Hematopoietic growth factor (CSF) prophylaxis

Primary prophylaxis is NOT indicated

See Chapter 43 for more information

Antimicrobial prophylaxis

Risk of fever and neutropenia is LOW

Antimicrobial primary prophylaxis to be considered:

• Antibacterial—not indicated

• Antifungal—not indicated

• Antiviral—not indicated unless patient previously had an episode of HSV

See Chapter 47 for more information

Diarrhea management

Latent or delayed onset diarrhea*:

Loperamide 4 mg orally initially after the first loose or liquid stool, *then*

Loperamide 2 mg orally every 2 hours during waking hours, *plus*

Loperamide 4 mg orally every 4 hours during hours of sleep

• Continue for at least 12 hours after diarrhea resolves

• Recurrent diarrhea after a 12-hour diarrhea-free interval is treated as a new episode

• Rehydrate orally with fluids and electrolytes during a diarrheal episode

• If a patient develops blood or mucus in stool, dehydration, or hemodynamic instability, or if diarrhea persists >48 hours despite loperamide, stop loperamide and hospitalize the patient for IV hydration

Alternatively, a trial of **Diphenoxylate hydrochloride** 2.5 mg **with Atropine sulfate** 0.025 mg (eg, Lomotil)

• Initial adult dose is 2 tablets 4 times daily until control has been achieved, after which the dose may be reduced to meet individual requirements. Control may often be maintained with as little as 2 tablets daily

• Clinical improvement of acute diarrhea is usually observed within 48 hours. If improvement of chronic diarrhea after treatment with a maximum daily dose of 8 tablets is not observed within 10 days, control is unlikely with further administration

*Abigerges D et al. J Natl Cancer Inst 1994;86:446–449

Rothenberg ML et al. J Clin Oncol 2001;19:3801–3807

Wadler S et al. J Clin Oncol 1998;16:3169–3178

Dose Modifications

Dosage Levels*

Initial dose	400 mg/day
First dose reduction	300 mg/day
Second dose reduction	200 mg/day

Hematologic*

G1/2	No modifications
Recurrence of a G2 toxicity	Hold imatinib until toxicity resolves to G ≤1, then restart at 1 lower dose level
First episode of a G3/4 toxicity	Hold imatinib until toxicity resolves to G ≤1, then restart at the same dose
Second episode of a G3/4 toxicity	Hold imatinib until toxicity resolves to G ≤1, then restart at 1 lower dose level
Recurrent G2/3/4 at a reduced dose	Hold imatinib until toxicity resolves to G ≤1, then restart at 1 lower dose level, or for recurrent G4, consider discontinuing imatinib

Nonhematologic

G1	No dose modifications
First episode of a G2 toxicity	Hold imatinib until toxicity resolves to G ≤1, then restart at the same dose
Recurrence of a G2 toxicity (second G2)	Hold imatinib until toxicity resolves to G ≤1, then restart at 1 lower dose level
G3/4	Hold imatinib until toxicity resolves to G ≤1, then restart at 1 lower dose level
Recurrent G2/3/4 at a reduced dose	Hold imatinib until toxicity resolves to G ≤1, then restart at 1 dose level lower, or for recurrent G4, consider discontinuing imatinib

*No dose modifications for anemia. Growth factors were allowed but not recommended

Efficacy (N = 359)
Median Follow-up for Surviving Patients = 19.7 Months

	Imatinib	Placebo	Hazard ratio Imatinib vs. Placebo
Estimated 1-year recurrence-free survival	98% (95% CI, 96–100)	83% (95% CI, 78–88)	0.35 (0.22–0.53) (p <0.0001)
Recurrence free survival tumor size >3 and <6 cm			0.23 (0.07–0.79) (p <0.011)
Recurrence free survival tumor size >6 and <10 cm			0.50 (0.25–0.98) (p <0.041)
Recurrence free survival tumor size >10 cm			0.29 (0.16–0.55) (p <0.0001)
Overall survival			0.66 (0.22–2.03) (p = 0.47)
Tumor recurrence or death at median follow-up of 19.7 months			30 (8%)

Adverse Events (N = 359)

Dose reduction or interruption, or both	59 (16%)
Dose reduction or interruption, because of adverse events	52 (15%)

(N = 337) Data are Number (%)*

	Grade 1	Grade 2	Grade 3	Grade 4
Toxicity, all patients, all toxicities	81 (24%)	148 (44%)	86 (26%)	15 (4%)
Neutropenia	23 (6%)	26 (7%)	7 (2%)	5 (1%)
Fatigue	117 (33%)	20 (5%)	5 (1%)	2 (<1%)
Dermatitis	54 (15%)	15 (4%)	11 (3%)	0
Abdominal pain	61 (17%)	25 (7%)	12 (3%)	0
Nausea	78 (22%)	14 (4%)	8 (2%)	0
Vomiting	37 (10%)	9 (2%)	8 (2%)	0
Diarrhea	79 (22%)	17 (4%)	10 (2%)	0
ALT	38 (11%)	9 (2%)	7 (2%)	2 (<1%)
AST	31 (9%)	4 (1%)	4 (1%)	3 (<1%)
Edema	220 (65%)	32 (9%)	7 (2%)	0
Hyperglycemia	27 (8%)	9 (2%)	2 (<1%)	0
Hypokalemia	28 (8%)	0	4 (1%)	0
Syncope	1 (<1%)	0	4 (1%)	0
Dyspnea	13 (3%)	1 (1%)	4 (1%)	0

ALT, alanine aminotransferase; AST, aspartate aminotransferase
*Grade 5:3 (1%)

Patient Population Studied

Randomized phase III, double-blind, placebo-controlled, multicenter trial. Eligible patients had complete gross resection of a primary GIST ≥3 cm in size and positive for the KIT protein by immunohistochemistry. Patients were randomly assigned to imatinib 400 mg (N = 359) or to placebo (N = 354) daily for 1 year after surgical resection. Patients and investigators were blinded to the treatment assignments. Patients assigned to placebo were eligible to crossover to imatinib treatment in the event of tumor recurrence. The primary end point was recurrence-free survival, and analysis was by intention-to-treat. Accrual was stopped early because the trial results crossed the interim analysis efficacy boundary for recurrence-free survival in favor of imatinib

Therapy Monitoring

1. *Day 7 and at least monthly for 6 months, then every 3 months:* History and physical examination
2. *Weekly:* Complete blood count with leukocyte differential count
3. *Twice monthly first 2 months, then monthly × 6, then every 3 months:* Liver function tests
4. *Every 3 months for the first 2 years, and every 6 months for the next 3 years:* CT scans with intravenous and oral contrast (or MRI with intravenous contrast) of the abdomen and pelvis

ADJUVANT REGIMEN

IMATINIB MESYLATE FOR 3 YEARS
(SSGXVIII/AIO)

Joensuu H et al. JAMA 2012;307:1265–1272

Starting dose: **Imatinib mesylate** 400 mg/day; administer orally with food and a large glass of water (total dose/week = 2800 mg)

Dose escalation: **Imatinib mesylate** 600–800 mg/day; administer orally with food and a large glass of water (total dose/week = 4200–5600 mg)

Notes:
- 400- and 600-mg doses may be given once daily, or, alternatively, may be split into 2 equal doses, one given during morning hours and a second dose during the evening
- 800-mg daily doses should be given as two 400-mg doses, one during morning hours and a second dose during the evening
- For patients unable to swallow the film-coated tablets, imatinib mesylate may be dispersed in a glass of water or apple juice. The required number of tablets should be placed in an appropriate volume of beverage (approximately 50 mL for a 100-mg tablet, and 200 mL for a 400-mg tablet) and stirred with a spoon. The suspension should be administered immediately after the tablets have completely disintegrated

Supportive Care
Antiemetic prophylaxis
Emetogenic potential is **LOW**
See Chapter 39 for antiemetic recommendations

Hematopoietic growth factor (CSF) prophylaxis
Primary prophylaxis is NOT indicated
See Chapter 43 for more information

Antimicrobial prophylaxis
Risk of fever and neutropenia is LOW
  Antimicrobial primary prophylaxis to be considered:
- Antibacterial—not indicated
- Antifungal—not indicated
- Antiviral—not indicated unless patient previously had an episode of HSV

See Chapter 47 for more information

Diarrhea management
Latent or delayed onset diarrhea*:
Loperamide 4 mg orally initially after the first loose or liquid stool, *then*
Loperamide 2 mg orally every 2 hours during waking hours, *plus*
Loperamide 4 mg orally every 4 hours during hours of sleep
- Continue for at least 12 hours after diarrhea resolves
- Recurrent diarrhea after a 12-hour diarrhea-free interval is treated as a new episode
- Rehydrate orally with fluids and electrolytes during a diarrheal episode
- If a patient develops blood or mucus in stool, dehydration, or hemodynamic instability, or if diarrhea persists >48 hours despite loperamide, stop loperamide and hospitalize the patient for IV hydration

Alternatively, a trial of **Diphenoxylate hydrochloride** 2.5 mg **with Atropine sulfate** 0.025 mg (eg, Lomotil)
- Initial adult dose is 2 tablets 4 times daily until control has been achieved, after which the dose may be reduced to meet individual requirements. Control may often be maintained with as little as 2 tablets daily
- Clinical improvement of acute diarrhea is usually observed within 48 hours. If improvement of chronic diarrhea after treatment with a maximum daily dose of 8 tablets is not observed within 10 days, control is unlikely with further administration

*Abigerges D et al. J Natl Cancer Inst 1994;86:446–449
Rothenberg ML et al. J Clin Oncol 2001;19:3801–3807
Wadler S et al. J Clin Oncol 1998;16:3169–3178

Dose Modifications

Dosage Levels*

Initial dose	400 mg/day
First dose reduction	300 mg/day
Second dose reduction	200 mg/day

Hematologic*

G1/2	No modifications
Recurrence of a G2 toxicity	Hold imatinib until toxicity resolves to G ≤1, then restart at 1 lower dose level
First episode of a G3/4 toxicity	Hold imatinib until toxicity resolves to G ≤1, then restart at the same dose
Second episode of a G3/4 toxicity	Hold imatinib until toxicity resolves to G ≤1, then restart at 1 lower dose level
Recurrent G2/3/4 at a reduced dose	Hold imatinib until toxicity resolves to G ≤1, then restart at 1 dose level lower, or for recurrent G4, consider discontinuing imatinib

Nonhematologic

G1	No dose modifications
First episode of a G2 toxicity	Hold imatinib until toxicity resolves to G ≤1, then restart at the same dose
Recurrence of a G2 toxicity (second G2)	Hold imatinib until toxicity resolves to G ≤1, then restart at 1 lower dose level
G3/4	Hold imatinib until toxicity resolves to G ≤1, then restart at 1 lower dose level
Recurrent G2/3/4 at a reduced dose	Hold imatinib until toxicity resolves to G ≤1, then restart at 1 dose level lower, or for recurrent G4, consider discontinuing imatinib

*No dose modifications for anemia. Growth factors were allowed but not recommended

Toxicity
(See Also Data from Imatinib for 1 Year and Imatinib in Metastatic Disease)

	Duration of Adjuvant Imatinib		
	12 Months N = 194*	36 Months N = 198*	p-Value
Any adverse event	192 (99%)	198 (100%)	0.24
G3/4 event	39 (20%)	65 (33%)	0.006
Cardiac event	8 (4%)	4 (2%)	0.26
Second cancer	14 (7%)	13 (7%)	0.84
Death, possibly imatinib-related	1 (1%)	0	0.49
Discontinued imatinib, no GIST recurrence	25 (13%)	51 (26%)	0.001

Most Frequent Adverse Events

	Any Grade			G3/4		
	% Any Grade		p-Value	% G3/4		p-Value
Duration of Imatinib	12 Months	36 Months		12 Months	36 Months	
Anorexia	72	80	0.08	1	1	1
Periorbital edema	59	74	0.002	1	1	1
Elevated LDH	43	60	0.001	0	0	—
Fatigue	48	48	1	1	1	0.62
Nausea	45	51	0.23	2	1	0.37
Diarrhea	44	54	0.044	1	2	0.37
Leukopenia	35	47	0.014	2	3	0.75
Muscle cramps	31	49	<0.001	1	1	1

*Safety cohort

Efficacy (Median Follow-up: 54 Months)

	Duration of Adjuvant Imatinib	
Efficacy End Points	12 Months N = 199*	36 Months N = 198*
Recurrence-free survival ITT population†	115 (57.8%)	148 (74.7%)
Recurrence-free survival ITT population 3 years†	60.1%	86.6%
	HR, 1.31; 95% CI, 0.65–2.62	
Recurrence-free survival ITT population 5 years†	47.9%	65.6%
	HR, 0.46; 95% CI; 0.32–0.65; P < .001)	
Overall survival at 3 years‡	94%	96.3%
Overall survival at 5 years‡	81.7%	92%
	HR, 0.45; 95% CI, 0.22–0.89; P = .02	

Cause of Death

GIST	25 (13%)	12 (6%)
Another cause with recurrence of GIST	6 (3%)	2 (1%)
Another cause, no GIST recurrence	5 (3%)	2 (1%)

*ITT cohort
†Hazard ratio 0.46 (95% CI, 0.32–0.65), p <0.0001
‡Hazard ratio 0.45 (95% CI, 0.22–0.89), p = 0.019

Patient Population Studied

A randomized phase III multicenter trial of adjuvant imatinib as treatment of operable GIST with a high risk of recurrence (SSGXVIII/AIO) according to the modified consensus criteria (Fletcher CDM et al. Hum Pathol 2002;33:459–465). Eligible patients had complete gross resection and of a primary GIST positive that was for the KIT protein by immunohistochemistry
Patients must also have a high risk of recurrence

• Tumor diameter >10 cm
• Tumor mitosis count >10/50 high-power fields, or
• Tumor rupture spontaneously or at surgery

Patients were randomly assigned to imatinib 400 mg daily for 1 or 3 years after surgical resection. Stratification: (a) R0 resection, no tumor rupture; (b) R1 resection or tumor rupture

Therapy Monitoring

First year:
1. *Every 1–3 months:* History and physical examination
2. *Every 2–12 weeks:* Complete blood counts with leukocyte differential and serum chemistry
3. *Every 6 months:* CT/MRI of abdomen and pelvis

Years 2 and 3:
1. *Every 6 months:* History and physical examination
2. *Every 6 months:* Complete blood counts with leukocyte differential and serum chemistry
3. *Every 6 months:* CT/MRI of abdomen and pelvis

METASTATIC REGIMEN

IMATINIB MESYLATE

Blanke CD et al. J Clin Oncol 2008;26:626–632
Verweij J et al. Lancet 2004;364:1127–1134

Starting dose: **Imatinib mesylate** 400 mg/day; administer orally with food and a large glass of water (total dose/week = 2800 mg)

Dose escalation: **Imatinib** 600–800 mg/day; administer orally with food and a large glass of water (total dose/week = 4200–5600 mg)

Notes:

- 400- and 600-mg doses may be given once daily, or, alternatively, may be split into 2 equal doses, one given during morning hours and a second dose during the evening
- 800-mg daily doses should be given as two 400-mg doses, one during morning hours and a second dose during the evening
- For patients unable to swallow the film-coated tablets, imatinib mesylate may be dispersed in a glass of water or apple juice. The required number of tablets should be placed in an appropriate volume of beverage (approximately 50 mL for a 100-mg tablet, and 200 mL for a 400-mg tablet) and stirred with a spoon. The suspension should be administered immediately after the tablets have completely disintegrated

Supportive Care

Antiemetic prophylaxis

Emetogenic potential is **LOW**

See Chapter 39 for antiemetic recommendations

Hematopoietic growth factor (CSF) prophylaxis

Primary prophylaxis is NOT indicated

See Chapter 43 for more information

Antimicrobial prophylaxis

Risk of fever and neutropenia is LOW

Antimicrobial primary prophylaxis to be considered:

- Antibacterial—not indicated
- Antifungal—not indicated
- Antiviral—not indicated unless patient previously had an episode of HSV

See Chapter 47 for more information

Diarrhea management

Latent or delayed onset diarrhea*:

Loperamide 4 mg orally initially after the first loose or liquid stool, *then*
Loperamide 2 mg orally every 2 hours during waking hours, *plus*
Loperamide 4 mg orally every 4 hours during hours of sleep

- Continue for at least 12 hours after diarrhea resolves
- Recurrent diarrhea after a 12-hour diarrhea-free interval is treated as a new episode
- Rehydrate orally with fluids and electrolytes during a diarrheal episode
- If a patient develops blood or mucus in stool, dehydration, or hemodynamic instability, or if diarrhea persists >48 hours despite loperamide, stop loperamide and hospitalize the patient for IV hydration

Alternatively, a trial of **Diphenoxylate hydrochloride** 2.5 mg **with Atropine sulfate** 0.025 mg (eg, Lomotil)

- Initial adult dose is 2 tablets 4 times daily until control has been achieved, after which the dose may be reduced to meet individual requirements. Control may often be maintained with as little as 2 tablets daily
- Clinical improvement of acute diarrhea is usually observed within 48 hours. If improvement of chronic diarrhea after treatment with a maximum daily dose of 8 tablets is not observed within 10 days, control is unlikely with further administration

*Abigerges D et al. J Natl Cancer Inst 1994;86:446–449
Rothenberg ML et al. J Clin Oncol 2001;19:3801–3807
Wadler S et al. J Clin Oncol 1998;16:3169–3178

Dose Modifications

Dose Levels*
800 mg
600 mg
400 mg
300 mg
200 mg

Hematologic*	
G1/2	No modifications
Recurrence of a G2 toxicity	Hold imatinib until toxicity resolves to G ≤1, then restart with dose decreased by 1 dose level
First episode of a G3/4 toxicity	Hold imatinib until toxicity resolves to G ≤1, then restart at the same dose
Second episode of a G3/4 toxicity	Hold imatinib until toxicity resolves to G ≤1, then restart with dose decreased by 1 dose level
Recurrent G2/3/4 at a reduced dose	Hold imatinib until toxicity resolves to G ≤1, then restart with dose decreased by 1 dose level, or, for recurrent G4 adverse effects, consider discontinuing imatinib

Nonhematologic	
G1	No dose modifications
First episode of a G2 toxicity	Hold imatinib until toxicity resolves to G ≤1, then restart at the same dose
Recurrence of a G2 toxicity (second G2)	Hold imatinib until toxicity resolves to G ≤1, then restart with dose decreased by 1 dose level
G3/4	Hold imatinib until toxicity resolves to G ≤1, then restart with dose decreased by 1 dose level
Recurrent G2/3/4 at a reduced dose	Hold imatinib until toxicity resolves to G ≤1, then restart with dose decreased by 1 dose level , or for recurrent G4 adverse effects, consider discontinuing imatinib

*No dose modifications for anemia. Hematopoietic growth factors are allowed but not recommended

Efficacy*,†

Response	400 mg/day‡		800 mg/day	
	Number	Percent	Number	Percent
Complete response	17	5	12	3
Partial response	137	40	148	42
Stable/no response	85	25	76	22
Progressive disease/early death	42	12	37	10
Assessment inadequate	34	10	52	15
Total	345	100	349	100

*Blanke CD et al. J Clin Oncol 2008;26:626–632
†RECIST (Response Evaluation Criteria in Solid Tumors; Therasse P et al. J Natl Cancer Inst 2000;92:205–216)
‡After progression on 400 mg/day, 33% of patients who crossed over to 800 mg/day achieved either an objective response or stable disease

Adverse Event*,†

Adverse Events	400 mg/day (n = 344)			800 mg/day (n = 347)		
	% G3	% G4	% G5	% G3	% G4	% G5
Death, cause undetermined	0	0	0	0	0	1
Allergy/immunology	0	0	0	<0.5	0	0
Auditory/hearing	0	0	0	<0.5	0	0
Blood/bone marrow	15	4	<0.5	19	8	0
Cardiovascular, Arrhythmia	2	0	0	1	0	<0.5
Cardiovascular, General	4	1	0	10	2	0
Constitutional symptoms	4	1	0	8	1	<0.5
Dermatology/skin	4	<0.5	0	7	<0.5	0
Gastrointestinal	8	1	0	15	1	0
Hemorrhage	4	1	1	8	2	1
Hepatic	4	0	0	2	1	<0.5
Infection/febrile neutropenia	4	1	0	5	1	1
Metabolic/laboratory	2	0	0	2	1	0
Musculoskeletal	1	0	0	1	0	0
Neurology	3	1	0	2	0	1
Ocular/visual	0	0	0	1	0	0
Pain	10	1	0	11	1	0
Pulmonary	2	1	0	4	0	0
Renal/genitourinary	1	0	0	1	1	0
Syndrome	0	0	0	<0.5	0	0

*Blanke CD et al. J Clin Oncol 2008;26:626–632
†National Cancer Institute (USA), Common Toxicity Criteria, version 2.0 (NCI CTC v2.0)

Patient Population Studied

Seven-hundred forty-six patients metastatic or surgically unresectable GIST were eligible for this phase III open-label clinical trial. At registration, patients were randomly assigned to either standard- or high-dose imatinib with close interval follow-up. If objective progression occurred by RECIST, patients on the standard-dose arm could reregister to the trial and receive the high-dose imatinib regimen. Patients were required to have measurable or nonmeasurable, visceral or intraabdominal, biopsy-proven GIST, which were not surgically curable. Tumors had to express CD117 by immunohistochemical staining. Any number of prior chemotherapy regimens was allowed

Best Overall Response to Treatment (Intention-to-Treat Analysis)*,†

	400 mg Once Daily (n = 473)	400 mg Twice Daily (n = 473)
Complete response	5%	6%
Partial response	45%	48%
No change	32%	32%
Progression	13%	9%
Not assessable	5%	5%

*Verweij J et al. Lancet 2004;364:1127–1134
†RECIST

Notes: These studies confirmed the effectiveness of imatinib as primary systemic therapy for patients with incurable GIST but showed limited advantage to higher dose (800 mg) treatment. The authors concluded:

- It appears reasonable to initiate therapy with 400 mg daily and to consider dose escalation on progression of disease (Blanke CD et al. J Clin Oncol 2008;26:626–632)
- If response induction is the only aim of treatment, a daily dose of 400 mg of imatinib is sufficient; however, a dose of 400 mg twice daily achieves significantly longer progression-free survival (Verweij J et al. Lancet 2004;364:1127–1134)

Adverse Event[*–‡]

	400 mg once daily (n = 470)				400 mg twice daily (n = 472)			
	% G1	% G2	% G3	% G4	% G1	% G2	% G3	% G4
Any side effect	21	46	26	6.2	8.7	40	43	7.6
Anemia	55	27	5.5	1.5	41	40	12	5.1
Leucopenia	27	13	2.7	—	29	16	2.1	0.4
Granulocytopenia	20	13	4.3	2.7	19	17	4.7	2.3
Thrombocytopenia	3.8	0.6	1	0.4	4	1.3	0.4	0.8
Edema	50	18	2.7	0.2	42	36	8.7	0.4
Fatigue	45	19	6	—	38	31	11	0.2
Fever	8.3	2.7	0.8	—	13	3.2	1.3	—
Pruritus	12	3.6	0.8	—	15	7.6	1.5	—
Rash	17	7.2	2.3	—	26	16	5.1	0.2
Anorexia	16	7.8	1.7	0.2	25	13	1.7	—
Constipation	11	3.8	0.8	0.2	13	4	1.5	—
Diarrhea	34	12	1.5	0.2	36	15	5.3	—
Nausea	36	10	2.5	—	36	21	3.2	—
Vomiting	18	5.3	2.5	0.2	23	13	2.8	—
Bleeding	7.2	<1	2.5	0.2	14	0.6	6.4	1.7
Infection	7.2	7.2	2.5	0.2	8.7	7.6	4.4	0.2
Dizziness	9.4	1.4	0.2	—	11	1.9	0.4	—
Arthralgia	11	2.3	—	—	12	3.2	0.8	—
Headache	13	3.2	0.2	—	11	1.7	0.8	—
Myalgia	19	5.7	0.2	—	19	7.4	1	—
Pleuritic pain	34	13	4	0.4	30	18	7	0.2
Cough	11	1.7	0.2	—	11	2.8	0.2	—
Dyspnea	—	8.3	3	0.2	—	13	3.4	1
Renal or genitourinary	9.1	3.4	0.4	0.2	10	4.7	2.1	0.6

*Verweij J et al. Lancet 2004;364:1127–1134
†NCI CTC v2.0
‡Data are the percentage of patients who started treatment per protocol

Therapy Monitoring

1. *Day 7 and at least monthly for 6 months, then every 3 months:* History and physical examination
2. *Weekly:* Complete blood count with leukocyte differential
3. *Twice monthly for the first 2 months, then monthly for 6 months, then every 3 months:* Liver function tests
4. *At the end of month 2, and every 3 months thereafter:* Radiographic assessments using the same modality as had been performed at baseline

METASTATIC REGIMEN
SUNITINIB

Demetri GD et al. Lancet 2006;368:1329–1338

Starting dose: **Sunitinib malate** 50 mg; administer orally, daily, continually for 4 consecutive weeks followed by a 2-week period without treatment, every 6 weeks (total dose/week = 350 mg; total dose per 6-week cycle = 1400 mg)

Notes:
- Dose interruption and dose modifications in 12.5-mg increments or decrements are recommended based on individual safety and tolerability
- Strong CYP3A4 inhibitors may increase sunitinib plasma concentrations
    - When medically appropriate, replace concomitant strong CYP3A4 inhibitors with medications that do not or minimally inhibit CYP3A4
    - A dose reduction for sunitinib to 37.5 mg/day should be considered if sunitinib must be co-administered with a strong CYP3A4 inhibitor
- CYP3A4 inducers such as rifampin may decrease sunitinib plasma concentrations
    - When medically appropriate, replace concomitant CYP3A4 inducers with medications that do not or minimally induce CYP3A4
    - A dose increase for sunitinib to a maximum of 87.5 mg/day should be considered if sunitinib must be co-administered with a CYP3A4 inducer

Supportive Care
Antiemetic prophylaxis
Emetogenic potential is **LOW**
See Chapter 39 for antiemetic recommendations

Hematopoietic growth factor (CSF) prophylaxis
Primary prophylaxis is NOT indicated
See Chapter 43 for more information

Antimicrobial prophylaxis
Risk of fever and neutropenia is LOW
Antimicrobial primary prophylaxis to be considered:
- Antibacterial—not indicated
- Antifungal—not indicated
- Antiviral—not indicated unless patient previously had an episode of HSV

See Chapter 47 for more information

Diarrhea management
Latent or delayed onset diarrhea*:
   Loperamide 4 mg orally initially after the first loose or liquid stool, *then*
   Loperamide 2 mg orally every 2 hours during waking hours, *plus*
   Loperamide 4 mg orally every 4 hours during hours of sleep
- Continue for at least 12 hours after diarrhea resolves
- Recurrent diarrhea after a 12-hour diarrhea-free interval is treated as a new episode
- Rehydrate orally with fluids and electrolytes during a diarrheal episode
- If a patient develops blood or mucus in stool, dehydration, or hemodynamic instability, or if diarrhea persists >48 hours despite loperamide, stop loperamide and hospitalize the patient for IV hydration

   Alternatively, a trial of **Diphenoxylate hydrochloride** 2.5 mg **with Atropine sulfate** 0.025 mg (eg, Lomotil)
- Initial adult dose is 2 tablets 4 times daily until control has been achieved, after which the dose may be reduced to meet individual requirements. Control may often be maintained with as little as 2 tablets daily
- Clinical improvement of acute diarrhea is usually observed within 48 hours. If improvement of chronic diarrhea after treatment with a maximum daily dose of 8 tablets is not observed within 10 days, control is unlikely with further administration

*Abigerges D et al. J Natl Cancer Inst 1994;86:446–449
Rothenberg ML et al. J Clin Oncol 2001;19:3801–3807
Wadler S et al. J Clin Oncol 1998;16:3169–3178

Hand-foot reaction (palmar-plantar erythrodysesthesia, PPE)
For patients who develop a hand-foot reaction, use topical emollients (eg, Aquaphor), topical or orally administered steroids, antihistamine agents (H_1-receptor antagonists), or pyridoxine
   Pyridoxine may provide relief for discomfort/pain associated with PPE, although the mechanism through which this occurs remains unclear
- The suggested pyridoxine starting dose is 50 mg/day, which may be increased to a maximum of 200 mg/day

Oral care
Prophylaxis and treatment for mucositis/stomatitis
   General advice:
- Encourage patients to maintain intake of non-alcoholic fluids
- Evaluate patients for oral pain and provide analgesic medications
- Consider histamine (H_2-subtype) receptor antagonists (eg, ranitidine, famotidine), or a proton pump inhibitor for epigastric pain
- *Lactobacillus* sp.-containing probiotics may be beneficial in preventing diarrhea

(continued)

(*continued*)

Patients with intact oral mucosa:

• Clean the mouth, tongue, and gums by brushing after every meal and at bedtime with an ultra-soft toothbrush with fluoride toothpaste

• Floss teeth gently every day unless contraindicated. If gums bleed and hurt, avoid bleeding or sore areas, but floss other teeth

• Patients may use saline or commercial bland, non-alcoholic rinses

  ▪ Do not use mouthwashes that contain alcohols

If mucositis or stomatitis is present:

• Keep the mouth moist utilizing water, ice chips, sugarless gum, sugar-free hard candies, or a saliva substitute

• Rinse mouth several times a day to remove debris

  ▪ Use a solution of ¼ teaspoon (1.25 g) each of baking soda and table salt (sodium chloride) in one quart (~950 mL) of warm water. Follow with a plain water rinse

  ▪ Do not use mouthwashes that contain alcohols

• Foam-tipped swabs (eg, Toothettes®) are useful in moisturizing oral mucosa, but ineffective for cleansing teeth and removing plaque

• Advise patients who develop mucositis to:

  ▪ Choose foods that are easy to chew and swallow

  ▪ Take small bites of food, chew slowly, and sip liquids with meals

  ▪ Encourage soft, moist foods such as cooked cereals, mashed potatoes, and scrambled eggs

  ▪ For trouble swallowing, soften food with gravies, sauces, broths, yogurt, or other bland liquids

  ▪ Avoid sharp, crunchy foods; hot, spicy or highly acidic foods (eg, citrus fruits and juices); sugary foods; toothpicks; tobacco products; alcoholic drinks

Hypertension Management

Persistent **CTCAE G1** = Prehypertension: SBP 120–139 mm Hg; DBP 80–89 mm Hg

Antihypertensive therapy: None
Blood pressure monitoring: Standard
Sunitinib dose modification: No change

Persistent **CTCAE G1** = Stage 1 (moderate) HTN: SBP 140–159 mm Hg; DBP 90–99 mm Hg

Antihypertensive therapy:
Step 1 Initiate DHP-CCB treatment, and, if needed, after 24–48 hours, increase the dose in incremental steps every 24–48 hours until BP is controlled or a maximum dose is reached
Step 2 If BP still not controlled, add another antihypertensive, a BB, ACEI, ARB, or ABB. Increase dose of the second drug as described in Step 1
Step 3 If BP still not controlled, add a third drug from the antihypertensives listed in Step 2; increase dose of this drug as described in Step 1
Step 4 If BP is still not controlled, consider either 1 dose level reduction or discontinuing sunitinib

Note: Stopping or decreasing sunitinib doses is expected to cause a decrease in BP. Treating clinicians should monitor the patient for hypotension and adjust the number and dose of antihypertensive medications accordingly

Blood pressure monitoring: BP should be monitored as recommended by the treating clinician
Sunitinib dose modification: No changes except as described for Step 4

Persistent **CTCAE G3** = Stage 2 (severe) HTN: SBP >160 mm Hg; DBP >100 mm Hg

Antihypertensive therapy: Withhold sunitinib until systolic BP <159 mm Hg and diastolic BP <99 mm Hg
BP management is identical to that for Grade 2 (see Steps 1–4 above) with 2 major exceptions:
1. If SBP >180 mm Hg or DBP >110 mm Hg and the patient is symptomatic:
   Optimal management with intensive IV support in ICU. Discontinue sunitinib and notify other medically responsible healthcare providers that stopping sunitinib may result in a decrease in BP, *and*
2. If SBP >180 mm Hg or DBP >110 mm Hg and the patient is asymptomatic:
   Two new antihypertensives must be given together in Step 1 (and dose escalated appropriately as in Step 1)

Note: Stopping or decreasing sunitinib dose is expected to cause a decrease in BP. Treating clinicians should monitor the patient for hypotension and adjust the number and dose of antihypertensive medications accordingly

Blood pressure monitoring: BP should be monitored as recommended by the treating clinician unless the patient is symptomatic with SBP >180 mm Hg or DBP >110 mm Hg in which case, monitoring should be intensive
Sunitinib dose modification:
1. Withhold sunitinib until SBP <159 mm Hg and DBP <99 mm Hg
2. In most circumstances, if BP cannot be controlled after an optimal trial of antihypertensive medications, consider either 1 dose level reduction or discontinuing sunitinib
3. If a patient requires hospitalization for management of symptomatic SBP >180 mm Hg or DBP >110 mm Hg, permanently discontinue sunitinib, or if BP is controlled, resume sunitinib with dose decreased by 1 dose level

(*continued*)

Hypertension Management (*continued*)

CTCAE G4 = Life-threatening consequences of hypertension

Antihypertensive therapy:
1. Optimal management with intensive parenteral support in ICU
2. Discontinue sunitinib and notify other medically responsible healthcare providers that stopping sunitinib may result in a decrease in BP

Blood pressure monitoring: Intensive
Sunitinib dose modification: Permanently discontinue sunitinib, or if BP is controlled, resume sunitinib with dose decreased by one dose level

ABB, α/β-Adrenergic blockers; ACEI, angiotensin-converting enzyme inhibitors; ARB, angiotensin II receptor blockers; BB, selective β-adrenergic blockers; CTCAE, National Cancer Institute (USA), Common Terminology Criteria for Adverse Events; DBP, diastolic blood pressure; DHP-CCB, dihydropyridine calcium-channel blockers; HTN, hypertension; SBP, systolic blood pressure
Notes: (Hypertension grading is based on the CTCAE, version 4.0)
• When SBP and DBP fall into different categories, the higher category should be selected in classifying an individual's blood pressure status
• Discontinue sunitinib if patients require delaying treatment >2 weeks for management of hypertension
• Discontinue sunitinib if patients require >2 dose reductions
• Patients may receive up to 2 drugs for managing hypertension prior to decreasing sunitinib dose
• Allow an interval of at least 24 hours between modifications of antihypertensive therapy

Commercially Available Orally Administered Antihypertensives

Pharmacologic Categories	Drug Name* (formulation)	Initial Dose	Intermediate Dose	Maximum Recommended Dose	Metabolism
Dihydropyridine calcium-channel blockers (DHP-CCB)	Nifedipine (extended release)	**30 mg daily**	**60 mg daily**	**90 mg daily**	CYP3A4 substrate
	Amlodipine besylate	**2.5 mg daily**	**5 mg daily**	**10 mg daily**	CYP3A4 substrate
	Felodipine (extended release)	2.5 mg daily	5 mg daily	10 mg daily	CYP3A4 substrate and inhibitor
Selective β-adrenergic blockers (BB)	Metoprolol tartrate	25 mg twice daily	50 mg twice daily	100 mg twice daily	CYP2D6 substrate
	Atenolol	**25 mg daily**	**50 mg daily**	**100 mg daily**	No
	Acebutolol HCl	100 mg twice daily	200–300 mg twice daily	400 mg twice daily	Yes (CYP450 unknown)
	Bisoprolol fumarate	2.5 mg daily	5–10 mg daily	20 mg daily	Yes (CYP450 unknown)
Angiotensin-converting enzyme inhibitors (ACEIs)	Captopril	12.5 mg 3 times daily	25 mg 3 times daily	50 mg 3 times daily	CYP2D6 substrate
	Enalapril maleate	5 mg daily	10–20 mg daily	40 mg daily	CYP3A4 substrate
	Ramipril	2.5 mg daily	5 mg daily	10 mg daily	Liver esterases and phase II metabolism; ie, not CYP450
	Lisinopril	**5 mg daily**	**10–20 mg daily**	**40 mg daily**	Minimally, not CYP450
	Fosinopril sodium	10 mg daily	20 mg daily	40 mg daily	Hydrolyzed by intestinal and hepatic esterases; ie, not CYP450
	Perindopril erbumine • rarely used	**4 mg daily**	None	**8 mg daily**	Hydrolysis and phase II metabolism; ie, not CYP450
	Quinapril • rarely used	**10 mg daily**	**20 mg daily**	**40 mg daily**	No
Angiotensin II receptor blockers (ARBs)	Losartan	25 mg daily	50 mg daily	100 mg daily	CYP3A4 substrate
	Candesartan	4 mg daily	8–16 mg daily	32 mg daily	CYP2C9 substrate
	Irbesartan	75 mg daily	150 mg daily	300 mg daily	CYP2C9 substrate
	Telmisartan	**40 mg daily**	None	**80 mg daily**	Phase II metabolism; ie, not CYP450
	Valsartan	**80 mg daily**	None	**160 mg daily**	Minimally, not CYP450
α/β-Adrenergic blocker	Labetalol HCl	100 mg twice daily	200 mg twice daily	400 mg twice daily	CYP2D6 substrate and inhibitor

CYP450, cytochromes P450 superfamily enzymes
*Drugs in bold are suggested as optimal choices to avoid or minimize potential drug interactions with sunitinib through CYP3A4

Dose Modifications

Dose Levels

Dose level +3	87.5 mg/day
Dose level +2	75 mg/day
Dose level +1	62.5 mg/day
Starting dose level	50 mg/day
Dose level −1	37.5 mg/day
Dose level −2	25 mg/day

Adverse Events	Treatment Modifications
G ≥3 hematologic or nonhematologic toxicity G ≥3 fatigue G ≥3 stomatitis G ≥3 abnormalities in liver functions/hepatic adverse event	Reduce by 1 dose level, or, if administering 25 mg/day, discontinue therapy
Clinical manifestations of congestive heart failure (CHF)	Discontinue sunitinib
Patients without clinical evidence of CHF but with an ejection fraction <50%, and >20% below baseline	Interrupt sunitinib treatment and/or reduce the dose or, if administering 25 mg/day, discontinue therapy
G2/3/4 serum lipase or serum amylase	Hold therapy until level G1, then resume therapy
Coadministration of potent CYP3A4 inhibitors (eg, ketoconazole, itraconazole, clarithromycin, atazanavir, ritonavir, telithromycin)*	Reduce sunitinib dose to a minimum of 37.5 mg daily
Coadministration of potent CYP3A4 inducers (eg, rifampin, phenytoin, phenobarbital, dexamethasone, carbamazepine, St. John's, wort)*	Increase sunitinib dose 1 level to a maximum of 87.5 mg daily

*If a medication with no effect on enzyme activity cannot be substituted

Patient Population Studied

Patients with histologically proven malignant gastrointestinal stromal tumor that was not amenable to surgery, radiation, or a combination of different approaches with curative intent. Patients also must have had confirmed objective failure of previous imatinib therapy based either on progression of disease or unacceptably severe toxic effects during imatinib therapy that precluded further treatment. The last imatinib should have been administered at least 2 weeks before randomization

Efficacy

Efficacy Endpoints

	Sunitinib	Placebo	Hazard Ratio
End point	Duration (95% CI)	Duration (95% CI)	HR (95% CI)
Median time to tumor progression for the ITT population (primary study end point)*	27.3 weeks (16–32.1)	6.4 weeks (4.4–10)	HR 0.33 (0.23–0.47) p <0.0001
Median duration of progression-free survival	24.1 weeks (11.1–28.3)	6 weeks (4.4–9.9)	HR 0.33 (0.24–0.47) p <0.0001
Percent progression-free ≥26 weeks[†]	16% (33)	1% (1)	—
Overall survival[‡]			HR 0.49 (0.29–0.83) p = 0.007
Median time to tumor response	10.4 weeks (9.7–16.1)		

Response Rates

	Partial Response	Stable Disease	Progressive Disease
Best tumor response (ITT population)	7% (14)[§,€]	58% (120)	19% (39)
Patients who entered study > disease progression on imatinib (N = 198)	5.1% (10)		
Patients who crossed over to sunitinib from placebo group (N = 59)	10.2% (3.8–20.8)	7% (4)[**]	
Patients classified as intolerant to imatinib and randomized to sunitinib (N = 9)	44% (4)[††]		11% (1)

*Central radiology assessment
[†]26 weeks (≈6 months) predefined as point most clinicians agree clinically meaningful
[‡]Despite option to cross over. Also note that since > half the patients in sunitinib group were still alive at interim analysis, a median overall survival value could not be calculated
[§]Although low, higher than with placebo (7% [14] vs. none; 95% CI 3.7–11.1%; p = 0.006)
[€]Only 3 of 14 had progression at interim analysis, so duration of response could not be reliably estimated; observed duration of response for the 3 patients: 15.9–29.9 weeks
[**]Stable disease for at least 26 weeks after crossover
[††]Although numbers small, seemed better in patients intolerant of imatinib than in those resistant to imatinib

Toxicity (N = 202)

Adverse Events That Occurred with a Frequency of at Least 5% Greater with Sunitinib Than Placebo in Per-Protocol Population*

	Number (%)		
	Grade 1/2	Grade 3	Grade 4
Nonhematologic			
Fatigue	58 (29%)	10 (5%)	0
Diarrhea	52 (26%)	7 (3%)	0
Skin discoloration	50 (25%)	0	0
Nausea	47 (23%)	1 (1%)	0
Anorexia	38 (19%)	0	0
Dysgeusia	36 (18%)	0	0
Stomatitis	30 (15%)	1 (1%)	0
Vomiting	30 (15%)	1 (1%)	0
Hand-foot syndrome	19 (9%)	9 (4%)	0
Rash	24 (12%)	2 (1%)	0
Asthenia	18 (9%)	6 (3%)	0
Mucosal inflammation	24 (12%)	0	0
Dyspepsia	22 (11%)	1 (1%)	0
Hypertension	15 (8%)	6 (3%)	0
Epistaxis	14 (7%)	0	0
Hair-color changes	14 (7%)	0	0
Dry mouth	13 (6%)	0	0
Glossodynia	11 (6%)	0	0
Hematologic			
Anemia	117 (58%)	7 (4%)	0
Leucopenia	104 (52%)	7 (4%)	0
Neutropenia	86 (43%)	17 (8%)	3 (2%)
Lymphopenia	80 (40%)	18 (9%)	1 (1%)
Thrombo-cytopenia	72 (36%)	8 (4%)	1 (1%)

*National Cancer Institute (USA), Common Terminology Criteria for Adverse Events, version 3.0

Therapy Monitoring

1. *Before initiation of treatment, during each cycle of treatment, and as clinically indicated:* History and physical examination. Complete blood count with leukocyte differential, liver and thyroid function tests

2. *As clinically indicated:* Monitor patients for signs and symptoms of congestive heart failure. Consider monitoring with on-treatment electrocardiograms and electrolytes

3. *Daily at first, then M-W-F, then biweekly, and then weekly:* Monitor blood pressure and treat as needed

Notes:

- Thyroid dysfunction may occur. Patients with signs and/or symptoms suggestive of hypothyroidism or hyperthyroidism should have laboratory monitoring of thyroid function performed and be treated as per standard medical practice

- Temporary interruption of therapy with sunitinib is recommended in patients undergoing major surgical procedures

- Adrenal hemorrhage was observed in animal studies. Monitor adrenal function in case of stress such as surgery, trauma or severe infection

- Patients who presented with cardiac events within 12 months prior to sunitinib administration, such as myocardial infarction (including severe/unstable angina), coronary/peripheral artery bypass graft, symptomatic CHF, cerebrovascular accident or transient ischemic attack, or pulmonary embolism, were excluded from clinical studies with sunitinib. It is unknown whether patients with these concomitant conditions may be at a greater risk for developing drug-related left ventricular dysfunction. Patients with preexisting cardiac pathologies should be carefully monitored for clinical signs and symptoms of CHF while receiving sunitinib. Baseline and periodic evaluations of LVEF should also be considered. In patients without cardiac risk factors, a baseline evaluation of ejection fraction should be considered

35. Testicular Cancer

Darren R. Feldman, MD and George J. Bosl, MD

Epidemiology

Incidence: 8,820 estimated new cases for 2014 in the United States 5.5 per 100,000 males per year

Deaths: Estimated 380 in 2014

Median age: 33 years

Siegel R et al. CA Cancer J Clin 2013;63:11–30
Surveillance, Epidemiology and End Results (SEER) Program, available from http://seer.cancer.gov (accessed in 2013)

Frequency of Stage at Presentation

	Seminoma	Nonseminoma
Stage I	85%	60%
Stage II	10%	20%
Stage III	5%	20%

Frequency of IGCCCG Risk Groups at Diagnosis for Patients Requiring Chemotherapy

IGCCCG Risk Group	Seminoma	Nonseminoma	All
Good	90%	56%	60%
Intermediate	10%	28%	26%
Poor	N/A	16%	14%

IGCCCG, International Germ Cell Cancer Collaborative Group; GCT germ cell tumor

Biggs M, Schwartz S. "Cancer of the Testis." In Ries SEER Survival Monograph: Cancer Survival Among Adults: U.S. SEER Program, 1988–2001. 2007:165–170
Bosl G et al. In Devita V, Lawrence T, Rosenberg S, eds. Cancer: Principles and Practice of Oncology. Philadelphia: Lippincott Williams and Wilkins, 2008:1463–1485
International Germ Cell Cancer Collaborative Group (IGCCCG). J Clin Oncol 1997;15:594–603
Siegel R et al. CA Cancer J Clin 2014;64:9–29

Pathology

Germ Cell Tumors (95%)	Non–Germ Cell Tumors (5%)

1. Seminoma
  a. Classic
  b. Spermatocytic
2. Nonseminoma
  a. Embryonal carcinoma
  b. Teratoma
    1. Teratoma (Mature or Immature)
    2. Teratoma with malignant transformation
  c. Choriocarcinoma
  d. Yolk sac (endodermal sinus) tumor
 	
Note: Most common nonseminoma histology is a mixture of ≥2 histologies. Pure teratoma represents a fully malignant GCT
	1. Sex cord-stromal (gonadal stromal) tumors
	  a. Leydig cell
	  b. Sertoli cell tumor
	  c. Granulosa cell
	2. Both germ cell and gonadal stromal elements
	  a. Gonadoblastoma
	3. Adnexal and paratesticular tumors
	  a. Mesothelioma
	  b. Carcinoma of rete testis
	4. Miscellaneous neoplasms
	  a. Carcinoid
	  b. Lymphoma
	  c. Sarcoma
	  d. Other

Work-up

Suspicious Testicular Mass (by History or Exam)	Confirmed Testicular Mass (by Ultrasound)	Seminoma or Nonseminoma (S/P Orchiectomy)
History and physical	STM if not yet done	STM
AFP, hCG, and LDH (serum tumor markers [STM])	CBC, complete metabolic profile	CBC, complete metabolic profile
CBC, complete metabolic profile	CT A/P + either CXR or CT chest	CT C/A/P if >4 weeks since prior
Scrotal ultrasound	Bone scan or MRI Brain, *only* if clinically indicated	Bone scan or MRI Brain, *only* if clinically indicated Discussion of sperm banking if further treatment (surgery, chemotherapy, or XRT) is required

Staging

T: Primary Tumor Staging

pTx	Primary tumor cannot be assessed
pT0	No evidence of primary tumor
pTis	Intratubular germ cell neoplasia (testicular intraepithelial neoplasia)
pT1	Tumor limited to testis and epididymis without lymphovascular invasion (LVI); tumor may invade tunica albuginea but not tunica vaginalis
pT2	Tumor limited to the testis and epididymis with LVI or tumor extending through the tunica albuginea with involvement of the tunica vaginalis
pT3	Tumor invades the spermatic cord with or without LVI
pT4	Tumor invades the scrotum with or without LVI

N: Regional Lymph Nodes Clinical Staging

NX	Regional lymph nodes (LN) cannot be assessed
N0	No regional LN metastasis
N1	LN mass ≤2 cm in greatest dimension; or multiple LN, none >2 cm
N2	LN mass >2 cm but not >5 cm in greatest dimension; or multiple LN, any 1 mass >2 cm but not >5 cm
N3	Lymph node mass >5 cm in greatest dimension

N: Regional Lymph Nodes Pathologic Staging

NX	Regional LN cannot be assessed
N0	No regional LN metastasis
N1	Metastasis with a lymph node mass ≤2 cm in greatest dimension and ≤5 lymph nodes positive, none >2 cm
N2	Positive LN >2 cm but <5 cm in greatest dimension; or >5 positive LN, none >5 cm; or evidence of extranodal extension
N3	Positive lymph node >5 cm in greatest dimension

M: Metastatic Disease Staging

Mx	Distant metastasis cannot be assessed
M0	No distant metastasis
M1	Distant metastasis
M1a	Nonregional nodal or pulmonary metastasis
M1b	Nonpulmonary visceral metastases

S: Serum Tumor Markers Staging

Sx	Markers not available or not performed
S0	Marker levels within normal limits
S1	LDH <1.5× upper limit of normal (ULN) and human chorionic gonadotropin, beta subunit (hCG) <5000 mIU/L and alpha-fetoprotein (AFP) <1000 ng/mL
S2	LDH 1.5–10× ULN or hCG 5000–50,000 mIU/L or AFP 1000–10,000 ng/mL
S3	LDH >10× ULN or hCG >50,000 mIU/L or AFP >10,000 ng/mL

Caveats Regarding Staging

1. Except for pTis and pT4, extent of tumor is classified by radical orchiectomy. Use pTx in absence of orchiectomy
2. Histology (seminoma vs. nonseminoma) is incorporated into the risk classification system but not AJCC stage
3. Serum tumor markers (STM) for staging and IGCCCG risk prognostication should be drawn after orchiectomy or other tissue diagnosis but before chemotherapy. Elevated preoperative STM must be repeated postorchiectomy after marker half-life has been evaluated

TNM Stage Grouping		IGCCCG Risk Group Classification		
Stage	TNM	Risk Group (5-Year DFS)	Seminoma (Criteria)	Nonseminoma (Criteria)
0	pTis, N0, M0, S0	Good	Any primary site. Absence of nonpulmonary visceral metastasis. Normal AFP, any level hCG or LDH	*Must fulfill all of the following criteria:* Primary site not mediastinum (Testis/retroperitoneal primary); absence of nonpulmonary visceral metastasis; markers S0 or S1
I	pT1–4, N0, M0, Sx	Nonseminoma (56% of cases)		
IA	pT1, N0, M0, S0	5-y PFS 89%		
IB	pT2–T4, N0, M0, S0	5-y survival 92%		
IS	Any pT/Tx, N0, M0, S1–3	Seminoma (90% of cases) 5-y PFS 82% 5-y survival 86%		
II	Any pT/Tx, N1–3, M0, Sx	Intermediate	Any primary site. Presence of nonpulmonary visceral metastasis Normal AFP, any level hCG or LDH	*Must fulfill all of the following criteria:* Primary site not mediastinum (Testis/retroperitoneal primary); absence of nonpulmonary visceral metastasis; and markers S2
IIA	Any pT/Tx, N1, M0, S0–1	Nonseminoma (28% of cases)		
IIB	Any pT/Tx, N2, S0–1	5-y PFS 75%		
IIC	Any pT/Tx, N3, S0–1	5-y survival 80%		
III	Any pT/Tx, Any N, M1a, Sx	Seminoma (10% of cases) 5-y PFS 67% 5-y survival 72%		
IIIA	Any pT/Tx, Any N, M1a, S0–1	Poor	N/A—Seminomas are never poor risk	*Must fulfill at least 1 of the following criteria:* Primary site mediastinum; or presence of nonpulmonary visceral metastases; or markers S3
IIIB	Any pT/Tx, Any N, M1a, S2 Any pT/Tx, N1–3, M0, S2	Nonseminoma (16% of cases) 5-y PFS 41%		
IIIC	Any pT/Tx, N1–N3, M0, S3 Any pT/Tx, Any N, M1a, S3 Any pT/Tx, Any N, M1b, Any S	5-y survival 48% Seminoma (seminomas are not classified as poor prognosis)		

International Germ Cell Cancer Collaborative Group (IGCCCG). J Clin Oncol 1997;15:594–603

Expert Opinion

I. Caveats

1. A testicular mass is malignant until proven otherwise. Radical inguinal orchiectomy is the indicated surgical procedure for all testicular masses; transscrotal orchiectomy and testicular biopsy are not recommended

2. Patients with seminoma and an elevated AFP level or any nonseminomatous histology, including teratoma, should be treated as a nonseminoma

3. Patients with pure testicular teratoma should be treated as a fully malignant nonseminoma

4. Primary mediastinal site and level of serum tumor markers (STMs) do not affect prognosis for seminoma patients

5. Sperm banking should be discussed with patients after orchiectomy before initiation of any further therapy

6. There is ≈2% lifetime risk of developing a contralateral testicular tumor; self-exam and MD exam are recommended at regular intervals. Such tumors are treated as new primary GCTs

II. Treatment Recommendations by AJCC Stage and Histology

A. Nonseminomas

Stage I

- Stage IA: surveillance is the preferred option for compliant patients. The risk of recurrence is ≈20% and if the disease recurs, >95% patients can be cured with chemotherapy (CT) using EP or BEP. For noncompliant patients, nerve-sparing retroperitoneal lymph node dissection (RPLND) may be preferred

- Stage IB: risk of relapse is ≈50%. RPLND, surveillance, or 1–2 cycles of BEP are all options. RPLND results in the least likelihood of patients receiving chemotherapy

- Stage IS: CT should be administered (EP × 4 or BEP × 3 for S1; BEP × 4 for S2–S3)

Stage II (S0 and S1 STM only; S2 and S3 STM qualify as Stage IIIB and IIIC, respectively)

- If adenopathy >2 cm or bilateral *or* STM are persistently elevated after orchiectomy, BEP × 3 or EP × 4 should be given

- If adenopathy <2 cm and unilateral/unifocal *and* STM are normal, RPLND or CT (EP × 4 or BEP × 3) can be considered depending on clinical circumstances. Following postchemotherapy RPLND, patients with complete resection should receive 2 cycles of EP or BEP if findings reveal pathologic stage IIB (pN2)

Stage III

- Treatment is based on IGCCCG risk classification

- Patients in the good-risk category should be given either EP × 4 or BEP × 3

- Patients in the intermediate- or poor-risk categories should be given BEP × 4

- VIP × 4 (etoposide, ifosfamide, cisplatin) is as effective as BEP × 4 in patients with poor-risk GCT, but VIP is associated with greater toxicity (primarily hematologic). VIP can be considered for patients in whom bleomycin is contraindicated (ie, pulmonary disease)

Residual masses

- In general, all sites of residual masses after completion of CT should be resected, if possible. PET is not routinely indicated for evaluation of post-CT residual masses

B. Seminomas

Stage I

- The risk of recurrence is 15–20%. The 3 treatment options are active surveillance, adjuvant radiation therapy (RT), and adjuvant carboplatin

- Surveillance is becoming the preferred option for compliant patients since RT and carboplatin overtreat ≥80% of patients. RT increases the risk of secondary cancers and data on the long-term risks with carboplatin are lacking

- RT, 2000–2500 cGy is an option for non-compliant patients but recognition of the increased incidence of secondary intra-abdominal malignancies has rapidly led to less frequent use. Carboplatin may be an alternative option for non-compliant patients but long-term follow-up is lacking such that the frequency of late relapses and late toxicity have not been established. For these reasons, the authors do not use carboplatin in their practice [Bosl SJ, Patil S. J Clin Oncol 2011;29:949]

Stage II

- Stage IIA: RT (3000–3500 cGy) to retroperitoneal and ipsilateral pelvic lymph nodes. CT (EP × 4 or BEP × 3) is an acceptable alternative to RT [Garcia-del-Muro X et al. J Clin Oncol 2008;26:5416]

- Small Stage IIB (single node <3 cm): either RT (≥3600 cGy) or CT with EP × 4 or BEP × 3

- Large (>3 cm) or multinodal Stage IIB, all Stage IIC and Stage III: Treatment is with chemotherapy based on IGCCCG risk stratification. EP × 4 or BEP × 3 are used for good-risk seminoma, BEP × 4 is used for intermediate-risk disease. Seminoma patients are never poor-risk

Residual masses

- Surgery is more difficult with seminoma and carries a higher complication rate

- PET scan is recommended to evaluate residual masses >3 cm. Additional treatment (surgical or medical) or diagnostic procedure may be indicated for PET-positive residual masses >3 cm. PET-negative lesions >3 cm require no further treatment, just active surveillance. Some patients with lesions <3 cm may benefit from PET scan evaluation. Since teratoma is rarely an issue with seminoma, false-negative results are uncommon

(continued)

Expert Opinion (continued)

III. Salvage Therapy
- We divide patients into 2 categories:
  1. *Patients with a favorable prognosis with conventional chemotherapy:* This group includes patients with a retroperitoneal or gonadal primary nonseminoma or a seminoma of any primary site who previously achieved a complete response (CR) or partial response (PR) with negative markers lasting >6 months to first-line therapy. We treat these patients with TIP, based on the 63% durable disease-free survival rate. These patients may be able to be cured without being subjected to the toxicity of high-dose chemotherapy. VIP and VeIP are additional options. Investigational treatments should also be considered
  2. *Patients with an unfavorable prognosis with conventional chemotherapy:* All patients who do not fit into the group above including (a) patients with mediastinal primary nonseminomas and (b) patients who do not achieve a CR or durable PR with negative markers. These patients should be treated with high-dose chemotherapy, which gives them the best chance of long-term survival (40–60%) [Feldman DR et al. J Clin Oncol 2010;28:1706]. Chance of cure with conventional chemotherapy is <10%. Investigational treatments should be considered

IV. Chemotherapy for Special Populations
- *Viable GCT upon resection after completing first-line chemotherapy:* Administer 2 additional cycles of adjuvant chemotherapy with EP
- *Late relapses:* defined as relapse after ≥2 years of being in remission after chemotherapy. These tumors tend to be more chemoresistant and difficult to cure than relapses occurring ≤2 years after completing treatment. Surgery is the treatment of choice when possible. When surgery is not possible, TIP (50% durable CR rate in 14 patients) and cisplatin plus epirubicin (30% durable CR rate in 21 patients) are 2 regimens that have shown promise. High-dose chemotherapy may be indicated in selected patients. Referral to a specialist center is recommended. Investigational treatments should be considered
- *Intermediate- or poor-risk patients with severe lung disease:* VIP can be substituted for BEP with equivalent efficacy but increased hematologic toxicity
- *Pulmonary toxicity developing during BEP × 3 for good-risk disease:* If DLCO or TVC decrease by ≥25% or there is physical exam or CXR evidence of bleomycin toxicity, then discontinuation of bleomycin is indicated with continuation of treatment with EP. Patients who require discontinuation of bleomycin prior to completing 3 full cycles of BEP can be given additional cycles of EP until a total of 4 cycles of chemotherapy have been administered (personal correspondence, Lawrence Einhorn, December 2008)

V. Mesna Dosing Schedules
- Ifosfamide 1200 mg/m² per day for 5 days
  a. Mesna 120 mg/m² by short intravenous infusion when ifosfamide administration commences, followed immediately afterward by Mesna 1200 mg/m² per day given by continuous intravenous infusion for 5 consecutive days (total dosage/5 days = 6120 mg/m²)
  b. Mesna 1200 mg/m² per day given intravenously for 5 consecutive days prepared as an admixture (in the same container) with ifosfamide (total dosage/5 days = 6000 mg/m²)
  c. Mesna 400 mg/m² per dose given intravenously when ifosfamide administration commences, and at 4 and 8 hours after ifosfamide for 3 doses per day such that equal total doses of mesna and ifosfamide are given daily; ie, 1200 mg/m² per day (total dosage/5 days = 6000 mg/m²)
- Ifosfamide 1500 mg/m² per day for 4 days
  a. Mesna 1500 mg/m² per day prepared as an admixture (in the same container) with ifosfamide (total dosage/4 days = 6000 mg/m²)
  b. Mesna 500 mg/m² per dose given intravenously with ifosfamide, and then at 4 hours and 8 hours after ifosfamide to equal the total amount of ifosfamide given daily; ie, 1500 mg/m² (total dosage/4 days = 6000 mg/m²)
  c. Mesna 500 mg/m² per dose given intravenously when ifosfamide administration commences followed by Mesna 1000 mg/m² per dose given orally at 4 and 8 hours after ifosfamide (for total of 2500 mg/m² mesna per day; total dosage/4 days from IV + oral routes = 10,000 mg/m²)

VI. Follow-up Schedules
- Follow-up guidelines based on disease stage, histology (seminoma vs. nonseminoma) and treatment type (radiation, chemotherapy, surgery, surveillance) have been published by various groups, primarily based on expert opinion rather than direct evidence from clinical trials. One commonly used set of guidelines is published by the National Comprehensive Cancer Network (NCCN) (http://www.nccn.org). Other guidelines are also available

For follow-up schedules, the authors consider the starting point to be the first day of definitive treatment (surgery, radiation, or chemotherapy) resulting in expected cure. For patients with metastatic disease who receive chemotherapy followed by surgery, the first day of the first cycle is considered to be the start of year 1 unless adjuvant therapy is required for persistent viable disease. When adjuvant chemotherapy is required, the start date of adjuvant therapy is used to mark the start of year 1

De Santis M et al. J Clin Oncol 2004;22:1034–1039
Einhorn LH et al. N Engl J Med 2007;357:340–348
Motzer RJ et al. Cancer 1991;67:1305–1310
Rabbani F et al. Urology 2003;62:1092–1096

FIRST-LINE TREATMENT REGIMENS
ETOPOSIDE + CISPLATIN (EP)

Bosl GJ et al. J Clin Oncol 1988;6:1231–1238

Hydration for cisplatin: Administer intravenously 0.9% sodium chloride injection, USP (0.9% NS) to insure a urine output of at least 100 mL/hour prior to each dose of cisplatin. Hydration should be continued until the patient has completed chemotherapy and is able to take adequate oral liquids to prevent dehydration. Monitor and replace electrolytes/magnesium as needed

Etoposide 100 mg/m^2 per day; administer intravenously diluted in 0.9% NS to a concentration within the range of 0.2–0.4 mg/mL over 60 minutes, for 5 consecutive days, days 1–5, every 21 days for 3–4 cycles (total dosage/cycle = 500 mg/m^2)

Cisplatin 20 mg/m^2 per day; administer intravenously in 25–250 mL 0.9% NS over 30–60 minutes for 5 consecutive days, on days 1–5, every 21 days for 3–4 cycles (total dosage/cycle = 100 mg/m^2)

EP × 3 indicates 3 treatment cycles; EP × 4 indicates 4 cycles

Supportive Care
Antiemetic prophylaxis
Emetogenic potential on days 1–5: **HIGH**. *Potential for delayed emetic symptoms*
See Chapter 39 for antiemetic recommendations

Hematopoietic growth factor (CSF) prophylaxis
Primary prophylaxis is indicated with one of the following:
  Filgrastim (G-CSF) 5 mcg/kg per day by subcutaneous injection, *or*
  Pegfilgrastim (pegylated filgrastim) 6 mg/0.6 mL by subcutaneous injection for 1 dose
  • Begin use from 24–72 hours after myelosuppressive chemotherapy is completed
See Chapter 43 for more information

Antimicrobial prophylaxis
Risk of fever and neutropenia is LOW
  Antimicrobial primary prophylaxis to be considered:
  • Antibacterial—not indicated
  • Antifungal—not indicated
  • Antiviral—not indicated, unless patient previously had an episode of HSV
See Chapter 47 for more information

Patient Population Studied

Patients with good-risk GCT not previously treated with chemotherapy

Bajorin D et al. J Clin Oncol 1993;11:598–606
Bosl GJ et al. J Clin Oncol 1988;6:1231–1238
Culine S et al. Ann Oncol 2007;18:917–924
Kondagunta GV et al. J Clin Oncol 2005;9290–9294

Treatment Modifications

Toxicity	MSKCC*	Indiana
Neutropenia day 1	Delay by 1 week unless WBC ≥2500/mm^3 *and* ANC ≥500/mm^3*; consider granulocyte colony-stimulating factor (G-CSF) with next cycle	No delay. Hold etoposide on day 5 if ANC still ≤2500/mm^3[†‡]; consider G-CSF with next cycle
Febrile Neutropenia (FN) or prior irradiation	Add G-CSF	Add G-CSF or reduce etoposide dosage by 25%[†]
FN despite G-CSF	Consider prophylactic antibiotic next cycle	Reduce etoposide dosage by 25%[‡]
Serum creatinine (Cr) ≥3.0 mg/dL (≥265.2 μmol/L)	Delay until Cr <3.0 mg/dL & CrCl creatinine clearance ≥50 mL/min (≥0.83 mL/s), then give full dose or substitute carboplatin if Cr does not return to <3.0 mg/dL or CrCl ≥50 mL/min	Delay until Cr <3.0 mg/dL[‡]

*Motzer R et al. Cancer 1990;66:857–861
†Einhorn L et al. J Clin Oncol 1989;7:387–391
‡Nichols CR et al. J Clin Oncol 1998;16:1287–1293

Efficacy (EP × 4 for Good-Risk Patients)*

Author	Year	N	CR/FR	DurFR	OS†	Median Follow-up (months)†
Bosl	1988	82	93%	82%	NR	26
Bajorin	1993	134	90%	87%	NR	22
Kondagunta*	2005	289	98%	92%	94%	92
Culine	2007	126	97%	86%	93%	53

CR/FR, complete or favorable response; DurFR, durable favorable response; OS, overall survival; NR, not reported
Favorable response: CR of any duration or PR with negative markers lasting ≥2 years
*Not a randomized controlled trial
†OS and Median Follow-up are 4-year actuarial rates

Toxicity

Bajorin D et al. J Clin Oncol 1993;11:598–606

Hematologic Toxicity	Percent (%)
Fever and neutropenia	23
Required RBC transfusion	13
Required platelets transfusion	3

Nonhematologic Toxicity

	% G1	% G2	% G3	% G4
Ototoxicity		23		
Neuropathy		31		
Mucositis		14		
Transaminitis		10		
Raynaud phenomenon*	None			

*Raynaud phenomenon reported in separate trial of EP × 4 for good-risk patients (de Wit R et al. J Clin Oncol 1997;15:1837–1843)

Therapy-Related Deaths N (%)	2 (1.5%)

Therapy Monitoring

1. *Every cycle:* CBC with differential, comprehensive metabolic profile, and serum tumor markers
2. *Response evaluation:* CT scan chest, abdomen, and pelvis and tumor markers after completion of cycle 4

REGIMEN

BLEOMYCIN, ETOPOSIDE, AND CISPLATIN (BEP)

Nichols CR et al. J Clin Oncol 1998;16:1287–1293

Hydration for cisplatin: 0.9% NS; administer intravenously to insure a urine output of ≥100 mL/hour prior to each dose of cisplatin and continue until the patient has completed chemotherapy and is able to take adequate oral liquids to prevent dehydration. We give 500 mL of 0.9% NS over 1 hour before cisplatin while premedications and etoposide are infused, and an additional 500 mL of 0.9% NS over 1 hour after cisplatin. Electrolytes/magnesium replaced as needed. Other hydration schedules are feasible

Bleomycin 30 units/week; administer by intravenous injection, weekly for 3–4 cycles (ie, 9–12 weeks; total dose/9-week course = 270 units; total dose/12-week course = 360 units)

Etoposide 100 mg/m² per day; administer intravenously diluted in 0.9% NS to a concentration within the range of 0.2–0.4 mg/mL over 30–60 minutes for 5 consecutive days on days 1–5, every 21 days for 3–4 cycles (total dosage/cycle = 500 mg/m²)

Cisplatin 20 mg/m² per day; administer intravenously in 25–250 mL 0.9% NS over 30–60 minutes for 5 consecutive days on days 1–5, every 21 days for 3–4 cycles (total dosage/cycle = 100 mg/m²)

BEP × 3 indicates 3 consecutive cycles; BEP × 4 indicates 4 consecutive cycles

Supportive Care

Antiemetic prophylaxis

Emetogenic potential on days 1–5: **HIGH**. *Potential for delayed symptoms*

Emetogenic potential on days with bleomycin alone: **MINIMAL**

See Chapter 39 for antiemetic recommendations

Hematopoietic growth factor (CSF) prophylaxis

Primary prophylaxis is indicated with one of the following:

Filgrastim (G-CSF) 5 mcg/kg per day by subcutaneous injection, *or*

Pegfilgrastim (pegylated filgrastim) 6 mg/0.6 mL by subcutaneous injection for 1 dose
 • Begin use from 24–72 hours after myelosuppressive chemotherapy is completed

See Chapter 43 for more information

Antimicrobial prophylaxis

Risk of fever and neutropenia is LOW

Antimicrobial primary prophylaxis to be considered:
 • Antibacterial—not indicated
 • Antifungal—not indicated
 • Antiviral—not indicated, unless patient previously had an episode of HSV

See Chapter 47 for more information

Patient Population Studied

Bleomycin, Etoposide, and Cisplatin × 3 (BEP × 3)

Indication/population studied: Good-risk GCT patients not previously treated with chemotherapy

Culine S et al. Ann Oncol 2007;18:917–924
de Wit R et al. J Clin Oncol 2001;19:1629–1640
Einhorn L et al. J Clin Oncol 1989;7:387–391
Loehrer P et al. J Clin Oncol 1995;13:470–476
Toner G et al. Lancet 2001;357:739–745

Bleomycin, Etoposide, and Cisplatin × 4 (BEP × 4)

Indication/population studied: Patients with intermediate- or poor-risk GCT not previously treated with chemotherapy

de Wit R et al. Br J Cancer 1995;71:1311–1314
Hinton S et al. Cancer 2003;97:1869–1875
Motzer R et al. J Clin Oncol 2007;25:247–256
Nichols C et al. J Clin Oncol 1991;9:1163–1172
Nichols CR et al. J Clin Oncol 1998;16:1287–1293

Toxicity (BEP × 4)

Hematologic Toxicity	% G3	% G4
Any hematologic toxicity	39	34

Nonhematologic Toxicity	% G3/G4
Nausea/vomiting	7
Neurologic	7
Infection	5
Pulmonary	5

Therapy-Related Deaths	N (%)
Pulmonary or pulmonary hemorrhage	3 (2)
Sepsis	3 (2)
Cerebral hemorrhage	1 (1)

Nichols CR et al. J Clin Oncol 1998;16:1287–1293

Toxicity (BEP × 3)

Hematologic Toxicity	Percent (%)
Leukocytes <1000/mm³	9
Fever and leukopenia (<2000/mm³ and T >38°C)	15
Platelet count is <25,000/mm³	3

Nonhematologic Toxicity	% G1	% G2	% G3	% G4
Pulmonary	13		1	
Ototoxicity	10	13	—	—
Sensory Neuropathy	20	4		—
Fatigue	39	21		—
Raynaud phenomenon*	8%			

*Raynaud phenomenon reported in regimen of BEP × 4 (not BEP × 3) for good-risk patients
(de Wit R et al. J Clin Oncol 1997;15:1837–1843)
de Wit R et al. J Clin Oncol 2001;19:1629–1640

Efficacy (BEP × 3; Good Risk)
Randomized Phase III Trials

Author	Year	N	CR/FR	DurFR	OS	Median Follow-up (months)
Einhorn	1989	88	98%	92%	94%	NR*
Loehrer	1995	86	94%	86%	95%	49
de Wit	2001	397	97%	90%	97%	NR[†]
Toner	2001	83	88%	90%	96%	33
Culine	2007	132	95%	91%	96%	53[‡]

CR/FR, complete or favorable response; DurFR, durable favorable response; OS, overall survival; NR, not reported
Favorable response: CR of any duration or PR with negative markers lasting 2 years
*All patients had ≥1 year follow-up
[†]DurFR and OS assessed at 2 years
[‡]DurFR and OS assessed at 4 years

Efficacy (BEP × 4: Intermediate- and Poor-Risk)
Randomized Phase III Trials

Author	Year	N	CR/FR	DurFR	OS	Median Follow-up (months)
Nichols	1991	77	73%	61%	74%	NR
de Wit	1995	105	72%	80%	80%	NR*
Hinton	2003	115	NR	55%	63%	88
Motzer	2007	111	55%	48%	72%	NR[†]

CR/FR, complete or favorable response; DurFR, durable favorable response; OS, overall survival; NR, not reported
Favorable response: CR of any duration or PR with negative markers lasting ≥2 years
*DurFR and OS assessed at 5 years
[†]DurFR assessed at 1 year and OS at 2 years

Treatment Modifications

Adverse Events	Treatment Modifications
Myelosuppression not improving during the first 4 days of therapy	Omit day 5 etoposide. Administer full dose cisplatin
Febrile neutropenia	Add filgrastim during ongoing cycle and subsequent cycles so as to administer full dose chemotherapy
Febrile neutropenia while receiving filgrastim	Reduce etoposide dosage by 25%
Clinical (rales or inspiratory lag) or radiographic evidence of pulmonary toxicity or fibrosis	Discontinue bleomycin

Repeated treatment cycles should begin on schedule without regard for the degree of myelosuppression noted on the day of scheduled treatment. Daily CBC is obtained to document marrow recovery

Therapy Monitoring

1. *Every cycle:* CBC with differential, comprehensive metabolic profile, serum tumor markers, and evaluation for bleomycin pulmonary toxicity (Indiana—lung exam[1,2], MSKCC—PFTs[3])
2. After completion of BEP × 3 or BEP × 4, repeat CT scan of chest, abdomen, and pelvis, and tumor markers

[1]Loehrer P et al. J Clin Oncol 1995;13:470–476
[2]Nichols CR et al. J Clin Oncol 1998;16:1287–1293
[3]Bosl GJ et al. J Clin Oncol 1988;6:1231–1238

SALVAGE TREATMENT REGIMENS REGIMEN

PACLITAXEL + IFOSFAMIDE + CISPLATIN (TIP × 4)

Kondagunta GV et al. J Clin Oncol 2005;23:6549–6555

Indications:
1. First-line salvage chemotherapy for patients who relapsed after a complete response or partial response with negative markers lasting >6 months
2. Other patients who are not candidates for high-dose chemotherapy or have progressed after high-dose therapy and have not received paclitaxel

Premedication for paclitaxel: **Dexamethasone** 20 mg/dose; administer orally or intravenously for 2 doses at 14 and 7 hours prior to paclitaxel, plus **diphenhydramine** 50 mg and **cimetidine** 300 mg; administer both intravenously 1 hour prior to paclitaxel
Paclitaxel 250 mg/m^2; administer intravenously in 0.9% sodium chloride injection (0.9% NS) or 5% dextrose injection (D5W) to yield a final concentration within the range of 0.3 and 1.2 mg/mL over 24 hours on day 1, every 21 days for 4 cycles (total dosage/cycle = 250 mg/m^2)
Hydration: 1000 mL 0.9% NS; administer intravenously over 2 hours on days 2–5 before or during ifosfamide administration. Consider additional intravenous fluid if medically appropriate until the patient has completed chemotherapy and is able to take adequate oral liquids to prevent dehydration. Monitor and replace electrolytes/magnesium as needed
Ifosfamide 1500 mg/m^2 per day; administer intravenously in 0.9% NS or D5W to produce a concentration within the range of 0.6 and 20 mg/mL, over 2–3 hours for 4 consecutive days on days 2–5, every 21 days for 4 cycles (total dosage/cycle = 6000 mg/m^2)
Mesna 500 mg/m^2 per dose; administer intravenously in D5W to yield a concentration of 20 mg/mL, for 3 doses/day starting just before or coincident with the start of ifosfamide, with repeated doses at 4 and 8 hours after ifosfamide for 4 consecutive days on days 2–5, every 21 days for 4 cycles (total daily dosage = 1500 mg/m^2; total dosage/cycle = 6000 mg/m^2) (See Expert Opinion for alternative administration schemes)
Cisplatin 25 mg/m^2 per day; administer intravenously in 25–250 mL 0.9% NS, over 30–60 minutes for 4 consecutive days on days 2–5, every 21 days for 4 cycles (total dosage/cycle = 100 mg/m^2)

Supportive Care
Antiemetic prophylaxis
Emetogenic potential on day 1: **LOW**
Emetogenic potential on days 2–5: **HIGH**. *Potential for delayed symptoms*
See Chapter 39 for antiemetic recommendations

Hematopoietic growth factor (CSF) prophylaxis
Primary prophylaxis is indicated with one of the following:
Filgrastim (G-CSF) 5 mcg/kg per day by subcutaneous injection, *or*
Pegfilgrastim (pegylated filgrastim) 6 mg/0.6 mL by subcutaneous injection for 1 dose
• Begin use from 24–72 hours after myelosuppressive chemotherapy is completed
• Discontinue daily filgrastim use if WBC >10,000/mm3 on 2 consecutive daily measurements
See Chapter 43 for more information

Antimicrobial prophylaxis
Risk of fever and neutropenia is INTERMEDIATE
Antimicrobial primary prophylaxis to be considered:
• Antibacterial—consider a fluoroquinolone or no prophylaxis; *P. jirovecii* prophylaxis is recommended (eg, cotrimoxazole)
• Antifungal—consider use during neutropenia
• Antiviral—antiherpes antivirals (eg, acyclovir)
See Chapter 47 for more information

Dose Modifications

Toxicity	Modification
ANC <450/mm^3 on day 1	Delay until ANC >450/mm^3
Platelet count <75,000/mm^3 on day 1	Delay until platelet count is >75,000/mm^3
Platelets <10,000/mm^3 or platelets <50,000/mm^3 with bleeding	Transfuse platelets to >10,000/mm^3 if no bleeding, and to >50,000/mm^3 if bleeding
Hgb <8 g/dL	Transfuse RBC to keep Hgb >8 g/dL

Kondagunta GV et al. J Clin Oncol 2005;23:6549–6555

Therapy Monitoring
1. CBC with differential weekly
2. Comprehensive metabolic profile and serum tumor markers once to twice per cycle
3. *Response assessment:* CT scan of chest, abdomen, and pelvis, and tumor markers after completion of 4 cycles

Patient Population Studied (N = 46)
GCT patients fulfilling *all* of the following 3 criteria:
1. Gonadal primary tumor
2. Prior therapy with cisplatin-based treatment totaling 6 or fewer cycles
3. Prior CR or PR with negative markers lasting >6 months from completion of first-line chemotherapy

Kondagunta GV et al. J Clin Oncol 2005;23:6549–6555

Toxicity

Hematologic Toxicity	Percent (%)
Febrile neutropenia	48

Nonhematologic Toxicity	Percent (%)
Grade 3 neuropathy	7
Grade 4 or 5 nephrotoxicity	7
Grade 3 elevation of transaminases	2
Therapy-related deaths	2

Kondagunta GV et al. J Clin Oncol 2005;23:6549–6555

Efficacy (N = 46)

	Percent (%)
CR	70
Chemotherapy alone	63
Chemotherapy + surgery	7
IR	30
PR, marker negative	4
Other	26
Relapse From CR	7
Continuously NED*	63
Two-year overall survival	78

CR (complete response): disappearance of all clinical, radiographic, and biochemical evidence of disease for at least 4 weeks
IR (incomplete response): failure to achieve CR to chemotherapy with or without surgery, including patients who were observed to have failure of serum tumor marker normalization
NED (no evidence of disease)
*Median follow-up of 68 months

SALVAGE TREATMENT REGIMENS REGIMEN

VINBLASTINE + IFOSFAMIDE + CISPLATIN (VeIP × 4)

Loehrer PJ Sr et al. J Clin Oncol 1998;16:2500–2504

Indications:

1. First-line salvage chemotherapy for patients who relapsed after achieving a complete response or partial response with negative markers lasting >6 months
2. Other patients who progressed on or after first-line therapy who are not candidates for high-dose chemotherapy or progressed after high-dose therapy

Vinblastine 0.11 mg/kg per day; administer by intravenous injection over 1–2 minutes on 2 consecutive days, on days 1 and 2, every 3 weeks for 4 cycles (total dosage/cycle = 0.22 mg/kg)
Hydration: Administer 0.9% NS intravenously to insure a urine output of ≥100 mL/hour prior to each dose of cisplatin. Continue intravenous hydration until a patient has completed chemotherapy and is able to take adequate oral liquids to prevent dehydration
Suggested: 0.9% NS 500 mL over 1 hour before cisplatin and an additional 500 mL of 0.9% NS over 1 hour after cisplatin. Electrolytes/magnesium replaced as needed. Other hydration schedules are feasible
Cisplatin 20 mg/m^2 per day; administer intravenously in 25–250 mL of 0.9% NS over 30–60 minutes for 5 consecutive days on days 1–5, every 3 weeks for 4 cycles (total dosage/cycle = 100 mg/m^2)
Ifosfamide 1200 mg/m^2 per day; administer intravenously in 0.9% NS or D5W sufficient to produce a concentration within the range of 0.6 and 20 mg/mL, over 30–60 minutes for 5 consecutive days on days 1–5, every 3 weeks for 4 cycles (total dosage/cycle = 6000 mg/m^2)
Mesna 500 mg/m^2 per dose; administer intravenously in 25–50 mL 0.9% NS or D5W, over 15–30 minutes starting simultaneously with ifosfamide, followed by **Mesna** 1200 mg/m^2 per day by continuous intravenous infusion in a volume of 0.9% NS, D5W (or dextrose and saline combinations) sufficient to produce a concentration of 20 mg/mL over 24 hours for 5 consecutive days on days 1–5, every 3 weeks for 4 cycles (total dosage/cycle = 6500 mg/m^2). (See Expert Opinion for alternative administration schemes)

Supportive Care
Antiemetic prophylaxis
*Emetogenic potential on days 1–5: **HIGH**. Potential for delayed symptoms*
See Chapter 39 for antiemetic recommendations

Hematopoietic growth factor (CSF) prophylaxis
Primary prophylaxis is indicated with one of the following:
  Filgrastim (G-CSF) 5 mcg/kg per day by subcutaneous injection, *or*
  Pegfilgrastim (pegylated filgrastim) 6 mg/0.6 mL by subcutaneous injection for one dose
  • Begin use from 24–72 hours after myelosuppressive chemotherapy is completed
  • Discontinue daily filgrastim use if WBC >10,000/mm^3 on 2 consecutive daily measurements
See Chapter 43 for more information

Antimicrobial prophylaxis
Risk of fever and neutropenia is INTERMEDIATE
  Antimicrobial primary prophylaxis to be considered:
  • Antibacterial—consider a fluoroquinolone or no prophylaxis; *P. jirovecii* prophylaxis is recommended (eg, cotrimoxazole)
  • Antifungal—consider use during neutropenia and for anticipated mucositis
  • Antiviral—antiherpes antivirals (eg, acyclovir)
See Chapter 47 for more information

Dose Modification

Toxicity	Modification
Neutropenia on day 1	No delay. Omit ifosfamide on day 5 if ANC still ≤2500/mm^3
Thrombocytopenia and bleeding, febrile neutropenia (FN), or prior irradiation	Reduce etoposide and vinblastine dosages by 25%*
Platelet count <100,000/mm^3 on day 5	Omit day 5 of ifosfamide*
Serum creatinine >2 mg/dL (>176.8 μmol/L)	Decrease ifosfamide dosage by 25%*
>10 RBCs/HPF	Hold ifosfamide and continue mesna and hydration until <10 RBCs/HPF

*Loehrer PJ Sr et al. J Clin Oncol 1998;16:2500–2504

Therapy Monitoring

1. Weekly CBC with differential
2. Comprehensive metabolic profile and serum tumor markers once to twice per cycle
3. *Response assessment:* CT scan of chest, abdomen, and pelvis, and tumor markers after completion of 4 cycles

Patient Population Studied (N = 145)

Second-line therapy for GCT patients who progressed during or after first-line chemotherapy

Loehrer PJ Sr et al. J Clin Oncol 1998;16:2500–2504

Toxicity

Hematologic Toxicity	Percent (%)
Febrile neutropenia	71
Required RBC transfusions	49
Required platelet transfusions	27

Nonhematologic Toxicity	Percent (%)
Renal insufficiency (Cr >4 mg/dL, 353.6 μmol/L)	6
Irreversible renal insufficiency	1
Secondary hematologic malignancies	1
Treatment-related deaths	2

Efficacy

Response	Percent (%)
CR	50
Chemotherapy alone	42
Chemotherapy + surgery	7
IR	50
Relapse From CR	24
Continuously NED	24

Progression-Free (PFS) and Overall Survival (OS)	
Median PFS	4.7 years
Median OS	1.3 years
OS at 2 years	38%
OS at 7 years	32%

CR (complete response): complete disappearance of all objective evidence of disease (clinical and radiographic) with normalization of hCG and AFP for at least 1 month
IR (incomplete response): any response that did not meet criteria of CR
NED (no evidence of disease) after VeIP + surgery

SALVAGE TREATMENT REGIMENS REGIMEN

ETOPOSIDE + IFOSFAMIDE + CISPLATIN (VIP × 4)

Nichols CR et al. J Clin Oncol 1998;16:1287–1293

Indication:
Initial therapy for intermediate- or poor-risk GCT patients who are not candidates for BEP (usually because of pulmonary compromise)

Order of administration: etoposide → cisplatin → ifosfamide/mesna
Hydration: 1000 mL 0.9% NS; administer intravenously over 2 hours. Consider additional intravenous fluid if medically appropriate until the patient has completed chemotherapy and is able to take adequate oral liquids to prevent dehydration. Monitor and replace electrolytes/magnesium as needed
Etoposide 75 mg/m^2 per day; administer intravenously diluted in 0.9% NS to a concentration within the range of 0.2–0.4 mg/mL over 60 minutes for 5 consecutive days on days 1 to 5, every 21 days for 4 cycles (total dosage/cycle = 375 mg/m^2)
Cisplatin 20 mg/m^2 per day; administer intravenously in 25–250 mL 0.9% NS over 30–60 minutes for 5 consecutive days on days 1–5, every 21 days for 4 cycles (total dosage/cycle = 100 mg/m^2)
Ifosfamide 1200 mg/m^2 per day; administer intravenously in 0.9% NS or D5W sufficient to produce a concentration within the range of 0.6 and 20 mg/mL, over 30–120 minutes for 5 consecutive days on days 1–5, every 21 days for 4 cycles (total dosage/cycle = 6000 mg/m^2)
Mesna 120 mg/m^2; administer by intravenous injection on day 1 just before or coincident with the start of ifosfamide administration, followed by **Mesna** 1200 mg/m^2 per day; administer by continuous intravenous infusion over 24 hours for 5 consecutive days on days 1–5, every 21 days for 4 cycles (total dosage/cycle = 6120 mg/m^2). (See Expert Opinion for alternative administration schemes)

Supportive Care
Antiemetic prophylaxis
Emetogenic potential on days 1–5: **HIGH**. *Potential for delayed symptoms*
See Chapter 39 for antiemetic recommendations

Hematopoietic growth factor (CSF) prophylaxis
Primary prophylaxis is indicated with one of the following:
  Filgrastim (G-CSF) 5 mcg/kg per day by subcutaneous injection, *or*
  Pegfilgrastim (pegylated filgrastim) 6 mg/0.6 mL by subcutaneous injection for 1 dose
  • Begin use from 24–72 hours after myelosuppressive chemotherapy is completed
  • Discontinue daily filgrastim use if WBC >10,000/mm^3 on 2 consecutive daily measurements
See Chapter 43 for more information

Antimicrobial prophylaxis
Risk of fever and neutropenia is INTERMEDIATE
  Antimicrobial primary prophylaxis to be considered:
  • Antibacterial—consider a fluoroquinolone or no prophylaxis; *P. jirovecii* prophylaxis is recommended (eg, cotrimoxazole)
  • Antifungal—consider use during neutropenia and for anticipated mucositis
  • Antiviral—antiherpes antivirals (eg, acyclovir)
See Chapter 47 for more information

Therapy Monitoring

1. *Every cycle:* CBC with differential, comprehensive metabolic profile, and serum tumor markers
2. *Response evaluation:* CT scan of chest, abdomen, and pelvis, and tumor markers after completion of cycle 4

Patient Population Studied (N = 135)

Primarily intermediate- or poor-risk GCT patients not previously treated with chemotherapy

Nichols C et al. J Clin Oncol 1998;16:1287–1293

Toxicity

Hematologic Toxicity	% G3	% G4	% G5
Any hematologic toxicity	28	60	1

Nonhematologic Toxicity	% G3/G4
Nausea/vomiting	9
Neurologic	8
Infection	6
Genitourinary	5

Therapy-Related Deaths	Percent (%)
Sepsis	3
Cerebral hemorrhage	1

Nichols CR et al. J Clin Oncol 1998;16:1287–1293

Dose Modification

Toxicity	MSKCC	Indiana
Neutropenia day 1	Delay cycle by 1 week	No delay. Hold etoposide on day 5 if ANC still $\leq$2500/mm^3*
Thrombocytopenia and bleeding (TB), febrile neutropenia (FN), or prior irradiation	TB—delay until platelet count is $\geq$100,000/mm^3 FN—add G-CSF	Reduce etoposide dosage by 25%*
Serum creatinine >3 mg/dL (>265.2 μmol/L)	Delay cisplatin until Cr <3 mg/dL, continue etoposide and ifosfamide on schedule.* Substitute carboplatin for cisplatin if Cr does not return to <3.0 mg/dL	

*Nichols CR et al. J Clin Oncol 1998;16:1287–1293

Efficacy

	Percent (%)
CR to chemotherapy alone	48
CR to chemotherapy + surgery	6
Partial response	22
Favorable response*	63
Failure-free survival at 2 years[†]	64
Overall survival at 2 years	74

*Includes patients with partial response and negative markers without relapse for $\geq$2 years
[†]Includes patients with partial responses (marker-negative or marker-positive) who did not have progression within 2 years

Nichols CR et al. J Clin Oncol 1998;16:1287–1293

	IGCCCG Classification		
	Good Risk (N = 13)	Intermediate Risk (N = 39)	Poor Risk (N = 92)
OS	92%	77%	62%
PFS	92%	72%	56%

Hinton S et al. Cancer 2003;97:1869–1875 (Long-term follow-up of patients in Nichols study (cited above) but with patients reclassified by IGCCCG risk status. Median follow-up for both OS and PFS was 7.3 years)

36. Thymic Malignancies

Arun Rajan, MD and Giuseppe Giaccone, MD, PhD

Epidemiology

Incidence: 0.13 cases per 100,000 (0.2–1.5% of all malignancies)
Median age: 40–60 years
Male to female ratio: 1:1

Engels EA, Pfeiffer RM. Int J Cancer 2003;105:546–551
Schmidt-Wolf IGH et al. Ann Hematol 2003;82:69–76
Tomiak EM, Evans WK. Crit Rev Oncol Hematol 1993;15:113–124

Stage at Presentation
(Masaoka Staging System)

Stage I:	32%
Stage II:	23%
Stage III:	34%
Stage IV:	11%

Pathology

Several histologic classifications of thymomas have been proposed. There is general agreement that the epithelial cells represent the malignant cells in this tumor type and the lymphocytic cells are considered benign

Classification of Thymic Epithelial Tumors

Muller-Hermelink	WHO Type	Levine and Rosai
Thymoma	Thymoma	Thymoma
Medullary type	Type A	Encapsulated
Mixed type	Type AB	—
Predominantly cortical	Type B1	Malignant type I (invasive)
Cortical type	Type B2	—
Well-differentiated carcinoma	Type B3	—
Thymic carcinoma	Type C	Malignant type II

Levine GD, Rosai J. Hum Pathol 1978;9:495–515
Müller-Hermelink HK, Marx A. Curr Opin Oncol 2000;12:426–433
Okumura M et al. Cancer 2002;94:624–632

Work-up

1. CT scan of the thorax
2. Extrathoracic disease such as metastases to the kidney, bone, liver, and brain are rare. Consequently, an extensive work-up for disease outside the thorax is not indicated in the absence of symptoms
3. Pleural or pericardial effusion represents the most common form of metastatic involvement
4. Proper intrathoracic staging is surgical

Ströbel P et al. Blood 2002;100:159–166
Thomas CR Jr et al. J Clin Oncol 1999;17:2280–2289

Five-Year Survival

Stage I	96–100%
Stage II	86–96%
Stage III	56–69%
Stage IV	11–50%

Schneider PM et al. Ann Surg Oncol 1997;4:46–56

Expert Opinion

- Despite their rarity as a group of cancers, thymic epithelial tumors are amongst the most common cancers of the anterior mediastinum in adults
- The clinical course can vary from relatively indolent in the case of some thymomas to highly aggressive in the case of thymic carcinomas
- Thymomas are often associated with a variety of autoimmune conditions; myasthenia gravis is the most common
- Complete surgical resection should be attempted whenever feasible
- Multimodality treatment is frequently required for locally advanced thymoma and thymic carcinoma
- Chemotherapy is offered to patients with advanced stages III to IV thymomas. The evidence for these recommendations is derived from small phase II studies in either the neoadjuvant or refractory/recurrent disease setting
- Platinum-based combination chemotherapy is the standard of care for unresectable, advanced disease. A combination of cisplatin, doxorubicin and cyclophosphamide (PAC) or cisplatin and etoposide (EP) are usually used as first-line regimens [Table]
- The molecular pathogenesis of thymic epithelial tumors and associated autoimmune conditions is gradually being unraveled and targeted therapy is being investigated for the management of advanced disease

Prospective Chemotherapy Trials in Extensive-Stage Inoperable Thymoma

Reference	Regimen	Stage	Patient #	CR+PR	mOS*
Anthracycline-Containing Regimen					
Loehrer et al.	CDDP + **DOX** + CTX	IV	30	50	3.2
Fornasiero et al.	CDDP + **DOX** + CTX + VCR	III/IV	32	90	1.25
Nonanthracycline-Containing Regimen					
Giaccone et al.	CDDP + VP-16	IV	16	56	4.3
Highley et al.	Ifosfamide	III/IV	13	46	N/R
Loehrer et al.	VP-16 + Ifosfamide + CDDP	IV	28	32	2.5
Grassin et al.	VP-16 + Ifosfamide + CDDP	IV	16	25	N/R
Lemma et al.	CDDP + Paclitaxel	IV	44	35	N/R
Loehrer et al.	Pemetrexed	IV	23	17	2.4

CDDP, cisplatin; CR, complete response; CTX, cyclophosphamide; mOS, median overall survival; OX, doxorubicin; PR, partial response; VCR, vincristine; VP-16, etoposide
*Median overall survival in years
Adapted from Kelly RJ et al. J Clin Oncol 2011;29:4820–4827

Fornasiero A et al. Cancer 1991;68:30–33
Giaccone G et al. J Clin Oncol 1996;14:814–820
Grassin F et al. J Thorac Oncol 2010;5:893–897
Highley MS et al. J Clin Oncol 1999;17:2737–2744
Lemma GL et al. J Clin Oncol 2008;26(Suppl):428s
Loehrer PJ et al. Cancer 2001;91:2010–2015
Loehrer PJ et al. J Clin Oncol 1994;12:1164–1168
Loehrer PJ et al. J Clin Oncol 2006;24(Suppl):383s

Clinical Staging of Thymic Epithelial Tumors

Masaoka Staging of Thymic Malignancies With Modifications by Koga et al. and WHO Classification of Thymic Malignancies

Stage/Type	Definition
Stage	
I	Grossly and microscopically completely encapsulated
II (a)	Microscopic transcapsular invasion
II (b)	Macroscopic invasion into thymic or surrounding fatty tissue or grossly adherent to but not breaking through mediastinal pleura or pericardium
III	Macroscopic invasion of neighboring organs (ie, pericardium, great vessel, or lung)
IV (a)	Pleural or pericardial dissemination
IV (b)	Lymphatic or hematogenous metastasis
Histologic Type	**Description**
A	Neoplastic oval or spindle cells; no atypia; no lymphocytes
AB	Type A with foci of lymphocytes
B1	Plump epithelioid cells resembling normal thymic medulla
B2	Scattered foci of atypical epithelial cells with lymphocytes
B3	Round or polygonal epithelial cells with mild atypia with minor component of lymphocytes
Thymic carcinoma	Histologic subtyping required

Kelly RJ et al. J Clin Oncol 2011;29:4820–4827
Masaoka A et al. Cancer 1981;48:2485–2492

REGIMEN

DOXORUBICIN + CISPLATIN + VINCRISTINE + CYCLOPHOSPHAMIDE (ADOC)

Berruti A et al. Br J Cancer 1999;81:841–845

Hydration before cisplatin: ≥1000 mL 0.9% sodium chloride injection (0.9% NS); administer intravenously over 2–4 hours before chemotherapy commences. Monitor and replace electrolytes/magnesium as needed

Doxorubicin 40 mg/m^2; administer by intravenous injection over 3–5 minutes, on day 1, every 3 weeks (total dosage/cycle = 40 mg/m^2)

Cisplatin 50 mg/m^2; administer intravenously in 50–250 mL 0.9% NS over 1 hour on day 1, every 3 weeks (total dosage/cycle = 50 mg/m^2)

Hydration after cisplatin: Administer intravenously 1000 mL 0.9% NS over a minimum of 2 hours. Monitor and replace magnesium and other electrolytes as needed

Vincristine 0.6 mg/m^2; administer by intravenous injection over 1–2 minutes, on day 2, every 3 weeks (total dosage/cycle = 0.6 mg/m^2)

Cyclophosphamide 700 mg/m^2; administer intravenously in 50–150 mL 0.9% NS or 5% dextrose injection over 15 minutes, on day 4, every 3 weeks (total dosage/cycle = 700 mg/m^2)

Supportive Care

Antiemetic prophylaxis
Emetogenic potential on day 1 is **HIGH***. Potential for delayed symptoms*
Emetogenic potential on day 2 is **MINIMAL**
Emetogenic potential on day 4 is **MODERATE**
See Chapter 39 for antiemetic recommendations

Hematopoietic growth factor (CSF) prophylaxis
Primary prophylaxis is NOT indicated
See Chapter 43 for more information

Antimicrobial prophylaxis
Risk of fever and neutropenia is LOW
   Antimicrobial primary prophylaxis to be considered:
   • Antibacterial—not indicated
   • Antifungal—not indicated
   • Antiviral—not indicated unless patient previously had an episode of HSV

See Chapter 47 for more information

Notes: Encourage patients to increase oral fluids intake on the days on which cisplatin and cyclophosphamide are administered

Use of steroids is discouraged, except for patients with myasthenia gravis who were previously receiving a stable dose of steroids

Patient Population Studied

A study of 16 patients with unresectable locally advanced nonmetastatic thymomas and locally advanced disease after radical surgery. Ten patients with stage III disease, and 6 patients with stage IVa disease. Three patients had recurrent disease after previous surgery

Efficacy (N = 16)*

Complete response	6.25%
Partial response	75%
Stable disease	12.5%
Progressive disease	6.25%

*WHO criteria

Toxicity*
(N = 16 patients/68 Cycles)

	% G3/4
Neutropenia	12.5
Anemia	—
Nausea/vomiting	6.25
Nephrotoxicity	—

*WHO criteria

Treatment Modifications

Adverse Event	Dose Modification
ANC <1500/mm^3 or platelet count <100,000/mm^3	Delay therapy a maximum of 2 weeks until ANC >1500/mm^3 or platelet count >100,000/mm^3
2-Week delay	Decrease dosage of all 4 drugs
Serum creatinine 1.6–2 mg/dL (141–177 μmol/L)	Hold therapy until serum creatinine <1.6 mg/dL (<141 μmol/L), then reduce cisplatin dosage by 25%
Serum creatinine ≥2 mg/dL (≥177 μmol/L)	Hold therapy until serum creatinine <1.6 mg/dL (<141 μmol/L), then reduce cisplatin dosage by 50%

Therapy Monitoring

1. *Pretreatment evaluation:* H&P, chest x-ray, CBC with differential, serum electrolytes, creatinine, LFTs, ECG, CT chest and abdomen, and anterior mediastinotomy with mediastinal biopsy
2. *Before each treatment cycle:* CBC with differential and serum creatinine
3. *Response evaluation:* Chest x-ray after 2 cycles. Complete restaging including CT of chest and abdomen after 4 cycles

Notes

1. Patients who achieve a CR or PR are referred for surgery after 4 cycles of ADOC chemotherapy
2. Additional ADOC is administered to patients with residual disease that is not surgically resectable for a maximum of 6 cycles
3. Patients with histologic evidence of malignancy at surgery receive fractionated RT (total dose = 45 Gy) followed by 2 additional cycles of ADOC

REGIMEN

CISPLATIN + ETOPOSIDE

Giaccone G et al. J Clin Oncol 1996;14:814–820

Hydration before cisplatin: 1000 mL 0.9% sodium chloride injection (0.9% NS); administer intravenously over a minimum of 1 hour. Complete infusion before commencing cisplatin administration

Cisplatin 60 mg/m^2; administer intravenously in 50–500 mL of 0.9% NS over 60 minutes on day 1, every 3 weeks (total dosage/cycle = 60 mg/m^2)

Hydration after cisplatin: 1000 mL 0.9% NS; administer intravenously over a minimum of 2 hours. Monitor and replace magnesium and other electrolytes as needed

Etoposide 120 mg/m^2 per day; administer intravenously over 60 minutes, diluted in 0.9% NS or 5% dextrose injection to a concentration within the range of 0.2–0.4 mg/mL, for 3 consecutive days, days 1–3, every 3 weeks (total dosage/cycle = 360 mg/m^2)

Notes: Patients who tolerate treatment well and do not progress can receive up to 8 consecutive cycles of therapy. Use of steroids is discouraged, except for patients with myasthenia gravis previously receiving a stable dose of steroids

Supportive Care

Antiemetic prophylaxis

Emetogenic potential on day 1 is **HIGH**. *Potential for delayed symptoms*

Emetogenic potential on days 2 and 3 is **LOW**

See Chapter 39 for antiemetic recommendations

Hematopoietic growth factor (CSF) prophylaxis

Primary prophylaxis is NOT indicated

See Chapter 43 for more information

Antimicrobial prophylaxis

Risk of fever and neutropenia is LOW

Antimicrobial primary prophylaxis to be considered:

- Antibacterial—not indicated
- Antifungal—not indicated
- Antiviral—not indicated unless patient previously had an episode of HSV

See Chapter 47 for more information

Treatment Modifications

Adverse Event	Dose Modification
ANC <1500/mm^3 or platelet count <100,000/mm^3	Delay therapy a maximum of 2 weeks until ANC >1500/mm^3 and platelet count >100,000/mm^3
>2-week delay	Decrease dosage of both drugs by 25%

Dose reductions are also made based on nadir counts. If the leukocyte nadir and/or platelet nadir was 1000–1999/mm^3 or 50,000–74,999/mm^3 respectively, the doses of both drugs were reduced by 25% for subsequent cycles; if the nadirs were <1000/mm^3 and/or <50,000/mm^3 respectively, the doses of both drugs were reduced by 50% for subsequent cycles

Serum creatinine 1.6–2 mg/dL (141–177 μmol/L)	Hold therapy until serum creatinine <1.6 mg/dL (<141 μmol/L), then reduce cisplatin dosage by 25%
Serum creatinine ≥1.5 mg/dL (≥133 μmol/L and remained elevated for more than 2 weeks after the scheduled time of the next cycle)	Hold therapy until serum creatinine <1.5 mg/dL (<133 μmol/L), then reduce cisplatin dosage by 50%

Patient Population Studied

A study of 16 patients with recurrent or metastatic malignant thymoma that was considered incurable by excision and/or radiation therapy. Patients who previously received chemotherapy were eligible if they had not received cisplatin or etoposide. Patients receiving corticosteroids were not eligible for the study of previous radiation therapy

Efficacy (N = 15)

Complete response	5 (33%)
Partial response	4 (27%)
Stable disease	6 (40%)
Progressive disease	0 (0%)
Median survival	51.6 months

Toxicity* (N = 28)

	% G3–4
Hematologic	
Leukopenia	51
Thrombocytopenia	—
Anemia	—
Hemorrhage	—
Nonhematologic	
Infection	6
Nausea and vomiting	81
Diarrhea	6
Alopecia	69
Mucositis	6
Peripheral neuropathy	—
Phlebitis	—

*CTC

Therapy Monitoring

1. *Pretreatment evaluation:* H&P, CBC with differential, serum creatinine, LFTs, electrolytes, chest x-ray; CT scan of the chest, and other tumor sites as indicated creatinine clearance if adequacy of renal function is in doubt

2. *Before each treatment cycle:* H&P, chest x-ray, CBC with differential, serum creatinine, LFTs, and electrolytes

3. *Response evaluation every 2 cycles:* CT scans of chest/abdomen

REGIMEN

CISPLATIN + DOXORUBICIN + CYCLOPHOSPHAMIDE (PAC)

Loehrer PJ Sr et al. J Clin Oncol 1997;15:3093–3099

Prechemotherapy hydration: ≥1000 mL 0.9% sodium chloride injection (0.9% NS); administer intravenously over a minimum of 2 hours. Monitor and replace magnesium and other electrolytes as needed

Cisplatin 50 mg/m²; administer intravenously in 50–150 mL of 0.9% NS over 15–30 minutes, on day 1, every 3 weeks (total dosage/cycle = 50 mg/m²)

Doxorubicin 50 mg/m²; administer by intravenous injection over 3–5 minutes, on day 1, every 3 weeks (total dosage/cycle = 50 mg/m²)

Cyclophosphamide 500 mg/m²; administer intravenously in 50–150 mL of 0.9% NS or 5% dextrose injection over 15–60 minutes, on day 1, every 3 weeks (total dosage/cycle = 500 mg/m²)

Postchemotherapy hydration: ≥1000 mL 0.9% NS; administer intravenously over a minimum of 2 hours on day 1, after chemotherapy is completed

Supportive Care

Antiemetic prophylaxis
Emetogenic potential on day 1 is HIGH. Potential for delayed symptoms
See Chapter 39 for antiemetic recommendations

Hematopoietic growth factor (CSF) prophylaxis
Primary prophylaxis is NOT indicated
See Chapter 43 for more information

Antimicrobial prophylaxis
Risk of fever and neutropenia is LOW
  Antimicrobial primary prophylaxis to be considered:
  • Antibacterial—not indicated
  • Antifungal—not indicated
  • Antiviral—not indicated unless patient previously had an episode of HSV
See Chapter 47 for more information

Note: Use of steroids is discouraged, except for patients with myasthenia gravis previously receiving a stable dose of steroids

Patient Population Studied

A study of 23 patients with limited-stage, unresectable thymoma or thymic carcinoma. Patients with limited-stage disease were defined as those patients with disease that could be encompassed by a single radiation therapy portal

Efficacy (N = 23)

Complete response	21.7%
Partial response	47.8%
Progressive disease	4.3%
Median survival	93 months

Treatment Modifications

Adverse Event	Dose Modification
ANC <1500/mm³ or platelet count <100,000/mm³	Delay therapy a maximum of 2 weeks until ANC >1500/mm³ or platelet count >100,000/mm³
2-Week delay	Decrease dosage of all 3 drugs
Serum creatinine 1.6–2 mg/dL (141–177 µmol/L)	Hold therapy until serum creatinine <1.6 mg/dL (<141 µmol/L) then reduce cisplatin dosage by 25%
Serum creatinine ≥2 mg/dL (≥ 177 µmol/L)	Hold therapy until serum creatinine <1.6 mg/dL (<141 µmol/L), then reduce cisplatin dosage by 50%

Therapy Monitoring

1. *Pretreatment evaluation:* H&P, CBC with differential, serum creatinine, LFTs, electrolytes, chest x-ray; creatinine clearance if adequacy of renal function is in doubt
2. *Before each treatment cycle:* H&P, CBC with differential, serum creatinine, LFTs, and electrolytes
3. *Disease evaluation every 2 cycles:* Response evaluated before starting RT

Notes

1. Patients who achieve a CR or PR after 2 or 4 cycles of chemotherapy are referred for RT (total dose = 5400 cGy) to primary tumor and mediastinal and bilateral hilar lymph nodes
2. A maximum of 6 additional cycles of PAC chemotherapy may be administered after completing RT

Toxicity* (N = 26)

	% G1	% G2	% G3	% G4
Hematologic				
Worst hematologic	19	23	12	42
Nonhematologic				
Emesis	15	23	15	—
Diarrhea	8	8	—	—
Infection	12	12	—	—
Cardiac	—	—	4	—
Mucositis	19	—	—	—
Neurologic/ clinical	19	—	4	—
Genitourinary	23	4	—	—
Hepatic	19	—	—	—
Worst nonhematologic	23	42	23	8

*Eastern Cooperative Oncology Group scale

REGIMEN

PACLITAXEL + CARBOPLATIN

Lemma GL et al. J Clin Oncol 2011;29:2060–2065

Premedication (primary prophylaxis against hypersensitivity reactions from paclitaxel):
Dexamethasone 20 mg intravenously 30–60 minutes before paclitaxel
Diphenhydramine 25 mg by intravenous injection 15–30 minutes before paclitaxel
Cimetidine 300 mg (or ranitidine 50 mg, or famotidine 20 mg, or an equivalent histamine receptor [H_2]-subtype antagonist); intravenously over 15–30 minutes, 30–60 minutes before starting paclitaxel administration

Paclitaxel 225 mg/m^2 intravenously in a volume of 0.9% sodium chloride injection or 5% dextrose injection (D5W) sufficient to produce a solution with concentration within the range 0.3–1.2 mg/mL over 3 hours, on day 1, every 3 weeks (total dosage/cycle = 225 mg/m^2)
Carboplatin [calculated dose] AUC = 6 mg/mL · min; intravenously in 50–150 mL D5W over 30 minutes, on day 1, every 3 weeks (total dosage/cycle calculated to produce an AUC = 6 mg/mL · min) (see equation below)
Dexamethasone 8 mg/dose orally every 12 hours for 6 doses after chemotherapy if G ≥2 arthralgias/myalgias occur
• In patients who develop arthralgia or myalgia, include dexamethasone as prophylaxis against recurrent symptoms during subsequent treatment cycles

Carboplatin dose calculation is based on formulae developed to achieve consistent drug exposure within and among patients. Area under the plasma concentration versus time curve (AUC) is the targeted pharmacokinetic end point used to obtain consistent exposure

The method of Calvert et al:
Current product labeling for carboplatin approved by the U.S. Food and Drug Administration describes dose calculation based on a formula described by Calvert et al:

$$\text{Total carboplatin dose (mg)} = (\text{target AUC}) \times (\text{GFR} + 25)$$

In practice, creatinine clearance (Clcr) is used in place of glomerular filtration rate (GFR). Clcr can be measured from a 24-hour urine collection or estimated from any among several equations, such as the method of Cockcroft and Gault:

$$\text{For males, Clcr} = \frac{(140 - \text{age [year]}) \times (\text{body weight [kg]})}{72 \times (\text{serum creatinine [mg/dL]})}$$

$$\text{For females, Clcr} = \frac{(140 - \text{age [year]}) \times (\text{body weight [kg]})}{72 \times (\text{serum creatinine [mg/dL]})} \times 0.85$$

Note: On October 8, 2010, the U.S. Food and Drug Administration (FDA) identified a potential safety issue with carboplatin dosing based on recent changes in the measurement of serum creatinine. By the end of 2010, all clinical laboratories in the United States will use the standardized Isotope Dilution Mass Spectrometry (IDMS) method to measure serum creatinine, which could result in an overestimation of the GFR in some patients with normal renal function. A carboplatin dose calculated with an IDMS-measured serum creatinine result using the Calvert formula could exceed an expected exposure (AUC) and result in increased drug-related toxicity
Provided actual GFR measurements are made to assess renal function, carboplatin can be safely dosed according to the Calvert formula described in product labeling
If GFR (or creatinine clearance) is estimated based on serum creatinine measurements by the IDMS method, the FDA recommended for patients with normal renal function capping an estimated GFR at 125 mL/min for any targeted AUC value. No greater estimated GFR values should be used
U.S. FDA. Carboplatin dosing. [online] May 23, 2013. Available from: http://www.fda.gov/AboutFDA/CentersOffices/OfficeofMedicalProductsandTobacco/CDER/ucm228974.htm

Calvert AH, Newell DR, Gumbrell LA et al. Carboplatin dosage: prospective evaluation of a simple formula based on renal function. J Clin Oncol 1989;7:1748–1756
Cockcroft DW, Gault MH. Prediction of creatinine clearance from serum creatinine. Nephron 1976;16:31–41
Jodrell DI, Egorin MJ, Canetta RM et al. Relationships between carboplatin exposure and tumor response and toxicity in patients with ovarian cancer. J Clin Oncol 1992;10:520–528
Sørensen BT, Strömgren A, Jakobsen P, Jakobsen A. Dose-toxicity relationship of carboplatin in combination with cyclophosphamide in ovarian cancer patients. Cancer Chemother Pharmacol 1991;28:397–401

(continued)

Patient Population Studied

A phase II study of carboplatin and paclitaxel in 46 patients with unresectable thymoma or thymic carcinoma. Patients previously treated with preoperative or adjuvant chemotherapy for thymic malignancy were allowed to enroll, if disease-free survival before recurrence was longer than 1 year

Toxicity (N = 46)

Adverse Event	G3	G4
Neutropenia	NR	24.4
Febrile neutropenia	2.2	2.2
Sensory neuropathy	13.3	0

National Cancer Institute Common Toxicity Criteria, version 2.0

(*continued*)

Supportive Care

Antiemetic prophylaxis
Emetogenic potential is at least **MODERATE**
See Chapter 39 for antiemetic recommendations

Hematopoietic growth factor (CSF) prophylaxis
Primary prophylaxis is NOT indicated
See Chapter 43 for more information

Antimicrobial prophylaxis
Risk of fever and neutropenia is LOW
  Antimicrobial primary prophylaxis to be considered:
  • Antibacterial—not indicated
  • Antifungal—not indicated
  • Antiviral—not indicated unless patient previously had an episode of HSV
See Chapter 47 for more information

Therapy Monitoring

1. *Pretreatment evaluation:* H&P, performance status (PS) evaluation, CBC with differential, metabolic profile including LFTs, CT scan of the chest and abdomen, pregnancy test (in females with childbearing potential)
2. *Before each cycle:* H&P, PS evaluation, CBC with differential, metabolic profile including LFTs, assessment of toxicity
3. *Response evaluation:* Every 2 cycles

Efficacy (N = 44)

Thymoma (N = 21)

ORR (N = 21)*	42.9% (9)	90% CI, 24.5% to 62.8%
CR (N = 21)*	14.3% (3)	
PR (N = 21)*	28.6% (6)	
Median PFS	16.7 months	95% CI, 7.2 to 19.8 months
Median OS	Not reached	Median follow up = 59.4 months
Median duration of response	16.9 months	95% CI, 3.1–22.0 months

Thymic Carcinoma (N = 23)

ORR (N = 22)	21.7% (5)	90% CI, 9.0–40.4%
CR (N = 22)	(0)	
PR (N = 22)	21.7 (5)	
Median PFS	5 months	95% CI, 3.0–8.3 months
Median OS	20 months	95% CI, 5.0–43.6 months
Median duration of response	4.5 months	95% CI, 3.4–9.9 months

*For patients with thymoma, no significant differences among various histologies were noted with respect to objective responses (A/AB v B1/B2 vs thymoma-NOS; $p = 0.49$), but the numbers were not large enough to make meaningful conclusions
Note: patients with thymoma have marginally improved PFS (logrank $p = 0.06$) and OS (logrank $p = 0.01$), compared with patients with thymic carcinoma. Cox regression analysis shows that the hazard ratio of thymic carcinoma over thymoma is 3.0 (95% CI, 1.2–7.8; $p = 0.02$) and 2.1 (95% CI, 1.0–4.5; $p = 0.06$) for OS and PFS, respectively

Treatment Modifications

Adverse Event	Treatment Modification
On day 1 of a cycle ANC $<$1500/mm^3 or platelet count $<$100,000/mm^3	Withhold paclitaxel and carboplatin until ANC $\geq$1500/mm^3 and platelet count $\geq$100,000/mm^3 for a maximum delay of 2 weeks
Delay of $>$2 weeks in reaching ANC $>$1500/mm^3 and platelet count $>$100,000/mm^3	Discontinue paclitaxel and carboplatin
After paclitaxel 225 mg/m^2 and carboplatin target AUC = 6 mg/mL · min: 1. Fever and neutropenia (ANC $<$500/mm^3 with fever $>$38°C) *or* 2. A delay of next cycle by $>$7 days for ANC $<$1500/mm^3, *or* 3. ANC $<$500/mm^3 $>$7 days	Reduce paclitaxel dosage to 175 mg/m^2 and carboplatin dose to target AUC = 5 mg/mL · min every 3 weeks
After paclitaxel 175 mg/m^2 and carboplatin target AUC = 5 mg/mL · min: 1. Fever and neutropenia (ANC $<$500/mm^3 with fever $>$38°C) *or* 2. A delay of next cycle by $>$7 days for ANC $<$1500/mm^3, *or* 3. ANC $<$500/mm^3 $>$7 days	Reduce paclitaxel dosage to 140 mg/m^2 and carboplatin dose to target AUC = 4 mg/mL · min every 3 weeks
After paclitaxel 140 mg/m^2 and carboplatin target AUC = 4 mg/mL · min: 1. Fever and neutropenia (ANC $<$500/mm^3 with fever $>$38°C) *or* 2. A delay of next cycle by $>$7 days for ANC $<$1500/mm^3, *or* 3. ANC $<$500/mm^3 $>$7 days	Discontinue paclitaxel and carboplatin
Platelet count $<$50,000/mm^3 at a paclitaxel dose of 225 mg/m^2 and carboplatin dose of AUC = 6 mg/mL · min every 3 weeks	Reduce paclitaxel dosage to 175 mg/m^2 and carboplatin dose to target AUC = 5 mg/mL · min every 3 weeks
Platelet count $<$50,000/mm^3 at a paclitaxel dose of 175 mg/m^2 and carboplatin dose of AUC = 5 mg/mL · min every 3 weeks	Discontinue paclitaxel and carboplatin
G3/4 sensory neuropathy at a paclitaxel dose of 225 mg/m^2 and carboplatin dose of AUC = 6 mg/mL · min every 3 weeks	Withhold paclitaxel and carboplatin until toxicity G $\leq$1, then reduce paclitaxel dosage to 175 mg/m^2 and carboplatin dose to target AUC = 5 mg/mL · min every 3 weeks
G2 Neurotoxicity	Reduce paclitaxel dosage to 200 mg/m^2
G3 Neurotoxicity	Reduce paclitaxel dosage to 175 mg/m^2
G3/4 Sensory neuropathy after paclitaxel 175 mg/m^2 and carboplatin dose of AUC = 5 mg/mL · min every 3 weeks	Withhold paclitaxel and carboplatin until toxicity G $\leq$1, then reduce paclitaxel dosage to 140 mg/m^2 and carboplatin dose to target AUC = 4 mg/mL · min every 3 weeks
G3/4 Sensory neuropathy after paclitaxel 140 mg/m^2 and carboplatin dose of AUC = 4 mg/mL · min every 3 weeks	Discontinue paclitaxel and carboplatin
G2 Arthralgia/myalgia despite dexamethasone	Reduce paclitaxel dosage to 200 mg/m^2
G3 Arthralgia/myalgia despite dexamethasone	Reduce paclitaxel dosage to 175 mg/m^2
G $\geq$2 AST or G $\geq$3 bilirubin	Hold paclitaxel
Moderate hypersensitivity	Patient may be retreated
Severe hypersensitivity	Discontinue therapy
Chest pain or arrhythmia during chemotherapy	Immediately stop chemotherapy and evaluate the patient
Symptomatic arrhythmias, or $\geq$ second-degree AV block, or an ischemic event	Discontinue therapy

REGIMEN

CAPECITABINE + GEMCITABINE

Palmieri G et al. Ann Oncol 2010;21:1168–1172

Capecitabine 650 mg/m^2 per dose orally twice daily with approximately 200 mL of water within 30 minutes after a meal for 28 doses on days 1–14 every 3 weeks (total dosage/cycle = 18,200 mg/m^2)

Gemcitabine 1000 mg/m^2 per dose; intravenously in 50–250 mL 0.9% sodium chloride injection over 30 minutes for 2 doses, on days 1 and 8, every 3 weeks (total dosage/cycle = 2000 mg/m^2)

Notes:
• Capecitabine is given for 2 consecutive weeks followed by 1 week without treatment
• Doses are given as combinations of 500-mg and 150-mg tablets
• If a dose is missed, do not double the next dose, continue with the original schedule
• Advise patients to stop taking capecitabine and to contact their medical care provider if they develop:
  1. Diarrhea: an additional 4 bowel movements per day in excess of what is normal, or any diarrhea at night
  2. Vomiting: more than once in a 24-hour period
  3. Nausea or anorexia
  4. Stomatitis
  5. Hand–foot syndrome
  6. Fever or infection

Supportive Care
Antiemetic prophylaxis
Emetogenic potential on days 1–14 is **LOW**
See Chapter 39 for antiemetic recommendations

Hematopoietic growth factor (CSF) prophylaxis
Primary prophylaxis is NOT indicated
See Chapter 43 for more information

Antimicrobial prophylaxis
Risk of fever and neutropenia is *LOW*
  Antimicrobial primary prophylaxis to be considered:
  • Antibacterial—not indicated
  • Antifungal—not indicated
  • Antiviral—not indicated unless patient previously had an episode of HSV
See Chapter 47 for more information

Diarrhea management
Latent or delayed onset diarrhea:
  Loperamide 4 mg orally initially after the first loose or liquid stool, *then*
  Loperamide 2 mg orally every 2 hours during waking hours, *plus*
  Loperamide 4 mg orally every 4 hours during hours of sleep
  • Continue for at least 12 hours after diarrhea resolves
  • Recurrent diarrhea after a 12-hour diarrhea-free interval is treated as a new episode
  • Rehydrate orally with fluids and electrolytes during a diarrheal episode
  • If a patient develops blood or mucus in stool, dehydration, or hemodynamic instability, or if diarrhea persists >48 hours despite loperamide, stop loperamide and hospitalize the patient for IV hydration
  Alternatively, a trial of **Diphenoxylate hydrochloride** 2.5 mg **with Atropine sulfate** 0.025 mg (eg, Lomotil)
  • Initial adult dose is 2 tablets 4 times daily until control has been achieved, after which the dose may be reduced to meet individual requirements. Control may often be maintained with as little as 2 tablets daily

(continued)

Patient Population Studied

A phase II study of capecitabine and gemcitabine in 15 patients with metastatic thymic epithelial tumors. All had previously received chemotherapy, including a platinum agent in first-line treatment

Patient Characteristics (N = 15)

	Number of Patients (percent)
Gender	
Male	10 (66.7)
Female	5 (33.3)
Median age (range), 63 years (43–77 years)	
Histology	
Thymoma	12 (80)
B2	6 (40)
B2-B3	3 (20)
B3	3 (20)
Thymic carcinoma	3 (20)
Stage IVB	15 (100)
ECOG performance status	
0	8 (53.3)
1	6 (40)
2	1 (6.7)
Prior therapy	
Thymectomy	7 (46.7)
Mediastinal radiotherapy	8 (53.3)
Neoadjuvant chemotherapy	2 (13.3)
Chemotherapy for metastatic disease	15 (100)
Two prior chemotherapeutic regimens	15 (100)
Two prior regimens	8 (53.3)
Previous chemotherapy*	
Cisplatin	15 (100)
Anthracyclines	15 (100)
Cyclophosphamide	15 (100)
Somatostatin analog	14 (93.3)
Prednisone	14 (93.3)
Etoposide	13 (86.7)
Carboplatin	6 (40)

(continued)

(continued)

- Clinical improvement of acute diarrhea is usually observed within 48 hours. If improvement of chronic diarrhea after treatment with a maximum daily dose of 8 tablets is not observed within 10 days, control is unlikely with further administration

Persistent diarrhea:
  Octreotide 100–150 mcg subcutaneously 3 times daily. Maximum total daily dose is 1500 mcg

Antibiotic therapy during latent or delayed onset diarrhea:
  A fluoroquinolone (eg, **Ciprofloxacin** 500 mg orally every 12 hours) if absolute neutrophil count <500/mm³ with or without accompanying fever in association with diarrhea
  - Antibiotics should also be administered if patient is hospitalized with prolonged diarrhea and should be continued until diarrhea resolves

*Abigerges D et al. J Natl Cancer Inst 1994;86:446–449
Rothenberg ML et al. J Clin Oncol 2001;19:3801–3807
Wadler S et al. J Clin Oncol 1998;16:3169–3178

Hand–foot reaction (palmar–plantar erythrodysesthesia, PPE)

For patients who develop a hand–foot reaction, use topical emollients (eg, Aquaphor), topically or orally administered steroids, antihistamine agents (H₁-receptor antagonists), or pyridoxine. Pyridoxine may provide relief for discomfort/pain associated with PPE although the mechanism through which this occurs remains unclear
- The suggested pyridoxine starting dose is 50 mg/day, which may be increased to a maximum of 200 mg/day
- Patients who develop G1/2 PPE while receiving doxorubicin HCl liposome injection may receive a fixed daily dose of pyridoxine 200 mg. This may allow for treatment to be completed without dosage reduction, treatment delay, or recurrence of PPE

Efficacy (N = 15)

Response After 6 Cycles	Number of Patients (percent)
Overall response rate	6 (40%)
ORR, thymic carcinoma (N = 3)	1 (33%)
Complete response	3 (20%) (95% CI 10–35)
Partial response	3 (20%)
Stable disease	6 (40%)
Progression	3 (20%)
Median number of cycles	6 (3–9)
Median progression-free survival	11 months (95% CI 4–17)
Median progression-free survival, thymoma	11 months
Median progression-free survival, thymic carcinoma	6 months
1-Year survival rate	12/15 (80%)
2-Year survival rate	10/15 (67%)

Patient Population Studied
(continued)

	Number of Patients (percent)
Time from end of previous chemotherapy to relapse	
≤2 months	12 (80)
>2 months	3 (20)
Sites of metastases	
Pleura	15 (100)
Lung	12 (80)
Lymph nodes	12 (80)
Soft tissues	4 (26.7)
Liver	5 (33.3)
Bone	4 (26.7)
Myocardial tissue	2 (13.3)
Brain	1 (6.7)
Paraneoplastic syndrome	
B lymphopenia	13 (86.7)
Hypogammaglobulinemia	11 (73.3)
Myasthenia gravis	7 (46.7)
Autoimmune diabetes	2 (13.3)
Psoriasis	1 (6.7)
Pure red cell aplasia	1 (6.7)

*Only those received by >33% of patients

Toxicity (N = 15)

Adverse Event	% G1/2	% G3	% G4
Neutropenia	46.7	20	0
Anemia	33.3	13.3	0
Thrombocytopenia	33.3	13.3	0
Nausea/vomiting	26.7	6.7	0
Diarrhea	26.7	6.7	0
Alopecia	20	0	0
Hand–foot syndrome	20	6.7	0

National Cancer Institute Common Terminology Criteria for Adverse Events, version 3.0

Treatment Modifications

Adverse Event	Dose Modification
First G2 nonhematologic toxicity	Hold capecitabine and gemcitabine and resume after adverse events resolve to G $\leq$1. No change in dosage required
Second G2 nonhematologic toxicity	Hold capecitabine and gemcitabine and resume after adverse events resolve to G $\leq$1. Reduce dosage of both drugs by 25%
Third G2 nonhematologic toxicity	Hold capecitabine and gemcitabine and resume after adverse events resolve to G $\leq$1. Reduce dosage of both drugs by 50%
Fourth G2 nonhematologic toxicity	Discontinue capecitabine and gemcitabine
First G3 or G4 hematologic or nonhematologic toxicity	Hold capecitabine and gemcitabine and resume after adverse events resolve to G $\leq$1. Reduce dosages of both drugs by 50%
Second G3 or G4 hematologic or nonhematologic toxicity	Discontinue capecitabine and gemcitabine
G3 or G4 toxicity persisting for >3 weeks	Discontinue capecitabine and gemcitabine
Diarrhea, nausea, and vomiting	Treat symptomatically. Resume previous dosage if toxicity is adequately controlled within 2 days after initiating treatment. If control takes longer, reduce the capecitabine dosage or if symptoms occur despite prophylaxis, reduce the capecitabine dosage by 25–50%
ANC 1000–1499/mm^3, WBC 1000–1999/mm^3, or platelets 50,000–99,999/mm^3 on day of treatment	Proceed with treatment, but decrease both drug dosages by 25%
ANC and WBC <1000/mm^3 or platelets <50,000/mm^3 on day of treatment	Hold treatment until ANC and WBC are >1000/mm^3 and platelets >50,000/mm^3. Resume treatment with gemcitabine dosage reduced by 50%
WHO G4 nonhematologic adverse events	Hold treatment until resolution to G $\leq$1, then resume with both drug dosages decreased by 50%

Adapted in part from NCI of Canada CTC

Therapy Monitoring

1. *Before each cycle:* H&P, PS evaluation, CBC with differential, metabolic profile including LFTs, assessment of toxicity
2. *Every week:* CBC with differential, metabolic profile including LFTs
3. *Response evaluation:* Every 2 cycles

37. Thyroid Cancer

Ann Gramza, MD and Sam Wells, MD

Epidemiology

Incidence: 62,980 (male: 15,190; female: 47,790. Estimated new cases for 2014 in the United States) (6.1 per 100,000 males 18.2 per 100,000 females)

Deaths: Estimated 1,890 in 2014 (male: 830; female: 1,060)

Median age: 50 years

Male to female ratio: 1:3

- One of the few cancers that has increased in incidence over the past several years
- Sixth most common cancer in women
- The number of new diagnoses is about double the number from 10 years ago
- Mainly affects young people. Nearly 2 of 3 cases are found in people between the ages of 20 and 55 years

Siegel R et al. CA Cancer J Clin 2014;64:9–29
Surveillance, Epidemiology and End Results (SEER) Program, available from http://seer.cancer.gov (accessed in 2013)

Pathology

Epithelial Carcinomas	Incidence	Other Cell Types	Incidence
Papillary carcinomas	75%	Medullary carcinoma	<8%
Usual papillary	(75)	Anaplastic carcinomas*	2%
Follicular variant	(15)	Lymphoma	Very rare
Tall cell variant	(4)	Angiomatoid neoplasms	Very rare
Columnar cell variant	(<1)	Mucoepidermoid carcinomas	Very rare
Diffuse sclerosing variant	(3)	Malignant adult thyroid teratomas	Very rare
Oxyphilic (Hürthle cell) variant	(2)	Carcinomas with thymic features	Very rare
Follicular carcinomas	10%	Paragangliomas	Very rare
Usual follicular	(76)		
Oxyphilic (Hürthle cell) variant	(20)		
Insular carcinoma	(4)		

*Evolved from papillary or follicular
Ain KB. Rev Endocr Metab Disord 2000;1:225–231
LiVolsi VA. Surgical Pathology of the Thyroid. Philadelphia, PA: WB Saunders, 1990

Papillary thyroid cancer (PTC)
1. Develops from the follicular cells in the normal thyroid
2. Usually found in 1 lobe; only 10–20% appear in both lobes
3. Considered a differentiated thyroid cancer
4. Together with follicular thyroid cancer, accounts for 80–90% of all thyroid cancers
5. Mutations in BRAF have been reported in 60–80% of patients with V600E (T1799A), the most common mutation

Follicular thyroid cancer (FTC)
1. Less common than PTC
2. Develops from the follicular cells in the normal thyroid
3. Considered a differentiated thyroid cancer
4. Together with PTC, accounts for 80–90% of all thyroid cancers
5. *Hürthle cell carcinoma* is usually assumed to be a variant of FTC, although its prognosis is worse
6. Mutations of codon 61 of N-*RAS* (N2) have been reported in as many as 19% of follicular tumors

Medullary thyroid cancer (MTC)
1. Accounts for 5–10% of thyroid cancers
2. Develops in the C cells of the thyroid; has very little, if any, similarity to normal thyroid tissue
3. Occurs with multiple endocrine neoplasia type 2 (MEN 2A and MEN 2B2), in familial medullary thyroid carcinoma (FMTC) and as a sporadic form (≈80% of cases are sporadic)
4. Germline mutations in the *RET* (REarranged during Transfection) protooncogene cause hereditary MTC (MEN 2A, MEN 2B, and FMTC). In addition, up to 50% of patients with sporadic MTC have somatic *RET* mutations
5. MEN 2B: RET mutations in codons 918, 883, or compound heterozygotes (V804M + E805K, Y806C or S904C)

(continued)

Pathology (continued)

6. MEN 2A and FMTC: RET mutations in codons 609, 611, 618, 620, 630, 634, 768, 790, 791, 804, or 891

7. The constitutively active RET oncoproteins associated with MTC are sensitive to agents that inhibit RET kinase providing a rationale for targeting RET in patients with MTC

Anaplastic thyroid cancer (ATC)

1. Rare and fast-growing tumors. The majority present with extensive local invasion. 15–50% have metastatic disease at presentation with lung and pleura most common sites of metastases followed by bone, brain, and other organs

2. A poorly differentiated thyroid cancer that starts from differentiated thyroid cancer or a benign tumor of the gland. Approximately 50% have either a prior or a coexistent differentiated carcinoma

3. Loss or mutation of the p53 tumor suppressor is commonly found

Work-up

Initial Work-up of Thyroid Nodule

Thyroid nodule in clinically euthyroid patient

1. TSH level

2. Ultrasound of thyroid and central neck area

3. Fine-needle aspiration (FNA) biopsy of thyroid nodule

Note: No role for thyroid scanning unless thyrotoxic (TSH suppressed):
- If thyrotoxic and palpated nodule is "hot" on scan, it is likely benign and biopsy is unnecessary. Refer to an endocrinologist
- If nodule is "cold," proceed to FNA

Neck lymph node

1. FNA biopsy is appropriate

Mass at site distant from neck

2. Biopsy (resection) and immunohistochemistry for thyroglobulin; calcitonin

Initial Work-up (Histologic Diagnosis Established)

Papillary or follicular carcinomas and their subtypes (usually iodine avid)

1. *Do not use iodinated contrast for radiography of any type of papillary or follicular carcinomas.* This stable iodine can interfere with ^{131}I scans and therapy for up to 10 months

2. *Preop:*
- Neck ultrasound or neck MRI
- Noncontrast chest CT
- CT or MRI for fixed, bulky substernal lesions
- Evaluate vocal cord mobility

3. *Postop:*
- ^{131}I scanning (see below)
- Thyroglobulin (TG) level

Dedifferentiated papillary/follicular cancers (iodine nonavid, often not apparent initially)

1. *CT scans (may use contrast if known to be nonavid for iodine):* Often "fused" with PET scans

2. *Preop:*
- Neck ultrasound or neck MRI
- Noncontrast chest CT
- CT or MRI for fixed, bulky substernal lesions
- Evaluate vocal cord mobility

3. *Postop:*
- ^{131}I scanning (see below)
- Thyroglobulin (TG) level

4. *PET scans (^{18}F-deoxyglucose):* Sensitivity enhanced with recombinant human TSH pretreatment

5. Radiographic bone surveys (may not need if PET scan is negative and all other scans do not demonstrate any obvious evidence of disease in bone)

(continued)

Work-up (continued)

Medullary thyroid carcinoma
1. Complete CT survey (with contrast)
2. Neck ultrasound
3. Evaluate vocal cord mobility
4. Calcitonin level
5. CEA level
6. Serum calcium
7. *MEN2A and MEN2B:* Pheochromocytoma screening. Evaluate and treat appropriately before continuing

Note: If a germline mutation is found, genetic counseling and testing of first-degree relatives are recommended

Anaplastic carcinoma
1. Complete CT survey (with contrast)
2. Consider bone scan or PET scan (may not need bone scan if PET scan is done)
3. May need restaging at 2- to 4-week intervals because of rapid rate of tumor progression

Follow-up (Histologic Diagnosis Established)

Papillary or follicular carcinomas (and their subtypes)
In patients who have had thyroidectomy and are receiving suppressive doses of levothyroxine (maintain TSH ≤ 0.1 mIU/L):

1. Serial TG levels every 6 months (monitor for presence of interfering anti-TG antibodies)
   Note: The "normal range" for TG in this situation is "undetectable"
2. Physical exams, patient neck self-exams
3. [131]I whole-body scans (WBS) every 6 months until scan and TG are negative. [131]I therapy is administered if WBS is positive (see Initial ^{131}I WBS below)
4. CT of chest (noncontrast only) (interval defined by disease status)
5. PET scans if ^{131}I WBS is negative but TG is positive. Sensitivity correlates with tumor dedifferentiation and hexokinase I expression (interval defined by disease status)
6. Radiographic bone survey (interval defined by disease status)
7. Neck ultrasonography (interval defined by disease status)

Initial ^{131}I WBS: Prepare with hypothyroid protocol:
- ≈ 6 *Weeks before scan:* Stop levothyroxine therapy. Continue without levothyroxine >6 weeks if needed until TSH >30 mIU/L (first 4 weeks on **liothyronine sodium** 25 mcg orally twice per day)
- *2 Weeks before and during scan:* Institute low-iodine diet

If the ^{131}I WBS is positive or if the TG level is above the lowest detectable limit*	Treat with [131]I. Obtain ^{131}I WBS (posttreatment WBS) 48–72 hours after ^{131}I therapy. Value of subsequent treatments is based on verifying uptake on posttreatment WBS and/or significant decrease of stimulated TG
If the ^{131}I WBS is negative *despite* hypothyroid protocol *and* if TG level is undetectable	Resume levothyroxine therapy and confirm absence of dedifferentiated disease (see nos. 4–7 above). If still negative, in subsequent studies, use recombinant human TSH preparation protocol (below)

*The lowest detectable limit differs considerably from one TG assay to another. Check with laboratory

Follow-up ^{131}I WBS: Prepare with recombinant human TSH (thyrotropin alfa, Thyrogen®) protocol:
- *2 Weeks before and during scan:* Institute low-iodine diet
- *Days 1 and 2:* Administer **recombinant human TSH** 0.9 mg/day intramuscularly for 2 consecutive days
- *Day 3:* Administer 4–5 mCi ^{131}I orally
- *Day 5:* Perform ^{131}I WBS (≥ 30 min/view; $\geq 140,000$ counts)
- *Day 5:* Obtain serum TG, antithyroglobulin autoantibody, and TSH levels

Note: Frequency of follow-up ^{131}I WBS and TG levels: Every 6 months until both ^{131}I WBS and TG levels are negative, then double the time interval between each negative study. Follow-up is life-long, considering current diagnostic modalities. Maximum interval between negative studies is 5 years

Note: A TG level greater than the lowest detectable limit is sufficient evidence for persistent/recurrent disease, even in the absence of positive ^{131}I WBS. Antithyroglobulin autoantibodies occur in 20% of patients and interfere with the TG assay making it insensitive, but can sometimes be a surrogate marker for persistent disease

Medullary carcinoma
1. Complete CT survey (with contrast)
2. Calcitonin and CEA levels

Staging

Separate stage groupings are recommended for papillary or follicular (differentiated), medullary, and anaplastic (undifferentiated) carcinoma

Papillary or Follicular (Differentiated)

Younger than 45 Years

Group	T	N	M
I	Any T	Any N	M0
II	Any T	Any N	M1

Papillary or Follicular (Differentiated)

45 Years and Older

Group	T	N	M
I	T1	N0	M0
II	T2	N0	M0
III	T3	N0	M0
	T1	N1a	M0
	T2	N1a	M0
	T3	N1a	M0
IVA	T4a	N0	M0
	T4a	N1a	M0
	T1	N1b	M0
	T2	N1b	M0
	T3	N1b	M0
	T4a	N1b	M0
IVB	T4b	Any N	M0
IVC	Any T	Any N	M1

Medullary Carcinoma (All Age Groups)

Group	T	N	M
I	T1	N0	M0
II	T2	N0	M0
	T3	N0	M0
III	T1	N1a	M0
	T2	N1a	M0
	T3	N1a	M0
IVA	T4a	N0	M0
	T4a	N1a	M0
	T1	N1b	M0
	T2	N1b	M0
	T3	N1b	M0
	T4a	N1b	M0
IVB	T4b	Any N	M0
IVC	Any T	Any N	M1

Anaplastic Carcinoma

All anaplastic carcinomas are considered Stage IV

Group	T	N	M
IVA	T4a	Any N	M0
IVB	T4b	Any N	M0
IVC	Any T	Any N	M1

Regional Lymph Nodes (N)

Regional lymph nodes are the central compartment, lateral cervical, and upper mediastinal lymph nodes

NX	Regional lymph nodes cannot be assessed
N0	No regional lymph node metastasis
N1	Regional lymph node metastasis
N1a	Metastasis to Level VI (pretracheal, paratracheal, and prelaryngeal/Delphian lymph nodes)
N1b	Metastasis to unilateral, bilateral, or contralateral cervical (Levels I, II, III, IV, or V) or retropharyngeal or superior mediastinal lymph nodes (Level VII)

Primary Tumor (T)

All categories may be subdivided: (s) solitary tumor and (m) multifocal tumor (the largest determines the classification)

TX	Primary tumor cannot be assessed
T0	No evidence of primary tumor
T1	Tumor 2 cm or less in greatest dimension, limited to the thyroid
T1a	Tumor 1 cm or less, limited to the thyroid
T1b	Tumor more than 1 cm but not more than 2 cm in greatest dimension, limited to the thyroid
T2	Tumor more than 2 cm but not more than 4 cm in greatest dimension, limited to the thyroid
T3	Tumor more than 4 cm in greatest dimension, limited to the thyroid, or any tumor with minimal extrathyroid extension (eg, extension to sternothyroid muscle or perithyroid soft tissues)
T4a	Moderately advanced disease. Tumor of any size extending beyond the thyroid capsule to invade subcutaneous soft tissues, larynx, trachea, esophagus, or recurrent laryngeal nerve
T4b	Very advanced disease. Tumor invades prevertebral fascia or encases carotid artery or mediastinal vessels

All anaplastic carcinomas are considered T4 tumors

T4a	Intrathyroidal anaplastic carcinoma
T4b	Anaplastic carcinoma with gross extrathyroid extension

Distant Metastasis (M)

M0	No distant metastasis (no pathologic M0; use clinical M to complete stage group)
M1	Distant metastasis

Edge SB, Byrd DR, Compton CC, Fritz AG, Greene FL, Trotti A, editors. AJCC Cancer Staging Manual. 7th ed. New York: Springer; 2010

Expert Opinion

Surgical Approach

1. *Cytologically (or clinically) suspicious or indeterminate thyroid nodule:* Ipsilateral complete lobectomy and isthmusectomy followed by completion (during initial or subsequent procedure) of total thyroidectomy if malignancy confirmed, *unless there is a solitary intrathyroidal papillary microcarcinoma with no lymphadenopathy*

2. *Thyroid biopsy or extrathyroidal site biopsy positive for cancer:* Total thyroidectomy with ipsilateral and central modified node dissection unless it is a solitary intrathyroidal papillary microcarcinoma (≤1.0 cm) with no lymphadenopathy (in which case perform a lobectomy only)

3. *Grossly invasive tumor or bilateral disease:* Total thyroidectomy with bilateral and central modified node dissection (exception: thyroidectomy not necessary for lymphomas)

4. Medullary thyroid carcinoma requires total thyroidectomy with bilateral and central neck dissections

5. Anaplastic carcinoma requires as complete a local resection as possible, often despite grossly invasive disease. Initially unresectable tumor might be resected after a partial course of external beam radiation therapy

Radioactive Iodine (^{131}I) for Papillary and Follicular Carcinomas Including Hürthle Cell Carcinoma
(*Note:* Prepare with **hypothyroid protocol** [see Work-up: Initial ^{131}I WBS])

Initial ablation for papillary and follicular carcinomas
1. *Intrathyroidal disease with no metastases:* 100 mCi empiric dosing
2. *N1M0 disease:* 140–200 mCi empiric dosing
3. *T3-4 or M1 disease:* 200 mCi empiric dosing or treat to maximal red marrow tolerance (200 REM, ascertain with whole body/blood dosimetry analysis)

Proven thyroid bed uptake or suspected residual disease based on pathology, postoperative thyroglobulin, and surgical findings
1. 30–100 mCi adjuvant dosing to destroy residual thyroid function and sites of uptake

Follow-up treatments for:
• Positive ^{131}I WBS
• TG level greater than the lowest detection limit (1 ng/mL)
• Stimulated TG >10 ng/mL and negative scans (including PET)
  1. 150–200 mCi empiric dosing with posttreatment ^{131}I imaging

Follow-up treatments for M1 disease
1. Single dose to maximal red marrow tolerance (200 REM; ascertain with whole-body/blood dosimetry analysis)
2. Adjuvant **lithium carbonate** to enhance ^{131}I tumor retention: **Lithium carbonate** 600 mg as loading dose orally, followed by **lithium carbonate** 300 mg orally every 8 hours. Begin lithium carbonate 2 days before the administration of ^{131}I and continue for an additional 5 days after ^{131}I (total 7 days)
3. *Note:* On the morning of ^{131}I therapy, obtain STAT trough lithium level. Titrate dose to a trough level of 0.6–1.2 mEq/L

Repeat Surgery
Indications:
1. Resection of macroscopic residual disease before ^{131}I
2. Localized non–iodine-avid tumor
3. Distant critical sites (eg, spinal cord, brain)
4. Bone metastases
5. Isolated distant metastases and palliation of recurrent disease

Suppression of TSH with Levothyroxine

Indication: Chronic (lifelong) tumorostatic therapy in all cases of papillary and follicular carcinomas
Goal: TSH ≤0.1 mIU/L, using minimal suppressive daily levothyroxine dosage
Note: May use a β-adrenergic blocker to mitigate tachycardia and risk of late left ventricular hypertrophy

(continued)

Three-Year Survival

Papillary Thyroid Cancer	
Stage I	100%
Stage II	100%
Stage III*	96%
Stage IV*	45%

Follicular Thyroid Cancer	
Stage I	100%
Stage II	100%
Stage III*	79%
Stage IV*	47%

Medullary Thyroid Cancer	
Stage I	100%
Stage II	97%
Stage III	78%
Stage IV	24%

Anaplastic Thyroid Cancer	
Stage IV†	9%

*All stages III and IV patients with follicular or papillary thyroid cancer are, by definition, more than 45 years old
†All anaplastic carcinomas are considered Stage IV

Expert Opinion (*continued*)

Bisphosphonate Therapy

Consider bisphosphonate therapy in patients with papillary, follicular, or medullary thyroid carcinoma who have symptomatic bone metastases or who have extensive disease that is not symptomatic, but who may need intervention if they progress

External Beam Radiation Therapy

Indications:

1. Localized non–iodine-avid disease (after surgical resection)
2. Protection of thoracic inlet after resection of anaplastic carcinoma (use hyperfractionation, if tolerated)
3. Palliation of distant sites of disease

Selected Multimodal Approaches

Anaplastic carcinoma: Complete primary resection followed by local external beam radiation. Restage to detect early recurrence or distant disease, then treat with chemotherapy using these sites to assess response

Systemic Chemotherapy

1. Clearly effective in thyroid lymphoma
2. Necessary (although usually futile) in anaplastic thyroid cancer
3. Should be considered in patients with symptomatic/metastatic MTC. See vandetanib regimen below
4. Despite reports of measured tumor shrinkage with some vascular endothelial growth factor (VEGF) tyrosine kinase inhibitors, evidence is still lacking that these therapies will either improve symptoms and quality of life or prolong survival. Consequently, because these therapies often have chronic and difficult side effects, patients with metastatic disease who have exhausted surgical and radiotherapy options and require systemic treatment should be referred for clinical trials
5. Inhibitors of Raf kinase have shown promising activity in preliminary reports and are undergoing extensive testing in patients with papillary thyroid carcinomas (as many as 80% of tumors harbor a mutant BRAF) with the expectation that they will likely be approved for this indication

^{18}F FDG PET Scans

As with most cancers, recommendations regarding the use of positron emission tomography (PET) scans in thyroid cancer are not evidence based at this time. In very few instances will a PET scan result alter management. General recommendations can be summarized as follows:

1. *Initial work-up of a thyroid nodule:* Although increased FDG accumulation may heighten suspicion and help identify a thyroid nodule as malignant, the poor sensitivity and high cost do not support the use of PET imaging as a tool for diagnosis
2. *DTC:* In patients considered intermediate- and high-risk, PET may have some utility in:
   - Assessing the extent of disease in patients with metastases, and
   - Assessing patients with high thyroglobulin (TG) levels and negative ^{131}I scans. In these patients, a positive PET may indicate dedifferentiation associated with tumor aggressiveness
3. *MTC:* The role of PET is limited
4. *ATC:* PET can help assess the extent of disease

REGIMEN

NEOADJUVANT + ADJUVANT DOXORUBICIN AND RADIATION WITH DEBULKING SURGERY

Nilsson O et al. World J Surg 1998;22:25–30
Tennvall J et al. Cancer 1994;74:1348–1354

TREATMENT A

Preoperative treatment:
Doxorubicin 20 mg/dose; administer by intravenous injection over 3–5 minutes starting 1–2 hours before radiation therapy, weekly, for 3 weeks (total dose/3-week course = 60 mg)
Radiation 100 cGy per fraction twice daily for 30 fractions with a minimum of 6 hours between fractions 5 days/week to a target dose of 3000 cGy in 3 weeks
Debulking surgery:
Around week 5 approximately 10–14 days after completing preoperative radiation therapy
Postoperative treatment:
Doxorubicin 20 mg/dose; administer by intravenous injection over 3–5 minutes, weekly, starting 1–2 hours before radiation therapy (total dose/week = 20 mg)
Radiation 100 cGy per fraction twice daily for 16 fractions with a minimum of 6 hours between fractions 5 days/week to a target dose of 1600 cGy (total cumulative radiation including preoperative dose = 4600 cGy over approximately 70 days)
Additional doxorubicin:
Doxorubicin 20 mg/dose; administer by intravenous injection over 3–5 minutes, weekly, in patients considered to be in "reasonably good condition" (maximum dosage/complete treatment = 750 mg/m^2)
Note: Doxorubicin is administered as a fixed dose (20 mg), but cumulative dosage is calculated as mg/m^2

Supportive Care
Antiemetic prophylaxis
Emetogenic potential on days doxorubicin is administered is **MODERATE**
See Chapter 39 for antiemetic recommendations

Hematopoietic growth factor (CSF) prophylaxis
Primary prophylaxis is NOT indicated
See Chapter 43 for more information

Antimicrobial prophylaxis
Risk of fever and neutropenia is LOW
  Antimicrobial primary prophylaxis to be considered:
  • Antibacterial—not indicated
  • Antifungal—not indicated
  • Antiviral—not indicated unless patient previously had an episode of HSV
See Chapter 47 for more information

TREATMENT B

Preoperative treatment:
Doxorubicin 20 mg/dose; administer by intravenous injection over 3–5 minutes, weekly, starting 1–2 hours before radiation therapy for 3 weeks (total dose/3-week course = 60 mg)
Radiation 130 cGy/per fraction twice daily for 23 fractions with a minimum of 6 hours between fractions, 5 days/week to a target dosage of 3000 cGy
Debulking surgery:
Around week 4 (approximately 2 weeks after completing preoperative radiation therapy)
Postoperative treatment:
Doxorubicin 20 mg/week; administer by intravenous injection over 3–5 minutes, weekly, starting 1 hour before radiation therapy (total dose/week = 20 mg)
Radiation 130 cGY/per fraction twice daily for 12 fractions with a minimum of 6 hours between fractions 5 days/week to a target dosage of 1600 cGY (total cumulative radiation dose including preoperative dose = 4600 cGY over approximately 50 days)
Additional doxorubicin:
Doxorubicin 20 mg/week; administer by intravenous injection over 3–5 minutes, weekly, in patients considered to be in "reasonably good condition" (maximum dosage/complete treatment = 400–440 mg)

Treatment Modifications

Postoperative doxorubicin was administered to patients with good performance status and in the absence of disease progression

Patient Population Studied

A study of 33 patients with anaplastic thyroid carcinoma treated with combined radiation, chemotherapy, and surgery. In later review, 160 patients were studied

Efficacy (N = 33)

	Treatment	
	A (n = 16)	B (n = 17)
Median survival	3.5 months	4.5 months
Local control	5 patients	11 patients
Local failure*	6 patients	2 patients
Persistent local disease*	5 patients	3 patients

*Cause of death

1. 24% of patient deaths attributed to local failure
2. 48% of patients had no signs of local recurrence
3. Preoperative doxorubicin and concomitant hyperfractionated radiation therapy converted unresectable tumors into a resectable state in 23 patients

Toxicity (N = 33)

1. WHO grades I and II mucosal and skin toxicity
2. Hematologic toxicity not observed
3. Treatment-related toxicities did not prevent any patient from completing planned treatment

Therapy Monitoring

1. *Weekly:* CBC with differential
2. *Before each treatment:* CBC with differential
3. *Every 2–3 cycles:* Imaging studies to evaluate response

Notes

Doxorubicin has been used historically; however, as a single agent, it is not considered an effective chemotherapeutic drug for anaplastic carcinoma

REGIMEN

96-HOUR CONTINUOUS-INFUSION PACLITAXEL AND WEEKLY PACLITAXEL

Ain KB et al. Thyroid 2000;10:587–594

Continuous 96-Hour IV Infusion

Optional premedication* (Primary prophylaxis against hypersensitivity reactions from paclitaxel):
Dexamethasone 20 mg/dose; administer orally for 2 doses on the evening before and the morning of chemotherapy before paclitaxel *plus*

Diphenhydramine 50 mg for 1 dose; administer by intravenous injection 30 minutes before paclitaxel *and*

Ranitidine 50 mg or **cimetidine** 300 mg for 1 dose; administer by intravenous infusion in 25–100 mL 0.9% sodium chloride injection (0.9% NS) or 5% dextrose injection (D5W) over 5–30 minutes given 30 minutes before paclitaxel

* The incidence of hypersensitivity reactions with 96-hour continuous infusion of paclitaxel is much lower than with other paclitaxel regimens, and in most patients premedication is not required. If a premedication regimen is not used, observe the patient carefully for at least 1 hour in the first cycle to ensure that no reaction occurs. If a reaction occurs, immediately stop paclitaxel infusion and administer the suggested premedication regimen, substituting intravenous dexamethasone

Paclitaxel 30–35 mg/m^2 per day; administer by continuous intravenous infusion in a volume of 0.9% NS or D5W sufficient to produce a solution with concentration within the range 0.3–1.2 mg/mL over 24 hours for 4 consecutive days, on days 1–4, every 3 weeks, for up to 6 cycles (total dosage/cycle for 30 mg/m^2 per day = 120 mg/m^2 for 35 mg/m^2 per day = 140 mg/m^2)

Supportive Care

Antiemetic prophylaxis
Emetogenic potential is **LOW**
See Chapter 39 for antiemetic recommendations

Hematopoietic growth factor (CSF) prophylaxis
Primary prophylaxis is NOT indicated
See Chapter 43 for more information

Antimicrobial prophylaxis
Risk of fever and neutropenia is LOW
    Antimicrobial primary prophylaxis to be considered:
    • Antibacterial—not indicated
    • Antifungal—not indicated
    • Antiviral—not indicated unless patient previously had an episode of HSV
See Chapter 47 for more information

Intermittent Weekly Administration

Note: Subsequent clinical experience suggests that optimal use of paclitaxel uses a 1-hour infusion of 175 mg/m^2 given weekly for 3 weeks every month, with restaging each month, and continuing until there is progressive disease or limiting toxicity. *This dose must be administered carefully with premedication against hypersensitivity reactions and growth factor support assessing patient before each dose with attention to occurrence of mucositis and neutropenia*

Primary prophylaxis against hypersensitivity reactions from paclitaxel:
Dexamethasone 20 mg/dose; administer orally for 2 doses on the evening before and the morning on which chemotherapy is given (eg, one dose 12 to 14 hours before paclitaxel plus a second dose 6 to 7 hours before paclitaxel):

Diphenhydramine 50 mg; administer by intravenous injection 30 minutes before paclitaxel, *and*:
Ranitidine 50 mg or **cimetidine** 300 mg; administer intravenously in 25–100 mL of 0.9% NS or D5W over 5–30 minutes, 30 minutes before paclitaxel

Paclitaxel 175 mg/m^2; administer by intravenous infusion in a volume of 0.9% NS or D5W sufficient to produce a solution with concentration of 0.3–1.2 mg/mL over 3 hours for 3 doses on 3 consecutive weeks every 28 days (monthly) (total dosage/cycle = 525 mg/m^2)

(continued)

Treatment Modifications

Adverse Event	Dose Modification
96-Hour Continuous Infusion Paclitaxel	
G2 hematologic adverse events	Hold paclitaxel until adverse events resolve to G1 or disappear, then resume paclitaxel with dosage reduced by 25%
G2/3 gastrointestinal, neurologic, cardiac, musculoskeletal toxicities, or mucositis	
G4 or unremitting G3 adverse events	Discontinue paclitaxel
ANC nadir <500/mm^3, platelet nadir <50,000/mm^3, or febrile neutropenia	Reduce paclitaxel dosage by 25%
Day 1 ANC <1500/mm^3 or platelets <100,000/mm^3	Delay chemotherapy until ANC > 1500/mm^3 and platelets >100,000/mm^3 for maximum delay of 2 weeks
Weekly Paclitaxel	
Day 1 ANC <1500/mm^3 or platelets <100,000/mm^3	Delay chemotherapy until ANC <1500/mm^3 and platelets >100,000/mm^3 for maximum delay of 2 weeks
Delay of <2 weeks in reaching ANC <1500/mm^3 and platelets >100,000/mm^3	Discontinue therapy
G2 neurotoxicity	Reduce paclitaxel dosage to 135 mg/m^2
G3 neurotoxicity	Discontinue paclitaxel
G2 arthralgia/myalgia despite dexamethasone prophylaxis	Reduce paclitaxel dosage to 135 mg/m^2
G3 arthralgia/myalgia despite dexamethasone prophylaxis	Discontinue paclitaxel
Moderate hypersensitivity	Patient may be retreated
Severe hypersensitivity	Discontinue therapy

(*continued*)

Supportive Care
Antiemetic prophylaxis
Emetogenic potential is LOW
See Chapter 39 for antiemetic recommendations

Hematopoietic growth factor (CSF) prophylaxis
Primary prophylaxis may be indicated
See Chapter 43 for more information

Antimicrobial prophylaxis
Risk of fever and neutropenia is LOW
   Antimicrobial primary prophylaxis to be considered:
   • Antibacterial—not indicated
   • Antifungal—not indicated
   • Antiviral—not indicated unless patient previously had an episode of HSV
See Chapter 47 for more information

Therapy Monitoring

1. *Before every cycle:* CBC with differential, platelet count, and LFTs
2. *Radiologic studies:* Every 2 cycles

Toxicity* (N = 11/8)

(Paclitaxel 140 mg/m², n = 11[†])

	G1	G2
Nausea	6	1
Alopecia	3	
Vomiting	2	
Diarrhea	3	
Fever	1	2

(Paclitaxel 120 mg/m², n = 8[‡])

	G1	G2
Nausea	1	
Alopecia	1	
Stomatitis	1	
Fatigue	1	
Neutropenia		1

*NCI Common Terminology Criteria for Adverse Events
[†]Patients who received paclitaxel 35 mg/m² per day for 4 days (total dosage/cycle = 140 mg/m²)
[‡]Patients who received paclitaxel 30 mg/m² per day for 4 days (total dosage/cycle = 120 mg/m²)

Patient Population Studied

A study of 20 patients with metastatic anaplastic thyroid cancer

Efficacy* (N = 19)

Partial responses	47%
Complete responses	5%
Disease stabilization	5%
Progressive disease	42%
Therapeutic response	Median survival: 32 weeks
No therapeutic response	Median survival: 10 weeks

*From WHO criteria

REGIMEN

MEDULLARY THYROID CANCER

VANDETANIB

Wells SA Jr et al. J Clin Oncol 2010;28:767–772
Wells et al. J Clin Oncol 2012;30:134–141

Vandetanib 100–300 mg per day; administer orally, continually (total dose/week = 700–2100 mg)

Note:

• Patients should take vandetanib once daily at the same time each day. Vandetanib absorption is not affected by a meal, so it may be administered with or without food. Tablets should be swallowed whole (without chewing)

  ▪ If a patient misses a scheduled dose of vandetanib, they may take the missed dose if the next scheduled dose is not due to be taken within the next 12 hours

  ▪ If <12 hours remain before the next scheduled dose is due, the patient should not take the missed dose but should wait and take the next regularly scheduled dose

  ▪ If the patient vomits ≤15 minutes after taking vandetanib, another dose may be administered. The dose may only be repeated only once

  ▪ If a patient vomits >15 minutes after an oral dose was administered, no attempt to supplement or replace the dose should be made

• If vandetanib tablets cannot be swallowed whole, they may be dispersed in a glass containing 2 ounces of non-carbonated water and stirred for approximately 10 minutes until the tablet is dispersed (tablets will not completely dissolve)

  ▪ No other liquids should be used

  ▪ The dispersion should be immediately swallowed or administered through nasogastric or gastrostomy tubes

  ▪ To ensure the full dose is received, any residue in the glass should be mixed again with an additional 4 ounces of non-carbonated water and swallowed

• Vandetanib should be withheld in patients who develop electrolyte abnormalities associated with diarrhea until the electrolyte abnormalities are corrected because of the risk of QTc prolongation and subsequent arrhythmias

Note: Patients receive once-daily oral doses of vandetanib 300 mg until disease progression, or unacceptable toxicity

Note: **Although the starting dose is 300 mg per day, a majority of patients will experience an adverse event making a dose reduction necessary.** In the study cited:

1. Vandetanib dose was reduced or interrupted in 24 patients because of adverse events, most commonly diarrhea (n = 7)

2. Among the 24 patients who required dose reduction or interruption, 21 patients had a combination of dose reduction and dose interruption and 3 patients had a dose interruption without dose reduction

3. Some patients required more than a single dose reduction

4. For patients who required dose reductions, vandetanib was decreased to:
   200 mg/day (60%, 18/30)
   150 mg/day (3%, 1/30)
   100 mg/day (23%, 7/30)
   50 mg/day (6.6%, 2/30)

5. The median time to first dose reduction was 4.9 months (95% CI, 2.7–8.4 months)

Supportive Care
Antiemetic prophylaxis
Emetogenic potential is **MINIMAL–LOW**
See Chapter 39 for antiemetic recommendations

Hematopoietic growth factor (CSF) prophylaxis
Primary prophylaxis is NOT indicated
See Chapter 43 for more information

(continued)

Patient Population Studied

Baseline Demographics and Patient Characteristics

Characteristic	Vandetanib (300 mg) (n = 231)		Placebo (n = 100)	
	No.	%	No.	%
Sex				
Male	134	58	56	56
Female	97	42	44	44
Mean age, years	50.7		53.4	
WHO performance status				
0	154	67	58	58
1	67	29	38	38
2	10	4	4	4
Disease type				
Hereditary	28	12	5	5
Sporadic or unknown	203	88	95	95
Locally advanced	14	6	3	3
Metastatic	217	94	97	97
Hepatic	154	67	64	64
Lymph nodes	135	58	68	68
Respiratory	126	54	60	60
Bone/locomotor	78	34	40	40
Neck	33	14	17	17
No. of organs involved (excluding thyroid)				
0 or 1	29	13	8	8
≥2	202	87	92	92
Prior systemic therapy for MTC				
0	141	61	58	58
≥1	90	39	42	42
***RET* mutation**				
Positive	137	59	50	50
Negative	2	1	6	6
Unknown	92	40	44	44

MTC, medullary thyroid cancer; *RET*, rearranged during transfection

(continued)

Antimicrobial prophylaxis
Risk of fever and neutropenia is LOW
  Antimicrobial primary prophylaxis to be considered:
  • Antibacterial—not indicated
  • Antifungal—not indicated
  • Antiviral—not indicated unless patient previously had an episode of HSV
See Chapter 47 for more information

Treatment Modifications

Vandetanib Dose Levels

Starting dose: Level 1	300 mg
Level −1	200 mg
Level −2	100 mg
Level −3	50 mg (100 mg every other day)

Adverse Event	Dose Modification
Cutaneous Toxicities	
Rash G ≥2	Hold vandetanib and provide *immediate* symptomatic treatment
If treatment held for more than 3 weeks because of cutaneous toxicity	Discontinue therapy
When toxicity resolves to G ≤1	Restart vandetanib at 1 dose level lower than that administered at the time the toxicity developed. Symptomatic treatment may continue indefinitely as a preventive measure
If cutaneous toxicity G3/4 recurs at a reduced doses of vandetanib	Again, hold vandetanib until the toxicity resolves to G ≤1 at which time vandetanib should be restarted at 1 dose level lower than that administered at the time the toxicity developed. Symptomatic treatment may continue indefinitely as a preventive measure
If cutaneous toxicity G3/4 recurs at dose level −2 or lower	Discontinue therapy
If with or without continued symptomatic treatment the cutaneous toxicity does not recur at the reduced doses of vandetanib	The dose of vandetanib may be increased 1 dose level to that which was being administered at the time the cutaneous toxicity developed. If toxicity recurs following this increase, then follow the guidelines above, with the exception that when drug is restarted the vandetanib dose should be reduced 1 dose level
Diarrhea	
G1/2 diarrhea	Focus on symptomatic treatment designed to resolve the diarrhea. No dose modifications will be made for G1/2 diarrhea unless G2 diarrhea persists for more than 2 weeks
If G2 diarrhea persists for more than 2 weeks	Then the guidelines below for G3/4 diarrhea should be followed

(continued)

Toxicity

Common Adverse Events (Safety Population)

Adverse Event	Vandetanib (300 mg) (n = 231)		Placebo (n = 99)	
	Number	%	Number	%
Any grade occurring with an incidence ≥10% overall				
Diarrhea	130	56	26	26
Rash	104	45	11	11
Nausea	77	33	16	16
Hypertension	73	32	5	5
Fatigue	55	24	23	23
Headache	59	26	9	9
Decreased appetite	49	21	12	12
Acne	46	20	5	5
Asthenia	34	14	11	11
Vomiting	34	14	7	7
Back pain	21	9	20	20
Dry skin	35	15	5	5
Insomnia	30	13	10	10
Abdominal pain	33	14	5	5
Dermatitis acneiform	35	15	2	2
Cough	25	10	10	10
Nasopharyngitis	26	11	9	9
ECG QT prolonged*	33	14	1	1
Weight decreased	24	10	9	9
Grade 3+ occurring with an incidence of ≥2% on either arm				
Diarrhea	25	11	2	2
Hypertension	20	9	0	
ECG QT prolonged*	18	8	1	1
Fatigue	13	6	1	1
Decreased appetite	9	4	0	
Rash	8	4	1	1
Asthenia	6	3	1	1
Dyspnea	3	1	3	3
Back pain	1	0.4	3	3
Syncope	0		2	2

*As defined according to the National Cancer Institute's Common Terminology Criteria for Adverse Events, v3 (and protocol-defined QTc prolongation)

Treatment Modifications *(continued)*		Therapy Monitoring
Diarrhea		1. *ECGs:* Unless additional ECGs are clinically indicated, 12-lead ECGs are performed before the start of treatment, weekly for the first 8 weeks, and then every 12 weeks thereafter. If the dose is increased then weekly monitoring is indicated for approximately 6 weeks
If the diarrhea cannot be controlled with the preventive measures outlined and is G3/4, or worsens by 1 grade level (G3 to G4) while on vandetanib and is not alleviated by symptomatic treatment within 48 hours	Hold vandetanib. Also, if persistent G2 diarrhea (persistent defined as lasting for more than 2 weeks) while on vandetanib is not alleviated by symptomatic treatment, hold vandetanib	2. *Response assessment:* Every 2–3 cycles
If vandetanib is held for more than 3 weeks and the diarrhea does not resolve to G ≤1	Discontinue therapy	
If within 3 weeks of holding therapy the diarrhea resolves to G ≤1	Restart vandetanib at 1 dose level lower than that administered at the time the toxicity developed	
If diarrhea that is G3/4 or persistent G2 (persistent defined as lasting for more than 2 weeks) recurs at the reduced doses of vandetanib and this is greater than dose level −1	Again, hold vandetanib until the toxicity resolves to CTCAE G ≤1, at which time vandetanib should be restarted at 1 dose level lower than that administered at the time the toxicity developed. Symptomatic treatment may continue indefinitely as a preventive measure	
If diarrhea that is G3/4 or persistent G2 (persistent defined as lasting for more than 2 weeks) recurs at dose level −2	Discontinue therapy	
If with or without continued symptomatic treatment the diarrhea does not recur at the reduced doses of vandetanib	The dose of vandetanib may be increased 1 dose level to that which was being administered at the time the diarrhea developed. If toxicity recurs following this increase, then follow the guidelines above, with the exception that when drug is restarted the vandetanib dose should be reduced 1 dose level	

Hypertension

Note: Patients should have their blood pressure checked once per week during their first 24 weeks of therapy or for any 8-week period after any adjustment is made in their vandetanib dose

G1 hypertension	Continue vandetanib at same dose and schedule
G2 asymptomatic	Treat with antihypertensive medications and continue vandetanib at same dose and schedule
G2 symptomatic or persistent G2 despite antihypertensive medications or diastolic BP >110 mm Hg or G3 hypertension	Treat with antihypertensive medications. Hold vandetanib (maximum 3 weeks until symptoms resolve and diastolic BP <100 mm Hg); then continue vandetanib at 1 dose level lower *Note:* If vandetanib is held more than 3 weeks, then discontinue therapy
G4	Discontinue therapy

QTc Abnormalities

ECGs and electrolytes should be checked 3 times per week if there are any QTc abnormalities noted

QTc prolongation defined as: • A single measurement of ≥550 milliseconds • An increase of ≥100 milliseconds from baseline • Two consecutive measurements (within 48 hours) ≥500 milliseconds but <550 milliseconds • An increase of ≥60 milliseconds but <100 milliseconds from baseline to a value ≥480 milliseconds	Hold vandetanib until QTc <480 milliseconds, then resume vandetanib at 1 dose level lower

Efficacy

Progression-Free Survival	Vandetanib		Placebo					
	# Events/ # Patients	%	# Events/ # Patients	%	HR	OR	95% CI	*P*
Primary analysis	73/231		51/100		0.46		0.31 to 0.69	<0.001
Predefined sensitivity analyses								
Cox proportional hazards model	73/231		51/100		0.46		0.32 to 0.68	<0.001
Per protocol analysis	71/215		48/91		0.45		0.30 to 0.68	<0.001
Whitehead's method	73/231		51/100		0.51		0.35 to 0.72	<0.001
Excluding data from open-label phase	64/231		59/100		0.27		0.18 to 0.41	<0.001
Investigator RECIST assessments	101/231		62/100		0.40		0.27 to 0.58	<0.001
Secondary efficacy end points								
Objective response rate		45		13		5.48	2.99 to 10.79	<0.001
Disease control rate		87		71		2.64	1.48 to 4.69	0.001
Calcitonin biochemical response rate		69		3		72.9	26.2 to 303.2	<0.001
CEA biochemical response rate		52		2		52.0	16.0 to 320.3	<0.001

HR, hazard ratio; OR, odds ratio; RECIST, Response Evaluation Criteria in Solid Tumors

Objective Response Rate: Summary of Subgroup Analyses (Randomized Phase)

Patient Subgroup and Randomized Treatment	No. of Patients	Responses	
		No.	%
Hereditary MTC			
Vandetanib, 300 mg	28	13	46.4
Placebo	5	0	
Sporadic *RET* mutation positive			
Vandetanib, 300 mg	110	57	51.8
Placebo	45	0	
Sporadic *RET* mutation negative			
Vandetanib, 300 mg	2	0	
Placebo	6	0	
Sporadic *RET* mutation unknown			
Vandetanib, 300 mg	91	31	34.1
Placebo	44	1	2.3
Sporadic *M918T* mutation positive			
Vandetanib, 300 mg	101	55	54.5
Placebo	41	0	
Sporadic *M918T* mutation negative			
Vandetanib, 300 mg	55	17	30.9
Placebo	39	1	2.6
Sporadic *M918T* mutation unknown			
Vandetanib, 300 mg	48	16	33.3
Placebo	17	0	

MTC, medullary thyroid cancer; *RET*, rearranged during transfection

MEDULLARY THYROID CANCER REGIMEN

CABOZANTINIB

Elsei et al. J Clin Oncol 2013;31:3639–3646

Cabozantinib 140 mg orally at least 2 hours after or at least 1 hour before after eating food, continually (total dose/week = 980 mg)

Notes:
- Capsules are swallowed whole (without opening or breaking)
- Do not take a missed dose within 12 hours of the next scheduled dose
- In light of the fact that 79% of patients starting at the 140-mg dose had a subsequent dose reduction and 27% discontinued the medication because of adverse effects, clinicians are advised to consider the following:

  ■ *Patients Taking CYP3A4 Inhibitors*
    ○ Avoid the use of concomitant strong CYP3A4 inhibitors (eg, atazanavir, clarithromycin, indinavir, itraconazole, ketoconazole, nefazodone, nelfinavir, ritonavir, saquinavir, telithromycin, voriconazole)
    ○ For patients who require treatment with a strong CYP3A4 inhibitor, reduce the daily cabozantinib dose by 40 mg. Resume the dose that was used prior to initiating the CYP3A4 inhibitor 2 to 3 days after discontinuing a strong inhibitor

  ■ *Patients Taking Strong CYP3A4 Inducers*
    ○ Avoid use of strong CYP3A4 inducers (eg, carbamazepine, phenobarbital phenytoin, rifabutin, rifampin, rifapentine) concomitantly with cabozantinib if alternative therapy is available
    ○ Inform patients not to ingest foods or nutritional supplements (eg, St. John's wort (*Hypericum perforatum*) known to induce cytochrome P450 activity
    ○ For patients who require treatment with a strong CYP3A4 inducer, increase the daily cabozantinib dose by 40 mg *only if tolerability on the dose without the inducer has been convincingly demonstrated*. Resume the dose that was used prior to initiating a CYP3A4 inducer 2 to 3 days after discontinuing a strong inducer. The daily cabozantinib dose should not exceed 180 mg

Supportive Care
Antiemetic prophylaxis
Emetogenic potential is **MINIMAL–LOW**
See Chapter 39 for antiemetic recommendations

Hematopoietic growth factor (CSF) prophylaxis
Primary prophylaxis is NOT indicated
See Chapter 43 for more information

Antimicrobial prophylaxis
Risk of fever and neutropenia is LOW
  Antimicrobial primary prophylaxis to be considered:
See Chapter 47 for more information

Diarrhea management
Latent or delayed onset diarrhea*:
  Loperamide 4 mg; administer orally initially after the first loose or liquid stool, *then*
  Loperamide 2 mg every 2 hours while awake; every 4 hours during sleep
  Alternatively, a trial of **Diphenoxylate hydrochloride** 2.5 mg **with Atropine sulfate** 0.025 mg (eg, Lomotil®) two tablets four times daily until control achieved.

Persistent diarrhea:
  Octreotide acetate (solution) 100–150 mcg; administer subcutaneously 3 times daily.

Antibiotic therapy during latent or delayed onset diarrhea:
  A fluoroquinolone (eg, **Ciprofloxacin** 500 mg orally every 12 hours) if absolute neutrophil count <500/mm³

Abigerges D et al. J Natl Cancer Inst 1994;86:446–449
Rothenberg ML et al. J Clin Oncol 2001;19:3801–3807
Wadler S et al. J Clin Oncol 1998;16:3169–3178

Hand-foot reaction (palmar-plantar erythrodysesthesia, PPE)
Use topical emollients (eg, Aquaphor®), topical or orally administered steroids, antihistamines, or pyridoxine 50 to 200 mg/day

Dose Modifications

Adapted in part from Cometriq (cabozantinib) capsules, for oral use; 11/2012 product label. Exelixis, Inc., South San Francisco, CA

Adverse Event	Dose Modification
G ≥3 or intolerable G2 nonhematologic adverse event at a 140-mg dose	Hold cabozantinib until return to baseline or resolution to G ≤1. Then, resume cabozantinib at a dose of 100 mg daily
G ≥3 or intolerable G2 nonhematologic adverse event at a 100-mg dose	Hold cabozantinib until return to baseline or resolution to G ≤1. Then, resume cabozantinib at a dose of 60 mg daily
G ≥3 or intolerable G2 nonhematologic adverse event at a 60-mg dose	Hold cabozantinib until return to baseline or resolution to G ≤1. Then, resume cabozantinib at a dose of 60 mg daily, and, if not tolerated, discontinue cabozantinib
G4 hematologic adverse event at a 140-mg dose	Hold cabozantinib until return to baseline or resolution to G ≤1. Then, resume cabozantinib at a dose of 100 mg daily
G4 hematologic adverse event at a 100-mg dose	Hold cabozantinib until return to baseline or resolution to G ≤1. Then, resume cabozantinib at a dose of 60 mg daily
G4 hematologic adverse event at a 60-mg dose	Hold cabozantinib until return to baseline or resolution to G ≤1. Then, resume cabozantinib at a dose of 60 mg daily

Patient Population Studied

Locally advanced on metastatic medullary thyroid cancer. All had RECIST documented progressive disease within 14 months before screening, although the interval between scans was not fixed. There were no limits on the number of prior therapies; 95% had ECOG 0/1 PS. RET mutation status was "positive" in 46%, "negative" in 14%, and unknown in 40%. Of the studied population, 51% had bone metastases at baseline

Efficacy

	Cabozantinib	Placebo	Statistics
Median PFS, independent review (months)	11.2	4.0	HR 0.28 (95% CI: 0.19–0.40) P <0.0001
Median PFS, investigator (months)	13.8	3.1	HR 0.29 (95% CI: 0.21–0.42) P <0.0001
1-Year PFS	47.3%	7.2%	
ORR, independent review	28%	0	P <0.0001
Median duration of response (months)	14.6	—	—
Mean calcitonin levels during first 3 months	↓ 45%	↑ 57%	

Toxicity

	Cabozantinib (N = 214)		Placebo (N = 109)	
Median Duration of Exposure	6.7 months		3.4 months	
Adverse Event (>25% incidence)	All Grades	G3/4	All Grades	G3/4
Diarrhea	135 (63%)	34 (16%)	36 (33%)	2 (2%)
Hand-foot skin reaction	107 (50%)	27 (13%)	2 (2%)	—
Decreased weight	102 (48%)	10 (5%)	11 (10%)	—
Decreased appetite	98 (46%)	10 (5%)	17 (16%)	1 (1%)
Nausea	92 (43%)	3 (1%)	23 (21%)	—
Fatigue	87 (41%)	20 (9%)	31 (28%)	3 (3%)
Dysgeusia	73 (34%)	1 (0.5%)	6 (6%)	—
Hair color changes	72 (34%)	1 (0.5%)	1 (1%)	—
Stomatitis	62 (29%)	4 (2%)	3 (3%)	—
Constipation	57 (27%)	—	6 (6%)	—
Hypertension	70 (33%)	18 (8%)	5 (5%)	1 (1%)
Hemorrhage	54 (25%)	7 (3%)	17 (16%)	1 (1%)
Venous thrombosis	12 (6%)	8 (4%)	3 (3%)	2 (2%)
GI perforation	7 (3%)	7 (3%)	0	0
Non–GI fistula	8 (4%)	4 (2%)	0	0
Death within 30 days of treatment	5.6%		2.8%	
Required dose reduction	79%		—	
Discontinued use	27%		—	

REGIMEN

SORAFENIB TOSYLATE
Late-stage (metastatic) differentiated thyroid cancer

Brose et al. ASCO 2013 Annual Meeting, J Clin Oncol 31, 2013 (Suppl; abstr 4)

Sorafenibtosylate 400 mg administer orally every 12 hours (eg, morning and evening) continually in 28-day cycles (total dose/day = 800 mg; total dose/cycle = 22,400 mg)

Notes:
• Patients should swallow tablets whole with approximately 250 mL (8 oz) of water. Tablets may be taken with or without food
• Special precautions: Sorafenib is metabolized by cytochrome P450 (CYP) CYP3A subfamily enzymes and has been shown in preclinical studies to inhibit multiple CYP isoforms. Therefore, all patients who are taking concomitant medications metabolized by CYP enzymes should be closely observed for side effects associated with concomitantly administered medications. Special caution should be used with any of the following medications: ketoconazole, itraconazole, voriconazole, ritonavir, clarithromycin, cyclosporine, carbamazepine, phenytoin, and phenobarbital. Furthermore, patients taking medications with a low therapeutic index (eg, warfarin, quinidine, digoxin) should be monitored proactively. *Patients using sorafenib should be advised to avoid consuming grapefruit products for as long as they continue to use sorafenib*

Supportive Care: Hand-foot reaction
For patients who develop a hand-foot reaction, use topical emollients (eg, Aquaphor®), topical and/or oral steroids, antihistamine agents (H₁-receptor antagonists), or pyridoxine 50–150 mg/day orally

Antiemetic prophylaxis
Emetogenic potential is **MINIMAL**
See Chapter 39 for antiemetic recommendations

Hematopoietic growth factor (CSF) prophylaxis
Primary prophylaxis is NOT indicated
See Chapter 43 for more information

Antimicrobial prophylaxis
Risk of fever and neutropenia is LOW
  Antimicrobial primary prophylaxis to be considered:
  • Antibacterial—not indicated
  • Antifungal—not indicated
  • Antiviral—not indicated unless patient previously had an episode of HSV
See Chapter 47 for more information

Diarrhea management
Latent or delayed-onset diarrhea:
  Loperamide 4 mg orally initially after the first loose or liquid stool, *then*
  Loperamide 2 mg orally every 2 hours during waking hours, *plus*
  Loperamide 4 mg orally every 4 hours during hours of sleep
• Continue for at least 12 hours after diarrhea resolves
• Recurrent diarrhea after a 12-hour diarrhea-free interval is treated as a new episode
• Rehydrate orally with fluids and electrolytes during a diarrheal episode
• If a patient develops blood or mucus in stool, dehydration, or hemodynamic instability, or if diarrhea persists >48 hours despite loperamide, stoploperamide and hospitalize the patient for IV hydration

Persistent diarrhea:
  Octreotide100–150 mcg subcutaneously 3 times daily. Maximum total daily dose is 1500 mcg

Antibiotic therapy during latent or delayed-onset diarrhea:
  A fluoroquinolone (eg, **Ciprofloxacin** 500 mg orally every 12 hours) if absolute neutrophilcount <500/mm3 with or without accompanying fever in association with diarrhea
  • Antibiotics should also be administered if patient is hospitalized with prolonged diarrhea and should be continued until diarrhea resolves

Abigerges D et al. J Natl Cancer Inst 1994;86:446–449
Rothenberg ML et al. J Clin Oncol 2001;19:3801–3807
Wadler S et al. J Clin Oncol 1998;16:3169–3178

Treatment Modifications

Sorafenib Dose Levels

Starting dose: Level 1	400 mg every morning; 400 mg every evening
Level −1	200 mg every morning; 400 mg every evening
Level −2	200 mg every morning; 200 mg every evening
Level −3	200 mg once daily

Adverse Event	Dose Modification
Cutaneous Toxicities	
Rash G ≥2	Hold sorafenib and provide immediate symptomatic treatment
If treatment is withheld for more than 3 weeks because of cutaneous toxicity	Discontinue therapy
When toxicity resolves to G ≤1	Restart sorafenib at one dose level less than the dose level administered at the time toxicity developed. Treatment for symptoms may continue indefinitely as a preventive measure
If cutaneous toxicity G3/4 recurs at reduced sorafenib doses	Again, hold sorafenib until the toxicity resolves to G ≤1, at which time sorafenib should be restarted at one dose level lower than the dose level administered at the time toxicity developed. Treatment for symptoms may continue indefinitely as a preventive measure
If cutaneous toxicity G3/4 recurs at dose levels −2 or lower	Discontinue therapy
If cutaneous toxicity does not recur at reduced sorafenib doses with or without continued treatment for symptoms	The dose of sorafenib may be increased one dose level to the dose level administered at the time cutaneous toxicity developed. If toxicity recurs following the increase, then follow the guidelines above, with the exception that when drug is restarted the sorafenib
Diarrhea	
G1/2 diarrhea	Focus on treatment for symptoms designed to resolve the diarrhea. No dose modifications will be made for G1/2 diarrhea unless G2 diarrhea persists for more than 2 weeks
If G2 diarrhea persists for more than 2 weeks	Follow the guidelines below for G3/4 diarrhea
If diarrhea cannot be controlled with the preventive measures outlined, and is G3/4 or worsens by one grade level (G3 to G4) while on sorafenib and is not alleviated within 48 hours by antidiarrheal treatment	Hold sorafenib. Also, withhold sorafenib if persistent G2 diarrhea is not alleviated by antidiarrheal treatment while sorafenib use continues (persistent is defined as lasting for >2 weeks)
If sorafenib is held for more than 3 weeks and diarrhea does not resolve to G ≤1	Discontinue therapy
If within 3 weeks of withholding sorafenib, diarrhea resolves to G ≤1	Restart sorafenib at one dose level less than the dose level administered at the time toxicity developed
If G3/4 diarrhea or persistent G2 diarrhea recurs at reduced doses of sorafenib (persistent is defined as lasting >2 weeks)	Again, withhold sorafenib until the toxicity resolves to CTCAE G ≤1, at which time sorafenib should be restarted at one dose level lower than the dose level administered at the time toxicity developed. Treatment for symptoms may continue indefinitely as a preventive measure

(continued)

Patient Population Studied

Multicenter, double-blind, placebo-controlled trial conducted in 417 patients with locally recurrent or metastatic, progressive differentiated thyroid carcinoma refractory to radioactive iodine treatment. Patients had papillary (57 percent), follicular (25 percent), and poorly differentiated (10 percent) carcinomas. Metastases were present in 96% of the patients: lungs in 86%, lymph nodes in 51%, and bone in 27%. Approximately half of the patients were male, the median age was 63 years, 68 percent had no uptake of radioactive iodine (RAI), and 34 percent had received a cumulative dose of at least 600 mCi of RAI. The median cumulative RAI activity administered prior to study entry was 400 mCi

Treatment Modifications (*continued*)

Adverse Event	Dose Modification
If G3/4 diarrhea or persistent G2 diarrhearecurs at dose level −2 (persistent defined as lasting for >2 weeks)	Discontinue therapy
If diarrhea does not recur at reduced sorafenib doses with or without continued treatment forsymptoms	The dose of sorafenib may be increased one dose level to the dose level administered at the time the diarrhea developed. If toxicity recurs following the increase, then follow the guidelines above, with the exception that when drug is restarted the sorafenib dose should be reduced one dose level

Hypertension

Note: Patients should have their blood pressure checked once weekly during their first 24 weeks of therapy and for an 8-week period after an adjustment in their sorafenib dose

G1 hypertension	Continue sorafenib at same dose and schedule
G2 asymptomatic	Treat with antihypertensive medications and continue sorafenib at same dose and schedule
G2 symptomatic, or persistent G2 despite antihypertensive medications, or diastolic BP >110 mm Hg, or G3 hypertension	Treat with antihypertensive medications. Hold sorafenib (maximum 3 weeks until symptoms resolve and diastolic BP <100 mm Hg); then continue sorafenib at one dose level lower. *Note:* Discontinue therapy if sorafenib is withheld >3 weeks
G4 hypertension	Discontinue therapy

Efficacy
(N = 417)

Variable	Sorafenib (N = 207)	Placebo (N = 210)
Progression-free survival (PFS)	10.8 months (95% CI 9.1–12.9)	5.8 months (95% CI 5.3–7.8)
	HR = 0.587 (95% CI, 0.46–0.76, p <0.001)	
Median treatment duration	40 weeks	20 weeks
Overall survival*	HR 0.88 (95% CI, 0.63–1.24, p = 0.47)	

	Percent of Patients	
Partial response[†]	12.2%	0.5%
Reduction in size of target lesions	73%	27%
Stable disease ≥6 months	42%	33.5%

CI, confidence interval

*Overall survival was not statistically significantly different in patients who received sorafenib tosylate compared with patients who received placebo. The analysis was performed after 33% of the patients had died. Note that following investigator-determined disease progression, 157 (75 percent) patients randomly assigned to receive the placebo crossed over to open-label sorafenib tosylate, and it remains uncertain if this may have impacted or will impact the OS analysis

[†]Duration of response = 10.2 months

Therapy Monitoring

1. Every 6 weeks to 3 months: Physical examination and routine laboratory tests
2. Response assessment: Every 2–3 cycles. A cycle defined as 28 days of oral therapy

Toxicity

	Percent of Patient	
	Sorafenib	Placebo
Palmar-plantar erythrodysesthesia syndrome (PPES)	69%	8%
Diarrhea	68%	15%
Alopecia	67%	8%
Weight loss	49%	14%
Fatigue	41%	20%
Hypertension	41%	12%
Rash	35%	7%
Decreased appetite	30%	5%
Stomatitis	24%	3%
Nausea	21%	12%
Pruritus	20%	11%
Abdominal pain	20%	7%
G3/4 adverse reactions	65%	30%
Squamous cell carcinoma	3%	—
Secondary malignancy	4.3%	1.9%
Hypocalcemia	36%	N/R

Dose modification due to adverse event	77.8%	30.1%
Dose interruptions	66%	
Dose reductions	64%	
Treatment discontinuation due to adverse event	18.8%	3.8%

N/R, not reported

38. Vaginal Cancer

Leslie Boyd, MD and Franco Muggia, MD

Epidemiology

Incidence: 3,170 (Estimated new cases for 2014 in the United States)
Incidence of clear cell adenocarcinoma as a result of in utero diethylstilbestrol (DES) exposure estimated at 1/1000

Deaths: Estimated 880 in 2014

Median age: Squamous cell cancer (60–65 years); DES-related adenocarcinoma/clear cell (19 years)

Stage at Presentation

Stage I:	28%
Stage II:	43%
Stage III:	16%
Stage IV:	13%

Daling JR et al. Gynecol Oncol 2002;84:263–270
Siegel R et al. CA Cancer J Clin 2014;64:9–29
Tedeschi C et al. J Low Genit Tract Dis 2005;9:11–18

Pathology

Histologic Classification of Vaginal Neoplasia

VAIN (VAginal Intraepithelial Neoplasms)

These are pre-malignant lesions of the vaginal squamous epithelium that can develop primarily in the vagina or as an extension from the cervix. Histologically, VAIN is defined in the same way as cervical intraepithelial neoplasia (CIN). Classification includes three grades: Grade 1 (VAIN I = mild dysplasia); Grade 2 (VAIN II = moderate dysplasia); and Grade 3 (VAIN III = severe dysplasia or carcinoma in situ)

Invasive carcinoma:

1. Squamous cell carcinoma	88%
2. Adenocarcinoma	5%
3. Other epithelial cell types (adenosquamous, adenoid cystic, undifferentiated)	1–2%
4. Mesenchymal tumors (leiomyosarcoma, sarcoma botryoides, endometrioid sarcoma)	2%
5. Mixed epithelial and mesenchymal tumors	<1%
6. Other histologies (melanoma, sarcoma, yolk sac tumors, lymphoma, carcinoid, small cell)	3–4%

Higinia R et al. Vagina. In: Hoskins WJ, Perez CA, Young RC, eds. Principles and Practice of Gynecologic Oncology. 4th ed. Philadelphia: Lippincott-Raven, 2005:707–742
Zaino RJ, Robboy SJ, Kurman RJ. Diseases of the vagina. In: Blaustein's Pathology of the Female Genital Tract. 5th ed. New York: Springer-Verlag, 2002:178–195

Work-up

VAIN (vaginal intraepithelial neoplasia):

1. H&P, including bimanual examination, palpation, and colposcopic examination of the vagina, vulva, and cervix
2. Multiple site-directed biopsies, including cervical and vulvar biopsies, to rule out invasive disease and metastatic lesions

Invasive carcinoma:

1. H&P including bimanual examination and palpation of vagina
2. Multiple site-directed biopsies, including cervical biopsies to rule out invasive disease and primary cervical cancer
3. Studies allowable for staging as per FIGO* guidelines: chest X-ray, cystoscopy, proctosigmoidoscopy, and intravenous pyelogram. Although not part of staging, pelvic MRI or CT scan may aid in planning of patient care
4. If clinically warranted, barium enema and CAT scan or MRI

Staging is best performed by gynecologic and radiation oncologists with the patient under general anesthesia. Additional biopsies of the vagina should be done to determine the limits of abnormal vaginal mucosa

*International Federation of Gynecology and Obstetrics (FIGO)
Hoskins WJ, Perez CA, Young RC, eds. Principles and Practice of Gynecologic Oncology. 2nd ed. Philadelphia: Lippincott-Raven, 1997

Staging

TNM Category	FIGO Stage	Primary Tumor (T)
TX		Primary tumor cannot be assessed
T0		No evidence of primary tumor
Tis	*	Carcinoma *in situ*
T1	I	Tumor confined to vagina
T2	II	Tumor invades paravaginal tissues but not to pelvic wall
T3	III	Tumor extends to pelvic wall[†]
T4	IVA	Tumor invades mucosa of the bladder or rectum and/or extends beyond the true pelvis (bullous edema is not sufficient evidence to classify a tumor as T4)

*FIGO staging no longer includes Stage 0 (Tis)
[†]Pelvic wall is defined as muscle, fascia, neurovascular structures, or skeletal portions of the bony pelvis

TNM Category	FIGO Stage	Regional Lymph Nodes (N)
NX		Regional lymph nodes cannot be assessed
N0		No regional lymph node metastasis
N1	III	Pelvic or inguinal lymph node metastasis

TNM Category	FIGO Stage	Distant Metastasis (M)
M0		No distant metastasis (no pathologic M0; use clinical M to complete stage group)
M1	IVB	Distant metastasis

Staging*

	T	N	M
0	Tis	N0	M0
I	T1	N0	M0
II	T2	N0	M0
III	T1–T3	N1	M0
	T3	N0	M0
IVA	T4	Any N	M0
IVB	Any T	Any N	M1

*FIGO staging no longer includes Stage 0 (Tis)

Edge SB, Byrd DR, Compton CC, Fritz AG, Greene FL, Trotti A, editors. AJCC Cancer Staging Manual. 7th ed. New York: Springer; 2010

Expert Opinion

General:

1. Vaginal neoplasms are quite rare and are considered primary only if neither the vulva nor the cervix is involved at the time of diagnosis
2. A carcinoma involving the upper vagina and cervix should be considered a cervical primary and managed accordingly
3. Histologically most vaginal carcinomas are squamous, and chemotherapeutic management is usually based on extrapolation from experience with cervical carcinoma, given similarities in location, pattern of spread, histologic appearance, relation to HPV, and response to radiation therapy

Therapeutic Principles:

1. *Vaginal intraepithelial neoplasia (VAIN):* Treated with local modalities such as CO_2 laser ablation, topical fluorouracil, local radiation, imiquimod, or surgical excision. Regression rates are excellent. Close cytologic surveillance is warranted
2. *Stages I and II:* Standard treatment by gynecologic or radiation oncologists is highly effective
3. *Stages III and IVA:* Radiation therapy alone has yielded suboptimal results. Reports of combined chemoradiation have been more encouraging, and because of similarities with cervical cancer, cisplatin-based chemoradiation has been advocated as standard therapy
4. *Stage IVB and recurrences are not amenable to locoregional therapy:* Anthracyclines and platinum compounds as single agents or in combinations have some activity, but experience is limited to small case series. Taxane-based therapy also is reasonable, particularly for adenocarcinoma. Considering the rarity of cases, care providers should consider clinical trials

Curtin JP et al. J Clin Oncol 2001;19:1275–1278
Dancuart F et al. Int J Radiat Oncol Biol Phys 1988;14:745–749
Davis KP et al. Gynecol Oncol 1991;42:131–136
Evans LS et al. Int J Radiat Oncol Biol Phys 1988;15:901–906
Grisbgy PW. Curr Treat Options Oncol 2002;3:125–130
Kucera H, Vavra N. Gynecol Oncol 1991;40:12–16
Piver MS et al. Am J Obstet Gynecol 1978;131:311–313
Vagina. In: Hoskins WJ, Perez CA, Young RC, eds. Principles and Practice of Gynecologic Oncology. 4th ed. Philadelphia: Lippincott-Raven Publishers, 2005:708–714

REGIMEN

DOXORUBICIN (SINGLE AGENT)

Piver MS et al. Am J Obstet Gynecol 1978;131:311–313

Doxorubicin 60–90 mg/m²; administer by slow intravenous injection over 3–5 minutes on day 1, every 4 weeks (total dosage/cycle = 60 to 90 mg/m²)

Supportive Care
Antiemetic prophylaxis
*Emetogenic potential: **MODERATE***
See Chapter 39 for antiemetic recommendations

Hematopoietic growth factor (CSF) prophylaxis
Primary prophylaxis is NOT indicated
See Chapter 43 for more information

Antimicrobial prophylaxis
Risk of fever and neutropenia is LOW
 Antimicrobial primary prophylaxis to be considered:
 • Antibacterial—not indicated
 • Antifungal—not indicated
 • Antiviral—not indicated unless patient previously had an episode of HSV
See Chapter 47 for more information

Toxicity

Myelosuppression	Dose-limiting toxicity. Leukopenia more common than thrombocytopenia or anemia. Nadir usually on days 10–14, with recovery by day 21 after treatment
Nausea and vomiting	Moderate severity on the day of treatment; delayed symptoms (>24 hours after treatment) uncommon
Mucositis and diarrhea	Common, but not dose limiting
Cardiotoxicity (acute)	Incidence not related to dosage. Presents within 3 days after treatment as arrhythmias, conduction abnormalities, ECG changes, pericarditis, and/or myocarditis. Usually transient and asymptomatic
Cardiotoxicity (chronic)	Dosage-dependent dilated cardiomyopathy associated with congestive failure. Risk increases with cumulative doses >550 mg/m²
Strong vesicant	Avoid extravasation
Skin	Hand-foot syndrome, with skin rash swelling, erythema, pain, and desquamation. Onset at 5–6 weeks after starting treatment. Hyperpigmentation of nails, rarely skin rash, urticaria. Potential for radiation recall
Alopecia	Common, but generally reversible within 3 months after discontinuing doxorubicin
Infusion reactions	Signs and symptoms include flushing, dyspnea, facial swelling, headache, back pain, chest and/or throat tightness, and hypotension. May occur with a first treatment. Symptoms resolve within several hours to a day after discontinuing doxorubicin
Urine discoloration	Red-orange discoloration usually within 1–2 days after drug administration

Chu E, DeVita VT Jr, eds. Physicians' Cancer Chemotherapy Drug Manual 2001. Sudbury, MA: Jones and Bartlett

Patient Population Studied

Cervical or vaginal malignancies; 7 of 100 patients with advanced vaginal squamous cell carcinoma

Efficacy

(N = 7 Patients with Vaginal Cancer)

Complete response	1 patient
Partial response	1 patient*

*Treated with combination doxorubicin, cyclophosphamide, and fluorouracil

Treatment Modifications

Adverse Events	Treatment Modifications
WBC <3000/mm³ and platelet counts <100,000/mm³	Delay start of next cycle until WBC >3000/mm³ and platelet counts >100,000/mm³
>2-week delay in start of cycle	Reduce doxorubicin dose by 15 mg/m²
Doxorubicin total cumulative lifetime dosage ≥550 mg/m²	Obtain frequent MUGA scans to monitor cardiac function

Therapy Monitoring

1. *Before each treatment with doxorubicin (every 4 weeks):* H&P, CBC with differential, serum electrolytes, LFTs, BUN, and serum creatinine
2. *After patients receive a total cumulative lifetime doxorubicin dose of 550 mg/m²:* Check radionuclide left ventricular ejection fraction periodically (every 2 cycles)

Piver MS et al. Am J Obstet Gynecol 1978;131:311–313

REGIMEN

CISPLATIN (SINGLE AGENT)

Thigpen JT et al. Gynecol Oncol 1986;23:101–104

Hydration before cisplatin: ≥1000 mL 0.9% sodium chloride injection (0.9% NS) administered intravenously over a minimum of 3–4 hours

Cisplatin 50 mg/m²; administer intravenously in 50–250 mL 0.9% NS at a rate of 1 mg/min on day 1, every 3 weeks, (total dosage/cycle = 50 mg/m²)

Hydration after cisplatin: ≥1000 mL 0.9% sodium chloride injection (0.9% NS) administered intravenously over a minimum of 3–4 hours. Encourage patients to increase oral intake of non-alcoholic fluids, and provide electrolyte replacement as needed (potassium, magnesium, sodium)

Supportive Care
Antiemetic prophylaxis
Emetogenic potential: **HIGH**. *Potential for delayed symptoms*
See Chapter 39 for antiemetic recommendations

Hematopoietic growth factor (CSF) prophylaxis
Primary prophylaxis is NOT indicated
See Chapter 43 for more information

Antimicrobial prophylaxis
Risk of fever and neutropenia is LOW
Antimicrobial primary prophylaxis to be considered:
- Antibacterial—not indicated
- Antifungal—not indicated
- Antiviral—not indicated unless patient previously had an episode of HSV

See Chapter 47 for more information

Patient Population Studied

Study of 22 patients with advanced or recurrent vaginal cancers

Efficacy (N = 22)

One complete response out of 22 evaluable patients with vaginal cancer (most were heavily pretreated)

Toxicity (N = 22)

Hematologic Toxicities

	% G1	% G2
Leukopenia*	9	13.6
Thrombocytopenia†	9	—

Nonhematologic Toxicities

	Mild	Moderate	Severe
Nephrotoxicity‡	27	—	—
Nausea/vomiting§	9	45	4.5
Fatigue	9	4.5	4.5

*Lowest WBC nadir = 2000 leukocytes/mm³
†Lowest platelet nadir = 126,000 platelets/mm³
‡Dose-limiting toxicity in 35–40%
§Most common adverse effect

Treatment Modifications

Adverse Events	Treatment Modifications
Serum creatinine ≥1.7 mg/dL (≥29.1 μmol/L)	Hold treatment until creatinine returns to pretreatment level, then reduce cisplatin dosage in subsequent cycles by 50%
G3/4 ototoxicity	Hold treatment until ≤ G2 then reduce cisplatin dosage in subsequent cycles by 50%
G3/4 neurotoxicity	Hold treatment until ≤ G2 then reduce cisplatin dosage in subsequent cycles by 50%

Toxicities Reported in other Studies

Neurotoxicity	Usually peripheral sensory neuropathy with bilateral paresthesia and anesthesia in a "stocking-and-glove" distribution. Risk increases with high individual doses and cumulatively. Motor and autonomic neuropathies may also occur. Neurotoxic effects may be irreversible
Ototoxicity	High-frequency hearing loss and tinnitus
Hypersensitivity	Facial edema, wheezing, bronchospasm, and hypotension within minutes of drug exposure
Hepatic	Transient increases in LFTs
Gustatory	Dysgeusia (metallic taste) and loss of appetite

Chu E, DeVita VT Jr, eds. Physicians' Cancer Chemotherapy Drug Manual 2001. Sudbury, MA: Jones and Bartlett; 100–105
Thigpen JT et al. Gynecol Oncol 1986;23:101–104

Therapy Monitoring

Before each treatment with cisplatin (every 4 weeks): H&P, paying attention to history and objective findings of neurotoxicity, CBC with differential, LFTs, serum electrolytes, and creatinine

REGIMEN

PACLITAXEL (SINGLE AGENT)

Curtin JP et al. J Clin Oncol 2001;19:1275–1278

Premedications:
Dexamethasone 20 mg per dose; administer orally or intravenously for 2 doses, 14 hours and 7 hours before starting paclitaxel
Diphenhydramine 50 mg; administer by intravenous injection 30 minutes before starting paclitaxel
Ranitidine 50 mg; administer intravenously in 25–100 mL of 0.9% sodium chloride injection (0.9% NS) or 5% dextrose injection (D5W), over 30–60 minutes, 30 minutes before starting paclitaxel
Paclitaxel 170 mg/m^{2*}; administer by continuous intravenous infusion diluted in 0.9% NS or D5W to a concentration within the range 0.3 and 1.2 mg/mL, over 24 hours on day 1, every 3 weeks (total dosage/cycle = 170 mg/m^{2*})

*Patients who previously received radiation treatment to the pelvis should be treated initially with a paclitaxel dosage of 135 mg/m^2. This may be increased according to the guidelines under dose modification

Supportive Care
Antiemetic prophylaxis
Emetogenic potential: LOW
See Chapter 39 for antiemetic recommendations

Hematopoietic growth factor (CSF) prophylaxis
Primary prophylaxis may be indicated
See Chapter 43 for more information

Antimicrobial prophylaxis
Risk of fever and neutropenia is LOW
Antimicrobial primary prophylaxis to be considered:
- Antibacterial—not indicated
- Antifungal—not indicated
- Antiviral—not indicated unless patient previously had an episode of HSV

See Chapter 47 for more information

Treatment Modifications

Paclitaxel dosage levels:
110 mg/m^2 (minimum dosage to be administered)
135 mg/m^2
170 mg/m^2
200 mg/m^2 (maximum dosage to be administered)

Adverse Events	Treatment Modifications*
ANC <1500/mm^3	Hold treatment until ANC ≥1500/mm^3
Platelet count <100,000/mm^3	Hold treatment until platelets ≥100,000/mm^3
G1 hematologic toxicity	Increase paclitaxel dosage by 1 level
G2/3 hematologic toxicity	Administer same paclitaxel dosage
G4 hematologic toxicity	Decrease paclitaxel dosage by 1 level
G2 nonobstructive renal toxicity	Decrease paclitaxel dosage by 1 level
G3 hepatic toxicity	
G3 mucositis	
G4 GOG nonhematologic toxicity	

*Based on adverse events during previous cycles

Patient Population Studied

Study of 42 patients with advanced nonsquamous cell cervical cancer who had either no benefit from or progressive disease on standard chemotherapy

Toxicity (N = 42)

Toxicity Grades*					
Toxicity[†]	0	1	2	3	4
Hematologic Toxicities					
Leukopenia	5	3	11	16	7
Neutropenia	7	1	3	5	26
Thrombocytopenia	35	5	1	1	0
Anemia	21	7	10	4	0
Nonhematologic Toxicities					
Nausea/vomiting	28	7	7	0	0
Gastrointestinal	31	5	5	0	1
Alopecia	16	7	19	0	0
Neurotoxicity	28	4	9	1	0
Edema	41	0	0	1	0

*Number of patients with toxicity
[†]The table identifies only toxicities where at least 1 patient experienced a G3 or G4 toxicity

Other Toxicities	
Febrile neutropenia	8 patients
Alopecia	26 patients
Mucositis	2 patients
Myalgia and arthralgia	Infrequent
Bradycardia grade 2	Incidence not specified

Efficacy

Complete response	9.5%
Partial response	21.5%
Median duration of response	4.8 months

Therapy Monitoring

Before each treatment: H&P, paying attention to history and objective findings of neurotoxicity, CBC with differential, LFTs, electrolytes, and creatinine

REGIMEN

CISPLATIN + FLUOROURACIL + RADIATION THERAPY

Roberts WS et al. Gynecol Oncol 1991;43:233–236

Hydration before cisplatin: 1000 mL 0.9% sodium chloride injection (0.9% NS); administer intravenously over a minimum of 2 hours
Cisplatin 50 mg/m²; administer intravenously in 100–1000 mL 0.9% sodium chloride injection (0.9% NS), over 6 hours on day 1, every 4 weeks for 2 cycles (total dosage/4-week cycle = 50 mg/m²)

Followed by:
Fluorouracil 1000 mg/m² per day; administer as a continuous intravenous infusion in 250–2000 mL 0.9% NS or 5% dextrose injection over 24 hours for 4 consecutive days, on days 1–4, every 4 weeks for 2 cycles (total dosage/4-week cycle = 4000 mg/m²)

Hydration after cisplatin: 1000 mL 0.9% sodium chloride injection (0.9% NS); administer intravenously over a minimum of 2 hours. Encourage patients to increase oral intake of non-alcoholic fluids, and provide electrolyte replacement as needed (potassium, magnesium, sodium)
Concurrent with chemotherapy administer radiation therapy as follows:
External beam radiation with 20-MeV linear accelerator, 180 cGy/day fractions to a total dose of 4000–5000 cGy to the whole pelvis, ± periaortic radiation to a dose of 3600–4500 cGy

±

Additional external pelvic irradiation to limited fields to a total dose of 6480 cGy

±

Additional brachytherapy starting 2–3 weeks after external beam radiation

Supportive Care
Antiemetic prophylaxis
Emetogenic potential on day 1: **HIGH**. *Potential for delayed symptoms*
Emetogenic potential on days 2–4: **LOW**
See Chapter 39 for antiemetic recommendations

Hematopoietic growth factor (CSF) prophylaxis
Primary prophylaxis is NOT indicated
See Chapter 43 for more information

Antimicrobial prophylaxis
Risk of fever and neutropenia is LOW
  Antimicrobial primary prophylaxis to be considered:
  • Antibacterial—not indicated
  • Antifungal—not indicated
  • Antiviral—not indicated unless patient previously had an episode of HSV
See Chapter 47 for more information

Patient Population Studied

Study of 67 patients with advanced carcinomas of the lower female genital tract that were not amenable to resection were eligible, among whom 7 had vaginal cancers. Of the 7 patients with vaginal cancer, 5 had Stage III disease and 2 had recurrent disease

Efficacy*

Complete clinical response (all histologies)	85%
Partial response (all histologies)	9%
Stable disease (all histologies)	3%

*Not stated for the subset of patients with vaginal cancer. However, 3 of 7 patients with vaginal cancer were without recurrence or failure of the treatment for a median follow-up of 13 months

Treatment Modifications

Roberts WS et al. Gynecol Oncol 1991;43:233–236
Whitney CW et al. J Clin Oncol 1999;17:1339–1348*

Adverse Events	Treatment Modifications
Serum creatinine ≥1.7 mg/dL (≥29.1 μmol/L)	Hold cisplatin until serum creatinine returns to pre-treatment level, then reduce dosage by 50% in subsequent cycles
WBC ≤3000/mm³ or platelet ≤100,000/mm³	Delay cisplatin and fluorouracil until WBC ≥3000/mm³ and platelet count ≥100,000/mm³
>2-week delay in start of cycle	Reduce cisplatin and fluorouracil dosages by 50% each
G3/4 hematologic toxicity	Hold radiation therapy until hematologic toxicity is G ≤2

*Whitney et al. utilized a similar regimen for patients with cervical cancer; 91% completed both chemotherapy courses and had similar completion rates for radiation therapy

Toxicity

Acute Toxicities	
Neutropenia and thrombocytopenia	1 patient*
Radiation enteritis	5 patients†
Nausea, vomiting, and diarrhea	Very common
Renal, hepatic, or neurologic	Not significant

Delayed Toxicities	
Rectovaginal fistula	3 patients‡
Radiation proctitis	1 patient‡
Small bowel fistula	2 patients‡
Soft tissue necrosis	2 patients‡
Hemorrhagic cystitis	1 patient

*Resulted in 8- to 14-day treatment delay
†Resulted in 8- to >14-day treatment delay
‡Required surgery

Therapy Monitoring

Weekly: CBC with differential, LFTs, electrolytes, and creatinine

REGIMEN

NEODAJUVANT CISPLATIN + EPIRUBICIN

Zanetta G et al. Gynecol Oncol 1997;64:431–435

Hydration before cisplatin with ≥1000 mL 0.9% sodium chloride injection intravenously over a minimum of 2 hours

Cisplatin 50 mg/m^2 per dose intravenously in 50–250 mL 0.9% NS over 30–60 minutes once weekly for 9 doses (total dosage/9-week course = 450 mg/m^2)

Hydration after cisplatin with ≥1000 mL 0.9% NS intravenously over a minimum of 2 hours
Notes: Encourage increased oral intake of nonalcoholic fluids. Goal is to achieve a urine output ≥100 mL/hour. Monitor and replace electrolytes as needed (potassium, magnesium, sodium)

Epirubicin HCl 70 mg/m^2 per dose intravenously by injection over 3–5 minutes *or* in 25–250 mL 0.9% NS or 5% dextrose injection over 15–20 minutes every 3 weeks, weeks 1, 4, and 7, for 3 doses (total dosage/9-week course = 210 mg/m^2)

Supportive Care

Antiemetic prophylaxis
Emetogenic potential is **HIGH**. *Potential for delayed symptoms*
See Chapter 39 for antiemetic recommendations

Hematopoietic growth factor (CSF) prophylaxis
Primary prophylaxis is indicated with:

Filgrastim (G-CSF) 5 mcg/kg per day by subcutaneous injection daily for 5 days
- Begin use on the day after cisplatin (± epirubicin) is administered
- Discontinue daily filgrastim use at least 24 hours before administering myelosuppressive treatment

See Chapter 43 for more information

Antimicrobial prophylaxis
Risk of fever and neutropenia is LOW

Antimicrobial primary prophylaxis to be considered:
- Antibacterial—not indicated
- Antifungal—not indicated
- Antiviral—not indicated unless patient previously had an episode of HSV

See Chapter 47 for more information

Oral care
Prophylaxis and treatment for mucositis/stomatitis
General advice:
- Encourage patients to maintain intake of nonalcoholic fluids
- Evaluate patients for oral pain and provide analgesic medications
- Consider histamine (H$_2$-subtype) receptor antagonists (eg, ranitidine, famotidine) or a proton pump inhibitor for epigastric pain
- *Lactobacillus* sp.-containing probiotics may be beneficial in preventing diarrhea

Patients with intact oral mucosa:
- Clean the mouth, tongue, and gums by brushing after every meal and at bedtime with an ultrasoft toothbrush with fluoride toothpaste
- Floss teeth gently every day unless contraindicated. If gums bleed and hurt, avoid bleeding or sore areas, but floss other teeth
- Patients may use saline or commercial bland, nonalcoholic rinses
  - Do not use mouthwashes that contain alcohols

If mucositis or stomatitis is present:
- Keep the mouth moist utilizing water, ice chips, sugarless gum, sugar-free hard candies, or a saliva substitute
- Rinse mouth several times a day to remove debris
  - Use a solution of ¼ teaspoon (1.25 g) each of baking soda and table salt (sodium chloride) in 1 quart (~950 mL) of warm water. Follow with a plain water rinse
  - Do not use mouthwashes that contain alcohol
- Foam-tipped swabs (eg, Toothettes) are useful in moisturizing oral mucosa, but ineffective for cleansing teeth and removing plaque

(continued)

Treatment Modifications

Adverse Event	Treatment Modification
ANC <2000/mm^3 or platelets <75,000/mm^3 on day of treatment	Delay treatment for 1 week

Patient Population Studied

The study population included 20 patients with locally advanced cervical adenocarcinoma (bulky IB–IIA, IIB) and 2 subjects with vaginal adenocarcinoma; mean age was 51 years (range: 15–67 years). Disease histology was adenocarcinoma in 18 subjects and adenosquamous in 4 subjects. Those with stages IB–IIA cervical carcinomas and those with vaginal adenocarcinoma were required to have tumors >4 cm in diameter, as assessed by alginate mold. All patients had a performance status <2 according to the World Health Organization criteria. Staging was done according to the International Federation of Gynecology and Obstetrics.

(*continued*)

- Advise patients who develop mucositis to:
  - Choose foods that are easy to chew and swallow
  - Take small bites of food, chew slowly, and sip liquids with meals
  - Encourage soft, moist foods such as cooked cereals, mashed potatoes, and scrambled eggs
  - For trouble swallowing, soften food with gravies, sauces, broths, yogurt, or other bland liquids
  - Avoid sharp, crunchy foods; hot, spicy, or highly acidic foods (eg, citrus fruits and juices); sugary foods; toothpicks; tobacco products; alcoholic drinks

Additional therapies given:

- In operable patients, Piver 3 radical hysterectomy with pelvic lymphadenectomy and aortic node sampling was performed within 30 days after the completion of chemotherapy
- Histologic analysis of all surgical specimens assessed the extent of cervical, vaginal, and parametrial disease and the status of all surgical margins and lymph nodes
- Patients with surgical detection of positive lymph nodes, parametrial infiltration, or peritoneal spread received adjuvant treatments
- Postoperative radiotherapy consisted of 4500 cGy with 18 MeV photons, given by means of a field up to L4–L5 in the case of negative nodes, and up to T11–T12 in the case of positive common iliac nodes for subjects with stable disease or minimal response
- Subjects achieving a good clinical response to neoadjuvant treatment received additional chemotherapy "in order to confirm this response"

Toxicity (N = 21*)

Grade	G0–1	G2	G3	G4
Leucopenia	5	6	8	2[†]
Thrombocytopenia	13	4	3	1
Anemia	11	6	4	—
Mucositis	18	2	1	—
Nephrotoxicity	4	—	1*	—
Neurotoxicity	18	3	—	—
Fever	17	2	2	—
Nausea/vomiting	—	12	9	—
Cardiac	—	—	—	—
Alopecia	—	9	12	—

Completed 9 courses of treatment	19/22 (86%)
No delays in administration	3/19
Delays in administration	16/19
Duration of delays in administration	1-5 weeks

*One patient refused further treatment after first course (*Note:* a course of therapy was inconsistently defined as "… the administration of cisplatin and epirubicin [weeks 1, 4, and 7] or the administration of cisplatin alone [weeks 2, 3, 5, 6, 8, and 9].")
[†]Two subjects requiring discontinuation of the treatment; 19 received the planned dose of drug without reduction

Efficacy

Number enrolled	22
Received more than 1 dose of therapy	21
Competed all planned therapy	19
Underwent surgery	18
Complete clinical response	2
Complete response at surgery	0
Microscopic residual tumor	4*
Macroscopic residual tumor	14

With median follow up of 22 months for surviving patients

Experienced recurrence	8[†]
Died of recurrent or persistent disease	5
Alive with tumor	3
Alive without evidence of recurrence	14

*At time of the report 2 were alive with no evidence of disease at 32 and 47 months; 1 was alive with tumor; and 1 died of disease at 33 months after first diagnosis
[†]In 4/8 patients with positive nodes at time of surgery, 2/10 without nodal metastases, and 2/4 not undergoing surgery

Treatment Monitoring

1. Weekly CBC with differential
2. Weekly serum electrolytes, BUN, and creatinine

SECTION II. Supportive Care, Drug Preparation, Complications, and Screening

39. Prophylaxis and Treatment of Chemotherapy-Induced Nausea and Vomiting

Thomas E. Hughes, PharmD, BCOP

Chemotherapy-Induced Nausea and Vomiting (CINV)

Neurotransmitters and their receptor targets implicated in CINV
- Serotonin and the serotonin subtype 3 (5-HT_3) receptor
- Dopamine and the dopamine subtype 2 (D_2) receptor
- Substance P and the neurokinin subtype 1 (NK_1) receptor
- Histamine, acetylcholine, opioids, and their respective receptors

Two Phases of CINV

Acute phase
- Occurs during the first 24 hours after exposure to emetogenic chemotherapy and is mediated by release of serotonin from enterochromaffin cells within GI tract
- Actual time of onset varies depending on the chemotherapeutic agent

Delayed phase
- Substance P and the NK_1 receptor may be more important than serotonin in delayed CINV
- Delayed CINV was initially described with cisplatin
- Delayed CINV has also been described with other chemotherapeutic agents, including carboplatin, cyclophosphamide, and the anthracyclines
- Although the onset of delayed emesis was initially defined as that which occurs 24 hours postchemotherapy, more recent evidence suggests that referable symptoms may occur as early as 16 hours after cisplatin
- The incidence of delayed vomiting after cisplatin is greatest during the 24-hour period from 48 to 72 hours after treatment, and, thereafter, declines progressively

Anticipatory Nausea and Vomiting

- Development is associated with poor emetic control during prior administration of chemotherapy
- Prevention is the best approach
- Pharmacologic interventions are usually not successful, but behavioral methods with systemic desensitization is effective and has been used with some success

Antiemetic Principles[1–7]

- 5-HT_3 receptor antagonists demonstrate comparable efficacy at equivalent doses. In general, they can be used interchangeably based on convenience, availability, and cost. Evidence from clinical trials suggests palonosetron may be more effective than other 5-HT_3-receptor antagonists in preventing delayed CINV. Clinical practice guidelines from the Multinational Association of Supportive Care in Cancer (2010), and the American Society of Clinical Oncology (2011 update) recommend palonosetron as the preferred 5-HT_3 receptor antagonist in prophylaxis for chemotherapy of moderate emetic potential when aprepitant is not included in the regimen.[2,4,6] The National Comprehensive Cancer Network antiemesis guideline (version 1.2012) recommends palonosetron as the preferred 5-HT_3 receptor antagonist in prophylaxis for both high and moderate emetic risk categories[3]
- The lowest established proven dose of each 5-HT_3 receptor antagonist should be used
- Single-dose prophylactic regimens of 5-HT_3 receptor antagonists and corticosteroids for acute phase CINV prophylaxis are effective and preferred
- At biologically equivalent doses, oral antiemetic regimens are equivalent to intravenous antiemetic regimens
- All patients receiving chemotherapy should have antiemetics available on a PRN basis for breakthrough nausea and vomiting. Rescue agents should be selected to complement, not duplicate the prophylactic regimen (ie, select drugs from a different pharmacologic class)
- For CINV prophylaxis where there is a high emetic potential (emetic incidence of >90%), an antiemetic regimen that includes a 5-HT_3 receptor antagonist, a corticosteroid, and aprepitant (NK_1 receptor antagonist) is recommended. This antiemetic regimen is also recommended for combination chemotherapy regimens that include an anthracycline (eg, doxorubicin, epirubicin) and cyclophosphamide (see Table 39-4)
- For CINV prophylaxis where there is a moderate emetic potential (emetic incidence of 30–90%), an antiemetic regimen that includes a 5-HT_3 receptor antagonist and a corticosteroid is recommended (see Table 39-4)
- A corticosteroid alone is the recommended prophylactic regimen for low or intermediate emetic potential chemotherapy (emetic incidence of 10–30%)

Table 39–1. Antiemetic Pharmacologic Classes and Class Side Effects

Pharmacologic Class	Agents/Generic Name (Trade Name) (U.S. FDA Approved)	Side-Effects Profile[8–13]
5-HT$_3$ receptor antagonists	Dolasetron (Anzemet) Granisetron (Kytril, Sancuso) Ondansetron (Zofran) Palonosetron (Aloxi)	Headache [C] Constipation [I] Light-headedness or dizziness [I] Transient elevations in liver enzymes [I] *ECG interval changes:* Prolongation of PR, QTc, and JT, and widening of QRS (especially dolasetron) [R]
Corticosteroids	Dexamethasone (Decadron, generic products) Methylprednisolone (Solu-Medrol, generic products)	Hyperglycemia Mood changes Increased appetite Diarrhea Perineal irritation with rapid IV administration of dexamethasone Fluid retention
NK$_1$ receptor antagonists	Aprepitant (Emend) Fosaprepitant (Emend)	In randomized trials, treatment side effects were similar with or without aprepitant
Dopaminergic antagonists: Phenothiazines	Chlorpromazine (Thorazine, generic products) Perphenazine (Trilafon, generic products) Prochlorperazine (Compazine, generic products) Promethazine (Phenergan, generic products) Thiethylperazine (Torecan, generic products)	Extrapyramidal side effects* Sedation Anticholinergic effects Hypotension with rapid IV administration, hypersensitivity Hepatotoxicity Cholestatic jaundice Leukopenia and agranulocytosis Hormonal dysfunction Neuroleptic malignant syndrome† Cardiovascular effects‡
Dopaminergic antagonists: Butyrophenones	Droperidol (Inapsine) Haloperidol (Haldol, generic products)	Extrapyramidal side effects* Sedation Agitation Dizziness Chills Hallucinations Hypotension or hypertension Prolongation of ECG intervals (QT prolongation) Arrhythmias (eg, torsades de pointes)
Substituted benzamides	Metoclopramide (Reglan) Trimethobenzamide (Tigan)	Sedation Diarrhea Extrapyramidal side effects* Neuroleptic malignant syndrome† Hypotension Arrhythmias
Benzodiazepines	Lorazepam (Ativan) Alprazolam (Xanax)	Sedation Lethargy Weakness Impaired coordination
Cannabinoids	Dronabinol (Marinol) Nabilone (Cesamet)	Mood changes Memory loss Euphoria Dysphoria Hallucinations Sedation Paranoid ideation Ataxia Motor incoordination Blurred vision Hunger Cardiovascular effects§ Syncope

(continued)

Table 39–1. (*continued*)

Pharmacologic Class	Agents/Generic Name (Trade Name) (U.S. FDA Approved)	Side-Effects Profile[8–13]
Atypical Antipsychotics	Olanzapine (Zyprexa) Mirtazapine (Remeron)	Sedation Extrapyramidal side effects* Neuroleptic malignant syndrome† Weight gain, hyperglycemia, and other features of metabolic syndrome may be seen with high doses and prolonged use
Antihistamines	Diphenhydramine (Benadryl, generic products) Hydroxyzine (Atarax, generic products) Meclizine (Antivert, generic products)	Sedation Dry mouth Constipation Blurred vision
Anticholinergics	Scopolamine (Transderm Scōp)	Dry mouth Somnolence Sedation Constipation

C, common; I, infrequent; R, rare. For other agents, order of frequency is less clear
*Extrapyramidal side effects: Akathisia, dyskinesias, parkinsonism, acute dystonias (oculogyric crisis, torticollis)
†Neuroleptic malignant syndrome: Hyperthermia, severe extrapyramidal dysfunction (eg, severe hypertonicity of skeletal muscles, altered mental status and/or level of consciousness, and autonomic instability)
‡Phenothiazine cardiovascular effects include hypotension, syncope, hypertension, bradycardia, and various ECG changes (nonspecific, reversible Q- and T-wave abnormalities). Cases of sudden death have also been reported, presumably secondary to ventricular arrhythmias
§The cardiovascular adverse effects of dronabinol are inconsistent but the following have been reported during therapy: hypotension, hypertension, syncope, tachycardia, palpitations, vasodilation, and facial flushing

Table 39–2. Pharmacokinetic Parameters of 5-HT$_3$ Receptor Antagonists[8–14]

Parameter	Ondansetron (0.15 mg/kg IV)	Granisetron (40 mcg/kg IV)	Dolasetron* (1.8 mcg/kg IV)	Palonosetron (10 mcg/kg IV)
Half-life (hours)	4.0†	8.95†	7.5†	40‡
Protein binding	70–76%	65%	69–77%	62%
Oral bioavailability	56%	60%	75%	NR
Metabolism CYP enzymes	Hepatic CYP3A4 (major) CYP2D6, CYP1A2	Hepatic CYP3A4	Hepatic CYP2D6 (major) CYP3A4 (minor)	Hepatic CYP2D6 (major) CYP3A4, 1A2
Urinary excretion (parent compound)	5%	12%	67%	40%
Decreased clearance in elderly Dosage adjustment in elderly	Yes No	Yes No	No No	No No
Decreased clearance in hepatic dysfunction Dosage adjustment in hepatic dysfunction	Yes Yes (in severe dysfunction)	Yes No	No (IV), Yes (PO) No	No No
Decreased clearance in renal dysfunction Dosage adjustment in renal dysfunction	Yes No	No No	Yes No	Yes No

*Dolasetron is rapidly converted to the active metabolite hydrodolasetron. All reported parameters refer to hydrodolasetron
†Data from cancer patients
‡Data from studies in healthy volunteers

Table 39–3. Classification of Emetic Risk[1-4]

Emetic Potential	Chemotherapy Drug	
High Frequency of emesis >90%	Carmustine (>250 mg/m^2)[1,3] Cisplatin (≥50 mg/m^2)[1,3,4] Cyclophosphamide (>1500 mg/m^2)[1-4] Dacarbazine[1-4] Lomustine (>60 mg/m^2)[1] Mechlorethamine[1-4] Streptozocin[1-4]	
Moderate Frequency of emesis 30–90%	Aldesleukin (IL-2) (>12–15 million IU/m^2)[3] Altretamine[3] Arsenic Trioxide[3] Azacitidine[3,4] Bendamustine[3,4] Busulfan (IV, oral >4 mg/kg per day)[3],* Carboplatin[1-4] Carmustine (≤250 mg/m^2)[1,3] Cisplatin (<50 mg/m^2)[1,3] Clofarabine[3,4] Cyclophosphamide (<1500 mg/m^2)[1-4] Cytarabine (>1000 mg/m^2)[1,2,4] Dactinomycin[3] Daunorubicin[2-4]	Doxorubicin[1-4] Epirubicin[2-4] Idarubicin[1-4] Interferon alfa (≥10 million IU/m^2)[3] Ifosfamide[1-4] Irinotecan[1-4] Melphalan (IV)[1,3] Methotrexate (>250 mg/m^2)[1,3] Oxaliplatin[2-4] Pentostatin* Procarbazine[1] Romidepsin* Temozolomide[3,4]
Low Frequency of emesis 10–30%	Aldesleukin (IL-2) (<12 million IU/m^2)[3] Bortezomib[2,4] Cabazitaxel[3] Capecitabine[4] Cetuximab[2,4] Cytarabine (<1000 mg/m^2)[1,2,4] Daunorubicin, Liposomal* Decitabine* Denileukin diftitox* Docetaxel[1-4] Doxorubicin, Liposomal[3,4] Eribulin[3] Etoposide[1-4] Everolimus[4] Fluorouracil[2-4] Gemcitabine[1-4] Imatinib* Interferon alfa (>5 to <10 million IU/m^2)[3] Ixabepilone[3,4]	Lapatinib[4] Lenalidomide[4] Methotrexate (>50 mg/m^2 to <250 mg/m^2)[1,3] Mitomycin[1-4] Mitoxantrone[2-4] Nelarabine* Paclitaxel[1-4] Paclitaxel, albumin-bound suspension[3] Panitumumab[4] Pazopanib* Pemetrexed[2-4] Pralatrexate[3] Sunitinib[4] Temsirolimus[4] Teniposide[1] Thalidomide[4] Thiotepa[1] Topotecan[1-4]
Minimal Frequency of emesis <10%	Alemtuzumab[3] Asparaginase[3] Bevacizumab[3,4] Bleomycin[1-4] Busulfan (oral, <4 mg/kg per day)[1] Chlorambucil[1,4] Cladribine[1-4] Dasatinib* Erlotinib[4] Fludarabine[1-4] Gefitinib[4] Hydroxyurea[1,4] Interferon alfa (≤5 million IU/m^2)[3] Ipilimumab[3]	Melphalan (oral)[1,4] Mercaptopurine[1] Methotrexate (<50 mg/m^2)[1,3,4] Nilotinib* Ofatumumab[3] Pegaspargase[3] Rituximab[2-4] Sorafenib[4] Thioguanine (oral)[1,4] Trastuzumab[3] Vinblastine[1-4] Vincristine[1-4] Vinorelbine[1-4]

Classifications are adapted from references 1–4. Each agent is referenced to a specific guideline. When discrepancies existed among guidelines, the author classified the agent on personal opinion and referenced the guideline that supported the classification chosen. If the agent was not classified by a clinical guideline or the clinical guideline classification was in doubt, the classification was based on the incidence of emesis documented in product labeling
*Classified based on the incidence of emesis documented in product labeling

Table 39–4. Antiemetic Regimens for Prophylaxis of CINV (Adults)[1–4]

Emetic Potential	Acute Nausea and Vomiting Antiemetic Regimen (First 24 Hours, Day 1)	Delayed Nausea and Vomiting Antiemetic Regimen (>24 Hours, Days 2–5)	Notes and Comments
High Frequency of emesis >90%	5-HT$_3$ antagonist + corticosteroid + aprepitant (all given as single doses 30–60 minutes prior to chemotherapy)	Aprepitant + corticosteroid	See Table 39-3 for emetic risk classification of chemotherapy agents and regimens Agents associated with delayed CINV include cisplatin, carboplatin, cyclophosphamide, anthracyclines (eg, doxorubicin, epirubicin) and drug combinations that include these agents See Table 39-5 for dosing recommendations for antiemetic agents Corticosteroids should *not* be used with regimens containing aldesleukin (IL-2)
Moderate Frequency of emesis 30–60%	5- HT$_3$ antagonist + corticosteroid ± aprepitant (all given as single doses 30–60 minutes prior to chemotherapy)	Aprepitant (if aprepitant is used for acute prophylaxis) *or* Corticosteroid *or* 5-HT$_3$ antagonist	See above Aprepitant should be utilized in patients treated with the combination of cyclophosphamide and an anthracycline (eg, doxorubicin or epirubicin). Aprepitant may be considered for other moderately emetogenic regimens, particularly in refractory patients
Low Frequency of emesis 10–30%	Corticosteroid (a single dose 30 minutes prior to chemotherapy *or* Dopaminergic antagonist (a single dose 30 minutes prior to chemotherapy) *Note:* Antiemetic prophylaxis may often be unnecessary	Not necessary	Dopaminergic antagonists include prochlorperazine, chlorpromazine, haloperidol, thiethylperazine, metoclopramide, perphenazine, and promethazine
Minimal Frequency of emesis <10%	Antiemetic prophylaxis is usually not necessary	Not necessary	See above

Table 39–5. Dosing Recommendations for CINV Prophylaxis (Adults) for Moderate to Highly Emetic Chemotherapy[1–4]

Agent	Acute CINV Prophylaxis (Day 1)*			Delayed CINV Prophylaxis (Days 2–5)	Dosage Forms
	Oral (PO)	Intravenous (IV)	Other		
5-HT$_3$ Receptor Antagonists					
Dolasetron mesylate (Anzemet)	100 mg PO	Not recommended		100 mg PO daily for 2–4 days	Injection Tablets: 50 mg, 100 mg
Granisetron HCl (Kytril)	2 mg PO	1 mg or 0.01 mg/kg IV		1 mg PO twice daily for 2–4 days	Injection Tablets: 1 mg
Granisetron HCl (Sancuso)	NA	NA	Apply 1 patch to the upper outer arm 24–48 hours before chemotherapy Patches are removed a minimum of 24 hours after emetogenic treatment is completed, and may be worn for up to 7 days		Transdermal system: 52-cm² patch delivers 3.1 mg/24 hours

(continued)

Table 39–5. (*continued*)

Agent	Acute CINV Prophylaxis (Day 1)*			Delayed CINV Prophylaxis (Days 2–5)†	Dosage Forms
	Oral (PO)	Intravenous (IV)	Other		
Ondansetron HCl (Zofran)	16–24 mg PO	8 mg or 0.15 mg/kg IV		8 mg PO twice daily for 2–4 days	Injection Tablets: 4 mg, 8 mg, 24 mg Oral solution: 4 mg/5 mL Orally disintegrating tablets: 4 mg, 8 mg
Ondansetron (Zuplenz)	8 mg PO, 30 minutes before emetogenic treatment, then 8 mg PO 8 hours after emetogenic treatment	NA		8 mg PO every 12 hours for 1–2 days	Oral soluble film: 4 mg, 8 mg
Palonosetron HCl (Aloxi)	0.5 mg PO, 60 minutes before emetogenic treatment	0.25 mg IV		NA	Injection Oral capsules‡: 0.5 mg

Notes:
- Because of its long half-life, palonosetron is usually given as a single dose prior to moderately and highly emetogenic chemotherapy with demonstrable efficacy against developing delayed CINV symptoms on subsequent days
- When utilized as prophylaxis in a multiple-day chemotherapy regimen, alternative palonosetron administration strategies have been employed (eg, days 1, 3, and 5, during a chemotherapy regimen in which cisplatin 20 mg/m² is given daily for 5 consecutive days)

Corticosteroids

Agent	Oral (PO)	Intravenous (IV)	Other	Delayed CINV	Dosage Forms
Dexamethasone phosphate (Decadron)	8–20 mg PO	8–20 mg IV		4 mg twice daily *or* 8 mg PO daily *or* 8 mg twice daily for 2–4 days	Injection Tablets: numerous tablet strengths
Methylprednisolone sodium succinate (Solu-Medrol)	NA	40–125 mg IV		NA	Injection

Notes:
- For highly emetogenic chemotherapy, dexamethasone doses of 20 mg have been shown to be more efficacious than lower doses. In moderately emetogenic chemotherapy, doses greater than 8 mg have not been shown superior to an 8-mg dose
- When combined with aprepitant, IV doses of dexamethasone should be reduced by 25%, and PO doses of dexamethasone should be reduced by 50%. A 12-mg dose of dexamethasone for acute prophylaxis in combination with aprepitant is the only dexamethasone dose evaluated in large randomized trials

NK₁ Receptor Antagonists

Agent	Oral (PO)	Intravenous (IV)	Other	Delayed CINV	Dosage Forms
Aprepitant (Emend)	125 mg PO	NA		80 mg PO daily for 2 days	Capsules: 80 mg, 125 mg
Fosaprepitant (Emend)	NA	115 mg IV *or* 150 mg IV		Not evaluated	Injection

Notes:
- Aprepitant has been evaluated only in single-day chemotherapy regimens, and, therefore, is recommended to be given for 3 days, with an initial dose of aprepitant 125 mg on the day of chemotherapy plus 80 mg/day on days 2 and 3 after emetogenic treatment. If utilized in a multiple-day chemotherapy regimen, longer durations may be indicated (80 mg/day); however, the safety of durations exceeding 5 days has not been studied
- Fosaprepitant has been evaluated in 2 dosing formats. It may be used in a 3-day regimen with fosaprepitant 115 mg IV on day 1, followed by 80 mg/day orally on days 2 and 3 after chemotherapy. It has also been studied in a single-dose regimen with fosaprepitant 150 mg on day 1 prior to chemotherapy with no additional aprepitant doses administered subsequently during the same course of emetogenic treatment. The single-dose fosaprepitant regimen was shown to be non-inferior to the alternative 3-dose aprepitant regimen in a randomized study of patients receiving a highly emetogenic, cisplatin-based chemotherapy regimen[17]

NA, Not applicable

*For chemotherapy/biologic regimens where emetogenic agents are given either multiple times within the same day or by continuous IV infusions, alternative multiple-dose antiemetic regimens may be indicated

†Delayed CINV has been associated with cisplatin, carboplatin, cyclophosphamide, and anthracyclines (eg, doxorubicin, epirubicin)

‡As of October 24, 2013, palonosetron capsules for oral administration are not commercially available in the United States

Table 39–6. Antiemetics for Treatment of Chemotherapy-Induced Nausea and Vomiting (Adults)

Pharmacologic Classes/Agents	Dosage Form	Adult Dosages, Routes, and Schedules
Dopaminergic Antagonists: Phenothiazines		
Chlorpromazine (Thorazine, others)	Oral solution	25–50 mg PO every 4–6 hours
	Tablets	25–50 mg PO every 4–6 hours
	Injection	25–50 mg IVPB/IM every 4–6 hours*
Perphenazine (Trilafon)	Tablets	2–4 mg PO every 8 hours
Prochlorperazine (Compazine, others)	Tablets	5–20 mg PO every 4–6 hours
	Sustained release capsules	15 mg PO every 8–12 hours, or 30 mg PO every 12 hours
	Suppositories	25 mg PR every 4–6 hours
	Injection	5–20 mg IVPB/IM every 4–6 hours*
Promethazine (Phenergan)	Tablets	12.5–25 mg PO every 4–6 hours
	Suppositories	12.5–25 mg PR every 4–6 hours
	Injection	12.5–25 mg IV every 4–6 hours†
Thiethylperazine (Torecan)	Tablets	10–20 mg PO every 4–6 hours
Dopaminergic Antagonists: Butyrophenones		
Haloperidol (Haldol, others)	Tablets	1–4 mg PO every 6 hours
	Injection	1–4 mg IVPB/IM every 6 hours*
Substituted Benzamide		
Metoclopramide (Reglan, others)	Tablets	20–40 mg (or 0.5 mg/kg) PO every 6 hours
	Injection	20–40 mg (or 0.5 mg/kg) IV every 6 hours‡
Corticosteroids		
Dexamethasone	Tablets/oral solution	4–10 mg PO every 6–12 hours
	Injection	4–10 mg IV every 6–12 hours
Methylprednisolone	Injection	20–125 mg IV/IM every 6 hours
Benzodiazepines§		
Alprazolam (Xanax)	Tablets	0.125–0.5 mg PO every 8 hours
Lorazepam (Ativan)	Tablets	0.5–1 mg PO every 6–12 hours
	Injection	0.5–1 mg IV every 6–12 hours
Cannabinoids		
Dronabinol (Marinol)	Capsules	2.5–10 mg PO every 6 hours
Nabilone (Cesamet)	Capsules	1–2 mg PO every 8–12 hours

IM, Intramuscular; IV, intravenously; IVPB, IV piggyback (IV infusion of short duration); PO, orally; PR, per rectum (suppository)

*Rapid IV administration may induce hypotension. Administer slowly by IV infusion (eg, over 30 minutes)

†Promethazine injection is a potential vesicant. Use caution with intravenous administration, particularly during administration into a peripheral vein. Drug dilution and administration by IV infusion are techniques that may reduce vascular irritation

‡Greater metoclopramide doses have been utilized for the prophylaxis of CINV for highly emetic chemotherapy

§Benzodiazepines lack intrinsic antiemetic effects and should not be used as single agents against emetogenic chemotherapy

References

1. ASHP therapeutic guidelines on the pharmacologic management of nausea and vomiting in adult and pediatric patients receiving chemotherapy or radiation therapy or undergoing surgery. Am J Health Syst Pharm 1999;56:729–764
2. Basch E, Prestrud AA, Hesketh PJ et al. Antiemetics: American Society of Clinical Oncology clinical practice guideline update. J Clin Oncol 2011;29:4189–4198
3. Antiemesis. NCCN Clinical Practice Guidelines in Oncology (NCCN Guidelines), version 1.2012, National Comprehensive Cancer Care Network, 20 July 2011. Available from: http://www.nccn.org
4. MASCC/ESMO Antiemetic Guidelines 2010, Multinational Association of Supportive Care in Cancer, Nov. 3, 2010, http://www.mascc.org/mc/page.do?sitePageId=88041
5. Kris MG, Tonato M, Bria E et al. Consensus recommendations for the prevention of vomiting and nausea following high-emetic-risk chemotherapy. Support Care Cancer 2010;19(Suppl 1):S25–S32
6. Herrstedt J, Rapoport B, Warr D et al. Acute emesis: moderately emetogenic chemotherapy. Support Care Cancer 2010;19(Suppl 1):S15–S23
7. Einhorn LH, Grunberg SM, Rapoport B et al. Antiemetic therapy for multiple-day chemotherapy and additional topics consisting of rescue antiemetics and high-dose chemotherapy with stem cell transplant: review and consensus statement. Support Care Cancer 2010;19(Suppl 1):S1–S4
8. Zofran (ondansetron hydrochloride) injection for intravenous use [package insert]. Research Triangle Park, NC: GlaxoSmithKline, September 2011
9. Zofran (ondansetron hydrochloride) Tablets, Zofran ODT (ondansetron) Orally Disintegrating Tablets, Zofran (ondansetron hydrochloride) Oral Solution [package insert]. Research Triangle Park, NC: GlaxoSmithKline, September 2011
10. Kytril (granisetron hydrochloride) Tablets, Oral Solution [package insert]. Nutley, NJ: Roche Laboratories, Inc., March 2010
11. Kytril (granisetron hydrochloride) injection for intravenous use [package insert]. Nutley, NJ: Roche Laboratories, Inc., April 2011
12. Anzemet (dolasetron mesylate) tablets [package insert]. Bridgewater NJ: Sanofi-Aventis, U.S., LLC, September 2011
13. Aloxi (palonosetron HCl) injection for Intravenous Use [package insert]. Woodcliff Lake, NJ: Eisai, Inc., September 2008
14. Aloxi (palonosetron HCl) Capsules [package insert]. Woodcliff Lake, NJ: Eisai, Inc., August 2008
15. Emend (aprepitant) Capsules [package insert]. Whitehouse Station, NJ: Merck & Co., Inc., March 2011
16. Davidson TG. Causes and prevention of chemotherapy-induced emesis. Philadelphia: Medical Education Systems, Inc., 1996;34–35
17. Emend (fosaprepitant dimeglumine) for Injection, for intravenous use [package insert]. Whitehouse Station, NJ: Merck & Co., Inc., March 2011

40. Drug Preparation and Administration

David R. Kohler, PharmD

The following tables describe appropriate handling and storage, and drug product preparation and administration procedures for antineoplastics and other selected medications often used concomitantly. The tables describe drug use under a variety of commonly encountered conditions, but do not identify all applications or conditions of product stability and compatibility. Likewise, the tables are not an exhaustive list of marketed products and should not be construed as an endorsement for any manufacturer's products or discriminating against products that were not specifically identified. Clinicians are advised to refer to product labeling for more complete information about individual products and up-to-date reference sources for information about drug compatibility and stability

The information contained in this chapter is derived from contemporary product labeling approved by the U.S. Food and Drug Administration (FDA), pharmaceutical manufacturers' websites, and, in some cases, from published studies and personal communications with pharmaceutical manufacturers

Occasionally, the package insert component of product labeling for drugs that have received FDA approval for commercial use is prefaced by prominent precautionary and warning summaries circumscribed by a rectangular border, commonly referred to as *black box warnings*, or, simply, *boxed warnings*. The boxed warnings reproduced in this chapter faithfully recapitulate the most current versions of manufacturers' product labeling available lacking only referent citations to information located elsewhere within product labeling. Referents are replaced here by an ellipsis (...). Health care providers are urged to consult the most current versions of product labeling and primary medical publications for more information

In 2001, the FDA Office of Generic Drugs requested manufacturers of sixteen similarly named drug pairs to voluntarily revise the appearance of those established drug names by enhancing distinguishing elements of otherwise very similar (look-alike) names. The Name Differentiation Project of 2001 encouraged manufacturers to supplement their applications with revised labeling that incorporated "Tall Man" letters within drug names to aid visual differentiation between those drug names with a goal toward minimizing medication errors by inappropriate drug selection, ie, capitalizing letters that aid in distinguishing between similar generic and proprietary drug names. With the exception of section titles, labeled identities, compendial names, and boxed warnings, drug names appear in this chapter with the Tall Man names and conventions established and recommended by the FDA (URL: http://www.fda.gov/Drugs/DrugSafety/MedicationErrors/ucm164587.htm [accessed February 14, 2014]) and the Institute for Safe Medication Practices, Horsham, PA. (URL: www.ismp.org [accessed, February 14, 2014])

Key to Abbreviations

0.45% NaCl	0.45% Sodium chloride injection, USP	D5W/0.9% NS	5% Dextrose and 0.9% sodium chloride injection, USP
0.9% NS	0.9% Sodium chloride injection, USP	D5W/LR	5% Dextrose injection in lactated Ringer's injection, USP
1/6-M SLI	Sodium lactate injection, USP (1/6 molar [1.9%] sodium lactate)	D5W/RI	5% Dextrose injection in Ringer's injection, USP
3% NaCl	3% Sodium chloride injection (hypertonic)	DEHP	di-2-ethylhexyl phthalate (a plasticizing ingredient commonly used in flexible PVC containers)
AKA	Also known as		
ANC	Absolute neutrophil count		
AUC	Area under the concentration versus time curve	LRI	Lactated Ringer's injection, USP
B0.9% NS	Bacteriostatic (antimicrobially preserved) 0.9% sodium chloride injection	NDC	National Drug Code
		NF	"National Formulary," a portion of the official American pharmaceutical compendia, *United States Pharmacopeia-National Formulary*
BSA	Body surface area		
BWFI	Bacteriostatic water for injection, USP		
CYP	A prefix denoting cytochrome P450 enzymes	PICC	Peripherally inserted central catheter
CSF	Cerebrospinal fluid	PK	Pharmacokinetic
D10W	10% Dextrose injection, USP	PVC	Polyvinyl chloride
D2.5W	2.5% Dextrose injection, USP	Q.S.	*Quantum sufficit* or *quantum satis* [Latin]: "As much as is sufficient"
D2.5W/0.45% NaCl	2.5% Dextrose and 0.45% sodium chloride injection, USP		
D5W	5% Dextrose injection, USP	RI	Ringer's injection, USP
D5W/0.2% NaCl	5% Dextrose and 0.20% sodium chloride injection, USP	SICC	Subclavian-inserted central catheter
		SWFI	(Sterile) Water for injection, USP
D5W/0.33% NaCl	5% Dextrose and 0.33% sodium chloride injection, USP	USP	United States Pharmacopeia/U.S. Pharmacopeial Convention
D5W/0.45% NaCl	5% Dextrose and 0.45% sodium chloride injection, USP	VAD	Vascular access device (eg, catheter, port, other cannula)

ado-TRASTUZUMAB

KADCYLA™ (ado-trastuzumab emtansine) for injection, for intravenous use; product label, May 2013. Manufactured by: Genentech, Inc. A Member of the Roche Group, South San Francisco, CA

Do Not Substitute KADCYLA for or with Trastuzumab

WARNING: HEPATOTOXICITY, CARDIAC TOXICITY, EMBRYO-FETAL TOXICITY

- Hepatotoxicity: Serious hepatotoxicity has been reported, including liver failure and death in patients treated with KADCYLA. Monitor serum transaminases and bilirubin prior to initiation of KADCYLA treatment and prior to each KADCYLA dose. Reduce dose or discontinue KADCYLA as appropriate in cases of increased serum transaminases or total bilirubin...
- Cardiac Toxicity: KADCYLA administration may lead to reductions in left ventricular ejection fraction (LVEF). Evaluate left ventricular function in all patients prior to and during treatment with KADCYLA. Withhold treatment for clinically significant decrease in left ventricular function...
- Embryo-Fetal Toxicity: Exposure to KADCYLA can result in embryo-fetal death or birth defects. Advise patients of these risks and the need for effective contraception...

Boxed Warning for "KADCYLA™ (ado-trastuzumab emtansine) for injection, for intravenous use; May 2013 product label. Genentech, Inc., A Member of the Roche Group, South San Francisco, CA

Product Identification, Preparation, Storage, and Stability

- Ado-trastuzumab emtansine contains the humanized anti-HER2 IgG1, trastuzumab, covalently linked to the microtubule inhibitory drug DM1 (a maytansine derivative) via the stable thioether linker MCC (4-[N-maleimidomethyl] cyclohexane-1-carboxylate). Emtansine refers to the MCC-DM1 complex
- The commercial product, KADCYLA™, is a sterile, white to off-white, preservative-free, lyophilized powder in individually packaged, single-use vials that contain ado-trastuzumab emtansine 100 mg (NDC 50242-088-01) or 160 mg (NDC 50242-087-01)
- Store intact vials under refrigeration at 2°–8°C (35.6°–46.4°F) until time of reconstitution
- *Do not freeze or shake* intact vials

Reconstitution:

- In order to prevent medication errors it is important to check the vial labels to ensure that the drug being prepared and administered is KADCYLA™ (ado-trastuzumab emtansine), *NOT* trastuzumab
- Using a sterile syringe, slowly inject SWFI diluent into vials containing ado-trastuzumab emtansine as follows:

Vial Contents (ado-trastuzumab emtansine)	SWFI Volume for Reconstitution	ado-Trastuzumab Emtansine Concentration after Reconstitution
100 mg	5 mL	20 mg/mL
160 mg	8 mL	

- Swirl vials gently until the drug substance is completely dissolved
  - *Do not shake* vials to aid dissolution to avoid foaming
- After reconstitution, each vial contains ado-trastuzumab emtansine 20 mg/mL, polysorbate 20 0.02% (w/v), sodium succinate 10 mmol/L, and sucrose 6% (w/v), with a pH = 5.0 and density = 1.026 g/mL
- Inspect the reconstituted drug product (20 mg/mL) for particulates and discoloration
  - The solution should be clear to slightly opalescent, free of visible particulates, and colorless to pale brown
  - *Do not use* the reconstituted solution if it contains visible particulates or is cloudy or discolored
- The reconstituted lyophilized drug product should be used immediately following reconstitution, or, if not used immediately, reconstituted product may be stored for up to 24 hours under refrigeration at 2°–8°C (35.6°–46.4°F). *Do not freeze*
- Discard all unused ado-trastuzumab emtansine stored under refrigeration after 24 hours

Note: The reconstituted product contains no preservative and is intended for single use only

Dilution:

- Calculate the volume of concentrated reconstituted ado-trastuzumab emtansine solution (20-mg/mL) needed to prepare a patient's dose
- With a syringe, aseptically transfer from one or more vials the volume needed to a parenteral product container prefilled with 250 mL 0.9% NS
  - *Do not use* 5% dextrose injection as a diluent/vehicle solution
- Mix the diluted drug product by repeated gentle inversion of the container to avoid foaming
- After dilution, ado-trastuzumab emtansine admixture should be used immediately, but if not used immediately, it may be stored under refrigeration (2°–8°C) for up to 24 hours prior to use
  - The time under refrigeration for storing diluted ado-trastuzumab emtansine (24 h) is in addition to the time allowed for storing the reconstituted concentrated solution (20 mg/mL) in vials (24 h)
- Do not freeze or shake the diluted drug product

Selected incompatibility:

- Do not mix ado-trastuzumab emtansine with other medicinal products in the same container

Recommendations for Drug Administration and Ancillary Care

General:

- In order to prevent medication errors it is important to check the vial labels to ensure that the drug being prepared and administered is KADCYLA™ (ado-trastuzumab emtansine) *NOT* trastuzumab
  - In order to improve traceability of biological pharmaceutical products and prevent medication errors, the complete generic name or a distinguishing proprietary (brand) name of the administered product should be clearly recorded in a patient's medical records

Administration:

- *Do not mix* ado-trastuzumab emtansine with other medicinal products in the same container or during administration
- *Do not substitute* ado-trastuzumab emtansine for trastuzumab *or* trastuzumab for ado-trastuzumab emtansine
- The recommended dose of ado-trastuzumab emtansine is 3.6 mg/kg, given as an intravenous infusion every 3 weeks (21-day cycles)
  - *Do not administer* KADCYLA at dosages greater than 3.6 mg/kg
  - *Do not administer* ado-trastuzumab emtansine by intravenous injection or bolus
  - *Do not re-escalate* ado-trastuzumab emtansine dosages after a dosage reduction is made

Event	Administration	Monitoring	
First infusion	• Administer intravenously over 90 minutes	• Observe patients closely during the infusion and for at least 90 minutes following the initial dose for fever, chills, and other infusion-related reactions	• Patients should be observed closely for infusion-related reactions, especially during the first infusion • Administration should be slowed or interrupted if a patient develops an infusion-related reaction • Permanently discontinue KADCYLA™ for life-threatening infusion-related reactions
Second and subsequent infusions	• Administer intravenously over 30 minutes if prior administrations were well tolerated • Subsequent doses may be administered at the dosage and rate previously tolerated during the most recently administered treatment	• Observe patients during the infusion and for ≥30 minutes after administration	

- Administer ado-trastuzumab emtansine intravenously only with a 0.22-micrometer, in-line, polyethersulfone filter
- If a planned dose is delayed or missed, it should be administered as soon as possible
  - *Do not wait* until the next planned cycle
  - The schedule of administration should be adjusted to maintain a 3-week interval between doses

Notes:

- FDA-approved product labeling for ado-trastuzumab emtansine includes recommendations for treatment modifications for concomitant use with potentially interacting medications, co-morbid conditions, and adverse effects associated with treatment, including: increased serum liver transaminases (AST and ALT), hyperbilirubinemia or both conditions, and hepatic toxicity including nodular regenerative liver hyperplasia; left ventricular dysfunction, thrombocytopenia, pulmonary toxicity, and peripheral neuropathy (refer to current product labeling for detailed recommendations)
  - Management may require temporary delays, interruption, dose reduction, or treatment discontinuation
- Infusion-related reactions associated with ado-trastuzumab emtansine reported in clinical trials were characterized by one or more of the following: flushing, chills, pyrexia, dyspnea, hypotension, wheezing, bronchospasm, and tachycardia, and one episode of a serious allergic/anaphylactic reaction
  - The overall frequency of infusion-related reactions reported in one randomized trial was 1.4%
  - In most patients, reactions resolved over the course of several hours to a day after ado-trastuzumab emtansine administration was discontinued
  - Interrupt ado-trastuzumab emtansine treatment in patients who develop severe infusion-related reactions
  - ado-Trastuzumab emtansine should be permanently discontinued in the event of life-threatening infusion-related reactions

ALDESLEUKIN

PROLEUKIN® (aldesleukin) for injection, for intravenous infusion; product label, July 2012. Manufactured by Prometheus Laboratories, Inc., San Diego, CA at Bayer HealthCare Pharmaceuticals, Emeryville, CA

WARNINGS

Therapy with Proleukin® (aldesleukin) should be restricted to patients with normal cardiac and pulmonary functions as defined by thallium stress testing and formal pulmonary function testing. Extreme caution should be used in patients with a normal thallium stress test and a normal pulmonary function test who have a history of cardiac or pulmonary disease

Proleukin should be administered in a hospital setting under the supervision of a qualified physician experienced in the use of anticancer agents. An intensive care facility and specialists skilled in cardiopulmonary or intensive care medicine must be available

Proleukin administration has been associated with capillary leak syndrome (CLS) which is characterized by a loss of vascular tone and extravasation of plasma proteins and fluid into the extravascular space. CLS results in hypotension and reduced organ perfusion which may be severe and can result in death. CLS may be associated with cardiac arrhythmias (supraventricular and ventricular), angina, myocardial infarction, respiratory insufficiency requiring intubation, gastrointestinal bleeding or infarction, renal insufficiency, edema, and mental status changes

Proleukin treatment is associated with impaired neutrophil function (reduced chemotaxis) and with an increased risk of disseminated infection, including sepsis and bacterial endocarditis. Consequently, preexisting bacterial infections should be adequately treated prior to initiation of Proleukin therapy. Patients with indwelling central lines are particularly at risk for infection with gram positive microorganisms. Antibiotic prophylaxis with oxacillin, nafcillin, ciprofloxacin, or vancomycin has been associated with a reduced incidence of staphylococcal infections

Proleukin administration should be withheld in patients developing moderate to severe lethargy or somnolence; continued administration may result in coma

---

Boxed Warning for "PROLEUKIN® (aldesleukin) for injection, for intravenous infusion"; July 2012 product label; Prometheus Laboratories, Inc., San Diego, CA

Product Identification, Preparation, Storage, and Stability

- Proleukin is supplied in individually boxed single-use vials containing aldesleukin 22 million IU as a sterile, white to off-white, preservative-free, lyophilized powder (equivalent to a protein mass of 1.3 mg). NDC 65483-116-07

  - Aldesleukin biologic potency is determined by a lymphocyte proliferation bioassay and is expressed in international units (IU) as established by the World Health Organization 1st International Standard for Interleukin-2 (human)

- Store intact vials and reconstituted and diluted aldesleukin under refrigeration at 2°C–8°C (35.6°F–46.4°F). Protect from light. *Do not* freeze aldesleukin

- Reconstitute the contents of a vial with 1.2 mL of SWFI to produce a clear, colorless to slightly yellow solution with a biologic potency of 18 million IU aldesleukin/mL (equivalent to 1.1 mg of aldesleukin protein per milliliter)

  - Each milliliter of the reconstituted product also contains 50 mg mannitol and 0.18 mg sodium dodecyl sulfate, buffered with approximately 0.17 mg monobasic and 0.89 mg dibasic sodium phosphate to a pH of 7.5 (range: 7.2–7.8)

- During reconstitution, direct the stream of SWFI at the side wall of a vial rather than directly into the drug powder and gently swirl vials to avoid excessive foaming

- *Do not shake* vials to dissolve aldesleukin

- For intraVENous administration, dilute aldesleukin *only* with D5W to a final concentration between 0.5 and 1.1 million IU/mL (30–70 mcg/mL; see chart below). Drug delivery may be adversely affected by aldesleukin concentrations <30 mcg/mL or >70 mcg/mL

Aldesleukin (million IU)	Diluent Volume (D5W)
5–11	10 mL
7.5–16.5	15 mL
12.5–27.5	25 mL
25–55	50 mL
50–110	100 mL

- If it is necessary to administer aldesleukin in a concentration <30 mcg/mL (<0.5 million IU/mL), the drug should be diluted in D5W that contains Albumin Human, USP, in a concentration of 0.1% (1 mg/mL)

- Either glass bottles or PVC bags are acceptable containers for aldesleukin, but plastic containers provide more consistent drug delivery than glass containers

- Reconstituted and diluted aldesleukin solutions are stable for up to 48 hours at 2°–25°C (35.6°–77°F), but the Proleukin product does not contain a preservative

- Store reconstituted and diluted solutions under refrigeration, but allow diluted aldesleukin to warm to room temperature before administering it to a patient

Selected incompatibility:

- *Do not combine* aldesleukin with other drugs in the same container

- *Do not reconstitute or dilute* aldesleukin with 0.9% NS or antimicrobially-preserved diluents, which may increase protein aggregation

Recommendations for Drug Administration and Ancillary Care

General:

- Dose modification for toxicity should be accomplished by withholding or interrupting a dose rather than reducing the dose to be administered
- See Chapter 41 for recommended use in renal dysfunction
- Bring aldesleukin solution to room temperature before administration
- Administer aldesleukin by intraVENous infusion over 15 minutes
- *Do not filter* aldesleukin either during preparation or administration
- Complete administration within 48 hours after reconstitution

Pharmacodynamic interactions:

- Aldesleukin may affect CNS function, which may be exacerbated by concomitant administration of drugs with psychotropic activity, for example, opioids, analgesics, antiemetics, sedatives, hypnotics
- Aldesleukin may increase the nephrotoxic, myelotoxic, cardiotoxic, or hepatotoxic effects of other drugs if given concurrently
- Impaired kidney and liver function associated with aldesleukin use may delay elimination and increase the risk of adverse events from concomitantly administered medications
- Hypersensitivity reactions that consisted of erythema, pruritus, and hypotension, have been reported in patients who received combination regimens containing sequential high-dose aldesleukin and antineoplastic agents, specifically: dacarbazine, CISplatin, tamoxifen, and interferon alfa. Adverse reactions occurred within hours after administration of chemotherapy, and required medical intervention in some patients[1]
- In patients who received aldesleukin and interferon alfa concurrently:
  - The incidence of myocardial injury, including myocardial infarction, myocarditis, ventricular hypokinesia, and severe rhabdomyolysis, appears to be increased[2]
  - Exacerbation or initial presentation of autoimmune and inflammatory disorders has been observed, including: crescentic IgA glomerulonephritis, oculobulbar myasthenia gravis, inflammatory arthritis, thyroiditis, bullous pemphigoid, and Stevens-Johnson syndrome
- Glucocorticoids have been shown to reduce aldesleukin-induced side effects, including fever, renal insufficiency, hyperbilirubinemia, confusion, and dyspnea, but concomitant use should be avoided to preclude compromising aldesleukin's antitumor effectiveness[3]
- Beta-blockers and other antihypertensives may potentiate aldesleukin's hypotensive effects
- Aldesleukin use followed by administration of iodinated radiographic contrast media is associated with acute, atypical adverse reactions, including fever, chills, nausea, vomiting, pruritus, rash, diarrhea, hypotension, edema, and oliguria, with onset commonly within 1–4 hours after the administration of contrast media. In some cases, the reactions resemble the immediate side effects caused by aldesleukin administration; however, other than a temporal relationship between aldesleukin and iodinated contrast media administration the cause of aldesleukin-associated contrast reactions is not known. Although most events were reported to occur when contrast media was given within 4 weeks after the last dose of aldesleukin, events were also reported to occur when contrast media was given several months after aldesleukin[4-9]

ALEMTUZUMAB

CAMPATH® (alemtuzumab) Injection for intravenous use; product label, August 2009. Manufactured and distributed by Genzyme Corporation, Cambridge, MA

> ### WARNINGS
> ### CYTOPENIAS, INFUSION REACTIONS, and INFECTIONS
>
> <u>Cytopenias</u>: Serious, including fatal, pancytopenia/marrow hypoplasia, autoimmune idiopathic thrombocytopenia, and autoimmune hemolytic anemia can occur in patients receiving Campath. Single doses of Campath greater than 30 mg or cumulative doses greater than 90 mg per week increase the incidence of pancytopenia…
>
> <u>Infusion Reactions</u>: Campath administration can result in serious, including fatal, infusion reactions. Carefully monitor patients during infusions and withhold Campath for Grade 3 or 4 infusion reactions. Gradually escalate Campath to the recommended dose at the initiation of therapy and after interruption of therapy for 7 or more days…
>
> <u>Infections</u>: Serious, including fatal, bacterial, viral, fungal, and protozoan infections can occur in patients receiving Campath. Administer prophylaxis against *Pneumocystis jirovecii* pneumonia (PCP) *[sic]* and herpes virus infections…
>
> *Boxed Warning* for "Campath® (alemtuzumab)", Injection for intravenous use"; August 2009 product label; Genzyme Corporation, Cambridge, MA

Change in Product Availability

- As of September 4, 2012, Campath (alemtuzumab) injection for treatment of B-cell chronic lymphocytic leukemia was withdrawn from commercial availability in the United States
- Genzyme Corporation, the American distributor, announced activation of the "US Campath Distribution Program," which "…was developed to ensure continued access to Campath (alemtuzumab) for appropriate patients"
- An announcement at http://www.campath.com/ advises visitors, "Campath will no longer be available commercially, but will be provided through the Campath Distribution Program free of charge. In order to receive Campath, the healthcare provider is required to document and comply with certain requirements."
- The website provides contact telephone numbers for more information:
  - Campath Distribution Program: 1-877-422-6728
  - Genzyme Medical Information: 1-800-745-4447, Option #2
  - URL: http://www.campath.com/ (Last accessed October 7, 2013)

Product Identification, Preparation, Storage, and Stability

- Campath is packaged in clear, glass, single-use vials containing 30 mg alemtuzumab/mL NDC 58468-0357-3 (3 vials per carton). NDC 58468-0357-1 (single vial per carton)
  - Campath is a sterile, clear, colorless, isotonic solution for injection containing alemtuzumab 30 mg/mL at pH 6.8–7.4
  - Each milliliter of the commercial product also contains 8 mg sodium chloride, 1.44 mg dibasic sodium phosphate, 0.2 mg potassium chloride, 0.2 mg monobasic potassium phosphate, 0.1 mg polysorbate 80, and 0.0187 mg disodium edetate dihydrate
- Store intact vials under refrigeration at 2°–8°C (35.6°–46.4°F); protect vials from direct sunlight
- *Do not freeze* alemtuzumab. If the product is accidentally frozen, thaw at 2°–8°C before use
- *Do not shake* vials before use

1. Withdraw from a vial into a syringe an amount of alemtuzumab needed to prepare a patient's dose
   a. 0.1 mL Campath solution for a 1-mg dose
   b. 0.33 mL Campath solution for a 10-mg dose
   c. 1 mL Campath solution for a 30-mg dose
2. Inject the amount of drug needed to prepare a patient's dose into 100 mL of 0.9% NS or D5W in a plastic parenteral product container
3. Gently invert the bag to mix the solution
- Diluted alemtuzumab solutions may be stored at room temperature (15°C–30°C; 59°F–86°F) or under refrigeration
- The commercial drug product contains no antimicrobial preservatives. Use the product within 8 hours after dilution

Selected incompatibility:
- Alemtuzumab is compatible with PVC bags, PVC- or polyethylene-lined PVC administration sets
- No data are available concerning the compatibility of alemtuzumab with other drugs. Do not add or simultaneously infuse other drugs through the same intraVENous line with alemtuzumab

Recommendations for Drug Administration and Ancillary Care

General:

- Administer alemtuzumab only by intraVENous infusion over ≥2 hours
- Do not administer alemtuzumab by direct intraVENous injection or bolus injection

Infusion reactions and dose escalation:

- Alemtuzumab administration can result in serious infusion reactions commonly including: pyrexia, chills, hypotension, urticaria, and dyspnea
  - G3 and G4 pyrexia and/or chills occurred in approximately 10% of previously untreated patients and in approximately 35% of previously treated patients
  - The occurrence of infusion reactions was greatest during the initial week of treatment and decreased with subsequent doses
  - All patients were pretreated with antipyretics and antihistamines; additionally, 43% of previously untreated patients received glucocorticoid prior to alemtuzumab
- Gradual escalation to the recommended maintenance dose/schedule is required when initiating therapy and after treatment interruptions ≥7 days. Generally, escalation to a 30-mg dose can be accomplished in 3–7 days as follows:

1. Initiate treatment with alemtuzumab 3 mg intraVENously over 2 hours
2. After a 3-mg DAILY dose is tolerated (ie, infusion-related toxicities are grades ≤2), escalate DAILY dose to 10 mg/day and continue until tolerated
3. After a 10-mg DAILY dose is tolerated (infusion-related toxicities grades ≤2), escalate to a maintenance dose and schedule of alemtuzumab 30 mg/dose on 3 nonconsecutive days for 3 doses per week (eg, Monday, Wednesday, and Friday) for a total treatment duration of 12 weeks, including the period of dose escalation

Concomitant medications:

- Give premedication 30 minutes before the first alemtuzumab dose, before dose escalations, and as clinically indicated, with:
  - **DiphenhydrAMINE** 50 mg orally or intraVENously
  - **Acetaminophen** 500–1000 mg orally

- Treat severe infusion-related events with:
  - **Hydrocortisone** intraVENously (anaphylactoid reactions)
  - **Meperidine** intraVENously (chills, rigors)
  - **Epinephrine 1:1000** (1 mg/mL) intraMUSCularly (preferred) or SUBCUTaneously (anaphylactoid reactions)
  - **Epinephrine 1:10,000** (0.1 mg/mL) intraVENously with cardiac monitoring (airway edema, severe bronchospasm, hypotension)
- Give antibacterial and antiviral primary prophylaxis during treatment and continue for at least 2 months after the last dose of alemtuzumab is administered or until CD4+ lymphocyte counts are ≥200/mm^3, whichever event occurs later, with:
  - **Cotrimoxazole** (trimethoprim 160 mg + sulfamethoxazole 800 mg) orally, twice daily for 3 days/week (or equivalent anti-PCP prophylaxis)
  - **Famciclovir** 250 mg orally twice daily (or equivalent anti-herpesvirus prophylaxis)

AMIFOSTINE

AMIFOSTINE FOR INJECTION; product label, May 2013. Manufactured by MedImmune Pharma B.V., Nijmegen, The Netherlands. Distributed by Bedford Laboratories, Bedford, OH

Product Identification, Preparation, Storage, and Stability

- Amifostine is packaged in 10-mL (capacity) single-use vials containing 500 mg (on an anhydrous basis) of amifostine trihydrate as a sterile lyophilized powder. NDC 55390-308-03 (3 vials per carton)
- Store intact vials at controlled room temperature, 20°–25°C (68°–77°F)
- Reconstitute amifostine with 9.7 mL of 0.9% NS to produce a solution with concentration of 500 mg amifostine/10 mL
- Amifostine may be further diluted in PVC containers with 0.9% NS to concentrations ranging from 5 to 40 mg/mL
- The reconstituted drug product (500 mg/mL) and diluted amifostine solutions are chemically stable for up to 5 hours at approximately 25°C and for up to 24 hours under refrigeration (2°–8°C; 35.6°–46.4°F)

Selected incompatibility:

- Product labeling advises admixture with solutions other than 0.9% NS with or without other (unspecified) additives is not recommended

Recommendations for Drug Administration and Ancillary Care

General:

- Administer intraVENously (see indication-specific recommendations below)
- Provide adequate hydration before amifostine infusion
- Administer antiemetic primary prophylaxis before amifostine
  - Emetic risk is related to amifostine dosage: low risk, ≤300 mg/m²; moderate risk, >300 mg/m² (NCCN Clinical Practice Guidelines in Oncology [NCCN Guidelines®]: Antiemesis, V.1.2014. National Comprehensive Cancer Network, Inc., 2013. [Accessed October 8, 2013, at http://www.nccn.org.])
- Monitor a patient's blood pressure every 5 minutes during amifostine administration, and thereafter as clinically indicated
- Keep patients in a supine position during the amifostine infusion. Interrupt amifostine administration if systolic blood pressure (SBP) decreases significantly from baseline as follows:

Baseline SBP (mm Hg)	Decrease in SBP That Warrants Interrupting Amifostine Infusion
<100	20 mm Hg
100–119	25 mm Hg
120–139	30 mm Hg
140–179	40 mm Hg
≥180	50 mm Hg

- If BP returns to normal within 5 minutes and the patient is asymptomatic, resume administration to complete the planned dose
- If the planned dose cannot be administered, decrease the amifostine dosage during subsequent chemotherapy cycles from 910 mg/m² to 740 mg/m²

To reduce cumulative renal toxicity with chemotherapy:

- Administer antiemetic primary prophylaxis before amifostine, including dexamethasone 20 mg intraVENously, a serotonin receptor (5-HT₃ subtype) antagonist, *plus* additional antiemetics as appropriate for the chemotherapy utilized
- Administer amifostine 910 mg/m² once daily by intraVENous infusion over 15 minutes, starting 30 minutes before chemotherapy
  - A 15-minute infusion is better tolerated than longer infusions

To decrease moderate-to-severe xerostomia from head and neck radiation:

- Administer antiemetic primary prophylaxis before amifostine, for example, a 5-HT₃ antagonist ± additional antiemetics if clinically appropriate
- Administer amifostine 200 mg/m² once daily by intraVENous infusion over 3 minutes, 15–30 minutes before standard-fraction radiation therapy (ie, 1.8–2 Gy/fraction)
- Monitor blood pressure at least before and immediately after the infusion, and thereafter as clinically indicated

ARSENIC TRIOXIDE

TRISENOX® (arsenic trioxide) injection, for intravenous use only; product label, June 2010. Manufactured for Cephalon Inc., Frazer, PA

WARNINGS

Experienced Physician and Institution: TRISENOX (arsenic trioxide) injection should be administered under the supervision of a physician who is experienced in the management of patients with acute leukemia

APL Differentiation Syndrome: Some patients with APL treated with TRISENOX have experienced symptoms similar to a syndrome called the retinoic-acid-Acute Promyelocytic Leukemia (RA-APL) or APL differentiation syndrome, characterized by fever, dyspnea, weight gain, pulmonary infiltrates and pleural or pericardial effusions, with or without leukocytosis. This syndrome can be fatal. The management of the syndrome has not been fully studied, but high-dose steroids have been used at the first suspicion of the APL differentiation syndrome and appear to mitigate signs and symptoms. At the first signs that could suggest the syndrome (unexplained fever, dyspnea and/or weight gain, abnormal chest auscultatory findings or radiographic abnormalities), high-dose steroids (dexamethasone 10 mg intraVENously BID) should be immediately initiated, irrespective of the leukocyte count, and continued for at least 3 days or longer until signs and symptoms have abated. The majority of patients do not require termination of TRISENOX therapy during treatment of the APL differentiation syndrome

ECG Abnormalities: Arsenic trioxide can cause QT interval prolongation and complete atrioventricular block. QT prolongation can lead to a torsade de pointes-type ventricular arrhythmia, which can be fatal. The risk of torsade de pointes is related to the extent of QT prolongation, concomitant administration of QT prolonging drugs, a history of torsade de pointes, preexisting QT interval prolongation, congestive heart failure, administration of potassium-wasting diuretics, or other conditions that result in hypokalemia or hypomagnesemia. One patient (also receiving amphotericin B) had torsade de pointes during induction therapy for relapsed APL with arsenic trioxide

ECG and Electrolyte Monitoring Recommendations: Prior to initiating therapy with TRISENOX, a 12-lead ECG should be performed and serum electrolytes (potassium, calcium, and magnesium) and creatinine should be assessed; preexisting electrolyte abnormalities should be corrected and, if possible, drugs that are known to prolong the QT interval should be discontinued. For QTc greater than 500 msec, corrective measures should be completed and the QTc reassessed with serial ECGs prior to considering using TRISENOX. During therapy with TRISENOX, potassium concentrations should be kept above 4 mEq/L and magnesium concentrations should be kept above 1.8 mg/dL. Patients who reach an absolute QT interval value >500 msec should be reassessed and immediate action should be taken to correct concomitant risk factors, if any, while the risk/benefit of continuing versus suspending TRISENOX therapy should be considered. If syncope, rapid or irregular heartbeat develops, the patient should be hospitalized for monitoring, serum electrolytes should be assessed, TRISENOX therapy should be temporarily discontinued until the QTc interval regresses to below 460 msec, electrolyte abnormalities are corrected, and the syncope and irregular heartbeat cease. There are no data on the effect of TRISENOX on the QTc interval during the infusion

Boxed Warning for "Trisenox® (arsenic trioxide) injection, For Intravenous Use Only"; June 2010 product label; Cephalon Inc., Frazer, PA

Product Identification, Preparation, Storage, and Stability

- Trisenox® is packaged in 10-mL, glass, single-use ampules containing 10 mg of arsenic trioxide (1 mg/mL). NDC 63459-600-10 (package of 10 ampules)
  - Trisenox® is formulated as a sterile, nonpyrogenic, clear, colorless, preservative-free solution of arsenic trioxide in water for injection. Sodium hydroxide and hydrochloric acid are used to adjust the pH to 7.5–8.5
- Store intact ampules at 25°C (77°F). Temperature excursions are permitted to 15°–30°C (59°–86°F)
- Dilute arsenic trioxide in 100–250 mL of 0.9% NS or D5W immediately after withdrawing the drug product from an ampule. Unused drug should be discarded in a manner appropriate for hazardous drugs
- Diluted arsenic trioxide solutions are chemically and physically stable for 24 hours when stored at room temperature and for up to 48 hours under refrigeration

Selected incompatibility:

Arsenic trioxide should not be mixed with other drugs

Recommendations for Drug Administration and Ancillary Care

General:

- See Chapter 41 for recommended use in renal and hepatic dysfunction
- Administer arsenic trioxide by intraVENous infusion over 1–2 hours. The duration of administration may be extended to 4 hours for patients who experience acute vasomotor reactions
- A central VAD is not required for administering arsenic trioxide

ECG changes:

- QT/QTc prolongation should be expected during treatment with arsenic trioxide, and torsade de pointes and complete heart block have been reported
- In >460 ECG tracings from 40 patients evaluated for QTc prolongation, 16 patients (40%) demonstrated at least 1 QTc interval >500 msec
- QTc prolongation was observed between 1 and 5 weeks after arsenic trioxide administration, and then returned towards baseline by the end of 8 weeks after arsenic trioxide administration
- Neither sex nor age factors correlated with QT prolongation events
- Complete AV block has also been reported in association with arsenic trioxide treatment, including a case in a patient with acute promyelocytic leukemia

ASPARAGINASE, *ERWINIA CHRYSANTHEMI* SOURCE

Asparaginase *Erwinia chrysanthemi* ERWINAZE™ for injection, intramuscular use; product label, November 2011. Manufactured by EUSA Pharma (USA), Inc., Langhorne, PA

Product Identification, Preparation, Storage, and Stability

Erwinaze™ is a sterile, white lyophilized powder supplied in clear, 3-mL, glass vials. Each carton of the commercial product contains 5 vials (NDC 57902-249-05). Each vial (NDC 57902-249-01) contains 10,000 IU of asparaginase *Erwinia chrysanthemi*
- Store intact vials and cartons under refrigeration at 2°–8°C (35.6°–46.4°F)
- Protect intact vials and the reconstituted drug product from light

Preparation for intraMUSCular use:

- Asparaginase *Erwinia chrysanthemi* is reconstituted by slowly injecting 1 or 2 mL of preservative-free 0.9% NS against the inner vial wall
- DO NOT forcefully inject the diluent solution directly into the drug powder

Diluent Volume	Product Concentration
1 mL	10,000 IU/mL
2 mL	5000 IU/mL

- Dissolve the drug powder by gentle mixing or swirling after adding preservative-free 0.9% NS diluent. DO NOT shake or invert vials to solubilize the drug product
- After reconstitution, asparaginase *Erwinia chrysanthemi* should be a clear, colorless solution
- Discard the reconstituted product if visible particles or protein aggregates are present
- DO NOT freeze or refrigerate asparaginase *Erwinia chrysanthemi* solutions

Recommendations for Drug Administration and Ancillary Care

General:

- See Chapter 41 for recommended use in hepatic dysfunction

IntraMUSCular administration:

- Asparaginase *Erwinia chrysanthemi* is administered ONLY by intraMUSCular injection
- Volumes for injection >2 mL should be distributed among 2 or more injection sites
- Withdraw from a vial into a polypropylene syringe within 15 minutes after reconstitution a volume of reconstituted asparaginase *Erwinia chrysanthemi* appropriate for a calculated dose
- Administer asparaginase *Erwinia chrysanthemi* within 4 hours after reconstitution

To substitute asparaginase *Erwinia chrysanthemi* for a dose of pegaspargase:

- For each planned dose of pegaspargase, the recommended dose of asparaginase *Erwinia chrysanthemi* is 25,000 IU/m² administered intraMUSCularly 3 times per week (eg, Monday, Wednesday, and Friday) for 6 doses

To substitute asparaginase *Erwinia chrysanthemi* for a dose of *Escherichia coli* asparaginase:

- The recommended dose is a single dose of asparaginase *Erwinia chrysanthemi* 25,000 IU/m² administered intraMUSCularly

ASPARAGINASE, *ESCHERICHIA COLI* SOURCE

ELSPAR (asparaginase) for injection, intravenous or intramuscular, product label, April 2010. Lundbeck, Inc, Deerfield, IL

Note: Information at http://www.lundbeck.com/us/products/customer-support [accessed January 11, 2014] states: As of January 18, 2013, Elspar was sold to Recordati Rare Diseases (Recordati). For access to Recordati's website for Elspar, go to http://www.recordatirarediseases.com/

Product Identification, Preparation, Storage, and Stability

Elspar® is packaged in individually boxed single-use vials containing asparaginase 10,000 IU as a sterile, white lyophilized plug or powder for intraVENous or intraMUSCular injection after reconstitution. NDC 67386-411-51

- Elspar® contains the enzyme L-asparagine amidohydrolase, type EC-2, derived from *Escherichia coli* and 80 mg of mannitol

  - One International Unit of asparaginase is defined as that amount of enzyme required to generate 1 μmol of ammonia per minute at pH 7.3 and 37°C

  - The product's specific activity is at least 225 IU/mg of protein

- Store intact vials under refrigeration at 2°–8°C (35.6°–46.4°F)

- After reconstitution, Elspar® is a clear, colorless solution

- Unused, reconstituted asparaginase should be stored at 2°–8°C and discarded after 8 hours or sooner if the reconstituted product becomes cloudy

- Asparaginase stability is dependent on solution pH and storage temperature[10]

- Asparaginase is relatively stable at pH = 4.5–11; drug activity is lost at greater extremes of pH

- Asparaginase also has a high stability to changes in temperature (37°–60°C), but both solution pH and storage temperature affect stability

- Asparaginase activity was preserved for at least 7 days after dilution in 0.9% NS and storage under refrigeration (8°C) in polyolefin or polyethylene containers

- Administer asparaginase by either intraVENous or intraMUSCular routes

For intraVENous use:

- Reconstitute vials containing asparaginase 10,000 IU with 5 mL of SWFI or 0.9% NS to produce a solution with concentration = 2000 IU/mL. Ordinary shaking during reconstitution does not inactivate the enzyme, but may cause foaming

- The reconstituted solution is suitable for direct intraVENous injection or may be diluted with 0.9% NS or LRI

- Asparaginase should be administered intraVENously over a period not less than 30 minutes

- Administer asparaginase within 8 hours after preparation and only if the solution remains clear

  1. Occasionally, a small number of gelatinous fiber-like particles may develop on standing

  2. Filtration through a 5-μm filter during administration removes the particles with no resultant loss in potency

  3. SOME LOSS OF POTENCY has been observed with the use of a 0.2-μm filter

For intraMUSCular use:

- Add 2 mL of 0.9% NS to a vial containing asparaginase 10,000 IU to produce a solution with concentration = 5000 IU/mL

- If a volume >2 mL is to be administered, 2 injection sites should be used

- Administer asparaginase within 8 hours and only if the solution remains clear

Recommendations for Drug Administration and Ancillary Care

General:

- See Chapter 41 for recommended use in hepatic dysfunction

Intradermal skin test:

- Asparaginase administration is associated with allergic reactions. An intradermal skin test may be performed before initial administration and when asparaginase is given after an interval ≥1 week has elapsed between doses

- Observe a skin test site for at least 1 hour for a wheal or erythema; either sign indicates a positive reaction

Note: A *negative* skin test reaction does not preclude the possibility of an allergic reaction to asparaginase treatment; that is, be wary of false-negative results

Prepare a skin test solution as follows:
1. Reconstitute asparaginase 10,000 IU with 5 mL of 0.9% NS
2. From the solution prepared in the previous step (containing 2000 IU/mL), withdraw 0.1 mL and inject it into a vial containing 9.9 mL of 0.9% NS, yielding a skin test solution of approximately 20 IU/mL
3. Inject intradermally 0.1 mL of the skin test solution (approximately 2 IU)

Note: In patients who demonstrate hypersensitivity by skin testing, and in any patient who previously completed a course of asparaginase, retreatment should be instituted only after successful desensitization

Desensitization should be performed before administering a first dose of asparaginase in positive reactors, and before retreating patients who have not received asparaginase for a period >1 week

(continued)

Recommendations for Drug Administration and Ancillary Care *(continued)*

Desensitization[11,12]:

- Rapid intraVENous desensitization may be attempted with progressively increasing amounts of asparaginase if adequate precautions are taken to treat an acute allergic reaction should it occur
- The following schedule begins with a total of 1 IU, intraVENously and, provided no reaction has occurred, doubles the dose every 10 minutes, until the accumulated total amount given equals the planned dose for that day

Injection Number	Asparaginase Dose (IU)	Accumulated Total Dose
1	1	1
2	2	3
3	4	7
4	8	15
5	16	31
6	32	63
7	64	127
8	128	255
9	256	511
10	512	1023
11	1024	2047
12	2048	4095
13	4096	8191
14	8192	16,383
15	16,384	32,767
16	32,768	65,535
17	65,536	131,071
18	131,072	262,143

Example: A patient weighing 20 kg who is to receive 4000 IU would receive desensitization injections 1 through 12

ELSPAR® (ASPARAGINASE) product label, December 2005. Merck & Co., Inc., Whitehouse Station, NJ

IntraVENous administration:

- Infuse over at least 30 minutes through the side arm of a running infusion of 0.9% NS or D5W

IntraMUSCular administration:

- Limit the volume at a single injection site to ≤2 mL

AZACITIDINE

VIDAZA® (azacitidine for injection) for SC or IV use; product label, December 2012. Manufactured by Ben Venue Laboratories, Inc., Bedford, OH, *or* Baxter Oncology GmbH, Halle/Westfalen, Germany, *or* BSP Pharmaceuticals S.r.l., Latina Scalo, Italy. Manufactured for Celgene Corporation, Summit, NJ

Product Identification, Preparation, Storage, and Stability

- Vidaza® is packaged in cartons with one single-use vial containing azaCITIDine 100 mg with 100 mg mannitol as a sterile, lyophilized, white to off-white powder for reconstitution as a suspension for SUBCUTaneous injection or as a solution for intraVENous infusion. NDC 59572-102-01
  - Store intact vials at 25°C (77°F); temperature excursions are permitted to 15°–30°C (59°–86°F)

Preparation for SUBCUTaneous administration:

1. Reconstitute lyophilized azaCITIDine powder by slowly injecting 4 mL of SWFI into a vial
2. Vigorously shake or roll the vial until a uniform cloudy suspension is formed. The resulting suspension contains 25 mg azaCITIDine per milliliter

Preparation for *immediate* SUBCUTaneous administration:

1. Divide doses >4 mL (>100 mg) equally into two syringes
2. Store reconstituted azaCITIDine suspension for up to 1 hour at room temperature, but the product must be administered within 1 hour after reconstitution

Preparation for *delayed* SUBCUTaneous administration:

1. Reconstituted azaCITIDine may be kept in the vial or drawn into a syringe
2. Divide doses >4 mL (>100 mg) equally into 2 syringes
3. Immediately place the product under refrigeration (2°–8°C; 35.6°–46.4°F)

where it may be maintained for up to 8 hours
  a. If refrigerated SWFI was used in reconstituting azaCITIDine, the reconstituted product may be stored under refrigeration (2°–8°C) for up to 22 hours
  b. If *non*-refrigerated SWFI was used in reconstituting azaCITIDine, the reconstituted product may be stored under refrigeration (2°–8°C) for up to 8 hours, or for one hour if stored at room temperature (25°C [77°F])
4. After removal from refrigeration, the suspension may be allowed to equilibrate to room temperature for up to 30 minutes before administration

Preparation for *delayed* intraVENous administration:

1. Reconstitute an appropriate number of vials to achieve the desired dose. Inject 10 mL SWFI into each vial and vigorously shake or roll the vial until all solids are dissolved. The resulting solution should be clear and will contain azaCITIDine 10 mg/mL
2. Withdraw a volume of azaCITIDine solution appropriate to deliver the desired dose and inject it into 50–100 mL of 0.9% NS or LRI
3. After reconstitution for intraVENous administration, azaCITIDine may be stored at 25°C, but administration must be completed within 1 hour after reconstitution

Selected incompatibilities:

- D5W, Hespan® (6% hetastarch [hydroxyethyl starch] in 0.9% NS), and solutions that contain bicarbonate have the potential to increase the rate of azaCITIDine degradation and should be avoided

Recommendations for Drug Administration and Ancillary Care

General:

- See Chapter 41 for recommended use in renal and hepatic dysfunction
- If patients experience an unexplained decrease in serum bicarbonate concentration to <20 mEq/L during or after treatment with azaCITIDine, the dosage should be decreased by 50% during the next treatment cycle
- If patients experience an unexplained increase in BUN or serum creatinine during treatment, the next cycle should be delayed until laboratory values return to normal or baseline and azaCITIDine dosage should be decreased by 50% on the next treatment course
- AzaCITIDine and its metabolites are substantially renally excreted. Elderly individuals and other patients with impaired renal function may be at increased risk of toxicity from azaCITIDine

For SUBCUTaneous administration only:

- Doses >4 mL (>100 mg) should be divided equally into 2 syringes and injected into 2 separate sites. Rotate sites for each injection (thigh, abdomen, or upper arm)
- New injections should be given at least 1 inch from an old site and never into areas where the site is tender, bruised, red, or hard
- For azaCITIDine suspension that is not administered immediately after preparation:
  - After removal from refrigeration, allow the suspension to equilibrate to room temperature for up to 30 minutes before administration
  - Resuspend the product before administration to provide a homogeneous suspension by vigorously shaking a vial or rolling syringes between the palms until a uniform cloudy suspension is formed

For IntraVENous administration:

- After reconstitution and further dilution, administer the total azaCITIDine dose over a period of 10–40 minutes
- Administration must be completed within 1 hour after initial reconstitution

BENDAMUSTINE HYDROCHLORIDE

TREANDA® (bendamustine hydrochloride) for Injection for Intravenous Infusion, product label, August 2013. Distributed by Teva Pharmaceuticals USA, Inc., North Wales, PA
TREANDA® (bendamustine hydrochloride) Injection for Intravenous Infusion; product label, September 2013. Distributed by Teva Pharmaceuticals USA, Inc., North Wales, PA
Note: Although "TREANDA® (bendamustine hydrochloride) Injection…" (product formulated in solution) received FDA approval in September 2013, it is not commercially available within the USA as of January 2014

Product Identification, Preparation, Storage, and Stability

Bendamustine HCl Injection (lyophilized product for reconstitution)

- TREANDA® is available in single-use, individually packaged, amber glass vials containing a sterile, non-pyrogenic, white to off-white, lyophilized powder available in two presentations:
  - 25 mg bendamustine HCl with 42.5 mg mannitol, USP; NDC 63459-390-08; *and*
  - 100 mg bendamustine HCl with 170 mg mannitol, USP; NDC 63459-391-20
- Store intact vials at temperatures up to 25°C (77°F); temperature excursions are permitted up to 30°C (86°F)
- Vials should be stored in the original packaging carton to protect bendamustine HCl from light
- Reconstitute the commercial products only with SWFI as follows:

Bendamustine HCl Content	SWFI (diluent) Volume	Resulting Bendamustine HCl Concentration
25 mg	5 mL	5 mg/mL
100 mg	20 mL	

- Shake well to yield a clear and colorless to pale yellow solution with pH of 2.5–3.5
- The lyophilized powder should completely dissolve within 5 minutes. If particulate matter is observed, the reconstituted product should not be used
- Within 30 minutes after reconstitution, transfer an amount of bendamustine HCl sufficient to prepare a patient's dose to a parenteral product container with a volume of 0.9% NS or D2.5W/0.45% NaCl sufficient to produce a clear and colorless to slightly yellow solution with a concentration within the range of 0.2–0.6 mg/mL
- Thoroughly mix the diluted product
- After reconstitution and dilution as described, the drug product is stable for 24 hours if stored under refrigeration (2°–8°C [35.6°–46.4°F]), or for 3 hours if stored at room temperature (15°–30°C [59°–86°F]) and exposed to room light
- Administration must be completed within the duration of known product stability
  - TREANDA® contains no antimicrobial preservatives. The admixture should be prepared as close as possible to the time of use

Bendamustine HCl Injection (product in solution)

- TREANDA® is packaged in single-use, individually cartoned, amber glass vials containing a clear, colorless-to-yellow solution of bendamustine HCl with a concentration of 90 mg/mL. The commercial product is available in two presentations:
  - Bendamustine HCl 45 mg/0.5 mL with propylene glycol, USP, 162 mg and 293 mg of *N,N*-dimethylacetamide, EP 293 mg; NDC 63459-395-02, *or*
  - Bendamustine HCl 180 mg/2 mL with propylene glycol, USP, 648 mg and 1172 mg of *N,N*-dimethylacetamide, EP 293 mg; NDC 63459-396-02
  - Each vial contains 0.2 mL of excess drug (overfill)
- Store intact vials under refrigeration at 2°–8°C (35.6°–46.4°F) in the original packaging carton to protect bendamustine HCl from light
- Aseptically transfer a volume of concentrated bendamustine HCl solution sufficient to prepare a patient's dose to a parenteral product container already containing a volume of 0.9% NS or D2.5W/0.45% NaCl sufficient to produce a clear colorless-to-yellow solution with a concentration within the range 0.2–0.7 mg/mL
- Thoroughly mix the diluted product
- After dilution, the admixture is stable for 24 hours if stored under refrigeration (2°–8°C), or for 2 hours if stored at room temperature (15°–30°C [59°–86°F]) and exposed to room light
- Administration must be completed within the duration of known product stability
  - TREANDA® contains no antimicrobial preservatives. The admixture should be prepared as close as possible to the time of use

Recommendations for Drug Administration and Ancillary Care

General:

- See Chapter 41 for recommended use in renal and hepatic dysfunction
- Dosages and administration rates vary between FDA-approved indications:
  - In treatment for chronic lymphocytic leukemia, administer bendamustine HCl (100 mg/m² per day for 2 consecutive days, days 1 and 2, during a 28-day cycle) by intraVENous infusion over 30 minutes
  - In treatment for non-Hodgkin lymphoma, administer bendamustine HCl (120 mg/m² per day for 2 consecutive days, days 1 and 2, during a 21-day cycle) by intraVENous infusion over 60 minutes

Potential drug interactions:

- CYP1A2 catalyzes bendamustine metabolism to its active metabolites, γ-hydroxy-bendamustine (M3) and *N*-desmethyl-bendamustine (M4)
  - CYP1A2 inhibitors (eg, fluvoxamine, ciprofloxacin) have a potential to increase bendamustine concentration and decrease concentrations of its active metabolites in plasma
  - Conversely, CYP1A2 inducers (eg, omeprazole, tobacco use) potentially may decrease plasma concentrations of bendamustine and its active metabolites
- *In vitro* studies suggest that P-glycoprotein (MDR1, ABCB1), breast cancer resistance protein (BCRP, ABCG2, MXR1), and other efflux transporters may have a role in bendamustine transport
- Based on *in vitro* data, bendamustine is not likely to inhibit metabolism via human CYP1A2, CYP2C9/10, CYP2D6, CYP2E1, or CYP3A4/5, or induce the metabolism of cytochrome P450 substrates

BEVACIZUMAB

AVASTIN® (bevacizumab) Solution for intravenous infusion; product label, December 2013. Manufactured by Genentech, Inc., A Member of the Roche Group, South San Francisco, CA

WARNING: GASTROINTESTINAL PERFORATIONS, SURGERY AND WOUND HEALING COMPLICATIONS, and HEMORRHAGE

<u>Gastrointestinal Perforations</u>
The incidence of gastrointestinal perforation, some fatal, in Avastin-treated patients ranges from 0.3 to 2.4%. Discontinue Avastin in patients with gastrointestinal perforation…

<u>Surgery and Wound Healing Complications</u>
The incidence of wound healing and surgical complications, including serious and fatal complications, is increased in Avastin-treated patients. Discontinue Avastin in patients with wound dehiscence. The appropriate interval between termination of Avastin and subsequent elective surgery required to reduce the risks of impaired wound healing/wound dehiscence has not been determined. Discontinue at least 28 days prior to elective surgery. Do not initiate Avastin for at least 28 days after surgery and until the surgical wound is fully healed…

<u>Hemorrhage</u>
Severe or fatal hemorrhage, including hemoptysis, gastrointestinal bleeding, central nervous systems (CNS) hemorrhage, epistaxis, and vaginal bleeding occurred up to five-fold more frequently in patients receiving Avastin. Do not administer Avastin to patients with serious hemorrhage or recent hemoptysis…

Boxed Warning for "AVASTIN® (bevacizumab) Solution for intravenous infusion"; December 2013 product label. Genentech, Inc., A Member of the Roche Group, South San Francisco, CA

Product Identification, Preparation, Storage, and Stability

- Avastin® is packaged in individually boxed, single-use, glass vials in 2 presentations containing either 100 mg or 400 mg bevacizumab preservative-free solution in a uniform concentration of 25 mg/mL. NDC 50242-060-01 (100 mg/4 mL). NDC 50242-061-01 (400 mg/16 mL)
- Store intact vials under refrigeration at 2°–8°C (35.6°–46.4°F) in the original carton to protect them from light
- *Do not freeze or shake* Avastin®
- The commercial product contains a clear to slightly opalescent, colorless to pale brown, sterile, solution of bevacizumab with pH = 6.2
  - The 100-mg product is formulated in 240 mg α,α-trehalose dihydrate, 23.2 mg sodium phosphate (monobasic, monohydrate), 4.8 mg sodium phosphate (dibasic, anhydrous), 1.6 mg polysorbate 20, and SWFI
  - The 400-mg product is formulated in 960 mg α,α-trehalose dihydrate, 92.8 mg sodium phosphate (monobasic, monohydrate), 19.2 mg sodium phosphate (dibasic, anhydrous), 6.4 mg polysorbate 20, and SWFI
- Withdraw from a vial an amount of bevacizumab sufficient to prepare a patient's dose and add it to a volume of 0.9% NS sufficient to produce a total volume of (Q.S.) 100 mL in a PVC or polyolefin container. Gently invert the container to mix diluted bevacizumab solution. Discard any unused bevacizumab that remains in a vial
- *Do not mix* bevacizumab with dextrose solutions
- After dilution, bevacizumab solutions may be stored at 2°–8°C for up to 8 hours
- After dilution in 0.9% NS, bevacizumab was stable for up to 24 hours under the following conditions:

Bevacizumab Concentrations (mg/mL)	Storage Temperatures	Container Composition	Results
0.9 2.25 3 6.6 7.5 16.5	30°C (86°F)	PVC, polyolefin, glass	No significant changes in protein concentration, pH, turbidity, or potency
1 12.5 25 (undiluted drug)	2°–8°C 30°C	Polyolefin	No change in protein concentration, turbidity, or potency

Genentech Medical Communications, Genentech, Inc., data on file, April 13, 2004

Selected incompatibility:

- Do not mix bevacizumab with dextrose solutions

Recommendations for Drug Administration and Ancillary Care

General:

- *Do not administer* bevacizumab by direct intraVENous injection or bolus injection
- Administer bevacizumab by intraVENous infusion after chemotherapy. The INITIAL DOSE is given over 90 minutes. If a dose given over 9 minutes was well tolerated, the administration duration may be decreased to 60 minutes during a subsequent infusion. If a 60-minute infusion was well tolerated, subsequent treatments may be administered over 30 minutes
- *Do not administer, mix, or flush* bevacizumab with dextrose solutions

BLEOMYCIN SULFATE

Bleomycin for Injection, USP; product label, July 2012. Product of Australia. Hospira, Inc. Lake Forest, IL
Bleomycin—bleomycin sulfate injection, powder, lyophilized, for solution; product label, April 2012. Manufactured by Teva Parenteral Medicines, Inc., Irvine, CA

WARNINGS

It is recommended that Bleomycin for Injection, USP, be administered under the supervision of a qualified physician experienced in the use of cancer chemotherapeutic agents. Appropriate management of therapy and complications is possible only when adequate diagnostic and treatment facilities are readily available

Pulmonary fibrosis is the most severe toxicity associated with bleomycin

The most frequent presentation is pneumonitis occasionally progressing to pulmonary fibrosis. Its occurrence is higher in elderly patients and in those receiving greater than 400 units total [cumulative] dose, but pulmonary toxicity has been observed in young patients and those treated with low doses

A severe idiosyncratic reaction consisting of hypotension, mental confusion, fever, chills, and wheezing has been reported in approximately 1% of lymphoma patients treated with bleomycin

Boxed Warning for "Bleomycin—bleomycin sulfate injection, powder, lyophilized, for solution"; April 2012 product label; Teva Parenteral Medicines, Inc., Irvine, CA

Product Identification, Preparation, Storage, and Stability

- Bleomycin is generically available as a lyophilized powder for reconstitution for injection in individually packaged vials
- Each vial contains sterile bleomycin sulfate equivalent to 15 units or 30 units of bleomycin
  - Sulfuric acid or sodium hydroxide are used, if necessary to adjust product pH
- Store intact vials under refrigeration at 2°–8°C (35.6°–46.4°F)
- One unit of bleomycin activity corresponds to 1 mg of bleomycin activity
  - Commercial products are a mixture of bleomycin glycopeptides. Measurement in activity units is a more precise indication of drug potency
- Reconstitute with 0.9% NS, SWFI, or BWFI as follows:

Bleomycin Content/ Vial	Diluent Volumes			
	0.9% NS for IntraVENous or Intrapleural Administration		0.9% NS, SWFI, or BWFI for SUBCUTaneous or IntraMUSCular Administration	
15 units	5 mL	Bleomycin concentration = 3 units/mL	1 mL	Bleomycin concentration = 15 units/mL
30 units	10 mL		2 mL	

- For *intrapleural administration* as a sclerosing agent, further dilute bleomycin 60 units in 50–100 mL of 0.9% NS
- *Do not reconstitute or dilute* bleomycin with dextrose-containing solutions
  - Bleomycins A_2 and B_2 potencies decrease after reconstitution or dilution in dextrose-containing solutions, which does not occur in 0.9% NS[13]
- After reconstitution in 0.9% NS, bleomycin is stable for 24 hours at room temperature
- Bleomycin is compatible with glass, PVC, and high-density polyethylene containers[13], and with polyethylene, PVC, and polybutadiene administration sets[14]

Recommendations for Drug Administration and Ancillary Care

General:

- See Chapter 41 for recommended use in patients with renal dysfunction
- Bleomycin is given by slow intraVENous injection over 10 minutes; by intraVENous infusion; and by the intraMUSCular, intrapleural, and SUBCUTaneous routes
- Bleomycin may be filtered during administration with filter membranes composed of cellulose ester[14,15], cellulose nitrate/cellulose acetate ester[16], or tetrafluoroethylene polymer (Teflon® [DuPont]), without a significant loss of drug potency

Idiosyncratic reactions:

- In approximately 1% of patients with lymphoma treated with bleomycin, a severe idiosyncratic reaction, similar to anaphylaxis, has been reported, consisting of: hypotension, mental confusion, fever, chills, and wheezing. Treatment is symptomatic including volume expansion, vasopressors, antihistamines, and glucocorticoids. The reaction may be immediate or delayed for several hours, and usually occurs after a first or second dose
  - Consequently, current FDA approved product labeling recommends because of the possibility of an anaphylactoid reaction, patients with lymphoma should receive not more than 2 units of bleomycin for the first 2 doses. If no acute reaction occurs, then the regular dosage schedule may be followed
    - The absence of hypersensitivity to test doses ($\leq$2 units bleomycin) does not preclude hypersensitivity phenomena during subsequent administration at full treatment dosages
- Renal insufficiency markedly alters bleomycin elimination. Bleomycin terminal elimination half-life increases exponentially as creatinine clearance decreases
  - Patients with impaired renal function should be treated with caution and their renal function should be carefully monitored during the administration of bleomycin. Bleomycin dosage reduction may be required in renally impaired patients
    - See Chapter 41 for modifying bleomycin dosage in renal impairment

For intrapleural administration:

- Administer bleomycin through a thoracostomy tube after excess pleural fluid drainage and confirming complete lung expansion. The thoracostomy tube is clamped after bleomycin instillation. The patient is moved from the supine to the left and right lateral positions several times during the next 4 hours. The clamp is then removed and thoracostomy tube suction is reestablished. The amount of time a thoracostomy tube remains in place following sclerosis is dictated by the clinical situation

BORTEZOMIB

VELCADE® (bortezomib) for Injection, for subcutaneous or intravenous use; product label, October 2012. Distributed and marketed by Millennium Pharmaceuticals, Inc., Cambridge, MA

Product Identification, Preparation, Storage, and Stability

- VELCADE® is packaged in individually packaged, single-use, 10-mL vials containing bortezomib 3.5 mg as a white to off-white, sterile, lyophilized cake or powder. NDC 63020-049-01
  - Each vial also contains 35 mg mannitol, USP
- Store unopened vials at controlled room temperature 25°C (77°F); temperature excursions are permitted from 15°–30°C (59°–86°F). Retain the product in its original packaging to protect it from light

Preparation for intraVENous injection (1 mg/mL solution)
- Reconstitute bortezomib powder with 3.5 mL of 0.9% NS to produce a clear, colorless solution with concentration = 1 mg bortezomib/mL

Preparation for SUBCUTaneous Injection (2.5 mg/mL solution)
- Reconstitute bortezomib powder with 1.4 mL of 0.9% NS to produce a clear, colorless solution with concentration = 2.5 mg bortezomib/mL

- The reconstituted product may be stored in its original vial or a syringe at 25°C (excursions are permitted from 15°–30°C), and should be administered within 8 hours after preparation
- Bortezomib solution must be used within 8 hours after reconstitution if the product is exposed to normal indoor lighting

Recommendations for Drug Administration and Ancillary Care

General:
- See Chapter 41 for recommended use in patients with renal and hepatic dysfunction

Caution:
- Exercise caution in calculating the volume of bortezomib to be administered
  - Different volumes of 0.9% NS diluent are used to reconstitute the product for the different routes of administration
  - The concentration of reconstituted bortezomib for SUBCUTaneous administration (2.5 mg/mL) is greater than the concentration of reconstituted bortezomib for intraVENous administration (1 mg/mL)
- Stickers that identify the intended route of administration are provided with

commercial VELCADE®, and should be placed on syringes containing prepared doses as a safeguard against administration via an unintended route
- The reconstituted product is suitable for direct injection

IntraVENous Administration:
- For administration by intraVENous injection over 3–5 seconds

SUBCUTaneous Administration:
- When administered SUBCUTaneously, rotate injection sites (thigh or abdomen). Administer repeated injections at least 1 inch from a previously injected site, and never where a site is tender, bruised, erythematous, or indurated

- If local injection site reactions occur after SUBCUTaneous administration of bortezomib prepared in a concentration of 2.5 mg/mL, a less-concentrated solution (1 mg/mL) may be administered SUBCUTaneously. Alternatively, consider intraVENous administration

Potential for drug interactions:
- Bortezomib is a substrate for metabolism by CYP3A4, CYP2C19, and CYP1A2
  - Concomitant administration with potent inhibitors or inducers of CYP3A subfamily enzymes has been shown to alter bortezomib's pharmacokinetic behavior
  - Avoid use of bortezomib with potent inhibitors or inducers of CYP3A subfamily enzymes

BRENTUXIMAB VEDOTIN

ADCETRIS™ (brentuximab vedotin) for Injection, For intravenous infusion; product label, September 2013. Manufactured by Seattle Genetics, Inc., Bothell, WA

WARNING: PROGRESSIVE MULTIFOCAL LEUKOENCEPHALOPATHY (PML)

JC virus infection resulting in PML and death can occur in patients receiving ADCETRIS…

Boxed Warning for "ADCETRIS™ (brentuximab vedotin) for Injection, For intravenous infusion"; September 2013 product label; Seattle Genetics, Inc., Bothell, WA

Product Identification, Preparation, Storage, and Stability

- ADCETRIS™ (brentuximab vedotin) for injection is supplied as a sterile, white to off-white, preservative-free, lyophilized cake or powder in individually boxed single-use vials containing 50 mg brentuximab vedotin. NDC 51144-050-01

  - The reconstituted product contains a solution of brentuximab vedotin 5 mg/mL with 70 mg/mL trehalose dihydrate, 5.6 mg/mL sodium citrate dihydrate, 0.21 mg/mL citric acid monohydrate, and 0.20 mg/mL polysorbate 80 and water for injection. The pH is approximately 6.6

- Store intact vials at 2°–8°C (35.6°–46.4°F) in the original carton to protect brentuximab vedotin from light

- *Caution:* Calculate a patient's dose and the number of ADCETRIS™ vials required to prepare a dose. A dose for patients weighing >100 kg should be calculated based on a weight of 100 kg

- *Reconstitution*
  1. Reconstitute brentuximab vedotin with 10.5 mL of SWFI, to produce a solution containing 5 mg brentuximab vedotin/mL
  2. Direct the stream of SWFI toward the vial wall, not directly into the drug product
  3. Gently swirl vial to aid drug dissolution. *Do not shake* a vial to aid dissolution
  4. The reconstituted solution should be clear to slightly opalescent, colorless, and free of visible particulates. Following reconstitution, dilute brentuximab vedotin immediately, or store the solution at 2°–8°C and use it within 24 hours after reconstitution. *Do not freeze* brentuximab vedotin
  5. Discard any unused portion of brentuximab vedotin left in a vial

- *Dilution*
  1. Immediately add reconstituted brentuximab vedotin (5 mg/mL) to a parenteral product container containing a minimum volume of 100 mL 0.9% NS, D5W, or LRI to achieve a final diluted concentration within the range, 0.4–1.8 mg/mL brentuximab vedotin
  2. Gently invert the product container to mix the solution
  3. Following dilution, administer brentuximab vedotin solution immediately, or store the solution at 2°–8°C and use the product within 24 hours after reconstitution. *Do not freeze* brentuximab vedotin

Recommendations for Drug Administration and Ancillary Care

General:

- The recommended initial dosage is brentuximab vedotin 1.8 mg/kg body weight administered intraVENously over 30 minutes every 3 weeks

  - Doses for patients whose body weight is >100 kg should be calculated based on a weight of 100 kg; that is, the maximum single brentuximab vedotin dose is 180 mg

  - *Do not administer* brentuximab vedotin by direct intraVENous injection or over a period <30 minutes

Cautions:

- In vitro, the binding of monomethyl auristatin E (MMAE, the microtubule disrupting portion of brentuximab vedotin)

to human plasma proteins ranged from 68–82%. MMAE is not likely to displace or to be displaced by highly protein-bound drugs

- *In vitro*, MMAE was a substrate but was not a potent inhibitor of the P-glycoprotein transport protein (P-gp, ABCB1, MDR1)

  - Avoid concomitant use of brentuximab vedotin with moderate and more potent inhibitors of the ABCB1 transport protein

- *In vitro* data indicate that MMAE is largely eliminated in urine and feces as unchanged drug; however, a small portion of MMAE is a substrate for metabolism by CYP3A4/5. *In vitro* studies using human liver microsomes indicate MMAE inhibits CYP3A4/5 but not other CYP isoforms

- Avoid concomitant use of brentuximab vedotin with potent inhibitors and inducers of CYP3A subfamily enzymes

- Concomitant use of brentuximab vedotin and bleomycin is contraindicated because of a greater incidence rate of noninfectious pulmonary toxicity with concurrent use than a historical comparison of the incidence of pulmonary toxicity reported with the ABVD (DOXOrubicin, bleomycin, vinBLAStine, dacarbazine) regimen

  - Patients typically reported cough and dyspnea. Interstitial infiltration and inflammation were observed on chest radiographs and CT. Most patients responded to steroids

(continued)

Recommendations for Drug Administration and Ancillary Care (*continued*)

Adverse events:

- Infusion-related reactions, including anaphylaxis, have occurred with brentuximab vedotin. Continually monitor patients during drug administration
  - If anaphylaxis occurs, immediately and permanently discontinue brentuximab vedotin administration and administer appropriate medical therapy
  - In the event of less-severe manageable infusion-related reactions, interrupt brentuximab vedotin administration and institute appropriate medical management
    - Patients who experience an infusion-related hypersensitivity reaction should receive prophylaxis against hypersensitivity reactions before retreatment with brentuximab vedotin
    - Medications for hypersensitivity prophylaxis may include acetaminophen, an antihistamine, and a glucocorticoid

- Peripheral neuropathy should be managed using a combination of dose delay and dosage reduction to 1.2 mg/kg
  - For new or worsening G2 or G3 neuropathy, withhold brentuximab vedotin until neuropathy improves to G1 or baseline, then restart treatment with brentuximab vedotin 1.2 mg/kg per dose
  - Discontinue brentuximab vedotin treatment for G4 peripheral neuropathy
- JC virus infection resulting in PML and death has been reported in patients treated with brentuximab vedotin
  - Other possible contributory factors include prior therapies and underlying disease that may cause immunosuppression
  - Consider a diagnosis of PML in any patient presenting with new-onset signs and symptoms of CNS abnormalities

  - Evaluation for PML includes, but is not limited to, consultation with a neurologist, brain MRI, and lumbar puncture or brain biopsy
  - Withhold brentuximab vedotin for any suspected case of PML and discontinue use if a diagnosis of PML is confirmed
- Neutropenia should be managed by dose delay and dosage reduction
  - Withhold brentuximab vedotin for neutropenia G $\geq$3 until ANC resolves to baseline or G $\leq$2 neutropenia
  - Hematopoietic growth factor support should be considered for subsequent cycles in patients who experience neutropenia G $\geq$3
  - Also consider dosage reduction to brentuximab vedotin 1.2 mg/kg in patients with recurrent G4 neutropenia despite the use of hematopoietic growth factors

BUSULFAN

BUSULFEX® (busulfan) injection; product label, May 2011. Manufactured by DSM Pharmaceuticals, Inc., Greenville, NC. Distributed and marketed by Otsuka America Pharmaceutical, Inc., Rockville, MD

WARNINGS

BUSULFEX® (busulfan) Injection is a potent cytotoxic drug that causes profound myelosuppression at the recommended dosage. It should be administered under the supervision of a qualified physician who is experienced in allogeneic hematopoietic stem cell transplantation, the use of cancer chemotherapeutic drugs and the management of patients with severe pancytopenia. Appropriate management of therapy and complications is only possible when adequate diagnostic and treatment facilities are readily available...

Boxed Warning for "BUSULFEX® (busulfan) Injection"; May 2011 product label; Otsuka America Pharmaceutical, Inc., Rockville, MD

Product Identification, Preparation, Storage, and Stability

- BUSULFEX® (busulfan) injection is supplied as a clear, colorless, sterile solution in 10-mL, single-use, clear, glass vials each containing busulfan 60 mg/10 mL (6 mg/mL) dissolved in *N,N*-dimethylacetamide (DMA) 33% (v/v) and polyethylene glycol 400, 67% (v/v). NDC 59148-070-90
- BUSULFEX® is distributed as a unit carton containing 8 vials. NDC 59148-070-91
- Store intact vials under refrigeration at 2°–8°C (35.6°–46.4°F)

Dilution for clinical use:
- The solubility of busulfan in water is 100 mg/L and the pH of BUSULFEX® diluted to approximately 0.5 mg busulfan/mL in 0.9% NS or D5W as recommended reflects the pH of the diluent used, and ranges from 3.4 to 3.9

- BUSULFEX® must be diluted for clinical use with either 0.9% NS or D5W
  - The volume of diluent should be 10-times the volume of BUSULFEX® solution, such that the final concentration of busulfan for clinical use is approximately 0.5 mg/mL
- Mix busulfan thoroughly by inverting the product container several times
- After dilution in 0.9% NS or D5W, BUSULFEX® is stable at room temperature, 25°C (77°F), for up to 8 hours, but administration must be completed within that time[17]
- After dilution in 0.9% NS, BUSULFEX® is stable under refrigeration at 2°–8°C for up to 12 hours, but administration must be completed within that time

Preparation and administration precautions:
- *Do not use* polycarbonate syringes or polycarbonate filter needles in transferring or administering busulfan solutions
- *Do not inject* BUSULFEX® solution (6 mg/mL) into a parenteral product container that does not contain 0.9% NS or D5W
  - Always add BUSULFEX® to a diluent (vehicle) solution, not the reverse

Selected incompatibility:
- *Do not mix* BUSULFEX® with another solution unless compatibility is known

Recommendations for Drug Administration and Ancillary Care

General:
- See Chapter 41 for recommended use in patients with hepatic dysfunction
- Select an administration set with minimal intraluminal priming volume (≤5 mL) to administer busulfan
- Prime the administration set tubing with diluted busulfan solution to allow accurate determination of the start of busulfan administration
  - It is important to accurately identify administration starting and completion times in order to modify busulfan dosage based on its pharmacokinetic behavior in individual patients

- A rate-controlling device (infusion pump) should be used to administer diluted busulfan by intraVENous infusion via a central VAD over 2 hours
  - More rapid administration has not been tested and is not recommended
- Before starting and after completing busulfan administration, flush the patient's VAD with approximately 5 mL of 0.9% NS or D5W. *Do not mix* BUSULFEX® with another solution unless compatibility is known
  - Flushing is particularly important if blood samples for pharmacokinetically guided busulfan dose adjustment must

be acquired from the same VAD used to administer the drug

Concomitant drug use:
- Busulfan crosses the blood–brain barrier and induces seizures. All patients should receive anticonvulsant prophylaxis with phenytoin prior to starting busulfan
  - Although phenytoin decreases busulfan AUC_{plasma} by 15%, other anticonvulsants may increase busulfan AUC_{plasma}, and increase the risk of venoocclusive disease or seizures
  - Busulfan pharmacokinetics were studied in patients treated with phenytoin, and its

(continued)

Recommendations for Drug Administration and Ancillary Care (*continued*)

clearance at the recommended dose may be less and exposure (AUC) greater in patients not treated with phenytoin
- Plasma busulfan exposure should be monitored in cases where other anticonvulsants must be used
- Acetaminophen use should be avoided within 72 hours before and concurrently with busulfan use
  - Busulfan is eliminated via conjugation with glutathione. Acetaminophen is known to decrease glutathione concentrations in blood and tissues. Concurrent use with busulfan may result in reduced busulfan clearance, potentially prolonged systemic exposure to busulfan, and enhanced adverse effects

Busulfan dosage as a component of the "BuCy" conditioning regimen before hematopoietic stem cell transplantation:
- The usual adult dosage is based on the lesser of either ideal or actual body weight, and is 0.8 mg/kg per dose, every 6 hours, for a total of 16 doses (total daily dosage = 3.2 mg/kg per day for 4 consecutive days, or a total dosage/4-day course = 12.8 mg/kg)
- Busulfan clearance is best predicted when doses are based on adjusted ideal body weight (AIBW)
  - Dose calculations based on actual body weight, ideal body weight, or other factors can produce significant differences in busulfan clearance among lean, normal, and obese patients

- Busulfan dosage in obese patients is based on adjusted ideal body weight as follows:

Ideal body weight and adjusted ideal body weight calculations (IBW and AIBW, respectively):
- IBW for men (kg) = 50 + 0.91 × ([height in cm] − 152)
- IBW for women (kg) = 45 + 0.91 × ([height in cm] − 152)
- AIBW men and women (kg) = IBW + 0.25 × ([actual body weight] − IBW)
- Where available, pharmacokinetic monitoring may be considered to optimize therapeutic targeting
  - Therapeutic target AUC_{plasma} = 1125 μmol · min

CABAZITAXEL

JEVTANA® (cabazitaxel) injection, 60 mg/1.5 mL, for intravenous infusion only; product label May 2013. sanofi-aventis U.S. LLC, Bridgewater, NJ

WARNING

Neutropenic deaths have been reported. In order to monitor the occurrence of neutropenia, frequent blood cell counts should be performed on all patients receiving JEVTANA. JEVTANA should not be given to patients with neutrophil counts of ≤1,500 cells/mm³

Severe hypersensitivity reactions can occur and may include generalized rash/erythema, hypotension and bronchospasm. Severe hypersensitivity reactions require immediate discontinuation of the JEVTANA infusion and administration of appropriate therapy… Patients should receive premedication… JEVTANA must not be given to patients who have a history of severe hypersensitivity reactions to JEVTANA or to other drugs formulated with polysorbate 80…

Boxed Warning for "JEVTANA® (cabazitaxel) Injection, 60 mg/1.5 mL, for intravenous infusion only"; May 2013 product label; sanofi-aventis U.S. LLC, Bridgewater, NJ

Product Identification, Preparation, Storage, and Stability

- JEVTANA® (cabazitaxel) injection 60 mg/1.5 mL (NDC 0024-5824-11) is supplied as a kit consisting of 2 vials in a blister pack in 1 carton, including:
  - one single-use vial contains 60 mg of cabazitaxel (anhydrous and solvent-free) in 1.5 mL of polysorbate 80 (1.56 g) as a sterile, nonpyrogenic, clear yellow to brownish-yellow, viscous solution. Each milliliter of the concentrated drug product contains cabazitaxel (anhydrous) 40 mg and 1.04 g of polysorbate 80
  - one vial contains Diluent for JEVTANA®, a clear, colorless, sterile, nonpyrogenic solution containing 13% (w/w) ethanol in water for injection, approximately 5.7 mL
- Both the JEVTANA® injection and Diluent for JEVTANA® vials contain excess drug and diluent solutions (overfill), respectively, to compensate for volume lost during preparation
- Store JEVTANA® injection and Diluent for JEVTANA® at 25°C (77°F); temperature excursions are permitted between 15°–30°C (59°–86°F)
- *Do not refrigerate* JEVTANA® Injection and Diluent for JEVTANA®
- JEVTANA® requires 2 dilutions before it may be administered to patients:
  - The concentrated drug product should be diluted only with the supplied Diluent for JEVTANA®, followed by dilution in either 0.9% NS or D5W
  - Do not use PVC infusion containers or polyurethane administration sets during preparation or administration of JEVTANA®

Initial dilution:
1. With a syringe, aseptically withdraw the entire contents of a Diluent for JEVTANA® vial and inject it into a vial containing the JEVTANA® drug product
   a. When transferring the diluent, direct the needle onto the inside wall of the drug product vial and inject slowly to limit foaming
2. Remove the syringe and needle and gently mix the initially diluted solution by repeated inversions for at least 45 seconds to assure a homogeneous mixture of the drug and diluent. *Do not shake* initially diluted JEVTANA® to avoid foaming
3. Let the solution stand for a few minutes to allow any foam to dissipate, and check that the solution is homogeneous and contains no visible particulate matter
   a. It is not required that all foam dissipate prior to continuing preparation
   b. The resulting initially diluted JEVTANA® solution (10 mg cabazitaxel/mL) requires further dilution before it may be given to patients

Caution: Secondary dilution must be completed within 30 minutes after completing initial dilution to obtain a product appropriate for administration to patients

Secondary dilution:
1. With a syringe, aseptically withdraw an amount of the initially diluted JEVTANA® solution (10 mg cabazitaxel/mL) appropriate for a patient's dose and transfer it to a volume of 0.9% NS or D5W to produce a cabazitaxel concentration within the range 0.1–0.26 mg/mL
   a. Product concentrations must not exceed 0.26 mg cabazitaxel/mL. Discard any unused portion of the initially diluted JEVTANA® solution
2. Thoroughly mix the secondarily diluted product by manual rotation and by gently inverting the container
3. After the second dilution in either 0.9% NS or D5W, JEVTANA® should be used within 8 hours if maintained at ambient temperatures (including the 1-hour administration time), or may be used within 24 hours after preparation (including the 1-hour administration time) if stored under refrigeration at 2°–8°C (35.6°–46.4°F)

Cautions: JEVTANA® should not be mixed with any other drugs

Chemical and physical stability of cabazitaxel solution has been demonstrated for 24 hours under refrigerated conditions; however, both the initially diluted and secondarily diluted solutions are supersaturated. Consequently, if crystals or particulates appear in either solution, the solutions must not be used and should be discarded

Recommendations for Drug Administration and Ancillary Care

General:

- See Chapter 41 for recommended use in patients with renal and hepatic dysfunction
- Cabazitaxel is administered intraVENously over 60 minutes in combination with predniSONE 10 mg/day administered orally, continually throughout treatment with cabazitaxel

Primary prophylaxis against hypersensitivity reactions:

- At least 30 minutes before each dose of cabazitaxel give the following medications intraVENously to decrease the risk or severity of hypersensitivity:
  - A histamine H_1-subtype receptor antagonist, for example, dexchlorpheniramine 5 mg, diphenhydramine 25 mg, or equivalent antihistamine, *plus*
  - A glucocorticoid, for example, dexamethasone 8 mg, or another steroid at a glucocorticoid-equivalent dose, *plus*
  - A histamine H_2-subtype receptor antagonist, for example, ranitidine 50 mg or equivalent

- After secondary dilution, JEVTANA® solution (concentration 0.1–0.26 mg cabazitaxel/mL) should be administered intraVENously over 60 minutes at room temperature through an in-line filter with nominal pore size of 0.22 μm
- Although it is recommended the secondarily diluted solution should be used immediately, storage time can be longer under specific conditions:
  - Up to 8 hours after preparation if maintained at ambient temperatures (including the 1-hour administration time), *or*
  - Up to 24 hours after preparation (including the 1-hour administration time) if stored under refrigeration at 2°–8°C

Caution with medications given concomitantly:

- Cabazitaxel is a substrate for metabolism catalyzed by CYP3A subfamily enzymes
  - *Avoid concomitant use* of moderate and more potent CYP3A subfamily enzyme inhibitors, which may increase systemic exposure to cabazitaxel (eg, atazanavir, clarithromycin, indinavir, itraconazole, ketoconazole, nefazodone, nelfinavir, ritonavir, saquinavir, telithromycin, voriconazole)
  - *Avoid concomitant use* of strong CYP3A subfamily enzyme inducers (eg, carbamazepine, phenobarbital, phenytoin, rifabutin, rifampin, rifapentine, St. John's wort), which may be expected to decrease cabazitaxel concentrations
- Cabazitaxel is a substrate of P-glycoprotein (P-gp, MDR1, ABCB1) in vitro, but is not a substrate of MRP1, MRP2, or the breast cancer resistance protein (BCRP, ABCG2, MXR1)
  - In vitro, cabazitaxel inhibited the transport of P-gp and BRCP, at concentrations at least 38-fold greater than what is observed clinically
- A risk of cabazitaxel perturbing the pharmacokinetic behavior of concurrently used medications by inhibiting P-gp or BCRP is unlikely at clinically used dosages

CARBOPLATIN

Carboplatin injection; product label, August 2007. Hospira, Inc., Lake Forest, IL
CARBOPLATIN–carboplatin injection, solution (50-, 150-, and 450-mg multidose vials); product label, October 2011. Manufactured by Pharmachemie B.V., Haarlem, The Netherlands. Manufactured for Teva Pharmaceuticals USA, Sellersville, PA, *and*
CARBOPLATIN INJECTION; product label, January 2008. APP Pharmaceuticals LLC, Schaumburg, IL

WARNINGS

Carboplatin injection should be administered under the supervision of a qualified physician experienced in the use of cancer chemotherapeutic agents. Appropriate management of therapy and complications is possible only when adequate treatment facilities are readily available

Bone marrow suppression is dose related and may be severe, resulting in infection and/or bleeding. Anemia may be cumulative and may require transfusion support. Vomiting is another frequent drug-related side effect

Anaphylactic-like reactions to carboplatin have been reported and may occur within minutes of carboplatin injection administration. Epinephrine, corticosteroids, and antihistamines have been employed to alleviate symptoms

---

Boxed Warnings for "Carboplatin Injection"; August 2007 product label; Hospira, Inc., Lake Forest, IL

Product Identification, Preparation, Storage, and Stability

- CARBOplatin is marketed as branded and generic products from several manufacturers in multidose (*or* multiuse) vials containing 50 mg, 150 mg, 450 mg, or 600 mg CARBOplatin per vial
- CARBOplatin injection is a sterile aqueous solution of CARBOplatin at a concentration of 10 mg/mL (1%); the pH of a 1% solution of CARBOplatin is 5–7
- Store unopened vials under temperature conditions indicated for individual products, generally within a range between 20°C and 25°C (68°F and 77°F). Available products often indicate temperature excursions to 15°–30°C (59°–86°F) are permitted. Protect unopened vials from light
- CARBOplatin injection in multidose vials maintain microbial, chemical, and physical stability for up to 14 days (Teva Pharmaceuticals USA product) or 15 days (Hospira, Inc. product) at 25°C following multiple needle entries

- CARBOplatin injection may be further diluted to concentrations as low as 0.5 mg/mL with either D5W or 0.9% NS. After dilution, CARBOplatin may be stored at room temperature (25°C [77°F]) for up to 8 hours before use

Selected incompatibility:

- Avoid admixture with solutions with pH >6.5 (eg, solutions containing fluorouracil or sodium bicarbonate)
- Avoid admixture with mesna
- Aluminum reacts with CARBOplatin, causing precipitation and loss of drug potency. *Do not prepare or administer* CARBOplatin with needles or administration sets that contain aluminum parts that may come into contact with the drug

Recommendations for Drug Administration and Ancillary Care

General:

- See Chapter 41 for recommended use in patients with renal dysfunction
- Administer CARBOplatin intraVENously over at least 15 minutes. Pre- or post-treatment hydration and forced diuresis are not required
- Prescriptions and medication orders should identify the drug by its complete generic name, "CARBOplatin", to prevent confusion with other platinum compounds

CARFILZOMIB

KYPROLIS™ (carfilzomib) for Injection, for intravenous use; product label, July 2012. Manufactured by Onyx Pharmaceuticals, Inc., South San Francisco, CA

Product Identification, Preparation, Storage, and Stability

- KYPROLIS™ (carfilzomib) for injection is supplied in individually cartoned single-use vials containing carfilzomib 60 mg as a sterile, white to off-white, lyophilized cake or powder with sulfobutylether beta-cyclodextrin 3000 mg, citric acid 57.7 mg, and sodium hydroxide sufficient to adjust the product pH to 3.5. NDC 76075-101-01
- Store unopened vials under refrigeration between 2°C and 8°C (35.6°F and 46.4°F) in the original packaging to protect carfilzomib from light
- Preparation:
  1. Remove a vial from refrigeration just prior to use
  2. Slowly inject 29 mL of SWFI by directing the solution onto the inside vial wall, not into the drug product to minimize foaming
  3. Gently swirl or slowly and repeatedly invert the vial for approximately 1 minute, or until the drug cake or powder has completely dissolved. DO NOT SHAKE carfilzomib to avoid generating foam
  4. If foaming occurs, set the vial aside for approximately 2–5 minutes, to allow the foam to dissipate
  5. After reconstitution, the resulting solution should be clear and colorless and contains carfilzomib at a concentration of 2 mg/mL
- Carfilzomib stability

Storage Conditions After Reconstitution (Carfilzomib 2 mg/mL)	Stability as a Function of Product Container*		
	Vial	Syringe	Diluted with D5W and Stored in a Plastic Container (Bag)
Refrigeration (2°–8°C)			24 hours
Room temperature (15°–30°C [59°–86°F])			4 hours

*Total time from reconstitution to administration should not exceed 24 hours

  6. Dilute carfilzomib in a parenteral product container with 50 mL of D5W
  7. Discard vials containing unused drug solution

Recommendations for Drug Administration and Ancillary Care

Supportive Care:

Hydration

- Prior to administering carfilzomib, evaluate a patient's fluid status to ensure they are well hydrated
- Patients should receive hydration with carfilzomib to reduce the risk of developing renal toxicity and tumor lysis syndrome (TLS)
  - Overall, TLS occurred in <1% of patients, but patients with multiple myeloma and a high tumor burden should be considered at greater risk for TLS
  - Monitor for evidence of TLS during treatment, and manage promptly
  - Interrupt carfilzomib treatments until TLS is resolved
- Maintain patients' fluid volume status and monitor blood chemistries closely throughout treatment with carfilzomib
  - During cycle 1:
    - Give 250–500 mL 0.9% NS or another fluid intraVENously as clinically appropriate before each carfilzomib dose
    - Give an additional 250–500 mL of fluids intraVENously as needed after completing each carfilzomib dose
  - During repeated treatment cycles, continue intraVENous hydration as needed
- Monitor patients for fluid overload

Prophylaxis against hypersensitivity/infusion-related reactions

- Hypersensitivity reactions may occur immediately after or during the first 24 hours after carfilzomib administration
- Infusion-related reactions may be characterized by any of the following: fever, chills, arthralgia, myalgia, facial flushing, facial edema, vomiting, weakness, shortness of breath, hypotension, syncope, chest tightness, angina
- To mitigate the incidence and severity of infusion reactions, administer **dexamethasone** 4 mg orally or intraVENously prior to each carfilzomib dose during cycle 1 and prior to each carfilzomib dose during the cycle in which carfilzomib dosage is escalated to 27 mg/m^2
- Continue or resume prophylaxis with **dexamethasone** 4 mg orally or intraVENously if symptoms develop or reappear during subsequent cycles

General:

- Carfilzomib is administered only by intraVENous infusion over 2–10 minutes, on 2 consecutive days, weekly, for three consecutive weeks every 28 days, that is administration on days 1, 2, 8, 9, 15, and 16, during a 28-day treatment cycle
- Flush with 0.9% NS or D5W the administration set tubing and VAD through which carfilzomib is given immediately before beginning and after completing carfilzomib administration
- Do not mix carfilzomib with other medicinal products or administer it through the same intraVENous VAD with other medicinal products

Carfilzomib dose calculation:

- Carfilzomib dose is calculated using a patient's actual BSA calculated at baseline. Patients with a BSA >2.2 m^2 should receive a dose based upon a BSA of exactly 2.2 m^2
- There is no need to make dose adjustments for changes in body weight ≤20%

Carfilzomib dosage escalation:

- During cycle 1, carfilzomib is administered at a dosage of 20 mg/m^2 each day of treatment
- If carfilzomib is well tolerated at 20 mg/m^2 per dose, the dosage during cycle 2 may be escalated to 27 mg/m^2 for each day of treatment, and continued at 27 mg/m^2 per dose during subsequent cycles

CARMUSTINE

BiCNU® (carmustine for injection); product label, May 2011. BiCNU® manufactured by Ben Venue Laboratories, Inc., Bedford, OH, *or* Emcure Pharmaceuticals Ltd., Hinjwadi, Pune 411057, INDIA. Diluent manufactured by Luitpold Pharmaceuticals, Inc., Shirley, NY. Distributed by Bristol-Myers Squibb Company, Princeton, NJ

WARNINGS

BiCNU® (carmustine for injection) should be administered under the supervision of a qualified physician experienced in the use of cancer chemotherapeutic agents

Bone marrow suppression, notably thrombocytopenia and leukopenia, which may contribute to bleeding and overwhelming infections in an already compromised patient, is the most common and severe of the toxic effects of BiCNU...

Since the major toxicity is delayed bone marrow suppression, blood counts should be monitored weekly for at least 6 weeks after a dose... At the recommended dosage, courses of BiCNU should not be given more frequently than every 6 weeks

The bone marrow toxicity of BiCNU is cumulative and therefore dosage adjustment must be considered on the basis of nadir blood counts from prior dose...

Pulmonary toxicity from BiCNU appears to be dose related. Patients receiving greater than 1400 mg/m² cumulative dose are at significantly higher risk than those receiving less

Delayed pulmonary toxicity can occur years after treatment, and can result in death, particularly in patients treated in childhood...

Boxed Warning for "BiCNU® (carmustine for injection)"; May 2011 product label; Bristol-Myers Squibb Company, Princeton, NJ

Product Identification, Preparation, Storage, and Stability[18]

- BiCNU®, NDC 0015-3012-60, packaging includes 2 containers, including:
  - One vial containing 100 mg of carmustine as sterile, lyophilized, pale-yellow flakes or a congealed mass
  - An ampule containing 3 mL of sterile dehydrated alcohol injection, USP, which is used to initially dissolve carmustine before attempting further dilution with aqueous media
- Dehydrated alcohol injection, USP, may be stored at room temperature 15°–30°C (59°–86°F) or under refrigeration at 2°–8°C (35.6°–46.4°F)
- Intact vials containing the drug product, carmustine, are stable for at least 3 years if stored under refrigeration at 2°–8°C, but for only 7 days if stored at room temperature (up to 25°C [≤77°F]). The lyophilized formulation does not contain a preservative and is intended for a single use
  - *Caution:* BiCNU® has a low melting point (30.5°–32°C [86.9°–89.6°F])
    - Exposure of the drug to this or greater temperatures will cause the drug to liquefy, becoming an oily film on the interior surface of a vial; a sign of decomposition indicating affected vials should be discarded
    - If upon receipt appropriate storage during transportation is in question, immediately examine the vial containing carmustine in each individual carton by holding it to a bright light for inspection
    - If carmustine appears as a very small amount of dry flakes or a dry congealed mass, the product is suitable for use and should be refrigerated immediately

Preparation
1. Dissolve carmustine with 3 mL of the supplied diluent (dehydrated alcohol injection, USP)
2. *Only after* the drug product has been completely dissolved, aseptically add 27 mL of SWFI
   a. The resulting solution is clear, colorless to yellowish, and contains 3.3 mg carmustine/mL in 10% ethanol
      - After reconstitution as recommended, carmustine is stable for 8 hours at room temperature (25°C) if it is protected from light exposure, and for at least 24 hours if stored under refrigeration and protected from light
        - Reconstituted vials should be examined for crystal formation prior to use
        - If crystals are observed, they may be re-dissolved by warming the vial to room temperature with agitation

Administration
- For administration to patients, carmustine should be further diluted to a concentration of 0.2 mg/mL with D5W and *stored only* in glass or polyolefin parenteral product containers[19]
- Carmustine adsorption to PVC, ethylene vinyl acetate (EVA), and polyurethane containers results in substantial drug loss as a result of drug adsorption to the container material

Stability as a Function of Carmustine Concentration and Storage Temperature[20, 21]

Diluent Solution	Carmustine Concentration	Storage Temperature	Duration of Stability
D5W	0.5–1 mg/mL	25°C (77°F)	4 hours
	0.1–1 mg/mL	4°C (39.2°F)	24 hours

- Initial solubilization with ethanol produces a carmustine solution that can be very irritating to vascular endothelium during intraVENous administration. Consequently, several investigators have evaluated alternative preparation schemes to decrease or eliminate ethanol from carmustine for intraVENous administration. Although these methods are not advocated by the product manufacturer, and may present some logistical challenges with respect to material resources, 2 methods for producing an ethanol-free solution for intraVENous administration are described below

Alternative Preparation Schemes

Method 1[22]:

- To a vial containing 100 mg carmustine, add 30 mL of preservative-free D5W
- Heat the vial to 60°C (140°F) in a water bath for 5 minutes, and, during heating, vigorously shake the vial 3 times
- The preparation scheme produces a solution with a carmustine concentration of 3.3 mg/mL and a stability half-life of 46 hours
  - The investigators demonstrated an 8% loss in concentration after product filtration
  - Although carmustine must be diluted before it is administered to patients, the investigators did not describe secondary dilution

Method 2[23]:

- To a vial containing 100 mg carmustine, add 25 mL of preservative-free D5W warmed to 37°C (98.6°F)
- Shake the vial by hand or in a water bath warmed to 37°C for approximately 5 minutes
- The preparation scheme produces a solution with a carmustine concentration of ~4 mg/mL and a mean stability half-life of 6.8 hours
  - When prepared with ethanol according to the manufacturer's instruction, carmustine must be diluted before it is administered to patients. Tepe et al. did not describe secondary dilution

Selected incompatibility:

- Avoid admixture with solutions of pH >6 (eg, solutions containing sodium bicarbonate)[24]
- Photodegradation occurs after exposure to strong light sources (>500 Lux; >46 foot-candles)

Recommendations for Drug Administration and Ancillary Care[25]

General:

- See Chapter 41 for recommended use in patients with renal and hepatic dysfunction
- Administer by intraVENous infusion over at least 1–2 hours
  - Carmustine is irritating to vascular endothelium largely because of the ethanol used to initially dissolve the drug. Administration over <1 hour may produce sensations of intense pain and burning at the site of administration
- *Use only* polyethylene or polyethylene-lined administration sets
  - A substantial amount of carmustine may be lost from solution as a result of adsorption to the surfaces of ethylene vinyl acetate, PVC, and polyurethane product containers and administration sets
- *Do not* mix carmustine with solutions containing sodium bicarbonate
- Carmustine should not be given more frequently than every 6 weeks

CETUXIMAB

ERBITUX® (cetuximab) injection, for intravenous infusion; product label, August 2013. Manufactured by ImClone LLC, a wholly owned subsidiary of Eli Lilly and Company, Branchburg, NJ. Distributed and marketed by Bristol-Myers Squibb Company, Princeton, NJ. Comarketed by Eli Lilly and Company, Indianapolis, IN

WARNING: SERIOUS INFUSION REACTIONS and CARDIOPULMONARY ARREST

Infusion Reactions: Serious infusion reactions occurred with the administration of Erbitux in approximately 3% of patients in clinical trials, with fatal outcome reported in less than 1 in 1000… Immediately interrupt and permanently discontinue Erbitux infusion for serious infusion reactions…

Cardiopulmonary Arrest: Cardiopulmonary arrest and/or sudden death occurred in 2% of patients with squamous cell carcinoma of the head and neck treated with Erbitux and radiation therapy in Study 1 and in 3% of patients with squamous cell carcinoma of the head and neck treated with European Union (EU)-approved cetuximab in combination with platinum-based therapy with 5-fluorouracil (5-FU) in Study 2. Closely monitor serum electrolytes, including serum magnesium, potassium, and calcium, during and after Erbitux administration…

Boxed Warning for "ERBITUX® (cetuximab) injection, for intravenous infusion"; August 2013 product label; Co-marketed by Bristol-Myers Squibb Company, Princeton, NJ, and Eli Lilly and Company, Indianapolis, IN

Product Identification, Preparation, Storage, and Stability

- ERBITUX® is supplied in individually packaged, single-use vials containing cetuximab 100 mg/50 mL (NDC 66733-948-23) or 200 mg/100 mL (NDC 66733-958-23) as a sterile, preservative-free, clear and colorless, injectable liquid with pH = 7.0–7.4
  - The commercial product contains cetuximab 2 mg/mL with 8.48 mg/mL sodium chloride, 1.88 mg/mL sodium phosphate dibasic heptahydrate, 0.41 mg/mL sodium phosphate monobasic monohydrate, and SWFI

- Store vials under refrigeration at 2°–8°C (35.6°–46.4°F). *Do not freeze* the product
- The product may contain a small amount of easily visible, white, amorphous cetuximab particulates
  - Increased particulate formation may occur at temperatures ≤0°C (≤32°F)
- Cetuximab stored in parenteral product containers is chemically and physically stable for up to 12 hours at 2°–8°C and for up to 8 hours at controlled room temperature (20°–25°C; 68°–77°F)

- Discard any unused cetuximab within 8 hours or within 12 hours after preparation for products maintained at controlled room temperature or under refrigeration (2°– 8°C), respectively
  - Discard any unused portions of cetuximab remaining in a vial
- *Do not shake or dilute* cetuximab solution

Recommendations for Drug Administration and Ancillary Care

General:

- Administer cetuximab by intraVENous infusion with an infusion pump or syringe pump
- *Do not administer* cetuximab by direct intraVENous injection or bolus injection

Premedication:

- Give primary prophylaxis against infusion-related reactions with an antihistamine (H$_1$-receptor) antagonist (eg, diphenhydrAMINE 50 mg IV, *or* equivalent H$_1$ antagonist) 30–60 minutes before a first dose of cetuximab
  - Infusion reactions have occurred in 15–21% of patients across studies, and included: pyrexia, chills, rigors, dyspnea, bronchospasm, angioedema, urticaria, hypertension, and hypotension
    - Grades 3 and 4 infusion reactions occurred in 2–5% of patients, and were fatal in 1 patient

- Premedication for subsequent cetuximab doses should be based upon clinical judgment and the presence and severity of infusion reactions during prior doses

Administration:

- Administer cetuximab through a low protein binding, 0.22-μm, inline filter (placed as proximal to the patient as practical)
- Administer cetuximab 400 mg/m^2 doses over 2 hours (120 min); administer 250 mg/m^2 doses over 1 hour (60 min)
  - The MAXIMUM INFUSION RATE should be ≤5 mL/min (≤10 mg/min), which is ≤300 mL/hour (≤600 mg/hour)
  - Use 0.9% NS to flush the line at the end of infusion

Patient monitoring:

- A 1-hour observation period is recommended after completing cetuximab administration in a setting with resuscitation equipment and other agents necessary to treat anaphylaxis (eg, epinephrine, bronchodilators, oxygen, and parenteral steroids and antihistamines)
  - Continue monitoring to confirm resolution of an acute event in patients who required treatment for infusion reactions
  - Longer observation periods may be required in patients who experience infusion reactions
- Patients should be periodically monitored for hypomagnesemia, hypocalcemia, and hypokalemia, during and following cetuximab administration. The same electrolyte analyses should be continually monitored for approximately 8 weeks after

(continued)

Recommendations for Drug Administration and Ancillary Care (*continued*)

the last dose administered, that is, a period of time commensurate with the half-life and persistence of cetuximab

• The onset of electrolyte abnormalities has been reported to occur from days to months after cetuximab administration. Electrolyte supplementation may be necessary in some patients and, in severe cases, intraVENous replacement may be required. The time to resolution of electrolyte abnormalities is not known

Patient counseling:

Advise patients:

• To report signs and symptoms of infusion reactions such as fever, chills, or breathing problems

• Of the potential risks of using cetuximab during pregnancy or breast-feeding and of the need to use adequate contraception in both males and females during treatment, and for 6 months following the last dose of cetuximab

• That breast-feeding is not recommended during, and for 2 months following the last dose of cetuximab therapy

• To limit sun exposure (use sunscreen, wear hats) while receiving cetuximab and for 2 months following the last dose of cetuximab

CISPLATIN

CISPLATIN INJECTION; product label, January 2008. APP Pharmaceuticals, LLC, Schaumburg, IL
PLATINOL–cisplatin injection, powder, lyophilized, for solution; product label, October 2010. Made in Italy. Manufactured for Bristol-Myers Squibb Company Princeton, NJ
CISPLATIN–cisplatin injection, solution; product label, February 2012 Teva Parenteral Medicines, Inc. Manufactured in The Netherlands by Pharmachemie B.V., Haarlem, The Netherlands. Manufactured for Teva Pharmaceuticals USA, Sellersville, PA

WARNINGS

[CISplatin] …should be administered under the supervision of a qualified physician experienced in the use of cancer chemotherapeutic agents. Appropriate management of therapy and complications is possible only when adequate diagnostic and treatment facilities are readily available

Cumulative renal toxicity associated with cisplatin is severe. Other major dose-related toxicities are myelosuppression, nausea, and vomiting

Ototoxicity, which may be more pronounced in children, and is manifested by tinnitus, and/or loss of high frequency hearing and occasionally deafness, is significant

Anaphylactic-like reactions to [CISplatin] …have been reported. Facial edema, bronchoconstriction, tachycardia, and hypotension may occur within minutes of [CISplatin] …administration. Epinephrine, corticosteroids, and antihistamines have been effectively employed to alleviate symptoms…

Exercise caution to prevent inadvertent [CISplatin] …overdose. Doses greater than 100 mg/m²/cycle once every 3 to 4 weeks are rarely used. Care must be taken to avoid inadvertent [CISplatin] …overdose due to confusion with… carboplatin …or prescribing practices that fail to differentiate daily doses from total dose per cycle

---

Boxed Warnings for "CISPLATIN INJECTION"; January 2008 product label; APP Pharmaceuticals, LLC, Schaumburg, IL; "PLATINOL—cisplatin injection, powder, lyophilized, for solution"; October 2010 product label; Bristol-Myers Squibb Company Princeton, NJ; and "CISPLATIN—cisplatin injection, solution"; February 2012 product label; Teva Pharmaceuticals USA, Sellersville, PA
• Prescriptions and medication orders should identify the drug by its complete generic name, "CISPLATIN", to prevent confusion with other platinum compounds
• Product labeling advises pharmacists to contact health care providers who prescribe CISplatin dosages >100 mg/m² per cycle for dose confirmation

---

Product Identification, Preparation, Storage, and Stability

• CISplatin is generically available from several manufacturers in multiuse vials in at least 2 presentations, including:
  ▪ A sterile, clear, light yellow, aqueous solution for injection (CISplatin injection)
    ○ Commercially available products contain 50 mg, 100 mg, or 200 mg CISplatin in individually packaged, multiple-dose, amber vials
      □ Each milliliter contains CISplatin 1 mg and sodium chloride 9 mg
      □ Additional excipients may be present in some product formulations
    ○ CISplatin Injection (1 mg/mL) must be diluted before it is administered to patients
  ▪ A white to light yellow lyophilized powder for reconstitution (CISplatin for injection)
    ○ Commercially available products contain 50 mg CISplatin in individually packaged, multiple-dose, amber vials
    ○ Reconstitute lyophilized CISplatin with 50 mL of SWFI to obtain a solution containing 1 mg CISplatin and sodium chloride 9 mg/mL
      □ Additional excipients may be present in some formulations

○ Reconstituted CISplatin (1 mg/mL) must be diluted before it is administered to patients
• Consult product labeling for manufacturer recommendations about acceptable storage temperatures for intact vials
  ▪ Acceptable storage temperatures for products in solution (CISplatin injection) vary within a range from 15°C (59°F) or 20°C (68°) for a lower temperature limit to an upper limit of 25°C (77°F)
  ▪ At least 1 commercial product formulated as a lyophilized powder for reconstitution (CISplatin for injection) specifies storage at controlled room temperature (25°C [77°F])
• *Do not store* CISplatin in solution (1 mg/mL) under refrigeration, under which condition it is more likely to precipitate
• Protect unopened containers from light
• Dilute CISplatin in a convenient volume of fluid. The diluting fluid MUST CONTAIN a chloride concentration ≥0.225% sodium chloride (≥38.5 mEq/L), for example, 0.45% NaCl, 0.9% NS, 3% NaCl, and

saline and dextrose solutions with chloride concentrations >0.225%[26]
• Mannitol is compatible and may be added to diluted CISplatin solutions
• Protect CISplatin solutions that are not used within 6 hours after preparation from exposure to light
• CISplatin that remains in an amber vial after initial entry is stable for 28 days if protected from light or for 7 days under fluorescent room lighting

Selected incompatibility:

• *Aluminum* reacts with CISplatin causing precipitation and loss of drug potency
  ▪ *Do not prepare or administer* CISplatin with needles or administration sets that contain aluminum parts that may come into contact with the drug
• *Do not dilute* CISplatin in solutions with chloride content less than the concentration found in 0.225% NaCl, that is, *not less than* 38.5 mEq/L
• CISplatin is incompatible in admixtures with mesna

Recommendations for Drug Administration and Ancillary Care

General:

- See Chapter 41 for recommended use in patients with renal dysfunction
- Hydration with 1000–2000 mL of fluid administered intraVENously is recommended starting at least 2 hours before CISplatin administration commences

- Consider continuing hydration during and after CISplatin administration is completed, particularly in patients who receive a diuretic before, during, or after CISplatin to augment urine formation
- Maintain increased hydration via oral, parenteral, or both routes, and urine

output for at least 24 hours after CISplatin administration
- Administer CISplatin intraVENously. Infusion duration generally is within a range of 15–120 minutes, but may be prolonged in some regimens (8–24 hours)

CLADRIBINE

CLADRIBINE INJECTION for intravenous infusion only; product label, January 2008. APP Pharmaceuticals, LLP, Schaumburg, IL
LEUSTATIN® (cladribine) injection, PRODUCT INFORMATION; product label, August 2, 2012. Janssen-Cilag Pty Ltd., Macquarie Park NSW, Australia
CLADRIBINE injection, Rx only, for intravenous infusion only; product label, August 2006. Manufactured by Ben Venue Laboratories, Inc., Bedford, OH. Manufactured for Bedford Laboratories, Bedford, OH

WARNINGS

Cladribine Injection should be administered under the supervision of a qualified physician experienced in the use of antineoplastic therapy. Suppression of bone marrow function should be anticipated. This is usually reversible and appears to be dose dependent. Serious neurological toxicity (including irreversible paraparesis and quadraparesis) has been reported in patients who received cladribine injection by continuous infusion at high doses (four to nine times the recommended dose for Hairy Cell Leukemia). Neurologic toxicity appears to demonstrate a dose relationship; however, severe neurological toxicity has been reported rarely following treatment with standard cladribine dosing regimens

Acute nephrotoxicity has been observed with high doses of cladribine (four to nine times the recommended dose for Hairy Cell Leukemia), especially when given concomitantly with other nephrotoxic agents/therapies

Boxed Warning for "CLADRIBINE INJECTION For Intravenous Infusion Only"; January 2008 product label; APP Pharmaceuticals, LLP, Schaumburg, IL

Product Identification, Preparation, Storage, and Stability

- Cladribine injection is generically available packaged in single-use, clear flint glass, 20-mL (capacity) vials containing cladribine 10 mg/10 mL (1 mg/mL) as a sterile, clear, colorless, preservative-free, isotonic solution
  - Each milliliter of commercially available products also contains 1 mg cladribine and 9 mg (0.15 mEq) of sodium chloride
  - The solution has a pH in the range of 5.5–8.0. Phosphoric acid and/or dibasic sodium phosphate may have been added to adjust the pH to 6.3 ± 0.3
- Presentations vary among manufacturers with respect to product packaging: vials may be packaged individually or in cases containing multiple vials
- Store intact vials under refrigeration 2°–8°C (35.6°–46.4°F) and protected from light during storage
- Cladribine *must be diluted* before administration

24-Hour drug supply (daily bag exchanges):
- Dilute in 500 mL of 0.9% NS an amount of cladribine needed to provide treatment for a single day
  - Compared with dilution in 0.9% NS, dilution in D5W increases the rate of cladribine degradation and is not recommended
  - Cladribine admixtures in 0.9% NS in PVC containers (eg, Viaflex Container, Baxter Healthcare Corporation, Deerfield, IL) are chemically and physically stable for at least 24 hours at room temperature under normal fluorescent lighting

(continued)

Recommendations for Drug Administration and Ancillary Care

General:
- See Chapter 41 for recommended use in patients with renal and hepatic dysfunction
- Administer only by intraVENous infusion over 2–24 hours
- Cladribine should be administered promptly, or, after dilution, stored under refrigeration (2°–8°C [35.6°–46.4°F]) for not more than 8 hours before starting administration
- Cladribine should not be mixed with other drugs or additives or administered simultaneously with other drugs via a common intraVENous line

Product Identification, Preparation, Storage, and Stability (*continued*)

7-Day drug supply:

- A 7-day infusion solution should only be prepared with B0.9% NS (preserved with 0.9% benzyl alcohol) as follows:

  1. Add to a plastic container an amount of cladribine needed for a 7-day supply of medication

  2. Add to the same plastic container a calculated amount of B0.9% NS sufficient to produce a total volume of (Q.S.) 100 mL

     a. Both cladribine and the diluent solution should be transferred into a parenteral product container through a sterile, disposable, hydrophilic syringe filter with pore size ≤0.22 μm to minimize the risk of microbial contamination

     b. Inject cladribine through the filter first followed by the B0.9% NS vehicle solution to flush into the product container any cladribine remaining in the filter

        ■ Solutions prepared with B0.9% NS for individuals weighing >85 kg may have reduced preservative effectiveness because of displacement of the benzyl alcohol-containing diluent by the volume of drug, that is, >53.6 mg in a total volume to deliver of 100 mL

        ■ Admixtures prepared with antimicrobially preserved diluent have demonstrated acceptable chemical and physical stability for at least 7 days in a SIMS Deltec, Inc., Medication Cassette Reservoir

  3. Aseptically connect to the drug product container (reservoir) any tubing that will be used to connect the reservoir to a patient's VAD during drug administration

  4. Aseptically remove air from the product container and any connected tubing

  5. Aseptically cap with a sterile Luer locking cap, closure, or seal any tubing attached to the drug reservoir for storage if the product is not immediately connected to a patient's VAD after preparation is completed

- Cladribine may precipitate when exposed to low temperatures, but can be resolubilized by warming at ambient room temperature and vigorous shaking

- *Do not* attempt to resolubilize cladribine by heating or microwaving

- Freezing does not adversely affect the solution. If freezing occurs, thaw at room temperature, but *do not* thaw cladribine by radiant thermal or microwave heating

- After thawing, vials are stable until the expiration date on the product label if stored under refrigeration

- *Do not* refreeze cladribine

- Any unused portion of cladribine remaining in a single-use vial should be discarded

CLOFARABINE

Clolar® (clofarabine) injection for intravenous use; product label, April 2013. Manufactured by Teva Pharmachemie, Haarlem, The Netherlands. Manufactured for Genzyme Corporation, Cambridge, MA. Distributed by Genzyme Corporation, Cambridge, MA

Product Identification, Preparation, Storage, and Stability

- Clolar® is packaged in 20-mL-capacity, flint glass, single-use vials containing 20 mL of a clear, practically colorless, preservative-free solution of clofarabine 1 mg/mL (20 mg/20 mL) (NDC 0024-5860-01)
  - The commercial product is formulated in 20 mL of unbuffered 0.9% NS. The pH range of the solution is 4.5–7.5

- Store intact vials at 25°C (77°F). Temperature excursions are permitted to 15°–30°C (59°–86°F)
- Clofarabine solution must be filtered before dilution. Use a sterile filter with a pore size equal to 0.2 μm either when aspirating the drug into a syringe *or* when expelling drug from the syringe into a diluent solution

- Dilute clofarabine with a volume of 0.9% NS or D5W sufficient to produce a concentration between 0.15 and 0.4 mg/mL before administering it to patients
- Diluted solutions may be stored at 15°–30°C, but must be used within 24 hours after preparation

Recommendations for Drug Administration and Ancillary Care

General:

- See Chapter 41 for comments about use in patients with renal and hepatic dysfunction
- Administer diluted clofarabine solutions by intraVENous infusion over 2 hours
- Provide supportive care, such as intraVENous fluids, allopurinol, and alkalinize urine throughout a 5-day treatment course to reduce the effects of tumor lysis and other adverse events
- Monitor patients taking medications known to affect blood pressure. Monitor cardiac function during clofarabine administration
  - Avoid medications that produce or exacerbate hypotension during the days on which clofarabine is administered
- Evaluate and monitor patients receiving clofarabine treatment for signs and symptoms of cytokine release (eg, tachypnea, tachycardia, hypotension, pulmonary edema) that could develop into systemic inflammatory response syndrome

(SIRS), capillary leak syndrome, and organ dysfunction
- Immediately discontinue clofarabine in the event of clinically significant signs or symptoms of SIRS or capillary leak syndrome and provide appropriate supportive measures, which may include steroids, diuretics, and albumin
  - Glucocorticoid prophylaxis (eg, hydrocortisone 100 mg/m² per day for 3 days [days 1–3]) may prevent signs or symptoms of SIRS or capillary leak syndrome
- Monitor renal and hepatic function closely during a 5-day treatment course with clofarabine
  - Although clofarabine has not been studied in patients with renal or hepatic impairment, 49–60% of a dose was renally eliminated as unchanged drug within 24 hours after administration to pediatric patients

- Avoid medications that adversely affect kidney and liver function during the days on which clofarabine is administered
- Clofarabine should be immediately discontinued if Grades ≥3 increases in serum creatinine or bilirubin are observed during treatment
  - Clofarabine treatment may resume after a patient's condition has stabilized and organ function has returned to baseline, generally with a 25% reduction in clofarabine dose
- Discontinue clofarabine administration if a Grade 4 noninfectious nonhematologic adverse event occurs

Selected incompatibility:

- Do not administer other medications through the same intraVENous line as clofarabine
  - Clofarabine compatibility with other drugs is not yet known

CYCLOPHOSPHAMIDE

Cyclophosphamide for injection, USP; product label, February 2013. Product made in Germany. Manufactured by Baxter Healthcare Corporation, Deerfield, IL

Product Identification, Preparation, Storage, and Stability

- Cyclophosphamide is available as a sterile white powder for reconstitution for injection in individually packaged single-use vials containing 500 mg (NDC 10019-955-01), 1000 mg (NDC 10019-956-01), or 2000 mg (NDC 10019-957-01) of cyclophosphamide monohydrate
- Store cyclophosphamide at temperatures ≤25°C (≤77°F)
- Cyclophosphamide may melt if exposed to high temperatures during transportation or storage
  - Melted cyclophosphamide appears as a clear or yellowish viscous liquid usually found in connection with portions of the drug that have remained in powdered form, or as droplets that have become separated from a portion of the drug that remains in powdered form
  - *Do not use* cyclophosphamide that exhibits signs of melting
- Commercially marketed cyclophosphamide products may not contain an antimicrobial preservative
- Reconstitute cyclophosphamide with 0.9% NS* or SWFI†, as follows:

Cyclophosphamide Content per Vial	Diluent Volume	Cyclophosphamide Concentration After Reconstitution
500 mg	25 mL	
1000 mg	50 mL	20 mg/mL
2000 mg	100 mL	

*After reconstitution with 0.9% NS, cyclophosphamide is suitable for direct intravenous, intraMUSCular, intraperitoneal, or intrapleural injection
†Reconstitution with SWFI yields a hypotonic product, which should not be administered by intraVENous injection, but may be administered by intraVENous infusion after further dilution with 1 of the following solutions: D5W, 0.45% NaCl, 0.9% NS, D5W/RI, D5W/0.9% NS, LRI, sodium lactate injection, USP (1/6 molar sodium lactate)

- After reconstituting cyclophosphamide with SWFI, the resulting solution is hypotonic. Reconstitution with SWFI and 0.9% NS to a concentration of 20 mg/mL yields solutions with the following osmolarity:

Cyclophosphamide and Diluent	Osmolarity
100 mg cyclophosphamide in 5 mL of SWFI	74 mOsm/L
100 mg cyclophosphamide in 5 mL of 0.9% NS	374 mOsm/L

- After adding a diluent solution, shake cyclophosphamide vials vigorously to dissolve the drug powder
  - If cyclophosphamide does not readily and completely dissolve, allow the vials to stand for a few minutes and, if necessary, resuming shaking
- Reconstitution to a concentration of 20 mg cyclophosphamide/mL yields a product that is chemically and physically stable for 24 hours at room temperature or for 6 days under refrigeration (2°–8°C [35.6°–46.4°F])
- After reconstitution with 0.9% NS or SWFI to a concentration of 20 mg cyclophosphamide per milliliter, the reconstituted solution may be further diluted
  - Product labeling identifies cyclophosphamide stability diluted with three vehicle solutions as follows:

Solution	Storage Temperature	
	Room Temperature	Refrigeration
0.45% NaCl	up to 24 hours	up to 6 days
D5W	up to 24 hours	up to 36 hours
D5W/0.9% NS	up to 24 hours	up to 36 hours

Recommendations for Drug Administration and Ancillary Care

General:

- After reconstitution with 0.9% NS to a concentration of 20 mg cyclophosphamide/mL the drug product is suitable for administration by direct intraVENous injection, intraVENous infusion, intraMUSCular intraperitoneal, or intrapleural injection
- Solutions prepared by reconstituting cyclophosphamide with SWFI are hypotonic, and *are not recommended* for intraVENous injection, but may be administered by intraVENous infusion if further diluted with any of the following solutions: D5W, 0.45% NaCl, 0.9% NS, D5W/RI, D5W/0.9% NS, LRI, sodium lactate injection, USP

CYTARABINE

Cytarabine injection for intravenous, intrathecal and subcutaneous use only; product label, April 2012. Manufactured by Zydus Hospira Oncology Private Ltd., Gujarat, India. Manufactured for Hospira, Inc. Lake Forest, IL

Cytarabine injection NOT FOR INTRATHECAL USE—CONTAINS BENZYL ALCOHOL FOR INTRAVENOUS OR SUBCUTANEOUS USE ONLY; product label, April 2012. Manufactured by Zydus Hospira Oncology Private Ltd., Gujarat, India. Manufactured for Hospira, Inc. Lake Forest, IL

Cytarabine injection PHARMACY BULK PACKAGE—NOT FOR DIRECT INFUSION; product label, April 2012. Manufactured by Zydus Hospira Oncology Private Ltd., Gujarat, India. Manufactured for Hospira, Inc. Lake Forest, IL

Cytarabine for injection USP, for intravenous, intrathecal, or subcutaneous use only; product label, September 2008. Manufactured by Ben Venue Laboratories, Inc., Bedford, OH. Manufactured for Bedford Laboratories, Bedford, OH

WARNING

Only physicians experienced in cancer chemotherapy should use Cytarabine Injection

For induction therapy patients should be treated in a facility with laboratory and supportive resources sufficient to monitor drug tolerance and protect and maintain a patient compromised by drug toxicity. The main toxic effect of Cytarabine Injection is bone marrow suppression with leukopenia, thrombocytopenia and anemia. Less serious toxicity includes nausea, vomiting, diarrhea and abdominal pain, oral ulceration, and hepatic dysfunction

The physician must judge possible benefit to the patient against known toxic effects of this drug in considering the advisability of therapy with Cytarabine Injection. Before making this judgment or beginning treatment, the physician should be familiar with... [all other elements of product labeling]

Boxed Warning for "Cytarabine Injection For Intravenous, Intrathecal and Subcutaneous Use Only"; April 2012 product label; Hospira, Inc., Lake Forest, IL

Product Identification, Preparation, Storage, and Stability

- Cytarabine is generically available from several manufacturers. Products are available in lyophilized (powdered) or solution formulations. Presentations include products packaged for a single use or multiple doses, and for pharmaceutical admixture and compounding (eg, *Pharmacy Bulk Package*)

Cautions: Among products in solution (ie, "cytarabine injection..."):
  - Cytarabine concentrations are not consistently the same among available products
  - Products may or may not contain an antimicrobial preservative
- In general, cytarabine products are stored at controlled room temperatures around 20°–25°C (68°–77°F), with temperature excursions permitted to 15°–30°C (59°–86°F)
  - Acceptable storage temperatures vary among products from different manufacturers
  - Refer to product packaging and labeling for storage conditions appropriate for different products
- *Do not use* bacteriostatically preserved drug and diluent products for intraTHECAL use and for preparing cytarabine for high-dose treatments (dosages ≥1000 mg/m²)
- Refer to product packaging and labeling for storage conditions appropriate for different products
- Reconstitute lyophilized cytarabine as follows
  - Diluent selection depends on route of administration (see below):

Cytarabine Content per Vial	Diluent Volume	Reconstituted Cytarabine Concentration
100 mg	5 mL	20 mg/mL
500 mg	10 mL	50 mg/mL
1000 mg	10 mL	100 mg/mL
2000 mg	20 mL	100 mg/mL

- Promptly use reconstituted cytarabine solutions that do not contain an antimicrobial preservative and those in which the concentration of preservatives is not adequate to inhibit microbial growth
- Solutions reconstituted with BWFI may be stored at controlled room temperature, 15°–30°C (59°–86°F), for up to 48 hours
- Discard solutions in which a slight haze develops

(continued)

Product Identification, Preparation, Storage, and Stability (*continued*)

For intraVENous or SUBCUTaneous use:

- Reconstitute cytarabine for injection with 0.9% NS, SWFI, or BWFI preserved with benzyl alcohol
  - *Do not use* bacteriostatically preserved diluents when preparing cytarabine doses ≥ 1000 mg/m^2
- The reconstituted product may be further diluted to a convenient volume in 0.9% NS or D5W

For intraTHECAL use:

- Reconstitute cytarabine *only* with PRESERVATIVE-FREE 0.9% NS to produce a solution with concentration ≤ 20 mg/mL. Typical administration volumes range from 5 to 10 mL, and should closely approximate the volume of cerebrospinal fluid removed
- Admixtures with hydrocortisone sodium succinate for intraTHECAL administration (with or without methotrexate) should be prepared just before use and administered as soon as possible (within minutes) after preparation because of the instability of the hydrocortisone component

Caution: **Do not use** an antimicrobially preserved diluent to prepare cytarabine for intraTHECAL use

Recommendations for Drug Administration and Ancillary Care

General:

- See Chapter 41 for recommended use in patients with renal and hepatic dysfunction
- Administer by intraVENous, intraTHECAL, or SUBCUTaneous routes
  - Use products prepared for intraTHECAL administration immediately after they are prepared
- If cytarabine is given intraMUSCularly, administration sites should be rotated
- Although the amount of drug administered is a modulating factor, patients generally can tolerate higher total doses given by rapid intraVENous injection than by slow infusion because of cytarabine's rapid inactivation and the relatively brief cellular exposure to cytotoxic concentrations that occur after rapid administration

CYTARABINE LIPOSOME INJECTION

DepoCyt®–cytarabine injection, lipid complex, for intrathecal use only DEPOCYT® (cytarabine liposome injection) for intrathecal use only, 50 mg vial; product label, September 2011. Manufactured by Pacira Pharmaceuticals, Inc. San Diego, CA. Distributed by Sigma-Tau Pharmaceuticals, Inc., Gaithersburg, MD

WARNINGS

DepoCyt® (cytarabine liposome injection) should be administered only under the supervision of a qualified physician experienced in the use of intrathecal cancer chemotherapeutic agents. Appropriate management of complications is possible only when adequate diagnostic and treatment facilities are readily available. In all clinical studies, chemical arachnoiditis, a syndrome manifested primarily by nausea, vomiting, headache and fever, was a common adverse event. If left untreated, chemical arachnoiditis may be fatal. The incidence and severity of chemical arachnoiditis can be reduced by coadministration of dexamethasone... Patients receiving DepoCyt should be treated concurrently with dexamethasone to mitigate the symptoms of chemical arachnoiditis...

Boxed Warning (excerpt) for "DepoCyt® - cytarabine injection, lipid complex, For Intrathecal Use Only DEPOCYT® (cytarabine liposome injection) For Intrathecal Use Only, 50 mg vial"; September 2011 product label; Sigma-Tau Pharmaceuticals, Inc., Gaithersburg, MD

Product Identification, Preparation, Storage, and Stability

- DepoCyt® is packaged in individually packaged, glass, 5-mL, single-use, vials containing a sterile, nonpyrogenic, white to off-white, ready-to-use, preservative-free suspension of cytarabine encapsulated into multivesicular lipid-based particles (liposomes). NDC 57665-331-01

  ▪ The liposome particles are suspended in sodium chloride 0.9% (w/v) in SWFI

  ▪ Cytarabine 50 mg is present at a concentration of 10 mg/mL. Inactive ingredients at their respective approximate concentrations, include cholesterol 4.4 mg/mL, triolein 1.2 mg/mL, dioleoylphosphatidylcholine 5.7 mg/mL, and dipalmitoylphosphatidylglycerol 1 mg/mL. The product pH is within the range 5.5–8.5

- The drug product does not contain a preservative and should be stored under refrigeration at 2°–8°C (35.6°–46.4°F). Protect DepoCyt® from freezing

- DepoCyt® is intended for direct administration without further dilution

- Allow vials to warm to room temperature before use

- Gently agitate or repeatedly invert a vial to resuspend drug particles before transferring its contents to a syringe. *Avoid* aggressively agitating the drug product

  ▪ DepoCyt® drug particles are denser than the solution in which they are suspended, and tend to settle with time and must be resuspended before use

- Administer a dose immediately after withdrawing the product from a vial. If treatment is delayed, do not use DepoCyt® more than 4 hours after withdrawing the product from a vial

- Any portion of vial contents not used to prepare a dose should be discarded

Selected incompatibility:

- *Do not mix* DepoCyt® with other medications

Recommendations for Drug Administration and Ancillary Care

General:

- Patients should receive dexamethasone 4 mg either orally or intraVENously twice daily for 5 days, beginning on the day of DepoCyt® injection to mitigate the symptoms of chemical arachnoiditis

- Inject DepoCyt® 50 mg slowly, over a period of 1–5 minutes directly into the cerebrospinal fluid via an intraventricular reservoir or by direct injection into the lumbar sac

  ▪ Do not use inline filters when administering DepoCyt®

- Patients should be instructed to lie flat for 1 hour after DepoCyt® administration by lumbar puncture

- Continually monitor patients for immediate adverse reactions after DepoCyt® injection

  ▪ If drug-related neurotoxicity develops, the dose should be reduced to 25 mg. If it persists, discontinue DepoCyt® treatment

- Advise patients about the expected adverse events of headache, nausea, vomiting, and fever, and about the early signs and symptoms of neurotoxicity

  ▪ Emphasize at the initiation of each treatment cycle the importance of concurrent dexamethasone use

  ▪ Patients should be instructed to seek medical attention if signs or symptoms of neurotoxicity develop, or if oral dexamethasone is not well tolerated

Note: DepoCyt® particles are similar in size and appearance to white blood cells: care must be taken in interpreting CSF examinations following DepoCyt® administration

DACARBAZINE

DACARBAZINE for injection, USP; product label, September 2007. Manufactured by Ben Venue Laboratories, Inc., Bedford, OH. Manufactured for
Bedford Laboratories, Bedford, OH
Dacarbazine for injection, USP; product label, July 2007. Hospira Inc., Lake Forest, IL
DACARBAZINE for injection, USP; product label, January 2008. APP Pharmaceuticals LLC, Schaumburg, IL

WARNINGS

It is recommended that dacarbazine be administered under the supervision of a qualified physician experienced in the use of cancer
chemotherapeutic agents

1. Hemopoietic depression is the most common toxicity with dacarbazine...
2. Hepatic necrosis has been reported...
3. Studies have demonstrated this agent to have a carcinogenic and teratogenic effect when used in animals
4. In treatment of each patient, the physician must weigh carefully the possibility of achieving therapeutic benefit against the risk of toxicity

---

Boxed Warning (excerpt) for "Dacarbazine for Injection, USP", labeling for products from:
   Bedford Laboratories™, Bedford, OH (dated, September 2007)
   Hospira Inc., Lake Forest, IL (dated, July 2007)
   APP Pharmaceuticals LLC, Schaumburg, IL (dated, January 2008)

Product Identification, Preparation, Storage, and Stability

- Dacarbazine is generically available from several manufacturers. In general, the drug is packaged in single-use, amber glass vials, containing either 100 mg or 200 mg dacarbazine per vial
  - Commercial formulations also include mannitol and citric acid
  - Packaging varies among manufacturers' products, including: individually packaged vials and boxes containing 10 vials
- Dacarbazine is a white to pale yellow solid that is sensitive to light
- Store intact vials under refrigeration at 2°–8°C (35.6°–46.4°F) and protect from light exposure
- Reconstitute dacarbazine with SWFI as follows:

Dacarbazine Content per Vial	Diluent (SWFI) Volume	Dacarbazine Concentration After Reconstitution
100 mg	9.9 mL	10 mg/mL
200 mg	19.7 mL	

- The resulting clear, yellowish solution has a pH from 3.0 to 4.0, and is highly sensitive to degradation as a result of exposure to light[27]
- The reconstituted solution is suitable for intraVENous injection, or it may be further diluted in up to 250 mL of D5W or 0.9% NS and given by intravenous infusion
- Product labeling includes the following stability information:
  - After reconstitution, dacarbazine solution (10 mg/mL) may be stored in the product vial at 4°C (39.2°F) for up to 72 hours or at normal room temperature and (fluorescent) lighting conditions for up to 8 hours[28]
  - After dilution in D5W or 0.9% NS, the resulting product may be stored at 4°C (39.2°F) for up to 24 hours or under normal room conditions (ambient temperature and artificial lighting) for up to 8 hours[28]
  - See comments under "Dacarbazine Degradation," below
- Change in solution color from pale yellow or ivory to pink or red is a sign of decomposition
  - Dacarbazine solutions that exhibit changes in color toward pink or red should not be used

Recommendations for Drug Administration and Ancillary Care

General:

- See Chapter 41 for recommended use in patients with renal and hepatic dysfunction
- Administer dacarbazine only by intraVENous routes:
  - By intraVENous injection over 1 minute *or* by intraVENous infusion over 15–30 minutes
- Cover parenteral product containers containing dacarbazine solutions with light-opaque materials (bags, aluminum foil)
- Use opaque or light-resistant (light -shielded) VAD to administer dacarbazine, or cover VAD used to administer dacarbazine to protect the drug from light; eg, with opaque sleeves or by wrapping tubing with aluminum foil

Dacarbazine degradation:

- Dacarbazine degrades to active and potentially toxic products, including 2-azahypoxanthine by photolysis[27,29] and hydrolysis
  - Photodegradation products are associated with adverse effects encountered during dacarbazine administration, including local venous pain, nausea, and vomiting
    - In small case series, venous pain ± other symptoms and signs of toxicity were eliminated or reduced during administration in a room illuminated by a red photographic lamp[30] and when the drug in vials and VAD tubing was protected from light exposure[31]
- Dacarbazine degradation is accelerated by light exposure and storage temperature
  - Sunlight causes more rapid photolysis than fluorescent lighting[32]
  - For dacarbazine exposed to sunlight during preparation or administration:
    - Cover parenteral containers with opaque material or foil during administration[32,33]
    - Use light-resistant or opaque administration sets, or wrap tubing with opaque material or foil during administration[32,33]
- Prepare dacarbazine just before it is used, or store reconstituted and diluted products under refrigeration and protected from light until used[28,32]

DACTINOMYCIN

Cosmegen® for Injection (dactinomycin for injection) (Actinomycin D); product label, February 2013. Manufactured by Baxter Oncology GmbH, Halle/Westfalen, Germany. Manufactured for Recordati Rare Diseases Inc., Lebanon, NJ
DACTINOMYCIN FOR INJECTION USP; product label, August 2012. Manufactured by Ben Venue Laboratories, Inc. Manufactured for Bedford Laboratories, Bedford, OH

WARNING

COSMEGEN® (dactinomycin for injection) should be administered only under the supervision of a physician who is experienced in the use of cancer chemotherapeutic agents. This drug is **HIGHLY TOXIC** and both powder and solution must be handled and administered with care. Inhalation of dust or vapors and contact with skin or mucous membranes, especially those of the eyes, must be avoided. Avoid exposure during pregnancy. Due to the toxic properties of dactinomycin (eg, corrosivity, carcinogenicity, mutagenicity, teratogenicity), special handling procedures should be reviewed prior to handling and followed diligently. Dactinomycin is extremely corrosive to soft tissue. If extravasation occurs during intravenous use, severe damage to soft tissues will occur. In at least one instance, this has led to contracture of the arms

---

Boxed warning for: Cosmegen® for Injection (dactinomycin for injection) (Actinomycin D); product label, February 2013. Manufactured by Baxter Oncology GmbH, Halle/Westfalen, Germany. Manufactured for Recordati Rare Diseases Inc., Lebanon, NJ

Product Identification, Preparation, Storage, and Stability

- DACTINomycin is marketed in individually packaged, single-use vials containing DACTINomycin 500 mcg (0.5 mg) and 20 mg mannitol as a sterile, yellow to orange, lyophilized powder. NDC 67386-811-55

- Store intact vials at 20°–25°C (68°–77°F). Temperature excursions to 15°–30°C (59°–86°F) are permitted. Protect vials from light and humidity

- Reconstitute the drug product by injecting 1.1 mL of SWFI (without preservative) into a vial to produce a clear, gold-colored solution that contains approximately 500 mcg (0.5 mg) DACTINomycin per milliliter

  - Reconstituted DACTINomycin is chemically stable, but the product does not contain an antimicrobial preservative

  - Diluents preserved with benzyl alcohol or parabens may cause drug precipitation and *should not* be used to reconstitute DACTINomycin

- *Do not filter* DACTINomycin during preparation. Filtration through cellulose ester filters may remove DACTINomycin from the solution being filtered

- DACTINomycin may be added to the tubing or side arm of a rapidly flowing intraVENous infusion of D5W or 0.9% NS. Alternatively, it may be prepared as an admixture in the same solutions for administration by intraVENous infusion or isolation perfusion techniques

  - DACTINomycin may be prepared as an admixture in 0.9 NS or D5W to concentrations ≥10 mcg/mL (≥0.01 mg/mL) in glass or PVC containers for intraVENous infusion

  - DACTINomycin is reported to be most stable at pH 5–7[34]

- Use a "2-needle technique" if DACTINomycin is to be injected percutaneously directly into a vein

  - DACTINomycin is corrosive to skin, irritating to the eyes and respiratory tract mucosa, highly toxic by the oral route, and a vesicant if extravasated

  - The "2-needle technique" prevents soft-tissue exposure to DACTINomycin

that remains on the external surfaces of needles used to reconstitute the drug product

Two-needle technique for preparing DACTINomycin for percutaneous administration:

1. Use 1 sterile needle to reconstitute and withdraw from a vial a measured amount of DACTINomycin needed to deliver a patient's dose

2. Aspirate all drug solution from the needle and needle hub into the syringe, and replace the first needle with a second sterile needle

3. With a second sterile needle on the syringe, carefully express air without expelling drug from the tip of the needle and inject DACTINomycin through an injection port into the tubing of a rapidly running intravenously administered solution

Recommendations for Drug Administration and Ancillary Care

General:

- See Chapter 41 for recommended use in patients with hepatic dysfunction
- For intraVENous administration *only*, by direct intraVENous injection over approximately 1 minute or intraVENous infusion over 15–30 minutes
- When diluted at concentrations of ≥10 mcg/mL in SWFI, 0.9% NS, or D5W in glass or PVC containers, DACTINomycin is chemically stable for up to 10 hours when stored at ambient room temperature
  - DACTINomycin should be diluted *only* with 0.9% NS or D5W for intraVENous infusion
  - *Caution*: After initial reconstitution with SWFI, further dilution with SWFI decreases DACTINomycin osmolality, which may result in an extremely hypotonic solution. Depending on administration rate and blood flow, administration of hypotonic solutions may result in some degree of intravascular hemolysis
- The dosage for DACTINomycin is calculated in micrograms (mcg)
  - The dose intensity per 2-week cycle for adults or children *should not exceed* 15 mcg/kg per day or 400–600 mcg/m² per day intraVENously for 5 days
  - Dosage calculations for obese or edematous patients should be performed on the basis of body surface area to more closely relate dosage to lean body mass
- Please review the 2-needle technique for direct intraVENous injection (see above). The procedure prevents soft-tissue exposure to DACTINomycin that remains on the external surfaces of needles used during drug preparation

- *Do not filter* DACTINomycin during administration
  - Filtration through 0.22-μm pore size filter membranes composed of cellulose ester (cellulose nitrate/cellulose acetate) or polytetrafluoroethylene (PTFE, Teflon) were shown to remove a substantial portion of DACTINomycin from the solution being filtered[16,35]
  - Filtration through a 0.22-μm pore size cellulose ester filter membranes resulted in approximately 13% of the total amount of filtered DACTINomycin bound by the filter[36]

Caution: DACTINomycin is a vesicant and may cause severe local soft-tissue necrosis if administered by injection into soft tissues or extravasated

DAUNORUBICIN HYDROCHLORIDE

CERUBIDINE (Daunorubicin HCl) FOR INJECTION; product label, February 2008. Manufactured by Ben Venue Laboratories, Inc., Bedford, OH. Manufactured for Bedford Laboratories, Bedford, OH
DAUNORUBICIN HYDROCHLORIDE injection; product label, June 2013. Manufactured by Ben Venue Laboratories, Inc., Bedford, OH. Manufactured for Bedford Laboratories, Bedford, OH
DAUNORUBICIN HYDROCHLORIDE–daunorubicin hydrochloride injection, solution; product label, September 2012. Manufactured by Teva Parenteral Medicines, Inc., Irvine, CA

WARNINGS

1. Daunorubicin hydrochloride injection must be given into a rapidly flowing intravenous infusion. It must never be given by the intramuscular or subcutaneous route. Severe local tissue necrosis will occur if there is extravasation during administration

2. Myocardial toxicity manifested in its most severe form by potentially fatal congestive heart failure may occur either during therapy or months to years after termination of therapy. The incidence of myocardial toxicity increases after a total cumulative dose exceeding 400 to 550 mg/m^2 in adults, 300 mg/m^2 in children more than 2 years of age, or 10 mg/kg in children less than 2 years of age

3. Severe myelosuppression occurs when used in therapeutic doses; this may lead to infection or hemorrhage

4. It is recommended that daunorubicin hydrochloride be administered only by physicians who are experienced in leukemia chemotherapy and in facilities with laboratory and supportive resources adequate to monitor drug tolerance and protect and maintain a patient compromised by drug toxicity. The physician and institution must be capable of responding rapidly and completely to severe hemorrhagic conditions and/or overwhelming infection

5. Dosage should be reduced in patients with impaired hepatic or renal function

Boxed Warning for "Daunorubicin Hydrochloride Injection"; September 2012 product label; Teva Parenteral Medicines, Inc., Irvine, CA; and "Daunorubicin Hydrochloride Injection"; July 1999 product label; Bedford Laboratories™, Bedford, OH

Product Identification, Preparation, Storage, and Stability

- DAUNOrubicin HCl injection (solution) and DAUNOrubicin HCl for injection (lyophilized powder) are generically available from several manufacturers. DAUNOrubicin is a sterile, deep red to red-orange product packaged in glass single-use vials
- Products are formulated either as a sterile, deep red to red-orange solution, or hygroscopic, crystalline lyophilized powder packaged in glass single-use vials
  - DAUNOrubicin HCl injection (solution) is available in vials containing 20 mg/4 mL (packaged in cartons containing 10 vials) or 50 mg (individually packaged) DAUNOrubicin base per milliliter
  - DAUNOrubicin HCl for Injection (lyophilized powder) is packaged in cartons containing 10 vials each containing 20 mg of DAUNOrubicin base
- Storage:
  - Store unreconstituted DAUNOrubicin HCl for injection (lyophilized powder) at controlled room temperature, 15°–30°C (59°–86°F)
  - Store DAUNOrubicin HCl injection (solution) under refrigeration at 2°–8°C (35.6°–46.4°F)
- Protect DAUNOrubicin from exposure to light by storing unused vials in their packaging carton

Reconstitution for lyophilized DAUNOrubicin:

- Reconstitute DAUNOrubicin HCl lyophilized powder with 4 mL of SWFI to produce a solution with concentration equal to 5 mg DAUNOrubicin base per milliliter

Stability (solution and lyophilized formulations):

- After reconstitution, DAUNOrubicin HCl (lyophilized powder formulation) is stable for 24 hours at 15°–30°C (59°–86°F) and 48 hours under refrigeration (2°–8°C [35.6°–46.4°F])
- DAUNOrubicin HCl injection (formulations already in solution) are stable for 24 hours at 15°–30°C (59°–86°F)
- DAUNOrubicin HCl diluted with D5W (pH = 4.36) or 0.9% NS (pH = 5.20 or 6.47) to a concentration of 98 µg/mL (estimated) in PVC containers stored at 25°C, 4°C or –20°C was stable for 43 days under all conditions evaluated[37]
  - DAUNOrubicin HCl for injection reconstituted with SWFI and diluted with 0.9% NS or D5W to an estimated concentration of 98 µg/mL stored in PVC containers for 43 days did not degrade during or after 11 repeated cycles of freezing (–20°C) and thawing at ambient temperature (25°C)[37]
- DAUNOrubicin HCl for injection reconstituted with SWFI to a concentration of 2 mg/mL was stable for at least 43 days when stored in polypropylene syringes at 4°C[37]

(continued)

Product Identification, Preparation, Storage, and Stability (*continued*)

- DAUNOrubicin solutions undergo photodegradation
  - The rate and extent of photodegradation are inversely related to DAUNOrubicin concentrations in solution[38]
    - At DAUNOrubicin concentrations ≥100 μg/mL (≥0.1 mg/mL) stored at 25°C for 168 h under artificial room lighting (four 65/80-Watt fluorescent tubes mounted approximately 1 m above the samples), little or no photodegradation occurred in clear or amber glass or opaque polyethylene containers[38]
    - At DAUNOrubicin concentrations ≥500 μg/mL (≥0.5 mg/mL), no special precautions are necessary to protect freshly prepared solutions from exposure to artificial light or sunlight[38]

Selected incompatibility:

- Product labeling recommends *not mixing* DAUNOrubicin with heparin or other drugs

Recommendations for Drug Administration and Ancillary Care

General:

- See Chapter 41 for recommended use in patients with renal and hepatic dysfunction
- A calculated dose is withdrawn into a syringe with 10–15 mL of 0.9% NS for intraVENous injection
- Inject DAUNOrubicin into the tubing or side-arm of a rapidly flowing intraVENous infusion of D5W or 0.9% NS
- Severe hepatic or renal impairment may enhance adverse effects associated with DAUNOrubicin
  - Clinical laboratory evaluation of hepatic and renal function should be completed before administering DAUNOrubicin. Consult recommendations for modifying DAUNOrubicin dosage and schedule in hepatic or renal impairment

Caution: DAUNOrubicin is a vesicant and can produce severe local soft-tissue necrosis if extravasation occurs. *NEVER inject DAUNOrubicin by the intraMUSCular, SUBCUTaneous, or intraTHECAL routes*

- The current standard of care for managing anthracycline extravasation, including extravasation of DAUNOrubicin, is a 3-day course of intraVENously administered dexrazoxane (Totect, Savene)
- Advise patients DAUNOrubicin HCl may transiently impart a red discoloration to urine after administration

DAUNORUBICIN CITRATE LIPOSOME INJECTION

DaunoXome® (daunorubicin citrate liposome injection); product label, December 2011. Manufactured for Galen US Inc, Souderton, PA

WARNINGS

1. Cardiac function should be monitored regularly in patients receiving DaunoXome (daunorubicin citrate liposome injection) because of the potential risk for cardiac toxicity and congestive heart failure. Cardiac monitoring is advised especially in those patients who have received prior anthracyclines or who have pre-existing cardiac disease or who have had prior radiotherapy encompassing the heart

2. Severe myelosuppression may occur

3. DaunoXome should be administered only under the supervision of a physician who is experienced in the use of cancer chemotherapeutic agents

4. Dosage should be reduced in patients with impaired hepatic function…

5. A triad of back pain, flushing, and chest tightness has been reported in 13.8% of the patients (16/116) treated with DaunoXome in the Phase III clinical trial, and in 2.7% of treatment cycles (27/994). This triad generally occurs during the first five minutes of the infusion, subsides with interruption of the infusion, and generally does not recur if the infusion is then resumed at a slower rate

---

Boxed Warning (excerpt) for "DaunoXome® (daunorubicin citrate liposome injection)"; December 2011 product label; Galen US Inc, Souderton, PA

Product Identification, Preparation, Storage, and Stability

- DaunoXome® is a translucent, red, liposomal dispersion of DAUNOrubicin citrate equivalent to 50 mg DAUNOrubicin base in 25 mL (2 mg/mL) packaged in single-use vials (NDC 10885-001-01)

- Store DaunoXome® under refrigeration at 2°–8°C (35.6°–46.4°F). Do not freeze DaunoXome. Protect it from exposure to light

- Withdraw the calculated volume of DaunoXome® needed for a patient's dose from a vial into a syringe, and transfer it into a sterile parenteral product container containing an equivalent volume of D5W (1:1 dilution) to produce a concentration after dilution = 1 mg DAUNOrubicin per milliliter of solution

- The product does not contain a preservative or bacteriostatic agent. Partially used vials should be discarded as hazardous waste

- If diluted DaunoXome® is not used immediately, it should be refrigerated at 2°–8°C (35.6°–46.4°F) for a maximum of 6 hours

Caution: The only fluid with which DaunoXome® may be mixed is D5W

Selected incompatibility:

- *Do not mix* DaunoXome® with any solution other than D5W

Recommendations for Drug Administration and Ancillary Care

General:

- See Chapter 41 for recommended use in patients with renal and hepatic dysfunction

- Administer DaunoXome® intraVENously over 60 minutes immediately after dilution

- *Do not filter* DaunoXome® during administration

- *Do not mix* DaunoXome® with other drugs

DECITABINE

DACOGEN® (decitabine) for INJECTION; product label, March 2010. Manufactured by Pharmachemie B.V. Haarlem, The Netherlands. Manufactured for Eisai Inc., Woodcliff Lake, NJ

Product Identification, Preparation, Storage, and Stability

- Decitabine is a sterile, lyophilized, white to almost-white powder, individually packaged in clear, colorless, single-use, 20-mL, glass vials containing 50 mg decitabine, 68 mg monobasic potassium phosphate (potassium dihydrogen phosphate), and 11.6 mg sodium hydroxide. NDC 62856-600-01
- Store intact vials at 25°C (77°F); temperature excursions are permitted to 15°–30°C (59°–86°F)
- Caution: BEFORE BEGINNING reconstitution, evaluate whether decitabine administration will begin within 15 minutes after the lyophilized product is reconstituted
  - Decitabine hydrolyzes spontaneously after reconstitution
  - If drug administration commences within 15 minutes after reconstitution began, there is no need to used prechilled diluents, but preparation should not commence until just before the drug is needed
  - If drug administration begins >15 minutes to within 7 hours after reconstitution, use prechilled solutions (2°–8°C [35.6°–46.4°F]) to reconstitute and dilute decitabine

- Reconstitution with 10 mL of SWFI produces a solution with concentration of 5 mg decitabine/mL at pH 6.7–7.3
- After powdered decitabine is completely dissolved, immediately withdraw with a syringe the calculated volume of drug needed for a patient's dose from a vial and transfer it into a sterile plastic or glass parenteral product container containing a volume of 0.9% NS, D5W, or LRI sufficient to produce a decitabine concentration between 0.1–1.0 mg/mL
  - If decitabine cannot be used within 15 minutes after diluent was introduced into a vial, the product should be promptly refrigerated and may be stored for up to 7 hours after reconstitution
  - Reconstituted and diluted products that have not been used within the time limits identified above and all materials potentially contaminated with decitabine during product preparation should be discarded as hazardous waste
- If a decitabine-containing solution was prepared and refrigerated as described (above) and used within 7 hours after reconstitution, administration should be completed within 3 hours after the product was transferred from refrigeration to room temperature conditions

Recommendations for Drug Administration and Ancillary Care

General:

- See Chapter 41 for recommended use in patients with renal and hepatic dysfunction
- If decitabine is not prepared with chilled solutions and promptly refrigerated after preparation, administration MUST BEGIN within 15 minutes after reconstitution
- If decitabine was prepared with chilled solutions and stored under refrigeration promptly after preparation, administration MAY BEGIN up to 7 hours after reconstitution
  - Drug administration should begin promptly after stored products are transferred from refrigeration to room temperature conditions
- Administer decitabine by intraVENous infusion over 3 hours

DENILEUKIN DIFTITOX

ONTAK® (denileukin diftitox) Injection for intravenous infusion; product label August 2011. Manufactured and Distributed by Eisai Inc., Woodcliff Lake, NJ

WARNING

SERIOUS INFUSION REACTIONS, CAPILLARY LEAK SYNDROME AND LOSS OF VISUAL ACUITY

The following adverse reactions have been reported:

- Serious and fatal infusion reactions. Administer Ontak in a facility equipped and staffed for cardiopulmonary resuscitation. Immediately stop and permanently discontinue Ontak for serious infusion reactions…
- Capillary leak syndrome resulting in death. Monitor weight, edema, blood pressure and serum albumin levels prior to and during Ontak treatment…
- Loss of visual acuity and color vision…

Boxed Warning (excerpt) for "ONTAK® (denileukin diftitox) Injection for intravenous infusion"; August 2011 product label, Eisai Inc., Woodcliff Lake, NJ

Product Identification, Preparation, Storage, and Stability

- ONTAK® is supplied in single-use vials as a sterile, frozen solution intended for intraVENous administration (6 vials/package; NDC 62856-603-01)
- Each vial contains 300 mcg of recombinant denileukin diftitox in 2 mL (150 mcg/mL) in a sterile solution of citric acid 20 mmol/L, EDTA 0.05 mmol/L, and polysorbate 20 (<1%) in SWFI. The solution has a pH range of 6.9–7.2
- Store ONTAK® at ≤ −10°C (≤14°F)
- Thaw vials either:
  1. Under refrigeration at 2°–8°C (35.6°–46.4°F) for not more than 24 hours, *or*
  2. At room temperature for 1–2 hours
     - *Do not heat* ONTAK® to thaw the product
     - *Do not refreeze* ONTAK® after thawing
- Allow ONTAK® to equilibrate with room temperature (up to 25°C [77°F]) before preparing a dose
- Mix ONTAK® solution in a vial by gentle swirling. *Do not shake* ONTAK® solution
  - After thawing, a haze may be visible. The haze should clear when the solution is at room temperature. Do not use the solution unless it is clear, colorless, and without visible particulate matter

- Prepare and contain diluted denileukin diftitox in plastic syringes or soft plastic parenteral product containers
  1. Do not use glass containers because an unpredictable portion of the drug may be lost because of adsorption to glass surfaces
  2. With a syringe, withdraw from 1 or more vials the amount of denileukin diftitox needed to prepare a patient's dose and inject it into an empty plastic parenteral product container (bag or syringe)
     - Denileukin diftitox concentration must be ≥15 mcg/mL during all preparation steps
  3. Add to the product container *no more than* 9 mL of preservative-free 0.9% NS for each 1 mL of denileukin diftitox in the container
- *Do not* mix denileukin diftitox with other drugs
- Partially used vials should be discarded immediately

Selected incompatibility:

- Product labeling recommends *not* mixing denileukin diftitox with other drugs

Recommendations for Drug Administration and Ancillary Care

Premedication:

- Premedicate with acetaminophen and an antihistamine (H$_1$-receptor antagonist) before each denileukin diftitox infusion

General:

- Withhold denileukin diftitox administration in a patient whose serum albumin is <3 g/dL
- Administer denileukin diftitox intraVENously over 30–60 minutes within 6 hours after preparation was completed
  - There is no clinical experience with prolonged infusion times (>80 minutes)
  - *Do not administer* denileukin diftitox by rapid or "bolus" intraVENous injection
- If infusion-related adverse events occur, denileukin diftitox administration should be discontinued, or the delivery rate should be decreased depending on the severity of the reaction
  - Immediately stop and permanently discontinue denileukin diftitox administration for serious infusion reactions
  - Resuscitative equipment should be available during denileukin diftitox administration
- *Do not mix* denileukin diftitox with other drugs
- *Do not filter* denileukin diftitox during administration

DEXRAZOXANE

Utilized as a Cardioprotectant

Zinecard® (dexrazoxane for injection); product label, June 2012. Distributed by Pharmacia & Upjohn Company, Division of Pfizer Inc., New York, NY
Dexrazoxane for injection; product label, June 2005. Manufactured by Ben Venue Laboratories, Inc., Bedford, OH. Manufactured for Bedford Laboratories, Bedford, OH
DEXRAZOXANE HYDROCHLORIDE; product label, September 2012. Manufactured by Gland Pharma Limited, Hyderabad-500 043, India. Manufactured for Mylan Institutional LLC, Rockford, IL

Product Identification, Preparation, Storage, and Stability

Product and Manufacturer	Dexrazoxane for Injection (generic)		Zinecard® (dexrazoxane for injection) Pharmacia & Upjohn
	Bedford Laboratories™	**Mylan Institutional LLC**	
Product presentation	Dexrazoxane for Injection is packaged in cartons containing two single-use vials: 1. A vial containing sterile, pyrogen-free, lyophilized dexrazoxane HCl equivalent to dexrazoxane 250 mg or dexrazoxane 500 mg 2. A vial containing 0.167 mol/L (0.167 M, 1/6 Molar, M/6) Sodium Lactate Injection, USP, for reconstitution		Zinecard® is packaged in cartons containing sterile, pyrogen-free, lyophilized dexrazoxane HCl equivalent to dexrazoxane 250 mg or dexrazoxane 500 mg
Formulation excipients	Hydrochloric Acid, NF, is added to adjust product pH		
Diluent	• 50 mL Sodium Lactate Injection, USP, 0.167 mol/L is packaged with dexrazoxane for injection 500 mg • 25 mL Sodium Lactate Injection, USP, 0.167 mol/L is packaged with dexrazoxane for injection 250 mg		• Reconstituted *only* with SWFI • Diluent is not included in Zinecard® products
NDC numbers			
500 mg/vial	55390-060-02	67457-208-50	0013-8727-89
250 mg/vial	55390-014-02	67457-207-25	0013-8717-62
Reconstitution	Dexrazoxane for Injection *must be* reconstituted with 0.167 M Sodium Lactate Injection, USP, to produce a solution with a concentration of 10 mg/mL, thus: 	Dexrazoxane Content per Vial	Diluent Volume (0.167 M Sodium Lactate, USP)	Zinecard® *must be* reconstituted with SWFI to produce a solution with a concentration of 10 mg/mL, thus: Dexrazoxane Content per Vial / Diluent Volume (SWFI) 250 mg / 25 mL 500 mg / 50 mL • pH for the reconstituted solution is within the range of 1.0–3.0
	250 mg	25 mL	
	500 mg	50 mL	
	• pH for the reconstituted solution is within the range of 3.5–5.5		
Dilution for clinical use	• The reconstituted solution may be transferred to a parenteral product container and diluted with either 0.9% NS or D5W to a concentration within the range of 1.3–5 mg/mL • All unused dexrazoxane solutions should be discarded		• The reconstituted solution may be transferred to a parenteral product container and diluted *only* with LRI to a concentration within the range of 1.3–3 mg/mL • The resulting solution pH is within the range of 3.5–5.5 • All unused dexrazoxane solutions should be discarded
Storage	• Store intact vials at 20°–25°C (68–77°F)		• Store intact vials at 25°C (77°F) • Temperature excursions are permitted to 15°–30°C (59°–86°F)
Stability	• Dexrazoxane (10 mg/mL) is stable for 6 hours after the time of reconstitution with 0.167 M Sodium Lactate Injection when stored at controlled room temperature, 20°–25°C, or under refrigeration, 2°–8°C (35.6°–46.4°F) • Diluted dexrazoxane is stable for 6 hours when stored at controlled room temperature or under refrigeration		• Dexrazoxane (10 mg/mL) is stable for 30 minutes after reconstitution with SWFI when stored at room temperature, or for up to 3 hours if stored under refrigeration, 2°–8°C (35.6°–46.4°F) • After dilution in LRI, dexrazoxane is stable for 1 hour at controlled room temperature, or for up to 4 hours if stored under refrigeration
Selected incompatibility	• Product labeling recommends *not* mixing dexrazoxane with other drugs		

Recommendations for Dexrazoxane Utilization as a Cardioprotectant

General:

• See Chapter 41 for recommended use in patients with hepatic dysfunction

Administration:

Product Source	Route and Rate of Administration
Bedford Laboratories™	Administer dexrazoxane by slow intraVENous injection *or* a rapid intraVENous infusion over a period of <30 minutes due to the temporal relationship between dexrazoxane and DOXOrubicin administration
Mylan Institutional LLC	
Pharmacia & Upjohn (Zinecard®)	Administer dexrazoxane *only* by intraVENous infusion over a period of <30 minutes

• DOXOrubicin administration must be completed within 30 minutes after dexrazoxane administration began
• Recommended dosage ratios of dexrazoxane to DOXOrubicin:
  ▪ Patients with creatinine clearance ≥40 mL/min (≥0.66 mL/s), dexrazoxane to DOXOrubicin ratio is 10 : 1; eg, 500 mg dexrazoxane/m² : 50 mg DOXOrubicin/m²
  ▪ Patients with creatinine clearance <40 mL/min (<0.66 mL/s), dexrazoxane to DOXOrubicin ratio is 5 : 1; eg, 250 mg dexrazoxane/m² : 50 mg DOXOrubicin/m²

DEXRAZOXANE

Utilized in Treating Anthracycline Extravasation

TOTECT® Kit (dexrazoxane) for injection, for intravenous infusion only; product label, May 2011. Manufactured by Ben Venue Laboratories, Inc., Bedford, OH, and Hameln Pharmaceuticals GmbH, Hameln, Germany. Manufactured for Topotarget A/S, Copenhagen, Denmark. Distributed by Integrated Commercialization Solutions, Brooks, KY. Marketed by Topotarget USA Inc., Rockaway, NJ
Savene 20 mg/mL powder for concentrate and diluent for solution for infusion. Summary of Product Characteristics, August 16, 2011. Last accessed: April 7, 2012, at: http://www.ema.europa.eu. Marketing authorization holder is SpePharm Holding B.V., Amsterdam, The Netherlands

Notes: On April 2, 2013, BIOCODEX USA (San Bruno, CA) announced acquisition of Totect® (at http://www.totect.com/ [accessed January 7, 2014]), and Totect® currently is not available
Norgine BV (Amsterdam, The Netherlands) has acquired the distribution rights of the product portfolio of SpePharm Holding, including Savene® (at: http://www.spepharm.com/ [accessed January 7, 2014])

Product Identification, Preparation, Storage, and Stability

- TOTECT® is packaged as a kit (NDC 38423-110-01) containing twenty 50-mL Type I glass vials, including:

  - 10 single-use vials, each containing 589 mg dexrazoxane hydrochloride (equivalent to 500 mg dexrazoxane) as a lyophilized powder, *plus*

  - 10 Vials each containing 50 mL of sodium lactate injection, USP, 0.167 mol/L (0.167 M, 1/6 M, M/6) diluent for reconstituting dexrazoxane hydrochloride

- Store the unreconstituted product in its carton to protect it from light at 25°C

(77°F). Temperature excursions are permitted to 15°–30°C (59°–86°F)

- Add 50 mL of 0.167 M sodium lactate injection, USP, to each vial of lyophilized dexrazoxane to produce a slightly yellow solution with dexrazoxane concentration of 10 mg/mL

  - The manufacturer recommends using reconstituted dexrazoxane solution within 2 hours after reconstitution

- Dilute the reconstituted product by injecting a volume of dexrazoxane

appropriate for a patient's dose into 1000 mL of 0.9% NS

- After dilution, TOTECT® is stable for 4 hours when stored at temperatures <25°C (<77°F)

- Discard any unused portion of dexrazoxane solutions

Selected incompatibility:

- Product labeling recommends *not* mixing or administering dexrazoxane with any other drugs

Recommendations for Drug Administration and Ancillary Care for Dexrazoxane

Utilized as an Antidote for Anthracycline* Extravasations
General:

- Dexrazoxane dosage should be decreased by 50% in persons whose creatinine clearance is <40 mL/min (<0.66 mL/s)

- Dimethylsulfoxide (DMSO) should not be applied topically to treat anthracycline extravasations in patients who are receiving dexrazoxane

  - Anecdotal clinical reports and experimental evidence in mice indicate concomitant use of topical DMSO at the site of anthracycline extravasation decreases the efficacy of systemically administered dexrazoxane

- Dexrazoxane is a cytotoxic drug and may produce myelosuppression additive to what is expected from antineoplastic treatments

- Reversible increases in liver enzymes (serum AST, ALT, bilirubin) may follow dexrazoxane use

Dosage and administration:

- Cooling packs (if used) should be removed from an extravasation site at least 15 minutes before dexrazoxane administration to improve blood flow to the affected site

  - Vasoconstriction caused by local hypothermia may compromise dexrazoxane distribution to the affected area

- **Dexrazoxane administration must begin within 6 hours** after an extravasation event to be optimally effective

- Administer dexrazoxane via a large-caliber vein:

  Day 1 Dexrazoxane 1000 mg/m² (maximum recommended single

dose = 2000 mg) in 1000 mL of 0.9% NS intraVENously over 1–2 hours, via an administration site not affected by the extravasation

Day 2[†] Dexrazoxane 1000 mg/m² (maximum recommended single dose = 2000 mg) in 1000 mL of 0.9% NS intraVENously over 1–2 hours via an administration site not affected by the extravasation

Day 3[†] Dexrazoxane 500 mg/m² (maximum recommended single dose = 1000 mg) in 1000 mL of 0.9% NS intraVENously over 1–2 hours via an administration site not affected by the extravasation (total dosage/3-day course = 2500 mg/m²; maximum recommended dose/3-day course = 5000 mg)

*Anthracyclines, including DAUNOrubicin, DOXOrubicin, epirubicin, and IDArubicin
[†]Product labeling recommends administering successive 24 hours (±3 hours) after a previously administered dose

DOCETAXEL

[*One- vial formulation*] TAXOTERE® (docetaxel) injection concentrate, intravenous infusion (IV); product label January 2013. sanofi-aventis U.S. LLC, Bridgewater, NJ
[*Two-vial formulation*] TAXOTERE® (docetaxel) injection concentrate, intravenous infusion (IV); product label January 2013. sanofi-aventis U.S. LLC, Bridgewater, NJ
Docetaxel injection, USP, for intravenous infusion only, product label May 2013. Manufactured by Zydus Hospira Oncology Private Ltd., Gujarat, India. Distributed by Hospira, Inc., Lake Forest, IL
Docetaxel injection for intravenous infusion only; product label June 2011. Manufactured for Sandoz, Princeton, NJ. Manufactured by EBEWE Pharma Ges.m.b.H. Nfg.KG, A-4866 Unterach, Austria
DOCEFREZ™ (docetaxel) for injection, intravenous infusion; product label, May 2011. Manufactured by Sun Pharmaceutical Ind. Ltd., Halol-389 350, Gujarat, India. Distributed by Caraco Pharmaceutical Laboratories, Ltd., Detroit, MI

Product-Specific Identification, Storage, and Stability

Product Name (Manufacturer or Distributor)	Product Identification	Product Storage
[*One-vial formulation*] TAXOTERE® (sanofi-aventis U.S. LLC)	[*One-vial formulation*] TAXOTERE® (docetaxel) Injection Concentrate, Intravenous infusion (IV) is a sterile, nonpyrogenic, pale yellow to brownish-yellow, nonaqueous solution in *single-use* vials containing 20 mg DOCEtaxel (anhydrous), 0.54 g polysorbate 80 and 0.395 g dehydrated alcohol solution per milliliter in three presentations: TAXOTERE® (docetaxel) Injection Concentrate 20 mg docetaxel in 1 mL in 50/50 (v/v) ratio polysorbate 80/dehydrated alcohol in a blister pack in 1 carton (NDC 0075-8003-01) *and* TAXOTERE® (docetaxel) injection concentrate 80 mg docetaxel in 4 mL in 50/50 (v/v) ratio polysorbate 80/dehydrated alcohol in a blister pack in 1 carton (NDC 0075-8004-04) *and* TAXOTERE® (docetaxel) Injection Concentrate 160 mg DOCEtaxel in 8 mL of 50/50 (v/v) ratio polysorbate 80 / dehydrated alcohol in a blister pack in one carton (NDC 0075-8005-01)	Store TAXOTERE® vials between 2° and 25°C (35.6° and 77°F) in the original packaging to protect the product from bright light Freezing does not adversely affect the product
[*Two-vial formulation*] TAXOTERE® (sanofi-aventis U.S. LLC)	[*Two-vial formulation*] TAXOTERE® (docetaxel) Injection Concentrate, intravenous infusion (IV) is a sterile, nonpyrogenic, clear, yellow to brownish-yellow, viscous solution in *single-use* vials Each milliliter of TAXOTERE® concentrate contains 40 mg DOCEtaxel (anhydrous) and 1040 mg polysorbate 80 TAXOTERE® injection concentrate *must be diluted twice:* (1) with a sterile, nonpyrogenic, diluent supplied for that purpose, and (2) with 0.9% NS or D5W before it is administered to a patient. The diluent packaged with concentrated TAXOTERE® contains 13% ethanol in water for injection, and is supplied in *single-use* vials Both drug and diluent components are blister packaged together in individual cartons in 1 of 2 presentations: • TAXOTERE® (docetaxel) Injection Concentrate 80 mg docetaxel in 2 mL of polysorbate 80 plus Diluent for TAXOTERE® 80 mg (NDC 0075-8001-80) *and* • TAXOTERE® (docetaxel) Injection Concentrate 20 mg DOCEtaxel in 0.5 mL of polysorbate 80 plus Diluent for TAXOTERE® 20 mg (NDC 0075-8001-20)	
Docetaxel Injection (Hospira, Inc.)	Docetaxel Injection is a sterile, nonpyrogenic, clear, colorless to pale yellow, nonaqueous solution, available in individually packaged vials in a *single-use* formulation: • DOCEtaxel 20 mg/2 mL (NDC 0409-0201-02); and in individually packaged *multi-use* vials in 2 presentations: • DOCEtaxel 80 mg/8 mL (NDC 0409-0201-10) *and* • DOCEtaxel (anhydrous) 160 mg/16 mL (NDC 0409-0201-20) Each milliliter of solution contains 10 mg DOCEtaxel (anhydrous) in 260 mg polysorbate 80, NF; 4 mg citric acid, USP; 23% (v/v) dehydrated alcohol, USP; and PEG 300, NF	Store at 20°–25°C (68°–77°F) in the original packaging carton to protect the product from bright light Freezing does not adversely affect the product. After first use and following multiple needle entries and product withdrawals, DOCEtaxel injection multiuse vials are stable for up to 28 days when stored between 2° and 8°C (35.6° and 46.4°F) and protected from light

(continued)

Product-Specific Identification, Storage, and Stability (*continued*)

Docetaxel Injection (Sandoz)	Docetaxel Injection is a sterile, nonpyrogenic, clear, colorless to pale yellow solution in *multiple dose* vials available in 3 presentations: • DOCEtaxel 20 mg/2 mL (NDC 66758-050-01), • DOCEtaxel 80 mg/8 mL (NDC 66758-050-02), *and* • DOCEtaxel 160 mg/16 mL (NDC 66758-050-03) Each milliliter of solution contains 10 mg DOCEtaxel 275.9 mg alcohol 96% (v/v), 4 mg citric acid, 648 mg polyethylene glycol 300, and 80 mg polysorbate 80	Store intact vials between 2° and 25°C (35.6° and 77°F) in the original packaging to protect from bright light Freezing does not adversely affect the product After initial entry, the multiple dose vials are stable for 28 days when stored between 2° and 8°C (35.6° and 46.4°F) and at room temperature, with or without protection from light
DOCEFREZ™ (Sun Pharmaceutical Ind. Ltd)	DOCEFREZ™ (docetaxel) for injection, intravenous infusion is a sterile, lyophilized, nonpyrogenic, white powder and is available in single-use vials available in 2 presentations: • DOCEtaxel (anhydrous) 20 mg (NDC 47335-285-41) *and* • DOCEtaxel (anhydrous) 80 mg (NDC 47335-286-41) Both product presentations are packaged with a sterile, nonpyrogenic, single-dose vial of diluent solution containing 35.4% (w/w) ethanol in polysorbate 80 in a tray packaged in a single carton	Store DOCEFREZ™ between 2° and 8°C (35.6° and 46.4°F) in the original packaging to protect from bright light

General Guidance

• Do not use plasticized PVC equipment or devices that will come into contact with DOCEtaxel solutions during drug preparation or administration
   ▪ Phthalate plasticizers (including DEHP; di-2-ethylhexyl phthalate) may be leached from PVC containers and administration sets
• Glass, polypropylene, and polyolefin devices and equipment, and containers and tubing with surfaces in contact with drug products composed of those materials are appropriate for use in manipulating, containing, and administering DOCEtaxel solutions and minimize patient exposure to phthalate plasticizers[19]

Product-Specific Preparation and Stability

Preparing the Following Products for Clinical Use:

Docetaxel Injection For Intravenous Infusion Only (Hospira, Inc.), **Docetaxel Injection For Intravenous Infusion Only** (Sandoz, Inc.), and *One-vial formulation* of **TAXOTERE®** (sanofi-aventis U.S. LLC)

• *Do not use* the one-vial formulation of TAXOTERE® with the two-vial formulation of TAXOTERE® (Injection Concentrate and diluent)
• After removing TAXOTERE® (one-vial formulation) from refrigeration, allow the vials to stand at room temperature for approximately 5 minutes before proceeding

Dilute the concentrated drug product:

1. Use only a 21-gauge needle to withdraw the drug product from a vial
   • Larger bore needles (eg, 18- and 19-gauge) may result in stopper coring and introduce particulate matter into the drug product
2. With a calibrated syringe, aseptically withdraw the an amount of concentrated

DOCEtaxel solution required for a patient's dose and transfer it into an appropriate parenteral product bag or bottle containing a volume of either 0.9% NS or D5W sufficient to produce a final DOCEtaxel concentration within the range 0.3–0.74 mg/mL

• *CAUTION: Product concentrations vary among commercial DOCEtaxel injection products:*
   ▪ The generic products from Hospira, Inc. and Sandoz, Inc. contain DOCEtaxel at a concentration of 10 mg/mL
   ▪ The concentration for the single-vial formulation of Taxotere® (sanofi-aventis U.S. LLC) is 2 times greater, that is 20 mg/mL
• Product concentrations *must not exceed* 0.74 mg DOCEtaxel per milliliter
3. Thoroughly mix the admixture by manual rotation and by gently inverting the product container
4. When prepared as described with the one-vial formulation of TAXOTERE® and stored between 2°–25°C (35.6°–77°F),

DOCEtaxel solutions are stable for 6 hours

• Physical and chemical in-use stability of TAXOTERE® (one-vial formulation) when prepared as recommended in non-PVC containers and stored at 2°–8°C has been demonstrated for up to 48 hours

Caution: Product labeling for the *one-vial formulation* of TAXOTERE® (only) includes a warning about product stability after dilution:

   ▪ TAXOTERE® infusion solution produced with the *one-vial formulation* (a solution diluted for administration to patients) is supersaturated; therefore, over time, crystals may appear in solution
   ▪ Solutions in which crystals or particulate matter appear should not be used but should be discarded
   ▪ A similar warning does not appear in product labeling for other DOCEtaxel products identified in this section

Preparing the *2-vial formulation* of TAXOTERE® (sanofi-aventis U.S. LLC)

• *Do not use* the 2-vial formulation (injection concentrate and diluent) with the 1-vial formulation

(*continued*)

Product-Specific Preparation and Stability (*continued*)

Prepare an initial dilution:

1. After removing TAXOTERE® and diluent vials from refrigeration, allow them to stand at room temperature for approximately 5 minutes before proceeding

2. Use only a 21-gauge needle to withdraw the drug product from a vial because larger-bore needles (eg, 18- and 19-gauge) may result in stopper coring and introduce particulate matter into the drug product

3. Aseptically withdraw the entire contents of an appropriate diluent vial (approximately 1.8 mL for Taxotere 20 mg and approximately 7.1 mL for Taxotere 80 mg) into a syringe by partially inverting the vial, and transfer the solution to the vial of TAXOTERE® concentrate with which it was co-packaged to produce an initially diluted solution containing 10 mg DOCEtaxel/mL

   - *CAUTION: Product concentrations vary among commercial docetaxel injection products:*
     - After initial dilution, the concentration of the 2-vial formulation of TAXOTERE® (sanofi-aventis U.S. LLC) is 10 mg/mL
     - In contrast, the concentration for the single-vial formulation of TAXOTERE® is 2 times greater, that is, 20 mg/mL

4. *Do not shake* the vials. Mix the initially diluted solution by repeatedly inverting for at least 45 seconds the Taxotere concentrate vials into which the ethanol-in-water diluent was injected

5. The initially diluted TAXOTERE® solution should be clear; however, there may be some foam on top of the solution caused by polysorbate 80. If foam is present, allow the vials to stand for a few minutes to allow any foam to dissipate. It is not necessary to wait for all foam to dissipate before continuing preparation

   - The initially diluted solution may be used immediately or stored under refrigeration or at room temperature for a maximum of 8 hours

Prepare a final dilution for administration to patients:

1. With a calibrated syringe, aseptically withdraw an amount of initially diluted TAXOTERE® solution (10 mg/mL) required for a patient's dose and transfer it into an appropriate parenteral product bag or bottle containing a volume of either 0.9% NS or D5W sufficient to produce a final DOCEtaxel concentration within the range, 0.3–0.74 mg/mL

   - Product concentrations *must not exceed* concentrations >0.74 mg docetaxel/mL

2. Thoroughly mix the infusion by manual rotation and by gently inverting the product container

3. When prepared as described with the two-vial formulation of DOCEtaxel and stored between 2° and 25°C (35.6° and 77°F), DOCEtaxel solutions are stable for 4 hours

Preparing DOCEFREZ™ (Sun Pharmaceutical Ind. Ltd)

Reconstitute the lyophilized drug product:

1. After removing DOCEFREZ™ and diluent from refrigeration, allow the drug product and diluent (35.4% ethanol in polysorbate 80) vials to stand at room temperature for approximately 5 minutes before proceeding

2. With a syringe, aseptically withdraw and transfer a volume of diluent solution appropriate for the amount of drug product used

DOCEFREZ™ Vial Content	Volume of Diluent Needed for Reconstitution
20 mg	1 mL
80 mg	4 mL

3. Shake the drug product vials well to completely dissolve the lyophilized drug

   CAUTION: The concentration of reconstituted Docefrez is not the same for the 20- and 80-mg products:

DOCEFREZ™ Vial Content	DOCEtaxel Concentration after Reconstitution
20-mg vials	25 mg/mL (20 mg in 0.8 mL)
80-mg vials	24 mg/mL

4. If air bubbles are present in the drug product after solubilization is complete, allow the solution to stand for a few minutes to allow suspended air bubbles to dissipate

5. The reconstituted solution may be used immediately or stored either in under refrigeration or at room temperature for a maximum of 8 hours

Prepare a final dilution for infusion:

1. Aseptically withdraw an amount of DOCEFREZ™ required for a patient's dose with a calibrated syringe and transfer it into an appropriate parenteral product bag or bottle containing a volume of either 0.9% NS or D5W sufficient to produce a final DOCEtaxel concentration within the range, 0.3–0.74 mg/mL

2. Product concentrations *must not exceed* 0.74 mg docetaxel/mL

3. Thoroughly mix the infusion by manual rotation and by gently inverting the product container

   - When prepared as described and stored between 2° and 25°C (35.6° and 77°F), DOCEtaxel solutions are stable for 4 hours

Recommendations for Drug Administration and Ancillary Care

Premedication:

- See Chapter 41 for recommended use in patients with renal and hepatic dysfunction
- FDA-approved product labeling recommends that all patients who are treated with DOCEtaxel should receive a steroid before, during, and after DOCEtaxel administration to reduce the incidence and severity of fluid retention and the severity of hypersensitivity reactions
  - For patients with hormone-refractory metastatic prostate cancer already receiving predniSONE concurrently:
    - **Dexamethasone** 8 mg/dose for 3 doses, at 12 hours, 3 hours, and 1 hour before DOCEtaxel administration
  - Other patients:
    - **Dexamethasone** 8 mg orally twice daily for 3 days (6 doses), starting 1 day before DOCEtaxel administration

General:

- Visually inspect the infusion product for particulate matter or discoloration prior to administration. All DOCEtaxel-containing solutions that are not clear or appear to contain a precipitate should be discarded
- When prepared as described to a concentration within the range of range 0.3–0.74 mg/mL and stored between 2°–25°C (35.6°–77°F), DOCEtaxel solutions are stable as follows:

Product (Manufacturer)	Duration of Stability*
TAXOTERE® one-vial formulation (sanofi-aventis U.S. LLC)	6 hours
DOCEtaxel injection (Hospira, Inc.)	4 hours
DOCEtaxel injection (Sandoz, Inc.)	
TAXOTERE® two-vial formulation (sanofi-aventis U.S. LLC)	
DOCEFREZ® (Sun Pharmaceutical Ind. Ltd)	

*Includes an administration duration of 60 minutes

- Administer DOCEtaxel by intraVENous infusion over one hour at ambient room temperature (<25°C; <77°F) and lighting conditions
- To minimize patient exposure to phthalate plasticizers (eg, DEHP), which may be leached from PVC containers and administration sets:
  - Administer DOCEtaxel *only* through polyethylene-lined administration sets

Potential drug interactions:

- DOCEtaxel is a substrate for metabolism by CYP3A4 and for extracellular transport by P-glycoprotein (MDR1, ABCB1)
  - Avoid concomitant use of DOCEtaxel with potent inhibitors and inducers of CYP3A subfamily enzymes and P-glycoprotein

Hypersensitivity reactions:

- Patients should be observed closely for hypersensitivity reactions, especially during the first and second infusions
  - Hypersensitivity reactions may occur within a few minutes after initiating DOCEtaxel administration
- Severe hypersensitivity reactions characterized by generalized rash/erythema, hypotension and/or bronchospasm, or very rarely fatal anaphylaxis, have been reported in patients who received steroid premedication
  - Severe hypersensitivity reactions require immediate discontinuation of the DOCEtaxel administration and aggressive supportive therapy
  - Patients with a history of severe hypersensitivity reactions should not be rechallenged with DOCEtaxel
- Minor events, including flushing, rash with or without pruritus, chest tightness, back pain, dyspnea, drug fever, or chills, have been reported and resolved after discontinuing DOCEtaxel administration and instituting appropriate therapy
- Treatment interruption is not required for minor reactions such as flushing or localized skin reactions

DOXORUBICIN HYDROCHLORIDE

ADRIAMYCIN® (DOXOrubicin HCl) for injection, USP, and ADRIAMYCIN® (DOXOrubicin HCl) injection, USP, for intravenous use only; product label, April 2012. Manufactured by Bedford Laboratories, Bedford, OH

DOXORUBICIN HYDROCHLORIDE–doxorubicin hydrochloride injection; product label, September 2011. Teva Parenteral Medicines, Inc., Irvine CA

Doxorubicin Hydrochloride Injection, USP (For IV Use Only); product label, January 2013. Made in India. Manufactured for SAGENT Pharmaceuticals, Schaumburg, IL

WARNING

1. Severe local tissue necrosis will occur if there is extravasation during administration... Doxorubicin must not be given by the intramuscular or subcutaneous route

2. Myocardial toxicity manifested in its most severe form by potentially fatal congestive heart failure (CHF) may occur either during therapy or months to years after termination of therapy. The probability of developing impaired myocardial function based on a combined index of signs, symptoms, and decline in left ventricular ejection fraction (LVEF) is estimated to be 1 to 2% at a total cumulative dose of 300 mg/m^2 of doxorubicin, 3 to 5% at a dose of 400 mg/m^2, 5 to 8% at 450 mg/m^2 and 6 to 20% at 500 mg/m^2. The risk of developing CHF increases rapidly with increasing total cumulative doses of doxorubicin in excess of 400 mg/m^2. Risk factors (active or dormant cardiovascular disease, prior [*or* previous] or concomitant radiotherapy to the mediastinal/pericardial area, previous therapy with other anthracyclines or anthracenediones, concomitant use of other cardiotoxic drugs) may increase the risk of cardiac toxicity. Cardiac toxicity with doxorubicin may occur at lower cumulative doses whether or not cardiac risk factors are present. Pediatric patients are at increased risk for developing delayed cardiotoxicity

3. Secondary acute myelogenous leukemia (AML) or myelodysplastic syndrome (MDS) have been reported in patients treated with anthracyclines, including doxorubicin... The occurrence of refractory secondary AML or MDS is more common when anthracyclines are given in combination with DNA-damaging anti-neoplastic agents or radiotherapy, when patients have been heavily pretreated with cytotoxic drugs, or when doses of anthracyclines have been escalated. The rate of developing secondary AML or MDS has been estimated in an analysis of 8563 patients with early breast cancer treated in 6 studies conducted by the National Surgical Adjuvant Breast and Bowel Project (NSABP), including NSABP B-15. Patients in these studies received standard doses of doxorubicin and standard or escalated doses of cyclophosphamide (AC) adjuvant chemotherapy and were followed for 61,810 patient years. Among 4483 such patients who received conventional doses of AC, 11 cases of AML or MDS were identified, for an incidence of 0.32 cases per 1000 patient years (95% CI 0.16 to 0.57) and a cumulative incidence at 5 years of 0.21% (95% CI 0.11 to 0.41%). In another analysis of 1474 patients with breast cancer who received adjuvant treatment with doxorubicin-containing regimens in clinical trials conducted at University of Texas M.D. Anderson Cancer Center, the incidence was estimated at 1.5% at 10 years. In both experiences, patients who received regimens with higher cyclophosphamide dosages, who received radiotherapy, or who were aged 50 or older had an increased risk of secondary AML or MDS. Pediatric patients are also at risk of developing secondary AML

4. Dosage should be reduced in patients with impaired hepatic function

5. Severe myelosuppression may occur

6. Doxorubicin should be administered only under the supervision of a physician who is experienced in the use of cancer chemotherapeutic agents

Boxed Warning (excerpt) for "ADRIAMYCIN® (DOXOrubicin HCl) for Injection, USP, ADRIAMYCIN® (DOXOrubicin HCl) Injection, USP, For Intravenous Use Only"; April 2012 product label; Bedford Laboratories™, Bedford, OH, and "Doxorubicin Hydrochloride Injection, USP (For IV Use Only)"; January 2013 product label. SAGENT Pharmaceuticals, Schaumburg, IL

Product Identification, Preparation, Storage, and Stability

• **DOXOrubicin Hydrochloride for Injection, USP** (ADRIAMYCIN® for injection, USP; Bedford Laboratories), is a sterile, red-orange, lyophilized powder packaged in single-dose vials as follows:

Content DOXOrubicin HCl	No. Vials/Package Unit	NDC No.
10 mg/vial	Carton of 10 vials	55390-231-10
20 mg/vial	Carton of 10 vials	55390-232-10
50 mg/vial	Individually boxed	55390-233-01

▪ Store intact vials (unreconstituted drug product) at controlled room temperature, 15°–30°C (59°–86°F) in the packaging carton to protect them from light

(continued)

Product Identification, Preparation, Storage, and Stability (continued)

- Reconstitute the lyophilized powder with 0.9% NS as follows to produce a final concentration of 2 mg DOXOrubicin HCl/mL:

DOXOrubicin HCl Content per Vial	Diluent Volume
10 mg	5 mL
20 mg	10 mL
50 mg	25 mL

- After adding the diluent, vials should be shaken and the contents allowed to dissolve
- After initially entering a sealed vial, DOXOrubicin solution is stable for 7 days at room temperature and under normal room light (100 foot-candles) and for 15 days at 2°–8°C (35.6°–46.4°F). Protect DOXOrubicin from exposure to sunlight. Promptly discard partially used vials
- One-hundred, twenty-four days after reconstitution to a concentration of 2 mg/mL and storage in the manufacturer's original glass vials at 4°C (39.2°F) and 23°C (73.4°F) DOXOrubicin retained >90% of its initial concentration, remained clear, and had exhibited no changes in pH or absorbance by ultraviolet-visible spectrophotometry[39]
  - ○ Mass balance analysis indicated approximately 3.5% of DOXOrubicin stored at 23°C and about 1% stored at 4°C had degraded at 124 days after reconstitution[39]
- Protect DOXOrubicin from exposure to sunlight. Promptly discard partially used vials
- **DOXOrubicin hydrochloride injection, USP**, is available from several manufacturers. The products contain a red-orange, sterile, isotonic solution with a concentration of 2 mg DOXOrubicin HCl/mL. Products may be packaged individually or are sold in cartons containing multiple vials:

DOXOrubicin HCl Content
10 mg in 5 mL, single-dose vials
20 mg in 10 mL, single-dose vials
50 mg in 25 mL, single-dose vials
150 mg in 75 mL, multiple-dose vials
200 mg in 100 mL, multiple-dose vials

- Store vials under refrigeration at 2°–8°C (35.6°–46.4°F) in their packaging carton to protect them from light
  - ○ Storage of DOXOrubicin HCl solution for injection under refrigeration can result in the formation of a gelled product. The gelled product will return to a slightly viscous to mobile solution after 2 hours to a maximum of 4 hours equilibration at controlled room temperature 15°–30°C (59°–86°F)
  - ○ After preparing a single dose, discard any unused portion of products formulated for a single use
  - ○ Unused solution remaining in multidose containers should be discarded after the recommended storage times
- DOXOrubicin HCl Injection (2 mg/mL), and DOXOrubicin HCl for Injection after reconstitution (2 mg/mL), are suitable for intraVENous injection but may also be diluted for administration to patients
  - Dilution in 0.9% NS, D5W, or LRI to concentrations as low as 0.01 mg/mL results in products stable for at least 24 hours when stored at room temperature under fluorescent lighting or in the dark
    - ○ DOXOrubicin stability is inversely related to solution concentration

Recommendations for Drug Administration and Ancillary Care

General:

- See Chapter 41 for recommended use in patients with hepatic dysfunction
- Administer DOXOrubicin by slow intraVENous injection into the tubing of a freely running intraVENous infusion of 0.9% NS or D5W. The tubing should be attached to a needle or cannula inserted preferably into a large vein. If possible, avoid veins over joints and in extremities with compromised venous or lymphatic drainage
- The rate of administration is dependent on vein size and DOXOrubicin dosage, but a dose should be administered over not less than 3–5 minutes
- *Caution*: DOXOrubicin is a powerful vesicant and can produce severe local soft tissue necrosis if extravasation occurs. DOXOrubicin *must not be given* by the intraMUSCular, SUBCUTaneous, or intraTHECAL routes
  - The current standard of care for managing anthracycline extravasation, including extravasation of DOXOrubicin, is a 3-day course of intraVENously administered dexrazoxane (Totect®, Savene®)
- Erythematous streaking along a vein as well as facial flushing may indicate an administration rate that is too rapid. Burning or stinging sensations may be indicative of perivenous infiltration and the infusion should be immediately terminated, and, if resumed, restarted in another vein. Extravasation also may occur painlessly

Inadvertent exposure:

- DOXOrubicin HCl spills and leaks on environmental surfaces should be treated with dilute sodium hypochlorite (1% available chlorine) solution, preferably by soaking, and then rinsing with water
- In case of skin contact, thoroughly wash the affected area with soap and water or sodium bicarbonate solution. *Do not abrade* the skin by using a scrub brush
- Treat accidental contact with the eyes immediately by copious lavage with water

(continued)

Product Identification, Preparation, Storage, and Stability (*continued*)

- DOXOrubicin has been shown to adsorb to PVC containers
  - The proportion of a dose lost to sorption may be expected to vary inversely with the surface area of a container with which the drug is in contact
  - The concentration of DOXOrubicin diluted with 0.9% NS (estimated concentration, 95.2 μg/mL) stored in 100-mL-capacity PVC containers at 4°C was shown to decrease over a period of 8 days, possibly representing initial adsorption to container surfaces followed by a protracted absorption and migration into the container matrix before equilibration was achieved, or adsorption of DOXOrubicin degradation products to container surfaces similar to the parent compound[37]
    - Loss of DOXOrubicin due to adsorption was [1] greater from solutions in which the vehicle solution was 0.9% NS in comparison with D5W, and [2] greatest at higher storage temperatures (25°C > 4°C > –20°C), and [3] greater at solution pH of 5.20 and 6.47 (0.9% NS) than at pH of 4.36 (D5W) at all temperatures conditions evaluated
- DOXOrubicin HCl solutions (estimated concentration, 95.2 μg/mL) stored in PVC containers at 25°C, 4°C, or –20°C was more stable at more acidic solution pH under the conditions of pH evaluated (4.36, 5.20, and 6.47)[37]
- DOXOrubicin HCl for injection reconstituted with SWFI and diluted with 0.9% NS or D5W to an estimated concentration of 95.2 μg/mL stored in PVC containers for 43 days did not degrade during or after 11 repeated cycles of freezing (–20°C) and thawing at ambient temperature (25°C)[37]
- DOXOrubicin HCl for injection reconstituted with SWFI to a concentration of 2 mg/mL was stable for at least 43 days when stored in polypropylene syringes at 4°C[37]
- DOXOrubicin solutions undergo photodegradation
  - The rate and extent of photodegradation are inversely related to DOXOrubicin concentrations in solution[38] and directly related to solution pH (rate of degradation increases at pH >5.0)[37]
  - At DOXOrubicin concentrations ≥100 μg/mL (≥0.1 mg/mL) stored at 25°C for 168 h under artificial room lighting (four 65/80-Watt fluorescent tubes mounted approximately 1 m above the samples), little or no photodegradation occurred in clear or amber glass or opaque polyethylene containers[38]
    - A 10-fold difference in lability to photodegradation was demonstrated for DOXOrubicin at a concentration of 0.01 mg/mL than a concentration of 0.1 mg/mL
  - At DOXOrubicin concentrations ≥500 μg/mL (0.5 mg/mL), no special precautions are necessary to protect freshly prepared solutions from exposure to artificial light or sunlight[38]

Selected incompatibility:

- Antimicrobially preserved diluents are not recommended for use in reconstituting DOXOrubicin for injection (lyophilized powder formulations)
- *Do not mix* DOXOrubicin with heparin or fluorouracil. The admixtures are incompatible and will precipitate
- *Do not mix* DOXOrubicin with alkaline solutions (eg, solutions containing sodium bicarbonate), which may cause hydrolytic degradation of DOXOrubicin

DOXORUBICIN HYDROCHLORIDE LIPOSOME INJECTION

DOXIL® (doxorubicin HCl liposome injection) for intravenous infusion; product label, March 2013. Manufactured by Ben Venue Laboratories, Inc., Bedford, OH. Manufactured for Janssen Products, LP, Horsham, PA
Doxorubicin Hydrochloride Liposome Injection for intravenous infusion; product label, September 2012. Manufactured by Sun Pharmaceutical Ind. Ltd., Gujarat, India. Distributed by Caraco Pharmaceutical Laboratories, Ltd., Detroit, MI

WARNING: INFUSION REACTIONS, MYELOSUPPRESSION, CARDIOTOXICITY, LIVER IMPAIRMENT, ACCIDENTAL SUBSTITUTION

1. The use of [doxorubicin hydrochloride liposome injection] may lead to cardiac toxicity. Myocardial damage may lead to congestive heart failure and may occur as the total cumulative dose of doxorubicin HCl approaches 550 mg/m^2. In a clinical study in patients with advanced breast cancer, 250 patients received [doxorubicin hydrochloride liposome injection] …at a starting dose of 50 mg/m^2 every 4 weeks. At all cumulative anthracycline doses between $450–500 \text{ mg/m}^2$ or between $500–550 \text{ mg/m}^2$, the risk of cardiac toxicity for patients treated with [doxorubicin hydrochloride liposome injection] …was 11%. Prior use of other anthracyclines or anthracenediones should be included in calculations of total cumulative dosage. Cardiac toxicity may also occur at lower cumulative doses in patients with prior mediastinal irradiation or who are receiving concurrent cyclophosphamide therapy…

2. Acute infusion-related reactions including, but not limited to, flushing, shortness of breath, facial swelling, headache, chills, back pain, tightness in the chest or throat, and/or hypotension have occurred in up to 10% of patients treated with… [doxorubicin hydrochloride liposome injection]. In most patients, these reactions resolve over the course of several hours to a day once the infusion is terminated. In some patients, the reaction has resolved with slowing of the infusion rate. Serious and sometimes life-threatening or fatal allergic/anaphylactoid-like infusion reactions have been reported. Medications to treat such reactions, as well as emergency equipment, should be available for immediate use. [Doxorubicin hydrochloride liposome injection doses >60 mg] …should be administered at an initial rate of 1 mg/min to minimize the risk of infusion reactions…

3. Severe myelosuppression may occur…

4. Dosage should be reduced in patients with impaired hepatic function…

5. Accidental substitution of [doxorubicin hydrochloride liposome injection] …for doxorubicin HCl has resulted in severe side effects. [Doxorubicin hydrochloride liposome injection] …should not be substituted for doxorubicin HCl on a mg per mg basis…

Boxed Warning (excerpts) from "DOXIL® (doxorubicin HCl liposome injection) for intravenous infusion"; March 2013 product label; Janssen Products, LP, Horsham, PA, and "Doxorubicin Hydrochloride Liposome Injection for intravenous infusion"; September 2012 product label. Caraco Pharmaceutical Laboratories, Ltd., Detroit, MI

Product Identification, Preparation, Storage, and Stability

Characteristics common to both products:

- Both products contain DOXOrubicin HCl, >90% of which is encapsulated in a proprietary liposome carrier
  - Both products are sometimes referred to as liposomal DOXOrubicin and "PEGylated DOXOrubicin", because the microscopic liposomes in which DOXOrubicin is encapsulated are formulated with surface-bound methoxypolyethylene glycol, which protects the liposomes from detection by the mononuclear phagocyte system and increases the circulation time in blood
- DOXOrubicin HCl liposome injection is a translucent, red, liposomal dispersion; it is neither clear nor a solution
- Store unopened vials at 2°–8°C (35.6°–46.4°F)
  - DOXOrubicin HCl liposome injection does not contain an antimicrobial preservatives or bacteriostatic agents
- Avoid freezing DOXOrubicin HCl liposome injection. Prolonged freezing may adversely affect liposomal drug products
  - Freezing for periods <1 month does not appear to adversely affect DOXOrubicin HCl liposome injection
- Dilute DOXOrubicin HCl liposome injection with D5W before administration as follows:

Note: Do not dilute DOXOrubicin HCl liposome injection with any solution other than D5W

Dose to Administer	Volume of D5W for Dilution
≤90 mg	250 mL
>90 mg	500 mL

- After dilution, the products will not clarify, but remain a translucent, red, liposomal dispersion
- After dilution, liposomal DOXOrubicin should be refrigerated (2°–8°C) and used within 24 hours
- *Do not filter* liposomal DOXOrubicin either before or after dilution

DOXIL®:

- Available products include six, individually packaged, vials containing DOXOrubicin HCl at a concentration of 2 mg/mL. Two presentations are available:
  - 20 mg DOXOrubicin HCl/10 mL in 10-mL (capacity) glass, single-use vials (NDC 59676-960-01), and
  - 50 mg DOXOrubicin HCl/25 mL in 30-mL (capacity) glass, single-use vials (NDC 59676-960-02)

(generic) DOXOrubicin Hydrochloride Liposome Injection:

- DOXOrubicin hydrochloride liposome injection is provided as a sterile, translucent, red, liposomal dispersion in individually cartoned, 10- or 30-mL capacity, glass, single-use vials
- Each vial contains DOXOrubicin hydrochloride, USP at a concentration of 2 mg/mL in two presentations:

(continued)

Product Identification, Preparation, Storage, and Stability (*continued*)

- DOXOrubicin HCl 20 mg in 10 mL; NDC 47335-049-40
- DOXOrubicin HCl 50 mg in 25 mL; NDC 47335-050-40

Characteristics and excipients common to both products:

- Each milliliter of both products also contains ammonium sulfate (approximately) 2 mg, histidine as a buffer, sucrose to maintain isotonicity, and hydrochloric acid and/or sodium hydroxide to maintain a pH of 6.5
- The pegylated liposome carriers are composed of cholesterol 3.19 mg/mL, fully hydrogenated soy phosphatidylcholine (HSPC) 9.58 mg/mL, and *N*-(carbonyl-methoxypolyethylene glycol 2000)-1,2-distearoyl-sn-glycero-3-phosphoethanolamine sodium salt (MPEG-DSPE) 3.19 mg/mL

Selected incompatibilities (both products):

- *Do not mix* liposomal DOXOrubicin with other drugs
- *Do not mix* liposomal DOXOrubicin with solutions that contain a bacteriostatic agent, such as benzyl alcohol

Recommendations for Drug Administration and Ancillary Care

General:

- See Chapter 41 for recommended use in patients with hepatic dysfunction
- Liposomal DOXOrubicin must be diluted before administration
- Administer liposomal DOXOrubicin by intraVENous infusion:
  - Give doses ≤60 mg over 60 minutes
  - Doses >60 mg should initially be administered no more rapidly than 1 mg/minute (60 mg/hour) to minimize the risk of adverse reactions during infusion
  - If no reactions are observed, the delivery rate may be increased to complete administration over one hour
  - Infusion reactions may respond to slowing the rate of administration or temporarily interrupting treatment, and resuming administration at a slower rate after signs and symptoms abate
    - Infusion-related adverse events have included life-threatening and fatal allergic or anaphylactoid reactions
    - Infusion-related adverse events have included one or more of the following:
      - Flushing, shortness of breath, facial swelling, headache, chills, chest pain, back pain, chest and throat tightness, fever, tachycardia, pruritus, rash, cyanosis, syncope, bronchospasm, asthma, apnea, hypotension
- *Do not filter* liposomal DOXOrubicin during administration
- *Do not rapidly flush* an administration set used to administer liposomal DOXOrubicin to complete drug delivery
  - Utilize a technique to empty an administration set containing liposomal DOXOrubicin that will not substantially increase the rate at which the dose was being administered
- *Caution*: liposomal DOXOrubicin has been associated with vesicant reactions after extravasation and may produce severe local necrosis if infiltration into soft tissues occurs[40]
  - Extravasation may occur during intravenous administration with or without an accompanying stinging or burning sensation, and in spite of easy blood aspiration (good blood return) from the vascular access device through which liposomal DOXOrubicin is administered
  - If signs or symptoms of extravasation occur during liposomal DOXOrubicin administration, the infusion should be immediately discontinued at the affected access site, but may be restarted in another vein
    - Liposomal DOXOrubicin *must never be given* by the intraMUSCular or SUBCUTaneous routes

Note:
- Advise patients that liposomal DOXOrubicin after treatment may impart a reddish-orange color to urine and other body fluids; a nontoxic reaction due to the color of the product that will dissipate as the drug is eliminated from the body

EPIRUBICIN HYDROCHLORIDE

ELLENCE® (epirubicin hydrochloride injection); product label, February 2013. Distributed by Pharmacia & Upjohn Co., Division of Pfizer Inc., New York, NY
EPIRUBICIN HYDROCHLORIDE—epirubicin hydrochloride injection, solution; product label, February 2013. Teva Parenteral Medicines, Inc., Irvine, CA
Epirubicin Hydrochloride injection; product label, January 2012. Product of Australia. Hospira, Inc., Lake Forest, IL
Epirubicin Hydrochloride for injection; product label, November 2007. Hospira, Inc., Lake Forest, IL

WARNING: RISK OF TISSUE NECROSIS, CARDIAC TOXICITY, SECONDARY ACUTE MYELOGENOUS LEUKEMIA, AND MYELOSUPPRESSION

1. Severe local tissue necrosis will occur if there is extravasation during administration. ELLENCE must not be given by the intramuscular or subcutaneous route…

2. Cardiac toxicity, including fatal congestive heart failure (CHF), may occur either during therapy with ELLENCE or months to years after termination of therapy. The probability of developing clinically evident CHF is estimated as approximately 0.9% at a cumulative dose of 550 mg/m², 1.6% at 700 mg/m², and 3.3% at 900 mg/m². In the adjuvant treatment of breast cancer, the maximum cumulative dose used in clinical trials was 720 mg/m². The risk of developing CHF increases rapidly with increasing total cumulative doses of ELLENCE in excess of 900 mg/m²; this cumulative dose should only be exceeded with extreme caution. Active or dormant cardiovascular disease, prior or concomitant radiotherapy to the mediastinal/pericardial area, previous therapy with other anthracyclines or anthracenediones, or concomitant use of other cardiotoxic drugs may increase the risk of cardiac toxicity. Cardiac toxicity with ELLENCE may occur at lower cumulative doses whether or not cardiac risk factors are present…

3. Secondary acute myelogenous leukemia (AML) has been reported in patients with breast cancer treated with anthracyclines, including epirubicin. The occurrence of refractory secondary leukemia is more common when such drugs are given in combination with DNA-damaging antineoplastic agents, when patients have been heavily pretreated with cytotoxic drugs, or when doses of anthracyclines have been escalated. The cumulative risk of developing treatment-related AML or myelodysplastic syndrome (MDS), in 7110 patients with breast cancer who received adjuvant treatment with ELLENCE-containing regimens, was estimated as 0.27% at 3 years, 0.46% at 5 years, and 0.55% at 8 years…

4. Severe myelosuppression may occur…

Boxed Warning (excerpt) from "ELLENCE® (epirubicin hydrochloride injection)"; February 2013 product label; Pharmacia & Upjohn Co., Division of Pfizer Inc., New York, NY

Product Identification, Preparation, Storage, and Stability

- **Epirubicin HCl injection** is available in individually packaged single-use vials containing a sterile, preservative-free, ready-to-use, clear, red solution containing 2 mg epirubicin hydrochloride/mL
  - Product presentations vary among manufacturers, but include vials containing 10 mg, 50 mg, 150 mg, and 200 mg epirubicin HCl
    - Inactive ingredients include sodium chloride, USP, and SWFI. Product pH is adjusted to 3.0 with hydrochloric acid, NF
- Store unopened vials under refrigeration between 2° and 8°C (35.6° and 46.4°F), but *do not freeze* epirubicin
  - Storage at refrigerated temperatures can result in the formation of a gelled product, which will return to a slightly viscous to mobile solution after 2 hours to a maximum of 4 hours equilibration at controlled room temperature (15°–25°C [59°–77°F])
- **Epirubicin Hydrochloride for injection** is a sterile, orange-red, lyophilized powder in single-use vials containing 50 mg or 200 mg of epirubicin hydrochloride
  - Each 50-mg and 200-mg vial also contains 250 mg and 1000 mg of lactose, respectively

- Epirubicin HCl for injection must be reconstituted prior to use with SWFI, resulting in a solution concentration of 2 mg/mL with a pH of 4.7 to 5.0

Epirubicin HCl Content per Vial	Diluent Volume
50 mg	25 mL
200 mg	100 mL

- Shake vials vigorously to aid dissolution
  - It may take up to 4 minutes for epirubicin hydrochloride to completely dissolve
  - The manufacturers' product labeling indicates reconstituted solutions are stable for 24 hours when stored at 2°–8°C (35.6–46.4°F) and protected from light, or 25°C (77°F) under normal lighting conditions
  - Epirubicin HCL for injection may be further diluted with sterile water for injection, USP
    - Epirubicin HCl for injection reconstituted with 0.9% NS to a concentration of 2 mg/mL stored in polypropylene syringes at either 4°C and protected from light exposure or stored at 25°C and either protected from light

or under illumination (~50 lumens/m²) was stable for 14 days at 25 ± 1°C (77° ± 1.8°F) and for 180 days at 4 ± 1°C (39.2° ± 1.8°F)[41]

  - Epirubicin HCl for injection reconstituted with SWFI to a concentration of 2 mg/mL was stable for at least 43 days when stored in polypropylene syringes at 4°C[37]
  - Epirubicin HCl for injection reconstituted with SWFI and diluted with D5W or 0.9% NS (to pH = 4.36 or 5.20, respectively) was stable for up to 43 days when stored in PVC containers at 25°C, 4°C, or –20°C (–4°F)[37]
    - Epirubicin HCl solutions (estimated concentration, 95.2 μg/mL) stored in PVC containers was more stable at more acidic solution pH under the conditions of pH evaluated (4.36, 5.20, and 6.47)
    - A significant loss in potency (≥10%) occurred at 20 days for epirubicin HCl admixtures in 0.9% NS (pH = 6.47) stored in PVC at 25°C, but not for epirubicin admixtures in 0.9% NS (pH = 5.20) stored in PVC at 25°C
  - Epirubicin HCl for injection reconstituted with SWFI and diluted

(continued)

Product Identification, Preparation, Storage, and Stability (*continued*)

with 0.9% NS or D5W to an estimated concentration of 95.2 µg/mL stored in PVC containers for 43 days did not degrade during or after 11 repeated cycles of freezing (–20°C) and thawing at ambient temperature (25°C)

- ○ Adsorption of epirubicin (diluted in D5W or 0.9% NS to a concentration of ~95.2 mg/mL) to PVC container surfaces during the 8 days after admixture preparation correlated inversely with solution pH (4.36 < 5.20 < 6.47) and directly with storage temperatures (25°C > 4°C > –20°C)[37]
  - ▫ Drug loss from PVC mini-bags appeared to be due to a combination of epirubicin degradation and adsorption to container surfaces

- Epirubicin solutions undergo photodegradation
  - ○ The rate and extent of photodegradation are inversely related to epirubicin concentrations in solution[38] and directly related to solution pH (rate of degradation increases at pH >5.0)[37]
  - ○ At epirubicin concentrations ≥100 µg/mL (≥0.1 mg/mL) stored at 25°C for 168 h under artificial room lighting (four 65/80-Watt fluorescent tubes mounted approximately 1 m above the samples), little or no photodegradation occurred in clear or amber glass or opaque polyethylene containers[38]
  - ○ At epirubicin concentrations ≥500 µg/mL (0.5 mg/mL), no special precautions are necessary to protect

freshly prepared solutions from exposure to artificial light or sunlight[38]

- Epirubicin HCl solution is suitable for direct intraVENous administration
- Use epirubicin HCl solution within 24 hours after first penetrating vial stoppers
- Discard partially used vials after dose preparation

Selected incompatibility:

- *Do not mix* epirubicin with other drugs in the same container
- Epirubicin is most stable at pH 4–5, and hydrolyzes spontaneously at alkaline pH
- Epirubicin is chemically incompatible with heparin and fluorouracil

Recommendations for Drug Administration and Ancillary Care

General:

- See Chapter 41 for recommended use in patients with renal and hepatic dysfunction
- Administer epirubicin by slow intraVENous injection into the tubing of a freely running intraVENous infusion of 0.9% NS or D5W over 3–20 minutes, depending on the dosage to be given and vein size
- Initial therapy within a dosage range of 100–120 mg/m² should generally be administered over 15–20 minutes
  - The administration time may be proportionally decreased, for lesser dosages, but SHOULD NOT BE <3 minutes
- Do *not* inject epirubicin directly into a vein because of the risk of extravasation, which may occur even in the presence of adequate blood return during aspiration. Venous sclerosis may result from injection into small vessels or repeated injections into the same vein
- Avoid administration into veins over joints or in extremities with compromised venous or lymphatic drainage
- *Caution*: Epirubicin is a vesicant and can produce severe local soft tissue necrosis if extravasation occurs. Epirubicin *must not be given* by the intraMUSCular. SUBCUTaneous, or intraTHECAL routes
  - The current standard of care for managing anthracycline extravasation, including extravasation of epirubicin, is a 3-day course of intraVENously administered dexrazoxane (Totect, Savene)

- Erythematous streaking along the vein through which epirubicin is administered and facial flushing may indicate too rapid an administration rate, and may precede local phlebitis or thrombophlebitis. Burning or stinging sensations may be indicative of perivenous infiltration and the infusion should be immediately terminated and resumed in another vein. Perivenous infiltration may occur painlessly

Caution:

- Do not administer epirubicin in combination with other cardiotoxic agents unless the patient's cardiac function is closely monitored
  - Administering epirubicin after stopping treatment with other cardiotoxic agents may also increase the risk of developing cardiotoxicity
  - Avoid when possible epirubicin therapy for up to 24 weeks after a last dose of trastuzumab
    - ○ Monitor cardiac function carefully if epirubicin is used within 24 weeks after stopping trastuzumab
  - Concomitant use of epirubicin with cardioactive compounds that could cause heart failure (eg, calcium channel blockers) requires close monitoring of cardiac function throughout treatment
- Coadministration of cimetidine increased epirubicin's mean AUC by 50% and decreased its plasma clearance by 30%
- Epirubicin administered immediately before or after DOCEtaxel did not affect the systemic exposure of epirubicin, but

increased the systemic exposure (mean AUC) of epirubicinol (~10% the cytotoxic activity of epirubicin) and 7-deoxydoxorubicin aglycone (inactive) when DOCEtaxel was administered immediately after epirubicin compared to epirubicin alone

- Epirubicin had no effect on the exposure of DOCEtaxel whether it was administered before or after DOCEtaxel
- Epirubicin administered immediately before or after PACLitaxel increased the systemic exposure of epirubicin, epirubicinol, and 7-deoxydoxorubicin aglycone
  - Epirubicin had no effect on the exposure of PACLitaxel whether it was administered before or after PACLitaxel
- It is likely that epirubicin use concurrently with radiotherapy may sensitize tissues to the cytotoxic actions of irradiation
- Epirubicin administration after ionizing radiation therapy may induce an inflammatory recall reaction involving previously irradiated tissues

Inadvertent exposure:

- Epirubicin HCl spills and leaks on environmental surfaces should be treated with dilute sodium hypochlorite (1% available chlorine) solution, preferably by soaking, and then rinsing with water
- In case of skin contact, thoroughly wash the affected area with soap and water or sodium bicarbonate solution. *Do not abrade* the skin by using a scrub brush
- Treat accidental contact with the eyes immediately by copious lavage with water

ERIBULIN MESYLATE

HALAVEN® (eribulin mesylate) injection for intravenous administration; product label, September 2013. Eisai Inc., Woodcliff Lake, NJ

Product Identification, Preparation, Storage, and Stability

- HALAVEN® is a clear, colorless, sterile solution for intraVENous administration. Each vial contains 1 mg of eribulin mesylate per 2 mL of solution (0.5 mg/mL) in ethanol:water (5:95)

- The commercial product is packaged in individually packaged single-use vials (NDC 62856-389-01)

- Store intact vials in their original cartons at 25°C (77°F). Temperature excursions are permitted to 15°–30°C (59°–86°F). *Do not* freeze eribulin mesylate. Store intact vials in their original cartons

- With a syringe, withdraw a volume of eribulin mesylate appropriate for a patient's dose

- Undiluted eribulin mesylate is suitable for direct intraVENous administration, or the drug product may be diluted in 100 mL of 0.9% NS

- Undiluted eribulin mesylate may be stored in a syringe for up to 4 hours at room temperature or for up to 24 hours under refrigeration 4°C (~40°F)

- Diluted solutions of eribulin mesylate may be stored for up to 4 hours at room temperature or for up to 24 hours under refrigeration 4°C (~40°F)

- Discard partially used and empty vials

Selected incompatibility:

- *Do not dilute or administer* eribulin mesylate through an administration set containing dextrose solutions

- *Do not administer* eribulin mesylate through an administration set with other medications

Recommendations for Drug Administration and Ancillary Care

General:

- See Chapter 41 for recommended use in patients with renal and hepatic dysfunction

- Administer eribulin mesylate by intraVENous injection over 2–5 minutes

Caution:

- ECG monitoring is recommended if therapy is initiated in patients with congestive heart failure, bradyarrhythmias, and drugs known to prolong the QT interval, including Class Ia and III antiarrhythmics, and electrolyte abnormalities

- The effect of eribulin mesylate on the QTc interval was assessed in an open-label, uncontrolled, multicenter, single-arm dedicated QT trial. A total of 26 patients with solid tumors received eribulin mesylate 1.4 mg/m² on days 1 and 8 of a 21-day cycle

  - A delayed QTc prolongation was observed on day 8, without prolongation observed on day 1

  - The maximum mean QTcF change from baseline (95% upper confidence interval) was 11.4 msec (19.5 msec; 95% upper confidence interval)

- Correct hypokalemia or hypomagnesemia prior to administering eribulin mesylate and monitor serum potassium and magnesium periodically during therapy

- Avoid administering eribulin mesylate to patients with congenital long QT syndrome

ETOPOSIDE

ETOPOSIDE INJECTION, USP; product label, October 2012. Manufactured for Bedford Laboratories, Bedford, OH
TOPOSAR® (etoposide injection, USP) product label, September 2011. Manufactured by Teva Parenteral Medicines, Inc., Irvine, CA
Information from Bristol-Myers Oncology Division. "VePesid stability above 0.4 mg/mL," April 26, 1993

WARNINGS

[Etoposide injection] …should be administered under the supervision of a qualified physician experienced in the use of cancer chemotherapeutic agents. Severe myelosuppression with resulting infection or bleeding may occur

---

Boxed Warning (excerpt) for "TOPOSAR® (etoposide injection, USP)"; September 2011 product label; Teva Parenteral Medicines, Inc., Irvine, CA; and "ETOPOSIDE INJECTION, USP"; October 2012 product label; Bedford Laboratories™, Bedford, OH

Product Identification, Preparation, Storage, and Stability

- Etoposide is generically available from several manufacturers. In general, etoposide injection, USP, is a viscous, clear, colorless to light yellow solution containing etoposide 20 mg/mL at pH 3–4
- Etoposide is sparingly soluble in water. Consequently, etoposide is made more miscible with water by means of organic solvent excipients, including: either polysorbate 80 or modified polysorbate 80, with polyethylene glycol 300, and dehydrated alcohol
  - Additional excipient components vary among manufacturers' products
- Available presentations include multidose vials containing 100, 500, or 1000 mg etoposide
- Store intact vials and diluted solutions at controlled room temperature of 20°–25°C (68°–77°F)
  - Unopened vials of etoposide injection are stable for 24 months at room temperature (25°C [77°F])
- Commercially marketed etoposide (20 mg/mL) MUST BE DILUTED before administration with either D5W or 0.9% NS to a concentration between 0.2 and 0.4 mg/mL in either glass or plastic containers
  - After dilution, product stability is affected by the concentration of etoposide and storage temperatures
  - Solutions with concentrations >0.1 mg/mL are supersaturated and potentially may precipitate
  - The time to precipitation at concentrations >0.4 mg/mL is unpredictable and may occur earlier than the times indicated in the following table, particularly if etoposide is stored at cool temperatures or is agitated, as may occur during administration with a peristaltic pump

Etoposide Concentration	Duration of Stability
0.1 mg/mL	96 hours
0.2 mg/mL	96 hours*
0.4 mg/mL	24–48* hours
0.6 mg/mL	8 hours
1 mg/mL	2 hours

*At 25°C (77°F), normal room fluorescent lighting, in both glass and plastic containers

Selected incompatibility:

- Devices made of acrylic or ABS plastic (acrylonitrile, butadiene, and styrene polymer) may crack and leak when used with undiluted etoposide injection

Recommendations for Drug Administration and Ancillary Care

General:

- See Chapter 41 for recommended use in patients with renal and hepatic dysfunction
- *Do not administer* etoposide by rapid intraVENous injection. Administer etoposide by intraVENous infusion over at least 30–60 minutes to prevent hypotension. Longer infusion durations may be used when clinically appropriate for the volume of fluid that must be administered

FLOXURIDINE (FUDR)

FLOXURIDINE for injection USP, for intraarterial infusion only; product label, February 2000. Manufactured by Ben Venue Laboratories, Inc., Bedford, OH. Manufactured for Bedford Laboratories, Bedford, OH
FLOXURIDINE for injection, USP, for intraarterial infusion only; product label, January 2008. APP Pharmaceuticals, LLC, Schaumburg, IL

WARNING

It is recommended that floxuridine be given only by or under the supervision of a qualified physician who is experienced in cancer chemotherapy and intra-arterial drug therapy and is well versed in the use of potent antimetabolites

Because of the possibility of severe toxic reactions, all patients should be hospitalized for initiation of the first course of therapy

---

Boxed Warning for "FLOXURIDINE FOR INJECTION USP, FOR INTRA-ARTERIAL INFUSION ONLY"; February 2000 product label; Bedford Laboratories™, Bedford, OH; and "FLOXURIDINE FOR INJECTION USP, FOR INTRA-ARTERIAL INFUSION ONLY"; January 2008 product label; APP Pharmaceuticals, LLC, Schaumburg, IL

Product Identification, Preparation, Storage, and Stability

- Floxuridine for injection USP is available generically as a sterile, nonpyrogenic, white to off-white, odorless, lyophilized powder for reconstitution packaged in individually packaged 5-mL vials containing 500 mg of floxuridine
- Storage temperature specifications for intact vials vary among different manufacturers' products, but include 15°–30°C (59°–86°F; Bedford Laboratories), and 20°–25°C (68°–77°F; APP Pharmaceuticals, LLC)
  - Consult product labels for product-specific recommendations
- Reconstitute floxuridine with SWFI 5 mL to yield a solution containing approximately 100 mg floxuridine/mL
- The reconstituted drug product (100 mg/mL) should be stored under refrigeration 2°–8°C (35.6°–46.4°F) for no longer than 2 weeks
- An appropriate amount of the reconstituted solution (100 mg/mL) is then diluted with a volume of 0.9% NS or D5W appropriate for delivery device used to administer the drug product intraarterially
  - Floxuridine administration is best achieved by utilizing a rate-controlling device able to overcome pressure in large arteries and ensure a uniform drug delivery rate

Selected incompatibility:

- Floxuridine is optimally stable at pH = 4–7. Avoid admixture with highly acidic or alkaline solutions

Recommendations for Drug Administration and Ancillary Care

General:

- See Chapter 41 for recommended use in patients with hepatic dysfunction
- Floxuridine has received FDA approval only for administration by continuous regional intraarterial infusion

FLUDARABINE PHOSPHATE

FLUDARABINE PHOSPHATE INJECTION, for intravenous use only; product label, December 2007. APP Pharmaceuticals, LLC, Schaumburg, IL
Fludarabine Phosphate for Injection, USP, for intravenous use only; product label, February 2013. Manufactured by Zydus Hospira Oncology Private Ltd., Gujurat, India. Manufactured for Hospira, Inc., Lake Forest, IL
Fludarabine Phosphate for Injection, USP (For IV Use Only); product label, October 2011. Made in Romania. Manufactured for SAGENT Pharmaceuticals, Schaumburg, IL

WARNING[A,B,C]

[Fludarabine phosphate] …should be administered under the supervision of a qualified physician experienced in the use of antineoplastic therapy.[A,B,C] [Fludarabine phosphate] …can severely suppress bone marrow function.[A,B,C] When used at high doses in dose-ranging studies in patients with acute leukemia, [fludarabine phosphate] …was associated with severe neurologic effects, including blindness, coma, and death.[A,B,C] This severe central nervous system toxicity occurred in 36% of patients treated with doses approximately four times greater (96 mg/m^2/day for 5 to 7 days) than the recommended dose.[A,B,C] Similar severe central nervous system toxicity[A,B,C] [...including coma, seizures, agitation, and confusion][B] has been[A,B] [rarely (0.2%)][A] [rarely (≤ 0.2%)[B] …reported in patients treated at doses in the range of the dose recommended for chronic lymphocytic leukemia.[A,B,C]

Instances of life-threatening and sometimes fatal autoimmune[A,B,C] [phenomena such as][B,C] [hemolytic anemia][A,B,C] [...autoimmune thrombocytopenia/thrombocytopenic purpura (ITP), Evan's syndrome, and acquired hemophilia][B,C] have been reported to occur after one or more cycles of treatment with [fludarabine phosphate].[A,B,C] Patients undergoing treatment with [fludarabine phosphate] …should be evaluated and closely monitored for hemolysis[A,B,C]

In a clinical investigation using [fludarabine phosphate] …in combination with pentostatin (deoxycoformycin) for the treatment of refractory chronic lymphocytic leukemia (CLL), there was an unacceptably high incidence of fatal pulmonary toxicity.[A,B,C] Therefore, the use of [fludarabine phosphate] …in combination with pentostatin is not recommended[A,B,C]

Boxed Warning for:
[A]"FLUDARABINE PHOSPHATE INJECTION, For Intravenous Use Only"; December 2007 product label; APP Pharmaceuticals, LLC, Schaumburg, IL
[B]"Fludarabine Phosphate for Injection, USP, For Intravenous Use Only"; May 2008 product label; Hospira, Inc., Lake Forest, IL
[C]"Fludarabine Phosphate for Injection, USP (For IV Use Only)"; October 2011 product label. SAGENT Pharmaceuticals, Schaumburg, IL

Product Identification, Preparation, Storage, and Stability

Fludarabine Phosphate for Injection, USP (lyophilized product for reconstitution)

- Fludarabine phosphate for injection, USP, is available generically in individually packaged, clear, glass, single-use vials containing a sterile, white, lyophilized, solid cake of fludarabine phosphate 50 mg with mannitol 50 mg and sodium hydroxide to adjust pH to 7.7

- Storage temperatures vary among the manufacturers' products, that is, storage at room temperature or under refrigeration

  - Consult product labeling for product specific recommendations for storage

- Reconstitute fludarabine with 2 mL of SWFI to produce a solution containing 25 mg fludarabine phosphate/mL at a pH within the range 7.2–8.2

- The solid cake should fully dissolve in ≤15 seconds

Fludarabine Phosphate Injection, USP (product in solution)

- Fludarabine phosphate injection is available generically in individually packaged, glass, single-use vials containing a clear, sterile solution of fludarabine phosphate 50 mg/2 mL (25 mg/mL), with mannitol, USP, 50 mg, SWFI (Q.S.), and sodium hydroxide to adjust pH to 6.8. The pH range for the final product is 6.0–7.1

- Store fludarabine phosphate injection under refrigeration at 2°–8°C (35.6°–46.4°F)

- After reconstitution, fludarabine phosphate is chemically stable for up to 16 days when stored at room temperature under ambient lighting

- Neither the lyophilized drug products nor products in solution contain an antimicrobial preservative and should be used within 8 hours after first entering a vial

- Fludarabine phosphate may be further diluted in 100–125 mL of D5W or 0.9% NS in glass or plastic containers

- *Do not mix* fludarabine phosphate with other drugs

Recommendations for Drug Administration and Ancillary Care

General:

- See Chapter 41 for recommended use in patients with renal dysfunction

- Administer fludarabine intraVENously over approximately 30 minutes

- *Caution:* The use of fludarabine phosphate, USP in combination with pentostatin (*AKA*, deoxycoformycin) for the treatment of refractory chronic lymphocytic leukemia in adults, is associated with an unacceptably high incidence of fatal pulmonary toxicity. Therefore, concomitant use of fludarabine phosphate with pentostatin is not recommended

Inadvertent exposure:

- In case of contact with skin or mucous membranes, thoroughly wash the affected area with soap and water. *Do not abrade* the skin by using a scrub brush

- Treat accidental contact with the eyes immediately by copious lavage with water

FLUOROURACIL

ADRUCIL® (fluorouracil injection, USP), PHARMACY BULK PACKAGE, NOT FOR DIRECT INFUSION; product label, August 2012. Manufactured by Teva Parenteral Medicines, Inc., Irvine CA
Fluorouracil Injection, USP, PHARMACY BULK PACKAGE—Not For Direct Infusion; product label, October 2008. APP Pharmaceuticals, LLC, Schaumburg, IL

WARNING

It is recommended that Fluorouracil Injection be given only by or under the supervision of a qualified physician who is experienced in cancer chemotherapy and who is well versed in the use of potent antimetabolites. Because of the possibility of severe toxic reactions, it is recommended that patients be hospitalized at least during the initial course of therapy...

Boxed Warning (excerpt) for "ADRUCIL® (fluorouracil injection, USP), PHARMACY BULK PACKAGE, NOT FOR DIRECT INFUSION"; August 2012 product label; Teva Parenteral Medicines, Inc., Irvine CA

Product Identification, Preparation, Storage, and Stability

- Fluorouracil Injection, USP, is available generically from several manufacturers. Presentations include products packaged for single use and for pharmaceutical admixture and compounding (*pharmacy bulk package*)
  - Fluorouracil injection, USP, is available in cartons of 10 single-use vials containing a sterile, nonpyrogenic, colorless to faint yellow solution of fluorouracil, 500 mg/10 mL
    - Each milliliter of the drug product contains fluorouracil 50 mg and water for injection. Sodium hydroxide may be added during manufacturing to adjust pH to approximately 9.2
  - Pharmacy bulk packages are *only* for use in a pharmacy admixture service
    - Pharmacy bulk package vials contain either 2500 mg (in 50 mL) or 5000 mg (in 100 mL)
    - Packaging varies among manufacturers, and includes individually packaged vials and cartons containing multiple vials
    - *Directions for proper use of a pharmacy bulk package (not for direct infusion) (excerpted and paraphrased)*
      - The 50- and 100-mL pharmacy bulk packages are for use in a pharmacy admixture service only in a suitable work area, such as a laminar flow hood
      - Container closures may be penetrated only 1 time, utilizing a suitable sterile transfer device or dispensing set that allows measured distribution of the contents
        - The use of a syringe with a needle is not recommended because multiple vial entries increase the potential of microbial and particulate contamination
      - Complete fluid transfers from a pharmacy bulk package within a maximum time of 4 hours after initial closure entry
- Fluorouracil should be stored at room temperature, but specific recommendations for storage temperature vary among manufacturers' products
  - Consult product labeling for product-specific storage instructions
  - Do not refrigerate or freeze fluorouracil
- Fluorouracil is subject to photodegradation and should be protected from light. Store the product in its original packaging carton until vials are used
  - Fluorouracil is characteristically colorless to faint yellow; the color results from the presence of free fluorine. Dark yellow indicates degradation and may result from prolonged storage in excessive heat or exposure to light. Discolored solutions should be discarded
  - Although fluorouracil solution may discolor slightly during storage, its potency and safety are not adversely affected
- If a precipitate occurs due to exposure to low temperatures, fluorouracil may be resolubilized by heating to 60°C (140°F) and vigorously shaking the solution
  - Allow fluorouracil to cool to body temperature before administering it to patients
- Fluorouracil may be given undiluted or diluted in a volume of dextrose or sodium chloride solutions, or solutions in which dextrose and sodium chloride are combined, appropriate for a particular application
- Discard any unused portion of fluorouracil remaining in single-use vials and in pharmacy bulk packages at 4 hours after initial vial entry

Selected incompatibility:

- Prepare, store, and administer fluorouracil with plastic containers and administration sets[42,43]
  - Fluorouracil adsorbs to glass surfaces more extensively than plastic surfaces (polyvinyl chloride, polyethylene, polypropylene)
- Fluorouracil and leucovorin calcium should not be combined in the same product container
- Fluorouracil should not be combined in the same product container with doxorubicin or simultaneously administered through the same administration set or VAD lumen

---

Recommendations for Drug Administration and Ancillary Care

General:

- See Chapter 41 for recommended use in patients with renal and hepatic dysfunction
- Fluorouracil injection, USP, may be given by direct intraVENous injection over ≤2 minutes or as an intraVENous infusion for durations of minutes to days
- Fluorouracil also has been given by prolonged infusion intraarterially and by regional venous perfusion (eg, via the portal vein)
- Fluorouracil solutions may be given via peripheral or central vascular access; however, the undiluted solution has an osmolality of 650 mOsm/kg, a pH of approximately 9.2 (range: 8.6–9.4) and can be irritating to small veins

GEMCITABINE HYDROCHLORIDE

Gemcitabine for injection, powder, lyophilized, for solution for intravenous use; product label, June 2013. Manufactured by Dr. Reddy's Laboratories Limited, Visakhapatnam-530 046 INDIA. Distributed by Bedford Laboratories, Bedford, OH

GEMZAR® (gemcitabine for injection) for intravenous use; product label, September 2013. Marketed by Lilly USA, LLC, Indianapolis, IN

Gemcitabine for injection. Gemcitabine for injection, USP, Powder, Lyophilized, For Solution For Intravenous Use; product label, April 2012. Manufactured by Intas Pharmaceuticals Limited, Ahmedabad–382 210. India. Manufactured for Accord Healthcare, Inc., Durham, NC

GEMCITABINE INJECTION, For Intravenous Use Only, Must Be Diluted Before Use; product label, August 2013. Manufactured by Zydus Hospira Oncology Private Ltd., Gujarat, India. Manufactured for Hospira, Inc., Lake Forest, IL

Product Identification, Preparation, Storage, and Stability

• Gemcitabine HCl is available generically from several manufacturers. Presentations vary among manufacturers' products

Gemcitabine for Injection, USP (lyophilized product for reconstitution)

• Gemcitabine For Injection is individually packaged in single-use vials containing 200 mg, 1000 mg, or 2000 mg of gemcitabine (expressed as free base) formulated as a sterile, white to off-white lyophilized powder with mannitol (200 mg, 1000 mg, or 2000 mg, respectively), and sodium acetate. Hydrochloric acid and/or sodium hydroxide may have been added to adjust product pH

• Store intact vials at controlled room temperature 20°–25°C (68°–77°F); temperature excursions between 15° and 30°C (59° and 86°F) are permitted

• Reconstitute gemcitabine with 0.9% NS (without preservatives) to produce a clear, colorless to light straw-colored solution with concentration equal to 38 mg/mL and pH within the range of 2.7–3.3

  ▪ Reconstitute gemcitabine as follows:

Gemcitabine Content per Vial	Volume of 0.9% NS Diluent per Vial	Total Volume After Reconstitution (see *Notes*, below)	Gemcitabine Concentration After Reconstitution
200 mg	5 mL	5.26 mL	
1000 mg	25 mL	26.3 mL	38 mg/mL
2000 mg	50 mL	52.6 mL	

Notes: The amount of gemcitabine powder within a vial is responsible for the apparent expansion of drug product volume after reconstitution; that is, the volume of the reconstituted product is greater than the volume of diluent added during reconstitution

Gemcitabine has limited solubility in aqueous media. Reconstitution to concentrations >40 mg/mL may prevent complete solubilization
• Shake vials to which 0.9% NS was added to aid gemcitabine dissolution

Gemcitabine Injection, USP (product in solution)

• Gemcitabine injection is individually packaged in single-use vials containing 200 mg, 1000 mg, or 2000 mg of gemcitabine (expressed as free base) at a concentration of 38 mg gemcitabine per milliliter formulated as a sterile, clear, colorless to light straw-colored solution in SWFI. Hydrochloric acid and/or sodium hydroxide may have been added to adjust product pH

• Store intact vials under refrigeration at 2°–8°C (35.6°–46.4°F)

Instructions common to both formulations

• *Do not refrigerate* reconstituted gemcitabine solutions to prevent crystallization
• Prior to administration the appropriate amount of drug must be further diluted with 0.9% NS to concentrations as low as 0.1 mg/mL
• When prepared as directed, diluted gemcitabine solutions are stable for 24 hours at 20°–25°C (68°–77°F)
• Discard any unused portion of gemcitabine solutions
• Gemcitabine is compatible with either glass or PVC containers and PVC administration sets

Recommendations for Drug Administration and Ancillary Care

General:

- See Chapter 41 for recommended use in patients with renal and hepatic dysfunction
- Administer gemcitabine by intraVENous infusion over 30 minutes

Treatment strategies and other factors affecting gemcitabine pharmacokinetics:

- Gemcitabine has been administered intraVENously at a fixed dose-rate (FDR) of 10 mg/m^2 per min

Notes: Experimental data have demonstrated that small increases in intracellular concentrations of gemcitabine's active triphosphate metabolite profoundly affect its intracellular AUC; the kinetics of interaction with deoxycytidine kinase, and a fixed gemcitabine administration rate of 10 mg/m^2 per minute maximizes the rate at which the metabolite accumulates in peripheral blood mononuclear cells

This observation is the basis for clinical trials with FDR gemcitabine administration, which attempt to correlate increases in intracellular gemcitabine triphosphate concentrations with improved objective treatment outcomes[44]

- Population pharmacokinetic analyses of combined single- and multiple-dose studies showed gemcitabine's volume of distribution (V_d) was significantly influenced by duration of administration and patients' sex
- Gemcitabine's V_d increases directly with its duration of administration (70–285-minute durations)
- Administration durations >60 minutes and administration at intervals more frequent than once weekly have been shown to increase the incidence of clinically significant adverse events
- Gemcitabine clearance is decreased in females[45] (vs. males) and the elderly,[46] resulting in higher concentrations of gemcitabine for any given dose

Caution:

- Enhanced tissue injury typically associated with radiation toxicity is associated with concurrent use of gemcitabine and radiation therapies given together or ≤7 days apart:
  - Gemcitabine has radiosensitizing activity. Toxicity associated with concurrent use of gemcitabine and radiation therapies is dependent on multiple factors, including gemcitabine dosage, the frequency of gemcitabine administration, radiation dose, radiotherapy planning technique, the type and target volume of irradiated tissues
- Gemcitabine clearance has been shown to be decreased by concurrent use of cisplatin
- If Gemcitabine Injection or diluted solutions contact the skin or mucosa, immediately wash the skin thoroughly with soap and water or rinse the mucosa with copious amounts of water
  - Acute dermal irritation has not been observed in animal studies, but 2 of 3 rabbits exhibited drug-related systemic toxicities (death, hypoactivity, nasal discharge, shallow breathing) due to dermal absorption

GLUCARPIDASE

VORAXAZE® (glucarpidase), for injection, for intravenous use; product label, March 2013. Manufactured by BTG International Inc., Brentwood, TN, Distributed by BTG International Inc., West Conshohocken, PA

Product Identification, Preparation, Storage, and Stability

- VORAXAZE® is marketed in individually packaged, single-use, glass vials as a sterile, preservative-free, white, lyophilized powder containing 1000 units of glucarpidase per vial, with lactose monohydrate 10 mg, Tris-HCl 0.6 mg, and zinc acetate dihydrate 2 mcg (NDC 50633-210-11)
  - Glucarpidase potency units correspond with the enzymatic cleavage of 1 micromol/L of methotrexate per minute at 37°C (98.6°F)

- Store glucarpidase under refrigeration at 2°–8°C (35.6°–46.4°F). *Do not freeze* glucarpidase
- Reconstitute the contents of a vial with 1 mL of 0.9% NS
- Gently roll and tilt vials to dissolve the lyophilized powder. *Do not shake* vials to aid dissolution
- Inspect the product to ensure product dissolution and discard vials in which the solution is not clear, colorless, and free of particulate matter
- Use reconstituted glucarpidase immediately, or store it under refrigeration at 2°–8°C (35.6°–46.4°F) for up to 4 hours if it is not used immediately
- Discard any unused reconstituted product

Recommendations for Drug Administration and Ancillary Care

General:

- Administer glucarpidase 50 units/kg of body weight as a single intraVENous injection over 5 minutes. Flush intraVENous lines through which glucarpidase is given before and after administering glucarpidase

Caution:

- Leucovorin is a substrate for glucarpidase. Do not administer leucovorin within 2 hours before or after glucarpidase
  - No dose adjustment is recommended for a continuing leucovorin regimen because leucovorin doses/dosages and schedules are based on a patient's methotrexate concentrations before glucarpidase is administered
- Glucarpidase is a carboxypeptidase produced by recombinant DNA technology in genetically modified *Escherichia coli*
  - Serious allergic reactions, including anaphylactic reactions, may occur. The most common adverse reactions (incidence >1%) associated with glucarpidase are paresthesia, flushing, nausea and/or vomiting, hypotension, and headache

Monitoring methotrexate concentration/interference with assay:

- Methotrexate concentrations within 48 hours following administration of glucarpidase can only be reliably measured by a chromatographic method
- DAMPA (4-deoxy-4-amino-N[10]-methylpteroic acid), an inactive metabolite of methotrexate resulting from treatment with glucarpidase, interferes with methotrexate concentration measurements using immunoassays, resulting in erroneous measurements that overestimate methotrexate concentrations
- Because of DAMPA's long half-life (approximately 9 hours), measurement of methotrexate using immunoassays is unreliable for samples collected within 48 hours after glucarpidase administration

Continuation and timing of leucovorin rescue:

- Continue to administer leucovorin after glucarpidase is administered. *Do not administer* leucovorin within 2 hours before or after a glucarpidase dose because leucovorin is a substrate for glucarpidase
- For the first 48 hours after administering glucarpidase, give the same leucovorin doses/dosages and schedules as had been given prior to glucarpidase
- Leucovorin doses/dosages and schedule at times >48 hours after glucarpidase are based on the measured methotrexate concentration
- Do not discontinue leucovorin therapy based on the determination of a single methotrexate concentration less than the threshold for starting or continuing leucovorin treatment
- Leucovorin rescue should be continued until methotrexate concentrations have been maintained below the leucovorin treatment threshold for a minimum of 3 days

IDARUBICIN HYDROCHLORIDE

Idamycin PFS® (idarubicin hydrochloride injection) product label, January 2006. Distributed by Pharmacia & Upjohn Company, Division of Pfizer, Inc., New York, NY
Idamycin® (idarubicin hydrochloride for injection, USP) product label, January 2006. Distributed by Pharmacia & Upjohn Company, Division of Pfizer, Inc., New York, NY
IDARUBICIN HYDROCHLORIDE—idarubicin hydrochloride injection; product label, September 2011. Teva Parenteral Medicines, Inc., Irvine CA
IDARUBICIN HYDROCHLORIDE *INJECTION*, For Intravenous Use Only; product label, December 2008. APP Pharmaceuticals LLC, Schaumburg, IL

WARNING

1. [IDArubicin hydrochloride] …should be given slowly into a freely flowing intravenous infusion. It must never be given intramuscularly or subcutaneously. Severe local tissue necrosis can occur if there is extravasation during administration

2. As is the case with other anthracyclines the use of [IDArubicin] …can cause myocardial toxicity leading to congestive heart failure. Cardiac toxicity is more common in patients who have received prior anthracyclines or who have preexisting cardiac disease

3. As is usual with antileukemic agents, severe myelosuppression occurs when [IDArubicin] …is used at effective therapeutic doses

4. It is recommended that [IDArubicin] …be administered only under the supervision of a physician who is experienced in leukemia chemotherapy and in facilities with laboratory and supportive resources adequate to monitor drug tolerance and protect and maintain a patient compromised by drug toxicity. The physician and institution must be capable of responding rapidly and completely to severe hemorrhagic conditions and/or overwhelming infection

5. Dosage should be reduced in patients with impaired hepatic or renal function…

Boxed Warnings for "Idamycin®" and "Idamycin PFS®"; January 2006 product labels. Pharmacia & Upjohn Company, Division of Pfizer, Inc., New York, NY

Product Identification, Preparation, Storage, and Stability

IDArubicin HCl is available generically from several manufacturers

IDArubicin Hydrochloride Injection (drug product in solution):

- IDArubicin HCl Injection is packaged in single-use vials containing a sterile, red-orange, isotonic parenteral preservative-free solution of IDArubicin at a uniform concentration of 1 mg/mL
- Product presentations include vials containing IDArubicin 5, 10, or 20 mg
- Store IDArubicin HCl injection (solution) under refrigeration 2°–8°C (35.6°–46.4°F) in their packaging carton to protect them from light

IDArubicin Hydrochloride for Injection, USP (lyophilized product for reconstitution):

- Idamycin® (IDArubicin hydrochloride for injection, USP) is packaged in single-use vials containing 20 mg IDArubicin HCl, USP, and Lactose, NF (hydrous), 200 mg as a red-orange lyophilized powder. NDC 0013-2526-86
- Store the lyophilized product at controlled room temperature (15°–30°C [59°–86°F]), and protect from light
- The vial contents are under negative pressure to minimize aerosol formation during reconstitution
- Reconstitute Idamycin lyophilized powder formulation with 20 mL of SWFI to produce a solution with a concentration of 1 mg/mL
- Reconstituted solutions are physically and chemically stable for 72 hours under refrigeration (2°–8°C) and at 15°–30°C (59°–86°F)

Instructions Common to Both Products

- IDArubicin HCl 1 mg/mL is suitable for direct administration to patients. It also may be diluted to a concentration as low as 0.01mg/mL in 0.9% NS or D5W, or to a concentration of 0.1 mg/mL in LRI
- IDArubicin is compatible with PVC, glass, and polypropylene containers
- *Note:* IDArubicin HCl solutions in 0.9% NS exhibit a low level of haziness that is visible under high-intensity light and measurable with a turbidimeter. The haziness increases to maximum with increasing drug dilution from a concentration of 1 mg/mL to 0.05 mg/mL. The haze is not indicative of drug instability or incompatibility[47]

Selected incompatibility:

- IDArubicin is subject to photodegradation, and its susceptibility is inversely related to the concentration of IDArubicin in solution. Protection from light is not necessary if IDArubicin is used promptly after preparation, but product containers should be protected from light exposure when IDArubicin is not administered within a few hours after preparation
- IDArubicin is physically incompatible with heparin (precipitation occurs)
- IDArubicin is degraded by contact with alkaline solutions

Recommendations for Drug Administration and Ancillary Care

General:

- See Chapter 41 for recommended use in patients with renal and hepatic dysfunction
- Administer IDArubicin by slow intraVENous injection over 10–15 minutes into the tubing of a freely running intraVENous infusion of 0.9% NS or D5W, or by intraVENous infusion after dilution (described above)

- *Caution*: IDArubicin is a vesicant and may produce severe local soft-tissue necrosis if extravasation occurs. IDArubicin *must not be given* by the intraMUSCular, SUBCUTaneous, or intraTHECAL routes
  - The current standard of care for managing anthracycline extravasation, including extravasation of IDArubicin, is a 3-day course of intraVENously administered dexrazoxane (Totect, Savene)

IFOSFAMIDE

IFEX (ifosfamide) for injection, intravenous use; product label, March 2012. Manufactured by Baxter Healthcare Corporation, Deerfield, IL
IFOSFAMIDE for injection, USP; product label, January 2008. APP Pharmaceuticals, LLC, Schaumburg, IL

WARNING

Ifosfamide Injection should be administered under the supervision of a qualified physician experienced in the use of cancer chemotherapeutic agents. Urotoxic side effects, especially hemorrhagic cystitis, as well as CNS toxicities such as confusion and coma have been associated with the use of ifosfamide. When they occur, they may require cessation of ifosfamide therapy. Severe myelosuppression has been reported...

Boxed Warnings for "IFOSFAMIDE for injection, USP"; January 2008 product label; APP Pharmaceuticals, LLC, Schaumburg, IL

WARNING: MYELOSUPPRESSION, NEUROTOXICITY, AND UROTOXICITY

Myelosuppression can be severe and lead to fatal infections. Monitor blood counts prior to and at intervals after each treatment cycle. CNS toxicities can be severe and result in encephalopathy and death. Monitor for CNS toxicity and discontinue treatment for encephalopathy. Nephrotoxicity can be severe and result in renal failure. Hemorrhagic cystitis can be severe and can be reduced by the prophylactic use of mesna...

Boxed Warnings for "IFEX (ifosfamide) for injection, intravenous use"; March 2012 product label; Baxter Healthcare Corporation, Deerfield, IL

Product Identification, Preparation, Storage, and Stability

Ifosfamide injection
- Ifosfamide injection is available in, individually boxed single-use vials containing a sterile solution of either 1000 mg/20 mL or 3000 mg/60 mL, in a concentration of 50 mg ifosfamide/mL
- Commercial formulations also contain monobasic sodium phosphate, dibasic sodium phosphate, and SWFI, but products vary in the amount of excipients present
- Store ifosfamide injection under refrigeration at 2°–8°C (35.6°–46.4°F)

Ifosfamide injection with Mesna injection kit
- Ifosfamide injection is copackaged in combination with Mesna injection in the following administration kit presentations:
  - Ten single-dose vials containing ifosfamide 1000 mg/20 mL + 10 multidose vials containing mesna 1000 mg/10 mL (NDC 0703-4116-48; Teva Parenteral Medicines, Inc.)
  - Two single-dose vials containing ifosfamide 3000 mg/60 mL + 6 multidose vials containing mesna 1000 mg/10 mL (NDC 0703-4106-48; Teva Parenteral Medicines, Inc.)

- Five single-dose vials containing ifosfamide 1000 mg/20 mL + 3 multidose vials containing mesna 1000 mg/10 mL (NDC 0703-4100-48; Teva Parenteral Medicines, Inc.)

Ifosfamide for injection
- Ifosfamide for injection, USP, is available in individually boxed single-use vials containing 1000 mg or 3000 mg ifosfamide without excipient ingredients
- Store intact vials at controlled room temperature 20°–25°C (68°–77°F). Protect ifosfamide from temperatures >30°C (>86°F)
- Reconstitute lyophilized ifosfamide with SWFI or BWFI (preserved with benzyl alcohol or parabens) as follows:

Ifosfamide Content per Vial	Diluent Volume	Ifosfamide Concentration After Reconstitution
1000 mg	20 mL	50 mg/mL
3000 mg	60 mL	

Benzyl alcohol-containing solutions can reduce the stability of ifosfamide

Instructions common to both products
- After adding a diluent solution, shake vials to dissolve ifosfamide powder
- Ifosfamide must be completely dissolved before the product may be used
- After reconstitution, ifosfamide may be diluted to obtain concentrations within the range of 0.6–20 mg/mL in any of the following fluids: D5W, 0.9% NS, LRI, D2.5W, 0.45% NaCl, or D5W/0.9% NS
  - Mesna may be prepared as an admixture with ifosfamide (both present in the same container) without compromising the stability of either product
- Ifosfamide is physically and chemically stable in a variety of parenteral product containers, including those made of glass, ethylene and propylene copolymers, PVC plasticized with phthalates, and other polyolefin materials
- Ifosfamide solutions should be refrigerated and used within 24 hours after preparation

Recommendations for Drug Administration and Ancillary Care

General:

- See Chapter 41 for recommended use in patients with renal and hepatic dysfunction
- On days when ifosfamide is administered, give intraVENous or oral fluid hydration consisting of *at least* 2000 mL/day greater than a patient's routine daily fluid consumption. Aggressive hydration has been shown to decrease the urothelial toxicity associated with ifosfamide
- Mesna should be used to reduce the incidence of urothelial hemorrhagic
  - When given concomitantly with ifosfamide, mesna protects the urinary tract from exposure to reactive ifosfamide metabolites that are highly concentrated in urine

- Mesna may be added to the same container as ifosfamide without compromising the stability of either product
- Administer ifosfamide by intraVENous infusion over a minimum of 30 minutes
- Ifosfamide is nephrotoxic and urotoxic
  - Evaluate glomerular and tubular kidney function before, during, and after ifosfamide treatment

Monitor:

- Urinary sediment for the presence of erythrocytes and other signs of urotoxicity/nephrotoxicity
- Serum and urine chemistries, including phosphorus and potassium
- Urinalysis prior to each ifosfamide dose

- If microscopic hematuria (>10 RBCs/HPF) is present, subsequent administration should be withheld until hematuria completely resolves. Further ifosfamide administration should be given with vigorous oral or parenteral hydration
- Use ifosfamide with caution, if at all, in patients with active urinary tract infections

Inadvertent exposure:

- In case of skin contact, thoroughly wash the affected area with soap and water. *Do not abrade* the skin by using a scrub brush
- Treat accidental contact with mucous membranes and the eyes immediately by copious lavage with water

INTERFERON ALFA-2b

INTRON® A interferon alfa-2b, recombinant for injection; product label, January 2014. Manufactured by Schering Corporation, a subsidiary of Merck & Co., Inc., Whitehouse Station, NJ

WARNING

Alpha interferons, including INTRON® A, cause or aggravate fatal or life-threatening neuropsychiatric, autoimmune, ischemic, and infectious disorders. Patients should be monitored closely with periodic clinical and laboratory evaluations. Patients with persistently severe or worsening signs or symptoms of these conditions should be withdrawn from therapy. In many but not all cases these disorders resolve after stopping INTRON A therapy…

Boxed Warnings for "INTRON® A Interferon alfa-2b, recombinant for Injection"; January 2014 product label; Schering Corporation, a subsidiary of Merck & Co., Inc., Whitehouse Station, NJ

Product Identification, Preparation, Storage, and Stability

- INTRON® A is available in several formulations and package formats. The products in solution packaged in vials and multidose pens are *not recommended* for intraVENous administration
- INTRON® A powder for injection is packaged as a kit containing two vials:
  - one single-use vial contains interferon alfa-2b as a white- to cream-colored powder, *plus*
  - one single-use vial contains Diluent for INTRON® A (Sterile Water for Injection, USP) 1.25 mL/vial
- The following presentations are available:

Amount of Recombinant Interferon Alfa-2b per Vial	Vial of Diluent (SWFI)	Interferon Alfa-2b Concentration After Reconstitution	NDC Number
10 million IU (0.038 mg/vial*)		10 million IU	0085-0571-02
18 million IU (0.069 mg/vial*)	1 mL	18 million IU	0085-1110-01
50 million IU (0.192 mg/vial*)		50 million IU	0085-0539-01

Each milliliter of the reconstituted solution also contains 20 mg glycine, 2.3 mg dibasic sodium phosphate, 0.55 mg monobasic sodium phosphate, and 1 mg albumin (human)†

*Based on the specific activity of approximately 2.6×10^8 IU/mg protein, as measured by HPLC assay
†The addition of albumin prevents drug adsorption to containers and administration set surfaces during drug preparation and administration

- Store recombinant interferon alfa-2b powder for injection between 2° and 8°C (35.6° and 46.4°F) both before and after reconstitution
- Prepare a solution for intraVENous infusion immediately before use by adding 1 mL of SWFI (diluent included in product packaging) to a vial containing Intron A powder for injection
  - Interferon alfa-2b products formulated as solutions are *not recommended* for intraVENous administration
- Vials may be gently swirled to hasten dissolving the powdered drug product
- Dilute an amount of interferon appropriate for a patient's dose in a bag containing 0.9% NS to produce a solution with an interferon alfa concentration ≥10 million IU/100 mL

Recommendations for Drug Administration and Ancillary Care

General:

- Premedication with acetaminophen my mitigate fever that often follows interferon alfa-2b administration
- Allow refrigerated solutions to come to room temperature before commencing administration
- Administration before sleep may mitigate a patient's experience of "flu-like" symptoms (fever, headache, chills, myalgias, fatigue) that are frequently associated with interferon alfa-2b administration
- Administer interferon alfa-2b by intraVENous infusion over 20 minutes

IPILIMUMAB

YERVOY® (ipilimumab) injection for intravenous infusion; product label, December 2013. Manufactured by Bristol-Myers Squibb Company, Princeton, NJ

WARNING: IMMUNE-MEDIATED ADVERSE REACTIONS

YERVOY (ipilimumab) can result in severe and fatal immune-mediated adverse reactions due to T-cell activation and proliferation. These immune-mediated reactions may involve any organ system; however, the most common severe immune-mediated adverse reactions are enterocolitis, hepatitis, dermatitis (including toxic epidermal necrolysis), neuropathy, and endocrinopathy. The majority of these immune-mediated reactions initially manifested during treatment; however, a minority occurred weeks to months after discontinuation of YERVOY

Permanently discontinue YERVOY and initiate systemic high-dose corticosteroid therapy for severe immune-mediated reactions…

Assess patients for signs and symptoms of enterocolitis, dermatitis, neuropathy, and endocrinopathy and evaluate clinical chemistries including liver function tests and thyroid function tests at baseline and before each dose…

Boxed Warning for "YERVOY® (ipilimumab) injection for intravenous infusion"; December 2013 product label; Bristol-Myers Squibb Company, Princeton, NJ

Product Identification, Preparation, Storage, and Stability

- YERVOY® is a sterile, preservative-free, clear to slightly opalescent, colorless to pale yellow solution for intraVENous infusion, which may contain a small amount of visible, translucent-to-white, amorphous ipilimumab particulates
- The commercial product is supplied in single-use vials containing either 50 mg/10 mL (NDC 0003-2327-11) or 200 mg/40 mL (NDC 0003-2328-22)
  - Each milliliter of solution contains 5 mg ipilimumab at a pH = 7, with the following inactive ingredients: diethylene triamine pentaacetic acid 0.04 mg, mannitol 10 mg, polysorbate 80 (vegetable origin) 0.1 mg, sodium chloride 5.85 mg, tris hydrochloride 3.15 mg (buffer), and SWFI
- Store unused vials under refrigeration at 2°–8°C (35.6°–46.4°F) protected from light. *Do not freeze* the product
- Ipilimumab *must be diluted* before administration

Preparation
- *Do not shake* ipilimumab
- Discard vials containing a cloudy solution, if there is pronounced discoloration (solution may have pale yellow color), or with the appearance of foreign particulate matter other than translucent-to-white, amorphous particles
- Allow vials to stand at room temperature for approximately 5 minutes before diluting the product for clinical use
- With a syringe, withdraw a volume of ipilimumab appropriate for a patient's dose and transfer it to a sterile parenteral product container
- Dilute the drug with 0.9% NS or D5W to a concentration within the range of 1–2 mg/mL. Mix the diluted solution by gently inverting the parenteral product container
  - Store the diluted solution for no more than 24 hours under refrigeration at 2°–8°C (35.6°–46.4°F) or at room temperature (20°–25°C [68°–77°F])
- Discard partially used and empty vials

Recommendations for Drug Administration and Ancillary Care

General:
- *Do not mix* ipilimumab during preparation or administration with fluids and medications other than 0.9% NS or D5W
- Administer diluted ipilimumab intraVENously over 90 minutes through a sterile, nonpyrogenic, low-protein-binding, 1.2 μm pore size inline filter
- Flush administration sets used to administer ipilimumab with 0.9% NS or D5W after completing drug administration

Risk Evaluation and Mitigation Strategy (REMS):
- As of April 2012, YERVOY® utilization is subject to a REMS
- REMS materials are designed to communicate to healthcare providers the risks of severe and fatal immune-mediated adverse reactions caused by YERVOY, including immune-mediated:
  - enterocolitis (including gastrointestinal perforation)
  - hepatitis (including hepatic failure)
  - dermatitis (including toxic epidermal necrolysis)
  - neuropathies
  - endocrinopathies
- Information about the REMS is available online at http://www.yervoy.com/hcp/rems.aspx [accessed February 14, 2014]

IRINOTECAN HYDROCHLORIDE

Camptosar® (Irinotecan) Injection, intravenous infusion; product label, July 2012. Distributed by Pharmacia & Upjohn Co., Division of Pfizer Inc, New York, NY
Camptosar® irinotecan hydrochloride injection, for intravenous use only; product label, June 2011. Distributed by Pharmacia & Upjohn Co., Division of Pfizer Inc, New York, NY
IRINOTECAN HYDROCHLORIDE- irinotecan hydrochloride injection, solution; product label, August 2010. Manufactured by Ebewe PHARMA, Unterach, Austria. Manufactured for SANDOZ, Princeton, NJ

WARNING: DIARRHEA AND MYELOSUPPRESSION

- Early and late forms of diarrhea can occur. Early diarrhea may be accompanied by cholinergic symptoms which may be prevented or ameliorated by atropine. Late diarrhea can be life threatening and should be treated promptly with loperamide. Monitor patients with diarrhea and give fluid and electrolytes as needed. Institute antibiotic therapy if patients develop ileus, fever, or severe neutropenia. Interrupt CAMPTOSAR and reduce subsequent doses if severe diarrhea occurs
- Severe myelosuppression may occur

Boxed Warning for "Camptosar® (Irinotecan) Injection, intravenous infusion"; July 2012 product label; Pharmacia & Upjohn Co., Division of Pfizer Inc, New York, NY

WARNINGS

CAMPTOSAR Injection should be administered only under the supervision of a physician who is experienced in the use of cancer chemotherapeutic agents. Appropriate management of complications is possible only when adequate diagnostic and treatment facilities are readily available. CAMPTOSAR can induce both early and late forms of diarrhea that appear to be mediated by different mechanisms. Both forms of diarrhea may be severe. Early diarrhea (occurring during or shortly after infusion of CAMPTOSAR) may be accompanied by cholinergic symptoms of rhinitis, increased salivation, miosis, lacrimation, diaphoresis, flushing, and intestinal hyperperistalsis that can cause abdominal cramping. Early diarrhea and other cholinergic symptoms may be prevented or ameliorated by atropine... Late diarrhea (generally occurring more than 24 hours after administration of CAMPTOSAR) can be life threatening since it may be prolonged and may lead to dehydration, electrolyte imbalance, or sepsis. Late diarrhea should be treated promptly with loperamide. Patients with diarrhea should be carefully monitored and given fluid and electrolyte replacement if they become dehydrated or antibiotic therapy if they develop ileus, fever, or severe neutropenia... Administration of CAMPTOSAR should be interrupted and subsequent doses reduced if severe diarrhea occurs...

Severe myelosuppression may occur...

Boxed Warning for "Camptosar® irinotecan hydrochloride injection, for intravenous use only"; June 2011 product label; Pharmacia & Upjohn Co., Division of Pfizer Inc, New York, NY

Product Identification, Preparation, Storage, and Stability

- Irinotecan Hydrochloride Injection is generically available
- Commercially available presentations include:
  - Individually packaged, single-use vials containing a sterile, pale yellow, clear, aqueous solution
  - Each milliliter of solution contains 20 mg of irinotecan hydrochloride (on the basis of the trihydrate salt), 45 mg of sorbitol, NF, and 0.9 mg of lactic acid, USP
  - Solution pH has been adjusted to 3.5 (range, 3.0–3.8) with sodium hydroxide or hydrochloric acid

Irinotecan Content

In Brown Glass Vials	In Amber-colored Polypropylene Vials
40 mg (2 mL)	40 mg (2 mL)
100 mg (5 mL)	100 mg (5 mL)
	300 mg (15 mL)

- Store intact vials at controlled room temperature (15°–30°C [59°–86°F]) in the original packaging carton to protect the drug product from light until it is used
- Irinotecan *must be diluted* before administration with D5W (preferred) or 0.9% NS to a concentration within the range of 0.12–2.8 mg/mL
- After dilution, irinotecan is physically and chemically stable for up to 24 hours at room temperature (approximately 25°C [77°F]) under ambient fluorescent lighting
- After dilution in D5W, solutions stored at approximately 2°–8°C (35.6°–46.4°F) and protected from light are physically and chemically stable for 48 hours

(continued)

Product Identification, Preparation, Storage, and Stability (continued)

- *Do not refrigerate* admixtures prepared with 0.9% NS to prevent the formation of visible particulates
- *Avoid* freezing irinotecan and admixtures containing irinotecan, which may result in drug precipitation
- Commercially available products contain no antimicrobial preservatives; therefore, product labeling recommends using irinotecan admixtures as follows:

Vehicle Solution	Storage Temperature (After Preparation)	Shelf-life/Expiry Time (After Preparation)
D5W	2°–8°C (35.6°–46.4°F)	24 hours
D5W *or* 0.9% NS	15°–30°C (59°–86°F)	6 hours
D5W *or* 0.9% NS*	15°–30°C (59°–86°F)	12 hours
	2°–8°C (35.6°–46.4°F)	24 hours

*Under strictly maintained aseptic conditions ["Camptosar® (Irinotecan) Injection, intravenous infusion" and "Camptosar® irinotecan hydrochloride injection, for intravenous use only" product labeling]

Selected incompatibilities:

- Irinotecan in its active lactone form is maximally stable at pH ≤6. *Avoid admixture* with neutral or alkaline solutions[48]
- Irinotecan is susceptible to photodegradation
  - Photodegradation occurs at any solution pH, but is accelerated at neutral and alkaline pH in comparison with acidic pH[49,50]
  - The extent of photodegradation appears to be inversely related to irinotecan concentration in solution[51]
  - Although there is experimental evidence that indicates light protection may not be necessary during clinical use,[52] given the compound's propensity for photodegradation, protection from light exposure is a simple and prudent measure to employ toward maintaining product quality[51]

Recommendations for Drug Administration and Ancillary Care

General:

- See Chapter 41 for recommended use in patients with renal and hepatic dysfunction
- Administer irinotecan intraVENously over 90 minutes
- Irinotecan has anticholinesterase activity
  - Patients may experience cholinergic symptoms during or shortly after receiving irinotecan, including rhinitis, increased salivation, miosis, lacrimation, diaphoresis, hypotension, flushing, bradycardia, and intestinal hyperperistalsis that may cause abdominal cramping and diarrhea
- Atropine 0.25–1 mg intraVENously or SUBCUTaneously may be administered prophylactically or therapeutically to patients who experience cholinergic symptoms in association with irinotecan

- Irinotecan is metabolically activated to SN-38 by carboxyl esterase enzymes primarily in the liver
- SN-38 is a substrate for phase 2 metabolism by polymorphically expressed uridine diphosphate glucuronosyltransferase enzymes, particularly UGT1A1
  - Approximately 10% of the North American population expresses homozygously *UGT1A1*28* alleles (also known as a UGT1A1 7/7 genotype) and, consequently, experiences greater exposure to SN-38 and is at greater risk for neutropenia from irinotecan than are persons who express wild-type *UGT1A1* alleles (*AKA* UGT1A1 6/6 genotype)
- Initial irinotecan dosage should be decreased for persons who homozygously express *UGT1A1*28* alleles
  - The degree to which irinotecan dosage should be decreased cannot be predicted

- Second and subsequent doses should be based on an individual's tolerance of prior treatment
- Irinotecan and SN-38 metabolism and elimination are susceptible to perturbation by potent CYP3A4 inducers (carbamazepine, phenobarbital, phenytoin, rifabutin, rifampin, St. John's wort) and inhibitors of CYP3A4 (ketoconazole), UGT1A1 (SORAfenib), or both CYP3A4 and UGT1A1 enzymes (atazanavir)

Inadvertent exposure:

- In case of skin contact, immediately and thoroughly wash the affected area with soap and water. *Do not abrade* the skin by using a scrub brush
- Treat accidental contact with mucous membranes immediately by thoroughly flushing the affected area with water

IXABEPILONE

IXEMPRA® Kit (ixabepilone) for injection, for intravenous infusion only; product label, October 2011. Manufactured by Baxter Oncology GmbH, Halle/Westfalen, Germany. Diluent for IXEMPRA® manufactured by Baxter Oncology GmbH. Distributed by Bristol-Myers Squibb Company, Princeton, NJ

WARNING: TOXICITY IN HEPATIC IMPAIRMENT

IXEMPRA (ixabepilone) in combination with capecitabine is contraindicated in patients with AST or ALT >2.5 × ULN or bilirubin >1 × ULN due to increased risk of toxicity and neutropenia-related death...

Boxed Warning for "IXEMPRA® *Kit* (ixabepilone) for Injection, for intravenous infusion only"; October 2011 product label; Bristol-Myers Squibb Company, Princeton, NJ

Product Identification, Preparation, Storage, and Stability

- IXEMPRA® is supplied as a kit containing 1 sterile, nonpyrogenic, single-use vial of ixabepilone as a lyophilized white powder, labeled: "IXEMPRA® for injection"
- The lyophilized drug product is packaged with a vial of a sterile, nonpyrogenic diluent solution of 52.8% (w/v) purified polyoxyethylated castor oil and 39.8% (w/v) dehydrated alcohol, USP, labeled: "Diluent for IXEMPRA®"
- The commercial product is marketed in 2 presentations:

1 Vial IXEMPRA® for Injection (Ixabepilone Content)	1 Vial of Diluent for IXEMPRA® (Diluent Volume)	NDC Number
15 mg	8 mL	0015-1910-12
45 mg	23.5 mL	0015-1911-13

Note: To compensate for withdrawal losses, vials labeled 15 mg Ixempra for injection contain 16 mg of ixabepilone and vials labeled 45 mg Ixempra for injection contain 47 mg of ixabepilone

- Commercial IXEMPRA® Kit must be stored under refrigeration at 2°–8°C (35.6°–46.4°F) and retained in the original packaging until time of use to protect it from light
- Prior to constituting Ixempra for injection, both drug and diluent vials should be removed from the refrigerator and allowed to stand at room temperature for approximately 30 minutes
  - When diluent vials are first removed from the refrigerator, a white precipitate may be observed within the vials. The precipitate will dissolve to form a clear solution after the diluent warms to room temperature
- Only the diluent supplied in a kit should be used to reconstitute Ixempra (ixabepilone) for injection

Reconstitution:
- With a syringe, aseptically withdraw the diluent and slowly inject it into the copackaged vial containing lyophilized ixabepilone:
  - To a vial containing 15 mg of ixabepilone, add 8 mL of diluent
  - To a vial containing 45 mg of ixabepilone, add 23.5 mL of diluent
- Gently swirl and invert the vial until the lyophilized powder is completely dissolved
- After reconstitution, concentrated ixabepilone solution (2 mg/mL) should be further diluted with an appropriate fluid as soon as possible, but may be stored in the vial (*not the syringe*) for a maximum of 1 hour at room temperature and room lighting

Dilution:
- Before administration, concentrated ixabepilone solution (2 mg/mL) must be further diluted in a DEHP-free parenteral product container (generally, non-PVC containers)
- Aseptically withdraw and measure with a calibrated syringe an amount of concentrated ixabepilone solution required for a patient's dose, and transfer it to a DEHP-free parenteral product bag or bottle containing a volume of solution sufficient to produce a final ixabepilone concentration within the range 0.2–0.6 mg/mL
- Fluids appropriate for diluting ixabepilone have in common a pH within the range of 6.0–9.0, which is required to maintain ixabepilone stability. Other infusion fluids should not be used
- The following parenteral fluids are appropriate for diluting ixabepilone:

Product Identification, Preparation, Storage, and Stability (*continued*)

- Lactated Ringer injection, USP
- Plasma-Lyte A injection pH 7.4 (multiple electrolytes injection, type 1, USP) (Baxter Healthcare Corporation)
- 0.9% Sodium chloride injection, USP, with pH adjusted with sodium bicarbonate injection, USP
  - When using 0.9% NS as a vehicle for clinical use, the solution pH must be adjusted to 6.0–9.0 *before* concentrated ixabepilone solution (2 mg/mL) is added to the vehicle solution
  - To 250 mL or 500 mL of 0.9% NS, add:

    2 mL of Sodium bicarbonate injection, USP 8.4% (w/v) solution, *or*

    4 mL of Sodium bicarbonate injection, USP 4.2% (w/v) solution
- Thoroughly mix diluted ixabepilone by manually rotating the product container

Recommendations for Drug Administration and Ancillary Care

Premedication:

- All patients must receive primary prophylaxis against hypersensitivity reactions approximately 1 hour before ixabepilone administration commences, including:
  - A histamine H_1-subtype receptor antagonist, for example, diphenhydrAMINE 50 mg or equivalent H_1 antihistamine administered orally, *plus*
  - A histamine H_2-subtype receptor antagonist, for example, ranitidine 150–300 mg or equivalent H_2 antihistamine administer orally
- In addition to pretreatment with H_1 and H_2 antihistamines, patients who previously experienced a hypersensitivity reaction associated with ixabepilone administration require steroid premedication, for example, dexamethasone 20 mg administered intraVENously 30 minutes before infusion, *or* dexamethasone 20 mg administered orally 60 minutes before starting ixabepilone administration

General:

- See Chapter 41 for recommended use in patients with renal and hepatic dysfunction
- DEHP-free administration sets must be used to administer ixabepilone
- Ixabepilone must be administered through an inline filter with a pore size within the range of 0.2–1.2 μm
- The durations of administration for recommended for 40 mg ixabepilone/m² is 3 hours, and 4 hours for 60 mg ixabepilone/m²
  - Other dosages, administration schedules, and durations of administration have been evaluated in clinical trials

LEUCOVORIN CALCIUM

LEUCOVORIN CALCIUM–leucovorin calcium injection, powder, lyophilized, for solution; product label, September 2012. Manufactured by Teva Parenteral Medicines, Inc., Irvine, CA
LEUCOVORIN CALCIUM for injection; product label, December 2009. APP Pharmaceuticals LLC, Schaumburg, IL
LEUCOVORIN CALCIUM injection USP; product label, September 2008. Manufactured by Ben Venue Laboratories, Inc., Bedford, OH. Manufactured for Bedford Laboratories, Bedford, OH
LEUCOVORIN CALCIUM INJECTION USP, LEUCOVORIN CALCIUM FOR INJECTION; product label, October 2013. Manufactured for Bedford Laboratories™, Bedford, OH

Product Identification, Preparation, Storage, and Stability

Leucovorin calcium for injection:

- Leucovorin calcium for injection is generically available in a variety of presentations, including:
  50 mg/vial packaged in cartons of 10 single-use vials
  100 mg/vial individually packaged in single-use vials *or* in cartons of 10 single-use vials
  200 mg/vial individually packaged in single-use vials
  350 mg/vial individually packaged in single-use vials

- Leucovorin calcium for injection is a sterile, lyophilized powder indicated for intraMUSCular or intraVENous administration. In general, the lyophilized powdered products do not contain an antimicrobial preservative
- Store leucovorin calcium for injection at room temperature
  - *Note:* Storage temperature requirements for leucovorin calcium for injection vary among different manufacturers' products
  - Consult product labeling for product-specific storage temperature recommendations
- Retain vials in their packaging carton to protect the drug product from light until they are used
- Reconstitute leucovorin calcium for injection with BWFI (preserved with benzyl alcohol)* or SWFI as follows:

Amount of Leucovorin Calcium per Vial	Volume of Diluent per Vial	Concentration After Reconstitution
50 mg	5 mL	10 mg/mL
100 mg	10 mL	
200 mg	20 mL	
350 mg	17.5 mL	20 mg/mL
500 mg	50 mL	10 mg/mL

*FDA-approved product labeling recommends reconstituting leucovorin with SWFI for dosages >10 mg/m² (for adult patients) because of the amount of benzyl alcohol present in BWFI. *Avoid* administering benzyl alcohol-containing products to adolescents and younger patients

- After reconstitution with BWFI, the resulting solution must be used within 7 days. If reconstituted with SWFI, use the product immediately and discard any unused portion

Leucovorin calcium injection:

- Leucovorin calcium injection, USP, is available in individually boxed, single-use vials containing leucovorin calcium 500 mg (per 50 mL) in a sterile, preservative-free solution indicated for intraMUSCular or intraVENous administration
- Each milliliter of solution contains leucovorin calcium equivalent to 10 mg leucovorin, USP, with sodium chloride and sodium hydroxide and/or hydrochloric acid to adjust solution to an alkaline pH which varies among different manufacturers' products (range: pH 6.5–8.5)
- Store leucovorin calcium injection under refrigeration at 2°–8°C (35.6°–46.4°F). Retain vials in their packaging carton to protect the drug product from light until they are used
- Discard any unused portion

Instructions common to both leucovorin calcium for injection and leucovorin calcium injection:

- Leucovorin calcium may be further diluted with D5W, 0.9% NS, D5W/0.9% NS, D10W, RI, or LRI for clinical use

Selected incompatibility:

- *Do not mix* leucovorin with fluorouracil. Admixture results in particulate formation

Recommendations for Drug Administration and Ancillary Care

General:

- For intraVENous or intraMUSCular administration
- Administer leucovorin intraVENously over *at least* 3 minutes
- *Do not administer* leucovorin intraVENously more rapidly than 160 mg/min because of the rate at which calcium will be injected
  - For solutions reconstituted from (lyophilized) leucovorin calcium for injection:

Leucovorin Concentration in Solution	Volume of Solution Containing 160 mg Leucovorin
10 mg/mL	16 mL
20 mg/mL	8 mL

  - One milligram of leucovorin calcium contains:

Calcium	0.004 mEq
Calcium	0.002 mmol
Leucovorin	0.002 mmol

Caution:

- In treating an accidental overdose of intraTHECALly administered folic acid antagonists, *do not administer* leucovorin intraTHECALly leucovorin may be harmful or fatal if given intraTHECALly
- Concomitant use of leucovorin with trimethoprim-sulfamethoxazole (cotrimoxazole) for the acute treatment of *Pneumocystis jirovecii* (formerly *Pneumocystis carinii*) pneumonia in patients with HIV infection was associated with increased rates of treatment failure and morbidity in a placebo-controlled study
- High doses of leucovorin by intraVENous, intraMUSCular, or oral routes may reduce the efficacy of intraTHECALly administered methotrexate

LEVOLEUCOVORIN CALCIUM

Fusilev® (levoleucovorin) for injection, powder, lyophilized, for solution for intravenous use; Fusilev® (levoleucovorin) injection, solution for intravenous use; product label, April 2011. Manufactured for Spectrum Pharmaceuticals, Inc., Irvine, CA

Product Identification, Preparation, Storage, and Stability

- LEVOleucovorin is the levorotatory isomeric form of racemic *d,l*-leucovorin, the pharmacologically active isomer of leucovorin [(6-*S*)-leucovorin], present as the calcium salt

Fusilev® Injection (product in solution):

- Fusilev® injection is provided in 50-mg single-use vials containing a sterile solution of either 175 mg LEVOleucovorin in 17.5 mL (NDC 68152-102-01) or 250 mg LEVOleucovorin in 25 mL (NDC 68152-102-02)
- Each milliliter of solution contains LEVOleucovorin calcium pentahydrate equivalent to 10 mg LEVOleucovorin and 8.3 mg sodium chloride. Sodium hydroxide is used to adjust solution pH to 8.0 (6.5–8.5). Fusilev® injection does not contain an antimicrobial preservative
- Store LEVOleucovorin in solution under refrigeration at 2°–8°C (35.6°–46.4°F) in its packaging carton to protect the drug product from light until vial contents are used
- Fusilev® injection (LEVOleucovorin in solution, 10 mg/mL) may be further diluted to a concentration = 0.5 mg/mL in 0.9% NS or D5W
- Fusilev® injection (LEVOleucovorin in solution) diluted in 0.9% NS or D5W stored at room temperature *must be used* within 4 hours after preparation

Fusilev® for injection (lyophilized product):

- Fusilev® for injection is provided in 50-mg single-use vials containing a sterile lyophilized powder consisting of 64 mg LEVOleucovorin calcium pentahydrate (equivalent to 50 mg LEVOleucovorin) and 50 mg mannitol per 50-mg vial. Sodium hydroxide and hydrochloric acid are used to adjust product pH during manufacture (NDC 68152-101-00).

- Fusilev® for injection does not contain an antimicrobial preservative
- Store lyophilized LEVOleucovorin at 25°C (77°F) in its packaging carton to protect the drug product from light until vial contents are used. Temperature excursions are permitted from 15° to 30°C (59°–86°F)
- Reconstitute the lyophilized product with 5.3 mL of sterile 0.9% NS to produce a solution with LEVOleucovorin concentration of 10 mg/mL
  - *Do not use* preserved diluent solutions
- The reconstituted solution (10 mg/mL) may be immediately diluted to concentrations within a range of 0.5–5 mg/mL in 0.9% NS or D5W
- After reconstitution (10 mg/mL), dilution in D5W, and storage at room temperature, LEVOleucovorin *must be used* within 4 hours after preparation
- After reconstitution (10 mg/mL) and dilution in 0.9% NS, LEVOleucovorin solutions stored at room temperature *must be used* within 12 hours after preparation
- *Do not use* LEVOleucovorin if cloudiness or a precipitate is observed in solution
- Do not administer LEVOleucovorin intraVENously at a rate greater than 160 mg/minute (not greater than 16 mL/min for the reconstituted solution without further dilution), because of the calcium content of the LEVOleucovorin solution

Selected incompatibility:

- *Do not mix* LEVOleucovorin with fluorouracil. Admixture results in particulate formation
- *Do not administer* LEVOleucovorin in an admixture with other drug products or in diluent or vehicle solutions other than 0.9 NS or D5W

Recommendations for Drug Administration and Ancillary Care

General:

- LEVOleucovorin dose or dosage is one-half (50%) the dose or dosage recommended for racemic *d,l*-leucovorin
- Fusilev® is indicated only for intraVENous administration. *Do not administer* LEVOleucovorin intraTHECALly
- *Do not inject* LEVOleucovorin intraVENously more rapidly than 160 mg/min because of the rate at which calcium will be injected
  - One milligram of LEVOleucovorin calcium contains:

Calcium	0.004 mEq
Calcium	0.002 mmol
Leucovorin	0.002 mmol

- Concomitant use of racemic leucovorin with trimethoprim-sulfamethoxazole (cotrimoxazole) for the acute treatment of *Pneumocystis jirovecii* (formerly *Pneumocystis carinii*) pneumonia in patients with HIV infection was associated with increased rates of treatment failure and morbidity in a placebo-controlled study

MECHLORETHAMINE HYDROCHLORIDE

Trituration of Mustargen® (mechlorethamine HCl for injection); product label, February 2013. Manufactured by Baxter Oncology, GmbH, 33790 Halle/Westfalen, Germany. Manufactured for Recordati Rare Diseases Inc., Lebanon, NJ

WARNINGS

MUSTARGEN® (mechlorethamine HCl) should be administered only under the supervision of a physician who is experienced in the use of cancer chemotherapeutic agents

This drug is **HIGHLY TOXIC** and both powder and solution must be handled and administered with care. Inhalation of dust or vapors and contact with skin or mucous membranes, especially those of the eyes, must be avoided. Avoid exposure during pregnancy. Due to the toxic properties of mechlorethamine (eg, corrosivity, carcinogenicity, mutagenicity, teratogenicity), special handling procedures should be reviewed prior to handling and followed diligently

Extravasation of the drug into subcutaneous tissues results in a painful inflammation. The area usually becomes indurated and sloughing may occur. If leakage of drug is obvious, prompt infiltration of the area with sterile isotonic sodium thiosulfate (1/6 molar) and application of an ice compress for 6 to 12 hours may minimize the local reaction. For a 1/6 molar solution of sodium thiosulfate, use 4.14 g of sodium thiosulfate per 100 mL of Sterile Water for Injection or 2.64 g of anhydrous sodium thiosulfate per 100 mL or dilute 4 mL of Sodium Thiosulfate Injection (10%) with 6 mL of Sterile Water for Injection

---

Boxed Warning for "Trituration of Mustargen® (mechlorethamine HCl for injection)"; February 2013 product label; Recordati Rare Diseases Inc., Lebanon, NJ

Product Identification, Preparation, Storage, and Stability

- Trituration of Mustargen® is a light yellow-brown, crystalline powder packaged in vials containing 10 mg mechlorethamine hydrochloride triturated with sodium chloride Q.S. 100 mg. NDC 55292-911-51 (package of 4 vials)
- Store intact vials at controlled room temperature (15°–30°C; 59°–86°F). Protect vials from light and humidity
- Mechlorethamine solution must be prepared *immediately before use* because it will rapidly and spontaneously decompose on standing
  - In neutral or alkaline aqueous solutions, mechlorethamine undergoes rapid chemical transformation and is highly unstable. Although solutions prepared

according to instructions are acidic and do not decompose as rapidly, they should be prepared immediately before each injection
- *Do not use* mechlorethamine solution if it is discolored or, if prior to reconstitution, droplets of water are visible within a vial
- When dissolved in 10 mL of SWFI or 0.9% NS, the resulting solution has a pH within the range of 3–5 at a concentration of 1 mg mechlorethamine HCl/mL

IntraVENous administration:

- Reconstitute by injecting 10 mL of SWFI or 0.9% NS into a vial containing mechlorethamine HCl 10 mg

Intracavitary administration:

- Reconstitute by adding 10 mL of SWFI or 0.9% NS to a vial containing mechlorethamine HCl 10 mg. The drug may be further diluted with 0.9% NS to a volume of 50–100 mL for intracavitary injection[53]
  - Refer to complete product labeling for more detailed information about intrapleural, intraperitoneal, and intrapericardial injection

---

Recommendations for Drug Administration and Ancillary Care

General:

- Mechlorethamine dosage varies with the clinical situation and pharmacodynamic responses to treatment (therapeutic and myelosuppression)
  - Dosage should be based on ideal dry body weight
  - The presence of edema or ascites must be considered so that dosage will be based on actual weight, not augmented by these conditions
- *Do not use* mechlorethamine solution if it is discolored

- After measuring a patient's dose in a syringe:
  1. Empty the needle lumen by withdrawing all mechlorethamine into the syringe barrel
  2. Remove the needle from the syringe used to withdraw mechlorethamine from a vial
  3. Replace it with a fresh needle before injecting the drug
  - Trace amounts of mechlorethamine may adhere to a needle's exterior surfaces when it is withdrawn from a vial

  - Replacing a needle used to aspirate mechlorethamine from a vial prevents tracking mechlorethamine adhering to a needle's exterior surface through soft tissue during venipuncture and from contaminating vascular access device surfaces when mechlorethamine is injected into the side arm of an administration set
- Mechlorethamine may be injected directly into any suitable vein, but preferably is injected into the side arm of a freely flowing intraVENous infusion

(continued)

Recommendations for Drug Administration and Ancillary Care (continued)

Caution: Mechlorethamine is a vesicant and may produce severe local soft-tissue necrosis if extravasation occurs

- Direct injection into the tubing rather than adding mechlorethamine to an infusion fluid minimizes the opportunity for a chemical reaction between the drug and the solution. The rate of injection is not critical provided it is completed within a few minutes

Intracavitary (intrapleural, intraperitoneal, intrapericardial) administration:

- The usual dose of nitrogen mustard for intracavitary injection is 0.4 mg/kg of body weight[53-56], though 0.2 mg/kg, or fixed doses of 10 and 20 mg (to 22 mg) have been used by the intrapericardial route[53,54]
- Mechlorethamine should be injected slowly, with frequent aspiration to ensure a free flow of fluid is present
  - If fluid cannot be aspirated, pain and necrosis due to injection of solution outside the cavity may occur

- Free flow of fluid also is necessary to prevent injection into a loculated space and to ensure adequate distribution within a cavity
- Have a patient change position every 5–10 minutes for 1 hour after injection to obtain uniform drug distribution throughout a serous cavity. The remaining fluid may be removed from the pleural or peritoneal cavity by paracentesis 24–36 hours after administration

Caution: Mechlorethamine is a vesicant and may produce severe local soft-tissue necrosis if extravasation occurs

Neutralization of equipment and unused solution:

- To clean rubber gloves, tubing, glassware, etc, after giving mechlorethamine, soak them in an aqueous solution containing equal volumes of sodium thiosulfate (5%) and sodium bicarbonate (5%) for 45 minutes. After soaking, excess reagents and reaction products may be easily washed away with water. Any unused mechlorethamine solution should be neutralized by mixing it with an equal volume of sodium thiosulfate + sodium bicarbonate solution. Allow the mixture to stand for 45 minutes. Vials that have contained mechlorethamine should be treated in the same way before disposal

Inadvertent exposures:

- Should accidental eye contact occur, immediately irrigate the eyes for at least 15 minutes with copious amounts of water, 0.9% NS, or a balanced salt ophthalmic irrigating solution, followed by prompt ophthalmologic consultation
- Should accidental skin contact occur, the affected part must be irrigated immediately with copious amounts of water, for at least 15 minutes, followed by 2% sodium thiosulfate solution. Medical attention should be sought immediately
- Contaminated clothing should be destroyed

MELPHALAN HYDROCHLORIDE

ALKERAN® (melphalan hydrochloride) for injection; product label, June 2011. ALKERAN® and diluent manufactured by GlaxoSmithKline, Research Triangle Park, NC. Distributed by ApoPharma USA Inc., Rockville, MD

Melphalan Hydrochloride for injection; product label, August 2008. Made in Italy. Manufactured for Bioniche Pharma USA LLC, Lake Forest, IL

WARNING

Melphalan should be administered under the supervision of a qualified physician experienced in the use of cancer chemotherapeutic agents. Severe bone marrow suppression with resulting infection or bleeding may occur. Controlled trials comparing intravenous (IV) to oral melphalan have shown more myelosuppression with the IV formulation. Hypersensitivity reactions, including anaphylaxis, have occurred in approximately 2% of patients who received the IV formulation. Melphalan is leukemogenic in humans. Melphalan produces chromosomal aberrations in vitro and in vivo and, therefore, should be considered potentially mutagenic in humans

---

Boxed Warning for "MELPHALAN HYDROCHLORIDE"; December 2011 product label; Mylan Institutional LLC, Rockford, IL

Product Identification, Preparation, Storage, and Stability

- Melphalan hydrochloride for injection is supplied in a carton containing (a) 1 single-use, clear, glass vial containing freeze-dried melphalan hydrochloride equivalent to 50 mg melphalan and the inactive ingredient povidone 20 mg as a sterile, nonpyrogenic, freeze-dried powder, and (b) one 10-mL, clear, glass vial of sterile, nonpyrogenic sterile diluent for melphalan hydrochloride for injection containing 200 mg sodium citrate, 6 mL of propylene glycol, 0.52 mL of ethanol (96%), and SWFI to a total of (Q.S.) 10 mL
- Store melphalan hydrochloride for injection at room temperature and protect from light
  - *Note:* Storage temperature requirements for Melphalan Hydrochloride for Injection vary among different manufacturers' products
  - Consult product labeling for product-specific storage temperature recommendations

Preparation for administration:

1. Reconstitute melphalan by *rapidly injecting* 10 mL of the supplied diluent directly into the vial of lyophilized powder using a sterile needle (≥20-gauge) and syringe
   a. Melphalan is practically insoluble in water and has a pKa₁ of ~2.5

   pKa_1 of ~2.5

2. Immediately *shake the vial vigorously* until a clear solution is obtained. This provides a 5-mg/mL solution of melphalan. Rapid addition of the diluent followed by immediate vigorous shaking is important for proper dissolution. The reconstituted solution is not stable at room temperature for more than 90 minutes
3. Immediately withdraw into a syringe an amount of reconstituted melphalan solution appropriate for a patient's dose and dilute it in 0.9% NS, to a concentration ≤0.45 mg/mL

a. The time between melphalan reconstitution, dilution, and administration should be kept to a minimum because the diluted solution is unstable
b. Within 30 minutes after melphalan reconstitution with sterile diluent for melphalan hydrochloride for injection, a citrate derivative of melphalan has been detected
c. After further dilution with 0.9% NS, nearly 1% of the labeled strength of melphalan hydrolyzes every 10 minutes
d. A precipitate forms if the reconstituted solution is stored at 5°C (41°F). *Do not refrigerate* the reconstituted product

---

Recommendations for Drug Administration and Ancillary Care

General:

- See Chapter 41 for recommended use in patients with renal dysfunction
- Administer melphalan by intraVENous infusion over 15–20 minutes (at least 15 minutes)
- *Complete melphalan administration within 60 minutes after reconstitution*, because reconstituted and diluted solutions are unstable

Caution:

- Severe renal failure has been reported in patients treated with a single dose of intraVENously administered melphalan

followed by standard oral doses of cycloSPORINE
- CISplatin may affect melphalan pharmacokinetics by inducing renal dysfunction and secondarily decreasing melphalan clearance
- IntraVENously administered melphalan may decrease the threshold for lung toxicity associated with carmustine
- The incidence of severe hemorrhagic necrotic enterocolitis has been reported to increase in pediatric patients when nalidixic acid and intraVENously administered melphalan are given simultaneously

Inadvertent exposure:

- If melphalan HCl contacts skin or mucosa, immediately wash the affected area with soap and water

MESNA

MESNA–mesna injection, solution; product label, October 2011. Manufactured for Mylan Institutional LLC, Rockford, IL
Mesna Injection 100 mg per mL (For IV Use); product label, September 2012. Made in India. Manufactured for SAGENT Pharmaceuticals, Schaumburg, IL
MESNEX–mesna injection, solution; product label, February 2009. Manufactured by Baxter Healthcare Corporation, Deerfield, IL
MESNA–mesna injection, solution; product label, July 2005. Manufactured by Ben Venue Laboratories, Inc., Bedford, OH. Manufactured for Amerinet Choice, St. Louis, MO
MESNA INJECTION; product label, March 2013. Manufactured for Bedford Laboratories, Bedford, OH
MESNA INJECTION; product label, January 2008. APP Pharmaceuticals LLC, Schaumburg, IL

Product Identification, Preparation, Storage, and Stability

- Mesna injection is a sterile, nonpyrogenic, clear, colorless, aqueous solution for intraVENous administration in clear, glass, multidose vials packaged individually or in greater quantities
- Each milliliter of mesna injection contains mesna 100 mg; edetate disodium 0.25 mg; benzyl alcohol 10.4 mg as a preservative, (Q.S.) SWFI, and sodium hydroxide to adjust solution to an alkaline pH that varies among different manufacturers' products (range: pH 6.5–8.5)
- Store mesna at room temperature, 20°–25°C (68°–77°F). Product-specific recommendations for storage temperatures may identify permissible temperature excursions
- Multidose vials may be stored and used for up to 8 days after initial vial entry
- For intraVENous administration mesna injection (100 mg/mL) may be diluted by admixture (1 mL of mesna injection added to 4 mL of a compatible solution) with any of the following fluids to produce a concentration of 20 mg mesna/mL: D5W, D5W/0.2% NaCl, D5W/0.33% NaCl, D5W/0.45% NaCl, 0.9% NS, LRI
- Diluted mesna solutions (20 mg/mL) are chemically and physically stable for 24 hours at 25°C (77°F)
- Additional compatibility and stability data indicate mesna is stable at room temperature for at least 24 hours when diluted to concentration of 1 mg/mL in 0.9% NS, D5W, D5W/0.45% NaCl, and LRI[57]
- Mesna is compatible in admixture (prepared in the same container) with both ifosfamide and cyclophosphamide

Selected incompatibility:

- Mesna is *not compatible* and should not be mixed in a container or in administration set tubing with cisplatin or carboplatin

Recommendations for Drug Administration and Ancillary Care

General:

- See Chapter 41 for comments about use in patients with renal and hepatic dysfunction
- Mesna may be administered by intraVENous injection, intermittent intravenous infusion over 15–30 minutes, or continuous intraVENous infusion during ifosfamide or cyclophosphamide administration and for periods afterward
- If mesna tablets are not available for use, the parenteral product also may be given orally, diluted just before use in a small volume (60–120 mL; 2–4 oz) of a chilled carbonated beverage to mask the drug's unpleasant flavor
- Avoid exposing mesna injection to the air. Mesna spontaneously oxidizes to dimesna on exposure to oxygen
- FDA-approved product labeling describes intermittent administration of mesna with ifosfamide as follows:

IntraVENous administration:

- Mesna in a dosage equal to 20% (w/w) of the ifosfamide dosage is given at the same time as ifosfamide, and then at 4 hours and 8 hours after ifosfamide administration began; that is, the total daily mesna dose is approximately 60% of the daily ifosfamide dose

IntraVENous and oral administration:

- Mesna in a dosage equal to 20% (w/w) of the ifosfamide dosage is given intraVENously at the same time as ifosfamide, and then mesna tablets are given orally at 2 hours and 6 hours after each ifosfamide dose with each oral doses equal to 40% of the ifosfamide dose; that is, the total daily mesna dose is approximately equal to the daily ifosfamide dose

Caution:

- Allergic reactions to mesna, ranging from mild hypersensitivity to systemic anaphylactic reactions, have been reported
- Mesna injection does not prevent urothelial toxicity in all patients
  - Advise patients who receive mesna with ifosfamide or cyclophosphamide who are not receiving parenterally administered fluids to drink at least one quart (≥1000 mL) per day on days of treatment and for several days afterward
  - A morning specimen of urine should be examined microscopically for the presence of hematuria each day prior to ifosfamide therapy
  - To reduce the risk of hematuria, mesna must be administered with each dose of ifosfamide
  - Mesna is not effective in reducing the risk of hematuria caused by other pathologic conditions, for example, thrombocytopenia,
- Multidose vials containing benzyl alcohol should not be used in neonates or infants and should be used with caution in older pediatric patients

Interaction with laboratory test:

- A false-positive test for urinary ketones may arise in patients treated with mesna injection. In this test, a red-violet color develops, which, with the addition of glacial acetic acid, will return to violet

METHOTREXATE

METHOTREXATE—methotrexate injection, powder, lyophilized, for solution [and]
METHOTREXATE—methotrexate injection, solution; product label, April 2012. Manufactured for Bedford Laboratories, Bedford, OH
METHOTREXATE—methotrexate sodium injection, solution; product label, December 2011. APP Pharmaceutical LLC, Schaumburg, IL
METHOTREXATE—methotrexate sodium injection, solution; product label, October 2011. Hospira, Inc., Lake Forest, IL
METHOTREXATE SODIUM—methotrexate sodium injection, solution; product label, December 2011. Manufactured for Sandoz Inc., Princeton, NJ. Manufactured by EBEWE Pharma Ges.m.b.H. Nfg.KG, A-4866 Unterach, AUSTRIA

WARNINGS

METHOTREXATE SHOULD BE USED ONLY BY PHYSICIANS WHOSE KNOWLEDGE AND EXPERIENCE INCLUDE THE USE OF ANTIMETABOLITE THERAPY. BECAUSE OF THE POSSIBILITY OF SERIOUS TOXIC REACTIONS (WHICH CAN BE FATAL):

METHOTREXATE SHOULD BE USED ONLY IN LIFE THREATENING NEOPLASTIC DISEASES, OR IN PATIENTS WITH PSORIASIS OR RHEUMATOID ARTHRITIS WITH SEVERE, RECALCITRANT, DISABLING DISEASE WHICH IS NOT ADEQUATELY RESPONSIVE TO OTHER FORMS OF THERAPY

DEATHS HAVE BEEN REPORTED WITH THE USE OF METHOTREXATE IN THE TREATMENT OF MALIGNANCY, PSORIASIS, AND RHEUMATOID ARTHRITIS

PATIENTS SHOULD BE CLOSELY MONITORED FOR BONE MARROW, LIVER, LUNG AND KIDNEY TOXICITIES...

PATIENTS SHOULD BE INFORMED BY THEIR PHYSICIAN OF THE RISKS INVOLVED AND BE UNDER A PHYSICIAN'S CARE THROUGHOUT THERAPY

THE USE OF METHOTREXATE HIGH DOSE REGIMENS RECOMMENDED FOR OSTEOSARCOMA REQUIRES METICULOUS CARE... HIGH DOSE REGIMENS FOR OTHER NEOPLASTIC DISEASES ARE INVESTIGATIONAL AND A THERAPEUTIC ADVANTAGE HAS NOT BEEN ESTABLISHED. METHOTREXATE FORMULATIONS AND DILUENTS CONTAINING PRESERVATIVES MUST NOT BE USED FOR INTRATHECAL OR HIGH DOSE METHOTREXATE THERAPY

1. Methotrexate has been reported to cause fetal death and/or congenital anomalies. Therefore, it is not recommended for women of childbearing potential unless there is clear medical evidence that the benefits can be expected to outweigh the considered risks. Pregnant women with psoriasis or rheumatoid arthritis should not receive methotrexate...

2. Methotrexate elimination is reduced in patients with impaired renal function, ascites, or pleural effusions. Such patients require especially careful monitoring for toxicity, and require dose reduction or, in some cases, discontinuation of methotrexate administration

3. Unexpectedly severe (sometimes fatal) bone marrow suppression, aplastic anemia, and gastrointestinal toxicity have been reported with concomitant administration of methotrexate (usually in high dosage) along with some non-steroidal antiinflammatory drugs (NSAIDs)...

4. Methotrexate causes hepatotoxicity, fibrosis and cirrhosis, but generally only after prolonged use. Acutely, liver enzyme elevations are frequently seen. These are usually transient and asymptomatic, and also do not appear predictive of subsequent hepatic disease. Liver biopsy after sustained use often shows histologic changes, and fibrosis and cirrhosis have been reported; these latter lesions may not be preceded by symptoms or abnormal liver function tests in the psoriasis population. For this reason, periodic liver biopsies are usually recommended for psoriatic patients who are under long-term treatment. Persistent abnormalities in liver function tests may precede appearance of fibrosis or cirrhosis in the rheumatoid arthritis population...

5. Methotrexate-induced lung disease, including acute or chronic interstitial pneumonitis, is a potentially dangerous lesion, which may occur acutely at any time during therapy and has been reported at low doses. It is not always fully reversible and fatalities have been reported. Pulmonary symptoms (especially a dry nonproductive cough) may require interruption of treatment and careful investigation

6. Diarrhea and ulcerative stomatitis require interruption of therapy; otherwise, hemorrhagic enteritis and death from intestinal perforation may occur

7. Malignant lymphomas, which may regress following withdrawal of methotrexate, may occur in patients receiving low-dose methotrexate and, thus, may not require cytotoxic treatment. Discontinue methotrexate first and, if the lymphoma does not regress, appropriate treatment should be instituted

8. Like other cytotoxic drugs, methotrexate may induce "tumor lysis syndrome" in patients with rapidly growing tumors. Appropriate supportive and pharmacologic measures may prevent or alleviate this complication

9. Severe, occasionally fatal, skin reactions have been reported following single or multiple doses of methotrexate. Reactions have occurred within days of oral, intramuscular, intravenous, or intrathecal methotrexate administration. Recovery has been reported with discontinuation of therapy...

10. Potentially fatal opportunistic infections, especially Pneumocystis carinii [*P. jirovecii*] pneumonia, may occur with methotrexate therapy

11. Methotrexate given concomitantly with radiotherapy may increase the risk of soft tissue necrosis and osteonecrosis

---

Boxed Warning for "METHOTREXATE - methotrexate injection, powder, lyophilized, for solution [and] METHOTREXATE - methotrexate injection, solution"; April 2012 product labels. Manufactured for Bedford Laboratories™, Bedford, OH

Product Identification, Preparation, Storage, and Stability

- Methotrexate is generically available in a variety of product strengths in liquid and lyophilized formulations
- Store methotrexate at room temperature and protected from light
  - *Note:* Storage temperature requirements for methotrexate vary among different manufacturers' products
  - Consult product labeling for product-specific storage temperature recommendations
- In general, reconstitute lyophilized products to a concentration not greater than 25 mg methotrexate/mL
- Protect methotrexate products from light. Methotrexate is susceptible to photodegradation, the extent of which correlates inversely with methotrexate concentration and is exacerbated by admixture with sodium bicarbonate
- After reconstitution, lyophilized formulations and methotrexate injection (product in solution) are suitable for direct intraVENous injection
- Methotrexate also may be further diluted for clinical use. A therapeutic indication often determines the volume in which a dose is prepared and administered; that is, whether dilution is necessary, or clinically or logistically appropriate. Compatible diluents include 0.9% NS, D5W, and combinations of saline and dextrose

For intraTHECAL injection and high-dose regimens:

- Use only preservative-free methotrexate and diluent solutions

For intraTHECAL injection:

- Use preservative-free 0.9% NS to dilute methotrexate for intraTHECAL injection to a concentration within the range of 1–2.5 mg/mL
- Admixtures with hydrocortisone sodium succinate for intraTHECAL administration (with or without cytarabine) should be prepared just before use and administered as soon as possible (within minutes) after preparation because of the instability of the hydrocortisone component

Recommendations for Drug Administration and Ancillary Care

General:

- See Chapter 41 for recommended use in patients with renal and hepatic dysfunction
- Methotrexate may be given parenterally by direct intraVENous injection, short intraVENous infusions over <1 hour, or continuous intraVENous infusions for periods up to 24–36 hours, and by the intraMUScular, intraarterial, and intraTHECAL routes

For intraVENous use:

- The duration of methotrexate administration varies among treatment protocols and published reports, and in the case of moderate- and high-dose regimens ($\geq$100 mg/m^2), often correlates with schemes for concomitant hydration, urinary alkalinization, serum level monitoring and expectations for the rate at which methotrexate will be eliminated, and leucovorin rescue

For intraTHECAL injection:

- Use *only products that do not contain antimicrobial preservatives* (eg, alcohols, parabens)
- Cerebrospinal fluid volume is dependent on age *not* body surface area (BSA); therefore, methotrexate doses for intraTHECAL use should be based on patient age, *not* BSA
- Administration should be completed as soon as possible after product preparation
- When possible, inject methotrexate in a volume equivalent to the volume of cerebrospinal fluid removed

Selected drug interactions:

- Avoid concomitant use of nonsteroidal antiinflammatory drugs (NSAIDs) or salicylates with methotrexate, particularly at dosages and treatment schedules used in oncology
  - NSAIDs and salicylates may compete for renal tubular secretion of methotrexate, thus decreasing the rate of methotrexate elimination and enhancing its toxicity
  - Use caution during concomitant use of NSAIDs or salicylates with methotrexate, such as doses and schedules used in immunologic and rheumatologic indications
- Penicillins and probenecid also diminish renal tubular transport and elimination of methotrexate. Serum or plasma methotrexate concentrations should be carefully monitored if methotrexate is given concurrently with these drugs
- Trimethoprim/sulfamethoxazole (cotrimoxazole) has been reported rarely to increase bone marrow suppression in patients receiving methotrexate, probably by competition for renal tubular secretion, additive antifolate effect, or a combination of factors
- Methotrexate increases concentrations of mercaptopurine in plasma during concomitant use
- Folate deficiency states may increase methotrexate toxicity; however, vitamin preparations containing folic acid or its derivatives may decrease responses to systemically administered methotrexate
- Methotrexate volume of distribution approximates the distribution of body water; that is, methotrexate distributes and slowly exits from third-space fluid compartments (eg, pleural or pericardial effusions or ascites), which may result in a prolonged elimination and unexpected toxicity. It is advisable to evacuate significant third-space fluid accumulations before treatment and to monitor serum or plasma methotrexate levels until they are no longer detectable (optimally, $\leq$0.01 μmol/L [$\leq$10^{-8} mol/L])
- Lesions of psoriasis may be aggravated by concomitant exposure to ultraviolet radiation. Radiation dermatitis and dermal inflammation and injuries associated with thermal and solar burns may be exacerbated and "recalled" by subsequent use of methotrexate

MITOMYCIN

MITOMYCIN FOR INJECTION, USP product label, March 2013. Manufactured for Bedford Laboratories, Bedford, OH
MITOMYCIN FOR INJECTION, USP, 5 mg vial, 20 mg vial and 40 mg vial product label, April 2011. Manufactured by Intas Pharmaceuticals Limited, Ahmedabad, India. Manufactured for Accord Healthcare, Inc., Durham, NC
Mitosol® (mitomycin for solution); product label, February 2012. Mobius Therapeutics, LLC. St. Louis, MO
Note: Mitosol® is indicated for use as an adjunct to *ab externo* glaucoma surgery, intended for topical application to the surgical site of glaucoma filtration surgery. *It is not intended* for intraocular administration

WARNINGS

Mitomycin should be administered under the supervision of a qualified physician experienced in the use of cancer chemotherapeutic agents. Appropriate management of therapy and complications is possible only when adequate diagnostic and treatment facilities are readily available

Bone marrow suppression, notably thrombocytopenia and leukopenia, which may contribute to overwhelming infections in an already compromised patient, is the most common and severe of the toxic effects of mitomycin…

Hemolytic Uremic Syndrome (HUS) a serious complication of chemotherapy, consisting primarily of microangiopathic hemolytic anemia, thrombocytopenia, and irreversible renal failure, has been reported in patients receiving systemic mitomycin. The syndrome may occur at any time during systemic therapy with mitomycin as a single agent or in combination with other cytotoxic drugs; however, most cases occur at doses ≥60 mg of mitomycin. Blood product transfusion may exacerbate the symptoms associated with this syndrome

The incidence of the syndrome has not been defined

Boxed Warning (excerpt) for "MITOMYCIN FOR INJECTION, USP"; March 2013 product label; Bedford Laboratories™, Bedford, OH

Product Identification, Preparation, Storage, and Stability

MitoMYcin for Injection

- MitoMYcin is available generically in individually packaged multiuse vials containing a dry mixture of mitoMYcin with mannitol
  - Available presentations include:
  MitoMYcin 5 mg with 10 mg of mannitol
  MitoMYcin 20 mg with 40 mg of mannitol
  MitoMYcin 40 mg with 80 mg of mannitol
- Store intact vials at 25°C (77°F), with temperature excursions permitted between 15° and 30°C (59° and 86°F)
  - MitoMYcin is heat stable and has a high melting point, but avoid exposure to temperatures >40°C (>104°F)
- Protect mitoMYcin from exposure to light by storing vials in their packaging cartons
- Reconstitute mitoMYcin as follows:

Amount of MitoMYcin per Vial	Volume of SWFI Diluent	MitoMYcin Concentration After Reconstitution
5 mg	10 mL	
20 mg	40 mL	0.5 mg/mL
40 mg	80 mL	

- After adding the diluent, shake the vials to dissolve mitoMYcin. If the product does not dissolve immediately, allow it to stand at room temperature until a solution is obtained
- After reconstitution with SWFI, the product is stable for 14 days under refrigeration or 7 days at room temperature
- Store reconstituted mitoMYcin solutions (0.5 mg/mL) under refrigeration 2°–8°C (35.6°–46.4°F)

(continued)

Recommendations for Drug Administration and Ancillary Care

MitoMYcin for Injection
General:
- See Chapter 41 for recommended use in patients with renal and hepatic dysfunction
- MitoMYcin may be injected directly into any suitable vein, but preferably is injected into the side arm of a freely flowing intraVENous infusion
- MitoMYcin diluted in 20–50 mL of SWFI or 0.9% NS has also been given intravesically into the urinary bladder as a treatment for transitional cell carcinoma

Caution:
- MitoMYcin is a powerful vesicant and may produce severe local soft-tissue necrosis if extravasation occurs
  - See Chapter 42 for recommendations on managing extravasation with mitoMYcin

Mitosol® (mitomycin for solution) for topical application to the surgical site of glaucoma filtration surgery

Method of Use
(Mitosol® Kits include detailed illustrated instructions for use):
- Mitosol® is a sterile lyophilized mixture of mitomycin and mannitol, which, after reconstitution with SWFI, provides a

(continued)

Product Identification, Preparation, Storage, and Stability (*continued*)

- Discard reconstituted solutions after 14 days if the product was stored under refrigeration. If unrefrigerated, discard after 7 days
- MitoMYcin stability is not adversely affected by exposure to fluorescent lighting
- Reconstituted mitoMYcin (0.5 mg/mL) is suitable for intraVENous administration, but the product may be further diluted to a concentration of 20–40 mcg/mL (0.02–0.04 mg/mL) in the following fluids at room temperature[58]:

Vehicle/Diluent Solution	Duration of Stability
D5W	3 hours
0.9% NS	12 hours
1/6-M SLI (sodium lactate injection, USP)	24 hours

- MitoMYcin stability is highly dependent on solution pH: it is most stable at pH ~7[59,60]

Mitosol® (mitomycin for solution)

- Mitosol® is a sterile lyophilized mixture of mitomycin and mannitol in a 1:2 ratio
- Mitosol® Kits include the following components:
  - An outer pack, which contains:
    1. One product package insert
    2. Detailed illustrated instructions for use
    3. One chemotherapy waste bag
    4. One sterile inner tray
  - A sterile inner tray, which contains:
    1. One vial containing 0.2 mg mitomycin
    2. One 1-mL syringe (prefilled with SWFI) with connector
    3. One plunger rod
    4. One vial adapter with spike
    5. One 1-mL Luer lock Tuberculin syringe
    6. One sponge container
    7. Six 3-mm absorbent sponges
    8. Six 6-mm absorbent sponges
    9. Six half-moon sponges
    10. One instrument wedge sponge
    11. One sterile alcohol prep pad
  - Three kits are supplied in each packaging carton (NDC 49771-002-03)
- Store lyophilized Mitosol® at controlled room temperature (20°–25°C [68°–77°F]). Avoid excessive heat. Protect from light
- Reconstitution:
  - Add 1 mL of SWFI, to the vial containing mitomycin, then shake to dissolve
  - If the product does not dissolve immediately, allow it to stand at room temperature until it dissolves into solution
  - Each milliliter of the reconstituted solution contains mitomycin 0.2 mg plus mannitol 0.4 mg and has a pH between 5.0 and 8.0
  - After reconstitution with SWFI and maintained at room temperature, the product (mitomycin 0.2 mg/mL) is stable for 1 hour

Recommendations for Drug Administration and Ancillary Care (*continued*)

solution for application in glaucoma filtration surgery
- Sponges provided with a Mitosol® Kit should be fully saturated with the entire reconstituted contents in the manner prescribed in the instructions for use
- A treatment area approximating 10 mm × 6 mm ± 2 mm should be treated with Mitosol®
- With the use of surgical forceps, apply fully saturated sponges equally to the treatment area in a single layer
- Retain the sponges on the treatment area for 2 minutes, then remove and return sponges to the inner tray for disposal in the chemotherapy waste bag provided

Precautions and Warnings:

- Mitomycin is cytotoxic. Use of mitomycin in concentrations >0.2 mg/mL or use for durations >2 minutes may lead to unintended corneal and scleral damage including thinning or perforation. Direct contact with the corneal endothelium will result in cell death
- The use of mitomycin has been associated with an increased instance of post-operative hypotony
- Use in phakic patients has been correlated to a higher instance of lenticular change and cataract formation

MITOXANTRONE HYDROCHLORIDE

MITOXANTRONE–mitoxantrone hydrochloride injection, solution, concentrate; product label, May 2012. Teva Parenteral Medicines, Inc., Irvine, CA
MITOXANTRONE–mitoxantrone hydrochloride injection, solution, concentrate; product label, June 2011. Hospira, Inc., Lake Forest, IL
MITOXANTRONE INJECTION, USP (concentrate); product label, January 2008. APP Pharmaceuticals, LLC, Schaumburg, IL
MITOXANTRONE–mitoxantrone hydrochloride injection, solution; product label, January 2006. Manufactured by Ben Venue Laboratories, Inc., Bedford, OH.
Manufactured for Bedford Laboratories, Bedford, OH

WARNING

Mitoxantrone injection USP (concentrate) should be administered under the supervision of a physician experienced in the use of cytotoxic chemotherapy agents

Mitoxantrone injection USP (concentrate) should be given slowly into a freely flowing intravenous infusion. It must NEVER be given subcutaneously, intramuscularly, or intra-arterially. Severe local tissue damage may occur if there is extravasation during administration…

NOT FOR INTRATHECAL USE. Severe injury with permanent sequelae can result from intrathecal administration…

Except for the treatment of acute nonlymphocytic leukemia, mitoxantrone injection USP (concentrate) therapy generally should not be given to patients with baseline neutrophil counts of less than 1,500 cells/mm^3. In order to monitor the occurrence of bone marrow suppression, primarily neutropenia, which may be severe and result in infection, it is recommended that frequent peripheral blood cell counts be performed on all patients receiving mitoxantrone injection USP (concentrate)

Cardiotoxicity:
Congestive heart failure (CHF), potentially fatal, may occur either during therapy with mitoxantrone injection USP (concentrate) or months to years after termination of therapy. Cardiotoxicity risk increases with cumulative mitoxantrone dose and may occur whether or not cardiac risk factors are present. Presence or history of cardiovascular disease, radiotherapy to the mediastinal/pericardial area, previous therapy with other anthracyclines or anthracenediones, or use of other cardiotoxic drugs may increase this risk. In cancer patients, the risk of symptomatic CHF was estimated to be 2.6% for patients receiving up to a cumulative dose of 140 mg/m^2. To mitigate the cardiotoxicity risk with mitoxantrone, prescribers should consider the following:

All Patients
• All patients should be assessed for cardiac signs and symptoms by history, physical examination, and ECG prior to start of mitoxantrone injection USP (concentrate) therapy
• All patients should have baseline quantitative evaluation of left ventricular ejection fraction (LVEF) using appropriate methodology (ex. Echocardiogram, multi-gated radionuclide angiography (MUGA), MRI, etc.)

Multiple Sclerosis Patient
• MS patients with a baseline LVEF below the lower limit of normal should not be treated with mitoxantrone injection USP (concentrate)
• MS patients should be assessed for cardiac signs and symptoms by history, physical examination and ECG prior to each dose
• MS patients should undergo quantitative reevaluation of LVEF prior to each dose using the same methodology that was used to assess baseline LVEF. Additional doses of mitoxantrone injection USP (concentrate) should not be administered to multiple sclerosis patients who have experienced either a drop in LVEF to below the lower limit of normal or a clinically significant reduction in LVEF during mitoxantrone injection USP (concentrate) therapy
• MS patients should not receive a cumulative mitoxantrone dose greater than 140 mg/m^2
• MS patients should undergo yearly quantitative LVEF evaluation after stopping mitoxantrone to monitor for late occurring cardiotoxicity

Secondary Leukemia
Mitoxantrone injection USP (concentrate) therapy in patients with MS and in patients with cancer increases the risk of developing secondary acute myeloid leukemia…

Boxed Warning (excerpt) for "MITOXANTRONE - mitoxantrone hydrochloride injection, solution, concentrate"; September 2011 product label; Teva Parenteral Medicines, Inc., Irvine, CA

Product Identification, Preparation, Storage, and Stability

- MitoXANTRONE injection, USP (concentrate) is available generically in individually packaged multidose vials containing a sterile, nonpyrogenic, dark blue, aqueous solution of mitoXANTRONE HCl

  - Available presentations include:
    MitoXANTRONE 20 mg/10 mL
    MitoXANTRONE 25 mg/12.5 mL
    MitoXANTRONE 30 mg/15 mL

- Each milliliter of the concentrated solution contains 2 mg mitoXANTRONE (free base equivalent), with sodium chloride 0.80% (w/v), sodium acetate anhydrous 0.005% (w/v), acetic acid 0.046% (w/v) and SWFI. The solution has a pH of 3–4.5 and contains sodium 0.14 mEq/ mL, but does not contain antimicrobial preservatives

- Store MitoXANTRONE injection, USP at room temperatures. *Do not* freeze mitoXANTRONE

  - *Note:* Storage temperature requirements for mitoXANTRONE vary among manufacturers' products. Consult product-specific storage temperature recommendations

- If vials are used to prepare >1 dose, the portion of undiluted mitoXANTRONE concentrate remaining in a vial should be stored no longer than 7 days at temperatures within the range of 15°–25°C (59°–77°F), or for up to 14 days under refrigeration (2°–8°C [35.6°–46.4°F])

- MitoXANTRONE concentrate *must be diluted* prior to use to at least 50 mL with either 0.9% NS, D5W, or 0.9% NS/ D5W, and used immediately

Selected incompatibility:

- MitoXANTRONE admixture with heparin may result in precipitation
- MitoXANTRONE should not be mixed in the same parenteral product container with other drugs

Recommendations for Drug Administration and Ancillary Care

General:

- See Chapter 41 for comments about use in patients with hepatic dysfunction
- MitoXANTRONE is usually given as a short, intraVENous infusion over 5–30 minutes into the side arm of a freely flowing intraVENous solution, or it may be given by continuous intraVENous infusion over 24 hours
- *Do not administer* a dose of MitoXANTRONE over <3 minutes
- *Caution:* MitoXANTRONE is a vesicant drug and may produce severe local soft-tissue necrosis if extravasation occurs

- MitoXANTRONE *must not be administered* intraTHECALly or intraarterially, or SUBCUTaneously, intraMUSCularly, or by other infiltrative routes into soft tissues
- Signs and symptoms of extravasation may include burning, pain, pruritus, erythema, swelling, blue discoloration, or ulceration at the injection site, but extravasation may occur with or without accompanying discomfort and even if blood returns well on aspiration of a patient's VAD
- See Chapter 42 for recommendation on managing extravasation with mitoXANTRONE

- Advise patients mitoXANTRONE may impart a blue-green color to their urine for 24 hours after administration, and discoloration of the sclera (blue) may also occur

Inadvertent exposure:

- Skin accidentally exposed to mitoXANTRONE should be rinsed copiously with warm water
- If the eyes are involved, standard irrigation techniques should be used immediately

NELARABINE

ARRANON® (nelarabine) Injection; product label, December 2011. GlaxoSmithKline, Research Triangle Park, NC

WARNING: NEUROLOGIC ADVERSE REACTIONS

Severe neurologic adverse reactions have been reported with the use of ARRANON. These adverse reactions have included altered mental states including severe somnolence, central nervous system effects including convulsions, and peripheral neuropathy ranging from numbness and paresthesias to motor weakness and paralysis. There have also been reports of adverse reactions associated with demyelination, and ascending peripheral neuropathies similar in appearance to Guillain-Barré syndrome...

Full recovery from these adverse reactions has not always occurred with cessation of therapy with ARRANON. Close monitoring for neurologic adverse reactions is strongly recommended, and ARRANON should be discontinued for neurologic adverse reactions of NCI Common Toxicity Criteria grade 2 or greater...

Boxed Warning for "ARRANON® (nelarabine) Injection"; December 2011 product label; GlaxoSmithKline, Research Triangle Park, NC

Product Identification, Preparation, Storage, and Stability

- ARRANON® is packaged in type I, clear, glass vials containing a clear, colorless solution of nelarabine 250 mg in 50 mL
- Each milliliter of solution contains 5 mg nelarabine with sodium chloride 4.5 mg and SWFI in a total volume of (Q.S.) 50 mL; solution pH is within the range 5.0–7.0. The product is packaged in cartons containing 6 vials. NDC 0007-4401-06
- Store ARRANON® at 25°C (77°F). Temperature excursions to 15°–30°C (59°–86°F) are permitted

- Preparation for Administration:
  - *Do not dilute* ARRANON® prior to administration. Transfer a volume of nelarabine appropriate for a patient's dose into a PVC or glass container
- Undiluted nelarabine is stable in PVC and glass containers for up to 8 hours at temperatures up to 30°C (86°F)

Recommendations for Drug Administration and Ancillary Care

General:

- See Chapter 41 for recommended use in patients with renal and hepatic dysfunction
- Administer nelarabine intraVENously over 2 hours for adult patients and over 1 hour for pediatric patients

OBINUTUZUMAB

GAZYVA™ (obinutuzumab) Injection, for intravenous infusion; product label, November 2013. Manufactured by Genentech, Inc., A Member of the Roche Group, South San Francisco, CA

WARNING: HEPATITIS B VIRUS REACTIVATION AND PROGRESSIVE MULTIFOCAL LEUKOENCEPHALOPATHY

- Hepatitis B Virus (HBV) reactivation, in some cases resulting in fulminant hepatitis, hepatic failure, and death, can occur in patients receiving CD20-directed cytolytic antibodies, including GAZYVA. Screen all patients for HBV infection before treatment initiation. Monitor HBV positive patients during and after treatment with GAZYVA. Discontinue GAZYVA and concomitant medications in the event of HBV reactivation…
- Progressive Multifocal Leukoencephalopathy (PML) including fatal PML, can occur in patients receiving GAZYVA…

Boxed Warning for "GAZYVA™ (obinutuzumab) Injection, for intravenous infusion"; November 2013 product label; Genentech, Inc., A Member of the Roche Group, South San Francisco, CA

Product Identification, Preparation, Storage, and Stability

- GAZYVA™ is supplied individually packaged, single-use vials that contain obinutuzumab as a sterile, clear, colorless to slightly brown, preservative-free, concentrated solution
  - Each vial of concentrated drug product contains 1000 mg obinutuzumab per 40 mL (25 mg/mL) formulated in L-histidine/L-histidine hydrochloride 20 mmol/L, trehalose 240 mmol/L, and poloxamer 188 0.02% at a pH = 6.0 (NDC 50242-070-01)
  - Store intact vials at 2°–8°C (35.6°–46.4°F) protected from light
  - *Do not freeze* and *do not shake* the drug product
- Preparation:

Cycles and Days of Treatment	Amount of Obinutuzumab per Dose	Instructions
Cycle 1: Dilution to a concentration within the range of 0.4–4 mg/mL			
Day 1	100 mg	1. With a sterile syringe, withdraw 40 mL of solution from a vial of GAZYVA™ (obinutuzumab)
		2. Transfer 4 mL (100 mg) of the concentrated drug product into a parenteral product container already containing 100 mL of 0.9% NS for immediate use
Day 2	900 mg	3. Transfer the remaining 36 mL (900 mg) of the concentrated drug product into a second parenteral product container already containing 250 mL of 0.9% NS for use on Day 2
		4. Mix the diluted drug products by repeated gentle inversion of the product container. *Do not shake* the drug product
		5. Store the second container under refrigeration (2°–8°C) for up to 24 hours; *do not freeze* the drug product
		6. After storage under refrigeration, allow diluted obinutuzumab to come to room temperature before use
Days 8 and 15	1000 mg	1. With a sterile syringe, withdraw 40 mL (1000 mg) of concentrated obinutuzumab from a vial
		2. Transfer 40 mL into a parenteral product container already containing 250 mL of 0.9% NS
		3. Mix the diluted drug product by repeated gentle inversion of the product container. *Do not shake* the drug product
		4. For microbiological stability, the solution may be stored under refrigeration (2°–8°C) for up to 24 hours; *do not freeze* the drug product
Cycles 2–6: Dilution to a concentration within the range of 0.4–4 mg/mL			
Day 1	1000 mg	1. With a sterile syringe, withdraw 40 mL (1000 mg) of concentrated obinutuzumab from a vial
		2. Transfer 40 mL into a parenteral product container already containing 250 mL of 0.9% NS
		3. Mix the diluted drug product by repeated gentle inversion of the product container. *Do not shake* the drug product
		4. For microbiological stability, the solution may be stored under refrigeration (2°–8°C) for up to 24 hours; *do not freeze* the drug product

- Product labeling recommends administering obinutuzumab solutions immediately after dilution; however, diluted products may be stored under refrigeration for up to 24 hours
- After dilution to concentrations within the range of 0.4–20 mg/mL in 0.9% NS in PVC or polyolefin infusion containers, obinutuzumab is stable for 24 hours at 2°–8°C followed by 48 hours (including infusion time) at room temperature (≤30°C [≤86°F])

Selected incompatibility:

- *Do not use* Dextrose solutions to dilute obinutuzumab
- *Do not mix* GAZYVA™ with other drugs

Recommendations for Drug Administration and Ancillary Care

Administration as Recommended in Product Labeling (version dated, November 2013)

Premedication:

• Premedication before each use to decrease the risk of infusion-related reactions (IRR)*

Cycle	Day	Patients Who Require Premedication	Premedication	Timing Relative to Obinutuzumab Administration
1	1	All patients	High-potency glucocorticoid†, intravenously; ie: **Dexamethasone** 20 mg, *or* **MethylPREDNISolone** 80 mg	Complete administration ≥1 hour before starting obinutuzumab
	2		**Acetaminophen** 650–1000 mg orally	≥30 minutes before starting obinutuzumab
			Antihistamine‡; eg: **DiphenhydrAMINE** 50 mg	
	8	All patients	**Acetaminophen** 650–1000 mg orally	≥30 minutes before starting obinutuzumab
	15	Patients with an IRR (G ≥ 1) during the previous infusion	Antihistamine‡; eg: **DiphenhydrAMINE** 50 mg	
2–6	1	Patients with a G3 IRR during the previous infusion *and* Patients with a lymphocyte count >25,000/mm³ before treatment	High-potency glucocorticoid†, intravenously; ie: **Dexamethasone** 20 mg, *or* **MethylPREDNISolone** 80 mg	Complete administration ≥1 hour before starting obinutuzumab

*Among 45 patients who received recommended premedication and obinutuzumab divided into two doses given on two consecutive days (100 mg followed by 900 mg on days 1 and 2, respectively), 21 patients (47%) experienced a reaction with the first 1000 mg and <2% thereafter
†Hydrocortisone is not recommended because it has not been effective in reducing the rate of infusion reactions
‡Antihistamine (H_1-receptor subtype antagonists)

Administration:

• *Administer* obinutuzumab only as an intravenous infusion through a dedicated line

  ▪ *Do not administer* as an intravenous push or bolus

  ▪ After storage under refrigeration, allow diluted obinutuzumab to come to room temperature before use

  ▪ No incompatibilities have been observed between GAZYVA™ and PVC or polyolefin containers and administration sets

• GAZYVA™ (obinutuzumab) should be administered only by healthcare professionals with appropriate medical support to manage severe infusion reactions that can be fatal if they occur

• Administration rates: initial rate and rate escalation

Cycle	Day	Obinutuzumab Dose	Administration Rate
1	1	100 mg	Administer at 25 mg/hour over 4 hours DO NOT increase the infusion rate
	2	900 mg	Initiate administration at 50 mg/hour If tolerated, the administration rate may be increased in increments of 50 mg/hour every 30 minutes to a maximum rate of 400 mg/hour
	8	1000 mg	Administration may begin at a rate of 100 mg/hour, and, if tolerated, may be increased by 100-mg/hour increments every 30 minutes to a maximum rate of 400 mg/hour
	15		
2–6	1		

  ▪ Obinutuzumab is administered for 6 cycles; each cycle is 28 days in duration

  ▪ If a planned dose is missed, administer the missed dose as soon as possible and adjust the dosing schedule accordingly

  ▪ If appropriate, patients who do not complete the Day 1, Cycle 1 dose may proceed to the Day 2, Cycle 1 dose

(continued)

Recommendations for Drug Administration and Ancillary Care (*continued*)

- Infusion-Related Reactions (IRR)
  - If a patient experiences an infusion reaction of any grade during obinutuzumab administration, adjust drug delivery as follows:

Reaction Grade (G)	Intervention
G4 (life threatening)	Immediately STOP administration and permanently discontinue treatment with obinutuzumab
G3 (severe)	1. Interrupt infusion and manage symptoms 2. After symptoms resolve, consider restarting obinutuzumab administration at no more than half the rate used at the time that an infusion reaction occurred 3. If the patient does not experience any further infusion reaction symptoms, rate escalation may again be attempted at increments and intervals appropriate for the treatment cycle and dose *Caution:* Permanently discontinue treatment with obinutuzumab if a patient experiences G3 infusion-related symptoms when re-challenged
GI–2 (mild–moderate)	1. Promptly decrease the rate, or interrupt administration and treat symptoms 2. After symptoms resolve, continue or resume administration 3. If the patient does not experience any further infusion reaction symptoms, rate escalation may again be attempted at increments and intervals appropriate for the treatment cycle and dose

- Additional recommendations for pharmacological support:
  - For patients with a high tumor burden or high circulating absolute lymphocyte counts ($>25,000/mm^3$), premedicate with **anti-hyperuricemics** (eg, allopurinol), and implement or ensure **hydration** appropriate for potential tumor lysis syndrome (TLS) starting 12–24 hours before obinutuzumab treatment begins
  - Hypotension may occur during obinutuzumab administration
    - Consider withholding antihypertensive medications for 12 hours before obinutuzumab administration, during treatment with obinutuzumab, and for the first hour after obinutuzumab administration until blood pressure is stable
    - For patients at increased risk of hypertensive crisis as a consequence of withholding antihypertensive medications, consider the benefits versus the risks of withholding hypertensive medications
  - **Antimicrobial prophylaxis** is strongly recommended for neutropenic patients throughout obinutuzumab treatment
    - Consider antiviral and antifungal prophylaxis
    - *Do not administer* obinutuzumab to patients with an active infection
    - Patients with a history of recurring or chronic infections may be at increased risk of infection
  - Immunization with live virus vaccines is not recommended during treatment and until B-cell recovery

Monitoring:

- Obinutuzumab can cause severe and life-threatening infusion reactions during and within 24 hours after administration
  - 47% of patients who received recommended premedication and the initial 1000 mg of obinutuzumab divided into two doses given on two consecutive days (100 mg and 900 mg on days 1 an 2, respectively) experienced an infusion reaction
    - A decrease from 89% of patients who did not receive premedication or "split dose" treatment experienced infusion reactions
  - Infusion reactions can also occur with subsequent infusions
  - Symptoms may include hypotension, tachycardia, dyspnea, and respiratory symptoms (eg, bronchospasm, larynx and throat irritation, wheezing, laryngeal edema)
  - Other common symptoms include nausea, vomiting, diarrhea, hypertension, flushing, headache, pyrexia, and chills
  - Institute medical management for infusion reactions as needed (eg, glucocorticoids, epinephrine, bronchodilators, oxygen)
  - Closely monitor patients throughout obinutuzumab administration
  - Patients with pre-existing cardiac or pulmonary conditions may be at greater risk of experiencing more severe reactions
    - Monitor more frequently during and after obinutuzumab administration
- Acute renal failure, hyperkalemia, hypocalcemia, hyperuricemia, and/or hyperphosphatemia associated with TLS also can occur within 12–24 hours after the first treatment
  - Correct electrolyte abnormalities, monitor renal function, fluid balance, and administer supportive care, including dialysis as indicated
- During the FDA registration trial, obinutuzumab in combination with chlorambucil caused:
  - G3/4 neutropenia in 34% of patients
    - Patients with G3/4 neutropenia should be monitored frequently until neutropenia resolves
    - Anticipate, evaluate, and treat any symptoms or signs of developing infection
    - Neutropenia onset can be >28 days after treatment completion and may persist >28 days
  - G3/4 thrombocytopenia in 12% of patients
    - In 5% of patients, an acute thrombocytopenia occurred within 24 hours after obinutuzumab administration
- Approximately 13% (9/70) of patients tested positive for anti-obinutuzumab antibodies at one or more time points during a 12-month follow-up period after obinutuzumab treatment
  - Neutralizing activity of anti-obinutuzumab antibodies has not been assessed

OFATUMUMAB

ARZERRA® (ofatumumab) injection, for intravenous infusion; product label, September 2013. Manufactured by Glaxo Group Limited, Greenford, Middlesex, UB6 0NN, United Kingdom. Distributed by: GlaxoSmithKline, Research Triangle Park, NC

WARNING: HEPATITIS B VIRUS REACTIVATION AND PROGRESSIVE MULTIFOCAL LEUKOENCEPHALOPATHY

- Hepatitis B Virus (HBV) reactivation can occur in patients receiving CD20-directed cytolytic antibodies, including ARZERRA, in some cases resulting in fulminant hepatitis, hepatic failure, and death...
- Progressive Multifocal Leukoencephalopathy (PML) resulting in death can occur in patients receiving CD20-directed cytolytic antibodies, including ARZERRA

Boxed Warning for "ARZERRA® (ofatumumab) Injection for intravenous infusion"; September 2013 product label; GlaxoSmithKline, Research Triangle Park, NC

Product Identification, Preparation, Storage, and Stability

- ARZERRA® is a sterile, clear to opalescent, colorless, preservative-free liquid concentrate (20 mg/mL) for dilution and intraVENous administration provided in single-use glass vials with a latex-free rubber stopper and an aluminum overseal
- Each vial contains either: 100 mg ofatumumab in 5 mL of solution, *or* 1000 mg ofatumumab in 50 mL of solution
  - The commercial product is available in the following presentations:
    - A carton containing 3, single-use, 100-mg/5 mL vials with 2 inline filter sets: NDC 0173-0821-33
      - single vials labeled NDC 0173-0821-02
    - A carton containing 1, single-use, 1000-mg/50 mL vials with 2 inline filter sets: NDC 0173-0821-01
- Store intact vials under refrigeration between 2° and 8°C (35.6° and 46.4°F), but do not freeze. Protect vials from light
- *Do not shake* vials containing ofatumumab
- The commercial product should be a colorless, but may contain a small amount of visible translucent-to-white, amorphous, ofatumumab particles. The solution should not be used if discolored or cloudy, or if foreign particulate matter is present
- Dilute *all* ofatumumab doses in 0.9% NS to deliver a volume of (Q.S.) 1000 mL, as follows:

Ofatumumab Dose	Volume of Ofatumumab Concentrate (20 mg/mL) Needed	Volume of 0.9% NS Needed
300 mg	15 mL	985 mL
2000 mg	100 mL	900 mL

- Mix the diluted product by gently inverting the container
- *Do not mix* ofatumumab with other drugs or fluids
- Store diluted ofatumumab solutions under refrigeration at 2°–8°C (35.6°–46.4°F)
- Ofatumumab should be administered through an inline filter supplied with the product

---

Recommendations for Drug Administration and Ancillary Care

Premedication:

- FDA-approved product labeling recommends all patients should receive from 2 hours to 30 minutes before each ofatumumab dose, the following premedication:
  - Acetaminophen 1000 mg (or equivalent) administer orally
  - An antihistamine (eg, cetirizine 10 mg, or equivalent) administer orally or intraVENously
  - A glucocorticoid (eg, prednisoLONE 100 mg, or equivalent) administer intraVENously
- *Do not decrease* glucocorticoid doses before administering ofatumumab doses 1, 2, and 9
- Glucocorticoid doses may be decreased as follows before ofatumumab doses 3, 4, 5, 6, 7, and 8, and doses 10, 11, and 12:

Ofatumumab Doses 3 through 8	Gradually decrease glucocorticoid doses with successive ofatumumab infusions if an infusion reaction grade ≥3 did not occur with the previously administered dose
Ofatumumab Doses 10 through 12	Administer prednisoLONE 50–100 mg (or equivalent) if an infusion reaction grade ≥3 did not occur with the 9th ofatumumab dose

(continued)

Recommendations for Drug Administration and Ancillary Care (*continued*)

Doses and schedules:

- Recommended doses and administration schedules for a total of 12 doses:
  - Dose 1 (initial dose)   Week 1   300 mg
  - Doses 2–8 (7 doses)   Weeks 2, 3, 4, 5, 6, 7, and 8   2000 mg/dose
  - Doses 9–12 (4 doses)   Weeks 12, 16, 20, and 24   2000 mg/dose

Escalating administration rates:

- If ofatumumab is well tolerated, administration rates may be escalated every 30 minutes as follows:

Interval After Starting Ofatumumab Administration (Minutes)	Administration Rates for the First, Second, Third, and Subsequent Ofatumumab Doses		
	Dose 1* (mL/hour)	Dose 2† (mL/hour)	Doses 3–12† (mL/hour)
0–30	12	12	25
31–60	25	25	50
61–90	50	50	100
91–120	100	100	200
>120	200	200	400

*Dose 1: Ofatumumab 300 mg in 1000 mL 0.9% NS (0.3 mg/mL)
†Doses 2–12: Ofatumumab 2000 mg in 1000 mL 0.9% NS (2 mg/mL)

General:

- Administer ofatumumab with an infusion pump, using PVC administration sets and the in-line filter provided with the product
- Flush the tubing through which ofatumumab is administered with 0.9% NS before and after each dose
- Start ofatumumab administration within 12 hours after product preparation
- Ofatumumab concentrate contains no antimicrobials preservatives
  - Discard diluted ofatumumab solutions within 24 hours after product preparation

Infusion-related hypersensitivity reactions:

- Ofatumumab can cause serious infusion reactions manifesting as bronchospasm, dyspnea, laryngeal edema, pulmonary edema, flushing, hypertension, hypotension, syncope, cardiac ischemia/infarction, back pain, abdominal pain, pyrexia, rash, urticaria, and angioedema
- Infusion reactions occur more frequently with the first 2 infusions:
  - Among 154 patients, infusion reactions occurred in 44% on the day of the first infusion (300 mg), 29% on the day of the second infusion (2000 mg), and less frequently during subsequent administration
- Intervene medically for severe infusion reactions, including angina and other signs and symptoms of myocardial ischemia

Modifying ofatumumab treatment for infusion reactions:

- Interrupt ofatumumab administration for infusion reactions of any severity
  - For G4 infusion reactions, *do not resume* ofatumumab administration
  - For G1–3 infusion reactions, if the infusion reaction resolves or remains G ≤2, resume infusion with the following modifications according to the initial grade of the reaction:
    - Grade 1 or 2: Resume administration at 50% the previous administration rate
    - Grade 3: Resume administration at a rate of 12 mL/hour
- After resuming ofatumumab administration, the infusion rate may be increased according to the table above ("Escalating Administration Rates"), based on patient tolerance

OMACETAXINE MEPESUCCINATE

SYNRIBO® (omacetaxine mepesuccinate) for injection, for subcutaneous use; product label, February 2014. Distributed by Teva Pharmaceuticals USA, Inc., North Wales, PA

Product Identification, Preparation, Storage, and Stability

- SYNRIBO® for injection is a sterile, preservative-free, white to off-white, lyophilized powder in individually packaged, clear, glass, 8-mL–capacity, single-use vials. Each vial contains 3.5 mg omacetaxine mepesuccinate and mannitol; NDC 63459-177-14
- Store unused vials at 20°–25°C (68°–77°F); temperature excursions are permitted from 15°–30°C (59°–86°F). Maintain omacetaxine mepesuccinate in its packaging carton until used to protect the drug from light

- Reconstitute omacetaxine mepesuccinate with 1 mL 0.9% NS
- After addition of the diluent, gently swirl the vial until a clear solution is obtained
- The lyophilized powder should be completely dissolved in <1 minute
- The resulting solution will contain 3.5 mg omacetaxine mepesuccinate per milliliter with pH between 5.5 and 7.0
- Protect the reconstituted solution from light
- Promptly discard any unused solution after completing dose preparation

- Avoid contact with the skin. If Synribo comes into contact with skin, immediately and thoroughly wash exposed areas with soap and water
- Use omacetaxine mepesuccinate within 12 hours after reconstitution when stored at room temperature and within 24 hours after reconstitution if the product is stored under refrigeration (2°–8°C [35.6°–46.4°F])

Recommendations for Drug Administration and Ancillary Care

General:

- Omacetaxine mepesuccinate is administered by SUBCUTaneous injection
- *Caution:*
  - FDA-approved recommendations for omacetaxine mepesuccinate use include different dose schedules for induction and maintenance dosing
  - In addition to hematologic adverse effects (decreased leukocyte, platelet, and erythrocyte counts), omacetaxine mepesuccinate can induce glucose intolerance, hyperglycemia, and in 1 patient during clinical development,

experienced hyperosmolar nonketotic hyperglycemia
  - Monitor blood glucose concentrations frequently, especially in patients with diabetes or risk factors for diabetes
  - Avoid omacetaxine mepesuccinate in patients with poorly controlled diabetes mellitus until good glycemic control has been established
- Omacetaxine mepesuccinate is not a substrate of CYP450 enzymes *in vitro*
  - Omacetaxine mepesuccinate and its primary metabolite, 4′-desmethylhomoharringtonine (4′-DMHHT), do not inhibit major

CYP450 enzymes *in vitro* at concentrations that can be expected clinically
  - The potential for omacetaxine mepesuccinate or 4′-DMHHT to induce CYP450 enzymes has not been determined
- Omacetaxine mepesuccinate is a substrate for transport by P-glycoprotein (P-gp, ABCB1, MDR1) *in vitro*
  - Omacetaxine mepesuccinate and 4′-DMHHT do not inhibit P-gp-mediated efflux of the P-gp substrate, loperamide, *in vitro* at concentrations that can be expected clinically

OXALIPLATIN

ELOXATIN® (oxaliplatin) injection for intravenous use; product label, August 2013. Manufactured by sanofi-aventis U.S. LLC, Bridgewater, NJ, A SANOFI COMPANY
Oxaliplatin for injection, powder for solution for intravenous use [and] Oxaliplatin injection, solution for intravenous use; product label, November 2011. Manufactured by Hospira Australia Pty Ltd, Mulgrave VIC 3170, Australia. Manufactured for Hospira, Inc., Lake Forest, IL
Oxaliplatin INJECTION, USP, concentrate, for solution for intravenous use; product label, MAY 2012. APP Pharmaceuticals LLC, Schaumburg, IL
Oxaliplatin for Injection, USP, for intravenous use for intravenous use; product label, FEBRUARY 2012. Manufactured at Sun Pharmaceutical Ind. Ltd., Gujarat, India. Distributed by Caraco Pharmaceutical Laboratories, Ltd., Detroit, MI

WARNING: ANAPHYLACTIC REACTIONS

Anaphylactic reactions to ELOXATIN [oxaliplatin] have been reported, and may occur within minutes of ELOXATIN [oxaliplatin] administration. Epinephrine, corticosteroids, and antihistamines have been employed to alleviate symptoms of anaphylaxis…

Boxed Warning for "ELOXATIN® (oxaliplatin) injection for intravenous use"; August 2013 product label; sanofi-aventis U.S. LLC, Bridgewater, NJ

Product Identification, Preparation, Storage, and Stability

Oxaliplatin for Injection (lyophilized powder):

- Oxaliplatin is supplied in individually packaged, clear, glass, single-use vials containing 50 mg oxaliplatin with lactose monohydrate 450 mg, *or* 100 mg of oxaliplatin with lactose monohydrate 900 mg as a sterile, preservative-free, lyophilized powder for reconstitution
- Store the lyophilized powder under normal lighting conditions at 20°–25°C (68°– 77°F); temperature excursions to 15°–30°C (59°–86°F) are permitted

Reconstitution of lyophilized oxaliplatin:
- *Important:* Reconstitution or final dilution must *never* be performed with a sodium chloride solution or other chloride-containing solutions
- Reconstitute oxaliplatin lyophilized powder for solution as follows:

Oxaliplatin Content per Vial	Volume of Diluent (SWFI *or* D5W)	Resulting Oxaliplatin Concentration
50 mg	10 mL	5 mg/mL
100 mg	20 mL	

- After reconstitution in the original vial, oxaliplatin solution (5 mg/mL) may be stored for up to 24 hours under refrigeration, 2°–8°C (35.6°–46.4°F)
- Reconstituted oxaliplatin (5 mg/mL) must be diluted in 250–500 mL of D5W before administration to patients
- After dilution in 250–500 mL of D5W, oxaliplatin solutions are stable for up to 6 hours if stored at room temperature, 20°–25°C, or up to 24 hours under refrigeration, 2°–8°C
- Oxaliplatin for injection is not light sensitive

Oxaliplatin concentrate (solution):

- Oxaliplatin concentrate is supplied in individually packaged, clear, glass, single-use vials
- Product formulations and presentations vary among manufacturers, but include vials containing 50 mg, 100 mg, or 200 mg of oxaliplatin as a sterile, preservative-free, aqueous solution at a concentration of 5 mg oxaliplatin/mL in SWFI ± additional excipients
- Store oxaliplatin solution at 25°C (77°F); temperature excursions to 15°–30°C are permitted. Do not freeze and protect from light (keep in original outer packaging carton)
- Oxaliplatin concentrate (5 mg/mL) must be diluted in 250–500 mL of D5W before administration to patients
- After dilution in 250–500 mL of D5W, oxaliplatin solutions are stable for up to 6 hours if stored at room temperature (20°–25°C), or up to 24 hours under refrigeration (2°–8°C)
- *Important:* Oxaliplatin concentrate dilution must never be performed with a sodium chloride solution or other chloride-containing solutions
- Protection from light exposure is not required after dilution

Selected incompatibility:

- Oxaliplatin in solution is incompatible and must not be mixed or administered simultaneously through the same infusion line with alkaline medications or media (eg, fluorouracil)
- Do not use aluminum needles or administration sets containing aluminum parts that may come into contact with oxaliplatin-containing solutions. Aluminum has been reported to cause degradation of platinum compounds

Recommendations for Drug Administration and Ancillary Care

General:

- See Chapter 41 for recommended use in patients with renal dysfunction
- Oxaliplatin administration does not require prehydration
- Oxaliplatin is usually given by intraVENous infusion over 2 hours
  - Increasing the infusion time for from 2 hours to 6 hours decreases maximum oxaliplatin concentrations by an estimated 32% and may mitigate acute toxicities
- Administration sets and VAD used to administer oxaliplatin should be flushed with D5W after completing oxaliplatin infusion before using them to administer any other medications
- Do not use aluminum needles or administration sets containing aluminum parts that may come into contact with oxaliplatin solutions. Aluminum has been reported to cause degradation of platinum compounds
- Prescriptions and medication orders should identify the drug by its complete generic name, oxaliplatin

Altered platinum exposure in renal impairment:

- The $AUC_{0-48\ hours}$ of platinum in plasma ultrafiltrate increases as renal function decreases. The $AUC_{0-48\ hours}$ of platinum in patients with mild (creatinine clearance 50–80 mL/min [Clcr 0.83–1.33 mL/s]), moderate (Clcr 30 to <50 mL/min [0.5 to <0.83 mL/s]), and severe renal (Clcr <30 mL/min [<0.5 mL/s]) impairment is increased by approximately 60%, 140%, and 190%, respectively, compared to patients with Clcr >80 mL/min (>1.33 mL/s)
- Consult recommendations for oxaliplatin use in renal impairment

Neuropathy associated with exposure to cold temperatures:

- Oxaliplatin is associated with 2 types of neuropathy, including an acute, reversible, primarily peripheral, sensory neuropathy
  - Onset is within hours or 1–2 days after administration; it characteristically resolves within 14 days, but frequently recurs with subsequent oxaliplatin treatment
- Symptoms may be precipitated or exacerbated by exposure to cold temperature or cold objects and usually present as transient paresthesia, dysesthesia, and hypoesthesia in the hands, feet, perioral area, or throat. Jaw spasm, abnormal tongue sensation, dysarthria, eye pain, and a feeling of chest pressure have also been observed
- Patients should be instructed to avoid cold drinks, use of ice (eg, prophylaxis against mucositis and palliation for pain with mucositis), and should cover skin exposed to cold temperatures

Inadvertent exposure:

- In case of skin contact, immediately and thoroughly wash the affected area with soap and water. *Do not abrade* the skin by using a scrub brush
- In case of contact with mucous membranes, thoroughly flush the affected area with water

PACLITAXEL

PACLITAXEL–paclitaxel injection, solution; product label, January 2012. Manufactured in The Netherlands by Pharmachemie B.V., Haarlem, The Netherlands. Manufactured for Teva Pharmaceuticals USA, Sellersville, PA
PACLITAXEL INJECTION, USP; product label, July 2013. Manufactured for Bedford Laboratories™, Bedford, OH
PACLITAXEL - paclitaxel injection, solution; product label, June 2011. Manufactured by EBEWE Pharma, Ges.m.b.H. Nfg.KG, Unterach, Austria. Manufactured for Sandoz, Princeton, NJ
PACLITAXEL *INJECTION, USP*; product label, September 2010. Made in India. APP Pharmaceuticals, LLC, Schaumburg, IL

WARNING

Paclitaxel injection should be administered under the supervision of a physician experienced in the use of cancer chemotherapeutic agents. Appropriate management of complications is possible only when adequate diagnostic and treatment facilities are readily available

Anaphylaxis and severe hypersensitivity reactions characterized by dyspnea and hypotension requiring treatment, angioedema, and generalized urticaria have occurred in 2 to 4% of patients receiving paclitaxel in clinical trials. Fatal reactions have occurred in patients despite premedication. All patients should be pretreated with corticosteroids, diphenhydramine, and H$_2$ antagonists... Patients who experience severe hypersensitivity reactions to paclitaxel injection should not be rechallenged with the drug

Paclitaxel injection therapy should not be given to patients with solid tumors who have baseline neutrophil counts of less than 1,500 cells/mm^3 and should not be given to patients with AIDS-related Kaposi's sarcoma if the baseline neutrophil count is less than 1000 cells/mm^3. In order to monitor the occurrence of bone marrow suppression, primarily neutropenia, which may be severe and result in infection, it is recommended that frequent peripheral blood cell counts be performed on all patients receiving paclitaxel

---

Boxed Warning for "PACLITAXEL INJECTION, USP"; July 2013 product label. Bedford Laboratories™, Bedford, OH

Product Identification, Preparation, Storage, and Stability

- PACLitaxel is generically available from several manufacturers. Available presentations vary among manufacturers' products, but include individually packaged, multidose, glass vials, containing: 30 mg (in 5 mL), 100 mg (in 16.7 mL), 150 mg (in 25 mL), or 300 mg (in 50 mL)

- PACLitaxel injection is a clear, colorless to slightly yellow, viscous, concentrated solution. Each milliliter contains PACLitaxel, USP, 6 mg formulated in a solvent system consisting of polyoxyl 35 castor oil, NF (*AKA*, polyoxyethylated castor oil; Cremophor EL), 527 mg; and dehydrated alcohol 49.7% (v/v). Some products may contain additional excipients

- Store unopened vials at 20°–25°C (68°–77°F) in the original package
  - Neither freezing nor refrigeration adversely affects PACLitaxel stability
  - Components in PACLitaxel injection may precipitate under refrigeration, but will redissolve upon reaching room temperature with little or no agitation
    - Precipitation and redissolution under these circumstances do not affect product quality

- Discard vials in which paclitaxel solution remains cloudy after warming to room temperature and gentle agitation, or if an insoluble precipitate is observed

- For clinical use, *concentrated PACLitaxel must be diluted* to a concentration within the range, 0.3–1.2 mg/mL with 0.9% NS, D5W, D5W/0.9% NS, or D5W/RI in a polyolefin container

- *Avoid bringing PACLitaxel into contact* with containers, syringes, tubing, and other materials made of PVC during drug preparation and administration

- PACLitaxel-containing solutions characteristically leach DEHP and other phthalate plasticizers from flexible PVC containers and infusion sets[61-64]
  - PACLitaxel solutions should be stored in stored in glass, polypropylene, or polyolefin[19] containers and administered through polyethylene- or polyolefin-lined administration sets
    - *Caution:* Use of vented administration sets with rigid (glass) parenteral product containers has been associated with PACLitaxel solution dripping from the air vent, presumably as a result of surfactant wetting the hydrophobic air vent (inlet) filter[65]
  - *Caution: Do not use* chemotherapy dispensing pins and similar solution transfer devices with spikes with PACLitaxel, because they can cause a vial's stopper to collapse and compromise the sterility of its contents

- After dilution in 0.9% NS or D5W, PACLitaxel solutions are physically and chemically stable for up to 48 hours at ambient temperature (20°–23°C [68°–73.4°F]) and fluorescent lighting[66-68]
  - Product labeling stipulates PACLitaxel solutions are stable at ambient temperature (approximately 25°C [77°F]) and lighting conditions for up to 27 hours after dilution to a concentration within the range 0.3–1.2 mg/mL in D5W/0.9% NS or D5W/RI

- PACLitaxel should be inspected visually for particulate matter and discoloration before administration whenever solution and container permit. After preparation, PACLitaxel solutions may show haziness, which is attributed to the presence of surfactant in the commercial product[69]

Recommendations for Drug Administration and Ancillary Care

General:

- See Chapter 41 for recommended use in patients with hepatic dysfunction
- Use non-PVC containers, administration sets, and filters to administer PACLitaxel. *Avoid vented* administration sets
  - Glass, polyethylene, and polyolefin containers and polyethylene- or polyolefin-lined administration sets are compatible
- After dilution within the recommended concentration range (0.3–1.2 mg/mL), PACLitaxel may unpredictably precipitate in a product container or administration set tubing. The mechanisms underlying spontaneous precipitation and predisposing conditions are not well defined. Consequently, care providers should remain vigilant for drug precipitation throughout the duration of PACLitaxel administration
- *Administer PACLitaxel through an inline filter* with a filter membrane pore size ≤0.22 μm. Filtration does not cause significant losses in potency
  - Use of filter devices that incorporate short inlet and outlet PVC-coated tubing has not resulted in significant leaching of DEHP
- Administer PACLitaxel by intraVENous infusion over periods from 1 to ≥24 hours (commonly, 3 hours)

Primary prophylaxis against hypersensitivity reactions:

- PACLitaxel treatment is contraindicated in patients who have a history of hypersensitivity reactions to PACLitaxel or other drugs formulated in polyoxyl 35 castor oil, NF (eg, cycloSPORINE, teniposide)
- All patients should receive primary prophylaxis against hypersensitivity reactions, particularly with PACLitaxel infusion duration ≤3 hours. Prophylaxis may consist of:
  1. **Dexamethasone** 20 mg; administer orally or intraVENously for 2 doses, at approximately 12 hours and 6 hours before PACLitaxel (in treatment of

Kaposi's sarcoma each dexamethasone dose is decreased to 10 mg per dose on the same administration schedule), *plus*
  2. **DiphenhydrAMINE** (or an equivalent H_1 antihistamine) 50 mg; administer intraVENously 30–60 minutes before PACLitaxel, *and*
  3. **Ranitidine** 50 mg *or* **cimetidine** 300 mg (or an equivalent H_2 antihistamine); administer intraVENously 30–60 minutes before PACLitaxel administration

Hypersensitivity reactions:

- Refer to the boxed "WARNING" (above) excerpted from current product labeling
- The most frequent hypersensitivity symptoms observed during severe reactions were dyspnea, flushing, chest pain, and tachycardia. Abdominal pain, pain in the extremities, diaphoresis, and hypertension were also noted
- Minor symptoms such as flushing, skin reactions, hypotension, dyspnea, or tachycardia do not require interruption of therapy
- Immediately discontinue PACLitaxel for severe reactions and utilize aggressive symptom-appropriate therapy

Selected drug interactions:

- In a phase I clinical trial in which PACLitaxel and CISplatin were given in sequence, myelosuppression was more profound when PACLitaxel was given after CISplatin than with the alternate sequence (ie, PACLitaxel before CISplatin). Pharmacokinetic data demonstrated a decrease in PACLitaxel clearance of approximately 33% when PACLitaxel was administered after CISplatin
- PACLitaxel metabolism is catalyzed by CYP2C8 and CYP3A4. Exercise caution when PACLitaxel is administered concomitantly with substrates, inhibitors, and inducers of either CYP2C8 or CYP3A4
- PACLitaxel has been shown to decrease the rate of DOXOrubicin metabolism when PACLitaxel is given concomitantly

in sequence before the other drug. A pharmacokinetic study in which the sequence of administration of PACLitaxel and DOXOrubicin alternated during 2 consecutive treatment cycles revealed DOXOrubicin plasma concentrations at the end of infusion were increased by an average of 70% and DOXOrubicin clearance was decreased approximately 30% when PACLitaxel is given first compared with the alternative sequence. Similarly, the incidence of G2/3 mucositis was 70% with the PACLitaxel-followed-by-DOXOrubicin sequence versus only 10% with the reverse sequence
- Patients exhibited an 80% mean increase in DOXOrubicin AUC and a mean decrease in clearance of 71% when liposomal DOXOrubicin hydrochloride DOXIL® was given concomitantly with weekly PACLitaxel
- PACLitaxel significantly increased the bioavailability of epirubicin and slowed recovery from neutropenia in patients with stages 2 or 3 breast cancer who received epirubicin either before or after a 3-hour infusion of PACLitaxel. Epirubicin AUC increased by 37% and maximum plasma concentration increased by 65%, while total clearance decreased by 25%. When epirubicin was given after PACLitaxel, ANC recovery occurred more slowly compared with the alternative administration sequence

Inadvertent exposure:

- If PACLitaxel injection solution contacts the skin, wash the skin immediately and thoroughly with soap and water
  - Following topical exposure, events have included tingling, burning, and redness
- If PACLitaxel injection contacts mucous membranes, thoroughly flush the affected area with water
- Upon inhalation, dyspnea, chest pain, burning eyes, sore throat, and nausea have been reported

PACLITAXEL PROTEIN-BOUND PARTICLES FOR INJECTABLE SUSPENSION

ABRAXANE® for Injectable Suspension (paclitaxel protein-bound particles for injectable suspension) (albumin-bound); product label, October 2013. Manufactured for Celgene Corporation, Summit, NJ

WARNING: NEUTROPENIA

- Do not administer ABRAXANE therapy to patients who have baseline neutrophil counts of less than 1,500 cells/mm³. In order to monitor the occurrence of bone marrow suppression, primarily neutropenia, which may be severe and result in infection, it is recommended that frequent peripheral blood cell counts be performed on all patients receiving ABRAXANE…
- *Note*: An albumin form of paclitaxel may substantially affect a drug's functional properties relative to those of drug in solution. DO NOT SUBSTITUTE FOR OR WITH OTHER PACLITAXEL FORMULATIONS

Boxed Warning for "ABRAXANE® for Injectable Suspension (paclitaxel protein-bound particles for injectable suspension) (albumin-bound)"; October 2013 product label; Celgene Corporation, Summit, NJ

Product Identification, Preparation, Storage, and Stability

- ABRAXANE® is available in individually packaged single-use vials containing 100 mg of PACLitaxel bound to human albumin and approximately 900 mg albumin human containing sodium caprylate and sodium acetyltryptophanate) as a sterile, white to yellow, lyophilized powder. NDC 68817-134-50
  - The product does not contain Cremophor or other solvents
- Store unopened vials at 20°–25°C (68°–77°F) in the original package to protect from light
- The following reconstitution procedure yields a suspension for intraVENous injection containing 5 mg PACLitaxel/mL:
  1. Slowly inject 20 mL of 0.9% NS against the inside wall of a product vial over a minimum of 1 minute. To prevent foaming, *do not inject* the diluent directly into the lyophilized drug
  2. After all diluent has been added to a vial, allow each vial to sit for a minimum of

5 minutes to ensure that the lyophilized drug is properly wetted, *then*
  3. Gently swirl and invert the vial slowly for at least 2 minutes until the drug is homogenously dispersed. Avoid aggressively agitating the vial contents to prevent foaming
  4. If foaming or clumping occurs, allow the solution to stand undisturbed for at least 15 minutes until foam subsides
- *Do not filter* ABRAXANE® during preparation or administration
- Reconstituted ABRAXANE® (5 mg PACLitaxel/mL) should be milky and homogenous without visible particulates. If particulates or drug settling are observed, gently invert affected product vials to completely resuspend the product before it is administered to a patient
- The reconstituted product may be stored under refrigeration at 2°–8°C (35.6°–46.4°F) for a maximum of 8 hours
  - Although freezing and refrigeration do not adversely affect product stability,

reconstituted ABRAXANE® suspension should be stored in its original carton and protected from bright light
- Discard the reconstituted suspension if precipitates are observed
- Inject an amount of reconstituted ABRAXANE® appropriate for a patient's dose into an empty, sterile, PVC container
  - DEHP-free solution containers and administration sets are not necessary to prepare or administer ABRAXANE®, but may be used
- After transfer to a parenteral product container, the ABRAXANE® suspension is stable at ambient temperature (approximately 25°C [77°F]) and lighting conditions for up to 4 hours
- Suspended particles may settle if the product is not used soon after reconstitution. Ensure complete resuspension by mildly agitating Abraxane before it is used
- Discard any unused reconstituted ABRAXANE® after preparing a patient's dose

---

Recommendations for Drug Administration and Ancillary Care

General:

- See Chapter 41 for recommended use in patients with hepatic dysfunction
- Premedication to prevent hypersensitivity reactions is not required before administering ABRAXANE®
- Administer ABRAXANE® suspension intraVENously over 30 minutes

  - Administration over 30 minutes may reduce the likelihood of infusion-related reactions in comparison with more protracted delivery durations
- It is not necessary to prepare or administer Abraxane with DEHP-free containers and administration sets, but they may be used
- *Do not filter* ABRAXANE® during administration

- If ABRAXANE® administration does not commence within 30 minutes after product preparation, the product container should be gently inverted (several repetitions) to resuspend the drug particles before commencing drug administration

PANITUMUMAB

Vectibix® (panitumumab) injection for intravenous infusion; product label, March 2013. Manufactured by Amgen Inc., Thousand Oaks, CA

WARNING: DERMATOLOGIC TOXICITY and INFUSION REACTIONS

__Dermatologic Toxicity:__ Dermatologic toxicities occurred in 89% of patients and were severe (NCI-CTC grade 3 and higher) in 12% of patients receiving Vectibix monotherapy…

__Infusion Reactions:__ Severe infusion reactions occurred in approximately 1% of patients. Fatal infusion reactions occurred in postmarketing experience…

Boxed Warning for "Vectibix® (panitumumab) Injection for intravenous infusion"; March 2013 product label; Amgen Inc., Thousand Oaks, CA

Product Identification, Preparation, Storage, and Stability

- Vectibix® is available in individually packaged single-use vials containing a sterile, colorless, preservative-free solution of panitumumab 20 mg/mL at a pH within the range 5.6–6.0 in the following presentations:

Panitumumab Content	Excipients Content	NDC Number
100 mg/5 mL	Sodium chloride 29 mg, sodium acetate 34 mg, and SWFI	55513-954-01
200 mg/10 mL	Sodium chloride 58 mg, sodium acetate 68 mg, and SWFI	55513-955-01
400 mg/20 mL	Sodium chloride 117 mg, sodium acetate 136 mg, and SWFI	55513-956-01

- Store vials in their packaging carton under refrigeration at 2°–8°C (35.6°–46.4°F) until time of use. Protect vials from direct exposure to sunlight and *do not freeze* the concentrated solution (20 mg/mL)
- The undiluted drug product may contain a small amount of visible translucent-to-white, amorphous, proteinaceous, panitumumab particulates
  - Particulates in solution will be removed by inline filtration during drug administration
- *Do not shake* concentrated panitumumab solution (20 mg/mL)
- *Do not use* panitumumab if it appears to be discolored
- Dilute panitumumab as follows:

Panitumumab Dose	Vehicle Solution	Total Product Volume After Dilution (Q.S.)
≤1000 mg	0.9% NS	100 mL
>1000 mg		150 mL

Do not exceed a final concentration of 10 mg/mL

- Mix diluted solutions by repeatedly but gently inverting the product container. *Do not shake* diluted solutions
- Use diluted panitumumab solutions within 6 hours after dilution if stored at room temperature, or within 24 hours after dilution if stored under refrigeration at 2°–8°C (35.6°–46.4°F). *Do not freeze* diluted panitumumab solutions
- Discard any unused panitumumab remaining in a vial

Recommendations for Drug Administration and Ancillary Care

Determining appropriate utilization:

- Detection of epidermal growth factor receptor (EGFR) protein expression is necessary in selecting patients for whom panitumumab treatment is appropriate
- The combination of panitumumab with oxaliplatin-based chemotherapy is contraindicated for patients with mutant KRAS metastatic colorectal carcinoma (mCRC) or for whom KRAS mCRC status is unknown

General:

- See Chapter 41 for comments about use in patients with renal and hepatic dysfunction
- *Caution: Do not administer* panitumumab as an intraVENous injection (IV push *or* bolus)
- Flush administration set tubing and a patient's VAD with 0.9% NS before and after panitumumab administration
  - *Do not mix or administer* panitumumab with other medications, or add other medications to solutions containing panitumumab
- Administer panitumumab intraVENously via a peripheral or central VAD with a rate controlling device; that is, an infusion pump
  - Administer doses ≤1000 mg over 60 minutes
  - Administer doses >1000 mg over 90 minutes
- During administration, the fluid pathway must include a low-protein-binding inline filter with pore size 0.2 or 0.22 μm

Infusion reactions:

- Severe infusion reactions including anaphylactoid and fatal reactions have occurred during panitumumab administration and on the day of administration
  - The utility of medications as prophylaxis against infusional toxicities is unknown
  - Appropriate medical resources for the treatment of severe infusion reactions should be available during panitumumab administration
- Dose modifications for infusion reactions
  - Decrease the administration rate by 50% in patients who experience a mild or moderate (grades 1 or 2) infusion reaction for the duration of that infusion
  - Terminate panitumumab administration in patients who experience more severe infusion reactions
  - Depending on the severity and/or persistence of a reaction, permanently discontinue panitumumab

Dermatologic Toxicities:

- Withhold panitumumab for intolerable dermatologic toxicities and those G ≥3 in severity
- If toxicity does not improve to G ≤2 within 1 month, permanently discontinue panitumumab
- If dermatologic toxicity improves to G ≤2, and the patient is symptomatically improved after withholding ≤2 doses, treatment may be resumed at 50% of the original dose

- If toxicities recur, permanently discontinue panitumumab
- If toxicities do not recur, subsequent panitumumab doses may be increased in increments of 25% of the original dose until the recommended dose of 6 mg/kg is reached

Additional selected potentially severe adverse effects:

- Interstitial lung disease (ILD), including fatalities, have been reported in patients treated with panitumumab
  - Interrupt panitumumab therapy for the acute onset or worsening of pulmonary symptoms
  - Discontinue panitumumab therapy if ILD is confirmed
- Hypomagnesemia has been associated with panitumumab therapy. Hypocalcemia has also been observed
  - Periodically monitor patients' electrolytes during and for 8 weeks after panitumumab therapy is discontinued
- Exposure to sunlight can exacerbate dermatological toxicities associated with panitumumab
  - Advise patients to wear sunscreen and hats and limit sun exposure while receiving panitumumab
- Keratitis and ulcerative keratitis, risk factors for corneal perforation, have been reported with panitumumab use
  - Monitor for evidence of keratitis or ulcerative keratitis, and interrupt or discontinue panitumumab for acute or worsening keratitis

PEGASPARGASE

Oncaspar® (pegaspargase) injection, for intramuscular or intravenous use; May 2011 product label. Manufactured by Sigma-Tau Pharmaceuticals, Inc., Gaithersburg, MD

Product Identification, Preparation, Storage, and Stability

- Oncaspar® (pegaspargase) is asparaginase (L-asparagine amidohydrolase; identical 34.5-kDa subunits) produced by *Escherichia coli* that is covalently conjugated to monomethoxypolyethylene glycol (mPEG; MW ~5 kDa). Approximately 69–82 molecules of mPEG are linked to L-asparaginase
  - Pegaspargase activity is expressed in International Units
  - One International Unit of L-asparaginase is defined as the amount of enzyme required to generate 1 micromole of ammonia per minute at pH 7.3 and 37°C
- The commercial product, Oncaspar®, is supplied in Type I, single-use vials containing a clear, colorless, preservative-free, isotonic, sterile solution in phosphate-buffered saline at pH 7.3
  - Each milliliter of solution contains pegaspargase 750 ±150 International Units, dibasic sodium phosphate, USP 5.58 mg, monobasic sodium phosphate, USP 1.20 mg, and sodium chloride, USP 8.50 mg in water for injection, USP
- Oncaspar® vials contain pegaspargase 3750 International Units (L-asparaginase) per 5 mL solution (NDC 54482-301-01)
- Store Oncaspar® under refrigeration at 2°–8°C (35.6°–46.4°F)
- *Do not shake or freeze* Oncaspar®. Protect vials from exposure to light

Recommendations for Drug Administration and Ancillary Care

Administration:

- The recommended dosage of pegaspargase is 2500 International Units/m² BSA for administration by intraMUSCular or intravenous routes not more frequently than every 14 days
- *IntraMUSCular administration*: Oncaspar® is suitable for intraMUSCular injection without further modification
  - The volume at a single injection site should be ≤2 mL. Dose volumes >2 mL should be administered in two or more injection sites
- *Intravenous administration*: Transfer a volume of pegaspargase appropriate for a patient's dose to a parenteral product container with 100 mL of 0.9% NS or D5W. Administer pegaspargase intravenously over 1–2 hours ('piggybacked' or as a secondary infusion) into a running intravenous fluid
  - Diluted pegaspargase should be used immediately. If immediate use is not possible, store diluted pegaspargase solutions under refrigeration at 2°–8°C
  - Storage after dilution should not exceed 48 hours from the time of preparation to completion of administration
  - Protect diluted pegaspargase from direct exposure to sunlight
- *Do not administer* Oncaspar® if the drug product has been frozen, stored at room temperatures 15°–25°C (59°–77°F) for >48 hours, or shaken or vigorously agitated

Potentially serious adverse events:

- Allergic reactions may occur in association with pegaspargase administration
  - Persons with known hypersensitivity to other forms of asparaginase are at increased risk of developing a serious allergic reaction
  - Observe patients for one hour after pegaspargase administration in a setting with resuscitation equipment and medications necessary for treating anaphylaxis (eg, oxygen and injectable epinephrine, steroids, antihistamines)
  - Discontinue pegaspargase in patients who experience serious allergic reactions
  - Patients should be informed of the possibility of serious allergic reactions, including anaphylaxis, and to immediately report any swelling or difficulty breathing
- Thrombotic events, including sagittal sinus thrombosis, can occur in persons who receive pegaspargase
  - Discontinue pegaspargase in patients who develop serious thrombotic events
  - Patients should be advised to immediately report a severe headache, swelling of extremities, acute shortness of breath, and chest pain after receiving pegaspargase

PEGINTERFERON ALFA-2b

SYLATRON™ (peginterferon alfa-2b) for injection, for subcutaneous use; product label, December 2013. Manufactured by Schering Corporation, a subsidiary of Merck & Co., Inc., Whitehouse Station, NJ

WARNING: DEPRESSION AND OTHER NEUROPSYCHIATRIC DISORDERS

The risk of serious depression, with suicidal ideation and completed suicides, and other serious neuropsychiatric disorders are increased with alpha interferons, including SYLATRON. Permanently discontinue SYLATRON in patients with persistently severe or worsening signs or symptoms of depression, psychosis, or encephalopathy. These disorders may not resolve after stopping SYLATRON…

Boxed Warning for "SYLATRON™ (peginterferon alfa-2b) for injection, for subcutaneous use"; December 2013 product label; Schering Corporation, a subsidiary of Merck & Co., Inc., Whitehouse Station, NJ

Product Identification, Preparation, Storage, and Stability

- SYLATRON™, peginterferon alfa-2b, is a covalent conjugate of recombinant alfa-2b interferon with monomethoxy polyethylene glycol (PEG)
  - The specific activity of pegylated interferon alfa-2b is approximately 0.7×10^8 IU/mg protein
- Each vial contains peginterferon alfa-2b as a sterile, white to off-white lyophilized powder, and dibasic sodium phosphate anhydrous 1.11 mg, monobasic sodium phosphate dihydrate 1.11 mg, polysorbate 80 0.074 mg, and sucrose 59.2 mg, in the following presentations:

Each SYLATRON™ package contains:

Labeled Peginterferon alfa-2b Content	Actual Product Contents	NDC No.
200 mcg	One vial of peginterferon alfa-2b powder (296 mcg), one vial containing 1.25 mL of SWFI, 2 syringes, and 2 alcohol swabs	0085-1388-01
300 mcg	One vial of peginterferon alfa-2b powder (444 mcg), one vial containing 1.25 mL of SWFI, 2 syringes, and 2 alcohol swabs	0085-1287-02
600 mcg	One vial of peginterferon alfa-2b powder (888 mcg), one vial containing 1.25 mL of SWFI, 2 syringes, and 2 alcohol swabs	0085-1312-01

Each SYLATRON™ PACK 4 Box contains:

Labeled Peginterferon alfa-2b Content	Actual Product Contents	NDC No.
200 mcg	Four vials of peginterferon alfa-2b powder (296 mcg), 4 vials containing 1.25 mL of SWFI, 8 syringes, and 8 alcohol swabs	0085-1388-02
300 mcg	Four vials of peginterferon alfa-2b powder (444 mcg), 4 vials containing 1.25 mL of SWFI, 8 syringes, and 8 alcohol swabs	0085-1287-03

- SYLATRON™ should be stored at 25°C (77°F); temperature excursions are permitted to 15°–30°C (59°–86°F). *Do not freeze* SYLATRON™

(continued)

Recommendations for Drug Administration and Ancillary Care

General:

- Give primary prophylaxis against febrile reactions with acetaminophen 500–1000 mg orally 30 minutes before a first dose of peginterferon alfa-2b, and as needed for subsequent doses
- *Do not withdraw* more than 0.5 mL of reconstituted solution from each vial
- Administer SYLATRON™ by SUBCUTaneous injection. Rotate injection sites

Contraindications:

- SYLATRON™ is contraindicated in patients with:
  - A history of anaphylaxis to peginterferon alfa-2b or interferon alfa-2b
  - Autoimmune hepatitis
  - Hepatic impairment (Child-Pugh scores >6 [classes B and C])

Potential for drug interactions:

- In healthy subjects who received peginterferon alfa-2b 1 mcg/kg once weekly for 4 weeks with metabolic probe drugs administered before the first dose and after the fourth dose, a measure of CYP2C9 activity increased to 1.25 times baseline, a measure of CYP2D6 activity decreased to 51% of baseline
  - The effects of pegylated interferon alfa-2b 3 mcg/kg per week and 6 mcg/kg per week on the pharmacokinetics of drug substrates for CYP enzymes have not been studied

(continued)

Product Identification, Preparation, Storage, and Stability *(continued)*

• Reconstitute SYLATRON™ products with SWFI as follows:

Labeled Peginterferon alfa-2b Content (actual content) per Vial	Volume of SWFI for Reconstitution	Deliverable Peginterferon alfa-2b	Reconstituted Product Concentration
200 mcg (296 mcg)		200 mcg in 0.5 mL	40 mcg/0.1 mL
300 mcg (444 mcg)	0.7 mL	300 mcg in 0.5 mL	60 mcg/0.1 mL
600 mcg (888 mcg)		600 mcg in 0.5 mL	120 mcg/0.1 mL

• Gently swirl vials to dissolve lyophilized peginterferon alfa-2b powder. *Do not shake* vials
• Visually inspect the solution for particulate matter and discoloration prior to administration. Discard vials containing a discolored or cloudy solution, or if particulates are present
• If the reconstituted solution is not used immediately, store it under refrigeration at 2°–8°C (35.6°–46.4°F) for no more than 24 hours. *Do not freeze* Sylatron
  ▪ Discard any unused reconstituted solution after 24 hours
• *Do not withdraw* more than 0.5 mL of reconstituted solution from each vial

Recommendations for Drug Administration and Ancillary Care *(continued)*

Advice and instructions for patients and their personal caregivers:

• Peginterferon alfa-2b may be administered with antipyretics at bedtime to minimize common "flu-like" symptoms (chills, fever, muscle aches, joint pain, headaches, tiredness)
• Maintain hydration with non-alcoholic fluids if patients are experiencing "flu-like" symptoms
• Immediately report any symptoms of depression or suicidal ideation to their health care provider during treatment and for up to 6 months after the last dose
• A female patient using peginterferon alfa-2b who becomes pregnant should promptly consult her health care provider for guidance about continuing use
• Do not re-use or share syringes and needles
• Instruct patients how to properly disposal of peginterferon alfa-2b vials, syringes, and hypodermic needles

PEMETREXED DISODIUM

ALIMTA® (pemetrexed for injection) for Intravenous Use; product label, September 2013. Marketed by Eli Lilly US LLC, Indianapolis, IN

Product Identification, Preparation, Storage, and Stability

- ALIMTA® is available in individually packaged, sterile, single-use vials containing PEMEtrexed disodium as a white to either light-yellow or green-yellow lyophilized powder in the following presentations:

PEMEtrexed Disodium Equivalent to PEMEtrexed (Labeled PEMEtrexed Content)	Excipients	NDC Number
100 mg	106 mg mannitol	0002-7640-01
500 mg	500 mg mannitol	0002-7623-01

Hydrochloric acid and/or sodium hydroxide may have been added to adjust pH

- PEMEtrexed for injection, should be stored at 25°C (77°F); temperature excursions are permitted to 15°–30°C (59°–86°F)
- Reconstitute PEMEtrexed disodium with preservative-free 0.9% NS as follows:

Labeled PEMEtrexed Content*	Diluent Volume	Resulting Concentration
100 mg	4.2 mL	25 mg/mL
500 mg	20 mL	

*Alimta vials contain an excess of PEMEtrexed to facilitate delivery of the labeled amount

- Gently swirl each vial until lyophilized PEMEtrexed powder is completely dissolved
- The resulting reconstituted solution (25 mg/mL) is clear, ranges in color from colorless to yellow or green-yellow without adversely affecting product quality, and has a pH within the range, 6.6 and 7.8
- Reconstituted PEMEtrexed solution (25 mg/mL) must be further diluted with preservative-free 0.9% NS to a total volume of (Q.S.) 100 mL
- ALIMTA® is compatible with standard PVC parenteral product containers and administration sets
- PEMEtrexed disodium is chemically and physically stable after reconstitution (25 mg/mL) and dilution in preservative-free 0.9% NS (to a volume of Q.S. 100 mL) for up to 24 hours after initial reconstitution, when stored under refrigeration at 2°–8°C (35.6°–46.4°F),[70] or ambient room temperatures and lighting
- ALIMTA® does not contain antimicrobial preservatives. Discard any unused portion

Selected incompatibility:

- ALIMTA® is physically incompatible with solutions containing calcium, including Ringer injection, USP, and lactated Ringer injection, USP
- Coadministration of PEMEtrexed with other drugs and diluents has not been studied, and, therefore, is not recommended

Recommendations for Drug Administration and Ancillary Care

General:

- See Chapter 41 for recommended use in patients with renal dysfunction
- Administer PEMEtrexed intraVENously over 10 minutes

Supportive ancillary care:

- To reduce treatment-related hematologic and gastrointestinal toxicities, patients treated with PEMEtrexed should take folic acid 400–1000 mcg orally daily. At least 5 daily doses of folic acid must be taken during the 7-day period before the first dose of PEMEtrexed. Folic acid supplementation should continue throughout treatment and for 21 days after the last dose of PEMEtrexed
- Give 1 intraMUSCular injection of vitamin B_{12} (cyanocobalamin) 1000 mcg during the week before the first dose of PEMEtrexed and every 3 cycles thereafter (ie, approximately every 9 weeks). Repeated vitamin B_{12} injections may be given the same day as PEMEtrexed
  - Do not substitute orally administered vitamin B_{12} for a vitamin B_{12} product administered intraMUSCularly
- Primary prophylaxis with dexamethasone (or an equivalent glucocorticoid) reduces the incidence and severity of cutaneous reactions in patients treated with PEMEtrexed. In clinical trials, dexamethasone 4 mg orally was given twice daily for 3 consecutive days: the day before, the day of, and the day after PEMEtrexed administration

Selected potential drug interactions:

Nonsteroidal antiinflammatory drugs (NSAIDs)

- Ibuprofen 400 mg administered 4 times daily decreases PEMEtrexed clearance by approximately 20% (and increases AUC by 20%) in patients with normal renal function. The effect of greater doses of ibuprofen on PEMEtrexed pharmacokinetics is unknown
  - Ibuprofen 400 mg 4 times daily may be administered with PEMEtrexed in patients with normal renal function (creatinine clearance ≥80 mL/min [≥1.33 mL/s])
  - PEMEtrexed dosage adjustment is not needed during concomitant NSAIDs use in patients with normal renal function
- Use caution when administering NSAIDs to patients with mild to moderate renal insufficiency (creatinine clearance 45–79 mL/min [0.75–1.31 mL/s]) concurrently with PEMEtrexed
- NSAIDs with short elimination half-lives (eg, diclofenac, indomethacin, tolmetin, ketoprofen, fenoprofen, mefenamic acid, meclofenamate) should be avoided for a 5-day period, that is, 2 days before, the day of, and for 2 days after PEMEtrexed administration
- There are no data regarding potential interaction between PEMEtrexed and NSAIDs with longer half-lives (eg, meloxicam, nabumetone, naproxen, oxaprozin). Patients taking these NSAIDs should interrupt dosing for at least 8 days, that is, 5 days before, the day of, and for 2 days after PEMEtrexed administration
- If NSAIDs use is necessary concomitantly with PEMEtrexed, patients should be monitored closely for toxicity, especially myelosuppression, renal, and gastrointestinal adverse effects

Competition for organic anion transporter 3

- In vitro studies indicate that PEMEtrexed is a substrate of OAT3 (organic anion transporter 3), which may play a role in active secretion of PEMEtrexed

Inadvertent exposure:

- In case of skin contact, immediately and thoroughly wash the affected area with soap and water. Do not abrade the skin by using a scrub brush
- In case of contact with mucous membranes, thoroughly flush the affected area with water

PENTOSTATIN

NIPENT® (pentostatin for injection); product label, April 2009. Product of Australia. Hospira, Inc., Lake Forest, IL
PENTOSTATIN FOR INJECTION; product label, August 2006. Manufactured by Ben Venue Laboratories, Inc., Bedford, OH. Manufactured for Bedford Laboratories, Bedford, OH

WARNING

[Pentostatin] …should be administered under the supervision of a physician qualified and experienced in the use of cancer chemotherapeutic agents. The use of higher doses than those specified… is not recommended. Dose-limiting severe renal, liver, pulmonary, and CNS toxicities occurred in Phase 1 studies that used [pentostatin] …at higher doses (20-50 mg/m^2 in divided doses over 5 days) than recommended.

In a clinical investigation in patients with refractory chronic lymphocytic leukemia using [pentostatin] …at the recommended dose in combination with fludarabine phosphate, 4 of 6 patients entered in the study had severe or fatal pulmonary toxicity. The use of [pentostatin] in combination with fludarabine phosphate is not recommended

---

Boxed Warning for "NIPENT® (pentostatin for injection)"; April 2009 product label; Hospira, Inc., Lake Forest, IL, *and* "PENTOSTATIN FOR INJECTION"; August 2006 product label; Bedford Laboratories™, Bedford, OH

Product Identification, Preparation, Storage, and Stability

- Pentostatin for injection is available in individually packaged single-dose vials containing 10 mg of pentostatin as a sterile, apyrogenic, lyophilized, white to off-white powder with mannitol, USP, 50 mg. The pH of the final product is maintained within the range 7.0–8.5 by addition of sodium hydroxide or hydrochloric acid
- Store intact vials under refrigeration at 2°–8°C (35.6°–46.4°F)
- Reconstitute pentostatin with 5 mL of SWFI to obtain a solution with concentration equal to 2 mg pentostatin/mL

- After reconstitution, pentostatin solution is suitable for direct intraVENous injection, or it may be diluted in 25–50 mL of D5W or 0.9% NS to concentrations within the range 0.18–0.33 mg/mL. Pentostatin does not interact with PVC parenteral product containers or administration sets
- Pentostatin in intact vials is stable when stored under refrigeration at 2°–8°C (36°–46°F) until the expiration date on package labeling

- After reconstitution (2 mg/mL) with or without further dilution (0.18–0.33 mg/mL) and storage at room temperature under ambient light, pentostatin manufacturers recommend using the product within 8 hours, because it does not contain antimicrobial preservatives
- Spills and wastes should be treated with a 5% sodium hypochlorite solution prior to disposal

---

Recommendations for Drug Administration and Ancillary Care

General:

- See Chapter 41 for recommended use in patients with renal dysfunction
- Administer pentostatin intraVENously by rapid injection over 5 minutes, or by infusion over 20–30 minutes
- Give intraVENous hydration with D5W/0.9% NS or D5W/0.45% NS, 500–1000 mL before pentostatin administration plus 500 mL of D5W after pentostatin is given

Selected potential drug interactions:

- Pentostatin has been shown to enhance the effects of vidarabine, a purine nucleoside with antiviral activity. The combined use of vidarabine and pentostatin may result in an increase in adverse reactions associated with each drug
- The combined use of pentostatin and fludarabine phosphate is not recommended because it may be associated with an increased risk of fatal pulmonary toxicity

- Acute pulmonary edema and hypotension, leading to death, have been reported in patients treated with pentostatin in combination with carmustine, etoposide, and high-dose cyclophosphamide as part of a conditioning regimen prior to hematopoietic stem cell transplantation

Inadvertent release:

- Spills and wastes should be treated with a 5% sodium hypochlorite solution prior to disposal

PERTUZUMAB

PERJETA® (pertuzumab) Injection, for intravenous use; product label, September 2013. Manufactured by Genentech, Inc., A Member of the Roche Group, South San Francisco, CA

WARNING: CARDIOMYOPATHY AND EMBRYO-FETAL TOXICITY

Cardiomyopathy
PERJETA administration can result in subclinical and clinical cardiac failure. Evaluate left ventricular function in all patients prior to and during treatment with PERJETA. Discontinue PERJETA treatment for a confirmed clinically significant decrease in left ventricular function...

Embryo-fetal Toxicity
Exposure to PERJETA can result in embryo-fetal death and birth defects. Studies in animals have resulted in oligohydramnios, delayed renal development, and death. Advise patients of these risks and the need for effective contraception...

"PERJETA® (pertuzumab) Injection, for intravenous use"; September 2013 product label. Genentech, Inc., A Member of the Roche Group, South San Francisco, CA

Product Identification, Preparation, Storage, and Stability

- PERJETA® is supplied in single-use vials containing a sterile, clear to slightly opalescent, colorless to pale brown, preservative-free solution of pertuzumab 420 mg/14 mL (30 mg/mL) with 20 mmol/L L-histidine acetate (pH 6.0), 120 mmol/L sucrose, and 0.02% polysorbate 20 (NDC 50242-145-01)
- Store vials under refrigeration at 2°–8°C (35.6°–46.4°F) until time of use in their outer packaging carton to protect pertuzumab from light. *Do not freeze* pertuzumab. *Do not shake* vials containing pertuzumab
- Preparation for clinical use:
  - Transfer to a PVC or non-PVC polyolefin parenteral product container containing 250 mL of 0.9% NS a volume of pertuzumab appropriate for a patient's dose
- *Do not use* dextrose solutions to dilute pertuzumab
- Mix the diluted solution by gentle inversion. *Do not shake* the admixture
- If pertuzumab solution is not used immediately after dilution, it can be stored under refrigeration (2°–8°C) for up to 24 hours
- Do not mix pertuzumab with other drugs

Recommendations for Drug Administration and Supportive Care

HER2 testing is prerequisite to using pertuzumab:

- Detection of HER2 protein overexpression is necessary in selecting patients for whom pertuzumab therapy is appropriate, because these are the only patients studied and for whom benefit has been shown
- HER2 status should be assessed by laboratories with demonstrated proficiency in the specific technology being utilized to avoid unreliable results

General:

- Pertuzumab is administered intraVENously every 3 weeks
- Dose for initial treatment, and if the interval between 2 consecutive pertuzumab doses is ≥6 weeks:
  - Pertuzumab 840 mg administered intraVENously over 60 minutes
- Dose for repeated treatments, and if the interval between consecutive pertuzumab doses is <6 weeks:
  - Pertuzumab 420 mg administered intraVENously over 30–60 minutes every 3 weeks
- Dosage recommendations for trastuzumab and DOCEtaxel given in combination with pertuzumab:

	Trastuzumab	DOCEtaxel
Initial dose	8 mg/kg over 90 minutes	75 mg/m²
Maintenance doses	6 mg/kg administered intraVENously over 30–90 minutes given 3 weeks after an initial dose, and every 3 weeks thereafter	Doses are repeated every 3 weeks Dosage may be escalated to 100 mg/m² if the initial docetaxel dose was well tolerated

- The order of administration when pertuzumab, trastuzumab, and DOCEtaxel are given together (on the same day):
  - When pertuzumab and trastuzumab are given together, they should be administered sequentially, and either drug may precede the other

(continued)

Recommendations for Drug Administration and Supportive Care (*continued*)

- Observe patients closely for 60 minutes after their first pertuzumab treatment before commencing treatment with either trastuzumab or DOCEtaxel and for 30–60 minutes after every subsequent treatment to monitor for infusion and hypersensitivity reactions, which may include anaphylaxis
  - If a significant infusion-associated reaction occurs, slow or interrupt pertuzumab administration and administer appropriate medical therapies
  - Immediately discontinue pertuzumab administration if a patient experiences a serious hypersensitivity reaction
  - Carefully monitor patients until signs and symptoms associated with hypersensitivity reactions completely resolve
  - Consider permanently discontinuing pertuzumab in patients who experience severe infusion reactions
  - Administer DOCEtaxel *after completing* pertuzumab and trastuzumab administration
  - If trastuzumab treatment is withheld or discontinued, pertuzumab also should be withheld or discontinued
- Observe patients closely for 60 minutes after their first pertuzumab treatment and for 30 minutes after subsequent treatments to monitor for infusion and hypersensitivity reactions, which may include anaphylaxis
  - If a significant infusion-associated reaction occurs, slow or interrupt pertuzumab administration and administer appropriate medical therapies
  - Immediately discontinue pertuzumab administration if a patient experiences a serious hypersensitivity reaction
- Carefully monitor patients until signs and symptoms associated with hypersensitivity reactions completely resolve
- Consider permanently discontinuing pertuzumab in patients who experience severe infusion reactions

Left ventricular ejection fraction (LVEF) monitoring:

- Assess LVEF prior to initiating treatment with pertuzumab and at regular intervals (eg, every 3 months) during treatment to ensure LVEF is within normal limits
  - Withhold pertuzumab and trastuzumab administration for ≥3 weeks for either:
    - LVEF decrease to <45%, *or*
    - LVEF = 45–49%, with an absolute decrease ≥10% from pretreatment values
  - Pertuzumab treatment may be resumed if the LVEF has recovered to >49%, or to 45–49% associated with an absolute decrease of <10% from pretreatment values
  - If, after a repeat assessment within approximately 3 weeks, LVEF has not improved or has declined further, discontinue pertuzumab and trastuzumab unless the benefits to be gained by a individual patient are considered to outweigh the risks of continuing treatment
- In combination treatment with trastuzumab and docetaxel:
  - Pertuzumab should be withheld or discontinued if trastuzumab treatment is withheld or discontinued
  - If docetaxel is discontinued, treatment with pertuzumab and trastuzumab may continue
- Pertuzumab dose reductions are not recommended
- Patients who received anthracyclines or radiotherapy to the chest area before starting treatment with pertuzumab may be at greater risk of decreased LVEF

PRALATREXATE

FOLOTYN® (pralatrexate injection) Solution for intravenous injection; product label, May 2012. Manufactured for Allos Therapeutics, Inc., Westminster, CO

Product Identification, Preparation, Storage, and Stability

- FOLOTYN® is available in individually packaged, single-use, clear, glass, vials (type I) containing a preservative-free, sterile, isotonic, nonpyrogenic, clear, yellow, aqueous solution of PRALAtrexate 20 mg in 1 mL (NDC 48818-001-01) *or* 40 mg in 2 mL (NDC 48818-001-02)
- Each milliliter of solution contains (racemic) PRALAtrexate 20 mg, sufficient

sodium chloride to produce an isotonic solution (280–300 mOsm), and sufficient sodium hydroxide and hydrochloric acid to adjust and maintain solution pH = 7.5
- The commercially marketed product does not contain antimicrobial preservatives: used vials including any unused drug should be discarded after withdrawing a dose

- Store intact vials of FOLOTYN® under refrigeration at 2°–8°C (35.6°–46.4°F) in the original packaging carton to protect the drug product from light
  - Unopened vials are stable at room temperature for up to 72 hours if stored in the original product carton, but should be discarded after that time

Recommendations for Drug Administration and Supportive Care

General:

- See Chapter 41 for recommendations for use in patients with renal and hepatic dysfunction
- PRALAtrexate 30 mg/m² per dose is administered by intraVENous injection over 3–5 minutes into a freely flowing solution of 0.9% NS once weekly for 6 consecutive weeks in 7-week cycles
- Before administering any dose of PRALAtrexate:
  - Mucositis if present should be G ≤1
  - Platelet count should be ≥100,000/mm³ for first dose and ≥50,000/mm³ for all subsequent doses
  - ANC should be ≥1000/mm³
- Omitted doses will not be made up at the end of a treatment cycle
- If PRALAtrexate dosage is decreased for toxicities, do not re-escalate dosage during subsequent treatments

Supportive care:

- Patients should receive folic acid 1–1.25 mg/day orally starting 10 days before first receiving PRALAtrexate, and continue use for 30 days after their last dose of PRALAtrexate

- Patients should receive cyanocobalamin (vitamin B₁₂) 1000 mcg by intraMUSCular injection within 10 weeks before they first receive PRALAtrexate. Doses should be repeated every 8–10 weeks thereafter
  - Repeated cyanocobalamin injections may be given on the same day when PRALAtrexate is given
  - Folic acid and cyanocobalamin supplementation potentially mitigate against treatment-related hematologic toxicity and mucositis

Potential drug interactions:

- Coadministration of increasing doses of probenecid resulted in delayed PRALAtrexate clearance and a commensurate increase in exposure
- In vitro studies using human hepatocytes, liver microsomes, S9 fractions, and recombinant human CYP enzymes showed PRALAtrexate is not significantly metabolized by CYP enzymes or phase II hepatic glucuronidases
- In vitro studies indicated that PRALAtrexate does not induce or inhibit the activity of CYP enzymes at clinically achievable concentrations

- In vitro, PRALAtrexate is a substrate for the breast cancer resistance protein (BCRP, ABCG2), MRP2 (ABCC2), multidrug resistance associated protein 3 (MRP3, ABCC3), and organic anion transport protein (OATP) OATP1B3 transporter systems at concentrations of PRALAtrexate that can be reasonably expected clinically
- PRALAtrexate is not a substrate for the P-glycoprotein (P-gp, ABCB1), OATP1B1, organic cation transporter 2 (OCT2), organic anion transporter (OAT) OAT1, and OAT3 transporter systems
- In vitro, PRALAtrexate inhibits MRP2 and MRP3 transporter systems at PRALAtrexate concentrations that can be reasonably expected clinically
  - MRP3 is a transport protein that may affect the transport of etoposide and teniposide
- In vitro, PRALAtrexate did not significantly inhibit the P-gp, BCRP, OCT2, OAT1, OAT3, OATP1B1, and OATP1B3 transporter systems at PRALAtrexate concentrations that can be reasonably expected clinically

RASBURICASE

ELITEK® (rasburicase) powder for solution, for intravenous infusion; product label, January 2011. Manufactured by sanofi-aventis U.S. LLC, Bridgewater, NJ

WARNING: ANAPHYLAXIS, HEMOLYSIS, METHEMOGLOBINEMIA, AND INTERFERENCE WITH URIC ACID MEASUREMENTS

Anaphylaxis
Elitek® can cause severe hypersensitivity reactions including anaphylaxis. Immediately and permanently discontinue Elitek in patients who experience a serious hypersensitivity reaction...

Hemolysis
Do not administer Elitek to patients with glucose-6-phosphate dehydrogenase (G6PD) deficiency. Immediately and permanently discontinue Elitek in patients developing hemolysis. Screen patients at higher risk for G6PD deficiency (eg, patients of African or Mediterranean ancestry) prior to starting Elitek...

Methemoglobinemia
Elitek can result in methemoglobinemia in some patients. Immediately and permanently discontinue Elitek in patients developing methemoglobinemia...

Interference with Uric Acid Measurements
Elitek enzymatically degrades uric acid in blood samples left at room temperature. Collect blood samples in pre-chilled tubes containing heparin and immediately immerse and maintain sample in an ice water bath. Assay plasma samples within 4 hours of collection...

Boxed Warning for "ELITEK® (rasburicase) Powder for solution, for intravenous infusion"; January 2011 product label; sanofi-aventis U.S. LLC, Bridgewater, NJ

Product Identification, Preparation, Storage, and Stability

- ELITEK® is available in 2 presentations, including:
  - Cartons containing 3 single-use, 3-mL, colorless, glass vials, each containing rasburicase 1.5 mg *plus* 3 ampules each containing 1 mL diluent (NDC 0024-5150-10)
  - Individually packaged, single-use, 10-mL, colorless, glass vials containing rasburicase 7.5 mg *plus* 1 ampule containing 5 mL diluent (0024-5151-75)
- ELITEK® is formulated as a sterile, white to off-white, lyophilized powder containing:

Rasburicase Content	Excipients	
	Rasburicase Vials	Diluent Ampules
1.5 mg	10.6 mg mannitol, 15.9 mg L-alanine, between 12.6 and 14.3 mg of dibasic sodium phosphate (lyophilized powder)	1 mL of SWFI and 1 mg poloxamer 188
7.5 mg	53 mg mannitol, 79.5 mg L-alanine, and between 63 and 71.5 mg dibasic sodium phosphate (lyophilized powder)	5 mL of SWFI and 5 mg poloxamer 188

- Store the copackaged drug product and diluent for reconstitution at 2°–8°C (35.6°–46.4°F) protected from light. *Do not freeze* rasburicase
- Reconstitute rasburicase as follows:

Rasburicase Content per Vial	Diluent Volume	Rasburicase Concentration After Reconstitution
1.5 mg	1 mL	1.5 mg/mL
7.5 mg	5 mL	

- Dissolve and mix rasburicase by gently swirling vials. *Do not shake* or vortex vials
- Inject a volume of reconstituted rasburicase (1.5 mg/mL) appropriate for a patient's dose into a volume of 0.9% NS sufficient to produce a total volume of (Q.S.) 50 mL
- Do not filter the diluents used to reconstitute rasburicase or when transferring reconstituted rasburicase during dilution
- Store reconstituted and diluted rasburicase solutions at 2°–8°C
- Discard unused rasburicase solutions within 24 hours after reconstitution

Recommendations for Drug Administration and Ancillary Care

General:

- Rasburicase is administered intraVENously over 30 minutes, and may be given daily for up to 5 days
- Dosing for periods >5 days or administration of >1 course of treatment are not recommended
- Administer rasburicase through a new administration set or VAD after flushing the tubing with at least 15 mL of 0.9% NS before starting and after completing rasburicase administration
- Do not filter rasburicase during administration
- Discard unused rasburicase solutions within 24 hours after reconstitution

Uric acid sample handling procedure:

- At room temperature, rasburicase causes enzymatic degradation of uric acid in blood, plasma, and serum samples potentially resulting in spuriously low plasma uric acid assay readings
- The following special sample handling procedure must be followed to avoid *ex vivo* uric acid degradation:
  1. Uric acid must be analyzed in plasma. Blood must be collected into prechilled tubes containing heparin anticoagulant
  2. Immediately after collecting samples for uric acid measurement, immerse samples in an ice water bath
  3. Plasma samples must be prepared by centrifugation in a precooled centrifuge (4°C [39.2°F])
  4. Plasma must be maintained in an ice water bath and analyzed for uric acid within 4 hours after collection

Contraindication:

- Rasburicase is contraindicated in patients with G6PD deficiency because hydrogen peroxide is one of the major by-products of the conversion of uric acid to allantoin
- Immediately and permanently discontinue rasburicase administration in any patient who develops hemolysis
  - Institute appropriate patient monitoring and support measures (eg, transfusion support)
- Screen patients at high risk for G6PD deficiency (eg, patients of African or Mediterranean ancestry) before administering rasburicase

RITUXIMAB

Rituxan® (rituximab) Injection for Intravenous Infusion; product label, September 2013. Manufactured by Genentech, Inc., A Member of the Roche Group, South San Francisco, CA

WARNING: FATAL INFUSION REACTIONS, SEVERE MUCOCUTANEOUS REACTIONS, HEPATITIS B VIRUS REACTIVATION and PROGRESSIVE MULTIFOCAL LEUKOENCEPHALOPATHY

Infusion Reactions

Rituxan administration can result in serious, including fatal infusion reactions. Deaths within 24 hours of Rituxan infusion have occurred. Approximately 80% of fatal infusion reactions occurred in association with the first infusion. Monitor patients closely. Discontinue Rituxan infusion for severe reactions and provide medical treatment for Grade 3 or 4 infusion reactions…

Severe Mucocutaneous Reactions

Severe, including fatal, mucocutaneous reactions can occur in patients receiving Rituxan…

Hepatitis B Virus (HBV) Reactivation

HBV reactivation can occur in patients treated with Rituxan, in some cases resulting in fulminant hepatitis, hepatic failure, and death. Screen all patients for HBV infection before treatment initiation, and monitor patients during and after treatment with Rituxan. Discontinue Rituxan and concomitant medications in the event of HBV reactivation…

Progressive Multifocal Leukoencephalopathy (PML), including fatal PML, can occur in patients receiving Rituxan…

Boxed Warning for "Rituxan® (rituximab) Injection for Intravenous Infusion"; September 2013 product label; Genentech, Inc., South San Francisco, CA

Product Identification, Preparation, Storage, and Stability

- Rituxan® is available in individually packaged single-use vials containing a sterile, preservative-free solution at a uniform concentration of 10 mg riTUXimab/mL in the following presentations:
  - RiTUXimab 100 mg in 10 mL (NDC 50242-051-21), *and*
  - RiTUXimab 500 mg in 50 mL (NDC 50242-053-06)
- Store intact vials under refrigeration at 2°–8°C (35.6°–46.4°F). Protect riTUXimab vials from direct sunlight. *Do not freeze or shake* vials containing riTUXimab
- Withdraw from a vial an amount of riTUXimab appropriate for a patient's dose and dilute it in either D5W or 0.9% NS to a concentration within the range of 1–4 mg/mL
- Gently invert the parenteral product container to mix the solution
- After dilution to a concentration within the range of 1–4 mg/mL, riTUXimab solutions may be stored under refrigeration for up to 24 hours after preparation, and may then be removed from refrigeration to room temperature conditions and used within 48 hours after preparation
- Discard any partially used vials
- No incompatibilities between riTUXimab and PVC or polyethylene bags have been observed
- *Do not mix* riTUXimab with other drugs

Recommendations for Drug Administration and Ancillary Care

General:

- Rate of administration is constrained by individual patient tolerance, and generally always proceeds through a series of escalating rates to a maximum of 400 mg/hour
  - Do not administer riTUXimab by rapid intraVENous injection

Premedication:

- Primary prophylaxis against adverse infusion-related reactions is indicated prior to administering riTUXimab
  - **Acetaminophen** 650–1000 mg orally 30–60 minutes before riTUXimab administration, and an antihistamine (H$_1$ receptor antagonist), for example, **diphenhydrAMINE** 50–100 mg (or equivalent) orally or intraVENously 30–60 minutes before riTUXimab administration

Other concomitant medications:

- Labeled indications for rheumatoid arthritis includes recommendations for premedication with glucocorticoids
- Glucocorticoids are given in combination with riTUXimab in treating Wegener granulomatosis and microscopic polyangiitis
- Recommendations for antibiotic prophylaxis are specific to indications for riTUXimab treatment, including:
  - *Pneumocystis jirovecii* pneumonia (PJP) and antiherpetic viral prophylaxis for patients with chronic lymphocytic leukemia during and for up to 12 months after completing treatment
  - PCP prophylaxis for patients with Wegener granulomatosis and microscopic polyangiitis during and for up to 6 months after completing treatment

(continued)

Recommendations for Drug Administration and Supportive Care (*continued*)

RiTUXimab dosage and administration:

- RiTUXimab dosages and administration schedules vary among its labeled indications
- Rate of administration is constrained by individual patient tolerance, and, at least during initial treatment, proceeds through a series of escalating rates to a standardized maximum rate:
  - If adverse reactions occur during riTUXimab administration, either decrease the administration rate or interrupt treatment depending on the type and severity of reaction
    - If riTUXimab administration was interrupted, and, after adverse symptoms resolve it is considered medically appropriate to resume treatment, restart riTUXimab at a rate decreased by at least 50% from the rate at which symptoms occurred
    - If riTUXimab is tolerated after resuming treatment, administration may continue without attempting to escalate the rate of administration, or rate escalation may be cautiously reattempted
- Initial treatment:
  - The recommended initial dose rate for first riTUXimab exposure and reexposure after a 3- to 6-month hiatus is 50 mg/hour. If no toxicity is seen, the dose rate may be escalated gradually in 50-mg/hour increments at 30-minute intervals to a maximum rate of 400 mg/hour
- Second and Subsequent Doses:
  - Standard Administration Scheme for Second and Subsequent Infusions
    - Patients who tolerate initial riTUXimab treatment without experiencing infusion-related adverse effects, but for whom the 90-minute infusion scheme during subsequent treatments is considered inappropriate, may receive subsequent riTUXimab doses at the standard rate for repeated treatments, which is as follows:
      - Begin at an initial rate of 100 mg/hour for 30 minutes. If administration is well tolerated, the administration rate may be escalated gradually in 100-mg/hour increments at 30-minute intervals to a maximum rate of 400 mg/hour
  - 90-minute Administration Scheme for patients with "...*previously untreated follicular NHL and DLBCL* [who] ...did not experience a Grade 3 or 4 infusion related adverse event during Cycle 1... [and who are receiving riTUXimab] ...with a glucocorticoid-containing chemotherapy regimen."*,†
    - If the first dose of riTUXimab was well tolerated, subsequent doses may be administered over 90 minutes with 20% of the total dose given during the first 30 minutes, and the remaining 80% of the total dose administered over the subsequent 60 minutes; eg:

Two-Step Rate Escalation	Volume to Administer (X mL)
First portion (0–30 minutes)	$\dfrac{\text{Total Dose (mg)}}{\text{RiTUXimab Concentration (mg/mL)}} \times 0.2 = \text{X mL (over 30 min)}$
Second portion (30–90 minutes)	$\dfrac{\text{Total Dose (mg)}}{\text{RiTUXimab Concentration (mg/mL)}} \times 0.8 = \text{X mL (over 60 min)}$

*Rituxan® (rituximab) Injection for Intravenous Infusion; September 2013 product label
†*Special Note:* The 90-minute administration scheme is not recommended for patients with clinically significant cardiovascular disease or high circulating lymphocyte counts (≥5000/mm³) before cycle 2

Caution:
- Do not administer riTUXimab as a rapid intraVENous injection or bolus
- Vaccination with live virus vaccines is not recommended during and for an unspecified period after completing riTUXimab treatment
  - Persons with impaired immunity receiving treatment with riTUXimab may be at increased risk of acquiring an infection from household contacts who receive live virus vaccinations
    - Examples of live vaccines, include intranasally administered influenza, measles, mumps, rubella, oral polio, BCG, yellow fever, varicella, and TY21a typhoid vaccines
- RiTUXimab is detectable in serum for up to 6 months after treatment is completed. Individuals of childbearing potential should use effective contraception during and for at least 6 months after completing treatment

ROMIDEPSIN

ISTODAX® (romidepsin) for injection, for intravenous infusion only; product label, June 2013. Manufactured by Ben Venue Laboratories, Inc., Bedford, OH or Baxter Oncology GmbH, Halle/Westfalen, Germany. Manufactured for Celgene Corporation, Summit, NJ

Product Identification, Preparation, Storage, and Stability

- The commercial product, ISTODAX® Kit (NDC 59572-983-01), includes in a single package 2 single-use vials
  - One vial contains romiDEPsin 10 mg and 20 mg of the bulking agent, povidone, USP, as a sterile, lyophilized, white powder
  - A second single-use vial contains 2 mL (deliverable volume) of a sterile clear solution of 80% (v/v) propylene glycol, USP and 20% (v/v) dehydrated alcohol, USP, to be used as a diluent in reconstituting romiDEPsin
- Store ISTODAX® Kit in its packaging carton at 20°–25°C (68°–77°F), temperature excursions are permitted between 15° and 30°C (59° and 86°F)

- Reconstitute romiDEPsin by slowly injecting 2 mL of the supplied diluent into the vial containing the lyophilized drug product
- Swirl the contents of the vial until there are no visible particles in the resulting solution. The reconstituted solution contains 5 mg romiDEPsin/mL, and is chemically stable for at least 8 hours at room temperature
- RomiDEPsin must be further diluted in 500 mL 0.9% NS before it may be given by intraVENous infusion (product label)
  - After dilution in 500 mL of 0.9% NS, romiDEPsin is chemically stable for at least 24 hours when stored at room temperature, but should be administered as soon as possible after dilution

- *Alternative dilution:* RomiDEPsin should be diluted before clinical use with 0.9% NS to a concentration within the range 0.02–0.16 mg/mL
  - RomiDEPsin solution (0.02–0.16 mg/mL) is stable for at least 24 hours when stored at room temperature, but when possible should be prepared within 4 hours before commencing administration
- After dilution, romiDEPsin is compatible with PVC, ethylene vinyl acetate, polyethylene, and glass parenteral product containers

Recommendations for Drug Administration and Ancillary Care

General:

- See Chapter 41 for comments about use in patients with renal and hepatic dysfunction
- Administer romiDEPsin intraVENously over 4 hours

Electrolytes and cardiac monitoring:

- Serum potassium and magnesium should be monitored and, if results are found less than the lower limits of normal values, supplemented and remeasured to ensure replacement was adequate to obtain serum potassium and magnesium results within the range of normal values before romiDEPsin is administered
- Several treatment-emergent morphologic changes in ECGs were reported in clinical studies, including T-wave and ST-segment changes; however, the clinical significance of ECG changes is unknown
- Consider ECG monitoring at baseline and periodically during treatment in patients:
  - With congenital long QT syndrome
  - With a history of significant cardiovascular disease
  - Who are taking antiarrhythmic medicines or medicinal products that lead to significant QT interval prolongation

- RomiDEPsin was associated with a delayed concentration-dependent increase in heart rate in patients with advanced cancer with a maximum mean increase in heart rate of 20 beats/min occurring at 6 hours after start of romiDEPsin 14 mg/m² administered intraVENously over 4 hours

Potential drug interactions:

- Concomitant use of romiDEPsin and warfarin was reported to prolong the PT and increase INR. The mechanism for an interaction between romiDEPsin and warfarin has not been determined
- RomiDEPsin is highly protein bound in both human serum (94–95%) and human plasma (92–94%) over the concentration range (50–1000 ng/mL). Specific binding to human serum albumin and α_1-acid-glycoprotein were 19.91% and 93.51%, respectively
- RomiDEPsin is a substrate for metabolism by CYP3A4
  - Avoid concomitant use of strong CYP3A4 inhibitors with romiDEPsin
    - Exercise caution during concomitant use of romiDEPsin with moderate CYP3A4 inhibitors

- Potent CYP3A4 inducers may decrease concentrations of romiDEPsin if used concomitantly and should also be avoided
  - Paradoxically, When given concomitantly with rifampin in a pharmacokinetic drug interaction trial, romiDEPsin exposure was increased by approximately 80% and 60% for $AUC_{0-\infty}$ and C_{max}, respectively; its clearance was decreased by 44% and volume of distribution was decreased by 52%
  - The increase in exposure is likely due to rifampin's inhibition of an undetermined hepatic uptake process that is predominantly responsible for romiDEPsin disposition
  - It is not known if other potent CYP3A4 inducers may also alter the romiDEPsin exposure
- RomiDEPsin is a substrate for the transport protein, ABCB1 (*AKA,* P-glycoprotein, P-gp, MDR1)
  - Concurrent use of romiDEPsin with drugs that inhibit ABCB1 may increase systemic exposure to romiDEPsin
- RomiDEPsin has also been found to inhibit BSEP (*AKA,* bile salt export pump, ABCB11, sister of P-glycoprotein [sPgp]) and OATP1B1

STREPTOZOCIN

ZANOSAR®–streptozocin powder, for solution; product label, May 2007. Manufactured by Teva Parenteral Medicines, Inc., Irvine, CA

WARNING

ZANOSAR should be administered under the supervision of a physician experienced in the use of cancer chemotherapeutic agents

A patient need not be hospitalized but should have access to a facility with laboratory and supportive resources sufficient to monitor drug tolerance and to protect and maintain a patient compromised by drug toxicity. Renal toxicity is dose-related and cumulative and may be severe or fatal. Other major toxicities are nausea and vomiting which may be severe and at times treatment-limiting. In addition, liver dysfunction, diarrhea, and hematological changes have been observed in some patients. Streptozocin is mutagenic. When administered parenterally, it has been found to be tumorigenic or carcinogenic in some rodents

The physician must judge the possible benefit to the patient against the known toxic effects of this drug in considering the advisability of therapy with ZANOSAR. The physician should be familiar with the following text before making a judgment and beginning treatment

---

Boxed Warning for "ZANOSAR® - streptozocin powder, for solution"; product label, May 2007. Teva Parenteral Medicines, Inc., Irvine, CA

Product Identification, Preparation, Storage, and Stability

- ZANOSAR® is available as individually packaged, single-use vials containing streptozocin 1000 mg as a sterile, pale yellow, freeze-dried powder (NDC 0703-4636-01)
- Store intact vials under refrigeration at 2°–8°C (35.6°–46.4°F) and protected from light in the original packaging
- Reconstitute the product with 9.5 mL of either D5W or 0.9% NS. Each milliliter of the resulting pale-gold solution contains streptozocin 100 mg and citric acid 22 mg. Sodium hydroxide may have been added to adjust product pH. After reconstitution as directed, the solution pH will range from 3.5–4.5
- Reconstituted streptozocin (10 mg/mL) is stable at room temperature, 15°–30°C (59°–86°F), for 48 hours or for 96 hours under refrigeration

- The reconstituted product may be further diluted to a volume convenient for clinical use in either D5W or 0.9% NS
  - After dilution to 2 mg/mL in D5W or 0.9% NS, streptozocin is stable for 48 hours at room temperature and 96 hours under refrigeration
- The commercial product does not contain an antimicrobial preservative and the manufacturer recommends storage for not greater than 12 hours after reconstitution
- At concentrations from 10–200 mcg/mL streptozocin exhibited no loss because of adsorption to filters made of mixed cellulose esters (nitrocellulose, Millex-GS; EMD Millipore Corporation, Billerica, MA) or PTFE (*AKA*, Teflon, poly[tetrafluoroethylene]; Millex-FG [EMD Millipore Corporation])[16,35]

Recommendations for Drug Administration and Ancillary Care

General:

- See Chapter 41 for recommendations for use in patients with renal and hepatic dysfunction
- Administer streptozocin either by rapid intraVENous injection (push) or by intraVENous infusion over a period within the range of 15 minutes to 6 hours
- Streptozocin does not contain an antimicrobial preservative, the manufacturer recommends storage for not greater than 12 hours after reconstitution

Inadvertent exposure:

- In case of contact with skin or mucous membranes, thoroughly wash the affected area with soap and water

TEMOZOLOMIDE

TEMODAR® (temozolomide) for Injection, administered via intravenous infusion; product label, June 2013. Manufactured by Baxter Oncology GmbH, Halle, Germany. Manufactured for Merck Sharpe & Dohme Corp., a Subsidiary of Merck & Co., Inc., Whitehouse Station, NJ

Product Identification, Preparation, Storage, and Stability

- TEMODAR® for Injection is supplied in single-use glass vials containing 100 mg temozolomide as a light tan to light pink, sterile, pyrogen-free, lyophilized powder with mannitol 600 mg, L-threonine 160 mg, polysorbate 80 120 mg, sodium citrate dihydrate 235 mg, and hydrochloric acid 160 mg (NDC 0085-1381-01)
- Store intact vials of TEMODAR® for Injection under refrigeration at 2°–8°C (35.6°–46.4°F)
- Allow vials of TEMODAR® for Injection to equilibrate to room temperature before reconstitution
- Reconstitute TEMODAR® for Injection with 41 mL of SWFI to produce a solution containing 2.5 mg temozolomide per milliliter
- Gently swirl but *do not* shake vials to aid dissolution
- After reconstitution, store reconstituted temozolomide (2.5 mg/mL) at room temperature (25°C [77°F]) for up to 14 hours
- TEMODAR® for Injection should not be diluted further after reconstituting the lyophilized drug product
  - Temozolomide is stable at acidic pH (<5) and labile at pH >7; therefore, it can be administered orally and intravenously
  - The prodrug, temozolomide, is rapidly hydrolyzed to its active metabolite, 5-(3-methyltriazen-1-yl) imidazole-4-carboxamide (MTIC); at neutral and alkaline pH values, hydrolysis occurs more rapidly at alkaline pH
- With a sterile syringe, aseptically transfer a volume of temozolomide appropriate for a patient's dose (up to 100 mg [40 mL] from each vial) into a plastic parenteral product container
- The dosage of temozolomide given intravenously is the same as the dosage given with orally administered capsules
- The reconstituted product must be used within 14 hours, including the time for administration

Recommendations for Drug Administration and Ancillary Care

General:

- See Chapter 41 for recommendations for use in patients with renal and hepatic dysfunction
- Flush administration set tubing with 0.9% NS both before and after temozolomide administration
  - Temozolomide may be administered through an administration set only with 0.9% NS
  - The compatibility of temozolomide solutions with other fluids and medications is not known
- Administer temozolomide intraVENously over 90 minutes using an infusion control device (pump)
  - Bioequivalence between oral and intravenous administration has been established only when temozolomide was administered intraVENously over 90 minutes
  - Administration over shorter or longer durations may result in suboptimal dosing, and potentially may alter the incidence of infusion-related adverse reactions
- Temozolomide must be used within 14 hours after reconstitution, which includes the administration time

Cautions:

- Administration of valproic acid decreases oral clearance of temozolomide by about 5%. The clinical implication of this effect is not known
- Temozolomide use is contraindicated in patients who have a history of hypersensitivity to dacarbazine because both drugs are metabolized to the active MTIC metabolite
- Adverse reactions probably related to treatment with intravenously administered temozolomide that were not reported in studies using orally administered temozolomide, include pain, irritation, pruritus, warmth, swelling, and erythema at the infusion site, petechiae, and hematoma
- Administration of valproic acid decreases oral clearance of temozolomide by about 5%. The clinical implication of this effect is not known

TEMSIROLIMUS

TORISEL® Kit (temsirolimus) injection, for intravenous infusion only; product label, May 2012. Distributed by Wyeth Pharmaceuticals, Inc., A subsidiary of Pfizer Inc., Philadelphia, PA

Product Identification, Preparation, Storage, and Stability

- Commercially available TORISEL® is packaged as a kit (NDC 0008-1179-01) consisting of 2 clear glass vials:
  - One single-use TORISEL® vial contains temsirolimus 25 mg/mL as a clear, colorless to light yellow, nonaqueous, ethanolic, sterile solution with dehydrated alcohol 39.5% (w/v), *dl-α*-tocopherol 0.075% (w/v), propylene glycol 50.3% (w/v), and anhydrous citric acid 0.0025% (w/v). The TORISEL® vial contains 0.2 mL of excess drug (5 mg overfill) to ensure the ability to withdraw from a vial the recommended dose
  - One single-use DILUENT for TORISEL® vial contains a sterile, solution of polysorbate 80 40.0% (w/v), polyethylene glycol 400 42.8% (w/v), and dehydrated alcohol 19.9% (w/v), in a deliverable volume of 1.8 mL. The DILUENT for TORISEL® vial also contains excess fluid to ensure the appropriate volume can be withdrawn from a vial
- Store TORISEL® kits at 2°–8°C (35.6°–46°F). Protect TORISEL® from light

TORISEL® Dilution

- TORISEL® (25 mg/mL) requires two dilutions before administration to patients
- During handling and preparation of admixtures, TORISEL® should be protected from excessive room light and sunlight
- *Do not add* undiluted TORISEL® injection to aqueous solutions without initially combining it with the provided DILUENT for TORISEL®

- Temsirolimus should be diluted only with the supplied DILUENT for TORISEL®
- Direct addition of TORISEL® injection to aqueous solutions will result in drug precipitation

Initial Dilution of TORISEL® Injection (25 mg/mL) with supplied DILUENT for TORISEL®

- Transfer 1.8 mL of solution from the vial containing DILUENT for TORISEL® to a vial containing the TORISEL® drug product
  - The resulting solution contains 30 mg temsirolimus in 3 mL (10 mg/mL)
- Mix the vial contents by repeatedly inverting the vial
- Allow time for air bubbles to subside. The solution should be clear to slightly turbid, colorless to light-yellow, and essentially free from visible particulates
  - The temsirolimus concentrate-diluent mixture (10 mg/mL) is stable at <25°C for up to 24 hours
  - After the contents of the TORISEL® injection vial have been diluted with DILUENT for TORISEL®, the resulting solution contains 35.2% alcohol
  - After admixture with the DILUENT for TORISEL®, the drug product contains polysorbate 80 (240 mg/mL), which is known to increase the rate of DEHP extraction from PVC
    - Avoid using phthalate-plasticized PVC transfer devices and containers when transferring DILUENT for TORISEL® for initial drug dilution and during all subsequent phases of temsirolimus preparation and administration

Secondary Dilution of the temsirolimus (10 mg/mL) concentrate-diluent mixture with 0.9% NS

- With a syringe, withdraw from a vial containing the required amount of temsirolimus concentrate-diluent mixture 10 mg/mL (the initially diluted product described above) and transfer it to an appropriate parenteral product container containing 250 mL of 0.9% NS
  - Parenteral product containers appropriate for preparing and administering temsirolimus should be composed of glass, polypropylene, or polyolefin
    - Non-PVC containers and administration sets are preferred, but if PVC materials must be used, they should not contain DEHP
- Mix the solutions by repeatedly inverting the product container, avoiding excessive shaking that may cause foaming
- Protect the temsirolimus admixture in 0.9% NS from excessive room light and sunlight

Selected incompatibilities:

- The stability of TORISEL® in solutions other than 0.9% NS has not been evaluated
- Temsirolimus is degraded by both acids and bases: avoid combinations of temsirolimus with agents capable of modifying solution pH
- Do not add other drugs or nutritional products to admixtures of TORISEL® after dilution in 0.9% NS

Recommendations for Drug Administration and Ancillary Care

General:

- See Chapter 41 for recommendations for use in patients with hepatic dysfunction
- After initial dilution with the DILUENT for TORISEL®, TORISEL® contains polysorbate 80, which is known to increase the rate of DEHP extraction from plasticized PVC devices in contact with the drug
- Administration sets in which the fluid pathway (the surface in contact with a fluid

or drug) is lined with polyethylene are appropriate for administering temsirolimus
  - Polyethylene-lined administration sets prevent excessive loss of temsirolimus and DEHP leaching into the drug-containing solution
  - Non-PVC administration sets are preferred, but if PVC materials must be used, they should not contain DEHP
- An inline polyethersulfone filter with a pore size ≤5 μm is recommended for

administration to avoid the possibility of particles >5 μm from being administered
- Polyethersulfone filters with pore sizes from 0.2–5 μm are acceptable
  - Administration sets that do not have an integral inline filter may be used with an appropriate polyethersulfone filter added to the fluid pathway (at the end of an administration set closest to a patient)
  - The use of dual inline and add-on filters is not recommended

(continued)

Recommendations for Drug Administration and Ancillary Care (continued)

Premedication:

- Patients should receive an antihistamine (H_1 receptor antagonist), for example, **diphenhydrAMINE** 25–50 mg (or equivalent) administered intraVENously approximately 30 minutes before the start of each temsirolimus dose

Temsirolimus administration:

- Administer temsirolimus intraVENously over 30–60 minutes with a rate-controlling device (eg, a pump); administration should be completed within 6 hours after dilution in 0.9% NS

Infusion-related reactions:

- Hypersensitivity reactions during temsirolimus administration have included, but are not limited to: flushing, chest pain, dyspnea, hypotension, apnea, loss of consciousness, and anaphylaxis
  - Infusion reactions can occur very early during a first exposure to temsirolimus, but may also occur with subsequent use
  - Monitor patients throughout temsirolimus administration and appropriate supportive care should be available
  - Interrupt temsirolimus administration in all patients who experience severe infusion reactions and administer medical interventions as appropriate
  - Give temsirolimus with caution to persons who have demonstrated hypersensitivity to temsirolimus, its metabolites (including sirolimus), polysorbate 80, any other component of the commercially available product, or to antihistamines (H_1 receptor antagonists), which are recommended as premedication for all persons who receive treatment with temsirolimus
- In patients who develops a hypersensitivity reaction during temsirolimus administration:
  - Interrupt the infusion and observe the patient for at least 30–60 minutes (duration depending on the severity of the reaction)
  - At the discretion of a treating physician, temsirolimus administration may resume after signs and symptoms of hypersensitivity abate and administering intraVENously an H_1 receptor antagonist, if one was not previously administered, and/or an H_2 receptor

antagonist (eg, famotidine 20 mg or ranitidine 50 mg) administered intraVENously approximately 30 minutes before restarting temsirolimus
  - Temsirolimus infusion may then be restarted at a slower rate (administration duration of up to 60 minutes)

Potential drug interactions:

- Temsirolimus has been shown to inhibit CYP2D6 and CYP3A4 in in vitro systems with human liver microsomes, but did not alter desipramine concentration in vivo when single 50-mg doses of desipramine (a CYP2D6 substrate) were administered to 26 healthy volunteers with and without temsirolimus 25 mg[71]
- Temsirolimus is a substrate of the efflux transporter P-glycoprotein (*AKA*, P-gp, ABCB1, MDR1) in vitro. It is not yet clear whether temsirolimus can modify the pharmacokinetic behavior or may itself be affected by concomitant use with other ABCB1 substrates or drugs that perturb expression or function of ABCB1[72]
- Use with CYP3A subfamily inducers
  - Concomitant administration of temsirolimus with rifampin, a potent CYP3A4/5 inducer, had no significant effect on temsirolimus C_{max} (maximum concentration) and AUC (area under the concentration versus time curve) after intraVENous administration, but decreased sirolimus C_{max} by 65% and AUC by 56% compared to temsirolimus treatment without rifampin
  - St. John's wort may decrease temsirolimus plasma concentrations unpredictably, and concomitant use with temsirolimus should be avoided
  - Strong CYP3A4/5 inducers such as dexamethasone, carbamazepine, phenytoin, phenobarbital, rifampin, and rifabutin may decrease sirolimus exposure
    - If a strong CYP3A4 inducer must be coadministered during treatment with temsirolimus, consider increasing temsirolimus dose from 25 to 50 mg/week
    - This temsirolimus dose is predicted to adjust the AUC to the range observed without inducers; however, there are no clinical data with this dose adjustment in patients receiving strong CYP3A4 inducers

- If a concomitantly administered strong inducer is discontinued, the temsirolimus dose should be returned to the dose used prior to initiation of a strong CYP3A4 inducer
- Use with CYP3A subfamily inhibitors:
  - Strong CYP3A4 inhibitors, such as atazanavir, clarithromycin, indinavir, itraconazole, ketoconazole, nefazodone, nelfinavir, ritonavir, saquinavir, and telithromycin, may increase sirolimus blood concentrations
  - Grapefruit juice may also increase sirolimus concentrations in plasma (a major metabolite of temsirolimus) and should be avoided
  - If a strong CYP3A4 inhibitor must be coadministered, consider temsirolimus dose reduction to 12.5 mg/week
    - This temsirolimus dose is predicted to adjust the AUC to the range observed without inhibitors; however, there are no clinical data with this dose adjustment in patients receiving strong CYP3A4 inhibitors
    - If a concomitantly administered strong inhibitor is discontinued, a washout period of approximately 1 week should be allowed before readjusting temsirolimus doses to what was used before strong CYP3A4 inhibitor was introduced or the recommended dose of temsirolimus with CYP3A subfamily inhibitors
- Combination treatment with temsirolimus and SUNItinib malate resulted in dose-limiting toxicities (G3/4 erythematous maculopapular rash, and gout/cellulitis requiring hospitalization) in 2 of 3 patients treated in a phase I study with temsirolimus 15 mg per week and SUNItinib 25 mg/day administered orally for 28 consecutive days, days 1–28, during a 6-week treatment cycle
- Persons receiving temsirolimus should not receive vaccination with live vaccines and should avoid close contact with persons who have received live vaccines during treatment
  - Examples of live vaccines, include intranasally administered influenza, measles, mumps, rubella, and polio (oral), BCG, yellow fever, varicella, and TY21a typhoid vaccines

TENIPOSIDE

VUMON® (teniposide injection); product label, October 2011. Made in Italy. Manufactured for Bristol-Myers Squibb Company, Princeton, NJ

WARNING

VUMON (teniposide injection) is a cytotoxic drug which should be administered under the supervision of a qualified physician experienced in the use of cancer chemotherapeutic agents. Appropriate management of therapy and complications is possible only when adequate treatment facilities are readily available

Severe myelosuppression with resulting infection or bleeding may occur. Hypersensitivity reactions, including anaphylaxis-like symptoms, may occur with initial dosing or at repeated exposure to VUMON. Epinephrine, with or without corticosteroids and antihistamines, has been employed to alleviate hypersensitivity reaction symptoms

---

Boxed Warning for "VUMON® (teniposide injection)"; October 2011 product label; Bristol-Myers Squibb Company, Princeton, NJ

Product Identification, Preparation, Storage, and Stability

- VUMON® (teniposide injection) is available in individually packaged, clear, colorless, glass ampules containing a clear, sterile, nonpyrogenic solution of teniposide in a nonaqueous medium intended for dilution with a suitable parenteral vehicle prior to intraVENous administration (NDC 0015-3075-19)
  - VUMON® ampules contain teniposide 50 mg in 5 mL. Each milliliter of solution contains 10 mg teniposide with 30 mg benzyl alcohol, 60 mg N,N-dimethylacetamide, 500 mg purified Cremophor EL (polyoxyl 35 castor oil)*, and 42.7% (v/v) dehydrated alcohol. Solution pH is adjusted to approximately 5 with maleic acid

*Cremophor EL is a registered trademark of BASF Aktiengesellschaft. Cremophor EL is further purified by a Bristol-Myers Squibb Company proprietary process before use

- Store unopened ampules under refrigeration at 2°–8°C (35.6°–46.4°F). Freezing does not adversely affect the product
- Retain ampules in their original packaging to protect teniposide from light
- Dilute teniposide (10 mg/mL) with either D5W or 0.9% NS to obtain products with teniposide concentrations of 0.1 mg/mL, 0.2 mg/mL, 0.4 mg/mL, *or* 1 mg/mL
  - *Do not permit plastic* equipment or devices to remain in contact with undiluted teniposide. Prolonged exposure may cause syringes and other plastic solution transfer devices, tubing, and containers to soften or crack, which may increase the risk of drug leakage. The effect has not been reported with teniposide solutions after dilution
  - Teniposide solutions may leach phthalate plasticizers from PVC containers and administration set tubing. The extent of leaching correlates directly with the concentration of drug and the duration of exposure[62,73]
  - *Use only non-DEHP* containers and administration sets (glass or polyolefin[19] containers, polyolefin-lined administration sets) to prepare and administer teniposide. Stability and use times are identical in glass and plastic containers
- Teniposide stability at ambient room temperature and lighting conditions after dilution in D5W or 0.9% NS is as follows:

Teniposide Concentration	Duration of Stability
0.1 mg/mL	24 hours
0.2 mg/mL	
0.4 mg/mL	
1 mg/mL	4 hours

- Do not refrigerate teniposide solutions after dilution. Stability and use times are identical in glass and plastic parenteral product containers

- Although the undiluted product is clear, solutions may exhibit a slight opalescence after dilution due to the its surfactant components
- Although solutions are chemically stable under the conditions indicated, precipitation still may occur unpredictably. Spontaneous precipitation has been reported during 24-hour infusions of teniposide diluted to the lowest recommended concentrations of 0.1–0.2 mg/mL, resulting in occlusion of central VAD
  - Precipitation depends upon the formation of crystallization nuclei. Once crystallization nuclei are formed, precipitation proceeds rapidly
  - Strategies to prevent precipitation, include:
    1. After diluting teniposide, gently invert product containers, agitating the solution as little as possible to ensure a homogeneous admixture
    2. *Minimize the storage time* between teniposide dilution and administration
    3. *Do not permit* diluted teniposide to come into contact with other drugs and fluids

Selected incompatibility:

- Teniposide admixture with heparin can cause precipitation

Recommendations for Drug Administration and Ancillary Care

General:

- See Chapter 41 for comments about use in patients with renal and hepatic dysfunction
- Administer teniposide as soon as possible after preparation to avoid precipitation
- Administer teniposide intraVENously over at least 30–60 minutes to avoid hypotension associated with more rapid administration
- In general, administration sets designed for infusing intraVENous fat emulsion or PACLitaxel, and low-DEHP-containing nitroglycerin sets, are suitable for use with teniposide
- Thoroughly flush an administration apparatus used to administer teniposide and a patient's VAD with D5W or 0.9% NS before and after teniposide administration
- *Do not permit* diluted teniposide to come into contact with other drugs and fluids

Hypersensitivity reactions:

- Teniposide treatment has been associated with a hypersensitivity reaction variably manifested by chills, fever, urticaria, tachycardia, bronchospasm, dyspnea, hypertension or hypotension, rash, and facial flushing
- Hypersensitivity reactions may occur with a first dose of teniposide and may be life-threatening if not treated promptly
- Patients who experience hypersensitivity reactions to teniposide are at risk for recurrence of symptoms if rechallenged, and should only be retreated with teniposide if the antileukemic benefit already demonstrated clearly outweighs the risk of a probable hypersensitivity reaction
- Patients who are retreated with teniposide in spite of an earlier hypersensitivity reaction should receive prophylaxis against recurrent hypersensitivity reactions with glucocorticoids and antihistamines (H_1 receptor antagonists) and remain under careful clinical observation during and after teniposide administration

- All patients who receive teniposide should be under continuous observation for at least the first 60 minutes after administration commences and at frequent intervals thereafter. If symptoms or signs of anaphylaxis occur, teniposide administration should be stopped immediately, followed by the administration of epinephrine, corticosteroids, antihistamines, vasopressor agents, or volume expanders as clinically appropriate at the discretion of a physician
  - An aqueous solution of epinephrine 1:1000 (1 mg/mL) and a source of oxygen should be available at the bedside during teniposide administration
    - Promptly administer epinephrine at the onset of anaphylaxis. IntraMUSCular administration is preferred to the SUBCUTaneous route because epinephrine is better absorbed after intraMUSCular administration. There are no absolute contraindications to epinephrine administration in anaphylaxis

Potential drug interactions:

- Patients with both Down syndrome (trisomy 21) and leukemia may be especially sensitive to myelosuppressive chemotherapy; that is, teniposide dosage initially should be reduced in these patients
  - Product labeling suggests teniposide should be given at half the usual dose

- Teniposide dosages during subsequent courses may then be modified in individual patients depending on the degree of myelosuppression and mucositis previously encountered in earlier courses
- In a study in which 34 different drugs were tested, therapeutically relevant concentrations of tolbutamide, sodium salicylate, and sulfamethizole displaced protein-bound teniposide in fresh human serum to a small but significant extent
  - Teniposide is very highly bound to plasma proteins (>99%); thus, small decreases in protein binding, whether because of hypoalbuminemia or displacement from plasma protein by other substances, may cause substantial increases in free drug levels that could result in potentiation of drug toxicity
  - Exercise caution when administering teniposide to hypoalbuminemic patients and those who are concomitantly receiving drugs implicated in protein displacement interactions
- Teniposide plasma kinetics were not altered when it was coadministered with methotrexate, but methotrexate clearance from plasma was slightly increased. An increase in intracellular levels of methotrexate was observed in vitro in the presence of teniposide

Inadvertent exposure:

- In case of skin contact, immediately and thoroughly wash the affected area with soap and water
- In case of contact with mucous membranes, thoroughly flush the affected area with water

THIOTEPA

THIOTEPA for injection USP; product label, April 2013. Manufactured for Bedford Laboratories, Bedford, OH

Product Identification, Preparation, Storage, and Stability

- Thiotepa for injection USP, is available in individually packaged single-use vials containing 15 mg of thiotepa as a nonpyrogenic, sterile, lyophilized powder for reconstitution for intraVENous, intracavitary, or intravesical administration (NDC 55390-030-10). The product does not contain an antimicrobial preservative

- Store intact vials under refrigeration at 2°–8°C (35.6°–46.4°F). Protect thiotepa from light at all times

- Reconstitute thiotepa with 1.5 mL SWFI to produce a solution with concentration of approximately 10.4 mg/mL, and pH within the range 5.5–7.5

  - Reconstitution with solutions other than SWFI may result in a hypertonic solution which can produce discomfort when injected

  - The actual amount of thiotepa present in a vial and the amounts that can be retrieved from vials are as follows:

Labeled content per vial	15 mg
Actual content per vial	15.6 mg
Approximate retrievable volume per vial	1.4 mL
Approximate retrievable amount (mass) per vial	14.7 mg

- Store reconstituted thiotepa (10.4 mg/mL) under refrigeration at 2°–8°C for up to 8 hours

- Reconstituted solutions should be clear. Solutions that are opaque or contain a precipitate should not be used

  - To eliminate haze in thiotepa solutions, filter the solutions through a 0.22-μm filter before or during administration (hydrophilic polyethersulfone or cellulose ester filter membranes [Acrodisc, Pall Corp.; MILLEX-GS, Millipore Corp.])

  - Filtering does not alter thiotepa potency

- Reconstitution with SWFI to 10.4 mg/mL and further dilution with 0.9% NS to concentrations ≥3 mg/mL produces a hypotonic solution. Greater dilution with 0.9% NS to concentrations of 0.5 mg/mL or 1 mg/mL produces nearly isotonic solutions (277 and 269 mOsm/kg, respectively)

- Dilution with 0.9% NS to concentrations <1.8 mg/mL are nearly isotonic; *but*

  - After dilution with 0.9% NS to a concentration <1 mg/mL, thiotepa solutions should be *used immediately* because of the formation of drug adducts with chloride[74]

    - Both the amount and rate of chloro-adduct formation are inversely related to the concentration of thiotepa in solution[74]

      - Storage under refrigeration slows the rate but does not eliminate chloro-adduct formation and loss of thiotepa potency[74]

- Dilute thiotepa (10.4 mg/mL) with 0.9% NS, D5W, D5W/0.9% NS, RI, or LRI before clinical use

  - Thiotepa is stable in alkaline medium, but unstable in acid medium in which it hydrolyzes

- Thiotepa diluted in D5W to 0.5 mg/mL and 5 mg/mL was stable in both PVC and polyolefin composition containers with no drug loss due to adsorption[75]

Recommendations for Drug Administration and Ancillary Care

General:

- See Chapter 41 for comments about use in patients with renal and hepatic dysfunction
- Thiotepa dosage must be carefully individualized. A slow response to thiotepa does not necessarily indicate a lack of effect. Increasing the frequency of repeated administration may only increase toxicity
- Initially, the higher dose in a given range is commonly administered. Maintenance dosages should be adjusted based on pretreatment blood counts (CBC with differential leukocyte and platelet counts)
- To eliminate haze in thiotepa solutions, a solution may be filtered through a 0.22-μm filter with hydrophilic polyethersulfone or cellulose ester filter membranes either before or during administration
  - Filtering does not alter thiotepa potency
- Thiotepa is usually given by rapid intraVENous administration, but has also been given by intravesical, intracavitary, intraTHECAL, intraMUSCular, and intratumoral routes

IntraVENous administration:

- Thiotepa 0.3–0.4 mg/kg body weight may be given by rapid intraVENous injection over 5 minutes at 1- to 4-week intervals

Intracavitary administration:

- Thiotepa 0.6–0.8 mg/kg body weight
- Tubing that is used to drain fluid from the body cavity often is used to instill thiotepa

Intravesical administration:

- Fluids are withheld for 8–12 hours before treatment. Thiotepa 60 mg in 30–60 mL of 0.9% NS is instilled into the bladder by a urethral catheter. For maximum effect, the solution should be retained for 2 hours. If it is not possible to retain 60 mL for 2 hours, the dose may be given in a volume of 30 mL. A patient is repositioned every 15 minutes for maximum area contact
- The usual course of treatment is once weekly for 4 consecutive weeks
- A treatment course may be repeated if necessary, but second and third courses must be given with caution since bone-marrow depression may be increased
- Deaths have occurred after intravesical administration, caused by bone-marrow depression from systemically absorbed drug

IntraTHECAL administration:

- Thiotepa 2–10 mg/m² per dose, or a fixed dose of 10 mg/dose administered by either intralumbar or intraventricular routes, diluted with 0.9% NS to a concentration of 1–5 mg/mL
- There is no PK advantage for intraTHECAL versus intraVENous administration[76]
  - Thiotepa clearance from the CSF is approximately 9 times greater than CSF bulk outflow which results in disproportionate distribution throughout the neuraxis[76]
  - TEPA (*N,N′,N″-*triethylenephosphoramide), thiotepa's active metabolite is formed only after systemic administration, after which, it readily crosses the blood–brain barrier[77]

Inadvertent exposure:

- In case of skin contact, immediately and thoroughly wash the affected area with soap and water
- In case of contact with mucous membranes, thoroughly flush the affected area with water

TOPOTECAN HYDROCHLORIDE

Topotecan Hydrochloride For Injection; product label, January 2011. Manufactured for Dr. Reddy's Laboratories Limited By Cipla Ltd, Verna-Salcette, Goa - 403722, INDIA. Distributed by Bedford Laboratories, Bedford, OH

Topotecan Hydrochloride For Injection; product label, February 2011. Made in Romania. Manufactured for SAGENT Pharmaceuticals, Inc., Shaumburg, IL

Topotecan Hydrochloride Injection; product label, February 2011. Made in India. Manufactured and distributed by Hospira Inc., Lake Forest, IL

HYCAMTIN® (topotecan hydrochloride) for injection; product label, August 2013. GlaxoSmithKline, Research Triangle Park, NC

WARNING: BONE MARROW SUPPRESSION

Do not give [topotecan hydrochloride for injection] …to patients with baseline neutrophil counts less than 1,500 cells/mm³. In order to monitor the occurrence of bone marrow suppression, primarily neutropenia, which may be severe and result in infection and death, monitor peripheral blood counts frequently on all patients receiving [topotecan hydrochloride for injection]…

Boxed Warning for "HYCAMTIN® (topotecan hydrochloride) for Injection"; August 2013 product label; GlaxoSmithKline, Research Triangle Park, NC

Product Identification, Preparation, Storage, and Stability

Topotecan for Injection (lyophilized powder):

- Topotecan for injection is available generically as a sterile, lyophilized, buffered, light yellow to greenish powder in single-dose vials containing topotecan hydrochloride equivalent to 4 mg of topotecan as the free base, with mannitol 48 mg and tartaric acid 20 mg. Hydrochloric acid and sodium hydroxide may be used to adjust the product pH. Available products do not contain an antimicrobial preservative
  - Presentations vary by manufacturer, but include individually packaged vials and packages containing 5 vials
- Store intact vials protected from light in the original cartons at controlled room temperature between 20° and 25°C (68° and 77°F)
- Reconstitute lyophilized topotecan HCl with 4 mL of SWFI to produce a yellow to yellow-green solution with concentration equal to 1 mg/mL and a pH within the range 2.5–3.5
- After reconstitution with SWFI to a concentration of 1 mg topotecan HCl per milliliter, topotecan HCl 1 mg/mL, stored for 28 days at 4°C (39.2°F) or 25°C and protected from light, the drug product was found to be physically and chemically stable by HPLC analysis without color change or visible precipitation[78]
- After reconstitution with SWFI to a concentration of 1 mg topotecan/mL in the original product vials, storage either upright or inverted for 28 days at 5°C (41°F), 25°C, or 30°C (86°F), and protected from light, the drug product was found to be physically and chemically stable by stability-indicating HPLC analysis without change in color or clarity
  - The amount of topotecan remaining was >98% of the initial concentration in all solutions stored at 5°C (41°F), 25°C, or 30°C
  - There was no significant difference in the total amount of impurities and degradation products for samples stored at 5°C. In comparison, the total amount of impurities and degradation products increased for samples stored at 25°C or 30°C, more so for samples stored at 30°C
- After reconstitution with BWFI (preserved with benzyl alcohol) to a concentration of 1 mg/mL and further diluted in a PVC container, topotecan HCl stability was as follows:

Diluting/Vehicle Solution	Diluted Concentration	Storage Conditions	% Loss of Topotecan
0.9% NS	10 mcg/mL	Room temperature × 4 days	<3%
	500 mcg/mL		
D5W	10 mcg/mL		
	500 mcg/mL		
BWFI	10 mcg/mL	Room temperature × 21 days	<4%

(continued)

Recommendations for Drug Administration and Ancillary Care

General:

- See Chapter 41 for recommendations for use in patients with renal dysfunction
- Administer topotecan doses intraVENously over 30 minutes

Inadvertent exposure:

- In case of skin contact, immediately and thoroughly wash the affected area with soap and water
- In case of contact with mucous membranes, thoroughly flush the affected area with water

Product Identification, Preparation, Storage, and Stability (*continued*)

- Dilute an amount of drug appropriate for a patient's dose in 50–250 mL of either 0.9% NS or D5W
- After dilution with 0.9% NS or D5W, solutions prepared with Topotecan for Injection are stable for at least 24 hours when stored at 20°–25°C
- Topotecan 0.05 mg/mL diluted in 0.9% NS or D5W was stable for up to 24 hours at 23°–24°C (73.4°–75.2°F) and for up to 7 days at 5°C (41°F) in PVC, polyolefin, and glass parenteral product containers[79]
- Topotecan 0.025 mg/mL diluted in 0.9% NS or D5W was stable for up to 24 hours at 23°–24°C and for up to 7 days at 5°C in PVC parenteral product containers.[79] At the topotecan concentrations and for the conditions studied:
  - There were no significant differences observed in stability between topotecan diluted in either 0.9% NS or D5W[79]
  - Topotecan hydrochloride did not contribute to significant leaching of DEHP from PVC containers[79]
- Topotecan is susceptible to photodegradation during storage:
  - *Protect stored solutions* from light exposure[78]
  - Protection from light is not necessary during topotecan administration

Topotecan Injection (solution):

- Topotecan Injection is available generically in individually packaged single-use vials containing a sterile, non-pyrogenic, clear, yellow to yellow-green solution of topotecan HCl
  - Each milliliter of solution contains topotecan hydrochloride equivalent to 1 mg of topotecan (free base), with 5 mg tartaric acid, NF, and SWFI. Hydrochloric acid and/or sodium hydroxide may be added to adjust product pH within the range 2.6–3.2
- Store intact vials under refrigeration at 2°–8°C (35.6°–46.4°F) and protected from light in the original packaging carton
- Dilute an amount of Topotecan Injection (1 mg/mL) appropriate for a patient's dose in a minimum volume of 50 mL of 0.9% NS or D5W
- After dilution with 0.9% NS or D5W, solutions prepared with Topotecan Injection are stable for 24 hours when stored at 20°–25°C under ambient lighting

Selected incompatibility:

- Topotecan is formulated with tartaric acid to maintain a pH between 2.5 and 3.5. Topotecan solubility and stability decrease with increasing pH; its lactone ring spontaneously hydrolyzes at pH >4

TRASTUZUMAB

HERCEPTIN® (trastuzumab) Intravenous Infusion; product label, November 2013. Manufactured by Genentech, Inc., A Member of the Roche Group, South San Francisco, CA

WARNING: CARDIOMYOPATHY, INFUSION REACTIONS, EMBRYO-FETAL TOXICITY, and PULMONARY TOXICITY

Cardiomyopathy
Herceptin administration can result in sub-clinical and clinical cardiac failure. The incidence and severity was highest in patients receiving Herceptin with anthracycline-containing chemotherapy regimens. Evaluate left ventricular function in all patients prior to and during treatment with Herceptin. Discontinue Herceptin treatment in patients receiving adjuvant therapy and withhold Herceptin in patients with metastatic disease for clinically significant decrease in left ventricular function…

Infusion Reactions; Pulmonary Toxicity
Herceptin administration can result in serious and fatal infusion reactions and pulmonary toxicity. Symptoms usually occur during or within 24 hours of Herceptin administration. Interrupt Herceptin infusion for dyspnea or clinically significant hypotension. Monitor patients until symptoms completely resolve. Discontinue Herceptin for anaphylaxis, angioedema, interstitial pneumonitis, or acute respiratory distress syndrome…

Embryo-Fetal Toxicity
Exposure to Herceptin during pregnancy can result in oligohydramnios and oligohydramnios sequence manifesting as pulmonary hypoplasia, skeletal abnormalities, and neonatal death…

Boxed Warning for "HERCEPTIN® (trastuzumab) Intravenous Infusion"; November 2013 product label; Genentech, Inc., A Member of the Roche Group, South San Francisco, CA

Product Identification, Preparation, Storage, and Stability

- HERCEPTIN® product package carton contains 2 vials, including:
  - One vial containing 440 mg trastuzumab as a sterile, white to pale yellow, preservative-free, lyophilized powder under vacuum with 400 mg α,α-trehalose dihydrate, 9.9 mg L-histidine HCl, 6.4 mg L-histidine, and 1.8 mg polysorbate 20, USP (NDC 50242-134-68)
  - A second vial containing 20 mL BWFI, preserved with 1.1% benzyl alcohol
- Store intact product vials under refrigeration at 2°–8°C (35.6°–46.4°F)
- Slowly inject 20 mL of BWFI *or* SWFI directly into the lyophilized powder cake to produce a solution containing 21 mg trastuzumab/mL, at a pH of approximately 6
  - Reconstitution with BWFI results in a solution useful for preparing ≥2 trastuzumab doses
    - Reconstitution with 20 mL of BWFI maintains product sterility for up to 28 days. Other diluents have not been shown to contain effective preservatives and should not be used

- Reconstitution with SWFI for persons with known hypersensitivity to benzyl alcohol results in a solution appropriate for preparing *only* one dose
  - After reconstitution with SWFI, the resulting trastuzumab should be used immediately and any unused portion discarded
- Gently swirl vials to aid reconstitution. *Do not shake* trastuzumab during reconstitution to avoid excessive foaming, which may make dissolution difficult and compromise the amount of solution that can be withdrawn from a vial
  - Trastuzumab may be sensitive to shear-induced stresses that can be produced during agitation or rapid expulsion from a syringe
  - Slight foaming is not unusual during reconstitution. After adding the diluent, allow vials to stand undisturbed for approximately 5 minutes
- Reconstituted trastuzumab (21 mg trastuzumab/mL) should be free of visible particulates, clear to slightly opalescent, and colorless to pale yellow
- After reconstitution, dilute an amount of trastuzumab appropriate for a patient's dose in 250 mL of 0.9% NS

- *Do not use* dextrose solutions to dilute trastuzumab
- Gently invert the container to mix the solution
- Trastuzumab is compatible with PVC and polyethylene containers
- For patients with known hypersensitivity to benzyl alcohol, trastuzumab may be reconstituted with SWFI, then diluted in 250 mL of 0.9% NS and used immediately. All partially used vials reconstituted in this manner must be discarded after a single use
- Trastuzumab solutions diluted in 0.9% NS in PVC or polyethylene bags may be stored at 2°–25°C (35.6°–77°F) for up to 24 hours before use, but the diluted solution will not inhibit microbial growth. Therefore, store reconstituted and diluted trastuzumab solutions under refrigeration at 2°–8°C (35.6°–46.4°F)

Selected incompatibility:
- *Do not use* D5W to dilute trastuzumab
- *Do not mix or dilute* trastuzumab with other drugs

Recommendations for Drug Administration and Ancillary Care

General:

- Administer doses intraVENously over 90 minutes. If administration over 90 minutes is well tolerated, subsequent doses may be administered over 30–90 minutes
  - *Do not administer* trastuzumab by rapid injection techniques (push or bolus)
  - Observe patients for fever and chills and other infusion-associated symptoms
- *Do not mix or dilute* trastuzumab with other drugs

Infusion reactions:

- Infusion reactions consist of a symptom complex characterized by fever and chills, and on occasion included nausea, vomiting, pain (in some cases at tumor sites), headache, dizziness, dyspnea, hypotension, rash, and asthenia
- Decrease the rate of infusion for mild or moderate infusion reactions
- Severe reactions, including bronchospasm, anaphylaxis, angioedema, hypoxia, and severe hypotension, were usually reported during or immediately after an initial treatment. However, the onset and clinical course were variable, including:
  - Progressive worsening
  - Initial improvement followed by clinical deterioration, *or*
  - Delayed postinfusion events with rapid clinical deterioration
- For fatal events, death occurred within hours to days following a serious infusion reaction
- Interrupt trastuzumab administration in all patients who experience dyspnea, clinically significant hypotension, and provide medical therapy appropriate for signs and symptoms, which may include epinephrine, corticosteroids, diphenhydramine, bronchodilators, and oxygen
- Evaluate and carefully monitor patients who experience moderate and more severe infusion reactions until associated signs and symptoms completely resolve
- Discontinue trastuzumab in all patients who experience severe or life-threatening infusion reactions
- There are no data to guide the most appropriate method for identifying patients who may safely be retreated with trastuzumab after experiencing a severe infusion reaction
- Prophylaxis against severe hypersensitivity reactions with antihistamines and/or steroids may or may not prevent recurrent severe infusion reactions

Cardiomyopathy:

- Trastuzumab can cause left ventricular cardiac dysfunction, arrhythmias, hypertension, disabling cardiac failure, cardiomyopathy, and cardiac death, and an asymptomatic decline in left ventricular ejection fraction (LVEF)
- There is a 4- to 6-fold increase in the incidence of symptomatic myocardial dysfunction among patients who receive trastuzumab as a single agent or in combination therapy compared with those who do not receive trastuzumab; the highest absolute incidence occurs when trastuzumab is administered with an anthracycline
- Assess left ventricular ejection fraction (LVEF) before administering trastuzumab and at regular intervals during treatment

Cardiac monitoring:

- Conduct thorough cardiac assessment, including history, physical examination, and determine LVEF by echocardiogram or MUGA scan. The following schedule is recommended:
  - Baseline LVEF measurement immediately before initiating trastuzumab
  - LVEF measurements every 3 months during and after completing trastuzumab treatments
  - Repeat LVEF measurement at 4-week intervals if trastuzumab is withheld for significant left ventricular cardiac dysfunction
  - LVEF measurements every 6 months for at least 2 years after completing trastuzumab as a component of adjuvant therapy

Treatment modification for cardiac toxicity:

- Withhold trastuzumab for at least 4 weeks for either of the following:
  - $\geq 16\%$ absolute decrease in LVEF from pretreatment values
  - LVEF below institutional limits of normal *and* $\geq 10\%$ absolute decrease in LVEF from pretreatment values
- Trastuzumab may be resumed if, within 4–8 weeks, LVEF returns to normal limits and the absolute decrease from baseline is $\leq 15\%$
  - Whether it is safe to continue or resume trastuzumab treatment in patients with trastuzumab-induced left ventricular cardiac dysfunction has not been studied
  - Permanently discontinue trastuzumab for a persistent (>8 weeks) LVEF decline or for suspension of trastuzumab dosing on >3 occasions for cardiomyopathy

Pulmonary toxicity:

- Trastuzumab use is associated with serious and fatal pulmonary toxicity, including dyspnea, interstitial pneumonitis, pulmonary infiltrates, pleural effusions, non-cardiogenic pulmonary edema, pulmonary insufficiency and hypoxia, acute respiratory distress syndrome, and pulmonary fibrosis
  - Pulmonary toxicity may occur as sequelae of infusion-related reactions
  - Patients with symptomatic intrinsic lung disease or with extensive tumor involvement of the lungs, resulting in dyspnea at rest, appear to have more severe toxicity

VALRUBICIN

VALSTAR® (valrubicin) Sterile Solution for Intravesical Instillation; product label, November 2012. Manufactured by BSP Pharmaceuticals Srl, Latina Scalo, Italy. Manufactured for Endo Pharmaceuticals Solutions Inc., Malvern, PA

Product Identification, Preparation, Storage, and Stability

- VALSTAR® Sterile Solution for Intravesical Instillation is available in, single-use, clear, glass vials packaged in cartons containing 4 vials (NDC 67979-001-01)
- Each vial contains a sterile, nonpyrogenic, clear, red, nonaqueous solution of valrubicin at a concentration of 40 mg/mL in 50% polyoxyl castor oil and 50% dehydrated alcohol, USP, without preservatives or other additives
- Store vials under refrigeration at 2°–8°C (35.6°–46.4°F) in the packaging carton. *Do not freeze* valrubicin. Unopened vials are stable until the date indicated on the packaging
- For each instillation, allow 4 vials (a total of 800 mg valrubicin) to warm slowly to room temperature, without heating

- *Notes:*
  1. Valstar sterile solution contains polyoxyl castor oil, which has been known to cause leaching of DEHP, a hepatotoxic plasticizer, from parenteral product containers and administration sets made from PVC
     a. Valstar solutions should be prepared and stored in glass, polypropylene, or polyolefin containers
     b. Only administration sets that do not contain DEHP in the fluid pathway (the surface in contact with a drug containing solution) should be used to administer valrubicin, for example, polyethylene-lined administration sets

  2. At temperatures <4°C (<39.2°F), polyoxyl castor oil may begin to form a waxy precipitate
     a. If a vial is found to contain a precipitate, warm the vial in one's hands until the solution is clear
     b. A vial in which particulate matter is still seen after warming should not be used to prepare a dose
- Withdraw 20 mL of valrubicin (800 mg) from the 4 vials and dilute the concentrated product with 55 mL of 0.9% NS to produce 75 mL of a diluted solution (10.7 mg/mL)
- After dilution in 0.9% NS for administration is stable for 12 hours at temperatures up to 25°C (77°F)

Compatibility:
- Valstar should not be mixed with other drugs

Recommendations for Drug Administration and Ancillary Care

General:
- See Chapter 41 for comments about use in patients with renal and hepatic dysfunction
- For intraVESICAL administration in the urinary bladder only
  - *Do not administer* by the intraVENous or intraMUSCular routes
- *Caution:* Delay administration ≥2 weeks after transurethral resection or fulguration
- Valrubicin is recommended at a dose of 800 mg administered intravesically once weekly for 6 weeks
  - A urethral catheter should be inserted into a patient's bladder under aseptic conditions, the bladder drained, and 75 mL of diluted valrubicin solution (10.7 mg/mL) instilled slowly via gravity flow over a period of several minutes. The urethral catheter should then be withdrawn
  - The patient should retain the drug for 2 hours before voiding. At the end of a 2-hour retention period, patients should void
- Some patients will be unable to retain the drug for a full two hours and may void earlier than planned

- Patients should be instructed to maintain adequate hydration following treatment

Information for patients:
- Advise patients the major acute toxicities from valrubicin are symptoms related to bladder irritation that may occur during drug instillation and retention and for a limited period following voiding
  - Use valrubicin with caution in patients with severe irritable bladder symptoms: bladder spasm and spontaneous discharge of the intravesical instillate may occur
  - Clamping the urinary catheter is not advised, but, if performed, should be executed with caution and under medical supervision
- Red-tinged urine is typical and should be expected during the first 24 hours after valrubicin administration
- Patients should immediately report to their physician prolonged irritable bladder symptoms or prolonged passage of red-colored urine

Contraindications:
- Valrubicin is contraindicated in patients with known hypersensitivity to anthracyclines or polyoxyl castor oil
- Patients with concurrent urinary tract infections should not receive valrubicin
- Valrubicin should not be administered to patients with a small bladder capacity, that is, unable to tolerate a 75-mL fluid instillation

Inadvertent exposure and release:
- Contact toxicity, common and severe with other anthracyclines, is not typical with valrubicin and, when observed, has been mild. Skin reactions may occur with accidental exposure
- Eye irritation has also been reported after accidental exposure
  - Immediately and thoroughly flush the affected eyes with water
- Spills on environmental surfaces should be cleaned with 5% sodium hypochlorite bleach

VINBLASTINE SULFATE

VINBLASTINE SULFATE–vinBLAStine sulfate injection; product label, October 2011. APP Pharmaceuticals LLC, Schaumburg, IL
VinBLAStine Sulfate for injection, USP; product label, May 2012. Manufactured for Bedford Laboratories, Bedford, OH

WARNINGS

Caution: This preparation should be administered by individuals experienced in the administration of vinblastine sulfate. It is extremely important that the intravenous needle or catheter be properly positioned before any vinblastine sulfate is injected. Leakage into surrounding tissue during intravenous administration of vinblastine sulfate may cause considerable irritation. If extravasation occurs, the injection should be discontinued immediately, and any remaining portion of the dose should then be introduced into another vein. Local injection of hyaluronidase and the application of moderate heat to the area of leakage help disperse the drug and are thought to minimize discomfort and the possibility of cellulitis

FOR INTRAVENOUS USE ONLY - FATAL IF GIVEN BY OTHER ROUTES...

[Treatment of patients given intrathecal vinBLAStine sulfate injection]

This product is for intravenous use only. It should be administered by individuals experienced in the administration of vinblastine sulfate. The intrathecal administration of vinblastine sulfate usually results in death. Syringes containing this product should be labeled, using the auxiliary sticker provided to state "FOR INTRAVENOUS USE ONLY – FATAL IF GIVEN BY OTHER ROUTES."

Extemporaneously prepared syringes containing this product must be packaged in an overwrap which is labeled "DO NOT REMOVE COVERING UNTIL MOMENT OF INJECTION. FOR INTRAVENOUS USE ONLY – FATAL IF GIVEN BY OTHER ROUTES."

After inadvertent intrathecal administration of vinca alkaloids, immediate neurosurgical intervention is required in order to prevent ascending paralysis leading to death. In a very small number of patients, life-threatening paralysis and subsequent death was averted but resulted in devastating neurological sequelae, with limited recovery afterwards

There are no published cases of survival following intrathecal administration of vinblastine sulfate to base treatment on. However, based on the published management of survival cases involving the related vinca alkaloid vincristine sulfate[81-83], if vinblastine sulfate is mistakenly given by the intrathecal route, the following treatment should be initiated **immediately after the injection:**

1. Remove as much CSF as is safely possible through the lumbar access
2. Insertion of an epidural catheter into the subarachnoid space via the intervertebral space above initial lumbar access and CSF irrigation with lactated Ringer's [Injection, USP] solution. Fresh frozen plasma should be requested and, when available, 25 mL should be added to every 1 liter of lactated Ringer's [Injection, USP] solution
3. Insertion of an intraventricular drain or catheter by a neurosurgeon and continuation of CSF irrigation with fluid removal through the lumbar access connected to a closed drainage system. Lactated Ringer's [Injection, USP] solution should be given by continuous infusion at 150 mL/hour, or at a rate of 75 mL/hour when fresh frozen plasma has been added as above

The rate of infusion should be adjusted to maintain a spinal fluid protein level of 150 mg/dL

The following measures have also been used in addition but may not be essential:

Glutamic acid, 10 grams, has been given intravenously over 24 hours, followed by 500 mg three times daily by mouth for 1 month. Folinic acid has been administered intravenously as a 100 mg bolus and then infused at a rate of 25 mg/hour for 24 hours, then bolus doses of 25 mg every 6 hours for 1 week. Pyridoxine has been given at a dose of 50 mg every 8 hours by intravenous infusion over 30 minutes. Their roles in the reduction of neurotoxicity are unclear

Boxed Warnings for "VinBLAStine Sulfate for Injection USP"; May 2012 product label; Bedford Laboratories™, Bedford, OH

Product Identification, Preparation, Storage, and Stability

VinBLAStine Sulfate for Injection, USP:
- VinBLAStine sulfate for injection, USP, is available generically in packages of 10 individually boxed vials containing a sterile, white to off-white, amorphous, solid, lyophilized, plug of vinBLAStine sulfate 10 mg (0.011 mmol) without excipients. After reconstitution with 0.9% NS or B0.9% NS

- Store under refrigeration 2°–8°C (35.6°–46.4°F) to assure extended stability
- Protect the lyophilized powder and vinBLAStine solutions from light
- Reconstitute vials containing 10 mg vinBLAStine sulfate with 10 mL of B0.9% NS (preserved with benzyl alcohol) or 0.9% NS to produce a solution with a concentration of 1 mg/mL

- VinBLAStine sulfate dissolves instantly to give a clear solution with a pH within the range 3.5–5
- After reconstitution with 10 mL of B0.9% NS (preserved with benzyl alcohol), vinBLAStine sulfate solution may be kept under refrigeration for 30 days without significant loss of potency

(continued)

Product Identification, Preparation, Storage, and Stability *(continued)*

- *Discard* partially used vials containing vinBLAStine sulfate reconstituted with 0.9% NS (without an antimicrobial preservative)

VinBLAStine Sulfate Injection:

- VinBLAStine sulfate injection (drug product in solution) is available generically in individually packaged multidose vials. Each milliliter contains vinBLAStine

sulfate 1 mg, sodium chloride 9 mg, benzyl alcohol 0.9% (v/v) as a preservative, Q.S. SWFI, at a pH within the range 3.5–5.0
- Store under refrigeration 2°–8°C (35.6°–46.4°F) to assure extended stability
- Protect vinBLAStine sulfate from light by retaining vials in their packaging carton until time of use
- *Discard* partially used vials within 28 days after initial use

VinBLAStine Sulfate for Injection, USP, and VinBLAStine Sulfate Injection:

- VinBLAStine sulfate may be further diluted with a volume of 0.9% NS, D5W, or LRI that is convenient for administration
- Maximum stability for vinBLAStine sulfate in aqueous solutions is within the pH range 2–4.[80] VinBLAStine (base) may precipitate in solutions with pH >6

Recommendations for Drug Administration and Ancillary Care

Special Dispensing Information: When dispensing vinBLAStine sulfate injection in other than its original container (eg, a syringe), it is imperative that it be packaged in the provided overwrap that bears the following statement: "DO NOT REMOVE COVERING UNTIL MOMENT OF INJECTION. FOR INTRAVENOUS USE ONLY— FATAL IF GIVEN BY OTHER ROUTES"

A syringe containing a specific dose must be labeled, using the auxiliary sticker provided to state: "FOR INTRAVENOUS USE ONLY—FATAL IF GIVEN BY OTHER ROUTES"

General:

- See Chapter 41 for recommendations for use in patients with hepatic dysfunction
- VinBLAStine is for intraVENous use only
  - VinBLAStine sulfate (1 mg/mL) is suitable for direct intraVENous injection, or it may be injected into the tubing of a running intraVENous solution. In either case, injection may be completed in about 1 minute
- Drug loss due to adsorption was demonstrated for vinBLAStine sulfate administration through nylon or positively-charged nylon filters[84]
  - VinBLAStine concentration was not affected by filtration through filter membranes made of cellulose acetate, cellulose nitrate/cellulose acetate ester, Teflon®, or polysulfone[15,16,35]
- FDA-approved labeling recommends rinsing the syringe and needle by aspirating blood into the syringe after completing drug injection before the needle is withdrawn. The procedure is intended to minimize the

possibility of vinBLAStine extravasation after administration by venipuncture
- VinBLAStine doses should not be further diluted after reconstitution or given intraVENously for prolonged periods (≥15 minutes), unless administration technique is based on continuous infusion through central VADs, SUBCUTaneously implanted "ports," or peripherally inserted central VADs (eg, PICC, SICC)
- Do not administer vinBLAStine by intraVENous injection into a lower extremity, or an extremity in which the circulation is impaired or potentially impaired by such conditions as compressing or invading neoplasm, phlebitis, or varicosity, because of the enhanced potential for treatment-related thrombosis
- *Caution:* VinBLAStine is a vesicant and may produce severe local soft-tissue necrosis if extravasation occurs
  - It is extremely important that the intraVENous needle or catheter be properly positioned before any vinBLAStine sulfate is injected
  - Leakage into surrounding tissue during intraVENous administration of vinBLAStine sulfate may cause considerable irritation
  - If extravasation occurs, the injection should be discontinued immediately, and any remaining portion of the dose should then be introduced into another vein
  - Local injection of hyaluronidase and the application of moderate heat to the area of leakage help disperse the drug and minimize discomfort and the possibility of cellulitis

  - See Chapter 42 for more information about vinBLAStine extravasation

Potential drug interactions:

- Concomitant administration of phenytoin and vinBLAStine sulfate has been associated with decreased blood concentrations of the anticonvulsant, and, consequently, increased seizure activity
  - Phenytoin dosage adjustment should be based on serial blood concentration monitoring
- VinBLAStine metabolism is mediated by CYP3A subfamily enzymes
  - Exercise caution in treating patients with vinBLAStine who are using drugs known to inhibit CYP3A subfamily enzymes and in patients with impaired hepatic function
    - Consult recommendations for vinBLAStine use in hepatic impairment
  - Enhanced toxicity has been reported in patients who received erythromycin, a CYP3A subfamily enzyme inhibitor, and vinBLAStine concomitantly

Inadvertent exposure:

- If accidental eye contamination occurs, severe irritation, or, if vinBLAStine was delivered under pressure, corneal ulceration may result
  - An exposed eye should be immediately and thoroughly irrigated with water
- 5% sodium hypochlorite bleach has been used to inactivate vinBLAStine sulfate spills on environmental surfaces[85]

VINCRISTINE SULFATE

VINCASAR PFS®–vincristine sulfate injection solution; product label, March 2013. Manufactured by Teva Parenteral Medicines, Inc., Irvine, CA
VinCRIStine Sulfate Injection, USP, PRESERVATIVE FREE SOLUTION; product label, March 2013. Hospira, Inc., Lake Forest, IL

WARNINGS

Caution—This preparation should be administered by individuals experienced in the administration of Vincristine Sulfate Injection, USP.. It is extremely important that the intravenous needle or catheter be properly positioned before any vincristine is injected. Leakage into surrounding tissue during intravenous administration of Vincristine Sulfate Injection, USP may cause considerable irritation. If extravasation occurs, the injection should be discontinued immediately, and any remaining portion of the dose should then be introduced into another vein. Local injection of hyaluronidase and the application of moderate heat to the area of leakage help disperse the drug and are thought to minimize discomfort and the possibility of cellulitis

FOR INTRAVENOUS USE ONLY. FATAL IF GIVEN BY OTHER ROUTES

See OVERDOSAGE section for the treatment of patients given intrathecal Vincristine Sulfate Injection, USP

WARNINGS

This preparation is for intravenous use only. It should be administered by individuals experienced in the administration of vincristine sulfate injection. The intrathecal administration of vincristine sulfate injection usually results in death

To reduce the potential for fatal medication errors due to incorrect route of administration, Vincristine Sulfate Injection should be diluted in a flexible plastic container and prominently labeled as indicated for intravenous use only

Syringes containing this product must be labeled, using the auxiliary sticker provided, to state "FOR INTRAVENOUS USE ONLY – FATAL IF GIVEN BY OTHER ROUTES."

Extemporaneously prepared syringes containing this product must be packaged in an overwrap which is labeled "do not remove covering until moment of injection. For intravenous use only fatal if given by other routes."

See OVERDOSAGE section for the treatment of patients given intrathecal Vincristine Sulfate Injection, USP

[Excerpted from "OVERDOSAGE" section:]

Treatment of patients following intrathecal administration of vincristine sulfate injection has included immediate removal of spinal fluid and flushing with Lactated Ringer's [Injection, USP], as well as other solutions and has not prevented ascending paralysis and death. In one case, progressive paralysis in an adult was arrested by the following treatment **initiated immediately after the intrathecal injection:**

1. As much spinal fluid was removed as could be safely done through lumbar access
2. The subarachnoid space was flushed with Lactated Ringer's [Injection, USP] …infused continuously through a catheter in a cerebral lateral ventricle at the rate of 150 mL/h. The fluid was removed through a lumbar access
3. As soon as fresh frozen plasma became available, the fresh frozen plasma, 25 mL, diluted in 1 L of Lactated Ringer's [Injection, USP] … was infused through the cerebral ventricular catheter at the rate of 75 mL/h with removal through the lumbar access. The rate of infusion was adjusted to maintain a protein level in the spinal fluid of 150 mg/dL
4. Glutamic acid, 10 [grams]…, was given intravenously over 24 hours followed by 500 mg 3 times daily by mouth for 1 month or until neurological dysfunction stabilized. The role of glutamic acid in this treatment is not certain and may not be essential

Boxed Warnings for "VinCRIStine Sulfate Injection, USP, PRESERVATIVE FREE SOLUTION"; March 2013 product label; Hospira, Inc., Lake Forest, IL

Product Identification, Preparation, Storage, and Stability

- VinCRIStine sulfate injection, USP, is available generically in individually packaged single-use vials in several presentations. In general, products are packaged in single-use vials containing either 1 mg or 2 mg of vinCRIStine sulfate, both in a concentration of 1 mg/mL

- Each milliliter of VinCRIStine sulfate injection, USP, contains vinCRIStine sulfate 1 mg (1.08 μmol), mannitol 100 mg, and Q.S. SWFI. Additional excipients potentially including acidic, basic, or buffering compounds, may have been added to maintain product pH within the range 3.5–5.5

- VinCRIStine sulfate injection, USP, does not contain antimicrobial preservatives
- Store VinCRIStine sulfate injection, USP, vials upright under refrigeration at 2°–8°C (35.6°–46.4°F) in the carton in which vials are packaged to protect the medication from light until it is used

(continued)

Product Identification, Preparation, Storage, and Stability (*continued*)

- VinCRIStine may be diluted with a volume of 0.9% NS or D5W that is convenient for administration, but *avoid admixture* with other solutions
  - Maximum stability for vinCRIStine sulfate in aqueous solutions is within the pH range 4–6[86]
  - Product labeling recommends not preparing vinCRIStine in solutions that

raise or lower the pH outside the range 3.5–5.5
  - After dilution with 0.9% NS to concentrations within the range, 0.0015–0.08 mg/mL, vinCRIStine sulfate solutions are stable for up to 24 hours when protected from light or for 8 hours under normal light at 25°C (77°F)

Selected incompatibility:
- When used in combination with asparaginase, vinCRIStine should be given 12–24 hours *before* asparaginase to minimize toxicity. Administering asparaginase before vinCRIStine may decrease vinCRIStine's hepatic clearance

Recommendations for Drug Administration and Ancillary Care

Special dispensing information:
When dispensed, the container or syringe (holding the individual dose prepared for administration to the patient) must be enclosed in an overwrap bearing the statement, "DO NOT REMOVE COVERING UNTIL MOMENT OF INJECTION. FOR INTRAVENOUS USE ONLY— FATAL IF GIVEN BY OTHER ROUTES"

A syringe containing a specific dose must be labeled, using the auxiliary sticker provided, to state:

"FOR INTRAVENOUS USE ONLY. FATAL IF GIVEN BY OTHER ROUTES"

The concentration of vinCRIStine sulfate contained in all vials is 1 mg/mL. Do not add extra fluid to the vial prior to removal of a dose. Withdraw the solution…into an accurate dry syringe, measuring the dose carefully. Do not add extra fluid to a vial in an attempt to empty it completely

General:
- See Chapter 41 for recommendations for use in patients with hepatic dysfunction
- VinCRIStine is *for intraVENous use only*
  - VinCRIStine sulfate (1 mg/mL) is suitable for direct intraVENous injection, or it may be injected into the tubing of a running intraVENous solution. In either case, injection may be completed in about 1 minute
- VinCRIStine sulfate injection *should not be given to patients* while they are receiving radiation therapy through fields that include the liver
- *Do not dilute* vinCRIStine sulfate doses or give the drug intraVENously for prolonged periods (≥15 minutes) unless administration technique is based on continuous infusion through central VADs, SUBCUTaneously implanted "ports," or peripherally inserted central VADs (eg, PICC, SICC)

- *Do not administer* vinCRIStine by intraVENous injection into a lower extremity, or an extremity in which the circulation is impaired or potentially impaired by such conditions as compressing or invading neoplasm, phlebitis, or varicosity, because of the enhanced potential for treatment-related thrombosis
- VinCRIStine sulfate diluted to a concentration of 25 mcg/mL in 0.9% NS exhibited a 9% loss of potency due to adsorption during the first 60 min of delivery through PVC administration set tubing, but negligible loss during delivery through a polyethylene administration set under identical conditions[84]
  - The concentration of vinCRIStine sulfate delivered through the PVC tubing returned to full concentration at 1.5 h after drug delivery began (samples for analysis were collected every 30 min)[84]
- *Do not filter* vinCRIStine solutions:
  - Administration through cellulose acetate, cellulose nitrate, cellulose ester, nylon, or Teflon filters has demonstrated variable drug loss because of absorption. In general, the extent of drug loss as a result of filtration is inversely proportional to the concentration of vinCRIStine in solution
- *Caution:* VinCRIStine is a vesicant and may produce severe local soft-tissue necrosis if extravasation occurs
  - It is extremely important that the intraVENous needle or catheter be properly positioned before any vinCRIStine sulfate is injected
  - Leakage into surrounding tissue during intraVENous administration of vinCRIStine sulfate may cause considerable irritation
  - If extravasation occurs, the injection should be discontinued immediately, and any remaining portion of the dose should then be introduced into another vein

  - Local injection of hyaluronidase and the application of moderate heat to the area of leakage help disperse the drug and minimize discomfort and the possibility of cellulitis
  - See Chapter 42 for more information about vinCRIStine extravasation

Potential drug interactions:
- Concomitant administration of phenytoin and vinCRIStine sulfate has been associated with decreased blood concentrations of the anticonvulsant, and, consequently, increased seizure activity
  - Phenytoin dosage adjustment should be based on serial blood concentration monitoring
- VinCRIStine metabolism is mediated by CYP3A subfamily enzymes
  - Concurrent administration of vinCRIStine sulfate with itraconazole (a known potent inhibitor of CYP3A subfamily enzymes) has been reported to cause an earlier onset and/or an increased severity of neuromuscular adverse effects presumably related to inhibition of vinCRIStine metabolism
  - Exercise caution in treating patients with vinCRIStine who are using drugs known to inhibit CYP3A subfamily enzymes and in patients with impaired hepatic function
    - Consult recommendations for vinCRIStine use in hepatic impairment

Inadvertent exposure:
- If accidental eye contamination occurs, severe irritation, or, if vinCRIStine was delivered under pressure, corneal ulceration may result
  - An eye exposed to vincristine should be washed with water immediately and thoroughly
- 5% sodium hypochlorite bleach has been used to inactivate vinCRIStine sulfate spills on environmental surfaces[85]

VINCRISTINE SULFATE LIPOSOME INJECTION

Marqibo® (vinCRIStine sulfate liposome injection) for intravenous infusion; product label, October 2012. vinCRIStine sulfate injection manufactured by Hospira Australia Pty Ltd., Mulgrave, Victoria 3170 Australia; Sphingomyelin/Cholesterol Liposome Injection manufactured by Cangene Corporation Winnipeg, Manitoba, Canada; Sodium Phosphate Injection manufactured by Jubilant HollisterStier Spokane, WA; Marqibo Kit for the Preparation of vinCRIStine sulfate LIPOSOME injection manufactured by Anderson Packaging, Inc Rockford, IL.; Distributed by Talon Therapeutics, Inc., South San Francisco, CA

WARNING

- For Intravenous Use Only — Fatal if Given by Other Routes…
- Death has occurred with intrathecal use
- Marqibo (vinCRIStine sulfate LIPOSOME injection) has different dosage recommendations than vinCRIStine sulfate injection. Verify drug name and dose prior to preparation and administration to avoid overdosage

---

Boxed Warnings for "Marqibo® (vinCRIStine sulfate LIPOSOME injection) for intravenous infusion"; October 2012 product label; Talon Therapeutics, Inc., South San Francisco, CA

Product Identification, Preparation, Storage, and Stability

- Marqibo® (vinCRIStine sulfate liposome injection) is vinCRIStine encapsulated in liposomes
  - The active ingredient in Marqibo® is vinCRIStine sulfate
  - The lipid components from which liposomes are formed are sphingomyelin and cholesterol at a molar ratio of approximately 60:40 (mol:mol)
- After preparation, each vial of Marqibo® contains 5 mg vinCRIStine sulfate with mannitol 500 mg, sphingomyelin 73.5 mg, cholesterol 29.5 mg, sodium citrate 36 mg, citric acid 38 mg, sodium phosphate 355 mg, and sodium chloride 225 mg
- Marqibo® appears as a white to off-white, translucent suspension, essentially free of visible foreign matter and aggregates
  - Approximate liposome mean diameter is 100 nm with >95% of vinCRIStine encapsulated in the liposomes
- A Marqibo® Kit (NDC 20536-322-01) includes the following components:
  - VinCRIStine sulfate injection, USP
    - Each vial contains 5 mg/5 mL vinCRIStine sulfate (equivalent to 4.5 mg/5 mL vinCRIStine base) and 100 mg/5 mL mannitol; NDC 20536-323-01
  - Sphingomyelin/cholesterol liposome injection (103 mg/mL)
    - Each vial contains sphingomyelin 73.5 mg/mL, cholesterol 29.5 mg/mL, citric acid 33.6 mg/mL, sodium citrate 35.4 mg/mL, and ethanol ≤0.1%; NDC 20536-324-01
  - Sodium phosphate injection
    - Each vial contains dibasic sodium phosphate 355 mg/25 mL

(14.2 mg/mL) and sodium chloride 225 mg/25 mL; NDC 20536-325-01
  - Flotation ring
  - Overlabel for sodium phosphate injection vial containing constituted Marqibo® (vinCRIStine sulfate liposome injection), 5 mg/31 mL (0.16 mg/mL)
  - Infusion bag label
- Store Marqibo® Kits under refrigeration at 2°–8°C (35.6°–46.4°F). *Do not freeze* the product

Product Preparation and Materials Required to Prepare Marqibo®

1. Marqibo Kit
2. Water bath*
3. Calibrated thermometer (scale graduations from 0°–100°C [32°–212°F)*
4. Calibrated electronic timer*
5. One sterile needle or another suitable venting device equipped with a sterile 0.2-μm (0.2-mcm, 0.2-micron) filter
6. One 1-mL- or 3-mL-capacity sterile syringe with needle
7. One 5-mL-capacity sterile syringe with needle

*The manufacturer will provide the water bath, calibrated thermometer, and calibrated electronic timer to the medical facility at the initial order of Marqibo® and will replace them every 2 years (statement reprinted from Marqibo® product label, October 2012; Talon Therapeutics, Inc.)

General instructions:

- Call [1-888-292-9617] with questions about preparing Marqibo®
- Aseptic technique must be strictly observed as no preservative or bacteriostatic agent is present in Marqibo®

- Marqibo® takes approximately 60–90 minutes to prepare
  - Persons who prepare Marqibo® should have adequate time to prepare the drug without interruption or distraction because of the extensive monitoring of temperature and time required for preparation
- Deviations in temperature, time, and preparation procedures may fail to ensure proper encapsulation of vinCRIStine sulfate into liposomes
  - In the event preparation deviates from the instructions that follow, the components of a kit affected by the deviation should be discarded and a new Marqibo® Kit used to prepare a dose

Engineering controls:

- The preparation steps that involve mixing sodium phosphate injection, sphingomyelin/cholesterol liposome injection, and VinCRIStine sulfate injection must be performed within a biologic safety cabinet or with engineering controls and by established safety procedures appropriate for the aseptic preparation of sterile injectable hazardous drugs
- The preparation steps that involve placing a vial in a water bath must be done outside of the aseptic preparation area
- *Do not use* with inline filters when preparing Marqibo®. *Do not mix* Marqibo® with other drugs

Preparation—nonaseptic environment:

1. Fill a water bath with water to a level ≥8 cm (≥3.2 inches) measured from

(continued)

Product Identification, Preparation, Storage, and Stability (continued)

the bottom and maintain this minimum water level throughout the procedure
- The water bath will remain outside of an aseptic product preparation environment

2. Place a calibrated thermometer in the water bath to monitor water temperature and leave it in the water bath until the procedure has been completed

3. Preheat the water bath to 63°–67°C (145.4°–152.6°F). Using the calibrated thermometer, maintain this water temperature until preparation is completed

Preparation—aseptic environment:

4. Visually inspect each vial in the Marqibo® Kit for particulate matter and discoloration prior to preparation, whenever solution and container permit. Do not use component products if a precipitate or foreign matter is present

5. Remove the caps from all vials and swab the vial septa (injection ports) with alcohol

6. Vent the vial containing sodium phosphate injection with a sterile needle equipped with a sterile 0.2-μm filter or another suitable venting device
- Position the venting needle tip well above the liquid level before adding sphingomyelin/cholesterol liposome injection and VinCRIStine sulfate injection

7. With a syringe, transfer 1 mL of sphingomyelin/cholesterol liposome injection into the vial labeled sodium phosphate injection

8. With a different syringe, transfer 5 mL of VinCRIStine sulfate injection into the vial labeled sodium phosphate injection

9. Remove the venting needle from the vial containing the mixture of vinCRIStine sulfate, sphingomyelin/cholesterol

liposome, and sodium phosphate, and gently invert the vial 5 times to mix. *Do not shake* the vial

10. Fit the flotation ring around the neck of the vial containing the mixture

Preparation—nonaseptic environment:

11. Confirm the water bath temperature is 63°–67°C (145.4°–152.6°F) using the calibrated thermometer

12. Remove from the aseptic preparation environment the vial containing the mixture of vinCRIStine sulfate, sphingomyelin/cholesterol liposome, and sodium phosphate, and place it into the water bath for 10 minutes using the calibrated electronic timer to measure the passage of time

13. Monitor the water bath temperature to ensure the temperature is maintained at 63°–67°C (145.4°–152.6°F)

14. After placing the vial containing the vinCRIStine sulfate, sphingomyelin/cholesterol liposome, and sodium phosphate mixture into the water bath, record the "constitution start time" and water temperature on the Marqibo® overlabel

15. At the end of 10 minutes, confirm the water temperature is 63°–67°C (145.4°–152.6°F) using the calibrated thermometer, remove the vial from the water bath (use tongs to prevent burns), and remove the flotation ring from the vial

16. Record the final constitution time and the water temperature on the Marqibo® overlabel

17. Dry the exterior of the vial containing the vinCRIStine sulfate, sphingomyelin/cholesterol liposome, and sodium phosphate mixture (subsequently referred to as "constituted Marqibo") with a clean paper towel, apply the Marqibo®

overlabel to the vial, and then, gently invert the vial 5 times to mix. *Do not shake* the vial

18. Permit constituted Marqibo® to equilibrate to controlled room temperature (15°–30°C [59°–86°F]) for at least 30 minutes

19. After preparation is completed, store constituted Marqibo® at controlled room temperature (15°–30°C [59°–86°F]) for no longer than 12 hours

Preparation—aseptic environment:

20. Return the vial containing constituted Marqibo® to the aseptic preparation environment and swab the vial septum with alcohol

21. Calculate a patient's Marqibo® dose based on their actual body surface area and the volume of Marqibo® that corresponds to that volume
- Constituted Marqibo® contains 5 mg of vinCRIStine sulfate per 31 mL of solution (0.16 mg/mL)

22. From a prefilled parenteral product container containing a nominal volume of 100 mL of either 0.9% NS or D5W, withdraw a volume of solution corresponding to a patient's Marqibo® dose

23. Transfer from a vial containing constituted Marqibo® the volume of drug needed for a patient's dose and inject it into the container of solution prepared in the previous step to produce a diluted solution of constituted Marqibo® with a total volume of 100 mL

24. Label the diluted drug product container according to applicable regulatory requirements

Preparation—nonaseptic environment:

25. Empty, clean, and dry the water bath after each use

Recommendations for Drug Administration and Ancillary Care

General:
- Dosage recommendations for VinCRIStine sulfate liposome injection (2.25 mg/m² administer intraVENously over 1 hour once every 7 days) are different than those for nonliposomal vinCRIStine sulfate injection
- Verify drug name and dose prior to preparation and administration to avoid overdose
  - *Warnings: For intraVENous use only. Fatal if given by other routes*

- Administration should be completed within 12 hours after preparation was initiated

Potential drug interactions:
- VinCRIStine is a substrate for CYP3A subfamily enzymes; therefore, concomitant use of strong CYP3A inhibitors and inducers should be avoided
- VinCRIStine is also a substrate for the MDR1 transport protein (*AKA*, ABCB1, P-glycoprotein [P-gp])

- In the absence of information to guide concomitant use of Marqibo® with potent MDR1 inhibitors or inducers, a conservative utilization strategy recommends avoiding concomitant use
- Marqibo® is expected to interact with drugs known to interact with nonliposomal VinCRIStine sulfate

VINORELBINE TARTRATE

Vinorelbine Injection, USP; product label, June 2009. Made in Romania. Manufactured for SAGENT Pharmaceuticals, Schaumburg, IL
NAVELBINE® (vinorelbine tartrate) Injection; product label, October 2007. Manufactured by Pierre Fabre Médicament, 92100 Boulogne, France. Pierre Fabre Pharmaceuticals Inc., Parsippany, NJ
VINORELBINE INJECTION, USP; product label, July 2005. Manufactured by Ben Venue Laboratories, Inc., Bedford, OH. Manufactured for Bedford laboratories, Bedford, OH

WARNING

Vinorelbine should be administered under the supervision of a physician experienced in the use of cancer chemotherapeutic agents. This product is for intravenous (IV) use only. Intrathecal administration of other vinca alkaloids has resulted in death. Syringes containing this product should be labeled "WARNING – FOR IV USE ONLY. FATAL if given intrathecally."

Severe granulocytopenia resulting in increased susceptibility to infection may occur. Granulocyte counts should be ≥1,000 cells/mm³ prior to the administration of vinorelbine. The dosage should be adjusted according to complete blood counts with differentials obtained on the day of treatment

Caution - It is extremely important that the intravenous needle or catheter be properly positioned before vinorelbine is injected. Administration of vinorelbine may result in extravasation causing local tissue necrosis and/or thrombophlebitis…

Boxed Warning for "Vinorelbine Injection, USP"; June 2009 product label; SAGENT Pharmaceuticals, Schaumburg, IL

Product Identification, Preparation, Storage, and Stability

- Vinorelbine injection, USP, is available in individually packaged single-use, clear, glass vials containing vinorelbine tartrate equivalent to 10 mg vinorelbine/mL as a sterile, nonpyrogenic, preservative-free, clear, colorless to pale yellow solution in SWFI at a pH of approximately 3.5
  - Commercially available presentations include vials containing 10 mg vinorelbine in 1 mL or 50 mg vinorelbine in 5 mL
- Store intact vials of vinorelbine injection, USP, under refrigeration at 2°–8°C

(35.6°–46.4°F), and in their packaging carton to protect the product from light. *Do not freeze* vinorelbine injection, USP
- Unused vials of vinorelbine injection, USP, are stable at temperatures up to 25°C (77°F) for up to 72 hours
- Vinorelbine injection, USP, must be diluted before administration with a compatible parenteral solution:
  - In a syringe, dilute vinorelbine tartrate to a concentration within the range 1.5–3 mg/mL with 0.9% NS or D5W

- In a parenteral product container (bag or bottle), dilute vinorelbine tartrate to a concentration within the range 0.5–2 mg/mL with 0.9% NS, D5W, 0.45% NaCl, D5W/0.45% NaCl, RI, or LRI
- Vinorelbine injection, USP, may be used for up to 24 hours under normal room light when stored at 5°–30°C (41°–86°F) in polypropylene syringes or PVC containers

Recommendations for Drug Administration and Ancillary Care

General:
- See Chapter 41 for recommendations for use in patients with hepatic dysfunction
- Diluted vinorelbine should be administered intraVENously into the side port of a freely flowing intraVENous solution closest to the parenteral product container as follows:[87]
  - In a syringe, diluted to 1.5–3 mg/mL, administer by intraVENous injection over 1–2 minutes
  - In a minibag, diluted to 0.5–2 mg/mL, administer by intraVENously over 6–10 minutes

- After vinorelbine administration is completed, flush the patient's VAD or administration set connected to a VAD with ≥75 mL to 125 mL of a solution compatible with vinorelbine (eg, 0.9% NS, D5W, 0.45% NaCl, D5W/0.45% NaCl, RI, or LRI)

Caution:
- Vinorelbine is a substrate for metabolism catalyzed by CYP3A subfamily enzymes. Concurrent vinorelbine tartrate use with an inhibitor of this metabolic pathway or in patients with impaired hepatic function

may cause an earlier onset and increased severity of adverse effects
- Administration of vinorelbine to patients who previously experienced soft-tissue damage from radiation therapy may result in radiation recall reactions within the areas that previously sustained injury

Inadvertent exposure:
- In case of contact with skin or mucous membranes, immediately wash the affected areas thoroughly with soap and water
- An eye exposed to vinorelbine tartrate should be washed with water immediately and thoroughly

ZIV-AFLIBERCEPT

ZALTRAP® (ziv-aflibercept) injection for intravenous infusion; product label, October 2013. Manufactured by sanofi-aventis U.S. LLC, Bridgewater, NJ

WARNING: HEMORRHAGE, GASTROINTESTINAL PERFORATION, COMPROMISED WOUND HEALING

Hemorrhage: Severe and sometimes fatal hemorrhage, including gastrointestinal (GI) hemorrhage, has been reported in the patients who have received ZALTRAP in combination with FOLFIRI. Monitor patients for signs and symptoms of GI bleeding and other severe bleeding. Do not administer ZALTRAP to patients with severe hemorrhage…

Gastrointestinal Perforation: Gastrointestinal (GI) perforation including fatal GI perforation can occur in patients receiving ZALTRAP. Discontinue ZALTRAP therapy in patients who experience GI perforation…

Compromised Wound Healing: Severe compromised wound healing can occur in patients receiving ZALTRAP/FOLFIRI. Discontinue ZALTRAP in patients with compromised wound healing. Suspend ZALTRAP for at least 4 weeks prior to elective surgery, and do not resume ZALTRAP for at least 4 weeks following major surgery and until the surgical wound is fully healed…

Boxed Warning for "ZALTRAP® (ziv-aflibercept) Injection for Intravenous Infusion"; October 2013 product label; sanofi-aventis U.S. LLC, Bridgewater, NJ

Product Identification, Preparation, Storage, and Stability

- ZALTRAP® is a sterile, clear, colorless to pale yellow, nonpyrogenic, preservative-free, solution supplied in single-use vials containing ziv-aflibercept 25 mg/mL in polysorbate 20 0.1%, sodium chloride 100 mmol/L, sodium citrate 5 mmol/L, sodium phosphate 5 mmol/L, and sucrose 20%, in SWFI, at a pH of 6.2
  - Commercial ZALTRAP® (ziv-aflibercept 25 mg/mL) is available in 3 presentations, including:
    - ziv-Aflibercept 100 mg/4 mL, carton containing 1 single-use vial, NDC 0024-5840-01

- ziv-Aflibercept 100 mg/4 mL, carton containing 3 single-use vials, NDC 0024-5840-03
- ziv-Aflibercept 200 mg/8 mL, carton containing 1 single-use vial, NDC 0024-5841-01
- Store unopened vials under refrigeration between 2° and 8°C (35.6° and 46.4°F) in the original packaging carton to protect ZALTRAP® from light
- *Do not* use the product if the solution is discolored or cloudy or the solution contains particles
- *Do not* reenter a vial after initial entry
- Withdraw an amount of drug appropriate for a patient's dose and dilute it in a volume

of 0.9% NS or D5W sufficient to produce a final concentration of ziv-aflibercept within the range 0.6–8 mg/mL
  - Discard any unused portion of drug left in a vial
- Compatible product containers include those made of polyolefin or PVC plasticized with DEHP
- Store diluted ziv-aflibercept under refrigeration (2°–8°C [35.6°–46.4°F]) for up to 4 hours
  - Discard any unused portion of a dose remaining at the end of treatment

---

Recommendations for Drug Administration and Ancillary Care

General:

- After dilution, ziv-aflibercept is administered intraVENously over 1 hour every 2 weeks before any component of the FOLFIRI combination chemotherapy regimen
- Administer ziv-aflibercept through an administration set made of 1 of the following materials:
  - PVC containing DEHP
  - DEHP-free PVC containing trioctyl-trimellitate (TOTM)
  - polypropylene
  - polyethylene-lined PVC
  - polyurethane
- Administer ziv-aflibercept through a polyethersulfone filter with pore size equal to 0.2 μm (0.2 microns)

- Do not use filters made of polyvinylidene fluoride (PVDF) or nylon
- Do not mix ziv-aflibercept in the same container with other medicinal products or administer it through an intraVENous VAD at the same time as other medicinal products
- Discontinue ziv-aflibercept for:
  - Severe hemorrhage
  - Gastrointestinal perforation
  - Compromised wound healing
  - Fistula formation
  - Hypertensive crisis or hypertensive encephalopathy
  - Arterial thromboembolic events
  - Nephrotic syndrome or thrombotic microangiopathy

- Reversible posterior leukoencephalopathy syndrome
- Temporarily suspend ziv-aflibercept:
  - At least 4 weeks prior to elective surgery
  - For recurrent or severe hypertension, until controlled. Upon resuming treatment, permanently decrease the ziv-aflibercept dosage to 2 mg/kg
  - For proteinuria of 2 g/24 hours. Resume when proteinuria is <2 g/24 hours. For recurrent proteinuria, withhold ziv-aflibercept until proteinuria is <2 g/24 hours, and then, permanently decrease the ziv-aflibercept dosage to 2 mg/kg
- For toxicities related to irinotecan, fluorouracil, or leucovorin, refer to current prescribing information for those products

General Reference

Trissel LA. Handbook on Injectable Drugs. 16th ed. Bethesda, MD: American Society of Health-System Pharmacists; 2011

Drug-Specific References

1. Heywood GR, Rosenberg SA, Weber JS. Hypersensitivity reactions to chemotherapy agents in patients receiving chemoimmunotherapy with high-dose interleukin 2. J Natl Cancer Inst 1995;87:915–922
2. Kruit WH, Punt KJ, Goey SH et al. Cardiotoxicity as a dose-limiting factor in a schedule of high dose bolus therapy with interleukin-2 and alpha-interferon. An unexpectedly frequent complication. Cancer 1994;74:2850–2856
3. Mier JW, Vachino G, Klempner MS et al. Inhibition of interleukin-2-induced tumor necrosis factor release by dexamethasone: prevention of an acquired neutrophil chemotaxis defect and differential suppression of interleukin-2-associated side effects [see comment]. Blood 1990;76:1933–1940. Comment in: Blood 1991;78:1389–1390
4. Oldham RK, Brogley J, Braud E. Contrast medium "recalls" interleukin-2 toxicity. J Clin Oncol 1990;8:942–943
5. Zukiwski AA, David CL, Coan J, Wallace S, Gutterman JU, Mavligit GM. Increased incidence of hypersensitivity to iodine-containing radiographic contrast media after interleukin-2 administration. Cancer 1990;65:1521–1524
6. Abi-Aad AS, Figlin RA, Belldegrun A, deKernion JB. Metastatic renal cell cancer: interleukin-2 toxicity induced by contrast agent injection. J Immunother 1991;10:292–295
7. Fishman JE, Aberle DR, Moldawer NP, Belldegrun A, Figlin RA. Atypical contrast reactions associated with systemic interleukin-2 therapy. AJR Am J Roentgenol 1991;156:833–834
8. Choyke PL, Miller DL, Lotze MT, Whiteis JM, Ebbitt B, Rosenberg SA. Delayed reactions to contrast media after interleukin-2 immunotherapy. Radiology 1992;183:111–114
9. Shulman KL, Thompson JA, Benyunes MC, Winter TC, Fefer A. Adverse reactions to intravenous contrast media in patients treated with interleukin-2. J Immunother Emphasis Tumor Immunol 1993;13:208–212
10. Stecher AL, de Deus PM, Polikarpov I, Abrahão-Neto J. Stability of L-asparaginase: an enzyme used in leukemia treatment. Pharm Acta Helv 1999;74:1–9
11. Clarkson B, Krakoff I, Burchenal J et al. Clinical results of treatment with E. coli L-asparaginase in adults with leukemia, lymphoma, and solid tumors. Cancer 1970;25:279–305
12. Tallal L, Tan C, Oettgen H et al. E. coli L-asparaginase in the treatment of leukemia and solid tumors in 131 children. Cancer 1970;25:306–320
13. Koberda M, Zieske PA, Raghavan NV, Payton RJ. Stability of bleomycin sulfate reconstituted in 5% dextrose injection or 0.9% sodium chloride injection stored in glass vials or polyvinyl chloride containers. Am J Hosp Pharm 1990;47:2528–2529
14. De Vroe C, De Muynck C, Remon JP, Sansom M. A study on the stability of three antineoplastic drugs and on their sorption by i.v. delivery systems and end-line filters. Int J Pharm 1990;65:49–56
15. Butler DL, Munson JM, DeLuca PP. Effect of inline filtration on the potency of low-dose drugs. Am J Hosp Pharm 1980;37:935–941
16. Pavlik EJ, van Nagell JR Jr, Hanson MB, Donaldson ES, Powell DE, Kenady DE. Sensitivity to anticancer agents in vitro: standardizing the cytotoxic response and characterizing the sensitivities of a reference cell line. Gynecol Oncol 1982;14:243–261
17. Xu QA, Zhang Y-p, Trissel LA, Martinez JF. Stability of busulfan injection admixtures in 5% dextrose injection and 0.9% sodium chloride injection. J Oncol Pharm Pract 1996;2:101–105
18. Arbus MH. Room temperature stability guidelines for carmustine. Am J Hosp Pharm 1988;45:531
19. Trissel LA, Xu QA, Baker M. Drug compatibility with new polyolefin infusion solution containers. Am J Health Syst Pharm 2006;63:2379–2382
20. Hadji-Minaglou-Gonzalvez MF, Gayte-Sorbier A, Airaudo CB, Verdier M. Effects of temperature, solution composition, and type of container on the stability and absorption of carmustine. Clin Ther 1992;14:821–824
21. Favier M, De Cazanove F, Coste A, Cherti N, Bressolle F. Stability of carmustine in polyvinyl chloride bags and polyethylene-lined trilayer plastic containers. Am J Health Syst Pharm 2001;58:238–241
22. Levin VA, Levin EM. Dissolution and stability of carmustine in the absence of ethanol. Sel Cancer Ther 1989;5:33–35
23. Tepe P, Hassenbusch SJ, Benoit R, Anderson JH. BCNU stability as a function of ethanol concentration and temperature. J Neurooncol 1991;10:121–127
24. Colvin M, Hartner J, Summerfield M. Stability of carmustine in the presence of sodium bicarbonate. Am J Hosp Pharm 1980;37:677–678
25. Fredriksson K, Lundgren P, Landersjö L. Stability of carmustine—kinetics and compatibility during administration. Acta Pharm Suec 1986;23:115–124
26. Cheung YW, Cradock JC, Vishnuvajjala BR, Flora KP. Stability of cisplatin, iproplatin, carboplatin, and tetraplatin in commonly used intravenous solutions. Am J Hosp Pharm 1987;44:124–130
27. Horton JK, Stevens MFG. A new light on the photo-decomposition of the antitumour drug DTIC. J Pharm Pharmacol 1981;33:808–811
28. Shetty BV, Schowen RL, Slavik M, Riley CM. Degradation of dacarbazine in aqueous solution. J Pharm Biomed Anal 1992;10:675–683
29. Dorr RT, Alberts DS, Einspahr J, Mason-Liddil N, Soble M. Experimental dacarbazine antitumor activity and skin toxicity in relation to light exposure and pharmacologic antidotes. Cancer Treat Rep 1987;71:267–272
30. Baird GM, Willoughby MLN. Photodegradation of dacarbazine [letter]. Lancet 1978;2:681
31. Shukla VS. A device to prevent photodegradation of dacarbazine (DTIC). Clin Radiol 1980;31:239–240
32. El Aatmani M, Poujol S, Astre C, Malosse F, Pinguet F. Stability of dacarbazine in amber glass vials and polyvinyl chloride bags. Am J Health Syst Pharm 2002;59:1351–1356
33. Kirk B. The evaluation of a light-protective giving set. The photosensitivity of intravenous dacarbazine solutions. Intensive Ther Clin Monit 1987;78, 81, 82, 85, 86
34. Crevar GE, Slotnick IJ. A note on the stability of actinomycin D. J Pharm Pharmacol 1964;16:429–432
35. Pavlik EJ, Kenady DE, van Nagell JR, et al. Properties of anticancer agents relevant to in vitro determinations of human tumor cell sensitivity. Cancer Chemother Pharmacol 1983;11:8–15
36. Rusmin S, Welton S, DeLuca P, DeLuca PP. Effect of inline filtration on the potency of drugs administered intravenously. Am J Hosp Pharm 1977;34:1071–1074
37. Wood MJ, Irwin WJ, Scott DK. Stability of doxorubicin, daunorubicin and epirubicin in plastic syringes and minibags. J Clin Pharm Ther 1990;15:279–289
38. Wood MJ, Irwin WJ, Scott DK. Photodegradation of doxorubicin, daunorubicin and epirubicin measured by high-performance liquid chromatography. J Clin Pharm Ther 1990;15:291–300
39. Walker S, Lau D, DeAngelis C, Iazzetta J, Coons C. Doxorubicin stability in syringes and glass vials and evaluation of chemical contamination. Can J Hosp Pharm 1991;44:71–78, 88
40. Lokich J. Doxil extravasation injury: a case report. Ann Oncol 1999;10:735–736
41. Pujol M, Munoz M, Prat J, Girona V, De Bolos J. Stability study of epirubicin in NaCl 0.9% injection. Ann Pharmacother 1997;31:992–995
42. Driessen O, de Vos D, Timmermans PJA. Adsorption of fluorouracil on glass surfaces. J Pharm Sci 1978;67:1494–1495
43. Benvenuto JA, Anderson RW, Kerkof K, Smith RG, Loo TL. Stability and compatibility of antitumor agents in glass and plastic containers. Am J Hosp Pharm 1981;38:1914–1918
44. Tempero M, Plunkett W, Ruiz Van Haperen V, et al. Randomized phase II comparison of dose-intense gemcitabine: thirty-minute infusion and fixed dose rate infusion in patients with pancreatic adenocarcinoma [see comment]. J Clin Oncol 2003;21:3402-8. Comment in: J Clin Oncol 2003;21:3383, 3384
45. Peters GJ, Clavel M, Noordhuis P, et al. Clinical phase I and pharmacology study of gemcitabine (2′, 2′-difluorodeoxycytidine) administered in a two-weekly schedule. J Chemother 2007;19:212–221
46. Gusella M, Pasini F, Bolzonella C, et al. Equilibrative nucleoside transporter 1 genotype, cytidine deaminase activity and age predict gemcitabine plasma clearance in patients with solid tumours. Br J Clin Pharmacol 2011;71:437–444
47. Trissel LA, Martinez JF. Idarubicin hydrochloride turbidity versus incompatibility. Am J Hosp Pharm 1993;50:1134, 1137
48. Li WY, Koda RT. Stability of irinotecan hydrochloride in aqueous solutions. Am J Health Syst Pharm 2002;59:539–544
49. Dodds HM, Craik DJ, Rivory LP. Photodegradation of irinotecan (CPT-11) in aqueous solutions: identification of fluorescent products and influence of solution composition. J Pharm Sci 1997;86:1410–1416

50. Thiesen J, Krämer I. Physicochemical stability of irinotecan injection concentrate and diluted infusion solutions in PVC bags. J Oncol Pharm Pract 2000;6:115–121

51. Akimoto K, Kawai A, Ohya K. Photodegradation reactions of CPT-11, a derivative of camptothecin. II. Photodegradation behaviour of CPT-11 in aqueous solution. Drug Stability 1996;1:141–146

52. Dodds HM, Robert J, Rivory LP. The detection of photodegradation products of irinotecan (CPT-11, Campto®, Camptosar®), in clinical studies, using high-performance liquid chromatography/atmospheric pressure chemical ionisation/mass spectrometry. J Pharm Biomed Anal 1998;17:785–792

53. Bonte FJ, Storaasli JP, Weisberger AS. Comparative evaluation of radioactive colloidal gold and nitrogen mustard in the treatment of serous effusions of neoplastic origin. Radiology 1956;67:63–66

54. Weisberger AS, Levine B. Use of nitrogen mustard in treatment of serous effusions of neoplastic origin. JAMA 1955;159:1704–1707

55. Weisberger AS. Direct instillation of nitrogen mustard in the management of malignant effusions. Ann N Y Acad Sci 1958;68:1091–1096

56. Bass BH. Nitrogen mustard in the palliation of lung cancer. Br Med J 1960;1:617–620

57. MESNA. In: Trissel LA, Davignon JP, Kleinman LM, et al., eds. NCI Investigational Drugs, Pharmaceutical Data 1987. NIH Publication 88-2141 ed. Bethesda (MD): U.S. Department of Health and Human Services, Public Health Service, National Institutes of Health, National Cancer Institute; 1987:57, 58

58. Dorr RT, Liddil JD. Stability of mitomycin C in different infusion fluids: compatibility with heparin and glucocorticosteroids. J Oncol Pharm Pract 1995;1:19–24

59. Beijnen JH, den Hartigh J, Underberg WJM. Qualitative aspects of the degradation of mitomycins in alkaline solution. J Pharm Biomed Anal 1985;3:71–79

60. Beijnen HN, Underberg WJM. Degradation of mitomycin C in acidic solution. Int J Pharm 1985;24:219–229

61. Waugh WN, Trissel LA, Stella VJ. Stability, compatibility, and plasticizer extraction of taxol (NSC-125973) injection diluted in infusion solutions and stored in various containers. Am J Hosp Pharm 1991;48:1520–1524

62. Pearson SD, Trissel LA. Leaching of diethylhexyl phthalate from polyvinyl chloride containers by selected drugs and formulation components. Am J Hosp Pharm 1993;50:1405–1409

63. Allwood MC, Martin H. The extraction of diethylhexylphthalate (DEHP) from polyvinyl chloride components of intravenous infusion containers and administration sets by paclitaxel injection. Int J Pharm 1996;127:65–71

64. Mazzo DJ, Nguyen-Huu J-J, Pagniez S, Denis P. Compatibility of docetaxel and paclitaxel in intravenous solutions with polyvinyl chloride infusion materials. Am J Health Syst Pharm 1997;54:566–569

65. Trissel LA, Xu Q, Kwan J, Martinez JF. Compatibility of paclitaxel injection vehicle with intravenous administration and extension sets. Am J Hosp Pharm 1994;51:2804–2810

66. Chin A, Ramakrishnan RR, Yoshimura NN, Jeong EWS, Nii LJ, DiMeglio LS. Paclitaxel stability and compatibility in polyolefin containers. Ann Pharmacother 1994;28:35–36

67. Xu Q, Trissel LA, Martinez JF. Stability of paclitaxel in 5% dextrose injection or 0.9% sodium chloride injection at 4, 22, or 32 °C. Am J Hosp Pharm 1994;51:3058–3060

68. Donyai P, Sewell GJ. Physical and chemical stability of paclitaxel infusions in different container types. J Oncol Pharm Pract 2006;12:211–222

69. Trissel LA, Bready BB. Turbidimetric assessment of the compatibility of taxol with selected other drugs during simulated Y-site injection. Am J Hosp Pharm 1992;49:1716–1719

70. Zhang Y, Trissel LA. Physical and chemical stability of pemetrexed in infusion solutions. Ann Pharmacother 2006;40:1082–1085

71. Boni J, Abbas R, Leister C, et al. Disposition of desipramine, a sensitive cytochrome P450 2D6 substrate, when coadministered with intravenous temsirolimus. Cancer Chemother Pharmacol 2009;64:263–270

72. Hofmeister CC, Yang X, Pichiorri F, et al. Phase I trial of lenalidomide and CCI-779 in patients with relapsed multiple myeloma: evidence for lenalidomide-CCI-779 interaction via P-glycoprotein [see comment]. J Clin Oncol 2011;29:3427-34. Comment in: J Clin Oncol 2012;30:340–342

73. Faouzi MA, Dinea T, Luyckxa M, et al. Leaching of diethylhexyl phthalate from PVC bags into intravenous teniposide solution. Int J Pharm 1994;105:89–93

74. Murray KM, Erkkila D, Gombotz WR, Pankey S. Stability of thiotepa (lyophilized) in 0.9% sodium chloride injection. Am J Health Syst Pharm 1997;54:2588–2591

75. Xu QA, Trissel LA, Zhang Y, Martinez JF, Gilbert DL. Stability of thiotepa (lyophilized) in 5% dextrose injection at 4 and 23 °C. Am J Health Syst Pharm 1996;53:2728–2730

76. Blaney SM, Balis FM, Poplack DG. Pharmacologic approaches to the treatment of meningeal malignancy. Oncology (Williston Park) 1991;5:107–116; discussion 123, 127

77. Strong JM, Collins JM, Lester C, Poplack DG. Pharmacokinetics of intraventricular and intravenous N,N',N''-triethylenethiophosphoramide (thiotepa) in rhesus monkeys and humans. Cancer Res 1986;46:6101–6104

78. Krämer I, Thiesen J. Stability of topotecan infusion solutions in polyvinylchloride bags and elastomeric portable infusion devices. J Oncol Pharm Pract 1999;5:75–82

79. Craig SB, Bhatt UH, Patel K. Stability and compatibility of topotecan hydrochloride for injection with common infusion solutions and containers. J Pharm Biomed Anal 1997;16:199–205

80. Vendrig DEMM, Smeets BPGM, Beijnen JH, van der Houwen OAGJ, Holthuis JJM. Degradation kinetics of vinblastine sulphate in aqueous solutions. Int J Pharm 1988;43:131–138

81. Dyke RW. Treatment of inadvertent intrathecal injection of vincristine. N Engl J Med 1989;321:1270–1271

82. Michelagnoli MP, Bailey CC, Wilson I, Livingston J, Kinsey SE. Potential salvage therapy for inadvertent intrathecal administration of vincristine. Br J Haematol 1997;99:364–367

83. Zaragoza MR, Ritchey ML, Walter A. Neurourologic consequences of accidental intrathecal vincristine: a case report. Med Pediatr Oncol 1995;24:61, 62

84. Francomb MM, Ford JL, Lee MG. Adsorption of vincristine, vinblastine, doxorubicin and mitozantrone to in-line intravenous filters. Int J Pharm 1994;103:87–92

85. Johnson EG, Janosik JE. Manufacturers' recommendations for handling spilled antineoplastic agents. Am J Hosp Pharm 1989;46:318, 319

86. Beijnen JH, Vendrig DEMM, Underberg WJM. Stability of vinca alkaloid anticancer drugs in three commonly used infusion fluids. J Parenter Sci Technol 1989;43:84–87

87. deLemos ML. Vinorelbine and venous irritation: optimal parenteral administration [see comment]. J Oncol Pharm Pract 2005;11:79–81. Comment in: J Oncol Pharm Pract 2006;12:123

41. Guidelines for Chemotherapy Dosage Adjustment

Pamela W. McDevitt, PharmD, BCOP and Tito Fojo, MD, PhD

Alphabetical Listing of Drugs by both Generic (bold) and Proprietary Names

Drug Names: Generic (in bold) or Proprietary	Drug Names: Generic (in bold) or Proprietary	Adjust if Function Impaired	
		Hepatic	Renal
Abiraterone acetate	Zytiga®	+	−
Abraxane®	**Paclitaxel protein bound particles**	+	−
Adcetris™	**Brentuximab vedotin**	−	−
ado-trastuzumab emtansine	Kadcyla™	±	±
Adriamycin®	**Doxorubicin HCl**	+	−
Afatinib	Gilotrif	±	±
Afatinib dimaleate	Gilotrif™	±	±
Afinitor®	**Everolimus**	+	±
Agrylin®	**Anagrelide HCl**	+	−
Aldesleukin	Proleukin®	−	+
Alemtuzumab	Campath®	−	−
Alimta®	**Pemetrexed disodium**	−	±
Alitretinoin	Panretin®	−	−
Alkeran®	**Melphalan (or Melphalan HCl)**	−	+
Altretamine	Hexalen®	−	−
Amifostine	Ethyol®	−	−
Aminoglutethimide	Cytadren®	−	−
Amsacrine	Amsidine®	+	+
Amsidine®	**Amsacrine**	+	+
Anagrelide HCl	Agrylin®	+	−
Anastrozole	Arimidex®	+	−
Aranesp®	**Darbepoetin alfa**	−	−
Aredia®	**Pamidronate disodium**	±	+
Arimidex®	**Anastrozole**	+	−
Aromasin®	**Exemestane**	−	−
Arranon®	**Nelarabine**	±	±
Arsenic trioxide	Trisenox™	+	+
Arzerra™	**Ofatumumab**	−	−
Asparaginase (*E. coli* source)	Elspar®	±	±
Asparaginase (*Erwinia chrysanthemi* source)	Erwinaze™	±	±
Atralin™	**Tretinoin**	+	+

(continued)

(continued)

Drug Names: Generic (in bold) or Proprietary	Drug Names: Generic (in bold) or Proprietary	Adjust if Function Impaired	
		Hepatic	Renal
Avastin®	**Bevacizumab**	−	−
Axitinib	Inlyta®	±	±
Azacitidine	Vidaza®	+	+
Bendamustine HCl	Treanda®	+	+
Bevacizumab	Avastin®	−	−
Bexarotene	Targretin®	±	±
Bexxar®	**Tositumomab**	−	±
Bicalutamide	Casodex®	±	−
BiCNU®	**Carmustine**	±	+
Blenoxane®	**Bleomycin sulfate**	±	+
Bleomycin sulfate	Blenoxane®	±	+
Bortezomib	Velcade®	+	±
Bosulif®	**Bosutinib**	±	±
Bosutinib	Bosulif®	±	±
Brentuximab vedotin	Adcetris™	−	−
Buserelin acetate	Suprefact®	−	−
Busulfan	Busulfex®	±	−
Busulfex®	**Busulfan**	±	−
Cabazitaxel	Jevtana®	±	±
Cabozantinib *S-malate*	Cometriq™	±	±
Campath®	**Alemtuzumab**	−	−
Camptosar®	**Irinotecan HCl**	+	−
Capecitabine	Xeloda®	±	+
Caprelsa®	**Vandetanib**	±	+
Carboplatin	Paraplatin−AQ®	−	+
Carfilzomib	Kyprolis™	±	−
Carmustine	BiCNU®	±	+
Casodex®	**Bicalutamide**	±	−
CeeNU®	**Lomustine**	±	+
Cerubidine®	**Daunorubicin HCl**	+	+
Cetuximab	Erbitux®	−	−
Chlorambucil	Leukeran®	±	+
Cisplatin	Platinol®	−	+
Cladribine	Leustatin®	±	+
Clofarabine	Clolar®	±	±
Clolar®	**Clofarabine**	±	±
Cometriq™	**Cabozantinib** *S-malate*	±	±
Cosmegen®	**Dactinomycin**	±	−

(continued)

(continued)

Drug Names: Generic (in bold) or Proprietary	Drug Names: Generic (in bold) or Proprietary	Adjust if Function Impaired	
		Hepatic	Renal
Crizotinib	Xalkori®	±	±
Cytadren®	**Aminoglutethimide**	−	−
Cytarabine	Cytosar-U®	+	+
Cytarabine lipid complex (liposome)	DepoCyt®	−	−
Cytosar-U®	**Cytarabine**	+	+
Dabrafenib	Tafinlar	±	±
Dabrafenib mesylate	Tafinlar®	±	±
Dacarbazine	DTIC-Dome®	±	+
Dacogen™	**Decitabine**	±	±
Dactinomycin	Cosmegen®	±	−
Denileukin diftitox	Ontak®	−	−
Denosumab	Xgeva®	±	±
Darbepoetin alfa	Aranesp®	−	−
Dasatinib	Sprycel®	±	±
Daunorubicin HCl	Cerubidine®	+	+
Daunorubicin citrate liposomal	DaunoXome®	+	+
DaunoXome®	**Daunorubicin citrate liposomal**	+	+
Decitabine	Dacogen™	±	±
DepoCyt®	**Cytarabine lipid complex (liposome)**	−	−
Dexrazoxane HCl	Totect®, Zinecard®	−	+
Docetaxel	Taxotere®	+	−
Doxil®	**Doxorubicin HCl liposomal**	+	−
Doxorubicin HCl	Adriamycin®	+	−
Doxorubicin HCl liposomal	Doxil®	+	−
Droxia®	**Hydroxyurea**	±	+
DTIC-Dome®	**Dacarbazine**	±	+
Ellence®	**Epirubicin HCl**	+	+
Eloxatin®	**Oxaliplatin**	−	+
Elspar®	**Asparaginase** (*E. coli* source)	±	±
Emcyt®	**Estramustine phosphate sodium**	−	−
Enzalutamide	Xtandi®	±	±
Epirubicin HCl	Ellence®	+	+
Epoetin alfa	Procrit®	−	−
Erbitux®	**Cetuximab**	−	−
Eribulin mesylate	Halaven™	+	+
Erivedge®	**Vismodegib**	±	±
Erlotinib HCl	Tarceva®	+	−
Erwinaze™	**Asparaginase** (*Erwinia chrysanthemi* source)	±	±

(continued)

(continued)

Drug Names: Generic (in bold) or Proprietary	Drug Names: Generic (in bold) or Proprietary	Adjust if Function Impaired	
		Hepatic	Renal
Estramustine phosphate sodium	Emcyt®	−	−
Ethyol®	**Amifostine**	−	−
Etopophos®	**Etoposide phosphate**	+	+
Etoposide	VePesid®	+	+
Etoposide phosphate	Etopophos®	+	+
Eulexin®	**Flutamide**	−	−
Everolimus	Afinitor®	+	±
Evista®	**Raloxifene HCl**	±	±
Exemestane	Aromasin®	−	−
Fareston®	**Toremifene citrate**	−	−
Faslodex®	**Fulvestrant**	+	−
Femara®	**Letrozole**	+	−
Filgrastim	Neupogen®	−	−
Floxuridine	FUDR®	+	±
Fludara®	**Fludarabine**	±	+
Fludarabine	Fludara®	±	+
Fluorouracil	Fluorouracil	±	±
Fluorouracil	**Fluorouracil**	±	±
Fluoxymesterone	Halotestin®	−	+
Flutamide	Eulexin®	−	−
Folotyn®	**Pralatrexate**	±	±
FUDR®	**Floxuridine**	+	±
Fulvestrant	Faslodex®	+	−
Gefitinib	Iressa®	−	−
Gemcitabine HCl	Gemzar®	+	−
Gemtuzumab ozogamicin	Mylotarg®	±	−
Gemzar®	**Gemcitabine HCl**	+	−
Gilotrif	**Afatinib**	±	±
Gilotrif™	**Afatinib dimaleate**	±	±
Gleevec®	**Imatinib mesylate**	+	+
Goserelin acetate	Zoladex®	−	−
Halaven™	**Eribulin mesylate**	+	+
Halotestin®	**Fluoxymesterone**	−	+
Herceptin®	**Trastuzumab**	−	−
Hexalen®	**Altretamine**	−	−
Hycamtin®	**Topotecan HCl**	−	+
Hydroxyurea	Droxia®	±	+
Ibritumomab tiuxetan	Zevalin®	−	−

(continued)

(continued)

Drug Names: Generic (in bold) or Proprietary	Drug Names: Generic (in bold) or Proprietary	Adjust if Function Impaired	
		Hepatic	Renal
Ibrutinib	Imbruvica	+	−
Iclusig™	**Ponatinib**	±	±
Idamycin®	**Idarubicin HCl**	+	+
Idarubicin HCl	Idamycin®	+	+
Ifex®	**Ifosfamide**	±	+
Ifosfamide	Ifex®	±	+
Imatinib mesylate	Gleevec®	+	+
Imbruvica	**Ibrutinib**	+	−
Interferon alfa-2b	Intron® A	−	−
Inlyta®	**Axitinib**	±	±
Intron® A	**Interferon alfa-2b**	−	−
Ipilimumab	Yervoy™	−	−
Iressa®	**Gefitinib**	−	−
Irinotecan	Camptosar®	+	−
Isotretinoin	Sotret®	±	−
Istodax®	**Romidepsin**	±	±
Ixabepilone	Ixempra®	+	±
Ixempra®	**Ixabepilone**	+	±
Jevtana®	**Cabazitaxel**	±	±
Kadcyla™	**ado-trastuzumab emtansine**	±	±
Kyprolis™	**Carfilzomib**	±	±
Lapatinib	Tykerb®	+	−
Lenalidomide	Revlimid®	−	+
Letrozole	Femara®	+	−
Leucovorin calcium	Leucovorin	−	−
Leucovorin	Leucovorin calcium	−	−
Leukeran®	**Chlorambucil**	±	+
Leukine®	**Sargramostim**	−	−
Leuprolide acetate	Lupron Depot®	−	−
Leustatin®	**Cladribine**	±	+
Lomustine	CeeNU®	±	+
Lupron Depot®	**Leuprolide acetate**	−	−
Lysodren®	**Mitotane**	−	−
Marqibo®	**Vincristine sulfate liposome**	±	±
Matulane®	**Procarbazine HCl**	−	+
Mechlorethamine HCl	Mustargen®		
Megace®	**Megestrol acetate**	−	−
Megestrol acetate	Megace®	−	−

(continued)

(continued)

Drug Names: Generic (in bold) or Proprietary	Drug Names: Generic (in bold) or Proprietary	Adjust if Function Impaired	
		Hepatic	Renal
Mekinist	Tramtetinib	±	±
Mekinist™	Trametinib dimethyl sulfoxide	±	±
Melphalan (*or* Melphalan HCl)	Alkeran®	−	+
Mercaptopurine	Purinethol®	±	+
Mesna	Mesnex®	±	±
Mesnex®	**Mesna**	±	±
Methotrexate	Methotrexate	+	+
Methotrexate	**Methotrexate**	+	+
Mitomycin	Mitozytrex®	±	+
Mitotane	Lysodren®	−	−
Mitoxantrone HCl	Novantrone®	±	−
Mitozytrex®	**Mitomycin**	±	+
Mozobil®	**Plerixafor**	−	+
Mustargen®	**Mechlorethamine HCl**	−	−
Mylotarg®	**Gemtuzumab ozogamicin**	±	−
Navelbine®	**Vinorelbine tartrate**	+	−
Nelarabine	Arranon®	±	±
Neulasta®	**Pegfilgrastim**	±	−
Neumega®	**Oprelvekin**	−	+
Neupogen®	**Filgrastim**	−	−
Neutrexin	**Trimetrexate glucuronate**	±	−
Nexavar®	**Sorafenib tosylate**	−	−
Nilandron®	**Nilutamide**	+	−
Nilotinib	Tasigna®	+	−
Nilutamide	Nilandron®	+	−
Nipent®	**Pentostatin**	−	±
Novantrone®	**Mitoxantrone HCl**	±	−
Nplate®	**Romiplostim**	±	±
Obinutuzumab	Gazyva	±	±
Octreotide acetate	Sandostatin® LAR®	+	+
Ofatumumab	Arzerra™	−	−
Omacetaxine mepesuccinate	Synribo™	±	±
Oncaspar®	**Pegaspargase**	−	−
Oncovin®	**Vincristine sulfate**	+	−
Ontak®	**Denileukin diftitox**	−	−
Oprelvekin	Neumega®	−	+
Oxaliplatin	Eloxatin®	−	+
Paclitaxel	Taxol®	+	−

(continued)

(continued)

Drug Names: Generic (in bold) or Proprietary	Drug Names: Generic (in bold) or Proprietary	Adjust if Function Impaired	
		Hepatic	Renal
Paclitaxel protein bound particles	Abraxane®	+	−
Pamidronate disodium	Aredia®	±	+
Panitumumab	Vectibix®	−	−
Panretin®	**Alitretinoin**	−	−
Paraplatin—AQ®	**Carboplatin**	−	+
Pazopanib HCl	Votrient™	+	−
Pegaspargase	Oncaspar®	−	−
Pegfilgrastim	Neulasta®	±	−
Pemetrexed disodium	Alimta®	−	±
Pentostatin	Nipent®	−	±
Perjeta®	**Pertuzumab**	±	±
Pertuzumab	Perjeta®	±	±
Platinol®	**Cisplatin**	−	+
Plerixafor	Mozobil®	−	+
Pomalidomide	Pomalyst®	±	±
Pomalyst®	**Pomalidomide**	±	±
Ponatinib HCl	Iclusig™	±	±
Pralatrexate	Folotyn®	±	±
Procarbazine HCl	Matulane®	−	+
Procrit®	**Epoetin Alfa**	−	−
Proleukin®	**Aldesleukin**	−	+
Provenge®	**Sipuleucel-T**	−	−
Purinethol®	**Mercaptopurine**	±	+
Raloxifene HCl	Evista®	±	±
Raltitrexed	Tomudex®	−	+
Regorafenib	Stivarga®	±	±
Revlimid®	**Lenalidomide**	−	+
Rituxan®	**Rituximab**	−	−
Rituximab	Rituxan®	−	−
Romidepsin	Istodax®	±	±
Romiplostim	Nplate®	±	±
Sandostatin® LAR®	**Octreotide acetate**	+	+
Sargramostim	Leukine®	−	−
Savene™	**Dexrazoxane HCl**	−	−
Sipuleucel-T	Provenge®	−	−
Stivarga®	**Regorafenib**	±	±
Soltamox™	**Tamoxifen citrate**	−	−
Sorafenib tosylate	Nexavar®	−	−

(continued)

(continued)

Drug Names: Generic (in bold) or Proprietary	Drug Names: Generic (in bold) or Proprietary	Adjust if Function Impaired	
		Hepatic	Renal
Sotret®	Isotretinoin	±	−
Sprycel®	Dasatinib	±	±
Streptozocin	Zanosar®	+	−
Sunitinib malate	Sutent®	±	±
Suprefact®	Buserelin acetate	−	−
Sutent®	Sunitinib malate	±	±
Synribo™	Omacetaxine mepesuccinate	±	±
Tabloid®	Thioguanine	±	−
Tafinlar	Dabrafenib	±	±
Tafinlar®	Dabrafenib mesylate	±	±
Tamoxifen citrate	Soltamox™	−	−
Tarceva®	Erlotinib HCl	+	−
Targretin®	Bexarotene	±	±
Tasigna®	Nilotinib	+	−
Taxol®	Paclitaxel	+	−
Taxotere®	Docetaxel	+	−
Tegafur-uracil	Uftoral®	±	−
Temodar®	Temozolomide	±	±
Temozolomide	Temodar®	±	±
Temsirolimus	Torisel®	+	−
Teniposide	Vumon®	±	±
Thalidomide	Thalomid®	−	−
Thalomid®	Thalidomide	−	−
Thioguanine	Tabloid®	±	−
Thiolex®	Thiotepa	±	−
Thiotepa	Thiolex®	±	−
Tomudex®	Raltitrexed	−	+
Topotecan HCl	Hycamtin®	−	+
Toremifene citrate	Fareston®	−	−
Torisel®	Temsirolimus	+	−
Tositumomab	Bexxar®	−	±
Totect®	Dexrazoxane HCl	−	+
Trabectedin	Yondelis®	±	+
Trametinib dimethyl sulfoxide	Mekinist™	±	±
Tramtetinib	Mekinist	±	±
Trastuzumab	Herceptin®	−	−
Treanda®	Bendamustine HCl	+	+
Tretinoin	Atralin™	+	+

(continued)

(continued)

Drug Names: Generic (in bold) or Proprietary	Drug Names: Generic (in bold) or Proprietary	Adjust if Function Impaired	
		Hepatic	Renal
Trimetrexate glucuronate	Neutrexin	±	−
Trisenox™	**Arsenic trioxide**	+	+
Tykerb®	**Lapatinib**	+	−
Uftoral®	**Tegafur-uracil**	±	−
Valrubicin	Valstar®	−	−
Valstar®	**Valrubicin**	−	−
Vandetanib	Caprelsa®	±	+
Vectibix®	**Panitumumab**	−	−
Velban®	**Vinblastine sulfate**	+	−
Velcade®	**Bortezomib**	+	±
Vemurafenib	Zelboraf®	±	±
VePesid®	**Etoposide**	+	+
Vidaza®	**Azacitidine**	+	+
Vinblastine sulfate	Velban®	+	−
Vincristine sulfate	Oncovin®	+	−
Vincristine sulfate liposome	Marqibo®	±	±
Vinorelbine tartrate	Navelbine®	+	−
Vismodegib	Erivedge®	±	±
Vorinostat	Zolinza®	+	−
Votrient™	**Pazopanib HCl**	+	−
Vumon®	**Teniposide**	±	±
Xalkori®	**Crizotinib**	±	±
Xeloda®	**Capecitabine**	±	+
Xgeva®	**Denosumab**	±	±
Xtandi®	**Enzalutamide**	±	±
Yervoy™	**Ipilimumab**	−	−
Yondelis®	**Trabectedin**	±	+
Zaltrap®	**ziv-aflibercept**	±	±
Zanosar®	**Streptozocin**	+	−
Zelboraf®	**Vemurafenib**	±	±
Zevalin®	**Ibritumomab tiuxetan**	−	−
Zinecard®	**Dexrazoxane HCl**	−	−
ziv-aflibercept	Zaltrap®	±	±
Zoladex®	**Goserelin acetate**	−	−
Zoledronic Acid	Zometa®	±	+
Zolinza®	**Vorinostat**	+	−
Zometa®	**Zoledronic Acid**	±	+
Zytiga®	**Abiraterone acetate**	+	−

Child-Pugh Liver Function Classification

Assessment	Degree of Abnormality	Score
Encephalopathy grade	None	1
	1 or 2	2
	3 or 4	3
Ascites	Absent	1
	Slight	2
	Moderate	3
Total bilirubin (mg/dL)	<2	1
	2–3	2
	>3	3
Serum albumin (g/dL)	>3.5	1
	2.8–3.5	2
	<2.8	3
Prothrombin time (seconds prolonged)	<4	1
	4–6	2
	>6	3

Mild hepatic impairment   =   Child-Pugh Class A   =   Score 5–6
Moderate hepatic impairment   =   Child-Pugh Class B   =   Score 7–9
Severe hepatic impairment   =   Child-Pugh Class C   =   Score 10–15

Calculation of Creatinine Clearance (CrCl)
Timed Urine Collection
(Often used to Approximate Glomerular Filtration Rate [GFR])
Requirements: Timed Urine Collection (Time, Urine Volume and Creatinine Concentration) and Serum Creatinine Concentration

Creatinine clearance (mL/min)	=	$\dfrac{U_{Cr} \times U_{Vol}}{Cr \times T_{min}}$
Corrected CrCl (mL/min · 1.73 m²)	=	$\dfrac{CrCl \times 1.73\ m^2}{BSA\ (m^2)}$

Calculation of Creatinine Clearance (CrCl)
Cockcroft and Gault Formula
Requirements: Weight, Age and Serum Creatinine Concentration

Males CrCL	=	$\dfrac{[IBW \times (140 - Age)]}{(72 \times Scr)}$
Females CrCL	=	$\dfrac{0.85 \times [IBW \times (140 - Age)]}{(72 \times Scr)}$

Cockcroft and Gault Formula:

• CrCL in mL/min

• BW = body weight in kg

• Age in years

• Scr in mg/dL

Note: Estimating ideal body weight in (kg)
Males: IBW = 50 kg + 2.3 kg for each inch over 5 feet
Females: IBW = 45.5 kg + 2.3 kg for each inch over 5 feet
Note: If the ABW (actual body weight) is less than the IBW use the ABW for calculating the CrCl

Guidelines for Chemotherapy Dosage Adjustments

Drug	Hepatic Dysfunction			Renal Dysfunction	
	Bilirubin (mg/dL and µmol/L)	AST/SGOT (units/L) ALT/SGPT (units/L)	Percent Dosage/Dose Administered	Creatinine Clearance (CrCL) (mL/min) or Serum Creatinine (SCr) (mg/dL and µmol/L)	Percent Dosage/Dose Administered
Abiraterone acetate[1]	Child-Pugh Class B (moderate hepatic impairment prior to starting treatment)		Reduce dose to 250 mg once daily	No Dosage Adjustments Necessary	
	Child-Pugh Class C (severe hepatic impairment prior to starting treatment)		Has not been studied in this population: avoid		
	Bilirubin >3 × ULN during treatment	ALT and/or AST >5 × ULN during treatment	Interrupt treatment. Restart 750 mg once daily after LFTs return to baseline or AST and ALT ≤2.5 × ULN and bilirubin <1.5 × ULN		
	Bilirubin >3 × ULN while receiving 750 mg once daily	ALT and/or AST >5 × ULN during treatment with 750 mg once daily	Interrupt treatment. Re-start 500 mg once daily after LFTs return to baseline or AST and ALT ≤2.5 × ULN and l bilirubin <1.5 × ULN		
	Bilirubin >3 × ULN while receiving 500 mg once daily	ALT and/or AST >5 × ULN during treatment with 500 mg once daily	Discontinue treatment		
ado-Trastuzumab emtansine[2]	Mild, moderate and severe hepatic impairment		No clinical trials have been conducted	Mild to moderate renal impairment (CrCL 30–90 mL/min [0.5–1.5 mL/s])	No dosage adjustments necessary
				Severe renal impairment (CrCL <30 mL/min [<0.5 mL/s])	No clinical trials have been conducted
Afatinib	Child-Pugh Class C (severe hepatic impairment)		Limited data available. Monitor closely for toxicity	CrCL <30 mL/min	No data
				CrCL 30–59 mL/min	Trough plasma concentration ↑85%
				CrCL 60–89 mL/min	Trough plasma concentration ↑27%
				CrCL >90 mL/min	No effect
Afatinib dimaleate[3]	Mild to moderate hepatic impairment		No dosage adjustment necessary	CrCL 60–89 mL/min [1–1.48 mL/s]	No dosage adjustment necessary
	Severe hepatic impairment		Monitor carefully and adjust dose if not tolerated	CrCL 30–59 mL/min [0.5–0.98 mL/s] CrCL <30 mL/min [<0.5 mL/s]	Monitor carefully and adjust dose if not tolerated

(continued)

(continued)

Drug	Hepatic impairment condition	Hepatic dosage adjustment	Renal impairment condition	Renal dosage adjustment
Aldesleukin[4-6]		No dosage adjustments necessary	SCr >4.5 mg/dL (>398 μmol/L)	Hold or discontinue treatment. Resume when SCr <4 mg/dL (<354 μmol/L)
			SCr ≥4.0 mg/dL (≥354 μmol/L) in presence of severe volume overload, acidosis, or hyperkalemia	Hold or discontinue treatment. Resume when SCr <4 mg/dL (<354 μmol/L) and fluid and electrolyte status are stable
			Renal failure requiring dialysis >72 hours while receiving an earlier course of therapy	Treatment contraindicated
			Persistent oliguria or urine output <10 mL/hour for 16–24 hours with rising serum creatinine	Withhold dose; may resume when urine output >10 mL/hour with serum creatinine decrease of >1.5 mg/dL (>133 μmol/L) or normalization
Alitretinoin[7]		No dosage adjustments necessary		No dosage adjustments necessary
Alemtuzumab[8]		No dosage adjustments necessary		No dosage adjustments necessary
Altretamine[9]		No dosage adjustments necessary		No dosage adjustments necessary
Amifostine[10]		No dosage adjustments necessary		No dosage adjustments necessary
Aminoglutethimide[11]		No dosage adjustments necessary		No dosage adjustments necessary
Amsacrine[12-14]	>2 mg/day (>34 μmol/L)	Administer 60–75% of dosage	SCr 1.2–1.8 mg/dL (106–159 μmol/L)	Administer 75–100% of dosage
	Severe hepatic impairment	Administer 50% of dosage	SCr 2–3 mg/dL, (177–265 μmol/L)	Administer 60–70% of dosage
			Oliguric patients	Adjust dosage based on toxicity
Anagrelide HCl[15]	Moderate hepatic impairment	Starting dose of 0.5 mg/day must be maintained for 1 week with cardiovascular monitoring. Do not increase dose more than 0.5 mg/day during any week. Measure liver function tests before and during treatment		No dosage adjustments necessary, but monitor renal function closely
	Severe hepatic impairment	Do not administer		
Anastrozole[16]	Mild-to-moderate hepatic impairment	No dosage adjustments necessary		No dosage adjustments necessary
	Severe hepatic impairment	No data available		

Drug	Hepatic Dysfunction			Renal Dysfunction	
	Bilirubin (mg/dL and μmol/L)	AST/SGOT (units/L) ALT/SGPT (units/L)	Percent Dosage/Dose Administered	Creatinine Clearance (CrCL) (mL/min) or Serum Creatinine (SCr) (mg/dL and μmol/L)	Percent Dosage/Dose Administered
Arsenic trioxide[17]	Child-Pugh Class C (severe hepatic impairment)		Limited data available. Monitor closely for toxicity	CrCl <30 mL/min	Monitor closely; may require dosage reduction
				Dialysis patients	Has not been studied
Axitinib[18]	Mild hepatic impairment		No dosage adjustment necessary	Mild to severe renal impairment (CrCl 15 to <89 mL/min [0.25 to <1.48 mL/s])	No dosage adjustment necessary
	Moderate hepatic impairment		Reduce starting dosage		
	Severe hepatic impairment		Not recommended as it has not been studied	End stage renal disease (CrCL <15 mL/min [<0.25 mL/s])	Use is not recommended as it has not been studied. Use only with caution
Azacitidine[19]	Hepatic impairment		No data available. Monitor closely for toxicity	Elevations of BUN or SCr	Delay next cycle until values return to normal or baseline and reduce dosage by 50%
Asparaginase[20]	Specific guidelines for dosage adjustments in hepatic impairment are not available; however, these patients may be at increased risk for toxicity. Evaluate hepatic enzymes and bilirubin pretreatment and periodically during treatment. Use caution in patients with a history of coagulopathy			Specific guidelines for dosage adjustments in renal impairment not available; it appears that no dosage adjustments are needed	
Bendamustine HCl[21]	Mild hepatic impairment		Use with caution	CrCl 40–60 mL/min	Use with caution
	1.5–3 × ULN	AST or ALT 2.5–10 × ULN	Do not administer	CrCl <40 mL/min	Do not administer
	>3 × ULN		Do not administer		
Bevacizumab[22]	No dosage adjustments necessary			No dosage adjustments necessary	
Bexarotene[23]	No specific studies have been conducted in patients with hepatic insufficiency. Less than 1% of a dose is excreted in the urine unchanged and there is in vitro evidence of extensive hepatic contribution to bexarotene elimination, thus hepatic impairment would be expected to lead to greatly decreased clearance. Use with great caution in this population			No formal studies have been conducted in patients with renal insufficiency. However, renal insufficiency may result in significant protein binding changes and may alter pharmacokinetics of bexarotene, so use caution	
Bicalutamide[24,25]	No adjustment required for mild, moderate, or severe hepatic impairment. Use caution with moderate-to-severe impairment. Consider periodic LFTs during long-term therapy. Discontinue if ALT >2 × ULN or jaundice develops			No dosage adjustment is necessary	

(continued)

(continued)

Drug	Hepatic impairment		Renal impairment	Dosage recommendations using Cockcroft and Gault formula
Bleomycin sulfate[26-28]	Not studied in patients with hepatic impairment; adjustment for hepatic impairment may be needed		CrCl >50 mL/min	Administer 100% of dosage
			CrCl 40–49 mL/min	Administer 70% of dosage
			CrCl 30–39 mL/min	Administer 60% of dosage
			CrCl 20–29 mL/min	Administer 55% of dosage
			CrCl 10–19 mL/min	Administer 45% of dosage
			CrCl 5–9 mL/min	Administer 40% of dosage
			Continuous renal replacement therapy (CRRT)	Administer 75% of dose
			Note: Terminal elimination half-life increases exponentially as the creatinine clearance decreases. Administration of nephrotoxic drugs with bleomycin may affect its renal clearance	
Bosutinib[29]	Mild, moderate and severe hepatic impairment	200 mg/day	CrCL <30 mL/min [<0.5 mL/s]	300 mg/day
Bortezomib[30]	1.5–3 × ULN	Reduce dosage to 0.7 mg/m² in the first cycle. Consider escalation to 1.0 mg/m² or further reduction to 0.5 mg/m² in subsequent cycles based on tolerability	No dosage adjustments necessary. *Note:* Dialysis may reduce concentrations, so the drug should be administered postdialysis	
Brentuximab vedotin[31]	No dosage adjustments necessary		No dosage adjustments necessary	
Buserelin acetate[32]	No dosage adjustments necessary		No dosage adjustment necessary	
Busulfan[33]	Has not been administered in clinical studies to patients with hepatic impairment. Has extensive hepatic metabolism. Dosage adjustment may be necessary, although specific guidelines are not available		No data in patients with renal impairment. Renal excretion is <3%	
Cabazitaxel[34]	No hepatic impairment data available. Patients with total bilirubin >ULN and/or ALT >1.5 × ULN were excluded from trials. Cabazitaxel is extensively metabolized by the liver and hepatic impairment is likely to increase cabazitaxel concentrations		CrCl <30 mL/min or end-stage renal disease	Use with caution
Cabozantinib S-malate[35]	Moderate to severe hepatic impairment	Avoid	Mild to moderate renal impairment (CrCL 30–90 mL/min [0.5–1.5 mL/s])	No dosage adjustment necessary
			Severe renal impairment (CrCL <30 mL/min [<0.5 mL/s])	Do not administer

Drug	Hepatic Dysfunction			Renal Dysfunction	
	Bilirubin (mg/dL and μmol/L)	AST/SGOT (units/L) ALT/SGPT (units/L)	Percent Dosage/Dose Administered	Creatinine Clearance (CrCL) (mL/min) or Serum Creatinine (SCr) (mg/dL and μmol/L)	Percent Dosage/Dose Administered
Capecitabine[36,37,39]	Mild-to-moderate hepatic dysfunction caused by liver metastases		No dosage adjustment necessary. Monitor carefully	CrCl 51–80 mL/min	No dosage adjustment necessary
	Severe hepatic dysfunction		No data available	CrCl 30–50 mL/min	Reduce dosage to 75%
				CrCl <30 mL/min	Do not administer
Carboplatin[27,28,38,39]	No dosage adjustments necessary for initial therapy			Patients with CrCl values less than 60 mL/min are at increased risk of severe bone marrow suppression. Incidence of severe leukopenia, neutropenia, or thrombocytopenia has been about 25% with the tiered dosage modifications shown below [Note: Dose modification for impaired renal function is not necessary for carboplatin doses based on systemic exposure (AUC) calculations, such as the methods described by Calvert et al, Chatelut et al, and Bénézét et al]	
				CrCl 41–59 mL/min	250 mg/m² (Day 1)
				CrCl 16–40 mL/min	200 mg/m² (Day 1)
				CrCl ≤15 mL/min	No guidelines available
				Hemodialysis	Administer 50% of dosage
				Continuous ambulatory peritoneal dialysis (CAPD)	Administer 25% of dosage
				Continuous renal replacement therapy (CRRT)	200 mg/m²
Carfilzomib[40]	Bilirubin ≥2 × ULN	ALT/AST ≥3 × ULN	Not recommended as it has not been studied and these were exclusion criteria from trials	Mild, moderate and severe renal impairment	No dosage adjustment necessary
				Hemodialysis	Administer after dialysis
Carmustine[27,28]	Dosage adjustment may be necessary, but no specific guidelines are available			CrCl 46–60 mL/min	Administer 80% of dosage
				CrCl 31–45 mL/min	Administer 75% of dosage
				CrCl <30 mL/min	Consider alternative therapy
Cetuximab[41]	No dosage adjustments necessary			No dosage adjustments necessary	
Chlorambucil	Hepatic metabolism into active and inactive metabolites. Dosage adjustment may be needed in patients with hepatic impairment			CrCl 10–50	Administer 75% of dosage
				CrCl <10 mL/min	Administer 50% of dosage
				Hemodialysis	Administer 50%; no supplemental dosing
				Peritoneal dialysis	Administer 50%; no supplemental dosing

(continued)

(continued)

Drug	Guideline	Condition	Recommendation
Cisplatin[27,28]	No dosage adjustments necessary	CrCl 10–50 mL/min	Administer 75% of dosage
		CrCl <10 mL/min	Administer 50% of dosage
		Hemodialysis	Administer 50% of dosage post-dialysis
		Peritoneal dialysis	Administer 50% of dosage
		Continuous renal replacement therapy (CRRT)	Administer 75% of dosage
Cladribine[42]	No specific dosage adjustment guidelines are available due to lack of data. Caution should be used in patients with hepatic impairment	*Note:* Clinicians have used the guidelines below. The manufacturer recommends repeat courses should not be given until SCr <1.5 mg/dL (<133 μmol/L) and/or BUN <25 (<8.9 mmol/L). No formal recommendation from FDA beyond use with caution	
		CrCl 10–50 mL/min	Adult: 75% of dosage
		CrCl <10 mL/min	Adult: 50% of dosage
Clofarabine[43]	Safety not established. Use with caution	Primary urinary excretion. Safety not established. Use with caution	
		CrCl 30–90 mL/min	No dosage adjustments necessary
		CrCl <30 mL/min	Starting dosage adjustments have not been determined; Use caution
		End-stage renal disease	No data; use caution[35]
Crizotinib[44]	Data are insufficient to determine if dosage adjustments are necessary. Use with caution. As crizotinib is extensively metabolized in the liver, hepatic impairment is likely to increase plasma crizotinib concentrations	Continuous ambulatory peritoneal dialysis (CAPD)	75% of normal dosage
		Continuous renal replacement therapy (CRRT)	No adjustment
Cytarabine[14,28,46]	Dosage adjustments may be necessary, but no specific guidelines are available. Some clinicians have used the guidelines below. Transaminases (any elevation); administer 50% of dose; may increase subsequent doses in the absence of toxicities	*Cytarabine 100–200 mg/m²*	No dosage adjustments necessary
		High-dose Cytarabine 1000–3000 mg/m² per dose	
		CrCl = 46–60 mL/min	Administer 60% of dosage
		CrCl = 31–45 mL/min	Administer 50% of dosage
		CrCl <30 mL/min	Consider use of alternative drug
		High-dose Cytarabine ≥2000 mg/m² per dose	
		SCr 1.5–1.9 mg/dL (133–168 μmol/L) or an ↑ from baseline of 0.5–1.2 mg/dL (44–106 μmol/L)	Administer 50% of dosage. May increase subsequent dosages in the absence of toxicities
		SCr ≥2 mg/dL (≥176 μmol/L) or ↑ from baseline of >1.2 mg/dL (>106 μmol/L)	Reduce dosage to 1000 mg/m² per dose
		>2 mg/dL (>34 μmol/L)	Reduce dosage to 100 mg/m² per day as a continuous infusion

Drug	Hepatic Dysfunction			Renal Dysfunction	
	Bilirubin (mg/dL and μmol/L)	AST/SGOT (units/L) ALT/SGPT (units/L)	Percent Dosage/Dose Administered	Creatinine Clearance (CrCL) (mL/min) or Serum Creatinine (SCr) (mg/dL and μmol/L)	Percent Dosage/Dose Administered
Cytarabine lipid complex (liposome)[47]	No dosage adjustments necessary			No dosage adjustments necessary	
Dabrafenib	Child-Pugh Class B-C (moderate to severe hepatic impairment)		Limited data available. Monitor closely for toxicity	Mild-moderate renal impairment	No dosage adjustment necessary
				Severe renal impairment	Limited data available. Monitor closely for toxicity
Dabrafenib mesylate[48]	Mild hepatic impairment		No dosage adjustments necessary	Mild to moderate renal impairment (CrCL 30–90 mL/min [0.5–1.5 mL/s])	No dosage adjustments necessary
	Moderate to severe hepatic impairment		No clinical trials have been conducted	Severe renal impairment (CrCL <30 mL/min [<0.5 mL/s])	No clinical trials have been conducted
Dacarbazine[49,50]		Dosage adjustments may be necessary but no specific guidelines are available		FDA-approved labeling does not contain dosage adjustment guidelines, but the following guidelines below have been used by some clinicians	
				CrCL 46–60 mL/min	Administer 80% of dosage
				CrCl 31–45 mL/min	Administer 75% of dosage
				CrCl <30 mL/min	Administer 70% of dosage
Dactinomycin[51,52]	Dosage adjustment is unlikely to be necessary			No dosage adjustments necessary	
	3 mg/dL (>51 μmol/L)		Administer 50% of dosage		
Darbepoetin alfa[53]	No dosage adjustments necessary			No dosage adjustments necessary	
Dasatinib[54]	No dosage adjustments necessary			Currently no clinical studies on renal insufficiency. Less than 4% of dasatinib and its metabolites are excreted via the kidney	
	Note: After administering a 70-mg dose, compared to subjects with normal liver function, patients with moderate hepatic impairment (Child-Pugh Class B) had decreases in dose normalized C_{max} and AUC of 47% and 8%, respectively; while patients with severe hepatic impairment (Child-Pugh Class C) had dose normalized C_{max} decreased by 43% and AUC decreased by 28% compared to normal controls. These differences in C_{max} and AUC are not clinically relevant				
Daunorubicin HCl[55]	1.2–3.0 mg/dL (21–51 μmol/L)		Administer 75% of dosage	SCr >3 mg/dL (>265 μmol/L)	Administer 50% of dosage
	>3 mg/dL (>51 μmol/L)		Administer 50% of dosage		
	>5 mg/dL (>85 μmol/L)		Hold therapy		

(continued)

(continued)

Drug	Hepatic criteria	Dosage adjustment (hepatic)	Renal criteria	Dosage adjustment (renal)
Daunorubicin citrate Liposomal[56]	1.2–3.0 mg/dL (21–51 μmol/L)	Administer 75% of dosage	SCr >3 mg/dL (>265 μmol/L)	Administer 50% of dosage
	>3 mg/dL (>51 μmol/L)	Administer 50% of dosage		
Decitabine[57]	No data exists on the use of decitabine in patients with hepatic dysfunction; therefore, it should be used with caution. If bilirubin and/or ALT is >2 × ULN temporarily hold until resolution		No data exists on the use of decitabine in patients with renal dysfunction; therefore, it should be used with caution. If SCr >2 mg/dL (>177 μmol/L) temporarily withhold decitabine until resolution	
Denosumab[58]	No clinical trials have been conducted		CrCl <30 mL/min	Use with caution. No dosage adjustment
Denileukin diftitox[59]	No dosage reductions necessary		No dosage reductions necessary	
Dexrazoxane HCl[60]	No dosage reductions necessary		CrCl <40 mL/min	Administer 50% of dosage
Docetaxel[61–66]	>ULN AST or ALT >1.5 × ULN and alkaline phosphatase >2.5 × ULN	Do not administer	No dosage reductions necessary. Note: Not removed by hemodialysis; may be administered before or after hemodialysis	
	AST or ALT 2.5–5 × ULN and alkaline phosphatase <2.5 × ULN	Administer 80% of dosage		
	AST or ALT 1.5–5 × ULN and alkaline phosphatase >2.5–5 × ULN	Administer 80% of dosage		
	AST or ALT >5 × ULN and/or alkaline phosphatase >5 × ULN	Do not administer		
Doxorubicin HCl[67–69]	1.2–3 mg/dL (21–51 μmol/L)	Administer 50% of dosage	No dosage reductions necessary	
	3.1–5 mg/dL (51–85 μmol/L)	Administer 25% of dosage		
	>5 mg/dL (>85 μmol/L)	Contraindicated		
Doxorubicin HCl liposomal[68,70]	1.2–3 mg/dL (21–51 μmol/L)	Administer 50% of dosage	No dosage reductions necessary	
	3.1–5 mg/dL (51–85 μmol/L)	Administer 25% of dosage		
	>5 mg/dL (>85 μmol/L)	Contraindicated		

Drug	Hepatic Dysfunction		Renal Dysfunction	
	Bilirubin (mg/dL and μmol/L) / AST/SGOT (units/L) ALT/SGPT (units/L)	Percent Dosage/Dose Administered	Creatinine Clearance (CrCL) (mL/min) or Serum Creatinine (SCr) (mg/dL and μmol/L)	Percent Dosage/Dose Administered
Enzalutamide[71]	Mild to moderate hepatic impairment	No dosage adjustments necessary	Creatinine clearance 30 to ≤89 mL/min [0.5 to ≤1.48 mL/s]	No dosage adjustment necessary
	Severe hepatic impairment	No clinical trials have been conducted	CrCL <30 mL/min [<0.5 mL/s]	No clinical trials have been conducted
Epirubicin HCl[39,72,73]	1.2–3 mg/dL (21–51 μmol/L) / AST 2–4 × ULN	Administer 50% of dosage	CrCl <50 mL/min	No dosage adjustments necessary[33]
	>3 mg/dL (>51 μmol/L) / AST >4 × ULN	Administer 25% of dosage	SCr >5 mg/dL (>442 μmol/L)	Dosage adjustment required; no specific guidelines
	Severe hepatic impairment	Use is contraindicated		
Epoetin Alfa[74]	No dosage adjustments necessary		No dosage adjustments necessary	
Eribulin mesylate[75]	Child-Pugh Class A (mild hepatic impairment)	Reduce dosage to 1.1 mg/m²	CrCl >50 mL/min	No dosage adjustments necessary
	Child-Pugh Class B (moderate hepatic impairment)	Reduce dosage to 0.7 mg/m²	CrCl 30–50 mL/min	Reduce dosage to 1.1 mg/m²
	Child-Pugh Class C (severe hepatic impairment)	Use has not been studied	CrCl <30 mL/min	No clinical trials have been conducted
Erlotinib HCl[76,77]	In vitro and in vivo data suggest erlotinib is cleared primarily by the liver. However, erlotinib exposure was similar in patients with moderately impaired hepatic function (Child-Pugh B) and patients with adequate hepatic function, including patients with primary liver cancer or hepatic metastases		No dosage adjustments necessary. Less than 9% of a single dose is excreted in the urine	
	1–7 mg/dL (17–120 μmol/L) / AST >3 × ULN	Administer 50% dosage. Escalate dosage if tolerated		
	>3 × ULN / ALT or AST >5 × ULN	Use extreme caution if at baseline, or D/C therapy if already in progress		
	>ULN / Child-Pugh A, B, and C (mild, moderate, and severe hepatic impairment)	Monitor closely		

Note: Erlotinib dosing should be interrupted or discontinued if changes in liver function are severe such as doubling of total bilirubin and/or tripling of transaminases in the setting of pretreatment values outside normal range

(continued)

(continued)

Drug	Hepatic function	Adjustment	Renal function	Adjustment
Estramustine phosphate sodium[78]	No dosage adjustments necessary		No dosage adjustments necessary	
Etoposide[39,79,80]	1.5–3.0 mg/dL (26–51 μmol/L); SGOT >180 units/L	Administer 50% dosage	CrCl 10–50 mL/min	Administer 75% dosage
			CrCl <10 mL/min	Administer 50% dosage
			Hemodialysis	Administer 50% dosage. No supplemental dosing needed
			Continuous ambulatory peritoneal dialysis (CAPD)	Administer 50% dosage. No supplemental dosing needed
			Continuous renal replacement therapy (CRRT)	Administer 75% dosage. No supplemental dosing needed
	Note: Decreased albumin increases unbound drug concentration and increases hematologic toxic effects			
Etoposide phosphate[45,80,81]	1.5–3.0 mg/dL (26–51 μmol/L); SGOT >180 units/L	Administer 50% dosage	CrCl 15–50 mL/min	Administer 75% dosage
			CrCl <15 mL/min	Data are not available; consider further dose reductions
Everolimus[82,83]	Child-Pugh Class A	No dosage adjustments necessary	No dosage adjustments necessary. Renal transplants should have daily doses decreased to 5 mg	
	Child-Pugh Class B	Reduce the dose to 5 mg daily		
	Child-Pugh Class C	Data not available. Do not administer		
Exemestane[84]	No dosage adjustments necessary		No dosage adjustments necessary	
Filgrastim[85]	No dosage adjustments necessary		No dosage adjustments necessary	
Floxuridine[86]	1.2 × ULN; Alkaline phosphatase 1.2 × ULN	Administer 80% of dosage	Dosage adjustment may be necessary. No specific guidelines are available	
	1.5 × ULN; AST or ALT 3 × baseline or alkaline phosphatase 1.5 × ULN	Administer 50% of dosage		
	2 × ULN; AST or ALT >3 × baseline or alkaline phosphatase 2 × ULN	No recommendations available[38]		

Drug	Hepatic Dysfunction			Renal Dysfunction	
	Bilirubin (mg/dL and µmol/L)	AST/SGOT (units/L) ALT/SGPT (units/L)	Percent Dosage/Dose Administered	Creatinine Clearance (CrCL) (mL/min) or Serum Creatinine (SCr) (mg/dL and µmol/L)	Percent Dosage/Dose Administered
Fludarabine[39,87]	Dosage adjustments may be necessary. No specific guidelines are available			CrCl 50–79 mL/min in adults	Administer 80% of IV dosage
				CrCl 30–49 mL/min in adults	Administer 60–75% of IV dosage
				CrCl <30 mL/min in adults	Administer 0–50% of IV dosage
				CrCl 30–50 mL/min in children	Administer 80% of IV dosage
				CrCl <30 mL/min in children	Do not administer
				Hemodialysis	Administer **IV** dose after dialysis
				Continuous ambulatory peritoneal dialysis (CAPD)	Administer 50% of IV dosage
				Continuous renal replacement therapy (CRRT)	Administer 75% of IV dosage
				CrCl 30–70 mL/min	Administer 80% of **ORAL** dosage Canadian PI: administer 50% of **ORAL** dosage
				CrCl <30 mL/min	Administer 50% of **ORAL** dose Canadian PI: contraindicated
Fluorouracil[39,45,88]	>5 mg/dL (>85 µmol/L)		Do not administer	Hemodialysis	Administer 50% dosage
	Increased bilirubin: no relation to toxic effects; no adjustment needed[74]				
Fluoxymesterone[89]	Severe hepatic impairment		Contraindicated	Severe renal impairment	Contraindicated
Flutamide[90,91]	Severe hepatic impairment		Contraindicated	No dosage adjustments necessary	
Fulvestrant[92]	Child-Pugh Class A (mild hepatic impairment)		No dosage adjustments necessary	No dosage adjustments necessary	
	Child-Pugh Class B (moderate hepatic impairment)		Reduce maintenance and initial doses to 250 mg		
	Child-Pugh Class C (severe hepatic impairment)		Use has not been evaluated		
Gefitinib[93]	Moderate-to-severe impairment as a result of metastases		No dosage adjustments necessary	No dosage adjustments necessary	
Gemcitabine HCl[52,94,95]		Elevated AST	No dosage adjustments necessary	No dosage adjustments necessary. Discontinue only if severe renal toxicity or hemolytic uremic syndrome (HUS) occur during treatment	
	>5 mg/dL (>85 µmol/L)		Reduce dosage by 20%		

(continued)

(continued)

Drug	Hepatic Impairment	Renal Impairment
Gemtuzumab ozogamicin[96]	Use extra caution when administering in patients with hepatic impairment	No dosage adjustments necessary
Goserelin acetate[97]	No dosage adjustments necessary	No dosage adjustments necessary
Hydroxyurea[45,98]	Moderate-to-severe hepatic impairment: Dosage adjustments may be necessary, but specific guidelines not available	CrCl <60 mL/min: Reduce initial dosage to 7.5 mg/kg/day. Titrate to response/avoidance of toxicity; CrCl 10–50 mL/min: Administer 50% dosage; CrCl <10 mL/min: Administer 20% dosage; Hemodialysis: Administer after dialysis. No supplemental dose necessary; Continuous renal replacement therapy (CRRT): Administer 50% dosage. It is recommended to reduce the initial dose in sickle cell anemia
Ibritumomab tiuxetan[99]	No dosage adjustments necessary	No dosage adjustments necessary
Ibrutinib	Metabolized in liver. Significant increases in exposure are expected with hepatic impairment. Insufficient data to recommend a dose in patients with baseline hepatic impairment	CrCL >25 mL/min: No dosage adjustment necessary; CrCL <25 mL/min or on dialysis: Limited data available. Monitor closely for toxicity
Idarubicin HCl[39,45]	1.5–3 mg/dL / AST/SGOT 60–180 units/L: Administer 75% dosage; 3–5 mg/dL (51–85 μmol/L) / AST/SGOT >180 units/L: Administer 50% dosage; >5 mg/dL (>85 μmol/L): Do not administer; Bilirubin >3 mg/dL (>85 μmol/L): Administer 25% of dosage	CrCl 10–50 mL/min: Administer 75% dosage; CrCl <10 mL/min: Administer 50% dosage
Ifosfamide[28,39,45,100]	Other dosage adjustments may be necessary, but no specific guidelines are available	CrCl 46–60 mL/min: Administer 80% of dosage; CrCl 31–45 mL/min: Administer 75% of dosage; CrCl <30 mL/min: Administer 70% of dosage; Hemodialysis: No supplemental dose needed
Imatinib mesylate[101,102]	>3–10 × ULN: Administer 75% of dose	CrCl 40–59 mL/min: 600 mg = maximum recommended dose; CrCl 20–39 mL/min: Decrease starting dose by 50%. 400 mg = maximum recommended dose; CrCl <20 mL/min: Dose adjustment may be necessary, specific guidelines not available. Two patients with severe renal impairment tolerated 100 mg/day
Interferon alfa[103]	No dosage adjustments necessary	No dosage adjustments necessary
Ipilimumab[104]	No formal recommendation, but dosage adjustment seems unnecessary	No formal recommendation, but dosage adjustment seems unnecessary

Drug	Hepatic Dysfunction			Renal Dysfunction	
	Bilirubin (mg/dL and μmol/L)	AST/SGOT (units/L) ALT/SGPT (units/L)	Percent Dosage/Dose Administered	Creatinine Clearance (CrCL) (mL/min) or Serum Creatinine (SCr) (mg/dL and μmol/L)	Percent Dosage/Dose Administered
Irinotecan HCl[105–108]	3-weekly irinotecan dosing (usual dose 350 mg/m² every 3 weeks)			Use caution; not recommended for use in patients on dialysis	
	<1.5 × ULN		350 mg/m²		
	1.5–3 × ULN		200 mg/m²		
	>3 × ULN		Not recommended		
	Once weekly irinotecan dosing (usual dose 125 mg/m² for 4 of 6 weeks)				
	1.5–3 × ULN	AST/ALT ≤5 × ULN	60 mg/m²		
	1.5–3 × ULN	AST/ALT 5.1–20 × ULN	40 mg/m²		
	3.1–5 × ULN	AST/ALT ≤5 × ULN	50 mg/m²		
	≤1.5 × ULN	AST/ALT 5.1–20 × ULN	60 mg/m²		
	Special Note: When administered in combination with other agents, or as a single-agent, a reduction in the starting dose by at least 1 level of irinotecan should be considered for patients known to be homozygous for the UGT1A1*28 allele				
Isotretinoin[109]	Empiric dose reductions are recommended in patients with hepatitis or abnormal liver enzymes			No dosage adjustments necessary	
Ixabepilone[110]	≤1 × ULN	AST and ALT ≤2.5 × ULN	No dosage adjustments necessary. If administering with capecitabine do not need a dosage adjustment	CrCl >30 mL/min	No dosage adjustment necessary
	≤1.5 × ULN	AST and ALT 2.5–10 × ULN	Reduce dosage to 32 mg/m²		
	1.5–3 × ULN	AST and ALT ≤10 × ULN	Reduce dosage to 20 mg/m² dosage in subsequent cycles may be escalated up to, but not exceed, 30 mg/m² if tolerated		
	>3 × ULN	AST or ALT >10 × ULN	Do not administer	CrCl <50 mL/min	Combination therapy with capecitabine has not been studied
	>1 × ULN	AST and ALT >2.5 × ULN	If administering with capecitabine, ixabepilone use is contraindicated		

(continued)

(continued)

Drug	Hepatic Dosage Adjustment	Renal Dosage Adjustment	Multiple Myeloma	MDS
Lapatinib[111]	Child-Pugh Class C (severe hepatic impairment) Dose reduction to 750 mg/day (HER2-positive metastatic breast cancer indication) or 1000 mg/day (hormone receptor-positive, HER 2-positive breast cancer indication)	Minimal renal elimination (<2%) Dosage adjustments may not be necessary		
Lenalidomide[112]	No dosage adjustments necessary	*Dosage recommendations using Cockcroft and Gault formula*		
		CrCl 30–60 mL/min	10 mg daily	5 mg daily
		CrCl <30 mL/min (not requiring dialysis)	15 mg every 48 hours	5 mg every 48 hours
		CrCl <30 mL/min (requiring dialysis)	5 mg daily after dialysis	5 mg 3 × per week after dialysis
Leucovorin calcium[113]	No dosage adjustments necessary	No dosage adjustments necessary		
Leuprolide acetate[114]	No dosage adjustments necessary	No dosage adjustments necessary		
Letrozole[115]	Child-Pugh Classes A and B (mild to moderate hepatic impairment) No dose adjustments necessary — Child-Pugh Class C (severe hepatic impairment) and cirrhosis Reduce dose to 2.5 mg every other day	CrCl >10 mL/min No dose adjustments necessary		
Lomustine[39,45,116]	Dosage adjustments may be necessary, but no specific guidelines are available. Use caution in patients with hepatic dysfunction	CrCl 10–50 mL/min Administer 75% dosage — CrCl <10 mL/min Administer 25–50% dosage		
Mechlorethamine HCl[117]	No dosage adjustments necessary	No dosage adjustments necessary		
Megestrol acetate[118]	No dosage adjustments necessary	No dosage adjustments necessary		
Melphalan *or* Melphalan HCl[39,119,120]	No dosage adjustments necessary	CrCl 10–50 mL/min Administer 75% dosage — CrCl <10 mL/min Administer 50% dosage — BUN ≥30 mg/dL (10.7 mmol/L) Administer 50% dosage		

Drug	Hepatic Dysfunction			Renal Dysfunction		
	Bilirubin (mg/dL and μmol/L)	AST/SGOT (units/L) ALT/SGPT (units/L)	Percent Dosage/Dose Administered	Creatinine Clearance (CrCL) (mL/min) or Serum Creatinine (SCr) (mg/dL and μmol/L)	Percent Dosage/Dose Administered Children	Adult
Mercaptopurine[39,121]	Dosage adjustment may be necessary, but no specific guidelines are available			CrCl <50 mL/min	Dose every 48 hours	
				Hemodialysis, continuous ambulatory peritoneal dialysis (CAPD), continuous renal replacement therapy (CRRT)	Administer every 48 hours	
Mesna[122]	Dosage adjustment may be necessary, but no specific guidelines are available			Dosage adjustment may be necessary, but no specific guidelines are available		
Methotrexate[39,45,52]	3.1–5.0 mg/dL (53–86 μmol/L)	ALT and AST >3 × ULN	Administer 75% dosage	CrCl 10–60 mL/min	Administer 50% dosage	Administer 50% dosage
	>5 mg/dL (>86 μmol/L)		Do not administer	CrCl <10 mL/min	Administer 30% dosage	Do not administer
				Hemodialysis	Administer 30% dosage	Administer 50% dosage
				Continuous renal replacement therapy (CRRT)	Administer 50% dosage	Administer 50% dosage
Mitomycin[39,123]	Dosage adjustment may be necessary, but no specific guidelines are available. Clearance is effected primarily by metabolism in the liver, but metabolism occurs in other tissues as well			CrCl <30 mL/min or SCr >1.7 mg/dL (>150 μmol/L)	Do not administer	
				Continuous ambulatory peritoneal dialysis (CAPD)	Administer 75% of dosage	
Mitotane[124]	Dosage adjustment may be necessary, but no specific guidelines are available. Monitoring serum levels is recommended			No dosage adjustments necessary		
Mitoxantrone HCl[125]	No laboratory measurement that allows for dose adjustment recommendations. Mitoxantrone is excreted in urine and feces as either unchanged drug or as inactive metabolites. Avoid in MS patients with hepatic impairment			No dosage adjustments necessary		
Nelarabine[126]	>3 × ULN		Monitor closely for toxicities	CrCl <50 mL/min	Monitor closely for toxicities	

(continued)

(continued)

Drug	Hepatic impairment		Recommendation	Renal impairment
Nilotinib[127]	Newly diagnosed Ph+ CML	Child-Pugh Class A, B, or C (mild, moderate or severe hepatic impairment)	200 mg twice daily. Increase to 300 mg twice daily if tolerated	Not studied in patients with serum creatinine >1.5 × ULN. Dosage adjustments for renal dysfunction may not be needed
	Resistant or intolerant Ph+ CML	Child-Pugh Class A or B (mild or moderate hepatic impairment)	300 mg twice daily. Increase to 400 mg twice daily if tolerated	
		Child-Pugh Class C (severe hepatic impairment)	200 mg twice daily; Increase to 300 mg twice daily and then further to 400 mg twice daily based on patient tolerability	
	During treatment	3 × ULN	Withhold treatment, monitor bilirubin; resume treatment at 400 mg once daily when bilirubin returns to ≤1.5 × ULN	
		ALT or AST >5 × ULN	Withhold treatment, monitor transaminases; Resume treatment at 400 mg once daily when ALT or AST return to <2.5 × ULN	
Nilutamide[128]	Dosage adjustment may be necessary, but no specific guidelines are available			No dosage adjustments necessary
	Severe hepatic impairment	Jaundice during treatment	Contraindicated	
		ALT >2 × ULN during treatment	Discontinue	
Obinutuzumab	No data			CrCL <30 mL/min: No data
				CrCL >30 mL/min: No effect on PK
Octreotide acetate[129]	Established liver cirrhosis		Initial dose: 10 mg IM every 4 weeks. Titrate based upon response	Non–dialysis-dependent renal impairment: No dosage adjustments necessary
				Dialysis-dependent renal impairment: Initial dose: 10 mg IM every 4 weeks. Titrate based upon response
Ofatumumab[130]	No formal studies in patients with hepatic impairment have been conducted			No formal studies in patients with renal impairment have been conducted
Omacetaxine mepesuccinate[131]	Hepatic impairment		No clinical trials have been conducted	Renal impairment: No clinical trials have been conducted

Drug	Hepatic Dysfunction			Renal Dysfunction	
	Bilirubin (mg/dL and μmol/L)	AST/SGOT (units/L) ALT/SGPT (units/L)	Percent Dosage/Dose Administered	Creatinine Clearance (CrCL) (mL/min) or Serum Creatinine (SCr) (mg/dL and μmol/L)	Percent Dosage/Dose Administered
Oprelvekin[132]	No dosage adjustments necessary			*Dosage recommendations using Cockcroft and Gault formula* CrCl <30 mL/min	Administer 25 mcg/kg (50% of dosage for CrCl ≥30 mL/min), once daily for 10–21 days
Oxaliplatin[133,134]	No dosage adjustments necessary			No formal recommendation for dose reduction. The AUC [0–48 hours] of platinum in patients with ClCr 50–80, 30–50, and <30mL/min increased by approximately 60, 140, and 190%, respectively, compared to patients with CrCl >80 mL/min. Consider omitting dose if CrCl <20 mL/min	
Paclitaxel[135,136]	**24-Hour infusion**			No dosage adjustments necessary	
	≤1.5 mg/dL (≤26 μmol/L)	AND <2 × ULN	135 mg/m²		
	≤1.5 mg/dL (≤26 μmol/L)	AND 2–10 × ULN	100 mg/m²		
	1.6–7.5 mg/dL (27–128 μmol/L)	AND <10 × ULN	50 mg/m²		
	>7.5 mg/dL (>128 μmol/L)	OR ≥10 × ULN	Do not administer		
	3-Hour infusion				
	≤1.25 × ULN	AND <10 × ULN	175 mg/m²		
	1.26–2.0 × ULN	AND <10 × ULN	135 mg/m²		
	2.0–5.0 × ULN	AND <10 × ULN	90 mg/m²		
	>5.0 × ULN	OR ≥10 × ULN	Do not administer		
Paclitaxel protein-bound particles[137]	>ULN to ≤1.25 × ULN	AND SGOT (AST) <10 × ULN	260 mg/m²	No dosage adjustments necessary	
	1.26–2.0 × ULN	AND SGOT (AST) <10 × ULN	200 mg/m²		
	2.01–5.0 × ULN	AND SGOT (AST) <10 × ULN	130 mg/m²		
	>5.0 × ULN	OR SGOT (AST) >10 × ULN	Do not administer		

(continued)

(continued)

Drug	Hepatic condition	Hepatic recommendation	Renal condition	Renal recommendation
Pamidronate disodium[138]	Mild-to-moderate hepatic impairment	No dosage adjustments necessary	CrCl <30 mL/min or SCr >3 mg/dL (265 mmol/L)	Do not administer or administer with caution
	Severe hepatic impairment	Not studied	Multiple myeloma: 90 mg over 4–6 hours unless renal impairment is preexisting then consider reduced initial dose	
Panitumumab[139]	No formal recommendation but dosage adjustment seems unnecessary		No formal recommendation but dosage adjustment seems unnecessary	
Pazopanib HCl[140,141]	Preexisting moderate dysfunction	Reduce to 200 mg once daily	No dosage adjustments necessary	
	Initial >3 × ULN AND Any ALT level	Do not administer		
	>2 times ULN — 3–8 × ULN during treatment	Continue treatment, monitor LFTs weekly until ALT G ≤1 or baseline		
	>8 × ULN during treatment	Interrupt treatment. Reinitiate when ALT G ≤1 or baseline at <400 mg/day		
	ALT >3 × ULN	Permanently discontinue. Monitor until resolution		
Pegaspargase[142]	No dosage adjustments necessary		No dosage adjustments necessary	
Pegfilgrastim[143]	No dosage adjustments seem to be necessary, but pharmacokinetic profiles in patients with hepatic insufficiency have not been assessed		No dosage adjustments necessary	
Pemetrexed disodium[144]	No dosage adjustments necessary		CrCl <80 mL/min	Use caution with concomitant NSAIDs
			CrCl <45 mL/min	Insufficient data. Do not administer
Pentostatin[145]	No dosage adjustments necessary		CrCl <60 mL/min	No recommendation but use caution
Pertuzumab[146]	Mild, moderate and severe hepatic impairment	No clinical trials have been conducted	Creatinine clearance 30 to ≤90 mL/min [0.5 to ≤1.5 mL/s]	No dosage adjustment necessary
			CrCL <30 mL/min [<0.5 mL/s]	No clinical trials have been conducted
Plerixafor[147]	No dosage adjustments necessary		CrCl >50 mL/min	No dosage adjustments necessary. 0.24 mg/kg; maximum dose: 40 mg/day
			CrCl ≤50 mL/min	0.16 mg/kg; maximum dose: 27 mg/day

Drug	Hepatic Dysfunction			Renal Dysfunction	
	Bilirubin (mg/dL and μmol/L)	AST/SGOT (units/L) ALT/SGPT (units/L)	Percent Dosage/Dose Administered	Creatinine Clearance (CrCL) (mL/min) or Serum Creatinine (SCr) (mg/dL and μmol/L)	Percent Dosage/Dose Administered
Pomalidomide[148]	Bilirubin >2 mg/dL [>34.2 μmol/L]	AST/SGOT >3 × ULN, ALT/SGPT >3 × ULN	Avoid since patients with bilirubin >2 mg/dL [>34.2 μmol/L] and AST/ALT >3 × ULN were excluded from trials	SCr >3 mg/dL [>265 μmol/L]	Avoid since patients with SCr >3 mg/dL were excluded from trials
Ponatinib HCl[149]	Moderate to severe hepatic impairment		Avoid unless benefits outweigh risks	Moderate to severe renal impairment (CrCL <60 mL/min [<1 mL/s])	Avoid unless benefits outweigh risks
Pralatrexate[150]	1.5 mg/dL (26 μmol/L)	ALT or AST >2.5 × ULN	No clinical trials have been conducted	moderate to severe renal function	No formal recommendation, but dosage reduction may be necessary with
Procarbazine HCl[46]	Dosage adjustment may be necessary, no specific guidelines are available			CrCL ≤30 mL/min	Do not administer
Raloxifene HCl[151]	Safety and efficacy have not been established in patients with hepatic impairment. Use with caution			Safety and efficacy have not been established in patients with moderate or severe renal impairment. Use with caution	
Raltitrexed[152]	No dosage adjustments necessary			CrCl 25–65 mL/min	Administer 50% dosage and increase dosage interval to 4 weeks
				CrCl <25 mL/min	Do not administer
Regorafenib[153]	Mild to moderate hepatic impairment		No dosage adjustments necessary	Mild renal impairment (CrCL 60–90 mL/min [1–1.5 mL/s])	No dosage adjustment necessary
	Severe hepatic impairment		Not recommended as it has not been studied	Moderate to severe renal impairment (CrCL <60 mL/min [<1 mL/s])	Not recommended as it has not been studied
Rituximab[154]	No dosage adjustments necessary			No dosage adjustments necessary	
Romidepsin[155]	Moderate-to-severe impairment		No formal recommendation, but dosage reduction may be necessary	End-stage renal disease	No formal recommendation, but dosage reduction may be necessary
Romiplostim[156]	No clinical studies have been conducted in patients with hepatic impairment. Use caution in this population			No clinical studies have been conducted in patients with renal impairment. Use caution in this population	
Sargramostim[157]	No dosage adjustments necessary			No dosage adjustments necessary	
Sipuleucel-T[158]	No dosage adjustments seem to be necessary, but no pharmacokinetic profiles in patients with hepatic insufficiency have been assessed			No dosage adjustments seem to be necessary, but no pharmacokinetic profiles in patients with renal insufficiency have been assessed	

(continued)

(continued)

Agent	Hepatic Dysfunction	Renal Dysfunction
Sorafenib tosylate[159,160]	≤1.5 × ULN: 400 mg BID; 1.5–3 × ULN: 200 mg BID; 3–10 × ULN: Do not administer	No dosage adjustments necessary if not on dialysis
Streptozocin[39,161]	No dosage adjustments seem to be necessary, but follow liver function tests carefully	CrCl 10–50 mL/min: Administer 75% of dosage; CrCl <10 mL/min: Administer 50% of dosage. *Note:* Renal toxicity is dose related and cumulative; may be severe or fatal. Minimize adverse effects by basing dosage on clinical, renal, hematologic, and hepatic responses and tolerance of the patient
Sunitinib malate[162]	Child-Pugh Class A or B (mild to moderate hepatic impairment): No dosage adjustments necessary; Child-Pugh Class C (severe hepatic impairment): No information available	No dosage adjustments necessary However, compared to subjects with normal renal function, the sunitinib exposure is 47% lower in subjects with ESRD on hemodialysis. Therefore, the subsequent dosages may be increased gradually up to 2-fold based on safety and tolerability
Tamoxifen citrate[163]	No dosage adjustments necessary	No dosage adjustments necessary
Tegafur-uracil	Data not available	No dosage adjustments necessary
Temozolomide[164]	No dosage adjustments necessary; Use caution in patients with severe hepatic impairment	No dosage adjustments necessary; Use caution in patients with severe renal impairment
Temsirolimus[165]	1–1.5 × ULN **or** AST >ULN **but** bilirubin ≤ULN: Reduce dose to 15 mg/week; >1.5 × ULN: Contraindicated	No dosage adjustments necessary
Teniposide[166]	Dosage adjustments may be necessary in patient with significant hepatic impairment	Dosage adjustment may be necessary, but no specific guidelines are available
Thalidomide[167]	No dosage adjustments necessary	No dosage adjustments necessary
Thioguanine[168]	No formal recommendation but dosage adjustments are recommended in patient with hepatic impairment	No dosage adjustments necessary
Thiotepa[169]	No formal recommendation, but dosage reduction may be necessary Monitor hepatic function tests	No formal recommendation, but dose reduction may be necessary Monitor renal function tests
Topotecan HCl[170,171]	No dosage adjustments necessary	>40 mL/min: No dosage adjustment necessary; 20–39 mL/min: Reduce dosage to 0.75 mg/m^2; <10 mL/min: Insufficient data
Toremifene citrate[172]	No dosage adjustments necessary	No dosage adjustments necessary

Drug	Hepatic Dysfunction			Renal Dysfunction	
	Bilirubin (mg/dL and μmol/L)	AST/SGOT (units/L) ALT/SGPT (units/L)	Percent Dosage/Dose Administered	Creatinine Clearance (CrCL) (mL/min) or Serum Creatinine (SCr) (mg/dL and μmol/L)	Percent Dosage/Dose Administered
Tositumomab[173]	No dosage adjustments necessary			No formal recommendation, but use with caution in presence of renal dysfunction	
Trabectedin (ET-743)[174]	Hepatic impairment may result in higher plasma concentrations but has not been sufficiently studied and is not recommended. Should not be used in patients with elevated bilirubin levels or clinically relevant liver disease such as hepatitis			CrCl <60 mL/min	Should not be used in combination with liposomal doxorubicin
				CrCl <30 mL/min	Do not administer
Trametinib	Child-Pugh Class C (severe hepatic impairment)		Limited data available. Monitor closely for toxicity	Mild-moderate renal impairment	No dosage adjustment necessary
				Severe renal impairment	Limited data available. Monitor closely for toxicity
Trametinib dimethyl sulfoxide[175]	Mild to moderate hepatic impairment		No dosage adjustment necessary	Mild to moderate renal impairment (CrCL 30–90 mL/min [0.5–1.5 mL/s])	No dosage adjustment necessary
	Moderate to severe hepatic impairment		No clinical trials have been conducted	Severe renal impairment (CrCL <30 mL/min [<0.5 mL/s])	No clinical trials have been conducted
Trastuzumab[176]	No dosage adjustments necessary			No dosage adjustments necessary	
Tretinoin[45]	3.1–5 mg/dL (53–86 μmol/L)		≤25 mg/m²	CrCl ≤60 mL/min	≤25 mg/m²
	>5 mg/dL (>86 μmol/L)		Do not administer		
		180 units/L	≤25 mg/m²		
Trimetrexate glucuronate[177]	No formal recommendation, but dosage adjustments may be necessary			No dosage adjustments necessary	
Valrubicin[178]	Dosage adjustments do not appear to be necessary, but no specific guidelines are available			Dosage adjustments do not appear to be necessary, but no specific guidelines are available	
Vandetanib[179]	Child-Pugh Classes B and C (moderate to severe hepatic impairment)		Data not available. Use is not recommended	CrCl <50 mL/min	Reduce starting dose to 200 mg
Vemurafenib[180]	1–3 × ULN		No dosage adjustments necessary	CrCl 30–89 mL/min	No dosage adjustments necessary
	>3 × ULN		Need for dosage adjustments has not been determined	CrCl <29 mL/min	Need for dosage adjustments has not been determined

(continued)

(continued)

Drug	Hepatic criteria			Hepatic adjustment	Renal criteria / adjustment
Vinblastine sulfate[45]	1.5–3 mg/dL (26–51 μmol/L)	AND	AST 60–180 units/L	Administer 50% dosage	No dosage adjustments necessary
	>3 mg/dL (>51 μmol/L)			Administer 50% dosage	
	>3 mg/dL (>51 μmol/L)	AND	AST >180 units/L	Do not administer	
Vincristine sulfate[45]	1.5–3 mg/dL (26–51 μmol/L)	AND	AST 60–180 units/L	Administer 50% dosage	No dosage adjustments necessary
	>3 mg/dL (>51 μmol/L)	AND	AST >180 units/L	Do not administer	
Vincristine sulfate liposome[181]	Mild to moderate hepatic impairment			No clinical trials have been conducted but dosage adjustments likely not necessary	Mild, moderate and severe renal impairment: No clinical trials have been conducted
	Severe hepatic impairment			Avoid unless benefits outweigh risks	
Vinorelbine tartrate[182,183]	2.1–3 mg/dL (36–51 μmol/L)			Administer 50% dosage	No dosage adjustments necessary
	3.1–5 mg/dL (53–85 μmol/L)			Administer 25% dosage	
	>5 mg/dL (>85 μmol/L)			Do not administer	
	Diffuse liver metastases			Administer 50% dosage	
Vismodegib[184]	Mild, moderate and severe hepatic impairment			No clinical trials have been conducted	Mild, moderate and severe renal impairment: No clinical trials have been conducted
Vorinostat[185,186]	1.5–3 × ULN			Use is not recommended	No dosage adjustments necessary
	>3 × ULN			Do not administer	
ziv-Aflibercept[187]	Mild to moderate hepatic impairment			No clinical trials have been conducted but dosage adjustments likely not necessary	Any renal impairment: No clinical trials have been conducted but dosage adjustments likely not necessary
	Severe hepatic impairment			Avoid unless benefits outweigh risks	

	Hepatic Dysfunction			Renal Dysfunction	
Drug	Bilirubin (mg/dL and μmol/L)	AST/SGOT (units/L) ALT/SGPT (units/L)	Percent Dosage/Dose Administered	Creatinine Clearance (CrCL) (mL/min) or Serum Creatinine (SCr) (mg/dL and μmol/L)	Percent Dosage/Dose Administered
Zoledronic Acid[188]			Data is not adequate to provide guidelines on dosage selection and adjustment or how to safely use zoledronic acid in patients with hepatic impairment	*Dose recommendations using Cockroft and Gault formula*	
				CrCl >60 mL/min	4 mg
				CrCl 50–59 mL/min	3.5 mg
				CrCl 40–49 mL/min	3.3 mg
				CrCl 30–39 mL/min	3 mg
				CrCl <30 mL/min	Use not recommended
				Hypercalcemia of malignancy with SCr >4.5 mg/dL (>398 μmol/L)	Consider treatment only after considering risks vs. benefits. Use not recommended
				Bone metastases with SCr >3.0 mg/dL (>265 μmol/L)	Use not recommended

References

1. Zytiga (abiraterone) prescribing information. Horsham, PA: Centocor Ortho Biotech, Inc., April 2011

2. http://www.gene.com/download/pdf/kadcyla_prescribing.pdf [ado-trastuzumab emtansine]

3. http://bidocs.boehringer-ingelheim.com/BIWebAccess/ViewServlet.ser?docBase=renetnt&folderPath=/Prescribing+Information/PIs/Gilotrif/Gilotrif.pdf [afatinib]

4. Lexi-Drugs Online: Aldesleukin. *LexiComp Online.* [Online] Lexi-Comp, Inc., 2011. [Cited: September 22, 2011.] http://online.lexi.com.soleproxy.hsc.wvu.edu/crlsql/servlet/crlonline

5. Aldesleukin, IL-2. Clin Pharmacol. [Online] June 22, 2010. [Cited: September 22, 2011.] www.clinicalpharmacology-ip.com.soleproxy.hsc.wvu.edu/Forms/Monograph/monograph.aspx?cpnum=12&sec=monindi

6. Proleukin (Aldesleukin for injection) product label. Emeryville, CA: Prometheus Laboratories Inc., August 2011

7. Panretin (alitretinoin) prescribing information. Woodcliff Lake, NJ: Eisai, Inc., July 2009

8. Campath (Alemtuzumab) product label. Cambridge, MA: Genzyme Corporation, 2009

9. Altretamine. *LexiComp Online.* [Online] Lexi-Comp, Inc., 2011. [Cited: September 22, 2011.] http://online.lexi.com.soleproxy.hsc.wvu.edu/crlsql/servlet/crlonline

10. Ethyol (Amifostine) product label. Bedford, OH: MedImmune Pharma BV, 2009

11. Cytadren (aminoglutethimide) tablet product label. East Hanover, NJ: Novartis, March 2002

12. Hornedo, DA and and Van Echo, J et al. Amsacrine (m-AMSA): a new antineoplastic agent. Pharmacology, clinical activity and toxicity. Pharmacotherapy 1985;5:78–90

13. Hall SW, Friedman J, Legha SS et al. Human Pharmacokinetics of a New Acridine Derivative, 4′-(9-Acridinylamino) methanesulfon-m-anisidide (NSC 249992). Cancer Res 1983;43:3422–3426

14. Koren G, Beatty K, Seto A et al. The effects of impaired liver function on the elimination of antineoplastic agents. Ann Pharmacother 1992;26:363–371

15. Agrylin (anagrelide HCl) prescribing information. Wayne, PA: Shire US, Inc., January 2011

16. Arimidex (Anastrozole) product label. Wilmington, DE: AstraZeneca Pharmaceuticals LP, April 2011

17. Trisenox (arsenic trioxide) product label. Frazer, PA: Cephalon, Inc., July 2010

18. http://labeling.pfizer.com/ShowLabeling.aspx?id=759 [axitinib]

19. Vidaza (azacitidine) product label. Summit, NJ: Celgene Corporation, August 2008

20. Elspar (asparaginase) package insert. Deerfield, IL: Lundbeck, April 2010

21. Treanda (bendamustine) product label. Frazer, PA: Cephalon, December 2010

22. Avastin (bevacizumab) package insert. South San Francisco, CA: Genentech Inc., February 2011

23. Targretin (bexarotene) prescribing information. Woodcliff Lake, NJ: Eisai, Inc., April 2011

24. Casodex (bicalutamide) product label. Wilmington, DE: AstraZeneca Pharmaceuticals LP, November 2009

25. Lexi-Drugs Online: Bicalutamide. *LexiComp Online.* [Online] Lexi-Comp, Inc., 2011. [Cited: September 22, 2011.] http://online.lexi.com.soleproxy.hsc.wvu.edu/crlsql/servlet/crlonline

26. Bleomycin (package insert). Princeton, NJ: Bristol-Myers Squibb Company, April 2010

27. Aronoff GR, Bennett WM, Berns JS et al. Drug Prescribing in Renal Failure: Dosing Guidelines for Adults and Children, 5th ed. Philadelphia, PA: American College of Physicians, 2007

28. Kintzel PE, Dorr RT. Anticancer drug renal toxicity and elimination: dosing guidelines for altered renal function. Cancer Treat Rev 1995;21:33–64

29. http://labeling.pfizer.com/ShowLabeling.aspx?id=884 [bosutinib]

30. Velcade (bortezomib) package insert. Cambridge, MA: Millennium Pharmaceuticals Inc., December 2010

31. Adcetris (brentuximab vedotin) prescribing information. Bothell, WA: Seattle Genetics, Inc., August 2011

32. Lexi-Drugs Online: Buserelin. *LexiComp Online.* [Online] Lexi-Comp, Inc., 2011. [Cited: September 22, 2011.] http://online.lexi.com.soleproxy.hsc.wvu.edu/crlsql/servlet/crlonline

33. Busulfex (busulfan) package insert. Rockville, MD: Otsuka America Pharmaceutical, Inc., April 2011

34. Jevtana (cabazitaxel) package insert. Bridgewater, NJ: Sanofi-Aventis, June 2010

35. http://www.exelixis.com/sites/default/files/pdf/COMETRIQ%20Prescribing%20Information.pdf [cabozantinib]

36. Xeloda (capecitabine) package insert. Nutley, NJ: Roche Pharmaceuticals, February 2011

37. Twelves C, Glynne-Jones R, Cassidy J et al. Effect of hepatic dysfunction due to liver metastases on the pharmacokinetics of capecitabine and its metabolites. Clin Cancer Res 1999;5:1696–1702

38. Paraplatin (carboplatin) product label. Princeton, NJ: Bristol-Myers Squibb, November 2010

39. Eklund JW, Trifilio S, Mulcahy MF. Chemotherapy dosing in the setting of liver dysfunction. Oncology (Williston Park) 2005;19:1057–1063

40. http://www.kyprolis.com/prescribing-information [carfilzomib]

41. Erbitux (cetuximab) product label. Branchburg, NJ: Bristol-Myers Squibb, March 2011

42. Leustatin (cladribine) package insert. Raritan NJ: Centocor Ortho Biotech Products L.P., January 2011

43. Clolar (clofarabine) product info. Charleston, SC: Genzyme Corporation, December 2010

44. Xalkori (crizotinib) prescribing information. New York, NY: Pfizer Inc., August 2011

45. Floyd J, Mirza I, Sachs B et al. Hepatotoxicity of chemotherapy. Semin Oncol 2006;33:50–67

46. Smith G, Damon LE, Rugo HS et al. High dose cytarabine dose modification reduces the incidence of neurotoxicity in patients with renal insufficiency. J Clin Oncol 1997;15:833–839

47. Depocyt (cytarabine) package insert. Gaithersburg, MD: Sigma-Tau Pharmaceuticals, January 2011

48. http://www.gsksource.com/gskprm/htdocs/documents/TAFINLAR-PI-MG.PDF [dabrafenib]

49. Lexi-Drugs Online: Dacarbazine. *LexiComp Online.* [Online] Lexi-Comp, Inc., 2011. [Cited: September 23, 2011.] http://online.lexi.com.soleproxy.hsc.wvu.edu/crlsql/servlet/crlonline

50. DTIC-Dome PI (dacarbazine) product label. West Haven, CT: Bayer Corporation, 1998

51. Cosmegen (dactinomycin) package insert. Deerfield, IL: Ovation Pharmaceuticals, 2008

52. Chu E, DeVita VT, eds. Cancer chemotherapy drug manual. Sudbury NA: Jones and Bartlett Publishers, 2006:379–386

53. Aranesp (darbepoetin alfa) prescribing information. Thousand Oaks, CA: Amgen Manufacturing Limited, June 2011

54. Sprycel (Dasatinib) package insert. Princeton, NJ: Bristol-Myers Squibb Company, October 2010

55. Cerubidine (daunorubicin HCl) package insert. Bedford, OH: Bedford Laboratories, February 2008

56. DaunoXome (daunorubicin liposomal) package insert. San Dimas, CA: Gilead Sciences, Inc., 2002

57. Dacogen (decitabine) prescribing information. Woodcliff Lake, NJ: Eisai, Inc., March 2010

58. Xgeva (denosumab) package insert. Thousand Oaks, CA: Amgen Inc., November 2010

59. Ontak (denileukin diftitox) product information. Woodcliff Lake, NJ: Eisai, Inc., August 2011

60. Totect (dexrazoxane) package insert. Bedford, OH: Ben Venue Laboratories, Inc., November 2009

61. Taxotere (docetaxel) package insert. Bridgewater, NJ: Sanofi Aventis Pharmaceuticals, June 2010

62. Lexi-Drugs Online: Docetaxel. *LexiComp Online.* [Online] Lexi-Comp, Inc., 2011. [Cited: September 22, 2011.] http://online.lexi.com.soleproxy.hsc.wvu.edu/crlsql/servlet/crlonline

63. Janus N, Thariat J, Boulanger H et al. Proposal for dosage adjustment and timing of chemotherapy in hemodialyzed patients Ann Oncol 2010;21:1395–403

64. Baker S, Ten Tije A, Carducci M et al. Evaluation of CYP3A activity as a predictive covariate for docetaxel clearance. Proc Am Soc Clin Oncol 2004;22, abstract 2006

65. Clarke SJ, Rivory LP. Clinical pharmacokinetics of docetaxel. Clin Pharmacokinet 1999;36:99–114

66. Hooker AC, Ten Tije AJ, Carducci MA et al. Population pharmacokinetic model for docetaxel in patients with varying degrees of liver function: incorporating cytochrome P4503A activity measurements. Clin Pharmacol Ther 2008;84:111–118

67. Adriamycin (doxorubicin) package insert. Bedford, OH: Bedford Laboratories, September 2010

68. Donelli MG, Zucchetti M, Munzone E et al. Pharmacokinetics of anticancer agents in patients with impaired liver function. Eur J Cancer 1998;34:33–46

69. Benjamin RS, Wiernik PH, Bachur NR. Adriamycin chemotherapy—efficacy, safety, and pharmacologic basis of an intermittent single high-dosage schedule. Cancer 1974;33:19–27

70. Doxil (doxorubicin liposomal) package insert. Bridgewater, NJ: Ortho Biotech, November 2010

71. https://www.astellas.us/docs/us/12A005-ENZ-WPI.pdf [enzalutamide]

72. Pharmorubicin PFS package insert. Kirkland, Quebec: Pfizer Canada Inc., May 2005

73. Dobbs NA, Twelves CJ, Gregory W et al. Epirubicin in patients with liver dysfunction: development and evaluation of a novel dose modification scheme. Eur J Cancer 2003;39:580–586

74. Procrit (epoetin alfa) prescribing information. Thousand Oaks, CA: Amgen, Inc., June 2011

75. Halaven (eribulin) package insert. Woodcliff Lake, NJ: Eisai Inc., November 2010

76. Tarceva (erlotinib) package insert. Melville, NY: OSI Pharmaceuticals, April 2010

77. Miller AA, Murry DJ, Owzar K et al. Phase I and pharmacokinetic study of erlotinib for solid tumors in patients with hepatic or renal dysfunction: CALGB 60101. J Clin Oncol 2007; 25:3055–3060

78. Emcyt (estramustine phosphate sodium) product info. New York, NY: Pfizer Inc., June 2007

79. Etoposide capsules (package insert). Rockford, IL: UDL Laboratories, Inc., October 2006

80. Joel SP, Shah R, Clark PI et al. Predicting etoposide toxicity: relationship to organ function and protein binding. J Clin Oncol 1996;14:257–267

81. Etopophos (etoposide phosphate) package insert. Princeton, NJ: Bristol-Myers Squibb, Co., March 2011

82. Afinitor (everolimus) package insert. East Hanover, NJ: Novartis Pharmaceutical Co, May 2011

83. Zortress (everolimus) package insert. East Hanover, NJ: Novartis Pharmaceutical Co, March 2010

84. Aromasin (exemestane) package insert. New York, NY: Pharmacia and UpJohn, April 2011

85. Neupogen (filgrastim) Prescribing Information. Thousand Oaks, CA: Amgen Manufacturing Limited, September 2007
86. Fudr (floxuridine) package insert. Bedford, OH: Bedford Laboratories, February 2000
87. Fludara (fludarabine) package insert. Cambridge, MA: Genzyme Corporation, July 2010
88. Fleming GF, Schilsky RL, Schumm LP et al. Phase I and pharmacokinetic study of 24-hour infusion 5-fluorouracil and leucovorin in patients with organ dysfunction. Ann Oncol 2003;14:1142–1147
89. Halotestin (fluoxymesterone) prescribing information. New York, NY: Pfizer Inc., May 2002
90. Flutamide prescribing information. Sellersville, PA: Teva Pharmaceuticals, January 2011
91. Flutamide package insert. Spring Valley, NY: Par Pharmaceutical Companies, October 2005
92. Faslodex (fulvestrant) prescribing information. Wilmington, DE: AstraZeneca Pharmaceuticals, September 2011
93. Iressa (gefitinib) package insert. Wilmington, DE: AstraZeneca, 2005
94. Venook AP, Egorin MJ, Rosner GL et al. Phase I and pharmacokinetic trial of gemcitabine in patients with hepatic or renal dysfunction: Cancer and Leukemia Group B 9565. J Clin Oncol 2000;18:2780–2787
95. Gemzar (gemcitabine) package insert. Indianapolis, IN: Eli Lilly, February 2011
96. Mylotarg (emtuzumab ozogamicin) product label. Philadelphia, PA: Wyeth Laboratories, April 2010
97. Zoladex (goserelin) product label. Wilmington, DE: AstraZeneca, January 2011
98. Droxia (hydroxyurea) package insert. Princeton, NJ: Bristol-Myers Squibb, April 2010
99. Zevalin (ibritumomab tiuxetan) prescribing information. Irvine, CA: Spectrum Pharmaceuticals, Inc., May 2010
100. Ifex (ifosfamide) package insert. Princeton, NJ: Bristol-Myers Squibb, July 2007
101. Gleevec (Imatinib) package insert. East Hanover, NJ: Novartis Pharmaceuticals, April 2011
102. Eckel F, von Delius S, Mayr M et al. Pharmacokinetic and clinical phase II trial of imatinib in patients with impaired liver function and advanced hepatocellular carcinoma. Oncology 2005;69:363–371
103. Intron A prescribing information. Whitehouse Station, NJ: Schering Corporation, February 2011
104. Yervoy (ipilimumab) prescribing information. Princeton, NJ: Bristol-Myers Squibb, March 2011
105. Camptosar (irinotecan) package insert. New York, NY: Pfizer Inc., May 2010
106. Venook AP, Enders Klein C, Fleming G et al. A phase I and pharmacokinetic study of irinotecan in patients with hepatic or renal dysfunction or with prior pelvic radiation: CALGB 9863. Ann Oncol 2003;14:1783–1790
107. Raymond E, Boige V, Faivre S et al. Dosage adjustment and pharmacokinetic profile of irinotecan in cancer patients with hepatic dysfunction. Clin Cancer Res 2006;20:4303–4312
108. Schaaf LJ, Hammond LA, Tipping SJ et al. Phase I and pharmacokinetic study of intravenous irinotecan in refractory solid tumor patients with hepatic dysfunction. Clin Cancer Res 2006;12:3782–3791
109. Sotret (isotretinoin) package insert. Jacksonville, FL: Ranbaxy Laboratories Inc., February 2010
110. Ixempra (ixabepilone) package insert. Princeton, NJ: Bristol-Myers Squibb Company, May 2010
111. Tykerb (lapatinib) package insert. Research Triangle Park, NC: GlaxoSmithKline, August 2011
112. Revlimid (lenalidomide) package insert. Summit, NJ: Celgene Corporation, October 2010
113. Leucovorin complete prescribing information. Kirkland, Quebec: s.n., September 2010
114. Lupron depot (leuprolide acetate) prescribing information. North Chicago, IL: Abbott Laboratories, June 2011
115. Femara (letrozole) package insert. East Hanover, NJ: Novartis, June 2010
116. CeeNU (lomustine) prescribing information. Princeton, NJ: Bristol-Myers Squibb Co., October 2010
117. Mustargen (mechlorethamine HCl) prescribing information. Deerfield, IL: Lundbeck, Inc., November 2010
118. Megace (megestrol acetate) prescribing information. Princeton, NJ: Bristol-Myers Squibb Co., March 2011
119. King, PD and Perry, MC. Hepatotoxicity of chemotherapy. Oncologist 2001;6:162–176
120. Alkeran (melphalan) package insert. Summit, NJ: GlaxoSmithKline, June 2011
121. Purinethol (mercaptopurine) package insert. Sellersville, PA: Teva Pharmaceuticals, May 2011
122. Mesnex (mesna) prescribing information. Deerfield, IL: Baxter Healthcare Corporation, February 2009
123. Mitozytrex (mitomycin for injection) package insert. Dublin, CA: SuperGen, Inc., November 2004
124. Lysodren (mitotane) package insert. Princeton, New Jersey: Bristol-Myers Squibb, June 2010
125. Novantrone (mitoxantrone) package insert. Rockland, MA: Serono, May 2010
126. Arranon (nelarabine injection) package insert. Research Triangle Park, NC: GlaxoSmithKline, Dec 2009
127. Tasigna (nilotinib) package insert. East Hanover, NJ: Novartis, January 2011
128. Nilandron (nilutamide) package insert. Bridgewater, NJ: Sanofi-Aventis US, June 2006
129. Sandostatin LAR (octreotide) Prescribing Information. East Hanover, NJ: Novartis Pharmaceutical Corporation, January 2010
130. Arzerra (ofatumumab) prescribing information. Research Triangle Park, NC: GlaxoSmithKline, September 2011
131. http://www.accessdata.fda.gov/drugsatfda_docs/label/2012/203585lbl.pdf [omacetaxine mepesuccinate]
132. Neumega (oprelvekin) prescribing information. Philadelphia, PA: Wyeth Pharmaceuticals, Inc., January 2011
133. Eloxatin (oxaliplatin) package insert. Bridgewater, NJ: Sanofi-Aventis, March 2009
134. Doroshow JH, Synold TW, Gandara D et al. Pharmacology of oxaliplatin in solid tumor patients with hepatic dysfunction: a preliminary report of the National Cancer Institute Organ Dysfunction Working Group. Semin Oncol 2003;30:14–19
135. Taxol (paclitaxel) package insert. Princeton, NJ: Bristol-Myers Squibb Oncology, April 2011
136. Venook AP, Egorin MJ, Rosner GL et al. Phase I and pharmacokinetic trial of paclitaxel in patients with hepatic dysfunction: Cancer and Leukemia Group B 9264. J Clin Oncol 1998;16:1811–1819
137. Abraxane (paclitaxel protein-bound particles) prescribing information. Bridgewater, NJ: Abraxis Bioscience, LLC, March 2010
138. Aredia (pamidronate disodium) prescribing information. East Hanover, NJ: Novartis, April 2011
139. Vectibix (panitumumab) prescribing information. Thousand Oaks, CA: Amgen, Inc., June 2011
140. Votrient (pazopanib) package insert. Research Triangle Park, NC: GlaxoSmithKline , April 2010
141. Lexi-Drugs Online: Pazopanib. LexiComp Online. [Online] Lexi-Comp, Inc., 2011. [Cited: September 26, 2011.] http://online.lexi.com.soleproxy.hsc.wvu.edu/crlsql/servlet/crlonline
142. Oncaspar® (pegaspargase) Injection, for intramuscular or intravenous use; May 2011 prescribing information. Sigma-Tau Pharmaceuticals, Inc., Gaithersburg, MD
143. Neulasta (pegfilgrastim) prescribing information. Thousand Oaks, CA: Amgen, Inc., June 2011
144. Alimta (Pemetrexed) prescribing information. Indianapolis, IN: Eli Lilly and Co, March 2011
145. Nipent (pentostatin for injection) product label. Bedford, OH: Ben Venue Laboratories, August 2006
146. http://www.gene.com/download/pdf/perjeta_prescribing.pdf [pertuzumab]
147. Mozobil (plerixafor) package insert. Cambridge, MA: Genzyme Corporation, June 2010
148. http://www.pomalyst.com/docs/prescribing_information.pdf [pomalidomide]
149. http://www.iclusig.com/pi/pdfs/Iclusig-Prescribing-Information.pdf [ponatinib]
150. Folotyn (pralatrexate) package insert. Westminster, CO: Allos Therapeutics Inc., August 2011
151. Evista (raloxifene) prescribing information. Indianapolis, IN: Eli Lilly and Company, January 2011
152. Judson. I, Maughan T, Beale P et al. Effects of impaired renal function on the pharmacokinetics of raltitrexed (Tomudex ZD1694). Br J Cancer 1998;78:1188–1193
153. http://labeling.bayerhealthcare.com/html/products/pi/Stivarga_PI.pdf [regorafenib]
154. Rituxan (rituximab) prescribing information. South San Francisco, CA: Genentech, Inc., April 2011
155. Istodax (romidepsin) package insert. Summit, NJ: Celgene Corps, June 2011
156. Nplate (romiplostim). Thousand Oaks, CA: Amgen, Inc., July 2011
157. Leukine (sargramostim) package insert. Seattle, WA: Bayer HealthCare, July 2009
158. Provenge (sipuleucel-T) package insert. Seattle, WA: Dendreon Corporation, June 2011
159. Nexavar (sorafenib) package insert. Wayne, NJ: Bayer HealthCare Pharmaceuticals, Inc., March 2011
160. Miller AA, Murray DJ, Owzar K et al. Pharmacokinetic (PK) and phase I study of sorafenib (S) for solid tumors and hematologic malignancies in patients with hepatic or renal dysfunction (HD or RD): CALGB 60301. Proc Am Soc Clin Oncol 2007;25, abstract 3538
161. Zanosar (streptozocin sterile powder) prescribing information. Irvine, CA: Teva Parenteral Medicines, Inc., May 2007
162. Sutent (sunitinib) prescribing information. New York, NY: Pfizer Inc., May 2011
163. Soltamox (tamoxifen) package insert. East Brunswick, NJ: Savient Pharmaceuticals, Inc., March 2006
164. Temodar (temozolomide) prescribing information. Whitehouse Station, NJ: Merck & Co., Inc., February 2011
165. Torisel (temsirolimus) package insert. Philadelphia, PA: Wyeth Pharmaceuticals, Inc., June 2011
166. Vumon (teniposide) prescribing information. Princeton, NJ: Bristol-Myers Squibb, Co., May 2011
167. Thalomid (thalidomide) package insert. Summit, NJ: Celgene Corporation, 2010
168. Tabloid (Thioguanine) package insert. Research Triangle Park, NC: GlaxoSmithKline, June 2009
169. Thiotepa package insert. Irvine, CA: Gensia Sicor Pharmaceuticals, Inc., December 2000
170. Hycamtin (topotecan) package insert. Research Triangle Park, NC: GlaxoSmithKline, June 2010
171. O'Reilly S, Rowinsky E, Slichenmyer W et al. Phase I and pharmacologic studies of topotecan in patients with impaired hepatic function. J Natl Cancer Inst 1996;88:817–824
172. Fareston (toremifene) prescribing information. Memphis, TN: GTx, Inc., December 2004
173. Bexxar (tositumomab) package insert. Research Triangle Park, NC: GlaxoSmithKline, October 2005
174. Yondelis (trabectedin). Toronto, Ontario: Janssen Inc., February 2011
175. https://www.gsksource.com/gskprm/htdocs/documents/MEKINIST-PI-PIL.PDF [trametinib]

176. Herceptin (trastuzumab) prescribing information. South San Francisco, CA: Genentech, Inc., October 2010

177. Neutrexin (trimetrexate) glucuronate for injection. Gaithersburg, MD: MedImmune Oncology Inc., 2000

178. Valstar (valrubicin) prescribing information. Bedford, OH: Ben Venue Laboratories, Inc., August 2011

179. Caprelsa (vandetanib) package insert. Wilmington, DE: AstraZeneca Pharmaceuticals, June 2011

180. Zelboraf (vemurafenib) prescribing information. South San Francisco, CA: Genentech USA, Inc., August 2011

181. http://www.accessdata.fda.gov/drugsatfda_docs/label/2012/202497s000lbl.pdf [vincristine sulfate liposome]

182. Navelbine (vinorelbine tartrate) package insert. Research Triangle Park, NC: GlaxoSmithKline, August 2005

183. Robieux I, Sorio R, Borsatti E et al. Pharmacokinetics of vinorelbine in patients with liver metastases. Clin Pharmacol Ther 1996;59:32–40

184. http://www.gene.com/download/pdf/erivedge_prescribing.pdf [vismodegib]

185. Zolinza (vorinostat) package insert. Whitehouse Station, NJ: Merck, October 2010

186. ZOLINZA® (vorinostat) Capsules; April 2013 prescribing information. Merck & Co., Inc., Whitehouse Station, NJ

187. http://products.sanofi.us/zaltrap/zaltrap.html [ziv-aflibercept]

188. Zometa (zoledronic acid) prescribing information. East Hanover, NJ: Novartis Pharmaceuticals Corporation, June 2011

42. Antineoplastic Drugs: Preventing and Managing Extravasation

David R. Kohler, PharmD

Irritants

Irritant drugs may produce any of the following reactions: erythema along a vein or phlebitis, with sensations of tenderness, warmth, or burning, and pain, and, as a consequence of extravasation, inflammatory reactions, which may include local swelling, erythema, induration with sensations of itching, warmth, aching, tightness, or pain, but generally not tissue necrosis. Drugs categorized as irritants are more or less irritating to soft tissues owing to intrinsic differences in their physical and chemical properties and the properties of excipient products with which they are formulated. The manifestations and severity of reactions after extravasation with irritant drugs often correlate with the concentration of drug, the amount of drug and volume extravasated, and the duration of exposure; that is, some irritants exhibit properties characteristic of vesicants if the amount of drug extravasated is large or highly concentrated. However, except for local changes in pigmentation at an extravasation site (often hyperpigmentation), symptoms associated with irritant drug extravasations are typically of short duration (days to weeks), and there are no lasting sequelae

Vesicants

Vesicant drugs may cause severe tissue injury, usually resulting in necrosis; consequently, vesicant extravasation is a medical emergency requiring prompt situationally appropriate action. Vesicant extravasation injuries may be subtle with a delayed onset of morbidity, or immediately apparent with a rapid onset of symptoms. The severity of lesions, the time over which they develop, and the likelihood of spontaneous healing without intervention, also vary among vesicant drugs. DNA-binding agents (eg, anthracyclines, anthracenediones, mitomycin, dactinomycin) tend to produce more severe and persistent lesions than drugs that do not bind to DNA (eg, Vinca alkaloids, taxanes). Over a period of days to weeks, erythema, swelling, induration, and pain may increase and progress to brawny discoloration, blistering, or dry desquamation. Lesions may ulcerate and form eschars. Ulcers are characteristically painful with erythematous borders and necrotic bases. Spontaneous reepithelialization typically does not occur. Lesions caused by DNA-binding agents may continue to expand laterally and deepen for weeks to months after an extravasation event, involving adjacent structures after cytolytic release of active drug from necrotic tissues

What to Avoid in Placement of Vascular Access Devices (VADs)

Peripheral VADs	Central VADs and Implanted Ports
• Fragile, small, or low-flow vessels such as the dorsal aspect of the wrist • Vessels overlying areas with little subcutaneous tissue such as the dorsum of the hand and wrist, and areas of flexion, such as the wrist and antecubital fossa, particularly for administering irritants or vesicants • Areas of hematoma, edema, impaired lymphatic drainage, frank lymphedema, or distal to lymphatic dissection, phlebitis, inflammation, induration or obvious infection, and sites previously irradiated or treated with irritating or sclerosing drugs • Veins in extremities with decreased sensation, paresthesia, or neurologic weakness. Impaired tactile sensation may prevent a patient from feeling and promptly reporting discomfort associated with extravasation • Sites distal to former venipuncture sites, particularly within the previous 24 hours • Sites distal to sites of previous extravasation or a site affected by previous extravasation • Probing during VAD insertion • A site that does not allow for continuous visual inspection • Inadequately secured VADs or administration (giving) sets	• Port placement in suboptimal locations, such as the groin or axillae • Areas where needle stability is compromised (eg, the side on which a patient prefers to sleep) • Deeply implanted ports

(continued)

What to Avoid in Placement of Vascular Access Devices (VADs) *(continued)*

Assessing VADs

New Peripheral VADs	Preexisting Peripheral VADs	Central VADs and Implanted Ports
• Obtain peripheral vascular access in a large vessel in the upper extremities. Peripheral venous access in a lower extremity is *not* recommended • Assess the length of percutaneously inserted VADs. A change in the length of the external portion of a catheter may indicate infiltration through a vein or migration (*backing*) out of a vein	• A new access site should be obtained before administering vesicant drugs peripherally • Assess preexisting peripheral VADs for patency by verifying a brisk blood return and ease of flushing. Flush solutions should flow freely to gravity • Assess site for swelling, erythema, pain, drainage • Assess for signs or symptoms of venous obstruction • Assess the length of percutaneously inserted VADs. A change in the length of the external portion of a catheter may indicate infiltration through a vein or migration (*backing*) out of a vein	• Radiographic confirmation of a central VAD catheter's tip location should be obtained immediately after device insertion and in the following clinical situations: 　1. Pain or discomfort after catheter placement; 　2. Inability to obtain positive aspiration of blood; 　3. Inability to flush the catheter easily; *or* 　4. After catheter migration is noted • Assess the length of percutaneously inserted VADs. A change in the length of the external portion of a catheter may indicate infiltration through a vein or migration (*backing*) out of a vein • Assess central VADs and ports for patency by verifying a substantial, free-flowing blood return (3–5 mL) and ease of flushing 　▪ A flash of blood on aspiration or blood-tinged flush solution are not sufficient to confirm appropriate VAD placement or function • Use noncoring needles of appropriate lengths for accessing implanted ports

Note: A new peripheral VAD placed just before drug administration is strongly recommended for administering vesicant drugs

General Principles for Irritant and Vesicant Drug Administration

1. For treatments administered peripherally through vascular access placed in the upper extremities, secure administration set tubing to the arm with tape. Have patients rest the arm through which treatment is administered on an armrest, across their lap, or on a bed rather than allowing the extremity to hang over the side of a chair or bed
   - Instruct patients to avoid moving a cannulated hand or arm during peripheral administration of irritant and vesicant drugs
2. Verify VAD patency by checking for a brisk blood return both before and after drug administration
   - Instruct patients to immediately report an incident in which tubing is pulled or tugged, and reevaluate VAD patency
3. Review with patients signs and symptoms commonly associated with drug extravasation. Encourage patients to immediately report sensations of swelling, itching, pain, burning, stinging, or other discomfort they experience during and after parenteral drug administration
   - Complaints of discomfort often occur during drug administration or promptly afterward, but may be delayed by ≥48 hours after completing drug administration. The onset of clinically apparent morbidity may be delayed by weeks after an extravasation incident
4. After drug administration is completed, flush the administration set with a compatible solution to ensure complete drug delivery

Intravenous Injection (Direct IV Injection *or* IV Push)

Peripheral VADs	Central VADs and Implanted Ports

- Administer intravenously a freely flowing compatible solution before beginning chemotherapy administration
- Introduce chemotherapy into an administration set at a Y-site or injection port most proximal to the patient
- Check for a blood return before starting chemotherapy administration, check during drug administration after every 1–2 mL of drug administered, and check after drug administration is completed. DO NOT check for VAD patency with a chemotherapy drug
- Flush the VAD and vein with the freely flowing compatible solution every 2–3 minutes when injecting large drug volumes, flush between different drugs, and flush after completing drug administration
- Advise patients to immediately report sensations of swelling, itching, pain, burning, stinging, or other discomfort they experience during and after parenteral drug administration
- Complaints of discomfort often occur during drug administration or promptly afterward, but may be delayed by ≥48 hours after completing drug administration. The onset of clinically apparent morbidity may be delayed by weeks after an extravasation incident
- Observe the vascular access site continuously during drug administration

Intravenous Piggyback (Secondary Infusions)

Peripheral VADs		Central VADs and Implanted Ports
• Administer a cytotoxic agent as a secondary infusion piggybacked into a primary line at a Y-site or injection port between the flush solution container and the infusion device (pump) used to control the rate of administration. If more than 1 injection port is available, use a port between the drug supply and a rate-controlling infusion device (*"above the pump"*) • Secure administration set tubing using tape or a secure locking device		• Secure administration set tubing using tape or a secure locking device • Administer as a secondary infusion piggybacked into a primary line at a Y-site or injection port • Every hour, observe the vascular access site for erythema or edema, and evaluate all fluid pathway connections • Advise ambulatory outpatients to monitor their VAD exit site or port entry site for redness and swelling, and sensations of warmth, tenderness, or discomfort, and instruct them whom to contact if complications arise

Irritant	Vesicant	
• Check for a brisk blood return before administering chemotherapy and after drug administration is completed • Observe the IV site every 15 minutes for erythema or edema until drug delivery is completed • An infusion pump should be used to administer irritant drugs through peripheral veins via continuous (prolonged) infusion	• DO NOT use an infusion pump to administer vesicant drugs • Check for a brisk blood return before administering chemotherapy, check every 5 minutes during administration, and check after drug administration is completed • Observe the vascular access site continuously for erythema or edema • DO NOT administer large volumes of vesicant drugs into peripheral veins unless using a peripherally inserted central catheter	

(continued)

General Principles for Irritant and Vesicant Drug Administration (continued)

Continuous or Prolonged (Primary Infusions)

Peripheral VADs	Central VADs and Implanted Ports
• Peripheral VADs should NOT be used to administer vesicant drugs	• A low-pressure infusion pump or controller is required • Every 1–4 hours, observe the vascular access site for erythema or edema, and monitor the connections • Advise ambulatory outpatients to monitor their VAD exit site or port entry site for redness and swelling, and sensations of warmth, tenderness, or discomfort, and instruct them whom to contact if complications arise

Extravasation is suspected if:

• A patient complains of swelling, pain, stinging, burning, or other discomfort at an injection site or in an area that is referable to the distal end of a catheter or implanted port
• There is erythema or blanching in the epidermis overlying an injection site, and swelling or induration around the site
• A blood return cannot be obtained from the VAD
• Parenteral fluids used to "carry" or flush the drug no longer flow freely

Note: Extravasation from a tunneled VAD may produce discomfort and edema along the subcutaneous track or erythema where the VAD exits the skin. Patients with tunneled VADs or implanted ports may complain of tingling, burning, aching, or other types of pain over the chest wall, the infraclavicular area, neck, or shoulder (sites referable to the location of the port body) ± fever

Dermal reactions that must be distinguished from extravasation include:

• *Flare reactions:* A local allergic reaction that occurs without pain or swelling, and blood return is unaffected. Flare reactions usually are characterized by red blotches along the vein through which a drug was administered, and typically subside within 30 minutes with or without treatment
• *Urticarial reactions:* Associated with pruritus along the vein through which a drug was administered
• *Other nonextravasation reactions:* Aching along the vein through which a drug was administered, supra- or perivascular hyperpigmentation, and wheals

If drug extravasation occurs or is suspected:

• STOP drug administration
• Remove the syringe used to administer push doses or disconnect the administration set at the point closest to the VAD, but do not dislodge, reposition, or remove the VAD or a needle used to access an implanted port
• With a fresh syringe, attempt to aspirate from the VAD (or a needle left in an implanted port) any drug it contains and any accessible drug that can be retrieved from the extravasation site
• Aspirate gently. Aggressive aspiration may cause the catheter to collapse or tissue to occlude the catheter or needle tip
• As a temporary VAD is removed, continue gentle aspiration until the cannula is removed from its insertion site
• With a soft-tipped indelible marker, mark the outside border (circumference) of the area of extravasation and identify in the patient's medical record what the marking represents (eg, erythema, swelling, induration)
  ▪ If possible the area of extravasation should be photographed as soon as possible after an extravasation event, and serially, thereafter to record and facilitate comparison of gross and subtle changes. Photographs should be dated to facilitate comparisons through time
• As appropriate for the situation, remove peripheral VADs (this does not include PICC, SICC, or midline catheters), or remove the needle from an implanted port before applying topical interventions
• Thermal interventions—topical warming or cooling—are based on considerations of whether an extravasated drug should be localized by cooling or dispersed by applying heat
  ▪ Cooling produces local vasoconstriction which may limit perfusion of local or systemic antidotes into an extravasation site; therefore, DO NOT use topical cooling within 15–30 minutes before or after or during administration of pharmacologic antidotes
• Implement appropriate pharmacologic and nondrug interventions as directed by a medically responsible care provider or as indicated by local policies, procedures, or standards of practice
  ▪ *Note:* If appropriate and practical, seek consultation with care providers experienced in managing extravasation of antineoplastic drugs. Nurses and pharmacists who are certified or experienced in oncology practice may be excellent resources for information about appropriate management
• Apply a dressing if indicated, but protect an extravasation site from unnecessary compression
• When extravasation occurs in an extremity, elevate the extremity
• Instruct patients to avoid exposing an extravasation injury site to sunlight and to report episodes of fever or chills, skin blistering, peeling, or sloughing, and worsening discomfort or pain

(continued)

(*continued*)

- Record in a patient's medical record details about the event and any interventions used in management
  Note: Documentation should identify the date and time of extravasation, the dimensions of the injured site (perpendicular length and width at their greatest dimensions), relevant patient complaints, identify what drugs were extravasated, an estimate of the amount of extravasated drugs, all interventions used in management, instructions given to the patient, and a record of subsequent evaluations and consultations. When recording measurements, identify what was measured (eg, swelling, erythema, induration, blistering, ulceration), and the time it was measured with respect to when extravasation occurred
- When vesicant extravasation occurs with a VAD placed in an extremity, the extremity should not be used for subsequent catheter placement. Treatment alternatives include discontinuation of therapy, use of the contralateral extremity, or use of a central VAD

VAD, vascular access device. In the present document, the term includes short peripherally inserted catheter (SICC); long-line, peripherally inserted, central catheter (PICC); and subcutaneously tunneled central catheter (CC)

The preceding recommendations are adapted from the following resources:

Camp-Sorrell D. Developing extravasation protocols and monitoring outcomes. J Intraven Nurs 1998;21:232–239

Extravasation. In: Polovich M, White JM, Olsen M, eds. Chemotherapy and Biotherapy Guidelines and Recommendations for Practice, 3rd ed. Pittsburgh, PA: Oncology Nursing Society (ONS), 2009:105–116, 360

Langer SW. Extravasation of chemotherapy. Curr Oncol Rep 2010;12:242–246

Schrijvers DL. Extravasation: A dreaded complication of chemotherapy. Ann Oncol 2003;14(Suppl 3):iii26–iii30

Schulmeister L, Camp-Sorrell D. Chemotherapy extravasation from implanted ports. Oncol Nurs Forum 2000;27:531–538

Society of Infusion Nursing. Infusion nursing standards of practice: infusion therapies: antineoplastic and biologic therapy. J Infus Nurs 2006;29(Suppl 1):S69–S71

Susser WS et al. Mucocutaneous reactions to chemotherapy. J Am Acad Dermatol 1999;40:367–398

The National Institutes of Health Clinical Center Nursing and Patient Care Services Department's Standard of Practice: Care of the Patient Receiving Intravenous Cytotoxic or Biologic Agents; revised, May 2010

Wengström Y, Margulies A. European Oncology Nursing Society extravasation guidelines. Eur J Oncol Nurs 2008;12:357–361

Table 42–1. Drug-Specific Extravasation Management Guidelines

Risk Category	Antidote Intervention and Preparation	Local Care	Comments
Actinomycin D	See guidelines for "Dactinomycin"		
Adriamycin	See guidelines for "Doxorubicin HCl"		
Alimta	See guidelines for "Pemetrexed disodium"		
Alkeran	See guidelines for "Melphalan HCl"		
BCNU	See guidelines for "Carmustine"		
Bendamustine HCl (Treanda; distributed by Cephalon, Inc., Frazer, PA)			
Irritant	No known antidotes	• Aspirate back through the VAD to remove any accessible extravasated drug • No specific local therapy is indicated	• Product labeling for Treanda (dated, July 2010) indicates extravasation has resulted in hospitalization with "…erythema, marked swelling, and pain. Precautions should be taken to avoid extravasation, including monitoring of the intravenous infusion site for redness, swelling, pain, infection, and necrosis during and after administration…"
Camptosar	See guidelines for "Irinotecan HCl"		
Carboplatin (available generically)			
Unclassified[a]	No known antidotes	No specific local therapy is indicated	
Carmustine (also called BCNU, BiCNU; distributed by Bristol-Myers Squibb Company, Princeton, NJ)[1]			
Irritant	No known antidotes	• Aspirate back through the VAD to remove any accessible extravasated drug • No specific local therapy is indicated	• Patients may complain of irritation and stinging pain during administration—a result of ethanol used to reconstitute carmustine ▪ Carmustine should be diluted in at least 250 mL fluid • Topical sodium bicarbonate solution inactivates carmustine spilled or splashed on the skin, but MUST NOT be injected locally in the event of carmustine extravasation
Cisplatin (available generically)[2–5]			
Irritant	See Comments	• No local therapy is indicated after extravasation with small volumes of dilute cisplatin solutions (see Comments) • Extravasation with large volumes or highly concentrated cisplatin solutions may be treated as an extravasation with mechlorethamine (see Comments)	• Injury to soft tissues has been reported after extravasation of cisplatin solutions with concentrations >0.4 mg/mL[3] • Product labeling for Cisplatin Injection (dated, January 2008; APP Pharmaceuticals, LLC, Schaumberg, IL) indicates administration of solutions with a cisplatin concentration >0.5 mg/mL may result in local soft-tissue toxicity with cellulitis, fibrosis, and necrosis • Although sodium thiosulfate has been recommended to chemically neutralize cisplatin, the conditions under which cisplatin extravasation will produce severe morbidity and tissue necrosis remain undefined (with respect to a threshold concentration or volume extravasated); therefore, the most appropriate use of sodium thiosulfate is not known
Cosmegen	See guidelines for "Dactinomycin"		
Dacarbazine (also called DTIC; available generically)[6,7]			
Irritant	No known antidotes	• Aspirate back through the VAD to remove any accessible extravasated drug • No local therapy is indicated • Protect exposed tissues from light following extravasation • Elevate an involved extremity • Avoid applying pressure to the extravasation site	• Increased skin toxicity was produced in some animal models when dacarbazine was administered intradermally followed by light exposure

(continued)

Table 42–1. (*continued*)

Risk Category	Antidote Intervention and Preparation	Local Care	Comments
Dactinomycin (also called actinomycin D; available generically)			
Vesicant	No known antidotes	• Conservative management[a] • Product labeling for Dactinomycin for Injection recommends applying ice to the site for 15 minutes four times daily for 3 days (alternatively, substitute circulating ice water, an ice pack, or other cold compress)	• Extravasation may occur with or without an accompanying burning or stinging sensation, even with a good blood return on aspiration from the injection site • Topical cooling has been inconsistently effective in animal studies • Blistering, ulceration, and persistent pain are indications for wide excision surgery, followed by skin grafting
Daunorubicin HCl (also called daunomycin. Cerubidine™; Bedford Laboratories, Bedford, OH; available generically)			
Vesicant	Dexrazoxane (see Comments)	• Aspirate back through the VAD to remove any accessible extravasated drug • Apply cold to an involved extremity with circulating ice water, an ice pack, or a cold compress for 15–60 minutes four times daily for at least 48 hours after extravasation[b] • Elevate an involved extremity • Avoid applying pressure to the extravasation site	Administer dexrazoxane for anthracycline extravasation[c, 8–10]: • **Dexrazoxane** 1000 mg/m² per day (maximum daily dose is 2000 mg) intravenously, diluted in 1000 mL 0.9% sodium chloride injection (0.9% NS) over 1–2 hours for 2 consecutive days, on days 1 and 2, *followed by:* • **Dexrazoxane** 500 mg/m² (maximum dose is 1000 mg) intravenously, diluted in 1000 mL 0.9% NS over 1–2 hours on day 3 after extravasation ▪ Effectiveness is decreased if dexrazoxane administration is initiated more than 6 hours after extravasation ▪ Repeated doses (days 2 and 3) should be administered 24 ± 3 hours after a previously administered dose ▪ Decrease dexrazoxane dosage by 50% for patients whose creatinine clearance is <40 mL/min (<0.66 mL/s)
Daunorubicin citrate liposome injection (also called DaunoXome®; Galen US Inc, Souderton, PA)[11–13]			
Irritant	No known antidotes	• Aspirate back through the VAD to remove any accessible extravasated drug • Apply cold to an involved extremity with circulating ice water, an ice pack, or a cold compress for 15–60 minutes 4 times daily for at least 48 hours after extravasation[b] • Elevate an involved extremity • Avoid applying pressure to the extravasation site	
DaunoXome	See guidelines for "Daunorubicin citrate liposome injection"		
Docetaxel (available generically)[14–16]			
Vesicant	No known antidotes	• Aspirate back through the VAD to remove any accessible extravasated drug • Apply cold to an involved extremity with circulating ice water, an ice pack, or a cold compress for 15–20 minutes at least 4 times daily for 24–48 hours after extravasation[b] • Elevate an involved extremity • Avoid applying pressure to the site	• Extravasation often presents acutely with erythema, swelling, and tenderness of the involved site, but onset may be delayed by several days. Blistering and onset or exacerbation of pain may be delayed by several days. Erythema and edema may increase markedly during the first week. Skin desquamation characteristically occurs within 2–3 weeks • It is not yet clear whether application of either cold or heat provides benefit in managing extravasation with taxoid drugs. In one case report, erythema and hyperpigmentation may have been exacerbated by warming after extravasation with the related drug, paclitaxel[17] • Locally altered tactile sensation (dysesthesia or loss of sensation) may persist for months after an extravasation event[15,18]

(*continued*)

Table 42–1. (*continued*)

Risk Category	Antidote Intervention and Preparation	Local Care	Comments
Doxil	See guidelines for "Doxorubicin HCl liposome injection"		

Doxorubicin HCl (available generically)[19–22]

| Vesicant | Dexrazoxane (see Comments for Daunorubicin HCl) | • Aspirate back through the VAD to remove any accessible extravasated drug
• Apply cold to an involved extremity with circulating ice water, an ice pack, or a cold compress for 15–60 minutes 4 times daily for at least 48 hours after extravasation[b]
• Elevate an involved extremity
• Avoid applying pressure to the extravasation site | • Administer Dexrazoxane as for extravasation with Daunorubicin HCl (see "Daunorubicin HCl," Comments)[8–10]
• Seek surgical consultation, especially if a patient reports pain at the extravasation site within 10 days after the event. Surgical debridement or excision may be required to remove nonviable tissues, release trapped drug, and prevent more extensive prolonged tissue injury
• Early surgical intervention should be reserved for patients with local uncontrolled pain, repeated infections, or limb restriction attributed to extravasation injury[23]
• Anecdotes and at least 1 prospective study suggest DMSO may mitigate local morbidity after extravasation with doxorubicin[d] |

Doxorubicin HCl liposome injection (Doxil; Centocor Ortho Biotech Products LP, Raritan, NJ)[24–27]

Irritant– Vesicant	No known antidotes	• Product labeling for Doxil (dated, November 2010) advises application of ice over the site of extravasation for approximately 30 minutes may be helpful in alleviating the local reaction • Elevate an involved extremity • Avoid applying pressure to the extravasation site	• Consider administering dexrazoxane[9,28] as for extravasation with daunorubicin HCl (see "Daunorubicin HCl," Comments) • The severity of tissue injury may be related to the volume and duration for which the extravasated drug remains in contact with the affected site[25]
Ellence	See guidelines for "Epirubicin HCl"		
Eloxatin	See guidelines for "Oxaliplatin"		

Epirubicin HCl (Ellence; Pharmacia & Upjohn Company, Division of Pfizer Inc., New York, NY)[29]

| Vesicant | Dexrazoxane (see Comments for daunorubicin HCl) | • Aspirate back through the VAD to remove any accessible extravasated drug
• Apply cold to an involved extremity with circulating ice water, an ice pack, or a cold compress for 15–60 minutes 4 times daily for at least 48 hours after extravasation[b]
• Elevate an involved extremity
• Avoid applying pressure to the extravasation site | • Administer dexrazoxane as for extravasation with daunorubicin HCl (see "Daunorubicin HCl," Comments)[8–10,30]
• Anecdotes and at least one prospective study suggest DMSO may mitigate local morbidity following extravasation with epirubicin[d] |

Etoposide (available generically)[31]

| Irritant (see Comments) | | • Treat as for vinblastine extravasation | • Skin ulceration is unlikely when etoposide injection is diluted to concentrations used clinically |

Fluorouracil (Adrucil; SICOR Pharmaceuticals, Inc, Irvine, CA)

| Irritant | | • No specific local therapy is indicated | |

(*continued*)

Table 42–1. (*continued*)

Risk Category	Antidote Intervention and Preparation	Local Care	Comments
Gemcitabine HCl (Gemzar; Eli Lilly and Company, Indianapolis, IN)			
Not well defined[a], but not a vesicant (see Comments)	No known antidotes	• No specific local therapy	• Product labeling for Gemzar (dated February 17, 2011) indicates gemcitabine is not a vesicant
Gemzar	See guidelines for "Gemcitabine HCl"		
Hycamtin	See guidelines for "Topotecan HCl"		
Idarubicin HCl (Idamycin; Pharmacia & Upjohn Company, Division of Pfizer Inc., New York, NY)[32]			
Vesicant	Dexrazoxane (see Comments for Daunorubicin HCl)	• Aspirate back through the VAD to remove any accessible extravasated drug	• Administer dexrazoxane as for extravasation with daunorubicin HCl (see "Daunorubicin HCl," Comments)[8–10]
Irinotecan HCl (Camptosar; Pharmacia & Upjohn Company, Division of Pfizer Inc., New York, NY)			
Unclassified[a]	No known antidotes	• Aspirate back through the VAD to remove any accessible extravasated drug • Apply cold to an involved extremity with circulating ice water, an ice pack, or a cold compress for 15–60 minutes at least 4 times daily for 24–48 hours after extravasation[b] • Elevate an involved extremity • Avoid applying pressure to the site	• The recommendations for local care are based on product labeling for Camptosar (dated August 2010), which specifies in the event of extravasation: "…flushing the site with sterile water [intradermally] and applications of ice [topically].…" Healthcare providers should note subcutaneous infiltration and intradermal irrigation with solutions as a means of diluting and removing an extravasated drug are experimental techniques
Mechlorethamine HCl (also called nitrogen mustard, HN_2; Trituration of Mustargen; Lundbeck Inc., Deerfield, IL)[33–36]			

Vesicant	Isotonic sodium thiosulfate 0.167 mol/L ($Na_2S_2O_3$ 1/6 M) solution	• Aspirate back through the VAD to remove any accessible extravasated drug
		• Inject 1/6 M $Na_2S_2O_3$ solution through IV access device: 2–5 mL for each milligram of mechlorethamine extravasated
		• Remove IV access device
		• With a 25G or smaller-gauge needle, inject subcutaneously 1/6 M $Na_2S_2O_3$ solution circumferentially around the perimeter of the involved site: 2 mL for each milligram of mechlorethamine extravasated
		• After sodium thiosulfate injection, apply an ice pack or cold compress for 6–12 hours to minimize the local reaction
		• Elevate an involved extremity
		• Avoid applying pressure to the site
			• Extravasation of the mechlorethamine into subcutaneous tissues results in painful inflammation
			• RAPID intervention is essential in treating mechlorethamine extravasation
			• $Na_2S_2O_3$ solution chemically neutralizes mechlorethamine
			• The intervention is clinically accepted, but reports confirming benefit are scant
			Preparation of a 1/6 M sodium thiosulfate ($Na_2S_2O_3$) solution
			• *Starting with* 10% $Na_2S_2O_3$ solution (1 g/10 mL):
			  ▪ In a syringe, mix 4 mL $Na_2S_2O_3$ with 6 mL water for injection, *or*
			• *Starting with* 25% $Na_2S_2O_3$ solution (2.5 g/10 mL):
			  ▪ In a syringe, mix 1.6 mL $Na_2S_2O_3$ with 8.4 mL water for injection, *or*
			• *Starting with* anhydrous $Na_2S_2O_3$ dilute 2.64 g in 100 mL water for injection

Melphalan HCl (also called L-PAM, L-phenylalanine mustard; Alkeran; GlaxoSmithKline, Research Triangle Park, NC)			
Vesicant	No known antidotes	• Aspirate back through the VAD to remove any accessible extravasated drug • Apply cold to an involved extremity with circulating ice water, an ice pack, or a cold compress for 15–60 minutes at least 4 times daily for 24–48 hours after extravasation[b] • Elevate an involved extremity • Avoid applying pressure to the site	• Product labeling for Alkeran for Injection (dated June 9, 2011) stipulates extravasation may cause local tissue damage, and reports among adverse reactions, skin ulceration at injection site, and skin necrosis rarely requiring skin grafting • An experimental study in mice inconsistently produced ulceration after intradermal injection of melphalan; doses, but not drug concentration were specified[5]

(*continued*)

Table 42–1. (*continued*)

Risk Category	Antidote Intervention and Preparation	Local Care	Comments
Mithramycin	See guidelines for "Plicamycin"		
Mitomycin (mitomycin-C, Mutamycin; Bristol-Myers Squibb Oncology, Bristol-Myers Squibb Company, Princeton, NJ. available generically)[37–42]			
Vesicant	No known antidotes	• Conservative management[a] • Aspirate back through the VAD to remove any accessible extravasated drug • Apply cold to an involved extremity with circulating ice water, an ice pack, or a cold compress for 15–60 minutes at least 4 times daily for 24–48 hours after extravasation[b] • Elevate an involved extremity • Avoid applying pressure to the extravasation site	• Extravasation is typically accompanied by pain and swelling, but initially may be painless • Mitomycin is associated with ulceration at areas of recent vascular damage, including venipuncture sites that are distant from the site of extravasation • Dermal injury after mitomycin extravasation may be delayed from 1 to 29 weeks after administration • Mitomycin extravasation injury may occur, may be exacerbated, or may recur after the affected area is exposed to sunlight[37] • Anecdotes and at least one prospective study suggest that topically applied DMSO may mitigate local morbidity after extravasation with mitomycin[d]
Mitoxantrone HCl (Novantrone; marketed by (osi)™ oncology, OSI Pharmaceuticals, Inc, Melville, NY)[5,43,44]			
Vesicant	Dexrazoxane (see Comments for Daunorubicin HCl)	• Aspirate back through the VAD to remove any accessible extravasated drug • Apply cold to an involved extremity with circulating ice water, an ice pack, or a cold compress for 15–60 minutes 4 times daily for at least 48 hours after extravasation[b] • Elevate an involved extremity • Avoid applying pressure to the extravasation site	• Consider administering dexrazoxane[28] as for extravasation with daunorubicin HCl (see "Daunorubicin HCl," Comments) ■ Dexrazoxane did not prevent ulceration after experimental mitoxantrone extravasation in a mouse model, but the size and duration of lesions was significantly decreased in comparison with controls[28] • May cause blue discoloration in soft tissues where infiltration occurs • Inconsistently produces tissue necrosis after extravasation • When ulceration occurs, lesions may spontaneously resolve with conservative management
Navelbine	See guidelines for "Vinorelbine tartrate"		
Nitrogen mustard	See guidelines for "Mechlorethamine HCl"		
Novantrone	See guidelines for "Mitoxantrone HCl"		
Oncovin	See guidelines for "Vincristine sulfate"		
Oxaliplatin (Eloxatin; Sanofi-Synthelabo Inc, New York, NY)[45–47]			
Irritant–Vesicant (see Comments)	No known antidotes	• Aspirate back through the VAD to remove any accessible extravasated drug • Apply cold to an involved extremity with circulating ice water, an ice pack, or a cold compress for 15–60 minutes at least 4 times daily for 24–48 hours after extravasation[b] • Elevate an involved extremity • Avoid applying pressure to the site • Orally administered nonsteroidal analgesics may be useful in managing pain and inflammation	• Product labeling for Eloxatin (dated March 2009) indicates necrosis associated with extravasation has been reported • Inflammatory reactions were reported after oxaliplatin extravasation (approximate amount extravasated: 40–104 mg)[47] • Clinical appearance within 2–3 days after extravasation is described as resembling erysipelas, with swelling, pain, induration, erythema, local heat, and impaired movement when joints are involved • Although there is concern that cold compresses may trigger the cold temperature-induced neuropathy associated with oxaliplatin,[46] both cold and warm compresses have been used to manage oxaliplatin extravasation without reports of deleterious effects from either intervention[47,48] • Induration, inflammation, and paresthesias may persist for weeks after an extravasation event[46]

(*continued*)

Table 42–1. (*continued*)

Risk Category	Antidote Intervention and Preparation	Local Care	Comments
Paclitaxel (available generically) [49–52]			
Vesicant (see Comments)	No known antidotes	• Aspirate back through the VAD to remove any accessible extravasated drug • Apply cold to an involved extremity with circulating ice water, an ice pack, or a cold compress for 15–20 minutes at least 4 times daily for 24–48 hours after extravasation[b] • Elevate an involved extremity • Avoid applying pressure to the site	• Onset of an injection site reaction may be delayed by up to 10 days • Paclitaxel administration after paclitaxel extravasation at a different site has been associated with recurrence of skin reactions at the site of prior extravasation, ie, a "recall" reaction • It is not yet clear whether application of either cold or heat provides benefit in managing paclitaxel extravasation. In 1 case report, blisters, erythema, and hyperpigmentation may have been exacerbated by warming[17] • Gross and microscopic examination of biopsied and excised tissues from paclitaxel extravasation injuries reveals tissue necrosis.[52,53] Anecdotal reports support product labeling which indicates extravasation reactions are usually mild, consisting of erythema, tenderness, skin discoloration, or swelling at the injection site. In general, administration procedures and extravasation management follow procedures developed for irritant (not vesicant) hazardous drugs • Skin overlying the extravasation site may become inflamed (mimicking a first-degree thermal burn) and desquamate • In 2 reported cases, subcutaneous perilesional infiltration with hyaluronidase after paclitaxel extravasation may have delayed healing[54] • Involved site dysesthesias or sensory loss are common sequelae; motor weakness also has been reported
Paraplatin See guidelines for "Carboplatin"			
Pemetrexed disodium (Alimta; Eli Lilly and Company, Indianapolis, IN)			
Unclassified[a] (see Comments)	No known antidotes	• No specific recommendations for local therapy	• Product labeling for Alimta (dated March 2011) indicates pemetrexed disodium is not a vesicant
Platinol See guidelines for "Cisplatin"			
Plicamycin (not currently marketed in the United States)			
Irritant	No known antidotes	• Aspirate back through the VAD to remove any accessible extravasated drug • No specific local therapy is indicated • Elevate an involved extremity • Avoid applying pressure to the site	
Taxol See guidelines for "Paclitaxel"			
Taxotere See guidelines for "Docetaxel"			
Teniposide (Vumon; Bristol Laboratories Oncology products, a Bristol-Myers Squibb Company, Princeton, NJ)			
Irritant–Vesicant (see Comments)		• Treat as for vinblastine extravasation	• Product labeling for Vumon (dated December 2010) indicates extravasation may result in local tissue necrosis

(*continued*)

Table 42–1. (*continued*)

Risk Category	Antidote Intervention and Preparation	Local Care	Comments
Topotecan HCl (Hycamtin; GlaxoSmithKline, Research Triangle Park, NC)			
Irritant	No known antidotes	• Aspirate back through the VAD to remove any accessible extravasated drug • Apply cold to an involved extremity with circulating ice water, an ice pack, or a cold compress for 15–20 minutes 4 times daily for 24 hours after extravasation[b] • Elevate an involved extremity • Avoid applying pressure to the site	• Product labeling for Hycamtin (dated April 2010) indicates "...most [extravasation] reactions have been mild but severe cases have been reported" • In 2 cases, extravasation was accompanied by pain, which resolved soon after discontinuing drug administration, and swelling that resolved within 24 hours without evidence of redness or ulceration. In one case, topical cooling was applied to mitigate swelling. There were no sequelae in either case. One patient received topotecan on the day after extravasation without adverse effects related to extravasation, and both patients received one or more additional courses of topotecan without morbidity related to the extravasation events[55]
Treanda	See guidelines for "Bendamustine HCl"		
Velban	See guidelines for "Vinblastine sulfate"		
Vinblastine sulfate (available generically)[56–59]			
Vesicant	No known antidotes	• Aspirate back through the VAD to remove any accessible extravasated drug • Consider dispersing the drug by administering hyaluronidase injection (150–300 units diluted in 1–6 mL 0.9% sodium chloride injection injected either into the VAD through which the extravasated drug was administered), by subcutaneous injection with a fine-gauge needle circumferentially around the perimeter of the involved site, or a combination of both techniques *Note:* Hyaluronidase is marketed in the United States in several formulations: solutions containing 150 USP units or 200 USP units/mL, and a lyophilized powder for reconstitution for injection • Apply warm packs for 15–20 minutes at least 4 times daily for 24–48 hours after extravasation[b] • Elevate an involved extremity • Avoid applying pressure to the site	• Warmth increases local blood flow, enhancing drug dispersal from the site • Hyaluronidase may further aid dispersing the drug from the site of extravasation ▪ Hyaluronidase injection currently marketed in the United States includes products from ovine and bovine sources, and recombinant (human) DNA technology. All products have received FDA approval for use as adjuvants to increase the absorption and dispersion of other injected drugs • DO NOT apply topical steroid products. Topical steroids have exacerbated extravasation injury associated with Vinca alkaloids in animal models
Vincristine sulfate (available generically)[59,60]			
Vesicant	No known antidotes	• Treat as for extravasation with vinblastine sulfate	
Vindesine sulfate (not currently marketed in the USA)[61,62]			
Vesicant	No known antidotes	• Treat as for extravasation with vinblastine sulfate	
Vinorelbine tartrate (available generically)[59,63–65]			
Vesicant	No known antidotes	• Treat as for extravasation with vinblastine sulfate	
VM-26	See guidelines for Teniposide		
VP-16, VP-16-213	See guidelines for Etoposide		

[a]**Conservative management**

When it is not known whether a drug is an irritant or a vesicant, and specific antidotes and other remedies have not been identified for mitigating toxicity after extravasation:

1. Aspirate back through the infiltrated VAD to remove any accessible extravasated drug

2. Apply topical cooling to an involved extremity with circulating ice water, an ice pack, or a cold compress for 15–60 minutes at least 4 times daily for 24–48 hours after extravasation[b]

3. When the site of extravasation is located on an extremity, elevate the involved extremity

4. Avoid applying pressure to an extravasation site

5. Closely monitor the site of extravasation serially (*watchful waiting*). The appearance of tissue injury related to extravasation becomes less likely with the passage of time

   • With the exception of mitomycin, for which the onset of acute extravasation injury may appear late, or after repeated exposure to the drug or after exposure of the injured site to ionizing or solar radiation[37,39,41,42,66]

6. Seek surgical consultation, especially if a patient reports pain at the extravasation site within 10 days after the event. Although recommendations for surgical treatment of tissue injury from extravasated drugs are not uniform with respect to standard techniques or interventional timing, surgical debridement or excision may be required to remove nonviable tissues and lesions complicated by secondary infection, remove active vesicant drug that remains sequestered in tissues to prevent more extensive prolonged tissue injury, and in skin grafting

   • Early surgical intervention should be reserved for patients with uncontrolled local pain, repeated infections, or limb restriction attributed to extravasation injury

   • Severe pain, blistering, and ulceration, at a site of extravasation have generally been considered indications for surgical excision[10]

   • If surgical excision is used to remove anthracycline drugs remaining in tissues after extravasation, the procedure may be guided intraoperatively by fluorescence microscopy. Fluorescence-positivity in tissue biopsies is indicative of the presence of anthracycline drugs, and facilitates differentiating between affected and drug-free tissues[67–72]

[b]**Heating and cooling**

Optimal temperatures and the frequency and duration for applying warm and cold compresses over areas of extravasation injury are not known. Heat produces vasodilation with local hyperemia, which facilitates drug absorption and dispersion,[10] but may also increase the cytotoxic effect of some drugs (eg, anthracyclines).[73,74] Cooling produces local vasoconstriction, which inhibits dispersion of a drug through extravascular tissues, thus, in an acute setting, potentially decreasing the extent of cytotoxic injury. Topical cooling also may decrease local swelling and provide an analgesic effect;[10] however, topical cooling should be used with caution around the time local or systemic antidotes are administered to avoid decreasing the distribution of antidote to tissues involved in an extravasation. When thermal interventions are utilized, caregivers should instruct patients to apply heat or cold intermittently for as long as possible during each application, but not with extremes of temperature or for durations that may compromise a patient's comfort or quality of life

[c]**Dexrazoxane (ICRF-187)**

Administer **dexrazoxane** in a large vein over 1–2 hours at a site remote from the site of anthracycline extravasation (eg, a contralateral extremity) Adverse effects commonly associated with dexrazoxane use, include decreased leukocyte, neutrophil, and platelet counts; decreased hemoglobin; and increased serum alanine and aspartate aminotransferases and bilirubin; injection site pain; fever; nausea; vomiting; diarrhea; and constipation After dexrazoxane use, monitor a patient's complete blood cell and leukocyte differential counts and hepatic transaminases in blood or serum DO NOT apply topical cooling to a site of extravasation within 15 minutes before or after, or during dexrazoxane administration DO NOT apply topical DMSO concurrently with dexrazoxane use

[d]**Dimethyl sulfoxide** (DMSO, CAS 67-68-5, NSC 763)

Topical application and intradermal injection of **DMSO** to treat extravasation injuries are controversial. Appropriate application settings and optimal strategies for utilizing DMSO after extravasation with particular antineoplastic drugs have not been defined Clinical anecdotes and at least 1 prospective study suggest dimethyl sulfoxide may prevent ulceration and mitigate local morbidity after extravasation of anthracyclines, mitomycin, and perhaps other drugs. However, in the majority of reports in which benefit was suggested, drug extravasation was suspected based on clinical observations but not confirmed (eg, by fluorescence microscopy-guided biopsy for anthracyclines); thus, neither extravasation nor clear attribution of benefit from DMSO use can be confirmed. In at least 2 anecdotal reports, a single application of DMSO and application 3-times-daily, respectively, were ineffective in preventing vesicant reactions[75,76] DMSO should NOT be used concomitantly with dexrazoxane for anthracycline extravasation[9,77,78]

Note: The following regimens are not ordered or ranked by either preference or effectiveness

Regimen 1. **Dimethyl sulfoxide 50%** (w/w) 1–2 mL applied topically over the involved site once, followed by cold compresses applied topically for 15–20 minutes every hour for 12–24 hours[42]

Regimen 2. **Dimethyl sulfoxide 99%** 4 drops/10 cm² of involved skin surface area, applied topically over an area 2-fold greater than the affected area (including the involved site) every 8 hours for 1 week. The solution is left to dry in air without a dressing, and its administration is followed by local cooling with a cold pack applied topically to the involved site for 60 minutes every 8 hours for the first 3 days after an extravasation event[79]

   • Treatment continued for up to 6 weeks in 29.3% of cases as a result of persistent symptoms

   • Fourteen of 127 evaluable patients sustained residual mild induration of perivascular tissues without functional impairment after a median follow-up duration of 18.5 months

Regimen 3. Dimethyl sulfoxide 99% applied topically over an area 2-fold greater than the affected area (including the involved site) every 6 hours for 14 days. The solution is left to dry in air without a dressing[80]

Regimen 4. Dimethyl sulfoxide 99% *or* 50% 15 mL *or* dimethylsulfoxide 75% volume not specified, applied topically over the involved site every 2–4 hours (at least every 6 hours) for at least 3 days after the extravasation event with topical cooling[81]
  • Among 4 patients treated, all received intradermal steroids injected into or around the site of suspected extravasation and topical cooling. One patient also received local injection of sodium bicarbonate
• *Note:* The U.S. Food and Drug Administration has approved dimethyl sulfoxide 50% (w/w) for administration to human subjects only for the symptomatic relief of interstitial cystitis. Dimethyl sulfoxide 99.0% is commercially marketed for cryopreservation, and is also available in various concentrations and purity grades for veterinary and laboratory use and as an industrial solvent. Dimethyl sulfoxide or particular product concentrations may not be commercially available in all countries. Healthcare providers are urged not to use DMSO products other than those labeled for clinical use. Although chemically equivalent, DMSO not formulated for use in human subjects may contain and facilitate systemic absorption of chemical impurities and contaminants during topical or parenteral use

Adverse Reactions From Dimethyl Sulfoxide

DMSO 50%	DMSO 99%	Reference
Unpleasant taste, halitosis, and body odor (often described as garlic-like)		79–81
Tingling, stinging, or burning sensation Histamine release with itching, erythema, rash, and urticaria • DMSO is hygroscopic. Application to moist or wet skin produces an exothermic reaction (heat)		82
	Erythema, itching, and scaling	80
	Blistering; severe if a dressing was applied over the site of DMSO application	80
	Local tingling, stinging, or burning	79, 80, 83–85
	Severe pain	86, 87
	Burning, swelling, and erythema	86

General References

Boyle DM, Engelking C. Vesicant extravasation: myths and realities. Oncol Nurs Forum 1995;22:57–67

Dorr RT. Antidotes to vesicant chemotherapy extravasations. Blood Rev 1990;4:41–60

Schulmeister L. Vesicant chemotherapy extravasation antidotes and treatments. Clin J Oncol Nurs 2009;13:395–398

Drug-Specific References

1. Colvin M, Hartner J, Summerfield M. Stability of carmustine in the presence of sodium bicarbonate. Am J Hosp Pharm 1980;37:677–678
2. Howell SB, Taetle R. Effect of sodium thiosulfate on *cis*-dichlorodiammineplatinum(II) toxicity and antitumor activity in L1210 leukemia. Cancer Treat Rep 1980;64:611–616
3. Lewis KP, Medina WD. Cellulitis and fibrosis due to *cis*-diamminedichloroplatinum(II) (Platinol) infiltration. Cancer Treat Rep 1980;64:1162–1163
4. Leyden M, Sullivan J. Full-thickness skin necrosis due to inadvertant interstitial infusion of cisplatin [letter]. Cancer Treat Rep 1983;67:199
5. Dorr RT, Alberts DS, Soble M. Lack of experimental vesicant activity for the anticancer agents cisplatin, melphalan, and mitoxantrone. Cancer Chemother Pharmacol 1986;16:91–94
6. Buesa JM, Gracia M, Valle M, Estrada E, Hidalgo OF, Lacave AJ. Phase I trial of intermittent high-dose dacarbazine. Cancer Treat Rep 1984;68:499–504
7. Dorr RT, Alberts DS, Einspahr J, Mason-Liddil N, Soble M. Experimental dacarbazine antitumor activity and skin toxicity in relation to light exposure and pharmacologic antidotes. Cancer Treat Rep 1987;71:267–272
8. Mouridsen HT, Langer SW, Buter J et al. Treatment of anthracycline extravasation with Savene (dexrazoxane): results from two prospective clinical multicentre studies. Ann Oncol 2007;18:546–550
9. Langer SW. Treatment of anthracycline extravasation from centrally inserted venous catheters. Oncol Rev 2008;2:114–116
10. Langer SW, Sehested M, Jensen PB. Anthracycline extravasation: a comprehensive review of experimental and clinical treatments. Tumori 2009;95:273–282
11. Cabriales S. Reader seeks clarification of the role of glucocorticoids and sodium bicarbonate. The author responds [comment, letter]. Oncol Nurs Forum 1998;25:654. Comment on: Oncol Nurs Forum 1998;25:653–654
12. Cabriales S, Bresnahan J, Testa D et al. Extravasation of liposomal daunorubicin in patients with AIDS-associated Kaposi's sarcoma: a report of four cases [see comments]. Oncol Nurs Forum 1998;25:67–70. Comment In: Oncol Nurs Forum 1998;25:653–654
13. Keenan A. Reader seeks clarification on the role of glucocorticoids and sodium bicarbonate [comment, see comments]. Oncol Nurs Forum 1998;25:653–654. Comment on: Oncol Nurs Forum 1998;25:67–70
14. Raley J, Geisler JP, Buekers TE, Sorosky JI. Docetaxel extravasation causing significant delayed tissue injury. Gynecol Oncol 2000;78:259–260
15. Ascherman JA, Knowles SL, Attkiss K. Docetaxel (Taxotere) extravasation: a report of five cases with treatment recommendations. Ann Plast Surg 2000;45:438–441
16. Berghammer P, Pöhnl R, Baur M, Dittrich C. Docetaxel extravasation. Support Care Cancer 2001;9:131–134
17. Goodman M, Stewart I, Lydon J et al. Use caution when managing paclitaxel and Taxotere infiltrations [see erratum]. Oncol Nurs Forum 1996;23:541–542. Erratum In: Oncol Nurs Forum 1996;23:847
18. Ho C-H, Yang C-H, Chu C-Y. Vesicant-type reaction due to docetaxel extravasation [letter]. Acta Derm Venereol 2003;83:467–468
19. Rudolph R, Stein RS, Pattillo RA. Skin ulcers due to Adriamycin. Cancer 1976;38:1087–1094
20. Larson DL. Treatment of tissue extravasation by antitumor agents. Cancer 1982;49:1796–1799
21. Linder RM, Upton J, Osteen R. Management of extensive doxorubicin hydrochloride extravasation injuries. J Hand Surg Am 1983;8:32–38
22. Loth TS, Eversmann WW Jr. Treatment methods for extravasations of chemotherapeutic agents: a comparative study. J Hand Surg Am 1986;11:388–396
23. Langstein HN, Duman H, Seelig D, Butler CE, Evans GRD. Retrospective study of the management of chemotherapeutic extravasation injury. Ann Plast Surg 2002;49:369–374
24. Madhavan S, Northfelt DW. Lack of vesicant injury following extravasation of liposomal doxorubicin [letter]. J Natl Cancer Inst 1995;87:1556–1557
25. Lokich J. Doxil extravasation injury: a case report [letter]. Ann Oncol 1999;10:735–736
26. Laufman LR, Sickle-Santanello B, Paquelet J. Liposomal doxorubicin extravasation. Community Oncol 2007;4:464–465
27. Masoorli S. Extravasation injuries associated with the use of central vascular access devices. J Vasc Access Device 2003;8:21–23
28. Langer SW, Thougaard AV, Sehested M, Jensen PB. Treatment of experimental extravasation of amrubicin, liposomal doxorubicin, and mitoxantrone with dexrazoxane. Cancer Chemother Pharmacol 2012;69:573–576
29. Wilson J, Carder P, Gooi J, Nishikawa H. Recall phenomenon following epirubicin. Clin Oncol 1999;11:424–425
30. Uges JWF, Vollaard AM, Wilms EB, Brouwer RE. Intrapleural extravasation of epirubicin, 5-fluouracil [*sic*], and cyclophosphamide, treated with dexrazoxane. Int J Clin Oncol 2006;11:467–470
31. Dorr RT, Alberts DS. Skin ulceration potential without therapeutic anticancer activity for epipodophyllotoxin commercial diluents. Invest New Drugs 1983;1:151–159
32. Lu K, Savaraj N, Kavanagh J et al. Clinical pharmacology of 4-demethoxydaunorubicin (DMDR). Cancer Chemother Pharmacol 1986;17:143–148
33. Hatiboglu I, Mihich E, Moore GE, Nichol CA. Use of sodium thiosulfate as a neutralizing agent during regional administration of nitrogen mustard: an experimental study. Ann Surg 1962;156:994–1001
34. Fasth A, Sörbo B. Protective effect of thiosulfate and metabolic thiosulfate precursors against toxicity of nitrogen mustard (HN$_2$). Biochem Pharmacol 1973;22:1337–1351
35. Owen OE, Dellatorre DL, Van Scott EJ, Cohen MR. Accidental intramuscular injection of mechlorethamine. Cancer 1980;45:2225–2226
36. Dorr RT, Soble M, Alberts DS. Efficacy of sodium thiosulfate as a local antidote to mechlorethamine skin toxicity in the mouse. Cancer Chemother Pharmacol 1988;22:299–302
37. Fuller B, Lind M, Bonomi P. Mitomycin C extravasation exacerbated by sunlight [letter]. Ann Intern Med 1981;94(4 pt 1):542
38. Johnston-Early A, Cohen MH. Mitomycin C-induced skin ulceration remote from infusion site [letter]. Cancer Treat Rep 1981;65:529
39. Argenta LC, Manders EK. Mitomycin C extravasation injuries. Cancer 1983;51:1080–1082
40. Khanna AK, Khanna A, Asthana AK, Misra MK. Mitomycin C extravasation ulcers. J Surg Oncol 1985;28:108–110
41. Aizawa H, Tagami H. Delayed tissue necrosis due to mitomycin C. Acta Derm Venereol 1987;67:364–366
42. Patel JS, Krusa M. Distant and delayed mitomycin C extravasation. Pharmacotherapy 1999;19:1002–1005
43. Peters FTM, Beijnen JH, ten Bokkel Huinink WW. Mitoxantrone extravasation injury [letter]. Cancer Treat Rep 1987;71:992–993
44. Luke E. Mitoxantrone-induced extravasation. Oncol Nurs Forum 2005;32:27–29
45. Baur M, Kienzer H-R, Rath T, Dittrich C. Extravasation of oxaliplatin (Eloxatin®)—clinical course. Onkologie 2000;23:468–471
46. Foo KF, Michael M, Toner G, Zalcberg J. A case report of oxaliplatin extravasation [letter]. Ann Oncol 2003;14:961–962
47. Kretzschmar A, Pink D, Thuss-Patience P, Dörken B, Reichert P, Eckert R. Extravasations of oxaliplatin [letter]. J Clin Oncol 2003;21:4068–4069
48. Kennedy JG, Donahue JP, Hoang B, Boland PJ. Vesicant characteristics of oxaliplatin following antecubital extravasation. Clin Oncol 2003;15:237–239
49. Lubejko BG, Sartorius SE. Nursing considerations in paclitaxel (Taxol®) administration. Semin Oncol 1993;20:26–30
50. Ajani JA, Dodd LG, Daugherty K, Warkentin D, Ilson DH. Taxol-induced soft-tissue injury secondary to extravasation: characterization by histopathology and clinical course [see comments]. J Natl Cancer Inst 1994;86:51–53. Comment in: Oncol Nurs Forum 1994;21:973
51. Rogers BB. An author responds [letter; comment]. Oncol Nurs Forum 1994;21:973. Comment on: J Natl Cancer Inst 1994;86:51–53
52. Herrington JD, Figueroa JA. Severe necrosis due to paclitaxel extravasation. Pharmacotherapy 1997;17:163–165
53. Bicher A, Levenback C, Burke TW et al. Infusion site soft-tissue injury after paclitaxel administration. Cancer 1995;76:116–120
54. du Bois A, Fehr MK, Bochtler H, Koechli OR. Clinical course and management of paclitaxel administration. Oncol Rep 1996;3:973–974
55. Oostweegel LMM, van Warmerdam LJC, Schot M, Dubbelman RC, Ten Bokkel Huinink WW, Beijnen JH. Extravasation of topotecan, a report of two cases. J Oncol Pharm Pract 1997;3:115–116
56. Britton RC, Habif DV. Clinical uses of hyaluronidase: a current review. Surgery 1953;33:917–940

57. Laurie SWS, Wilson KL, Kernahan DA, Bauer BS, Vistnes LM. Intravenous extravasation injuries: the effectiveness of hyaluronidase in their treatment. Ann Plast Surg 1984;13:191–194

58. Dorr RT, Alberts DS. Vinca alkaloid skin toxicity: antidote and drug disposition studies in the mouse. J Natl Cancer Inst 1985;74:113–120

59. Bertelli G, Dini D, Forno GB et al. Hyaluronidase as an antidote to extravasation of *Vinca* alkaloids: clinical results. J Cancer Res Cin Oncol 1994;120:505–506

60. Bellone JD. Treatment of vincristine extravasation [letter]. JAMA 1981;245:343

61. Dorr RT, Jones SE. Inapparent infiltrations associated with vindesine administration. Med Pediatr Oncol 1979;6:285–288

62. Mateu J, Llop C. Delayed treatment of vindesine extravasation [letter]. Ann Pharmacother 1994;28:967–968

63. Bertelli G, Garrone O, Bighin C, Dini D. Correspondence re: Cicchetti S, Jemec B, Gault DT: two case reports of vinorelbine extravasation: management and review of the literature. Tumori, 86:289–292, 2000 [comment, letter]. Tumori 2001;87:112–113. Comment on: Tumori 2000;86:289–292

64. Moreno de Vega MJ, Dauden E, Abajo P, Bartolome B, Fraga J, Garcia-Diez A. Skin necrosis from extravasation of vinorelbine. J Eur Acad Dermatol Venereol 2002;16:488–490

65. Heijmen L, Vehof J, van Laarhoven HWM. Blistering of the hand in a breast cancer patient. Extravasation. Neth J Med 2011;69:82, 85

66. Prados M, Faruqui S, Blackmon AM. Delayed tissue necrosis to chemotherapy—a case report. J La State Med Soc 1982;134:5–7

67. Cohen FJ, Manganaro J, Bezozo RC. Identification of involved tissue during surgical treatment of doxorubicin-induced extravasation necrosis. J Hand Surg Am 1983;8:43–45

68. Bleicher JN, Haynes W, Massop DW, Daneff RM. The delineation of Adriamycin extravasation using fluorescence microscopy. Plast Reconstr Surg 1984;74:114–116

69. Duray PH, Cuono CB, Madri JA. Demonstration of cutaneous doxorubicin extravasation by rhodamine-filtered fluorescence microscopy. J Surg Oncol 1986;31:21–25

70. Dahlstrøm KK, Chenoufi H-L, Daugaard S. Fluorescence microscopic demonstration and demarcation of doxorubicin extravasation. Experimental and clinical studies. Cancer 1990;65:1722–1726

71. Andersson AP, Dahlstrøm KK. Clinical results after doxorubicin extravasation treated with excision guided by fluorescence microscopy. Eur J Cancer 1993;29A:1712–1714

72. Hooke MC. Clinical nurse specialist and evidence-based practice: managing anthracycline extravasation. J Pediatr Oncol Nurs 2005;22:261–264

73. Dorr RT, Alberts DS, Stone A. Cold protection and heat enhancement of doxorubicin skin toxicity in the mouse. Cancer Treat Rep 1985;69:431–437

74. Soble MJ, Dorr RT, Plezia P, Breckenridge S. Dose-dependent skin ulcers in mice treated with DNA binding antitumor antibiotics. Cancer Chemother Pharmacol 1987;20:33–36

75. Herrera D, Burnham N. DMSO and extravasation of mitomycin [letter, comment]. Oncol Nurs Forum 1989;16:155. Comment on: Oncology Nursing Society guidelines: module V—Recommendations for the management of extravasation and anaphylaxis, Pittsburgh, PA, 1988

76. Schrijvers DL. Extravasation: a dreaded complication of chemotherapy. Ann Oncol 2003;14(Suppl 3):iii26–iii30

77. El Saghir N, Otrock Z, Mufarrij A et al. Dexrazoxane for anthracycline extravasation and GM-CSF for skin ulceration and wound healing. Lancet Oncol 2004;5:320–321

78. Langer SW, Thougaard AV, Sehested M, Jensen PB. Treatment of anthracycline extravasation in mice with dexrazoxane with or without DMSO and hydrocortisone. Cancer Chemother Pharmacol 2006;57:125–128

79. Bertelli G, Gozza A, Forno GB et al. Topical dimethylsulfoxide for the prevention of soft tissue injury after extravasation of vesicant cytotoxic drugs: a prospective clinical study. J Clin Oncol 1995;13:2851–2855

80. Olver IN, Aisner J, Hament A, Buchanan L, Bishop JF, Kaplan RS. A prospective study of topical dimethyl sulfoxide for treating anthracycline extravasation. J Clin Oncol 1988;6:1732–1735

81. Lawrence HJ, Walsh D, Zapotowski KA, Denham A, Goodnight SH, Gandara DR. Topical dimethylsulfoxide may prevent tissue damage from anthracycline extravasation. Cancer Chemother Pharmacol 1989;23:316–318

82. Kligman AM. Dimethyl sulfoxide—part 2. JAMA 1965;193:923–928 CONCL

83. Alberts DS, Dorr RT. Case report: topical DMSO for mitomycin-C-induced skin ulceration. Oncol Nurs Forum 1991;18:693–695

84. Bertelli G, Dini D, Forno G et al. Dimethylsulphoxide and cooling after extravasation of antitumour agents [letter]. Lancet 1993;341:1098–1099

85. St. Germain B, Houlihan N, D'Amato S. Dimethyl sulfoxide therapy in the treatment of vesicant extravasation. Two case presentations. J Intraven Nurs 1994;17:261–266

86. Creus N, Mateu J, Massó J, Codina C, Ribas J. Toxicity to topical dimethyl sulfoxide (DMSO) when used as an extravasation antidote. Pharm World Sci 2002;24:175–176

87. Llinares ME, Bermúdez M, Fuster JL, Díaz MS, González CM. Toxicity to topical dimethyl sulfoxide in a pediatric patient with anthracycline extravasation. Pediatr Hematol Oncol 2005;22:49–52

43. Indications for Growth Factors in Hematology-Oncology

Pamela W. McDevitt, PharmD, BCOP, James N. Frame, MD, FACP, and Lee S. Schwartzberg, MD, FACP

Febrile Neutropenia

Epidemiology

Febrile neutropenia is a major dose-limiting toxicity of chemotherapy. Studies have demonstrated that selective use of colony-stimulating factors (CSFs) in patients at high-risk for complications of neutropenia can enhance cost-effectiveness by reducing the risk, severity and duration of febrile neutropenia

NCI Common Terminology Criteria for Adverse Events (CTCAE) Version 4.0 Neutrophil Count Decreased[3]

Grade	ANC/AGC
0	Normal
1	$\geq 1500/mm^3$ to LLN
2	≥ 1000 to $<1500/mm^3$
3	≥ 500 to $<1000/mm^3$
4	$<500/mm^3$

AGC, absolute granulocyte count; ANC, absolute neutrophil count; LLN, lower limit of normal range

WHO Toxicity Criteria

Grade	ANC/AGC
0	$2000/mm^3$
1	$1500–1900/mm^3$
2	$1000–1400/mm^3$
3	$500–900/mm^3$
4	$<500/mm^3$

AGC, absolute granulocyte count; ANC, absolute neutrophil count; WHO, World Health Organization

Examples of Regimens with >20% Risk of Febrile Neutropenia[2]

(The list is not comprehensive)

Cancer Type	Regimen
Bladder	MVAC (methotrexate, vinblastine, doxorubicin
Breast	Dose Dense AC→T (doxorubicin, cyclophosphamide, paclitaxel)
	Docetaxel, trastuzumab
	TAC (docetaxel, doxorubicin, cyclophosphamide)
Esophageal and gastric	DCF (docetaxel, cisplatin, fluorouracil)
Hodgkin lymphoma	BEACOPP (bleomycin, etoposide, doxorubicin, cyclophosphamide, vincristine, procarbazine, prednisone)
Kidney	Doxorubicin, gemcitabine
Non-Hodgkin lymphoma	ICE (ifosfamide, carboplatin, etoposide)
	CFAR (cyclophosphamide, fludarabine, alemtuzumab, rituximab)
	RICE (rituximab, ifosfamide, carboplatin, etoposide)
	CHOP-14 (cyclophosphamide, doxorubicin, vincristine, prednisone ± rituximab)
	MINE (mesna, ifosfamide, mitoxantrone, etoposide)
	ESHAP (etoposide, methylprednisolone, cisplatin, cytarabine)
	Hyper-CVAD + rituximab (cyclophosphamide, vincristine, doxorubicin, dexamethasone, + rituximab)
	DHAP (dexamethasone, cisplatin, cytarabine)
	ESHAP (etoposide, methylprednisolone, cisplatin, cytarabine)
Melanoma	Dacarbazine-based combinations (with: cisplatin, vinblastine, aldesleukin [IL-2])
Myelodysplastic syndromes	Antithymocyte globulin, rabbit/cyclosporine
	Decitabine
Ovarian	Topotecan
	Paclitaxel
	Docetaxel

(continued)

Examples of Regimens with >20% Risk of Febrile Neutropenia[2] (continued)

Cancer Type	Regimen
Soft tissue sarcoma	MAID (mesna, doxorubicin, ifosfamide, dacarbazine)
	Doxorubicin
	Doxorubicin/ifosfamide
Lung, small cell	Topotecan
Testicular	VeIP (vinblastine, ifosfamide, cisplatin)
	VIP (etoposide, ifosfamide, cisplatin)
	BEP (bleomycin, etoposide, cisplatin)
	TIP (paclitaxel, ifosfamide, cisplatin)

NCI Common Terminology Criteria for Adverse Events (CTCAE) Version 4.0 Febrile Neutropenia[3]

Grade	
3	ANC <1000/mm^3 with a single temperature >38.3°C (>101°F) or a sustained temperature ≥38°C (≥100.4°F) for more than 1 hour
4	Life-threatening consequences; urgent intervention indicated
5	Death

Treatment Overview

NCCN Guidelines® (V.1.2013)[2] and ASCO Guidelines (2006 Update)[5] recommend routine use of CSFs support for patients at high risk (defined >20%) of developing febrile neutropenia who are receiving treatment with curative intent, adjuvant therapy, or treatment expected to prolong survival or to improve quality of life (QOL)[2,5]

ASCO Guidelines also recommends CSFs for:
• Patients with diffuse aggressive lymphomas aged ≥65 years treated with curative chemotherapy (CHOP or more aggressive regimens)
• Patients exposed to lethal doses of total-body irradiation (TBI) (CSFs or pegylated G-CSF)[5]

NCCN Guidelines (V.1.2013) also recommend evaluation of patients for the use of myeloid growth factors before every cycle of cytotoxic chemotherapy
• If febrile neutropenia or a dose-limiting neutropenic event previously occurred during chemotherapy without CSFs use, the guidelines recommend considering CSFs use during repeated treatment cycles
• If fever with neutropenia or a dose-limiting neutropenic event occurred during prior chemotherapy in spite of appropriate CSFs use, the guidelines recommend considering decreasing the dosages of myelosuppressive treatment, or changing the treatment regimen

The chemotherapy regimens given as examples increase a patient's risk of developing febrile neutropenia. Additional risk factors to be considered when evaluating a patient's overall risk of febrile neutropenia include:
• Age (>65 years)
• Previous chemotherapy or radiation therapy
• Preexisting neutropenia or bone marrow involvement with tumor
• Preexisting conditions including:
  ▪ Neutropenia
  ▪ Infection/open wounds
  ▪ Recent surgery
• Poor performance status
• Poor renal function
• Liver dysfunction, most notably elevated bilirubin

Radiation Therapy Oncology Group (RTOG) Cooperative Group Common Toxicity Criteria[4]

Grade	Granulocyte/Band
0	≥2000
1	1500–1900
2	1000–1200
3	500–900
4	<500

Preparations

1. Filgrastim (granulocyte-colony stimulating factor, G-CSF)
2. Pegfilgrastim (pegylated G-CSF)
3. Sargramostim (granulocyte macrophage-colony stimulating factor, GM-CSF)

REGIMEN

FILGRASTIM (G-CSF, NEUPOGEN®)

Patients with cancer receiving myelosuppressive chemotherapy:
Filgrastim 5 mcg/kg per day; administer by subcutaneous or intravenous injection or by subcutaneous or intravenous infusion beginning 1–3 days after completion of chemotherapy and continuing until ANC reaches 10,000/mm³ or clinically sufficient neutrophil count is achieved after nadir

Notes:
- Calculated doses may be rounded to use the most economical combination of available products (commercial vials and syringes contain either 300 mcg or 480 mcg
- FDA-approved labeling indicates subcutaneous or intravenous administration for up to 2 weeks after expected chemotherapy-induced ANC nadir)
- It is recommended not to use filgrastim within 24 hours before or 24 hours after chemotherapy administration

Dose Adjustment:
- Dosages may be increased in increments of 5 mcg/kg per dose for each chemotherapy cycle, according to the duration and severity of the ANC nadir

Patients with cancer receiving bone marrow/peripheral blood cell transplants (BMT/PBPCT):
Filgrastim 10 mcg/kg per day; administer by intravenous infusion over 4 or 24 hours or as a continuous 24-hour subcutaneous infusion
Note: Administer at least 24 hours after cytotoxic chemotherapy, and at least 24 hours after bone marrow infusion

Dosage Adjustment:
- When ANC >1000/mm³ for 3 consecutive days, reduce dose to 5 mcg/kg per day
- If ANC remains >1000/mm³ for 3 more consecutive days, discontinue G-CSF
- If ANC decreases to <1000/mm³, resume at 5 mcg/kg per day
- If ANC decreases to <1000/mm³ at any time during administration of 5 mcg/kg per day, increase G-CSF dosage to 10 mcg/kg per day and follow dose adjustment guidelines

Peripheral blood progenitor cells (PBPCs) collection:
Filgrastim 10 mcg/kg/day; administer by subcutaneous injection or continuous infusion

Notes:
- The optimal timing and duration of growth factor stimulation have not been determined
- Administration is recommended to begin 4 days before the first leukapheresis and continued until the last leukapheresis

Severe chronic neutropenia (SCN):
Congenital neutropenia
Filgrastim 6 mcg/kg per dose; administer by subcutaneous injection twice daily, continually
Idiopathic or cyclic neutropenia
Filgrastim 5 mcg/kg per day; administer by subcutaneous injection, continually

Notes:
- Chronic daily administration is needed to maintain clinical benefit
- ANC should not be used as the sole indication of efficacy
  - Dosages should be individually adjusted based on a patient's clinical course as well as ANC
- In a postmarketing surveillance study, median daily doses were 6 mcg/kg (congenital neutropenia), 2.1 mcg/kg (cyclic neutropenia), and 1.2 mcg/kg (idiopathic neutropenia). In rare instances patients with congenital neutropenia have required dosages ≥100 mcg/kg per day

Notes on dosing:
- The recommendations listed apply only to adult patients
- Doses for obese patients should be calculated on actual body weight, including morbidly obese patients
- Do not empirically reduce doses in elderly patients because of patient age

Preparation for intravenous administration:
- Filgrastim may be diluted in 5% dextrose injection (D5W) to a concentration within the range of 5–15 mcg/mL
  - Dilution to concentrations <5 mcg/mL is not recommended

(continued)

Efficacy

- In a phase III placebo-controlled trial of patients with small cell lung cancer, filgrastim use reduced the incidence of febrile neutropenia after chemotherapy by 36% (76% vs. 40%, P <0.001)
- An increase in ANC is seen approximately 24 hours after beginning filgrastim administration
- A 50% decrease in circulating neutrophils occurs within 1–2 days after discontinuing filgrastim use, which returns to pretreatment levels within 4–7 days
- In patients with AML receiving induction chemotherapy, filgrastim use reduced the median time to ANC recovery by 5 days (P <0.0001), the median duration of fever by 1.5 days (P = 0.009), and resulted in a statistically significant reduction in duration of intravenous antibiotic use and hospitalization
- In patients with AML receiving consolidation therapy, filgrastim significantly reduced the incidence of severe neutropenia, time to neutrophil recovery, the incidence and duration of fever, and the duration of intravenous antibiotic use and hospitalization
- After BMT, patients who received filgrastim support had a statistically significant reduction in the median number of days of severe neutropenia (21.5 vs. 10 days) and in the number of days of febrile neutropenia (13.5 vs. 5 days)
- In mobilized PBPCs, both CFU-GM and CD34+ cells were increased by more than 10-fold from baseline on day 5, and remained increased with leukapheresis. During engraftment, filgrastim-treated patients had significantly fewer days of platelet transfusion (median 6 vs. 10 days), fewer days of RBC transfusion (median 2 vs. 3 days), and significantly shorter time to recover a sustained ANC ≥500/mm³
- In 120 patients with severe chronic neutropenia, filgrastim treatment resulted in significant benefits in the incidence and duration of infection, fever, antibiotic use, and oropharyngeal ulcers[6]

(*continued*)

- The diluted product must be protected from adsorption to container and administration set surfaces by adding albumin (human) to the vehicle solution (D5W) to a final concentration of 2 mg/mL BEFORE adding filgrastim
- *Do not* dilute filgrastim with sodium chloride-containing solutions
  - Admixture in saline solutions may cause precipitation
- The needle cover of prefilled syringes contains dry natural rubber (a latex derivative), which may cause allergic reactions in sensitive individuals

Adverse Events

Adverse Events Reported Among Patients with Cancer Receiving Myelosuppressive Chemotherapy and GCSF Support in Clinical Trials[6]

Allergic reactions (<1 in 4000)	Dyspnea (9%)	Fever and neutropenia (13%)
Alopecia (18%)	Fatigue (11%)	Pain, unspecified (2%)
Anorexia (9%)	Fever (12%)	Skeletal pain (22%)
Chest pain (5%)	Generalized weakness (4%)	Skin rash (6%)
Constipation (5%)	Headache (7%)	Sore throat (4%)
Cough (6%)	Mucositis (12%)	Stomatitis (5%)
Diarrhea (14%)	Nausea/Vomiting (57%)	

- Bone pain was reported more frequently in patients treated at high dosages, 20–100 mcg/kg per day administered intravenously compared with low dosages of 3–10 mcg/kg per day administered subcutaneously. Bone pain is generally controlled with nonopioid analgesics but may infrequently require opioids
- Spontaneously reversible, mild-to-moderate increases in serum uric acid, lactate dehydrogenase, and alkaline phosphatase, occurred in 27–58% of 98 patients receiving cytotoxic chemotherapy

Adverse Events Reported Postmarketing
1. Splenomegaly and splenic rupture, including fatalities
2. Acute respiratory distress syndrome (ARDS)
3. Alveolar hemorrhage and hemoptysis
4. Sickle cell crisis, including fatalities
5. Cutaneous vasculitis
6. Sweet's syndrome (acute febrile neutrophilic dermatosis)
7. Decreased bone density and osteoporosis in pediatric patients with severe chronic neutropenia (SCN) receiving chronic CSF treatment[6]

Indications

Patients with neoplastic diseases
- Use after myelosuppressive chemotherapy to reduce the incidence of febrile neutropenia
- Patients with acute myeloid leukemia receiving induction or consolidation chemotherapy

BMT
- Peripheral blood progenitor cell (PBPC) collection

Patients with non-neoplastic diseases
Severe chronic neutropenia[6]

Therapy Monitoring

1. *During G-CSF therapy after cytotoxic chemotherapy:* CBC with differential, before chemotherapy and twice weekly
2. *After BMT:* CBC with differential at least 3 times per week
3. *During initiation of therapy for severe chronic neutropenia:* CBC with differential twice weekly for the first 4 weeks and for 2 weeks following dose adjustment, then monthly if ANC is stable during the first year of treatment. Thereafter, regular CBC evaluation is recommended as clinically indicated and at least quarterly
4. *PRBC collection:* ANC after 4 days of G-CSF, and consider dose modifications if WBC is >100,000/mm^3

Notes

1. The manufacturer recommends against CSF use 24 hours before or after cytotoxic chemotherapy, as well as simultaneous CSF use with chemotherapy and radiation
2. Patients must be instructed to report abdominal or shoulder tip pain, prompting evaluation for splenomegaly or splenic rupture, especially healthy donors receiving filgrastim for mobilization of PBPC
3. Patients must be instructed to report symptoms associated with respiratory distress, prompting evaluation for acute respiratory distress syndrome (ARDS)
4. Use with caution in patients with sickle cell disease; sickle cell crises have been reported following therapy. Only physicians qualified by specialized training or experience in the treatment of patients with sickle cell disorders should prescribe filgrastim for such patients, and only after careful consideration of the potential risks and benefits
5. Safety has not been established in patients with chronic myeloid leukemia (CML) or myelodysplastic syndromes (MDS), in patients receiving chemotherapy associated with delayed myelosuppression, or those receiving mitomycin or myelosuppressive doses of antimetabolites such as fluorouracil
6. In all clinical studies of the use of G-CSF for PBPC collection, G-CSF was administered after reinfusion of the collected cells
7. G-CSF is contraindicated in patients with a hypersensitivity to *Escherichia coli*–derived proteins, filgrastim, or any component of the formulation (sorbitol, polysorbate 80)
8. Patients should be referred to the "Information for Patients and Caregivers" portion of product labeling which provides information about neutrophils, neutropenia, safety, and efficacy. If home administration is desired, a puncture-resistant container for the disposal of used syringes and needles should be provided[6]

REGIMEN

PEGFILGRASTIM (PEGYLATED G-CSF, NEULASTA®)

Patients with cancers receiving myelosuppressive chemotherapy:
Pegfilgrastim 6 mg; administer subcutaneously once per chemotherapy cycle

Notes:
- A 6 mg fixed dose is recommended for adult patients whose body weight is ≥45 kg
- Administer doses at least 24 hours after cytotoxic chemotherapy is completed and at least 14 days before the next administration of cytotoxic chemotherapy
- Recommended injection sites are outer upper arm, abdomen >2 inches from the umbilicus, the front of the middle thighs, and upper outer area of the buttocks

Indications

Patients with neoplastic diseases:
To reduce the incidence of febrile neutropenia after myelosuppressive chemotherapy in patients with non-myeloid malignancies, NCCN Guidelines® (V.1.2013) recommend *routine use* of CSF support as primary prophylaxis for patients at high risk (defined >20%) and *consideration* of CSF support in patients at intermediate risk (10–20%) of developing febrile neutropenia who are receiving treatment with curative intent, adjuvant therapy, or treatment expected to prolong survival or improve QOL[2]

NCCN Guidelines® (V.1.2013) also recommend:
1. Evaluation of patients for the use of myeloid growth factors before each cycle of cytotoxic chemotherapy
2. If febrile neutropenia or dose-limiting neutropenia occurred in cycles with no CSF support, consider using a CSF
3. If febrile neutropenia or dose-limiting neutropenia occurred during a cycle in which a CSF was used, consider decreasing the dose/dosage of the myelosuppressive drugs in use or a change in the antineoplastic treatment regimen

ASCO Guidelines also recommend CSF support for:
1. Patients aged ≥65 years with diffuse aggressive lymphomas treated with curative chemotherapy (CHOP or more aggressive regimens)
2. Patients exposed to lethal doses of TBI[5]

Therapy Monitoring

Recommended only with regard to patient's hematologic status and ability to tolerate myelosuppressive chemotherapy[7]

Efficacy

- In a phase III trial in patients with breast cancer (Stages II–IV) who received combination chemotherapy with doxorubicin 60 mg/m^2 and docetaxel 75 mg/m^2, the efficacy of pegfilgrastim was similar to that of filgrastim based on the duration of severe neutropenia (1.8 days vs. 1.6 days) and the incidence of febrile neutropenia (13% vs. 20%)[7,8]
- Pegfilgrastim is primarily eliminated by neutrophil receptor binding. Consequently, pegfilgrastim concentrations decline rapidly at the onset of neutrophil recovery[7]
- In two randomized controlled trials, pegfilgrastim was similar to filgrastim in the number of days of severe neutropenia during cycles 2–4 of chemotherapy[7]
- In a placebo-controlled trial, pegfilgrastim was found to lower the incidence of febrile neutropenia compared to placebo (1% vs. 17% P <0.001), decrease hospitalizations (1% vs. 14%), and decrease anti-infective use (2% vs. 10%)[7]

Adverse Events

Adverse Events Reported in Clinical Trials[7]

≥10% of patients	
Bone pain*	31%

<10% of patients	
Pain in extremity	9%
Leukocytosis (WBC >100,000/mm^3)	<1%

*Bone pain is generally controlled with nonopioid analgesics but may infrequently require opioid use

Adverse Events Reported Postmarketing

1. Splenic rupture
2. Sickle cell crisis
3. Allergic reactions, including urticaria, rash, generalized erythema, flushing, or anaphylaxis
4. ARDS
5. Sweet syndrome
6. Cutaneous vasculitis
7. Injection-site reactions[7]

Notes

1. Safety and efficacy have not been established for PBPC mobilization
2. Allergic reactions including anaphylaxis, skin rash, generalized erythema, flushing, and urticaria have been reported. In rare cases, allergic reactions including anaphylaxis recurred within days after initial anti-allergic treatment was discontinued. Patients should report flushing, dizziness, rash, and any signs or symptoms of infection
3. Patients must be instructed to report upper left abdominal or shoulder tip pain, prompting evaluation for splenomegaly or splenic rupture
4. Patients must be instructed to report symptoms of respiratory distress including shortness of breath, prompting evaluation for acute respiratory distress syndrome
5. Use with caution in patients with sickle cell disease; sickle cell crises have been reported following therapy with filgrastim, the active component of pegfilgrastim. Only physicians qualified by specialized training or experience in the treatment of patients with sickle cell disorders should administer pegfilgrastim
6. The needle cover of prefilled syringes contains dry natural rubber (a latex derivative), which may cause allergic reactions in sensitive individuals
7. The G-CSF receptor through which pegfilgrastim and filgrastim act has been found on tumor cell lines. The possibility that pegfilgrastim acts as a growth factor for any tumor type, including myeloid malignancies and myelodysplasia, diseases for which pegfilgrastim is not approved, cannot be excluded[7]

REGIMEN

SARGRAMOSTIM (GM-CSF, LEUKINE®)

Following induction chemotherapy in AML (adults):
Sargramostim 250 mcg/m^2 per day; administer by intravenous infusion over 4 hours until ANC >1500/mm^3 for 3 consecutive days or a maximum of 42 days is reached
Notes:
- Start therapy on day 11 of cycle or 4 days after completion of induction chemotherapy if the bone marrow on day 10 is hypoblastic with <5% blasts
- This regimen may be repeated if a second cycle of induction chemotherapy is needed
- Interrupt or reduce the dose by half if ANC is >20,000 cells/mm^3
- Discontinue immediately if leukemia regrows

Mobilization of peripheral blood progenitor cells (PBPCs):
Sargramostim 250 mcg/m^2 per day; administer by intravenous infusion over 24 hours or by subcutaneous injection once daily throughout the entire course of PBPC collection
Note:
Reduce dose by 50% if WBC >50,000 cells/mm^3

Following transplantation of autologous PBPCs:
Sargramostim 250 mcg/m^2 per day; administer by intravenous infusion over 24 hours or by subcutaneous injection once daily beginning immediately after the infusion of PBPCs and continuing until ANC >1500 cells/mm^3 for 3 consecutive days

Myeloid reconstitution after autologous or allogeneic BMT:
Sargramostim 250 mcg/m^2 per day; administer by intravenous infusion over 2 hours beginning 2–4 hours after bone marrow infusion and ≥24 hours after the last dose of chemotherapy or radiation therapy. Patients should not receive sargramostim until the postmarrow infusion ANC is <500 cells/mm^3. Continue therapy until ANC >1500 cells/mm^3 for 3 consecutive days
Notes:
1. If blast cells appear or progression of the underlying disease occurs, discontinue use immediately
2. Interrupt or reduce the dosage by half if ANC is >20,000 cells/mm^3

BMT failure or engraftment delay:
Sargramostim 250 mcg/m^2 per day; administer by intravenous infusion over 2 hours for 14 consecutive days
Notes:
- If engraftment has not occurred within 7 days after completing sargramostim therapy, repeat the course of **Sargramostim** 250 mcg/m^2 per day by intravenous infusion over 2 hours for 14 consecutive days
- If engraftment has not occurred within 7 days after completing a second course of sargramostim, administer **Sargramostim** 500 mcg/m^2 per day by intravenous infusion over 2 hours for 14 consecutive days. If there is still no improvement, it is unlikely that further dose escalation will be beneficial
- If blast cells appear or progression of the underlying disease occurs, discontinue use immediately
Notes on dosing:
- If a severe adverse reaction occurs, temporarily reduce the sargramostim dosage by 50% or temporarily interrupt administration until the reaction abates
- Doses recommended are for adult patients
- Doses for obese patients should be calculated on actual body weight, including use in morbidly obese patients
- Do not empirically reduce doses in elderly patients because of patient age

Preparation of solution:
Sargramostim for intravenous infusion must be diluted with 0.9% sodium chloride injection (0.9% NS). If the final concentration of sargramostim is less than 10 mcg/mL, albumin (human) must be added to the vehicle solution (0.9% NS) to produce a final albumin concentration of 0.1% BEFORE adding sargramostim to prevent sargramostim adsorption to the product container and administration set tubing
- To produce a vehicle solution with an albumin concentration of 0.1% suitable for diluting sargramostim:

    Add 1 mL 5% albumin (human) to 49 mL 0.9% NS, *or*
    Add 0.2 mL 25% albumin (human) to 49.8 mL 0.9% NS

When administered by subcutaneous injection, sargramostim should be used without further dilution

Efficacy

- After AML 7+3 induction therapy consisting of daunorubicin 60 mg/m^2 per day for 3 consecutive days plus cytarabine 100 mg/m^2 per day for 7 consecutive days, sargramostim significantly shortened the duration of neutropenia compared to placebo[9] (ANC <500/mm^3 by 4 days, ANC <1000/mm^3 by 7 days), decreased the incidence of grades III–V infection (10% vs. 36%, respectively) and death from infection (6% vs. 15%, respectively), and significantly shortened the time to neutrophil recovery[10]
- A retrospective review of PBPC collections from patients with cancer treated with sargramostim 250 mcg/m^2 per day showed significantly higher numbers of granulocyte-macrophage colony-forming units (CFU-GM) than those collected without mobilization (11.41 × 10^4 CFU-GM/kg vs. 0.96 × 10^4 CFU-GM/kg, respectively)[9]
- In a historical controlled study of patients with lymphoma or myeloid leukemia who experienced BMT failure or engraftment delay, patients who received sargramostim with autologous transplantation achieved a median survival of 474 days versus 161 days for historical controls who had not received GM-CSF[9]
- Similarly, after failure of allogeneic hematopoietic progenitor cell transplantation, the median survival was 97 days in a group of patients who received sargramostim versus 35 days for the historical control patients who had not received GM-CSF[9]

Indications

1. Following induction chemotherapy in AML
2. Mobilization of PBPCs for collection and myeloid reconstitution after autologous PBPC transplantation
3. Myeloid reconstitution after autologous or allogeneic BMT
4. BMT failure or engraftment delays[9]

Therapy Monitoring

CBC with differential twice weekly during therapy. Monitoring of renal and hepatic function is recommended at least biweekly in patients displaying renal or hepatic dysfunction prior to initiation of treatment. Body weight and hydration status should be carefully monitored during administration. Interrupt therapy or reduce dose by half for excessive leukocytosis as defined by manufacturer: ANC >20,000 cells/mm^3 or WBC >50,000 cells/mm^3

Notes

1. Use with caution in patients with:
   a. Pre-existing cardiac disease
   b. Hypoxia, lung disease, or pulmonary symptoms
   c. Fluid retention
   d. Renal or hepatic impairment
   e. Rapid increase in peripheral blood counts
2. Use with caution in children
3. Discontinue GM-CSF immediately if blast cells appear after bone marrow infusion. It is possible that GM-CSF may act as a growth factor for tumor cells; use caution with patients with any malignancy with myeloid characteristics
4. Contraindications
   a. Patients with known hypersensitivity to GM-CSF, yeast-derived products, or any component of the sargramostim formulations, including:
      i. Mannitol, sucrose, tromethamine in both liquid and lyophilized formulations
      ii. Benzyl alcohol in the liquid formulation (do not administer to neonates, infants, pregnant women, and nursing mothers, as benzyl alcohol may cause "Gasping Syndrome")
   b. Concomitant sargramostim use with cytotoxic chemotherapy and radiation therapy
      i. Commence administering sargramostim at least 24 hours after completing myelosuppressive chemotherapy or radiation therapy, and discontinue use at least 24 hours before resuming myelosuppressive chemotherapy or radiation therapy administration
   c. Patients with >10% leukemic myeloid blasts in the bone marrow or peripheral blood
5. Efficacy of GM-CSF has not been assessed in AML patients <55 years of age[9]

Expert Opinion

According to the *ASCO 2006 Update of Recommendations for the Use of White Blood Cell Growth Factors*:
1. A reduction in febrile neutropenia (FN) is an important clinical outcome that justifies the use of CSFs when the risk of febrile neutropenia is approximately 20%
2. Primary prophylaxis with CSFs is recommended for the prevention of FN in patients who are at high-risk based on age, medical history, disease characteristics, and myelotoxicity of the chemotherapy regimen
3. Prophylactic CSF should be utilized for patients ≥65 years of age with diffuse aggressive lymphoma receiving curative chemotherapy[5]

Patient risk factors for development of febrile neutropenia include[11]:
Greatest risk factors include:
• Age >65 years
1. Types of chemotherapy, with the anthracyclines, topotecan, mitomycin, docetaxel, etoposide, gemcitabine, cisplatin, carboplatin, cyclophosphamide, ifosfamide, vinorelbine causing highest risk
2. Combination chemotherapy with more than 2 myelosuppressive agents
3. >85% of standard dose intensity
4. No myeloid growth factor

Intermediate risk factors include:
1. Type of cancer, specifically small cell lung cancer, lymphoma, and breast cancer
2. Poor renal or liver function
3. Previous chemotherapy or radiotherapy
4. Preexisting infection or neutropenia

Lower risk factors include:
1. Diabetes mellitus
2. Immunosuppressive agents such as carbamazepine, phenothiazine, diuretics
3. Recent surgeries

Adverse Events

Adverse Events Reported in >10% of Patients Receiving GM-CSF Support in Clinical Trials[9]

Fever*	Stomatitis
Nausea	Alopecia
Diarrhea	Edema
Vomiting	Anorexia
Chills*	Hypertension
Dyspnea	Hemorrhage
Peripheral edema	Rash
Asthenia*	GI hemorrhage

Pain (bone pain, headache, arthralgia, myalgia)*

*These systemic events were generally mild-moderate, and were usually prevented or reversed by the administration of analgesics and antipyretics such as acetaminophen

Adverse Events Associated with the First Administration of Sargramostim[9]

1. Respiratory distress
2. Hypoxia
3. Flushing
4. Hypotension
5. Syncope
6. Tachycardia

These signs have been reported to occur following the first administration of sargramostim in a particular cycle, and have resolved with symptomatic treatment. They usually do not recur with subsequent doses in the same cycle of treatment

Adverse Events Reported Postmarketing[9]

1. Arrhythmia
2. Fainting
3. Eosinophilia
4. Dizziness
5. Hypotension
6. Tachycardia
7. Thrombosis
8. Pain (abdominal, back, chest, and joint)
9. Transient liver function abnormalities
10. Injection-site reactions

References: Febrile Neutropenia

1. Ozer H et al. J Clin Oncol 2000;18:3558–3585
2. Myeloid growth factors. Version 2.2013. NCCN Clinical Practice Guidelines in Oncology (NCCN Guidelines™). National Comprehensive Cancer Network, Inc., 2013. At: http://www.nccn.org [accessed December 31, 2013]
3. NCI, CTCAE, National Cancer Institute (USA) Common Terminology Criteria for Adverse Events, version 4.0. At: http://ctep.cancer.gov/protocolDevelopment/electronic_applications/ctc.htm [accessed December 7, 2013]
4. RTOG® Radiation Therapy Oncology Group Cooperative Group Common Toxicity Criteria. At: http://www.rtog.org/ResearchAssociates/AdverseEventReporting/CooperativeGroupCommonToxicityCriteria.aspx [accessed December 31, 2013]
5. Smith TJ et al. 2006 update of recommendations for the use of white blood cell growth factors: an evidence-based clinical practice guideline. J Clin Oncol 2006;24:3187–3205
6. Neupogen® (filgrastim); September 2013 product label. Amgen Manufacturing, Limited, a subsidiary of Amgen, Inc. Thousand Oaks, CA
7. Neulasta® (pegfilgrastim) injection for subcutaneous use; June 2011 product label. Amgen, Inc. Thousand Oaks, CA
8. Green MD et al. Ann Oncol 2003;14;29–35
9. Leukine® (sargramostim); June 2012 product label. sanofi-aventis U.S., LLC, Bridgewater, NJ. A SANOFI COMPANY
10. Rowe JM et al. Blood 1995;86:457–462
11. Lyman GH et al. Proc Am Soc Clin Oncol 2006;24:483s [abstract 8561]

Chemotherapy-Induced Anemia

Epidemiology

Incidence rates of 50–60% for chemotherapy-induced anemia have been reported in retrospective reviews of patients with non-myeloid malignancies who were receiving myelosuppressive chemotherapy and who have required red blood cell (RBC) transfusion during therapy[1]

Agent/Regimen	Malignancy	Anemia Cases	
		% G1/2	% G3/4[2]
Paclitaxel	Breast cancer	93	7
Docetaxel	NSCLC	73–85	2–10
Docetaxel	Ovarian cancer	58–60	27–42
CHOP	Non-Hodgkin lymphoma	49	17
Topotecan	Ovarian cancer	67	32
Cisplatin/Etoposide	SCLC	59	16–55
Fluorouracil	Colorectal cancer	50–54	5–8
Vinorelbine	Breast cancer	67–71	5–14
Cisplatin/Cyclophosphamide	Ovarian cancer	43	9
Fluorouracil/Carboplatin	Head and neck	42	14
Paclitaxel-Doxorubicin	Breast cancer	78–84	8–11
Paclitaxel-Carboplatin	NSCLC	10–59	5–34

NCI, CTCAE, Version 4.0 Criteria, Anemia[3]

Grade	Severity	Hemoglobin
0	None	WNL
1	Mild	10.0 g/dL to < lower limit of normal
2	Moderate	8.0 to <10 g/dL
3	Severe	6.5 to <8 g/dL; transfusion indicated
4	Life-threatening	<6.5g/dL; urgent intervention indicated

Preparations

1. Epoetin alfa (Procrit®, Epogen®)
2. Darbepoetin alfa (Aranesp®)

Treatment Overview[4–6]

- In patients with cancer, use erythropoiesis-stimulating agents (ESAs) only for treatment of anemia associated with myelosuppressive chemotherapy
- ESAs are not indicated for patients receiving myelosuppressive therapy when the anticipated outcome is cure
- ESAs are not indicated for use in treating anemia associated with hormonal agents, therapeutic biologic products, or radiotherapy, unless a patient is also receiving myelosuppressive chemotherapy concomitantly
- Discontinue ESAs following the completion of a chemotherapy course (no plan to resume treatment)
- ESA use has not been demonstrated to improve symptoms of anemia, quality of life, fatigue, or patient well-being in controlled clinical trials
- Patients should be instructed to read the manufacturer supplied "Medication Guide and Patient Instructions for Use" and should be informed that this is not a disclosure of all possible side effects
  - According to the manufacturers' product information, "patients should be informed of the increased risks of mortality, serious cardiovascular events, thromboembolic reactions, stroke, and tumor progression"
- The possibility that ESAs can act as a growth factor for any tumor type, particularly myeloid malignancies, cannot be excluded. ESAs shortened overall survival and/or increased the risk of tumor progression or recurrence in some clinical studies in patients with breast, non–small cell lung, head and neck, lymphoid, and cervical cancers.[4–7] To decrease these risks, as well as the risk of serious cardio- and thrombo-vascular events, use the lowest dose needed to avoid red blood cell transfusion[2,5]

(continued)

Treatment Overview[4–6] (continued)

- Blood pressure in patients with a history of hypertension or cardiovascular disease should be carefully monitored and controlled prior to initiation and during treatment with ESAs
- Epoetin alpha increases the reticulocyte count within 10 days of initiation, followed by increases in the RBC count, Hgb, and Hct, usually within 2–6 weeks
- A lack of response or failure to maintain a hemoglobin response with ESAs within the recommended dosing range may be due to deficiencies of folic acid, iron, or vitamin B_{12}, which should be excluded or corrected. Baseline and periodic monitoring of iron, total iron-binding capacity, transferrin saturation ($\geq$20%), ferritin ($\geq$100 ng/mL), folate, and vitamin B_{12} levels are recommended
- Iron supplementation should be instituted as necessary to provide for increased requirements during ESA therapy
- In a prospective, randomized trial of 157 patients with cancer- or chemotherapy-related anemia, patients were randomly assigned to receive:
  1. No iron
  2. Ferrous sulfate 325 mg orally twice daily
  3. Iron dextran 100 mg intravenously at each weekly visit until the calculated dose for iron replacement was reached
     - The first 3 doses required a 25-mg iron dextran test dose administered by intravenous injection over 1–2 minutes, *followed by:*
     - Iron dextran 75 mg as a short intravenous infusion
     - A test dose was not given if allergic reactions had not occurred during the first 3 weekly doses
  4. Total dose infusion (TDI) of iron dextran calculated to achieve a desired hemoglobin concentration
     - Methylprednisolone 125 mg/dose was given before and after iron dextran to ameliorate arthralgias and myalgias associated with this method of iron administration
     - Iron dextran was given as a 25-mg test dose by intravenous injection over 1–2 minutes. If the test dose was tolerated, it was followed after a 1-hour observation period with:
     - Iron Dextran diluted in 500 mL 0.9% sodium chloride injection administered at a rate of 175 mL/h
     - Iron dextran TDI was calculated as follows for patients with body weight >15 kg:

     Dose of Iron Dextran (mL) = 0.0442 (desired Hgb − measured Hgb) × (IBW + [0.26 × IBW])

     Where:

	Hgb = hemoglobin (g/dL)
	IBW = ideal body weight (kg)
Females	IBW = 45.5 kg + 2.3 kg per inch in height >60 inches
Males	IBW = 50 kg + 2.3 kg per inch in height >60 inches

- Mean increases in Hgb levels were 0.9 g/dL, 1.5 g/dL, 2.5 g/dL, and 2.4 g/dL for the no iron, oral ferrous sulfate, weekly iron dextran, and TDI iron dextran groups, respectively. The percentage of patients who had a Hgb response was also significantly better ($P <0.01$) in both groups given iron dextran (68%) than patients who received oral therapy (36%), or no iron therapy (25%)
- Pure red blood cell aplasia (PRCA) has been reported in a limited number of patients. If a patient shows evidence of PRCA (severe anemia and low reticulocyte count), withhold treatment and evaluate patient for neutralizing antibodies to erythropoietin, contact Amgen (1-800-772-6436) to perform assays for binding and neutralizing antibodies. If PRCA is detected, do not restart or switch to any other ESA[2,4–6]
- There have been rare reports of potentially serious allergic reactions to ESAs
- Contraindications to ESA therapy are uncontrolled hypertension PRCA that begins after ESA treatment, and serious allergic reactions to ESAs.
- If home use is prescribed for a patient, the patient should be thoroughly instructed in the importance of proper disposal and cautioned against reusing needles, syringes, or drug product. A puncture-resistant container should be available for the disposal of used syringes and needles, and guidance provided on disposal of full containers

References

1. Groopman JE, Itri LM. J Natl Cancer Inst 1999;91:1616–1634
2. Cancer- and chemotherapy-induced anemia. Version 2.2014. NCCN Clinical Practice Guidelines in Oncology (NCCN Guidelines™). National Comprehensive Cancer Network, Inc., 2014. At: http://www.nccn.org [accessed December 30, 2013]
3. NCI, CTCAE, National Cancer Institute (USA) Common Terminology Criteria for Adverse Events, version 4.0. At: http://ctep.cancer.gov/protocolDevelopment/electronic_applications/ctc.htm [accessed December 7, 2013]
4. Aranesp® (darbepoetin alfa) injection, for intravenous or subcutaneous use; July 2012 product label. Amgen Inc., Thousand Oaks, CA
5. PROCRIT® (epoetin alfa) injection, for intravenous or subcutaneous use; July 2012 product label. Manufactured by Amgen Inc., Thousand Oaks, CA. Manufactured for Janssen Products, LP, Horsham, PA
6. Epogen® (epoetin alfa) injection, for intravenous or subcutaneous use; July 2012 product label. Amgen Inc., Thousand Oaks, CA
7. Bennett CL et al. JAMA 2008;299:914–924
8. Auerbach M et al. J Clin Oncol 2004;22:1301–1307
9. Rizzo JD et al. American Society of Clinical Oncology/American Society of Hematology clinical practice guideline update on the use of epoetin and darbepoetin in adult patients with cancer. J Clin Oncol 2010;28:4996–5010
10. Canon J-L et al. J Natl Cancer Inst 2006;98:273–284
11. Centers for Medicaid & Medicare Services (Accessed December 30, 2013, at cms.gov)
12. European Medicine Agency Press Release: Doc. Ref. EMEA/CHMP/333963/2008 –corr. London, 26 June. At: www.ema.europa.eu/docs/en_GB/document_library/Press_release/2009/11/WC500015069.pdf [accessed December 30, 2013]

REGIMEN

EPOETIN ALFA (EPOGEN®, PROCRIT®)

In patients with non-myeloid malignancies where anemia is due to the effect of myelosuppressive chemotherapy, and, after initiating epoetin therapy, there are planned at least two additional months of chemotherapy:

- Therapy *should not* be initiated if Hgb ≥10 g/dL
- ESA treatment should target the lowest Hgb level that will avoid RBC transfusion
- ESA therapy is not indicated for patients receiving chemotherapy with curative intent

Adult cancer patients receiving myelosuppressive chemotherapy[3]:
Epoetin alfa 40,000 units; administer by subcutaneous injection once weekly*, *or*
Epoetin alfa 150 units/kg; administer by subcutaneous injection 3 times per week

Note: NCCN Guidelines® list alternative regimens with extended dosing intervals[2]:
Epoetin alfa 80,000 Units; administer by subcutaneous injection every 2 weeks *or*
Epoetin alfa 120,000 Units; administer by subcutaneous injection every 3 weeks

*This schedule is more convenient and more practical than a 3-times-weekly regimen

Pediatric patients (ages 5–18 years) with cancer who are receiving myelosuppressive chemotherapy:
Epoetin alfa 600 Units/kg; administer by intravenous injection once weekly (maximum weekly dose = 40,000 Units)

Treatment Modifications
Reduce epoetin alfa dose by 25% when Hgb reaches a level needed to avoid transfusion or Hgb increases >1 g/dL during any 2-week period
Hold dose if Hgb exceeds a level needed to avoid transfusion. Resume epoetin alfa use at 25% less than the dose previously administered when Hgb approaches a level at which transfusions may be required
Increase epoetin alfa dose if Hgb increase is ≤1 g after 4 weeks of therapy without RBC transfusion:
For **adults patients with cancer** increase doses to either 60,000 units by subcutaneous injection weekly, *or*
300 units/kg three times weekly
For **pediatric patients with cancer** increase doses to 900 units/kg by intravenous injection (maximum weekly dose = 60,000 units)
Discontinue *epoetin alfa* if Hgb response after 8 weeks of use is <1 g/dL, or transfusion is still required
Discontinue *epoetin alfa* following completion of a chemotherapy course

Therapy Monitoring

Until a maintenance dose is established and after any dose adjustment: Monitor Hgb weekly until the hemoglobin level is stable and sufficient to minimize the need for RBC transfusion
After Hgb stabilizes: Monitor Hgb at regular intervals
Monitor iron, folate, and vitamin B_{12} status before and during treatment. Supplementation is recommended if serum ferritin <100 mcg/L or serum transferrin saturation <20%, or folate or vitamin B_{12} are less than the range of normal concentrations

Efficacy

- Among anemic patients with cancer receiving epoetin alfa or placebo concomitantly with chemotherapy, 14% vs. 28%, respectively, required transfusion support during weeks 5–16 after starting ESA treatment (59/344 were receiving cisplatin-containing regimens)[5]
- In a randomized, placebo-controlled study in patients with anemia who received chemotherapy, epoetin alfa was shown to significantly reduce transfusion requirements (24.7% vs. 39.5%, $P = 0.0057$) and raise Hgb levels (2.2 g/dL vs. 0.5 g/dL, $P = 0.001$)[2]
- A double-blind, placebo-controlled, randomized, phase III study found patients who received darbepoetin alfa 2.25 mcg/kg per week required fewer transfusions (27% vs. 52%, $P < 0.001$) than patients receiving placebo[2]

Indications

Patients with neoplastic diseases
- Anemia from concomitantly administered chemotherapy for non-myeloid, metastatic malignancies receiving chemotherapy for a minimum of 2 months
- In addition to the FDA-approved indications, ASCO/ASH 2007 guidelines recognize ESA use in low-risk myelodysplasia[9]

Patients with non-neoplastic diseases
- Anemia from chronic kidney disease (CKD)
- Zidovudine-related anemia in HIV patients
- Reduction of allogeneic blood transfusion in patients who receive elective, noncardiac, nonvascular surgery

Adverse Events

Adverse Events Reported Among Patients with Cancer Receiving Chemotherapy and Epoetin Alfa Support in Clinical Trials[6]

≥10% of Patients

Nausea (35%)	Arthralgia (10%)
Vomiting (20%)	Stomatitis (10%)
Myalgia (10%)	

1%–9% of Patients

Cough (9%)	Weight decrease (9%)
Leukopenia (8%)	Bone pain (7%)
Rash (7%)	Hyperglycemia (6%)
Insomnia (6%)	Headache (5%)
Depression (5%)	Dysphagia (5%)
Hypokalemia (5%)	Thrombosis (5%)

Adverse Events Reported Postmarketing

Seizures	Serious allergic reactions
PRCA	Porphyria

Injection-site reactions, including irritation and pain

Notes

1. Epoetin alpha increases the risk of seizures in patients with CKD. Patients should be monitored closely and contact their prescriber for new-onset seizures, premonitory symptoms, or change in seizure frequency.

2. Epoetin alfa is contraindicated in patients with hypersensitivity to any component of the formulation:

Epogen® and Procrit®

- Single-dose vials containing preservative-free epoetin alfa 2000, 3000, 4000 or 10,000 units/mL also contain the following excipients: albumin (human), sodium citrate, sodium chloride, and citric acid in water for injection, USP

- Single-dose vials containing preservative-free epoetin alfa 40,000 units/mL also contain albumin (human), sodium phosphate monobasic monohydrate, sodium phosphate dibasic anhydrate, sodium citrate, sodium chloride, and citric acid in water for injection, USP

- Multi-dose vials containing 10,000 units/mL or 20,000 units/mL of epoetin alfa also contain albumin (human), sodium citrate, sodium chloride, ± citric acid, and 1% benzyl alcohol as preservative in water for injection, USP

3. Patients with uncontrolled hypertension should not receive epoetin alfa

4. Epoetin alfa should be discontinued after completion of a course of chemotherapy

5. ESA therapy increased the risks for myocardial infarction, stroke, congestive heart failure and fatal thrombotic events (1.1% in patients with cancer participating in clinical trials). An increase in Hgb >1 g/dL over 2 weeks may contribute to these risks

6. Multi-dose vials contain benzyl alcohol, which is contraindicated in neonates, infants, pregnant women, and nursing mothers, as it may cause "Gasping Syndrome"

REGIMEN

DARBEPOETIN ALFA (ARANESP®)

In adult patients with metastatic, nonmyeloid malignancies receiving myelosuppressive chemotherapy:
- Therapy *should not* be initiated if Hgb is ≥10 g/dL
- ESA treatment should target the lowest Hgb level that will avoid RBC transfusion
- ESA therapy is not indicated for patients receiving chemotherapy with curative intent

Patients with cancer who are receiving myelosuppressive chemotherapy:
Darbepoetin 2.25 mcg/kg; administer by subcutaneous injection, once weekly, *or*
Darbepoetin alfa 500 mcg; administer by subcutaneous injection, once every 3 weeks

NCCN guidelines list alternative dosing schedules for consideration:
Darbepoetin 100 mcg weekly
Darbepoetin 200 mcg biweekly
Darbepoetin 300 mcg every three weeks

Notes:
- NCCN Guidelines® include alternative fixed dose schedules for consideration:[2]
  - **Darbepoetin alfa** 100 mcg; administer by subcutaneous injection, once weekly, *or*
  - **Darbepoetin alfa** 200 mcg; administer by subcutaneous injection, once every 2 weeks, *or*
  - **Darbepoetin alfa** 300 mcg; administer by subcutaneous injection, once every 3 weeks
- For patients who receive weekly darbepoetin, if Hgb increases <1 g/dL and remains <10 g/dL after 6 weeks of therapy, increase the darbepoetin dosage to 4.5 mcg/kg per week
- If Hgb increases >1 g/dL in a 2-week period or Hgb reaches a level needed to avoid transfusion, reduce the dosage by 40% of dose previously administered
- If Hgb exceeds a level needed to avoid transfusion, hold therapy until Hgb approaches a level where transfusion may be required, then reinitiate at a dosage decreased by 40% from the dose previously administered
- Discontinue darbepoetin following completion of a chemotherapy course, or, if after 8 weeks of therapy there is no response as measured by Hgb levels or if transfusions are still required

Therapy Monitoring[4]

Until a maintenance dose established and after any dose adjustment: Monitor Hgb weekly until hemoglobin is stable and sufficient to minimize the need for RBC transfusion
After Hgb stabilized: Monitor Hgb at regular intervals
Monitor iron, folate, and vitamin B_{12} status before and during treatment. Supplementation is recommended if serum ferritin <100 mcg/L or serum transferrin saturation <20%, or folate or vitamin B_{12} are less than the range of normal concentrations

Indications[4]

Patients with neoplastic diseases
Anemia from concomitantly administered chemotherapy that is expected to continue for a minimum of 2 months (non-curative intent) in patients with metastatic, nonmyeloid malignancies

Patients with non-neoplastic diseases
Anemia associated with chronic renal failure, including patients on dialysis and patients not on dialysis

Efficacy

Darbepoetin once weekly dosing was studied in advanced lung cancer patients (both SCLC and NSCLC) with Hgb values <11g/dL who were receiving platinum containing chemotherapy regimens. At 12 weeks, a significantly lower proportion of patients who received darbepoetin vs. placebo required a RBC transfusion (26% vs. 50%, respectively)[4]

Efficacy of darbepoetin 500 mcg administered once every 3 weeks versus 2.25 mcg/kg weekly was studied in patients with a Hgb <11g/dL undergoing cytotoxic chemotherapy. Seventy-two percent of patients required dose reductions in the every-3-weeks group whereas 77% required dose reductions in the once weekly group. Twenty-three percent of patients in the once-every-3-weeks group required RBC transfusion and 28% of the weekly group required RBC transfusion[4,10]

Adverse Events

Adverse Events Reported in Clinical Trials[4]

≥10% of Patients

Edema (12.8%)	Abdominal pain (13.2%)

<10% of Patients

Thrombotic adverse reactions (6.1%)	Arterial adverse reactions (1.2%)
Myocardial infarction (0.6%)	Venous adverse reactions (5%)
Pulmonary embolism (1.3%)	Cerebrovascular disorders* (1.7%)

*Cerebrovascular disorders encompass CNS hemorrhages and cerebrovascular accidents (ischemic and hemorrhagic)

Adverse Events Reported Postmarketing[4]

1. Seizures

2. Pure red cell aplasia

3. Serious allergic reactions

Expert Opinion

The Epogen®/Procrit® and Aranesp® revised package inserts include two additional documents: a "Medication Guide" and "A Patient Instructions for Use." The Medication Guide provides patients with important information necessary for safe and effective use of Epogen®/Procrit® and Aranesp®. Under FDA regulations, a Medication Guide must be distributed to all patients to whom the products are dispensed[2]

Prescribers should discuss with their patients the benefits of treatment with ESAs and the potential and demonstrated risks of ESAs for thrombovascular events (myocardial infarction, stroke, venous thromboembolism, thrombosis of vascular access), increased risk of tumor progression or recurrence, and shortened survival time of cancer patients before starting or continuing therapy with ESAs

In the United States, the Centers for Medicare and Medicaid Services (CMS) has ruled that Medicare will not underwrite the cost of ESAs for patients whose Hgb concentration is >10 g/dL, as stated in the July 2007 National Coverage Determination on ESAs. Currently, CMS does not make a distinction in ESA coverage between curative and palliative goals[11]

In June 2008, the European Medicines Agency recommended that the ESAs prescribing information state that "blood transfusion should be the preferred method of correcting anemia in patients suffering cancer"[12]

Randomized, Controlled Trials with Decreased Survival and/or Decreased Locoregional Control[4,7]

Tumor Type	Hgb Target	Primary End Point	Adverse Outcome in ESA Arm
Chemotherapy Trials			
Metastatic breast cancer (BEST Study)	12–14 g/dL	12-Month overall survival	Decreased 12-month survival
Lymphoid (20000161)	13–15 g/dL (M) 13–14 g/dL (F)	Proportion of patients achieving a Hgb response	Decreased overall survival
Early breast cancer (PREPARE Study)	12.5–13 g/dL	Relapse-free and overall survival	Decreased 3-year relapse-free and overall survival
Cervical cancer (GOG 191)	12–14 g/dL	Progression-free and overall survival and locoregional control	Decreased 3-year progression-free and overall survival and locoregional control

Source: Adapted from Bennett CL et al. JAMA 2008;299:914–924

Notes

1. Darbepoetin alfa increases the risk of seizure in patients with CKD; monitor patients for changes in seizure frequency or premonitory symptoms
2. Patients with uncontrolled hypertension, PRCA, or allergy to any component of Aranesp® should not receive darbepoetin alfa
   - Aranesp®, packaged in vials and prefilled syringes contains darbepoetin alfa and polysorbate 80, sodium chloride, sodium phosphate dibasic anhydrous, and sodium phosphate monobasic monohydrate, in Water for Injection, USP
3. Darbepoetin alfa should be discontinued after completion of a chemotherapy course
4. The needle cover of the prefilled syringe contains dry natural rubber (a derivative of latex), which may cause allergic reactions in individuals sensitive to latex
5. Rare cases of allergic reactions, including skin rash, anaphylactic reactions, angioedema, bronchospasm, and urticaria have been reported
6. *Do not use* darbepoetin alfa that has been shaken or frozen

Conversion of Epoetin Alfa to Darbepoetin Alfa in Adult Patients[4]

Epoetin Alfa (Units/wk)	Darbepoetin Alfa (mcg/wk)
<2,499	6.25
2,500–4,999	12.5
5,000–10,999	25
11,000–17,999	40
18,000–33,999	60
34,000–89,999	100
≥90,000	200

Chemotherapy-Induced Thrombocytopenia

Epidemiology

Among patients receiving dose-intensive myelosuppressive chemotherapy for solid tumors or lymphoma, 20–25% develop clinically significant platelet counts with nadirs $<50,000/mm^3$; nadir platelet counts $\leq 20,000/mm^3$ may occur in 10–15% of these patients[1]

NCI, CTCAE, Version 4.0 Criteria[2]

Grade	Platelet Count
0	Normal
1	$75,000/mm^3$ to normal
2	50,000 to $<75,000/mm^3$
3	25,000 to $<50,000/mm^3$
4	$<25,000/mm^3$

Preparations

Oprelvekin (Neumega®)

References

1. Dutcher JP et al. Cancer 1984;53:557–562
2. NCI, CTCAE, National Cancer Institute (USA) Common Terminology Criteria for Adverse Events, version 4.0. At: http://ctep.cancer.gov/protocolDevelopment/electronic_applications/ctc.htm [accessed December 7, 2013]
3. NEUMEGA® (oprelvekin); January 2011 product label. Wyeth Pharmaceuticals Inc., A subsidiary of Pfizer Inc. Philadelphia, PA
4. Gordon MS et al. Blood 1996;87:3615–3624

REGIMEN

OPRELVEKIN (recombinant human interleukin-11 [rhIL-11] NEUMEGA®)

Therapy Monitoring[3]

1. *Platelet counts:* Monitor during the time of the expected nadir and until adequate recovery has occurred. Discontinue oprelvekin when postnadir platelet counts are $\geq$50,000/mm^3

2. *Fluid and electrolytes:* Monitor especially in patients receiving chronic diuretic therapy. In clinical trials, 2 patients died from severe hypokalemia after high-dose ifosfamide and use of daily diuretics. A CBC should be obtained prior to chemotherapy and at regular intervals during oprelvekin therapy

Notes[3]

1. Not indicated after myeloablative chemotherapy. In a phase II trial of women who received myeloablative chemotherapy and autologous bone marrow transplant, the incidence of platelet transfusions and time to neutrophil and platelet engraftment were similar between patients who received oprelvekin or placebo. The incidence of adverse events was increased with oprelvekin use

2. *Severe or fatal adverse reaction reported postmarketing in BMT setting:* Fluid retention that may lead to pulmonary edema, capillary leak syndrome, peripheral edema, dyspnea on exertion, atrial arrhythmias, exacerbation of pre-existing pleural effusion, and papilledema

3. Safety and efficacy for oprelvekin use has also not been established in the following settings:
   a. Agents that cause delayed myelosuppression such as nitrosoureas or mitomycin
   b. Myelosuppressive regimens of >5 days' duration
   c. Chronic administration
   d. Children

4. Use with caution in patients who have a history of atrial arrhythmia or CHF, in patients at risk of developing fluid retention or CHF, patients receiving aggressive hydration, and in patients whose clinical condition can be exacerbated by fluid retention

5. Patients with a history of stroke or TIA may be at increased risk for nervous system events

6. Oprelvekin is contraindicated in patients with a history of hypersensitivity to the drug or any component of the formulation, including: glycine, dibasic sodium phosphate heptahydrate, monobasic sodium phosphate monohydrate, and water for injection

Indications

Prevention of severe thrombocytopenia (platelet count $\leq$20,000/mm^3) and the reduction of the need for platelet transfusion in adult patients who are at high risk for thrombocytopenia after myelosuppressive chemotherapy for non-myeloid malignancies

Efficacy[3]

1. In a randomized placebo-controlled trial of 93 patients with various nonmyeloid malignancies who had recovered from an episode of severe chemotherapy-induced thrombocytopenia (platelet counts $\leq$20,000/mm^3), the number of patients who required platelet transfusions was significantly less for patients who received oprelvekin (50 mcg/kg per day) than for patients who received placebo (72% versus 93%, respectively; P <0.05)

2. Oprelvekin should be reserved for patients who experienced therapy-limiting thrombocytopenia; it is not recommended for routine primary prophylaxis against thrombocytopenia

3. Platelet increases are seen within 5–9 days. After cessation of treatment, platelet counts continue to increase for up to 7 days, then return toward baseline within 14 days

Adverse Events

Adverse Events Reported Among Patients Receiving Oprelvekin in Clinical Trials[3]

Boxed warning: Allergic or hypersensitivity reactions, including anaphylaxis, have been reported in the postmarketing setting

$\geq$10% of Patients

Anemia*		Fever	36%	Palpitations†	14%
Asthenia†	14%	Headache	41%	Pharyngitis	25%
Atrial fibrillation/flutter†	12%	Increased cough	29%	Pleural effusion†	10%
Conjunctival injection†	19%	Insomnia	33%	Rash	25%
Diarrhea	43%	Mucositis	43%	Rhinitis	42%
Dizziness	38%	Nausea/vomiting	77%	Syncope	13%
Dyspnea†	48%	Neutropenia and fever	42%	Tachycardia†	20%
Edema†	59%	Oral moniliasis†	14%	Vasodilation	19%

*Probably a dilutional phenomenon; appears within 3–5 days after initiating therapy and resolves in about 1 week after discontinuing oprelvekin use
†Occurred in significantly more in oprelvekin-treated patients than in placebo-treated patients

(continued)

Adverse Events (continued)

<10% of Patients

Antibody development (1%)

Papilledema (2%)

Stroke (unknown rate)

Note: In clinical studies, most adverse events resolved within 7 days of oprelvekin discontinuation[4]

Sudden death (two patients): Investigator considered "possibly or probably related to oprelvekin." Both deaths occurred in patients with severe hypokalemia (serum concentrations <3mEq/L [<3 mmol/L]) who had received high-dose ifosfamide and were receiving daily doses of a diuretic

Serious and/or Frequent Adverse Events Reported Postmarketing[3]

Allergic reactions and anaphylaxis/anaphylactoid reactions	Ventricular arrhythmias
Papilledema	Capillary leak syndrome
Visual disturbances ranging from blurred vision to blindness	Renal failure
Injection-site reactions (dermatitis, pain, and discoloration)	Optic neuropathy

Dosage

Patients with cancer receiving myelosuppressive chemotherapy:
Oprelvekin 50 mcg/kg per day; administer by subcutaneous injection, beginning 6–24 hours after completion of chemotherapy until platelet count is $\geq$50,000/mm^3 or for a maximum of 21 days

Notes:
- Product concentration after reconstitution is 5 mg/mL
- Do not round doses
- Administer oprelvekin for a maximum of 21 days for up to 6 cycles
- Discontinue oprelvekin at least 2 days before starting myelosuppressive chemotherapy
- Administer subcutaneously in the abdomen, thighs, hips, or upper arms
- In renal impairment (creatinine clearance <30 mL/min [<0.5 mL/s]), reduce dosage to 25 mcg/kg per day
- Recommended dosage in obese adults does not differ from the standard adult dose of 50 mcg/kg per day, which is based on actual body weight. The maximum patient weight treated with oprelvekin in clinical trials was 147 kg

44. Indications for Bone-Modifying Agents in Hematology-Oncology

Reem Abozena Shalabi, PharmD, BCOP and James N. Frame, MD, FACP

Primary Indications in Patients with Cancer

1. To protect bone from new metastatic lesions
2. To treat hypercalcemia of malignancy
3. To prevent treatment-related bone demineralization, osteolysis, and pathologic fractures
4. To treat osteolytic lesions, decrease the incidence of pathologic fractures, prevent skeletal deformities, and prevent and decrease the severity of pain

Intravenous Versus Oral Bisphosphonates

Intravenous

1. Much more effective than oral agents at reversing hypercalcemia and relieving bone pain, particularly in patients with breast cancer and multiple myeloma
2. Can overcome disadvantages associated with oral agents, including poor absorption from the GI tract (<3% oral bioavailability); have a lower incidence of adverse GI events
3. Require clinic/hospital administration

Oral

1. Convenient
2. Absorption can be impaired by food and beverages other than water
3. Associated with greater incidence of upper GI toxicity than with intravenous administration, including dysphagia; esophagitis; and esophageal, gastric, or duodenal erosion; ulceration; and perforation

Body JJ et al. J Clin Oncol 1998;16:3890–3899
Riccardi A et al. Tumori 2003;89:223–236

Hypocalcemic Effects

Bisphosphonate	Median Time to Normocalcemia	Duration of Normocalcemia	% Achieving Normocalcemia
Zoledronic acid[1]	4 days	32 days	87
Pamidronate[2,3]	4 days	28 days	70–100
Clodronate[3]	3 days	14 days	80
Alendronate[4]	4 days	15 days	74
Ibandronate[5]	4 days	14 days	76.5
Etidronate[6]	4 days	29 days	63

References

1. Major P et al. J Clin Oncol 2001;19:558–567
2. Body JJ, Dumon JC. Ann Oncol 1994;5:359–363
3. Purohit OP et al. Br J Cancer 1995;72:1289–1293
4. Nussbaum SR et al. J Clin Oncol 1993;11:1618–1623
5. Pecherstorfer M et al. Support Care Cancer 2003;11:539–547
6. Singer FR et al. Arch Int Med 1991;151:471–476

Notes

Osteonecrosis of the Jaw

1. The American Society of Bone and Mineral Research Task Force has defined osteonecrosis of the jaw (ONJ) as the presence of exposed bone in the maxillofacial region that does not heal within 8 weeks after identification by a healthcare professional[1]

2. Potential risk factors for developing ONJ in patients with cancer[2]:

   a. Poor oral hygiene and periodontal disease[3]

   b. History of dental procedures for extractions or denture use (that may cause soft tissue injury)

   c. Prolonged exposure to high doses of intravenous bisphosphonates

   d. Intravenous bisphosphonate use poses greater risk than oral bisphosphonates

   e. Zoledronic acid seems to cause more ONJ compared to pamidronate[4]

   f. ONJ developed in 7% to 10% of patients with myeloma and 4% of patients with breast cancer

   g. Among patients on oral bisphosphonates (eg, alendronate), there is a very low risk (estimated at 0.7 cases of per 100,000 person-years exposure) of developing bone osteonecrosis[5]

   h. Radiation-induced damage with head and neck cancer or oral cancer[3]

   i. Concomitant therapy with corticosteroids; chemotherapy[3]

3. Clinical presentation and diagnosis of ONJ

   a. Signs and symptoms include localized pain, soft-tissue swelling and inflammation, loosening of previously stable teeth, drainage, and exposed bone. These symptoms most commonly occur at the site of previous tooth extraction or other dental surgical procedures but may also occur spontaneously. Objective signs before overt clinical presentation may include a sudden change in the health of periodontal or mucosal tissues, failure of the oral mucosa to heal, oral pain, loose teeth, or soft-tissue infection[3]

4. Supportive treatment[2]

   a. Antiseptic oral rinses (eg, 0.12% chlorhexidine gluconate)

   b. The decision to treat with an antibiotic is a clinical judgment and should be made by an oral maxillofacial surgeon or other dental specialist with the treating physician/oncologist. If an antibiotic is used, cultures should be collected to determine appropriate antimicrobial intervention. Cultures should include assessment of aerobic and anaerobic bacteria, viral, and fungal species[3]

   c. Limited surgical debridement as needed, which usually leads to healing

5. The bisphosphonates class of medications have clearly enhanced care of patients with oncologic disease. ONJ is an unforeseen and unfortunate potential adverse effect associated with these medications[6]

   a. All oncology patients should receive a comprehensive dental examination to include a panoramic jaw radiograph and appropriate preventive dentistry before starting bisphosphonate therapy

   b. At a minimum, oncologists should perform a visual inspection of the oral cavity at baseline and at each follow-up visit to look for the presence of necrotic or exposed bone[3]

   c. Good oral hygiene along with regular dental care is the best way to lower risk

   d. Active oral infections should be treated, and sites at high risk for infection should be eliminated

   e. While on therapy, patients should maintain excellent oral hygiene along with regular dental care[5], and, if possible, avoid invasive dental procedures[6]

   f. Patients should be instructed to contact their dentist if any problem develops in the oral cavity[5]

   g. Patients should be instructed to inform their dentist if they are taking bisphosphonate medications[5]

   h. The decision to defer or discontinue bisphosphonate therapy must be made by the treating oncologist in consultation with an oral maxillofacial surgeon or other dental specialist[3]

Role of Bone-modifying Agents (Bisphosphonates) in Multiple Myeloma

The American Society of Clinical Oncology (ASCO) first published evidence-based clinical practice guidelines in 2002, which were reviewed and expanded in 2007. Below is a summary of the updated guidelines[6]:

1. For patients with lytic bone disease on plain radiographs, a bisphosphonate is recommended. **Pamidronate** 90 mg administered intravenously over at least 2 hours every 3 to 4 weeks may be preferable to **zoledronic acid** 4 mg intravenously over at least 15 minutes due to an increased risk of ONJ with the latter[4]

2. Monitoring: Renal adverse events have resulted in increased caution with regard to dosing. New dosing guidelines were added to recommendations for zoledronic acid use in patients with pre-existing renal impairment

   a. Practitioners should monitor patients receiving pamidronate or zoledronic acid for albuminuria every 3 to 6 months

   b. In patients experiencing unexplained albuminuria (>500 mg albumin in urine per 24 hours), discontinuation of the drug is advised until renal problems are resolved. Reassessment is recommended every 3 to 4 weeks (with a 24-hour urine collection for total protein and urine protein electrophoresis). If treatment with pamidronate resumes after renal function returns to baseline, the drug should be administered over a longer infusion duration (≥4 hours) and at doses and treatment intervals not greater than 90 mg every 4 weeks

   c. The ASCO practice guidelines 2007 Update Committee supported the use of screening urinalysis for proteinuria, but underscores that a 24-hour urine collection for determination of total protein and electrophoresis is required if the screening test is positive. Similar guidelines are not available for zoledronic acid; however, some Update Committee members recommended that treatment with zoledronic acid when resumed should be administered over durations greater than 15 minutes (eg, ≥30 minutes)

(continued)

Notes *(continued)*

3. Duration of therapy: the ASCO 2007 Update Committee recommended monthly bisphosphonate for a maximum of 2 years after tandem transplant for multiple myeloma[6]

   a. The Update Committee also recommended that physicians should seriously consider discontinuing bisphosphonate therapy in patients with responsive or stable disease, but continued use remains at the discretion of a treating physician. For patients in whom bisphosphonate therapy is discontinued after 2 years of treatment, bisphosphonate therapy may be resumed upon relapse with new-onset skeletal-related events

4. Bisphosphonate therapy is reasonable in a patient with multiple myeloma with osteopenia without evidence of lytic bone lesions on radiographs

5. Bisphosphonate therapy is not recommended in a patient with indolent myeloma or solitary plasmacytoma with no lytic bone lesions

6. Bisphosphonate therapy is not recommended for patients with monoclonal gammopathy of undetermined significance (MGUS)

7. Measuring biochemical markers to monitor bisphosphonate use is not recommended

8. Pamidronate or zoledronic acid is recommended for management of pain as a result of osteolytic disease and as adjunct for patients receiving radiation, analgesics, or surgical intervention to stabilize fractures

9. A discussion related to osteonecrosis of the jaw was added to the guidelines

The International Myeloma Working Group reviewed data published through August 2012, and developed additional recommendations for the management of multiple myeloma-related bone disease[7]:

1. Bisphosphonates should be considered in all patients who are receiving first-line anti-myeloma therapy

2. Zoledronic acid or pamidronate is recommended for preventing skeletal-related events in patients with multiple myeloma

3. Zoledronic acid is preferred over oral clodronate because of potential anti-myeloma effect and survival benefit

Role of Bone-modifying Agents in Metastatic Breast Cancer

On February 22, 2011, the American Society of Clinical Oncology (ASCO) published an "Executive Summary of the Clinical Practice Guideline Update on Bone-modifying Agents in Metastatic Breast Cancer."[8] The guideline updates previously published guidance for use of bisphosphonates in patients with breast cancer (2003) and changed the term, "bisphosphonates," to "bone-modifying agents" (BMA). A separate ASCO update will address the role of BMA for adjunctive treatment of breast cancer and for the management of treatment-associated bone loss. A summary of the 2011 guideline update follows:

1. For patients with breast cancer and bone metastases with evidence of bone destruction on radiographs, CT scans, or MRI, treatment with BMA, including: **Denosumab** 120 mg administered subcutaneously every 4 weeks, *or* **Pamidronate** 90 mg intravenously administered over not less than 2 hours every 3 to 4 weeks, *or* **Zoledronic** acid 4 mg administered intravenously over not less than 15 minutes every 3 to 4 weeks is recommended

   a. Treatment with BMA for an abnormal bone scan without bone destruction is not recommended outside of a clinical trial

   b. The Update Committee determined that there is insufficient evidence comparing efficacy between BMA to prefer one over another

2. For women with breast cancer and extra-skeletal metastases without evidence of bone metastases, treatment with BMA is not recommended

3. Recommendations relative to renal safety concerns with BMA (see sections in this chapter about individual BMA and consult current product labeling for guidance about dose/dosage modifications in renally impaired persons):

   a. In patients with a CrCl >60 mL/min (>1 mL/s), doses/dosages, infusion times, and dosing intervals are not modified for pamidronate or zoledronic acid

      i. Product labeling for zoledronic acid includes guidance for use when CrCl is ≥30 mL/min (≥0.5 mL/s) but <60 mL/min

      ii. Infusion times <2 hours for pamidronate or <15 minutes for zoledronic acid are to be avoided

   b. The Update Panel recommended that serum creatinine should be monitored prior to each dose of pamidronate or zoledronic acid in accordance with FDA-approved labeling. In addition, serum electrolytes, including calcium, phosphate, and magnesium, and hemoglobin and hematocrit should be monitored regularly

      i. The risk of hypocalcemia with denosumab 120 mg every 4 weeks has not been evaluated in patients with a CrCl <30 mL/min or undergoing dialysis. Patients with impaired CrCl who receive treatment with denosumab should be closely monitored for evidence of hypocalcemia

   c. For patients treated with denosumab, pamidronate, or zoledronic acid there is no evidence to guide the interval for monitoring serum electrolytes, hemoglobin, and hematocrit

4. Recommendations/observations relative to osteonecrosis of the jaw (ONJ) and BMA:

   a. ONJ is an uncommon but potentially serious complication associated with the use of BMA

   b. The Update Committee concurs with revised FDA labeling for pamidronate, zoledronic acid, and denosumab, and recommends that all patients with cancer receive a dental examination and necessary preventive dentistry prior to initiating therapy with an inhibitor of osteoclast function unless there are mitigating factors that preclude a dental assessment

      i. Patients should maintain optimal oral hygiene, and, if possible, avoid invasive dental procedures that involve manipulation of the jawbone or periosteum while receiving inhibitors of osteoclast function. Good oral hygiene includes brushing and flossing teeth after meals and use of a fluoride mouth rinse

(continued)

Notes (continued)

ii. Therapy initiation with BMA should be delayed whenever possible in a setting of invasive dental procedures until the initial bone healing process of the tooth socket bone has taken place. The Update Committee consensus recommendation for initiating bone-modifying therapy after invasive manipulation of bone underlying the teeth is that it should ideally be delayed for 14 to 21 days to allow for wound healing, if the clinical situation permits

c. Most cases of ONJ have occurred in patients receiving intravenously administered bisphosphonates who have undergone invasive dental procedures. However, ONJ has been reported to occur spontaneously, and in patients treated with other BMA, including oral bisphosphonates and direct osteoclast inhibitors

5. Once initiated, the optimal duration of BMA is to continue therapy until, based on clinical judgment, there is evidence of substantial decline in a patient's general performance status

a. There is no evidence addressing the consequences of stopping BMA after ≥1 adverse skeletal-related events

6. The optimal intervals between dosing for BMA are every 4 weeks for denosumab 120 mg, subcutaneously; and every 3 to 4 weeks for pamidronate 90 mg, intravenously over 2 hours, and for zoledronic acid 4 mg intravenously, over 15 minutes

7. For patients with pain secondary to bone metastases, BMA are an adjunctive therapy for controlling bone pain, and are not recommended as first-line treatment for cancer-related pain

8. The use of biochemical markers of bone metabolism to guide or monitor BMA use is not recommended outside of a clinical trial

Vitamin D Deficiency

1. If a patient is receiving a bisphosphonate for osteoporosis, healthcare providers are likely to check a patient's vitamin D level. If the indication is metastatic bone disease, a vitamin D level is often overlooked

2. A 25-hydroxyvitamin D (25-OHD) level of approximately 30 ng/mL (~75 nmol/L) is an acceptable target

3. An appropriate dose of Vitamin D supplementation in oncology patients is 1000 International Units daily as endorsed by the Dietary Guidelines for Americans[9]

Musculoskeletal Pain

1. An FDA Alert issued in January 2008 highlighted the possibility of severe and sometimes incapacitating bone, joint, and/or muscle (musculoskeletal) pain in patients taking bisphosphonates[10]

2. Severe musculoskeletal pain may occur within days, months, or years after starting a bisphosphonate. Some patients have reported complete relief of symptoms after discontinuing the bisphosphonate, whereas others have reported slow or incomplete resolution. The risk factors and incidence of severe musculoskeletal pain associated with bisphosphonates are unknown

3. The severe musculoskeletal pain associated with bisphosphonates is in contrast to the acute phase response characterized by fever, chills, bone pain, myalgias, and arthralgias that sometimes accompanies initial intravenous administration of bisphosphonates and may occur with initial exposure to once-weekly or once-monthly doses of oral bisphosphonates

a. The symptoms related to the acute phase response tend to resolve within several days with continued drug use

4. Healthcare professionals should consider whether bisphosphonate use may be responsible for severe musculoskeletal pain in patients who present with these symptoms and consider temporary or permanent discontinuation of the drug

References

1. Khosla S et al. J Bone Miner Res 2007;22:1479–1491
2. Drake MT et al. Mayo Clin Proc 2008;83:1032–1045
3. Ruggiero S et al. J Oncol Pract 2006;2:7–14
4. Zervas K et al. Br J Haematol 2006;134:620–623
5. American Dental Association Council on Scientific Affairs. J Am Dent Assoc 2006;137:1144–1150
6. Kyle RA et al. J Clin Oncol 2007;25:2464–2472
7. Terpos E et al. J Clin Oncol 2013;31:2347–2357
8. Van Poznak CH et al. [see erratum] J Clin Oncol 2011;29:1221–1227. Erratum in: J Clin Oncol 2011;29:2293
9. Wang-Gillam A et al. Oncologist 2008;13:821–827
10. Information for Healthcare Professionals: Bisphosphonates (marketed as Actonel, Actonel+Ca, Aredia, Boniva, Didronel, Fosamax, Fosamax+D, Reclast, Skelid, and Zometa). U.S. Department of Health & Human Services, U.S. Food and Drug Administration, 2008. (Accessed January 28, 2014, at http://www.fda.gov/Drugs/DrugSafety/PostmarketDrugSafetyInformationforPatientsandProviders/ucm124165.htm)

REGIMENS

Key to abbreviations and symbols: 0.9% NS, 0.9% sodium chloride injection; 0.45% NS, 0.45% sodium chloride injection; D5W, 5% dextrose injection; ASCO, American Society of Clinical Oncology; AUC, area under the plasma concentration versus time curve; CrCl, creatinine clearance; SCr, serum creatinine

ZOLEDRONIC ACID (ZOMETA®)

Oncology-Related Indications	Usual Dosages	Dose Adjustments for CrCl ≤60 mL/min[†]	
Multiple myeloma and patients with documented bone metastases from solid tumors, in conjunction with standard anti-neoplastic therapy[1,2] Prostate cancer should have progressed after treatment with at least one hormonal therapy[1,2]	**Zoledronic acid** 4 mg; administer intravenously in 100 mL 0.9% NS or D5W* over at least 15 minutes every 3–4 weeks (4 mg is recommended for patients with CrCl >60 mL/min [>1 mL/s]) Supplementation for myeloma and bone metastases from solid tumors: **Calcium** 500 mg/day orally, *plus* **vitamin D** 400 IU/day orally	**Pre-Treatment CrCl**	**Recommended Dose**
		50–60 mL/min (0.83–1 mL/s)	3.5 mg
		40–49 mL/min (0.66–0.81 mL/s)	3.3 mg
		30–39 mL/min (0.5–0.65 mL/s)	3 mg

[†]Doses are calculated to produce an AUC (0.6 mg · hour/L) similar to that achieved in patients with CrCl = 75 mL/min (1.25 mL/s)

		Baseline SCr	SCr Increase	Action
Hypercalcemia of malignancy: Serum Ca[2+] ≥12 mg/dL (≥3 mmol/L)[1]	**Zoledronic acid** 4 mg intravenously in 100 mL 0.9% NS or D5W* over at least 15 minutes every 3–4 weeks	Within normal limits	≥0.5 mg/dL (≥44.2 µmol/L)	Withhold zoledronic acid until SCr decreases to within 10% of baseline, then resume with the same dose given previously
		Abnormal	≥1 mg/dL (≥88.4 µmol/L)	
	Notes: Avoid mixing zoledronic acid with calcium- or other divalent cation-containing solutions, such as Lactated Ringer's Injection *Do not* administer zoledronic acid through a common intravenous line or the same fluid pathway through which other drugs are being administered	Dose adjustments of zoledronic acid are not necessary in treating patients for hypercalcemia of malignancy presenting with mild-to-moderate renal impairment prior to the initiation of therapy (ie, with SCr <4.5 mg/dL; <400 µmol/L) *Note:* Patients with SCr ≥4.5 mg/dL (≥400 µmol/L) were excluded from trials of hypercalcemia of malignancy		

Toxicity

>10%	Fever (30–40%), nausea/vomiting (29%), constipation (26.7%), hypomagnesemia (10.5%), hypotension (10.5%)
1–10%	Bone/back pain (10%), flulike syndrome, injection site reaction, dyspepsia, hypocalcemia, hypophosphatemia, hypermagnesemia, increased serum creatinine
<1%	Rash, pruritus, increased liver transaminases, chest pain, ocular inflammation, uveitis, iritis, scleritis, episcleritis, conjunctivitis, osteonecrosis of jaw

References

1. Ibrahim A et al. Clin Cancer Res 2003;9:2394–2399
2. Zometa (zoledronic acid) Injection product label, October 2009 (revised). Novartis Pharmaceuticals Corporation, East Hanover, NJ

Efficacy

Zometa Compared to Placebo in Patients with Bone Metastases from Prostate Cancer or Other Solid Tumors

		I. Analysis of Proportion of Patients with a SRE*			II. Analysis of Time to the First SRE		
Study	Study Arm & Patient No.	Proportion	Difference[†] & 95% CI	P-Value	Days (Median)	Hazard Ratio[‡] & 95% CI	P-Value
Prostate cancer	Zometa 4 mg (n = 214 Placebo (n = 208)	33% 44%	−11% (−20%, −1%)	0.02	Not reached 321	0.67 (0.49, 0.91)	0.011
Solid tumors (other than breast or prostate)	Zometa 4 mg (n = 257) Placebo (n = 250)	38% 44%	−7% (−15%, 2%)	0.13	230 163	0.73 (0.55, 0.96)	0.023

*SRE: skeletal-related event
[†]Difference for the proportion of patients with a SRE for Zometa 4 mg vs. placebo
[‡]Hazard ratio for the first occurrence of a SRE for Zometa vs. placebo
Note: In these studies, Zometa infusion duration was increased from 5 to 15 minutes every 3–4 weeks due to renal toxicity; the median treatment durations for the prostate cancer group and solid tumors group were 10.5 mo and 3.8 mo, respectively

Zometa Compared to Pamidronate in Patients with Multiple Myeloma or Bone Metastases from Breast Cancer

		I. Analysis of Proportion of Patients with a SRE*			II. Analysis of Time to the First SRE		
Study	Study Arm & Patient No.	Proportion	Difference[†] & 95% CI	P-Value	Days (Median)	Hazard Ratio[‡] & 95% CI	P-Value
Multiple myeloma and breast cancer	Zometa 4 mg (n = 561) Pamidronate (n = 555)	44% 46%	−2% (−7.9, 3.7%)	0.46	373 363	0.92 (0.77, 1.09)	0.32

*SRE: skeletal-related event
[†]Difference for the proportion of patients with a SRE for Zometa 4 mg vs. pamidronate 90 mg
[‡]Hazard ratio for the first occurrence of a SRE for Zometa vs. pamidronate 90 mg
Note: In these studies, Zometa infusion duration was increased from 5 to 15 minutes every 3–4 weeks due to renal toxicity; pamidronate 90 mg was administered intravenously every 3–4 weeks; the median treatment duration was 12 months

Pooled Study Data[†] of Zometa Compared to Pamidronate in Patients with Hypercalcemia of Malignancy[‡]

Variable[§]	Zometa 4 mg		Pamidronate 90 mg	
Complete response[ϵ]	Patient numbers	Response rates	Patient numbers	Response rates
By Day 4	86	45.3%	99	33.3%
By Day 7	86	86.2%*	99	63.6%
Duration of response	Patient numbers	Median duration (d)	Patient numbers	Median duration (d)
Time to relapse	86	30*	99	17
Duration of CR	76	32	69	18

*P-value <0.05 vs. pamidronate 90 mg
[†]Data were derived from two identical multicenter, randomized, double-blind, double-dummy studies of Zometa 4 mg given intravenously over 5 minutes or pamidronate 90 mg given intravenously over 2 h. The two multicenter trials of hypercalcemia of malignancy were combined in a preplanned analysis. The most common tumor types were lung, breast, head and neck, and renal; median patient age is 59 years. The Zometa infusion duration of 5 minutes, as performed in this study, is not recommended due to an increased risk of renal failure. Zometa should be administered intravenously over not less than 15 minutes
[‡]Hypercalcemia of malignancy was defined as a corrected serum calcium (CSC) concentration of ≥12.0 mg/dL (≥3.00 μmol/L)
[§]Primary efficacy variable was the proportion of patients who had a complete response (defined as the lowering of the CSC to ≤10.8 mg/dL (≤2.70 μmol/L) within 10 days after Zometa administration
[ϵ]The proportion of patients whose CSC normalized by Day 10 were 88% and 70% for Zometa 4 mg and pamidronate 90 mg, respectively (P = 0.002)

Monitoring Therapy

1. Prior to therapy: See *Guidance, Caveat, and Comments* section for Zometa dosage adjustments relative to renal function (creatinine clearance may be calculated using the Cockcroft Gault formula)

   a. Patients treated with Zometa should not be treated with Reclast (contains same active ingredient as Zometa)

   b. Caution is advised when Zometa is used in conjunction with loop diuretics (may increase hypocalcemia), thalidomide (may increase risk of renal dysfunction), and other potentially nephrotoxic drugs

2. For patients with hypercalcemia of malignancy:

   a. Initiate treatment only after: (1) adequate hydration with 0.9%NS; (2) adequate urine output of $\approx$2 L/d throughout therapy; and (3) avoidance of over-hydration, especially in patients with CHF

   b. Encourage ambulatory patients to maintain hydration orally

   c. If hypercalcemia persists or recurs, there should be $\geq$7 days between consecutive treatments

3. Supplementation for myeloma and bone metastases from solid tumors: calcium 500 mg/day, administer orally + Vitamin D 400 International Units/day, administer orally

4. During therapy:

   a. Standard hypercalcemia-related metabolic parameters, such as levels of calcium, phosphate, magnesium, and serum creatinine, should be carefully monitored. Short-term supplemental therapy may be necessary if hypokalemia, hypophosphatemia, or hypomagnesemia occurs

   b. For patients with multiple myeloma and metastatic bone lesions of solid tumors, the serum creatinine should be measured before each dose of zoledronic dose and treatment withheld for renal deterioration (see *Guidance, Caveats, and Comments* section for dose adjustments)

5. Patient counseling information:

   a. Patients should be instructed to tell their healthcare provider if they have kidney problems before being given Zometa

   b. Patients should be informed of the importance of getting their blood tests (eg, serum creatinine) during the course of their Zometa therapy

   c. Female patients should not be given Zometa if they are pregnant or breast feeding, or plan to become pregnant

   d. Patients should be advised to have a dental examination prior to treatment with Zometa and should avoid invasive dental procedures during treatment

   e. Patients should be informed of the importance of good dental hygiene and routine dental care

   f. Patients with multiple myeloma and bone metastases should be advised to take an oral calcium supplement of 500 mg and a multiple vitamin containing 400 IU of vitamin D daily

   g. Patients should be aware of the most common side effects of Zometa, including anemia, nausea, vomiting, constipation, diarrhea, fatigue, pyrexia, weakness, lower limb edema, anorexia, decreased weight, bone pain, myalgia, arthralgia, back pain, worsening of their malignancy, headache, dizziness, insomnia, paresthesia, dyspnea, cough, and abdominal pain

ZOLEDRONIC ACID (RECLAST®)

Indications	Usual Doses, Administration Routes, and Schedules	Guidance, Caveats, and Comments
Treatment of osteoporosis in postmenopausal women	Zoledronic acid 5 mg; administer intravenously in 100 mL ready to infuse solution over at least 15 minutes through a separate vented infusion line every 12 months (up three doses in clinical trials)	Exclusions: patients with baseline creatinine clearance <30 mL/min (<0.5 mL/s); urine dipstick ≥2+ or increase in serum creatinine >0.5 mg/dL (>44.2 μmol/L) during screening visits; pregnant women; patients being treated with Zometa for oncology indications
Prevention of osteoporosis in postmenopausal women	**Zoledronic acid** 5 mg; administer intravenously in 100 mL ready to infuse solution over at least 15 minutes through a separate vented infusion line every 2 years	Supplementation: elemental calcium orally, 1000–1500 mg/d and vitamin D orally, 400–1200 IU/d
Treatment to increase bone mass in men with osteoporosis	**Zoledronic acid** 5 mg; administer intravenously in 100 mL ready to infuse solution over at least 15 minutes through a separate vented infusion line once annually up to a total of 2 doses	All osteoporosis patients should be instructed on the importance of calcium and vitamin D supplementation in maintaining serum calcium levels
Treatment and prevention of glucocorticoid-induced osteoporosis in patients expected to be using glucocorticoids for at least 12 mo (≥7.5 mg of prednisone or equivalent per day in clinical trial)	**Zoledronic acid** 5 mg; administer intravenously in 100 mL ready to infuse solution over at least 15 minutes through a separate vented infusion line	Pre-existing conditions: pre-existing hypocalcemia and disturbances of mineral metabolism (eg, hypo-parathyroidism, thyroid surgery, parathyroid surgery, malabsorption syndromes, excision of small intestine) must be treated before initiating therapy with Reclast. Clinical monitoring of calcium, phosphorus, and magnesium levels is highly recommended for these patients

EFFICACY: Treatment Summary of Osteoporosis in Postmenopausal Women (Reclast vs. Placebo)

Outcome	Reclast (N = 3875) Event Rate*, n (%)	Placebo (N = 3861) Event Rate*, n (%)	Absolute Risk Reduction in Fracture Incidence, % (95% CI)	Relative Risk Reduction in Fracture Incidence % (95% CI)
Any clinical fracture§	308 (8.4)	456 (12.8)	4.4 (3.0, 5.8)	33 (23, 42)†
Clinical vertebral fracture℃	19 (0.5)	84 (2.6)	2.1 (1.5, 2.7)	77 (63, 86)†
Non-vertebral fracture**	292 (8.0)	388 (10.7)	2.7 (1.4, 4.0)	25 (13, 36)‡

*Event rates based on Kaplan-Meier estimates at 36 mo
†P-value <0.001
‡P-value <0.0001
§Excludes finger, toe, and facial fractures
§Includes clinical thoracic and clinical lumbar vertebral fractures
**Excludes finger, toe, facial, and clinical thoracic and lumbar fractures

EFFICACY: Prevention of Osteoporosis in Postmenopausal Women with Osteopenia (Reclast vs. Placebo)*

Outcome	Clinical study: 581 women with osteopenia; 2-year randomized, multi-center, double-blind, placebo-controlled study. Age ≥45 years, stratified by years after menopause: Stratum I (<5 years after menopause; n = 224) and Stratum II (≥5 years after menopause; n = 357). Strata I and II patients were randomized to one of three groups: (1) Reclast given at randomization and at month 12 (Stratum I, n = 77; Stratum II, n = 121); (2) Reclast given at randomization and placebo at month 12 (Stratum I, n = 70; Stratum II, n = 111); and (3) Placebo given at randomization and month 12 (n = 202)
Change in BMD relative to baseline, %	Reclast given at randomization and placebo at month 12: (1) Resulted in a 6.3% increase in BMD (Stratum I) and a 5.4% increase in BMD (Stratum II) over 24 months as compared to placebo (both P <0.0001) (2) Resulted in a 4.7% increase in total hip BMD (Stratum I) and a 3.2% increase in total hip BMD (Stratum II) over 24 months as compared to placebo (both P <0.0001)

*All participants received 500 to 1200 mg of elemental calcium plus 400 to 800 IU of vitamin D supplementation per day

EFFICACY: Treatment to Increase Bone Mass in Men with Osteoporosis (Reclast vs. Control)*

Outcome	Clinical study: 302 men, ages 25–86 years (mean age, 64 years) with osteoporosis or significant osteoporosis secondary to hypogonadism assessed in a randomized, multicenter, double-blind, active controlled study for 2 years. Patients were randomly assigned to Reclast 5 mg administered intravenously over at least 15 minutes once annually for up to two doses, or to an oral weekly bisphosphonate (active control) for up to 2 years
Change in BMD relative to control, %	Annual infusion of Reclast was non-inferior to oral weekly bisphosphonate active control based on the percentage change in lumbar spine BMD at month 24 relative to baseline (Reclast: 6.1% increase; active control: 6.2% increase)

*All participants received 1000 mg of elemental calcium plus 800–1000 IU of vitamin D supplementation daily

EFFICACY: Treatment and Prevention of Glucocorticoid-induced Osteoporosis (GIO) in Patients Expected to be Using Glucocorticoids for at Least 12 Months (Reclast vs. Control)*

Outcome	Clinical Study: 833 women and men, aged 18–85 years (mean age, 54.4 years) treated with prednisone ≥7.5 mg/day, orally (or equivalent) assessed in a randomized, multicenter, double-blind, stratified, active controlled study. Patients were stratified by their duration of pre-study corticosteroid use (≤3 months [prevention subpopulation] vs. >3 months [treatment subpopulation]), and randomized to either Reclast administered intravenously over at least 15 minutes or to an oral daily bisphosphonate (active control) for 1 year
Change in BMD relative to control, %	*GIO treatment subpopulation:* Reclast demonstrated a significant mean increase in lumbar spine BMD compared to active control at 1 year (Reclast 4.1%, active control 2.7%) with a treatment difference of 1.4% ($p < 0.001$) *GIO prevention subpopulation:* Reclast demonstrated a significant mean increase in lumbar spine BMD compared to active control at 1 year (Reclast 2.6%, active control 0.6%) with a treatment difference of 2.0% ($p < 0.001$)

*All participants received 1000 mg of elemental calcium plus 400–1000 IU of vitamin D supplementation daily

Adverse Reactions in Women with Postmenopausal Osteoporosis (Select)

>10%	Arthralgia (18%–24%), fever (18%), headache (8%–12.4%), pain in extremity (5.9%–11%), myalgia (4.9%–11%)
2%–10%	Flu-like symptoms (8%), dizziness (7.6%), headache (7%), general pain (1.5%–3%)
<2%	Transient increase in serum creatinine within 10 days after dosing (1.8%), atrial fibrillation (1.3%), injection site reaction (0%–0.7%), decline in serum calcium to <7.5 mg/dL (0.2%), iritis/uveitis/episcleritis (<0.1%–0.2%), osteonecrosis of the jaw (1/3862 in Study 1)

Adverse Reactions in Women with Postmenopausal Osteopenia (Select)

>10%	Arthralgia (18.8%–27.3%), generalized pain (14.9%–24.2%), pyrexia (21%), headache (14.6%–20.4%), back pain (16.6%–18.2%), chills (18.2%), nausea (11.6%–17.1%), fatigue (9.9%–14.6%), hypoesthesia (2.2%–5.6%)
2%–10%	Pain in extremity (3.9%), influenza-like illness (1.5%–3.3%),
<2%	Malaise (1.0%–2.2%), abdominal distension (0.6–2.0), iritis/episcleritis/conjunctivitis (1.1%)

Adverse Reactions in Men with Osteoporosis (Select)

>10%	Myalgia (19.6%), fatigue (17.6%), headache (15.0%), musculoskeletal pain (12.4%)
2%–10%	Chills (9.8%), influenza-like illness (9.2%), abdominal pain (7.9%), malaise (7.2%), increased serum creatinine (2%)
<2%	No reports on osteonecrosis of the jaw in this cohort

Reclast® (zoledronic acid) Injection product label, Revised 01/2010. Novartis Pharmaceuticals Corporation; East Hanover, NJ

PAMIDRONATE DISODIUM (AREDIA)

Oncology-Related Indications	Usual Doses, Administration Routes and Schedules	Guidance, Caveats, and Comments		
Multiple myeloma with osteolytic bone lesions on plain radiographs[1,2] Metastatic breast cancer with abnormal bone radiographs ± pain[1,2]	**Pamidronate** 90 mg intravenously in 250–500 mL 0.9% NS, 0.45% NS, or D5W, over 1–4 hours, every 3–4 weeks	In patients with Bence-Jones proteinuria and dehydration, ensure adequate hydration with 0.9% NS before administering pamidronate		
		Baseline	**Retreatment**	**Action**
		Normal SCr	SCr increased ≥0.5 mg/dL (≥44 μmol/L)	Hold until SCr is within 10% of baseline[†]
		Abnormal SCr	SCr increased ≥1.0 mg/dL (≥88 μmol/L)	Hold until SCr is within 10% of baseline[†]
Steroid-induced osteoporosis*[,3,4]	**Pamidronate** 60 mg intravenously in 250 mL 0.9% NS, 0.45% NS, or D5W over 2 hours every 12 weeks for 48 weeks, *or* **pamidronate** 150 mg orally, daily for 12–24 months[‡]	Pamidronate is available outside the United States in a tablet formulation containing 150 mg of the active drug		

Toxicity

>10%	Nausea/vomiting (27%), injection site reaction (18%), abdominal pain/GI complaints (15%), hypertension (15%), constipation (12.6%), and fever
1–10%	Anemia (6%), tachycardia (6%), hypothyroidism (6%), hypomagnesemia (4.9%), leukopenia (4%), hypophosphatemia (1.9%), hypotension (1.9%), rash (1%), flulike syndrome, bone/back pain, anorexia, hypocalcemia, fluid overload
<1%	Allergic reaction (dyspnea, angioedema, anaphylaxis), hypokalemia, transient proteinuria, ocular inflammation, uveitis, iritis, scleritis, episcleritis, jaw osteonecrosis

*Not an FDA-approved indication
[†]When resuming treatment after a hiatus for renal impairment, administer pamidronate over at least 2 hours at doses not >90 mg and not more frequently than every 4 weeks after renal function returns to baseline
[‡]An oral formulation is not available for commercial use in the United States

References

1. Hillner BE et al. American Society of Clinical Oncology guideline on the role of bisphosphonates in breast cancer. American Society of Clinical Oncology Bisphosphonates Expert Panel. J Clin Oncol 2000;18:1378–1391
2. Aredia product label, October 2003. Novartis Pharmaceutical Corporation, East Hanover, NJ
3. Smith MR et al. N Engl J Med 2001;345:948–955
4. Reid IR et al. Lancet 1988;331:143–146

CLODRONATE DISODIUM (BONEFOS, OSTAC)*

Oncology-Related Indications	Usual Doses, Administration Routes and Schedules	Guidance, Caveats, and Comments
Treatment of hypercalcemia of malignancy:[†,1,14] serum $Ca^{2+} \geq 12$ mg/dL (≥ 3 mmol/L)[1]	Clodronate 300 mg/day; administer intravenously in 500 mL 0.9% NS or D5W over 2 hours for up to 5 days, *or* Clodronate 1500 mg single dose; administer intravenously in 500 mL 0.9% NS or D5W over not less than 4 hours	Treatment with intravenous clodronate may continue for >5 days but should not exceed 10 days for a single hypercalcemic episode
Maintenance treatment after effective IV treatment for hypercalcemia[†,2–5,14]	Clodronate 1600 mg/day (range: 400–3200 mg); administer orally, indefinitely *Note:* Typical treatment duration of 6 mo may be extended depending on the course of the disease; it may be necessary to restart after interruption	Clodronate disodium is available outside the United States in: 400-mg capsules; 520-mg tablets (higher bioavailability); 800-mg tablets. The oral bioavailability of one 520-mg tablet approximately equals two 400-mg capsules or one 800-mg tablet. Clodronate should be taken with water at least 2 hours before or 2 hours after eating, drinking, or taking other medications
Multiple myeloma (regression of bone lesions)[†,5–7]	Clodronate 1600–3200 mg/day; administer orally, *or* Clodronate 1040–2080 mg/day; administer orally	
Metastatic bone disease[†,5,7–13]	Clodronate 300 mg/day; administer intravenously in 250–500 mL D5W or 0.9% NS over 2–3 hours, for 8–14 consecutive days, *followed by:* Clodronate 1040–2080 mg/day; administer orally, indefinitely, *or* Clodronate 1600 mg 2 times daily or 1600 mg/day (as a single 1600-mg dose, 800 mg twice daily, or 400 mg 4 times daily); administer orally, indefinitely *Note:* Studies have examined treatment durations of 4–11 weeks. Treatment likely will continue for longer durations with clodronate or another agent	Oral clodronate should not be taken with milk or food containing calcium or other divalent cations. It is important to establish and maintain full hydration with oral or IV fluids prior to the infusion of clodronate disodium

Intravenous Clodronate Dose Modifications in Renal Impairment

CrCl (mL/min)	Dose Reduction
50–80 (0.83–1.33 mL/s)	25%
12–50 (0.2–0.83 mL/s)	25–50%
<12 (<0.2 mL/s)	50%

ORAL Clodronate Dose Modifications in Renal Impairment

CrCl (mL/min)	Dose Reduction
50–80	No dose reduction
30–50	25%
<30	50%

Toxicity

>10%	Dysgeusia (50%)
1–10%	Bone/back pain, nausea/vomiting, constipation, diarrhea, dyspepsia, abdominal pain, flatulence, abdominal distention, dysphagia, transient proteinuria (IV form)
<1%	Hyperparathyroidism (0.6%), increased serum creatinine, gastritis, gastric ulceration, increase in liver transaminases, ocular inflammation, uveitis, respiratory impairment in aspirin sensitive patients, hypersensitivity (respiratory symptoms), rash, hypocalcemia, hypomagnesemia

*Clodronate is not available for commercial use in the United States
[†]Not an FDA-approved indication

References

1. Bonefos (disodium clodronate) product label. Bayer Inc. Toronto, Ontario, Canada. Revised January 18, 2010
2. Percival RC et al. Br J Cancer 1985;51:665–669
3. Rastad J et al. Acta Med Scand 1987;221:489–494
4. Ziegler R, Scharla SH. Recent Results Cancer Res 1989;116:46–53
5. Clodronic acid. In: Sweetman SC, ed. Martindale, the Complete Drug Reference, 33rd ed. Grayslake (IL): Pharmaceutical Press; 2002:751–752
6. Coleman RE. Am J Clin Oncol 2002;25(6 Suppl 1):S32–S38
7. Diel IJ et al. N Engl J Med 1998;339:357–363
8. Adami S et al. J Urol 1985;134:1152–1154
9. Heidenreich A et al. J Urol 2001;165:136–140
10. Rizzoli R et al. Bone 1996;18:531–537
11. Kanis JA et al. Bone 1996;19:663–667
12. Body J-J et al. J Clin Oncol 1998;16:3890–3899
13. McCloskey EV et al. Br J Haematol 1998;100:317–325
14. Clasteon® (clodronate disodium) product label. Sepacor Pharmaceuticals, Inc., Mississauga, Ontario, Canada. Revised April 14, 2009

ALENDRONATE SODIUM (FOSAMAX)

Oncology-Related Indication (s)	Usual Doses, Administration Routes and Schedules	Guidance, Caveats, and Comments	
Treatment and prevention of osteoporosis in postmenopausal women	Alendronate 5 mg; administer orally, daily	**Dose Adjustments**	
Treatment to increase bone mass in men with osteoporosis		**Elderly patients**	**No adjustments**
For the treatment of steroid-induced osteoporosis in men and women receiving a daily dose equivalent to ≥7.5 mg prednisone and who have low bone mineral density*	Alendronate 10 mg; administer orally, daily	CrCl ≥35 mL/min (≥0.58 mL/s)	No adjustments
		CrCl <35 mL/min (<0.58 mL/s)	Do not administer drug
		Contraindications: • Abnormalities of the esophagus that delay esophageal emptying, such as stricture or achalasia • Inability to stand or sit upright for at least 30 minutes • Patients at increased risk of aspiration • Hypocalcemia	
	Alendronate 5, 10, or 15 mg; administer intravenously† over 2 hours	Not recommended if CrCl <35 mL/min (<0.58 mL/s)	

Toxicity

>10%	Fever (intravenous formulation)
1–10%	Constipation (3.1%), diarrhea (3.1%) headache (2.6%), gastritis/gastric ulceration (1.5%), nausea/vomiting, abdominal pain, flatulence, abdominal distention, dysphagia, hypocalcemia, hypophosphatemia
<1%	Increases in liver transaminases (intravenous formulation), iritis, scleritis, episcleritis, osteonecrosis of the jaw

*Not an FDA-approved indication
†A parenteral formulation is not available for commercial use in the United States

References

1. Fosamax tablets and oral solution product label, September 2003. Merck & Co., Inc., Whitehouse Station, NJ
2. Nussbaum SR et al. J Clin Oncol 1993;11:1618–1623

RISEDRONATE SODIUM (ACTONEL)

Oncology-Related Indications	Usual Doses, Administration Routes and Schedules	Guidance, Caveats, and Comments	
For the prevention and treatment of steroid-induced osteoporosis in men and women receiving a daily dose equivalent to ≥7.5 mg prednisone	Risedronate 5 mg; administer orally daily	Dosage Adjustments	
		Elderly Patients	**No Adjustments**
		CrCl ≥30 mL/min (≥0.5 mL/s)	No adjustments
		CrCl <30 mL/min	Do not administer drug

Toxicity

>10%	Arthralgia (32.8%), bone/back pain (26.1%), headache (18%), nausea/vomiting (10.9%), abdominal pain (11.6%), diarrhea (10.6%)
1–10%	Flulike syndrome (9.8%), rash (7.7%), chest pain (5%), asthenia (4.9%), hypercholesterolemia (4.8%), flatulence (4.6%), gastritis/gastric ulceration (4.1%), conjunctivitis (3.1%), pruritus (3%), abdominal distention, dysphagia
<1%	Iritis, scleritis, episcleritis, osteonecrosis of jaw

Actonel product label, March 2003. Proctor and Gamble Pharmaceuticals, Cincinnati, OH
Brooks JK et al. Oral Surg Oral Med Oral Pathol Oral Radiol Endod 2007;103:780–786

IBANDRONATE SODIUM (BONIVA)

Indications	Usual Doses, Administration Routes and Schedules	Guidance, Caveats, and Comments		
Treatment of postmenopausal osteoporosis[1]	**Ibandronate** 2.5 mg; administer orally daily, *or* **Ibandronate** 150 mg; administer orally once a month, *or* **Ibandronate** 3 mg; administer intravenously every 3 months	Dose Adjustments		
		Elderly Patients	No Adjustments	
		CrCl ≥30 mL/min (≥0.5 mL/s)	No adjustments	
		CrCl <30 mL/min	Use is not recommended	
Prevention of postmenopausal osteoporosis[1]	**Ibandronate** 2.5 mg; administer orally daily, *or* **Ibandronate** 150 mg; administer orally once a month	CrCl <30 mL/min in oncologic indications	**Ibandronate** 50 mg; administer orally once weekly, *or* **Ibandronate** 2 mg; administer intravenously over 1 hour every 3 weeks	
Hypercalcemia of malignancy[*,2–4] serum Ca^{2+} ≥12 mg/dL (≥3 mmol/L)	**Ibandronate** 4–6 mg; administer intravenously over 2 hours	Ibandronate should be taken orally 60 minutes before the first food or drink of the day, and any oral medications (including antacids, vitamins or supplements). Ibandronate should be taken in an upright position with a full glass (6–8 oz) of plain water and the patient should avoid lying down for 60 minutes to minimize the possibility of GI side effects		
Metastatic bone disease[*,5–7]	**Ibandronate** 50 mg; administer orally daily, *or* **Ibandronate** 6 mg; administer intravenously over 1 hour every 3–4 weeks	Contraindications: 1. Abnormalities of the esophagus that delay esophageal emptying such as stricture or achalasia; 2. Inability to stand or sit upright for at least 60 min.; 3. Hypocalcemia; Hypersensitivity to ibandronate sodium		

Effect of Ibandronate on the Incidence of Vertebral Fracture in the 3-Year Osteoporosis Study*

Outcome	Proportion of Patients with Fracture (%)			
	Placebo (n = 975)	Ibandronate 2.5 mg Daily (n = 977)	Absolute Risk Reduction % (95% CI)	Relative Risk Reduction % (95% CI)
New vertebral fracture 0–3 years	9.6	4.7	4.9 (2.3, 7.4)	52[†] (29, 68)
New and worsening vertebral fracture 0–3 years	10.4	5.1	5.3 (2.6, 7.9)	52 (30, 67)
Clinical (symptomatic) vertebral fracture 0–3 years	5.3	2.8	2.5 (0.6, 4.5)	49 (14, 69)

*The endpoint value is the value at the study's last endpoint, 3 years, for all patients who had a fracture identified at that time; otherwise, the last post-baseline value prior to the study's last time point is used

[†]p = 0.0003 vs. placebo

EFFICACY: Mean Percent Change in BMD from Baseline to Endpoint in Patients Treated Daily with Ibandronate 2.5 mg or Placebo in the 3-year Osteoporosis Treatment Study[‡]

	Placebo	Ibandronate 2.5 mg Daily
Lumbar spine	1.4 (n = 693)	6.4 (n = 712)
Total hip	−0.7 (n = 638)	3.1 (n = 654)
Femoral neck	−0.7 (n = 683)	2.6 (n = 699)
Trochanter	0.2 (n = 683)	5.3 (n = 699)

[‡]The endpoint value is the value at the study's last time point, 3 years, for all patients who had BMD measured at that time; otherwise, the last post-baseline value prior to the study's last time point is used

EFFICACY: Mean Percent Change in Lumbar Spine BMD from Baseline in Osteoporosis Patients Treated Monthly with Ibandronate 150 mg or Daily with Ibandronate 2.5 mg

Clinical study: Randomized, double-blind, multinational, non-inferiority trial of 1602 women aged 54–81 years, who were on average postmenopausal for 18 years and had L2–L4 lumbar spine BMD T-score less than −2.5 SD at baseline. The main outcome measure was the comparison of the percentage change from baseline in lumbar BMD after 1 year of treatment with once-monthly ibandronate (100 mg, 150 mg) or daily ibandronate. All patients received 400 IU Vitamin D and 500 mg calcium supplementation daily
Exclusions: Patients with dyspepsia or concomitant use of NSAIDS, proton pump inhibitors, and H_2-receptor antagonists

	Ibandronate 150 mg Monthly n = 327	Ibandronate 2.5 mg Daily n = 318	Mean Difference
Lumbar spine BMD 1 year	4.85% (95% CI: 4.41%, 5.29%)	3.86% (95% CI: 3.40%, 4.32%)	0.99%§ (95% CI: 0.38%, 1.60%)

§p = 0.002

EFFICACY: Prevention of Postmenopausal Osteoporosis (Ibandronate 2.5 mg Daily or 150 mg Monthly)

Clinical study: Randomized, double-blind, placebo-controlled 2-year study (Prevention Study) of 653 postmenopausal women without osteoporosis at baseline. Patient ages were 41–82 years, were on average postmenopausal for 8.5 years, and had lumbar BMD T-scores greater than −2.5 SD. Women were stratified to time since menopause (1–3 years, >3 years) and baseline BMD (T-score, greater than −1, −1 to −2.5). The study compared ibandronate at three dose levels (0.5 mg, 1 mg · 2.5 mg) with placebo. All women received 500 mg of supplemental calcium daily
Primary efficacy measure: change in BMD of lumbar spine (LS) after 2 years of treatment (Ibandronate 2.5 mg daily)
Results: (1) Ibandronate treatment resulted in a mean increase in LS BMD of 3.1% compared with placebo at 6 months and all later time points. (2) Ibandronate treatment resulted in a higher BMD response at the LS compared with placebo, irrespective of time since menopause or degree of pre-existing bone loss across all four baseline strata (time since menopause; baseline LS BMD). (3) Compared to placebo, ibandronate increased BMD of the total hip by 1.8%, the femoral neck by 2.0%, and the trochanter by 2.1%

Clinical study: Randomized, double-blind, placebo-controlled 1-year study (Monthly Prevention Study) of 160 post-menopausal women with low bone mass (T-score of −1 to −2.5 SD). Women, aged 46–60 years, were on average postmenopausal for 5.4 years. All women received 400 IU of vitamin D and 500 mg calcium supplementation daily
Primary efficacy measure: Relative change in BMD at the lumbar spine (LS) after 1 year of treatment (Ibandronate 150 mg monthly)
Results: (1) Ibandronate treatment resulted in a mean increase in LS BMD of 4.12% (95% CI: 2.96, 5.28) compared to placebo following 1 year of treatment (p <0.0001), based on a 3.73% and −0.39 mean change in BMD from baseline in the ibandronate and placebo groups, respectively; (2) BMD at other skeletal sites was also increased relative to baseline values

Toxicity

>10%	Fever (11%), with oral administration: nausea and vomiting (20%), epigastric pain and dyspepsia (25%)
1–10%	Abdominal pain, diarrhea, and constipation. Joint pain, backache, muscle aches, arthritis, arthropathy, hypertension, and hypercholesterolemia
<1%	Ocular inflammation, uveitis, scleritis
Post-marketing experience	Voluntarily reported adverse reactions post-approval (difficult to reliably determine incidence due to population of uncertain size): Hypersensitivity (anaphylaxis, angioedema, bronchospasm, and rash), hypocalcemia, musculoskeletal pain (severe or incapacitating), osteonecrosis of the jaw

References

1. Boniva tablets product label, Revised January, 2010. Genentech USA, Inc. South San Francisco, CA
2. Pecherstorfer M et al. J Clin Oncol 1996;14:268–276
3. Ralston SH et al. Br J Cancer 1997;75:295–300
4. Pecherstorfer M et al. Support Care Cancer 2003;11:539–547
5. Diel IJ et al. Eur J Cancer 2004;40:1704–1712
6. Body J-J et al. Ann Oncol 2003;14:1399–1405
7. Heidenreich A et al. Prostate Cancer Prostatic Dis 2002;5:231–235

ETIDRONATE SODIUM (DIDRONEL)

Indications	Usual Doses, Administration Routes and Schedules	Guidance, Caveats, and Comments	
Treatment of postmenopausal osteoporosis*	**Etidronate** 200 mg; administer orally daily for 2 weeks, followed by a 13-week period with no etidronate Then repeat the cycle Maintain adequate calcium and vitamin D intake during the 15-week cycle	**Dose Adjustments**	
		Elderly patients	No specific dosage adjustments. Evaluate renal function carefully and consider reduction
		SrCr >2.5 mg/dL (>221 μmol/L)	Use cautiously
		SrCr >5 mg/dL (>442 μmol/L)	Use is not recommended
Hypercalcemia of malignancy[2,3] serum Ca^{2+} ≥12 mg/dL (≥3 mmol/L)	**Etidronate** 7.5 mg/kg per day; administer intravenously over 2 hours for 3 consecutive days[†] Normocalcemia can be maintained after IV therapy with **Etidronate** 20 mg/kg; administer orally daily for 30–90 days		

Toxicity

>10%	Headache, gastritis, arthralgia (low-grade fever, myalgias, arthralgias, headache)
1–10%	Diarrhea, nausea, hyperphosphatemia
<1%	Arthritis, glossitis, esophagitis, pruritus, agranulocytosis, pancytopenia

*Not an FDA-approved indication
[†]An IV formulation is not available for commercial use in the United States

References

1. Didronel product label, October 2007. Proctor and Gamble Pharmaceutical, Inc., Cincinnati, OH
2. Ralston SH et al. Lancet 1989;334:1180–1182
3. Saunders Y et al. Palliat Med 2004;18:418–431

Monitoring Bisphosphonate Therapy*,†

Tests	Zoledronic Acid[1,2,9]	Pamidronate[1,3,9]	Clodronate[1,4,5]	Alendronate[1,6]	Risedronate[1,7]	Ibandronate[8,9]	Etidronate[10]
SCr prior to single-dose	+	Renal impairment‡	+	+	+	+	+
SCr prior to repeated treatments	+		+	+	+	+	+
Serum albumin and BUN	Unexplained albuminuria or azotemia§⁌		−	−	−	−	−
CBC with differential	−	+	+	−	−	−	−
Calcium	+	+	+	+	+	+	+
Phosphorus	+	+	+	−	+	+	+
Magnesium	+	+	−	−	−	+	−
Hemoglobin and hematocrit	+	+	+	−	−	−	−
Oral exam; preventive dentistry	+	+	+	+	+	+	+

+, Complete the test or evaluation before drug administration; −, No need to test

*Evaluation is recommended before initial treatment with parenterally administered bisphosphonates, each repeated administration, and at the time of routine repeated visits for patients receiving oral agents (eg, monthly to quarter annually)

†Product labeling for some products warns about a potential for fetal harm if pregnant females receive bisphosphonate treatment during gestation

‡When resuming treatment after a hiatus for renal impairment, administer pamidronate over at least 2 hours, at doses not greater than 90 mg, and at administration frequencies not greater than every 4 weeks after renal function returns to baseline

§In patients with multiple myeloma, discontinue bisphosphonate treatment until renal problems resolve in patients with:
- Unexplained albuminuria >500 mg/24 h, or
- Azotemia (an increase in SCr ≥0.5 mg/dL (>44 μmol/L), or an absolute SCr value >1.4 mg/dL (>124 μmol/L), among patients with normal baseline creatinine[1]
- Reassess every 3 to 4 weeks with a 24-hour urine collection for total protein and urine protein electrophoresis

⁌In patients with multiple myeloma for whom pamidronate treatment was withheld for renal dysfunction, reinstitute pamidronate only after renal function returns to baseline, with infusion durations >2 h and at doses/schedules ≤90 mg every 4 weeks[1]

References

1. Berenson JR. J Clin Oncol 2002;20:3719–3736; Kyle RA et al. J Clin Oncol 2007;25:2464–2472
2. Zometa (zoledronic acid) Injection product label, October 2009. Novartis Pharmaceuticals Corporation, East Hanover, NJ
3. Aredia product label, October 2003. Novartis Pharmaceutical Corporation, East Hanover, NJ
4. Bonefos® (disodium clodronate); product label, January 18, 2010. Bayer Inc., Toronto, Ontario, Canada
5. Clasteon® (clodronate disodium); product label, April 14, 2009. Sepracor Pharmaceuticals, Inc., Mississauga, Ontario; Licensed by ABIOGEN PHARMA S.p.A Italy
6. Fosamax® (alendronate sodium) capsules & oral solution; product label, March 2010. Merck & Co., Inc., Whitehouse Station, NJ
7. Actonel® (risedronate sodium); product label, March 2010. Warner Chilcott Puerto Rico LLC, Manati, PR; Norwich Pharmaceuticals, Inc., North Norwich, NY; Chinoin Pharmaceutical and Chemical Works Private Co Ltd, Veresegyhaz, Hungary
8. Boniva® (ibandronate sodium); product label, January 2010. Genentech USA, Inc. South San Francisco, CA
9. Van Poznak CH et al. J Clin Oncol 2011;29:1221–1227
10. Didronel® (etidronate disodium); product label, 2005. Procter & Gamble Pharmaceuticals; Cincinnati, OH

REGIMEN

RANK LIGAND INHIBITOR DENOSUMAB (XGEVA®)

Oncology-Related Indications	Usual Doses, Administration Routes, and Schedules	Guidance, Caveats, and Comments
• Prevention of skeletal-related events in patients with bone metastases from solid tumors • Denosumab is not indicated for the prevention of skeletal-related events in patients with multiple myeloma Mechanism of action: • Denosumab is a genetically engineered human IgG_2 monoclonal antibody that binds to human release receptor activator of nuclear factor kappa B ligand (RANKL) preventing activation of the RANK receptor on osteoclasts • Osteoclast inhibition results in reduced bone resorption, tumor-induced bone destruction, and skeletal-related events (SRE)	Denosumab 120 mg; administer by subcutaneous injection every 4 weeks in the upper arm, upper thigh, or abdomen Denosumab (as XGEVA®) is available in single-use vials containing 120 mg/1.7 mL (70 mg/mL): 1. Prior to administration, denosumab is removed from refrigeration (2°C–8°C; 35.6°F–46.4°F) and left standing in its original packaging at room temperature (≤25°C; ≤77°F) for 15–30 minutes • XGEVA® should not be warmed in any other way 2. Using a 27-gauge needle, the entire contents of the vial are withdrawn into a syringe and injecte *Do not* vigorously shake the vial *Do not* expose vials to direct light or heat *Do not* re-enter vials after withdrawing the drug product	**Dose adjustments** No dose adjustments for renal impairment (denosumab is not eliminated by the kidney) No clinical trials have been conducted to evaluate the effect of hepatic impairment on the pharmacokinetics of denosumab Exclusion criteria in clinical trials: 1. A history of ONJ or osteomyelitis of the jaw 2. An active dental or jaw condition requiring oral surgery 3. Any planned invasive dental procedure 4. Non-healed dental/oral surgical wounds or lesions 5. Previous intravenous bisphosphonate therapy 6. Current or previous oral bisphosphonates for treatment of bone metastases

Efficacy

Denosumab* Compared to Zoledronic Acid[†]

	Trial 1 Metastatic Breast Cancer		Trial 2 Metastatic Solid Tumors or Multiple Myeloma		Trial 3 Metastatic Castration-Resistant Prostate Cancer	
Regimen	Denosumab	Zoledronic acid	Denosumab	Zoledronic acid	Denosumab	Zoledronic acid
Patient number	1026	1020	886	890	950	951
1st on study SRE						
Number of patients with SRE (%)	315 (30.7)	372 (36.5)	278 (31.4)	323 (36.3)	341 (35.9)	386 (40.6)
Components of 1st SRE						
Radiation to bone	82 (8.0)	119 (11.7)	119 (13.4)	144 (16.2)	177 (18.6)	203 (21.3)
Pathologic fracture	212 (20.7)	238 (23.3)	122 (13.8)	139 (15.6)	137 (14.4)	143 (15.0)
Surgery to bone	12 (1.2)	8 (0.8)	13 (1.5)	19 (2.1)	1 (0.1)	4 (0.4)
SC[§] compression	9 (0.9)	7 (0.7)	24 (2.7)	21 (2.4)	26 (2.7)	36 (3.8)
Median time to SRE	NR[‡]	26.4 mo	20.5 mo	16.3 mo	20.7 mo	17.1 mo
Hazard ratio (95% CI)	0.82 (0.71, 0.95)		0.84 (0.71, 0.98)		0.82 (0.71, 0.95)	
Non-inferiority P-value	<0.001		<0.001		<0.001	
Superiority P-value[ϵ]	0.010		0.060		0.008	

*Denosumab 120 mg by subcutaneous injection every 4 weeks (median duration of exposure, 12 mo [range 0.1–41 mo]; 75% received chemotherapy concomitantly)
[†]Zoledronic acid 4 mg by intravenous infusion every 4 weeks with CrCl ≥30 mL/min and dose-adjusted based on CrCl
[‡]Not reached
[§]Spinal cord
[ϵ]Superiority testing performed only after denosumab was demonstrated non-inferior to zoledronic acid within trial. Survival: OS and PFS were similar in all three trials; mortality was higher with denosumab in a subgroup analysis of patients with multiple myeloma (hazard ratio 2.26; n = 180)

Toxicity

Selected Per-patient Incidence of Any Severity From Trials 1, 2, and 3

Variable	Denosumab (n = 2841) %	Zoledronic Acid (n = 2836) %
Fatigue/Asthenia	45	46
Nausea/Diarrhea	31/20	32/19
Hypocalcemia* Hypophosphatemia[†]	18 32	9 20
Dyspnea/Cough	21/15	18/15
Headache	13	14
Bone: Osteonecrosis of the jaw[‡]	1.8 (2.2 with 4-mo trial extension phase)	1.3

*Hypocalcemia (corrected, <7 mg/dL [<1.75 mmol/L]): 3.1% of denosumab cohort (33% experienced ≥2 episodes) vs. 1.3% of zoledronic acid cohort
[†]Hypophosphatemia (<2 mg/dL [<0.65 mmol/L]): 15.4% of denosumab cohort vs. 7.4% of zoledronic acid cohort
[‡]Median time to ONJ was 14 months (range, 4–25 mo)

Adverse Events
Denosumab cohort:
• The most common (≥25%), included fatigue/asthenia, hypophosphatemia, and nausea
• The most common serious event was dyspnea
• The most common events that resulted in discontinuing treatment were osteonecrosis of the jaw and hypocalcemia

Monitoring Therapy

Prior to treatment:
1. Measure serum calcium, vitamin D, magnesium, and phosphorus
2. Correct pre-existing hypocalcemia and other levels as necessary prior to treatment
3. Perform an oral examination and appropriate preventive dentistry prior to the initiation of denosumab

Supplementation:
Daily oral administration of calcium (≥500 mg) and vitamin D (≥400 IU) is strongly recommended

During treatment:
1. Monitor serum levels of calcium, magnesium, and phosphorus, and replace as necessary
2. Avoid invasive dental procedures during treatment
3. Perform periodic oral examination and preventive dentistry
4. Patients who are suspected of having or who develop osteonecrosis of the jaw (ONJ) while receiving treatment with denosumab should receive care by a dentist or an oral surgeon (extensive dental surgery to treat ONJ may exacerbate the condition)

Advise patients to contact a healthcare professional for any of the following:
1. Symptoms of hypocalcemia, including paresthesias, muscle stiffness, twitching, spasms, or cramps
2. Symptoms of ONJ including pain, numbness, swelling of or drainage of the jaw, mouth, or teeth
3. Persistent pain or slow healing of the mouth or jaw after dental surgery
4. Pregnancy or nursing (women who become pregnant during Xgeva® are encouraged to enroll in Amgen's Pregnancy Surveillance Program; 1-800-772-6436)

Advise patients of the need for:
1. Proper oral hygiene and routine dental care
2. Informing their dentist they are receiving denosumab
3. Avoiding invasive dental procedures during treatment with denosumab
4. Informing their healthcare provider if they are taking Xgeva® (denosumab is also marketed under the proprietary name, Prolia®)

Lipton A et al. Comparison of denosumab versus zoledronic acid (ZA) for treatment of bone metastases in advanced cancer patients: an integrated analysis of 3 pivotal trials [abstract]. Ann Oncol 2010;21(Suppl 8):viii380
Stopeck AT et al. Denosumab compared with zoledronic acid for the treatment of bone metastases in patients with advanced breast cancer: a randomized, double blind study. J Clin Oncol 2010;28(35):5132–5139
Xgeva® (denosumab) injection, for subcutaneous use; product label, August 2013. Amgen Manufacturing Limited, a subsidiary of Amgen Inc., Thousand Oaks, CA

DENOSUMAB (PROLIA®)

Indication	Usual Doses, Administration Routes, and Schedules	Guidance, Caveats, and Comments
Treatment of postmenopausal women with osteoporosis at high risk for fracture (defined as a history of osteoporotic fracture, multiple risk factors for fracture, or patients who have failed or are intolerant to other available osteoporosis therapy)	**Denosumab** 60 mg; administer as a single subcutaneous injection in the upper arm, upper thigh; or the abdomen once every 6 months. If a dose is missed, administer the injection as soon as the patient is available and thereafter, every 6 months from the last injection **Denosumab** (as Prolia®) is available in single-use prefilled syringes and single-use vials containing 1 mL of a 60-mg/mL solution 1. Prior to administration, denosumab is removed from refrigeration (2°C–8°C; 35.6°F–46.4°F) and left standing in its original packaging at room temperature (≤25°C; ≤77°F) for 15–30 minutes • Prolia® should not be warmed in any other way 2. From a single-use vial, using a syringe with a 27-gauge needle, withdraw the entire contents of the vial and administer the drug by subcutaneous injection *Do not* vigorously shake vials or syringes *Do not* expose vials or syringes to direct light or heat *Do not* re-enter vials after withdrawing the drug product	**Dose adjustments** No dose adjustments are necessary in patients with renal impairment Pre-existing hypocalcemia must be corrected prior to initiating therapy with Prolia® People sensitive to latex should not handle the gray needle cap on the single-use prefilled syringe, which contains dry natural rubber (a latex derivative)

The Effect of Prolia on the Incidence of New Vertebral Fractures

	Proportion of Women with Fracture (%)*		Absolute Risk Reduction, % (95% CI)	Relative Risk Reduction, % (95% CI)
	Placebo (N = 3691)	Prolia (N = 3702)		
0–1 year	2.2	0.9	1.4 (0.8, 1.9)	61 (42, 74)
0–2 years	5.0	1.4	3.5 (2.7, 4.3)	71 (61, 79)
0–3 years	7.2	2.3	4.8 (3.9, 5.8)	68 (59, 74)

*Absolute risk reduction and relative risk reduction base on Mantel-Haenszel method adjusting for age group variable

The Effect of Prolia on the Incidence of Non-vertebral Fractures at Year 3

Outcome	Proportion of Women with Fracture, %†		Absolute Risk Reduction, % (95% CI)	Relative Risk Reduction, % (95% CI)
	Placebo (N = 3906)	Prolia (N = 3902)		
Non-vertebral fracture‡	8.0	6.5	1.5 (0.3, 2.7)	20 (5, 33)*

*P-value = 0.01
†Event rates based on Kaplan-Meier estimates at 3 years
‡Excluding those of the vertebrae (cervical, thoracic, and lumbar), skull, facial, mandible, metacarpus, finger/toe phalanges

Toxicity

>10%	Back pain (34.7%; same rate as control), dermatitis/eczema/rashes (10.8%)
1–10%	Musculoskeletal pain (7.6%), sciatica (4.6%), non-fatal serious infections (4%), hypocalcemia <8.5 mg/dL (1.7%; occurred at approximately day 10 after Prolia® in patients with normal renal function), patients who withdrew from study due to ADR (2.4%; control 2.1%; most common reasons: breast cancer [causality has not been established], back pain, and constipation)
<1%	Skin infections (0.4%), pancreatitis (0.2%), infections resulting in death (0.2%; same rate as control)

Monitoring Therapy

Prior to treatment:
1. Measure serum calcium, vitamin D, magnesium, and phosphorus
2. Correct pre-existing hypocalcemia and other levels as necessary prior to treatment
3. Perform an oral examination and appropriate preventive dentistry prior to the initiation of denosumab

Supplementation:
Daily oral administration of calcium (at least 1000 mg) and vitamin D (≥400 International Units) is advised

During treatment:
1. Monitor serum levels of calcium, magnesium, and phosphorus, and replace as necessary
2. Avoid invasive dental procedures during treatment
3. Perform periodic oral examination and preventive dentistry
4. Patients who are suspected of having or who develop ONJ while on denosumab should receive care by a dentist or an oral surgeon (in these patients, extensive dental surgery to treat ONJ may exacerbate the condition)

Advise patients to contact a healthcare professional for any of the following:
1. Symptoms of hypocalcemia, including paresthesias, muscle stiffness, twitching, spasms, or cramps
2. Symptoms of ONJ including pain, numbness, swelling of or drainage of the jaw, mouth, or teeth
3. Persistent pain or slow healing of the mouth or jaw after dental surgery
4. Pregnancy or nursing (women who become pregnant during Xgeva are encouraged to enroll in Amgen's Pregnancy Surveillance Program; 1-800-772-6436)

Advise patients of the need for:
1. Proper oral hygiene and routine dental care
2. Informing their dentist that they are receiving denosumab
3. Avoiding invasive dental procedures during treatment with denosumab
4. Informing their healthcare provider if they are taking Prolia® (denosumab is also marketed as Xgeva®)

Prolia® (denosumab) Injection, for subcutaneous use; product label, July 2013. Amgen Manufacturing Limited, a subsidiary of Amgen Inc., Thousand Oaks, CA

45. Transfusion Therapy

Ashok Nambiar, MD and Joseph E. Kiss, MD

PRODUCT

WHOLE BLOOD[1–3]

Administration

Whole blood is given over a maximum of 4 hours through a 170-μm filter

Notes

1. Whole blood is not routinely available and is rarely required in hematology-oncology patients. It is not a source of viable white blood cells (WBCs) or platelets
2. *Shelf life:* 21 days in CPD (citrate-phosphate-dextrose); 35 days in CPDA-1 (citrate-phosphate-dextrose-adenine) preservatives

Preparation/Composition

1. Donor blood 450–550 mL containing red blood cells (RBCs), plasma, clotting factors, and anticoagulant
2. Platelets and granulocytes are not functional

Indications

RBC replacement in acute blood loss with pronounced hypovolemia

PRODUCT

RED BLOOD CELLS[1–3]

Preparation/Composition

1. RBCs obtained by apheresis collection or prepared from whole blood by centrifugation
2. RBCs collected in CPDA-1 anticoagulant have a hematocrit of 65–80% and a storage volume of 250–400 mL
3. RBC collections from which plasma has been removed and 100 mL of adenine-containing RBC nutrient solution (eg, AS-1) has been added, have a hematocrit of 55–60% and a volume of 300–350 mL

Notes

1. Patients with febrile nonhemolytic transfusion reactions benefit from leukoreduced blood products
2. Premedication with **acetaminophen** 650–1000 mg orally, may also be given
3. Patients with allergic transfusion reactions are treated with **diphenhydramine** 25–50 mg orally or intravenously
4. *Shelf life:* 35 days in CPDA-1; 42 days if stored in additive solutions like AS-1 (contains sodium chloride 154 mmol/L, adenine 2 mmol/L, glucose 111 mmol/L, and mannitol 41.2 mmol/L)

Administration

1. RBCs are administered over a maximum period of 4 hours through a 170-μm filter
2. Do not add medications to blood products. If needed to decrease viscosity, 0.9% sodium chloride injection is the only compatible intravenous solution that may be added to RBCs; however, this is rarely needed with current additive solutions

Indications

1. Improves oxygen carrying capacity in anemic patients
2. In most stable asymptomatic patients without cardiovascular disease, transfusion is initiated if hemoglobin is <7 g/dL
3. Transfusion thresholds in patients with cardiovascular disease who are asymptomatic are not well defined; results of clinical trials are awaited. Higher transfusion thresholds (9–10 g/dL) may be appropriate for patients with symptomatic cardiac disease[3–6]

PRODUCT

WASHED RED BLOOD CELLS[1,2]

Preparation/Composition

Washing RBCs with 1 L 0.9% sodium chloride injection (0.9% NS) removes more than 98% of plasma proteins. RBCs are then resuspended in 0.9% NS at an approximate *hematocrit* of 75%

Indications

1. Patients with a history of severe or recurrent allergic reactions
2. For patients with paroxysmal nocturnal hemoglobinuria, routine washing of group-specific RBCs is not required
3. Washed RBCs are used to decrease potassium load in neonates with cardiac or renal disease

Administration

Washed RBCs must be transfused within 24 hours

Notes

1. RBCs washed with larger volumes of 0.9% NS ($\geq$2 L) or units collected from IgA-deficient donors are required for patients with severe IgA deficiency
2. *Shelf life:* Washed RBCs have a shelf life of only 24 hours

PRODUCT

LEUKOCYTE-REDUCED RED BLOOD CELLS[1,2]

Preparation/Composition

Contains <5 × 10^6 WBCs per unit. Leukocyte reduction filters remove >99.9% of the contaminating leukocytes

Administration

The product is transfused over a maximum period of 4 hours through a 170-μm filter

Indications

1. Patients with recurrent febrile nonhemolytic transfusion reactions (FNHTR)
2. To decrease the likelihood of HLA alloimmunization and platelet transfusion refractoriness
3. To decrease the risk of transmission of cytomegalovirus (CMV) infection in high-risk CMV-seronegative patients

Notes

1. Prestorage leukoreduction is superior to bedside filtration
2. The use of bedside leukoreduction filters has been associated with "hypotensive" reactions and facial flushing
3. *Shelf life:* Depends on the preservative added; 35 days for CPDA-1; 42 days for additive solutions such as AS-1

PRODUCT

FROZEN DEGLYCEROLIZED RED BLOOD CELLS[1,2]

Preparation/Composition

Goal: Remove glycerol in which RBCs are suspended

1. RBCs are frozen with glycerol as the cryoprotectant to maintain integrity after thawing
2. Deglycerolization is achieved by first thawing RBCs and then washing them with saline solutions of decreasing osmolarity to remove the glycerol
3. The final product has few leukocytes and <0.1% of the original plasma; however, it does not meet requirements of leukoreduced components

Administration

Deglycerolized RBCs must be transfused within 24 hours

Indications

Indications for use include:

1. Storing units with rare blood types
2. Storing autologous collections

Notes

1. As shelf life of deglycerolized RBCs is limited, transfusion of rare, frozen RBCs should be carefully planned to avoid wastage
2. *Shelf life:* Deglycerolized RBCs have a shelf life of only 24 hours

PRODUCT

PLATELETS[1,2,7]

Preparation/Composition

1. *Single-donor apheresis platelets:* Collected from single donors by apheresis. Contain $\geq 3 \times 10^{11}$ platelets in 250–300 mL plasma

2. *Platelet concentrates (PC):* Platelet concentrates prepared from units of whole blood. PCs contain $\geq 5.5 \times 10^{10}$ platelets suspended in 45–60 mL of plasma. Pooled platelets (4–6 PC) have a shelf-life of 4 hours. An FDA-approved closed system for pre-storage pooled platelets with a shelf-life of 5 days from time of whole blood collection is available now

Administration

1. When administering PCs, an adult dose is obtained by pooling 4–6 units into a single pack
2. Use a standard 170-μm filter or a leukocyte reduction filter, and infuse within 4 hours

Notes

1. Platelets are not routinely recommended for correction of thrombocytopenia in patients with ITP or TTP in the absence of a risk for severe bleeding

2. Washed, irradiated, and leukoreduced platelets have indications similar to those described under RBCs

3. *Platelet increments and HLA-matched platelets[9]*

   Among chronically transfused patients, 20–30% will develop alloimmunization to HLA antigens and will not experience an increment in their platelet count when platelets from randomly selected donors are administered. Platelet count should be obtained 15–60 minutes after transfusion, and the corrected count increments (CCIs; see equation) should be calculated. CCIs should be obtained for 2 consecutive transfusions. In the absence of clinical causes such as splenomegaly, fever, or ongoing bleeding to explain a poor increase in the platelet count, patients with poor CCIs are usually found to have an immune-mediated cause for the poor increments. In these patients, platelet cross-matching is carried out to select compatible products. Alternatively, HLA and platelet antibody screening tests are done. If the HLA antibody screen is positive, patients are supported with HLA-matched platelet products. Rarely, antibodies may be directed against platelet-specific antigens, in which case phenotype-matched platelet donors are recruited. Immune globulin (human) does not produce sustained responses; its routine use in alloimmunized patients is not recommended

$$\text{Corrected Count Increment (CCI)} = \frac{((\text{posttransfusion platelet count } [\mu L]) - (\text{pretransfusion platelet count } [\mu L])) \times (\text{body surface area } [m^2])}{\text{number of platelets transfused (multiples of } 10^{11})}$$

Note: The number of apheresis units transfused can be entered as the denominator in the formula above. For example, if a patient (70 kg, 167.6 cm, BSA = 1.8 m^2) has an incremental increase of 10,000/μL in platelet count following transfusion of a platelet product containing 3×10^{11} platelets, the calculated CCI would be 6000. A CCI of <5000–7500/μL suggests platelet refractoriness

4. *Shelf life:* 5 days. Pooled platelets must be transfused within 4 hours

Indications[8]

1. Actively bleeding patients with thrombocytopenia

2. Actively bleeding patients with congenital or acquired platelet function disorders, regardless of platelet counts

3. Prophylactic treatment when:

   • Platelet counts are <10,000/μL in stable afebrile patients with hematologic disease without underlying coagulopathy

   • Platelet counts are <20,000/μL in patients with active mucosal bleeding or fever

   • Platelet counts are <50,000/μL in patients requiring line placement, invasive procedures or surgery

   • Platelet counts are <100,000/μL in patients requiring ophthalmic surgery, or surgical procedures involving the upper airway, brain, or spinal cord

PRODUCT

FRESH-FROZEN PLASMA (FFP)[1,2]

Preparation/Composition

Fresh-frozen plasma (FFP) (200–250 mL) is:
- Obtained by apheresis, *or*
- Prepared by centrifugation of whole blood and frozen within 8 hours after collection
- Plasma frozen within 24 hours (FP24) may be separated and frozen up to 24 hours after collection. Except for containing slightly lower levels of the labile factors V and VIII, FP24 is considered clinically equivalent to FFP

Administration

When replacing coagulation factors, a dose of 10–20 mL/kg is recommended, with periodic monitoring of coagulation tests to determine efficacy and appropriate dosing intervals. Attention to volume status and judicious use of a diuretic is essential to avoid volume overload ("TACO"—transfusion-associated circulatory overload)

Indications

1. Replacement of coagulation factors in patients with coagulopathy of liver disease, massive transfusion, warfarin overdose, and DIC. The INR should be >1.5, or the PT/PTT must be increased by at least 1.5 times the upper limit of normal ranges
2. Therapeutic plasma exchange in patients with TTP. Cryo-poor plasma is FFP from which the cryoprecipitate fraction has been removed through cold precipitation. This may also be used as the plasma exchange replacement fluid in patients with TTP
3. Patients with rare disorders, such as isolated factor (V, X, XI) deficiencies or C-1 esterase inhibitor deficiency

Notes

1. Vitamin K therapy should be used to correct altered PT/PTT in patients who are not actively bleeding. Similarly, FFP is unnecessary for patients with warfarin overdose in the absence of active bleeding or risk for bleeding from an emergent procedure. Patients with INR ≤5 are initially managed with cessation of therapy for 48 hours with watchful return of coagulation tests to baseline levels
2. FFP from IgA-deficient donors is indicated for patients with IgA-deficiency
3. *Shelf life:* One year when FFP is stored frozen at ≤−18°C (≤−0.4°F); 24 hours when thawed and kept at 1°–6°C (33.8°–42.8°F). Plasma can be relabeled as Thawed Plasma and stored for an additional 4 days at 1°–6°C. While ADAMTS13 levels are well preserved, Thawed Plasma prepared from FFP and stored for 5 days contains reduced levels of Factor V (>60%) and Factor VIII (>40%)

PRODUCT

CRYOPRECIPITATE[1,2]

Preparation/Composition

1. Cryoprecipitate is the cold-insoluble precipitate formed when FFP is thawed at 1°–6°C (33.8°–42.8°F)
2. Cryoprecipitate contains 200–250 mg fibrinogen, 100–150 units factor VIII, as well as 40–70% of the VWF and 20–30% of the factor XIII present in a unit of FFP

Notes

1. Cryoprecipitate is no longer used to treat patients with hemophilia A or von Willebrand disease (VWD)
2. *Shelf life:* 1 Year when kept frozen at ≤−18°C (≤−0.4°F); 6 hours after thawing when kept at 20°–24°C; (68°–75.2°F); 4 hours after pooling

Indications

1. Fibrinogen replacement during dilutional coagulopathy
2. The hypofibrinogenemia/dysfibrinogenemias of liver disease, DIC, and asparaginase therapy
3. Factor XIII deficiency

Administration

Each unit (bag) of cryoprecipitate increases fibrinogen level by 5–10 mg/dL. Six to 10 bags are pooled and infused as a single dose in a 70-kg adult

PRODUCT

GRANULOCYTE TRANSFUSIONS[1,2]

Preparation/Composition

1. Large numbers of granulocytes can be collected from healthy donors by means of granulocyte colony-stimulating factor (G-CSF) plus corticosteroid marrow stimulation followed by large-volume leukapheresis
2. Product contains $\geq 1 \times 10^{10}$ granulocytes suspended in 200–300 mL plasma

Indications

1. Severely neutropenic patients (ANC $<500/mm^3$) with bacterial sepsis without improvement despite 48–72 hours of optimum antibiotic therapy, provided there is a reasonable expectation of bone marrow recovery
2. Possible role in severely neutropenic patients with serious fungal infection not responding to antifungal therapy
3. Patients with granulocyte function disorders such as chronic granulomatous disease with refractory bacterial or fungal infections may also benefit from granulocyte transfusions

Administration

1. Transfusions are given daily until clinical improvement or neutrophil recovery occurs
2. Given the large number of RBCs in the product, donors should be RBC crossmatch-compatible with a recipient
3. Granulocyte products are routinely irradiated
4. The product is stored at room temperature (outdated in 24 hours), and is preferably infused soon after its collection
5. *Do not use* leukocyte reduction filters; use standard 170-μm filters

Notes

1. HLA-matched granulocyte donors should be considered for HLA alloimmunized patients
2. CMV-seronegative donors should be selected for CMV-seronegative recipients
3. Severe febrile and pulmonary reactions may occur, especially in HLA alloimmunized patients. Amphotericin administration should be temporally separated by at least 2 hours separated from either before or after granulocyte infusion
4. *Shelf life:* 24 Hours

PRODUCT

IRRADIATED CELLULAR BLOOD PRODUCTS[1,2]

Preparation/Composition

RBCs, platelets, and granulocytes are irradiated with 25 Gy of gamma radiation

Indications

1. Patients at risk for transfusion-associated graft-versus-host disease (TA-GVHD) must receive irradiated cellular products. These include:
   - Patients with a hematologic malignancy receiving myeloablative chemoradiotherapy
   - Patients undergoing autologous or allogeneic peripheral blood stem cell and bone marrow transplantation
   - Patients with Hodgkin and non-Hodgkin lymphoma
   - Patients with congenital severe immunodeficiency
   - Patients receiving fludarabine/cladribine
2. HLA-matched or cross-matched platelets and directed donations from blood relatives should be irradiated
3. Blood products are routinely irradiated for infants <4 months in age

Administration

The guidelines for administering irradiated products are similar to those described earlier for nonirradiated products

Notes

1. Plasma products such as FFP and cryoprecipitate need not be irradiated
2. Leukoreduction does not prevent TA-GVHD and should not be substituted for irradiation
3. *Shelf life:* RBCs must be used within 28 days after they are irradiated or before their original outdate, whichever is earlier. The shelf life of platelets and granulocytes is not affected by irradiation

PRODUCT
RH$_O$(D) IMMUNE GLOBULIN (RH$_O$(D) IgG)[1,2]
Preparation/Composition

High-titer IgG, anti-D immunoglobulin derived from pooled human plasma

Administration

1. Rh$_o$(D)-negative mothers receive a standard fixed dose of RH$_o$(D) immune globulin (human) 1500 IU (300 mcg) intravenously or intramuscularly at 28 weeks antepartum. A second fixed dose of RH$_o$(D) immune globulin (human) 1500 IU (300 mcg) intravenously or intramuscularly within 72 hours after delivery of an Rh$_o$(D)-positive infant, protects against up to 15 mL of Rh$_o$(D)-positive RBCs

2. Rh$_o$(D) immune globulin (human) for treatment of incompatible blood transfusion:

Route of Administration	RH$_o$(D) Immune Globulin (Human) Dose	
	If Exposed to Rh$_o$(D)-Positive Whole Blood	If Exposed to Rh$_o$(D)-Positive Red Blood Cells
Intravenous	45 IU (9 mcg)/mL blood	90 IU (18 mcg)/mL of red blood cells
	Administer 3000 IU (600 mcg) every 8 hours via the intravenous route, until the total dose, calculated from the above table, is administered	
Intramuscular	60 IU (12 mcg)/mL blood	120 IU (24 mcg)/mL of red blood cells
	Administer 6000 IU (1200 mcg) every 12 hours via the intramuscular route, until the total dose, calculated from the above table, is administered	

Note: Patients receiving an incompatible transfusion and those with ITP, who receive doses of anti-D immunoglobulin >300 IU/kg (>60 mcg/kg), are at an increased risk of developing chills, fever, and headache, as well as a larger hemoglobin decrease and intravascular hemolysis

Initial dosing after confirming a patient is Rho (D)-positive
RH$_o$(D) immune globulin (human) 250 IU/kg (50 mcg/kg) of body weight
In patients whose hemoglobin is between 8 and 10 g/dL, a reduced dose of RH$_o$(D) immune globulin (human), 125–200 IU/kg (25–40 mcg/kg), should be given to minimize the risk of increasing the severity of anemia
Note: Initial doses may be administered in 2 divided doses given on separate days, if desired. In patients with a hemoglobin <8 g/dL, alternative treatments should be used because of the risk of increasing the severity of the anemia

Subsequent dosing
If subsequent therapy is required to increase platelet counts, give RH$_o$(D) immune globulin (human) 125–300 IU/kg (25–60 mcg/kg) body weight
Note: Doses and the frequency of repeated doses administered should be based on a patient's clinical response by assessing platelet counts, red cell counts, hemoglobin, and reticulocyte counts

Indications

Prophylaxis against alloimmunization to Rh$_o$(D) antigen in Rh$_o$(D)-negative individuals, especially children and women of childbearing age who have been exposed to Rh$_o$(D)-positive RBCs via RBC, platelet, or granulocyte transfusions

Notes

1. RH$_o$(D) immune globulin (human) is also given after miscarriage, termination of pregnancy, amniocentesis, chorionic villous biopsy, or other obstetric manipulations/trauma. Optimal RH$_o$(D) immune globulin (human) dosages vary with indication/gestation
2. RH$_o$(D) immune globulin (human) 250–375 IU/kg (50–75 mcg/kg) is FDA approved for use in RH$_o$(D)-positive nonsplenectomized patients with ITP. A 1–2-g/dL drop in hemoglobin may occur after therapy; patients should be monitored for hemolysis

PRODUCT

CMV-NEGATIVE CELLULAR BLOOD PRODUCTS[1,2]

Preparation/Composition

1. RBCs, platelets, and granulocytes are collected from CMV-seronegative donors
2. Only 30–50% of donors are CMV-seronegative; hence, this product is frequently in short supply
3. Leukoreduced products are provided when CMV-seronegative products are unavailable

Indications

1. CMV-seronegative patients undergoing myelosuppressive chemotherapy and/or radiation therapy
2. CMV-seronegative, hematopoietic progenitor cell transplantation candidates, when the donor is CMV-seronegative. For T-cell–depleted transplants, CMV-seronegative products may be indicated even if the donor is CMV-seropositive
3. CMV-seronegative patients with immunodeficiency disorders
4. CMV-seronegative patients receiving solid-organ transplantations from CMV-seronegative donors
5. CMV-negative products are recommended for pregnant women, for all intrauterine transfusions, and transfusions in infants with very low birth weight
6. CMV-negative products are not indicated for CMV-seronegative, immunocompetent patients
7. CMV-negative products are not indicated for immunosuppressed patients, if they are CMV-seropositive

Administration

CMV-seronegative products are infused following the same guidelines described earlier for RBCs, platelets, and granulocytes

Notes

1. CMV is a cell-associated virus; hence, plasma products such as FFP and cryoprecipitate do not transmit CMV infection
2. Blood products that have been leukoreduced with third-generation filters are considered to be equivalent to CMV seronegative products. Several centers routinely use leukoreduced products in lieu of CMV-negative components[10]
3. *Shelf life:* Not affected by the CMV status of the blood product

TRANSFUSION COMPLICATIONS[11,18]
ACUTE HEMOLYTIC TRANSFUSION REACTION (AHTR)

General
1. The estimated risk per unit transfused is 1 in 25,000
2. Infusion of ABO-incompatible blood is the leading cause of AHTR. Phlebotomy errors and blood administration errors account for the majority of cases
3. *Immune-mediated AHTR can* result in intravascular or extravascular hemolysis
   Donor RBCs may be lysed by naturally occurring anti-A/anti-B alloantibodies, drug-induced antibodies, or RBC autoantibodies present in recipient plasma
   Recipient RBCs may undergo destruction if incompatible antibodies are present in plasma-containing products such as FFP and platelets, or plasma-derived products such as immune globulin (human)
4. *Non–immune-mediated* hemolysis may mimic AHTR:
   Donor RBCs may be lysed by the addition of medications or hypotonic solutions to a blood bag, malfunctioning blood warmers, and membrane damage in an extracorporeal circuit
   Recipient RBCs may be lysed by the administration of large amounts of hypotonic replacement fluids
5. Hemolytic transfusion reactions must be distinguished from episodes of hemolysis in patients with glucose-6-phosphate dehydrogenase (G6PD) deficiency or sickle cell disease

Pathophysiology
1. Antigen-antibody complexes are formed on the surface of RBCs, complement is activated, and RBCs are lysed
2. The free hemoglobin, C3a and C5a anaphylatoxins, TNF-α, IL-1, IL-6, and IL-8, when liberated, mediate hypotension, bronchospasm, renal ischemia, and activation of the coagulation cascade seen in AHTR

Clinical picture
1. Signs and symptoms include fever; rigors; severe anxiety; vomiting; pain in the chest, abdomen, flank or infusion site; dyspnea; hypotension; hemoglobinuria; and diffuse bleeding
2. Clinical presentation is more severe in immune-mediated compared with non–immune-mediated hemolysis. In general, the clinical course of intravascular hemolysis is more severe than extravascular hemolysis
3. Severity depends on the volume and rate of infusion of incompatible RBCs, and on the nature of the antigen and titers of antibody involved

Management
Clinical
1. Stop the transfusion. Replace the infusion set and keep intravenous line open with 0.9% sodium chloride injection
2. Assess cardiopulmonary status and provide support as necessary
3. Notify the blood bank, check the patient's identity with identifiers on the issued blood unit, and return the remaining blood product along with attached labels and infusion set
4. Draw and send to the blood bank fresh blood samples. Send additional samples to evaluate CBC, plasma hemoglobin, bilirubin, LDH, haptoglobin, electrolytes, BUN, and creatinine. A delayed urine sample is preferred for hemoglobin testing
5. Achieve brisk diuresis using furosemide 20–40 mg intravenously, dosed as needed to achieve and maintain a urine output >100 mL/hour
6. Provide maintenance intravenous fluid administered at a rate of 3000 mL/m^2 per day, and monitor fluid balance. Deteriorating renal function may require dialysis
7. Monitor for ongoing hemolysis and DIC

Blood bank
1. Clerical check is carried out to verify that all labels on the blood unit match the recipient
2. The posttransfusion plasma sample is visually inspected for hemoglobinemia
3. A direct antiglobulin test (DAT, direct Coombs test) is done on the posttransfusion sample. If positive, the eluate is examined to identify the coating antibody. However, the direct antiglobulin test may be negative if all incompatible RBCs have been hemolyzed
4. Additional testing may include reconfirmation of the ABO and Rh type of the patient (using both pre- and post-transfusion specimens) and of the donor unit. The antibody screen and cross-match may also be repeated to confirm donor-patient compatibility
5. Nonimmune hemolysis must be excluded when a work-up is negative for antibody-mediated RBC destruction

TRANSFUSION COMPLICATIONS
DELAYED HEMOLYTIC TRANSFUSION REACTION (DHTR)

General
1. A newly formed alloantibody or an anamnestic increase in the titer of a previously undetectable antibody results in the destruction of transfused RBCs 3–14 days after a serologically compatible RBC transfusion
2. Patients have typically been previously alloimmunized through transfusion or pregnancy

Pathophysiology
1. Antibodies are commonly directed against the Rh/Kell antigens and rarely fix complement
2. RBC destruction occurs extravascularly with minimal cytokine release

Clinical picture
1. Patients may be asymptomatic or may present with fever, jaundice, or malaise. Decreased hematocrit, reticulocytosis, hyperbilirubinemia, or elevated LDH may be seen on testing
2. In patients with sickle cell disease, DHTR may mimic a painful crisis or present with severe hemolysis
3. Intravascular hemolysis, renal dysfunction, and progression to DIC are rare with DHTR

Management
Clinical
1. Future RBC transfusions must be negative for the antigen against which the patient has made an antibody

Blood bank
1. A DAT is performed on the posttransfusion sample and any coating antibody identified. The antibody screen is also repeated on this sample

TRANSFUSION COMPLICATIONS
FEBRILE NONHEMOLYTIC TRANSFUSION REACTION (FNHTR)

General
1. FNHTRs are fairly common (0.5% per unit transfused), with higher rates seen in frequently transfused patients and multiparous women
2. Other causes of fever, including bacterial contamination and AHTR must be ruled out

Pathophysiology
1. Antibodies in a patient's plasma directed against HLA/platelet/granulocyte antigens form antigen-antibody complexes on the surface of transfused platelets and granulocytes. Less commonly, such antibodies in the donor plasma can complex with corresponding antigens present on recipient cells. Complement activation follows with release of complement components and inflammatory cytokines
2. During the storage process, leukocytes can elaborate IL-1, IL-6, IL-8, and TNF-α, which are known to mediate FNHTR. Prestorage leukoreduction decreases the concentration of inflammatory mediators in the product

Clinical picture
1. An increase in temperature of $\geq 1°C$ ($\geq 1.8°F$) occurring during or for up to 4 hours after a transfusion
2. In addition to fever, the patient may have chills, rigors, headache, and severe anxiety
3. With continued infusion, high fever and debilitating symptoms may develop

Management
Clinical
1. Stop the transfusion, keep the line open with 0.9% sodium chloride injection, perform all clerical checks, and return the remaining product to the blood bank
2. Fever is usually self-limited and responds to antipyretics
3. Control of rigors may require **Meperidine** 25–50 mg by intravenous injection
4. Complete a work-up of AHTR if hemolysis cannot be ruled out
5. Obtain blood cultures if bacterial contamination is being considered in the differential diagnosis
6. Individuals with FNHTR benefit from premedication with **Acetaminophen** 650–1000 mg administered orally

Blood bank
1. Patients with frequent febrile reactions should receive leukoreduced products

TRANSFUSION COMPLICATIONS
ALLERGIC TRANSFUSION REACTION

General
1. Similar to FNHTR, allergic transfusion reactions are fairly common, especially in chronically transfused patients
2. Severe IgA deficiency should be ruled out in patients with anaphylactic reactions
3. Rare cases of anaphylaxis mediated by antibodies to haptoglobin or complement component C4 have been reported in patients with deficiencies of these proteins

Pathophysiology
1. Hypersensitivity to allergens (eg, plasma proteins) or drugs in donor plasma

Clinical picture
1. Symptoms range from mild uncomplicated urticaria to fatal anaphylaxis
2. Mild allergic reactions are very common, limited to localized rash, pruritus, and flushing, and do not require detailed work-up
3. Infrequently, patients present with severe bronchospasm, tongue and laryngeal swelling, hypotension, vomiting, diarrhea, and shock

Management
Clinical: For uncomplicated allergic reactions
1. Stop transfusion. Administer **Diphenhydramine** 50 mg intravenously or another histamine (H_1) receptor antagonist. If symptoms improve, restart the transfusion
2. If symptoms reappear and progress on restarting the transfusion, stop the transfusion and do not restart
3. For future transfusions, premedicate the patient with **Diphenhydramine** 50 mg administered by intravenous injection or orally or another H_1-receptor antagonist, 30–45 minutes before a transfusion
4. For patients with recurrent reactions, in addition to prophylaxis with a H_1-receptor antagonist, consider administering intravenously a **Histamine (H_2) receptor antagonist** and **Hydrocortisone** 50–100 mg prior to the start of a transfusion
5. For patients with severe reactions to platelets, use volume-reduced or washed platelets; for severe reactions to RBCs, use saline-washed products

Clinical: For anaphylactoid and anaphylactic reactions
1. Stop transfusion; maintain intravenous access and initiate resuscitation with fluids, vasopressors, bronchodilators, and respiratory support as needed
2. Investigate whether the recipient is severely IgA deficient
3. If an allergen has not been identified, cellular components for future transfusions must be extensively washed. Adequate preparation of the patient is recommended with H_1- and H_2-receptor antagonists and steroids
4. For patients with severe IgA deficiency, all cellular products must be extensively washed and plasma must be obtained from IgA-deficient donors (see next section)

TRANSFUSION COMPLICATIONS

ALLERGIC TRANSFUSION REACTION: PATIENTS WITH IgA DEFICIENCY
(TRANSFUSION STRATEGY FOR PATIENTS WITH IgA DEFICIENCY)

General
1. IgA deficiency affects approximately 1 in 600 people
2. IgA deficiency must be excluded when anaphylactic reactions develop to blood products
3. Patients with known IgA deficiency are usually managed with washed RBCs to avoid sensitization and subsequent anaphylaxis
4. Patients with severe IgA deficiency and anti-IgA antibodies are at risk for developing an anaphylactic reaction when receiving blood products containing IgA

Pathophysiology
1. IgA exists as 2 subclasses, IgA1 and IgA2; the IgA2 subclass is associated with 2 allotypic determinants, 2m [1] and 2m [2]
2. Anti-IgA antibodies may be class-specific (anti-IgA), subclass-specific (anti-IgA1 or IgA2) or allotype-specific (anti-IgA2m [1] or anti-IgA2m [2])

Clinical picture
1. Patients may present with severe bronchospasm, tongue and laryngeal swelling, hypotension, vomiting, diarrhea, and shock

Management
Clinical: For anaphylactoid and anaphylactic reactions
1. Stop transfusion; maintain IV access and initiate resuscitation with fluids, vasopressors, bronchodilators, and respiratory support as needed
2. For patients with severe IgA deficiency, all cellular products must be extensively washed, and plasma must be obtained from IgA-deficient donors

Blood bank: Guide to selecting components for patients at risk for IgA-anaphylaxis
RBCs
1. RBC units washed with 1–2 L of 0.9% sodium chloride injection have a 99% reduction in their plasma protein content. For IgA-sensitized individuals, it is recommended that RBCs be washed with greater volumes of saline (2–3 L) for satisfactory removal of IgA
2. Frozen deglycerolized RBCs are essentially free of IgA and are probably as safe as RBCs collected from IgA-deficient donors
3. Freezing of autologous units should be considered for IgA-sensitized individuals who have recurrent reactions with washed RBCs

Platelets
• Platelets can be rendered IgA-deficient by washing them free of the plasma IgA. Some hospital blood banks may not provide this service

Fresh-frozen plasma and cryoprecipitate
• Plasma-derived components such as FFP and cryoprecipitate should be obtained only from IgA-deficient donors

Immunoglobulins and plasma derivatives
• IgA-deficient products, chosen after scrutiny of a manufacturer's product insert and confirmed to contain <0.05 mg/dL of IgA, can be safely transfused in IgA-sensitized patients

TRANSFUSION COMPLICATIONS

TRANSFUSION-ASSOCIATED CIRCULATORY OVERLOAD (TACO)[12]

General
1. TACO, an under-recognized complication, occurs in up to 1% of transfusions. Elderly patients are at increased risk

Pathophysiology
1. A rapid increase in the intravascular volume in patients with severe chronic anemia or in those with compromised cardiorespiratory or renal function can precipitate acute pulmonary edema

Clinical picture
1. Signs and symptoms are those of congestive heart failure

Management
Clinical
1. The transfusion should be stopped
2. Provide supplemental oxygen, administer intravenous diuretics, and reassess fluid balance
3. Further transfusions may require more diuresis and slower infusion rates (1 mL/kg per hour)
4. The differential diagnosis includes transfusion-related acute lung injury (TRALI)

TRANSFUSION COMPLICATIONS
TRANSFUSION-RELATED ACUTE LUNG INJURY (TRALI)[11,13,14]

General
Estimated incidence: 1 in 5000 transfusions of plasma-containing components

Pathophysiology
1. TRALI results from the transfusion of plasma containing blood components (RBCs, platelets, FFP, cryoprecipitate, or granulocytes) or plasma-derivatives like immune globulin (human)
2. Antibodies (HLA class I/II, antineutrophil) in donor plasma react with a patient's WBCs or antibodies in the recipient plasma to form complexes with donor leukocytes
3. Antigen–antibody complex formation and complement activation lead to aggregation, margination, and sequestration of neutrophils in the pulmonary microvasculature
4. Tissue-disruptive enzymes and free radicals released from neutrophils damage the vascular endothelium, and fluid extravasates into the interstitium and alveolar spaces
5. Alternatively, a lipid-priming agent in stored blood acting in concert with a "priming" lung injury that preceded the transfusion has been proposed in the two-hit hypothesis for the development of TRALI

Clinical picture
1. Signs and symptoms occur within 1–6 hours after starting transfusion
2. Fever and mild-to-moderate hypotension are frequently seen. Less frequently, hypertension is present
3. Respiratory distress can rapidly progress to severe hypoxemia and respiratory failure
4. *Chest x-rays:* Bilateral extensive whiteout pattern or more patchy changes
5. The pulmonary edema is noncardiogenic in origin. Central venous and pulmonary capillary wedge pressures are normal
6. A transient drop in WBC count has also been described

Management
Clinical
1. Achieve optimum oxygenation with rapid and intensive respiratory support
2. Exclude AHTR, anaphylaxis, bacterial contamination, and fluid overload
3. Most patients improve clinically and radiologically in 72–96 hours
4. Blood products may continue to be used cautiously. Leukoreduced components might be beneficial where TRALI is mediated by anti-HLA or antineutrophil antibodies present in the recipient

Blood bank
1. Other blood components prepared from an implicated donor are quarantined, and the blood donor center is notified
2. Donors are evaluated for anti-HLA and antineutrophil antibodies. If a specific antibody is identified, the patient is typed for HLA and neutrophil antigens to look for a match with the cognate antigen
3. Antibody-positive donors implicated in fatal TRALI are permanently deferred
4. Rarely, anti-HLA and anti-neutrophil antibodies present in the recipient may mediate TRALI
5. TRALI mitigation measures implemented by blood centers in the United States include the decision to minimize the preparation of high plasma-volume components like FFP and apheresis platelets from donors known to be leukocyte-alloimmunized or at increased risk of leukocyte alloimmunization

TRANSFUSION COMPLICATIONS
TRANSFUSION-ASSOCIATED GRAFT-VERSUS-HOST-DISEASE (TA-GVHD)

General
1. The provision of gamma-irradiated cellular blood components for all patient groups at risk for TA-GVHD effectively prevents this frequently fatal complication of transfusion

Pathophysiology
1. Similar to GVHD seen in the hematopoietic transplant setting, immunocompetent lymphocytes in a donor unit proliferate in a susceptible (immunodeficient or immunosuppressed) host and launch a destructive immune response against host tissues expressing foreign HLA antigens
2. In rare instances, a directed donation from a family member (donor with a homozygous haplotype) has caused TA-GVHD in an immunocompetent host (recipient heterozygous for the donor haplotype)

Clinical picture
1. Symptoms and signs appear 10–14 days after transfusion
2. Marrow hypoplasia is a distinguishing hallmark of TA-GVHD
3. The fulminant cutaneous, gastrointestinal, and hepatic manifestations of acute GVHD are also seen with TA-GVHD
4. More than 90% of patients have a fatal outcome

Management
Clinical
1. Unlike transplant-associated GVHD, TA-GVHD responds poorly to interventions
2. Responses have been reported to combination therapies involving lymphocyte immune globulin, antithymocyte globulin (ATG); cyclosporine; methylprednisolone; anti-CD3 monoclonal antibodies; nafamostat mesylate (not available in the United States); and filgrastim
3. Prevention of TA-GVHD is achieved by identifying all groups at risk and by the meticulous attention to irradiation of all cellular components transfused to these patients

Blood bank
1. The blood bank should be notified about all patients at risk for TA-GVHD even before any blood products are ordered
2. HLA-matched and cross-matched platelets and granulocyte products are irradiated
3. Patients receiving fludarabine or other purine analogs like cladribine for illnesses other than hematologic malignancies (eg, SLE) should also receive irradiated blood products
4. All cellular components from blood relatives are irradiated
5. HLA typing of patients' circulating lymphocytes may aid in the diagnosis of TA-GVHD

TRANSFUSION COMPLICATIONS
POST-TRANSFUSION PURPURA (PTP)

General
1. PTP is a rare complication, presenting as sudden onset of severe thrombocytopenia 7–10 days after transfusion in a previously transfused or pregnant patient
2. Approximately 200 cases have been reported worldwide

Pathophysiology
1. In >90% of cases, platelet destruction is mediated by an alloantibody directed against the human platelet specific antigen, HPA-1a
2. Rapid destruction of the autologous HPA-1a–negative platelets by a poorly defined "innocent bystander" mechanism contributes to the thrombocytopenia

Clinical picture
1. Severe unexplained thrombocytopenia developing 7–10 days after transfusion of a blood product should raise the suspicion of PTP
2. Patients may be asymptomatic or may present with purpura, ecchymoses, mucosal bleeding, or life-threatening hemorrhage

Management
Clinical
1. The thrombocytopenia is usually self-limiting and spontaneously resolves in 2–3 weeks
2. Routine platelet transfusions do not improve platelet counts, may in fact be detrimental, and should be avoided if there is time to begin specific treatment
3. For patients with life-threatening hemorrhage, high-dose intravenous immune globulin (IVIG) (0.4 g/kg/day for 2–5 days or 1 g/kg per day for 2 days) is preferred over therapeutic plasma exchange as the first line of therapy. Platelet counts typically recover in 3–4 days. A second course of IVIG may be required in some patients

Blood bank
1. Antibody studies may show the presence of anti–HPA-1a platelet antibody. Rarely, other specificities like anti–HPA-1b and anti–HPA-5a have been implicated in PTP
2. Patients should preferably receive appropriate antigen-negative platelets
3. Transfused platelets from random donors may successfully increase platelet counts after IVIG therapy has been initiated
4. RBC requirements are best met by providing washed products

TRANSFUSION COMPLICATIONS
BACTERIAL CONTAMINATION[15]

General
1. Until recently, an important cause of transfusion-related mortality
2. Mandatory bacterial testing of platelets in the United States, beginning March 2004, has significantly reduced this risk
3. *Risk of bacterial contamination of platelets:* Bacterial contamination is detected in approximately 1 in 5000 apheresis platelet collections using culture methods. However, current methods fail to detect all contaminated units. Using data from passive surveillance of transfusion reactions, this residual risk was estimated as approximately 1 in 75,000 septic reactions per distributed component.[15]
4. RBC units have a much lower risk of bacterial contamination

Pathophysiology
1. Bacteria enter donor units during collection process/component preparation
2. Components (eg, platelets) stored at room temperature are commonly associated with Gram-positive organisms such as *Staphylococcus*
3. Components (eg, RBCs) stored at 4°C (39.2°F) are associated with Gram-negative organisms, such as *Enterobacter, Yersinia, Pseudomonas,* and *Serratia*

Clinical picture
1. High fever, chills, rigors, dyspnea, hypotension, and shock may develop rapidly
2. Milder presentations, particularly in a previously febrile patient may go unrecognized

Management
Clinical
1. Stop the transfusion and resuscitate aggressively
2. Send the remaining product for bacterial culture; send patient samples for blood cultures
3. Commence broad-spectrum antibiotics to cover both Gram-positive and Gram-negative organisms; modify therapy based on culture results

Blood bank
1. The implicated product should be sent immediately for Gram's staining and culture
2. All other components (RBC, FFP, cryoprecipitate) made from the same donation should be quarantined
3. Depending on the identity of the organism, donor follow-up may be indicated. A review of all donor collection and processing procedures might also be appropriate in certain instances

TRANSFUSION COMPLICATIONS
OTHER INFECTIOUS RISKS OF TRANSFUSION[16,17]

Viruses

1. All blood donations in the United States are tested for human immune deficiency virus (HIV-1/2), human T-cell lymphotropic virus (HTLV-I/II), hepatitis B virus (HBV), hepatitis C virus (HCV), West Nile virus (WNV), and Chagas infections

2. Routine testing for hepatitis A virus and parvovirus B19 is not done

3. On rare occasions, donors with window-phase infections can still transmit disease

4. Currently, the estimated risks of viral transmission from a blood unit are:

   HIV: 1 in 2.14 million
   HTLV: 1 in 3 million
   HBV: 1 in 488,800
   HCV: 1 in 1.94 million

Parasites

1. Posttransfusion malaria and babesiosis have been reported in the United States

2. Routine screening of donor blood for these agents is not carried out

Prions

1. A screening test for variant Creutzfeldt-Jakob disease (vCJD) is not currently available

2. Donor exclusion criteria are based on a history of travel and residence in Europe

3. Transfusion-transmitted vCJD has been reported from the United Kingdom[17]

References

1. Roback JD et al., eds. Technical Manual, 17th ed. Bethesda, MD: American Association of Blood Banks, 2011
2. Simon TL et al., eds. Rossi's Principles of Transfusion Medicine. 4th ed. Bethesda, MD: AABB Press and Hoboken, NJ: Blackwell Publishing Ltd, 2009
3. Goodnough LT et al. Concepts of blood transfusion in adults. Lancet 2013;381:1845–1854
4. Hébert PC et al. A multicenter, randomized, controlled clinical trial of transfusion requirements in critical care. N Engl J Med 1999;340:409–417
5. Hébert PC et al. Is a low transfusion threshold safe in critically ill patients with cardiovascular diseases? Crit Care Med 2001;29:227–234
6. Carson JL et al. Red blood cell transfusion: a clinical practice guideline from the AABB. Ann Intern Med 2012;157:49–58
7. Stroncek DF, Rebulla P. Platelet transfusions. Lancet 2007;370:427–438
8. Schiffer CA et al. Platelet transfusion for patients with cancer: clinical practice guidelines of the American Society of Clinical Oncology. J Clin Oncol 2001;19:1519–1538
9. Sacher RA et al. Management of patients refractory to platelet transfusion. Arch Pathol Lab Med 2003;127:409–414
10. Blajchman MA et al. Proceedings of a consensus conference: prevention of post-transfusion CMV in the era of universal leukoreduction. Transfus Med Rev 2001;15:1–20
11. Popovsky MA et al., eds. Transfusion Reactions. 4th ed. Bethesda, MD: American Association of Blood Banks, 2012
12. Alam A et al. The prevention of transfusion-associated circulatory overload. Transfus Med Rev 2013;27:105–112
13. Kleinman S et al. Toward an understanding of transfusion-related acute lung injury: statement of a consensus panel. Transfusion 2004;44:1774–1789
14. Sachs UJ. Recent insights into the mechanism of transfusion-related acute lung injury. Curr Opin Hematol 2011;18:436–442
15. Eder AF et al. Bacterial screening of apheresis platelets and the residual risk of septic transfusion reactions: the American Red Cross experience (2004–2006). Transfusion 2007;47:1134–1142
16. Stramer SL. Current risks of transfusion-transmitted agents: a review. Arch Pathol Lab Med 2007;131:702–707
17. Zou S et al. Transfusion transmission of human prion diseases. Transfus Med Rev 2008;22:58–69
18. The National Healthcare Safety Network (NHSN) Manual. Biovigilance Component. Protocol v2.0. 2013 [cited 2013 August 29].
    Available from: http://www.cdc.gov/nhsn/PDFs/Biovigilance/BV-HV-protocol-current.pdf

46. Oncologic Emergencies

Mauricio Burotto Pichun, MD and Tito Fojo, MD, PhD

Spinal Cord Compression (SCC)[1–36]

Etiology

Lifetime incidence of SCC in cancer patients:	1–6%
Median overall survival of patients with SCC:	3–16 months
SCC as the initial manifestation of cancer:	20–30% of all cases of SCC
SCC as the initial manifestation of cancer:	Lung cancer Cancer of unknown primary Non-Hodgkin lymphoma Multiple myeloma

SCC distribution along spine:
        Thoracic spine:
        Lumbar spine:
        Cervical spine:
	
	60–80%
	15–30%
	4–13%

Sites of Involvement	Percentage of SCC	Histology (% Among All Cases)
Extradural metastases:*	90–95	Prostate cancer (15–20%) Breast cancer (15–20%) Lung cancer (15–20%) Non-Hodgkin lymphoma (5–10%) Multiple myeloma (5–10%) Renal cancer (5–10%)
Intradural masses:	5–10	Meningioma Nerve sheath tumors Large leptomeningeal metastases
Transforaminal progression of paravertebral tumor:	Uncommon	Lymphomas Neuroblastomas
Primary hematogenous seeding to epidural space:	Rare	

*The most common mechanisms are:
- Direct extension into the epidural space of a hematogenous metastasis to a vertebral body
- Pathologic fracture of a vertebral body infiltrated by a metastatic deposit resulting in cord injury by a bone fragment or spinal instability

Work-up

- Spinal cord compression has been associated with most cancers. Consequently, any patient with cancer and new back pain or a change in character of preexisting back pain should receive appropriate evaluation
- Differential diagnosis of SCC:
  1. Epidural abscess
  2. Subdural abscess
  3. Hematoma
  4. Herniated disc
  5. Leptomeningeal disease
  6. Hypertrophic arthritic changes
  7. Radiation myelopathy
  8. Myelopathy secondary to intrathecal chemotherapy
- Suspected spinal cord compression requires immediate imaging studies and consultation with a radiation oncologist and a neurosurgeon
- Because multiple spinal epidural metastasis are found in one-third of patients it is recommended that the entire spinal cord be imaged, or at least the thoracic and lumbar spine in addition to the symptomatic region

Symptoms

Back pain	95%
Weakness	60–85%
Sensory deficits	40–90%
Autonomic dysfunction	50%
Ataxia	5%

Imaging Studies

Gadolinium-enhanced MRI	• The standard for diagnosis of spinal cord compression • Sensitivity: 93%; specificity: 97%; overall diagnostic accuracy: 95%
CT scan	• Useful for assessing the degree of bone destruction and whether bone or tumor is causing spinal cord compression
Myelography	• Myelography and postmyelogram CT is used for patients in whom MRI is contraindicated (such as patients with pacemakers, mechanical valves, and other metal implants) • Myelography is contraindicated in the presence of brain masses, thrombocytopenia, or coagulopathy, and has a small risk of worsening the neurologic deficit from pressure shifts in the event of complete spinal subarachnoid block

Treatment Strategies

1. Supportive care

- Pain frequently is resistant to standard analgesics. Pain control with opioids as clinically indicated
- Steroids to lessen pain, reduce vasogenic cord edema, and avoid radiation-induced spinal edema

Dexamethasone 96 mg; administer intravenously over 15–30 min, *followed by:*

Dexamethasone 24 mg/dose; administer orally for 4 doses per day (approximately every 6 hours) for 3 days. Gradually decrease doses and increase administration intervals (taper) to discontinue use after 10 days

Note: This regimen was used in a randomized controlled trial in which high-dose dexamethasone was compared to no therapy in 57 patients with metastatic SCC treated with RT alone. Eighty-one percent of the participants in the intervention arm were ambulatory after treatment compared with 63% in the control group. Significant side effects were reported in 11% of those who received high-dose dexamethasone

Sørensen PS et al. Eur J Cancer 1994;30A:22–27

or

Dexamethasone 10 mg; administer as a short intravenous infusion over 10–20 minutes, *followed 6 hours later by:*

Dexamethasone 4 mg; administer orally every 6 hours. Taper to discontinue use within 2 weeks

Note: Used because of an increased incidence in side effects observed with higher doses

Heimdal K et al. J Neurooncol 1992;12:141–144
Vecht CJ et al. Neurology 1989;39:1255–1257

2. Radiation therapy

a. Preferred treatment for most patients with metastatic SCC

b. If surgery is contraindicated, external beam radiotherapy with corticosteroids remains first-line therapy

c. Indications for postoperative radiation are not clear: Treatment of tumor relapses versus combining radiotherapy with surgery to improve local control (Lutz et al. 2011); however, RT may increase the risk of pathologic fracture in cases of spinal instability

d. Important variables:

    (1) Early diagnosis

    (2) Favorable histology

Radiosensitive tumors:	Lymphoma Multiple myeloma Seminoma Ewing sarcoma
Moderately radiosensitive tumors:	Breast cancer Prostate cancer Lung Cancer
Relatively radio-resistant tumors:	Melanoma Renal cell cancer Osteosarcoma Colon cancer

Maranzano E, Latini P. Int J Radiat Oncol Biol Phys 1995;32:959–967

A prospective analysis of 209 patients treated with radiation and steroids

- Among patients who were ambulatory, nonambulatory, or paraplegic before treatment, 98%, 60%, and 11%, respectively, were able to ambulate
- Early diagnosis was the most important predictor of success, so a majority of patients able to walk and with good bladder function maintained these capacities
- When diagnosis was late, tumors with favorable histologies (ie, multiple myeloma, and breast and prostate carcinomas) responded best to radiation therapy
- Duration of response was also influenced by histology. A favorable histology was associated with high median response durations: for multiple myeloma, and breast and prostate carcinomas, 16, 12, and 10 months, respectively
- Median survival time was 6 months, with a 28% probability of survival at 1 year
- There was a correlation between patient survival and duration of response, with systemic relapse of disease generally being the cause of death

Notes:

- Transient myelopathy can develop 2–6 months after radiation therapy secondary to transient demyelination of the posterior columns
- The symptoms of transient myelopathy often resolve spontaneously within a year in most cases
- Chronic progressive myelitis is a late delayed complication of radiation

Conventional radiation:

- Efficacy of conventional radiotherapy is well established with complete or partial responses observed in 65–86% of patients
- There is no difference in efficacy and tolerance between different radiation schema but a short schema (8 Gy in 1 fraction) may be preferred in patients with long bone metastases or an estimated life expectancy ≤3 months

(continued)

Treatment Strategies (continued)

Different Radiation Therapy Schema: Comparison of Efficacy and Tolerance

Sze WM et al. Cochrane Database Syst Rev 2004;CD004721
(N = 11 trials; 3435 Patients)

	Radiation Schema		OR (95% CI)
	Single RT	Multifraction RT	
Overall pain response rates	60%	59%	1.03 (0.89–1.30; NS)
Complete pain response rate	34%	32%	1.11 (0.94–1.19; NS)
Probability of re-irradiation*	21.5%	7.4%	3.44 (2.67–4.43)
Fractures at site of RT	3%	1.6%	1.82 (1.06–3.11)

Hartsell WF et al. J Natl Cancer Inst 2005;97:798–804 (N = 898)

	Radiation Schema		Significance
	8 Gy × 1	3 Gy × 10	
CR + PR	15% + 50%	18% + 48%	NS
Median survival	9.1 months	9.5 months	NS
G2–4 acute complications†	10%	17%	$p = 0.002$
Late toxicity	4%	4%	NS
Fractures at site of RT	5%	4%	NS
Probability of re-irradiation‡	18%	9%	$p < 0.001$

Foro Arnalot P et al. Radiother Oncol 2008;89:150–155 (N = 160)

	Radiation Schema		Significance
	8 Gy × 1	3 Gy × 10	
CR + PR at 3 weeks	15% + 60%	13% + 73%	NS
CR + PR at 12 weeks	13% + 52%	11% + 51%	NS
Pan progression	28%	43%	NS
Net pain relief	68%	71%	NS
Acute toxicity	12%	18%	NS
Probability of re-irradiation‡	28%	2%	$p < 0.001$

NS, Not significant; OR, overall response
*Estimated
†Primarily gastrointestinal symptoms
‡Uncertain if a result of an increased recurrence rate at a lower dose and/or reluctance of radiation therapists to re-irradiate after a dose of 30 Gy previously administered to the spinal cord

(continued)

Treatment Strategies (*continued*)

Stereotactic radiosurgery (also called stereotactic body radiation therapy [SBRT])

• A growing body of literature supports its efficacy in treating spine lesions

• Used to deliver a high dose of RT to the target volume while protecting organs at risk, usually with a single fraction

• Advocates claim it can partially overcome intrinsic tumor resistance to ionizing radiation, but solid data supporting the strategy is not available

• May be applied to any part of the body with stereotactic techniques such as Volumetric-Modulated Arc Therapy (VMAT) or CyberKnife

• For a single lesion, 8–24 Gy may be given depending on the distance to the spinal cord

• More protracted regimens can deliver 20–30 Gy in 2–6 fractions

• The best candidates include: (a) solitary lesion or oligometastatic disease; (b) ≥5 mm between lesion and spinal cord; (c) good general health status; (d) no spinal cord compression; and (e) life expectancy ≥6 months (Chawla S et al. Bone 2009;45:817–821)

• Exclusion criteria: Canal narrowing >25%, instability requiring surgical treatment, and a life expectancy =3 months (Lutz S et al. Int J Radiat Oncol Biol Phys 2011;79:965–976)

• May be valuable when considering treatment of a recurrence after RT such as spinal tumors where retreatment is limited by tolerance of the spinal cord

Salvage Stereotactic Body Radiation Therapy (Salvage SBRT)

	No. of Tumors/No. of Patients		Retreat for Salvage (n)		
Author	Total Number	Number Retreated	Number	Follow-up Months (Range)	Local Control
Milker-Zabel et al.	19/18	19/18	18	Median 12 (4–33)	95%
Hamilton et al.	5/5	5/5	5	Median 6 (1–12)	100%
Mahan et al.	8/8	8/8	8	Mean 15.2	100%
Gerszten et al.	500/393	344/NR	51	Median 21 (3–53)	88%
Sahgal et al.	60/38	37/26	31	Median 7 (1–48)	90% (96% 1 year*)
Garg et al.	63/59	63/59	59	Median 17.6	76% 1 year[†]

*Progression-free probability
[†]Of the tumors that progressed, 13/16 (81%) patients had tumors within 5 mm of the spinal cord, and six eventually developed spinal cord compression

Intensity modulated radiotherapy (IMRT)

• Can significantly reduce the incidence and severity of iatrogenic complications by improving radiation conformation around the target volumes, with more accurate dose distributions using intensity modulation of multiple-beam irradiation (Veldeman L et al. Lancet Oncol 2008;9:367–375)

• Because IMRT requires precise repositioning devices and correction of setup errors (particularly for spinal or paraspinal lesions), it must be associated with repositioning techniques guided by imaging (IGRT) (Guckenberger M et al. Radiother Oncol 2007;84:56–63)

• IMRT can deliver high doses of radiation within a few fractions, mimicking stereotactic radiosurgery

• Single-fraction image-guided IMRT may also be used

• A retrospective analysis of 62 patients reported fracture progression in 39% of patients treated with IMRT. Risk factors for fracture were: (a) Lesions located between T10 and sacrum; (b) lytic features; and (c) percent involvement of a vertebral body. Local tumor progression occurred in only 7 patients (Rose PS et al. J Clin Oncol 2009;27:5075–5079)

3. Surgery ± Radiation

Surgery should be considered in patients with:

• Spinal instability

• Paraplegia at diagnosis

• Retropulsion of bones within the vertebral canal

• Radioresistant tumors

• Deterioration during RT

• Prior radiation therapy in the same areas

• No tissue diagnosis

(*continued*)

Treatment Strategies (*continued*)

Note:

(Patchell R et al. Proc Am Soc Clin Oncol 2003;22:1 [abstract 2])

The first phase III randomized trial in which the efficacy of direct decompressive surgery was evaluated in patients with metastatic SCC compared the standard 30 Gy in 3-Gy, uninterrupted, daily fractions with decompressive and stabilization surgery within 24 hours after diagnosis followed by the same radiotherapy started within 2 weeks. The trial was terminated early at interim analysis when early stopping rules were met regarding the primary end points of ambulatory rate and time ambulatory after treatment. Regarding the primary end point of ambulation, the combined treatment had a median ambulation time of 126 days, compared with 35 days for radiation alone ($P = 0.006$). Furthermore, baseline ambulatory and nonambulatory patients who had surgery and radiation had one-half the likelihood of being nonambulatory compared with those who had radiation alone. For nonambulatory patients, the combined-treatment patients had a significantly higher chance of regaining the ability to walk after therapy (56% vs. 19%; $P = 0.03$). Although the study included only 101 patients the results of this study challenges the accepted status quo of radiation alone in the management of metastatic SCC

Note:

(Shehadi JA et al. Eur Spine J 2007;16:1179–1192)

One-hundred twenty-five interventions in 87 patients with vertebral metastases in a population of 479 patients with breast cancer. Indications for spinal surgery (in patients able to tolerate it, and a life expectancy ≥3 months):

• Spinal deformity with major pain

• Spinal cord compression

• Previous irradiation of the site concerned

• Uncontrollable pain

Results:

• Of 76 patients who were ambulatory before surgery, 98% were also ambulatory after surgery

• 6/10 with pain before spinal surgery reduced to 2/10 with pain control for ≥12 months ($p <0.001$, significant compared to the population of patients without intervention)

• Median follow-up of 13 months

• Median survival after the first spinal surgery was 21 months (95% CI, 16–27 months)

• 39% of patients had complications; 26% considered significant

4. **Chemotherapy ± Radiation**

Chemotherapy can be used in combination with radiotherapy for treatment of SCC or alone for chemosensitive tumors including neuroblastoma, Ewing sarcoma, osteogenic sarcoma, germ cell tumors, and lymphomas in patients who are not candidates for surgery or radiation

5. **Vertebroplasty** (injecting cement percutaneously to treat a spinal metastasis with a risk of fracture [Anselmetti GC et al. Cardiovasc Intervent Radiol 2007;30:441–447; Bròdano GB et al. Eur Rev Med Pharmacol Sci 2007;11:91–100])

• Effective at relieving pain

• Increases spinal stability

• Can help prevent the risk of fracture

• Allows for radiotherapy to be delivered within a few days

6. **Balloon kyphoplasty**

(Berenson J et al. Lancet Oncol 2011;12:225–235)

• For painful vertebral compression fractures, can provide rapid pain relief

• Can improve neurological function when compared with a nonsurgical strategy

• Allows for radiotherapy to be delivered within a few days

Superior Vena Cava (SVC) Syndrome (SVCS)[37–59]

Etiology

- Obstruction of the SVC affects approximately 15,000 people per year in the United States

Causes of SVC Syndrome

Malignant Causes	85–95% of All Cases
Bronchogenic carcinoma*	80%
Non-Hodgkin lymphoma†	15%
Metastatic cancers‡	5–10%
Nonmalignant causes§	**10–15%**

*Small cell lung cancer accounts for up to 60% of all cases of SVC obstruction
†Diffuse large cell and lymphoblastic lymphomas are the most common subtypes associated with SVC syndrome. Despite a common presentation with mediastinal lymphadenopathy, Hodgkin disease rarely causes SVC syndrome
‡*Most common primary tumor sites:* Breast cancer >>> germ cell malignancies and gastrointestinal cancers
§Causes include granulomatous infections, goiter, aortic aneurysms, fibrosing mediastinitis, tension pneumothorax, and SVC thrombosis. Many cases of SVC thrombosis are caused by the presence of indwelling central venous access devices

Work-up

- Appropriate management of SVC syndrome requires identification of the condition and its antecedent cause
- As many as 60% of patients with SVC syndrome secondary to cancer present without a known diagnosis of cancer
- The rapidity of onset of symptoms and signs from SVC obstruction is dependent upon the rate at which complete obstruction of the SVC occurs in relation to the recruitment of venous collaterals. Patients with malignant disease develop symptoms of SVC syndrome within weeks to months because the rapidity of tumor growth does not allow adequate time to develop collateral flow

Symptoms

Dyspnea:	60%	Dysphagia:	9%
Facial swelling:	50%	Dizziness:	<5%
Cough:	20%	Headache:	<5%
Arm swelling:	18%	Lethargy:	<5%
Chest pain:	15%	Syncopal attacks:	<5%

1. Contrast-enhanced chest CT:
   - Preferred imaging modality once the diagnosis is suspected
   - Defines the level and extent of venous blockage
   - Maps collateral pathways of venous drainage
   - Often permits identification of the underlying cause of venous obstruction
2. Bilateral upper extremity venography:
   - Can define the site and extent of SVC obstruction and visualize collateral pathways
   - Does not identify the cause of SVC obstruction unless thrombosis is the sole etiology
3. Biopsy:
   - To confirm malignancy and establish histologic diagnosis
   - Bronchoscopy, mediastinoscopy, or thoracotomy may be indicated when less invasive procedures do not provide a definitive diagnosis

Treatment Strategies

General Principles
- Treatment should be selected according to the histologic disorder and stage of the primary process
- Goals of treatment are to relieve symptoms and attempt the cure of the primary malignant process
- Deferring therapy until a full diagnostic work-up has been completed does not pose a hazard for most patients, provided the evaluation completed expeditiously and the patient is clinically stable
- Treatment recommendations should be determined by a multidisciplinary team to include a radiation oncologist, medical oncologist, radiologist, and a surgeon or pulmonologist, when appropriate
- Prognosis and life expectancy are related to the histologic type and stage of the underlying malignancy at presentation
- Despite the favorable outcomes with stents, chemotherapy and/or radiotherapy comprise the basis of treatment for obstruction of the SVC
- Chemotherapy and radiotherapy are effective in relieving obstruction of the SVC in a variable proportion of patients, depending on tumor histology
- Stents can relieve symptoms rapidly in 80–95% of patients; however, severe bleeding, cardiopulmonary complications, and stent migration remain significant problems. Use of thrombolytics following stent insertion increase morbidity
- Recurrence of obstruction following stent placement occurs in 4–45% of cases
- Stents are useful in patients with diseases that respond less well to chemotherapy or radiotherapy such as mesothelioma
- Optimal timing of stent insertion—whether at diagnosis or following failure of other modalities—is currently uncertain, although they are most frequently used after chemotherapy and/or radiotherapy
- No study has described the effectiveness of steroids in SVC obstruction; their value remains uncertain but use is widespread

A Cochrane Database analysis (Rowell NP, Gleeson FV. Cochrane Database Syst Rev 2001;CD001316) reported the results of 2 randomized and 44 nonrandomized controlled trials. Studies examined enrolled patients with *carcinoma of the bronchus* and a diagnosis of SVC obstruction who had been treated with any combination of the following treatment modalities: (a) steroids, (b) chemotherapy, (c) radiotherapy, or (d) insertion of an expandable metal stent

Small cell lung cancer (SCLC):
- SVC obstruction is present at diagnosis in 10% of patients
- *One randomized trial:* The rate of recurrence of SVC obstruction was not significantly reduced by giving radiotherapy after completion of chemotherapy
- Chemotherapy and/or radiotherapy relieved SVC obstruction in 77%; 17% of those treated had a recurrence of SVC obstruction
- Data support the use of stenting when obstruction of the SVC recurs or when it persists following initial chemotherapy and radiotherapy

Non–small cell lung cancer (NSCLC):
- SVC obstruction is present at diagnosis in 1.7% of patients
- *One randomized trial:* Addition of induction chemotherapy to synchronous chemoradiotherapy did not increase the rates of relief of SVC obstruction
- 60% had relief of SVC obstruction following chemotherapy and/or radiotherapy; in 19% of those treated, obstruction of the SVC recurred
- Data support both stenting as part of initial therapy, and stenting when SVC obstruction recurs or persists after initial chemotherapy and/or radiotherapy

1. **Radiation Therapy**
   a. Most often chosen as the initial modality of treatment
   b. Provides quick relief of symptoms, often within 72 hours
   c. 70–90% of patients are free of symptoms by 2 weeks
   d. Complications:
      - Esophagitis
      - Nausea and vomiting
      - Skin irritation
      - Possible worsening of symptoms secondary to edema
   e. Recurrence of SVC syndrome is reported in 10–19% of patients treated with RT; causes include:
      - Tumor recurrence
      - Radiation fibrosis
      - Thrombosis
   f. The optimal total dose fraction has not been established and dosage must be individualized to a patient and the underlying malignancy
2. **Chemotherapy**
   a. An acceptable alternative. Choice of therapy is guided by evaluation

(continued)

Treatment Strategies (*continued*)

Radiotherapy vs. Chemotherapy
(Rowell NP, Gleeson FV. Clin Oncol [R Coll Radiol] 2002;14:338–351)
- A systematic review of 2 randomized and 44 nonrandomized studies to determine the effectiveness of different treatment modalities for SVC obstruction in patients with carcinoma of the bronchus
- *Small cell lung cancer:* Chemotherapy and/or radiotherapy relieved SVC obstruction in 77%; 17% had a recurrence of obstruction
- *Non–small cell lung cancer:* Chemotherapy and/or radiotherapy relieved SVC obstruction in 60%; 16% had a recurrence of obstruction
- *Conclusions:* It is reasonable to choose between RT and chemotherapy treatment on the basis of stage and performance status. Effectiveness was not clearly related to any particular radiotherapy fractionation schedule or chemotherapy regimen

3. **Endovascular therapies: expandable wire stents**
   a. Successfully used to open and maintain the patency of SVC obstruction resulting from malignant causes
   b. Complete resolution of SVC syndrome occurs in 68–100% of patients treated with a metallic stent
   c. Prompt resolution is achieved regardless of the stent type
      - Several investigators reported immediate relief of disabling headaches caused by SVC syndrome
      - Facial cyanosis and facial edema usually resolve within 1–2 days
      - Truncal and upper extremity edema usually resolve within 2–3 days, but may take up to 1 week
   d. Recurrence rates range from 4–45%; secondary to:
      - Tumor in-growth through the interstices of the stent
      - Tumor growth around the ends of the stent leading to thrombosis
   e. Recurrence can be treated with anticoagulation, angioplasty of the stented area, or repeated stenting
   f. Thrombolysis is often an integral part of the endovascular management of SVCs, because thrombosis is frequently a critical component of the obstruction and lysis is necessary to allow the passage of the wire. Using these techniques, technical success can be achieved in 90–100% of cases
   g. Indications:
      - Patients with reduced life expectancy
      - SVC obstruction recurring after first-line therapy
      - Patients with symptoms that are acute and so severe that immediate treatment is needed
   Note: Thrombus or complete SVC obstruction are not contraindications for stent placement although in one study thrombosis of the superior vena cava was the only independent factor for failure of the endovascular prosthesis
   (Fagedet D et al. Cardiovasc Intervent Radiol 2013;36:140–149)

   h. Complication (rates) of endovascular therapy:
      - Stent misplacement (10%)
      - Stent migration (5%)
      - Stent occlusion (10%)
      - Cardiac arrhythmias (rare)
   i. There is no consensus for anticoagulation use (warfarin/aspirin) after stent placement
   Notes:
   - Used especially in patients with the presence of a thrombus visualized on venography
   - Autopsy studies: 30–50% of patients with SVC syndrome have evidence of thrombosis
   - Suspect an obstructing thrombus if symptoms do not improve within the first week after starting radiotherapy or chemotherapy
   - Many patients have large, necrotic, friable tumor masses, and the area of tumor is under increased pressure. For these patients, anticoagulant or fibrinolytic therapy poses a considerable risk of bleeding

Guidelines That May Influence the Choice Among the Most Common Stents Used for the Treatment of Superior Vena Cava Syndrome*

Stent	Characteristics of the Stenosis
Gianturco Z-stent	Short, straight stenosis involving large diameter vessel
Wallstent and Memotherm stent	Long, curved stenosis involving vessel with small diameter
Palmaz stent	Short stenosis in locations where stent migration may pose a problem

*Adapted from Nguyen NP et al. Thorax 2009;64:174–178

Tumor Lysis Syndrome (TLS)[60–68]

Etiology

1. TLS describes the metabolic derangements that occur with tumor breakdown following the initiation of cytotoxic therapy and is characterized by:
   a. Hyperkalemia
   b. Hyperphosphatemia with secondary hypocalcemia
   c. Hyperuricemia
2. TLS may also occur spontaneously prior to cytotoxic therapy, but is less common and usually is associated with normal phosphorus levels
3. TLS can lead to acute renal failure and can be life-threatening
4. Risk factors for TLS
   a. Bulky disease
      • Bulky adenopathy
      • Hepatosplenomegaly
      • High leucocyte count ($>25,000/mm^3$)
      • Elevated pre-treatment LDH (LDH >500 units/L)
      • Elevated pretreatment uric acid
      • Chemosensitive tumors
   b. Compromised renal function
      • Biochemical abnormalities
        Elevated pre-treatment uric acid (>8.1 mg/dL; >0.48 mmol/L)
      • Decreased urine output
      • Use of potentially nephrotoxic drugs
   c. Effective cytoreductive therapies

Degree of Risk	Tumor Type	Supporting Data
Highest	• Burkitt lymphoma • Lymphoblastic lymphoma • T-cell acute lymphoblastic leukemia • Other acute leukemias	Frequent cases
Moderate	• Low-grade lymphoma treated with chemotherapy, RT, or steroids • Multiple myeloma • Breast carcinoma treated with chemotherapy or hormonal therapy • Small cell carcinoma • Germ cell cancers	Recognized complication, but few occurrences
Lowest	• Low-grade lymphoma treated with interferons • Merkel cell carcinoma • Medulloblastoma • Adenocarcinoma of the gastrointestinal tract	Case reports only

Work-up

• It is essential to maintain a high index of suspicion to identify patients at risk of developing TLS
• Patients at high risk should receive preventive measures and proactive interventions

Cairo-Bishop Definition of Tumor Lysis Syndrome (TLS) in Adults

Laboratory Tumor Lysis Syndrome (LTLS)

Present when ≥2 baseline measurements exceed maximum values or when ≥2 results change within 3 days before or within 7 days after cytotoxic therapy

Test (Serum or Plasma)	Baseline Values	Changes from Baseline
Uric acid	≥8.1 mg/dL (≥0.48 mmol/L, or ≥478 µmol/L)	25% increase
Potassium	≥6 mEq/L (≥6 mmol/L)	
Phosphorus	• Ages 1 to <18 years: ≥2.1 mmol/L (≥6.5 mg/dL) • Ages ≥18 years: ≥1.45 mmol/L (≥4.5 mg/dL)	
Calcium	≤7 mg/dL (≤3.5 mEq/L; ≤1.75 mmol/L)	25% decrease

Clinical Tumor Lysis Syndrome (CTLS)

Presence of LTLS, plus 1 or more of the 3 below

Increased serum creatinine	Cardiac arrhythmias/sudden death	Seizures

Cairo MS, Bishop M. Br J Haematol 2004;1127:3–11
Coiffier B et al. J Clin Oncol 2008;26:2767–2778

Clinical Tumor Lysis Syndrome: Severity Grades

Grade	0	1	2	3	4	5
LTLS present	No	Yes	Yes	Yes	Yes	Yes
Serum creatinine*	≤1.5 × ULN	1.5 × ULN	>1.5–3 × ULN	>3–6 × ULN	>6 × ULN	Death
Cardiac arrhythmia	None	Intervention not indicated	Nonurgent medical intervention indicated	Symptomatic and incompletely controlled medically or controlled with device (eg, defibrillator)	Life-threatening (eg, arrhythmias associated with CHF, hypotension, syncope, shock)	
Seizures	None	—	• One brief generalized seizure • Seizure well-controlled by anticonvulsants • Infrequent focal motor seizures not interfering with ADL	• Seizures in which consciousness is altered • Poorly controlled seizure disorder, with breakthrough • Generalized seizure despite medical intervention	Seizures of any kind that are prolonged, repetitive, or difficult to control (eg, status epilepticus, intractable epilepsy)	

LTLS, Laboratory tumor lysis syndrome; ULN, upper limit of normal range laboratory results; CHF, congestive heart failure; ADL, activities of daily living
The maximal clinical manifestations (renal, cardiac, neurological) define graded severity of TLS
*Upper limit of normal is based on institutional values (ULN) for age- and gender-defined normal ranges. If not specified by an institution, ULN serum creatinine may be defined as:

Age	Sex	Serum Creatinine ULN
>1 to <12 years	Males and females	0.7 mg/dL (61.9 µmol/L)
≥12 to <16 years	Males and females	1.0 mg/dL (88 µmol/L)
≥16 years	Females	1.19 mg/dL (105.2 µmol/L)
≥16 years	Males	1.29 mg/dL (114 µmol/L)

Cairo MS, Bishop M. Br J Haematol 2004;1127:3–11

Treatment Strategies

1. **Hydration and diuresis: mainstays of therapy**
   a. **Hydration with 3000 mL/m² per day** unless a patient presents with signs of acute renal dysfunction and oliguria
      - Maintain urine specific gravity ≤1.010
      - *Do not add* potassium, calcium, or phosphorus to fluids so as to avoid hyperkalemia, hyperphosphatemia, and calcium phosphate precipitation
   b. Diuresis with **furosemide 20–40 mg/dose**; administer intravenously
      - To maintain a urine output ≥100 mL/m² per hour if there is no evidence of acute obstructive uropathy and/or hypovolemia

2. **Correction of hyperkalemia**
   - Hyperkalemia may develop within 12–24 hours following initiation of chemotherapy
   - Emergent treatment is indicated if cardiac toxicity or muscular paralysis is present, or if hyperkalemia is severe (serum potassium >6.5–7 mEq/L [>6.5–7 mmol/L]), even in the absence of electrocardiographic changes
      a. Glucose and insulin
         - **50% glucose**, 25 g (*or* 1 g/kg); administer intravenously, *plus*
         - **Regular insulin** 5–10 units (*or* 0.1 unit/kg); administer by intravenous injection
            - Effective therapy usually leads to a 0.5- to 1.5-mEq/L decrease in plasma potassium concentrations, an effect that begins within 15 minutes, peaks at 60 minutes, and lasts for 4–6 hours
      b. Sodium bicarbonate
         - **Sodium bicarbonate** ($NaHCO_3$), 44–88 mEq (3.7–7.4 g); administer intravenously
            - Onset of action within 15–30 minutes with a duration of action of 1–2 hours
            - Sodium bicarbonate-containing solutions may or may not be compatible with solutions containing calcium salts depending on the concentrations of the additives
      c. Calcium infusions
         - **Calcium gluconate** 10%, 5–30 mL (*or* 50–200 mg/kg); administer intravenously at a rate not greater than 0.7–1.8 mEq/min, *or*
         - **Calcium chloride** 5%, 5–30 mL; administer intravenously at a rate not greater than 0.7–1.8 mEq/min
            - Indicated when it is potentially dangerous to wait for 30–60 minutes for a response to insulin and glucose or sodium bicarbonate
            - May be repeated after 5 minutes if ECG does not improve
            - The protective effect of calcium begins within minutes, but is relatively short-lived (<60 minutes)
      d. Nebulizer therapy
         - **Nebulized albuterol** 10–20 mg in 4 mL 0.9% sodium chloride injection; administer by inhalation over 10–15 minutes
      e. Potassium-binding cation exchange resins
         - **Sodium polystyrene sulfonate** 15–50 g (*or* 1000 mg/kg); administer orally or rectally mixed in 50–70% sorbitol solution. May be *repeated every 6 hours* until serum potassium is within normal limits
      f. Dialysis
         - Definitive therapy for patients with severe hyperkalemia
         - May be indicated if pharmacologic measures are ineffective, and in patients with renal failure and other metabolic derangements

3. **Correction of hyperphosphatemia (and hypocalcemia)**
   - Hyperphosphatemia develops within 24–48 hours following the initiation of chemotherapy
   - Hyperphosphatemia may result in precipitation of calcium phosphate in tissues resulting in hypocalcemia, intrarenal calcifications, nephrocalcinosis, and acute obstructive uropathy

   Note: Treatment of hyperphosphatemia will usually correct any related hypocalcemia; thus, calcium administration should be given only to patients with symptoms related to hypocalcemia
   a. Oral phosphate binders
      - **Aluminum hydroxide** 15–30 mL (*or* 12.5–37.5 mg/kg); administer orally every 6 hours
   b. Hemodialysis
      - The most effective therapeutic strategy
      - Consider if hyperphosphatemia is severe, especially in settings of renal failure and symptomatic hypocalcemia
      - The clearance of phosphorus is better following hemodialysis versus continuous venovenous hemofiltration versus continuous peritoneal dialysis

(*continued*)

Treatment Strategies (*continued*)

4. Correction of hyperuricemia
   - Hyperuricemia develops within 24–48 hours following the initiation of chemotherapy when the excretory capacity of the renal tubules is exceeded
   - In the presence of an acidic urine pH, uric acid crystals form in the renal tubules, leading to intraluminal renal tubular obstruction and the development of acute renal obstructive uropathy and renal dysfunction

   a. **Xanthine oxidase inhibitor**
      - **Allopurinol** 100 mg/m^2; administer orally every 8 hours (maximum 800 mg/day), *or*
      - **Allopurinol** 3.3 mg/kg per dose; administer orally every 8 hours (maximum 800 mg/day), *or*
      - **Allopurinol** 200–400 mg/m^2 per day; administer intravenously as a single dose or in up to 3 divided doses (maximum 600 mg/day)

   Notes:
   - Patients who have no evidence of laboratory or clinical tumor lysis syndrome and a low risk for developing TLS are candidates for allopurinol

Allopurinol Dose Adjustments in Patients with Renal Impairment

Creatinine Clearance	Oral Allopurinol Dose
10–20 mL/min	200 mg/day
3–10 mL/min	100 mg/day
<3 mL/min	100 mg every 36–48 hours

   - Both allopurinol and its active metabolite, oxypurinol, inhibit xanthine oxidase, the enzyme responsible for converting hypoxanthine to xanthine and, in turn, xanthine to uric acid. Because both allopurinol and oxypurinol inhibit uric acid synthesis, but have no effect on preexisting uric acid, serum levels usually do not fall until after 48–72 hours of treatment
   - Allopurinol inhibits the metabolism of **azathioprine** and **mercaptopurine**: azathioprine and mercaptopurine doses *must be decreased* by 65–75% if they are used concomitantly with allopurinol
   - Side effects include rash (1.5%), nausea (1.3%), vomiting (1.2%), and renal insufficiency (1.2%)
   - The incidence of allergic reactions is increased in patients receiving amoxicillin, ampicillin, or thiazide diuretics
   - Discontinue allopurinol if allergic reactions such as skin rashes and urticaria occur

   b. **Recombinant urate oxidase**
      - **Rasburicase** (recombinant urate oxidase) appears beneficial in children with hematologic malignancies, and is cost-effective in adults with ALL, NHL, and possibly AML, although randomized controlled trials in adults have been less convincing
      - Chemotherapy should be initiated within 4–24 hours after the first rasburicase dose

   Notes:
   - Because urate oxidase degrades uric acid rather than preventing its synthesis as does allopurinol, rapid reduction in uric acid occurs following its administration without precursor accumulation
   - The manufacturer recommends a rasburicase dose 0.2 mg/kg for up to 5 days. However, except in rare patients with very high serum levels of uric acid, much less is usually sufficient and can confer substantial cost savings. A recommended strategy is as follows:
     (1) Evaluate patients for their TLS risk
     (2) Administer rasburicase to patients at high risk for TLS or with clinical manifestations of TLS
     (3) Begin by initially administering a single 3-mg dose of rasburicase
     (4) Follow uric acid levels and administer additional rasburicase doses only if uric acid levels remain greater than an arbitrarily selected serum uric acid concentration such as 5 mg/dL 24 hours after a rasburicase dose. The half-life of rasburicase in serum is approximately 18–21 hours, so that about one-half of the administered dose is still present 24 hours after administration
   - Rasburicase does not require dosage or schedule adjustment for patients with decreased creatinine clearance
   - Side effects include skin rash, nausea and vomiting, and, rarely, hypersensitivity reactions, including anaphylaxis. Antibodies against rasburicase or its epitopes occur in approximately 6–18% of patients
   - Commercial product labeling stipulates only a single course of rasburicase, and use not exceeding 5 days to prevent developing an allergic reaction on repeated exposure

(*continued*)

Treatment Strategies *(continued)*

- **Rasburicase is contraindicated in patients with G6PD deficiency and/or methemoglobinemia**
  - Screen patients who are at high risk for G6PD deficiency before administering rasburicase, particularly persons with African or Mediterranean ancestry, because hydrogen peroxide, a byproduct of the urate oxidase reaction, can lead to hemolysis
  - Onset of severe hemolytic reactions is within 2–4 days after administering rasburicase
  - Permanently discontinue rasburicase in any patient who develops hemolysis and implement appropriate monitoring and supportive interventions (eg, transfusion)
- **Important: Rasburicase enzymatically degrades uric acid in blood samples left at room temperature.** To monitor serum/plasma uric acid concentrations after rasburicase treatment:
  - (1) Collect blood samples in pre-chilled tubes containing heparin,
  - (2) Immediately immerse and maintain samples in an ice water bath, and
  - (3) Assay uric acid in plasma samples within 4 hours after collection

5. **Alkalinization of the urine**

  a. **Sodium bicarbonate** administered intravenously continuously (preferred) or intermittently, every 4–6 hours
  - The amount of sodium bicarbonate added to intravenously administered fluids should produce a solution with sodium content not greater than the concentration of sodium in 0.9% sodium chloride injection ($\leq$154 mEq/L)

Sodium Bicarbonate Is Added to a Solution to Maintain Urine pH 6.5 to $\leq$7.0

Base Solution Sodium Content	Sodium Bicarbonate Additive	Total Sodium Content
0.45% Sodium Chloride Injection (0.45% NS)		
77 mEq/L	50–75 mEq	127–152 mEq/L
0.2% Sodium Chloride Injection (0.2% NS)		
34 mEq/L	100–125 mEq	134–159 mEq/L
5% Dextrose Injection (D5W)		
0	125–150 mEq	125–150 mEq/L
D5W/0.45% NS		
77 mEq/L	50–75 mEq	127–152 mEq/L
D5W/0.2% NS		
34 mEq/L	100–125 mEq	134–159 mEq/L

Notes:
- Administration of as little as 100 mEq sodium bicarbonate will maintain urine pH above 7.5, a pH that is needed not because of uric acid, which has a pKa of 5.4, but because of its diprotic oxypurine precursors, xanthine (pKa = 7.74 and 11.86) and hypoxanthine (pKa 8.94 and 12.1). Thus alkalinization is not a means to avoid uric acid crystallization, as at pH 6.4 more than 90% already exists as soluble urate, but as a means to avoid xanthine and hypoxanthine crystallization
- Discontinue sodium bicarbonate administration (while continuing hydration) if serum bicarbonate concentration is >30 mEq/L (>30 mmol/L) or urine pH >7.5
- However, urinary **alkalinization is not uniformly recommended and in a majority of cases should be avoided** because:
  - (1) It favors precipitation of calcium/phosphate complexes in renal tubules, a concern in patients with concomitant hyperphosphatemia
  - (2) A metabolic alkalemia may result from bicarbonate administration, which can worsen the neurologic manifestations of hypocalcemia

Syndrome of Inappropriate Secretion of Antidiuretic Hormone (SIADH)[69-73]

Etiology

- Of patients with cancer, 1–2% develop SIADH
- Hyponatremia is initially mediated by ADH-induced water retention
- The ensuing volume expansion activates secondary natriuretic mechanisms resulting in sodium and water loss and the restoration of near euvolemia
- The combination of water retention caused by inappropriate ADH secretion and secondary solute loss (sodium and potassium) accounts for a decrease in plasma sodium concentration
- Thus, patients with SIADH have normal volume status, hyponatremia with hypoosmolality, increased renal excretion of sodium (>40 mEq/L [>40 mmol/L]), and urine osmolality in excess of plasma osmolality

Causes of SIADH

Tumors	• *Small-cell lung cancer (SCLC)* is the tumor most commonly associated with SIADH. Hyponatremia caused by SIADH occurs in 10% of persons with SCLC • Other tumors
Pulmonary conditions	• Pneumonia • Tuberculosis • Pulmonary abscess • Acute respiratory failure • Positive pressure ventilation
Central nervous system disease	• Stroke • Acute psychosis • Inflammatory and demyelinating disorders • Trauma • Mass lesions • Seizures • Infection • Hemorrhage
Drugs	• *Cytotoxic drugs:* cyclophosphamide, ifosfamide, vinca alkaloids • *Other drugs:* phenothiazines, tricyclic antidepressants, chlorpropamide, clofibrate, oxytocin, desmopressin, opioids, serotonin reuptake inhibitors
Miscellaneous	• Severe pain • Postoperative state

Work-up

1. Careful history with attention to excluding other possible causes, including:
   - Diuretic administration
   - Preexisting renal disease
   - Adrenal insufficiency
   - Hypothyroidism
2. Review of recent chemotherapy agents and ancillary medications used in looking for a causative agent (see above)
3. Search for pulmonary or CNS disease if clinically indicated
4. Serum sodium as part of serum electrolytes, including BUN and creatinine
5. Urine sodium, urine osmolality, plasma osmolality
6. Thyroid function tests
7. Morning serum cortisol and ACTH, if clinically indicated

Treatment Strategies

General Principles
- The first step focuses on deciding whether sodium depletion secondary to either reduced intake, gastrointestinal losses, or renal losses is present. After excluding these 3 causes, physicians often proceed with a presumptive diagnosis of SIADH
- Correction of hyponatremia is guided by the severity of the clinical presentation and the pace with which hyponatremia developed. If hyponatremia developed slowly, correct over several days
- The rate of correction should not exceed an 8- to 10-mmol/L change in serum sodium on any day of treatment. The initial rate of correction can be 1–2 mmol/L per hour for several hours in patients with severe symptoms

1. **Water restriction: the mainstay in asymptomatic hyponatremia: 500–1000 mL/24 hours**
   - The associated negative water balance raises the plasma sodium concentration toward normal. It can also lead to volume depletion due to unmasking of the sodium deficit
2. **Salt (sodium) administration:**
   - Severe symptomatic or resistant hyponatremia often requires the administration of salt. Whereas both sodium and water are retained in hypovolemia, sodium handling is intact in patients with SIADH. Thus, when isotonic saline is administered, the sodium will be excreted in the urine while some of the water may be retained, leading to the possible worsening of hyponatremia. Consequently, in order to elevate the plasma sodium in patients with SIADH, hypertonic saline may need to be administered
   - Measure the serum sodium concentration every 4 hours during fluids administration

Formula used to estimate the effect of 1 L of any infusate on serum Na^+

$$\text{Change in serum } Na^+ = \frac{(\text{infusate } Na^+ \text{ concentration}) - (\text{serum } Na^+ \text{ concentration})}{(\text{total body water}) + 1}$$

Infusate	Na^+ Content in mmol/L
5% Sodium chloride, hypertonic (in water)	855
3% Sodium chloride, hypertonic (in water)	513
0.9% Sodium chloride injection	154
Ringer lactate injection	130
0.45% Sodium chloride injection*	77
5% Dextrose injection*	0

Estimated Total Body Water (in Liters)*	
Patient	Fraction of Body Weight
Nonelderly men	0.6
Nonelderly women	0.5
Elderly men	0.5
Elderly women	0.45

*Calculated as a fraction of body weight

*Should *never* be used in management of hyponatremia

Notes: The initial goal is to increase the serum sodium concentration by 4–5 mmol/L over the first 12 hours. One liter of 3% sodium chloride injection will increase the serum sodium concentration by 10.9 mmol/L. To increase serum sodium concentration by 5 mmol/L, only 0.46 L are required, *thus:*

$$5 \text{ mmol/L} \times \frac{1 \text{ L 3\% Sodium Chloride}}{10.9 \text{ mmol/L}} = 0.46 \text{ L 3\% Sodium Chloride}$$

Therefore, 460 mL 3% sodium chloride, hypertonic solution is administered intravenously over the first 12 hours (at a rate of 38 mL/hour). Twelve hours after starting the 3% sodium chloride administration, the patient's clinical condition improved and his serum sodium increased to 114 mmol/L. Consequently, the hypertonic sodium chloride infusion was stopped, but fluid restriction continued

3. **Salt plus loop diuretics**
   - The effect of hypertonic saline can be enhanced by being given with a loop diuretic. This lowers the urine osmolality and increases water excretion by impairing the renal responsiveness to ADH
   a. **Furosemide 20–40 mg; administer by intravenous injection**

Note: If saline and furosemide prove inadequate and hyponatremia fails to improve or worsens after 72–96 hours of fluid restriction, plasma levels of arginine vasopressin (AVP) and atrial natriuretic peptide (ANP) should be measured to discriminate between SIADH (SIAVP) and SIANP, especially in patients with SCLC. Unlike patients with SIADH and hyponatremia, patients whose tumors produce ANP experience a persistent decline in serum sodium following fluid restriction, especially if sodium intake is not concomitantly increased. If plasma levels of AVP support the diagnosis of SIADH, consider the use of demeclocycline, or an aquaretic agent (AVP-receptor antagonist)

(continued)

Treatment Strategies (*continued*)

4. Demeclocycline

- Use if the above measures fail to induce nephrogenic diabetes insipidus
  a. Demeclocycline 600–1200 mg/day; administer orally

Notes:

- Monitoring of renal function is required because demeclocycline has nephrotoxic effects
- Side effects: nausea, vomiting, diarrhea, glossitis, dysphagia, hepatotoxicity, nephrotoxicity
- Contraindications: hypersensitivity to tetracyclines

5. Aquaretic agents, arginine vasopressin (AVP)-receptor antagonists

- Have demonstrated efficacy and safety in clinical trials and represent additional options for managing hyponatremia
- Indicated to raise serum sodium in hospitalized patients with clinically significant hypervolemic and euvolemic hyponatremia (serum sodium <125 mEq/L) or less marked hyponatremia that is symptomatic and has resisted correction with fluid restriction
- Ensure frequent monitoring of serum sodium and volume status
- Beware an overly rapid rise in serum sodium (>12 mEq/L [>12 mmol/L] per 24 hours) as this may result in serious neurologic sequelae. In the event of an undesirably rapid rate of rise of serum sodium, discontinue treatment and monitor carefully

Note: Additional studies are needed to determine benefits in terms of disease outcome and length of hospital stays to justify their use

a. **Conivaptan HCl:** Nonselective AVP antagonist available for intravenous use in hospitalized patients only

- Administer through large veins and change the infusion site every 24 hours to minimize the risk of vascular irritation
- Administration:
  - *Loading dose:* **Conivaptan HCl** 20 mg; administer intravenously over 30 minutes
  - *Initial dose:* **Conivaptan HCl** 20 mg; administer by continuous intravenous infusion over 24 hours
  - *Additional dosing:* **Conivaptan HCl** 20 mg/day; administer by continuous intravenous infusion over 24 hours for an additional 1–3 days

Notes:

- If serum sodium is not rising at the desired rate, conivaptan HCl may be titrated upward to a dose of 40 mg daily, administered in a continuous intravenous infusion
- The total duration of infusion for conivaptan HCl after a loading dose should not exceed 4 days
- The maximum daily dose of conivaptan HCl after a loading dose is 40 mg/day
- Conivaptan HCl is a sensitive substrate of CYP3A subfamily enzymes and should not be coadministered with potent CYP3A inhibitors
- Conivaptan HCl is a potent *mechanism-based* inhibitor of CYP3A subfamily enzymes, and can alter the pharmacokinetics of other CYP3A substrates
- Coadministration of digoxin 0.5 mg, a substrate for the transport protein, P-glycoprotein (P-gp, MDR1, ABCB1) with conivaptan 40 mg twice daily resulted in a 30% reduction in digoxin clearance and 79% and 43% increases in maximum digoxin plasma concentration and exposure (area under the plasma concentration vs. time curve), respectively

Vaprisol (conivaptan hydrochloride) injection, for intravenous use, product label 02/2012. Marketed by Astellas Pharma US, Inc., Deerfield, IL; manufactured by Baxter Healthcare Corporation, Deerfield, IL

b. **Tolvaptan:** Selective vasopressin (V_2) receptor antagonist available as 15- and 30-mg tablets for oral use

- *Usual starting dose:* **Tolvaptan** 15 mg; administer orally once daily without regard to meals
- Titration as needed:
  - *At least 24 hours after initiating treatment:* The daily dose may be increased to **tolvaptan** 30 mg; administer orally once daily without regard to meals
  - The daily dose may be increased to a maximum of **tolvaptan** 60 mg; administer orally once daily without regard to meals, as needed to achieve a desired level of serum sodium

Notes:

- During initiation and titration, frequently monitor for changes in serum electrolytes and volume
- Avoid fluid restriction during the first 24 hours of therapy
- Advise patients receiving tolvaptan to continue ingestion of fluid in response to thirst
- Tolvaptan treatment is associated with an acute reduction of the extracellular fluid volume that could result in increased serum potassium. Serum potassium concentration should be monitored serially after initiating tolvaptan treatment in patients with a serum potassium >5 mEq/L (>5 mmol/L) and persons who are using drugs known to increase serum potassium concentrations
- In clinical trials, tolvaptan has been continued for ≥6 months
- Tolvaptan is metabolized by CYP3A subfamily enzymes, and use with strong CYP3A inhibitors causes a marked (5-fold) increase in exposure. Avoid coadministration of tolvaptan with potent and moderate CYP3A subfamily enzyme inhibitors
- Coadministration of tolvaptan with potent CYP3A subfamily enzyme inducers (eg, rifampin) reduces tolvaptan plasma concentrations by 85%

Samsca (tolvaptan) tablets for oral use, product label 02/2012. Otsuka America Pharmaceutical, Inc., Rockville, MD

Hypercalcemia Associated with Cancer[74–84]

Etiology

- Hypercalcemia is the most common metabolic complication of malignancy, overall occurring in 10–30% of persons with cancer
- Hypercalcemia of malignancy is a grave complication with median survival rates between 6 and 10 weeks

Most Common Types of Hypercalcemia Associated with Cancer

Type	Frequency	Bone Metastasis	Causative Factors	Typical Tumor
Humoral	80%	Absent—minimal	PTHrP	SCC of lung SCC of esophagus SCC of cervix SCC of head and neck Renal cell carcinoma Breast cancer Ovarian cancer
Local osteolytic	20%	Common—extensive	Cytokines Chemokines PTHrP	Breast cancer Multiple myeloma Lymphoma

PTH, Parathyroid hormone (parathormone); PTHrP, PTH-related protein; SCC, squamous cell cancer
Notes:
- Circulating PTHrP levels are increased in virtually all patients with humoral hypercalcemia of malignancy and up to two-thirds of patients with bone metastases
- Although PTHrP shares only limited homology with PTH, the common amino terminus binds to the same cell surface receptor in bone and kidney and stimulates an increase in bone resorption together with an increase in renal tubular calcium reabsorption leading to hypercalcemia. In addition, PTHrP can synergize local (paracrine) factors, including IL-1, IL-6, and TNF-α, further contributing to hypercalcemia

Work-up

The tumors in a patient with hypercalcemia associated with malignant disease are generally large and readily apparent. However, a further evaluation should consider not only mechanisms potentially related to a cancer but also causes of calcium elevation that are unrelated to cancer
Evaluate:
1. Serum calcium as part of serum electrolyte, mineral, and hepatic panels that include serum albumin
2. Ionized calcium (see **Notes** below)
3. Levels of intact PTH should be measured routinely
4. PTHrP only in selected cases

(Although most patients with typical humoral hypercalcemia of malignancy have increased levels of circulating PTHrP, the diagnosis is usually obvious on clinical grounds. Therefore, PTHrP should only be measured in occasional cases in which the diagnosis of humoral hypercalcemia of malignancy cannot be made on clinical grounds or when the cause of hypercalcemia is obscure)

Notes: Approximately 55% of total serum calcium is bound to serum proteins (primarily albumin) and is biologically inert; approximately 45% is in the active ionized form. In general, the portion of unbound calcium varies inversely with changes in the plasma albumin concentration. Because of the high prevalence of low protein levels in persons with cancer, direct measurement of ionized serum calcium is preferred because it avoids the uncertainty about how much calcium is metabolically available as a result of variability in serum protein concentrations. However, if ionized calcium measurement is not available, serum total calcium can be estimated for decreases in serum albumin by the formulas:
1. Corrected total calcium (mg/dL) = Measured total calcium (mg/dL) + 0.8 × [4 − measured albumin (g/dL)]
   - Correction assumes each 1 g/dL decrease of albumin will decrease measured serum Ca 0.8 mg/dL and thus 0.8 must be added to the measured calcium to get a corrected calcium value
2. Corrected total calcium (mmol/L) = Measured total calcium (mmol/L) + 0.2 × [4 − measured albumin (g/dL)]
   - Correction assumes each 1 g/dL decrease of albumin will decrease measured serum Ca 0.2 mmol/L and thus 0.2 must be added to the measured calcium to get a corrected calcium value
3. Corrected total calcium (mEq/L) = Measured total calcium + 0.4 × [4 − measured albumin (g/dL)]
   - Correction assumes each 1 g/dL decrease of albumin will decrease measured serum Ca 0.4 mEq/L and thus 0.4 must be added to the measured calcium to get a corrected calcium value

Treatment Strategies

General Principles

- Therapeutic interventions depend on the presentation. Asymptomatic patients with a serum calcium level of 3.25 mmol/L (13 mg/dL) or less can be managed conservatively, whereas symptomatic patients or those with a serum calcium level above 3.25 mmol/L (>13 mg/dL) require immediate aggressive measures
- Several agents commonly used before the introduction of bisphosphonates are now used infrequently, usually when bisphosphonates are ineffective or contraindicated

1. Hydration

- Extracellular volume deficits exist in all patients with symptomatic hypercalcemia of malignancy. Therefore, the first intervention should be intravenous hydration with isotonic saline
- The volume deficit, and, therefore, volume needed for replacement, depends on assessment of a patient's baseline level of dehydration, renal function, cardiovascular status, degree of mental impairment, and severity of hypercalcemia
  - a. **Hydration** with 1000–2000 mL 0.9% sodium chloride injection (0.9% NS); administer intravenously over 2–4 hours

  Note: This will result at most in a decrease in serum calcium levels of 0.5 mmol/L (1–2 mg/dL)

2. Diuretics

  - a. **Furosemide** 20–40 mg; administer by intravenous injection

  Notes:
  - The use of diuretics should be avoided until the volume deficit has been fully corrected. Loop diuretics (such as furosemide) cause calciuresis and may be effective in acutely decreasing calcium levels after volume repletion
  - Thiazide diuretics decrease renal calcium excretion and should be avoided

3. Bisphosphonates (first-line therapy; see Chapter 44 for more information about bisphosphonates)

- Bisphosphonates should be initiated as soon as hypercalcemia is diagnosed
- Initiate treatment only after (a) adequate hydration with 0.9% NS; (b) adequate urine output; and (c) with doses appropriate for a patient's creatinine clearance (CrCl) or measured serum creatinine
- Encourage ambulatory patients to maintain hydration orally
- If hypercalcemia persists or recurs, there should be ≥7 days between consecutive treatments

See Chapter 44 for more information about bisphosphonates utilization

Hypocalcemic Effects of Bisphosphonates

Adapted from Riccardi A et al. Tumori 2003;89:223–236, and Body J-J. Semin Oncol 2001;28(4 Suppl 11):49–53

Bisphosphonate	Median Time to Normocalcemia	Duration of Normocalcemia	% Achieving Normocalcemia
Pamidronate disodium[81,82]	4 days	28 days	70–100%
Zoledronic acid[83]	4 days	32 days	87%
Clodronate disodium[81]	3 days	14 days	80%
Alendronate sodium[84]	4 days	15 days	74%

  a. **Pamidronate disodium** 90 mg; administer intravenously in 250–1000 mL 0.9% NS, 0.45% NS, or D5W, over 2–24 hours, every 3–4 weeks
  - Durations of administration >2 hours may decrease the risk for renal toxicity, particularly in patients with preexisting renal impairment

Dose Modifications for Renal Impairment for Doses After the First Dose

Baseline	Retreatment	Action
Normal SCr	SCr increased ≥0.5 mg/dL (≥44 μmol/L)	Hold until SCr is within 10% of baseline
Abnormal SCr	SCr increased ≥1 mg/dL (≥88 μmol/L)	

  b. **Zoledronic acid:** 4–8 mg; administer intravenously in 100 mL 0.9% NS or D5W over at least 15 minutes, every 3–4 weeks

Dose Adjustments for Patients with Baseline CrCl ≤60 mL/min

Baseline CrCl	Recommended Doses*
50–60 mL/min (0.83–1 mL/s)	3.5 mg
40–49 mL/min (0.66–0.81 mL/s)	3.3 mg
30–39 mL/min (0.5–0.65 mL/s)	3 mg

*Doses are calculated to produce an AUC (0.6 mg · hours/L) similar to that achieved in patients with CrCl = 75 mL/min

(*continued*)

Treatment Strategies (*continued*)

c. **Clodronate disodium** 300 mg/day; administer intravenously in 500 mL 0.9% NS or D5W over at least 2 hours for up to 5 days (treatment with intravenous clodronate may continue for >5 days but should be limited to not more than 10 days for a single hypercalcemic episode), *or*

Clodronate disodium 1500 mg single dose; administer intravenously in 500 mL 0.9% NS or D5W over 4 hours

Clodronate disodium has not received FDA approval for use outside clinical trials and is not commercially available in the United States

Dose Modifications for Renal Impairment for Doses After the First Dose

CrCL	Dose Reduction
50–80 mL/min (0.83–1.33 mL/s)	25%
12–50 mL/min (0.2–0.83 mL/s)	25–50%
<12 mL/min (<0.2 mL/s)	50%

d. **Alendronate sodium** 5, 10, or 15 mg; administer intravenously over 2 hours

Note: A parenteral formulation is not commercially available in the United States

Treatment Modification for Renal Impairment

Elderly patients	No adjustments
CrCl ≥35 mL/min (≥0.58 mL/s)	No adjustments
CrCl <35 mL/min (<0.58 mL/s)	Do not administer drug

4. **Calcitonin-Salmon (first-line therapy)**

1. **Calcitonin** 4 units/kg; administer intramuscularly or by subcutaneous injection every 12 hours. *If ineffective or effectiveness begins to wane (developing tachyphylaxis):*

2. **Calcitonin** 8 units/kg; administer intramuscularly or by subcutaneous injection every 12 hours. *If ineffective or effectiveness begins to wane (developing tachyphylaxis):*

3. **Calcitonin** 8 units/kg; administer intramuscularly or by subcutaneous injection every 6 hours. *Discontinue if ineffective or effectiveness begins to wane, and seek an alternative intervention*

Notes:

- Calcitonin's value is the rapid onset of its hypocalcemic effect, typically within 2–6 hours after administration. The need for frequent administration and the occurrence of tachyphylaxis within a few days after instituting therapy limits its utility to the acute setting where it should be used in combination with longer-acting agents

- Calcitonin may be used concomitantly with bisphosphonates to augment and compensate for the slower onset of hypocalcemic effect characteristic of bisphosphonate compounds

- *Adverse effects:* Flushing, nausea, vomiting, local inflammatory reaction at the site of injection

5. **Gallium nitrate (second-line therapy)**

Gallium nitrate 100–200 mg/m^2 per day; administer intravenously in 1000 mL 0.9% NS or D5W over 24 hours, daily for 5 consecutive days

Notes:

- Results in a gradual reduction of serum calcium over the 5-day infusion. If the serum calcium levels are lowered into normal range before 5 days of gallium nitrate administration are completed, treatment may be discontinued

- Hydration must be maintained throughout the period of gallium nitrate administration

- The 5-day schedule of administration is more cumbersome than single-day administration associated with bisphosphonates such as zoledronic acid and pamidronate disodium

- *Contraindications:* Renal impairment (serum creatinine >2.5 mg/dL; >221 μmol/L)

- *Adverse effects:* Renal failure, hypophosphatemia, hypocalcemia, respiratory alkalosis, vomiting, hypotension, tachycardia, nausea, vomiting, diarrhea, acute optic neuritis

6. **Glucocorticoids (second-line therapy, with limited applications)**

- May be useful in patients with steroid-sensitive cancers such as lymphomas or multiple myeloma by decreasing the 1,25-dihydroxycholecalciferol levels

  a. **Prednisone** 60 mg; administer orally, daily for 7–10 days (or equivalent steroid dose)

Note: Steroids have a slow onset of action (7 days) and short duration of action (3–4 days)

(*continued*)

Treatment Strategies (*continued*)

7. **Plicamycin (third-line therapy)**

   a. **Plicamycin** 25 mcg/kg; administer intravenously in 1000 mL 0.9% NS or D5W over 4–6 hours
   - Plicamycin is a highly toxic antibiotic antineoplastic with hypocalcemic activity that acts by blocking RNA synthesis in osteoclasts. **Plicamycin is not available in the United States** outside the context of a clinical trial
   - Plicamycin lowers serum calcium levels within 12 hours, with a maximum effect at about 48 hours, *therefore:*
   - Repeated doses should *not* be given more frequently than every 48 hours to prevent excessive iatrogenic decreases in serum calcium

   Notes:
   - Although widely used in the past, the occurrence of side effects, including thrombocytopenia, myelosuppression, hepatotoxicity, nephrotoxicity, coagulopathy including hemorrhagic diathesis, nausea, and vomiting, the availability of other effective less-toxic agents, and limited availability worldwide, currently limit plicamycin use
   - *Contraindications:* Bone marrow suppression, thrombocytopenia, coagulation disorder, bleeding

8. **Phosphorus**

   a. **Neutral phosphate salts** 500–1500 mg/day of elemental phosphorus; administer orally in 2–4 divided doses

   Caution: Intravenous phosphorus administration in a setting of hypercalcemia may result in deposition of calcium phosphate in renal tubules and soft tissues

   Notes:
   - Hypophosphatemia develops in most patients with hypercalcemia associated with cancer, and the presence of hypophosphatemia increases the difficulty of treating hypercalcemia
   - Phosphorus should be replaced orally or administered through a nasogastric tube
   - *Avoid* intravenous phosphorus administration except in the presence of severe hypophosphatemia (serum phosphorus <1.5 mg/dL [<0.48 mmol/L]) and when oral phosphorus cannot be administered
   - Intravenously administered phosphorus should be used with extreme caution and with continual serial observation of serum phosphorus and creatinine concentrations

9. **Denosumab**

   - **Denosumab**, a fully human monoclonal antibody with a high affinity and specificity for RANK ligand (RANKL)
   - Two Denosumab products have received U.S. Food and Drug Administration (FDA) **approval** for different indications:
     - Proprietary name, Xgeva, denosumab is approved for the prevention of skeletal-related events (SREs) in patients with bone metastases from solid tumors (Xgeva [denosumab] injection, for subcutaneous use, product label 11/2010. Amgen Manufacturing Limited, a subsidiary of Amgen Inc., Thousand Oaks, CA)
     - Proprietary name, Prolia, denosumab is approved for (a) use in patients who are at high risk for fracture, including patients receiving androgen-deprivation therapy (ADT) for nonmetastatic prostate cancer, (b) treatment of bone loss in women receiving adjuvant aromatase inhibitor (AI) therapy for breast cancer to increase bone mass, and (c) for the treatment of postmenopausal women with osteoporosis who are at high risk for fracture (Prolia [denosumab] injection, for subcutaneous use, product label 09/2010. Amgen Manufacturing Limited, a subsidiary of Amgen Inc., Thousand Oaks, CA)

       Notes: Denosumab is *not* indicated for the prevention of SREs in patients with multiple myeloma
     - Although **denosumab** may garner FDA approval for hypercalcemia associated with malignancy, it is likely that delineation of optimal doses and schedules will evolve over time as has happened with the bisphosphonates. Its use in acute hypercalcemia must be demonstrated in clinical trials before it can be recommended. A single-arm, open-label, proof-of-concept study, evaluated patients with hypercalcemia of malignancy with albumin-corrected serum calcium (CSC) levels ≥12.5 mg/dL despite recent intravenous bisphosphonate treatment. They received subcutaneous denosumab on days 1, 8, 15, and 29, and then every 4 weeks. By day 10, 12/15 patients (80%; 95% confidence interval [CI] = 52–96%) had achieved a CSC ≤11.5 mg/dL, the primary endpoint. However, the median response duration was only 26 days

       Hu et al. J Natl Cancer Inst 2013; 105:1417–1420

     - *Administration:*

       Denosumab 120 mg; administer by subcutaneous injection in the upper arm, upper thigh, or abdomen every 4 weeks
       Ancillary medicines: Administer calcium and vitamin D as necessary to treat or prevent hypocalcemia
       Caution: The risk of hypocalcemia at the recommended dosing schedule of 120 mg every 4 weeks has not been evaluated in patients with a creatinine clearance of less than 30 mL/min (<0.5 mL/s) or in persons receiving dialysis
     - *Adverse effects:* Hypocalcemia and osteonecrosis of the jaw (ONJ)
     - In a recent statistical analysis comparing the rates of skeletal-related events (SREs) "observed with denosumab to those with placebo based on the results of the registrational studies of zoledronic acid and pamidronate, denosumab reduced the risk of developing a first skeletal related event (SRE) by 48%". The number needed to treat (NNT) "with denosumab compared with placebo was 4 patient-years, indicating that, on average, treatment of 4 patients with denosumab for one year is expected to prevent one additional first SRE compared with no treatment"

       Martin et al. Clin Cancer Res 2012;18:4841–4849

Randomized Phase III Trial of Denosumab versus Zoledronic Acid
Selected Baseline Disease Characteristics

Martin et al. Clin Cancer Res 2012;18:4841–4849

Characteristic	Zoledronic Acid ($N = 1,020$) 4 mg IV Q4W	Denosumab ($N = 1,026$) 120 mg sc Q4W
Age, y, median (Q1, Q3)	56 (49, 65)	57 (48, 65)
Postmenopausal status, n (%)	831 (82%)	839 (82%)
ECOG status, n (%)		
0	488 (48%)	504 (49%)
1	444 (445)	451 (44%)
2	82 (85)	68 (75)
Median time from primary cancer diagnosis to initial diagnosis of bone metastases	35 months	33 months
Presence of visceral metastases, n (%)	525 (515)	552 (54%)
Prior SREs, n (%)		
No prior SREs	647 (63%)	648 (63%)
One or more prior SREs	373 (37%)	378 (37%)
Prior radiation therapy to bone, n (%)	280 (285)	258 (25%)
Pain scores on BPI-SF, n (%)*		
No or mild pain (0–4)	500 (49%)	542 (53%)
Moderate or severe pain (>4)	451 (44%)	433 (425)
FACT-G total score, median (Q1, Q3)[†]	74 (61, 86)	74 (61, 85)

*BPI-SF scores range from 0 to 10, with a higher score indicating greater pain severity. Baseline BPI-SF data were missing for 69 patients (7%) of patients in the zoledronic acid group and 51 patients (5%) in the denosumab group; these patients were not included in the HRQoL analyses
[†]FACT-G total score ranges from 0 to 108

Bone-Related Complications and Quality of Life in Advanced Breast Cancer
Results from a Randomized Phase III Trial of Denosumab Versus Zoledronic Acid

Martin et al. Clin Cancer Res 2012;18:4841–4849

Event or Assessment	Denosumab (1,020/1,026)[†]	Zoledronic Acid (1,013/1,020)[†]	*P* Value and NNT
Proportion of pts with ≥1 SRE on study	31%	36%	$P = 0.006$
First on-study SRE [in patient-years (pt-yrs)]	315 events [In 1065 pt-yrs]	372 events [In 1040 pt-yrs]	NNT=16 patient-years[‡]
First and subsequent on-study SREs	660 events [In 1353 pt-yrs]	835 events [In 1353 pt-yrs]	NNT=7 patient-years[‡]
Proportion of pts with ≥2 SREs on study amongst patients with ≥1 SRE on study	33%	38%	$P = 0.16$
Proportion of pts with ≥1 SRE while on study amongst those with SRE prior to study	36%	44%	$P = 0.021$
Proportion of pts with ≥1 SRE while on study amongst those without SRE prior to study	28%	32%	$P = 0.085$

(continued)

Bone-Related Complications and Quality of Life in Advanced Breast Cancer
Results from a Randomized Phase III Trial of Denosumab versus Zoledronic Acid (*continued*)

Event or Assessment	Denosumab (1,020/1,026)[†]	Zoledronic Acid (1,013/1,020)[†]	P Value and NNT
Incidence of first radiation therapy to bone	123 (12%)	162 (16%)	
Time to radiation therapy to bone	Time prolonged by denosumab HR, 0.74; 95% CI, 0.59–0.94		P = 0.012
Risk of SRE or hypercalcemia of malignancy	Risk reduced by denosumab 18% HR, 0.82; 95% CI, 0.70–0.95		P = 0.007
Median time to first on-study SRE or hypercalcemia	NR	25.2 months	P = 0.007
	HR, 0.82; 95% CI, 0.70–0.95		
Hypercalcemia events	28 events	58 events	P = 0.036
	Rate ratio = 0.48; 95% CI, 0.24–0.95		
Patients with first on-study SREs[§]			
Pathologic fractures	21%	23%	—
Radiation to bone	82 (8%)	119 (12%)	—
Median FACT-G total score: Clinically meaningful improvement in HRQoL[ϵ]	34%	31%	—
ECOG performance status			
Maintained during study	59%	55%	—
Worsened during study	36%	41%	—
Improved during study	5%	4%	—
Incidence of renal toxicity AEs	50 (4.9%)	86 (8.5%)	P = 0.001
Withdraw for renal toxicity	0	3 (0.3%)	—
Acute-phase AEs ≤3 days after treatment[**,‡‡]	10.4%	27.3%	P < 0.0001
Pyrexia	0.9%	11.5%	—
Fatigue	2.4%	4.0%	—
Bone pain	1.3%	3.6%	—
Chills	0.3%	3.6%	—
Arthralgia	1.5%	3.2%	—
Headache	0.7%	3.1%	—
Serious acute-phase AEs ≤3 days after treatment[††,‡‡]	0	10 (1%)	—

SRE, skeletal-related event; ZA, zoledronic acid; pt, patient; pts, patients; NNT, number-needed-to-treat; HRQoL, health-related quality of life; FACT-G questionnaire, functional assessment of cancer therapy–general questionnaire

*Dosing: Denosumab 120 mg as a single subcutaneous injection and intravenous placebo every 4 weeks. No dose adjustment or dose withholding for renal dysfunction was required for denosumab

*Dosing: Zoledronic acid 4 mg (adjusted for renal function per zoledronic acid prescribing information) as an intravenous infusion over at least 15 minutes and subcutaneous placebo every 4 weeks. As required per zoledronic acid prescribing information, doses were adjusted to <4 mg in 131 patients (13%) and 245 doses were withheld in 56 patients (6%) on study because of serum creatinine increases

[†]Numbers represent the number that received at least one dose of drug/number randomized

[‡]Treatment of 16 patients *per year* with denosumab rather than zoledronic acid is expected to prevent one additional first SRE (or 7 patients *per year* to prevent one additional first or subsequent SRE)

[§]First SREs of surgery to bone and spinal cord compression ≈1% of patients in each group

[ϵ]≥5-point increase in FACT-G total score; the positive effect of denosumab treatment on HRQoL was observed regardless of pain severity at baseline

[**]Acute-phase reactions associated with a flu-like syndrome within the first 3 days after treatment, including pyrexia, fatigue, bone pain, chills, arthralgia, and headache

[††]Including pyrexia (n = 7), bone pain (n = 2), asthenia, back pain, chest pain, chills, headache, and malaise (one patient each). Some patients experienced more than one event

[‡‡]Eight of the 10 patients in the zoledronic acid group with serious acute-phase reaction AEs were hospitalized or had their hospitalization prolonged as a result of these events. Three patients with serious acute-phase reaction AEs discontinued zoledronic acid treatment after the first dose. Over the 34 months of treatment included in this analysis, the patient incidence of pyrexia in denosumab-treated patients (16.7%) was approximately half the incidence of pyrexia in the placebo groups in a 12-month study of zoledronic acid in patients with advanced breast cancer (32.7%) and in 3 studies of pamidronate versus placebo (32%–38%), suggesting that the acute-phase reaction events observed with denosumab represent the background rate expected in this population

Anaphylaxis[85-89]

Etiology

- An acute hypersensitivity reaction is an unpredictable and potentially catastrophic complication of treatment with chemotherapeutic agents and can occur at any time during the administration of therapy
- Almost all the antineoplastic drugs have been reported to cause hypersensitivity reactions
- Certain classes of chemotherapeutic agents commonly associated with hypersensitivity reactions include the **taxanes, platinum compounds, asparaginases, and epipodophyllotoxins (etoposide, teniposide)**
- Despite prophylactic measures with steroids or antihistamines to reduce the incidence of hypersensitivity reactions, hypersensitivity reactions still occur and severe reactions may require immediate medical management with the drugs listed below

Work-up

1. Focused physical examination
2. Establishment of a stable airway
3. Establishment of intravenous access
4. Administration of epinephrine

Note: **Parenteral epinephrine is the cornerstone of management**

Treatment Strategies

Drug	Dose	Route	Frequency
Epinephrine 1:1000 (1 mg/mL)	0.3–0.5 mL	IM, SC*	Immediately, then every 5–15 minutes
Epinephrine 1:10,000 (0.1 mg/mL)	0.5–1 mL	IV†	Immediately, then every 5–10 minutes
	3–5 mL	ET‡	Immediately
Diphenyhydramine§	25–50 mg	IV, PO, or IM	Immediately, then every 4–6 hours as needed
Cimetidine *or*	300 mg	IV	Every 8–12 hours as needed
Ranitidine	50 mg	IV	Every 8–12 hours as needed
Hydrocortisone∈	100 mg	IV	Every 6 hours as needed
Albuterol**	2.5–5 mg	Via nebulizer	Every 20 minutes up to 3 doses
Glucagon††	1–2 mg	IV	Immediately, then every 5–15 minutes

ET, Via endotracheal tube; IM, intramuscularly; IV, intravenously; PO, orally; SC, subcutaneously
Notes:
*Promptly administer epinephrine at the onset of anaphylaxis. Intramuscular (IM) administration is preferred over subcutaneous (SC), because IM epinephrine is better absorbed. There are no absolute contraindications to epinephrine administration in anaphylaxis
†Patients with severe airway edema, severe hypotension, or severe bronchospasm should receive IV epinephrine. Administer 0.5–1 mL of a 1:10,000 dilution (0.1 mg/mL) at intervals of 5–10 minutes with cardiac monitoring
- Give fluids intravenously (colloid or crystalloid) to hypotensive patients with anaphylaxis who do not quickly respond to epinephrine. Aggressive fluid resuscitation with rapid volume expansion may be required initially and for patients who develop vasogenic shock
‡If IV access cannot be obtained administer 3–5 mL of a 1:10,000 epinephrine (0.1 mg/mL) via an endotracheal tube
§Antihistamines should be given to all patients with anaphylaxis and continued until symptoms resolve completely
∈Steroids are administered to prevent recurrent or protracted anaphylaxis. Use hydrocortisone or a glucocorticoid equivalent dose of another steroid; for example:

(continued)

Treatment Strategies (*continued*)

Drug	Glucocorticoid Equivalent Doses
Hydrocortisone	100 mg
Prednisone or prednisolone	25 mg
Methylprednisolone	20 mg

**Persistent respiratory distress or wheezing requires the use of nebulized beta-adrenergic agents. Administer albuterol by inhalation if bronchospasm does not adequately respond to epinephrine

††Patients on beta-adrenergic blockers may be resistant to treatment with epinephrine and can develop refractory hypotension and bradycardia. Glucagon has inotropic and chronotropic effects that are not mediated through beta-adrenergic receptors and should be administered in this subset of patients

References

1. Gabriel K, Schiff D. Semin Neurol 2004;24:375–383
2. Schiff D. Neurol Clin 2003;21:67–86, viii
3. Prasad D, Schiff D. Lancet Oncol 2005;6:15–24
4. Schiff D et al. Neurology 1997;49:452–456
5. Bilsky MH et al. Oncologist 1999;4:459–469
6. Yalamanchili M, Lesser GJ. Curr Treat Options Oncol 2003;4:509–516
7. Loblaw DA et al. J Clin Oncol 2005;23:2028–2037
8. Loblaw DA, Laperriere NJ. J Clin Oncol 1998;16:1613–1624
9. Sze WM, Clin Oncol (R Coll Radiol) 2003;15:345–352
10. Hardy JR, Huddart R. Clin Oncol (R Coll Radiol) 2002;14:132–134
11. Maranzano E et al. J Clin Oncol 2005;23:3358–3365
12. Kwok Y, Regine WF. J Clin Oncol 2005;23:3308–3310
13. Greenberg HS et al. Ann Neurol 1980;8:361–366
14. Sørensen PS et al. Eur J Cancer 1994;30A:22–27
15. Heimdal K et al. J Neurooncol 1992;12:141–144
16. Vecht CJ et al. Neurology 1989;39:1255–1257
17. Lutz S et al. Int J Radiat Oncol Biol Phys 2011;79:965–976
18. Maranzano E, Latini P. Int J Radiat Oncol Biol Phys 1995;32:959–967
19. Sze WM et al. Cochrane Database Syst Rev 2004;(2):CD004721
20. Hartsell WF et al. J Natl Cancer Inst 2005;97:798–804
21. Foro Arnalot P et al. Radiother Oncol 2008;89:150–155
22. Chawla S et al. Bone 2009;45:817–821
23. Milker-Zabel S et al. Int J Radiat Oncol Biol Phys 2003;55:162–167
24. Hamilton AJ et al. Neurosurgery 1995;36:311–319
25. Mahan SL et al. Int J Radiat Oncol Biol Phys 2005;63:1576–1583
26. Gerszten PC et al. Spine (Phila, Pa 1976) 2007;32:193–199
27. Sahgal A et al. Int J Radiat Oncol Biol Phys 2009;74:723–731
28. Garg AK et al. Cancer 2011;117:3509–3516
29. Veldeman L et al. Lancet Oncol 2008;9:367–375
30. Guckenberger M et al. Radiother Oncol 2007;84:56–63
31. Rose PS et al. J Clin Oncol 2009;27:5075–5079
32. Patchell R et al. Proc Am Soc Clin Oncol 2003;22:1[abstract 2]
33. Shehadi JA et al. Eur Spine J 2007;16:1179–1192
34. Anselmetti et al. Cardiovasc Intervent Radiol. 2007;30:441–447
35. Bròdano GB et al. Eur Rev Med Pharmacol Sci 2007;11:91–100
36. Berenson J et al. Lancet Oncol 2011;12:225–235
37. Rowell NP, Gleeson FV. Cochrane Database Syst Rev 2001;CD001316
38. Rowell NP, Gleeson FV. Clin Oncol (R Coll Radiol) 2002;14:338–351
39. Wudel LJ Jr et al. Curr Treat Options Oncol 2001;2:77–91
40. Markman M, Cleve Clin J Med 1999;66:59–61
41. Ostler PJ et al. Clin Oncol (R Coll Radiol) 1997;9:83–89
42. Armstrong BA et al. Int J Radiat Oncol Biol Phys 1987;13:531–539
43. Spiro SG et al. Thorax 1983;38:501–505
44. Pignon J-P et al. N Engl J Med 1992;327:1618–1624
45. Hochrein J et al. Am J Med 1998;104:78–84
46. Yim CD et al. Radiol Clin North Am 2000;38:409–424
47. Schindler N, Vogelzang RL. Surg Clin North Am 1999;79:683–694, xi
48. Rowell NP, Gleeson FV. Cochrane Database Syst Rev 2001;(4):CD001316
49. Nguyen NP et al. Thorax 2009;64:174–178
50. Nagata T et al. Cardiovasc Intervent Radiol 2007;30:959–967
51. Barshes NR et al. Vascular 2007;15:314–321
52. Shah R et al. J Thorac Cardiovasc Surg. 1996;112:335–340
53. Gross CM et al. AJR Am J Roentgenol 1997;169:429–432
54. Thony F et al. Eur Radiol 1999;9:965–971
55. Smayra T et al. Cardiovasc Intervent Radiol 2001;24:388–394
56. de Gegorio Ariza MA et al. Eur Radiol 2003;13:853–862
57. Urruticoechea A et al. Lung Cancer 2004;43:209–214
58. Lanciego C et al. AJR Am J Roentgenol 2009;193:549–558
59. Duvnjak S, Andersen PE. Int Angiol 2011;30:458–461
60. Cairo MS, Bishop M. Br J Haematol 2004;127:3–11
61. Coiffier B et al. J Clin Oncol 2008;26:2767–2778
62. Arrambide K et al. Semin Nephrol 1993;13:273–280
63. Cairo MS et al. Clin Lymphoma 2002;3 Suppl 1:S26–S31
64. Baeksgaard L, Sørensen JB. Cancer Chemother Pharmacol 2003;51:187–192
65. Nicolin G et al. Eur J Cancer 2002;38:1365–1377; discussion 1378–1379
66. Davidson MB et al. Am J Med 2004;116:546–554
67. Locatelli F, Rossi F. Contrib Nephrol 2005;147:61–68
68. Yarpuzlu AA. Clin Chim Acta 2003;333:13–18
69. Adrogue HJ et al. Int J Biochem Cell Biol 2003;35:1495–1499
70. Androgué HJ, Madias NE. N Engl J Med 2000;342:1581–1589
71. Silverman P, Distelhorst CW. Semin Oncol 1989;16:504–515
72. Flombaum CD et al. Semin Oncol 2000;27:322–334
73. Goh KP et al. Am Fam Physician 2004;69:2387–2394
74. Stewart AF et al. N Engl J Med 2005;352:373–379
75. Davidson TG. Am J Health Syst Pharm 2001;58 Suppl 3:S8–S15
76. Mundy GR. Am J Med 1997;103:134–145
77. Ralston SH et al. Calcif Tissue Int 2004;74:1–11
78. Ratcliffe WA et al. Lancet 1992;339:164–167
79. Riccardi A et al. Tumori 2003;89:223–236
80. Body J-J. Semin Oncol 2001;28(4 Suppl 11):49–53
81. Purohit OP. Br J Cancer 1995;72:1289–1293
82. Body JJ. Ann Oncol 1994;5:359–363
83. Major P. J Clin Oncol 2001;19:558–567
84. Nussbaum SR et al. J Clin Oncol 1993;11:1618–1623
85. Zanotti KM, Markman M. Drug Saf 2001;24:767–779
86. Shepherd GM. Clin Rev Allergy Immunol 2003;24:253–262
87. Ellis AK, Day JH. CMAJ 2003;169:307–311
88. Tang AW. Am Fam Physician 2003;68:1325–1332
89. Simons FER et al. J Allergy Clin Immunol 2001;108:871–873

47. Fever and Neutropenia

Jennifer Cuellar-Rodriguez, MD and Juan C. Gea-Banacloche, MD

Definitions According to the Infectious Diseases Society of America's Current Recommendations[1]

Fever: Single oral temperature ≥38.3°C (≥101°F) or a temperature ≥38.0°C (≥100.4°F) for 1 hour or longer

Neutropenia: Absolute neutrophil count (ANC) of <500 cells/mm³, or a count expected to decrease to <500 cells/mm³ during the next 48 hours

Etiology

In patients with fever and neutropenia:
- 10–20%: Microbiologically documented infection (most commonly bacteremia)
- 20–30%: Clinically documented infection (eg, cellulitis, pneumonia, typhlitis)
- 50–70%: No clinically or microbiologically documented infection

Infectious etiology:
1. Bacteria are the most commonly documented etiology
2. Gram-positive bacteria predominate in recent series; however, the frequency of Gram-negative bacteria is increasing
3. Gram-negative bacteremia may be associated with faster clinical deterioration and death as compared to Gram-positive bacteremia. Hence empirical treatment is targeted to cover Gram-negative pathogens, particularly *Pseudomonas aeruginosa*
4. *Candida* and *Aspergillus* species are the most common causes of invasive fungal infections in neutropenic patients. They are uncommon early or during short episodes of neutropenia but increase in frequency with longer duration of neutropenia

Factors contributing to immune compromise of an individual patient:
1. Corticosteroids, fludarabine, and alemtuzumab (Campath-1H) produce severe defects in cellular immunity
2. Myeloma and CLL are accompanied by defects in humoral immunity
3. Patients without a spleen are at risk of overwhelming sepsis caused by encapsulated bacteria, mainly *Streptococcus pneumoniae*
4. Obstruction (biliary obstruction, ureteral obstruction, bronchial obstruction) facilitates local infection (cholangitis, pyelonephritis, postobstructive pneumonia)
5. Intravascular devices, drainage tubes, or stents may become colonized and lead to local infection, bacteremia, or fungemia

General Management

1. Expeditious evaluation is mandatory, with special attention to skin, mouth, perianal region, and lungs
2. Cultures of blood*, urine, and sputum should be obtained in all patients
3. In case of diarrhea, stool culture with a test to rule out *Clostridium difficile* (PCR is most sensitive) should be obtained
4. In case of signs or symptoms of upper respiratory tract infection, a nasopharyngeal wash to screen for viruses should be obtained
5. CBC with differential count, chemistry panel, and chest radiograph should be obtained at baseline
6. Antimicrobial treatment should be instituted without delay (for dosage, route of administration, dose adjustment for renal and hepatic impairment of specific agents, see Appendix I)
7. High-risk patients have ANC <100 cells/mm³ and expected duration >7 days, and/or significant comorbidities (hypotension, pneumonia, new-onset abdominal pain, or neurologic changes). They should be admitted and treated with IV antibiotics. Low-risk patients have anticipated brief neutropenia periods and no or few comorbidities, and may be considered for oral or outpatient therapy, provided they have good access to a health care system

*Standard practice in obtaining blood cultures:
- Adequate volume of blood drawn is critical for successful isolation of microorganisms
- Aerobic and anaerobic blood culture bottles should be obtained with 10 mL of blood collected in each bottle (adult)
- Minimum 2 sets of cultures (2 aerobic and 2 anaerobic blood culture bottles) should be obtained
- In case of a vascular access device with multiple lumens, each lumen should be sampled
- Peripheral cultures are helpful mainly to establish the diagnosis of catheter-related bacteremia; they are not mandatory if enough blood may be obtained from a central line

Antibiotic Therapy

A flow diagram with suggested antibiotic therapy for inpatients with fever and neutropenia is presented in **Figure 47–1**. We recommend a systematic approach in which specific questions are answered in order:

1. **In a clinically stable patient:**

   In a clinically stable patient who does not need vancomycin (uncomplicated fever and neutropenia), intravenous monotherapy with an antipseudomonal β-lactam (cefepime, piperacillin-tazobactam, imipenem, or meropenem)* is recommended. Combination therapy with a β-lactam + aminoglycoside has been associated with more toxicity and no better outcome, and is not recommended in uncomplicated fever and neutropenia[5,6]

   • **Piperacillin sodium** 4000 mg + **Tazobactam sodium** 500 mg, intravenously every 6 hours

   • **Cefepime** 2000 mg, intravenously every 8 hours

   • **Imipenem** 500 mg + **Cilastatin sodium** 500 mg, intravenously every 6 hours

   • **Meropenem** 1000 mg, intravenously every 8 hours

   Note: **Ceftazidime** 2000 mg intravenously every 8 hours, is no longer recommended by the Infectious Diseases Society of America Guidelines because of concerns regarding antimicrobial resistance. Institutional discretion based on local patterns of resistance is advised

   *It is critically important for clinicians to be familiar with the pattern of resistance to the various β-lactam antibiotics in their institutions. In vitro susceptibility may vary widely among different institutions, making some of these alternatives unacceptable

2. **When is vancomycin required as part of the initial regimen?**

   • Severe sepsis or septic shock

   • Clinically apparent catheter-related infection

   • Known colonization with methicillin-resistant *Staphylococcus aureus* (MRSA) or penicillin-resistant *Streptococcus pneumoniae*

   • Severe mucositis (risk of infection with viridans group *Streptococcus*)

   • Pneumonia

   Dose: **Vancomycin HCl** 1000 mg intravenously every 12 hours, aim for trough* concentrations ≥15 mcg/mL

   *Trough concentrations in body fluids (most often serum or plasma) are the concentration of a drug at the end of a dosing interval (ie, just before another dose is given), and may also be known as minimum concentrations

3. **Is sepsis or septic shock present?**

   In the presence of severe sepsis or septic shock, broad-spectrum coverage for Gram-negative bacilli and viridans group streptococci should be instituted. Many authorities recommend dual therapy targeting Gram-negative bacteria (β-lactam + aminoglycoside or β-lactam + fluoroquinolone or β-lactam + colistin) to try to maximize the antimicrobial spectrum. Vancomycin is typically added in this situation.[1] Common regimens include:

   β-Lactam + **Aminoglycoside** + vancomycin   *or*   β-lactam + **fluoroquinolone** + vancomycin

β-Lactam	**Ceftazidime** 2000 mg intravenously every 8 hours *or* **Cefepime** 2000 mg intravenously every 8 hours *or* **Meropenem** 1000 mg intravenously every 8 hours *or* **Imipenem** 500 mg + **Cilastatin** 500 mg intravenously every 6 hours **Piperacillin** 4000 mg + **Tazobactam** 500 mg intravenously every 6 hours
Aminoglycoside	**Gentamicin** 4–7 mg/kg intravenously every day *or* **Tobramycin** 4–7 mg/kg intravenously every day *or* **Amikacin** 15 mg/kg intravenously every day
Fluoroquinolone	**Ciprofloxacin** 400 mg intravenously every 8 hours *or* **Levofloxacin** 750 mg intravenously every day
Polymyxin	**Colistin (colistimethate sodium)** 5 mg/kg per day intravenously in 2–4 divided doses *or* **Polymyxin B** 7500 to 12,500 units/kg intravenously every 12 hours
Vancomycin	**Vancomycin** 1000 mg intravenously every 12 hours

4. **Is oral therapy acceptable?**

   If a patient has a MASCC (Multinational Association for Supportive Care in Cancer) index ≥21,[2] oral antibiotics may be used. This scoring system has good sensitivity and specificity to identify patients at low risk for complications. A recommended regimen is:

   • **Ciprofloxacin** 750 mg + **amoxicillin/clavulanic acid** 875 mg/125 mg orally twice daily.[3] Moxifloxacin 400 mg orally every day is an alternative.[17]

   (Start oral treatment in an inpatient setting. After 24 hours of observation, selected patients with support from a personal caregiver [friend, relative, or health care professional], reliable telecommunications, readily available transportation, and close access to emergency medical care may be discharged)

(continued)

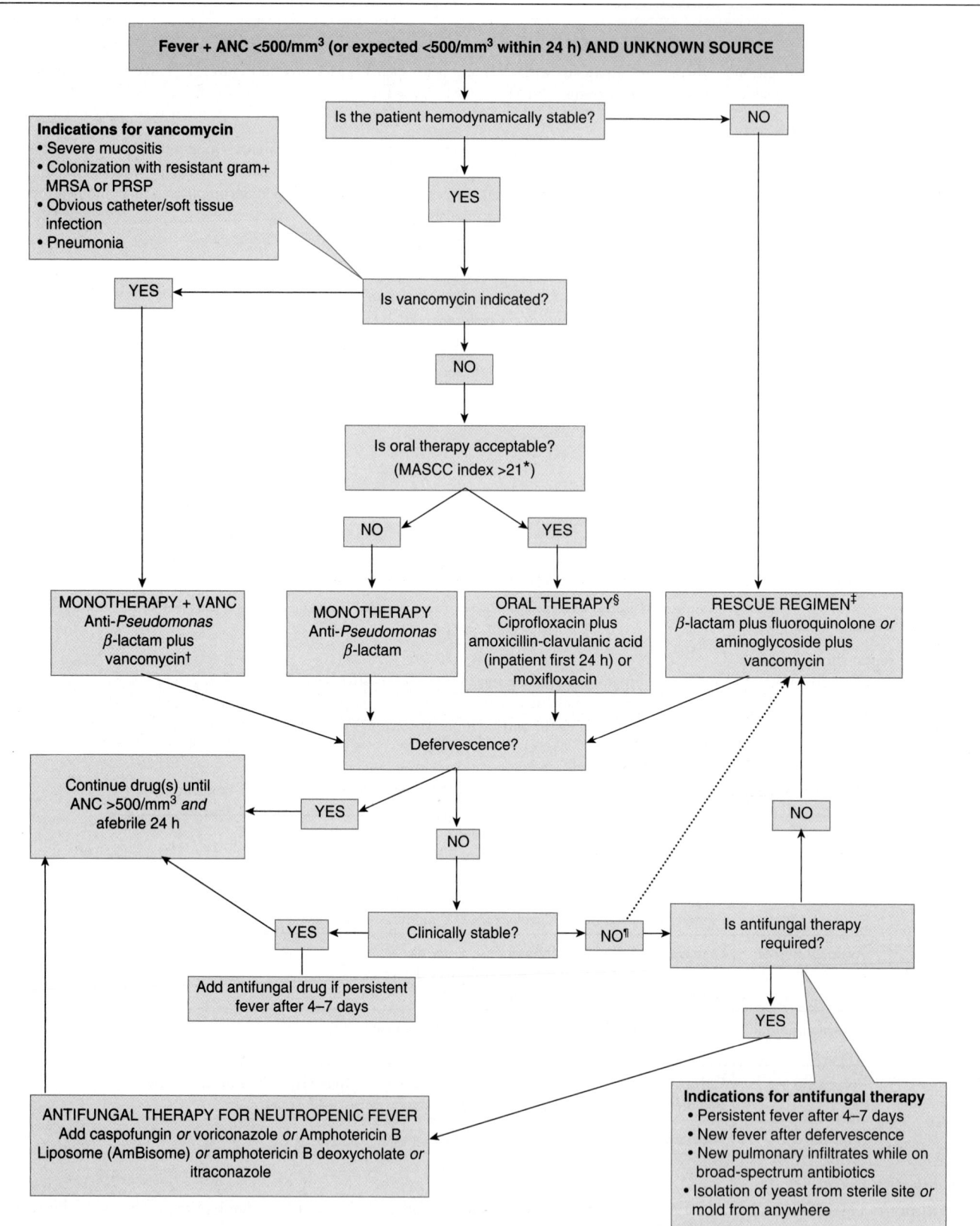

Figure 47–1. MRSA, methicillin (oxacillin)-resistant *Staphylococcus aureus*; PRSP, penicillin-resistant *Streptococcus pneumoniae*

*MASCC Index (Multinational Association of Supportive Care in Cancer). Burden of illness: no or mild symptoms, +5; moderate symptoms, +3; no hypotension, +5; no chronic obstructive pulmonary disease, +4; solid tumor or no previous fungal infection, +4; no dehydration, +3; outpatient status, +3; age <60 years, +2. A MASCC Index ≥21 has been associated with a relatively low risk of severe complications

†Vancomycin should be discontinued after 48 hours if there is no bacteriologic documentation of a pathogen requiring its use, except in soft tissue or tunnel infections

‡This "rescue" antibacterial regimen varies among institutions depending on the local patterns of antibiotic resistance. β-lactum + fluoroquinolone/ aminogylcoside + vancomycin is typical, but it may be broader depending on the prevalence of multiresistant pathogens

§We recommend initiating oral therapy in the hospital (see text for a detailed discussion)

¶Dashed line used to indicate that a change in antibacterial agents may not be needed

Antibiotic Therapy (continued)

Scoring System for Risk of Complications Among Febrile Neutropenic Patients, Based on the Multinational Association for Supportive Care in Cancer (MASCC) Predictive Model

Characteristic	Point Score
Burden of illness • No or mild symptoms • Moderate symptoms	5 3
No hypotension	5
No chronic obstructive pulmonary disease	4
Solid tumor or no previous fungal infection in hematologic tumor	4
Outpatient status	3
No dehydration	3
Aged <60 years	2

Scoring note: The maximum value in this system is 26, and a score of ≤21 predicts a <5% risk for severe complications and a very low mortality (<1%) in febrile neutropenic patients

Antoniadou A, Giamarellou H. Fever of unknown origin in febrile leukopenia. Infect Dis Clin North Am 2007;21:1055–1090
Klastersky J. Management of fever in neutropenic patients with different risks of complications. Clin Infect Dis 2004;39 Suppl 1:S32–S37

5. **Further management depends on the presence/absence of fever and the clinical stability of the patient:**
- If fever resolves, then antibiotics are continued until ANC ≥500/mm³
- For a **clinically or microbiologically documented** bacterial infection, antibiotics should be continued for the standard amount of time typically used to treat such infections or until resolution of neutropenia, whichever is longer
- For uncomplicated fever and neutropenia **of uncertain etiology**, antibiotics should be continued until fever has resolved and ANC is >500/mm³ for 24 hours. If there was no documented fungal infection, antifungal agents can also be discontinued at this time
- **Persistent fever:** If fever persists and the patient remains neutropenic but there are no other clinical changes, continue the initial regimen, performing daily meticulous physical exam and cultures and adding an antifungal agent after 4 days of fever. In many of these cases, a fever will abate with neutrophil recovery and no infection will be documented. The common practice of empirically adding vancomycin in this setting has been shown to be ineffective in a randomized, placebo-controlled clinical trial,[4] and should be discouraged
- If fever persists and the patient's condition deteriorates, change the antibacterial agents and evaluate exhaustively for the presence of an invasive fungal infection. In some cases, an automatic change in antibacterial agents may not be needed (indicated by the dashed line in the figure). The introduction of antifungal agents has been made easier by the availability of less toxic drugs
- **Recrudescent fever:** If fever resolved for more than 24–48 hours and then reoccurs, the risk of a new bacterial or fungal infection is high. Antibacterial agents should be changed, antifungal agents should be modified or added and diagnostic tests (preferably CT) should be implemented to look for occult infection

Antibiotic Choices in Special Clinical Circumstances

1. Penicillin-allergic patient:
- **Aztreonam** 2000 mg intravenously every 6 hours + **vancomycin** 1000 mg intravenously every 12 hours
or
- **Ciprofloxacin** 400 mg intravenously every 12 hours + **clindamycin** 900 mg intravenously every 8 hours
2. Abdominal pain (consider neutropenic enterocolitis):
- **Piperacillin** 4000 mg + **Tazobactam** 500 mg intravenously every 6 hours
or
- **Imipenem** 500 mg + **Cilastatin** 500 mg intravenously every 6 hours
or
- **Meropenem** 1000 mg intravenously every 8 hours
or
- **Ceftazidime** 2000 mg intravenously every 8 hours + **metronidazole** 500 mg intravenously every 6 hours*
or
- **Cefepime** 2000 mg intravenously every 8 hours + **metronidazole** 500 mg intravenously every 6 hours*

(continued)

Antibiotic Choices in Special Clinical Circumstances (*continued*)

3. Pulmonary infiltrates in the setting of neutropenia + fever[†]:

- **Imipenem-cilastatin** *or* **meropenem** *or* **ceftazidime** *or* **cefepime** intravenously + **Levofloxacin** 750 mg intravenously every 24 hours

or

- **Imipenem-cilastatin** *or* **meropenem** *or* **ceftazidime** *or* **cefepime** intravenously + **Moxifloxacin** 400 mg intravenously every 24 hours

or

- **Imipenem-cilastatin** *or* **meropenem** *or* **ceftazidime** *or* **cefepime** intravenously + **Moxifloxacin** 400 mg intravenously every 24 hours

[*]The addition of metronidazole may be the preferred approach until *Clostridium difficile* is ruled out
[†]Early CT and bronchoalveolar lavage (BAL) is recommended,[7] as the vast array of potential pathogens in these patients makes empirical management of pneumonia particularly risky. The inclusion of a fluoroquinolone in this situation aims to provide adequate coverage for the common causes of community-acquired pneumonia

Antifungal Agents

Drug Name	Administration	Spectrum of Activity	Toxicity		Refs
Amphotericin B Deoxycholate	0.6–1 mg/kg intravenously over 2–6 hours, daily	Amphotericin B (as deoxycholate or in a lipid formulation) has activity against most yeasts, *Aspergillus* and agents of mucormycosis. It is not active against *Scedosporium*, *Fusarium*, and dematiaceous molds	Most toxic. High incidence of renal insufficiency. One liter of 0.9% sodium chloride injection before or around the infusion may prevent nephrotoxicity		8, 9
	Acetaminophen 650 mg orally ± **diphenhydramine** 12.5–50 mg orally or intravenously may be given prior to amphotericin. Additional doses of acetaminophen and diphenhydramine may be given PRN or on a preset schedule. Alternatively one can observe a patient's response to an initial dose of amphotericin and give premedication only if amphotericin was not tolerated. **Meperidine** 25 mg/dose may be given IV for rigors (oral administration is not effective). An additional 2 doses of meperidine may be administered at 10-minute intervals (total 3 doses) if rigors persist. Decreasing the rate of amphotericin administration may mitigate infusion-related effects				
AmBisome (liposomal amphotericin B)	3–7.5 mg/kg intravenously over 120 minutes, daily (may be reduced to 60 minutes if infusion over 120 minutes was tolerated)	See above	Less toxic than amphotericin B deoxycholate, but not more effective		10
Voriconazole	*Initial dose:* 6 mg/kg intravenously every 12 hours for 24 hours (2 doses), followed by *Maintenance dose:* 4 mg/kg intravenously every 12 hours	Treatment of choice for aspergillosis. No significant activity against agents of mucormycosis. May be preferable to lipid formulations of amphotericin B against *Fusarium* and *Scedosporium*	Interact with multiple drugs metabolized by cytochrome P450 enzymes, so that the dose of other drugs may need to be adjusted. Liver enzyme abnormalities have been described with all the azoles, and hepatic failure has been reported. **Monitor LFT's** weekly to biweekly, then monthly	No need for adjustment in renal insufficiency. Monitor levels and aim for 2–5 mcg/mL	11
Posaconazole	*Initial and maintenance doses:* 400 mg or 200 mg orally every 6 hours always with food	Active against yeast, *Aspergillus*, and some dematiaceous molds		There is NO intravenous formulation. Therapeutic levels are not reached for 5 to 7 days	12
Fluconazole	400 mg intravenously or orally once or twice daily	Inactive against molds. Empirical administration for persistent fever and neutropenia should be considered only where a risk of aspergillosis is very low		Adjust dose in renal insufficiency: 50% doses for creatinine clearance <50 mL/min	13
Caspofungin	*Loading dose:* 70 mg intravenously on the first day of treatment followed on subsequent days by *Maintenance dose:* 50 mg intravenously daily	Active only against *Candida* and *Aspergillus*	Caspofungin has been shown to be equivalent to AmBisome in the management of persistent fever during neutropenia, but its efficacy compared to other agents in the treatment of established fungal infections in neutropenic patients is unknown		14, 15

(*continued*)

Antifungal Agents (continued)

Drug Name	Administration	Spectrum of Activity	Toxicity	Refs
Micafungin	100–150 mg daily intravenously	Active only against *Candida* and *Aspergillus*	Micafungin has been shown to be effective for the management of candidemia and disseminated candidiasis, and equivalent to fluconazole as antifungal prophylaxis. Its efficacy compared to other agents in the treatment of established fungal infections in neutropenic patients is unknown	
Anidulafungin	*Loading dose:* 200 mg intravenously on the first day of treatment followed on subsequent days by *Maintenance dose:* 100 mg intravenously daily	Active only against *Candida* and *Aspergillus*	Anidulafungin has been shown to be effective for the management of candidemia and disseminated candidiasis, and equivalent to fluconazole as antifungal prophylaxis. Its efficacy compared to other agents in the treatment of established fungal infections in neutropenic patients is unknown	

Management of Specific Clinical Syndromes During Neutropenia

Diagnostic Considerations	Management

Skin/Soft-Tissue Infections

1. Prompt biopsy with histologic staining and culture for bacteria, mycobacteria, viruses, and fungi
2. A vesicle should be unroofed and a scraping of the base examined by direct fluorescence assay (DFA) to make the diagnosis of VZV. The scrapings should also be sent for HSV testing

Pathogens:
- Gram-negative bacilli (eg, *Pseudomonas aeruginosa*, *Aeromonas* spp., *Plesiomonas shigelloides*, Enterobacteriaceae)
- *Streptococcus pyogenes*
- *Staphylococcus aureus*

Management:
- Empirical management should include coverage against MRSA:
  - **Vancomycin** 1000 mg intravenously every 12 hours *or*
  - **Daptomycin** 4 mg/kg intravenously every 24 hours *or*
  - **Linezolid** 600 mg intravenously or orally every 24 hours (can prolong the duration of neutropenia)
- For ecthyma gangrenosum include coverage of *Pseudomonas*:
  - **Ceftazidime** 2000 mg intravenously every 8 hours *or*
  - **Cefepime** 2000 mg intravenously every 8 hours *or*
  - **Ciprofloxacin** 400 mg intravenously every 8 hours
- Treat *Streptococcus pyogenes* infections aggressively with:
  - **Penicillin G** 4 million units intravenously every 4 hours +
  - **Clindamycin** 600–900 mg intravenously every 8 hours +
  - Surgical debridement
- In case of streptococcal shock syndrome, intravenous immune globulin, human (IVIG) may be helpful:
  - **IVIG** 1000 mg/kg of body weight on day 1 followed by
  - **IVIG** 500 mg/kg on days 2 and 3
- Treat perianal cellulitis with broad-spectrum coverage including anaerobes:
  - **Imipenem** 500–1000 mg + **Cilastatin** 500–1000 mg administer intravenously every 6 hours *or*
  - **Meropenem** 1000 mg administer intravenously every 8 hours *or*
  - **Piperacillin** 4000 mg + **Tazobactam** 500 mg, intravenously every 6 hours

---

- Varicella zoster virus (VZV)
- Herpes simplex virus (HSV)

- VZV: **Acyclovir** 10 mg/kg intravenously every 8 hours
- HSV: **Acyclovir** 5 mg/kg intravenously every 8 hours

- *Candida* spp.
- Agents of mucormycosis (eg, *Rhizopus*, *Mucor*)
- **Fusarium and dematiaceous molds**

- Treat multiple discrete lesions in patients at high risk for invasive mold infections with antifungals until etiologic diagnosis is established
  - **Voriconazole** 6 mg/kg intravenously every 12 hours for 24 hours (2 doses), followed by 4 mg/kg intravenously every 12 hours—*preferred*—or
  - **Amphotericin B formulation** (deoxycholate or liposomal)

(continued)

Management of Specific Clinical Syndromes During Neutropenia (*continued*)

Diagnostic Considerations	Management

Sinusitis

1. Evaluate with CT scan and examination by otolaryngologist
2. Tissue should be biopsied if there is suspicion of fungal infection or no response to antibiotic therapy after 72 hours

Diagnostic Considerations	Management

Pathogens:
• *Pseudomonas aeruginosa*
• *Staphylococcus aureus*
• *Streptococcus pneumoniae*
• *Haemophilus influenzae*
• *Moraxella catarrhalis*
• *Enterobacteriaceae*
	Management:
	• Broad-spectrum coverage including *Pseudomonas* and *Staphylococcus aureus*:
	  ▪ **Imipenem** 500–1000 mg + **Cilastatin sodium** 500–1000 mg intravenously every 6 hours *or*
	  ▪ **Meropenem** 1000 mg intravenously every 8 hours *or*
	  ▪ **Cefepime** 2000 mg intravenously every 8 hours
	  ▪ **Piperacillin sodium** 4000 mg + **Tazobactam sodium** 500 mg intravenously every 6 hours

Fungi:
• *Aspergillus* spp.
• Invasive fungal infections (*Aspergillus, Zygomycetes, Fusarium*)
• Dematiaceous molds
	• Consider fungal coverage:
	  ▪ **Amphotericin B sodium deoxycholate** 1 mg/kg intravenously every day *or*
	  ▪ An **amphotericin B lipid formulation** 5 mg/kg intravenously every day

Pulmonary Infections

1. CT scan and bronchoalveolar lavage should be performed early
2. Pneumonia during neutropenia is often caused by Gram-negative bacilli and *Staphylococcus aureus* but can also be caused by community-acquired pneumonia pathogens
3. Neutropenic patients are at risk for invasive fungal infections particularly aspergillosis

Diagnostic Considerations	Management

Pathogens:
• Gram-negative bacilli
• *Staphylococcus aureus*
• *Streptococcus pneumoniae*
• *Haemophilus influenzae*
• *Legionella* spp
• *Chlamydophila pneumoniae*
	Management:
	• Cefepime, imipenem, and meropenem have better activity than ceftazidime against *Streptococcus pneumoniae*:
	  ▪ **Cefepime** 2000 mg intravenously every 8 hours *or*
	  ▪ **Imipenem** 500–1000 mg + **Cilastatin** 500–1000 mg intravenously every 6 hours *or*
	  ▪ **Meropenem** 1000 mg intravenously every 8 hours *or*
	  ▪ **Piperacillin** 4000 mg + **Tazobactam** 500 mg intravenously every 6 hours
	• Adding coverage for atypical pathogens (mainly *Legionella*) is recommended:
	  ▪ **Levofloxacin** 750 mg intravenously every day *or*
	  ▪ **Moxifloxacin** 400 mg intravenously every day *or*
	  ▪ **Azithromycin** 500 mg intravenously every day
	• Adding coverage for MRSA in severely hypoxic or extensive infiltrates is recommended:
	  ▪ **Vancomycin** 1000 mg intravenously every 12 hours

• Invasive fungal infections (*Aspergillus, Zygomycetes, Fusarium*)	• If pneumonia develops while a patient is receiving antibiotics, antifungal coverage should be added:
	  ▪ **Amphotericin B deoxycholate** 1 mg/kg intravenously every day *or*
	  ▪ **Amphotericin B lipid formulation** 5 mg/kg intravenously every day *or*
	  ▪ **Voriconazole** 6 mg/kg intravenously every 12 hours × 2 loading doses, followed by 4 mg/kg intravenously every 12 hours *or*
	  ▪ **Caspofungin** 70 mg intravenously loading dose, followed by 50 mg intravenously daily

Gastrointestinal Tract Infections

Mucositis or esophagitis: Lesions associated with mucositis or esophagitis can become superinfected

Diagnostic Considerations	Management

Pathogens:
• *Candida* (oral mucositis and esophagitis)
• HSV (oral mucositis and esophagitis)
• CMV (esophagitis)
	Management:
	• Mucositis or esophagitis:
	  ▪ **Fluconazole** 400 mg intravenously every day *and*
	  ▪ **Acyclovir** 5 mg/kg intravenously every 8 hours
	• Treatment of documented CMV esophagitis:
	  ▪ **Ganciclovir** 5 mg/kg intravenously every 12 hours

(*continued*)

Management of Specific Clinical Syndromes During Neutropenia (*continued*)

Diagnostic Considerations	Management
Diarrhea: most commonly caused by *Clostridium difficile* (send toxin assay) but can also be caused by other organisms	
Pathogens: • *Salmonella* spp • *Shigella* spp • *Aeromonas* spp • *Campylobacter* spp • Viruses (rotavirus, adenovirus, astrovirus, calicivirus) • Parasites (*Giardia, Cryptosporidium*)	For diarrhea caused by *Clostridium difficile:* ■ **Metronidazole** 500 mg intravenously or orally every 6–8 hours for 10–14 days ■ **Vancomycin** 125–250 mg orally every 6 hours if refractory to metronidazole or severe disease ■ **Fidaxomicin** 200 mg orally every 12 hours for 10 days[18] *Note:* For *Clostridium difficile*, no follow-up testing is recommended, as up to one-third of patients remain carriers, and treatment of carriers is not recommended
Enterocolitis: Enterocolitis in neutropenic patients (**typhlitis**) is most commonly caused by a mix of bowel organisms including *Clostridium* species and *Pseudomonas*	
Pathogens: • Enteric Gram-negative bacilli • *Clostridium* species • *Pseudomonas aeruginosa*	• For enterocolitis in neutropenic patients, use broad-spectrum coverage including *Pseudomonas* coverage: ■ **Imipenem** 500–1000 mg + **Cilastatin** 500–1000 mg intravenously every 6 hours *or* ■ **Meropenem** 1000 mg intravenously every 8 hours *or* ■ **Piperacillin** 4000 mg + **Tazobactam** 500 mg intravenously every 6 hours *or* ■ **Ceftazidime** 2000 mg intravenously every 8 hours + ■ **Metronidazole** 500 mg intravenously every 6 hours

Urinary Tract Infections

1. Treat bacteriuria in neutropenic patients
2. Consider whether candiduria may represent disseminated candidiasis

Pathogens: • Enteric Gram-negative bacilli (*Escherichia coli, Klebsiella* spp.) • *Pseudomonas aeruginosa* (prior antibiotics, instrumentation, stents) • *Enterococcus* spp. (including VRE) • *Candida* spp.	Management: • Remove Foley catheter to clear colonization • In a neutropenic patient, treat bacteriuria/candiduria regardless of symptoms • Treat bacteriuria according to susceptibility testing • Candiduria may be treated with **fluconazole** 400 mg intravenously or orally every day

CNS Infections

Bacteria cause most cases of meningitis (*Streptococcus pneumoniae, Listeria monocytogenes, Neisseria meningitidis*, other Gram-negative bacilli, *Rothia mucilaginosa* [formerly *Stomatococcus mucilaginosus*])
In patients with cell-mediated immunodeficiency, also consider *Listeria* or *Cryptococcus neoformans*

Pathogens: • *Streptococcus pneumoniae* • *Listeria monocytogenes* • *Neisseria meningitidis* • Gram-negative bacilli • *Enterococcus* spp.	Management: Bacterial meningitis during neutropenia should be treated with combination therapy: • **Ceftazidime** 2000 mg intravenously every 8 hours *or* • **Cefepime** 2000 mg intravenously every 8 hours *or* • **Meropenem** 2000 mg intravenously every 8 hours (can lower seizure threshold) + • **Vancomycin** 1000 mg intravenously every 12 hours + • **Ampicillin** 2000 mg intravenously every 4 hours
Encephalitis: Most commonly caused by HSV but consider other viruses	
• Herpes simplex • Human herpesvirus 6 (HHV-6) (after allogeneic stem cell transplantation)	Encephalitis: • **Acyclovir** 10 mg/kg intravenously every 8 hours until HSV encephalitis has been ruled out • For HHV-6: **Ganciclovir** 5 mg/kg every 12 hours *or* **foscarnet** 90 mg/kg every 12 hours (some experts recommend both)
Brain abscesses: During neutropenia are almost always caused by fungi	
• *Candida* spp., *Aspergillus* spp. (brain abscess during neutropenia) • *Cryptococcus* (meningitis in T-cell immunodeficiency)	Cryptococcal meningitis: • **Amphotericin B deoxycholate** 1 mg/kg intravenously every day for at least 2 weeks *or* • An **amphotericin B lipid formulation** 6 mg/kg intravenously every day for at least 2 weeks *with* • **Flucytosine** 25 mg/kg per dose orally every 6 hours (adjust dosage for renal insufficiency) for at least 2 weeks *followed by* • Fluconazole 400–800 mg orally every 24 hours

Viral Infections During Neutropenia

Herpes Simplex Virus (HSV)

1. HSV may reactivate during neutropenia, and worsen chemotherapy or radiation therapy-induced mucositis 2. Suspicious oral and genital lesions should be cultured for HSV 3. Pending culture results, empirical treatment of suspicious lesions should be initiated 4. Reactivation during 1 cycle of chemotherapy does not imply HSV recurrence will follow each cycle, and prophylactic treatment is not necessary. If reactivation occurs after several cycles of chemotherapy, attempt prevention with **valacyclovir** 500 mg per dose, orally twice daily or acyclovir 800 mg orally twice daily 5. When to use IV versus oral therapy? Oral agents may be as effective as intravenous acyclovir; the decision is based on the presence of nausea, vomiting, or clinical situations that make absorption questionable	• **Acyclovir** 5 mg/kg per dose intravenously every 8 hours *or* • **Valacyclovir** 500–1000 mg per dose orally twice daily *or* • **Famciclovir** 250 mg per dose orally twice daily

Varicella Zoster (VSZ)

1. VZV reactivation is related more to defects in cell-mediated immunity than to neutropenia 2. A maculopapular and vesicular rash in a dermatomal distribution suggests VZV infection, although HSV may have a similar presentation 3. A vesicle should be unroofed and a scraping of the base examined by direct fluorescence assay (DFA) to establish a diagnosis 4. The main risk of VZV in immunocompromised patients is visceral dissemination. If infection is documented, respiratory precautions should be instituted and treatment started with high-dose intravenous acyclovir	• **Acyclovir** 10 mg/kg per dose intravenously every 8 hours *or* • **Acyclovir** 500 mg/m^2 per dose intravenously every 8 hours

Cytomegalovirus (CMV)

1. CMV is an uncommon pathogen during neutropenia, but can occur in the setting of coexisting severe defects of cell-mediated immunity 2. Determination of pp65 antigenemia cannot be used during neutropenia, as the test requires an ANC >1000/mm^3 to quantify the number CMV-infected white blood cells 3. CMV disease (organ damage caused by CMV, as opposed to CMV reactivation determined by PCR or pp65 antigenemia) is unusual except in HIV (retinitis, colitis) and after allogeneic stem cell transplantation (pneumonitis, enterocolitis) 4. Diagnosis of CMV colitis requires rectosigmoidoscopy or colonoscopy with biopsy. The tissue sample should be processed both for viral culture and immunohistochemistry, as there are cases diagnosed by one modality and not the other. A common differential diagnosis includes acute graft versus host disease, *Clostridium difficile* colitis, and neutropenic enterocolitis (typhlitis). Tissue examination is mandatory, as more than 1 process may be present 5. The diagnosis of CMV pneumonitis requires an appropriate host (typically an allogeneic stem cell transplant recipient), a consistent clinical presentation, and the presence of CMV in the respiratory secretions[16] or lung biopsy 6. For CMV pneumonitis, the treatment of choice is **ganciclovir**	**CMV pneumonitis:** • **Ganciclovir** 5 mg/kg intravenously every 12 hours for 21 days (adjust dose for renal insufficiency). Consider adding **IVIG** 500 mg/kg intravenously every 48 hours for 3 weeks *or* • **Foscarnet** 90 mg/kg intravenously every 12 hours (May be substituted for ganciclovir to avoid the potential bone marrow toxicity of ganciclovir)

References

1. Freifeld AG et al. Clin Infect Dis 2011;52:e56–e93
2. Klastersky J et al. J Clin Oncol 2000;18:3038–3051
3. Freifeld A et al. N Engl J Med 1999;341:305–311
4. Cometta A et al. Clin Infect Dis 2003;37:382–389
5. Furno P et al. Lancet Infect Dis 2002;2:231–242
6. Paul M et al. BMJ 2003;326:1111–1115
7. Maschmeyer G et al. Ann Hematol 2003;82(Suppl 2):S118–S126
8. Pizzo PA et al. Am J Med 1982;72:101–111
9. European Organization for Research on Therapy of Cancer International Antimicrobial Therapy Cooperative Group. Am J Med 1989;86(6 Pt 1):668–672
10. Walsh TJ et al. N Engl J Med 1999;340:764–771
11. Walsh TJ et al. N Engl J Med 2002;346:225–234
12. Boogaerts M et al. Ann Intern Med 2001;135:412–422
13. Winston DJ et al. Am J Med 2000;108:282–289
14. Walsh TJ et al. N Engl J Med 2004;351:1391–1402
15. Klastersky J [Editorial]. N Engl J Med 2004;351:1445–1447
16. Ljungman P et al. Clin Infect Dis 2002;34:1094–1097
17. Kern et al. J Clin Oncol 2013;31:1149–1156
18. Louie TJ et al. N Engl J Med 2011;364:422–431

48. Catheter-Related Bloodstream Infections: Management and Prevention

Naomi P. O'Grady, MD

Epidemiology and Microbiology

Most Common Organisms[1]

Organism	Frequency	Antimicrobial Resistance
Coagulase-negative staphylococci	31%	
Enterococci	9%	Dramatic rise in enterococcal isolates resistant to vancomycin—from 0.5% in 1989 to 25.9% in 1999
Staphylococcus aureus	20%	>50% of all *S. aureus* nosocomial isolates are oxacillin resistant[1]
Gram-negative bacilli	20%	Increasing prevalence of Enterobacteriaceae with extended-spectrum β-lactamases (ESBLs), and carbapenemase-producing organisms particularly *Klebsiella pneumoniae*. Such organisms may be resistant to many commonly used cephalosporins and carbapenems
Candida infections		Growing resistance of *Candida albicans* to antifungals; 50% of *Candida* bloodstream infections are caused by non-*albicans* species including *Candida glabrata* and *Candida krusei*, which are more likely than *C. albicans* to demonstrate resistance to fluconazole and itraconazole. Resistance to voriconazole has not been reported thus far, although continued surveillance is need

Definitions[2]

- **Catheter colonization:** Significant growth of a microorganism in a quantitative or semiquantitative culture of the catheter tip, subcutaneous catheter segment, or catheter hub
- **Exit-site infection:** Erythema, induration, and/or tenderness within 2 cm of the catheter exit site; may be associated with other signs and symptoms of infection, such as fever or pus emerging from the exit site with or without concomitant bloodstream infections
- **Tunnel infection:** Tenderness, erythema, and/or induration within 12 cm from the catheter exit site along the subcutaneous tract of a tunneled catheter (eg, Hickman or Broviac) with or without concomitant bloodstream infections
- **Pocket infection:** Infected fluid in the subcutaneous pocket of a totally implanted intravascular device; often associated with tenderness, erythema, and/or induration over the pocket; spontaneous rupture and drainage, or necrosis of the overlying skin, with or without concomitant bloodstream infection, may also occur
- **Catheter-related bloodstream infection:** Bacteremia or fungemia in a patient who has an intravascular device and 1 positive result from culture of blood samples from the peripheral vein, clinical manifestations of infection (eg, fever, chills, and/or hypotension), and no apparent source for bloodstream infection (except for the catheter). One of the following should be present: a positive result of semiquantitative (>15 CFU per catheter segment) or quantitative (>10^2 CFU per catheter segment) catheter culture, whereby the same organism (species and antibiogram) is isolated from a catheter segment and a peripheral blood sample; simultaneous quantitative cultures of blood samples with a ratio of >5:1 (central venous catheter [CVC] versus peripheral catheter); differential time to positivity (ie, a positive result of culture from a CVC is obtained at least 2 hours earlier than a positive result from a culture from peripheral blood)

Diagnosis

1. **Blood cultures**
   - Clinical findings for establishing the diagnosis of catheter-related infection are unreliable because of poor sensitivity and specificity
   - When catheter infection is suspected, 2 sets of blood cultures should be sent with at least 1 drawn percutaneously[2]
   - Paired quantitative or qualitative blood cultures with continuously monitored differential time to positivity are recommended when long-term catheters cannot be removed[3–5]

2. **Catheter cultures**
   - Culture catheters only when catheter-related bloodstream infection is suspected[2]
   - Quantitative or semiquantitative cultures are recommended[2]
   - When culturing a catheter segment, catheter tip should be cultured rather than the subcutaneous segment[6]
   - For suspected pulmonary artery catheter infection, the introducer tip should be cultured[2]

Management[2]

Nontunneled central venous catheters (CVCs) (see Figures 48–1 and 48–2)

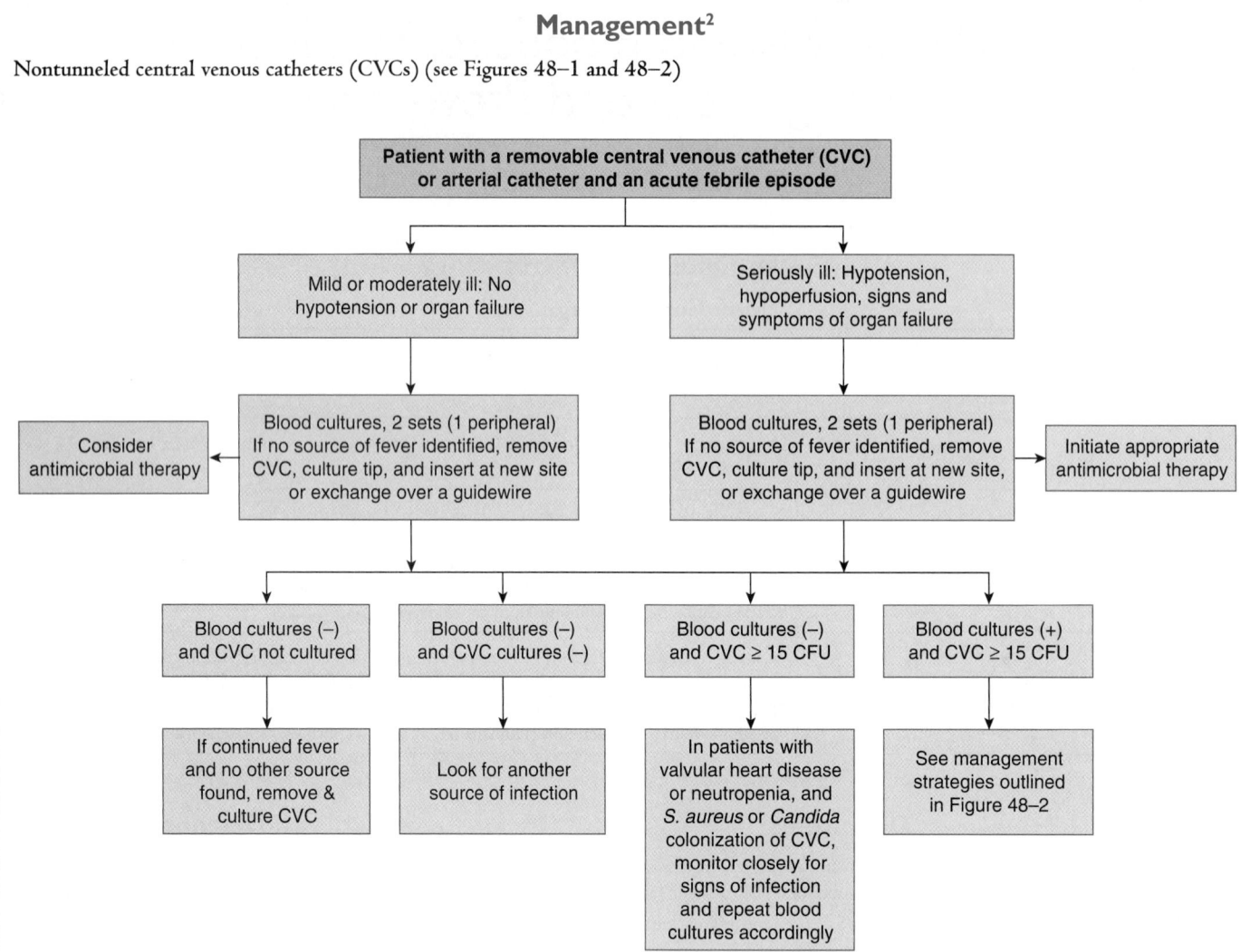

Figure 48–1. CFU, Colony-forming unit. (From Guidelines for the Management of Intravascular Catheter-Related Infections)

- CVCs in patients with fever and mild to moderate symptoms do not need to be routinely removed
- CVCs should be removed and cultured if the patient has a tunnel infection (erythema or purulence overlying the catheter exit site) or clinical signs of sepsis
- If blood culture results are positive or if the CVC is exchanged over the guidewire and has significant colonization according to results of quantitative or semiquantitative cultures, the catheter should be removed and placed into a new site
- In some patients without evidence of persistent bloodstream infection, or if the infecting organism is a coagulase-negative staphylococci and if there is no suspicion of local or metastatic complications, the CVC may be retained
- A transesophageal echocardiogram (TEE) should be obtained to rule out vegetations (endocarditis) in patients with a catheter-related *S. aureus* bloodstream infection if less than 4 weeks of therapy is being considered
- If a TEE is not available and the results of transthoracic echocardiography are negative, the duration of therapy for *S. aureus* bacteremia should be 4–6 weeks
- After removal of a colonized catheter associated with bloodstream infection, if there is persistent bacteremia or fungemia or a lack of clinical improvement, aggressive evaluation for septic thrombosis, infective endocarditis, and other metastatic infections should commence
- Febrile patients with valvular heart disease or patients with neutropenia whose catheter tip culture reveals significant growth of *S. aureus* or *Candida* species on semiquantitative or quantitative culture with no bloodstream infection should be followed up closely for development of infection, and samples of blood for culture should be obtained accordingly
- After a catheter is removed from a patient with a catheter-related bloodstream infection, nontunneled catheters may be reinserted after appropriate systemic antimicrobial therapy is begun

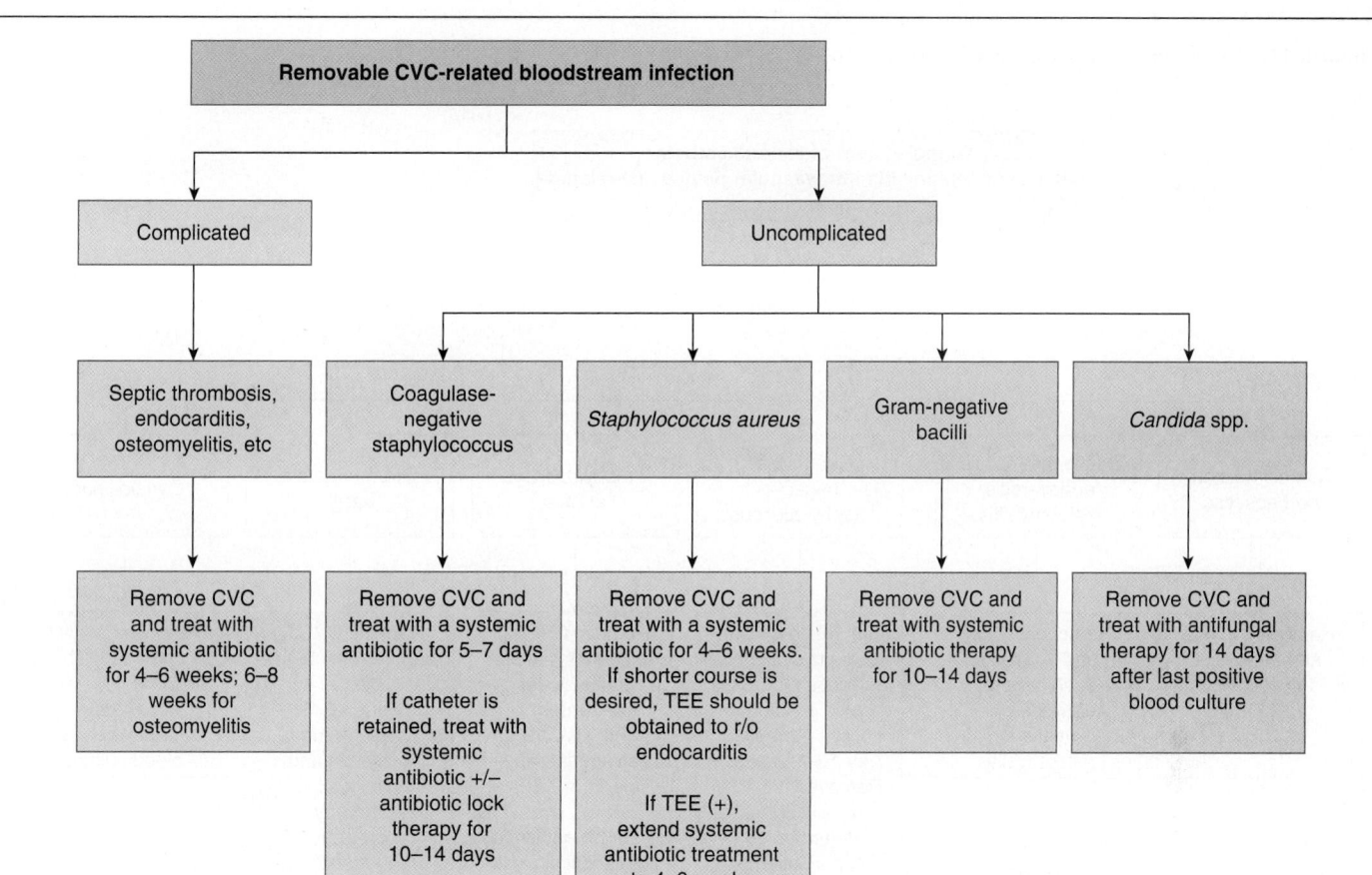

Figure 48–2. CVC, Central venous catheter; TEE, transesophageal echocardiography. (From Guidelines for the Management of Intravascular Catheter-Related Infections)

Tunneled CVCs and intravascular devices (see Figure 48–3)

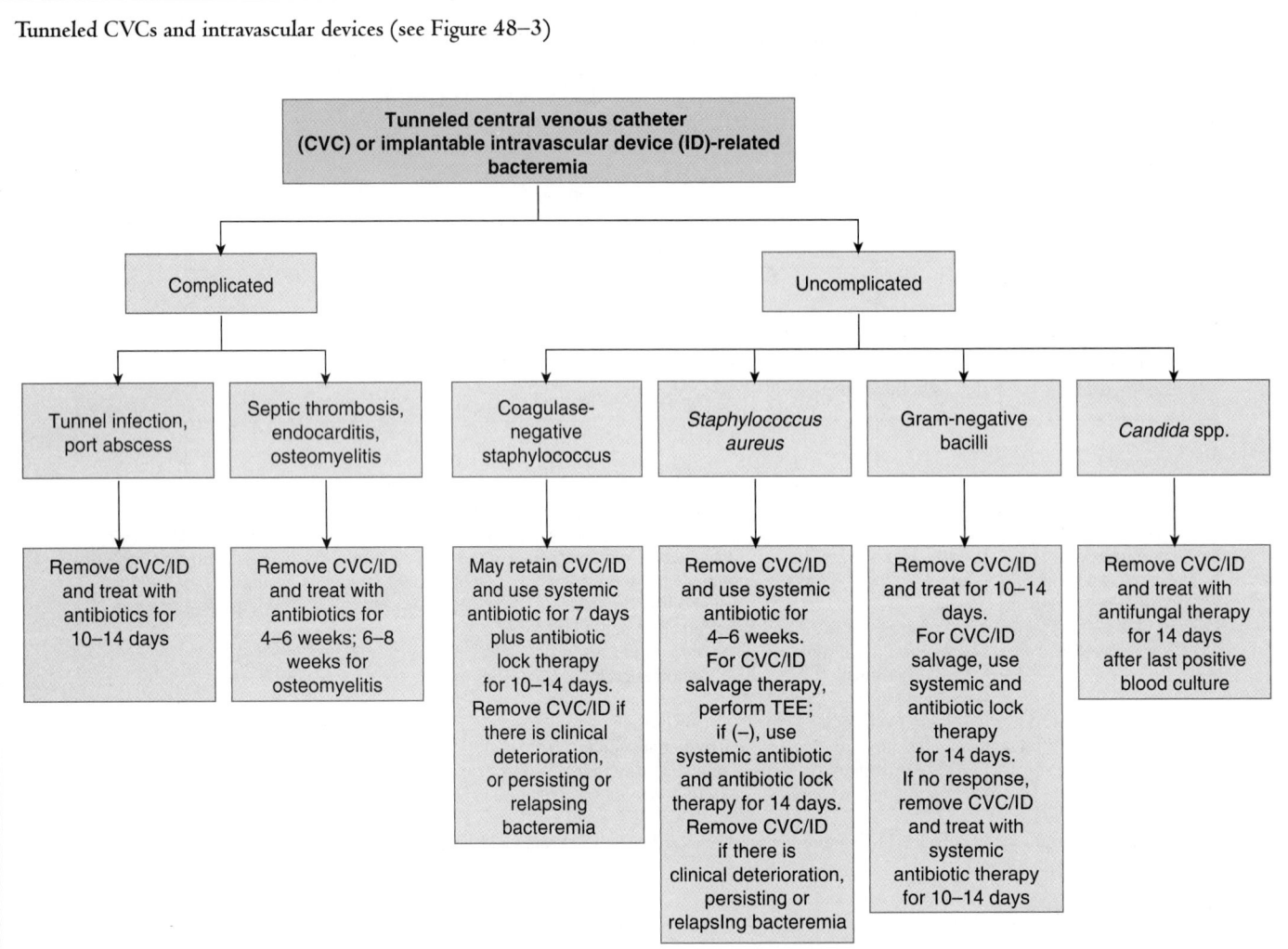

Figure 48–3. CVC, Central venous catheter; TEE, transesophageal echocardiography. (From Guidelines for the Management of Intravascular Catheter-Related Infections)

- Clinical assessment is recommended to determine whether the CVC or the ID is the source of infection or bloodstream infection
- For complicated infections, the CVC or the ID should be removed
- For salvage of the CVC or the ID in patients with uncomplicated infections, antibiotic lock therapy should be used for 2 weeks with standard systemic therapy for treatment of catheter-related bacteremia caused by *S. aureus*, coagulase-negative staphylococci, and Gram-negative bacilli for suspected intraluminal infection in the absence of tunnel or pocket infection
- Tunneled catheter pocket infections or port abscess require removal of a catheter and usually 7–10 days of appropriate antibiotic therapy
- Reinsertion of tunneled intravascular devices should be postponed until after appropriate systemic antimicrobial therapy is begun, based on susceptibilities of the bloodstream isolate and after repeated cultures of blood samples yield negative results

Prevention[7]

1. **Site of catheter insertion**
   - Subclavian site has lowest rate of infectious complications
   - Catheters inserted into an internal jugular vein have been associated with higher risk of infection than that of those inserted into a subclavian or femoral veins[8,9]
   - Femoral catheters are at high risk for thromboembolic disease
2. **Skin antisepsis**
   - Chlorhexidine (>0.5%) should be used in adult and adolescent patients, unless there is a contraindication to its use
3. **Catheter-site dressing regimens**
   - Transparent, semipermeable polyurethane dressings are reliable, secure, and convenient

(*continued*)

Prevention (*continued*)

- **Chlorhexidine-impregnated sponge dressings** can reduce the risk of bacteremia with CVCs in place >4 days. This small disk can be placed over the insertion site and left in place for up to 7 days
- **Mupirocin ointment** applied at the insertion sites of CVCs prevents catheter-related bloodstream infections, but it has also been associated with mupirocin resistance and selection for fungal organisms. This ointment may adversely affect the integrity of polyurethane catheters and is therefore not recommended
- Mupirocin ointment has been used intranasally to decrease nasal carriage of *S. aureus* and reduce the risk of catheter-related bloodstream infections. However, this practice is not recommended because of the development of resistance

4. **Antimicrobial/antiseptic impregnated catheters**
   - Certain antimicrobial or antiseptic-impregnated or antiseptic-coated catheters have been shown to decrease the risk of catheter-related bloodstream infection[10]
   - Catheters coated with **chlorhexidine/silver sulfadiazine** on the external luminal surface only reduced the risk of bacteremia compared with standard noncoated catheters.[11,12] Selection of resistance to chlorhexidine/silver sulfadiazine is a concern; however, this has not yet been demonstrated. These catheters may be cost-effective in the ICU and in burn patients, neutropenic patients, and patients who have had catheters placed under emergency conditions
   - Catheters impregnated on the internal and external surfaces with **minocycline/rifampin** are associated with lower rates of bacteremia when compared with chlorhexidine/silver sulfadiazine-impregnated catheters.[13] No minocycline/rifampin-resistant organisms were reported, although this is a theoretical risk
   - A second-generation catheter is now available with a chlorhexidine coating on both the internal and external luminal surfaces
   - The decision to use chlorhexidine/silver sulfadiazine- or minocycline/rifampin-impregnated catheters should be based on the need to enhance prevention of catheter-related bloodstream infections and balanced against the concern for possible emergence of resistant pathogens and the cost of implementing this strategy

5. **Antibiotic lock prophylaxis**
   - Antibiotic lock prophylaxis can be useful in neutropenic patients with long-term catheters using a solution containing heparin plus 25 mcg/mL of vancomycin
   - This practice can increase the risk of VRE.[14] Antibiotic lock prophylaxis is not recommended routinely, although in patients with difficult access who have had multiple episodes of bacteremia, it is not an unreasonable strategy

6. **Replacement of catheters**
   - There are no studies that show an advantage of routine catheter replacement at scheduled time intervals as a method to reduce catheter-related bloodstream infections[15–17]
   - Replacement of temporary catheters over a guidewire in the setting of bacteremia is not an acceptable replacement strategy, because the source of infection is usually colonization of the skin tract from the insertion site to the vein[18,19]

7. **Chlorhexidine baths:**
   - Chlorhexidine baths daily have been shown to reduce the risk of hospital acquired infection, including catheter-related infections

References

1. Wisplinghoff H et al. Nosocomial bloodstream infections in US hospitals: analysis of 24,179 cases from a prospective nationwide surveillance study. Clin Infect Dis 2004;39(3):309–317
2. Mermel LA et al. Guidelines for the management of intravascular catheter-related infections 2009 Update by the Infectious Diseases Society of America. Clin Infect Dis 2009;49(1):1–45
3. Maki DG et al. N Engl J Med 1977;296:1305–1309
4. DesJardin JA et al. Ann Intern Med 1999;131:641–647
5. Blot F et al. Lancet 1999;354:1071–1077
6. Sherertz RJ et al. J Clin Microbiol 1997;35:641–646
7. O'Grady NP et al. Guidelines for the prevention of intravascular catheter-related infections. Clin Infect Dis 2011;52(9):e162–e193
8. Merrer J et al. JAMA 2001;286:700–707
9. Mermel LA et al. Am J Respir Crit Care Med 1994;149:1020–1036
10. Raad I et al. Ann Intern Med 1997;127:267–274
11. Mermel LA. Ann Intern Med 2000;132:391–402
12. Veenstra DL et al. JAMA 1999;281:261–267
13. Darouiche RO et al. NEJM 1999;340:1–8
14. Centers for Disease Control and Prevention. Recommendations for preventing the spread of vancomycin resistance. Recommendations of the Hospital Infection Control Practices Advisory Committee (HICPAC). MMWR Morb Mortal Wkly Rep 1995;44:1–13
15. Eyer S et al. Crit Care Med 1990;18:1073–1079
16. Uldall PR et al. Lancet 1981;1:1373
17. Cook D et al. Crit Care Med 1997;25:1417–1424
18. Mermel LA et al. Am J Med 1991;91:197S–205S
19. Cobb DK et al. N Engl J Med 1992;327:1062–1068

49. Venous Catheter-Related Thrombosis

Roy E. Smith, MD, MS

Incidence[1–5]

	Central Venous Catheter (CVCs)	Peripherally Inserted Central Catheters (PICCs)
Symptomatic DVT	1–10%	1–4%
Asymptomatic DVT (documented by venography)	~30%	~20%
Catheter occlusion (without DVT)	~10%	

Evaluation[5–7]

Differential diagnosis:
1. Cellulitis
2. Fluid retention
3. Local vein compression by tumor

Upper extremity DVT predication score[8]

Parameter Category	Point Designation
Presence of catheter or access device in a subclavian or jugular vein or a pacemaker	+1
Unilateral pitting edema in catheterized extremity	+1
Localized pain in catheterized extremity	+1
Another diagnosis at least as plausible	−1
Probability Category (Prevalence)	**Risk Score**
Low (9–13%)	−1 or 0
Intermediate (20–38%)	+1
High (64–70%)	>1

Imaging procedures:
1. *Ultrasound:* Use for jugular, axillary, and subclavian veins (sensitivity and specificity 80%)
2. *Venography:* Use for more central veins including innominate and vena cava, and when high clinical suspicion despite negative ultrasound

Complications of Upper Limp DVT[5]
1. *Pulmonary embolism (PE):* The incidence of clinical overt PE is estimated at 12%; the incidence of PE in persons with cancer is higher at 15–25%
2. Postphlebitic syndrome occurs in ~15%

Risk Factors Associated with Central Venous Catheter-Related Thromboembolism Among Patients with Cancer[9]

Technical

Thrombogenicity of catheter material (polyethylene > polyurethane or silicone)
Large catheter diameter and number of lumens
Malpositioned catheter tip
Percutaneous insertion > cut down
More than 1 insertion attempt
Prior CVC insertion
Left-sided placement
Subclavian vein insertion > internal jugular insertion

Patient and Vascular

Catheter-associated infection
Fibrinous catheter lumen occlusion
Extrinsic vascular compression (enlarged cervical and/or mediastinal lymph nodes, etc)
Factor V Leiden mutation (and perhaps other thrombophilias)
Prior venous thromboembolism
Ovarian cancer

Treatment-Related

Asparaginase
Estrogens and/or progesterone
Growth factors (ie, epoetin, GM-CSFs, G-CSFs)
Aldesleukin (IL-2)
Thalidomide
Lenalidomide
Heparin-induced thrombocytopenia and thrombosis (HIT, HITT)
Chemical irritation

Treatment of Catheter-Related Venous Thrombosis[10-13]

1. If a CVC is functioning and does not appear to be infected, there is no imperative to remove it
2. If CVC removal is planned, consider full anticoagulation with unfractionated *or* low-molecular-weight heparin for 5–7 days prior to removal to reduce the risk embolization with device extraction
3. Clinicians should keep in mind patients with active malignancy may require prolonged anticoagulation after catheter removal should it be determined that the event occurred independent of the presence of CVC (eg, an additional thrombotic event distant to catheter site)
4. Catheter-related thrombosis occurring in patients with HIT/HITT is a special circumstance. These patients should receive a direct thrombin inhibitor or fondaparinux for acute anticoagulation with a transition to warfarin or fondaparinux for a total of 3 months of anticoagulation, or for as long as a catheter remains in place

	Acute Care	Subacute Care
CVC-related DVT; restoring patency is not imperative	1. Standard doses of **unfractionated heparin:** *Loading dose:* 80 units/kg by IV injection *Maintenance dose:* 18 units/kg per hour by continuous IV infusion for 5–7 days, *or* a low-molecular-weight heparin (LMWH) **enoxaparin** 1 mg/kg subcutaneously every 12 hours for a total of 5–7 days, *or* An alternative LMWH	**Warfarin** orally to maintain an INR of 2–3 for a total duration of anticoagulation of 3 months, or for as long as the catheter is in place, or (a LMWH) **Enoxaparin** 1 mg/kg subcutaneously once daily for a total duration of 3 months, or for as long as the catheter is in place
CVC-related DVT; restoring patency is imperative	1. **Alteplase** (tPA) by direct injection into a clot under fluoroscopic guidance, *or* 2. **Urokinase** by direct injection into a clot under fluoroscopic guidance 3. Standard doses of **unfractionated heparin** *Loading dose:* 80 units/kg by IV injection *Maintenance dose:* 18 units/kg per hour by continuous IV infusion for 5–7 days, *or* **Enoxaparin** 1 mg/kg subcutaneously every 12 hours for a total of 5–7 days, *or* An alternative LMWH	**Warfarin** orally to maintain an INR of 2–3 for 3 months, *or* **Enoxaparin** 1 mg/kg subcutaneously once daily (or an alternative LMWH) for 3 months
SVC thrombosis	1. **Alteplase** by direct injection into a clot under fluoroscopic guidance 2. **Urokinase** by direct injection into a clot under fluoroscopic guidance 3. Standard doses of **unfractionated heparin** *Loading dose:* 80 units/kg *Maintenance dose:* 18 units/kg per hour for 5–7 days, *or* **Enoxaparin** 1 mg/kg subcutaneously every 12 hours for a total of 5–7 days, *or* An alternative LMWH	**Warfarin** orally to maintain an INR of 2–3 for 3 months, *or* **Enoxaparin** 1 mg/kg subcutaneously once daily (or an alternative LMWH) for 3 months
Internal jugular vein thrombosis	1. Apply heat topically 2. Systemic antiinflammatory agents 3. If symptoms are severe or progressive, standard doses of **unfractionated heparin** *Loading dose:* 80 units/kg *Maintenance dose:* 18 units/kg per hour for 5–7 days, *or* **Enoxaparin** 1 mg/kg subcutaneously every 12 hours for a total of 5–7 days, *or* An alternative LMWH	If treatment with heparin is required then **Warfarin** orally to maintain an INR of 2–3 for 3 months, *or* **Enoxaparin** 1 mg/kg subcutaneously once daily (or an alternative LMWH) for 3 months
Peripheral vein thrombophlebitis	1. Apply heat topically 2. Oral and/or topical antiinflammatory agents 3. VAD removal is almost always indicated	Patients at risk for the development of deep vein thrombosis (superficial phlebitis close to a deep vein or the presence thrombophilia) and patients with proximal basilic or cephalic thrombosis who remain symptomatic 1. Full-dose anticoagulation can be considered 2. The duration of anticoagulation should be individualized based upon the risk of bleeding and improvement in symptoms

IV, intravenous; VAD, vascular access device
*Urokinase is not available in the United States

Prevention of Catheter-Related Venous Thrombosis[3,14-18]

1. Randomized controlled studies have not established the efficacy of prophylaxis with low-molecular-weight heparin or low-dose warfarin (1 mg/day). The 8th Annual American College of Chest Physicians Practice Guidelines for Antithrombotic and Thrombolytic Therapy do not recommend the use of prophylactic anticoagulation in this setting
2. If used, it is likely that therapeutic or near-therapeutic levels of anticoagulation and close monitoring will be required for the successful prevention of catheter-associated incident thrombosis and reduction of bleeding risk
3. When considering pharmacologic prophylaxis, clinicians must take into consideration an individual patient's risk for developing catheter-related thrombosis. Some experts have suggested that thromboprophylaxis should be considered for patients believed to be at high risk

Notes

Common Venous Access Devices[19]

Design	Use			Duration of Use	Routine Flush[†]
	Blood Draw	IV Fluid	Blood Product[*]		
Tunneled					
Open-ended (eg, Hickman)	++++	++++	++++	Weeks to years	Daily
Valved[‡] (eg, Groshong)	++++	++++	++++	Weeks to years	Weekly
Ports (open or valved end)	++++	++++	++++	Months to years	Monthly
Nontunneled					
Peripheral (PICC, open or valved)	+	++++	+	<3 months	Daily or weekly
Midline	+	++++	+	<6 weeks	Daily
Central	++++	++++	++++	<3 months	Daily

*The ability to administer packed red blood cells depends on the internal diameter of a catheter lumen
†Either unfractionated heparin or 0.9% sodium chloride injection may be used. Heparin is contraindicated in patients with a history of heparin allergy or heparin-induced thrombocytopenia
‡Valved catheters reduce or eliminate the need for heparinization and the risk of air embolism and blood reflux

Contraindications for the Placement of Central Venous Access Devices[20]
Absolute:
1. An uncooperative patient
2. Availability of appropriate alternative peripheral insertion site
3. Significant coagulopathy in a stable patient
4. Obstruction of target vein (eg, venous thrombosis, anatomical defect, external compression)

Relative:
1. Infection or burn at insertion site
2. Sepsis (unless blood cultures were deemed sterile during prior 36–48 hours)
3. Significant coagulopathy in an unstable patient
4. Decreased platelet count associated with an increased bleeding risk (ie, platelets <50,000/mm^3)

Incidence of Complications of Venous Access Devices[21]

Arrhythmia	13%
Arterial puncture	2.8–3.8%
Inappropriately positioned reservoir	2%
Pneumothorax	1–1.8%
Wound dehiscence	1.5%
Hemorrhage	1.1–1.2%
Failure of insertion	1.2%

(continued)

Notes (*continued*)

Optimal Catheter Placement
The catheter tip should be in the mid-superior vena cava, just outside the right atrium. Opinions differ about the risks and benefits of placing the tip within the right atrium

Management of Catheter Tip occlusion with a Fibrin Sheath[4,22–25]
Mechanism:
Accumulation of a fibrin coating (sheath) at the tip of a catheter, forming a one-way valve that blocks withdrawal from the CVC but allows infusion

Differential diagnosis:
1. Catheter migration out of the superior vena cava into a smaller vein where it abuts the vein wall more easily
2. Perpendicular abutment of the catheter tip against the wall of the superior vena cava
3. Catheter compression by kinking or a suture
4. Catheter lumen occlusion with precipitated salts or lipid

Evaluation:
1. Reposition the patient to relieve a reversible malposition of the catheter tip
2. Obtain chest x-ray to identify catheter tip location
3. Inject x-ray contrast material through the occluded lumens to identify pericatheter backtracking indicative of a fibrin sheath, and to rule out an extensive fibrin sheath that could lead to extravasation of infused fluids

Treatment:
1. If an occlusive fibrin sheath is identified but there is no evidence that infused fluid will extravasate, the catheter can be used for infusion
2. *To restore the ability to withdraw (aspirate) fluid through a catheter:* Instill **alteplase** 2 mg (2 mL of a 1-mg/mL solution) (Cathflo Activase, Genentech, Inc., South San Francisco, CA) into each occluded lumen and allow it to dwell for 2 hours. If this does not restore lumen patency, the same alteplase treatment may be repeated once
3. If available, **urokinase** offers another alternative. Doses ranging from 5000 units in each affected lumen with a dwell time of 15–60 minutes, which may be repeated for a second instillation if patency was not restored after a single instillation. **Urokinase** 10,000-unit boluses up to 2 times have been successful. Also, for refractory occlusions, slow infusions of **urokinase** (diluted to 5000 units/mL) 40,000 units (8 mL)/hour for 6–12 hours may restore function[26–29]

References

1. Chemaly RF et al. Venous thrombosis associated with peripherally inserted central catheters: a retrospective analysis of the Cleveland Clinic experience. Clin Infect Dis 2002;34:1179–1183
2. Horne MK et al. Venographic surveillance of tunneled venous access devices in adult oncology patients. Ann Surg Oncol 1995;2:174–178
3. Kuriakose P et al. Risk of deep venous thrombosis associated with chest versus arm central venous subcutaneous port catheters: a 5-year single-institution retrospective study. J Vasc Interv Radiol 2002;13:179–184
4. Stephens LC et al. Are clinical signs accurate indicators of the cause of central venous catheter occlusion? JPEN J Parenter Enteral Nutr 1995;19:75–79
5. Verso M et al. Venous thromboembolism associated with long-term use of central venous catheters in cancer patients. J Clin Oncol 2003;21:3665–3675
6. Baarslag HJ et al. Prospective study of color duplex ultrasonography compared with contrast venography in patients suspected of having deep venous thrombosis of the upper extremities. Ann Intern Med 2002;136:865–872
7. Haire WD et al. Limitations of magnetic resonance imaging and ultrasound-directed (duplex) scanning in the diagnosis of subclavian vein thrombosis. J Vasc Surg 1991;13:391–397
8. Constans J et al. A clinical prediction score for upper extremity deep venous thrombosis. Thromb Haemost 2008;99:202–207
9. Linenberger ML. Catheter-related thrombosis: risks, diagnosis, and management. J Natl Compr Canc Netw 2006;4:889–901
10. Becker DM et al. Axillary and subclavian venous thrombosis. Prognosis and treatment. Arch Intern Med 1991;151:1934–1943
11. Chang R, Horne MK 3rd, Mayo DJ, Doppman JL. Pulse-spray treatment of subclavian and jugular venous thrombi with recombinant tissue plasminogen activator. J Vasc Interv Radiol 1996;7:845–851
12. Gould JR et al. Groshong catheter-associated subclavian venous thrombosis. Am J Med 1993;95:419–423
13. Mayo DJ et al. Superior vena cava thrombosis associated with a central venous access device: a case report. Clin J Oncol Nurs 1997;1:5–10
14. Agnelli G, Verso M. Is antithrombotic prophylaxis required in cancer patients with central venous catheters? No. J Thromb Haemost 2006;4:14–15
15. Bern MM et al. Very low doses of warfarin can prevent thrombosis in central venous catheters. A randomized prospective trial. Ann Intern Med 1990;112:423–428
16. Cunningham MS et al. Primary thromboprophylaxis for cancer patients with central venous catheters—a reappraisal of the evidence. Br J Cancer 2006;94:189–194
17. Hirsh J et al. American College of Chest P: Antithrombotic and thrombolytic therapy: American College of Chest Physicians Evidence-Based Clinical Practice Guidelines (8th edition). Chest 2008;133:110S–112S
18. Monreal M et al. Upper extremity deep venous thrombosis in cancer patients with venous access devices--prophylaxis with a low molecular weight heparin (Fragmin). Thromb Haemost 1996;75:251–253
19. Horne MK, Mayo DJ, Freifeld AG. In: Beutler E, Lichtman MA, Coller BS, Kipps TJ, Seligsohn U, eds. Williams Hematology, 6th ed. New York: McGraw-Hill, 2001:887–898
20. Bishop L et al. Guidelines on the insertion and management of central venous access devices in adults. Int J Lab Hematol 2007;29:261–278
21. Kuter DJ. Thrombotic complications of central venous catheters in cancer patients. Oncologist 2004;9:207–216
22. Crain MR et al. Fibrin sheaths complicating central venous catheters. AJR Am J Roentgenol 1998;171:341–346
23. Mayo DJ et al. Chemotherapy extravasation: a consequence of fibrin sheath formation around venous access devices. Oncol Nurs Forum 1995;22:675–680
24. Semba CP et al. Treatment of occluded central venous catheters with alteplase: results in 1,064 patients. J Vasc Interv Radiol 2002;13:1199–1205
25. Tschirhart JM, Rao MK. Mechanism and management of persistent withdrawal occlusion. Am Surg 1988;54:326–328
26. Haire WD et al. Urokinase versus recombinant tissue plasminogen activator in thrombosed central venous catheters: a double-blinded, randomized trial. Thromb Haemost 1994;72:543–547
27. Haire WD et al. Recombinant urokinase for restoration of patency in occluded central venous access devices. A double-blind, placebo-controlled trial. Thromb Haemost 2004;92:575–582
28. Haire WD, Lieberman RP. Thrombosed central venous catheters: restoring function with 6-hour urokinase infusion after failure of bolus urokinase. JPEN J Parenter Enteral Nutr 1992;16:129–132
29. Monturo CA et al. Efficacy of thrombolytic therapy for occlusion of long-term catheters. JPEN J Parenter Enteral Nutr 1990;14:312–314

50. Complications and Follow-Up After Hematopoietic Cell Transplantation

Michael M. Boyiadzis, MD, MHSc, Juan C. Gea-Banacloche, MD, and Michael R. Bishop, MD

Multifactorial etiology of posttransplant hematopoietic cell transplantation (HCT) complications
- Chemotherapy and/or radiation therapy used as conditioning regimen
- Immunodeficiency state following HCT
- Immunosuppressive therapy and adverse events related to medications
- Graft-versus-host disease (after allogeneic HCT)

Infectious Complications Following Autologous and Allogeneic HCT

Freifeld AG et al. Clin Infect Dis 2011;52:e56–e93
Tomblyn M et al. Biol Blood Marrow Transplant 2009;15:1143–1238
Wingard JR. Transpl Infect Dis 1999;1:3–20

Preengraftment Period (Before Neutrophil Recovery)

Autologous and allogeneic transplant recipients are similar with respect to early infectious complications. The risk of infection during this period is related to neutropenia and mucositis resulting from the conditioning regimen

Bacterial	Principal causes of sepsis • Gram-negative bacilli (eg, *Pseudomonas aeruginosa*, Enterobacteriaceae) • Gram-positive bacteria (eg, viridans group *Streptococcus*, coagulase-negative staphylococci) • Common sources include gastrointestinal tract and intravascular devices
Fungal	Fungal infections become more common with prolonged and profound neutropenia *Candida* infections occur early and are often prevented with fluconazole (*see table below for doses and duration of prophylaxis*) *Aspergillus* infections occur later (generally after 10–14 days of neutropenia) • There is no proven effective prophylaxis for *Aspergillus* infections after hematopoietic cell transplantation. The best evidence supports posaconazole; some experts recommend voriconazole, caspofungin, or micafungin
Viral	Herpes simplex virus (HSV) commonly reactivates during this period, and can worsen mucositis Prophylaxis with acyclovir or valacyclovir reduces **HSV** reactivation (*for dose and duration of prophylaxis see table below*)

Early Postengraftment Period (30–100 Days After HCT)

The risk of infection is greater and different for allogeneic recipients than autologous recipients during this period

Autologous HCT

There is some degree of immunodeficiency, but opportunistic infections are the exception rather than the rule

Bacterial	Related to an intravascular device
Fungal	Uncommon Some centers continue prophylaxis against *Pneumocystis jirovecii* (formerly *Pneumocystis carinii*) for 6 months after transplantation
Viral	VZV reactivation and community respiratory virus infections

(continued)

Early Postengraftment Period (30–100 Days After HCT) (continued)
Allogeneic HCT

The infection risk during this period is related to severely impaired cell-mediated immunity, acute GVHD and its treatment, and CMV reactivation. The latter two increase the risk of viral and fungal infections

Factors That Increase Risks	Factors That Lower Risks
• Haplo-identical stem-cell transplantation	• Transplants from an HLA-identical sibling
• Unrelated donor	
• Cord blood	
• T-cell depletion (CD34 selection)	

Bacterial	In the absence of acute GVHD and its treatment, the most common pathogens are related to use of an intravascular device and include: • Gram-positive organisms (eg, coagulase-negative staphylococci) • Nonfermentative Gram-negative bacilli (including *Pseudomonas* spp., *Acinetobacter*, and *Stenotrophomonas*) Respiratory infections are also commonly seen, frequently following upper respiratory viral infections In the presence of acute GVHD and its treatment, the most common pathogens are: • Enteric Gram-negative bacilli (eg, *Escherichia coli*, *Klebsiella*, *Enterobacter*, *Citrobacter*, *Serratia*) and *Pseudomonas*
Fungal	*Aspergillus* is the most common mold, but prophylaxis with voriconazole increases the risk of infection with other molds, including *Fusarium* and the agents of mucormycosis (*Mucor*, *Rhizopus*) *Risk factors* • CMV disease • Steroid use (≥1 mg/kg of prednisone equivalent for ≥1 week) Non-albicans *Candida* infections, which may be resistant to fluconazole, are increasing
Viral	CMV reactivation occurs in up to 70% of recipients at risk The risk of CMV varies depending on recipient/donor serostatus: R+/D− > R+/D+ > R−/D+ >> R−/D−. If both recipient and donor are CMV seronegative (R−/D−) the incidence is <5% VZV and HSV can be prevented with acyclovir, which may be administered safely long-term HHV6 commonly reactivates following allogeneic hematopoietic transplantation. In most cases, reactivation is asymptomatic. However, in some cases it has been associated with fever, rash, pneumonitis, and limbic encephalitis
	Respiratory viruses: Adenovirus, RSV, and parainfluenza cause significant morbidity and mortality Coinfections (particularly *Aspergillus*) have been documented with parainfluenza and other respiratory viruses

Bowden RA. Am J Med 1997;102(3 Suppl 1):27–30; discussion 42–43
Fukuda T et al. Blood 2003;102:827–833
Hentrich M et al. Br J Haematol 2005;128:66–72
Kumar D, Humar A. Infect Dis Clin North Am 2010;24:395–412
Ljungman P et al. Bone Marrow Transplant 2008;42:227–240
Nichols WG et al. Blood 2001;98:573–578

Late Postengraftment Period (>100 Days After HCT)

The risk of infection is higher for allogeneic recipients than autologous recipients

Allogeneic HCT

Risk of sepsis from bacterial pathogens after an allogeneic **hematopoietic** transplantation persists, particularly in patients with chronic graft-versus-host disease, which induces a state of functional hyposplenism. The treatment of chronic GVHD consists of immunosuppressive agents that increase the risk of infection. There is also persistent humoral immunodeficiency

Bacterial	Encapsulated bacteria, particularly *Streptococcus pneumoniae*, are significant pathogens
Fungal	Fungal infections are uncommon except in the presence of active immunosuppression
Viral	CMV reactivation is an ever-present risk, higher if the patient received ganciclovir prophylaxis or treatment • Up to 25% of patients will have a VZV reactivation in the first few months after discontinuing acyclovir prophylaxis • Respiratory virus infections continue to be a problem for months. Influenza vaccination should be restarted 6 months after transplantation

Boeckh M et al. Blood 2003;101:407–414
Kulkarni S et al. Blood 2000;95:3683–3686

Prophylactic Agents Commonly Used to Reduce the Rates of Infections and Virus Reactivation Posttransplantation

Tomblyn M et al. Biol Blood Marrow Transplant 2009;15:1143–1238

FLUCONAZOLE

Indication:
- To prevent invasive disease with *Candida* species
- Administration of fluconazole should commence at the time of transplant and should continue for at least 75 days following HCT

Dose: Fluconazole 400 mg; administer orally or intravenously daily for at least 75 days following HCT

ACYCLOVIR

Indication:
- Acyclovir prophylaxis reduces **HSV** reactivation by 75%
- Acyclovir prophylaxis in adults can also be administered in HSV-negative patients
- Administration of acyclovir or valacyclovir should commence at the time of transplant
- Acyclovir prophylaxis can be continued safely for at least 1 year and reduces the incidence of HSV and VZV

Doses:
Acyclovir 800 mg; administer orally every 12 hours, *or*
Acyclovir 250 mg/m^2 per dose; administer intravenously every 12 hours, *or*
Valacyclovir 500 mg; administer orally once daily

COTRIMOXAZOLE (TRIMETHOPRIM + SULFAMETHOXAZOLE IN A 1:5 RATIO)

Indication:
- Cotrimoxazole (trimethoprim + sulfamethoxazole; TMP + SMZ) is the agent of choice for prophylaxis against *Pneumocystis jirovecii* and confers some degree of protection against toxoplasmosis
- *Pneumocystis jirovecii* prophylaxis is recommended from the time of engraftment until 6 months after HCT and after 6 months if the patient has GVHD or is receiving immunosuppressive therapy

Prophylaxis:
Cotrimoxazole (TMP 160 mg + SMZ 800 mg); administer orally, daily, *or*
Cotrimoxazole (TMP 80 mg + SMZ 400 mg); administer orally, daily, *or*
Cotrimoxazole (TMP 160 mg + SMZ 800 mg); administer orally, 3 days per week

Alternatively:
Dapsone 50 mg; administer orally, twice daily, *or*
Dapsone 100 mg; administer orally, once daily
Aerosolized pentamidine 300 mg; administer by inhalation every 3–4 weeks
Rule out G6PD deficiency before starting dapsone. Methemoglobinemia may develop in up to 5% of patients on dapsone prophylaxis

VARICELLA-ZOSTER IMMUNOGLOBULIN (VariZIG)

Indication:
- Prevention of varicella-zoster viral disease after exposure of HCT recipients (<24 months after HCT, or >24 months after HCT if patient is receiving immunosuppressives, or has chronic GVHD) to a person with chickenpox or shingles

Dose: VariZIG is supplied in 125-IU vials and should be administered intramuscularly. The recommended dose is 125 IU/10 kg of body weight, up to a maximum of 625 IU (five vials). The minimum dose is 62.5 IU (0.5 vial) for patients weighing ≤2.0 kg and 125 IU (one vial) for patients weighing 2.1–10.0 kg

IMMUNE GLOBULIN INTRAVENOUS (IVIG)

Indication: IgG levels <400 mg/dL and severe infections

Dose: IVIG 400–500 mg/kg; administer intravenously, every 2–4 weeks until the patient is able to maintain a level of IgG ≥400 mg/dL on his or her own

Cytomegalovirus Surveillance and Treatment During the Posttransplantation Period

Tomblyn M et al. Biol Blood Marrow Transplant 2009;15:1143–1238

Ganciclovir prophylaxis (the systematic administration of ganciclovir to all patients at risk for CMV reactivation) reduces the incidence of CMV disease to 2–4%, but does not improve outcome and is associated with late CMV reactivation. The preferred approach is "preemptive," based on monitoring CMV reactivation by measuring pp65 antigenemia or CMV DNA by PCR, and intervening with ganciclovir or foscarnet only when reactivation is detected, before active disease occurs

Indications for monitoring:
HCT recipients who are CMV IgG-positive or received a graft from a donor who is CMV IgG-positive

Monitoring (the choice of CMV PCR or antigenemia is based on laboratory test availability):
Weekly CMV antigenemia, *or*
Weekly CMV PCR (CMV PCR should be performed in patients with ANC $<500/mm^3$)

Duration of monitoring:
Continue beyond posttransplantation day +100 if immune suppression continues (excluding immune suppression produced by cyclosporine or tacrolimus) or there is a history of late CMV reactivation (after day +75)

Treatment indications:
A patient with positive CMV antigenemia or 2 consecutive PCR assays positive for CMV

Treatment:
• **Ganciclovir** 5 mg/kg per dose; administer intravenously, every 12 hours for 7 days, *followed by:*
• **Ganciclovir** 5 mg/kg per dose; administer intravenously, once daily, 5 days per week

Alternative:
• **Foscarnet** 60 mg/kg per dose; administer intravenously, every 12 hours for 7 days, *followed by:*
• **Foscarnet** 60 mg/kg per dose; administer intravenously, once daily, 5 days per week

Alternative:
• **Valganciclovir** 900 mg; administer orally, every 12 hours, *followed by:*
• **Valganciclovir** 900 mg; administer orally, once daily, 5 days per week

Discontinue acyclovir when either ganciclovir or foscarnet is used

Ganciclovir and foscarnet are equally effective; the choice is usually made based on the risk of toxicity (myelosuppression with ganciclovir, nephrotoxicity and electrolyte disturbances with foscarnet. Valganciclovir, the prodrug of ganciclovir, has the advantage of oral administration. However, the difficulty of properly adjusting the dose may result in higher rate of myelotoxicity

Duration of treatment:
Continue treatment until 2 consecutive weekly CMV antigenemia tests or PCR for CMV are negative

Boeckh M et al. Blood 2003;101:407–414

Recommended Vaccinations for Adult Hematopoietic Stem-Cell Transplantation Recipients, Including Both Autologous and Allogeneic Recipients

Type (Dose and Administration Route)	3–6 Months	12[‡‡] Months	14–18 Months	24 Months
Influenza virus	Lifelong, annually (seasonal), starting before HCT and resuming after 6 months			
Pneumococcal 13-valent conjugate (0.5 mL, intramuscularly)	X	X	X (18 months)	
Pneumococcal 23-valent Vaccine (0.5 mL subcutaneously or intramuscularly)				X[††]
DTaP* (0.5 mL intramuscularly)		X	X	X
Hib[†] conjugate (0.5 mL intramuscularly)		X	X	X
IPV[‡] (0.5 mL subcutaneously or intramuscularly)		X	X	X
Hepatitis A (1 mL intramuscularly)		X	X	
Hepatitis B (1 mL intramuscularly)		X	X	X

(continued)

Recommended Vaccinations for Adult Hematopoietic Stem-Cell Transplantation Recipients, Including Both Autologous and Allogeneic Recipients (continued)

Type (Dose and Administration Route)	3–6 Months	12[‡‡] Months	14–18 Months	24 Months
Meningococcal[§] (0.5 mL subcutaneously)		X		
MMR[€] (0.5 mL subcutaneously)				X
VZV[**] (0.5 mL subcutaneously)				X

*Diphtheria toxoid, tetanus toxoid, and acellular pertussis vaccine, absorbed (DTaP, Tdap)

[†]Haemophilus b conjugate vaccine

[‡]Poliovirus vaccine, inactivated (IPV). Consult product labeling for specific recommendations about revaccinating previously unvaccinated, incompletely vaccinated, and completely vaccinated subjects

[§]Meningococcal polysaccharide-protein conjugate vaccine (Menactra) is recommended for patients in appropriate high-risk groups (ages 11–18 years, college students living in dormitories, other age groups with functional or anatomic asplenia or complement component deficiency. Refer to the CDC website for further guidance)

[€]Measles, mumps, and rubella vaccine, live, attenuated; only given if patient is immunocompetent at 24 months; that is, NOT on immune suppression AND NO GVHD for 6 months

[**]Varivax is the only varicella virus vaccine that should be used in post-HCT recipients because of the higher plaque-forming unit content in Zostavax and a lack of safety data with Zostavax. HCT recipients who have not had chicken pox (including those who have previously received a varicella vaccine) should receive post-HCT vaccination. For patients with a history of chicken pox, varicella vaccination may be considered but it should be noted that efficacy in preventing zoster has not been established

[††]For patients with chronic GVHD who are likely to respond poorly to the 23-valent pneumococcal vaccine, a fourth dose of the 7-valent conjugate should be considered

[‡‡]Initiation of nonlive vaccination series can begin as early as 6 months postallogeneic transplantation if patients are off immunosuppression and do not have active GVHD. If early vaccination is given, consider monitoring for response. At any time point, if vaccination is initiated in a patient who remains on immunosuppression, consider monitoring for response

Hilgendorf I et al. Vaccine 2011;29:2825–2833
Tomblyn M et al. Biol Blood Marrow Transplant 2009;15:1143–1238

Noninfectious Complications Following Allogeneic HCT

Antin JH. N Engl J Med 2002;347:36–42
Ferrara JLM et al. Lancet 2009;373:1550–1561
Majhail NS et al. Biol Blood Marrow Transplant 2012;18:348–371
Savani BN et al. Blood 2011;17:3002–3009
Socié G et al. Blood 2003;101:3373–3385
Wingard JR et al. Hematology 2002:422–444

ACUTE GRAFT-VERSUS-HOST DISEASE FOLLOWING ALLOGENEIC HCT

Ferrara JLM et al. Lancet 2009;373:1550–1561
Glucksberg H et al. Transplantation 1974;18:295–304
Jagasia M et al. Blood 2012;119:296–307
Martin PJ et al. Biol Blood Marrow Transplant 2012;18:1150–1163
Thomas ED et al. NEJM 1975;292:895–902

Incidence at 100 Days*

HLA identical sibling donors

    Grades B–D: 39%

    Grades C–D: 16%

Unrelated donors

    Grades B–D: 59%

    Grades C–D: 32%

Risk Factors

HLA mismatch

Female donor to male recipient

Disease status other than early

Ineffective GVHD prophylaxis

Organ Involvement

Organ Involved	Percent of Patients
Skin	81%
Gastrointestinal	54%
Liver	50%

*Incidence of acute GVHD from a study of adults receiving allogeneic HCT from HLA-identical sibling donors (n = 3191) and unrelated donors (n = 2370) using the International Bone Marrow Transplant Registry (IBMTR) grating system (A–D)

Jagasia M et al. Blood 2012;119:296–307

Staging of Acute GVHD

Skin, liver, and gastrointestinal tract are staged independently and these are combined for an overall grade

Stage	Skin*	Liver	Gastrointestinal Tract†
Stage I	Rash on <25% of skin	Total bilirubin 2–3 mg/dL (34.2–51.3 μmol/L)	Diarrhea >500 mL/day
Stage II	Rash on 25–50% of skin	Total bilirubin 3.1–6 mg/dL (53–102.6 μmol/L)	Diarrhea >1000 mL/day
Stage III	Generalized erythroderma	Total bilirubin 6.1–15 mg/dL (104.3–256.5 μmol/L)	Diarrhea >1500 mL/day
Stage IV	Bullae	Total bilirubin >15 mg/dL (>256.5 μmol/L)	Severe abdominal pain, bleeding, ± ileus

*A maculopapular rash initially involving the face, ears, palms, soles, and upper trunk. If GVHD advances, rash spreads to the rest of the body, generally sparing the scalp. Histologic examination is needed to establish diagnosis
†A pan-intestinal process that can present with nausea, vomiting, anorexia, diarrhea, and/or abdominal pain

The diagnosis of gastrointestinal GVHD must be made by mucosal biopsy

Grading for Acute GVHD

Grade	Skin	Liver		Gut
I	1–2	0		0
II	1–3	1	and/or	1
III	2–3	2–4	and/or	2–3
IV	2–4	2–4	and/or	2–4

Glucksberg H et al. Transplantation 1974;18:295–304
Przepiorka D et al. Bone Marrow Transplant 1995;15:825–828
Thomas ED et al. NEJM 1975;292:895–902

International Bone Marrow Transplant Registry Severity Index for grading acute GVHD

A–Stage 1 skin involvement; no liver or gut involvement
B–Stage 2 skin involvement; Stage 1 to 2 gut or liver involvement
C–Stage 3 skin, liver, or gut involvement
D–Stage 4 skin, liver, or gut involvement

Rowlings PA et al. Br J Haematol 1997;97:855–864

REGIMEN FOR PROPHYLAXIS

CYCLOSPORINE + METHOTREXATE AND TACROLIMUS + METHOTREXATE

Storb R et al. Blood 1989;73:1729–1734
Storb R et al. Blood 1992;80:560–561
Storb R et al. N Engl J Med 1986;314:729–735

Cyclosporine + Methotrexate

Cyclosporine 2–5 mg/kg per dose; administer intravenously or orally twice daily (every 12 hours) starting 1–2 days prior to graft infusion, and continuing for a total of 6 months
Methotrexate 15 mg/m²; administer intravenously on day +1 after transplantation, (total dosage: 15 mg/m²), *followed by:*
Methotrexate 10 mg/m² per dose; administer intravenously for 3 doses, on days 3, 6, and 11, after transplantation (total dosage = 30 mg/m²)

Treatment Modifications

General guidance:

1. Cyclosporine dose modifications may be guided by pharmacokinetics when these are available. Often, however, therapeutic targets can be effectively achieved by making small, incremental changes of 10–25%
2. If levels are high, or in the presence of toxicity, withhold cyclosporine and resume a lower dose after:
   • Demonstrating a concentration within the targeted range
   • Adverse events have diminished or resolved

Adverse Event	Dose Modification
Baseline serum creatinine within normal limits and serum creatinine increases to 1.5–2 mg/dL (133–177 μmol/L)	Reduce cyclosporine dose by 50%
Baseline serum creatinine within normal limits and serum creatinine increases to >2 mg/dL (>177 μmol/L)	Hold cyclosporine and check daily creatinine and cyclosporine levels. Restart cyclosporine at 50% of the initial dose after creatinine is <2 mg/dL (<177 μmol/L)
Hypertension develops while on cyclosporine	Consider calcium channel blockers or β-adrenergic blockers as first-line therapy
Voriconazole therapy in a patient with therapeutic cyclosporine levels	Reduce cyclosporine dose by ≈50%

Notes

1. Begin with intravenous administration, convert to oral administration, and then continue
2. Oral cyclosporine is incompletely absorbed. Changing from intravenous to oral administration (or the reverse) requires a conversion

Approximate IV-to-Oral Dose Ratio (mg:mg)	
Cyclosporine (Sandimmune)	Cyclosporine, Modified (Neoral)
1:2–3	1:1–2

3. Cyclosporine may also be given once daily; however, an intermittent 12-hour dose interval increases trough concentrations and decreases peak concentrations

Toxicity

Cyclosporine

Common
Headache
Hirsutism, hypertrichosis
Nausea, vomiting, diarrhea
Tremor
Hypertension
Nephrotoxicity
Hyperlipidemia

Serious
Reversible posterior leukoencephalopathy syndrome (RPLS): a neurologic syndrome defined by clinical and radiologic features. The typical clinical syndrome includes headache, confusion, visual symptoms, and seizures. Typical MRI findings are consistent with vasogenic edema and are predominantly localized to the posterior cerebral hemispheres. Although RPLS is most often reported with cyclosporine use, it has also been associated with other agents, including tacrolimus and sirolimus

Gingival hyperplasia
Hepatotoxicity
Hypomagnesemia
Anaphylaxis with intravenously administered products (rare)
Hyperkalemia (rare)
Pancreatitis (rare)
Paresthesia (rare)

Methotrexate

Common
Alopecia, photosensitivity, rash
Anorexia, diarrhea
Nausea, vomiting
Stomatitis

Serious
Cirrhosis
Elevated liver function test
Hepatic fibrosis, atrophy, necrosis, and failure
Gastrointestinal bleeding
Mucositis, ulceration
Hyperuricemia
Nephropathy, renal failure
Interstitial pneumonitis (acute, chronic)
Methotrexate-induced lung disease
Myelosuppression

Efficacy

Storb R et al. N Engl J Med 1986;314:729–735

In a seminal randomized trial comparing the effect of a methotrexate and cyclosporine combination to cyclosporine alone, there was a significant reduction in the cumulative incidence of grades II–IV acute GVHD in patients who received the combination regimen (33%) compared with those who received cyclosporine alone (54%) (p = 0.014)

Therapy Monitoring

1. *Daily cyclosporine concentration measurements:*
   - When clinical toxicity is encountered
   - When potentially interacting agents are added or withdrawn
2. *Check cyclosporine concentrations 24–72 hours after changes in:*
   - Dose/dosage
   - Administration schedule
   - Route of administration
   - Product formulation
3. *Weekly to every 2 weeks:*
   - Check BUN and serum creatinine

Notes:

1. *Be wary* when comparing cyclosporine concentration results performed by different laboratory facilities. Cyclosporine assay methodologies vary among clinical laboratories
2. Therapeutic target concentrations also vary with:
   - Type of sample assayed (if specimen other than whole blood is analyzed)
   - Dosing interval
   - Temperature
   - Clinician preferences
3. Therapeutic monitoring strategies also vary. Sample collection times may be expressed in any of the following ways:
   - For a sample collected before a cyclosporine dose is given: "predose," "trough," or "C0"
   - For a sample collected 2 hours after a cyclosporine dose is given: "2-hour postdose," "C2," or "absorption profiling"
4. Verify whether aberrant cyclosporine measurements are correct before altering a cyclosporine regimen, particularly when they occur unexpectedly. Factors that perturb cyclosporine levels include:
   - Noncompliance with an oral regimen
   - The introduction, modification, and discontinuation of drugs that potentially interfere with cyclosporine absorption (after oral administration), metabolism, and elimination
   - Incorrect sampling time
   - Blood drawn through an intravenous catheter lumen previously used to administer cyclosporine
   - Drawing specimens while administering cyclosporine intravenously
5. Cyclosporine is extensively metabolized by cytochrome P450 (CYP) CYP3A subfamily enzymes; its metabolism and elimination may be markedly perturbed by drugs that induce or inhibit CYP3A enzymes

Tacrolimus + Methotrexate

Nash RA et al. Blood 2000;96:2062–2068
Ratanatharathorn V et al. Blood 1998;92:2303–2314

Tacrolimus 0.03 mg/kg per day; administer by continuous IV infusion over 24 hours starting on the day before transplantation
- Tacrolimus dosage is altered to achieve a concentration measurement within a targeted range of concentrations
- Treatment is continued for 8 weeks (2 months after transplantation), after which the dose rate is slowly decreased (tapered) by 20% per month and discontinued 6 months after transplantation

Methotrexate 15 mg/m^2; administer intravenously on day 1 after marrow transplantation, *followed by:*
Methotrexate 10 mg/m^2 per dose; administer intravenously for 3 doses on days 3, 6, and 11

Notes: Tacrolimus was converted from IV to oral administration at the ratio of 1 mg (IV) to 4 mg (orally). The total daily dose was given orally in 2 divided doses per day when the patients were able to tolerate oral intake. Tacrolimus dose was reduced by 25% when a serum creatinine measurement was increased 2-times greater than baseline, and decreased by 50% for patients whose creatinine increased to 3-times greater than baseline. Tacrolimus concentrations were maintained within the range 10–30 ng/mL (10–30 mcg/L).

Tacrolimus Adverse Effects
Common: Constipation, diarrhea, nausea, vomiting, headache, insomnia, tremor
Serious: Hyperglycemia (frequent), hyperkalemia, hypomagnesemia, hypertension, myocardial, hypertrophy, cardiac QT interval prolongation, torsades de pointes, nephrotoxicity

In comparison with cyclosporine and methotrexate, the combination of tacrolimus and methotrexate is associated with a greater reduction of acute GVHD and severe acute GVHD; however, there is no difference in all-cause mortality between the 2 approaches

Ram R et al. Bone Marrow Transplant 2009;43:643–653

REGIMEN FOR TREATMENT OF ACUTE GVHD

Martin PJ et al. Biol Blood Marrow Transplant 2012;18:1150–1163
Martin PJ et al. Blood 1990;76:1464–1472
Weisdorf D et al. Blood 1990;75:1024–1030

Whenever possible, a clinical diagnosis of acute GVHD (aGVHD) should be confirmed by biopsy of an affected end organ

First-line treatment:
Methylprednisolone 2 mg/kg per day; administer intravenously, *or*
Prednisone 2–2.5 mg/kg per day; administer orally
(aGVHD of the upper GI tract, a distinct clinical entity of anorexia, nausea, vomiting, and dyspepsia is responsive to low-dose systemic and topical steroid therapy; initial approach to treatment of aGVHD of the upper GI tract is methylprednisolone or prednisone at 1 mg/kg per day)
• Efficacy: ~50% of patients who develop acute GVHD show durable improvement after initial steroid treatment
• Decisions to begin systemic treatment depend not only on the severity of GVHD manifestations but also on their rate of progression
• The survival and response data from studies combining the use of other immunosuppressive agents together with glucocorticoid treatment do not support this approach as the standard of care
• Tapering steroid doses should begin as soon as GVHD manifestations show major improvement. Inappropriately rapid taper rates carry a risk of GVHD exacerbation or recurrence, whereas inappropriately slow taper rates increase the risk of steroid-related complications. Taper rates should be slowed after the daily prednisone dose has been decreased to <20–30 mg

Second-line therapy for acute graft-versus-host disease:
Criteria and indications for secondary systemic therapy of aGVHD have not been systematically defined. Both the severity and duration of manifestations should be taken into account in deciding that initial glucocorticoid treatment has not adequately controlled GVHD. In general, decisions to initiate secondary therapy should be made sooner for patients with more severe GVHD. For example, secondary therapy may be indicated after 3 days with progressive manifestations of GVHD, after 1 week with persistent, nonimproving grade III GVHD or after 2 weeks with persistent, nonimproving grade II GVHD
Because comparative data demonstrating superior efficacy for particular agents are not available, the choice of a second-line regimen should be guided by the effects of any previous treatment and by considerations of potential toxicity and interactions with other agents, including those used for prophylaxis, convenience, expense, the familiarity of the physician with the agent, and the prior experience of the physician

Agents used for second-line therapy include: methotrexate, basiliximab, daclizumab, denileukin diftitox, etanercept, infliximab, antithymocyte globulin, sirolimus

CHRONIC GRAFT-VERSUS-HOST DISEASE FOLLOWING ALLOGENEIC HCT

Ferrara JLM et al. Lancet 2009;373:1550–1561
Filipovich AH et al. Biol Blood Marrow Transplant 2005;11:945–956
Savani BN et al. Blood 2011;17:3002–3009
Wolff D et al. Biol Blood Marrow Transplant 2010;16:1611–1628
Wolff D et al. Biol Blood Marrow Transplant 2011;17:1–17

Incidence

HLA-identical sibling donor	~40%
HLA-matched unrelated donor	~70%

Risk Factors

- Higher degree of HLA mismatching
- Older age of donor and/or recipient
- Donor and recipient gender disparity
- Prior acute GVHD
- Cytomegalovirus seropositivity (donor and recipient)
- The use of peripheral blood precursor cells rather than bone marrow

Timing of Onset of Chronic GVHD

HCT Source	Median Time to Diagnosis
HLA-identical sibling donor	201 days
HLA-non-identical related donor	159 days
Unrelated donor	133 days

Organ Involvement

Organ Involved	Percent of Patients
Skin	65–80%
Mouth	48–72%
Liver	40–73%
Eye	18–47%
Gastrointestinal	16–26%
Lung	10–15%
Joints	2–12%

- The diagnosis of chronic GVHD requires the following:
  i. Distinction from acute GVHD
  ii. Presence of at least one diagnostic clinical sign of chronic GVHD or presence of at least one distinctive manifestation confirmed by pertinent biopsy or relevant tests
  iii. Exclusion of other possible diagnoses
- Scoring of organ manifestations requires careful assessment of signs, symptoms, laboratory values, and other study results

Categories of Chronic GVHD

	Time of Symptoms after HCT or DLI	Presence of Acute GVHD Features	Presence of Chronic GVHD Features
Classic chronic GVHD	No time limit	No	Yes
Overlap syndrome	No time limit	Yes	Yes

Signs and Symptoms of Chronic GVHD

Organ or Site	Diagnostic Sufficient to Establish the Diagnosis of Chronic GVHD	Distinctive Seen in Chronic GVHD, but Insufficient Alone to Establish a Diagnosis of Chronic GVHD
Skin	Poikiloderma Lichen-type features Sclerotic features Morphea-like features Lichen-sclerosis	Depigmentation
Nails		Dystrophy Longitudinal ridging, splitting, or brittle Onycholysis Pterygium unguis Nail loss (usually symmetric, affects most nails)
Scalp and body hair		New onset of scarring or nonscarring scalp alopecia (after recovery from chemoradiotherapy) Alopecia; scaling, papulosquamous lesions
Mouth	Lichen-type features Hyperkeratotic plaques Restriction of mouth opening from sclerosis	Xerostomia Mucocele Mucosal Atrophy
Eyes		New onset dry, gritty, or painful eyes Cicatricial conjunctivitis Keratoconjunctivitis sicca Confluent areas of punctuate keratopathy
Genitalia	Lichen-type features Vaginal stricture or stenosis	Erosions Fissures Ulcers
GI tract	Esophageal web Strictures or stenosis in the upper to mid-third of the esophagus	Pancreatic insufficiency
Lung	Bronchiolitis obliterans diagnosed with lung biopsy	Bronchiolitis obliterans diagnosed with PFTs and radiology
Muscles, fascia, joints	Fasciitis Joint stiffness or contractures secondary to sclerosis	Myositis or polymyositis

Treatment of Chronic GVHD

Mild **chronic** GVHD may be treated either with topical immunosuppressive agents or with systemic steroids alone. With respect to treatment limited to topical immunosuppression, close follow-up and screening for potential manifestations of **chronic** GVHD is crucial to detect systemic progression of **chronic** GVHD during topical treatment. Mild manifestations of **chronic** GVHD that cannot be sufficiently treated by topical treatment such as hepatic manifestations or fasciitis may be treated with systemic corticosteroids alone

Treatment of moderate chronic GVHD requires systemic immunosuppression. Standard treatment is prednisone 1 mg/kg per day, *or a* glucocorticoid equivalent dose of **methylprednisolone** (0.8 mg/kg per day). Dose intensity should be maintained for 2 weeks, then decreased (tapered) to 1 mg/kg every other day over a period of 6–8 weeks if symptoms are stable or improving, and then either maintain this dose for 2–3 months or continue to taper by dose decrements of 10–20% per month. Patients with complete responses (CRs) should have doses decreased further by 10–20% monthly, whereas persons without a CR who are still responding should stay on 1 mg/kg for about another 3 months after achieving maximum response, and then doses should be slowly tapered. If symptoms flare during tapering, increasing the steroid dose may again induce a favorable response

Treatment of severe **chronic** GVHD (cGVHD) follows the same rules as treatment of moderate **chronic** GVHD. Severe cGVHD has been associated with an increased mortality and may require prolonged immunosuppression

Refractory **chronic** *GVHD:* Generally, accepted criteria for steroid-refractory **chronic** GVHD, include:
1. Progression despite immunosuppressive treatment using prednisone 1 mg/kg per day for 2 weeks,
2. Stable disease after 4–8 weeks of prednisone ≥0.5 mg/kg per day, *and*
3. Inability to taper prednisone to <0.5 mg/kg per day

Although different treatment options are available for salvage therapy of steroid refractory cGVHD, the "trial-and-error system" remains, to date, the only way to identify the drug or drug combination effective in an individual patient. In principle, initial secondary treatment should include agents with an adequate safety profile and well-documented activity. Patients should be treated for an adequate length of time (at least 4 weeks) before concluding treatment failure

Treatment modalities are the use of steroids and calcineurin inhibitors as well as immunomodulating modalities (photopheresis, mTOR-inhibitors, thalidomide, hydroxychloroquine, vitamin A analogs, clofazimine), and cytostatic agents (mycophenolate mofetil, methotrexate, cyclophosphamide, pentostatin), rituximab, alemtuzumab, and etanercept

Antimicrobial Prophylaxis for Patients with Chronic GVHD

Infections are a common cause of death in chronic GVHD. Recommendations regarding prophylaxis are based on expert opinion rather than controlled trials (Couriel D et al. Biol Blood Marrow Transplant 2006;12:375–396; Vogelsang GB. Blood 2001;97:1196–1201). A common practice is to start antimicrobial prophylaxis once the diagnosis of chronic GVHD is made, or at least once active immunosuppression for the treatment of chronic GVHD is started

First Choice	Alternative
Antibiotic Prophylaxis	
Penicillin V potassium 500 mg; administer orally, twice daily	*Penicillin allergy:* **Cotrimoxazole** (trimethoprim 80 mg + sulfamethoxazole 400 mg); administer orally, once daily *Penicillin and sulfonamide allergy:* **Clarithromycin** 500 mg; administer orally, daily Be wary of potential interactions with CYP3A subfamily substrates
Antiviral Prophylaxis	
Valacyclovir 500 mg; administer orally, once daily *or* **Acyclovir** 200 mg; administer orally every 12 hours	Most experience is with acyclovir; valacyclovir is more convenient and is an acceptable alternative
Antifungal Prophylaxis	
It is unknown if administering antifungal prophylaxis during GVHD is efficacious in terms of decreasing the incidence of invasive fungal infections or improving outcome. Some experts, concerned with the risk of invasive aspergillosis advocate the use of voriconazole in this setting, but the approach is off-label and must be considered experimental. Emerging data regarding long-term toxicities of voriconazole (osteopathy-fluorosis and carcinogenesis) make this approach questionable	
***Pneumocystis Jirovecii* Prophylaxis**	
Prophylaxis for ***Pneumocystis jirovecii*** should be administered to all patients undergoing treatment of chronic GVHD and for 6 months after immunosuppressive medications are discontinued	
Cotrimoxazole (trimethoprim 160 mg + sulfamethoxazole 800 mg) per day; administer orally, 3 days/week	**Aerosolized pentamidine** 300 mg; administer by inhalation, every 4 weeks

ORAL COMPLICATIONS

Majhail NS et al. Biol Blood Marrow Transplant 2012;18:348–371

Sicca Syndrome Caries

Risk factors: GVHD, TBI/radiation exposure to head and neck

Follow-up: Clinical oral evaluations should be performed at 6 months and 1 year and yearly thereafter. More frequent evaluations may be needed in patients at high risk of oral complications (eg, chronic GVHD, exposure to TBI)

All HCT recipients should receive a thorough evaluation by a dentist or oral medicine specialist at 1 year after HCT and yearly thereafter. More frequent dental consultations may be considered in patients with oral GVHD

Notes: The mouth is one of the most frequently affected organs in chronic GVHD. Changes involving the oral mucosa, salivary glands, oral and lingual muscles, taste buds, and gingiva may completely regress, but some long-term sequelae may continue despite the resolution of chronic GVHD

Salivary gland dysfunction and xerostomia increase the risk of dental caries, periodontal disease, and oral cancer. Particular attention to oral malignancies should be paid to patients with previous severe chronic GVHD of the oral and pharyngeal mucosa

Even in patients who have never had GVHD, some degree of salivary gland hypofunction may persist for prolonged periods of time after receiving chemotherapy, and especially after local irradiation

Patients with GVHD can be treated with topical oral steroids, systemic treatments for GVHD, and supportive care for xerostomia symptoms

Among HCT recipients who require dental procedures antimicrobial prophylaxis against endocarditis should be followed

OCULAR COMPLICATIONS

Majhail NS et al. Biol Blood Marrow Transplant 2012;18:348–371

Keratoconjunctivitis sicca syndrome
Cataract
Retinopathy
Optic disc edema
Infectious retinitis

Risk factors: TBI/radiation exposure to head and neck, corticosteroids, GVHD

Follow-up: Routine clinical evaluation of visual history and symptoms, with attention to sicca syndrome, is recommended at 6 months, 1 year, and yearly thereafter for all HCT recipients

Measurement of visual acuity and fundus examination at 1 year after transplantation is recommended for all HCT recipients. Patients with cGVHD may be referred for an ophthalmologic exam sooner than 1 year after transplantation. Subsequent frequency of routine screening should be individualized according to recognized defects, ocular symptoms, or the presence of cGVHD

Notes:

Ocular sicca syndrome: reduced tear flow, keratoconjunctivitis sicca, sterile conjunctivitis, corneal epithelial defects, and corneal ulceration. The incidence is approximately 40–60% in patients with cGVHD. Artificial tears can provide symptomatic treatment of dry eyes. Temporary or permanent occlusion of the tear duct puncta for drainage control may provide benefit. Corticosteroids or calcineurin inhibitors may improve symptoms but can cause sight-threatening complications when inappropriately used in herpes simplex virus or bacterial keratitis

Cataract: After myeloablative single-dose TBI, almost all patients develop cataracts within 3–4 years. Fractionation of TBI delays the onset and reduces the incidence of cataract to 40–70% at 10 years after transplantation. In patients who receive conditioning without TBI, the probability of cataract formation at 10 years is 5–20%. Cataracts are effectively treated surgically

Ischemic microvascular retinopathy presents with cotton wool spots and optic disc edema. Retinopathy is observed almost exclusively after allogeneic transplantation, particularly in patients conditioned with TBI and in patients receiving cyclosporine for GVHD prophylaxis. In most cases, retinal lesions resolve with withdrawal or reduction of immunosuppressive therapy, even in cases where visual acuity is decreased

ENDOCRINE COMPLICATIONS

Majhail NS et al. Biol Blood Marrow Transplant 2012;18:348–371

Hypothyroidism
Gonadal dysfunction
Adrenal failure

Risk factors: TBI/radiation exposure, corticosteroids, young age at time of HCT, chemotherapy exposure

---

Follow-up:

Thyroid function tests (TSH, T_3, and free T_4) should be performed at 1 year after HCT and yearly thereafter in all transplantation recipients and additionally if relevant symptoms develop

Clinical and endocrinologic gonadal assessment at 1 year after HCT is recommended for all women who were postpubertal at the time of transplantation. Frequency of subsequent assessments should be guided by clinical need (eg, menopausal status). Women should have annual gynecologic evaluations as part of general health screening, at which time, hormone replacement therapy should be addressed for those who are postmenopausal

Gonadal function in men, particularly FSH, LH, and testosterone, should be assessed if symptoms warrant (lack of libido or erectile dysfunction). Consider referral to an endocrinologist for men who may need testosterone replacement therapy

---

Notes:

Subclinical, compensated hypothyroidism: elevated TSH and normal serum-free T_4 levels, occurs in 7–15% of patients in the first year after transplantation. Single-dose ablative TBI is associated with a 50% incidence of overt hypothyroidism, whereas fractionated TBI is associated with an incidence of approximately 15%. The incidence reported after busulfan and cyclophosphamide conditioning is 11%. The median time to diagnosis of hypothyroidism is nearly 4 years after HCT or TBI exposure

Gonadal dysfunction is highly prevalent in HCT recipients, with rates as high as 92% for males and 99% for females. Although the risk of gonadal failure is high in all individuals, women generally experience higher rates of failure than do men. Hypogonadism is nearly universal after high-dose irradiation or busulfan. Fractionation of radiation reduces the risk compared with unfractionated radiation. The risk is lower with cyclophosphamide alone. In general, ovarian endocrine failure is irreversible in adult women

Adult women should be evaluated by a gynecologist and may require hormone replacement therapy to maintain libido, sexual function, and bone density. Vaginal GVHD may result in strictures and synechiae

Most men have normal testosterone levels after transplantation, although germ cell damage (infertility) is a near-universal finding in men exposed to high doses of radiation or chemotherapy

Adrenal failure: Greater durations and intensity of exposure generally are associated with longer persistence of adrenal suppression. Patients with prolonged exposure to corticosteroids after HCT should have adrenal axis testing when withdrawing corticosteroids, particularly if symptoms of adrenal insufficiency develop

PULMONARY COMPLICATIONS

Majhail NS et al. Biol Blood Marrow Transplant 2012;18:348–371

Idiopathic pneumonia syndrome
Bronchiolitis obliterans syndrome
Cryptogenic organizing pneumonia
Sinopulmonary infections
Diffuse alveolar hemorrhage
Pulmonary thromboembolism
Pulmonary venoocclusive disease
Pleural effusions

Risk factors: TBI/radiation exposure to chest, GVHD, infectious agents, allogeneic HCT, exposure to busulfan or carmustine (BCNU)

Follow-up: clinical assessment by history and physical exam for pulmonary complications at 6 months, 1 year, and yearly thereafter
In patients with symptoms or signs of lung compromise, PFTs and focused radiologic assessment should be performed as clinically indicated. Follow-up evaluations should be guided by clinical circumstances for patients with recognized defects

---

Notes:

Bronchiolitis obliterans syndrome (BOS): Occurs with an incidence of 2–14% among allogeneic HCT recipients and is almost exclusively seen among patients with cGVHD. Treatment of BOS includes immunosuppressive agents such as corticosteroids, calcineurin inhibitors, sirolimus, and antithymocyte globulin. The prognosis of BOS is poor, and 5-year survival rates are <20% if patients do not respond to initial treatment

Cryptogenic organizing pneumonia (previously known as bronchiolitis obliterans organizing pneumonia): Presents typically in the first 6–12 months posttransplantation. Pulmonary function tests typically show a restrictive pattern. Corticosteroids are the mainstay of treatment and 80% of patients can be expected to recover, but relapses are common if steroids are rapidly tapered

Sinopulmonary infections can occur in patients with delayed immune reconstitution and cGVHD. Appropriate vaccinations are recommended, and in patients with ongoing immune deficiency and infections, immune globulin levels should be monitored and replacement should be considered

CARDIAC AND VASCULAR ABNORMALITIES

Majhail NS et al. Biol Blood Marrow Transplant 2012;18:348–371

Cardiomyopathy
Congestive heart failure
Arrhythmias
Valvular anomaly
Coronary artery disease
Cerebrovascular disease
Peripheral arterial disease

Risk factors: Anthracycline exposure, TBI/radiation exposure to neck or chest, older age at HCT, allogeneic HCT, cardiovascular risk factors before/after HCT, chronic kidney disease, metabolic syndrome

Follow-up: Routine clinical assessment and cardiovascular risk factor evaluation for all HCT recipients at 1 year and yearly thereafter. More frequent assessments and if clinically appropriate, extended cardiac evaluations (eg, electrocardiogram, echocardiogram) may be indicated in patients at high risk for cardiac complications (eg, patients with Hodgkin lymphoma who have received mediastinal radiation therapy, patients with amyloidosis, and patients with preexisting cardiac and vascular abnormalities)

LIVER COMPLICATIONS

Majhail NS et al. Biol Blood Marrow Transplant 2012;18:348–371

GVHD
Hepatitis B
Hepatitis C
Iron overload
Venoocclusive disease

Risk factors: Cumulative transfusion exposure, risk factors for viral hepatitis transmission

Follow-up: LFTs (serum total bilirubin, alkaline phosphatase, and transaminases) should be performed every 3–6 months for the first year, and then at least yearly thereafter. More frequent assessments may be needed based on an individual patient's medical status (eg, patients with GVHD) and particularly in allogeneic transplantation survivors

Serum ferritin should be measured at 1 year after transplantation in patients who received RBC infusions pre- or posttransplantation. Subsequent monitoring with serum ferritin should be considered among patients with elevated levels, especially in the presence of abnormal LTFs, continued RBC transfusions, or HCV infection. Additional diagnostic testing (eg, liver biopsy, MRI, or superconducting quantum interference device [SQUID]) may be indicated if therapy is contemplated for suspected iron overload

Notes:
Chronic GVHD is a major cause of liver dysfunction after transplantation and can manifest with elevations of serum alanine transaminase, alkaline phosphatase, and gamma-glutamyl transferase. Evaluation should exclude other causes of liver dysfunction (eg, viral infections, drug-related injury). Liver biopsy should be performed to confirm the diagnosis when liver dysfunction occurs as the only manifestation of cGVHD and systemic immunosuppression is being considered

The cumulative incidence of HCV progressing to cirrhosis is 11% at 15 years and 24% at 20 years, being more rapid in transplantation than in nontransplantation patients (18 vs. 40 years). In patients with known HCV infection, liver biopsy can be considered at 8–10 years after transplantation to assess for the presence of cirrhosis

When iron overload is suspected, the hepatic iron content should be estimated by appropriate imaging (specialized magnetic resonance imaging [MRI] protocols or superconducting quantum interference device [SQUID]) or liver biopsy. Patients with significant iron overload (eg, >7 mg/g dry weight liver iron) and liver dysfunction are candidates for phlebotomy or iron-chelation therapy

• Hepatic sinusoidal obstruction syndrome (hepatic SOS, previously called hepatic veno-occlusive disease) is associated with hepatomegaly, right upper quadrant pain, jaundice, and ascites, and usually begins within 6 weeks after HCT. Not all features may be present, and the severity of signs and symptoms can vary. The incidence following high-dose chemotherapy and TBI is 20–50%

For patients suspected to have hepatic SOS, perform ultrasound and Doppler studies to determine whether there is attenuation or reversal of venous flow or portal vein thrombosis. Prophylaxis with ursodiol (ursodeoxycholic acid) is recommended in HCT recipients to reduce hepatic complications:

   Ursodiol 600 mg/day (eg, 300 mg twice daily); administer orally, from transplantation day −1 to day +80 after transplantation

RENAL COMPLICATIONS

Majhail NS et al. Biol Blood Marrow Transplant 2012;18:348–371

Chronic Kidney Disease

Risk factors: older age at HCT, diagnosis (eg, myeloma) and pretransplantation renal function and therapy exposures (eg, platinum compounds), acute GVHD and cGVHD, use of TBI in conditioning regimen, exposure to medications to prevent or treat GVHD (eg, calcineurin inhibitors), and certain antimicrobials (eg, acyclovir, amphotericin, aminoglycosides)

Blood pressure should be checked at every clinic visit, and hypertension should be investigated and managed appropriately in all HCT recipients
Renal function should be evaluated at 6 months, 1 year, and at least yearly thereafter for all HCT recipients. Screening should include assessment of BUN, serum creatinine, and urine protein. Further work-up (eg, renal ultrasound, renal biopsy), as clinically indicated should be pursued in patients with late-onset acute renal failure or chronic kidney disease posttransplantation

Notes: The incidence of chronic kidney disease defined as sustained decrease in glomerular filtration rate <60 mL/min per 1.73 m^2, has been reported to range from 5–65%. The majority of patients have an idiopathic form of chronic kidney disease which is not associated with thrombotic microangiopathy or nephrotic syndrome and has a multifactorial etiology

MUSCULOSKELETAL COMPLICATIONS

Majhail NS et al. Biol Blood Marrow Transplant 2012;18:348–371

Avascular necrosis
Osteoporosis
Osteopenia
Myopathy
Fasciitis/scleroderma
Polymyositis

Risk factors: inactivity, TBI, corticosteroids, GVHD, hypogonadism, allogeneic HCT

Follow-up: A screening dual-photon densitometry should be performed 1 year after transplantation in adult women, all allogeneic HCT recipients, and patients who are at high risk for bone loss after transplantation (eg, prolonged treatment with corticosteroids or calcineurin inhibitors). Repeat densitometry should be performed in those with recognized defects, ongoing risk factors, or to follow-up response to therapy. Physicians should evaluate gonadal and other related endocrine abnormalities in patients with a decline in bone density

Notes:
Rapid loss of bone usually takes place within 6–12 months after transplantation with incidence rates as high as 25% for osteoporosis and 50% for osteopenia. Treatment choices for patients with established osteopenia and osteoporosis include active exercise, calcium and vitamin D supplementation, use of estrogen replacement in women, and minimizing the total exposure and duration of steroid and other immune-suppressive therapies. Bisphosphonate therapy should be considered for treatment of patients with established osteopenia and osteoporosis, patients with evidence of progressive bone density loss, and patients at high risk for bone loss (eg, patients with GVHD on extended steroid therapy). Osteonecrosis of the jaw has been reported in patients who receive bisphosphonates for osteoporosis, especially among those undergoing oral procedures while on these agents. If appropriate, dental evaluation should be performed before starting bisphosphonates in order to detect and correct dental problems
Avascular necrosis (AVN) has been described in 4–19% of HCT survivors. Although the hip is the most frequently affected joint ($>80\%$ of cases; bilateral in $>60\%$), other joints can be affected, including the knees, wrists, and ankles. Most adult patients with advanced AVN will require surgical intervention
Myopathy after HCT is one of the most frequent complications of long-term steroid therapy for cGVHD. Myopathy progresses insidiously in most cases. Proximal lower extremity muscles are commonly involved, with quadriceps muscles affected most severely
Myositis or polymyositis is a rare distinctive feature of cGVHD as defined by National Institutes of Health consensus criteria. Chronic GVHD-associated polymyositis or myopathy usually occurs 2–5 years after HCT. The common presenting symptoms are moderate to severe proximal muscle weakness and/or myalgia; lower extremities are commonly involved. This syndrome may be hard to distinguish from steroid-induced myopathy. The majority of patients have increased serum creatine kinase (creatine phosphokinase, CK) levels, a myopathic pattern on electromyography, a largely perifascicular lymphocytic infiltration on muscle biopsy, and a very favorable response to immunosuppressive therapy
Sclerosis can affect the skin and subcutaneous tissues including fasciae, joints, and the musculoskeletal system with varying degrees of severity and is a diagnostic feature of cGVHD. Aggressive and prolonged immunosuppressive therapy is necessary to prevent progression of contractures, but is usually ineffective at reversing established contractures. Early intervention and rehabilitation become essential to restore range of motion and strength
For patients on corticosteroids, frequent clinical evaluation is recommended for steroid-induced myopathy by manual muscle tests or by assessing patients' ability to rise from a seated to a standing position

MUCOCUTANEOUS COMPLICATIONS

Majhail NS et al. Biol Blood Marrow Transplant 2012;18:348–371

Cutaneous sclerosis
GVHD

Risk factors: GVHD, TBI/radiation exposure to pelvis

Follow-up: All women recipients of allogeneic HCT should undergo clinical screening for symptoms of genital GVHD. Women who have established chronic GVHD should have gynecologic examination to screen for genital involvement

Late complications involving skin and appendages are frequent after HCT. Nearly 70% of patients with chronic GVHD experience skin involvement. Early changes of lichen planus-like or papulosquamous lesions may progress to sclerosis or poikiloderma and can be associated with skin ulcers and subsequent infections

Severe genital GVHD may develop in ~12% of women with or without associated systemic GVHD

Patients may present with excoriated or ulcerated mucosa, fissures, narrowing of introitus, or vaginal scarring and obliteration that may lead to hematocolpos. Treatment of vaginal GVHD includes topical steroids, topical cyclosporine and vaginal dilators. Surgical intervention can be used to treat severe cases. Genital involvement with GVHD is less common in men

NEUROPSYCHOLOGICAL DEFICITS

Majhail NS et al. Biol Blood Marrow Transplant 2012;18:348–371

Leukoencephalopathy
Late infections
Neuropsychological and cognitive deficits
Calcineurin neurotoxicity
Peripheral neuropathy
Depression
Anxiety
Fatigue

Risk factors: TBI/radiation fields that include the head, GVHD, exposure to fludarabine, intrathecal chemotherapy, hypogonadism, long-term corticosteroid administration

Follow-up: All HCT recipients should undergo clinical assessment for symptoms or signs of neurologic dysfunction 1 year after HCT, and at least yearly thereafter. Earlier and more frequent evaluations may be considered in high-risk patients, which includes allogeneic HCT recipients; patients who receive prolonged immune suppression with calcineurin inhibitors, TBI, cranial radiation, or intrathecal chemotherapy; and patients with chronic GVHD

Clinical assessment is recommended throughout the recovery period, at 6 months, at 1 year, and at least yearly thereafter, with assessment by a mental health professional for those with recognized deficits

Notes:
Neuropsychological deficits have been described in nearly 20% of recipients and cognitive deficits in ~10% of HCT recipients
Neurocognitive function generally improves over time, but long-term deficits may persist in more than 40% of survivors

SECONDARY MALIGNANCIES

Majhail NS et al. Biol Blood Marrow Transplant 2012;18:348–371

Patients who receive allogeneic HCT have a 2- to 3-fold increased risk of developing solid tumors, compared with an age-, gender-, and region-adjusted population. Risk of secondary leukemia or myelodysplasia after autologous HCT is also greater than anticipated, with an overall incidence of approximately 4% 7 years after transplantation, with a median onset of 2.5 years (range: 3 months to 7 years) posttransplantation

Risk factors: GVHD, TBI/radiation exposure, T-cell depletion, exposure to alkylating agents or etoposide

Follow-up: All patients should at least receive country-specific general population recommendations for cancer screening. Screening for breast cancer is recommended at an earlier age (25 years or 8 years after radiation, whichever occurs later) but no later than age 40 years among recipients of TBI or chest irradiation

Notes:
Nearly all cancer types are described after allogeneic and autologous transplantation
Posttransplantation lymphoproliferative disorder (PTLD) is a rare complication of allogeneic HCT that is associated with donor–recipient HLA disparity, T-cell depletion, and GVHD. Overall incidence is 1% at 10 years after HCT. Although PTLD usually occurs early (within 6 months after transplantation), it is reported as late as 8 years after HCT. The majority of PTLDs are associated with Epstein-Barr virus infection

51. Radiation Complications

Ramesh Rengan, MD, PhD, Diana C. Stripp, MD, and Eli Glatstein, MD

The ultimate determinant of the efficacy of any anticancer therapy is the *therapeutic ratio*. The therapeutic ratio for a given dose of radiation therapy (RT) is defined as the ratio of the tumor control rate to the observed normal tissue toxicity. The larger this ratio is, the better tolerated the treatment is at any given dose. Indeed, the "definitive" therapeutic dose for most solid tumors has been determined by the clinically observed radiotolerance of the surrounding normal tissues, not the dose required for tumor sterilization. Therefore, with an understanding of acute and chronic toxicities of radiation, one can potentially improve the therapeutic ratio through effective intervention

Factors Affecting Side-Effect Profile

Clinical:
- The location of the primary tumor and its proximity to critical structures
- The tolerance of the surrounding normal tissue to RT
- The associated use of other modalities of therapy such as surgery or chemotherapy

Physical:
- The arrangement and energy of the radiation beams and the anatomic structures in their path

Biologic:
- The tissue response to RT at the molecular level
- The individual's biological sensitivity to radiation

Radiation Side Effects: Acute and Late Phases

Early or acute side effects
- Largely represent killing of rapidly proliferating cells, such as the epithelial lining of mucosal surfaces, skin, and bone marrow
- Occur during or shortly after RT
- Usually begin 2–3 weeks into RT, increase progressively, and resolve after completion of radiotherapy
- A majority recover without long-term sequelae because of the repopulation of normal stem cells
- The use of concomitant chemotherapy may significantly prolong and worsen acute reactions

Late or chronic side effects
- Probably represents cell loss from microvascular injury (perhaps secondary to endothelial apoptosis) and organ or tissue atrophy. Inflammation is rarely seen unless infection becomes superimposed
- Occur months or years after RT
- Generally progress slowly and are usually irreversible
- Can result in permanent undesirable effects of RT without sacrificing tumor control

Morbidity Scoring

Common Terminology Criteria for Adverse Events version 3.0 (CTCAE v3.0)[1]

Tolerance Dose (TD)

- Refers to the normal tissue tolerance of each organ to radiation
- TD 5/5 is the dose that results in a 5% rate of major complications within 5 years after treatment (presumes that RT is given with the conventional fraction size of 1.8–2 Gy/day). TD 50/5 is the dose that results in a 50% rate of major complications within 5 years after treatment
- Attempts have been made to define the TD 5/5 for each organ[2]
- The defined TD 5/5 should be used only as a guideline and not as an absolute. In the current era of combining chemotherapy and radiation or using altered fractionation schedules, adjustments in the tolerance doses are necessary

Radiation Complications
Normal Tissue Tolerance to Therapeutic Irradiation

Organ	Selected End Point	TD 5/5 Volume*			TD 50/5 Volume*		
		1/3	2/3	3/3	1/3	2/3	3/3
Kidney	Clinical nephritis	5000	3000†	2300		4000†	2800
Bladder	Symptomatic bladder contracture and volume loss		8000	6500		8500	8000
Bone							
Femoral head	Necrosis			4200–5200³			6500
TM joint	Marked limitation of joint function	6500	6000	6000	7700	7200	7200
Rib cage	Pathologic fracture	5000			6500		
Skin	Telangiectasias			100 cm²/5000			100 cm²/6500
	Necrosis, ulceration	10 cm²/5000	30 cm²/5000	100 cm²/5500			100 cm²/7000
Brain	Necrosis, infarction	6000	5000	4500	7500	6500	6000
Brain stem	Necrosis, infarction	6000	5300	5000			6500
Optic nerve	Blindness			5000			6500
Chiasma	Blindness			5000			6500
Spinal cord	Myelitis, necrosis	5 cm/5000	10 cm/5000	20 cm/7000	5 cm/7000	10 cm/7000	
Cauda equina	Clinically apparent nerve damage			6000			7500
Brachial plexus	Clinically apparent nerve damage	6200	6100	6000	7700	7600	7500
Eye lens	Cataract requiring intervention			1000			1800
Retina	Blindness			4500			6500
Ears Mid/external	Acute serous otitis	3000	3000	3000†	4000	4000	4000†
Mid/external	Chronic serous otitis	5500	5500	5500†	6500	6500	6500†
Parotid†	Xerostomia‡		3200†	3200†		4600†	4600†
Larynx	Cartilage necrosis	7900†	7000†	7000†	9000†	8000†	8000†
	Laryngeal edema		4500	4500†			8000†
Lungs	Pneumonitis	4500	3000	1750	6500	4000	2450
Heart	Pericarditis	6000	4500	4000	7000	5500	5000
Esophagus	Clinical stricture/perforation	6000	5800	5500	7200	7000	6800
Stomach	Ulceration, perforation	6000	5500	5000	7000	6700	6500
Small intestine	Obstruction, perforation/fistula	5000		4000†	6000		5500
Colon	Obstruction, perforation/ulceration/fistula	5500		4500	6500		5500
Rectum	Severe proctitis/necrosis/fistula, stenosis			6000			8000
Liver	Liver failure	5000	3500	3000	5500	4500	4000

*Values shown are tolerance doses for 1/3, 2/3, and 3/3 partial volumes of all listed organs
†<50% of volume doesn't make a significant change
‡TD 100/5 is 5000

Unless otherwise indicated, data is from Emami B et al. Int J Radiat Oncol Biol Phys 1991;21:109–122

SKIN

Skin: Early (Acute) Side Effects

Presentation

1. Seen as early as 7–10 days after starting RT
2. Clinical characteristics include erythema (as early as the second week) → increased dryness → hyperpigmentation → loss of hair (epilation) → dry desquamation at 4–5 weeks
3. Moist (wet) desquamation is seen 5–7 days after dry desquamation with continuation of RT dose
4. Important to rule out infection (cellulitis). Examine the patient carefully for any signs of lymphangitic streaking and a careful examination of regional nodal stations must be performed
5. The patient should be questioned about the presence of any pain or pruritus

Management

1. Erythema, dryness, hyperpigmentation, and epilation

   General

   • Avoid topical products on the skin within the RT portal *during radiation delivery*

   • When topical products, such as **Eucerin** Original Moisturizing Lotion or **Keri** Original Moisture Therapy lotion are used, they must be washed off prior to delivery of radiotherapy

   • Avoid shaving, if possible

   • Specifically avoid any topical products containing metals (**silver sulfadiazine**) until after completion of radiotherapy as scatter from the metals can exacerbate the skin reaction to radiation

   • Wash skin gently with lukewarm water and pat it dry

   • Keep skin well moisturized[4] and encourage regular moisturization after RT with nonirritating, fragrance-free topically applied lotions such as **Eucerin** Original Moisturizing Lotion or **Keri** Original Moisture Therapy lotion

   • *Pruritus*: Add **hydrocortisone cream 1% or 2.5%** to the moisturizer; apply topically to intact skin twice daily

2. Moist desquamation

   General

   • A treatment break from radiotherapy may be required to allow for skin healing

   • Serial examinations must be performed to assess response to therapy and healing (granulation tissue identified at wound site)

   • Apply compresses topically with **0.9% sodium chloride** or **aluminum acetate solution** (**Burow or modified Burow solution**) 3 or 4 times daily to clean and remove dead skin

   • Use **nonionic moisturizers** such as **Aquaphor** Healing Ointment or a **vitamin A and E ointment** topically to provide a barrier to infection and loss of body fluid

   • Use a nonadhesive dressing when necessary to prevent added irritation

   • *Antibiotics:* Use a topical antibiotic cream if infection occurs

     ▪ Apply triple antibiotic ointment (**polymyxin B sulfate + neomycin sulfate + bacitracin zinc**) topically twice daily to affected area, *or*

     ▪ Apply **silver sulfadiazine** topically twice daily to affected area. This must be discontinued prior to reinitiation of radiotherapy

   • *Analgesia:* Use systemic medications for pain control as needed: **Oxycodone, hydromorphone,** or **morphine**

Skin: Late (Chronic) Side Effects

Presentation

1. Hyper- or hypopigmentation/increased risk of basal cell carcinoma and melanoma
2. Telangiectasias
3. Permanent alopecia
4. Chronic ulceration, cutaneous atrophy
5. Fibrosis
6. Edema
7. Photosensitivity
8. Increased risk of basal cell carcinoma and melanoma

Management

• Hyper- or hypopigmentation/increased risk of basal cell carcinoma and melanoma

  ▪ Permanent use of **skin moisturizers with SPF >15 and protection from the sun** are advised

• Chronic ulceration not responding to conservative therapy

  ▪ Usually requires surgical repair

  ▪ **Hyperbaric oxygen** treatment can lead to reepithelialization and eliminate the need for surgical intervention. Hyperbaric oxygen is considered after the failure of conservative management

  ▪ **Pentoxifylline** 400 mg orally 2–3 times daily. May increase blood flow and promote healing[5]

• Radiation-induced fibrosis: **Pentoxifylline and α-tocopherol** (D-α-tocopherol or DL-α-tocopherol acetate; vitamin E) can potentially reduce fibrosis[4]

  ▪ **Pentoxifylline** 400 mg orally 2–3 times per day

  ▪ **α-Tocopherol** 1000 units/day orally

SOFT TISSUES AND BONE

Soft Tissues and Bone: Early (Acute) Side Effects

Presentation

1. Soft-tissue edema can develop especially in treatment of the head and neck regions
2. Bony fractures can develop potentially in any site of irradiation (pelvic radiation is of particular concern)

Management

1. Soft-tissue edema
   - A temporary tracheostomy may be required when a patient develops laryngeal edema (when the possibility of laryngeal edema is high, a prophylactic tracheostomy can be performed before starting RT)
   - Short course of steroids:
     - **Dexamethasone** orally 2–4 times per day. Begin with a dose of 4 mg per day, gradually decreasing doses and administration frequency toward discontinuation over 14 days, with dose and duration of treatment depending on response
2. Bony fractures
   - Consult an orthopedic surgeon. Consider prophylactic intervention

Soft Tissues and Bone: Late (Chronic) Side Effects

Presentation

1. Soft-tissue edema
   - Common late effect; more common with RT + neck dissection
   - Edema can occur in the neck, oral cavity, pharynx, or larynx
2. Soft-tissue necrosis
   - Rare late complication. May present as an unhealed wound, chronic ulceration
3. Soft-tissue fibrosis of the neck
   - Common late effect, especially with RT + neck dissection
   - Woody fibrosis of cervical soft tissues with limited range of motion
4. Trismus
   - Caused by temporomandibular joint (TMJ) fibrosis and/or masticator fibrosis
5. Osteoradionecrosis (ORN) of the mandible
   - Uncommon late effect of RT to head and neck. This is most commonly observed in the molar and premolar regions.[6] Clinical presentation is typified by erythema of the mucosa overlying the area of necrosis. This can progress to ulceration and ultimately the underlying necrotic bone is exposed. Risk increased by xerostomia and poor dental/oral hygiene
6. Long bone fractures
   - Most typically occurs after high-dose radiotherapy treatment used in the management of extremity sarcoma. The risk is significantly increased after periosteal stripping[7]
7. Pelvic/hip fractures
   - *Pelvis:* Increased likelihood after pelvic radiation, particularly in women after age 65 years irradiated for pelvic malignancies.[8] Anal cancer is of particular concern with an approximate 3-fold increased incidence
   - *Hip:* The most vulnerable location for fracture within the pelvic skeletal architecture is the femoral neck. The best available data suggests that cigarette use may contribute. Although there is no clear predictive dose response correlation with femoral neck fractures, it is rarely seen when the total dose is kept below 42 Gy[3]

Management

1. Soft-tissue edema
   - Elevation of head and neck while in bed
   - Short course of steroids:
     - **Dexamethasone** orally 2–4 times per day. Begin with 4 mg per day, gradually decreasing doses and administration frequency toward discontinuation over 14 days, with dose and duration of treatment depending on response
2. Soft-tissue necrosis
   - Conservative management:
     - Good oral hygiene
     - **Pentoxifylline** 400 mg orally 2–3 times per day
     - **α-Tocopherol** 1000 units per day orally
     - **Antibiotics** for possible underlying infection that prevents healing. Choice of agents depends on the sites of infection. Use anaerobic coverage for mucosal lesions; Gram-positive coverage for skin ulcers
   - Hyperbaric oxygen, and, if necessary, surgical intervention with planned hyperbaric oxygen in persistent cases is recommended after failure of conservative management

3. Soft-tissue fibrosis of neck
   - Range-of-motion exercises of the neck and shoulder for prevention
4. Trismus
   - Preventive jaw stretching exercise
5. Osteoradionecrosis (ORN) of the mandible
   - Xerostomia and poor dental and oral hygiene increase the risk of developing ORN. See "Head and Neck: Salivary Gland and Taste Buds" for recommendations
   - *Prevention:*
     - Full dental evaluation with correction of periodontal disease before starting RT is necessary
     - *To maintain healthy teeth:* Daily **topical fluoride application using a fluoride tray:** 1.1% w/w sodium fluoride toothpaste (PreviDent 500 Plus) topically for 10–15 minutes twice daily during and after completion of RT
6. Long bone fracture
   - If suspected, an orthopedic surgeon should be contacted immediately. Additionally, tumor recurrence must be ruled out. Surgical stabilization may be appropriate. In rare cases, for example with tumors located within the anterior thigh compartment, prophylactic placement of a femoral rod may be considered in consultation with the surgeon[9]
7. Pelvic/hip fractures
   - *Pelvis:* Preventive measures such as ensuring that a patient has had the current standard screening for osteoporosis and appropriate treatment is important. Usual treatment after identification of an insufficiency fracture is physical therapy and pain control. This regimen will usually result in an improvement in symptoms within 1–2 months, often with a complete resolution within 12 months.[10] An orthopedic surgeon should be consulted for recommendations regarding management
   - *Hip:* The best therapy is obviously prevention. Care must be taken to minimize the femoral neck/head dose as much as possible using blocking or through identification of the femoral head and neck as a separate avoidance structure, if intensity modulated radiation therapy (IMRT) is being used. Upon diagnosis of the fracture, the patient must be referred to an orthopedic surgeon. Special mechanical reinforcement, for example with the use of acetabular reinforcement rings, may be required due to poor bone healing after irradiation[11]

EARS

Ears: Early (Acute) Side Effects

Presentation
1. Otitis externa
2. Serous otitis media, or infectious otitis externa or media
   - Usually occurs after the third or fourth week of RT and can persist after completion of RT

Management
1. Otitis externa
   - **Hydrocortisone** otic drops; instill into the ear 3 times daily, or
   - **Hydrocortisone 1% + neomycin 5 mg + polymyxin B 10,000 units** otic drops: Instill solution into the ear 3 times daily, *or*
   - **Anesthetic otic drops:** Instill into the ear 3 times daily for pain in the external ear canal
   - In the case of tympanic perforation, or in the treatment of otitis media in a patient with myringotomy tubes, use **ciprofloxacin hydrochloride/dexamethasone otic drops**
2. Serous otitis media or infectious otitis externa or media
   - Decongestants or antihistamines:
     - **Diphenhydramine** 12.5–50 mg orally 3 times per day
     - **Loratadine** 10 mg orally once per day, or another **nonsedating antihistamine** (eg, cetirizine HCl, levocetirizine dihydrochloride, desloratadine, or fexofenadine HCl)
   - If medical therapy is not effective, consult an otolaryngologist for consideration of myringotomy tube insertion
   - If infection is suspected, oral antibiotics should be used:
     - **Amoxicillin** 500 mg orally every 8 hours for 10 days

Ears: Late (Chronic) Side Effects

Presentation
1. Permanent sensorineural hearing loss
   - Can occur in patients who receive a high dose to the cochlea (>60 Gy)[12,13]

Management

1. Permanent hearing loss

- Prevention is the best treatment. However, in a situation in which a high dose to the cochlea is unavoidable, such as with posterior fossa radiation, a hearing aid may be needed. Limit the cochlear dose to <60 Gy when possible. The use of chemotherapy concomitantly may increase the risk of sensorineural hearing loss. When the posterior fossa is being treated to high dose, the use of conformal techniques, such as intensity modulated radiation therapy (IMRT) may be of benefit[14]

HEAD AND NECK: ORAL AND ORAL PHARYNGEAL MUCOSA

Oral and Oral Pharyngeal Mucosa: Early (Acute) Side Effects

Presentation

1. Mucositis

- Starts approximately 1–2 weeks after commencing RT
- Oral discomfort → injected mucosa → patch ulceration → confluent mucositis at about the fourth to fifth weeks
- Plateaus for approximately 1–2 weeks
- Recovery starts close to the end of the treatment course
- Complete mucosal healing usually occurs within 2–3 weeks after RT completion
- Concomitant chemoradiation can be associated with a severe and long-lasting mucositis

2. Oral/mucosal candidiasis

- The most common infection of the oropharynx in patients who have received radiotherapy
- May exacerbate the symptoms of mucositis

3. Bacterial infection

- May also occur, but less common than candidiasis
- Usually occurs early in the course of head and neck irradiation

Management

1. Mucositis

General:

- Minimize exposure to mechanical or chemical irritants (such as poorly fitting dentures, alcohol, and chewing tobacco)
- **Baking soda or saline (0.9% sodium chloride for irrigation) oral rinses:** 1 tsp baking soda or 1 tsp table salt in 1 quart (~946 mL) of water. Gargle a minimum of 3 times per day and after all meals
- Use a water flosser (eg, Waterpik) to remove sticky materials from the mucosa
- **Sucralfate suspension** 1000 mg/10 mL orally 3–4 times daily, *or*
- Other mucosal coating products (with emollient properties to soothe irritated tissues but without an anesthetic component). These rinses relieve the pain of oral lesions by adhering to injured tissue of the oral mucosa and protecting it from further injury while providing a moist wound environment necessary for healing:

  - **Gelclair** bioadherent oral gel (polyvinylpyrrolidone, sodium hyaluronate, and glycyrrhetinic acid): mix Gelclair with 1–3 tbsp (15–45 mL) tap water (it may also be used undiluted): Swish the product around the oral cavity or gargle with it for at least 1 minute. Use as needed. The product is usually expectorated, but is harmless if swallowed

  - **Biotene Mouthwash** (glucose oxidase, lactoperoxidase, and lysozyme): Administer by swishing the product around the oral cavity or gargling with it for at least 30 seconds, and then expectorate. Use as needed

  - **RadiaCare (Carrington) Oral Wound Rinse:** mix the powder with the specified amount of water. A usual dose is approximately 1 tbsp (15 mL) that should be swished or gargled in the mouth for about 1 minute (safe if swallowed). Repeat 4 times per day or as needed

Analgesia:

- Topical anesthetics

  - **Viscous lidocaine 2%/simethicone liquid/with or without diphenhydramine liquid (12.5 mg/5 mL)** in a 1:1:1 mixture, 1 tbsp (15 mL) every 4–6 hours as needed

Note: This may be swallowed, but the lidocaine component can numb the hypopharynx, increasing the risk of aspiration

  - **Topical morphine** rinse, 1 tbsp (15 mL) of a 2% morphine solution every 3 hours, 6 times per day, swished in the mouth or gargled and then expectorated

    ○ 15 mL of a 2% solution contains 300 mg morphine and should NOT be swallowed

Note: Topical morphine has been shown to be superior to other topical anesthetics in a small, randomized trial. It has better pain control with decreased duration of functional imparment[15]

- Oral or parenteral opioids: Medication for pain control is used as needed: **Oxycodone, hydromorphone, fentanyl, or morphine.** See Chapter 52

Note: Systemic opioids are mostly used to control pain associated with mucositis

2. Oral/mucosal candidiasis
   - Topical antifungal agents: Continue treatment for at least 48 hours after perioral symptoms resolve and cultures no longer demonstrate growing yeast
     - **Nystatin suspension** 500,000–1,000,000 units (5–10 mL) orally 4 times per day
     - **Clotrimazole troche** 10 mg slowly dissolved in the mouth 5 times per day for 14 consecutive days
   Notes:
   (1) Patients with esophageal candidiasis require systemic antifungal treatment
   (2) Topical antifungal agents such as nystatin require contact with the affected area, and results among patients may be inconsistent
   - Oral antifungal agents:
     - **Fluconazole** 200 mg orally on day 1, followed by **fluconazole** 100 mg per day orally for 13 days on days 2–14
3. Bacterial infection
   - Antibiotics that provide good anaerobic coverage:
     - **Amoxicillin with or without clavulanic acid** orally every 12 hours until symptoms resolve, typically 7–10 days (co-amoxiclav: amoxicillin 825 mg + clavulanic acid 125 mg)
     - **Metronidazole** 500 mg orally every 6 hours
   - A culture should be obtained if a patient fails to benefit from antimicrobial therapy or if there are systemic symptoms, such as fevers/chills, etc. Culture directed therapy should then be initiated based upon isolate sensitivities

Oral and Oral Pharyngeal Mucosa: Late (Chronic) Side Effects

Presentation
1. Pallor, telangiectasia, thinning of mucosa
2. Persistent ulceration of soft tissue
   - Can be very painful

Management
1. Pallor, telangiectasia, thinning of the mucosa
   - Maintain meticulous oral hygiene
2. Persistent ulceration of soft tissue
   - *Analgesia:* Adequate pain control, may need opioids
     - **Morphine, hydromorphone, oxycodone,** or **fentanyl.** See Chapter 52
   - Exposed bone needs prompt attention
   - Hyperbaric oxygen may promote soft tissue and bony healing. If bone remains exposed, surgical repair with or without planned hyperbaric oxygen is needed to prevent osteomyelitis

HEAD AND NECK: SALIVARY GLANDS AND TASTE BUDS

Salivary Glands and Taste Buds: Early (Acute) Side Effects

Presentation
1. Acute sialadenitis
   - Tenderness and swelling of the salivary glands
   - May occur within hours after the first RT session and subside within a few days
2. Xerostomia
   - Progressive thickening of saliva with decrease in salivary output within the first 2–3 days
3. Loss of taste
   - Common side effect of head and neck RT
   - Return of taste, with or without some degree of permanent impairment 4–6 months after completion of RT

Management
1. Acute sialadenitis and xerostomia
   General:
   - Hydration during RT is essential, especially in symptomatic patients
   - Oral rinses with any of the following products, 3–4 times per day:
     - Baking soda 1 teaspoonful in 1 quart (~946 mL) of water
     - Guaifenesin
     - Carbonated drinks (sugar and alcohol-free)
   - Papain
   Note: All these have been tried with variable results

- **Pilocarpine** 5–10 mg/dose orally 3–4 times/day up to a total daily dose of 30 mg

Note: Compared with placebo, pilocarpine maintains significantly better salivary function in patients undergoing RT, although quality of life is not different[16]

Prevention:

- Radioprotector for the salivary gland during postoperative RT for head and neck cancer: **Amifostine** 200 mg/m² by intravenous infusion over 3 minutes 15–30 minutes before daily RT.[17] An alternate route of administration is 1000 mg subcutaneously 20 minutes before daily RT, which may be a better tolerated method of delivery[18]

Salivary Glands and Taste Buds: Late (Chronic) Side Effects

Presentation

1. Permanent xerostomia

- Occurs in patients who receive high doses of RT to both parotid glands

Management

1. Permanent xerostomia

- Mixed results have been achieved with either:
  - **Artificial saliva products** may be used as often as needed to moisten and lubricate the mouth and throat in xerostomia (products are available in spray and moistened swab forms), *or*
  - **Pilocarpine** 5–10 mg/dose orally 3–4 times/day up to a maximum daily dose of 30 mg
- Surgery may present a possible option. A prospective study by Jha et al. evaluated the efficacy of surgical transfer of a submandibular gland to the submental space in order to protect the transferred gland prior to initiation of RT. At a median follow-up of 14 months, 81% experienced minimal to no xerostomia, with the remaining 19% having moderate/severe xerostomia. There were no surgery-related complications[19]

HEAD AND NECK: PHARYNX AND ESOPHAGUS

Pharynx and Esophagus: Early (Acute) Side Effects

Presentation

1. Pharyngitis/esophagitis

- Dysphagia and odynophagia occur in the second or third week of RT; resolve 2–3 weeks after completion of RT
- Characterized by somatic pain when swallowing
- Severe oropharyngitis → intermittent aspiration. Silent aspiration occurs in >60% of patients[20]

Management

1. Pharyngitis/esophagitis

General:

- Soft diet to maintain nutritional intake
- **Sucralfate suspension** 1000 mg/10 mL orally 3–4 times per day
- **Biotene Mouthwash** (glucose oxidase, lactoperoxidase, and lysozyme): Swish the product around the oral cavity or gargle with it for at least 30 seconds, and then expectorate. Use as needed
- **Gelclair** bioadherent oral gel (polyvinylpyrrolidone, sodium hyaluronate, and glycyrrhetinic acid): Mix Gelclair with 1–3 tbsp (15–45 mL) tap water (or may be used undiluted); swish the product around the oral cavity or gargle with it for at least 1 minute. The product is usually expectorated, but is harmless if swallowed
- **RadiaCare (Carrington) Oral Wound Rinse:** Mix the powder with the specified amount of water. A usual dose is approximately 1 tbsp (15 mL), which should be swished or gargled in the mouth for about 1 minute (safe if swallowed). Repeat 4 times per day or as needed

Analgesia:

- Topical anesthetics
  - **Viscous lidocaine 2%/simethicone liquid/with or without diphenhydramine** solution (sugar-free and alcohol-free, 12.5 mg/5 mL) in a 1:1:1 mixture, 1 tbsp (15 mL) swished around the oral cavity or gargled and then expectorated every 4–6 hours as needed
  - *Note:* This product may be swallowed, but the lidocaine component can numb the hypopharynx, increasing the risk of aspiration
  - **Topical morphine** rinse, 1 tbsp (15 mL) of a 2% morphine solution every 3 hours, 6 times daily, swished around the oral cavity or gargled and then expectorated
    - 15 mL of a 2% solution contains 300 mg morphine and should NOT be swallowed
    - *Note:* This has been shown to be superior to other topical anesthetics in a small, randomized trial. Better pain control with decreased duration of functional impairment[5]

- Oral or parenteral opioids: For pain control to maintain comfort: **Morphine, oxycodone, hydromorphone, fentanyl.** See Chapter 52

Note: Systemic opioids are often used to control pain associated with pharyngitis/esophagitis

Prevention in patients at risk for severe mucositis, pharyngitis, and esophagitis:

- Placement of a feeding tube before starting RT is recommended
- *Note:* Many patients who receive chemotherapy and radiation concurrently become dependent on enteral tube feeding for nutritional support. Most patients will eventually regain swallowing ability, however, as many as 20% of patients treated with concurrent chemoradiation may still be PEG tube dependent after 1 year[21]
- Recent data suggest that the radiotherapy dose to the pharyngeal constrictor muscles as well as the glottic and supraglottic larynx have the greatest deleterious effects in the development of esophagitis. Eisbruch et al. demonstrated, using IMRT, that the dose to these structures could be limited to <50 Gy without compromising tumor coverage. This approach reduced the dose to these critical structures by 20% on average when compared to conventional 3D-conformal techniques[22]

Rehabilitation:

- Speech and swallowing therapy aid in recovery

Pharynx and Esophagus: Late (Chronic) Side Effects

Presentation

1. Soft-tissue changes, including pallor, telangiectasia, and fibrosis, which may lead to stricture formation
2. Persistent inability to swallow
3. Chronic aspiration

Management

1. Strictures
   - Surgical dilation
2. Persistent inability to swallow
   - Speech and swallowing therapy
   - Severe cases that persist despite speech and swallowing therapy may require a permanent feeding tube
3. Chronic aspiration
   - Nothing by mouth with nutritional support via a permanent feeding tube
   - Severe cases may need a laryngectomy for airway protection

LUNGS

Lungs: Early (Acute) Side Effects

Presentation

1. Dry, nonproductive cough. Likely caused by transient injury to the airway mucosa soon after completing RT

Management

1. Dry, nonproductive cough
   - Symptomatic treatment, including cough suppressants, bronchodilators, and humidification

Lungs: Subacute Side Effects

Presentation

1. Radiation pneumonitis (RP)
   - Uncommon side effect, usually seen 1–5 months after RT
   - Can be lethal if it involves sufficient lung volume
   - *Acute symptoms of RP:* Dry cough, low-grade fever, congestion, dyspnea, pleuritic chest pain, and, rarely, hemoptysis
   - *Findings on imaging studies:* Classically, the changes generally correspond to the RT portal; however, these changes do not correlate with clinical severity of the presentation. Additionally, a sporadic form of radiation pneumonitis has been previously described. In this syndrome, unirradiated lung may show changes on the chest x-ray. This is believed to represent an immune mediated hypersensitivity pneumonitis[23]
   - Relevant predictive factors
     - Poor performance status[24]
     - Ongoing smoking may *decrease* the frequency of radiation-induced pneumonitis[25]
     - Comorbid pulmonary disease may *increase* risk
     - The greater the lung volume irradiated the greater the risk

Notes:

1. Risk starts when >22% of total lung volume is exposed to 20 Gy,[11] RP is generally not seen if <22% of total lung volume is exposed to 20 Gy compared with an 8% frequency when 22–31% of lung is exposed to 20 Gy[26]

2. RP is a clinical diagnosis of exclusion. Typical imaging findings in the absence of clinical symptoms does not warrant the diagnosis of RP

3. No solid data to indicate that chemotherapy used in combination with thoracic radiation (as in lung or esophageal cancer) leads to increased RP. However, if one uses chemotherapy agents that have known toxicity to lung, such as bleomycin, mitomycin, or cyclophosphamide, the risk increases dramatically

Management

1. Radiation pneumonitis (RP)

   Prevention:
   - Limit the lung volume exposed to <22% of total lung volume and <20 Gy[26]

   General:
   - Superinfection: Use antibiotics including **penicillin-based, cephalosporin, macrolides, or fluoroquinolones.** See Chapter 47
   - Supplemental **oxygen** as needed
   - Inhaled corticosteroids, such as **fluticasone** or **fluticasone + salmeterol**
     - **Fluticasone Inhalation Aerosol** (Flovent HFA) 44 mcg per metered dose, 2 puffs for a total of 88 mcg by oral inhalation twice daily, *or* **Fluticasone Inhalation Aerosol Powder** (Flovent Diskus) 100 mcg by oral inhalation twice daily
     - **Fluticasone propionate/salmeterol xinafoate** (Advair Diskus) 250/50 (250 mcg microfine fluticasone propionate + 50 mcg salmeterol base) by 1 oral inhalation twice daily
       - Care must be taken to gargle with salt water after each inhalation to prevent oropharyngeal fungal infection
   - *Corticosteroids:* **Prednisone** 30–60 mg/dose orally every day for 2–3 weeks, followed by a dose and administration schedule gradually decreasing (tapering) toward discontinuation
     - Reduce daily dose by 5–10 mg/day each week or every other week, depending on a patient's symptoms

   Note: Initiate corticosteroids only when symptoms are associated with hypoxemia. It is often very difficult to taper steroids in the setting of RP because of persistent symptoms. The rate of tapering should depend on the response of the patient

Lungs: Late (Chronic) Side Effects

Presentation

1. Pulmonary fibrosis
   - May occur anywhere from several months to years after radiation
   - May or may not be preceded by radiation pneumonitis. Usually develops silently in radiated area
   - Most patients are asymptomatic when small volumes of the lung are affected
   - If a sufficient or significant amount of lung is involved → dyspnea → progressive cor pulmonale. This process is irreversible

   Note: Occurs nearly always in the radiated area. In general, consider the area of the lung that receives >30–35 Gy as functionless and likely to develop fibrosis.[27] Therefore, it is prudent for the radiation oncologist to select patients and to minimize lung exposure to radiation

Management

1. Pulmonary fibrosis
   - Supportive care
   - Supplemental **oxygen**
   - Bronchodilators
     - **Ipratropium bromide inhalation aerosol** (18 mcg/actuation) 4 times per day. Additional doses may be given as required to a maximum of 12 inhalations/24 hours, *or*
     - **Ipratropium bromide inhalation solution** 0.02%. The usual dose is 500 mcg by nebulization every 6–8 hours
   - Prevention

   Note: It has been reported that **amifostine** is effective in reducing acute severe esophagitis and pneumonitis in persons with locally advanced non–small cell lung cancer treated with chemoradiation.[28,29] Although, a recent RTOG report failed to confirm objective improvement in esophagitis, patient self-assessment showed statistically improved swallowing function with amifostine[30]

HEART

Heart: Early (Acute) Side Effects

Presentation
1. Cardiac damage
   - Uncommon when <30% of the heart receives <40 Gy
2. Acute pericarditis
   - Rare

Management
2. Pericarditis
   - Observation
   - **Nonsteroidal antiinflammatory agents:** Aspirin, ibuprofen, naproxen, or indomethacin
   - Steroids: **Prednisone** 30–60 mg/dose orally daily for 2–3 weeks, followed by a dose and administration schedule gradually decreasing (tapering) toward discontinuation
     - Reduce daily dose by 5–10 mg either each week or every other week, depending on a patient's symptoms

Heart: Late (Chronic) Side Effects

Presentation
1. Pericarditis
   - May develop 6 months to years after RT
   - Presentation: Chest pain, dyspnea, fever, and abnormalities on ECG
   - Pericardial effusion with tamponade may develop
2. Cardiomyopathy or pancarditis
   - Uncommon but can occur if RT + cardiotoxic chemotherapy such as doxorubicin is administered
3. Other cardiac effects of uncertain etiology: Coronary artery disease, valvular defects, conduction abnormalities

Management
1. Pericarditis
   - Pericardiocentesis and pericardiotomy are necessary for impending tamponade; both visceral and parietal pericardium must be removed
2. Cardiomyopathy or pancarditis
   - Avoid cardiomyopathy by adjusting anthracycline dosages and meticulously designing radiation portals. Special care should be taken when treating a patient with left-sided breast cancer as they may be at increased risk. In the Stockholm trial, a 6.8% incidence of excess cardiac morbidity was reported with left-sided tumors treated with deep tangent fields. The average volume of heart receiving at least 25 Gy in that study was 25%, whereas with conformal techniques, this can be reduced to 6% or less[31]

GASTROINTESTINAL SYSTEM: ESOPHAGUS

Esophagus: Early (Acute) Side Effects

Presentation
1. *Esophagitis:* Sensation of food getting stuck while swallowing (contrast with somatic pain that occurs when swallowing with pharyngitis from head and neck RT)
2. Gastroesophageal reflux disease (GERD)
3. Colonization by *Candida* species

Management
1. Esophagitis
   General:
   - Soft diet to maintain nutritional intake
   - **Sucralfate suspension** 1000 mg/10 mL orally 3–4 times per day
   Analgesia:
   - Topical anesthetics
     - **Viscous lidocaine 2%/simethicone liquid/with or without diphenhydramine liquid** (12.5 mg/5 mL) in 1:1:1 mixture, 1 tbsp (15 mL) every 4–6 hours as needed

Note: This may be swallowed, but the lidocaine component can numb the hypopharynx, increasing the risk of aspiration
- **Topical morphine** rinse 1 tbsp (15 mL) of a 2% morphine solution every 3 hours, 6 times daily, swished in the mouth or gargled and then expectorated
  - 15 mL of a 2% solution contains 300 mg morphine and should NOT be swallowed

Note: Topical morphine has been shown to be superior to other topical anesthetics in a small, randomized trial. Better pain control with decreased duration of functional impairment[15]

- *Oral or parenteral opioids:* For pain control to maintain comfort: **Morphine, oxycodone, hydromorphone, fentanyl.** See Chapter 52

Note: Systemic opioids are often used to control pain associated with pharyngitis/esophagitis

Prevention in patients at risk for severe mucositis, pharyngitis, and esophagitis:
- Placement of a feeding tube before starting RT is recommended
- *Note:* Many patients who receive chemotherapy and radiation concurrently become dependent on enteral tube feeding for nutritional support. Most patients will eventually regain swallowing ability
- Recent data suggests that the radiotherapy dose to the pharyngeal constrictor muscles as well as the glottic and supraglottic larynx have the greatest deleterious effects in the development of esophagitis. Eisbruch et al. demonstrated with the use of IMRT, the dose to these structures can be limited to <50 Gy without compromising tumor coverage. This approach reduced the dose to these critical structures by 20% on average when compared to conventional 3D-conformal techniques[22]

Rehabilitation:
- Speech and swallowing therapy aid in recovery

2. GERD
- Antacids and proton pump inhibitors

3. Colonization by *Candida* species
- *Topical antifungal agents:* Continue treatment for at least 48 hours after perioral symptoms resolve and cultures return to normal
  - **Nystatin suspension** 500,000–1,000,000 units (5–10 mL) orally 4 times per day
  - **Clotrimazole troches** 10 mg dissolved slowly in the mouth 5 times per day

Notes:
- Patients with esophageal candidiasis require systemic antifungal treatment
- Topical antifungal agents such as nystatin and clotrimazole require contact with the affected area and results among patients may be inconsistent
- *Oral antifungal agents:* **Fluconazole** 200 mg orally on day 1, followed by **fluconazole** 100 mg per day orally for 13 consecutive days on days 2–14

Esophagus: Late (Chronic) Side Effects

Presentation
1. Persistent esophagitis
2. Stricture
3. Chronic ulceration
4. Fistula

Management
1. Persistent esophagitis
- Symptomatic relief, supportive care, similar to management of acute esophagitis
2. Stricture
- Esophageal dilation
3. Chronic ulceration
- Surgical intervention may be needed

GASTROINTESTINAL SYSTEM: STOMACH

Stomach: Early (Acute) Side Effects

Presentation
1. Nausea and vomiting
- Occurs frequently with gastric RT. Resolves after the completion of RT
2. Acute gastritis with ulceration
- 2–3 weeks after the start of RT. Resolves after the completion of RT

Management

1. Nausea and vomiting
   - *Antiemetics before RT:*
     - **Ondansetron** 4–8 mg orally 30–60 minutes before RT. For intractable nausea: 4–8 mg orally twice daily continually
       - Outpatients who are not able to retain swallowed medications may benefit from oral disintegrating tablet or oral soluble film formulations
     - **Granisetron** 2 mg orally 30–60 minutes before RT. For intractable nausea: 1 mg twice daily continually if needed
       - Outpatients who are not able to retain swallowed medications may benefit from a transdermal patch formulation
     - **Tropisetron** 5 mg/day either as needed, or, if administered prophylactically, start use 1 day before initiating RT, then 1–2 hours before each RT fraction, and after completion of RT once daily for 7 days
       - In the United States, tropisetron has not received FDA approval for use outside a clinical trial
     - **Metoclopramide** 40 mg orally 30–60 minutes before RT. For intractable nausea: 20–40 mg 4-times daily, continually
     - **Prochlorperazine** 20 mg orally 30–60 minutes before RT. For intractable nausea 5–20 mg orally every 4–6 hours, continually
     - **Lorazepam** 1 mg orally 30–60 minutes before RT. For intractable nausea: 0.5–1 mg orally every 6–12 hours, continually
     - **Dronabinol** 10 mg orally 30–60 minutes before RT. For intractable nausea 2.5–10 mg orally every 6 hours, continually
     - **Chlorpromazine** 50 mg orally 30–60 minutes before RT. For intractable nausea: 25–50 mg orally every 4–6 hours, continually
2. Nausea and vomiting and acute gastritis with ulceration
   - Smaller daily RT fraction sizes

Stomach: Late (Chronic) Side Effects

Presentation (a few months to years after the completion of RT)

1. Dyspepsia, chronic gastritis
2. Persistent ulceration
3. Gastric outlet obstruction
4. Perforation

Management

1. Dyspepsia, chronic gastritis
   - H_2-blockers
     - **Ranitidine HCl** 150 mg orally 2 times per day, or 300 mg orally at bedtime, *or*
     - **Famotidine** 40 mg orally at bedtime, or 20 mg orally 2 times per day, *or*
     - **Cimetidine** 300 mg orally 4 times per day, or 400 mg orally 2 times per day
   - Proton pump inhibitors:
     - **Rabeprazole sodium** 20 mg orally daily, or
     - **Esomeprazole magnesium** 20 mg orally daily, or
     - **Lansoprazole** 15 mg orally daily, or
     - **Pantoprazole sodium** 30 mg orally daily
   - *Note:* The proton pump inhibitors doses and schedules vary by indication. Dose adjustment and duration of administration must be tailored to individual patients
   - **Sucralfate suspension** (1000 mg/10 mL) 1500 mg orally 3–4 times per day
2. Persistent ulceration, gastric outlet obstruction, and perforation
   - Urgent referral for surgical evaluation. In the event of bleeding ulceration, endoscopy with argon laser coagulation may provide temporary control[32]

GASTROINTESTINAL SYSTEM: SMALL AND LARGE INTESTINE

Small and Large Intestine: Early (Acute) Side Effects

Presentation

1. Fatigue, nausea, vomiting, early satiety, anorexia, and diarrhea
2. Enteritis
   - Crampy abdominal pain and watery diarrhea
3. Proctocolitis
   - Occurs 2–3 weeks after the start of pelvic RT
   - Frequent bowel movement with or without watery diarrhea; rectal urgency; and tenesmus
4. Proctitis

Management

1. Fatigue, nausea, vomiting, early satiety, anorexia, and diarrhea
   - Antidiarrheal medications
     - **Psyllium fiber** 1 tsp in 8 oz water orally 3–4 times per day
     - **Cholestyramine** 1000 mg orally 1–4 times per day as needed
     - **Loperamide** 4 mg orally at the first onset of loose stools, followed by loperamide 2 mg orally every 2 hours around the clock until the patient is diarrhea-free for 12 hours
     - **Diphenoxylate-atropine** 2 tablets orally after each bowel movement
       - The commercially available combination product contains diphenoxylate 2.5 mg hydrochloride + atropine sulfate 0.025 mg per tablet
       - The maximum dose of diphenoxylate per 24-hour interval is 20 mg
     - **Octreotide acetate** injection 100–500 mcg/dose subcutaneously 2 or 3 times daily, doubling the dose at 3- to 4-day intervals until maximum control of symptoms is achieved
       - Maximum total daily octreotide dose is 1500 mcg
     Note: Octreotide has been shown to be more effective compared with conventional treatments mentioned above in the control of radiation induce diarrhea[34]
     - **Oral sucralfate** has been shown to reduce acute and late toxicity from pelvic irradiation in a prospective study[33]
2. Enteritis and proctocolitis
   - Low-residue diet
3. Mild proctitis
   - **Topical anesthetic products** (eg, pramoxine cream, lotion, gel, spray, foam, wipes) externally to the affected area up to 5 times daily
   - **Hydrocortisone-containing preparations**, including creams, lotions, gels, suppositories, and aerosol foam
     - Creams, lotions, gels, and aerosol foam products often include an applicator for rectal administration
     - Apply topically by insertion into the rectum twice daily as needed
4. Severe proctitis
   - **Mesalamine rectal** suppositories 1000 mg inserted rectally twice daily
     - Retain in the rectum for 1–3 or more hours to increase exposure, and, potentially, beneficial response
     - Response may occur within days, but the usual duration of use is 3–6 weeks, depending on symptoms and endoscopic findings
   - **Mesalamine rectal** enema 4000 mg/60 mL instilled into the rectum once daily and retained for approximately 8 hours
     - Response may occur within days, but the usual duration of use is 3–6 weeks, depending on symptoms and endoscopic findings
   - Glucocorticoid retention enemas
     - **Hydrocortisone Rectal Suspension retention enema** 100 mg in 60 mL of an aqueous suspension once daily at bedtime
       - The enema should be retained for at least 1 hour, and preferably during hours of sleep. Overcoming the urge to evacuate may be facilitated by concurrent use of sedatives and antidiarrheal medications
       - Instructions for use often recommend patients lie on their left side during administration and for 30 minutes afterward to improve fluid distribution throughout the left colon
     - **Prednisolone retention enema** 20 mg/100 mL of prednisolone (as sodium phosphate) in an aqueous solution once daily at bedtime
       - Instructions for use as for Hydrocortisone Rectal Suspension (above)
     - **Sucralfate Suspension** 3000 mg as a retention enema in 15–30 mL water for 10–20 minutes once daily from the start of RT, until 2 weeks after RT is completed
     Note: In the United States, rectal use is "off-label" for both prednisolone and sucralfate, which are not marketed in the United States in formulations intended for rectal administration. Instead, the liquid products formulated for oral use are used as an enema

Small and Large Intestine: Late (Chronic) Side Effects

Presentation

1. Radiation injury to small bowel
   - Malabsorption of fat, diarrhea, persistent bleeding, ulceration, perforation, and fistulas
   - *Small bowel obstruction:* Uncommon, occurs 1–5 years after RT. Obstruction may be preceded by episodic, crampy, abdominal pain
2. Radiation injury to colon
   - Strictures, persistent painless bleeding, ulceration, tenesmus, obstipation, diarrhea, and rectal urgency
3. Rectovaginal fistulas may occur because of a high local RT dose from a brachytherapy implant

Management
1. Radiation injury to small bowel: Malabsorption
   • **Lactase enzyme** (eg, Lactaid) orally with dairy products
   • Pancreatic or lactase enzyme preparations: **Pancrelipase**—start with 400 units lipase/kg per meal orally and titrate to 2500 units lipase/kg per meal orally
   • *Note:* In some patients, enteric-coated pancrelipase enzyme tablets may not dissociate as intended and may pass through the bowel intact
   Note: Administer pancrelipase with meals or snacks. Individualize dosage by giving the number of tablets or capsules that optimally minimizes steatorrhea. Adjust doses slowly; monitor symptoms and response
     ▪ Select products with a high lipase content to avoid steatorrhea
     ▪ Do not crush or chew enteric-coated products or the enteric-coated contents of opened capsules
     ▪ Capsules may be opened and shaken onto a small quantity of soft food that is not hot and does not require chewing
     ▪ Pancrelipase should be swallowed immediately without chewing to prevent mucosal irritation
     ▪ Ingested doses should be followed with a glass of juice or water to ensure complete ingestion
     ▪ Avoid mixing pancrelipase with foods that have a pH >5.5, which can dissolve enteric coatings
   • **Parenteral nutrition** can improve outcome and delay surgery in some patients[35]
2. Radiation injury to small bowel, colon, and rectovaginal fistulas
   • Surgical intervention for persistent symptoms should be considered as a last resort

LIVER

Liver: Early (Acute) Side Effects

Presentation
1. *Acute hepatitis:* This is initially heralded by a relatively silent period, because more extensive radiation injury is required before the onset of clinically significant acute inflammation of hepatic tissues. Usually, symptoms occur subacutely

Management
1. Acute hepatitis:
   • Expectant

Liver: Subacute to Late (Chronic) Side Effects

Presentation
1. Radiation-induced liver disease (RILD)
   • The incidence of these severe toxicities is related to dose and treatment volume
   • The risk of liver damage is increased in patients who receive >30 Gy to the whole liver
     ▪ Liver dose <30 Gy; the incidence is <5%
   • Volume of liver irradiated plays a significant role. Some studies suggest if <25% of the liver is irradiated, there may be no dose-dependent risk of RILD[36]
   • Development of anicteric ascites 2–4 months after RT
   • Venoocclusive disease of the lobular central veins occurs
     ▪ Vague to intense right upper quadrant discomfort
     ▪ Ascites
     ▪ Jaundice occurs later; alkaline phosphatase level ≫ bilirubin and other LFTs[37,38]
   • *Computed tomography findings:* Low-density changes
2. Combined-modality-induced liver disease (CMILD) occurs with bone marrow preparative regimens
   • Occurs early, usually within 4–6 weeks after RT
   • Venoocclusive disease of the lobular central veins:
     ▪ Vague to intense right upper quadrant discomfort
     ▪ Ascites
     ▪ Jaundice occurs early; bilirubin ≫ alkaline phosphatase
   • There are no imaging findings in CMILD patients

Management

1. Radiation-induced liver disease (RILD) and combined-modality-induced liver disease (CMILD)
   - No specific therapy exists for treatment of RILD or CMILD
   - No proven benefit to anticoagulants or corticosteroids
   - Conservative management of ascites using diuretics, including spironolactone

GENITOURINARY SYSTEM: BLADDER

Urinary Bladder: Early (Acute) Side Effects

Presentation:

Usually begins 2 weeks after starting RT

1. Cystitis with dysuria
2. Urinary frequency and urgency
3. Obstructive urinary symptoms

Management

1. Dysuria
   - Topical analgesics
     - **Phenazopyridine hydrochloride** 200 mg orally 3 times daily
     - NSAIDs:
       - **Ibuprofen** 200 mg orally 3–4 times per day as needed
       - **Naproxen** 220 mg orally 1–2 times per day as needed
2. Urinary frequency and urgency
   - Antispasmodics
     - **Oxybutynin chloride** 5 mg orally 2–3 times per day as needed
     - **Flavoxate hydrochloride** 100–200 mg orally 3–4 times per day as needed
     - **Hyoscyamine sulfate** 0.125–0.30 mg orally 3–4 times per day as needed
3. Obstructive urinary symptoms
   - **Terazosin hydrochloride** start 1 mg orally at bedtime; titrate as needed over 4–6 weeks to a maximum of 20 mg/day
   - **Doxazosin mesylate** start 1 mg orally once a day; titrate as needed over 4–6 weeks to a maximum of 8 mg/day
   - **Tamsulosin hydrochloride** start 0.4 mg orally once a day; increase to 0.8 mg daily after 1–2 weeks
   - **Finasteride** 5 mg orally once daily

Urinary Bladder: Late (Chronic) Side Effects

Presentation

1. Persistent dysuria
2. Persistent frequency and urgency
3. Obstructive urinary symptoms
4. Hematuria or hemorrhage caused by telangiectasia or ulceration
5. Decreased bladder capacity
6. Urethral stricture, especially in patients with a history of transurethral resection of the prostate
7. Fistula
8. Sphincter insufficiency is less common; injury to ureters is rarely seen

Management

1. Persistent dysuria, frequency, urgency, and obstructive symptoms:
   - Symptomatic relief is the goal
   - Use agents recommended for acute management, as above
2. Hematuria or hemorrhage:
   - May require cystoscopy with bladder irrigation
   - Intravesical treatment with prostaglandins or silver nitrate can be used
   - Embolization of the hypogastric arteries may be a consideration
3. Severely decreased bladder capacity:
   - May require cystectomy

GENITOURINARY SYSTEM: KIDNEY

Kidneys: Early (Acute) Side Effects

Presentation
1. Acute radiation nephropathy
   - Rarely symptomatic
   - Symptoms are similar to those with nephropathy of other causes
   - *Note:* Renal damage is rarely reversible

Management
1. Acute radiation nephropathy
   - Limit the volume of kidney irradiated
   - TD 5/5 (5% incidence at 5 years) is 20 Gy if both kidneys are irradiated

Kidneys: Late (Chronic) Side Effects

Presentation
1. Chronic radiation nephropathy–chronic renal failure
   Note: The incidence of renal toxicity is dose-and volume-dependent. With increased volume irradiated and increased radiation dose, there is an increased risk of renal toxicity
   - When both kidneys are irradiated to 20 Gy, the rate of renal failure is 5% at 5 years
   - When both kidneys are irradiated to 28 Gy, the rate of renal failure is 50% at 5 years
   Note: Renal damage is rarely reversible. Progression to chronic radiation nephropathy can occur ≈1–2 years after completion of RT. Associated symptoms include:
   - Hyperreninemic hypertension
   - Nephrotic syndrome

Management
1. Chronic radiation nephropathy–chronic renal failure
   - Limit the volume of kidney irradiated. TD 5/5 (5% incidence at 5 years) is 20 Gy if both kidneys are irradiated
   - Low-protein diet and salt restriction may reduce kidney workload
   - For end-stage renal disease, dialysis or transplantation is needed

GENITOURINARY SYSTEM: TESTIS AND ERECTILE FUNCTION

Testis and Erectile Function: Early (Acute) Side Effects

Presentation
1. Azoospermia, oligospermia, and hormonal changes
   - Can occur even in patients receiving low-dose testicular RT
   Note: Sperm count may recover; however, recovery may take months or years after RT

Management
1. Azoospermia and oligospermia
   - Sperm banking before starting RT is recommended in men with fertility concerns

Testis and Erectile Function: Late Side Effects

Presentation
1. Erectile dysfunction
   - Can occur with high RT dose to the prostate
   - Radiation dose to the penile bulb appears to be a predictive factor for erectile dysfunction[39]

Management
1. Erectile dysfunction:
   - **Sildenafil citrate** 25–100 mg orally once daily 1 hour before sexual activity
   - **Vardenafil hydrochloride** 5–20 mg orally once daily 1 hour before sexual activity
   - **Tadalafil** 5–20 mg orally once daily 1 hour before sexual activity
   - Local therapy (consult a urologist):
     - **Alprostadil** (prostaglandin E_1) for intracavernosal injection or pellets for intraurethral insertion
     - Urethral implants

GENITOURINARY SYSTEM: VULVA

Vulva: Early (Acute) Side Effects

Presentation

1. Skin reactions
   - Vulvar reactions to radiation are essentially skin reactions but are more severe because of the location

Management

1. Skin reactions
   - Attention to personal hygiene
   - Topical steroids for symptoms of pruritus: **Hydrocortisone** cream 1–2.5%; apply locally twice daily
   - **Topical antibiotics** may be necessary if signs of infection are present: **Triple antibiotic ointment (polymyxin B sulfate + neomycin sulfate + bacitracin zinc)** apply twice daily to affected area
   - A treatment break from RT may be warranted if confluent grade 4 (moist desquamation) reaction occurs
   - Areas of moist desquamation may be treated topically with an aqueous solution of gentian violet (crystal violet) 1% which has an antimicrobial effect, but it dries and stains the dermis and may cause irritation and interfere with wound healing[40]

Vulva: Late (Chronic) Side Effects

Presentation

1. Skin atrophy
2. Ulceration
3. Fibrosis with associated dyspareunia
4. Pruritus
5. Pain
6. Telangiectasia
7. Pigmentation changes
8. Hair loss

Management

1. Atrophy of the skin
   - Topical estrogen or testosterone creams:
     - **Estradiol gel** 0.06% (eg, EstroGel) metered-dose pump 1.25 mg (1 metered application) topically to intact skin once daily, at the same time each day
   Note: The recommended area of application is the arm, from shoulder to wrist
     - **Estrace** cream topically once daily
   - Maintaining dose of radiation delivered to the vulvar region to 180 cGy/fraction or less may minimize the likelihood of long-term vulvar complications
2. Persistent ulceration
   - Surgical intervention
3. Fibrosis with narrowing of the introitus
   - Daily use of a dilator

GENITOURINARY SYSTEM: VAGINA

Vagina: Early (Acute) Side effects

Presentation

1. Vaginitis
2. Vaginal candidiasis

Management

1. Vaginitis

   • Vaginal douching with water or a 1:10 mixture of 1 part hydrogen peroxide with 9 parts water 2–3 times daily

2. Vaginal candidiasis

   • **Miconazole nitrate**

      ▪ *Intravaginal suppositories:* Insert 1 suppository intravaginally once daily at bedtime for 1 day (1200 mg/suppository), for 3 consecutive days (200 mg/suppository) or for 7 consecutive days (100 mg/suppository)

      ▪ *Intravaginal cream:* Insert 1 applicator-full intravaginally once daily at bedtime for 3 consecutive days (4% miconazole cream) or 7 consecutive days (2% miconazole cream)

      ▪ *Topical cream:* Apply to affected areas daily (morning and evening) for up to 7 consecutive days, or as needed

   • **Clotrimazole**

      ▪ *Intravaginal suppositories:* Insert 1 suppository intravaginally once daily at bedtime for 3 consecutive days (200 mg/suppository) or for 7 consecutive days (100 mg/suppository)

      ▪ *Topical cream:* Apply to affected areas twice daily (morning and evening) for up to 7 consecutive days or as needed

   • **Nystatin**

      ▪ *Vaginal tablets:* Insert 2 tablets using an applicator, high in the vagina daily for 2 weeks (100,000 units/tablet)

      ▪ *Topical cream:* Apply to affected external areas 2–3 time daily until healing is complete

      ▪ *Topical powder:* Apply to affected external areas 2–3 times daily until healing is complete

   • **Fluconazole** 150 mg orally for 1 dose

Vagina: Late (Chronic) Side Effects

Presentation

1. Adhesion, dyspareunia, fibrosis
2. Ulceration, fistula formation
3. Atrophy
4. Telangiectasia

Management

1. Adhesion formation and fibrosis

   • Daily vaginal dilation to prevent adhesion formation and fibrosis

   • Topical estrogen creams to promote healing and prevent atrophy and dyspareunia

      ▪ **Estradiol gel** 0.06% (eg, EstroGel) metered-dose pump 1.25 mg (1 metered application) topically to intact skin once daily, at the same time each day

   Note: The recommended area of application is the arm, from shoulder to wrist

      ▪ **Estradiol vaginal cream** (eg, Estrace) topically once daily

2. Persistent ulcer or fistula

   • Tumor recurrence must be ruled out

   • Surgical intervention may be necessary

GENITOURINARY SYSTEM: UTERINE CERVIX AND UTERUS

Uterine Cervix and Uterus: Early (Acute) Side Effects

Presentation

1. Ulceration of the uterine cervix

   • Unavoidable with RT for curative treatment of cervical cancer

   • May present with persistent clear watery discharge

Management:

1. Ulceration of the uterine cervix

   • Personal hygiene is essential to prevent super-infection

   • Vaginal douching with water or a 1:10 mixture of 1 part hydrogen peroxide and 9 parts water 2–3 times per day

   • If ulceration persists, the patient may require surgical intervention

Uterine Cervix and Uterus: Late (Chronic) Side Effects

Presentation

1. Hematometra
   - Rare complication caused by residual functioning endometrium and a stenotic cervical os
2. Cervical ulceration
   - Necrosis of the cervix (or uterus) can be seen with high-dose brachytherapy used in the treatment of gynecologic cancers

Management

1. Hematometra
   - Cervical os dilation and surgical debridement may be necessary

GENITOURINARY SYSTEM: OVARIES

Ovaries; Late (Chronic) Side Effects

Presentation

1. Permanent menopause develops in premenopausal women who receive high-dose RT to the ovaries
2. Sexual dysfunction with dyspareunia frequently follows treatment for pelvic malignancies. The causes are both physical and psychological

Management

1. Permanent menopause
   - When fertility is an issue, one can surgically move ovaries out of the RT portal before starting RT
   - To reduce hot flashes: **Venlafaxine extended release** 37.5 mg orally once daily[41]
2. Sexual dysfunction with dyspareunia
   - Attention to personal hygiene
   - Hormone replacement therapy. Many commercial preparations are available. Consult a gynecologist before initiation
   - Lubrication and daily dilation of the vagina may aid in prevention of dyspareunia

CENTRAL NERVOUS SYSTEM: BRAIN

Brain: Early (Acute) Side Effects

Presentation

1. Increased intracranial pressure (ICP) caused by RT-induced edema with the first few fractions of RT leads to:
   - Nausea
   - Vomiting
   - Increased headache
   - Changes in mental status (less commonly seen)
   - Worsening of neurologic signs (less commonly seen)
   - Seizures (less commonly seen)

Management

1. Increased ICP
   - **Dexamethasone** 10 mg orally or intravenously as a loading dose, followed by 4–6 mg intravenously or orally 4 times per day. The dose can be tapered after symptoms have stabilized for 3–4 days

   Note: A fast tapering schedule with a reduction in dose of 50% every 3–4 days is recommended if a patient has been receiving dexamethasone less than 1 week

Brain: Subacute Side Effects

Presentation

1. Somnolence syndrome
   - Often noted ≈1–4 months after cranial RT
   - Characterized by drowsiness, fatigue, nausea, irritability, anorexia, apathy, and dizziness without focal neurologic abnormalities
   - Resolves spontaneously within 2–5 weeks

   Note: Focal neurologic signs seen after RT may be related to intralesional or local reaction, such as edema, demyelination, or bleeding into a tumor

Management

1. Somnolence syndrome may be alleviated by corticosteroids
   - **Dexamethasone** 10 mg orally or intravenously as a loading dose followed by 4–6 mg intravenously or orally 4 times per day. The dose can be tapered after symptoms have stabilized for 3–4 days

   Note: May need a slow taper depending on a patient's symptoms
   - **Methylphenidate** may be used with some efficacy after whole brain radiotherapy. Dose is usually started at 10 mg twice daily and then increased to 30 mg twice daily as tolerated with 2-week intervals between increases in dose[42]

Brain: Late (Chronic) Side Effects

Presentation

1. Focal necrosis of the brain
   - Occurs 6 months to several years after RT
   - Occurs in 1–5% of patients who received ≥60 Gy to the brain
   - Associated with focal symptoms as well as symptoms associated with increased ICP
   - Abnormalities can be seen on CT scan or magnetic resonance imaging
   - A void of metabolic activity on PET (positron emission tomography) scan can confirm the clinical diagnosis
2. Leukoencephalopathy
   - Diffuse white matter injury
   - Characterized by lethargy, seizures, spasticity, paresis, ataxia, dementia, or even death
   - More severe forms are seen in patients who received combined chemotherapy and RT
   - The incidence of leukoencephalopathy has been reported to be as high as 45% when RT and intravenous or intrathecal methotrexate were given together and <1% when RT is given alone[43]
3. Neuropsychological and intellectual deficits
   - Memory deficits and learning disabilities can be seen in children 6 months after RT
   - Global IQ decline can be observed 1–2 years after RT[44]
   - Risk factors for more severe deficits,[45] include:
     - Young age when exposed to RT
     - High RT doses
     - Large volume of brain irradiated
4. In adults, memory loss, confusion, dementia, ataxia, and psychomotor retardation can also be seen
5. RT-induced glioma
   - Well documented in pediatric medical literature
   - 15-year cumulative risk is estimated to be 2.7%[46]

Management

1. Focal necrosis
   - May be alleviated by corticosteroids: **Dexamethasone** 10 mg orally or intravenously as a loading dose, followed by 4–6 mg intravenously or orally 4 times per day. The dose can be tapered after symptoms have stabilized for 3–4 days

   Note: May need a slow taper, depending on a patient's symptoms
   - Symptomatic treatment with anticonvulsant drugs
   - Surgical resection may be needed
2. Leukoencephalopathy
   - Supportive care
3. Neuropsychological and intellectual deficits
   - A phase II study conducted by Shaw et al. suggests that 6 months of treatment with **donepezil** improved long-term cognitive function, mood, and health-related quality of life with minimal toxicity. Patients were treated with 5 mg for the initial 6 weeks and then 10 mg for the remaining 24 weeks

CENTRAL NERVOUS SYSTEM: SPINAL CORD

Spinal Cord: Early (Acute) Side Effects

Presentation

1. Demyelination
   - Transient radiation effects on the spinal cord may be seen within 2–4 months after RT
   - Incidence is as high as 15% after mantle RT for Hodgkin disease
   - Presumed to be the result of the transient demyelination within the RT portal[47]
   - Lhermitte sign: Electric-like shock radiating down the spine to the extremities with flexion of the neck
   - Spontaneous resolution expected within 6 months. No relationship to late injury reported

Management

1. Demyelination
   - Symptoms may be alleviated by corticosteroids: **Dexamethasone** 10 mg orally or intravenously as a loading dose followed by 4–6 mg intravenously or orally 4 times per day. The dose can be tapered after symptoms have stabilized for 3–4 days
   - *Note:* May need a slow taper, depending on a patient's symptoms
   - **Gabapentin** 100–600 mg orally 3 times per day can be used for pain

Spinal Cord: Late (Chronic) Side Effects

Presentation

1. Chronic progressive radiation myelitis (CPRM)
   - Rare but devastating late effect. Symptoms start 9–15 months after RT is completed
   - Caused by intramedullary vascular damage that progresses to hemorrhagic necrosis or infarction and extensive demyelination with white matter necrosis
   - Presents with progressive paresthesias, sensory changes, and weakness
   - Risk of developing CPRM varies directly with:
     - Radiation fraction size
     - Length of the cord treated
     - Total dose: A cord dose of 45 Gy in 1.8- to 2-Gy daily fractions has <0.2% chance of developing CPRM[48]
   - The majority of patients die of secondary complications

Management

1. CPRM
   - High-dose corticosteroids: **Dexamethasone** 10 mg orally or intravenously 4 times per day. The dose can be tapered slowly after symptoms have stabilized or improved for several days
   - Use of **hyperbaric oxygen** may lead to remission

ENDOCRINE SYSTEM

Endocrine System: Early (Acute) Side Effects

Presentation

1. Hyperthyroidism
   - Thyrotoxicosis has rarely been reported after mantle or cervical RT for Hodgkin disease
   - Subsequently evolves into hypothyroidism
2. Diffuse, symmetric thyroid enlargement resembling Hashimoto thyroiditis has been reported but is a rare reaction to RT

Management

1. Hyperthyroidism
   - Antithyroid agents may be needed, such as **methimazole or propylthiouracil.** In addition, a β-blocker may also be needed. Consult an endocrinologist for help in management

Endocrine System: Late (Chronic) Side Effects

Presentation

1. Hypothyroidism
   - Late RT effect, 1–2 years after RT
   - As high as 63% at 10 years after treatment of head and neck region and thorax[49]
   - Can also be seen in patients who receive a moderate dose to the pituitary that leads to the decreased production of thyroid stimulating hormone
   - Risk factors
     - *Dose:* Some studies show a relationship between dose and RT-induced hypothyroidism
     - *Age:* Young children tend to be more susceptible
     - *Chemotherapy:* Some studies show chemotherapy increases the risk of hypothyroidism when used in combination with moderate doses of RT

2. Thyroid cancer
   - A late effect of radiation exposure
   - Risk after RT is about 1.7% in adults[50]
   - Risk is increased in children and young adults[51]

Management

1. Hypothyroidism
   - TSH and thyroxin (T_4) levels should be measured every 6 months after head and neck and upper thoracic RT
   - If hypothyroidism develops, treat accordingly

References

1. Trotti A, Colevas AD, Setser A et al. CTCAE v3.0: development of a comprehensive grading system for the adverse effects of cancer treatment. Semin Radiat Oncol 2003;13:176–181
2. Emami B, Lyman J, Brown A et al. Tolerance of normal tissue to therapeutic irradiation. Int J Radiat Oncol Biol Phys 1991;21:109–122
3. Grigsby PW, Roberts HL, Perez CA. Femoral neck fracture following groin irradiation. Int J Radiat Oncol Biol Phys 1995;32:63–67
4. Momm F, Weißenberger C, Bartelt S et al. Moist skin care can diminish acute radiation-induced skin toxicity. Strahlenther Onkol 2003;179:708–712
5. Delanian S, Porcher R, Balla-Mekias S, Lefaix J-L. Randomized, placebo-controlled trial of combined pentoxifylline and tocopherol for regression of superficial radiation-induced fibrosis. J Clin Oncol 2003;21:2545–2550
6. Thorn JJ, Hansen HS, Specht L, Bastholt L. Osteoradionecrosis of the jaws: clinical characteristics and relation to the field of irradiation. J Oral Maxillofac Surg 2000;8:1088–1093; discussion 1093–1095
7. Lin PP, Schupak KD, Boland PJ et al. Pathologic femoral fracture after periosteal excision and radiation for the treatment of soft tissue sarcoma. Cancer 1998;82:2356–2365
8. Baxter NN, Habermann EB, Tepper JE et al. Risk of pelvic fractures in older women following pelvic irradiation. JAMA 2005;294:2587–2593
9. Helmstedter CS, Goebel M, Zlotecki R, Scarborough MT. Pathologic fractures after surgery and radiation for soft tissue tumors. Clin Orthop Relat Res 2001;389:165–172
10. Konski A, Sowers M. Pelvic fractures following irradiation for endometrial carcinoma. Int J Radiat Oncol Biol Phys 1996;35:361–367
11. Massin P, Duparc J. Total hip replacement in irradiated hips. A retrospective study of 71 cases. J Bone Joint Surg Br 1995;77:847–852
12. Pan CC, Eisbruch A, Lee JS et al. Prospective study of inner ear radiation dose and hearing loss in head-and-neck cancer patients. Int J Radiat Oncol Biol Phys 2005;61:1393–1402
13. Bhandare N, Antonelli PJ, Morris CG et al. Ototoxicity after radiotherapy for head and neck tumors. Int J Radiat Oncol Biol Phys 2007;67:469–479
14. Huang E, Teh BS, Strother DR et al. Intensity-modulated radiation therapy for pediatric medulloblastoma: early report on the reduction of ototoxicity. Int J Radiat Oncol Biol Phys 2002;52:599–605
15. Cerchietti LCA, Navigante AH, Bonomi MR et al. Effect of topical morphine for mucositis-associated pain following concomitant chemoradiotherapy for head and neck carcinoma. Cancer 2002;95:2230–2236
16. Fisher J, Scott C, Scarantino CW et al. Phase III quality-of-life study results: impact on patients' quality of life to reducing xerostomia after radiotherapy for head-and-neck cancer–RTOG 97–09. Int J Radiat Oncol Biol Phys 2003;56:832–836
17. Brizel DM, Wasserman TH, Henke M et al. Phase III randomized trial of amifostine as a radioprotector in head and neck cancer. J Clin Oncol 2000;18:3339–3345
18. Koukourakis MI, Simopoulos C, Minopoulos G et al. Amifostine before chemotherapy: improved tolerance profile of the subcutaneous over the intravenous route. Clin Cancer Res 2003;9:3288–3293
19. Jha N, Seikaly H, Harris J et al. Prevention of radiation induced xerostomia by surgical transfer of submandibular salivary gland into the submental space. Radiother Oncol 2003;66:283–289
20. Eisbruch A, Lyden T, Bradford CR et al. Objective assessment of swallowing dysfunction and aspiration after radiation concurrent with chemotherapy for head-and-neck cancer. Int J Radiat Oncol Biol Phys 2002;53:23–28
21. Kies MS, Haraf DJ, Athanasiadis I et al. Induction chemotherapy followed by concurrent chemoradiation for advanced head and neck cancer: improved disease control and survival. J Clin Oncol 1998;16:2715–2721
22. Eisbruch A, Schwartz M, Rasch C et al. Dysphagia and aspiration after chemoradiotherapy for head-and-neck cancer: which anatomic structures are affected and can they be spared by IMRT? Int J Radiat Oncol Biol Phys 2004;60:1425–1439
23. Holt JAG. The acute radiation pneumonitis syndrome. J Coll Radiol Australas 1964;8:40–47
24. Robnett TJ, Machtay M, Vines EF et al. Factors predicting severe radiation pneumonitis in patients receiving definitive chemoradiation for lung cancer. Int J Radiat Oncol Biol Phys 2000;48:89–94
25. Johansson S, Bjermer L, Franzen L, Henriksson R. Effects of ongoing smoking on the development of radiation-induced pneumonitis in breast cancer and oesophagus cancer patients. Radiother Oncol 1998;49:41–47
26. Graham MV, Purdy JA, Emami B et al. Clinical dose-volume histogram analysis for pneumonitis after 3D treatment for non-small cell lung cancer (NSCLC). Int J Radiat Oncol Biol Phys 1999;45:323–329
27. Rosen II, Fischer TA, Antolak JA et al. Correlation between lung fibrosis and radiation therapy dose after concurrent radiation therapy and chemotherapy for limited small cell lung cancer. Radiology 2001;221:614–622

28. Komaki R, Lee JS, Kaplan B et al. Randomized phase III study of chemoradiation with or without amifostine for patients with favorable performance status inoperable stage II-III non–small cell lung cancer: preliminary results. Semin Radiat Oncol 2002;12:46–49
29. Antonadou D, Throuvalas N, Petridis A et al. Effect of amifostine on toxicities associated with radiochemotherapy in patients with locally advanced non–small-cell lung cancer. Int J Radiat Oncol Biol Phys 2003;57:402–408
30. Movsas B, Scott C, Langer C et al. Randomized trial of amifostine in locally advanced non-small-cell lung cancer patients receiving chemotherapy and hyperfractionated radiation: radiation therapy oncology group trial 98–01. J Clin Oncol 2005;23:2145–2154
31. Gyenes G, Gagliardi G, Lax I et al. Evaluation of irradiated heart volumes in stage I breast cancer patients treated with postoperative adjuvant radiotherapy. J Clin Oncol 1997;15:1348–1353
32. Morrow JB, Dumot JA, Vargo JJ 2nd. Radiation-induced hemorrhagic carditis treated with argon plasma coagulator. Gastrointest Endosc 2000;51:498–499
33. Henriksson R, Franzén L, Littbrand B: Effects of sucralfate on acute and late bowel discomfort following radiotherapy of pelvic cancer. J Clin Oncol 1992;10:969–975
34. Yavuz MN, Yavuz AA, Aydin F et al. The efficacy of octreotide in the therapy of acute radiation-induced diarrhea: a randomized controlled study. Int J Radiat Oncol Biol Phys 2002;54:195–202
35. Silvain C, Besson I, Ingrand P et al. Long-term outcome of severe radiation enteritis treated by total parenteral nutrition. Dig Dis Sci 1992;37:1065–1071
36. Dawson LA, Ten Haken RK, Lawrence TS. Partial irradiation of the liver. Semin Radiat Oncol 2001;11:240–246
37. Ganem G, Saint-Marc Girardin M-F, Kuentz M et al. Venoocclusive disease of the liver after allogeneic bone marrow transplantation in man. Int J Radiat Oncol Biol Phys 1988;14:879–884
38. Piedbois P, Ganem G, Cordonnier C et al. Interstitial pneumonitis and venoocclusive disease of the liver after bone marrow transplantation. Radiother Oncol 1990;18(Suppl 1):125–127
39. Merrick GS, Butler WM, Wallner KE et al. The importance of radiation doses to the penile bulb vs. crura in the development of postbrachytherapy erectile dysfunction. Int J Radiat Oncol Biol Phys 2002;54:1055–1062
40. Mak SSS, Molassiotis A, Wan W-M et al. The effects of hydrocolloid dressing and gentian violet on radiation-induced moist desquamation wound healing. Cancer Nurs 2000;23:220–229
41. Loprinzi CL, Kugler JW, Sloan JA et al. Venlafaxine in management of hot flashes in survivors of breast cancer: a randomised controlled trial. Lancet 2000;356:2059–2063
42. Weitzner MA, Meyers CA, Valentine AD. Methylphenidate in the treatment of neurobehavioral slowing associated with cancer and cancer treatment. J Neuropsychiatry Clin Neurosci 1995;7:347–350
43. Bleyer AW, Griffin TW. White matter necrosis, mineralizing microangiopathy, and intellectual abilities in survivors of childhood leukemia: associations with central nervous system irradiation and methotrexate therapy. In: Gilbert HA, Kagan AR, eds. Radiation Damage to the Nervous System: A Delayed Therapeutic Hazard. New York: Raven Press; 1980:225
44. Palmer SL, Goloubeva O, Reddick WE et al. Patterns of intellectual development among survivors of pediatric medulloblastoma: a longitudinal analysis. J Clin Oncol 2001;19:2302–2308
45. Mulhern RK, Kepner JL, Thomas PR et al. Neuropsychologic functioning of survivors of childhood medulloblastoma randomized to receive conventional or reduced-dose craniospinal irradiation: a Pediatric Oncology Group study. J Clin Oncol 1998;16:1723–1728
46. Tsang RW, Laperriere NJ, Simpson WJ et al. Glioma arising after radiation therapy for pituitary adenoma. A report of four patients and estimation of risk. Cancer 1993;72:2227–2233
47. Jones A. Transient radiation myelopathy (with reference to Lhermitte's sign of electrical paraesthesia). Br J Radiol 1964;37:727–744
48. Marcus RB Jr, Million RR. The incidence of myelitis after irradiation of the cervical spinal cord. Int J Radiat Oncol Biol Phys 1990;19:3–8
49. Pai HH, Thornton A, Katznelson L et al. Hypothalamic/pituitary function following high-dose conformal radiotherapy to the base of skull: demonstration of a dose-effect relationship using dose-volume histogram analysis. Int J Radiat Oncol Biol Phys 2001;49:1079–1092
50. Hancock SL, Cox RS, McDougall IR. Thyroid diseases after treatment of Hodgkin's disease. N Engl J Med 1991;325:599–605
51. Hanford JM, Quimby EH, Frantz VK. Cancer arising many years after radiation therapy. Incidence after irradiation of benign lesions in the neck. JAMA 1962;181:404–410

52. Cancer Pain: Assessment and Management

Ann Berger, MSN, MD

Definition of Pain

Pain is "an unpleasant sensory and emotional experience associated with actual or potential tissue damage" (IASP Subcommittee on Taxonomy, p. 250). What this tells us is that pain is far more than a physical phenomenon; it clearly has a sensory and emotional component. A very important definition of pain is: "Pain is whatever the experiencing person says it is, existing whenever he/she says it does" (McCaffery, p. 95). This is important in that it is critical to always believe the patient with cancer who says that he/she has pain

Pain terms: a list with definitions and notes on usage. Recommended by the IASP Subcommittee on Taxonomy. Pain 1979;6:249–252
McCaffery M. Nursing Practice theories related to cognition, bodily pain, and man–environment interactions. Los Angeles, UCLA Student Store, 1968

Prevalence

- More than 70% of patients with advanced cancer report having moderate-to-severe pain
- At time of diagnosis and during active treatment, 30–50% of patients have cancer pain
- In the advanced stages, 70–90% have pain (Levy)
- 40–50% of patients report their pain as being moderate or severe
- 25–30% of patients report very severe or excruciating pain
- In a large series of 2000 patients, one-third had 1 site of pain, one-third had 2 sites of pain, and one-third had 3 or more sites (Twycross)

Levy MH. N Engl J Med 1996;335:1124–1132
Twycross R. In: Sykes N, Fallon MT, Patt RP, eds. Clinical Pain Management: Cancer Pain/Practical Applications & Procedures. London, UK: Hodder & Stoughton Educational; 2003:3–21

Table 52–1. Etiology of Cancer Pain

1. Pain secondary to tumor involvement

Invasion into cutaneous, deep tissues and bone, resulting in somatic pain:
- Bone pain
- Muscle and soft tissue pain
- Headache

Injury to sympathetically innervated organs, resulting in visceral pain:
- Hepatic distention syndrome
- Midline retroperitoneal syndrome
- Chronic intestinal obstruction
- Peritoneal carcinomatosis
- Malignant perineal pain
- Adrenal pain syndrome
- Ureteric obstruction

Aberrant somatosensory processes caused by injury to nervous system, resulting in neuropathic pain:
- Cranial neuralgias
- Radiculopathies
- Brachial plexopathy
- Lumbosacral plexopathy
- Peripheral mononeuropathies
- Spinal cord compression

2. Pain after diagnostic and therapeutic procedures
- Lumbar puncture
- Needle biopsy
- Bone marrow biopsy
- Paracentesis/thoracentesis

3. Treatment-related pain

Surgical removal of tumor or metastases:
- Postoperative pain
- Postmastectomy pain
- Post–radical neck dissection pain
- Postthoracotomy pain
- Stump and phantom limb pain
- Lymphedema

Chemotherapy:
- Mucositis
- Peripheral neuropathy
- Arthralgia and myalgia caused by paclitaxel
- Hand/foot syndrome (capecitabine)
- Flare of bone pain with hormonal therapy for breast and prostate cancer

Radiation therapy:
- Mucositis/esophagitis
- Enteritis and proctitis
- Myelitis
- Chronic myelopathy
- Plexopathy (brachial and lumbosacral)
- Osteoradionecrosis
- Skin "burns"

Other:
- Growth factor-induced bone pain
- Postherpetic neuralgia
- Aldesleukin (IL-2)- and interferon-related myalgias

Portenoy RK, Conn M. Cancer pain syndromes. In: Bruera ED, Portenoy RK, eds. Cancer Pain: Assessment and Management. New York, NY: Cambridge University Press; 2003:89–108
McGuire DB. Occurrence of cancer pain. J Natl Cancer Inst Monogr 2004;32:51–56

Table 52–2. Physical Pain Assessment

Where is it most painful now?

How long have you been in pain?

Has this changed from your initial complaint?

What is the temporal pattern of your pain? Is it continuous, or is it intermittent?

What are the characteristics of the pain: aching, cramping, burning, throbbing, numb, tingling, shooting?

What is its intensity: at present, at its lowest, and at its highest level? Scale: 0–10; or mild, moderate, severe

What is an acceptable or tolerable level of pain?

What factors aggravate the pain, such as moving, standing, or sitting?

What factors relieve pain, such as heat, cold, massage, or medications?

What treatments have you tried, what has been their effectiveness, and what side effects have you experienced? (Include over-the-counter medications and alternative and complementary therapies.)

Table 52–3. Types of Pain

Type	Description	Examples	Treatment
Somatic	Localized, aching, throbbing	Bone, joint pain Gnawing feeling	NSAIDs, opioids
Visceral	Pressure, tightening, aching	Pleural, hepatic disease Pulling, stretching	NSAIDs, opioids, steroids
Neuropathic	Severe, sharp, shooting, stabbing, burning, hot, numbing, tingling	Peripheral neuropathy Postherpetic neuralgia	Opioids, steroids, neuroleptics, tricyclic antidepressants, acupuncture
Myofascial	Tightness, pulling, spasm	Upper back, neck	NSAIDs, heat, stretching, TENS trigger point release

TENS, Transcutaneous electrical nerve stimulation

Note: Suffering and pain issues: Total pain is more than just physical pain. Total pain can involve a suffering component as well as a physical component. Suffering involves psychological and coping factors, social support and loss issues, fear of death, financial concerns, and spiritual concerns

Table 52–4. Assessment of Pain: Psychosocial Assessment

Initial Assessment	Reassessment
What are you most hoping for?	How do you feel things are going?
What are your goals, and how can we best achieve it?	What is the hardest part of your treatment?
What do you fear the most?	Are you having good days? Are you finding enjoyment in things?
Who do you turn to for support?	How is your family/spouse/significant other doing?
Why do you think this disease has occurred? What other losses have you endured during your life?	What helps you meet the challenges you endure?
Do you want others to be involved in decision making about your care?	Who would speak on your behalf if complications arise?

Reproduced, with permission, from Baker K, Berger A. Cancer Pain Assessment: Where Does It Hurt? In: Berger A, ed. Advances in Cancer Pain: A Bedside Approach. The Oncology Group, CMP Healthcare Media, ©2004

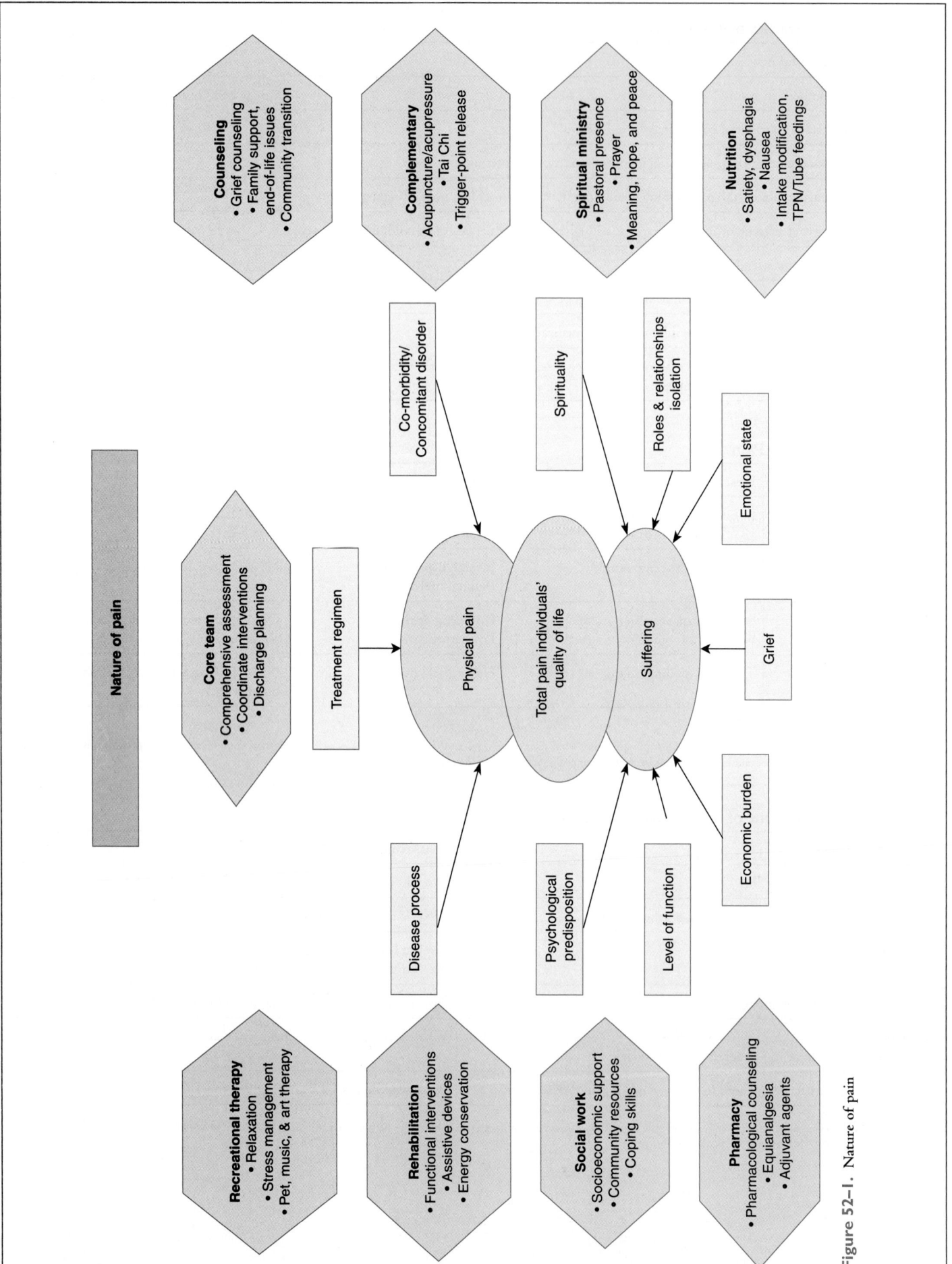

Figure 52–1. Nature of pain

Table 52–5. Other Issues to Address in Pain Assessment

- Current mood state
- History of psychiatric disorders
- Social support
- Financial stress/insurance issues
- Access to healthcare/medications
- Current use of illicit drugs/alcohol
- Past history of substance abuse
- Coping skills
- Home environment (physical layout, who is living in the home)
- Primary language spoken, literacy
- Conflict within the family
- Loss/grief issues
- Fears
- Comorbidities
- Concurrent symptoms (fatigue, nausea, diarrhea/constipation, insomnia)
- Concurrent medications
- Cultural influences/preferences
- Functional status
- Patient goals
- Family concerns/issues

Table 52–6. Pain: The Spiritual History

- *Faith*: Is spirituality a part of your life?
- *Meaning*: What meaning do you place on having this cancer pain?
- What is your meaning of being?
- *Importance*: What significance does your belief have on your disease?
- *Community*: Do you have a supportive spiritual community?
- *Care*: How can we attend to these spiritual needs in your care?

Ambuel B. Taking a spiritual history #19. J Palliat Med 2003;6:932–933

Table 52–7. Important Terms with Opioid Use

- *Tolerance*: The need to escalate doses of opioids despite a lack of change in the pain being treated. This is a rare occurrence. Opioid doses usually require escalation because of worsening pain in the face of disease progression
- *Physical dependence*: After approximately 1 week on steady dosing of opioids, the body becomes physically dependent on the medication. If one were to abruptly stop the opioids, withdrawal symptoms would occur. Hence, all opioids should be tapered over time. Note that the experience of withdrawal can often be confused with addiction
- *Addiction*: A psychological and behavioral process that encompasses 3 types of aberrant phenomenon: loss of control over drug use, compulsive drug use, and continued use despite harm. There is a craving for the opioid, and extreme measures will be taken to gain access, for example, theft, prostitution, and so on. The risk involves those who take opioids for reasons other than pain. The risk of addiction is very low in individuals who take opioids for pain
- *Pseudoaddiction:* Occurs when pain is being undertreated. The individual monitors very closely the timing of the opioids and is frequently asking for opioids more frequently than ordered and/or for a higher dose. They are striving to get better pain control, not an inappropriate amount of opioids for other intentions

---

Table 52–8. Principles of Opioid Management

I. Dosing and dose titration

  A. Consider prior exposure to opioids and dosing requirement

  B. Dose according to pain intensity

  C. Perform ongoing reassessment and titrate to therapeutic effect or toxicity

  D. Titrate upward by 25–50%

  E. Begin with as-needed (PRN) dosing to determine opioid requirement

  F. Should frequent PRN dosing be required, pain is constant or severe, consider long-acting agent

  G. Determine 24-hour opioid requirement and convert to long-acting agent

  H. Provide short-acting agent for breakthrough dosing (5–15% of long-acting opioid dose)

II. Monitoring and treatment of side effects

  A. Sedation

    1. May develop tolerance 2–3 days after initiation of an opioid or dose adjustment

    2. Assess use of other centrally acting agents

    3. Check organ function

    4. Adjust opioid dose by 30–50%

    5. May consider use of a stimulant such as **methylphenidate HCl** 5–20 mg orally for 2 doses/day at 8 am and 12 noon, or one dose after waking and a second dose approximately 4 hours later

    6. Reassure staff and family that this might be secondary to sleep deprivation in the past

  B. Respiratory depression

    1. Monitor sedation in opioid-naïve patients

    2. Slow and safe titration

  C. Nausea

    1. Consider other causative factors

    2. Assess bowel function

    3. Review concurrent medications

    4. Rotate opioids

    5. If other opioids are not an option:

      a. Medicate with an antiemetic to help central and peripheral mechanisms such as:

       • **Metoclopramide** 10–40 mg (or 0.5 mg/kg per dose) orally 4 times daily, *or*

      b. Medicate with an antiemetic to help vestibular (motion-related) nausea such as:

       • **Meclizine HCl** 6.25–25 mg orally 4 times per day, *or*

       • **Scopolamine** 1.5-mg patch applied to intact skin behind an ear every 72 hours

    Note: Although scopolamine is also available in products formulated for oral and parenteral administration, such products are less useful for continuous symptom management than the transdermal patch system because of a shorter duration of action and a greater incidence of anticholinergic adverse effects associated with transiently high systemic concentrations after intermittent use

    6. Consider use of acupressure bands

  D. Constipation

    1. Tolerance does not develop

    2. Prevent constipation with a daily bowel regimen that includes **docusate** and **senna**

St. Germaine D, Berger A. Cancer pain management. In: Berger A, ed. Handbook of Supportive Oncology. Hackensack, NJ: Cambridge Medical Publications (in press)

Table 52–9. Opioid Equianalgesic Dosing

Drug	Oral (mg)	IV (mg)	Ratio (PO:IV)
Codeine	200	—	—
Fentanyl*	—	80–100 mcg	—
Hydrocodone	20	—	—
Hydromorphone	7.5	1.5	5:1
Methadone†	3	1.5	2:1
Morphine	30	10	3:1
Oxycodone	20	—	—
Oxymorphone	10	1	10:1

*Morphine 1 mg IV is equivalent to fentanyl 10 mcg IV
†Methadone equianalgesic potency varies relative to dose of opioid

Morphine Equivalence

From	↔	To	Ratio					
			Oral	↔	Oral	IV	↔	IV
Morphine	↔	Hydromorphone	4	↔	1	6	↔	1
Morphine	↔	Oxycodone	1.5	↔	1	—	↔	—
Morphine	↔	Methadone*	10	↔	1	6	↔	1
Morphine	↔	Fentanyl**	—	↔	—	100	↔	1

Morphine/Fentanyl Equivalence

Morphine 1 mg/hour intravenously	≈	Fentanyl 10 mcg/hour intravenously
Fentanyl 10 mcg/hour intravenously	≈	Fentanyl 10 mcg/hour transdermally
Transmucosal fentanyl (Actiq) 200 mcg	≈	2 mg morphine intravenously

Daily Oral Morphine Equivalents (DOME) → Transdermal Fentanyl

DOME (mg)	→	Transdermal Fentanyl (mcg/hour)
60–134	→	25
135–224	→	50
225–314	→	75
315–404	→	100
405–494	→	125
495–585	→	150

Transdermal Fentanyl → DOME (Daily Oral Morphine Equivalents)

25 mcg/hour patch	→	50 mg DOME
100 mcg/hour patch	→	200 mg DOME

Notes regarding fentanyl transdermal system (commonly known as "fentanyl patches"; Duragesic and generic products): Analgesic onset begins in 6–12 hours with peak effect in 24–72 hours. Change patches every 72 hours. The analgesic effect decreases by 50% at 17 hours after discontinuation. DO NOT use a fentanyl transdermal system in *opioid-naïve patients* (ie, persons taking <45 mg oral morphine daily)

(*continued*)

Table 52–9. *(continued)*

Actiq (oral transmucosal fentanyl) → Fentora (fentanyl buccal tablets)
Actiq 200 mcg is equivalent to 2 mg IV morphine
Actiq 800 mcg is equivalent to 8 mg IV morphine

Actiq (mcg) (Oral Transmucosal Fentanyl)	→	Fentora (mcg) (Fentanyl Buccal Tablets)
200	→	100
400	→	100
600	→	200
800	→	200
1200	→	400
1600	→	400

Notes regarding Actiq (oral transmucosal fentanyl citrate):
- Analgesic onset begins in 5–15 minutes with peak effect in 20–40 minutes and lasts 2–4 hours. Twirl between cheek and gum until dissolved. Doses may be repeated every 4 hours as needed
- Actiq is indicated only for the management of breakthrough cancer pain in patients *who are already receiving and who are tolerant to around-the-clock opioid therapy for their underlying pain*. Patients considered opioid tolerant are those who are taking around-the-clock medicine consisting of at least 60 mg of oral morphine daily, or an equianalgesic dose of another opioid daily for a week or longer. Patients must remain on around-the-clock opioids when taking Actiq
- Substantial differences exist in the pharmacokinetic profile of Actiq compared to other fentanyl products that result in clinically important differences in the extent of absorption of fentanyl. As a result of these differences, the substitution of Actiq for any other fentanyl product may result in a fatal overdose
- The initial dose of Actiq is always 200 mcg. The medication should be titrated to a dose that provides adequate analgesia and minimizes side effects
- If a breakthrough pain (BTP) episode is not relieved 15 minutes after completion of an Actiq unit (30 minutes after the start of the unit), patients may take ONLY 1 additional dose using the same strength for that BTP episode
- Patients must wait at least 4 hours before taking another dose
- Once titrated to an effective dose, patients should limit their consumption of Actiq to 4 or fewer units per day

PCA guidelines for opioid-naïve patients:
No basal rate (continuous infusion) until basal analgesic requirements are established
Usual lockout period ranges from 6 to 12 minutes
Examples
Morphine: no basal, 1 mg per dose, lockout 10 minutes
Hydromorphone: no basal, 0.2 mg per dose, lockout 10 minutes
Fentanyl: no basal, 10–15 mcg per dose, lockout 10 minutes

Table 52–10. Principles of Adjuvant Medication Use

I. Choose Appropriate Analgesics
  A. Introduce adjuvant therapy when:
    1. Opioids/analgesics are ineffective or produce unacceptable side effects
    2. Mechanism of pain is identified
  B. Select adjuvant agent with lowest adverse-effect profile
  C. Consider drug–drug interactions
  D. Anticipate therapeutic response time
  E. Discuss goals of therapy with patient:
    1. Titration process
    2. Anticipated response time
  F. Begin at lowest recommended dose
  G. Titrate 1 agent at a time to effectiveness or dose-limiting toxicities:
    1. Titrate no sooner than every 72 hours
    2. Titration schedule is dependent on half-life of agent
  H. If partial response obtained with dose-limiting toxicities:
    1. Lower existing dose by 25%
    2. Add agent from a different drug class
  I. If partial response obtained at maximum dosing without toxicities: add agent from a different drug class

II. Reevaluate
  A. Determine response and side effects
  B. Decrease opioid dose as adjuvant agents reach effectiveness
  C. Consider combining adjuvant drugs with different mechanisms of action
  D. Introduce complementary modalities to optimize pain management

---

St. Germaine D, Berger A. Cancer pain management. In: Berger A, ed. Handbook of Supportive Oncology. Hackensack, NJ: Cambridge Medical Publications (in press).

Table 52-11. Neuropathic Pain Medications

Note on dosing: For some of the drugs, the maximum daily doses specified may produce systemic concentrations that are associated with pharmacologic toxicities, particularly in patients with impaired end-organ function. For these, information about toxic concentrations for the drug and relevant metabolites are provided as follows: TDM Toxic: [*analyte name*], concentrations at which drug-related toxicities typically occur (specimen in which the concentration is measured). TDM, Therapeutic drug monitoring

Drug	Analgesic Indication	Dosing (*see note above*)	Special Considerations	Side Effects
Anticonvulsants				
Carbamazepine	Trigeminal neuralgia Diabetic neuropathy	300 mg TID orally Max. 300 mg QID orally	Obtain CBC and LFTs before administration Monitor for agranulocytosis	Somnolence, dizziness, gait disturbance
Note: TDM Toxic: *carbamazepine* (blood) ≥15 mg/L (≥64 µmol/L)				
Gabapentin	Postherpetic neuralgia Diabetic neuropathy Migraine headaches	300 mg TID orally Max. 1200 mg TID orally	Somnolence may require lower initial dosing Night-time dosing may facilitate sleep	Somnolence, diarrhea, mood swings, fatigue nausea, dizziness
Note: TDM Toxic: *gabapentin* (blood) ≥25 mcg/mL (≥25 mg/L)				
Lamotrigine	HIV neuropathy Trigeminal neuralgia Cold-induced allodynia	25–50 mg/day orally Max. 200 mg BID orally	Titrate slowly For pain refractory to phenytoin and carbamazepine Valproic acid reduces clearance	Rash, dizziness, ataxia, constipation, nausea, diplopia, somnolence
Note: TDM Toxic: not established. Be wary of *lamotrigine* (blood) >20 mcg/mL (>20 mg/L)				
Oxcarbazepine	Trigeminal neuralgia	300–600 mg/day orally Max. 2400 mg/day orally	Similar to carbamazepine with less-severe side effects	Skin sensitivity, hyponatremia
Phenytoin	Trigeminal neuralgia Diabetic neuropathy	300 mg/day orally 1000 mg initial loading dose orally or intravenously	Weak to moderate analgesic effect Obtain CBC and LFTs before administration	Gingival hyperplasia, hirsutism
Note: TDM Toxic: *total phenytoin* (blood) >20 mg/L (>79 µmol/L); TDM Toxic: *free phenytoin* (blood) ≥2.5 mg/L (≥9.9 µmol/L). Phenytoin is available in a variety of formulations and strengths for oral administration, including prompt-release capsules containing 100 mg phenytoin sodium (equivalent to 92 mg phenytoin); extended-release capsules containing 30 mg or 100 mg phenytoin sodium (equivalent to 27.6 mg and 92 mg phenytoin, respectively); extended-release capsules containing 200 mg or 300 mg phenytoin sodium (equivalent to 184 mg and 276 mg phenytoin, respectively); chewable tablets containing 50 mg phenytoin; and a liquid suspension containing 125 mg phenytoin/5 mL and ≤6% alcohol				
Topiramate	Postthoracotomy Reflex sympathetic dystrophy Headaches, intercostal neuralgia	25–50 mg/day orally Max. 200 mg BID orally	Prolonged use may cause renal calculi Absorption slowed by food	Anorexia, weight loss
Valproic acid	Migraine headaches Cluster headaches Tension headaches	250 mg/day orally Max. 600 mg TID orally	Multiple drug interactions	CNS depression, hepatic, hematologic toxicity
Note: TDM Toxic: *total valproic acid* (blood) >120 mg/L (>832 µmol/L); TDM Toxic: *free valproic acid* (blood) >15 mg/L (>104 µmol/L)				

Tricyclic Antidepressants

Drug	Indication	Dosage	Comments	Side Effects
Amitriptyline (Elavil, and many generic products)	Neuropathic pain Musculoskeletal pain	10–25 mg orally at bedtime Max. 150 mg orally at bedtime	Take 10 hours before planned waking to decrease side effects	Dry mouth, sedation, cardiac arrhythmias, urinary retention

Note: TDM Toxic: *amitriptyline* (blood) ≥500 mcg/L (≥1805 nmol/L)

Drug	Indication	Dosage	Comments	Side Effects
Desipramine (Norpramin, and many generic products)	Neuropathic pain Musculoskeletal pain	10–25 mg orally at bedtime Max. 50–100 mg orally at bedtime	Less sedative and anticholinergic effects than amitriptyline	Dry mouth, sedation, cardiac arrhythmias, urinary retention

Note: TDM Toxic: *desipramine* (blood) ≥500 mcg/L (≥1880 nmol/L)

Drug	Indication	Dosage	Comments	Side Effects
Nortriptyline (Pamelor, and many generic products)	Neuropathic pain Musculoskeletal pain	10–25 mg orally at bedtime Max. 100–150 mg orally at bedtime		Dry mouth, sedation, cardiac arrhythmias, urinary retention

Note: TDM Toxic: *nortriptyline* (blood) ≥500 mcg/L (≥1900 nmol/L)

Neuroleptic Agents

Drug	Indication	Dosage	Comments	Side Effects
Olanzapine	Opioid-induced cognitive impairment	2.5–5 mg/day orally Max 20 mg/day orally	Safer neuroleptic, with reduced extrapyramidal effects, drug interactions, and neutropenia	Agitation, headache, insomnia, somnolence

NMDA (*N*-methyl-d-aspartate) Receptor Antagonists (a glutamate receptor)

Drug	Indication	Dosage	Comments	Side Effects
Ketamine	Refractory neuropathic pain	0.1–1.5 mg/kg per hour, intravenously Use as continuous infusion in hospice setting; or intermittently for less-severe pain	Poorly absorbed orally Do not use with increased ICP, hypertension, or psychosis Ketamine is hepatically metabolized Pharmacodynamic effects may be prolonged in patients with impaired liver function	Confusion, hallucinations
Methadone	Somatic pain Neuropathic pain	2.5 mg QD or BID orally or intravenously	May reduce opioid tolerance	
Dextromethorphan polistirex oral suspension, extended-release equivalent to 30 mg dextromethorphan HBr/5 mL (Delsym)	Polyneuropathy	15 mg BID orally Maximum dose can vary and is determined empirically	Slow-release dextromethorphan Product contains 0.26% alcohol	Pharmacokinetic interaction between dextromethorphan and serotonin reuptake inhibitors or MAO inhibitors may result in serotonin syndrome

(*continued*)

Table 52–11. (*continued*)

Antiarrhythmics			
Mexiletine	Refractory neuropathic pain	50 mg TID orally Max. 10 mg/kg per day orally	May worsen preexisting cardiac arrhythmias. Do not use in second- and third-degree AV blocks Monitor ECG at high doses

Note: TDM Toxic: mexiletine (blood) >2 mcg/mL (>11.2 μmol/L)

Lidocaine	Refractory neuropathic pain	Administer intravenously	Do not use with compromised cardiac contractility or conduction Avoid use of tricyclic antidepressants

Note: TDM Toxic: lidocaine (blood) ≥6 mcg/mL (≥25.6 μmol/L)

Nausea, anxiety, dizziness

Local/Cutaneous Anesthetics			
Eutectic mixture of lidocaine 2.5% and prilocaine 2.5% (EMLA)	Peripheral neuropathy allodynia	Apply topically to intact skin QID and cover with an occlusive dressing (eg, OpSite film dressing; Smith & Nephew Inc., Memphis, TN)	
Lidocaine patch 5% (Lidoderm)	Postherpetic neuralgia	Apply topically to intact skin for up to 12 hours every 24 hours	

Topical Agents			
Capsaicin	Peripheral neuropathy Arthropathy Mucositis	Apply topically to intact skin QID	
Polyvinylpyrrolidone, sodium hyaluronate, and glycyrrhetinic acid bioadherent oral gel (Gelclair)	Mucositis	Dilute the contents of 1 Gelclair packet with 1–3 tablespoons (15–45 mL) tap water (or may be used undiluted); "swish" the product around the oral cavity or gargle with it for at least 1 minute, QID. The product is usually expectorated, but is harmless if swallowed	

Corticosteroids				
Dexamethasone	Oncologic emergency (spinal cord or nerve compression) Refractory neuropathic pain Increased ICP Organ distention Bone metastasis	80–100 mg intravenously × 1, then 10–12 mg intravenously QID; or 1 mg–4 mg orally QID	Improves pain, nausea, appetite, and malaise Longer duration of action (36–72 hours) No mineralocorticoid effects (edema) Taper dosing to discontinue	Myopathy, delirium, depression
Prednisone		5–10 mg BID orally	Use to reduce myopathy Taper dose to discontinue Improves pain, nausea, and appetite	Hypotension, dry mouth, somnolence
***α*₂-Adrenergic Agonists**				
Clonidine	Diabetic neuropathy Cancer-related neuropathy Chronic headache	0.1 mg/day orally max. 2 mg/day orally; *or* Apply and replace topical patches to intact hairless skin every 7 days	Beneficial in less opioid-responsive patients May reduce opioid requirement	Hypotension, dry mouth, somnolence

BID, twice per day; ICP, intracranial pressure; QD, once per day; QID, 4 times per day; TID, 3 times per day

Table 52–12. Nonsteroidal Anti-inflammatory Agents

Agent	Typical Starting Dose	Maximum Daily Dose	Comments
Aspirin	650 mg orally every 4 hours	4000 mg	Irreversibly inhibits platelet aggregation
Celecoxib (**Celebrex**)	100–200 mg orally every 12 hours	400 mg	Contraindicated in patients who are allergic to sulfonamides
Choline magnesium trisalicylate (**Trilisate**, and others)	500–1000 mg orally every 12 hours	3000 mg	Inexpensive Does not interfere with platelet aggregation Less gastric upset than aspirin and other salicylates
Diclofenac (**Voltaren**)	50–75 mg orally every 8–12 hours orally	225 mg	Available in sustained-release form
Diflunisal (**Dolobid**, and others)	250–500 mg orally every 8–12 hours	1500 mg	Causes less gastric irritation than aspirin Increases acetaminophen level 50% when both drugs are administered concomitantly
Etodolac (**Lodine**, and others)	200 mg orally every 6 hours to 400 mg orally every 8 hours	400 mg	Causes less gastric irritation, especially in the elderly Antacids reduce peak concentration by 20%
Fenoprofen (**Nalfon**, and others)	300–600 mg orally every 6 hours	3200 mg	Associated with higher incidence of renal toxicity compared with other NSAIDs
Flurbiprofen (**Ansaid**, and others)	50–100 mg orally every 6–8 hours	300 mg/day	May cause CNS stimulation
Ibuprofen (**Motrin**, and others)	200–800 mg orally every 6–8 hours	3200 mg	Associated with less gastric toxicity compared with other NSAIDs
Indomethacin (**Indocin**, and others)	25–50 mg orally every 6–8 hours, *or* 25–50 mg rectally every 6–8 hours	200 mg	Associated with greater incidence and severity of toxicities than other NSAIDs
Ketoprofen (**Orudis**, and others)	50–75 mg orally every 6–8 hours	300 mg	Associated with higher incidence of dyspepsia compared with other NSAIDs
Ketorolac (**Toradol**, and others)	15–30 mg intramuscularly (IM) every 6 hours 15–30 mg intravenously (IV) every 6 hours 10 mg orally every 4–6 hours	120 mg IM 120 mg IV 40 mg orally	Used only for pain (minor antipyretic properties) *An NSAID available in injectable form (indomethacin sodium trihydrate is also available in injectable form)* Not to be used for more than 5 days because of potential toxicity
Meclofenamate sodium	50–100 mg orally every 6 hours	400 mg	Rarely used owing to gastric and neurologic toxicities Associated with high incidence of diarrhea
Meloxicam (**Mobic**)	7.5–15 mg orally daily	15 mg	Preferential COX-2 activity Less selective than other COX-2 inhibitors
Nabumetone (**Relafen**, and others)	1000–2000 mg orally daily, *or* 500–750 mg orally 2 times per day	2000 mg	Associated with higher incidence of diarrhea than other NSAIDs
Naproxen (**Naprosyn**, and others)	250 every 8–500 mg every 12 hours, orally	1250 mg	May increase effects of phenytoin, warfarin, and sulfonylureas
Oxaprozin (**Daypro**, and others)	600–1200 mg orally daily	1800 mg	
Piroxicam (**Feldene**, and others)	10–20 mg orally daily	20 mg	Optimum efficacy may not occur for 1–2 weeks Associated with high incidence of dyspepsia Increases the effect of phenytoin, warfarin, and sulfonylureas
Sulindac (**Clinoril**, and others)	150–200 mg orally every 12 hours	400 mg	Associated with less renal toxicity than other NSAIDs

Data from Mosby's Drug Consult. St. Louis, MO: CV Mosby; 2004.

Table 52–13. Visceral Pain Syndromes

Agent	Dosing	Comments
Bladder Spasm		
Opium tincture	Starting dose: 3 drops orally every 6 hours Titrate to therapeutic response or side effects	Shares the toxicities associated with opiate agonists; used commonly to inhibit gastric motility, but can provide analgesia for bladder spasms
Opium tincture, deodorized contains 10 mg anhydrous morphine equivalents/mL and 19% ethanol		
Belladonna and opium rectal suppository	30–60 mg per rectum 1–2 times/day Maximum of 4 doses per day	Analgesic and antispasmodic agent Decreased effect with phenothiazines; increased effect with central nervous system depressants, tricyclic antidepressants
Belladonna and opium rectal suppositories are manufactured in at least 2 product formulations, including suppositories for rectal insertion containing powdered belladonna extract 16.2 mg and powdered opium 30 mg, or powdered belladonna extract 16.2 mg and powdered opium 60 mg. The product is marketed as a schedule II (CII) controlled		
Oxybutynin chloride (**Ditropan**, and many generic products)	Starting dose: 5 mg orally 2–3 times per day Maximum dose of 5 mg 4 times per day	Antimuscarinic agent Use cautiously in individuals also receiving belladonna; may result in excessive anticholinergic activity
Phenazopyridine hydrochloride (**Pyridium**, and many generic products)	100–200 mg orally 3 times per day	Produces topical analgesia on urinary tract mucosa Decreases urinary pain, burning, urgency, and frequency
Bowel Obstruction		
Octreotide acetate (Sandostatin)	*Solution:* 50–300 mg per dose intravenously or subcutaneously for 2–4 doses per day *Suspension:* 10–40 mg per dose intramuscularly (gluteal muscles ONLY) every 4 weeks	Very costly Useful in bowel obstruction for its antisecretory properties
Octreotide acetate injectable solution is a short-acting product for administration by intravenous or subcutaneous injection. Octreotide acetate for injectable suspension (Sandostatin LAR) is a long-acting formulation for *intragluteal administration only*		
Transdermal scopolamine	One patch delivers 1 mg scopolamine over 3 days Apply 1 patch to the hairless (intact) skin behind the ear every 3 days	Peak levels achieved within 24 hours Reduces motility and intraluminal secretions
Hyoscyamine sulfate (**Levsin**, and other generic products)	*Prompt-release products* 0.125 mg orally or sublingually 2 times per day; maximum dose: 0.25 mg, 3 times per day *Extended- and sustained-release products* 0.375–0.75 mg orally every 12 hours	Individual must be well hydrated to receive maximum dose
Glycopyrrolate (**Robinul**, and other generic products)	1–2 mg orally 2–3 times per day	Anticholinergic and antispasmodic
Corticosteroids	Variable dosing	Useful for analgesia and inflammation

Data from Mosby's Drug Consult. St. Louis, MO: CV Mosby; 2004

53. Hospice Care and End-of-Life Issues

Charles F. von Gunten, MD, PhD and David E. Weissman, MD

Hospice Care

The number one complaint about hospice care from patients and families is that no one told them about it sooner. Referral for hospice care is appropriate when the most important goal is comfort rather than making the cancer better. If patients improve or resume anticancer therapy, they can be discharged (graduate) and resume services later without penalty

Eligibility: Prognosis of less than 6 months *if a patient's disease runs its usual course.* Individual patients can continue to be eligible if they live longer than 6 months as long as their physician believes death is *more likely than not* within 6 months. A patient does not need a DNR order. There is no limit to the number of days a patient can receive hospice care. There is no penalty if a physician is wrong about a patient's longevity

Prognosis: Oncologists overestimate prognosis when compared with actual survival. Referral for hospice care is associated with an *increase* in survival as compared with controls

General Indicators of Poor Prognosis	Specific Indicators of Poor Prognosis
Performance status: Karnofsky 10 or 20 (ECOG/Zubrod 4): <1 month Karnofsky 30 or 40: 1–2 months Karnofsky 50 (or ECOG/Zubrod 3): 2–3 months	*Hypercalcemia:* 6 weeks *Multiple brain metastases:* 3–6 months *Anorexia:* <2 months *Delirium/confusion:* <1 month *Dyspnea:* <1 month
Nutritional status: *Serum albumin <2.5 mg/dL:* <6 months	**Specific cancers:** *Stage IV non–small cell lung cancer:* 6–12 months *Unresectable pancreas cancer:* 4–7 months *Stage IV esophagus cancer:* 3–6 months *Stage IV gastric cancer:* 7 months

Discussing Hospice Care

One of the biggest barriers to timely referral for hospice care is physician discomfort with the discussion
Clinical pearl: Discuss hospice care after determining broad goals of care (if focus of care is comfort, to be as independent and comfortable as possible, hospice helps achieve the goals)

Steps	Suggested Phrases
1. Establish the setting: privacy, time	"I'd like to talk with you about our overall goals for your care"
2. What does the patient understand? Get the patient talking	"What do you understand about your current health situation?" *or* "What have the doctors told you about your cancer?"
3. What does the patient expect? Correct misperceptions	"What do you expect in the future?" *or* "What goals do you have for the time you have left—what is important to you?"
4. Discuss hospice care	"You've told me you want to be as independent and comfortable as possible. Hospice care is the best way I know to help you achieve those goals." **Never say, "There's nothing more we can do"**
5. Respond to emotions	Be quiet. The most profound initial response a physician can make is silence, providing a reassuring touch, and offering facial tissues. The most frequent mistake is to talk too much
6. Establish a plan	"I'll ask the hospice to come by to give information, then you and I can discuss it"

Discussing DNR (Do Not Resuscitate) Orders

Discuss DNR orders *after* discussions of overall goals of care, following a stepwise approach

Steps	Suggested Phrases
1. Establish the setting: privacy, time	"I'd like to talk with you about our overall goals for your care"
2. What does the patient understand? Get the patient talking	"What do you understand about your current health situation?" *or* "What have the doctors told you about your cancer?"
3. What does the patient expect? Correct misperceptions. An informed decision about DNR status is only possible if patients have a clear understanding of their illness and prognosis	"What do you expect in the future?" *or* "What goals do you have for the time you have left—what is important to you? "Do you ever think about dying?" "How do you want it to be?"
4. Discuss DNR Order *Clinical pearl:* Start general and become specific later in the conversation	**Never say, "Do you want us to do everything?"** "You have said you want to be comfortable when you die and you hope you'll just slip away in your sleep. Therefore, I recommend that I write a 'DNR' order which means that we won't try artificial or heroic means to keep you alive when that time comes"
5. Respond to emotions	Be quiet. The most profound initial response a physician can make is silence, providing a reassuring touch, and offering facial tissues. The most frequent mistake is to talk too much
6. Establish a plan. A DNR order does not address any aspect of care other than preventing the use of CPR	"We will continue maximal medical therapy"

When the Patient Will Not Be DNR

The seemingly unreasonable persistent request for CPR typically stems from one of several themes:

Steps	Suggested Phrases
1. Inaccurate information about CPR For patients with advanced cancer, who undergo CPR in the hospital, the survival to discharge is zero	"What do you know about CPR?"
2. Hopes, fears, and guilt Some need an explicit recommendation or permission to stop all efforts to prolong life, that death is coming and that they no longer have to continue "fighting"	"What do you expect to happen? What do you think would be done differently, after the resuscitation, that wasn't being done before?"
3. Distrust of the medical care system	"What you said makes me wonder if you may not trust the doctors and nurses to do what is best for you—will you tell me about your concerns?"

If patients are not ready for a DNR order, don't let it distract you from other important end-of-life care needs; emphasize the goals that you are trying to achieve; save a repeat discussion for a future time; good care, relationship building, and time will help resolve most conflicts

Managing Persistent Requests for CPR

Decide if you believe that CPR represents a futile medical treatment—that is, if CPR cannot be expected to either restore cardiopulmonary function or to achieve the expressed goals of the patient. Physicians are not legally or ethically obligated to participate in a futile medical treatment. Some facilities have a policy that a physician may enter a DNR order in the chart against patient wishes. Your options at this time include:

• Transfer care to another physician chosen by the patient/family

• Plan to perform CPR at the time of death—**but don't end the discussion**. Tell them that you need guidance if the patient survives because it is very likely the patient will be on life support in the ICU, and the patient may not be able to make decisions for themself; ask the patient (or the family) to help you determine guidelines for deciding whether to continue life-support measures. If not already done, clarify if there is a legal surrogate decision maker

Normal Dying	
Weakness/fatigue	Give permission to patient, family, and other caregivers to accept weakness/fatigue. This does not represent loss of will, the patient is dying
Decreasing appetite/food intake, wasting	Loss of appetite and weight loss are normal at the end of life. Parenteral or enteral feeding neither improves symptom control nor lengthens life: The patient is dying of cancer—it is the cancer that is making the patient thin
Decreasing fluid intake, dehydration	Blood pressure or weak pulse is normal. Peripheral edema or ascites means excess body water and salt. Low oncotic pressure means parenteral fluids cause peripheral or pulmonary edema, worsened breathlessness, cough, and orotracheobronchial secretions
Decreasing blood perfusion, renal failure	Tachycardia, hypotension, peripheral cooling, peripheral and central cyanosis, and mottling of the skin (livedo reticularis) are normal. Venous blood may pool along dependent skin surfaces. Urine output falls as perfusion of the kidneys diminishes. Oliguria or anuria is normal. Parenteral fluids will not reverse this circulatory shutdown: The body is shutting down
Neurologic dysfunction: 2 patterns	Brain failure—the "usual road" with decreased level of consciousness that leads to coma and death. The "difficult road" that a few patients follow presents as an agitated delirium caused by central nervous system (CNS) excitation, with or without myoclonic jerks that leads to coma and death
Pain	There is no evidence that there is a crescendo of pain near death. Terminal delirium frequently is misdiagnosed as pain
Changes in respiration	Diminished tidal volume. Periods of apnea and/or Cheyne-Stokes pattern respirations are normal. Accessory respiratory muscle use may become prominent
Loss of ability to swallow	Gurgling, crackling, or rattling sounds with each breath may be heard. Some have called this the "death rattle." For unprepared families and professional caregivers, it may sound like the patient is choking
Loss of ability to close eyes	Wasting leads to loss of the retroorbital fat pad, and the orbit falls posteriorly within the orbital socket. Eyelids are of insufficient length
Loss of sphincter control	Urinary and fecal incontinence are frequent. A marked increase in need for direct care giving is required to keep patient clean

End-of-Life Issues

Medications at the End of Life

Limit medications to those needed to manage symptoms, such as pain, breathlessness, excess secretions, terminal delirium, and seizures and their prevention. Choose the least-invasive route of administration: the buccal mucosa or oral routes first, the subcutaneous or intravenous routes only if necessary, and the intramuscular route almost never

Indication	Drug	Utilization*
Terminal Delirium	Lorazepam	1–2 mg orally or sublingually every 1 hour until settled
	Midazolam	1–2 mg subcutaneously or intravenously every 15 min until settled
	Haloperidol	1–5 mg (haloperidol *lactate*) orally or subcutaneously every 1 hour until settled *Caution:* Haloperidol *decanoate* is formulated in sesame seed oil, and is administered *only* by intramuscular injection
	Chlorpromazine	10–25 mg orally, per rectum (suppository), or intravenously every 2–6 hours
Seizures	Any benzodiazepine	Lorazepam 2–5 mg orally, sublingually, subcutaneously, or intravenously every 1 hour, *or* Midazolam 2–4 mg by subcutaneous or intravenous injection every 15 minutes
	Fosphenytoin	10–20 mg PE/kg body weight intravenously at a maximum rate of 150 mg PE/min *Note:* 1.5 mg Fosphenytoin sodium is equivalent to 1 mg phenytoin sodium, and is referred to as "1 mg PE (phenytoin equivalents)" Maintenance dosage, initially: 4–6 mg PE/kg per day with fosphenytoin sodium (intravenously) or phenytoin sodium (orally)
	Phenobarbital	60–120 mg by intravenous or intramuscular injection, or per rectum (suppository) every 20 minutes until settled

(continued)

(continued)

Indication	Drug	Utilization*
Rattle	Scopolamine	0.2–0.4 mg subcutaneously every 4 hours, *or* 0.1–1 mg/hour, by continuous intravenous or subcutaneous infusion, *or* one to three 1.5-mg transdermal patches, apply to intact skin every 72 hours
	Glycopyrrolate	0.2 mg subcutaneously, intravenously, or intramuscularly every 4–6 hours, *or* 0.4–1.2 mg/day by continuous intravenous or subcutaneous infusion
Bowel obstruction	Octreotide	50 mcg subcutaneously every 12 hours, *or* 10 mcg/hour, by continuous intravenous or subcutaneous infusion and titrate to response *Note:* Range of doses in anecdotal reports is 50–220 mg twice daily *Caution:* Octreotide acetate *solution* is appropriate for subcutaneous or intravenous administration. Octreotide acetate *suspension* is administered *only* by intramuscular injection

Breathlessness	Morphine	*Opioid-naïve patients:*
		    5–10 mg orally every 1 hour, *or*
		    1–2 mg subcutaneously every 20 minutes, *or*
		    1–2 mg intravenously every 15 minutes
		 Opioid-tolerant patients:
		    Increase analgesic dose by 50%

*Some of the products identified or formulations appropriate for a particular route of administration may not be available worldwide

Care at the Time of Death

Answer questions and review the signs and potential events that can be expected. For many families and caregivers, knowing ahead of time decreases anxiety. Most people do not know much about death

Signs of death discussed with family:

The heart stops beating; breathing stops; pupils become fixed; body color becomes pale and waxen as blood settles; body temperature drops; muscles and sphincters relax, urine and stool may be released; eyes may remain open; the jaw can fall open; the trickling of fluids internally may be heard

After expected death occurs:

Go to the bedside to comfort family members who are distressed and appreciate that the doctor shows "he or she cared." This need not take more than 5–10 minutes

Participate with nursing to create a visually peaceful and accessible environment. A few moments spent alone in the room positioning the patient's body, disconnecting any lines and machinery, removing catheters, and cleaning up any mess will allow the family closer access to the patient's body. If eyes remain open, eyelids can be manually held closed for a few minutes and will usually remain closed once they dry. If they remain open, a small amount of surgical tape or a short Steri-Strip will hold them closed for longer without pulling on eyelashes when they are removed. If the jaw falls open as muscles relax, a rolled-up towel placed under the chin with the head elevated on pillows will usually hold the jaw closed until muscles stiffen some 4–6 hours later

The doctor may need to tell the "bad news" of a patient's death to someone who didn't have previous warning. Follow the guidelines for communicating bad news. Avoid breaking unexpected news by telephone, as communicating in person provides much greater opportunity for assessment and support. Tell them what to expect before they see the body (eg, changes in body color, temperature, and the scene they will see)

Writing a Condolence Note

A note or letter from the doctor after the death has been widely reported to be helpful to the bereaved. Such a note has 2 goals: to offer tribute to the deceased as someone who was important, and to be a source of comfort to the survivors. It should be handwritten and sent promptly, generally within 2 weeks after the death. Use any standard stationery

Steps	Suggested Phrases
Acknowledge the loss and name the deceased	"The hospice called to let me know that your mother, Mary Smith, died on Thursday"
Express your sympathy	"I was so sad to hear the news"
Note special qualities of the deceased	"I will miss her sense of humor"
Recall a memory about the deceased	"I particularly remember when she had all of us in the office laughing at one of her jokes about the examination gown"

(continued)

(continued)

Steps	Suggested Phrases
Name personal strengths of the bereaved	"I was impressed by the devotion you and your family showed your mother during her illness. I remember when she commented on it herself"
Offer help, but be specific. Don't say, "If there is anything I can do, please call"	"I'd be happy to answer any questions you or your family might have about her illness and her care. Just make an appointment with the office—no charge"
End with a word or phrase of sympathy	"I'll never forget your mother or the care you gave her"

Telephone Notification

There will be cases where the people who need to know about the death are not present. In some of these cases, you may choose to tell someone by phone that the patient's condition has "changed," and wait for them to come to the bedside in order to tell them the news. Factors to consider in weighing this include family member advice, whether death was expected, the anticipated emotional reaction, if the person is alone, if the person is able to understand, distance, availability of transportation, and time of day. Inevitably, there are times when notification of death by telephone is unavoidable. If this is anticipated, prepare for it. Determine who should be called and in what fashion. Some families will prefer not to be awakened at night if there is an expected death

Steps	Suggested Phrases
1. Get the setting right	Ask to speak to the person closest to the patient
2. Ask what the person understands	"What have the doctors told you about M's condition?"
3. Provide a "warning shot"	"I'm afraid I have some bad news"
4. Tell the news	"I'm sorry to have to give you this news, but M just died"
5. Respond to emotions	Active listening is best initial approach. "I can hear how sad you are"
6. Conclude with a plan	If the family chooses to come to see the body, arrange to meet them personally

References

Buckman R. How to Break Bad News: a Guide for Health Care Professionals. Baltimore, MD: The Johns Hopkins University Press; 1992:65–97
Diem SJ et al. Cardiopulmonary resuscitation on television. Miracles and misinformation. N Engl J Med 1996;334:1578–1582
Emanuel LL, von Gunten CF, Ferris FD (eds). The EPEC Curriculum. 1999. The EPEC Project, www.epec.net
Fast Facts and Concepts. End of Life/Palliative Education Resource Center, Medical College of Wisconsin. Available at: www.eperc.mcw.edu/EPERC/FastFactsandConcepts. Last accessed, August 1, 2013
Medical futility in end-of-life care, Report of the Council on Ethical and Judicial Affairs (American Medical Association). JAMA 1999;281:937–941
Warm, E. Improving EOL care—internal medicine curriculum project. J Palliat Med 1999;2:339–340

54. Cancer Screening

Kathleen A. Calzone, PhD, RN, APNG, FAAN, Jennifer Eng-Wong, MD, MPH, and Sheila Prindiville, MD, MPH

American Cancer Society (ACS) Recommendations for the Early Detection of Cancer in Average-Risk, Asymptomatic People[1]

Cancer Site	Population	Test or Procedure	Frequency
Breast	Women >20 years	Breast self-examination (optional)	Monthly, starting at age 20
		Clinical breast examination	Every 3 years from ages 20–39 Annually, starting at age 40*
		Mammography	Annually, starting at age 40
Colorectal	Men and women, age 50+ years	Fecal occult blood test (FOBT)[†] *or*	Annually, starting at age 50
		Stool DNA test (sDNA) *or*	Interval uncertain, starting at age 50
		Flexible sigmoidoscopy *or*	Every 5 years, starting at age 50
		Fecal occult blood test (FOBT) *and* flexible sigmoidoscopy[‡] *or*	Annual FOBT and flexible sigmoidoscopy every 5 years, starting at age 50
		Double-contrast barium enema (DCBE) *or*	Every 5 years, starting at age 50
		Colonoscopy *or*	Every 10 years, starting at age 50
		CT colonography	Every 5 years starting at age 50
Prostate	Men >50 years	Digital rectal examination (DRE) *and* prostate-specific antigen test (PSA)	The PSA test and the DRE should be offered annually, starting at age 50, for men who have a life expectancy of at least 10 years[§]
Cervix[€]	Women age <21	None	
	Women age 21–29	Cytology alone	Every 3 years. HPV testing for screening should not be used
	Women age 30–65	Preferred: HPV and cytology contesting	Every 5 years. HPV testing for screening not recommended for most clinical settings
		Acceptable: Cytology alone	Every 3 years
	Women age 65+	None following adequate prior negative screening	History of CIN2 or greater diagnosis should continue screening for 20 years
	Women following hysterectomy and NO history of CIN2 or greater diagnosis	None	Applies only to women with: • No cervix • Without a history of CIN2 or greater diagnosis in the past 20 years • No history of cervical cancer
	Women following hysterectomy and history of CIN2 or greater diagnosis	Continue age specific screening for at least 20 years	
	Women HPV vaccinated	Continue to follow age specific guidelines above for non-vaccinated women	
Cancer-related checkup	Men and women age 20+ years		On the occasion of a periodic health exam, the cancer-related check-up should include examination for cancers of thyroid, testicles, ovaries, lymph nodes, oral cavity, and skin, as well as health counseling about tobacco, sun exposure, diet and nutrition, risk factors, sexual practices, and environmental and occupational exposures

*Beginning at age 40, annual clinical breast examination
[†]FOBT or FIT as sometimes done in the physician's office, with the single stool sample on fingertip during a DRE is NOT recommended. Toilet bowl FOBT tests also are not recommended. In comparison with guaiac-based tests for the detection of occult blood, immunochemical tests are more patient-friendly and are likely to be equal or better in sensitivity and specificity. There is no justification for repeating FOBT in response to an initial positive finding
[‡]Flexible sigmoidoscopy together with FOBT is preferred compared with FOBT or flexible sigmoidoscopy alone
[€]Screening for cervical cancer should not be performed annually by any method

ACS Guidelines for Screening and Surveillance for Individuals at Increased Risk of Colon Cancer[1-3]

Risk Category	When to Begin	Recommendation	Comment
Small rectal hyperplastic polyps		Colonoscopy or other screening modality at intervals for average risk people	Patients with hyperplastic polyposis syndrome have an increased risk for adenomas and colorectal cancer and need more intensive follow-up
1–2 small tubular adenoma(s) with low-grade dysplasia	5–10 years after the initial polypectomy	Colonoscopy	If exam is normal, the patient can thereafter be screened as per average-risk guidelines
Single small (<1cm) adenoma	3–6 years after the initial polypectomy	Colonoscopy	The interval timing is based on prior colonoscopy, family history, physician judgment and patient preference
3–10 adenomas or 1 adenoma >1 cm or any adenoma with villous features or high grade dysplasia	3 years after the initial polypectomy	Colonoscopy	Adenomas must be completely removed. Colonoscopy interval every 5 years IF follow-up colonoscopy that is normal or only 1–2 small tubular adenomas with low grade dysplasia
More than 10 adenomas on a single exam	Less than 3 years after initial polypectomy	Colonoscopy	Consider possibility of a familial polyposis syndrome
Sessile adenoma removed piecemeal	2–6 months following removal to verify complete removal	Colonoscopy	Following complete removal based on both endoscopic and pathologic assessment, colonoscopy interval based on endoscopist's judgment

Increased Risk-Patients with Family History

Risk Category	When to Begin	Recommendation	Comment
Either colorectal cancer or adenomatous polyps in any first degree relative before age 60 or in 2 or more first degree relatives at any age	Age 40, or 10 years before the youngest case in the immediate family	Colonoscopy	Every 5 years
Either colorectal cancer or adenomatous polyps in any first degree relative ≥60 or in 2 or more second degree relatives at any age	Age 40	Screening modality at intervals for average risk people	Screening should initiate at an earlier age however individuals may choose to be screened with any recommended form of testing
Genetic diagnosis of familial adenomatous polyposis (FAP) or suspected FAP without genetic testing evidence	Age 10–12	Annual flexible sigmoidoscopy to determine whether individual has evidence of FAP Genetic counseling for consideration of genetic testing	Patients with a confirmed FAP associated mutation should be considered for colectomy
Genetic or clinical diagnosis of Lynch Syndrome*† (previously called Hereditary Non-Polyposis Colon Cancer [HNPCC]) or individuals at increased risk of Lynch Syndrome	Age 20–25 or 10 years prior to the youngest case in the immediate family	Colonoscopy every 1–2 years Genetic counseling for consideration of genetic testing	Lynch Syndrome genetic testing should be offered to all first degree relatives of known MMR mutation carriers. Genetic testing should also be offered when 1 or 3 of the modified Bethesda criteria are present and no familial mutation has been identified
Inflammatory bowel disease, Chronic ulcerative colitis, Crohn's disease	Significant cancer risk 8 years after onset of pancolitis, or 12–15 years after onset of left sided colitis	Colonoscopy with biopsies for dysplasia	Every 1–2 years. These patients are best referred to a center with experience in the surveillance and management of inflammatory bowel disease

(continued)

ACS Guidelines for Screening and Surveillance for Individuals at Increased Risk of Colon Cancer[1-3] (continued)

Risk Category	When to Begin	Recommendation	Comment
Increased Risk-Patients with Colorectal Cancer			
Diagnosis of colon and rectal cancer	3–6 months following cancer resection	Colonoscopy	Undergo high quality perioperative clearing
Personal history of curative intent resection of colorectal cancer	1 year after cancer resection (or 1 year following colonoscopy to clear colon of synchronous disease)	Colonoscopy	If normal, repeat exam in 3 years. If normal then, repeat examination every 5 years. Interval may be shortened if there is evidence of Lynch Syndrome or adenomas warrant earlier colonoscopy

*See Genetics of Common Inherited Cancer Syndromes Chapter 55, Table 3 for definition
†See Genetics of Common Inherited Cancer Syndromes Chapter 55, Table 4 for complete Lynch Syndrome cancer screening guidelines

For screening of individuals with genetic syndromes that increase risk of colorectal cancer, see Chapter 55

Modified NCCN Guidelines for Screening and Treating Women at Increased Risk of Breast Cancer[4,†]

Risk Category	Breast Awareness (including BSE) Encouraged	Clinical Breast Exam	Mammogram	Breast MRI	Risk Reduction Strategy
Prior thoracic radiation therapy, age <25	Yes	Every 6 to 12 months starting eight to ten years after radiation	None	None	No data on chemoprevention in this population
Prior thoracic radiation therapy, age ≥25	Yes	Every 6 to 12 months starting eight to ten years after radiation or age 25, whichever occurs last	Every 12 months	Consider every 12 months	No data on chemoprevention in this population
Gail Model risk ≥1.7% over next 5 years and 35 years old or older*	Yes	Every 6 to 12 months	Every 12 months	None	Life Expectancy >10 years: • Risk reducing mastectomy if desired • Risk reduction bilateral salphingo oophorectomy (Limited to those with a documented or strongly suspected *BRCA1/2* mutation†) • Risk reducing agent (gynecology assessment for all women with an intact uterus and ophthalmology exam if history of cataracts or vision problems) Premenopausal women: 1. Tamoxifen 20 mg, orally, daily for 5 yrs Postmenopausal women: 1. Clinical Trial or 2. Tamoxifen 20 mg orally, daily for 5 yrs or 3. Raloxifene or 4. Exemestane
LCIS	Yes	Every 6 to 12 months	Every 12 months	None	
Lifetime risk >20% based on models dependent mostly on family history (ie, Claus, BRCAPro, BOADICEA, Tyer-Cuzick)	Yes	Every 6 to 12 months starting at age 30	Every 12 months starting at age 30	Consider every 12 months starting at age 30	

*Determine Gail model risk at: http://bcra.nci.nih.gov/brc/
†See Genetics of Common Inherited Cancer Syndromes Chapter 55, Table 3 for definition
‡See Genetics of Common Inherited Cancer Syndromes Chapter 55, Table 4 for complete *BRCA1/2* mutation cancer screening guidelines

References

1. Smith RA et al. Cancer screening in the United States: A review of current American Cancer Society guidelines and current issues in cancer screening. CA Cancer J Clin 2012;62:129–142
2. Saslow D et al. (2012). American Cancer Society, American Society for Colposcopy and Cervical Pathology, and American Society for Clinical Pathology Screening guidelines for the prevention and early detection of cervical cancer. CA Cancer J Clin 2012;62:147–172
3. Levin B et al. Screening and surveillance for the early detection of colorectal cancer and adenomatous polyps, 2008: A joint guidelines from the American Cancer Society, the US Multi-Society Task Force on Colorectal Cancer, and the American College of Radiology, CA Cancer J Clin 2008;58:130–160
4. NCCN, NCCN Practice Guidelines for Prevention, Detection and Risk Reduction. Breast Screening and Diagnosis (1.2012). http://www.nccn.org/professionals/physician_gls/pdf/breast-screening.pdf (2012)

55. Genetics of Common Inherited Cancer Syndromes

Kathleen A. Calzone, PhD, RN, APNG, FAAN and Sheila Prindiville, MD, MPH

Table 55–1. Indications for Genetic Testing for Cancer Susceptibility American Society of Clinical Oncology (ASCO)[1,2]

1. Personal and/or family history suggestive of a known cancer susceptibility syndrome
2. The genetic test can be adequately interpreted
3. Genetic test results will aid in diagnosis and/or influence medical or surgical management

Testing should be performed only in the context of both pre- and posttest genetic counseling including risks, benefits and limitations of testing, early detection, and risk reduction options[1,3]

ASCO also recommends that the evidence of clinical utility of any genetic test (including multiplex tests and low or moderate disease genes or SNP tests) be considered when either ordering or making medical recommendations based on a test result

---

Table 55–2. Selected Hereditary Cancer Syndromes[4]

Syndrome	Gene	Mode of Inheritance	Clinical Manifestations
Basal cell nevus syndrome (Gorlin syndrome)	PTCH	Autosomal dominant	Basal cell carcinoma, medulloblastoma, ovarian fibrosarcoma, odontogenic keratocyst, palmar/plantar pits, ectopic calcification
Breast/ovarian cancer syndrome	BRCA1	Autosomal dominant	Breast, ovary, fallopian tube, prostate, pancreas, and possibly gastric, as well as other sites
	BRCA2	Autosomal dominant	Breast, ovary, fallopian tube, prostate, pancreas, melanoma, and possibly gastric, as well as other sites
Cowden syndrome	PTEN	Autosomal dominant	Multiple mucocutaneous lesions, vitiligo, angiomas, benign proliferative disease of multiple organ systems, macrocephaly, breast cancer, thyroid (nonmedullary) cancer, endometrial cancer, and renal cancer, as well as other possible sites
Familial adenomatous polyposis (FAP)	APC	Autosomal dominant	Multiple colon and/or rectal adenomatous polyps (>100 polyps = FAP; <100 polyps = attenuated FAP), polyps in the upper gastrointestinal tract, osteomas, epidermoid cysts, desmoid tumors, congenital hypertrophy of retinal pigment, dental abnormalities and cancers of the thyroid, small bowel, hepatoblastoma, and brain tumors
Familial juvenile polyposis	BRIP1A SMAD4	Autosomal dominant	Hamartomatous polyps of the stomach, small intestine, colon and rectum. Colon cancer, as well as cancers of the stomach, duodenum, and pancreas
Fanconi anemia	FANCA FANCB/FAAP95 FANCC FANCD1?BRCA2 FANCD2 FANCE FANCF FANCG/XRCC FANCI/KIAA1784 FANCJ/BACH1/ BRIP1 FANCL/PHF9/ FAAP43/POG FANCM/ FAAP250/Hef FANCCN/PALB2	Autosomal recessive	Leukemia, hepatocellular carcinomas, squamous cell carcinomas—head/neck, esophagus, cervix, vulva, anus, hepatic adenoma, myelodysplastic syndrome, aplastic anemia

(continued)

Table 55–2. (*continued*)

Syndrome	Gene	Mode of Inheritance	Clinical Manifestations
Li-Fraumeni syndrome	*TP53*	Autosomal dominant	Breast cancer, sarcoma, brain tumors, leukemia, adrenocortical carcinoma, as well as other possible cancers
Lynch syndrome (also known as hereditary nonpolyposis colorectal cancer)	*MLH1* *MSH2* *MSH6* *MSH3* *PMS1* *PMS2*	Autosomal dominant	Cancers of the colon, rectum, stomach, small intestine, biliary tract, brain, endometrium, and ovary, and transitional cell carcinoma of the ureters and renal pelvis
Melanoma	*CDKN2A* *CDK4*	Autosomal dominant	Melanoma, astrocytoma, pancreatic cancer, ocular melanoma, as well as possibly breast cancer
Multiple endocrine neoplasm type I	*MEN1*	Autosomal dominant	Pancreatic and neuroendocrine tumors, gastrinomas, insulinomas, parathyroid disease, carcinoids, as well as adrenal cortical tumors, malignant schwannomas, ovarian tumors, pancreatic islet cell cancers, and gastrointestinal stromal tumors
Multiple endocrine neoplasm type II	*RET*	Autosomal dominant	Medullary thyroid cancer, pheochromocytoma, papillary thyroid cancer, ganglioneuromas
MYH-associated polyposis (MAP)	*MYH*	Autosomal recessive	Cancers of the colon and duodenum, colon, duodenal and gastric fundic gland polyps, osteomas, sebaceous gland adenomas, and pilomatricomas
Neurofibromatosis type 1	*NF1*	Autosomal dominant	Malignant peripheral neural sheath tumors, neurofibromas, benign pheochromocytomas, meningiomas, hamartomatous intestinal polyps, gastrointestinal stromal tumors, optic gliomas, café-au-lait macules, axillary or inguinal freckles, iris hamartomas, sphenoid wing dysplasia or congenital bowing/thinning of long bones, as well as other malignancies
Neurofibromatosis type 2	*NF2*	Autosomal dominant	Neurofibromas, gliomas, vestibular schwannoma, schwannomas of other cranial and peripheral nerves, meningioma, ependymomas, astrocytomas
Prostate cancer	*BRCA1* *BRCA2* *HOXB13* *RNASEL* *ELAC2/HPC2* *MSR1* *EMSY* *AMACR* *KLM6* *NBS1* *CHEK2* *MMR genes (MLH1, MSH2, MSH6, PMS2)* *Several other loci under study*	Varied: Autosomal dominant, autosomal recessive, X-Linked	Prostate cancer, other cancers not fully defined
Retinoblastoma	*RB1*	Autosomal dominant	Retinoblastoma, soft tissue and osteosarcoma, melanoma, brain tumors and nasal cavity cancers, lung cancer, bladder cancer, retinomas, lipomas
von Hippel-Lindau	*VHL*	Autosomal dominant	Renal cell cancer, hemangioblastoma of brain, spinal cord, and retina, renal cysts, pheochromocytomas, endolymphatic sac tumors, pancreatic islet cell tumors
Wilms tumor	*WT1*	Autosomal dominant	Wilms tumor, nephrogenic rests
Xeroderma pigmentosum	*XPA* *ERCC3* *XPC* *ERCC2* *DDB2* *ERCC4* *ERCC5* *POLH*	Autosomal recessive	Basal and squamous cell skin cancer, melanoma, sarcoma, brain, lung, breast, uterus, kidney, and testicle cancers, leukemia, conjunctival papillomas, actinic keratosis, lid epithiomas, keratoacanthomas, angiomas, fibromas

Table 55–3. Selected Criteria for Referring a Patient to a Genetics Professional[4–6,*]

1. General indications:
   a. Family member with documented deleterious mutation in a cancer susceptibility gene
   b. Cancer in two or more close relatives (on same side of family)
   c. Early age at cancer diagnosis
   d. Multiple primary tumors
   e. Bilateral cancer in paired organs
   f. Multiple rare cancers in biologically related relatives
   g. Constellation of tumors consistent with known hereditary syndrome (eg, medullary thyroid cancer and pheochromocytoma)
   h. Rare histology

2. Breast and/or ovarian genetic syndrome assessment if patient has 1 or more of the following:
   a. Member of a family with a known mutation in a breast cancer susceptibility gene
   b. Age ≤45 years at diagnosis of breast cancer (including ductal carcinoma in situ [DCIS])
   c. Age ≤50 years at diagnosis of breast cancer (including DCIS) and/or ≥1 first-, second-, or third-degree relative with epithelial ovarian cancer at any age
   d. Two primary breast cancers with first breast cancer diagnosed at age ≤50 years
   e. Triple-negative (ER, PR, HER2) breast cancer diagnosed at age ≤60 years
   f. Breast cancer at any age with ≥2 first-, second-, or third-degree relatives with breast and/or epithelial ovarian cancer at any age
   g. Breast cancer at any age with ≥2 first-, second-, or third-degree relatives with pancreatic cancer or aggressive prostate cancer (Gleason score > or = 7) at any age
   h. Breast cancer at any age with first-, second-, or third-degree relatives with male breast cancer
   i. Breast cancer at any age in populations at risk, for example, Ashkenazi Jewish descent
   j. Epithelial ovarian cancer at any age
   k. Male breast cancer at any age
   l. Pancreatic cancer or aggressive prostate cancer (Gleason score > or = 7) at any age with ≥2 first-, second-, or third-degree relatives with breast cancer and/or ovarian and/or pancreatic cancer or aggressive prostate cancer (Gleason score > or = 7)
   m. No history of cancer but family history consistent with any of the above criteria

3. Li-Fraumeni syndrome criteria:
   a. Member of a kindred with a known positive *TP53* mutation
   b. Individual diagnosed with a sarcoma younger than 45 years of age and with a first-degree relative diagnosed at younger than 45 years of age with any cancer and an additional first- or second-degree relative in the same lineage with any cancer diagnosed at younger than age 45 years of age or a sarcoma at any age

4. Li-Fraumeni–like syndrome criteria:
   a. Individual with
      i. Any childhood tumor
      ii. Any sarcoma, brain tumor or adrenocortical carcinoma diagnosed at younger than age 45 years *and*
      iii. A first- or second-degree relative with a typical Li-Fraumeni syndrome at any age and another first- or second-degree relative with any cancer diagnosed at younger than the age of 60 years

5. Colorectal cancer (FAP/Lynch) syndrome criteria:
   a. Family with known hereditary syndrome associated with cancer with or without mutation (eg, polyposis)
   b. Early age onset colorectal cancer (younger than age 50 years)
   c. Presence of synchronous or metachronous colon cancer diagnosed at any age
   d. Colon cancer at any age with ≥1 first-, second-, or third-degree relatives with a Lynch syndrome-associated cancer with 1 cancer diagnosed at younger than age 50 years
   e. Colon or endometrial cancer with MSI-H histology
   f. Colon cancer at any age with ≥2 first-, second-, or third-degree relatives with a Lynch syndrome–associated cancer at any age
   g. Endometrial cancer at <50 years of age
   h. Clustering of same or related cancer in close relative
      i. Colorectal
      ii. Endometrial
      iii. Ovarian
      iv. Duodenal/small bowel
      v. Stomach
      vi. Ureteral/renal pelvis
      vii. Sebaceous adenomas or sebaceous carcinoma OR
   i. Multiple colorectal carcinomas or >10 adenomas in same individual OR
   j. History of a desmoid tumor

*Testing is most informative when testing an affected family member first. Testing unaffected individuals can be considered when no affected family member is available but this limits test interpretation

Table 55–4. Management Guidelines for Selected Inherited Cancer Syndromes

Cancer Risk Management Options for Selected Cancers Associated with Hereditary Breast/Ovarian Cancer Syndrome[5]

Cancer	Test or Procedure	Frequency	Considerations
FEMALE			
Breast	Mammography	Every 12 months starting at age 25 years or individualized based on the earliest breast cancer case in family, whichever is earlier	Consider offering participation in ongoing high-risk screening studies using novel imaging modalities
	Breast MRI	Every 12 months starting at age 25 years or individualized based on the earliest breast cancer case in family, whichever is earlier	
	Risk-reducing mastectomy	Consider once childbearing/breast-feeding is complete	
	Clinical breast exam	Every 6–12 months starting at age 25 years	
	Breast awareness	Training and education starting at age 18 years	
	Chemoprevention	Consider on a case-by-case basis	Cancer Screening, Chapter 54 for a summary of breast chemoprevention from the table: Modified ACS Guidelines for Screening and Treating Women at Increased Risk for Breast Cancer
Ovarian	Transvaginal ultrasound with color flow Doppler	Every 6 months starting at age 30 years or 5–10 years prior to the earliest ovarian cancer case in the family	Optimal to perform on days 1–10 of menstrual cycle in premenopausal women
	CA-125	Every 6 months starting at age 30 years or 5–10 years prior to the earliest ovarian cancer case in the family	Optimal to perform after day 5 of menstrual cycle in premenopausal women
	Risk-reducing bilateral salpingo oophorectomy	Recommended when childbearing complete, ideally between ages 35 and 40 years or individualized based on earliest ovarian cancer case in the family	
	Chemoprevention: oral contraceptive	Consider on a case-by-case basis	Evidence is unclear about whether this is associated with a small increased breast cancer risk
MALE			
Prostate	Digital rectal exam	Consider every year starting at age 40 years	
	PSA	Consider every year starting at age 40 years	
Breast	Mammography	Consider baseline mammogram at age 40 years; annual mammogram if baseline exam shows gynecomastia or parenchymal glandular breast density	
	Clinical breast exam	Consider every 6–12 months starting at age 35 years	
	Breast awareness	Training and education starting at age 35 years	

American Cancer Society Guidelines should be followed for cancer screening other than that outlined above
Refer to Chapter 54 for more information

(*continued*)

Table 55–4. (*continued*)

Cancer Risk Management Options for Lynch Syndrome (Hereditary Nonpolyposis Colorectal Cancer [HNPCC])[6]

Cancer	Test or Procedure	Frequency	Considerations
Colon	Colonoscopy	Every 1–2 years starting at age 20–25 years or 2–5 years prior to the earliest age of diagnosis in the family if earlier than age 25 years	
Ovarian	Transvaginal ultrasound with color flow Doppler	No evidence to support this screening but can be considered every year	
	CA-125	No evidence to support this screening but can be considered every year	
	Risk-reducing bilateral salpingo oophorectomy	Consider when childbearing complete	
Endometrial	Transvaginal ultrasound with color flow Doppler	No evidence to support this screening but can be considered every year	
	Endometrial aspirate	No evidence to support this screening but can be considered every year	
	Risk-reducing hysterectomy	Consider when childbearing complete	
Stomach and small bowel	Upper endoscopy	No evidence to support this screening but EGD with extended duodenoscopy can be considered every 2–3 years starting at age 30–35 years. Consider capsule endoscopy for small bowel every 2–3 years starting at age 30–35 years	
Urinary tract	Urinalysis	Every year starting at age 25–30 years	
Central nervous system	Physical examination	Every year starting at age 25–30 years	
Pancreas	None	Data insufficient to recommend screening modality	
Breast	None	There is emerging evidence that Lynch Syndrome increases breast cancer risk. Data is insufficient to recommend screening beyond American Cancer Society Guidelines for breast cancer screening	

Table 55–5. Key Elements of Informed Consent for Genetic Testing for Cancer Susceptibility[1,3,4]

Topic	Content	
Purpose of test	*No prior history of cancer:* 1. Potential clarification of personal cancer risk 2. Risk for other family members *History of cancer:* 1. Establishing the basis for existing cancer 2. Identifying risk for other cancers 3. Risk for other family members	
Practical aspects of test	1. Type of analysis being performed 2. Cost 3. Insurance coverage 4. Biosample required (blood, buccal swab, etc.) 5. Timeframe for results to be available 6. Plan for result disclosure	
Possible test outcomes	Specificity and sensitivity of test *Known deleterious mutation in family:* 1. Negative/informative 2. Positive for deleterious mutation in family *No known mutation in family:* 1. Negative/uninformative 2. Variant of uncertain significance 3. Positive for deleterious mutation 4. Cancer risks associated with gene if deleterious mutation identified	
Psychosocial implications	*Psychological:* 1. Relief 2. Anxiety 3. Vulnerability 4. Anger 5. Depression 6. Guilt 7. Regret over prior decisions	*Social:* 1. Family implications 2. Patterns of transmission 3. Family dissemination plan for results 4. Testing other family members 5. Insurance risks (health, life, disability and long-term care insurance) and the protections provided by the Genetic Information Non-Discrimination Act (GINA) 6. Employment discrimination 7. Military discrimination
Options for medical follow-up	Benefits, limitations, and recommendations for: 1. Surveillance options 2. Prophylactic surgery options 3. Chemoprevention options 4. Risk avoidance options 5. Participation in clinical research	
Privacy and confidentiality	1. Where test report will be stored 2. Who has access to test report 3. Process and considerations in disclosing to third parties	
Tissue storage and reuse	Laboratories policy on: 1. Additional testing of identifiable samples 2. Length of storage of sample	
Alternatives to testing	Options for: 1. Decline testing 2. Empiric risk calculations 3. Delay of testing 4. Delay in receiving results once tested 5. Research participation	

Table 55–6. Resources

Organization	Contact Information	Resource
American Society of Clinical Oncology	http://www.asco.org	Policy statements on genetic testing for cancer susceptibility
Center for Disease Control	http://www.cdc.gov/genomics	Genomics and Disease Prevention at CDC online information resource and listserve
Gene tests	http://www.ncbi.nlm.nih.gov/sites/GeneTests/	Genetics web-based information resource on genetic syndromes, genetic testing and laboratory and clinical directories
NCI Cancer Genetic Services Directory	http://www.cancer.gov/cancertopics/genetics/directory	List of healthcare professionals who provide cancer genetic services and who meet specified criteria
OMIM Online Mendelian Inheritance in Man	http://www.ncbi.nlm.nih.gov/omim	An online catalog of information on human genes and genetic disorders
Physician's Database Query (PDQ)	http://www.cancer.gov/cancertopics/pdq/genetics	PDQ—an NCI database that contains the latest information about genetics

References

1. ASCO. American Society of Clinical Oncology policy statement update: genetic testing for cancer susceptibility. J Clin Oncol 2003;21:2397–2406
2. Robson ME, Storm CD, Weitzel J, Wollins DS, Offit K. American Society of Clinical Oncology policy statement update: genetic and genomic testing for cancer susceptibility. J Clin Oncol 2010;28(5):893–901
3. Riley BD, Culver JO, Skrzynia C et al. Essential elements of genetic cancer risk assessment, counseling, and testing: updated recommendations of the National Society of Genetic Counselors. J Genet Couns 2012;21(2):151–161
4. Lindor NM, McMaster ML, Lindor CJ, Greene MH. Concise handbook of familial cancer susceptibility syndromes—2nd edition. Journal of the National Cancer Institute Monographs, 2008;38:1–93
5. NCCN. NCCN Practice Guidelines for Prevention, Detection and Risk Reduction. Genetic/Familial High-Risk Assessment: Breast and Ovarian (2.2013). [Cited June 5, 2013] Available from: http://www.nccn.org/professionals/physician_gls/pdf/genetics_screening.pdf (2013)
6. NCCN. NCCN Practice Guidelines for Prevention, Detection and Risk Reduction. Colorectal Cancer Screening (1.2013). [Cited June 5, 2013] Available from: http://www.nccn.org/professionals/physician_gls/pdf/colorectal_screening.pdf (2013)

SECTION III. Selected Hematologic Diseases

56. von Willebrand Disease

Pier M. Mannucci, MD

von Willebrand disease (VWD)
- A congenital bleeding disorder resulting from a quantitative or qualitative deficiency of von Willebrand factor (VWF)
- VWF is a plasma glycoprotein with essential platelet-dependent function in primary hemostasis and a carrier for factor VIII (FVIII) in the circulation
- Acquired von Willebrand syndrome presents as a similar bleeding disorder

Epidemiology

Prevalence:
Inherited: 0.01–1%
- 0.01% of population using the number of patients seen at specialized hemostasis centers
- 1% of population using population-based screening (the most common inherited bleeding disorder)
Acquired: 0.04–0.13%

Male to female ratio: 1:1

Rodeghiero F et al. Blood 1987;69:454–459
Sadler JE et al. Thromb Haemost 2000;84:160–174
Werner EJ et al. J Pediatr 1993;123:893–898

Classification of Inherited VWD

	Percent of Cases	Defect	Inheritance
Type 1 (classic)	70–80%	*Quantitative* deficiency of VWF	AD
Type 2 (variant)	15–30%	*Qualitative* defect of VWF	AD or AR
Type 2A	10–20%	Decreased platelet-dependent VWF function, with lack of high-molecular-weight VWF multimers	AD Rarely AR
Type 2B	5–10%	Increased VWF affinity for platelet receptor (leading to decreased plasma levels of VWF). Patients may or may not lack high-molecular-weight VWF multimers. They may have thrombocytopenia from clearance of platelet aggregates formed by the heightened binding of VWF to platelets	AD
Type 2M	Uncommon	Decreased platelet-dependent VWF function, with normal high-molecular-weight VWF multimers	AD
Type 2N	Uncommon	Decreased affinity for FVIII. Lack of protection of FVIII by VWF leads to rapid clearance and low levels of FVIII, with normal or low borderline levels of VWF	AR
Type 3	Rare (1–5/10^6)	Complete (*quantitative*) deficiency of VWF	AR

VWF, von Willebrand factor; AD, autosomal dominant; AR, autosomal recessive
Sadler JE et al. J Thromb Haemost 2006;4:2103–2114

Work-up

Diagnostic Test		Role/Comment
Abbreviation	**Name**	
aPTT	Activated partial thromboplastin time	Not a sensitive measure for VWD
VWF:Ag	Plasma VWF antigen	
VWF:RCo	Plasma VWF activity (ristocetin **co**factor activity and **co**llagen binding activity	ELISA; limited availability
FVIII*	Factor VIII activity*	
Bleeding time	Bleeding time	Not sensitive or specific measures for VWF function
PFA-100	Automated platelet function analyzer testing	

Perform tests below:
1. To determine the VWD subtype after the diagnosis is established
2. If there is a high index of suspicion for VWD, and some of the tests above are normal

VWF multimers	VWF multimers	Gel electrophesis for size distribution of plasma multimers
RIPA	*Ristocetin-induced platelet aggregation*	Use to determine if a patient's VWF has an abnormally high affinity for platelet receptors; it is a necessary and specific for the diagnosis of type 2B VWD

VWF, von Willebrand factor; VWD, von Willebrand disease
*Note: FVIIIC is the coagulant component of FVIII, which, in normal people, circulates in the plasma complexed with von Willebrand factor

Type	VWF:Ag	VWF:RCo	RIPA	Plasma Multimer Distribution	Factor VIII:C*	Bleeding Time
1	↓	↓	N/↓	N	↓/N	↑/N
2A	↓/N	↓↓/↓	↓	↓ HMW	N/↓	↑/N
2B	↓/N	↓/N	↑↑	↓ HMW (sometimes normal)	N/↓	↑/N
2M	↓/N	↓↓/↓	↓	N	N/↓	↑/N
2N	N/↓	N	N	N	↓↓	N
3	↓↓↓	↓↓↓	↓↓↓	Not detectable	↓↓↓	↑↑

N, Normal; HMW, high molecular weight
*Note: Factor VIII:C (*or* factor VIIIC) is the coagulant component of factor VIII, which, in normal people, circulates in the plasma complexed with von Willebrand factor

Treatment Principles

Background:
1. Until 2001, cryoprecipitate was the therapeutic mainstay for bleeding in VWD
2. After 2001, concerns for potential transmission of bloodborne pathogens, led to use of plasma-derived factor VIII (pdFVIII) products enriched in VWF

Indications:
1. Unlike patients with hemophilia in whom treatment may be administered regularly to prevent bleeding, *patients with VWD* generally have less frequent and less severe clinical bleeding and *usually receive treatment only in anticipation of an invasive procedure or for trauma*
2. An *exception* may be patients with *type 3 VWD* who *might receive replacement therapy regularly* particularly if they bleed repeatedly into the joints (secondary prophylaxis)

Rationale:
1. Replace the primary hemostasis defect (VWF deficiency)
2. FVIII synthesis is not defective in VWD, but its half-life is severely reduced because VWF is its natural carrier and stabilizer. Consequently, FVIII is also deficient *but* the intrinsic coagulation defect is secondary to that of VWF

(continued)

Treatment Principles (continued)

3. Satisfactory hemostasis in VWD depends on achieving adequate plasma levels of both VWF (mediating primary hemostasis) and FVIII (responsible for fibrin formation in secondary hemostasis)
4. Hemostasis is satisfactory when the ristocetin cofactor activity (VWF:RCo)—a measure of VWF activity—is more than 0.6 IU/mL (60% of normal)

Determinants of therapeutic efficacy:
1. **FVIII:C levels:** Main determinants for the control of *soft tissue and surgical bleeding*
2. **Functional VWF levels:** Main determinants for the control of *mucosal tract hemorrhages*

Mannucci PM. Blood 2001;97:1915–1919
Mannucci PM. N Engl J Med 2004;351:683–694

Treatment Options

1. Desmopressin acetate (DDAVP; 1-deamino-8-D-arginine vasopressin). Perform therapeutic trial before use
2. *Replacement therapy:* Virally inactivated concentrates containing factor VIII/VWF or VWF only
   - Most products are intermediate purity pdFVIII concentrates that also contain VWF, and thus may be used in the treatment of either hemophilia A or VWD
   - Wilfactin a human plasma-derived product that is considered to be a highly purified VWF-containing concentrate is the exception (protocols using highly purified VWF may recommend a single supplemental dose of high-purity FVIII concentrate at the onset of therapy)
3. Antifibrinolytic agents
4. Topical agents
5. Platelet concentrates (rarely used)

Mannucci PM. Blood 2001;97:1915–1919
Mannucci PM. N Engl J Med 2004;351:683–694

Management of Different Types of Inherited VWD

Type	Treatments of Choice		Alternative and Adjuvant Therapies
	First Choice	Second Choice	
1	Desmopressin acetate	FVIII/VWF concentrates*	Antifibrinolytic agents
2A	FVIII/VWF concentrates	Desmopressin acetate	Antifibrinolytic agents
2B	FVIII/VWF concentrates	Desmopressin acetate[†]	Antifibrinolytic agents
2M	FVIII/VWF concentrates	Desmopressin acetate	Antifibrinolytic agents
2N	Desmopressin acetate[‡]	FVIII/VWF concentrates	Antifibrinolytic agents
3	FVIII/VWF concentrates	—	Antifibrinolytic agents and platelet concentrates

*Especially in patients with severe type 1 variants
[†]May decrease the platelet count and aggravate bleeding in patients with type 2B VWD
[‡]Increase in FVIII levels may be shorter in duration than expected

Mannucci PM. N Engl J Med 2004;351:683–694
Nichols WL et al. Haemophilia 2008;14:171–232

von WILLEBRAND DISEASE— THERAPEUTIC OPTIONS

DESMOPRESSIN ACETATE (DDAVP, 1-DEAMINO-8-D-ARGININE VASOPRESSIN)

Mannucci PM. Blood 2001;97:1915–1919
Mannucci PM. N Engl J Med 2004;351:683–694
Rodeghiero F et al. Blood 1989;74:1997–2000

Intravenous Administration

Note: Intravenous administration is preferred for treatment of acute bleeding episodes

Test dose

1. Measure VWF:RCo and FVIII levels before administering desmopressin acetate
2. **Desmopressin acetate** 0.2–0.3 mcg/kg (not to exceed 20 mcg) intravenously in 50 mL 0.9% sodium chloride injection (0.9% NS) over 20–30 minutes
3. Measure VWF:RCo and FVIII levels at 1 and 4 hours after administration. Expect 2–4-fold increases in VWF and FVIII levels at 30–60 minutes, falling over 6–12 hours

Therapeutic dose

1. **Desmopressin acetate** 0.2–0.3 mcg/kg (not to exceed 20 mcg) intravenously in 50 mL 0.9% NS over 30 minutes; may be repeated every 12–24 hours for 3–4 doses

Intranasal Administration (eg, Stimate Nasal Spray, 1.5 mg/mL)

Test dose

1. Measure VWF:RCo and FVIII levels before administration
2. Administer according to patient weight:
   Patient weight ≤ 50 kg: **Desmopressin acetate** 1 spray (150 mcg) intranasally in 1 nostril
   Patient weight > 50 kg: **Desmopressin acetate** 2 sprays (300 mcg) intranasally, 1 spray in each nostril
3. Measure VWF:RCo and FVIII levels at 1 and 4 hours after administration. Expect 2- to 4-fold increases in VWF:RCo and FVIII levels at 1 hour after administration, falling over 6–12 hours

Therapeutic dose

1. Administer according to patient weight:
   Patient weight ≤ 50 kg: **Desmopressin acetate** 1 spray (150 mcg) intranasally in 1 nostril
   Patient weight > 50 kg: **Desmopressin acetate** 2 sprays (300 mcg) intranasally, 1 spray in each nostril. Repeat every 12–24 hours for 2–4 doses

Toxicity

Symptom	Frequency	Comment
Facial flushing	Common but mild	Etiology: Vasodilation
Headache	Common but mild	Often controlled by decreasing infusion rate
Tachycardia	Common but mild	
Hypotension	Common	
Hypertension	Uncommon	
Volume overload	Uncommon	
Hyponatremia	Rare	Unlikely if excessive fluid intake is avoided and not more than 4–5 doses are administered
Hyponatremia and seizures	Rare	Tachyphylaxis with serious hyponatremia and seizures can occur with ≥4 doses*

*If desmopressin acetate is to be administered for more than 4 doses:
1. Limit doses to once daily
2. Restrict water intake
3. Monitor daily serum sodium levels, and measure VWF:RCo levels for evidence of tachyphylaxis (or follow response clinically)

Efficacy

Type	Response
1	Usually effective; most effective in mild or moderate disease
2A	Effective only if FVIII levels are low
2B	**Contraindicated**, because it may cause transient thrombocytopenia and worsening of bleeding in some patients
2M	Limited experience; use if test dose indicates a response
2N	May be effective, but the duration of FVIII increase will be shortened owing to a decreased survival of the FVIII
3	Ineffective

Notes

1. Advantage: Unlimited availability and avoidance of plasma concentrates
2. Response is generally consistent. Perform a test dose at the time of diagnosis to establish the individual pattern of response and to predict clinical efficacy
3. Tachyphylaxis may develop with repeated doses. Follow patients clinically, and/or measure VWF:RCo levels to assess response after >3–4 doses or after >3–4 days of use
4. **Contraindicated in type 2B VWD,** because the platelet count may drop to a level that might contribute to bleeding (<30,000–50,000/mm³)
5. Adults should limit fluid intake to 1 L during the 24-hour period after receiving desmopressin acetate
6. Avoid desmopressin acetate use in patients with known atherosclerosis or unstable coronary artery disease
7. Desmopressin acetate is not absolutely contraindicated in children, but usually it is not administered to children ≤2 years old
8. Desmopressin acetate has little oxytocic activity, and hence, may be used during pregnancy

Mannucci PM. Blood 2001;97:1915–1919
Mannucci PM. Blood 2005;105:3382
Mannucci PM. N Engl J Med 2004;351:683–694

von WILLEBRAND DISEASE— THERAPEUTIC OPTIONS VIRALLY INACTIVATED FVIII/VWF CONCENTRATES

ANTIHEMOPHILIC FACTOR/von WILLEBRAND FACTOR COMPLEX (HUMAN) (HUMATE-P, ALPHANATE, FANHDI)

Mannucci PM. Blood 2001;97:1915–1919
Mannucci PM. N Engl J Med 2004;351:683–694

Indications for FVIII/VWF concentrates:
1. Demonstration of inadequate response to a test dose of DDAVP ("severe" type 1, type 2, type 3)
2. Patients in whom DDAVP is contraindicated
3. Prediction of prolonged treatments with desmopressin (potential or actual tachyphylaxis)

Problem with FVIII/VWF concentrates:
1. High plasma levels of FVIII are a strong risk factor for venous thrombosis
   - *Venous thrombosis in VWD:* 4 cases after treatment with a VWF/FVIII concentrate used to ensure competent hemostasis during invasive and surgical procedures
   - *Venous thromboembolism in VWD:* 7 cases in 12,640 yearly treatments over 10 years

Makris M et al. Thromb Haemost 2002;88:387–388
Mannucci PM. Thromb Haemost 2002;88:378–379

Virally Inactivated Antihemophilic Factor/von Willebrand Factor Complex (Human) (FVIII/VWF) Concentrates
Humate-P, Alphanate, and Fanhdi are approved in the United States and in some European countries for use in VWD and are labeled with VWF:RCo units. Ristocetin cofactor units are used to calculate dose (refer to product-specific labeling)

Humate-P (CSL Behring)
1. Pasteurized
2. *Average VWF:RCo-to-factor VIII ratio:* 2.4:1
3. Efficacy and safety established in 2 prospective and several retrospective studies

Lethagen S et al. J Thromb Haemost 2007;5:1420–1430
Thompson AR et al. Haemophilia 2004;10:42–51

Alphanate (Grifols) and Fanhdi (Grifols)
1. Virally inactivated by solvent/detergent and heating
2. *VWF:RCo-to-FVIII ratio:* varies by product lot (Alphanate)
3. Efficacy and safety established by 2 prospective studies and a few retrospective studies

Bello IF et al. Haemophilia 2007;13(Suppl 5):25–32
Mannucci PM et al. Blood 2002;99:450–456

Other FVIII/VWF concentrates
1. Various products, virus-inactivated
2. Several small retrospective studies

(continued)

Monitoring Replacement Therapy

1. *Surgical procedures:* Measure plasma levels of FVIII and/or VWF:RCo every 12 hours on the day of surgery, then every 24 hours or as dictated by clinical circumstances
2. It is not usually necessary to monitor replacement therapy in patients with spontaneous minor bleeding
3. *Every physician encounter:* Careful clinical follow-up because bleeding may not correlate well with factor levels; careful clinical monitoring is needed

Notes

1. Fresh-frozen plasma contains both FVIII and VWF, but the large amounts that are needed to attain hemostatic concentrations may cause volume overload. In addition, plasma is not generally inactivated for infectious agents and is not recommended
2. Eight to 12 bags of cryoprecipitate (each bag contains 80–100 units of FVIII, a 5–10-times greater concentration than fresh-frozen plasma) can normalize FVIII and VWF levels and stop or prevent bleeding. However, methods for inactivating infectious agents are not routinely applicable to this plasma fraction. Thus, cryoprecipitate is not recommended. Use only for very serious bleeding when virally inactivated concentrates are not available

(continued)

General Guidelines for All Virally Inactivated FVIII/VWF Concentrates
(*Note:* Specific Guidelines from Package Inserts Listed Under Each Preparation Represent Only Minor Variations Over These General Guidelines)
Dosing Replacement Therapy*

Clinical Situation	Dose of VWF:RCo and/or Factor VIII:C	Number of Infusions	VWF:RCo Target Plasma Level†
Major surgery	40–60 units/kg	Every 12 hours initially, then once daily until wound healing is complete	50–100 units/dL Maintain levels for 3–10 days
Minor surgery	30–50 units/kg	Once daily (may require only 1–3 days)	>30 units/dL
Dental extraction	20–30 units/kg	Usually 1 dose prior to procedure	>30 units/dL for >12 hours
Spontaneous minor bleeding	20–30 units/kg	One dose is usually sufficient. Monitor clinically	>30 units/dL

*Monitor patients clinically, and give replacement according to the clinical setting and judgment of the physician
†Factor levels can be predicted based on pharmacokinetic data; 40–50 units/kg (VWF:RCO) will increase plasma VWF levels to 80–100% depending on baseline levels and hematocrit

REGIMEN

ANTIHEMOPHILIC FACTOR/von WILLEBRAND FACTOR COMPLEX (HUMAN) PRODUCTS
HUMATE-P

1. *General:* A stable, purified, sterile, lyophilized concentrate of human antihemophilic Factor (FVIII) *and* human von Willebrand Factor (VWF) to be administered by the intravenous route in the treatment of patients with classical hemophilia (hemophilia A) and von Willebrand disease (VWD). Factor VIII is an essential cofactor in activation of Factor X, leading ultimately to formation of thrombin and fibrin. The VWF promotes platelet aggregation and platelet adhesion on damaged vascular endothelium; it also serves as a stabilizing carrier protein for the procoagulant protein FVIII. The activity of VWF is measured as VWF:RCo

2. *Indications:* Adult and pediatric patients with severe von Willebrand disease and mild-to-moderate von Willebrand disease where use of desmopressin is known or suspected to be inadequate for:
   • Treatment of spontaneous and trauma-induced bleeding episodes
   • Prevention of excessive bleeding during and after surgery

3. *Administration and dosage (see also tables below):*
   • The dosage should be adjusted according to the extent and location of bleeding
   • As a rule, 40–80 IU VWF:RCo (corresponding to 17–33 IU factor VIII in Humate-P) per kg body weight are given every 8–12 hours
   • Repeat doses are administered for as long as needed based on repeated monitoring of appropriate clinical and laboratory measures
   • Expected levels of VWF:RCo are based on an expected in vivo recovery of 2 IU/dL rise per 1 IU/kg VWF:RCo administered
   • The administration of 1 IU of factor VIII per kg body weight can be expected to lead to a rise in circulating VWF:RCo of approximately 5 IU/dL

4. *Properties:*
   • Humate-P has been demonstrated in several studies to contain the high-molecular-weight multimers of VWF. This component is considered to be important for correcting the coagulation defect in patients with VWD. Bleeding time decreased when Humate-P was administered to patients with VWD (types 1, 2, and 3). This effect was correlated with the presence of a multimeric composition of VWF similar to that found in normal plasma
   • The virus-reduction steps in the manufacturing process include: (a) cryoprecipitation, (b) $Al(OH)_3$ adsorption, glycine precipitation, and sodium chloride precipitation, and (c) pasteurization in aqueous solution at 60°C (140°F) for 10 hours

Humate-P
VWF:RCo Dosing Recommendations for Treatment of von Willebrand Disease
(Source: Humate-P Package Insert)

Classification of VWD	Hemorrhage	Dosage (IU VWF:RCo/kg body weight)
Type 1, mild, if desmopressin is inappropriate (Baseline VWF:RCo activity typically >30%)	Major (eg, severe or refractory epistaxis, GI bleeding, CNS trauma, or traumatic hemorrhage)	• *Loading dose:* 40–60 IU/kg • *Maintenance dose, days 1–3:* 40–50 IU/kg every 8–12 hours for 3 days to keep the trough level of VWF:RCo >50% • *Maintenance dose, days 4–7:* 40–50 IU/kg daily for a total of up to 7 days of treatment
Type 1, moderate or severe (baseline VWF:RCo activity typically <30%)	Minor (eg, epistaxis, oral bleeding, menorrhagia)	40–50 IU/kg (1 or 2 doses)
	Major (eg, severe or refractory epistaxis, GI bleeding, CNS trauma, hemarthrosis, or traumatic hemorrhage)	• *Loading dose:* 50–75 IU/kg • *Maintenance dose, days 1–3:* 40–60 IU/kg every 8–12 hours for 3 days to keep the trough level of VWF:RCo >50% • *Maintenance dose, days 4–7:* 40–60 IU/kg daily for a total of up to 7 days of treatment *Note:* Monitor and maintain factor VIII:C levels as recommended below*

(continued)

(continued)

Types 2 (all variants) and 3	Minor (eg, epistaxis, oral bleeding, menorrhagia)	40–50 IU/kg (1 or 2 doses)
	Major (eg, severe or refractory epistaxis, GI bleeding, CNS trauma, hemarthrosis, or traumatic hemorrhage)	• *Loading dose:* 60–80 IU/kg • *Maintenance dose, days 1–3:* 40–60 IU/kg every 8–12 hours for 3 days to keep the trough level of VWF:RCo >50% • *Maintenance dose, days 4–7:* 40–60 IU/kg daily for a total of up to 7 days of treatment *Note:* Monitor and maintain factor VIII:C levels as recommended below*

*Recommendations for maintaining Factor VIII:C levels:

Minor hemorrhage: Monitor closely to achieve FVIII:C plasma level approximately 30% of normal range

Moderate hemorrhage: Monitor closely to achieve FVIII:C plasma level approximately 30% of normal range using the same dose once or twice daily for a total of up to 7 days, or until adequate wound healing

Severe/life-threatening hemorrhage: Monitor closely to achieve FVIII:C plasma level at 80–100% of normal for 7 days, then continue the same dose once or twice daily for another 7 days in order to maintain the FVIII:C level at 30–50% of normal range

VWF:RCo and FVIII:C Target Trough Plasma Levels and Minimum Duration of Treatment Recommendations for Subsequent Maintenance Doses for the Prevention of Excessive Bleeding During and After Surgery (Humate-P Antihemophilic Factor/von Willebrand Factor Complex (Human) Lyophilized Powder for Reconstitution for Intravenous Use Only, product labeling, January 2010. Manufactured by CSL Behring GmbH, Marburg, Germany)

Type of Surgery	VWF:RCo Target Trough Plasma Levels*		FVIII:C Target Trough Plasma Levels*		Minimum Duration of Treatment
	Up to 3 Days Following Surgery	After Day 3	Up to 3 Days Following Surgery	After Day 3	
Major	>50 IU/dL	>30 IU/dL	>50 IU/dL	>30 IU/dL	72 hours
Minor	≥30 IU/dL	—	—	>30 IU/dL	48 hours
Oral†	≥30 IU/dL	—	—	>30 IU/dL	8–12 hours‡

*Trough levels for either coagulation factor should not exceed 100 IU/dL

†Oral surgery is defined as removal of fewer than 3 teeth, if the teeth are nonmolars and have no bony involvement. Removal of more than 1 impacted wisdom tooth is considered major surgery because of the expected difficulty of the surgery and the expected blood loss, particularly in subjects with type 2A or type 3 VWD. Removal of more than 2 teeth is considered major surgery in all patients

‡Administer at least 1 maintenance dose following surgery based on individual pharmacokinetic values. Subsequent therapy with an antifibrinolytic agent is usually administered until adequate healing is achieved

Efficacy*

Summary of Efficacy for Bleeding Episodes—All Subjects

	Diagnosis							
	Type 1 VWD		Type 2A VWD		Type 2B VWD		Type 3 VWD	
Number of subjects	13	—	2	—	10	—	21	—
Excellent/good	13	100%	2	100%	10	100%	18	86%
Poor/none	—	—	—	—	—	—	3	14%
Number of events	32	—	17	—	60	—	208	—
Excellent/good	32	100%	17	100%	60	100%	198	95%
Poor/none	—	—	—	—	—	—	10	5%

*Clinical efficacy of Humate-P in the control of bleeding in subjects with VWD was determined by a retrospective review of clinical safety and efficacy data obtained from 97 Canadian subjects with VWD who received the product under an Emergency Drug Release Program. Dosage schedule and duration of therapy were determined by the judgment of the medical practitioner. Humate-P was administered to the 97 subjects in 530 treatment courses: 73 for surgery, 344 for treatment of bleeding, and 20 for prophylaxis of bleeding. For 93 "other" uses, the majority involved dental procedures, diagnostic procedures, prophylaxis prior to a procedure, or a test dose

(continued)

Efficacy* (continued)

Summary of Hemostatic Efficacy Among Subjects in American (U.S.) and European Clinical Studies

	Study	
	U.S. (N = 35)	European (N = 27)
Patient Characteristics and Procedures Performed		
Number of subjects (female/male)	35 (21/14)	27
Type 1	12	10
Type 2A	2	9
Type 2B	3	—
Type 2M	5	1
Type 3	13	7
Major surgical procedures (eg, orthopedic joint replacement, hysterectomy, intracranial surgery, multiple tooth extractions, laparoscopic adnexectomy, laparoscopic cholecystectomy, basal cell carcinoma excision)	28	16
Minor surgical procedures (eg, placement of intravenous access device)	4	—
Oral surgery	3	—
Investigator's Overall Hemostatic Efficacy Assessments†		
Effective (excellent/good)	35 (100%)	26 (96.3%)
95% CI for effective proportion‡	91.3–100%	82.5–99.8%
Assessments of Hemostatic Efficacy at End of Surgery		
Effective at end of surgery	32 (91.4%)	25 (96%)
Effective end of surgery 95% CI	78.5–97.6%	82–99.8%
Median Duration of Treatment		
Minor surgery	5 days	3.5 days
Range for minor surgery	3–7 days	1–17 days
Major surgery	5.5 days	9 days
Range for major surgery	2–26 days	1–17 days
Oral surgery	1 day	—
Range for oral surgery	1–2 days	—

*Adapted from **Humate-P** product labeling, January 2010
†In the U.S. study, overall hemostatic efficacy was assessed 24 hours after the last infusion of Humate-P or 14 days after surgery, whichever came first. In the European study, overall hemostatic efficacy was not prospectively defined; the efficacy result displayed is the least-efficacious ranking assigned by an investigator between surgery and day 14
‡The 95% CIs according to Blyth-Still-Casella

Toxicity and Adverse Effects

1. The most serious adverse reaction observed is *anaphylaxis*. The most commonly reported are allergic-anaphylactic reactions (including urticaria, chest tightness, rash, pruritus, edema, and shock) reported in 6 of 97 (6%) subjects in a Canadian retrospective study

2. *Thromboembolic events* have also been observed

3. Other adverse events that were considered to have a possible or probable relationship to the product in 4/97 (4%) subjects included chills, phlebitis, vasodilation, paresthesia, pruritus, rash, and urticaria. All were mild in intensity with the exception of a moderate case of pruritus

4. For patients undergoing surgery, the most common adverse reactions are postoperative wound or injection-site bleeding

5. In a prospective, open-label, safety and efficacy study of Humate-P in VWD patients with serious life- or limb-threatening bleeding or who were undergoing emergency surgery, 7 of 71 (10%) subjects experienced 9 adverse reactions, including mild vasodilation (1/9), allergic reactions (2/9), pruritus (1/9), and paresthesia (2/9)

6. Among 63 VWD patients who received Humate-P during and after surgery, the most common adverse events were postoperative hemorrhage (35 events in 19 patients with 5 patients experiencing bleeding at up to 3 different sites), postoperative nausea (15 patients), and postoperative pain (11 patients)

REGIMEN

ANTIHEMOPHILIC FACTOR/von WILLEBRAND FACTOR COMPLEX (HUMAN) PRODUCTS ALPHANATE/FANHDI

Alphanate (Antihemophilic Factor/von Willebrand Factor [AHF/VWF] Complex [Human]) Sterile, lyophilized powder for injection, product labeling, dated June 2011. Manufactured and distributed by Grifols Biologicals Inc., Los Angeles, CA
• Grifols manufactures both Alphanate and Fanhdi. The latter is marketed outside the United States

1. *General:* Alphanate contains a labeled amount of FVIII expressed in IU FVIII/vial and Willebrand factor:Ristocetin cofactor activity in IU VWF:RCo/vial. The ratio of VWF:RCo to FVIII in Alphanate varies by lot, so dosage should be reevaluated whenever lot selection is changed. Dosage and duration of treatment depend on the severity of the VWF deficiency, the location and extent of bleeding, and a patient's clinical condition. Overdosage resulting in FVIII levels above 150% should be avoided
2. *Indications:* Adult and pediatric patients with severe von Willebrand disease as well as patients with mild-to-moderate von Willebrand disease where use of desmopressin is known or suspected to be inadequate for:
   • Treatment of spontaneous and trauma-induced bleeding episodes
   • Prevention of excessive bleeding during and after surgery
   Note: The products are not indicated for patients with severe VWD (Type 3) who are undergoing major surgery
3. *Administration:*
   • Replacement therapy is given intravenously over 15–20 minutes within 10–30 minutes before a planned procedure by a slow intravenous infusion at a rate not greater than 10 mL/min
4. *Dosage (see tables below):*
   • *Adults:* Preoperative dose of 60 IU VWF:RCo/kg of body weight; subsequent doses of 40–60 IU VWF:RCo/kg of body weight at 8–12-hour intervals postoperatively as clinically needed for 1–3 days
   • *Pediatric:* Preoperation dose of 75 IU VWF:RCo/kg body weight; subsequent doses of 50–75 IU VWF:RCo/kg body weight at 8–12-hour intervals postoperatively as clinically needed for 1–3 days
5. *Properties:*
   • Alphanate is prepared from pooled human plasma by cryoprecipitation of FVIII, fractional solubilization, and further purification employing heparin-coupled, cross-linked agarose, which has an affinity for the heparin-binding domain of VWF/FVIII:C complex
   • The product is (a) treated with a mixture of tri-*n*-butyl phosphate (TNBP) and polysorbate 80 to inactivate enveloped viruses and (b) subjected to heating at 80°C (176°F) for 72 hours to inactivate enveloped and nonenveloped viruses

Alphanate Dosage and Administration
Guidelines for Prophylaxis During Surgery and Invasive Procedure of von Willebrand Disease (Except Type 3 Subjects Undergoing Major Surgery)*

Minor Surgery/Bleeding		
	VWF:RCo	**Target FVIII:C Activity Levels**
Preoperative, *or* Preprocedure dose	*Adults:* • 60 IU VWF:RCo/kg body weight *Pediatrics:* • 75 IU VWF:RCo/kg body weight	40–50 IU/dL
Maintenance dose	*Adults:* • 40–60 IU VWF:RCo/kg body weight • 8–12-hour intervals • As clinically needed for 1–3 days *Pediatrics:* • 50–75 IU VWF:RCo/kg body weight • 8–12-hour intervals • As clinically needed for 1–3 days	40–50 IU/dL
Safety monitoring	Peak and trough concentrations at least once daily	Peak and trough concentrations at least once daily
Therapeutic goal†	Trough >50 IU/dL for 3–5 days	
Safety parameter‡	Should not exceed 150 IU/dL	Should not exceed 150 IU/dL

(continued)

(continued)

	VWF:RCo	Target FVIII:C Activity Levels
	Major Surgery/Bleeding	
Preoperative, *or* Preprocedure dose	*Adults:* • 60 IU VWF:RCo/kg body weight *Pediatrics:* • 75 IU VWF:RCo/kg body weight	100 IU/dL
Maintenance dose	*Adults:* 40–60 IU VWF:RCo/kg body weight 8–12-hour intervals As clinically needed for at least 3–7 days *Pediatrics:* 50–75 IU VWF:RCo/kg body weight 8–12-hour intervals As clinically needed for at least 3–7 days	100 IU/dL
Safety monitoring	Peak and trough concentrations at least once daily	Peak and trough concentrations at least once daily
Therapeutic goal†	Trough >50 IU/dL for 7–14 days	
Safety parameter‡	Should not exceed 150 IU/dL	Should not exceed 150 IU/dL

General Guidelines:

Replacement therapy is given intravenously over 15–20 minutes within 10–30 minutes before a planned procedure by a slow intravenous infusion at a rate not greater than 10 mL/minute

General calculations:

• Dosage (units) = body weight (kg) × desired FVIII rise (IU/dL) × 0.5 (IU/kg × dL/IU)
• Dosage (units) = body weight (kg) × desired FVIII rise (% normal) × 0.5 (IU/kg)

Thus, an administered antihemophilic factor dose of 50 IU/kg will be expected to increase the circulating FVIII level to 100% of normal or 100 IU/dL

*Adapted from Alphanate product labeling, dated June 2011
†The therapeutic goal is recommended in the NHLBI Guidelines (NIH von Willebrand Disease Expert Panel. The Diagnosis, Evaluation, and Management of von Willebrand Disease. Bethesda, MD: U.S. Department of Health and Human Services, National Institutes of Health, National Heart, Lung, and Blood Institute December 2007; NIH Publication No. 08–5832)
‡The safety parameter is extracted from Mannucci PM et al. Blood Transfus 2009;7:117–126

Toxicity and Adverse Effects

1. Anaphylaxis and severe hypersensitivity reactions are possible. Should symptoms occur, treatment with Alphanate should be discontinued, and emergency treatment should be sought
2. Development of activity-neutralizing antibodies has been detected in patients receiving FVIII containing products. Development of alloantibodies to VWF in type 3 VWD patients have been occasionally reported in the literature
3. Thromboembolic events may be associated with AHF/VWF Complex (Human) use in VWD patients, especially in the setting of known risk factors
4. Intravascular hemolysis may be associated with infusion of massive doses of AHF/VWF Complex (Human)
5. Rapid administration of a FVIII concentrate may result in vasomotor reactions
6. Plasma products carry a risk of transmitting infectious agents, such as viruses, and, theoretically, the Creutzfeldt-Jakob disease (CJD) agent, despite steps designed to reduce this risk
7. The most frequent adverse effects reported with Alphanate in >5% of patients, include:
   • Respiratory distress
   • Pruritus, rash
   • Urticaria
   • Facial edema
   • Paresthesia
   • Pain
   • Fever
   • Chills
   • Joint pain
   • Fatigue

Efficacy*

Prophylaxis with Alphanate (A-SD/HT)† in Surgery

Number of patients	18
Number of surgical procedures	24
Median number of infusions per surgical procedure (range)	4 (1–18)
Median dosage IU VWF:RCo/kg infusion #1 (range)	59.9 (40.6–75)
Median dosage IU VWF:RCo/kg infusion ≥ #2 combined (range)	40 (10–63.1)

Effect of Treatment on Surgical Prophylaxis (Referee Evaluation) Analysis per Treated Event with Alphanate (A-SD/HT)†

	Referee 1	Referee 2
Number of treated subjects	18	18
Number of treated events	24	24
Success (absolute number [proportion])	22 (0.9166)	21 (0.8750)
95% CI for the proportion‡	0.7300–0.9897	0.6763–0.9734

*Adapted from Alphanate product labeling, dated June 2011, and Federici AB et al. Clinical efficacy of highly purified, doubly virus-inactivated factor VIII/von Willebrand factor concentrate (Fanhdi) in the treatment of von Willebrand disease: a retrospective clinical study. Haemophilia 2002;8:761–767

†Distinguishes Alphanate (A-SD/HT, Alphanate Solvent Detergent/Heat Treated) from an earlier formulation designated Alphanate (A-SD, Alphanate Solvent Detergent)

‡95% confidence interval for the proportion of subjects with successful prophylaxis, exact estimation

REGIMEN

VWF CONCENTRATE
WILFACTIN (HUMAN von WILLEBRAND FACTOR)
(LICENSED IN A FEW EUROPEAN COUNTRIES)

Borel-Derlon A et al. J Thromb Haemost 2007;5:1115–1124

1. *General:* A pure VWF concentrate almost devoid of FVIII developed and used in France since 1989 to correct the primary von Willebrand factor (VWF) defect and avoid supraphysiologic plasma levels of factor VIII

2. *Indications:*
   - Prevention and treatment of hemorrhages or surgical bleeding in von Willebrand Disease (VWD) when desmopressin acetate treatment alone is ineffective or contraindicated
   - Elective major surgery, particularly when repeated infusions are foreseen and patients are at high risk for thrombosis (old age, cancer surgery, orthopedic surgery)
   - Long-term secondary prophylaxis in von Willebrand patients when indicated
     - Target joints
     - Recurrent GI bleeding
     - Recurrent epistaxis in children

3. *Administration:*
   - A concomitant priming dose of FVIII concentrate (30–40 IU/kg) is recommended in patients with severe bleeding episodes and to those with baseline plasma FVIII levels below 20 IU/dL (Only 38% of spontaneous bleeding episodes needed a priming dose of FVIII)
     Borel-Derlon A et al. J Thromb Haemost 2007;5:1115–1124
   - When a priming dose of FVIII is needed, recombinant or plasma-derived FVIII concentrates may be used. Infuse Wilfactin first, immediately followed by the FVIII product in the same venous access
   - *Scheduled procedures:* Administer Wilfactin only 12–24 hours before surgery in order to allow endogenous FVIII to attain plasma levels of at least 60 IU/dL at the time of surgery
   - *Emergency procedures:* Administer a priming does of FVIII together with Wilfactin before surgery in order to attain a FVIII peak of at least 60 IU/dL

4. *Dosage:*
   See table below

5. *Properties:*
   - Treated with 3 virus-inactivation/removal methods: solvent/detergent, 35-nm nanofiltration, dry heat treatment (80°C [176°F] for 72 hours)
   - VWF:RCo (IU/mg protein) ≥50
   - VWF:RCo-to-FVIII ratio = 1

Dosage and Administration
Treatment Schedule in 2 Studies

Clinical Situation	French Study	European Study
Mucosal Bleeding		
First dose	Wilfactin 50 IU/kg, plus FVIII concentrate (30–40 IU/kg) when baseline FVIII levels are <20 IU/dL *or* in case of severe bleeding	Wilfactin 60 IU/kg
Subsequent doses (if necessary)	Wilfactin 30–50 IU/kg every 12–24 hours, to be repeated as clinically necessary	Wilfactin 60 IU/kg, twice daily for 48 hours, then daily or every other day to maintain VWF:RCo and FVIII levels ≥30 IU/dL as clinically necessary
Muscle or Joint Bleeding		
	Dosing identical to mucosal bleeding	Dosing identical to mucosal bleeding plus FVIII concentrate in case of severe bleeding (dose adjusted to obtain a peak FVIII level ≥80 IU/dL)
Scheduled Surgery		
First preoperative dose	Wilfactin 50 IU/kg, 12–24 hours before surgery if baseline FVIII levels <60 IU/dL	Wilfactin 60 IU/kg, 12 hours before surgery if baseline FVIII levels are <60 IU/dL

(continued)

(continued)

Second preoperative dose	Wilfactin 50 IU/kg, 1 hour before surgery	Wilfactin 60 IU/kg, 1 hour before surgery
Subsequent doses	Wilfactin 50 IU/kg, twice daily (3 times daily for type 3); dosage of injections adapted to target levels	Wilfactin 60 IU/kg, twice daily, then daily or every other day; dosage of injections adapted to target levels
Target levels	VWF:RCo and FVIII (monitoring once daily) ≥60 and 40 IU/dL, respectively, until complete healing	VWF:RCo and FVIII (monitoring once a day) ≥50 IU/dL until suture removal (7–10 days)

Unscheduled Surgery

	Same treatment regimen as above but infuse first Wilfactin dose 1 hour prior to surgery together with a FVIII concentrate (dose adjusted to obtain peak FVIII levels ≥60 IU/dL)	

Secondary Prophylaxis

	Wilfactin 50–60 IU/kg, 2 or 3 times per week	

Efficacy

Spontaneous Bleeding Episodes: Relationship Between Dosage and Site of Bleed

Borel-Derlon A et al. J Thromb Haemost 2007;5:1115–1124

Musculoskeletal	Nasopharyngeal	Genital	Gastrointestinal	Oral Cavity	Other	Total
Number of Patients						
13	8*	6	6*	8	1	26*
Number of Bleeding Episodes						
44 (32%)	41 (29%)	29 (21%)	11 (8%)	13 (9%)	1 (1%)	139
Total Number of Infusions						
291	93	258	72	18	1	733
Median Infusion Dosage VWF:RCo IU/kg (Range)						
37.5 (24.3–57.3)	39.7 (14.2–74.5)	53.2 (35.6–68.3)	41 (20.8–72.8)	38.3 (24.9–71.1)	17.1	41.8 (14.2–74.5)
Median Number of Infusions Per Bleeding Episode (Range)						
4 (1–46)	2 (1–7)	9 (1–32)	5 (1–18)	1 (1–3)	1	3 (1–46)
Median Exposure Days Per Bleeding Episode (Range)						
3.5 (1–37)	2 (1–5)	5 (1–21)	3 (1–13)	1 (1–2)	1	3 (1–37)
Number of FVIII Coadministrations With First VWF Infusion						
25	9	11	6	2	0	53
Excellent/Good Efficacy Responses (%)[†]						
77.3	95.1	92.9	90.9	100	100	89.1

*Two patients had a total of 4 and 6 hemorrhages during the European and the French study, respectively
[†]Twenty-four hours postinfusion (home treatment) or at the time of hospital discharge (hospitalization)

(continued)

Efficacy (continued)

Prevention of Surgical Bleeding
Relationship Between Dosage and Surgical or Invasive Procedure

Borel-Derlon A et al. J Thromb Haemost 2007;5:1115–1124

	Surgical Procedures							Total
	Ortho	Gyn/OB	Gnl	Dental	GI	Liver Bx	Inv Pro	
Number of patients	11*	8	6	12	9	8	17	44
Number of procedures	14	10	7	14	12	8	43	108[†]
Total number of infusions administered	341	142	67	68	98	37	72	825
Median infusion dosage VWF:RCo IU/kg (range)[†]	43.7 (30.4–68.7)	41.3 (35.4–59.4)	46.8 (33.2–69.3)	53.2 (24.7–62.4)	43.2 (25.5–67.6)	46.4 (33.3–59.6)	45 (11.1–100)	45.5 (11.1–100)
Median number of infusions (range)[†]	22 (3–65)	15 (1–29)	9 (1–18)	2.5 (1–20)	5.5 (3–21)	4 (3–8)	2 (1–4)	3 (1–65)
Median exposure days (range)[†]	19 (2–57)	11.5 (1–18)	7 (1–17)	2 (1–10)	4 (2–16)	3 (2–4)	1 (1–3)	3 (1–57)
Excellent/good response at hospital discharge (%)	100	100	100	100	100	100	NAB	—
Median consumption during hospitalization (VWF:RCo IU/kg)[†]	577	411	245	100	187	191	63	133
Thrombotic complication	None							
anti-VWF antibodies	None							

Ortho, Orthopedic; Gyn/OB, gynecologic/obstetrical; Gnl, general; GI, gastrointestinal; Liver Bx, needle liver biopsy; Inv Pro, invasive procedures; NAB, no abnormal bleeding
*Thirteen unscheduled and 95 scheduled procedures (48 performed with only 1 preoperative VWF infusion)
[†]Includes all perioperative infusions and infusions given after surgical interventions, for example, physical therapy after joint surgery

Adverse Events

Patient characteristics:
- Fifty patients followed over a median of 21 months (range: 1–42 months)
  - Thirty-five patients were followed for ≥12 months; 25 patients were followed for ≥2 years
- At the end of the studies, 6.7 million IU of VWF concentrate had been administered during 2389 infusions over 2046 exposure days
- Fifteen patients also received 150,000 IU of recombinant or plasma-derived FVIII

Adverse events:
- *Possible or probable (4%):* Mild pruritus and chills
- *Doubtful:* Vein inflammation and malaise
- *Clinically overt thrombosis:* None
- *anti-VWF:RCo antibodies detected:* None

REGIMEN

von WILLEBRAND DISEASE—THERAPEUTIC OPTIONS
ANTIFIBRINOLYTIC AGENTS
AMINOCAPROIC ACID (EACA), TRANEXAMIC ACID

Mannucci PM. N Engl J Med 1998;339:245–253
Mannucci PM. N Engl J Med 2004;351:683–694

1. *General:*
   - The manifestations of bleeding that are most frequently seen in von Willebrand's disease—such as epistaxis and menorrhagia—are sustained, in part, by the rich fibrinolytic activity of mucosal tracts. Local fibrinolytic activity in the buccal mucosa and gums also compromises hemostasis during dental extractions. These findings are the basis for the therapeutic use of antifibrinolytic amino acids in von Willebrand's disease
   - These synthetic agents inhibit the activation of plasminogen to plasmin, and, at high doses, inhibit plasmin
2. *Indications:*
   - Less-severe forms of mucosal bleeding, menorrhagia, epistaxis, dental procedures
   - Adjuncts to desmopressin acetate or replacement therapy with virally inactivated FVIII/VWF concentrate
3. *Contraindications:*
   - Contraindicated in patients bleeding from the upper urinary tract because of a risk that clots that do not lyse will be retained in the ureter and bladder and may cause ureteral obstruction
   - Long-term use as this may lead to thrombosis. Use only intermittently for bleeding episodes
   - Patients with evidence of an active intravascular coagulation process
4. *Administration and dosage:*
   - **Aminocaproic acid** (*also,* epsilon-aminocaproic acid, EACA, 6-aminohexanoic acid, Amicar)
     Aminocaproic acid 50–60 mg/kg orally every 4–6 hours, *or*
     Aminocaproic acid 50–60 mg/kg intravenously over 30–60 minutes diluted in 0.9% sodium chloride injection (0.9% NS) or 5% dextrose injection (D5W) to a concentration within the range 10–100 mg/mL, every 4–6 hours, *or*
     Aminocaproic acid 200–360 mg/kg by continuous intravenous infusion over 24 hours diluted in 0.9% NS or D5W to a concentration within the range 10–100 mg/mL (maximum dose of 24,000 mg/day)
   - **Tranexamic acid**
     Tranexamic acid 20–25 mg/kg orally every 8–12 hours, *or*
     Tranexamic acid 20–25 mg/kg intravenously in 25–500 mL 0.9% NS or D5W every 8–12 hours at a rate NOT greater than 1 mg/min to prevent hypotension
     Notes: These agents should be used intermittently for bleeding episodes. Long-term use may lead to thrombosis. The duration of use for episodes of bleeding in VWD patients is usually 3–5 days
     Both aminocaproic acid and tranexamic acid accumulate in persons with impaired renal function; that is, dosages and administration schedules must be modified in renally impaired patients

     Notes on Monitoring Antifibrinolytic Therapy:
     Aminocaproic acid or tranexamic acid
       Renal function tests at baseline and periodically, thereafter, for the duration of use
       Clinically assess antifibrinolytic response

     Tranexamic acid
       Retinal changes or focal retinal degeneration developed in 4 different animal models following oral or intravenous tranexamic acid at doses from 3–40-times recommended usual human doses for durations of several days or longer. The incidence of lesions has varied from 25–100% of animals treated and was dose-related. At low doses, some lesions appeared to be reversible
       No retinal changes have been reported or noted in patients treated with tranexamic acid for weeks to months in clinical trials. However, visual abnormalities, often poorly characterized, represent the most frequently reported postmarketing adverse reaction in Sweden
5. *Practical considerations:*
   - May be sufficient in managing the less-severe forms of mucosal bleeding
   - More often, these are prescribed as adjuncts to replacement therapy with desmopressin and plasma concentrates during both minor and major surgery
   - Aminocaproic acid and tranexamic acid use is contraindicated in patients with coexisting bleeding originating in the upper urinary tract or urinary bladder
   - Antifibrinolytics should not be administered with factor IX complex or antiinhibitor coagulant concentrates, because the risk of thrombosis may be increased

(continued)

(continued)

6. *Adverse effects:*
The side effects of tranexamic acid and aminocaproic acid are dose dependent
- *Nausea:* Common
- *Vomiting:* Occasional
- *Abdominal pain:* Occasional
- *Headache:* Occasional
- *Thrombotic complications:* Rare. The incidence of thrombotic events secondary to the inhibition of the fibrinolytic system is unknown, but may be particularly increased in those patients who have some underlying predisposition to develop thrombosis
- *Less-common side effects:*
  1. Hypotension
  2. Cardiac arrhythmias
  3. Rhabdomyolysis
  4. Retinal changes and focal retinal degeneration in animal models following oral or intravenous tranexamic acid
  5. Hypotension, bradycardia, and arrhythmia after rapid intravenous administration of aminocaproic acid

Note: Aminocaproic acid is a derivative and analog of the amino acid, lysine, which makes it an effective inhibitor for enzymes that bind lysines. Such enzymes include proteolytic enzymes like plasmin, the enzyme responsible for fibrinolysis. These synthetic agents inhibit the activation of plasminogen to plasmin and at high doses, inhibit plasmin

REGIMEN

von WILLEBRAND DISEASE—THERAPEUTIC OPTIONS
TOPICAL AGENTS

Mannucci PM. N Engl J Med 1998;339:245–253
Mannucci PM. Blood 2001;97:1915–1919

Topical therapies can be placed locally on accessible bleeding sites, such as oral or nasal bleeding; they may be used until bleeding is controlled

1. **Absorbable gelatin sponge** (eg, Gelfoam) soaked with topical thrombin
   - Water-insoluble, off-white, nonelastic, porous, pliable product prepared from purified pork skin gelatin, USP, granules and water for injection, USP
   - Able to absorb and hold within its interstices, many times its weight of blood and other fluids
   - Gelfoam sterile sponge may be cut without fraying
   - There is a theoretical risk for antigenicity given they are derived from nonhuman sources, but to date no adverse events have been linked to gelatin formulations

   Note: Thrombin bypasses all steps in the coagulation cascade and helps to convert fibrinogen to fibrin which forms a clot

   Topical thrombin (eg, Thrombostat, Thrombin-JMI)
   - Derived from bovine thrombin
   - Can be saturated into absorbable gelatin sponge

   Topical thrombin (Recothrom, other products)
   - Recombinant thrombin
   - Available in vials containing 5000 or 20,000 units of sterile recombinant topical thrombin powder for solution
   - Can be saturated into absorbable gelatin sponge

2. **Topical fabric soaked with topical thrombin**

3. **Microfibrillar collagen hemostat** (eg, Avitene, other products)
   - Active absorbable topical hemostatic agent
   - Bovine collagen is processed and purified into water-insoluble acid salts that initiate platelet activation
   - Easy removal with irrigation and suction
   - Various products available in pads, foam sponge, and powder formulations
     a. Avitene Flour (powder) microfibrillar collagen hemostat
     b. Avitene microfibrillar collagen hemostat
        Benefits:
        - Effective in controlling arterial bleeding
        - Conforms and adheres to irregular spaces
        - Available in 0.5-, 1-, and 5-g containers
     c. Avitene Sheets
        Benefits:
        - Cut to any shapes or sizes
        - Clings tenaciously to hemorrhages
        - Ideal for use on flat surfaces or to wrap vessels and anastomosis sites
        - Available in 3 sizes of nonwoven web sheets
     d. Avitene Ultrafoam Collagen Sponge
        Benefits:
        - Active absorbable topical hemostatic agent
        - Reduced thrombin usage may lower costs
        - Available in 4 sizes

REGIMEN

von WILLEBRAND DISEASE—THERAPEUTIC OPTIONS
PLATELET CONCENTRATES

Castillo R et al. Blood 1991;77:1901–1905
Mannucci PM. N Engl J Med 2004;351:683–694

1. Used infrequently in VWD patients

2. Use when mucosal tract hemorrhages are not controlled despite adequate factor VIII and VWF:RCo levels

3. Platelet concentrates [4×10^{11} to 5×10^{11}] are given together with factor VIII/VWF concentrates in an attempt control bleeding

4. Transfused normal platelets are thought to be hemostatically effective because they contain VWF that they transport and localize from flowing blood into sites of vascular injury

5. Platelets from human leukocyte antigen-compatible donors should be used if repeated or frequent use is likely

von WILLEBRAND DISEASE

SPECIAL THERAPEUTIC SETTINGS
MANAGEMENT OF PATIENTS WITH von WILLEBRAND
DISEASE DURING PREGNANCY AND DELIVERY

Mannucci PM. Blood 2001;97:1915–1919
Mannucci PM. Blood 2005;105:3382
Mannucci PM. N Engl J Med 2004;351:683–694

General:

- No evidence that VWD, even severe type 3, impairs fertility in affected women or that miscarriages are more frequent in these patients than in women without VWD
- Patients with VWD have a higher rate of postpartum hemorrhage compared with 3–5% among the general population
  - 16–29% in the first 24 hours
  - 22–29% after 24 hours
- *Type 1 or 2 VWD:* Levels of VWF and FVIII rise 2–3-fold greater than baseline during the second and third trimesters of pregnancy, but fall rapidly after delivery
- *Type 2 VWD:* Although levels of VWF and factor VIII increase, complete normalization of hemostasis may not occur because part of the increased VWF is **qualitatively abnormal** but may not sustain VWF activity
- *Type 2B VWD:* Thrombocytopenia may develop or worsen
- *Type 3 VWD:* The risk of bleeding is greater because there is no physiologic increase in the FVIII:C and VWF levels
- FVIII levels are the best predictor of bleeding during and after delivery
  - The risk of bleeding at delivery is minimal when FVIII level >50 units/dL
  - The risk of bleeding at delivery is increased if FVIII level <20 units/dL
- Monitor patients for VWF and FVIII levels:
  - Once during the second and third trimesters of pregnancy
  - Within 10 days before the expected delivery date
  - For 2 weeks after delivery
- Monitor clinically for at least 2–4 weeks after delivery when the risk of bleeding is increased
- During and after delivery, measures aimed at rapid and complete contraction of the uterus are of utmost importance to prevent excessive bleeding

Therapy:

- *Indications for treatment intervention:*
  - FVIII level <20 units/dL: Administer **desmopressin acetate** *or* **factor VIII/VWF concentrates** at the time of delivery and for 3–4 days thereafter
  - Generally, 3–4 doses of factor VIII/VWF concentrates (40–60 IU VIII:C per kg, *or* 40–60 IU VWF:RCoF per kg) per day are needed to avoid postpartum bleeding
  - VWF and FVIII activity should be >50 units/dL for caesarean section or epidural anesthesia; replacement therapy should also be given if an episiotomy is required
  - *Type 3 disease:* Because VWF levels remain low, daily doses of factor VIII/VWF concentrates during and after delivery are needed to prevent bleeding
- *Cesarean section:* Reserve for usual obstetrical indications
- Desmopressin acetate may be used in pregnancy because it does not cause uterine contractions

(continued)

(*continued*)

Considerations in Pregnancy According to the Classification of Inherited VWD

Type	Defect	Changes During Pregnancy	Comments
Type 1 (classic)	Quantitative	Levels of VWF and FVIII rise 2–3-fold greater than baseline during the second and third trimesters, but fall rapidly after delivery	• VIII:C levels are the best predictor of bleeding risk at parturition and in the postpartum period • Monitor VIII:C levels in days before parturition and for 1–2 weeks postpartum: times when plasma levels fall rapidly and late bleeding may occur
Type 2 (variant)	Qualitative		• Although levels of VWF and FVIII ↑, a complete normalization of hemostasis may not occur because part of the increased VWF is **qualitatively** abnormal and may not sustain VWF activity
Type 2B			• Thrombocytopenia may develop or worsen
Type 3	Quantitative	• No physiologic increase in FVIII:C and VWF levels • VIII:C levels are low and remain low or unmeasurable throughout pregnancy	• Risk of bleeding higher because FVIII:C and VWF levels do not ↑ • Monitoring of little use during pregnancy • Replacement therapy with plasma concentrates and VIII:C monitoring necessary *during and after parturition*

VWD, von Willebrand disease; VWF, von Willebrand factor

Recommendation for Treatment During Pregnancy and in Postpartum Period According to the Classification of Inherited VWD

Type	Previously Shown to Respond to Desmopressin Acetate by a Therapeutic Trial	Excessive Bleeding Despite Desmopressin Acetate *or* Previously *not* Shown to Respond to Desmopressin Acetate by a Therapeutic Trial
After Delivery with FVIII Level of <20 units/dL		
Type 1	**Desmopressin acetate** at 12-hour intervals for 2–3 doses	Virally inactivated **FVIII/VWF concentrate** as indicated
Type 2		
After Delivery with FVIII Level of 20–50 units/dL		
Type 1	**Desmopressin acetate** at 12-hour intervals for 2–3 doses to ↑ factor VIII levels >50 units/dL	Virally inactivated **FVIII/VWF concentrate** as indicated to ↑ factor VIII levels >50 units/dL
Type 2		
Type 3	No therapeutic role for desmopressin acetate	Replacement with **FVIII/VWF concentrate** is necessary during and after parturition Two to 4 doses of **FVIII/VWF concentrate**/day (40–60 units/kg VWF:RCoF) may be needed to prevent postpartum bleeding*

VWD, von Willebrand disease; VWF, von Willebrand factor
*The risk for bleeding may be increased if the dosage is less or with shorter durations of treatment. Patients must be monitored clinically and may require additional replacement for up to 3–7 days in unusual cases

Kouides PA. Best Pract Res Clin Haematol 2001;14:381–399
Kouides PA. Haemophilia 1998;4:665–676
Mannucci PM. Blood 2001;97:1915–1919
Mannucci PM. N Engl J Med 2004;351:683–694

von WILLEBRAND DISEASE
SPECIAL THERAPEUTIC SETTINGS
ACQUIRED von WILLEBRAND DISEASE

Federici AB. Expert Opin Investig Drugs 2000;9:347–354
Veyradier A et al. Thromb Haemost 2000;84:175–182

General:
- Acquired VWD is associated with a number of disease states including:
  - Lymphoproliferative diseases
  - Autoimmune diseases
  - Malignancies
  - Essential thrombocythemia
  - Hypothyroidism
  - Valvular heart disease particularly aortic stenosis, and may also occur with mitral valve prolapse
  - Drugs
- Putative mechanisms include:
  - Accelerated clearance of von Willebrand factor from plasma because of its absorption on the surface of abnormal cells
  - Formation of complexes with other plasma proteins
  - Heightened in vivo proteolysis
  - Inactivating autoantibodies
- When possible, successful treatment of the underlying disease associated with acquired VWD usually leads to resolution of a bleeding diathesis
- The choice among therapeutic options is often determined by an increase in plasma factor levels after the administration of test doses
- Most frequently used options for therapy include:
  - Desmopressin acetate
  - Factor VIII/VWF concentrates
  - Immune globulin intravenous (human) (IVIG)

Therapy:
For life-threatening bleeding:
- FVIII/VWF concentrates should be used initially to attempt to reach therapeutic levels of VWF (and factor VIII) quickly
- Although specific recommendations are not published, it is reasonable to administer **FVIII/VWF concentrate** 50–70 units/kg (VWF activity) and follow the response both clinically and with FVIII and VWF activity levels at 1–2 hours, 4–6 hours, and 8–12 hours to assess response
- If not contraindicated, **desmopressin acetate** may also be administered

Bleeding that is not life-threatening:
- A trial of **desmopressin acetate** is recommended in all patients with acquired VWD
- Measure VWF and factor VIII at baseline, and monitor levels at intervals over the 4–6 hours after desmopressin acetate administration to evaluate the response

Bleeding that is not life-threatening, but did not respond to a trial of desmopressin acetate:
- Administer either **IVIG** or virally inactivated **FVIII/VWF concentrates**
- The choice between FVIII/VWF concentrates and IVIG should be based on the underlying cause of the acquired VWD

Immune globulin intravenous (human) (IVIG):
- Patients with demonstrable antibodies to VWF with underlying lymphoproliferative disorders and IgG monoclonal gammopathies are more likely to respond to IVIG than those without antibodies
- Administer 1 g/kg body weight per day for 2 consecutive days
- Monitor FVIII and VWF activity before and at intervals for 7–15 days after infusion for IVIG
  Notes:
  - IVIG may have a longer duration of action than desmopressin acetate or FVIII/VWF concentrates
  - Response to IVIG may not be observed until 2–3 days after a dose is administered

Virally inactivated factor VIII/VWF:
- Administer intravenously **virally inactivated FVIII/VWF concentrate** 50–60 units/kg
- Monitor FVIII coagulant activity and VWF factor levels at baseline and at intervals over the next 12 hours to assess the half-life of the infused factor
  Note:
  - Patients with demonstrable circulating antibodies (6–15% of cases) may require larger doses of FVIII/VWF concentrate (50–100 units/kg)

Additional treatment options used in small numbers of patients with acquired VWD:
- Plasmapheresis or extracorporeal immunoadsorption for life-threatening bleeding unresponsive to other measures
- Glucocorticoids, such as prednisone, beginning at 1 mg/kg per day orally, *or* prednisolone 1 mg/kg per day intravenously, and gradually decrease (*taper*) the dose over several weeks
- Other immunosuppressive agents, such as cyclophosphamide or rituximab

von WILLEBRAND DISEASE

SPECIAL THERAPEUTIC SETTINGS
ALLOANTIBODIES TO von WILLEBRAND FACTOR

Mannucci PM. Blood 2001;97:1915–1919
Mannucci PM. N Engl J Med 2004;351:683–694

General:

• Ten to 15% of patients with type 3 VWD develop anti-VWF alloantibodies after transfusion of FVIII/VWF concentrates

• In some patients, FVIII/VWF concentrates may not be effective and may cause serious or fatal anaphylaxis

• Patients with type 3 VWD are generally not screened for alloantibodies unless there is suspicion of an antibody suggested by:

▪ A lack of response to replacement therapy

▪ Occurrence of anaphylaxis with replacement therapy

▪ Another family member with VWD who developed an antibody

Therapy:

• There is limited experience in the treatment of patients with alloantibodies to VWF

• Treatment options include:

▪ Recombinant activated FVII (F7): 90 mcg/kg by intravenous injection over 2–5 minutes every 2 hours for 2–3 doses. Assess response clinically

▪ Recombinant FVIII by continuous intravenous infusion to maintain FVIII levels at approximately 0.5 units/dL. This approach may require huge doses to displace antibodies and restore hemostatic competency (eg, 5000–8000 units/hour in an adult). Monitor FVIII levels

von WILLEBRAND DISEASE

SPECIAL THERAPEUTIC SETTINGS
PREPARATION AND MANAGEMENT OF PATIENTS WITH von WILLEBRAND DISEASE FOR DENTAL PROCEDURES

General:
Prophylactic treatment depends on the type of dental procedure to be performed

Therapy:
Routine examinations and cleaning:
- Can generally be performed without increasing FVIII/VWF levels
- Patients with a history of excessive bleeding with dental prophylaxis or nonserious procedure-related bleeding:
  - **Desmopressin acetate** may be given prior to a procedure, *and/or*
  - **Aminocaproic acid** may be administered usually for 1–3 days

Special circumstances in which factor concentrate and/or antifibrinolytic therapy should be given before and possibly after a dental appointment:
- *Deep cleaning:*
  - Patients who have heavy plaque and/or calculus accumulation in which bleeding is likely to be induced with scaling
- *Block local anesthesia or mandibular block:*
  - Dependent on the severity of a patient's VWD
- *Dental extractions:*
  - Before an extraction, virally inactivated **FVIII/VWF concentrate** is administered to raise the level to ~50 IU/dL for uncomplicated extractions or to 50–100 IU/dL for difficult or multiple extractions
    - Usually, further administration of FVIII/VWF concentrate is not required
  - **Aminocaproic acid** starting 4–8 hours before surgery and continuing with 2–3 g orally 4 times daily for 5–7 days after dental work is completed
    Tranexamic acid may also be used

57. Hemophilia

Steven J. Jubelilirer, MD and Margaret Ragni, MD, MPH

Hemophilia A

Epidemiology

1. Hemophilia A is a congenital X-linked recessive bleeding disorder characterized by deficient or defective coagulation factor VIII
2. Overall incidence: 1 in 10,000 males
3. Annual incidence estimated at approximately 500 male births
4. Hemophilia A observed in all ethnic and racial groups

Work-up

1. Bleeding time of PFA-100—usually normal
2. Prothrombin time (PT)—normal
3. Activated partial thromboplastin time (aPTT)—usually prolonged except in certain cases of mild hemophilia; it is corrected by the addition of an equal volume of normal plasma
4. Factor VIII coagulant activity—low
   a. Classification of severity

Factor VIII Coagulant

Activity	Severity	Bleeding Episodes
<1%	Severe	Spontaneous and traumatic bleeding, predominately in joints/muscles
1–4%	Moderate	Severe bleeding after trauma
≥5%	Mild	Bleeding, infrequent, usually after surgery or trauma

5. Factor VIII von Willebrand Factor antigen (FVIII VWF:Ag) and FVIII Ristocetin cofactor (FVIII VWF:RCo)—normal
6. The 1-stage FVIII coagulant assay is the most widely used method for the determinations of the FVIII clotting activity because of its reproducibility, simplicity, and low cost. In many centers, particularly in Europe, use for the chromogenic assay to determine FVIII levels is more frequent. The results obtained with both assays usually correlate with each other. No significant differences in the results between the 2 methods have been detected in normal donors and in those with chronic liver disease (Chandler WL et al. Am J Clin Pathol 2003;120:34–39). However, discrepancies in the assays are observed in patients with mild hemophilia who have missense mutations (Verbruggen B et al. Haemophilia 2008;14(Suppl 3):76–82). Very low FVIII coagulant activities can sometimes be better diagnosed by a chromogenic assay
7. Differential diagnosis of an isolated prolongation of a PTT (Ragni MV, Kessler CM, Lozier JN. Clinical aspects and therapy for hemophilia. In Hoffman R, Benz EJ, eds. Hematology Basic Principles and Practice. Philadelphia, PA: Church Livingstone Elsevier; 2009:1918)
   a. Heparin use
   b. Factor VIII deficiency or inhibitor to factor VIII
   c. von Willebrand disease (VWD)—especially the type II-N variant of VWD
   d. Factor IX deficiency or inhibitor to factor IX
   e. Factor XI deficiency or inhibitor to factor XI
   f. Factor XII deficiency
   g. Contact factor deficiency or inhibitor
   h. Lupus anticoagulant
   i. Factor VIII and factor XI deficiency; factor VIII and factor XII deficiency

Treatment Options

1. Factor VIII replacement
2. Desmopressin acetate
3. Antifibrinolytic therapy
4. Topical agents
5. Platelet concentrates
6. Recombinant Factor VIIIa
7. Prothrombin complex concentrates (PCC)

Acute bleeds should be treated early (immediately, or as soon as possible within 2 hours of onset). Home therapy should be used to manage uncomplicated mild bleeding episodes (eg, hemarthrosis, small muscle bleeds), while more severe bleeds should be evaluated in the clinic or hospital setting, if needed, with subsequent management as needed under the care of a hematologist with expertise in hemophilia care. Patients should avoid use of drugs affecting platelet function;—that is, aspirin or aspirin-containing compounds, or nonsteroidal antiinflammatory drugs (NSAIDs). Use of acetaminophen-containing analgesics is a safe alternative. If possible, intramuscular injections should be avoided, unless performed under coverage of clotting factor VIII

REGIMEN FOR FACTOR VIII REPLACEMENT

1. Factor VIII concentrates available in the United States

Recombinant Factor VIII Products
Product (Manufacturer)
Recombinate (Baxter Healthcare Corporation)
ReFacto (Wyeth Pharmaceuticals Inc.)
Kogenate FS (Bayer HealthCare LLC)
Helixate FS (CSL Behring LLC)
Advate (Baxter Healthcare Corporation)
Xyntha (Wyeth Pharmaceuticals Inc.)

Plasma-derived FVIII Products
Hemophil-M (Baxter Healthcare Corporation)
Monoclate-P (CSL Behring LLC)

Plasma-derived FVIII Products with Von Willebrand Factor
Alphanate (Grifols Biologicals Inc.)
Humate-P (CSL Behring LLC)
Koāte-DVI (Talecris Biotherapeutics, Inc.)

Toxicity

1. *Infection—HIV and hepatitis C with chronic liver disease*: Seen in most patients who received factor VIII and IX concentrates before 1985
2. *Development of an inhibitor*: 25–30%
3. *Redness at injection site*: <1%
4. *Dizziness*: <1%
5. *Hypersensitivity reaction (hives, urticaria, wheezing, chest tightness, and arthralgia)*: Rare
6. *Hypertension*: Rare

Notes

Recombinant products are the preferred products for treatment of patients with hemophilia A. All recombinant products appear to be comparable in efficacy, risk of infection, and risk of inhibitor development

The potential advantage of second-generation recombinant products is higher specific activity and stability without added serum albumin, further reducing the potential risk of transmissible infectious agents

With third-generation recombinant products, animal components have been removed from the culture media. ReFacto and rAHF-PFM Advate are manufactured and formulated without human or animal proteins

If recombinant factor VIII is not available, a plasma-derived concentrate can be used, but with an inherent risk of potential infection from transmissible agents. Whenever possible, patients should store their own products at home and bring them to emergency facilities for immediate treatment of trauma

Indications

To prevent bleeding and limit existing hemorrhage in patients with hemophilia A or factor VIII deficiency

Efficacy

Eighty-five percent of bleeding episodes are treated successfully with 1–2 infusions (rated excellent or good hemostasis) (Keeling D et al. Haemophilia 2008:14:671–684). Of course, target joints, that is, joints in which repeated hemorrhages occur, may require more aggressive or longer treatment

Administration Guidelines (REF)

1. *Loading dose:* Administer over a period of up to 5 minutes (maximum infusion rate 10 mL/min)
2. *Maintenance doses:* Administer over a period of up to 5 minutes (maximum infusion rate 10 mL/min)
3. *Reconstitution:* Reconstitute factor VIII according to a product manufacturer's instructions

Calculating the Amount of Factor VIII Required

1. Initial dose

	100% Plasma Factor VIII = 1 Unit Factor VIII/mL Plasma
Method 1:	0.5 unit factor VIII/kg → increases factor VIII levels 1% Amount of factor VIII required = weight (kg) × desired level (%) × 0.5
Example:	Weight = 70 kg. Amount of factor VIII desired = 0.5 units/mL (50% plasma factor VIII) 70 × 50 × 0.5 = 1750*
Method 2:	Plasma volume = 40 mL/kg Amount of factor VIII required = 40 mL/kg × weight (kg) × desired units/mL plasma
Example:	Weight = 70 kg. Amount of factor VIII desired = 0.5 units/mL (50% plasma factor VIII) 40 × 70 × 0.5 = 1400 units*

*Note: Results would be similar if, for Method 2, one assumes plasma volume of 50 mL/kg instead of 40 mL/kg

2. *Maintenance dose:* One-half the loading dose every 12 hours (biologic half-life of factor VIII is ≈12 hours. Thus, at 12 hours the plasma factor VIII level will decrease to one-half the initial level; infusion of one-half the initial dose restores the plasma factor VIII to the initial level)

Treatment of Specific Types of Bleeding Episodes

Type of Hemorrhage	Dose	% Desired Level	Dose (units/kg)*	Comments
Superficial laceration	None	None	None	Local pressure + apply adhesive skin closure products
Deep laceration	Single dose	50–100	25–50	Sutures after factor given
Joint	Single dose	54–100	25–50	Second infusion (10 units/kg) may be required in 12 hours if target joint, or if pain and/or swelling persist. If target joint, may require 50–100 units/kg Adjunctive car mnemonic is "RICE": rest, ice, compression, and elevation Mobilize joint when pain subsides
Muscle (except iliopsoas)	Single dose	50–100	25–50	Depends on the severity of bleed, and on the severity of hemophilia. May require up to 1–2 weeks if large; eg, in thigh
Iliopsoas muscle	Initial bolus	100	50	Limit activity until pain resolves
	Maintenance	50	25	Every 12 hours for ≥3 days until pain or disability is resolved
CNS head	Initial bolus	100	50	Emergency neurology/neurosurgery consultation; consider CNS bleed in patients with change in mental status, severe headache, recent fall with head injury, or in infant with change in eating or sleeping habits
	Maintenance	50	25	For ≥10–14 days or longer if still bleeding
Throat/neck	Initial bolus	100	50	Assure patency of airway; maintain sitting rather than supine position
	Maintenance	50	25	Every 12 hours for ≥7–10 days if still bleeding
Gastrointestinal	Initial bolus	100	50	Treat origin of GI bleed as indicated
	Maintenance	50	25	Every 12 hours for ≥5–7 days if still bleeding
Renal	Single dose	100	50	Avoid aminocaproic acid.† Order bed rest, oral or IV hydration
Ophthalmic	Single dose	100	50	Obtain emergency room ophthalmology consultation

*Dose calculation based on Method 1 above

†Aminocaproic acid should not be used to treat hematuria because blood loss from the upper urinary tract can provoke painful clot retention and even renal failure associated with bilateral ureteral obstruction

Adapted, with permission, from Protocols for the treatment of hemophilia and von Willebrand disease. Hemophilia of Georgia. World Federation of Hemophilia (Georgia USA). April 2008 (no. 14)

REGIMEN

DESMOPRESSIN ACETATE (DDAVP)
DDAVP (DESMOPRESSIN ACETATE)
(1-DEAMINO-8-D-ARGINE VASOPRESSIN)
STIMATE (INTRANASAL PREPARATION)

Dunn AL et al. Haemophilia 2000;6:11–14
Hemophilia of Georgia (Georgia, USA). April 2008 (no 14) World Federation of Hemophilia monograph
Lethagen S. Semin Thromb Hemost 2003;29:101–105

Intravenous Use

Test dose:
1. Measure factor VIII levels before the infusion
2. **Desmopressin acetate**, 0.3 mcg/kg (not to exceed 20 mcg) intravenously in 50 mL 0.9% sodium chloride injection (0.9% NS) over 15–30 minutes
   • Rapid administration may be accompanied by hypotension
3. Measure factor VIII levels 1–2 and 4 hours after the infusion. Expect a 2–5-fold increase in factor VIII levels, persisting for 6–12 hours

Therapeutic dose:
Desmopressin acetate, 0.3 mcg/kg (not to exceed 20 mcg) intravenously in 50 mL 0.9% NS over 30 minutes. Infusion may be repeated every 12–24 hours for 2–4 doses
Note: Tachyphylaxis with serious hyponatremia can occur with repeated doses. If possible, limit use to 1 dose daily to avoid tachyphylaxis. If administering more than 4 doses, monitor daily serum sodium levels and measure VWF levels

Intranasal Use
Desmopressin acetate nasal spray, 1.5 mg/mL
Test dose:
Because of marked variability in response to desmopressin acetate nasal spray, all patients should be tested before therapeutic use
1. Measure factor VIII levels before administration
2. Patient weight <50 kg: desmopressin acetate 1 spray (150 mcg) intranasally in 1 nostril
   Patient weight ≥50 kg: desmopressin acetate 2 sprays (300 mcg) intranasally; 1 spray in each nostril
3. Measure factor VIII levels 2 and 4 hours after administration. Expect a 2–5-fold increase in factor VIII levels, persisting for 6–12 hours

Therapeutic dose:
Patient weight ≤ 50 kg: Desmopressin acetate 1 spray (150 mcg) intranasally in 1 nostril
Patient weight ≥ 50 kg: Desmopressin acetate 2 sprays (300 mcg) administer intranasally, 1 spray into each nostril
Administer desmopressin acetate nasal spray before a procedure, and repeat every 12–24 hours for 2–4 doses
Note: Tachyphylaxis with serious hyponatremia can occur with repeated doses. If possible, limit use to 1 dose daily to avoid tachyphylaxis

Subcutaneous Use*
Test dose:
1. Measure factor VIII levels before the infusion
2. Desmopressin acetate 0.2–0.3 mcg/kg (not to exceed 20 mcg) subcutaneously
3. Measure factor VIII levels 1 hour and 4 hours after administration. Expect a 2–5-fold increase in factor VIII levels, persisting for 6–12 hours

Therapeutic dose:
Desmopressin acetate 0.2–0.3 mcg/kg (not to exceed 20 mcg) subcutaneously
Note: Tachyphylaxis with serious hyponatremia can occur with repeated doses. If possible, limit use to 1 dose daily to avoid tachyphylaxis

*Used infrequently

Indications

1. Synthetic analog of vasopressin indirectly release factor VIII/VWF from endothelial cell storage sites
2. dDAVP is useful in patients with mild hemophilia with factor VIII levels >5% who have shown through pretesting to be responsive to its infusion

Efficacy

On the basis of 3 small studies, a rise in factor VIII coagulant activity to >3 times baseline and normal hemostasis were seen in 80% of patients

Toxicity

Usually well tolerated, desmopressin acetate has the advantage of posing no risk of transmitting bloodborne viruses

1. *Vasodilation with associated flushing and hypotension after rapid administration:* Occasional
2. *Headache:* Usually transient and probably dose-related, and may resolve with dose reduction
3. *Tingling:* Occasional
4. *Hypotension:* Uncommon and usually mild
5. *Hypertension:* Uncommon and usually mild
6. *Tachycardia:* Uncommon
7. *Volume overload:* Uncommon
8. *Hyponatremia:* Caused by ADH

Note: Tachyphylaxis with serious hyponatremia can occur with repeated doses if desmopressin acetate is administered over a prolonged period:
1. Limit administration to once daily or less frequently
2. Restrict water intake
3. Monitor daily serum sodium levels

Notes

A trial of desmopressin acetate at the time of diagnosis assesses an individual's response pattern

Once a test dose is known to be successful, desmopressin acetate can be used without subsequently testing for responsiveness

Adults should be advised to limit fluid intake to 1000 mL for 24 hours after desmopressin acetate use

Adverse event reports describe thrombosis including MI after DDAVP administration; thus, it should be used with caution in patients with unstable angina, MI, etc

ANTIFIBRINOLYTIC THERAPY

ANTIFIBRINOLYTIC AGENT
(EPSILON-AMINOCAPROIC ACID, EACA AMICAR)

Cooksey MW et al. Br Med J 1966;2:1633–1634
Djulbegovic B et al. Am J Hematol 1996;51:168–170
Mannucci PM. N Engl J Med 1998;339:245–253
Mannucci PM. Blood 2001;97:1915–1919
Reid WO et al. Am J Med Sci 1964;248:184–188
Stajčić A. Int J Oral Surg 1985;14:339–345

Aminocaproic acid 50 mg/kg orally* every 6 hours for 7–10 days (maximum dosage: 24 g/24 hours) after dental surgery or extraction

*Tablets (500 mg and 1000 mg) and a syrup (25%, 250 mg/mL) for oral administration are commercially available

Indications

1. As an antifibrinolytic agent that is often used along with factor VIII products for invasive dental work or for the treatment of mouth bleeds
2. Not recommended for treatment of most internal hemorrhages

Efficacy

In small case studies in which aminocaproic acid is given after factor VIII replacement in patients undergoing dental extractions, hemostasis was excellent in 90% of cases and good in 10%. In the studies in which aminocaproic acid is given alone in patients undergoing dental extractions, only 8% required subsequent factor replacement

Toxicity

1. *Nausea:* Common
2. *Vomiting:* Common
3. *Abdominal pain:* Occasional
4. *Diarrhea:* Occasional
5. *Thrombotic complications:* Rare

Notes

1. Aminocaproic acid should not be administered to a patient with evidence of an active intravascular clotting process or hematuria of upper urinary tract origin, or when taken at the same time as factor IX complex concentrates or antiinhibitor coagulant concentrates
2. Contraindicated in patients with bleeding from the upper urinary tract because clots that do not lyse may cause ureteral obstruction
3. For intermittent use only, because long-term use may lead to thrombosis

SUPPORTIVE CARE

Topical agents: A wide variety of topical hemostatic agents are available to help control surgical bleeding. These include gelatin sponges, collagens, fibrin sealants, and thrombin preparations (see table: adapted from Kessler CM, Ortel TL. Thromb Haemost 2009;101:15–24)

Purified human plasma-derived thrombin (Evithrom; J&J Wound Management) and recombinant thrombin (Recothrom; Bristol-Myers Squibb) are approved for use as topical adjunctives to achieve surgical hemostasis. Clinical trials have demonstrated that these human-thrombin products possess equivalent efficacy and safety; with an improved immunogenicity profile (ie, antithrombin, anti-V antibodies and bleeding/thromboembolic complications) compared to bovine-derived thrombin products

Platelet concentrates: Platelet concentrates are not used in hemophilia except rarely in patients with inhibitors in high titers who are bleeding and do not respond to factor concentrates rituximab, desmopressin acetate, or other interventions. Platelets also are used in patients with ITP, HIV, or portal hypertension secondary to hepatitis C liver disease especially if there is active bleeding

Special Therapeutic Approaches

DENTAL CARE

Considerations before dental procedures:

1. Routine examinations and cleaning generally can be performed without prophylactically increasing factor VIII levels

2. Adequate coverage (ie, factor VIII concentrate, antifibrinolytic therapy, or both) should be given before and possibly after a dental appointment in patients who need the following

    a. Deep cleaning or scaling because of heavy plaque and/or calculus accumulation in which bleeding would be induced

    b. Block local anesthesia or mandibular block

    c. Dental extractions, especially multiple procedures or other surgery

Suggested therapy:

1. Multiple dental extractions or other surgery:

    a. *Loading dose:* Calculate the units of factor VIII needed to raise the level to ≈50% in plasma. Factor VIII products should be reconstituted according to a manufacturer's instructions. The loading dose should be diluted according to a manufacturer's instructions and administered over a period of ≤5 minutes (maximum infusion rate 10 mL/min) 1 hour before a dental extraction or other surgery

    b. *Maintenance dose:* Further administration of factor VIII is usually not required, but can be repeated every 12 hours if bleeding recurs. Factor VIII products should be dissolved according to a manufacturer's instructions and administered over a period of ≤5 minutes (maximum infusion rate 10 mL/min)

2. When surgery is performed, in addition to factor VIII:

    a. *Initial dose:* Aminocaproic acid 3000 mg orally 4–6 hours after a dental procedure

    b. *Maintenance dose:* Aminocaproic acid 50 mg/kg every 6 hours or 4 times per day for 7 days after dental work is completed

For additional information and indications, refer to notes in Hemophilia A: Factor VIII Replacement

Brewer AK et al. Haemophilia 2003;9:673–677
Brewer AK. Haemophilia 2008;14(Suppl 3):119–121
Stajčić A. Int J Oral Surg 1985;14:339–345

ELECTIVE SURGERY

Considerations before surgery:

1. *Preadmission studies:* CBC, inhibitor screen

2. Mini-PK study to establish response to factor VIII concentrate

3. At least 1 week before a surgical procedure, notify the Blood Bank about approximate amounts of factor VIII required

4. Notify special Hematology Department that frequent assays will be required during the week of surgery

Suggested therapy:

1. Factor VIII bolus administration protocol

    Hemophilia of Georgia (Georgia, USA): Protocols for the treatment of hemophilic and Von Willebrand disease April 2008(14). World Federation of Hemophilia Monograph

    a. *Loading dose (approximately 2 hours before surgery):* Calculate the units of factor VIII needed to raise plasma levels to ≈80–100% of normal, prepare products according to the manufacturer's instructions, and administer over a period of ≤5 minutes (maximum infusion rate = 10 mL/min)

    b. *Maintenance dose:* Begin with approximately one-half the loading dose of factor VIII. Prepare products according to the manufacturer's instructions and administer over a period of ≤5 minutes (maximum infusion rate = 10 mL/min) every 12 hours. Adjust dose according to measured factor VIII levels to maintain factor VIII levels >50% for the next 10–14 days or until general healing is complete. Factor VIII levels should be checked daily. Since the half-life of factor VIII is 8–12 hours, assays should be performed near the end of a 12-hour dose interval

2. Factor VIII continuous infusion administration protocol

Hay CR et al. Blood Coagul Fibrinolysis 1996;7(Suppl 1):15–19
Martinowitz U et al. Br J Haematol 1992;82:729–734

Rationale for adjusted continuous infusion is by avoiding the peaks and troughs in clotting factor levels seen with bolus injection regimens, a steady-state concentration of the factor may reduce the amount of concentrate used and be more convenient. However, dosing guidelines for continuous infusion of factor VIII are not currently established, and no products are currently licensed for this route of administration

Suggested protocol:

    a. *Loading dose (approximately 2 hours before surgery):* Factor VIII 40–50 units/kg prepared according to the manufacturer's instructions and administered by intravenous injection

(continued)

(*continued*)

Maintenance dose (begin continuous infusion immediately after a loading dose):

    a. Factor VIII 4 units/kg per hour intravenously as a continuous infusion. Dissolve factor VIII in 0.9% sodium chloride injection (0.9% NS). Mix an amount of factor VIII sufficient for infusion over 8 hours. Use a pump with compatible disposable (administration sets) capable of accurately administering small volume rates

    b. One hour after a continuous infusion is started, measure the patient's plasma factor VIII

    c. Ensure the patient's factor VIII level is ≥70% before sending to surgery

    d. Monitor with daily factor VIII assays

    e. Maintain factor VIII level at >70% for the first 48 hours after surgery

    f. 48 hours after surgery, decrease infusion to maintain a factor VIII level of 50–60%

    g. On postoperative day 5, discontinue the continuous infusion. The factor VIII level should be between 40–60% when infusion is discontinued

    h. When infusion is discontinued, begin intravenous bolus administration every 12 hours over a period of ≤5 minutes (maximum infusion rate = 10 mL/min) to keep levels between 40% and 50%. Continue for ≥5–7 days, depending on surgery (*example:* hip replacement in which physical therapy required)

MINOR INVASIVE PROCEDURES

Considerations before procedure:

Factor VIII concentrate should be administered to achieve a factor VIII level ≥50% before invasive diagnostic procedures such as lumbar punctures, arterial blood gas measurements, bronchoscopy with brushings or biopsy, colonoscopy with biopsy, upper gastrointestinal endoscopy, or cardiac catheterization

Suggested therapy:

Loading and maintenance doses: Calculate the amount of factor VIII needed to raise the level to ≥50% in plasma, prepare products according to the manufacturer's instructions, and administer over a period of ≤5 minutes (maximum infusion rate = 10 mL/min). The dose may be repeated hours later if bleeding ensues

Hermans C et al. Haemophilia 2009;15:639–658

Surgical Procedure	Preoperative Factor Levels	Postoperative Factor Levels	Adjunctive Treatment	Levels of Evidence
Major orthopedic surgery (eg, open synovectomy, knee replacement)	80–100%	≥50%	Continuous infusion factor VIII safe and effective thromboprophylaxis should be considered in certain settings	IV
Liver biopsy	≥80%	Replacement therapy (≥50%) for at least 3 days; biopsy method selected dependent upon local experience	—	III
Children undergoing tonsillectomy, subcutaneously implanted reservoir catheter ("port") placement, circumcision	≥80%	Replacement therapy (≥50%) Tonsillectomy: 7–10 days Port placement: ≥3 days Circumcision: 3–4 days	Antifibrinolytic therapy, fibrin glue	III
Dental extraction	≥50%	—	Antifibrinolytic therapy for 7 days	IV, I for fibrinolytic therapy

(*continued*)

PROPHYLAXIS

Definition of prophylaxis

1. *Primary prophylaxis:* long-term continuous factor VIII administration started after the first joint bleed and before the age of 2 years, or before the age of 2 years in the absence of clinically evident joint bleeds

2. *Secondary prophylaxis:* long-term continuous factor VIII administration started after 2 or more joint bleeds or at an age >2 years. Short-term prophylaxis is defined as intermittent continuous ("around-the-clock") administration for patients with frequent bleeds

3. *On-demand therapy:* treatment given when bleeding occurs

Prophylaxis in children

1. A number of retrospective cohort or prospective observational studies and two recent randomized controlled studies gave indicated benefit of primary or early secondary prophylaxis

   a. On the U.S. Joint Outcome Study (JOS), the efficacy of prophylaxis (25 units/kg) every other day in preventing joint damage was compared with an enhanced episodic infusion schedule (factor VIII 40 units/kg at joint bleed onset, 20 units/kg at 24 and 72 hours, and 20 units/kg every 48 hours thereafter until complete recovery) in 65 children (mean age: 1.6 years). Early prophylaxis resulted in 93% of patients having normal index-joint structure on MRI at 6 years compared with 55% of those in the on-demand treatment group

   b. The Evaluation Study on Prophylaxis—a randomized Italian trial (Espirit) compared children on prophylaxis (factor VIII 25 units/kg 3 times per week) with dose adjustments to maintain trough FVIII levels >1% with patients who received on demand treatment (factor VIII ≥25% units/kg per day until recovery). At 10 years follow-up, there was a lower median frequency of joint bleeds among those who received prophylaxis

Prophylaxis in adults

1. Prophylaxis in adults has been less well studied than prophylaxis in children. There have been 6 published studies (preliminary results from 4 of 6 studies) on the effects of secondary prophylaxis in adolescent or adult hemophiliacs. All have studies indicated secondary prophylaxis markedly reduces the number of bleeding episodes in the joints and other sites[1]

2. Regimens used for prophylaxis in adults[1–4]

   a. FVIII at a dose of 25–40 units/kg 3 times per week, or every other day

   b. FVIII 15–25 units/kg 2 to 3 times per week

   c. FVIII 50 units/kg weekly initially; increase the dose or frequency according to a patient's bleeding pattern

   d. Factor IX (hemophilia B patients) 25–40 units/kg twice per week

3. The Medical and Scientific Advisory Council of the U.S. National Hemophilia Foundation (MASAC has recommended prophylaxis as the standard of care for severe hemophilia in all age groups)

4. The optimal and most cost-effective dosage, administration interval, and duration of prophylaxis are still unknown

References

1. Coppola A et al. Thromb Haemost 2009;101:674–681
2. Tagliaferri A et al. Haemophilia 2008;14:945–951
3. National Hemophilia Foundation. MASAC Recommendation #179, Recommendations concerning prophylaxis (regular administration of clotting factor concentrate to prevent bleeding). November 2007. Available at: www.hemophilia.org/NHFWeb/MainPgs/MainNHF.aspx?menuid=57&contentid=1007
4. Valentino LA. Haemophilia 2009;15(Suppl 2):5–22

HEMOPHILIA CARRIERS AND PRENATAL DIAGNOSIS

Detection[1,2]

1. Only females can be carriers

2. Obligatory carriers

   a. All daughters of a man with hemophilia

   b. Mothers of 1 son with hemophilia and at least 1 other family member with hemophilia (brother, maternal grandfather, uncle, nephew, or cousin)

   c. Mother of 1 son with hemophilia and a family member who is a carrier of hemophilia gene (ie, mother, sister, maternal grandmother, aunt, niece, or cousin)

   d. Mothers of 2 or more sons with hemophilia

3. Possible carriers

   a. Daughters of a carrier

   b. Mothers of 1 son with hemophilia who have no other family members who either have or are carriers of hemophilia

   c. Sisters, mothers, maternal grandmothers, aunts, nieces, and female cousins of carriers

4. Clotting factor levels in hemophilia carriers

   a. The expected mean clotting factor levels in hemophilia carriers is 50% of the concentration found in the unaffected population. However, because of exonization (ie, random suppression of one of the two X chromosomes) a wide range in clotting factor levels is found (ie, <1% to >150%)

   b. Other factors (eg, ABO blood types, pregnancy, stress hormones, etc) may influence the level of FVIII activity

5. Bleeding symptoms in carriers (reference 1, below)

   a. Carriers with clotting factor levels of <50% may have an increased risk of bleeding. The risk of bleeding roughly correlates inversely with levels of FVIII/IX, the lower the level, the greater the risk of bleeding. In most cases, clinical symptoms are comparable to those with mild hemophilia, except that carriers may bleed excessively after menstruation or after surgery or delivery. When bleeding occurs, carriers must be treated similarly as those with hemophilia

Prenatal diagnosis

1. Invasive methods[3,4]

   a. Chorionic villus sampling

      a. Method of choice for prenatal diagnosis of hemophilia

      b. Performed at 11–14 weeks gestation under ultrasound guidance

      c. Permits diagnosis in first trimester

      d. DNA obtained from sample screened for FVIII intron 22 inversion. If negative, direct gene sequencing is performed

      e. FVIII/IX concentrates should be given prior to the procedure to raise factor level to ≥50%

   b. Amniocentesis

2. Noninvasive methods[1,2]

   a. Modern ultrasound assessment in the second and third trimesters can accurately determine fetal sex

   b. The use of quantitative real-time polymerase chain reaction (RT-PCR) to assess free fetal DNA in the maternal circulation for the presence or absence of Y-chromosome specific DNA sequences

   c. Knowledge of fetal gender precludes a need for invasive testing in pregnancy

Antenatal management

1. Check FVIII/IX levels at 28 and 34 weeks of gestation, especially in carriers with low pre-pregnancy levels <50%[1,2]

2. Treatment with factor concentrates usually is not necessary during pregnancy because of the significant rise of the FVIII level. Hemophilia B carriers with a low level of factor IX are more likely to require factor concentrate for delivery, as factor IX does not significantly rise in pregnancy[1,2,5]

3. The use of desmopressin (DDAVP) to increase FVIII during pregnancy is controversial because of the theoretical risk of placental insufficiency associated with arterial vasoconstriction. This may result in a miscarriage or preterm labor. However, several studies have indicated its safety during pregnancy[1,6]

Labor/delivery

1. There is no contraindication for an epidural block if the APTT and platelet count are normal, and factor VIII/IX is raised to ≥50%

2. The risk of serious bleeding during a normal vaginal delivery is small and is considered standard of care. However, vacuum extraction, midcavity forceps, scalp sampling, and prolonged labor should be avoided. If a difficult delivery is anticipated then an early recourse to caesarian section should be considered[1,7]

3. Arrange for cord blood sampling at delivery. Cord blood should be collected from all male offspring of hemophilia carriers to assess clotting factor levels for identification and early management of newborns at risk

4. Avoid intramuscular vitamin K administration and circumcision until results of cord blood sampling are known

5. Factor levels should be monitored postdelivery and maintained >50% for at least 3 days (or 5 days if a C-section was performed)

References

1. Mauser-Bunschoten EP. Symptomatic carriers of hemophilia. World Federation of Hemophilia Publication Dec. 2008, no. 46
2. Kasper CK, Buzin CH. Genetics of hemophilia A and B: an introduction for clinicians. 2007
3. Lee CA et al. Haemophilia 2006;12:301–336
4. Street AM et al. Haemophilia 2008;14(Suppl 3):181–187
5. United Kingdom Haemophilia Centre Doctors' Organisation. Haemophilia 2003;9:1–23
6. Mannucci PM. Blood 1997;90:2515–2521
7. Kadir RA et al. Br J Obstet Gynaecol 1997;104:803–810

COMPLICATIONS OF HEMOPHILIA

Factor VIII Inhibitors

Epidemiology (Van Helden PMW et al. Br J Haematol 2008;142:644–652)

1. FVIII inhibitors are IgG antibodies, predominantly of the IgG_4 subclass which interfere with the interaction of FVIII with its cofactors and activators

2. An estimated 22–52% of patients with severe hemophilia A and 3–13% of patients with moderate or mild hemophilia develop inhibitors

Risk factors for inhibitor development

1. Genetic risk factors (Astermark J et al. Haemophilia 2008;14[Suppl 3]:36–42)
   a. Hemophilia severity
   b. FVIII mutations, for example, nonsense mutations, intron 22/intron 1 inversions
   c. Major histocompatibility complex (MHC)
   d. Polymorphisms of cytokine genes (tumor necrosis factor-alpha [TNF-α], interleukin-10 [IL-10], cytotoxic T-lymphocyte associated protein-4 [CTLA-4])
   e. Family history of inhibitors
   f. Race/ethnicity (African American and Latino descent)

2. Environmental risk factors (Oldenburg J et al. Semin Hematol 2004;41[1 Suppl 1]:82–88)
   a. Intensive FVIII exposure (particularly during the first 50 exposure days)
   b. Immunologic/inflammatory/or infectious events, for example, vaccination, surgery, illness
   c. Some studies have suggested a higher incidence of inhibitor with the use for recombinant products. However, the role of product type in the occurrence of an inhibitor is unresolved

Laboratory Diagnosis (Hay CRM et al. Br J Haematol 2006;133:591–605)

1. When an inhibitor is suspected, the Bethesda assay is performed to both confirm and quantify the anti-FVIII antibody. In this assay, normal pooled plasma is incubated with undiluted patient plasma for 2 hours at 37°C (98.6°F) and then assayed for residual FVIII

2. Bethesda unit = log[% residual FVIII in test mixture]

3. One Bethesda unit (1 BU) = amount of inhibitor needed to inactivate 50% of FVIII in pooled normal plasma after incubation

4. Typical sensitivity of Bethesda assay = 0.5–0.6 BU

5. Nijmegen modification of the above assay
   a. May better allow the detection of very-low-titer inhibitors
      (1) The Bethesda assay may result in false positives at very-low-titer inhibitors (<1 BU)
      (2) In contrast, the Nijmegen modified assay would result zero inhibition levels
   b. The control consists of normal plasma incubated with immunodepleted FVIII-deficient plasma
   c. The normal plasma used in the incubation mixture is buffered to a pH of 7.4 with 0.1 M imidazole buffer

Classification of inhibitors (White GC II et al. Thromb Haemost 2001;85:560)

1. *Low-titer inhibitor:* Inhibitor levels ≤5 BU

2. *Low-responding inhibitor:* An inhibitor titer that never increases to >5 BU despite immunologic challenge with FVIII; may be transient

3. *High-titer inhibitor:* Inhibitor levels >5 BU

4. *High-responding inhibitor:* Inhibitor that increases markedly in response to FVIII concentrate within a few days (anamnesis); the inhibitor titer may become low titer over time

TREATMENT OF ACUTE BLEEDING EPISODES IN PATIENTS WITH FVIII INHIBITORS

Treatment of acute bleeding in a patient with a factor VIII inhibitor depends on
1. Whether the patient has a high-response or low-response inhibitor
2. The current inhibitor titer
3. The severity of a bleeding episode

Both recombinant and plasma-derived factor VIII products can be used in treatment

DiMichele DM et al. Haemophilia 2007;13(Suppl 1):1–22
Lloyd Jones M et al. Haemophilia 2003;9:464–520

Bleeding in a patient with a low-response and/or low-titer inhibitor
Suggested therapy: Attaining a therapeutic plasma level ≥50% is recommended

1. Loading dose
Factor VIII 100 units/kg; prepare according to the manufacturer's instructions and administer intravenously over <5 minutes (maximum infusion rate = 10 mL/min)

2. Maintenance dose
Factor VIII 50–100 units/kg prepare according to the manufacturer's instructions and administer intravenously over ≤5 minutes (maximum infusion rate = 10 mL/min) every 8–12 hours for 5 days

3. Continuous infusion
Factor VIII 10 units/kg per hour administered intravenously in 0.9% sodium chloride injection for 5 days

Note: Factor VIII doses should be great enough to saturate the inhibitor and increase the plasma factor VIII activity to hemostatic levels. With an inhibitor expressed in BU (Bethesda units), the dose needed to saturate the inhibitor can be calculated according to the following formula:

$$\text{Units factor VIII} = \frac{2 \times \text{body weight (kg)} \times [80 \times (100 - \text{Hematocrit})]}{100 \times \text{inhibitor titer (BU)}}$$

4. In addition to factor VIII bolus or infusion regimens for the management of a low-response inhibitor, **aminocaproic acid** 50 mg/kg per dose can be administered orally every 6 hours for 3–10 days for patients with oral mucosal dental bleeding
5. If a patient is known to respond to **desmopressin acetate** (mild hemophilia A), one may give **desmopressin acetate** 300 mcg intranasally (150 mcg for patients <50 kg) for minor bleeding

Metijan A, Konkle BA. Inhibitors in hemophilia A and B. In: Hoffman R, Benz EJ Jr, Shattil SJ et al., eds. Hematology: Basic Principles and Practice, 5th ed. Philadelphia, PA: Churchill Livingstone Elsevier; 2009

Bleeding in a patient with a high-response and/or high-titer inhibitor

Suggested therapy
1. Factor VIIa bolus dose protocol
Bolus dose*: Coagulation factor VIIa (recombinant) (NovoSeven RT; Novo Nordisk, Inc.) 90 mcg/kg per dose, prepared according to the manufacturer's instructions and administered by slow intravenous injection over 2–5 minutes
Additional bolus doses[†]: Coagulation factor VIIa (recombinant) (NovoSeven RT) 90 mcg/kg per dose, prepared according to the manufacturer's instructions, and administered by slow intravenous injection over 2–5 minutes every 2–3 hours for at least 3–4 doses or more if bleeding continues
Recent evidence from a number of studies supports the administration of single doses of 270 mcg/kg and has shown the dose is both effective and safe

*Although evidence is accumulating that high bolus doses of recombinant factor VIIa (>200–300 mcg/kg) may be more efficacious for the treatment of acute bleeding, further studies are needed to test this in a prospective manner and to clarify the frequency of thrombotic events
Abshire T, Kenet G. J Thromb Haemost 2004;2:899–909
[†]Most patients who reported adverse experiences (ie, allergic reactions or thrombotic events) received more than 12 doses

2. Factor VIIa bolus dose followed by continuous infusion protocol
Bolus dose*: Coagulation factor VIIa (recombinant) (NovoSeven RT) 90–150 mcg/kg; prepared according to the manufacturer's instructions, and administered by slow intravenous injection over >2–5 minutes
Continuous infusion: Coagulation factor VIIa (recombinant) (NovoSeven RT); prepared according to the manufacturer's instructions and administered by continuous infusion at a rate of 20–50 mcg/kg per hour

(continued)

(continued)

Note: NovoSeven RT is labeled to be used within 3 hours after preparation. Continuous administration for longer periods will require additional preparation steps to replace expired drug supplies

NovoSeven RT Coagulation factor VIIa (Recombinant) Room Temperature Stable product labeling, May 9, 2008. Novo Nordisk Inc., Princeton, NJ

*In studies in which factor VII levels were maintained immediately after surgery by continuous intravenous factor VIIa administration after an initial bolus dose, treatment was likely to provide a margin of safety sufficient to prevent bleeding. No thrombotic events were noted in those studies

Ludlam CA et al. Br J Haematol 2003;120:808–813
Santagostino E et al. Thromb Haemost 2001;86:954–958

Antiinhibitor Coagulant Complex (AICC)
Antiinhibitor Coagulant Complex (Activated prothrombin complex concentrate; Feiba NF or Feiba VH, Baxter Healthcare Corporation) 50–100 units/kg of body weight; prepare according to the manufacturer's instructions, and administer intravenously every 12 hours for 3–4 doses as needed, or longer if there is continued bleeding. AICC should be infused slowly, at a rate not greater than 2 mL/kg of body weight per minute

Note: If headache, flushing, changes in pulse rate, or changes in blood pressure appear to be infusion-related, the rate should be decreased. In such instances, it is advisable to initially stop the infusion until the symptoms disappear, then to resume at a slower rate

Hay CRM et al. Br J Haematol 2006;133:591–605

General rules for treating acute bleeding in patients with inhibitors

(Dargaud Y et al. Haemophilia 2008;14(Suppl 4):20–27)

The choice of bypassing agent (FVIIa or AICC) used as first-line treatment is left up to treating physicians. A recent randomized study comparing AICC and rFVIIa in hemophilia with inhibitors showed these 2 products appeared to exhibit a similar beneficial effect on joint bleeds (Astermark J et al. Blood 2007;109:546–551)

Some favor the use of rFVIIa in "plasma-naïve patients, especially children." The use of rFVIIa does not usually induce an anamnestic response, a beneficial attribute in the context of immune tolerance

If the hemostatic response is unsatisfactory with the first bypassing agent, one could increase the administration frequency of the product used in treatment. If still no improvement results in spite of increasing the dose or administration frequency, consider using the alternative product (rFVIIa or AICC)

If hemorrhage still persists under monotherapy with either class of bypassing agents, one may consider sequential therapy with both types of bypassing agents. However, the clinical benefit of this approach requires confirmation. The optimal time period between sequential administration of each product has not been identified

Antifibrinolytic agents (eg, aminocaproic acid) may be used concomitantly with either of the bypassing agents for oral or muscle bleeds. Antifibrinolytics ideally should not be given within 12 hours of AICC administration because of a potential risk of thrombosis. Patients who receive sequential therapy with rFVIIa and AICC should not receive antifibrinolytic therapy

Neither bypassing agent is able to effect hemostasis in all patients or in all bleeds. Product effectiveness should be assessed early after administration and products switched or doses increased promptly when a patient shows signs of insufficient or lacking response to treatment. A consensus guideline recommends re-evaluating treatment response every 8–12 hours for 1 day, and every 24 hours thereafter for limb bleeding, and every 2–4 hours for life-threatening bleeds

Aledort LM. Management of inhibitors in patients with hemophilia A (monograph). December 2008
Astermark J et al. Blood 2007;109:546–551
Berntorp E. Haemophilia 2009;15:3–10
Teitel J et al. Haemophilia 2007;13:256–263

SURGERY IN A PATIENT WITH A HIGH-RESPONSE INHIBITOR

Examples of surgical procedures:

1. *Minor procedures:* Arthrocentesis, endoscopy/colonoscopy, dental extractions
2. *Intermediate procedures:* Arthroscopy, removal of osteophytes or small cysts
3. *Major procedures:* Bone fixation for fractures, hip/knee replacement, arthrodeses (joint fusion), open synovectomy, pseudotumor removal, hardware removal (plates, intramedullary nails), neurosurgery (craniotomy), general surgery (eg, appendectomy, colectomy, gastrectomy)

Antiinhibitor Coagulant Complex (Activated Prothrombin Complex Concentrates; Feiba)

	Preoperatively	Days 1–5	Days 6–14
Minor procedures	50–75 units/kg	50–75 units/kg every 12–24 hours for 1–2 doses	No recommendation
Intermediate or major procedures	75–100 units/kg	75–100 units/kg every 8–12 hours	75–100 units/kg every 12 hours

Coagulation rFVIIa (NovoSeven RT)

	Preoperatively	Days 1–5	Days 6–14
Minor procedures	Adult: 90–120 mcg/kg	90–120 mcg/kg every 2 hours up to 4 doses	No recommendation
	Pediatric:120–150 mcg/kg	90–120 mcg/kg every 3–6 hours for up to 24 hours	
Intermediate or major procedures	Adult: 120 mcg/kg every 2 hours	90–120 mcg/kg Day 1: every 2 hours Day 2: every 3 hours Days 3–5: every 4 hours	90–120 mcg/kg every 6 hours
	Pediatric: 150 mcg/kg every 2 hours		
Continuous infusion	15–50 mcg/kg per hour	15–50 mcg/kg per hour	15–50 mcg/kg per hour

Adapted with permission from Rodriguez-Merchan EC et al. Haemophilia 2004;10(Suppl 2):50–52

CONSENSUS RECOMMENDATIONS FOR IMMUNE TOLERANCE INDUCTION (ITI)

DiMichele DM et al. Haemophilia 2007;13(Suppl 1):1–22

Recommendations for when to start ITI

1. Postpone initiating ITI until the inhibitor titer has decreased to at least <10 Bethesda units (BU) although an inhibitor titer substantially <10 BU may correlate with a better response
   a. The waiting time is usually short, and most children are young at the start of ITI
   b. Closely monitor inhibitor levels during the waiting period to ensure ITI is promptly started
   c. Avoid FVIII exposure during a waiting period
2. Consider starting ITI regardless of the inhibitor titer if:
   d. The inhibitor titer does not decrease to <10 BU during a 1–2-year period of close observation
   e. Severe life- or limb-threatening bleeding occurs

Recommendations for ITI dosing

1. Among good-risk patients (ie, peak historical inhibitor titers <200 BU, pre-ITI titer <10 BU, <5 years since diagnosis), no dosing regimen has been shown superior to another. These patients may be eligible to participate in the I-ITI study (International Immune Tolerance Induction Study). This study is an evaluation of the effect of FVIII dose on the overall ITI success rate and time to success by randomly assigning 150 patients with severe hemophilia A to receive FVIII doses of either 200 IU/kg daily or 50 IU/kg 3 times weekly for up to 33 months
2. Among poor-risk patients (ie, peak historical titer >200 BU, pre-ITI titer >10 BU, >5 years since inhibitor diagnosis) evidence suggests a higher success rate with the use of high-dose FVIII regimens. These patients may be eligible to participate in the Resist Study (Rescue Immune Tolerance Study), which randomly assigned patients to receive high-dose FVIII (200 units/kg per day) with either recombinant FVIII or a plasma-derived FVIII concentrate containing von Willebrand factor (VWF)

Recommendations in favor of using FVIII products

1. ITI is successful using FVIII products with or without VWF
2. No data supports the superiority of any FVIII product
3. There is no evidence to support switching from one FVIII product to another for de novo ITI
4. There is no role for immunoabsorption as a first-line treatment for ITI

(continued)

(continued)

Recommendations for prophylaxis during ITI

1. Prophylaxis should be considered if patients continue to bleed frequently while awaiting or receiving ITI

2. Recombinant FVIIa (NovoSeven RT) 90–270 mcg/kg daily is preferred for prophylaxis when ITI is delayed to allow time for inhibitor titers to decline to <10 BU

3. Prophylaxis with AICC (Feiba NF) 50–200 units/kg daily or twice weekly, or recombinant FVIIa 90–270 mcg/kg daily may be considered for patients undergoing ITI who experience early joint bleeding or intracranial hemorrhage

Note: The total daily AICC dosage should not exceed 200 units/kg

4. Monitor FVIII recovery when the inhibitor titer drops to 10 BU

5. Discontinue bypassing therapy at any level of FVIII recovery

Recommendations for central venous access devices (CVAD)

1. Use peripheral venous access whenever possible

2. Subcutaneously implanted vascular access ports (infusion ports) are preferable to external catheters because of their significantly lower risk of infection

3. Follow published guidelines for catheter care and infection prevention

    a. A CVAD with the smallest possible catheter diameter should be used; the tip of the catheter should be positioned in the lower third of the superior vena cava (SVC)

    b. Refrain from using a CVAD in the first week after surgery to prevent the introduction of bacteria through the surgical wound

    c. Remove the residual lipid of anesthetic creams from the skin by scrubbing with soap and water before accessing an implanted port

    d. Use of topical antiseptics to reduce infection is encouraged (eg, chlorhexidine)

4. Instruct families on techniques for accessing and caring for CVADs before starting ITI

5. If a CVAD-related deep venous thrombosis (DVT) occurs, discontinue bypassing prophylaxis (if used) and review infusion techniques with the family in addition to the following:

    a. Consider removing the catheter and switch to a peripheral vascular access device

    b. Consider modifying the ITI regimen and future bypass therapy regimens

    c. Monitor closely for clot resolution

    d. If a severe clot fails to resolve or progresses, consider catheter-directed thrombolysis or a short-term course of anticoagulation

Valentino LA et al. Haemophilia 2004;10:134–146

6. An AV fistula (AVF) is an option for venous access in children ≥1 year of age who have experienced CVAD failure

    a. Long-term follow-up of an AVF with ultrasound (duplex) is important

    b. Dismantle an AVF as soon as peripheral veins provide adequate vascular access

    c. If an AVF-related thrombosis occurs, ITI can continue but stop prophylactic bypassing therapy access

DiMichele DM et al. Haemophilia 2007;13(Suppl 1):1–22
Santagostino E et al. Br J Haematol 2003;123:502–506

Recommendations for managing incomplete or lack of response to ITI

1. Continue initial ITI regimen particularly if a low-dose regimen is being used for reasons of preferential use of peripheral vascular access

2. Maximize the ITI dose if a low-dose regimen is being used and adequate venous access exists

3. Consider switching to a FVIII/VWF product if ITI was initiated with a recombinant product

Gringeri A et al. J Thromb Haemost 2005;3(Suppl 1):A207

4. Consider adding rituximab or another immunomodulating drug to the current regimen (rituximab dosage: 375 mg/m² weekly for 4 consecutive weeks)

Franchini M et al. Haemophilia 2008;14:903–912

Recommendations for defining ITI outcome

1. Pharmacokinetic parameters of success

    a. Disappearance of the inhibitor (ie, undetectable using Bethesda assay)

    b. Normal FVIII recovery (≥66% of predicted)

    c. Normal FVIII half-life (≥6 hours after a 72-hour FVIII washout period)

    d. Absence of anamnesis upon further FVIII exposure

DiMichele DM et al. Haemophilia 2007;13(Suppl 1):1–22

(continued)

(*continued*)

2. Pharmacokinetic parameters of partial success
   a. An inhibitor titer of <5 BU
   b. FVIII recovery <66% of predicted
   c. FVIII half-life <6 hours after a 72-hour FVIII washout period
   d. Clinical response to FVIII
   e. No increase in the inhibitor titer >5 BU over a 6-month period of on-demand therapy or a 12-month period of prophylaxis

DiMichele DM et al. Haemophilia 2007;13(Suppl 1):1–22

3. Pharmacokinetic parameters of failure
   a. Failure to fulfill criteria for full or partial success within 33 months
   b. Less than a 20% reduction in the inhibitor titer for any 6-month period during ITI after the first 3 months of treatment which implies:
      • 9 months is the minimum period for an ITI
      • 33 months is the maximum duration of ITI, although the decision may be made to continue immune tolerance

DiMichele DM et al. Haemophilia 2007;13(Suppl 1):1–22

4. If the criteria for success are met
   a. Treatment can be terminated by tapering the FVIII dose by 10–50% each month
   b. If there is no inhibitor, subsequent interventions include prophylaxis (eg, AICC 20–40 units/kg 3 times weekly) or on-demand treatment
   c. Participation in prospective randomized national or international trials if available

HEMOPHILIC ARTHROPATHY

Monitoring by radiographic imaging:
1. A plain x-ray is a well-tested and reliable technique to image bones and soft tissues, but it cannot directly visualize the cartilage that is lost early in hemophilia arthropathy
2. Ultrasound can visualize cartilage synovium blood and fluid but does not visualize bone

Klukowska A et al. Haemophilia 2001;7:286–292

3. Magnetic resonance imaging (MRI) has been shown to detect early signs of arthropathy such as synovial hypertrophy or early cartilage damage that is not identified on x-rays

Yu W et al. Haemophilia 2009;15:1090–1096

Management of chronic hemophilic arthropathy:
1. Primary or secondary prophylaxis to prevent recurrent bleeds
2. Radiosynovectomy (synoviorthesis)
   a. Developed as a simple, noninvasive alternative to arthroscopic or open surgical synovectomy
   b. The radioisotopes utilized are pure β-emitting radioisotopes that avoid whole-body irradiation: they are large enough to avoid leakage from the joint space and have a short half-life

   Bossard D et al. Haemophilia 2008;14(Suppl 4):11–19

   c. Are used as a colloidal suspension allowing homogenous distribution into the joint space Bossard D et al. Haemophilia 2008;14(Suppl 4): 11–19
   d. Radioactive phosphorus (^{32}P) single agent licensed in the United States
      (1) *Indication:* Chronic/progressive arthropathy with recurrent bleeding and synovial hypertrophy of a "target" joint with few cartilage and bone lesions
      (2) *Safety issues:* Little cartilage or bone toxicity, two cases of acute lymphoblastic leukemia reported in pediatric patients

      Dunn AL et al. J Thromb Haemost 2005;3:1541–1542

      (3) No standard guidelines for the use of this procedure

Surgical procedures:
1. Open surgical synovectomy
   a. Effective for removing hypertrophied synovium and thus decrease recurrence of hemarthroses
   b. The procedure can be complicated by a reduction in range of motion and cannot stop progressive joint damage

   Montane I et al. J Bone Joint Surg Am 1986;68:210–216

(*continued*)

(continued)

    c. Above rarely performed and may be indicated when there is limited access to the synovial hypertrophia under arthroscopy or when bone surgery is necessary

        Bossard D et al. Haemophilia 2008;14(Suppl 4):11–19

2. Arthroscopic synovectomy

    a. Most frequent procedure for decreasing pain and improving range of motion

    b. Indicated for knee arthropathy but increasing experience is being gained within ankles, elbows, and shoulders

        Pasta G et al. Haemophilia 2008;14(Suppl 3):170–176
        Wiedel JD. Haemophilia 2002;8:372–374

3. Joint replacement and prosthesis

    a. Orthopedic surgery is higher risk surgery for hemophiliacs than for nonhemophiliacs because of

      • The increased wear or loosening of a prosthesis since implantation is often done in patients younger than those undergoing surgery for osteoarthritis

      • The necessity for a revision of the prosthesis 10–20 years after initial implantation

      • The difficulty in performing surgery in persons with hemophilia as a result of stiffness and potentially severe joint deformities

      • Increased postoperative complications such as sepsis or bleeding

        Beeton K et al. Haemophilia 2000;6:474–481
        Bossard D et al. Haemophilia 2008;14(Suppl 4):11–19

4. *Total knee replacement (TKR):* TKR is the most frequent surgery performed in patients with advanced hemophilic arthropathy of the knee. In general, surgical outcomes are less than those achieved in nonhemophiliac persons with respect to mobility

    a. TKR surgery in hemophiliac patients with inhibitors is feasible, especially with the use of recombinant factor VIIa (NovoSeven RT) and antiinhibitor coagulant complex (activated prothrombin complex concentrate; Feiba NF)

      • The EUREKA (European Register on Knee Arthroplasty) Study is ongoing in order to provide additional information, including long-term outcome data on TKR surgery in hemophiliacs with inhibitors receiving first line or FVIIa

        Laurain YD et al. J Thromb Haemost 2007;5(Suppl 2):abstract PM 140

    b. With respect to hip surgery, synovectomy in hemophiliacs is limited a result of difficult anatomic access. Total hip replacement (THR) is the best option, provided it is performed in a center in which hematologists and orthopedic surgeons work together frequently

    c. Mann et al. described a relatively noninvasive technique for ankle arthropathy; that is, medial malleolar osteotomy bone graft and compression with staples

        Mann HA et al. Haemophilia 2009;15:458–463

5. *Orthotics:* A foot-supporting device or insole, or a more complex device to control joint motion

    a. Can serve as an interim measure before definitive reconstructive surgery

    b. Ankle guards and arch supports useful in patients with ankle arthropathy and can assist in maintaining and improving gait and weight bearing

    c. Shoe lifts can equalize the lengths of lower extremities and improve gait

    d. Orthotics often applied to knees and occasionally elbows

CARDIOVASCULAR DISEASE (CVD) RISK MANAGEMENT

Data are often lacking on the risk of cardiovascular disease in persons with hemophilia largely because of the early death of the previous generations of patients. However, the number of hemophiliacs with cardiovascular disease, although lower than the general population, appears to be increasing

Strategies for optimally managing hemophiliacs with CVD

1. Emphasize the importance of exercise

2. Despite the cardiovascular concerns that lead to the recall of the COX-2 inhibitors, many healthcare providers who treat patients with hemophilia believe that the benefits of this class of nonsteroidal antiinflammatory drugs (NSAIDs) outweigh the risks. NSAIDs may be effective in relieving the pain of hemophilic arthropathy, and, consequently assisting older hemophiliac patients maintain an active lifestyle

3. Although hemophilia is associated with increased morbidity from bleeding, it has been found to have a protective effect on cardiovascular disease. It is unclear whether long-term prophylaxis mitigates this benefit. Also, it may argue for lower prophylactic doses in hemophilia patients with CVD risk factors, particularly those that adversely affect cardiovascular health

   Highly active antiretroviral therapy (HAART) increases the risk of hyperepidemia, whereas active HCV is associated with early atherosclerosis

4. Cardiovascular risk factors such as hypertension, diabetes, and renal disease, should be managed as aggressively as for individuals without hemophilia (opinion, not evidence based)

5. Anecdotal studies of cardiac surgery in patients with hemophilia have demonstrated surgery can safely be performed with pre- and postoperative factor VIII or IX replacement, use of antifibrinolytic agents, and postoperative thromboprophylaxis (if required)

   Tang M et al. Haemophilia 2009;15:101–107

6. Although drug-eluting stents appear superior to bare-metal stents in preventing reocclusion, antiplatelet therapy with aspirin and clopidogrel is recommended for 12 months after placement of a drug-eluting stent compared with up to 4 weeks after insertion of a bare-metal stent

   Dolan G et al. Haemophilia 2009;15(Suppl 1):20–27
   Schutgens REG et al. Haemophilia 2009:15:952–958
   Smolka G et al. Haemophilia 2007;13:428–431
   Tuinenburg A et al. J Thromb Haemost 2009;7:247–254

   Thus, a bare metal stent is more appropriate for hemophiliacs, particularly since the longer duration of antiplatelet therapy increases the risk of bleeding

   Dolan G et al. Haemophilia 2009;15(Suppl 1):20–27

   However, there are no randomized trials to confirm the best approach

DIALYSIS IN PATIENTS WITH HEMOPHILIA

In a meta-analysis of medical records of 3422 patients with hemophilia, 52% were documented to have chronic renal disease

Most common causes of renal disease in hemophiliacs

1. HIV infection

2. Hypertension

3. Diabetes

4. Chronic hepatitis B and C, which may cause membranous nephropathy and membranoproliferative glomerulonephritis

5. Nephrotic syndrome in patients with hemophilia B undergoing immune tolerance therapy for inhibitors

Types of dialysis:

1. Small studies have suggested peritoneal dialysis (PD) is safer because it minimizes bleeding risk of bad IV access for dialysis treatment. However, patients with coexisting hepatitis C with liver involvement may not be the best candidates for PD, because complications of liver disease such as ascites may impair PD clearance

2. Patients with HIV may be at risk of peritonitis. If a peritoneal dialysis catheter is to be placed, factor VIII or IX infusion ($\geq$50% level) should be given preoperatively and for 2–3 days postoperatively

3. Hemodialysis

   a. During the decision process for permanent access, an external catheter or Vas-Cath is placed as a temporary measure. Factor correction to 100% for 24–48 hours after catheter placement is recommended

   b. An AV fistula is recommended for more permanent access

   c. There are no standard recommendations for the factor replacement target level in an undialyzed patient or for the use of heparin. The target factor level prior to dialysis should be the lowest amount of factor replacement required to reduce the bleeding risk without increasing the dialysis machine clotting risk. The clearance of FVIII is not affected by dialysis

   d. Several studies suggest that low-dose FVIII infusions of 1000 units before dialysis (to maintain FVIII level between 10% and 20%) and through the arterial dialysis line at the end of dialysis is sufficient to minimize bleeding, but not great enough to exacerbate clot formation in the extracorporeal dialysis circuit without heparin

Lambing A et al. Haemophilia 2009;15:33–42

Hemophilia B

Epidemiology

Hemophilia B is a congenital X-linked, recessive bleeding disorder, characterized by deficient or defective factor IX or coagulation factor IX

Incidence: An X-linked disorder, estimated to occur in one of 25,000–30,000 male births

Classification: [100% plasma factor IX = 1 unit factor IX/mL plasma]
Severe hemophilia (factor IX level ≤1%)
Moderate hemophilia (factor IX level 2–4%)
Mild hemophilia (factor IX level ≥5%—50%)

Bolton-Maggs PHB, Pasi KJ. Lancet 2003;361;1801–1809
White GC II et al. Thromb Haemost 2001;85:560

Work-up

1. *Elevated aPTT:* This is corrected by the addition of an equal volume of normal plasma. If the APTT remains prolonged after the addition of an equal volume of normal plasma, consider the presence of an inhibitor to factor IX
2. Prothrombin time is usually normal but may be prolonged in some patients if ox-brain thromboplastin is used
3. A specific assay of factor IX levels is necessary for diagnosis

Treatment Options

1. Factor IX concentrates
2. Coagulation factor VIIa (recombinant)

REGIMEN FOR FACTOR IX REPLACEMENT

Low-purity plasma-derived human antihemophilic factor IX complex concentrates (Feiba NF, Bebulin VH, Profilnine D, and Proplex T)

Very-High Purity Plasma-Derived Factor IX (AlphaNine SD or Mononine) Recombinant Ultrapure Coagulation factor IX (BeneFIX)

Cohen AJ, Kessler CM. In: Kitchens CS, Alving BM, Kessler CM, eds. Consultative Hemostasis and Thrombosis. Philadelphia, PA: WB Saunders; 2002:43
Kasper CK. Haemophilia 2000;6(Suppl 1):13–27
Kasper CK. Hemophilia of Georgia, USA. Haemophilia 2000;6(Suppl 1):84–93
National Hemophilia Foundation, MASAC (Medical and Scientific Advisory Council) recommendation concerning the treatment of hemophilia and other bleeding disorders. 2003; No. 141
Srivastava A. Br J Haematol 2004;127:12–25

Indications

For control and prevention of bleeding episodes in patients with hemophilia B (congenital factor IX deficiency) including control and prevention of bleeding in surgical settings

Efficacy

More than 90% of success in controlling bleeding on an on demand basis or for prevention of bleeding including soft tissue or muscle bleed and hemarthroses

Notes

1. Previously untreated and minimally treated patients should receive the recombinant product (BeneFIX). If the recombinant product is not available, then a very-high-purity plasma-derived product can be used
2. Factor IX concentrates can also be given by continuous infusion in a similar manner as that described for factor VIII for those undergoing major surgery

Toxicity

1. Phlebitis/cellulitis at IV site
2. Alteration of taste
3. Inhibitor formation (3–5% of patients)
4. *Hypersensitivity reactions (rare):* Urticaria, dyspnea, wheezing, hypotension, tachycardia, anaphylaxis
5. Thrombosis (rare)
6. Nausea (rare)
7. Nephrotic syndrome if used for immune tolerance

Factor IX Products*

Product Class	Examples	Advantage	Disadvantage
Low-purity antihemophilic factor IX complex concentrate	Feiba (Baxter Healthcare Corp)	Only advantage is for use in the treatment of patients with inhibitor	Less pure, higher viral risk, prothrombotic
Monoclonal product; very-high-purity plasma-derived human coagulation factor IX	Mononine (CSL Behring LLC) AlphaNine SD (Grifols Biologicals, Inc)	High purity	Not recombinant derived
Recombinant factor IX	BeneFIX (Baxter)	Recombinant, effective	Only recombinant product available; high cost per unit

*All currently available factor IX concentrates are treated to inactivate viruses

Administration Guidelines

Loading dose:	**Administer over a period of ≤5 minutes**
Maintenance doses:	Administer over a period of ≤5 minutes
Reconstitution:	Reconstitute factor IX preparations according to the manufacturer's instructions

(continued)

(continued)

Calculating the Amount of Factor IX Required

Initial dose

100% Plasma Factor IX = 1 Unit Factor IX/mL Plasma

Method 1:	Use for plasma-derived factor IX concentrates 1 unit factor IX/kg → increases factor IX levels 1% Amount of factor IX required = Body Wt (kg) X desired factor IX increase (% increase or IU/dL normal) × 1 IU/kg
Example:	Weight = 70 kg. Amount of factor IX desired = 0.5 units/mL (50% plasma factor IX) 70 × 50 = 3500 IU
Method 2:	Use for Ultrapure Recombinate Factor IX (BeneFIX) Amount of factor IX required = Body Wt (kg) × desired factor IX increase (IU/dL or % of normal) × (1.2)*
Example:	Weight = 70 kg. Amount of factor IX desired = 0.5 units/mL (50% plasma factor IX) 70 × 50 × 1.2 = 4200 IU

*The difference in volume of distribution between the recombinant and plasma-derived products is primarily caused by a difference in charge conferred by decreased or absent phosphorylation and sulfation at 2 sites

Maintenance dose
One-half the loading dose every 18–24 hours
(Biologic half-life of factor IX is ≈18–24 hours. Thus, at 18–24 hours the plasma factor IX level will decrease to one-half the initial level; infusion of one-half the initial dose restores the plasma factor IX to the initial level)

Treatment of Specific Types of Bleeding Episodes with Factor IX

Type of Hemorrhage	Dose	% Desired Level	Dose (units/kg)	Comments
Superficial laceration	None	None	None	Local pressure + apply adhesive skin closure products
Deep laceration	Single dose	40	40	Sutures after factor given
Joint	Single dose	40	40	A second infusion (10 units/kg) may be required in 24 hours if persistent pain and/or swelling *Adjunctive care:* Ice, rest, and elevation Mobilize joint when pain subsides
Muscle (not iliopsoas)	Single dose	40	40	
Iliopsoas muscle	Initial bolus	60–80	60–80	Limit activity until pain resolves
	Maintenance	30–60	30–60	Every 18–24 hours for 3 days or more until pain or disability is resolved
CNS head	Initial bolus	60–80	60–80	Consult neurology/neurosurgery
	Maintenance	30	30	For 10–14 days or longer if still bleeding
Throat/neck	Initial bolus	60–80	60–80	
	Maintenance	30	30	Every 18–24 hours for ≥7–10 days if still bleeding
Gastrointestinal	Initial bolus	60–80	60–80	Treat origin of GI bleed as indicated
	Maintenance	30	30	Every 18–24 hours for ≥5–7 days if bleeding continues
Renal	Single dose	40	40	Order bed rest, IV hydration
Ophthalmic	Single dose	60–80	60–80	Obtain ophthalmology consult
Surgery (major)	Initial bolus	60–80	60–80	
	Maintenance	30	30	Every 18–24 hours for 10–14 days depending on the type of surgery

Adapted, with permission, from Protocols for the treatment of hemophilia and von Willebrand disease. Hemophilia of Georgia, USA. Haemophilia 2000;6(Suppl 1):84–93

INHIBITORS IN HEMOPHILIA B

Epidemiology:
1. 1.5–3% of all patients with hemophilia B
2. 9–23% of severe hemophilia B
3. High-affinity neutralizing IgG antibody
4. Possible hypotheses explain the lower incidence of inhibitors in factor IX compared to FVIII deficiency
   a. Lower proportion of severe phenotype (<1%) in hemophilia B compared to hemophilia A (30–40% to 60%, respectively, in the United States)
   b. More patients with factor IX than FVIII deficiency are cross-reactive material (CRM) positive (ie, have a detectable factor IX antigen)
   c. Higher prevalence of masseuse Mutations (thus less-severe disease) in patients with factor IX than FVIII deficiency
5. A strong association between absent endogenous factor IX protein as a result of gross or complete gene mutations and inhibitor development

Risk factors for factor IX inhibitor development:
1. Positive family history
2. African ethnicity
3. Hemophilia B genotype (large deletion)

Clinical manifestations:
1. Allergic, anaphylactic reaction prior or concomitant with antibody development occurs characteristically in conjunction with inhibitor development
   a. Factor IX (55,000 kDa) accounts for its extracellular distribution and thus the potential for mast-cell activation and IgE-mediated hypersensitivity response
2. Antibody development occurs in all ethnic groups and in response to therapy with both plasma-derived and recombinant factor IX concentrates

Laboratory detection:
1. Factor IX inhibitors are IgG antibodies, predominately of the IgG_4 subclass (κ light chain) that interfere with the interaction of factor IX with its cofactors and activators. Most of these inhibitors can be detected when the PTT is prolonged on a mixture of normal and patient's plasma. In contrast to inhibitors in hemophilia A, antibodies to factor IX are neither time-dependent nor temperature-dependent; thus, it is not necessary to incubate the mixture for 2 hours at 37°C (98.6°F). Inhibitors to factor IX can be quantified by modifying the Bethesda method for detecting factor VIII inhibitors
2. There is no international consensus on the definition of a negative antibody titer, by either Bethesda or Nijmegen assay

Treatment/prevention of hemorrhage:
1. Few retrospective or prospective studies of treatment or prevention of bleeding in inhibitor patients have involved those with factor IX inhibitors. Thus, current standards of care for the treatment of hemorrhage in patients with factor IX inhibitors derive from those of FVIII inhibitor patients
2. Treatment of hemorrhage in patients with low titer (<5 BU) or low responder inhibitors
   a. High-dose factor IX therapy (eg, twice the dose as in standard therapy) bolus or continuous infusion of factor IX. Frequent monitoring of factor IX levels is crucial for accurately estimating a patient's daily factor IX requirement
   b. If there is a poor therapeutic response, the factor IX dose can be increased based on measured plasma IX activity, or, alternatively, bypass therapy (AICC or recombinant VIIIa)
3. Treatment of hemorrhage in patients with a high titer (≥5 BU)
   a. Antiinhibitor coagulant complex (AICC; activated prothrombin complex concentrates)
      (1) Feiba (Baxter Healthcare Corporation, Westlake, CA, USA) is the only currently licensed product within this class of bypass agents
      (2) *Dose:* 50–100 units/kg and subsequent infusions as needed to a maximum of 200 units/kg per day
   b. Recombinant activated factor VII (rFVIIa; NovoSeven)
      (1) *Dose:* 90 mcg/kg every 2–3 hours until bleeding stops. Several studies have indicated that a single dose of 270 mcg/kg can be used safely and can rapidly relieve pain (especially in hemarthrosis)
   c. Recombinant FVIIa is the treatment of choice in those with a history of anaphylaxis to factor IX concentrate

Bypass therapy bleeding prophylaxis:
1. There have been no controlled trials to assess optimal dosing or treatment efficacy/safety
2. *Feiba:* 50–100 units/kg twice daily or 3–4 times/week
3. *rFVIIa:* 90-mcg/kg or 270-mcg/kg regimens have been used
4. Whenever possible, patients with factor IX inhibitors should be enrolled in prospective, randomized, well-designed national or international studies

5. Use of plasmapheresis or protein A Sepharose column immunoabsorption can result in a rapid and efficient reduction of inhibitor titer if bypass agents fail to control hemostasis or if there is life- or limb-threatening bleeding. It can be used also for the initiation of immune tolerance for a high-titer inhibitor

6. Immune tolerance induction (ITI)

   a. Experience with factor IX inhibitors is quite limited

   b. ITI therapy associated with frequent development of allergic reactions or nephrotic syndrome

   c. Less successful than in patients with factor VIII inhibitors

DiMichele D. Br J Haematol 2007;138:305–315

Roth DA et al. Human recombinant factor IX: safety and efficacy studies in hemophilia B patients previously treated with plasma-derived factor IX concentrates [see comment]. Blood 2001;98:3600–3606. Comment in: Blood 2002;100:4242–4243

58. The Hypercoagulable State

Jeffrey I. Zwicker, MD and Kenneth A. Bauer, MD

Risk Factors for Venous Thromboembolism (VTE)

Acquired* Risk Factors	Established Inherited Risk Factors
1. Malignancy-associated	1. Antithrombin deficiency
2. Antiphospholipid antibody syndrome	2. Protein C deficiency
3. Pregnancy-associated	3. Protein S deficiency
4. Estrogen therapy	4. Factor V Leiden mutation
5. Immobilization	5. Prothrombin G20210A mutation
6. Trauma	6. Dysfibrinogenemia (rare)
7. Nephrotic syndrome	
8. Heparin-induced thrombocytopenia	
9. Myeloproliferative neoplasms	
10. Paroxysmal nocturnal hemoglobinuria	
11. Prolonged air travel	
12. Major surgery	

*Some acquired risk factors may be transient

Evaluation of a Patient After a VTE

Routine Evaluation

1. History and examination to identify acquired risk factors (see above). This should include obstetric history in women because recurrent second- or third-trimester fetal loss may suggest antiphospholipid antibody syndrome or hereditary thrombophilia
2. Detailed family history with inquiry regarding female family members who have taken oral contraceptives or suffered any venous thrombotic events during pregnancy
3. CBC and peripheral smear to evaluate for underlying disease (eg, myeloproliferative disorder such as essential thrombocythemia, polycythemia vera or microangiopathic hemolysis)
4. Other laboratory tests as indicated (eg, antibody testing to evaluate for heparin-induced thrombocytopenia if applicable)
5. Extensive screening for malignancy not recommended. Perform age-appropriate screening as indicated. Lower threshold to search for malignancy based on symptoms or signs, especially in older patients with a smoking history, recurrent or bilateral VTE
6. Thrombophilia screen as outlined below for idiopathic deep vein thrombosis

Who should be tested for hereditary thrombophilia?

Yes
- VTE at age <50 years with positive family history (first-degree relatives)
- Cerebral venous thrombosis
- Portal/mesenteric vein thrombosis (rule out myeloproliferative neoplasms such as polycythemia vera, essential thrombocythemia, and paroxysmal nocturnal hemoglobinuria)
- Pregnancy loss (second and third trimester)

Reasonable
- VTE in association with oral contraceptives/hormone replacement therapy or pregnancy
- Patients >50 years with first spontaneous VTE

No
- Arterial thrombosis (except for paradoxical emboli)
- Asymptomatic patients with no personal or familial history of VTE

(continued)

Evaluation of a Patient After a VTE (*continued*)

- Women using oral contraceptives with no familial history of VTE
- Venous thromboembolism in patients with active cancer
- Elderly patients with postoperative venous thromboembolism
- Retinal vein thrombosis

Laboratory Evaluation for Recurrent Arterial Thrombosis

1. Only the presence of a lupus anticoagulant/elevated cardiolipin antibody levels are risk factors for *arterial thrombosis;* the hereditary thrombophilias are not risk factors
2. Consider other disease states, including paroxysmal nocturnal hemoglobinuria, heparin-induced thrombocytopenia, occult malignancy, myeloproliferative disorders, and cocaine abuse

Acquired Risk Factors

1. Malignancy-Associated Thrombosis

General:

1. Accounts for approximately 20% of all cases of VTE
2. In some prospective studies, the incidence of malignancy in the first year after diagnosis of an idiopathic VTE is >7%. However, trials have not demonstrated improved patient outcomes and cost-effectiveness of extensive screening beyond age-appropriate or symptom-directed cancer screening

Pathogenesis:

1. Etiology not clearly established
2. May be related to tissue factor elaborated by tumor cells

Management of thrombosis:

1. *Acute thrombosis:* **Heparin or low-molecular-weight heparin (LMWH)**
2. *Long-term therapy:* Patients with cancer have a higher risk of recurrence than individuals who suffer an unprovoked VTE in the absence of cancer. Anticoagulate a minimum of 6 months and as long as the malignancy is active. Chronic anticoagulation can be considered with **LMWH** owing to high recurrence rates and potential for increased bleeding complications during anticoagulation with warfarin. In a randomized trial comparing LMWH (dalteparin) with warfarin, recurrence at 6 months was 17% in warfarin-treated patients compared with 8% in the dalteparin group ($P = 0.0017$), although there was no significant difference in major bleeding rates

Lee AYY et al. N Engl J Med 2003;349:146–153
Prandoni P et al. N Engl J Med 1992;327:1128–1133

2. Antiphospholipid Antibody Syndrome

General:

1. A clinical diagnosis characterized by a thrombotic event (venous or arterial thrombosis or recurrent fetal loss) in association with a persistent lupus anticoagulant (LA) in specialized coagulation assays and/or persistently elevated titers of cardiolipin antibodies (IgG and IgM)
2. LAs are rarely associated with bleeding, but confer an increased risk for recurrent thrombosis
3. Clinical manifestations include thrombocytopenia, recurrent fetal loss, and arterial or venous thrombosis

Pathogenesis:

1. LAs result from antibodies that bind to phospholipids and plasma proteins (β_2-glycoprotein I, prothrombin) in vitro, and prolong clotting times (critically dependent on the amount of phospholipid in assay)
2. LAs are often associated with:
   a. Systemic lupus erythematosus
   b. Drugs (usually not prothrombotic)
   c. Cancer
   d. Idiopathic
   e. Infections (often transient)

Management of thrombosis:

1. *Acute thrombosis:* **Unfractionated heparin or low-molecular-weight heparin (LMWH)**
2. *Long-term therapy:* **Warfarin** administered orally. Retrospective studies suggested that patients with antiphospholipid antibody syndrome required a target INR >3 to obtain adequate antithrombotic protection. However, subsequent prospective studies showed that an INR = 2–3 is adequate in patients with venous thrombosis

Crowther MA et al. N Engl J Med 2003;349:1133–1138
Finazzi G et al. J Thromb Haemost 2005;3:848–853

(*continued*)

Acquired Risk Factors (*continued*)

3. Pregnancy-Associated Thrombosis

General:

1. Thrombosis is a leading cause of maternal mortality in developed countries
2. The risk of thrombosis increases 5- to 6-times during pregnancy and the increased risk persists up to 6 weeks postpartum
3. Most (80%) of DVTs are located in the left leg because of iliac vein compression by the right iliac artery

Management (antepartum):

Warfarin is absolutely contraindicated between the 6th and 12th weeks of pregnancy when the risk of warfarin embryopathy is greatest

1. *Acute thrombosis:*
   - LMWH are preferred for long-term anticoagulation over unfractionated heparin because of increased bioavailability, longer half-life, and a lower incidence of osteoporosis and heparin-induced thrombocytopenia
   - When therapeutic doses are used, monitor anti-Xa levels monthly to adjust for pregnancy-associated weight changes
   - With twice-daily dosing, therapeutic anti-Xa levels are between 0.6 and 1.0 unit/mL, and should be assessed 4–6 hours after LMWH administration
2. *Prophylaxis:* See **Anticoagulant prophylaxis during pregnancy** below

Management (peripartum):

Prepartum:
   - Discontinue LMWH at least 24 hours before delivery to minimize bleeding risks associated with epidural anesthesia and delivery
   - The decision to bridge with intravenous unfractionated heparin should be based on perceived risk of thrombosis during the time off anticoagulation
   - Intravenous unfractionated heparin should be administered *if:*
     - The time interval from the episode of thrombosis has been <1 month
     - Additional prothrombotic risk factors exist or the patient is otherwise perceived as having a high risk of thrombosis
   - Discontinue unfractionated heparin 4–6 hours before delivery (usually at the start of labor) to allow for normalization of aPTT

Management (postpartum):

1. Barring any bleeding complications, therapeutic anticoagulation can usually be resumed 12–18 hours after a vaginal delivery and 24 hours after cesarean section delivery

Restarting Anticoagulation Postpartum

	Vaginal Delivery	Cesarean Delivery
Prophylactic dosing	6 hours	12 hours
Therapeutic dosing	12–24 hours	24–36 hours

2. **Warfarin or LMWH,** depending on patient preference
   - Anticoagulation is recommended for at least 6 weeks postpartum (minimum 3–6 months in total after a diagnosis of VTE)

Anticoagulant prophylaxis during pregnancy:

1. In women with a history of thrombosis associated with a transient risk factor, anticoagulant prophylaxis is generally not required antepartum because of the low rate of recurrent thrombosis. However, short-term anticoagulation for 6–8 weeks postpartum should be considered
2. In women with a history of thrombosis and a hereditary thrombophilic disorder (see below), the risk of recurrence without anticoagulation appears to be increased and anticoagulation antepartum is justified. However, the intensity of anticoagulation—therapeutic versus prophylactic—has not been established and should be based on perceived risk of thrombosis. During the postpartum period, therapeutic anticoagulation should be administered for 6–8 weeks
3. The management of asymptomatic carriers of hereditary thrombophilias is controversial. Considering that the estimated risk of thrombosis in women with the prothrombin G20210A mutation or factor V Leiden mutation is only 0.2–0.5% during pregnancy, prophylactic anticoagulation antepartum is generally not recommended but may be considered. During the postpartum period, anticoagulation likely needs to be considered only for high risk patients (eg, following cesarean section, complicated delivery with prolonged immobilization, pre-eclampsia) and can be administered for 6–8 weeks
4. In recurrent adverse pregnancy outcomes, some evidence suggests that hereditary thrombophilia is a risk factor for recurrent fetal loss and prophylactic LMWH may result in improved pregnancy outcomes. Additional studies are required

Bates S et al. Chest 2008;133;844S–886S
Brill-Edwards P et al. N Engl J Med 2000;343:1439–1344
Dudding TE, Attia J. Thromb Haemost 2004;91:700–711
Freedman et al. Blood Coagul Fibrinolysis 2008;19:55–59
Gerhardt A et al. N Engl J Med 2000;342:374–380
Gris J-C et al. Blood 2004;103:3695–3699

Inherited Risk Factors

Prevalence of Defects in Patients with Idiopathic VTE

Hereditary Thrombophilia	General Population	Outpatients with DVT	Relative Risk of Thrombosis (CI)	
Antithrombin Type I Type II	 1 in 2000 1 in 600	1.1%	5.0	(0.7–34)
Protein C deficiency	0.2–0.5%	4%	3.8	(1.3–10)
Protein S deficiency	0.03–0.13%	1–7%	2.4	(0.8–7.9)
Factor V Leiden	5–6%	21%	6.6	(3.6–12.0)
Prothrombin G20210A	2%	6%	2.8	(1.4–5.6)
Elevated factor VIII (≥90th percentile)	10%	25%	4.8	(2.3–10)

Adapted from Bauer KA, Zwicker JI. Natural anticoagulants and the prethrombotic state. In: Handin RI, Lux SE, Stossel TP, eds. Blood: Principles and Practice of Hematology. 2nd ed. Philadelphia, PA: Lippincott Williams & Wilkins; 2003:1307

1. Antithrombin Deficiency

General:

Synthesized in liver and neutralizes thrombin, factors IXa, Xa, XIa, XIIa

Diagnostic assays:

Antithrombin–heparin cofactor assay to measure factor Xa inhibition (preferred); antithrombin antigen

Types of deficiency states:

1. Quantitative deficiency

2. Functional deficiency—reactive center or heparin-binding site defect

Acquired antithrombin deficiency:

1. DIC

2. Sepsis

3. Liver disease

4. Nephrotic syndrome

5. Occasionally, acute thrombosis

6. Heparin therapy

Management:

1. *Acute thrombosis:* **Heparin, LMWH, rarely antithrombin concentrate with either heparin or LMWH**

   • **Heparin or LMWH.** High doses may be required to achieve a therapeutic aPTT. Most individuals can be successfully treated with heparin or LMWH without the addition of antithrombin concentrate

   • **Antithrombin (human) concentrate** can be used to normalize antithrombin levels in chronically anticoagulated patients in special situations that present an unacceptably high risk of bleeding with concomitant anticoagulant use, such as neurosurgery, trauma, and obstetric intervention

   • **Antithrombin (recombinant)** concentrate produced by transgenic technology was recently approved for the prevention of perioperative and peripartum VTE in patients with familial antithrombin deficiency

   • **Antithrombin (human) concentrate with either heparin or LMWH,** in cases of extensive or life-threatening thrombosis

2. *Asymptomatic carriers:* Anticoagulation is not routinely recommended except in high-risk situations such as surgery and possibly pregnancy. Based on familial penetrance of VTE, long-term prophylactic anticoagulation can be considered

2. Protein C Deficiency

General:

Protein C: A vitamin K-dependent protein synthesized in the liver that exerts anticoagulant activity after activation by thrombin

Diagnostic assays:

1. Protac (Technoclone GmbH, Vienna, Austria) direct activation of protein C anticoagulant assay

2. Protac amidolytic assay to measure active site activity

3. Protein C antigen

Types of deficiency states:

1. Quantitative deficiency

2. Functional deficiency—based on abnormal amidolytic or anticoagulant activity

(continued)

Inherited Risk Factors (continued)

Acquired protein C deficiency:

1. Warfarin
2. Liver disease
3. DIC
4. Sepsis
5. Occasionally, acute thrombosis

Management:

1. *Acute thrombosis:* **Heparin, LMWH, fondaparinux,** or **warfarin**

   Warfarin can be used, but caution is necessary with the initiation of warfarin because of rare occurrence of warfarin-induced skin necrosis. Keep a patient fully anticoagulated with heparin when starting warfarin. The initial warfarin dose should be fairly low (2 mg for 3 days) with 2- to 3-mg increments until a therapeutic INR is achieved

2. *Asymptomatic carriers:* anticoagulation is not routinely recommended except in high-risk situations such as surgery

Griffin JH et al. J Clin Invest 1981;68:1370–1373

3. Protein S Deficiency

General:

Protein S: A vitamin K-dependent protein that enhances the anticoagulant effect of activated protein C

Diagnostic assays:

1. APC anticoagulant assay
2. Total and free protein S antigen quantification

Types of deficiency states:

	Total Protein S	Free Protein S	Protein S Activity
I	↓	↓	↓
II	↔	↔	↓
III	↔	↓	↓

Acquired protein S deficiency:

1. Warfarin
2. Pregnancy (>first trimester)
3. Oral contraceptives, DIC
4. Acute thrombosis
5. Liver disease
6. Inflammatory disorders

Management:

Standard therapy with **heparin and warfarin**

Comp PC, Esmon CT. N Engl J Med 1984;311:1525–1528
Schwarz HP et al. Blood 1984;64:1297–1300

4. Factor V Leiden

General:

Arginine-506 to glutamine substitution renders factor Va relatively resistant to activated protein C

Diagnostic assays:

1. Genotyping or
2. Activated protein C (APC) resistance assay with confirmation by genotyping

Management:

1. *Acute thrombosis:* Standard therapy with **LMWH, fondaparinux,** or **unfractionated heparin** and **warfarin**
2. *Asymptomatic carriers:*
   - 5% of white population are carriers of the mutation, but it is not found among native Asian and African populations
   - Chronic anticoagulation without a history of thrombosis is not recommended
   - Prophylactic measures should be considered during high-risk situations such as major surgery or trauma
   - Oral contraceptives containing estrogen are not recommended because of a 30-fold increased risk of thrombosis in asymptomatic carriers
   - Large-scale population screening for factor V Leiden is not cost-effective (approximately 8000 women would need to be screened to prevent a single DVT)

Bertina RM et al. Nature 1994;369:64–67
Dahlback B et al. Proc Natl Acad Sci U S A 1993;90:1004–1008

(continued)

Inherited Risk Factors (continued)

5. Prothrombin G20210A Mutation

General:

Mutation at position 20210 in the 3′-untranslated region of prothrombin leads to increased efficiency of prothrombin biosynthesis without affecting the rate of transcription

Diagnostic assay:

Genotyping

Management:

1. *Acute thrombosis:* Standard therapy with **LMWH, fondaparinux,** or **unfractionated heparin** and **warfarin**

2. *Asymptomatic carriers:*

   • Approximately 2% of the white population are carriers of the mutation, but it is not found among native Asian and African populations

   • Chronic anticoagulation for asymptomatic carriers not recommended (see Factor V Leiden above)

Poort SR et al. Blood 1996;88:3698–3703

Management issues:

Although case-control studies have demonstrated that hyperhomocysteinemia is a modest risk factor for arterial and venous thrombosis, prospective studies have failed to show a clinical benefit in reducing homocysteine levels. We do not recommend testing for hyperhomocysteinemia

Bønaa KH et al. N Engl J Med 2006;354:1578–1588
Ray JG et al. Ann Intern Med 2007;146:761–767

Treatment of Thrombotic Events

Acute Treatment of Acute Thrombosis

1. Initial management not generally affected by the presence of hereditary risk factors

2. Unfractionated heparin, low-molecular-weight heparin, fondaparinux for at least 5 days and until the INR is ≥2.0 for 24 hours

3. Unfractionated heparin should be administered in adequate dose-rates because failure to reach a therapeutic level of anticoagulation within the first 24 hours increases the risk for recurrence

   • Weight-based dosing for unfractionated heparin with an intravenously administered loading dose, followed by a continuous intravenous infusion

4. Warfarin can be started on day 1 with target INR = 2.0–3.0. Standard starting dose is 5–10 mg daily. Variants of CYP2C9 and VKORC1 genes contribute to variability in therapeutic warfarin dosing. Genotype-influenced warfarin dosing algorithms may offer benefit over standard dosing; however, its applicability in nonresearch settings has yet to be determined. (Klein TE et al. N Engl J Med 2009;360:753–764)

5. Rivaroxaban, an oral direct factor Xa inhibitor, is approved for initial treatment (3–12 months) of deep venous thrombosis and/or pulmonary embolism (N Engl J Med 2010;363:2499–2510, N Engl J Med 2012;366:1287–1297)

   • It does not require laboratory monitoring

   • Rivaroxaban use has not been adequately evaluated in prophylaxis or treatment for initial or recurrent episodes of DVT or PE in persons with creatinine clearance <30 mL/min (<0.5 mL/s)

   • Rivaroxaban is not specifically indicated for patients with malignancy-associated thrombosis

   • For initial treatment of acute DVT or PE: Rivaroxaban 15 mg, orally, twice daily with food for 21 days, then:
   Rivaroxaban 20 mg, orally, once daily with food at approximately the same time every day

   • For decreasing the risk of DVT or PE recurrence: Rivaroxaban 20 mg, orally, once daily with food at approximately the same time every day

Long-Term Therapy Following an Acute Thrombosis:

Balancing Risk of Recurrence Against Risk of Prolonged Anticoagulation

Risk of recurrence

1. Following an idiopathic event after discontinuing 3–12 months of anticoagulation: ~5–15% in the first year (25% at 5 years; 30% at 8 years)

2. After a provoked event such as surgery, pregnancy, or oral contraception, the rate of recurrence is lower (Christiansen SC et al. JAMA 2005; 293:2352–2361; Baglin T et al. Lancet 2003;262:523–266)

3. Generally considered increased in the following situations (increased risk of recurrence appended parenthetically):

   • Malignancy (~3 ×)

   • Antiphospholipid antibody syndrome (~2 ×)

   • Compound heterozygosity for factor V Leiden and prothrombin G20210A mutations (~2.5 ×)

   • Homozygosity for factor V Leiden or prothrombin G20210A mutations (~2 ×)

(continued)

Treatment of Thrombotic Events (*continued*)

• Selected kindreds with strong clinical penetrance for antithrombin, protein C, or protein S deficiency
• The presence of 2 or more prothrombotic risk factors (eg, factor V Leiden and protein C deficiency)
(Prandoni P et al. Blood 2002;100:3484–3488)
4. Not increased in heterozygosity for factor V Leiden or prothrombin G20210A mutation alone

De Stefano V et al. N Engl J Med 1999;341:801–806
Heit JA et al. Arch Intern Med 2000;160:761–768
Prandoni P et al. Ann Intern Med 1996;125:1–7

Bleeding risk with prolonged oral anticoagulation
1. Rate of major bleed is ~1–2% per year with a 0.4% per year fatality rate
2. The risk of bleeding is greater in patients with a history of GI bleeding, renal or liver failure, diabetes, or uncontrolled hypertension, or in those with advanced age (>75 years)

Beyth RJ et al. Am J Med 1998;105:91–99
Fitzmaurice DA et al. BMJ 2002;325:828–831
Palareti G et al. Lancet 1996;348:423–428

Long-Term Therapy: Indications and Guidelines

Indications	Duration/Intensity of Therapy
Provoked first event with reversible or time-limited risk factor (eg, pregnancy, surgery)	3 months. Target INR = 2.0–3.0
Idiopathic (unprovoked) VTE, first event	3–6 months. Target INR = 2.0–3.0 After 6 months, consider indefinite anticoagulation
• Recurrent idiopathic VTE • High recurrence rate situations (eg, combined hereditary defects) • After a life-threatening pulmonary embolism • Thrombosis at unusual sites (eg, cerebral, mesenteric, or hepatic vein thrombosis) • Active malignancy • Antiphospholipid antibodies	Indefinite anticoagulation Target INR = 2.0–3.0 (see below) Consider low-molecular-weight heparin in malignancy-associated VTE

Factors that may identify individuals with a lower risk for recurrence include:
• Female sex (RR = 0.7)
• Isolated calf DVT (RR = 0.5)
• Normal D-dimer (usually <500 ng/mL using validated ELISA) measured 1 month following discontinuation of anticoagulation (RR = 0.4)
• Absence of residual deep vein thrombosis (RR = 0.7)
• Asian ethnicity (RR = 0.8)

Kearon C et al. Chest 2008;133:454S–545S

Notes: Duration and intensity of long-term therapy
Recent randomized trials evaluating strategies to prevent recurrent events after an initial idiopathic VTE have demonstrated:
• Efficacy of longer-duration therapy
• Lower intensity better than placebo but inferior to higher target INR anticoagulation after therapeutic anticoagulation for 3–6 months
• If patients prefer less frequent INR monitoring, low-intensity anticoagulation (INR 1.5–1.9) can be considered

	PREVENT Trial		ELATE Trial	
	Placebo	INR 1.5–2.0	INR 1.5–1.9	INR 2.0–3.0
Recurrence	7.2%	2.6%	1.9%	0.7%
Major bleed	0.4%	0.9%	1.1%	0.9%

Kearon C et al. N Engl J Med 1999;340:901–907
Ridker P et al. N Engl J Med 2003;348:1425–1434

Therapeutic Options for Venous Thromboembolic Events (VTEs)

REGIMEN

UNFRACTIONATED HEPARIN SODIUM

Hirsh J et al. Circulation 2001;103:2994–3018

Intravenous (unfractionated) heparin sodium
Loading dose:
Heparin sodium 80 units/kg by intravenous push, *followed by:*
Maintenance dose:
Heparin sodium, begin with 18 units/kg per hour; administer by continuous intravenous infusion, diluted in a convenient volume of 0.9% sodium chloride injection (0.9% NS) or 5% dextrose injection (D5W)

Weight-Based Nomogram for Intravenous Heparin Administration

aPPT	Bolus	Maintenance Dose-Rate*
<35 s (<1.2 × control)	80 units/kg	Increase infusion by 4 units/kg per hour
35–45 s (1.2–1.5 × control)	40 units/kg	Increase infusion by 2 units/kg per hour
46–70 s (1.5–2.3 × control)	No bolus	No change in maintenance dose
71–90 s (2.3–3 × control)	No change	Decrease infusion rate by 2 units/kg per hour
>90 s (>3 × control)	Hold infusion for 1 hour	Decrease infusion rate by 3 units/kg per hour

*Begin with 18 units/kg per hour by continuous intravenous infusion

Check aPTT every 6 hours until therapeutic range (1.5–2.3 × aPTT control) is sustained. When therapeutic range is achieved, check aPTT for 2 consecutive measurements 6 hours apart; then check aPPT every 24 hours

Note: Prepare heparin infusions in a standardized concentration that facilitates converting administration rates of "units/hour" to "volume/time (mL/hour)"; for example, heparin sodium 25,000 units in 250 mL 0.9% NS produces a concentration of 100 units/mL

Note: Intravenous (unfractionated) heparin sodium should be used with caution in patients who have baseline abnormal aPTT

Treatment Monitoring

Check aPTT 6 hours after starting continuous intravenous infusion and after each change in rate of administration. Maintain aPTT 1.5–2.3 × the upper limit of normal

Treatment Modifications

Adverse Event	Dose Modification
Heparin-induced thrombocytopenia (see Chapter 59)	Discontinue all heparin (including flushes). If not otherwise contraindicated, initiate therapy with a direct thrombin inhibitor
Life-threatening bleeding	Discontinue heparin

Adverse Effects

1. HIT: 1–3% of patients receiving unfractionated heparin for >1 week (see Chapter 59)
2. Non–immune-mediated, heparin-associated thrombocytopenia (HAT): 1–30%
   - Decreased platelet count usually mild and transient
   - Onset typically 2–4 days after start of heparin
   - Thrombocytopenia resolves despite continuing heparin administration
3. Osteopenia/osteoporosis
4. Hypoaldosteronism/hyperkalemia: 7–8% of patients
5. Increased serum free T_4 and T_3 with normal TSH
6. Increased hepatic AST and ALT
7. Increased serum triglycerides
8. Hypersensitivity reactions (rarely), including vasospasm, cutaneous effects around the injection site, conjunctivitis
9. Fever

REGIMEN: LOW-MOLECULAR-WEIGHT HEPARINS (LMWHs)

ENOXAPARIN SODIUM, TINZAPARIN SODIUM

Caution:
- Doses for LMWHs or unfractionated heparin cannot be used interchangeably
- Do not use any LMWH in a patient with heparin-induced thrombocytopenia

Enoxaparin sodium 1 mg/kg twice daily or 1.5 mg/kg once daily; administer *only* by subcutaneous injection

Tinzaparin sodium 175 anti-Xa units/kg; administer *only* by subcutaneous injection once daily

Dalteparin sodium 200 Units/kg (maximum daily dose = 18,000 Units); administer by subcutaneous injection
In patients with cancer treated long term:
- Days 1–30: 200 Units/kg once daily (maximum daily dose = 18,000 Units)
- Months 2–6: 150 Units/kg once daily (maximum daily dose = 18,000 Units)
- Dose recommendations for use beyond 6 months are not established

Toxicity

1. Increased risk of bleeding in patients who use drugs that may affect hemostasis and in those with comorbid pathologies that predispose to hemorrhage
2. Thrombocytopenia*

Incidence of HIT is less than with unfractionated heparin

Platelet Count	Incidence	LMWH Implicated
50,000–100,000/mm³	1.3%	Enoxaparin
	1%	Tinzaparin
<50,000/mm³	0.1%	Enoxaparin
	0.13%	Tinzaparin

*Discontinue LMWH if a platelet count decreases to <100,000/mm³

3. Pain at injection sites/injection site hematoma
4. Reversible increase in AST, ALT + alkaline phosphatase, LDH, and CK
5. Decreases in bone mineral density and osteoporosis (but less frequent than with unfractionated heparin)

Treatment Modifications

There is cumulative anti–factor Xa activity of LMWH in patients with renal impairment, which can increase the bleeding complications of therapy. In patients with severe renal failure, anticoagulation with unfractionated heparin is recommended. If LMWH is selected, close monitoring of anti-Xa activity is recommended

Notes

- Enoxaparin, Dalteparin, and Tinzaparin clearance is decreased in persons with creatinine clearance <30 mL/min and anti-Factor Xa concentrations are inversely increased
  - Dose adjustments may be needed to maintain anti-Xa concentrations within a targeted therapeutic range
- LMWH doses in persons with severe renal impairment, extremes of body weight, and those at high risk for bleeding are guided by monitoring anti-Xa levels

Treatment Monitoring

In most patients, no monitoring is necessary. In some circumstances, such as pregnancy, renal dysfunction, obesity, and long-term therapy, a dose adjustment may be necessary. For twice-daily administration, the target therapeutic anti-Factor Xa concentration range is between 0.6 and 1.0 units/mL 4–6 hours after subcutaneous dose, but for once-daily dose the target range is less-well established (usually between 1.0 and 2.0 units/mL)

Notes

Advantages of LMWHs over unfractionated heparin:
1. Increased bioavailability
2. Lower incidence of osteoporosis
3. Lower incidence of heparin-induced thrombocytopenia

REGIMEN
WARFARIN SODIUM

Warfarin sodium; administer orally once daily, continually to maintain an INR of 2–3

Initiate therapy with an oral dose of 5–10 mg/day in the evening and increase doses in increments of 1–2 mg/day guided by laboratory values

Treatment Monitoring

Monitor INR initially 2 times per week. When stabilized, gradually reduce frequency to once per week. Less frequent testing can safely be performed in patients who are stable and/or receiving lower-intensity anticoagulation

Adverse Effects

1. Hemorrhage: Patients with a variant polymorphism for the cytochrome P450 CYP2C9 enzyme may have an increased risk of an exaggerated response to warfarin and hemorrhage
2. Warfarin embryopathy or fetal warfarin syndrome with congenital abnormalities after exposure in utero. *Warfarin is absolutely contraindicated between the 6th and 12th weeks of pregnancy*
3. Abdominal pain, cramping, flatulence, bloating, nausea, vomiting, diarrhea
4. Increased LFTs, cholestatic liver injury, jaundice
5. Nephritis with acute renal failure
6. Urolithiasis (calcium oxalate)
7. Increased liver enzymes, hepatitis, and a syndrome that mimics viral hepatitis
8. Skin necrosis (risk factors include protein C and heparin-induced thrombocytopenia; case reports of protein S deficiency and factor V Leiden)
9. Rash, dermatitis, bullous eruptions, urticaria, pruritus, and purpuric skin eruption
10. Alopecia
11. Osteoporosis

Notes

Numerous drug and food interactions can occur with oral administration of warfarin

Drug interactions:
- Antibiotics (eg, erythromycin, metronidazole, rifampin, fluconazole)
- Antiepileptics (carbamazepine, barbiturates)
- Lipid-lowering agents (eg, clofibrate, cholestyramine, lovastatin)

Food interactions:
- Many vegetables contain high levels of vitamin K, but patients do not need to specifically avoid such foods
- Patients should be instructed to keep diet fairly uniform and adjust the warfarin dose according to INR
- Alcohol in small quantities is usually tolerated without affecting prothrombin time

Recommendations for Managing Elevated INRs or Bleeding in Patients Receiving Vitamin K Antagonists*

Condition	Description
INR above therapeutic range, but <5.0; no significant bleeding	Lower dose or omit dose, monitor more frequently, and resume at lower dose when INR is therapeutic; if only minimally above therapeutic range, no dose reduction may be required
INR ≥5.0, but <10.0; no significant bleeding	Omit next 1 or 2 doses, monitor more frequently, and resume at lower dose when INR is in therapeutic range. Alternatively, omit dose and give vitamin K_1 (≤5 mg orally), particularly if at increased risk of bleeding. If more rapid reversal is required because the patient needs urgent surgery, vitamin K_1 (2–4 mg orally) can be given with the expectation that a reduction of the INR will occur in 24 hours. If the INR is still high, additional vitamin K_1 (1–2 mg orally) can be given. However, a recent randomized study failed to demonstrate a reduction in bleeding in patients with asymptomatic increase in INR (4.5–10) treated with oral vitamin K compared with placebo (Crowther MA et al. Ann Intern Med 2009;150[5]:293–300)
INR ≥10.0; no significant bleeding	Hold warfarin therapy and give higher dose of vitamin K_1 (5–10 mg orally) with the expectation that the INR will be reduced substantially in 24–48 hours. Monitor more frequently and use additional vitamin K_1 if necessary. Resume therapy at lower dose when INR is therapeutic
Serious bleeding at any elevation of INR	Hold warfarin therapy and give vitamin K_1 (10 mg by slow IV infusion), supplemented with fresh plasma or prothrombin complex concentrate†, depending on the urgency of the situation. Vitamin K_1 can be repeated every 12 hours
Life-threatening bleeding	Hold warfarin therapy and give prothrombin complex concentrate† supplemented with vitamin K_1 (10 mg over 15 minutes). The factor IX complex, Profilnine SD, is currently available in the United States. It can be administered at 30 IU/kg over 10 minutes but because of low factor VII activity, additional fresh-frozen plasma should be administered (eg, 2 units)

*If continuing warfarin therapy is indicated after high doses of vitamin K_1, then heparin or LMWH can be given until the effects of vitamin K_1 have been reversed and the patient becomes responsive to warfarin therapy. Note that INR values >4.5 are less reliable than values within or near the therapeutic range. Consequently, these guidelines represent an approximate guide for high INRs
†Prothrombin Complex Concentrate (eg, Beriplex® P/N, Confidex®, Kcentra®) is the treatment of choice when normal plasma levels of vitamin K must be urgently restored in a bleeding emergency
Adapted from Ansell J et al. The pharmacology and management of the vitamin K antagonists. Chest 2004;126:204S–233S

- Most anticoagulation management questions have not been adequately studied
- Kcentra® (prothrombin complex concentrate [human]) is the first nonactivated 4-factor prothrombin complex concentrate approved in the USA for the urgent reversal of vitamin K antagonist (eg, warfarin) therapy in adult patients with acute major bleeding or needing an urgent surgery or other invasive procedure

Holbrook A et al. Evidence-based management of anticoagulant therapy antithrombotic therapy and prevention of thrombosis, 9th ed: American College of Chest Physicians evidence-based clinical practice guidelines. Chest 2012;141(2 Suppl):e152S–e184S

REGIMEN

ANTITHROMBIN III (HUMAN) (THROMBATE III®)

- Antithrombin III (AT-III units required*) intraVENously over 10–20 minutes, followed by:
- Antithrombin III (60% of initial dose) every 24 hours as needed (typically 2–8 days)
- Loading doses and maintenance intervals should be individualized for each patient
- Dose should be individually determined to increase plasma antithrombin III concentration (desired $[\text{AT-III}]_{plasma}$) to within a range of normal from the pre-therapy level (baseline $[\text{AT-III}]_{plasma}$)
  - Dosage may be calculated from the following formula:

$$*\text{Units required (IU)} = \frac{(\text{desired \% } [\text{AT-III}]_{plasma} - \text{baseline \% } [\text{AT-III}]_{plasma}) \times \text{weight (kg)}}{1.4 \text{ \%/International units per kg (body weight)}}$$

- AT-III levels should initially be drawn at baseline and 20 minutes after AT-III administration
  - After an initial dose of THROMBATE III, plasma AT-III levels should be initially monitored at least every 12 hours and before the next dose with the goal of maintaining plasma AT-III levels >80%
- Subsequent doses may be calculated based on the level achieved with the first dose

*Expressed as % normal $[\text{AT-III}]_{plasma}$ based on functional AT-III assay. The formula is based on an expected incremental in vivo recovery greater than baseline $[\text{AT-III}]_{plasma}$ of 1.4% per IU/kg administered

ANTITHROMBIN III (RECOMBINANT) (ATryn®)

- Dosage is individualized based on a patient's pretreatment functional AT-III activity level (expressed as percentage of normal) and body weight (kg), and using therapeutic drug monitoring
- The goal of treatment is to restore and maintain functional AT-III activity levels between 80 and 120% of normal (0.8–1.2 IU/mL)
- Administer a loading dose intraVENously over 15 minutes, immediately followed by a maintenance dose given by continuous intraVENous infusion

	Loading Dosage (International Units)	Maintenance Dosage (International Units/hour)
Surgical patients	$\left(\frac{100 - \text{baseline AT-III activity}}{5.4}\right) \times \text{body weight (kg)}$	$\left(\frac{100 - \text{baseline AT-III activity}}{10.2}\right) \times \text{body weight (kg)}$
Pregnant females	$\left(\frac{100 - \text{baseline AT-III activity}}{1.3}\right) \times \text{body weight (kg)}$	$\left(\frac{100 - \text{baseline AT-III activity}}{5.4}\right) \times \text{body weight (kg)}$

- Plasma AT-III activity monitoring is required for appropriate treatment. Check plasma AT-III activity once or twice daily with dose adjustments as suggested by the following table:

Initial Monitor Time	AT Level	Dose Adjustment	Recheck AT Level
2 hours after initiation of treatment	<80%	Increase 30%	2 hours after each dose adjustment
	80–120%	None	6 hours after initiation of treatment or dose adjustment
	>120%	Decrease 30%	2 hours after each dose adjustment

(continued)

(continued)

Recombinant antithrombin has a shorter half-life and more rapid clearance than plasma-derived antithrombin
• Mean elimination half-life ($t_{1/2}$) of antithrombin III products:

Antithrombin-III Product	Half-life
Plasma-derived (Thrombate III®)	22 h (plasma $t_{1/2}$) 2.5–3.8 d (biological $t_{1/2}$)
Recombinant (ATryn®)	
50 Int. Units/kg	11.6 h
100 Int. Units/kg	17.7 h

The half-life of AT-III may be decreased following surgery, and in settings of hemorrhage, acute thrombosis, and during intravenous heparin administration

In such conditions, plasma AT-III levels should be monitored more frequently, and repeated AT-III doses administered as necessary

Adverse Effects

Infusion-related events:
1. Dizziness/light-headedness
2. Chest tightness or pain
3. Nausea
4. Dysgeusia
5. Chills
6. Cramps
7. Shortness of breath
8. Urticaria
9. Fever

Treatment Monitoring

1. Monitor peak antithrombin levels 20 minutes after infusion and trough levels just prior to next dose and adjust to keep levels above 80% of normal
2. Also recommended to check antithrombin levels 12 hours after the initial infusion
3. Simultaneous heparin administration can affect half-life and more frequent monitoring may be necessary

Treatment Modifications

Infusion-related reactions	Decrease the rate of administration, or interrupt administration until symptoms abate; then resume administration at a slower rate

59. Heparin-Induced Thrombocytopenia

James N. Frame, MD, FACP and John R. Bartholomew, MD, FACC, MSVM

Heparin-induced thrombocytopenia is a prothrombotic disorder mediated by IgG antibodies that bind to conformational epitopes on PF4 when it is complexed with heparin. Typically, the platelet counts are only moderately reduced. Occasionally patients do not have thrombocytopenia, but their platelet counts decrease by 50% from pretreatment levels

Kelton JG et al. N Engl J Med 2013;368:737–744

Epidemiology

A. **Frequency**: Determined by heparin type (UFH > LMWH), patient type (surgery > medical), patient gender (F > M); odds ratio 17.4 for postoperative thromboprophylaxis (UFH > LMWH), and duration of heparin therapy (10–14-day course >1 day: >2% vs. 0.02%)

   1. *>1%:* Postoperative patients: UFH at prophylactic or therapeutic dose (1–5%); cardiac surgery (1–3%)

   2. *0.1–1%:* Postoperative patients: UFH flushes or LMWH in prophylactic or therapeutic dosages (0.1–1%); Medical patients: cancer (1%), UFH at prophylactic or therapeutic dose (0.1–1%), LMWH at prophylactic or therapeutic dose (0.6%), intensive care patients (0.4%)

   3. *<0.1%:* UFH flushes, obstetrics patients (non-surgical)

B. **Thrombotic risk**: Isolated HIT (untreated): 30-day cumulative rate ~50% after stopping heparin; initial rate of thrombosis per day over the first 1–2 days after discontinuing heparin: 5–10%

C. **Mortality** (9 studies, 876 patients): Overall population, ~20%; among patients with thrombosis, ~46%

Lee DH, Warkentin TE. Frequency of heparin-induced thrombocytopenia. In: Warkentin TE, Greinacher A, eds. Heparin-Induced Thrombocytopenia. 4th ed. New York, NY: Informa Healthcare USA; 2007:67–116
Linkins L-A et al. Chest 2012;141(Suppl 2):e495S–e530S
Warkentin TE. Clinical picture of heparin-induced thrombocytopenia. In: Warkentin TE, Greinacher A, eds. Heparin-Induced Thrombocytopenia. 4th ed. New York, NY: Informa Healthcare USA; 2007:21–66
Warkentin TE et al. Chest 2008;133(Suppl 6):340S–380S

Work-up

The diagnosis of HIT is based on both clinical and serologic findings and thus should be considered a clinicopathologic syndrome (Warkentin TE et al. Thromb Haemost 1998;79:1–7)

A. The work-up section for HIT outlines an approach for making or excluding a diagnosis of HIT and when to consider the initiation of alternative anticoagulation therapy for heparin/low-molecular-weight heparin that incorporates the following considerations:

   1. **Clinical suspicion** (determining the magnitude and pattern of platelet count fall correlated with the clinical setting, presence or absence of arterial/venous thromboembolic events and presence of other HIT manifestations). The authors recommend a review of the peripheral blood smear to exclude pseudothrombocytopenia and assess for other abnormalities (eg, TTP) that may influence the differential consideration for HIT (*see* Table B)

   2. **Pretest Probability** (determining the likelihood of HIT with 4Ts score; *see* Table C)

   3. **HIT laboratory testing** (*see* Table D)

   4. **Posttest Probability** (determining the likelihood of HIT that incorporates results of the pretest probability with the strength of the quantitative value from HIT testing; when indicated and where clinically feasible, additional testing for the presence of HIT antibodies with a washed-platelet functional assay) (*see* Table B)

   5. **Other considerations** that have a bearing on HIT management/treatment:

      a. Weight of the patient in kilograms

      b. Determination of the patient's renal and hepatic status

      c. Presence or absence of any clinical bleeding

      d. Whether or not the patient requires an invasive procedure in the near-term (eg, "next few days")

      e. Determination of any non-HIT indications for anticoagulation

Alving BM. Blood 2003;101:31–37
Cuker A et al. Blood 2012;120:4160–4167

(continued)

Work-up (continued)

Greinacher A et al. Thromb Haemost 2005;94:132–135
Linkins L-A et al. Chest 2012;141(2 Suppl):e495S–e530S
Wallis DE et al. Am J Med 1999;106:629–635
Warkentin TE. Br J Haematol 2003;121:535–555
Warkentin TE. Clinical picture of heparin-induced thrombocytopenia. In: Warkentin TE, Greinacher A, eds. Heparin-Induced Thrombocytopenia. 4th ed. New York, NY: Informa Healthcare USA; 2007:21–66
Warkentin TE. Hematology Am Soc Hematol Educ Program 2011;143–149
Warkentin TE. Thromb Haemost 1999;82:439–447
Warkentin TE et al. Ann Intern Med 1997;127:804–812
Warkentin TE et al. Chest 2008;133(6 Suppl):340S–380S
Warkentin TE et al. N Engl J Med 1995;332:1330–1335
Watson H et al. Br J Haematol 2012;159:528–540

B. Summary Guidelines for Establishing or Excluding a Diagnosis of HIT

Parameter	ACCP Guidelines 9th ed. (2012)*	British Committee for Standards in Haematology (2012)‡
Clinical Suspicion	• Investigating for a diagnosis of HIT is recommended if the platelet count decreases by ≥50%, and/or a thrombotic event occurs, between days 5 and 14 (inclusive) following heparin initiation, even if the patient is no longer receiving heparin when thrombosis or thrombocytopenia occurs† • Investigating for HIT antibodies in postoperative cardiac surgery patients is recommended if the platelet count falls by ≥50%, and/or a thrombotic event occurs between postoperative days 5 and 14 (inclusive; day 0 = day of cardiac surgery)	HIT should be considered and clinical assessment made for platelet count decreases ≥30% and/or a patient develops a new thrombosis or skin allergy or any of the more rare manifestations of HIT between days 4 and 14 after starting heparin
Pretest probability of HIT (4Ts)	Low probability 4Ts assumed not to have HIT	HIT can be excluded by a low pretest probability score without need for laboratory testing
	Discontinue heparin in patients with a moderate or high 4Ts score or confirmed HIT, order an ELISA, and start alternative anticoagulation (eg, argatroban)	If pretest probability of HIT is not low, heparin should be stopped and alternative anticoagulation started in full doses while laboratory tests are performed
HIT laboratory Testing	The washed platelet SRA and HIPA are generally accepted as the reference standard assays for HIT	Platelet activation assays using washed platelet HIPA and SRA are regarded as the reference standard (use should be restricted to expert laboratories)
	For laboratories using the GTI-PF4 ELISA, reporting of the quantitative test value with threshold for a (+) result is recommended over reporting as (+) or (−)	Nonexpert laboratories should use an antigen assay of high sensitivity (only IgG class). Useful information to report: actual OD, % of inhibition by high-dose heparin, cutoff value for a (+) test
Posttest probability of HIT	A (−) ELISA or PaGIA in a patient with a low pretest probability probably excludes the diagnosis of HIT	HIT can be excluded in all patients by a (−) antigen assay of high sensitivity
	For clinicians using the GTI-PF4 ELISA to determine HIT, it is suggested to take into account the pretest probability for HIT and quantitative level of results. A threshold OD between 0.4 and 1.0 in a patient with a low or intermediate probability of HIT should be confirmed with a functional assay	HIT can be excluded in patients with an intermediate probability score who have a (−) particle gel assay; a (+) alternative anticoagulant while more specific tests are performed (eg, washed platelet assay, if accessible)
	A threshold >1.0 OD with a high clinical suspicion for HIT (eg, intermediate or high 4Ts score) may have a similar accuracy for diagnosing HIT as the reference standard (SRA) (this strategy requires validation in prospective studies)	The pretest probability estimate of HIT, together with the type of assay used and its quantitative value (ELISA only) and information on reversal using higher doses of heparin should be used to determine the posttest probability of HIT

*Linkins L-A et al. Chest 2012;141(2 Suppl):e495S–e530S
†Warkentin TE et al. Chest 2008;133(6 Suppl):340S–380S (8th edition of ACCP Guidelines for Treatment and Prevention of HIT; no change in criteria for when to consider HIT from 8th to 9th editions)
‡Watson H et al. Br J Haematol 2012;159:528–540

(continued)

Work-up (continued)

C. The Four Ts: Estimating the Pretest Probability of HIT*

Category	Point Score for Each of 4 Categories (Maximum Possible Score = 8)[†]		
	2	1	0
Acute thrombocytopenia	>50% Fall (nadir ≥20,000/mm³)	30–50% Platelet fall (or >50% fall as a result of surgery) or nadir 10–19,000/mm³	<30% Platelet fall or nadir ≤10,000/mm³
Timing[‡] of platelet count fall, thrombosis, or other sequelae (first day of heparin use = day 0)	Clear onset between days 5 and 10 or ≤1 day (if heparin exposure within past 30 days)	Consistent with days 5–10 fall, but not clear (eg, missing platelet counts) or ≤1 day (heparin exposure with past 31–100 days) or if platelet fall after day 10	Platelet count fall ≤4 days without recent heparin exposure
Thrombosis or other sequelae (eg, skin lesions, acute systemic reactions)	New thrombosis; skin necrosis, acute systemic reaction after an intravenous heparin bolus	Progressive or recurrent thromboses; erythematous skin lesions	None
Other cause of thrombocytopenia not evident	No explanation (besides HIT) for platelet count fall is evident	Possible other cause is evident • Sepsis without proven microbial source • Thrombocytopenia associated with initiation of ventilator	Probable other cause is present • Confirmed bacteremia/fungemia • Chemotherapy or radiation within past 20 days • DIC due to non-HIT causes • Post-transfusion purpura • Platelet count <20,000/mm³ and given a drug causing drug-induced thrombocytopenia • Non-necrotizing skin lesions at LMWH injection sites

*Format adapted from Warkentin TE. Clinical picture of heparin-induced thrombocytopenia. In: Warkentin TE, Greinacher A, eds. Heparin-Induced Thrombocytopenia. 4th ed. New York, NY: Informa Healthcare USA; 2007:21–66, and Appendix 2; and Estimating the pretest probability of HIT: The four Ts. In: Warkentin TE, Greinacher A, eds. Heparin-Induced Thrombocytopenia. 4th ed. New York, NY: Informa Healthcare USA; 2007:531. Linkins LA et al. Chest 2012;141(2 Suppl):e495S–e530S

[†]*Pretest probability score:* High = 6–8 points; intermediate = 4–5 points; low = 0–3 points

[‡]The first day of immunizing heparin exposure = day 0; the day the platelet count begins to fall is considered the day of onset of thrombocytopenia as it generally takes 1–3 more days until an arbitrary threshold that defines thrombocytopenia is passed. In general, giving heparin during or soon after surgery is most likely to induce immunization. The scoring system shown here has undergone minor modifications from previously published scoring systems (Appendix 2. Estimating the pretest probability of HIT: The four Ts. In: Warkentin TE, Greinacher A, eds. Heparin-Induced Thrombocytopenia. 4th ed. New York, NY: Informa Healthcare USA; 2007:531)

1. The 4Ts score is the best studied of currently developed pretest clinical prediction rules to assist physicians in determining the probability of HIT. A recently reported systematic review and metaanalysis estimated the predictive value of the 4Ts in patients with suspected HIT. In this report, 3068 patients* identified with suspected HIT were evaluated both by the 4Ts and a reference standard (functional assay for HIT in all but 1 study) against which the 4Ts could be compared. The results of these analyses showed the following:

4Ts Probability Category	Patient Number (%)	PPV (95% CI)	NPV (95% CI)
Low (score: 1–3)	1712 (55.8)	—	0.998 (0.970–1.000)
Intermediate (score: 4–5)	1103 (36.0)	0.14 (0.009–0.22)	—
High (score: 6–8)	253 (8.2)	0.64 (0.400–0.82)	—

CI, confidence interval; NPV, negative predictive value; PPV, positive predictive value

Cuker AA et al. Blood 2012;120:4160–4167

*Twelve of 43 screened full-text articles met review inclusion criteria from which the study patients were identified

Notes:
1. The pooled estimates of sensitivity and specificity with 95% CI of 4Ts at a cut off of ≥4 were 0.99 (0.86–1.00) and 0.54 (0.43–0.66), respectively
2. The authors make the conclusion that "a low probability 4Ts score appears to be a robust means of excluding HIT"
3. Based on the results of this study, the authors propose an algorithm for the initial evaluation and management of patients with suspected HIT using the 4Ts pretest probability score: (a) score ≥4: discontinue heparin; start alternative anticoagulant; obtain HIT laboratory testing; (b) score ≤3: continue heparin; consider alternative diagnoses
4. While integrating 4Ts in the evaluation and initial management of suspected HIT may reduce overtesting, overdiagnosis, and overtreatment of HIT, the authors emphasize, "that this approach requires investigation in a randomized comparison with institution-based diagnosis"

(continued)

Work-up (continued)

2. **Timing of platelet fall** (additional considerations relative to pattern of platelet fall):
   - *Typical onset HIT* (approximately 67% of presentations): thrombocytopenia occurs 5–10 days after initial exposure to immunizing doses of UFH or LMWH
   - *Rapid-onset HIT* (approximately 25–30% of presentations): platelet count falls unexpectedly within 24 hours after reexposure to UFH or LMWH. Typically, these patients have had prior UFH or LMWH exposure in the preceding 100 days with circulating HIT antibodies at the time of reexposure
   - *Delayed-onset HIT* (approximately 3–5% of presentations): thrombocytopenia and/or associated thrombosis that occurs within several days (9–40 days) after stopping UFH or LMWH when given in a perioperative setting or inflammatory states
   - *For postoperative cardiac surgery patients*, a diagnosis of HIT should be excluded if the platelet count falls ≥50% (and/or a thrombotic events occurs) from the highest postoperative days 4 and 14 (day 0 = day of cardiac surgery) or thrombocytopenia that persists for >4 days after surgery. Following cardiopulmonary bypass (CPB), the platelet count falls by approximately 38% and continues to fall for the first 1–2 days postoperatively before rising in a continuous fashion to a level above the preoperative platelet count
   - *No single definition of thrombocytopenia in HIT is appropriate in all clinical situations*

3. **Evaluation for thrombosis**

   In cases of strongly suspected or confirmed HIT, routine venous ultrasonography of the lower limb veins for investigation of DVT is recommended (whether or not there is clinical evidence of lower-limb DVT). In addition, upper-arm venous ultrasonography should be considered in patients who have or recently had indwelling venous catheters (authors' opinion)

4. **Clinical manifestations of HIT**

Common	Uncommon
• DVT (lower > upper extremity) ± PE (~17–55%) • Thrombosis preceding thrombocytopenia (~25%) • Acute limb ischemia (~5–10%) • Acute stroke/MI (~3–5%)	• Acute systemic reactions post-IV UFH bolus (~25% of sensitized patients) • Erythematous plaques/skin necrosis at UFH/LMWH injection sites (~10–20%) • Venous limb gangrene (~5–10% of HIT with DVT acutely treated with a VKA) • Decompensated DIC (~5–10%)

"Rare"
• Adrenal hemorrhagic infarction/necrosis due to adrenal vein thrombosis • Warfarin-induced skin necrosis • Cerebral dural sinus thrombosis • Thrombosis involving arteries of upper limb, renal, mesenteric, spinal, and other sites • Cardiac arrest

Greinacher A et al. Thromb Haemost 2005;94:132–135
Linkins L-A et al. Chest 2012;141(2 Suppl):e495S–e530S
Warkentin TE. Clinical picture of heparin-induced thrombocytopenia. In: Warkentin TE, Greinacher A, eds. Heparin-Induced Thrombocytopenia. 4th ed. New York, NY: Informa Healthcare USA; 2007:21–66
Warkentin TE et al. Ann Intern Med 1997;127:804–812
Warkentin TE et al. N Engl J Med 1995;332:1330–1335

(continued)

Work-up (continued)

D. Antigen Assays for the Detection of HIT Antibodies*

Assay	Sensitivity	Specificity	PPV	NPV
GTI-PF4	100%	81–88%	28–43%	100%
ID-PaGIA Heparin/PF4 antibody test	94–95%	88–92%	37–57%	99%

GTI-PF4 (Genetics Testing Institute), ELISA; ID-PaGIA Heparin/PF4 antibody test (DiaMed), gel filtration assay that uses the binding of antibodies to antigen-coated (PF4/heparin) high-density, red polystyrene beads; NPV, negative predictive value; PPV, positive predictive value
*Adapted from Linkins L-A et al. Chest 2012;141(2 Suppl):e495S–e530S using data from the following references: Bakchoul T et al. J Thromb Haemost 2009;7:1260–1265, Pouplard C et al. J Thromb Haemost 2007;5:1373–1379, Warkentin TE et al. J Thromb Haemost 2008;6:1304–1312 (these studies met the criteria for comparison with at least 1 reference standard functional assay and blood samples collected from consecutive patients with suspected HIT)

Notes:
1. Both of these assays can exclude a diagnosis of HIT. Neither test is ideal as a stand-alone test to confirm a diagnosis of HIT. A (+) ELISA or PaGIA in a patient with a low 4Ts pretest probability of HIT should not be interpreted as diagnostic for HIT and requires confirmation with a functional assay (eg, washed platelet SRA or HIPA)
   Linkins L-A et al. Chest 2012;141(2 Suppl):e495S–e530S
2. Washed platelet SRA and HIPA are generally accepted as the reference standard assays for HIT. Both assays have sensitivities of 90–98% and specificities of >95% (early platelet fall within 4 days after starting heparin) and 80–97% (late platelet fall ≥5 days after starting heparin)
   Warkentin TE, Greinacher A. Chest 2004;126(3 Suppl):311S–337S

E. Summary Guidelines on the Treatment/Management and Prevention of HIT

Parameter	ACCP Guidelines 9th ed (2012)*	British Committee for Standards in Haematology (2012)†
Platelet monitoring on heparin with risk of HIT >1%	Every 2 or 3 days from days 4–14 or until heparin is stopped, whichever occurs first	• Baseline platelet count in any patient to receive heparin (UFH)
Platelet monitoring on heparin with risk of HIT ≤1%	No monitoring	• Postoperative patients (including obstetric cases) receiving UFH or post-CPB receiving LMWH: monitor platelets every 2–3 days from days 4–14, or until heparin is stopped • Postoperative and CPB patients exposed to UFH in last 100 days, *and* are receiving any type of heparin: platelet count 24 hours after starting UFH • Medical and obstetric patients receiving UFH do not need routine platelet monitoring
Treatment of HITT	Nonheparin anticoagulants, in particular lepirudin, argatroban, and danaparoid	Lepirudin, argatroban, danaparoid at therapeutic doses, or fondaparinux (not licensed for this indication)
Treatment of isolated HIT or HITT and normal renal function	Argatroban over lepirudin or danaparoid over other nonheparin anticoagulants	Lepirudin, argatroban, danaparoid at therapeutic doses, or fondaparinux (not licensed for this indication)
Treatment of isolated HIT or HITT and renal insufficiency	Argatroban over other nonheparin anticoagulants	Regimen choice in this scenario not specifically addressed
Use of platelet transfusion with HIT and severe thrombocytopenia	Only if bleeding or during performance of an invasive procedure with a high risk of bleeding	May be used in the event of bleeding and not for prophylaxis
Platelet count threshold for initiation of VKA in strongly suspected or confirmed HIT	Usually a platelet count ≥150,000/mm³ with VKA in low doses (maximum: 5 mg of warfarin or 6 mg phenprocoumon)	Not until the platelet count has recovered to normal range
Countermeasures for VKA started when a patient is diagnosed with HIT	Administration of vitamin K	Administration of vitamin K

(continued)

	Work-up (continued)	
Parameter	**ACCP Guidelines 9th ed (2012)***	**British Committee for Standards in Haematology (2012)†**
Duration of VKA overlap with nonheparin anticoagulant in confirmed HIT	Minimum of 5 days and until the INR is within the target range, *and* the INR rechecked after resolution of nonheparin anticoagulant effect	Minimum of 5 days between nonheparin anticoagulants and VKA therapy is recommended
Treatment of isolated HIT	Lepirudin, or argatroban, or danaparoid	Alternative full-dose nonheparin anticoagulant
Nonheparin anticoagulant use with acute HIT or subacute HIT (platelets recovered, HIT Ab+) for patients who require *urgent* cardiac surgery	Bivalirudin over other nonheparin anticoagulants and over heparin plus antiplatelet agents	Bivalirudin is suggested where urgent surgery is required
Patients with acute HIT who require *nonurgent* cardiac surgery	Delay surgery (if possible) until HIT has resolved and HIT antibodies are negative	Delay surgery until the patient is antibody negative if possible
Requirement for percutaneous coronary interventions with acute or subacute HIT	Bivalirudin or argatroban over other nonheparin anticoagulants	Bivalirudin is recommended
Requirement for renal replacement therapy in acute or subacute HIT	Argatroban or danaparoid over other nonheparin anticoagulants	Argatroban and danaparoid have been used (regimens provided in reference†)
Requirement for ongoing renal replacement therapy or catheter locking in patients with a past history of HIT	Regional citrate over the use of heparin or LMWH	Regimen choice in this scenario not specifically addressed
Treatment of pregnant patients with acute or subacute HIT	Lepirudin‡ or fondaparinux *only* IF danaparoid is not available	Danaparoid where available; fondaparinux also considered
Requirement for cardiac surgery in patients with a history of HIT without heparin Ab	Heparin (short-term use only) over nonheparin anticoagulants	Intraoperative heparin in preference to other anticoagulants
Requirement for cardiac surgery in patients with a history of HIT with heparin antibodies present	Nonheparin anticoagulants over heparin or LMWH	Delay surgery until antibody negative if possible and then intraoperative heparin
Requirement for cardiac catheterization or PCI with a history of HIT with absent heparin Ab	Bivalirudin or argatroban over other nonheparin anticoagulants	Bivalirudin is recommended in patients with previous or present HIT
Acute thrombosis (not related to HIT) with a past history of HIT and normal renal function	Fondaparinux at full therapeutic doses until transition to VKA can be achieved	Fondaparinux (therapeutic dose) or danaparoid have been used
Duration of anticoagulation for HIT or HITT	Isolated HIT: VKA therapy or alternative anticoagulant for 4 weeks; HITT: VKA therapy or alternative anticoagulant for 3 months	Isolated HIT: 4 weeks; HITT: 3 months

Ab, antibody; CPB, cardiopulmonary bypass; h, hour; HITT, HIT with thrombosis; LMWH, low-molecular-weight heparin; PCI, percutaneous coronary artery intervention; UFH, unfractionated heparin; VKA, vitamin K antagonist
*Linkins L-A et al. Chest 2012;141(2 Suppl):e495S–e530S
†Watson H et al. [Haemostasis and Thrombosis Task Force of the **British Committee** for **Standards** in **Haematology**] Guidelines on the diagnosis and management of **heparin-induced thrombocytopenia: second edition.** Br J Haematol 2012;159:528–540

Notes:
‡1. Since the publication of the ninth edition of the ACCP Guidelines on the treatment of HIT and prior to the publication of the second edition of the British Committee on the Standards in Haematology's guidelines for the diagnosis and management of HIT, Refludan (lepirudin [rDNA] for injection) manufacturing has been permanently discontinued unrelated to safety concerns. Lepirudin is no longer being supplied in the European Union as of April 1, 2012, and no further product is expected to be shipped to wholesalers in the United States as of May 31, 2012
2. Danaparoid sodium is the most widely used treatment for HIT outside the United States (it has not been available in the United States since 2002)

REGIMEN

ARGATROBAN

Bartholomew JR. J Thromb Thrombolysis 2005;19:183–188
Lewis BE et al. Argatroban in heparin-induced thrombocytopenia. In: Warkentin TE, Greinacher A, eds. Heparin-Induced Thrombocytopenia. 4th ed. New York, NY: Informa Healthcare USA; 2007:379–408
Lewis BE et al. Arch Intern Med 2003;163:1849–1856
Lewis BE et al. Circulation 2001;103:1838–1843
Linkins L-A et al. Chest 2012;141(2 Suppl):e495S–e530S
Verme-Gibboney CN, Hursting MJ. Ann Pharmacother 2003;37:970–975
Warkentin T. Thromb Res 2003;110:73–82

ARGATROBAN injection prescribing information. GlaxoSmithKline. April 2012

Mechanism of action: Direct thrombin inhibitor
Half-life: 39–51 minutes
Metabolism: Hepatic clearance (major); 16% unchanged drug eliminated renally

Prior to initiating therapy: Discontinue heparin (if ongoing administration). Do not start if PTT ratio is ≥2.5; baseline CBC, chemistry (eg, LFTs and serum creatinine), and coagulation studies (eg, PT, INR, aPTT)

HIT or HITTS (normal liver function):
Loading dose: None
Maintenance dose: **Argatroban** 2 mcg/kg per minute; administer intravenously. Dilute **argatroban** in 0.9% sodium chloride injection (0.9% NS), 5% dextrose injection (D5W), or lactated Ringer injection (LRI), to produce a solution with a concentration = 1 mg/mL (eg, 250 mg in 250 mL diluent)

Note: Renal impairment in the absence of hepatic impairment (see below), initial dose: 2 mcg/kg per min

HIT or HITTS (hepatic impairment):
Loading dose: None
Maintenance dose: **Argatroban** 0.5 mcg/kg per minute; administer intravenously. Dilute **argatroban** in 0.9% NS, D5W, or LRI to produce a solution with a concentration = 1 mg/mL
• Child-Pugh score >6, total serum bilirubin >1.5 mg/dL (initial dose: 0.5 mcg/kg per minute)
• CHF, multiorgan failure, severe anasarca, postcardiac surgery (initial dose: 0.5–1.2 mcg/kg per minute)

Antidote: None. The drug generally disappears from the circulation within 2–4 hours, or longer in the setting of liver disease. Discontinue the drug if life-threatening bleeding and/or excessive anticoagulation (with or without bleeding) occurs and obtain aPTT and other coagulation tests. rVIIa and FFP have been used to treat patients with severe bleeding
Comment: Above argatroban dosing recommendations per 2012 9th ed ACCP HIT Guidelines

Conversion to Warfarin

1. Initiate warfarin at a modest daily dose (≤5 mg/day) while argatroban is continued
2. If the INR is >4 on co-therapy and *assuming a minimum 5-day overlap* on an average argatroban dose of ≤2 mcg/kg per minute, discontinue argatroban and repeat the INR after 4–6 hours
   a. If the repeated INR is within the therapeutic range (2–3) for 2 consecutive days, warfarin therapy alone is indicated
   b. If the repeated INR is less than the therapeutic range, resume argatroban and repeat the process daily until the target INR is achieved
3. When the INR is ≥4 in patients receiving warfarin and argatroban >2 mcg/kg per minute, decrease the argatroban dose-rate to 2 mcg/kg per minute for 4–6 hours, then remeasure the INR
   a. If the INR has fallen to <4, argatroban should be resumed to keep the aPTT in the therapeutic range
   b. If the INR is >4 on combination therapy with warfarin and argatroban >2 mcg/kg per minute and assuming a minimum 5-day overlap, discontinue argatroban and repeat the INR after 4–6 hours
      (1) If the repeated INR is within the therapeutic range (2–3) for 2 consecutive days, continue warfarin therapy alone
      (2) If the repeated INR is less than the therapeutic range, resume argatroban and repeat the process daily until the target INR is achieved

Adverse Events*

Major Hemorrhagic Events (Study 1 and Study 2)[†]; n = 568	Minor Hemorrhagic Events (Study 1 and Study 2)[†]; n = 568
• Overall bleeding (5.3%)	• Gastrointestinal (14.4%)
• Gastrointestinal (2.3%)	• Genitourinary and hematuria (11.6%)
• Decrease in Hgb/Hct (0.7%)	• Groin (5.4%)
• Multisystem hemorrhage and DIC (0.5%)	• Hemoptysis (2.9%)
• Limb and below-knee amputation stump (0.5%)	• Brachial (2.4%)
• Intracranial hemorrhage (0; n = 1 ICH 4 days after stopping argatroban and following therapy with urokinase and oral anticoagulation)	

*Argatroban injection; April 2012 product label. GlaxoSmithKline, Research Triangle Park, NC
[†]Study 1: historically controlled efficacy and safety study; Study 2: follow-on efficacy and safety study (these studies were comparable with regard to study design, study objectives, and dosing regimens, as well as study outline, conduct, and monitoring)
Note: See Efficacy Results Table for Study 1 and Study 2 treatment outcomes

Efficacy Results of Study 1*

Parameter, N (%)	HIT		HITTS		HIT/HITTS	
	Control n = 147	Argatroban n = 160	Control n = 46	Argatroban n = 144	Control n = 193	Argatroban n = 304
Composite end point†	57 (38.8)	41 (25.6)	26 (56.5)	63 (43.8)	83 (43.0)	104 (34.2)
Death	32 (21.8)	27 (16.9)	13 (28.3)	26 (18.1)	45 (23.3)	53 (17.4)
Amputation	3 (2.0)	3 (1.9)	4 (8.7)	16 (11.1)	7 (3.6)	19 (6.2)
New thrombosis	22 (15.0)	11 (6.9)	9 (19.6)	21 (14.6)	31 (16.1)	32 (10.5)

*Argatroban injection; April 2012 product label. GlaxoSmithKline, Research Triangle Park, NC
In this study, 568 adult patients were treated with argatroban and 193 adult patients comprised the control group. Patients were required to have a diagnosis of HIT ± thrombosis, age 18–80 years, a platelet count fall to <100,000/mm³ or a 50% decrease in platelets after the initiation of heparin therapy with no apparent explanation other than HIT (HIT laboratory testing with HIPA or SRA was positive in 174 of 304 [57%] of argatroban-treated patients and in 149 of 193 [77%] historical controls). The initial argatroban dosage rate was 2 mcg/kg per min (not to exceed 10 mcg/kg per min) with an aPTT obtained 2 hours after treatment initiation with dose adjustments made to achieve a steady-state aPTT of 1.5- to 3-times baseline. At first assessment during treatment: HIT patients, the mean aPTT was 64 seconds (baseline: 38 seconds); HITTS patients, the mean aPTT was 70 seconds (baseline: 34 seconds). Overall, the mean aPTT during argatroban infusion was 64.5 seconds
†Death (all causes), amputation (all causes), or new thrombosis within a 37-day study period

Note: Study 2 (follow-on and safety study): 264 patients with HIT (125/264, 47.3%) or HITTS (139/264, 52.7%) were treated with argatroban versus the same historical control group from Study 1. The composite end point (argatroban vs. historical control) showed the following: HIT (25.6% vs. 38.8%); HITTS (41.0% vs. 56.5%); and HIT/HITTS (33.7% vs. 43.0%)

Therapy Monitoring

aPTT 2 hours after starting infusion (and after each dose change), adjust dose (± 0.5 mcg/kg per minute, or less in the setting of hepatic impairment) to give an aPTT 1.5–3 times a patient's baseline aPTT. Monitor aPTT at least daily after the argatroban infusion is at a steady-state level

REGIMEN

LEPIRUDIN

Greinacher A et al. Blood 2000;96:846–851
Greinacher A et al. Circulation 1999;99:73–80
Greinacher A et al. Circulation 1999;100:587–593
Greinacher A. Lepirudin for the treatment of heparin-induced thrombocytopenia. In: Warkentin TE, Greinacher A, eds. Heparin-Induced Thrombocytopenia. 4th ed. New York, NY: Informa Healthcare USA; 2007:345–378
Linkins L-A et al. Chest 2012;141(2 Suppl):e495S–e530S
Lubenow N et al. J Thromb Haemost 2005;3:2428–2436
Refludan® (lepirudin [rDNA] for injection); October 2004 product label. BERLEX®, Montville, NJ
Refludan® (lepirudin [rDNA] for injection); December 2006 product label. Bayer HealthCare Pharmaceuticals Inc., Wayne, NJ
Willey ML et al. Pharmacotherapy 2002;22:492–499

Mechanism of action: Direct thrombin inhibitor; a recombinant hirudin analog
Half-life: Terminal; mean 1.3 hours (range: 0.8–1.7 hours) in young healthy volunteers
Metabolism: Predominantly renal clearance

Prior to initiating therapy:
Discontinue heparin (if ongoing administration) and allow the patient's aPTT ratio (patient aPTT/median of normal aPTT range) to decline to <2.5 (per PI)

Dose for HIT or HITTS
Loading dose: Either omit or, in the case of perceived life- or limb-threatening thrombosis, give **lepirudin** 0.2 mg/kg; administer by intravenous injection over 15–20 seconds

Lepirudin preparation for intravenous injection
1. Reconstitute the freeze-dried powder by injecting 1 mL Sterile Water for Injection, USP (SWFI) or 0.9% Sodium Chloride Injection, USP (0.9% NS) into a vial containing lepirudin 50 mg
2. Gently shake the vial to aid dissolution and to obtain a clear, colorless solution with a concentration of 50 mg/mL
3. With a sterile syringe (15–30-mL capacity), aspirate the contents of the vial (reconstituted lepirudin 50 mg in 1 mL)
4. Draw up into the same syringe an additional volume of 0.9% NS or 5% Dextrose Injection, USP (D5W), sufficient to produce a total volume of 10 mL
   a. The resulting solution has a concentration of 5 mg/mL and is administered by intravenous injection
   b. The diluted product (5 mg/mL) should be used immediately, but remains stable at room temperature for up to 24 hours
   c. The diluted product should be warmed to room temperature before use
   Lepirudin is administered by direct intravenous injection at a dosage based on a patient's body weight

Lepirudin infusion rate is determined by the patient's serum creatinine level and body weight with slower infusion rates for patients with higher serum creatinine levels (See table below)

Lepirudin preparation for intravenous injection
1. Reconstitute two vials of lepirudin by injecting into each vial 1 mL SWFI or 0.9% NS
2. Gently shake the vials to aid dissolution and to obtain a clear, colorless solution with a concentration of 50 mg/mL
3. With a syringe, transfer the contents of both vials to a parenteral product container containing 500 mL (final concentration = 0.2 mg/mL) or 250 mL (final concentration = 0.4 mg/mL) of 0.9% NS or D5W
   Lepirudin is administered by intravenous infusion at a dosage based on body weight at a rate adjusted for a patient's serum creatinine

(continued)

Therapy Monitoring

1. Check aPTT ratio (using the patient's baseline or mean of laboratory normal range) 4 hours after starting lepirudin infusion and 4 hours after the rate of infusion has been changed until it is apparent that a steady state aPTT is achieved within the therapeutic range

Target aPTT Ratio

HIT	1.5–2.0
HITTS	1.5–2.0

Dose Adjustments

aPTT ratio >2.0*	Stop infusion for 2 hours; restart at 50% of previous dose
aPTT ratio <1.5	Increase infusion rate in 20% increments; remeasure aPTT ratio 4 hours after a dose-rate change

*Any aPTT value out of target should be confirmed before drawing conclusions with respect to dose modifications, unless there is a critical need to react immediately

A follow-up aPTT should be measured at least once daily as long as lepirudin is ongoing. More frequent aPTT measurements are highly recommended in patients with renal impairment or serious liver injury ~40% of patients develop antilepirudin IgG antibodies after ≥5 days of use and may require dose adjustment; usually a reduction

Conversion to Warfarin

1. Once the patient is scheduled to begin a vitamin K antagonist for oral anticoagulation, the dose of lepirudin should be gradually reduced to result in an aPTT ratio just above 1.5 before initiating oral anticoagulation
2. After the platelet count has substantially recovered (eg, usually to >150,000/mm³) initiate warfarin at a modest daily dose (≤5 mg/day) while lepirudin is continued maintaining an aPTT ratio of 1.5–2.0
3. After not less than 5 days on combined therapy and with INR in the target range (2–3) for 2 consecutive days on the combined anticoagulants, discontinue lepirudin and repeat INR ~4 hours later to confirm that it is still within the target range. If the INR falls below the target range, resume lepirudin (maintaining an aPTT ratio to just above 1.5, but between 1.5–2.0) for another 24 hours and repeat the process

(*continued*)

Initial Infusion Rate of Lepirudin

Serum Creatinine	Lepirudin Dose (mg/kg per hour)
<90 μmol/L (<1.0 mg/dL)	0.10
90–140 μmol/L (1.0–1.6 mg/dL)	0.05
140–400 μmol/L (1.6–4.5 mg/dL)	0.01
>400 μmol/L (>4.5 mg/dL)	0.005

Note: As noted in the 9th ed ACCP guidelines for the Treatment and Prevention of Heparin-Induced Thrombocytopenia, the dosing guidelines reflect modifications of the U.S. Food and Drug Administration (FDA) labeling dosing guidelines due to concern about an increased risk of bleeding

Current product labeling recommends limiting the maintenance dose to a maximum of 16.5 mg/hour (0.15 mg/kg per hour for a patient with body weight = 110 kg)

In case of overdose (suggested by excessively high aPTT values), the risk of bleeding is increased. If life-threatening bleeding occurs and excessive plasma levels of lepirudin are suspected: a) immediately stop lepirudin; b) determine aPTT and other coagulation levels as appropriate; c) determine hemoglobin level and prepare for blood transfusion and d) follow guidelines for treating patients with shock

Antidote: None. Individual clinical case reports and in vitro data suggest that either hemofiltration or hemodialysis (using high-flux dialysis membrane with a cutoff point of 50,000 daltons, may be useful in this situation (Refludan® (lepirudin [rDNA] for injection); October 2004 product label. BERLEX®, Montville, NJ)

Efficacy

Parameter: From Start of Treatment	HAT 1,2,3 Studies* (n = 403)	Historical Control (n = 120)	Risk Reduction (%)
Death	47 (11.7%)	21 (17.5%)	36.0
Amputation	22 (5.5%)	8 (6.7%)	17.9
New TEC	30 (7.4%)	30 (25.0%)	70.4

*Includes patients with HIT ± thrombosis; median platelet recovery to 150,000/mm³ in 4 days (isolated HIT; HAT 1,2,3 Meta-Analysis)

The risk for new thromboembolic events decreased by 92.9%: from 5.1% per patient day during the 1.3 day period between the diagnosis of HIT and the beginning of treatment with lepirudin to 0.4% during the period of active treatment with lepirudin

Lubenow N et al. J Thromb Haemost 2005;3:2428–2436

Adverse Events*

	HAT 1, 2, 3 Studies[‡] (n = 403)	Control[§] (n = 120)
Major bleeding[†]	71 (17.6%)	7 (5.8%)

*Lubenow N et al. J Thromb Haemost 2005;3: 2428–2436
[†]Fatal or life-threatening, requiring surgical intervention, intracranial, permanently or significantly disabling, or requiring transfusion of ≥2 units of packed red blood cells
[‡](a) Study participants with renal impairment (serum creatinine >1.0 mg/dL [>90 μmol/L]; (b) one-third of participants) compared with those with a serum creatinine of >1.0 mg/dL (≤90 μmol/L) had an increased rate of bleeding (p <0.001); (c) death secondary to bleeding complications: among 5 patients (1.2%) death was in 1 patient attributed to intracranial bleeding during treatment with thrombolytics; (d) allergic reactions: among 17 patients (4.2%), a relationship with lepirudin was considered in 9 (1 participant required termination of lepirudin; the authors recommend "that lepirudin treatment should be started in a setting appropriate for dealing with allergic/anaphylactic reactions, especially those during repeated treatment courses"); (e) antihirudin IgG antibodies developed in 30% (121) of lepirudin-treated patients at the end of the first treatment cycle (exposure) and in 70% (21) after the second treatment cycle
[§]Treated for HIT according to the practices of individual participating hospitals before lepirudin or other hirudins were available

Notes:
1. *Hemorrhagic events* (HAT 1 & 2, n = 198 [all patients] vs. historical control, n = 91 with thromboembolic events): bleeding from puncture sites/wounds: 14.1% vs. 4.4%; anemia or isolated drop in Hgb (13.1% vs. 1.1%); other hematoma/unclassified bleeding: 11.1% vs. 4.4%; hematuria: GI/rectal bleeding: 5.1% vs. 6.6%; hemothorax: 3.0% vs. none; epistaxis: 3.0% vs. 1.1%; intracranial bleeding: none vs. 2.2%
2. *Airway reactions* (cough, bronchospasm, stridor, dyspnea) have been reported in 1% to <10% of populations other than HIT patients
   • Refludan (lepirudin [rDNA] for injection); December 2006 product label. Bayer HealthCare Pharmaceuticals Inc., Wayne, NJ

Notes

The rationale for the revised lepirudin dose and monitoring recommendations is based on further analyses of prospective and retrospective studies, and increasing clinical experience. These analyses provide evidence that the lepirudin dosages used in the approval studies was too high

REGIMEN

BIVALIRUDIN

Angiomax (bivalirudin) for injection, product label: May 2013. The Medicines Company; Parsippany, NJ
Bartholomew JR. Bivalirudin for the treatment of heparin-induced thrombocytopenia. In: Warkentin TE, Greinacher A, eds. Heparin-Induced Thrombocytopenia. 4th ed. New York, NY: Informa Healthcare USA; 2007:409–439
Francis JL et al. Blood 2003;102:571 (abstract)
Kiser TH et al. Pharmacotherapy 2008;28:1115–1124
Koster A et al. Anesth Analg 2003;96:1316–1319
Reed MD et al. Pharmacotherapy 2002;22:105S–111S
Robson R. J Invasive Cardiol 2000;12(Suppl F): 33F–36F
Robson R et al. Clin Pharmacol Ther 2002;71:433–439

Mechanism of action: Direct thrombin inhibitor
Half-life: 25–36 minutes
Metabolism: 80% proteolytic cleavage by plasma proteases; 20% renal mechanisms

Prior to initiating therapy:
Discontinue heparin (if administration is ongoing) and allow the patient's aPTT ratio to decline to <2.5 (patient aPTT/median of normal aPTT range)

Dose for HIT or HITTS: (off-label experience)
Loading dose: None
Maintenance dose: **Bivalirudin** 0.15–0.20 mg/kg per hour; administer as a continuous intravenous infusion using a solution containing 250 mg bivalirudin in 500 mL 0.9% sodium chloride or 5% dextrose injection.
Antidote: None. Large amounts of bivalirudin can be removed by hemofiltration (65,000-kDa large-pore filter) or plasmapheresis

Initial Dose-Rates are Based on Renal Function

	Bivalirudin Dosages, Distribution of Patients in Relation to aPTT Goals, and Outcomes by Varying Creatinine Clearance Groups Among Patients (n = 37) with Clinical or Prior History of HIT[*,†]		
	Clcr (mL/min)[‡] Groups		
Variable	≥60 (>1 mL/s) n = 12	30–60 (0.5–1 mL/s) n = 11	<30 (<0.5 mL/s) or RRT[§] n = 14
Initial dosage, mg/kg • hour[ϵ]	0.15 (0.14–0.15)	0.08 (0.04–0.18)	0.05 (0.02–0.05)
Dosage achieving aPTT goal, mg/kg • hour[ϵ]	0.15 (0.13–0.15)	0.1 (0.05–0.14)	0.03 (0.02–0.05)
Dosage over study period, mg/kg • hour[ϵ]	0.15 (0.13–0.15)	0.10 (0.05–0.13)	0.03 (0.02–0.04)
Therapy duration, days	8 ± 7	16 ± 19	11 ± 11
aPTT with initial dose, n (% in group)			
• At goal[**]	6/12 (50)	7/11 (64)	6/14 (43)
• Above	2/6 (33)	2/4 (50)	4/8 (50)
• Below	4/6 (67)	2/4 (50)	4/8 (50)
aPTT (s)[††]			
• Baseline	31.8 ± 2.4	31.1 ± 3.3	31.0 ± 3.0
• During therapy	72 ± 11	74 ± 18	62 ± 17
• After achieving goal	67 ± 8	68 ± 8	60 ± 9
INR[††]			
• Baseline	1.2 ± 0.2	1.6 ± 0.3	1.5 ± 0.4
• During therapy	2.1 ± 0.9	2.0 ± 0.4	1.8 ± 0.6
Outcome, n			
• All-cause mortality[‡‡]	1 (8%)	2 (18%)	5 (36%)
• New thrombosis on therapy	0	0	1
• Clinically significant bleeding[§§]	0	1	1
• Limb amputation	0	0	0

aPTT, activated partial thromboplastin time; Clcr, creatinine clearance; INR, international normalized ratio; RRT, renal replacement therapy; s, seconds
*Kiser TH et al. Pharmacotherapy 2008;28:1115–1124 (retrospective study)
[†]Clinical HIT diagnosis: new in 78%, prior admission in 22%; H-PF4 (+) in 14/34 (41%); baseline thrombosis (n = 10); ages ≥18 y
[‡]Creatinine clearance; Cockcroft-Gault method (weight descriptor not stated, eg, actual vs. ideal vs. adjusted body weight)
[§]Clcr estimated before start of RRT (continuous venovenous ultrafiltration [n = 9]; continuous venovenous hemofiltration [n = 4])
[ϵ]Values expressed as median (interquartile range; 25th–75th percentile)
[**]aPTT 1.5- to 2.5-times baseline, or upper limit of normal laboratory standard (mean goal: 47–78 s)
[††]Values expressed as mean ± SD
[‡‡]Attributed to acute or underlying disease rather than HIT; all-cause mortality = 22% (8/37); no death as a result of thrombosis
[§§]Attributable to bivalirudin with therapeutic aPTTs requiring treatment cessation, the use of blood product support and survived

Efficacy

Parameter	Francis, 2003 n = 45	Skrupkey, 2010 n = 92	Runyan, 2011 n = 64		Tsu, 2012 n = 135
(+) H-PF4 antibody (%)	80	33	22/53 (41.5)		47
Clinical features, n (%)					
• Baseline VTE	18 (40)	34 (37)	18 (28)		61 (45)
• Clcr (mL/min):					
• ≤60	—	59 (64)	47 (73)		42 (31)
• <30 or RRT	—	17 (18)	26 (41)		21 (15.6)
• Platelets (×10³/mm³)	<100 in 23 patients	105 ± 66	71 (IQR 52–107)		62.8 ± 35.5
• Initial treatment in ICU	—	80 (87)	53 (83)		96 (71)

Bivalirudin dosage (mg/kg · hour)
Mean, initial
• Mean, during infusion

Francis, 2003: 0.17 (0.01 – 0.40)[‡]

Skrupkey, 2010: 0.07 ± 0.08* / 0.07 ± 0.05[§]

Runyan, 2011:

Clcr*	Dosage-Rate
>60	0.15**
Any	0.09[††]
>60	0.15 (n = 17)[††]
30–60	0.10 (n = 21)[††]
<30	0.08 (n = 11)[††]
CVVH	0.06 (n = 4)[††]
HD	0.04 (n = 11)[††]

Tsu, 2012: 0.07 ± 0.02[†] / 0.1 ± 0.07[‡]

Parameter	Francis, 2003	Skrupkey, 2010	Runyan, 2011	Tsu, 2012
Mean treatment duration	8 (3–24) days	148 (77–262) h	—	8 days
Platelet recovery	3.2 (1–5) days	—	50 (78%)	—
New thrombosis, n (%)	1 (2.2)	7 (8)	2 (3)	1 (<0.01)
Amputation, n (%)	0	0	None reported	—
Major bleeding, (%)	0	8 (9)[ε]	4 (6)[‡‡]	52 (38.5)[‡‡]
All-cause mortality, n (%)	6 (13.3)	18 (20)	14 (22)	33 (24)

Clcr, creatinine clearance (mL/min); CVVH, continuous venovenous hemofiltration; HD, hemodialysis; IQR, interquartile range; RRT, renal replacement therapy; VTE, venous thromboembolism

*Ideal body weight used to estimate Clcr (Cockcroft-Gault method)

[†]Total body weight (mean ± SD) used to estimate Clcr (Cockcroft-Gault method)

[‡]Dosage that resulted in an aPTT goal of 1.5- to 2.5-times baseline

[§]Dosage that resulted in an aPTT goal of 1.5- to 2.5-times control (aPTT 45–75 seconds) as measured at time of first therapeutic aPTT; the authors recommended initial bivalirudin dosage within a range of 0.06–1.0 mg/kg · hour for most patients and 0.02–0.06 mg/kg · hour in persons with renal dysfunction

[ε]Defined as a decrease in Hgb by ≥2 g/dL over <72 hours and need for transfusion

**No initial protocol for dosage recommendations for persons with Clcr <60 mL/min; bivalirudin was dosed empirically by prescribers

[††]Medians of steady-state conditions (constant dose for ≥12 hours with ≥2 aPTTs at 60–80 seconds obtained 4 hours apart for 2 measurements

[‡‡]Defined in reference: Shulman S, Kearon C. J Thromb Haemost 2005;3:692–694

Francis JL et al. Blood 2003;102:[abstract 571] *Note:* weight descriptor for dose calculations was not provided
Runyan CL et al. Pharmacotherapy 2011;31:850–856 (retrospective study)
Skrupky LP et al. Pharmacotherapy 2010;30:1229–1238 (retrospective study)
Tsu LV, Dager WE. Pharmacotherapy 2012;32:20–26 (retrospective study)

Conversion to Warfarin

1. Initiate warfarin at a modest daily dose (≤5 mg/day) while bivalirudin is continued maintaining an aPTT ratio of 1.5–2.0

2. After not less than 5 days on combined therapy and with INR in the target range (2–3) for 2 consecutive days on combined therapy, stop bivalirudin and repeat INR ~4 hours later to confirm that it is still within the target range. If the INR falls below the target range, resume bivalirudin (maintaining an aPTT ratio of 1.5–2.0) for another 24 hours and repeat the process daily until the INR is within therapeutic range (2–3), then discontinue bivalirudin

Notes

1. Drugs incompatible with bivalirudin when administered through the same IV tubing: alteplase, amiodarone hydrochloride, amphotericin B, chlorpromazine hydrochloride, diazepam, prochlorperazine edisylate, reteplase, streptokinase, vancomycin hydrochloride

2. Bivalirudin was conditionally compatible with dobutamine concentrations ≤4 mg/mL, but incompatible with dobutamine 12.5 mg/mL

3. Labeled indications for bivalirudin include (doses for the labeled indication are not shown):

   a. Use as an anticoagulant in patients with unstable angina undergoing percutaneous transluminal coronary angioplasty

   b. For patients with or at high-risk of HIT/HITTS undergoing percutaneous coronary intervention

Infusion Dose Adjustment with Impaired Renal Function*

Normal renal function or mild renal impairment (Clcr ≥60 mL/min [≥1 mL/s])	No dose reduction
Moderate renal impairment (Clcr = 30–59 mL/min [0.5–1 mL/s])	20% dose reduction
Severe renal impairment (10–29 mL/min [0.2–0.5 mL/s])	60% dose reduction

*Bivalirudin dosing adjustment recommendations based on glomerular filtration rate (GFR) for percutaneous coronary interventions. In practice, an estimated or measured creatinine clearance (Clcr) may be used in place of GFR

Adverse Events

Bleeding is the major adverse effect and occurs more frequently in patients with renal impairment

Allergic reactions: 1/3639 patients (0.03%) reported in clinical trials from 1993–1995

Therapy Monitoring

1. Titrate bivalirudin to maintain a therapeutic aPTT (1.5 to 2.5-times a patient's baseline aPTT or mean of laboratory range)

2. Repeat aPTT at 6-hour intervals and adjust bivalirudin in increments of 0.05 mg/kg per hour until a therapeutic aPTT is achieved

3. Once a therapeutic aPTT is achieved and confirmed on a subsequent aPTT obtained at 6 hours, then monitor aPTT daily

4. In the event there is a significant reduction or improvement in renal function while on bivalirudin therapy, more frequent aPTT monitoring is suggested (eg, every 6 hours) to determine that a therapeutic range aPTT is being maintained with subsequent dose adjustments (decrements or increments) as indicated

5. Once a steady state therapeutic aPTT is achieved, monitor aPTT daily

REGIMEN

DANAPAROID SODIUM

(Danaparoid Sodium is not Currently Available in the United States)

Chong BH et al. Blood 1989;73:1592–1596
Chong BH et al. Thromb Haemost 2001;86:1170–1175
Chong BH, Magnani HN. Danaparoid for the treatment of heparin-induced thrombocytopenia. In: Warkentin TE, Greinacher A, eds. Heparin-Induced Thrombocytopenia, 4th ed. New York, NY: Informa Healthcare USA;2007:319–343
Chong BH, Magnani HN. Haemostasis 1992;22:85–91
de Valk HW et al. Ann Intern Med 1995;123:1–9
Farner B et al. Thromb Haemost 2001;85:950–957
Greinacher A et al. Thromb Haemost 1992;67:545–549
Magnani HN, Gallus A. Thromb Haemost 2006;95:967–981
ORGARAN®, Danaparoid Sodium Injection, 750 anti-Xa units/ampoule (1250 anti-Xa units/mL); April 14, 2011 product label. Merck Canada Inc., Kirkland, Quebec

Mechanism of action: Factor Xa inhibitor; weak inhibitor of Factor IIa
Anti-Xa terminal half-life: ≈25 hours
Metabolism: Predominantly renal clearance

Prior to initiating therapy:
Discontinue heparin (if ongoing administration) and allow the patient's aPTT ratio (patient aPTT/median of normal aPTT range) to decline to <2.5
plasma anti-Xa level ~0.8 Units/mL (see Therapy Monitoring below)

HIT and HITTS with normal renal function

Subcutaneous regimen
Loading dose: None
Maintenance dose:
≥60 kg: Danaparoid sodium 2250 anti-Xa units (approx. 165 mg); administer by subcutaneous injection every 12 hours
<60 kg: Danaparoid sodium 1500 anti-Xa units (approx. 110 mg); administer by subcutaneous injection every 12 hours

HIT and HITTS with normal renal function

IV regimen
Loading dose: According to weight as follows:

<60 kg	**Danaparoid sodium**	1500 anti-Xa units
60–75 kg	**Danaparoid sodium**	2250 anti-Xa units
75–90 kg	**Danaparoid sodium**	3000 anti-Xa units
>90 kg	**Danaparoid sodium**	3750 anti-Xa units

Adverse Effects

Population: 1478 patients from compassionate use program, ADRs, and published literature:
• Composite of new/extended thrombosis, new/persistent platelet count reduction, unplanned amputation (follow-up duration: up to 3 months): 16.4%
• Frequency of thrombotic events: 11%
• Major bleeding: 8.1%

Therapy Monitoring

Monitoring is not required in most situations. However, anti-Xa levels, using a standard calibration curve for danaparoid, should be followed in patients with:
• Low or high body weights
• Substantial renal impairment
• Life- or limb-threatening thrombosis
• High bleeding risk
• A critical illness or clinical instability

In these patients, obtain anti-Xa levels at approximately 6 hours after a change in dose until a plasma anti-Xa level of 0.5–0.8 units/mL is achieved, then daily

A higher target anti-Xa level (approximately 1 unit/mL) should be sought for a patient with life- or limb-threatening venous or arterial thrombosis or clotting during renal replacement therapy

A lower target anti-Xa level (eg, approximately 0.3 units/mL) may be appropriate for a patient judged to have a high risk of bleeding

Efficacy				
	HIT/HITTS, n (%)		HIT/HITTS, n (%)	
Parameter	Dan (n = 24)	Dextran-70 (n = 17)	Dan (n = 53)	Lepirudin (n = 144)
New thrombosis	3 (12.5)	7 (41.2)	5 (9.4)	9 (7.9)
Amputation	1 (4.2)	3 (17.6)	4 (7.5)	7 (6.1)
Major bleed	0	0	2 (3.8)	7 (6.1)

Dan, Danaparoid (therapeutic dosing); lepirudin (therapeutic dosing)
Dan vs. Dextran-70 (Chong BH et al. Thromb Haemost 2001;86:1170–1175)
Dan vs. lepirudin (baseline thromboses: 88.7% vs. 92.1%) (Farner B et al. Thromb Haemost 2001;85:950–957)

Maintenance dose: Administer **danaparoid sodium** by continuous intravenous infusion. Dilute danaparoid in 0.9% sodium chloride injection and administer as follows:

    400 anti-Xa units/hour for 4 hours, *then*
    300 anti-Xa units/hour for 4 hours, *then*
    150 – 200 anti-Xa units/hour for ≥5 days

In selected patients, such as those with any evidence of renal dysfunction the administration rate should be titrated to achieve a plasma anti-Xa level of 0.5–0.8 Units/mL (see Therapy Monitoring)

Venous thromboembolism prophylaxis (prior HIT): **Danaparoid sodium** 750 units; administer by subcutaneous injection every 8 or 12 hours

Antidote: None

Protamine sulfate is not a neutralizing agent for danaparoid sodium overdose. In cases of major bleeding, danaparoid sodium should be discontinued or temporarily interrupted (with subsequent continuation at a lower dose). Routine hematological counts and other coagulation parameters should be measured. Transfusion with fresh frozen plasma, or, if bleeding is uncontrolled, plasmapheresis or surgery should be considered

Note:
For patients with strongly suspected or confirmed HIT, use a therapeutic regimen
In selected patients, such as those with any evidence of renal dysfunction, the administration rate should be titrated to achieve a plasma anti-Xa level of 0.5–0.8 Units/mL (see Therapy Monitoring)
In elderly patients, danaparoid sodium dosage-rate reduction is not necessary unless kidney or liver function is impaired

Conversion to Warfarin

1. Initiate warfarin in low doses (maximum daily doses: warfarin 5 mg *or* phenprocoumon 6 mg) while danaparoid sodium is continued at therapeutic dosages
2. After not less than 5 days on combined therapy and the INR is in the target range (2–3) for 2 consecutive days on co-therapy discontinue danaparoid therapy
3. In addition, if an acute thrombosis is present, overlapping danaparoid-warfarin should be continued until the thrombosis is controlled on clinical grounds

REGIMEN
FONDAPARINUX

ARIXTRA™ (fondaparinux sodium injection) Solution for subcutaneous injection; September 2003 product label. GlaxoSmithKline, Research Triangle Park, NC

Bradner JE, Eikelboom JW. Emerging anticoagulants and heparin-induced thrombocytopenia: Indirect and direct Factor Xa inhibitors and oral thrombin inhibitors. In: Warkentin TE, Greinacher A, eds. Heparin-Induced Thrombocytopenia. 4th ed. New York, NY: Informa Healthcare USA; 2007:441–461

Efird LE, Kockler DR. Ann Pharmacother 2006;40:1383–1387

Lobo B et al. Thromb Haemost 2008;99:208–214

Papadopoulos S et al. Pharmacotherapy 2007;27:921–926

Savi P et al. Blood 2005;105:139–144

Warkentin TE. Thromb Haemost 2008;99:2–3

Mechanism of action: Synthetic pentassaccharide that is a selective factor Xa inhibitor

Anti-Xa terminal half-life: 17–21 hours

Metabolism: Renally eliminated

Prior to initiating therapy:
Discontinue heparin (if administration is ongoing) and allow the patient's aPTT ratio (patient aPTT/median of normal aPTT range) to decline to <2.5

Dose for HIT and HITTS with normal renal function (off-label experience)
Subcutaneous regimen
(Do not use if creatinine clearance <30 mL/min)
Loading dose: None
Maintenance doses:

Weight (kg)	Fondaparinux Dose (Subcutaneous, Once-Daily Administration)
<50	5 mg
≥50–100	7.5 mg
>100	10 mg

Venous thromboembolism prophylaxis (prior HIT): **Fondaparinux** 2.5 mg every 24 hours

Antidote: None available. If an overdose with bleeding has occurred, discontinue fondaparinux, search for the primary cause of bleeding and initiate appropriate therapy (eg, surgical hemostasis, blood replacement, fresh plasma transfusion, or plasmapheresis). Recombinant factor VIIa with tranexamic acid has been used to manage hemorrhagic shock in an orthopedic patient complicating fondaparinux use (Huvers F et al. Neth J Med 2005;63:184–186)

Comments:

1. Antiplatelet factor 4 heparin antibodies are as likely to form with fondaparinux as with enoxaparin. Fondaparinux is less likely to cause HIT, however, in part because it forms poorly with the PF4 antigens recognized by HIT antibodies and is less likely to induce platelet activation (Warkentin TE et al. Blood 2005;106:3791–3796)

2. *Potential strategy for fondaparinux to avoid problems during the transition from direct thrombin inhibitors (DTI) to warfarin therapy:* After platelet counts normalize on a DTI, replace the DTI with fondaparinux and begin transition to warfarin (avoids fondaparinux use in acute HIT for which efficacy and safety not yet established). 8th ACCP Guidelines on HIT (Warkentin TE et al. Chest 2008;133(6 Suppl):340S–380S)

3. One case of HIT associated with fondaparinux has been reported

Warkentin TE. N Engl J Med 2007;356:2653–2654

Adverse Effects

Major bleeding reported as between 1.2% for treatment of venous thromboembolism and 2.7% for prophylaxis of patients undergoing orthopedic surgery; non-HIT thrombocytopenia; elevations in ALT and AST

Buller HR et al. Ann Intern Med 2004;140:867–873
Turpie AGG et al. Arch Intern Med 2002;162: 1833–1840

Therapy Monitoring

Monitoring is not required in most situations. However, anti-Xa levels, using a standard calibration curve for fondaparinux, should be considered in patients with low body weights (<50 kg) or renal impairment

- In these patients, obtain anti-Xa levels to fondaparinux. These should be expressed in milligrams and cannot be compared to anti-Xa levels of UFH or LMWH. The mean peak steady-state plasma concentration is in the range of 1.2–1.26 mg/L per the package insert

Efficacy

Prospective Pilot Trial of Fondaparinux in Patients with Acute HIT (n = 7)

Patient Characteristics	Treatment Outcomes
Mean age: 65 years (M 57%) Platelets (mean; /mm³) • Pre-heparin: 241,000 • Nadir: 66,000 • Baseline pre-fondaparinux: 73,000 Baseline thrombosis: 6/7 High 4 Ts score: 6/7 (+) H-PF4 EIA: 7/7 Median OD: 0.7 (0.5 to >3)	Median treatment duration: 7–9 days Mean ↑ platelet counts by day 7: 52.5% (platelet count recovery in 7 of 7 [100%]) New TEC: 0; Death: 0, Major bleeding: 0 ≥2 g/dL ↓ Hgb: 3/7 (no clinical bleeding) Transfusion: 4/7 without evidence of bleeding Amputation: 1/7 as a result of progression of prior TEC

Fondaparinux dosing*,†

Body weight	Dose
<50 kg	5 mg
50–100 kg	7.5 mg
>100 kg	10 mg

*Doses administered by subcutaneous injection for patients with thrombosis; patients without thrombosis received 2.5 mg by subcutaneous injection
†Patients with creatinine clearance ≥30 mL/min

Lobo B et al. Thromb Haemost 2008;99:208–214

Conversion to Warfarin

1. Initiate warfarin co-therapy with fondaparinux as outlined in the section on Oral Therapy: Warfarin

2. Overlap both anticoagulants for at least 5 days ensuring that the INR is in the target range (2–3) for at least 2 consecutive days before discontinuing fondaparinux therapy

3. Fondaparinux may cause only subtle prolongation of the prothrombin time (1 second); thereby, simplifying bridging to warfarin (Bijsterveld NR et al. Circulation 2002;106:2550–2554)

Comment: FDA-approved indications for fondaparinux include venous thromboembolism prevention in hip fracture, elective hip or knee replacement, abdominal surgery, and acute treatment of DVT or PE in conjunction with warfarin, management of unstable angina or non-ST segment elevation myocardial infarction (MI) for the prevention of death and subsequent MI, and management of ST segment elevation MI for the prevention of death and MI in patients who are managed with thrombolytics or who initially are to receive no form of reperfusion therapy

Special Therapeutic Approaches

HIT in dialysis patients

Heparin must not be added to any flushing solution and no heparin-coated devices should be used in this population. LMWH is also to be avoided. Argatroban is theoretically an ideal agent for use in this patient population because of its predominant hepatic elimination with no initial dose adjustments required based on renal dysfunction alone. Regimens using lepirudin and danaparoid have also been published (Fischer K-G. Hemodial Int 2007;11:178–189)

Alternative Anticoagulants During Hemodialysis of HIT Patients

Agent	Procedure	Timing	Other Parameters	Dosage		Monitoring Test	Target Range
				Bolus	Continuous Infusion		
Danaparoid*	Intermittent HD (QOD)	Before first 2 HDs		3750 U (2500)‡	—	Anti-Xa activity	0.5–0.8 U/mL§§
		Subsequent HD	Pre-HD Anti-Xa activity‡: <0.3 0.3–0.35 0.35–0.4 >0.4	3000 U (2000)§ 2500 U (1500)§ 2000 U (1500)§ 0ᶜ	— — — —		
	Intermittent HD (daily)	First HD Second HD Subsequent HD		3750 U (2500)§ 2500 U (2000)§ See above	— — —	Anti-Xa activity	0.5–0.8 U/mL§§
	Continuous HD/HF		Initial bolus First 4 h Next 4 h Subsequently	2500 U (2000)§ — — —	600 (600) 400 (400) 200–600†† (150–400)††	Anti-Xa activity Anti-Xa activity	0.5–0.8 U/mL§§ 0.5–1.0 U/mL§§
Argatroban†	Continuous HD			100 mcg/kg**	0.5 mcg/kg · min‡‡	aPTT	1.5–3.0ᶜᶜ
	Intermittent HD			250 mcg/kg	2.0 mcg/kg/min	ACT	170–230 s***

ACT, activated clotting time; aPTT, activated partial thromboplastin time; h, hour; HD, hemodialysis; HF, hemofiltration; m, minutes; QOD, every other day; s, seconds; U, units
*Adapted in part from: Fisher K-G. Hemodialysis in heparin-induced thrombocytopenia. In: Warkentin TE, Greinacher A, eds. Heparin-Induced Thrombocytopenia, 4th ed. New York, NY: Informa Healthcare USA; 2007:463–485 and Watson H et al. Br J Haematol 2012;159:528–540
†Alatri A et al. Thromb Res 2012;129:426–433
‡Determined 30–60 min before beginning respective HD session
§Danaparoid dosage (anti-Xa units) in parentheses for patients whose body weight is <55 kg
ᶜAddition of 1500 anti-Xa units as bolus if fibrin deposition in dialyzer or clots in extracorporeal circuit
**When a patient is already being treated with argatroban, no bolus dose is required
††Maintenance dosage depends on anti-Xa activity determined every 12 h (if no bleeding/clotting occurs)
‡‡Dose of argatroban should be adjusted according to SOFA (sequential organ failure assessment)-II score, APACHE (acute physiology and chronic health assessment)-II or SAPS (simplified acute physiology score)-II or to a critically ill hepatic nomogram (see reference † in this table)
§§Peak activity determined after approximately 30 min of HD; this level is not required throughout HD procedure
ᶜᶜaPTT 1.5- to 3.0-times a patient's baseline (not to exceed 100 s)
***The infusion should be discontinued 1 hour before the end of a HD procedure

HIT in cancer patients

1. Establishing a diagnosis of HIT among patients with cancer is complex due to the multiple potential causes of thrombocytopenia (eg, cancer treatment-, non-cancer treatment- and disease-related mechanisms), timing of treatment-related myelosuppressive effects that have the potential to mimic HIT platelet-pattern declinations and a population enriched for thromboembolic risk

2. While the current NCCN Guidelines Version 2.2013 for Venous Thromboembolic Disease (section on HIT) utilizes the 4T's Score to calculate the pre-test probability for the cancer patient with suspected HIT, applying the 4T's Score in this population has potential inherent biases. For example, the 4T's may lead to both under-scoring (score of "0" for "probable other causes present" giving a potential maximum score of 6 of 8 OR a score of "1" for progressive or recurrent thrombosis that may be attributable to HIT) or over-scoring (scores of "2" in each of the domains for ">50% platelet decline" or "timing of platelet decline" or "presence of thrombosis" that may be related to the malignancy and/or its treatment temporarily occurring with, but unrelated to the use of UFH or LMWH; authors' comment). With these considerations in mind and in lieu of a HIT pre-test probability scoring system validated in the cancer patient population, the 4T's score provides a framework from which to guide clinical reasoning and management considerations for the cancer patient in whom HIT is suspected (See: NCCN Clinical Practice Guidelines in Oncology [NCCN Guidelines®]. Venous Thromboembolic Disease: Heparin Induced Thrombocytopenia [HIT]. Version 2.2013; www.NCCN.org Miriovsky BJ, Ortel TL. J Natl Compr Canc Netw 2011;9:781–787)

(continued)

Special Therapeutic Approaches (continued)

HIT in pregnancy

1. The incidence of HIT is reported to be lower during pregnancy than in the nonpregnant population, particularly when LMWH is used for thromboprophylaxis or at therapeutic doses (1 in 1167 pregnancies [3 studies]; zero in 2777 pregnancies [systematic review])

2. With HIT development, heparin (LMWH) should be discontinued and treatment initiated with a nonheparin anticoagulant for HIT (see Table E. *Summary Guidelines on the Treatment/Management and Prevention of HIT*)

3. There is limited data describing the treatment of HIT developing during pregnancy. The quality of evidence on the safety and efficacy of nonheparin anticoagulants in this patient population is low (Linkins LA et al. Chest 2012;141(2 suppl):e495S–e530S)

4. **Danaparoid**

   a. The largest experience for danaparoid use in pregnancy with HIT comes from a retrospective review of 18 case reports including 30 women who presented up to 120 days of HIT diagnosis ("current HIT" group). The report also includes the experience of danaparoid use during pregnancy in "past HIT" (n = 17 pregnancies; 9 case reports) and "non-HIT" (n = 44 pregnancies; 15 case reports) groups. These 3 groups will be collectively referred to as the *all-group* cohort. All patients had previously failed heparin or LMWH. *The following information presented pertains exclusively to the "current HIT" group except where otherwise specified*

      i. *HIT diagnosis confirmation.* HIT diagnosis evaluation among the "current HIT" and "past HIT" groups was reported as *group-nondesignated* compiled data and included (+) serology (n = 38; functional test: n = 29; ELISA: n = 9), "rechallenge" thrombocytopenia (n = 2), and "highly likely" HIT with (−) serology/no information (remaining patients)

      ii. *Thrombotic history.* Seventy percent had at least 1 acquired (n = 10) or inherited (n = 11) clotting disorder among other important comorbidities. Ninety-three percent had a thromboembolic event presenting ≤5 days (n = 15), >5 days earlier (n = 13), or in a previous or "outside" pregnancy (n = 7) in relation to initiating danaparoid treatment

      iii. *Danaparoid use and pregnancy outcome.* Danaparoid was started during the first, second, and third trimesters in 50%, 28.6%, and 21.4% of pregnancies, respectively. Danaparoid was administered intravenously or subcutaneously at various daily doses, including: <1500 units (n = 1), 1500–2500 units (n = 11), and >2500 units (n = 16) (doses not identified, n = 2). The median durations of danaparoid administration during the intrapartum and postpartum periods were 14 weeks (range: <1–33 weeks) and 7 days (range: 2–56 days), respectively. Danaparoid was administered until delivery in 96.3% (vaginal deliveries: n = 17; C-section deliveries: n = 9). From the *all-groups* cohort experience in this report, danaparoid was usually stopped a median of <12 hours before vaginal delivery and a median of 24 hours before C-section (only known for 19 patients). In the same *all-group* cohort, danaparoid was restarted (postpartum) in 37 (49.3%) of 75 patients who received it until live delivery. Among them, 14 and 10 patients, respectively, restarted it a median of <12 hours (but within 24 hours) and >24 hours to 3 days after vaginal delivery, respectively, and a median approximately 9 hours after C-section (n = 13; range: 2–72 hours) when hemostasis was achieved. The live birth rate was 96.3% (26/27) among individuals for whom the outcome of pregnancy was known. One fetal death occurred as a result of prematurity

      iv. *Intrapartum maternal adverse events (AEs)* included:

         (a) *New venous thromboembolic events* (n = 5; at least 2 responded to increased danaparoid dosing);

         (b) *Nonfatal bleeding event* (n = 2; 1 patient with a small placental hematoma during C-section use of dextran after danaparoid discontinuation; 1 patient with injection site bleeding that stopped after danaparoid dose reduction);

         (c) *Maternal death* (n = 2; 1 patient on day 2 danaparoid resulting from severe bleeding during emergency C-section for full placenta previa; 1 patient 5 days after danaparoid cessation for elective C-section who developed placental abruption, severe bleeding, heart failure and refused blood transfusion); and

         (d) *Emergency below-knee amputation* resulting from pre–danaparoid-treatment gangrene as a result of phlegmasia cerulea dolens that did not improve with thrombolytic or danaparoid treatment (pregnancy terminated during the same operation; n = 1)

      v. *Postpartum AEs* (1 each) included *major bleeding* and *skin necrosis* at previous danaparoid injection sites (3 days after completing transition to VKA with normal protein C antigen levels)

      vi. *Cord blood and breast milk.* Anti-Xa activity was absent from 3 infants' cord blood tested after delivery and none or <0.07 units/mL in breast milk samples from 3 mothers given danaparoid postpartum (which would be deactivated in a neonate's or infant's stomach)

      vii. The reviewer concluded the successful birth rate and adverse event profile indicates that danaparoid "can be a safe alternative antithrombotic in pregnancies complicated by HIT" (Magnani HN. Thromb Res 2010;125:297–302)

5. **Fondaparinux**

   a. Indirect evidence for the safety of subcutaneously administered fondaparinux during pregnancy (without HIT) is derived from 1 small prospective cohort study of 12 pregnancies (1 with twins) among 10 patients. All patients were treated initially with a LMWH for a history of DVT attributed to oral contraceptives use (n = 6), idiopathic venous thromboembolism (n = 3), or recurrent fetal loss (n = 1). Fondaparinux 2.5 mg subcutaneously, twice daily, was administered as a result of hypersensitivity skin reactions to LMWH in all patients (n = 8 during second trimester; n = 2 during third trimester). Fondaparinux was discontinued at the start of spontaneous labor, restarted 4–8 hours after delivery (when blood loss was normal), and discontinued 6 weeks postpartum. *The results of this study showed:* (a) no hypersensitivity skin reactions during fondaparinux; (b) no early or late fetal loss; (c) a mean gestational age of 39 weeks at delivery; (d) mean blood loss during delivery of 450 mL (3 patients experienced blood loss >1000 mL); (e) no bleeding or thrombosis during pregnancy or upon restarting fondaparinux in the postpartum period; and (f) none among 13 infants with congenital anomalies or neonatal bleeding (Knol HM et al. J Thromb Haemost 2010;8:1876–1879)

(continued)

Special Therapeutic Approaches (*continued*)

b. Fondaparinux has been shown to cross the human placenta. In 1 study of 5 pregnant women with allergy to heparin who were subsequently treated with fondaparinux, low measureable anti-Xa levels in the umbilical cord blood (n = 4) were observed (at approximately 1/10 the concentration in maternal plasma). Neonatal bleeding did not occur in the infants of these women (Dempfle CE. N Engl J Med 2004;350:1914–1915)

c. One case report describes the successful use of fondaparinux in the treatment of HIT in a 24-year-old pregnant woman. At 34 weeks' gestation the patient developed dyspnea and was found to have bilateral pulmonary emboli by spiral CT and a saddle embolus on transthoracic echocardiogram. Following initial therapeutic heparinization and transition to LMWH, platelet counts fell by >50% from baseline over 7 days, a H-PF4 ELISA was (+), and a diagnosis of HIT was made (other diagnoses excluded). Fondaparinux 7.5 mg once daily was administered subcutaneously with subsequent platelet count normalization by 37 weeks gestation followed by treatment cessation 24 hours prior to C-section. After a complication-free delivery (with normal neonate platelet counts) fondaparinux was reintroduced on POD-1, warfarin overlap began on POD-2, and discharge on POD-8 with therapeutic warfarin alone (with her neonate) (Ciurzyński M et al. Med Sci Monit 2011;17:CS56–CS59)

HIT in cardiac patients undergoing percutaneous coronary interventions

In patients with acute or subacute HIT the 2012 ACCP Evidence-based guidelines for HIT recommends the use of bivalirudin (Grade 2B) or argatroban (Grade 2C) over other non-heparin anticoagulants. The 2012 British Committee for Standards in Haematology guidelines on the diagnosis and management of HIT (second edition) recommends the use of bivalirudin (2B) in patients with previous or present HIT who require coronary intervention including angiography and PCI

Linkins L-A et al. Chest 2012;141(2 Suppl):e495S–e530S
Watson H et al. Br J Haematol 2012;159:528–540

	Argatroban	Bivalirudin
Dosing	*Loading dose:* 350 mcg; administer intravenously over 3–5 min without hepatic impairment *Maintenance infusion:* 25 mcg/kg per minute; administer intravenously	*Loading dose:* 0.75 mg/kg; administer intravenously just prior to angioplasty *Infusion for duration of procedure:* 1.75 mg/kg per hour; administer intravenously
Monitoring therapy and dose adjustment	• Infusion dose-adjusted (15–40 mcg/kg per minute) to achieve an ACT of 300–450 seconds • *Additional boluses:* 150 mcg/kg; administer intravenously as needed. The ACT should be checked 5–10 minutes following an initial bolus and after any additional bolus dose or change in infusion rate	Dose adjustments based on renal function: *CrCl <30 mL/min:* *Bolus:* No change *Infusion:* 1 mg/kg per hour; administer intravenously Dialysis-dependent: *Bolus:* No change *Infusion:* 0.25 mg/kg per hour; administer intravenously
Comments	Following the procedure, the sheaths should be removed no sooner than 2 hours after discontinuing argatroban and when the ACT is <160 seconds	Postinfusion IV infusion duration: • Usually continued for the duration of the procedure • Continuation of post-bolus infusion for up to 4 hours after the procedure is optional; additional infusion beyond this point may be given at a rate of 0.2 mg/kg per hour; administer intravenously, for up to 20 hours (normal renal function)
Efficacy in patients with HIT/HITTS or previous HIT	Among 112 PCIs performed in 91 patients, a satisfactory PCI outcome (subjectively assessed) occurred in 94.5% (86/91) of patients undergoing initial PCI and in all 21 patients undergoing repeated PCI. One patient (1.1%) experienced peri-procedural major bleeding (major bleeding defined as Hgb decrease ≥5 g/dL that led to a transfusion ≥2 units, or that was intracranial, retroperitoneal or into a prosthetic joint). Death, MI, and emergent bypass occurred in 0, 4, and 2 patients, respectively Lewis BE et al. Catheter Cardiovasc Interv 2002;57:177–184	Among 52 patients, procedural success (TIMI grade 3 flow and <50% stenosis) and clinical success were achieved in 98% and 96%, respectively. No abrupt closures or thrombus formation occurred during or after the procedure. One death from cardiac arrest occurred 46 hours after successful PCI Mahaffey KW et al. J Invasive Cardiol 2003;15:611–616

Catheter flushes in patients with HIT

• There are no published trials specifically evaluating the use of bivalirudin as a flush solution. In the EVOLUTION-ON and CHOOSE-ON/OFF trials, bivalirudin 0.1-mg/mL flushes were used before and after cardiopulmonary bypass per protocol. The frequency of flushing arterial lines and the quantity of solution used each time was at the discretion of the physician (Veale JJ et al. J Extra Corpor Technol 2005;37:296–302)

• Among non-HIT patients, Horne et al randomly assigned 49 patients undergoing or who had received bone marrow transplantation to receive either lepirudin 3 mL (300 mcg; n = 25) or heparin 3 mL (300 units; n = 24) to prevent withdrawl occlusion of double- or triple-lumen central line catheters. Withdrawl occlusion and alteplase instillation occurred in 20% of patients who received lepirudin and 12.5% of patients treated with heparin (Horne MK et al. Pharmacotherapy 2006;26:1262–1267)

• Lepirudin use for dialysis port flush was reported in a trauma patient who developed HIT. From a 50-mg vial reconstituted to 0.5 mg/mL, 0.5 mg was administered intravenously and 1.3 mL into each dialysis port. The strategy was repeated for 10 dialysis sessions without catheter occlusion (Patel VB et al. Thromb Haemost 1999;82:1205–1206)

60. Autoimmune Hemolytic Anemia

James N. Frame, MD, FACP

Autoimmune hemolytic anemia (AIHA) is an acquired immunologic disease in which a patient's red blood cells are selectively destroyed or hemolyzed by autoantibodies (auto-Ab) produced by the patient's own immune system

Mack P, Freedman J. Transfus Med Rev 2000;14: 223–233

Etiology

		Percent of Cases	
1. **Idiopathic**	58%		
2. **Secondary**	42%		
Neoplasia		18%	
Carcinomas			25%
CLL			22%
NHL			18%
MDS			9%
Hodgkin disease			5%
Drug-induced		8%	
Other immune based/or miscellaneous		7%	
Infection		5%	
Unspecified			38%
Mycoplasma pneumoniae			33%
Viral/unspecified pneumonia			17%
Mononucleosis			7%
Collagen vascular diseases		4%	
Rheumatoid arthritis			61%
Systemic lupus erythematosus			37%

Gehrs BC, Friedberg RC. Am J Hematol 2002;69: 258–271
Pirofsky B. Semin Hematol 1976;13:251–265
Sokol RJ et al. J Clin Pathol 1992;45:1047–1052

Epidemiology

- Idiopathic AIHA is more common in women than men (2:1) with a peak incidence in the fourth and fifth decades of life. Idiopathic AIHA is not associated with any demonstrable underlying disease
- Secondary causes have been reported in 20–80% of case series

	United Kingdom*		United States
	Incidence/Year	Percent of Cases	Percent of Cases
Overall	1/25,600	—	—
Warm antibody AIHA	1/40,800	63	48–78
Cold antibody AIHA	1/87,500	29	16–32
Paroxysmal cold hemoglobinuria (PCH)	1/2,470,000	1	7–8
Mixed-type AIHA	1/370,000	7	3

*Data from a 10-year study (1982–1991) of 1834 patients evaluated for suspected AIHA or because of RBC interference in blood grouping or typing from a 4.7 million population base at the Regional Blood Transfusion Center, Sheffield, UK (Sokol RJ et al. J Clin Pathol 1992;45:1047–1052)

Spectrum of Drug-Induced Immune Hemolytic Anemia (DIIHA)

Variable	Johnson ST et al. (2007)	Garratty G et al. (2003)
Retrospective study period, number of patients	20-year experience, 71 patients with 73 drug-dependent antibodies Blood Center of Wisconsin, Inc Milwaukee, WI, USA*	25-year experience (1978–2003), 114 American Red Cross Blood Services Los Angeles, CA, USA[†]
Agents, number (%)		
Cephalosporins	37 (51)	84 (74)
Cefotetan/ceftriaxone	27 (37)/5 (7)	72 (63)/10 (9)
Penicillin and/or derivatives	12 (16)	17 (15)
Piperacillin	5	4
Piperacillin + tazobactam	5	—
Tazobactam	—	5
Clavulanate	—	3
Sulbactam	—	1
Ticarcillin	—	1
Ampicillin	1	—
Nafcillin	1	1
NSAIDs (various)	11 (15)	—
Quinine/quinidine	7;6/1 (10)	
Others	6 (8); 1 each: carboplatin, levofloxacin, cefoxitin, oxaliplatin, probenecid	13 (11); 2 each: fludarabine, probenecid, rifampin; 1 each: chlorpropamide, erythromycin, mefloquine, oxaliplatin, phenacetin, procainamide, tolmetin
(+) DAT results, number (%)		
IgG + C3	46/68 (68)	81/113 (70)
IgG only	17/68 (25)	11/113 (10)
C3 only	5/68 (7)	11/113 (10)

*DAT results were (+) in 68 patients (96%) of whom 51 (75%) had ≥2+ hemagglutination reactions; the initial RBC eluate was (−) in 52 patients, <2+ in 14 patients, and 4+ in 2 patients; 1 patient was (+) for antibodies to cefotetan, cefuroxime, and cefotaxime

[†]DAT results were (+) in 113 patients (1 patient with a [−] DAT at 17 days postdrug had a strongly [+] eluate with drug-coated RBCs); 19 (17%) deaths were reported: cefotetan (13), ceftriaxone (4), piperacillin (1), tazobactam (1)

Arndt PA, Garratty G. Semin Hematol 2005;42:137–144
Garratty G et al. Blood 2003;560a [abstract 2059]
Johnson ST et al. Transfusion 2007;47:697–702

Case Reports of DIIHA Relevant to the Care of the Hematology/Oncology Patient (Selected Examples)

Ceftriaxone (Seltsam A, Salama A. Intensive Care Med 2000;26:1390–1394)
Cladribine (2-chloro-2′-deoxyadenosine) (Aslan DL et al. 2000;37:125–130 and Fleischman RA, Croy D. Am J Hematol 1995;48:293)
Diclofenac (Ahrens N et al. Am J Hematol 2006;81:128–131)
Efalizumab (for plaque psoriasis) (Kwan JM et al. J Am Acad Dermatol 58:1053–1055)
Fludarabine (Myint H et al. Br J Haematol 1995;91:341–344)
Hydrocortisone (Martinengo M et al. Transfusion 2008;48:1925–1929 [reported to be the first case])
Immune globulin (human) intravenous (Okubo S et al. Transfusion 1990;30:436–438)

Interferon alfa (Andriani A et al. Haematologica 1996;81:258–260)
Lenalidomide (Darabi K et al. J Clin Oncol 2006;24:e59)
Levofloxacin and other fluoroquinolones (Oh YR et al. Ann Pharmacother 2003;37:1010–1013)
Omeprazole (Butt MI et al. Ir Med J 2007;100:372)
Oxaliplatin (Arndt P et al. Transfusion 2009;49:711–718)
Pemetrexed (Park GM et al. J Thorac Oncol 2008;3:196–197)
Pentostatin (Byrd JC et al. Ann Oncol 1995;6:300–301)
Ribavirin (Massoud OI et al. J Clin Gastroenterol 2003;36:367–368)
Rituximab (Jourdan E et al. Leuk Lymphoma 2003;44:889–890 [reported to be the first case])

Classification

Warm antibody AIHA
1. Idiopathic or primary type (no recognized underlying disease is present)
2. Secondary type:
   a. Lymphoproliferative disorders (eg, CLL, HD, NHL, and others)
   b. Autoimmune disorders (eg, SLE, RA, ulcerative colitis, Sjögren syndrome)
   c. Infections (eg, EBV, hepatitis C infection)
   d. Tumors (Kaposi sarcoma, various carcinomas, teratoma, ovarian dermoid cyst), thymoma
   e. Immunodeficiency disorders (eg, AIDS, dys- or hypo-gammaglobulinemia)
   f. Posttransplantation (recipients of allogeneic BMT or peripheral blood stem cells; solid organs)

Cold antibody AIHA
1. Idiopathic or primary type (no recognized underlying disease is present)
2. Secondary type (cold agglutinin syndrome):
   a. Infection (eg, *Mycoplasma pneumoniae*, mononucleosis, CMV, VZV, HIV)
   b. Clinically evident lymphoproliferative disorders (eg, CLL, the lymphomas including Waldenström macroglobulinemia)
   c. Tumors (eg, squamous cell carcinoma of the lung, metastatic adenocarcinomas of the lung and adrenal gland; mixed parotid tumor)

Paroxysmal cold hemoglobinuria (PCH)
1. Idiopathic or primary type (no recognized underlying disease is present)
2. Secondary type
   a. Donath-Landsteiner hemolytic anemia, usually associated with an acute viral syndrome in children (eg, measles, mumps, EBV, CMV, VZV, adenovirus, influenza A, *M. pneumoniae*, *Haemophilus influenzae*)
   b. Late-onset or congenital syphilis

Mixed-type AIHA
1. Idiopathic or primary type (no recognized underlying disease is present)
2. Secondary type:
   a. Autoimmune disorders (eg, SLE, lymphoproliferative disorders)

Drug-induced IHA (DIIHA; classified by absence or presence of drug-dependent antibodies)
1. Drug-independent antibodies
   a. *"True" autoantibody type:* Only antibodies are detectable and does not require the presence of drug for detection (eg, cladribine, fludarabine, levodopa, methyldopa, procainamide)
   b. *Antibodies that react like "true" autoantibodies in vitro but found in combination with drug-dependent antibodies* (eg, some cephalosporins, streptomycin, teniposide, zomepirac)
2. Drug-dependent antibodies
   a. *Antibodies that react with drug-treated (ie, drug-coated) RBCs:* Also referred to as "penicillin type," "drug-adsorption type," or "hapten type" DIIHA. These agents bind covalently to the RBC membrane, are not easily washed off RBCs, and are inhibited by the in vitro addition of soluble drug (eg, penicillin [PCN] ± PCN derivatives; cephalosporins: cefotetan, cefuroxime, cefotaxime, cefoxitin, cefazolin)
   b. *Antibodies that react with RBCs in the presence of soluble drug* (when drug, antibody [patient serum] and RBCs are mixed): also referred to as "nonpenicillin type," "immune complex type," or "neoantigen type" DIIHA. These agents do not bind covalently to the RBC membrane, are easily washed off RBCs and can activate complement and lead to severe intravascular hemolysis (eg, carboplatin, ceftriaxone, ceftazidime, levofloxacin, cefoxitin, nonsteroidal antiinflammatory drugs, piperacillin-tazobactam, quinine, quinidine)

Laboratory Testing

CBC with differential (review of peripheral blood smear), reticulocyte count, comprehensive metabolic profile with direct bilirubin, lactate dehydrogenase (LDH), haptoglobin, direct/indirect Coombs testing

Additional goal-oriented work-up: infection (eg, mycoplasma, mononucleosis, HIV, syphilis, viral syndromes), plasma/urine Hgb, RBC eluate, serum and urine protein electrophoresis with immunofixation, bone marrow aspiration and biopsy (infiltrative disorder/clarification of cytopenias), Hgb electrophoresis, pregnancy test, autoimmune disease, antiphospholipid antibody syndrome malignancy, CD55/59 for paroxysmal nocturnal hemoglobinuria

Findings indicating hemolysis:
- *Elevated:* Reticulocyte count (typical cases), LDH, unconjugated bilirubin levels (total bilirubin rarely >5 mg/dL)
- *Decreased:* Hemoglobin, haptoglobin levels

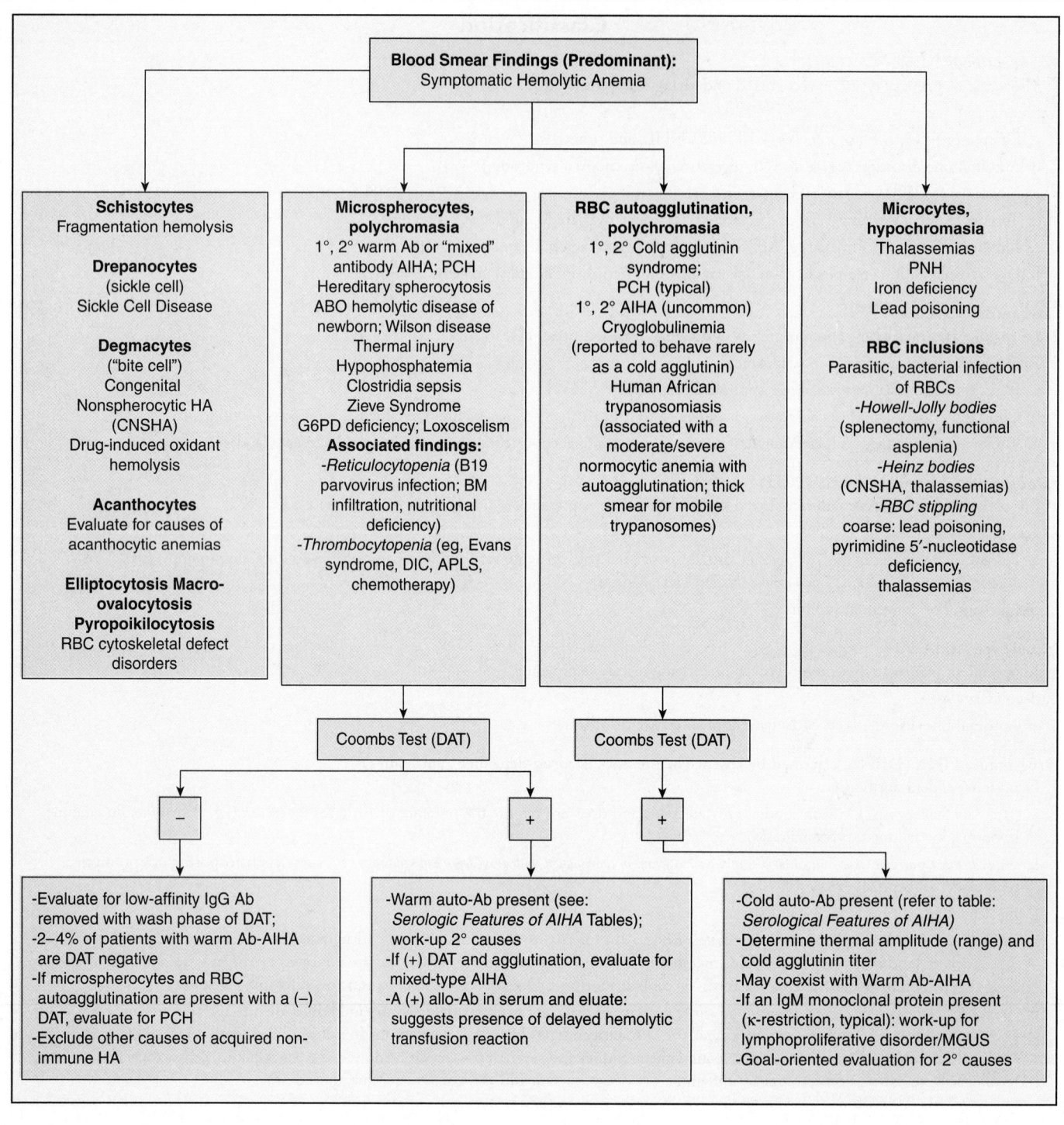

Blood Smear Findings (Predominant):
Symptomatic Hemolytic Anemia

Schistocytes
Fragmentation hemolysis

Drepanocytes
(sickle cell)
Sickle Cell Disease

Degmacytes
("bite cell")
Congenital
Nonspherocytic HA
(CNSHA)
Drug-induced oxidant
hemolysis

Acanthocytes
Evaluate for causes of
acanthocytic anemias

**Elliptocytosis Macro-
ovalocytosis
Pyropoikilocytosis**
RBC cytoskeletal defect
disorders

**Microspherocytes,
polychromasia**
1°, 2° warm Ab or "mixed"
antibody AIHA; PCH
Hereditary spherocytosis
ABO hemolytic disease of
newborn; Wilson disease
Thermal injury
Hypophosphatemia
Clostridia sepsis
Zieve Syndrome
G6PD deficiency; Loxoscelism
Associated findings:
-*Reticulocytopenia* (B19
parvovirus infection; BM
infiltration, nutritional
deficiency)
-*Thrombocytopenia* (eg, Evans
syndrome, DIC, APLS,
chemotherapy)

**RBC autoagglutination,
polychromasia**
1°, 2° Cold agglutinin
syndrome;
PCH (typical)
1°, 2° AIHA (uncommon)
Cryoglobulinemia
(reported to behave rarely
as a cold agglutinin)
Human African
trypanosomiasis
(associated with a
moderate/severe
normocytic anemia with
autoagglutination; thick
smear for mobile
trypanosomes)

**Microcytes,
hypochromasia**
Thalassemias
PNH
Iron deficiency
Lead poisoning

RBC inclusions
Parasitic, bacterial infection
of RBCs
-*Howell-Jolly bodies*
(splenectomy, functional
asplenia)
-*Heinz bodies*
(CNSHA, thalassemias)
-*RBC stippling*
coarse: lead poisoning,
pyrimidine 5'-nucleotidase
deficiency,
thalassemias

Coombs Test (DAT)

Coombs Test (DAT)

−

+

+

-Evaluate for low-affinity IgG Ab
removed with wash phase of DAT;
-2–4% of patients with warm Ab-AIHA
are DAT negative
-If microspherocytes and RBC
autoagglutination are present with a (−)
DAT, evaluate for PCH
-Exclude other causes of acquired nonimmune HA

-Warm auto-Ab present (see:
Serologic Features of AIHA Tables);
work-up 2° causes
-If (+) DAT and agglutination, evaluate for
mixed-type AIHA
-A (+) allo-Ab in serum and eluate:
suggests presence of delayed hemolytic
transfusion reaction

-Cold auto-Ab present (refer to table:
Serological Features of AIHA)
-Determine thermal amplitude (range) and
cold agglutinin titer
-May coexist with Warm Ab-AIHA
-If an IgM monoclonal protein present
(κ-restriction, typical): work-up for
lymphoproliferative disorder/MGUS
-Goal-oriented evaluation for 2° causes

1°, primary; 2°, secondary; Ab, antibody; APLS, Antiphospholipid syndrome; BM, bone marrow; PCH, paroxysmal cold hemoglobinuria; CNSHA, congenital non-spherocytic hemolytic anemia; PNH, paroxysmal nocturnal hemoglobinuria; RBC, red blood cell; MGUS, monoclonal gammopathy of undetermined significance
Berentsen S et al. Hematology 2007;12:361–370
Gehrs BC, Friedberg RC. Am J Hematol 2002;69:258–271
Gertz MA. Br J Haematol 2007;138:422–429
Jeng MR et al. In: Greer JP et al., eds. Wintrobe's Clinical Hematology. 11th ed. Philadelphia, PA: Lippincott; 2004:1223–1246
Neff AT. In: Greer JP et al., eds. Wintrobe's Clinical Hematology. 11th ed. Philadelphia, PA: Lippincott; 2004:1157–1182
Packman CH. Blood Rev 2008;22:17–31
Petz LD. Blood Rev 2008;22:1–15

Serologic Features: Autoimmune Hemolytic Anemia (AIHA)

Variable	Warm Antibody	Cold Antibody	PCH	Mixed
DAT	>95% DAT (+): Polyclonal IgG; ↑reactivity at 37°C (98.6°F) IgG only: 20–66% IgG + C3: 24–63% C3: 7–14% IgG ± IgA or IgM: uncommon IgA or IgM only: rare 2–4% DAT (−)	All DAT (+): C3 more reactive at 0°–4°C (32°–39.2°F) IgM autoantibody: dissociates after C3 binding IgG or IgA auto-Ab: rare	All DAT (+): C3 (IgG positive if done at lower temperatures) Thermal amplitude is usually <20°C (<68°F) (ie, Donath-Landsteiner [DL] test is (+) at <20°C (<68°F); rare reports of thermal amplitude extending to 32°C [89.6°F])	DAT (+): "Mixed" with warm antibody AIHA AND a cold antibody Warm hemolysin: IgG, C3, and occasionally IgM or IgA
RBC eluate	Mostly IgG₁ > IgG₃	Nonreactive	Nonreactive (usually)	Variable
Antigen targets	Rh (e, E, C) Band 4.1 Band 3 Glycophorin A	Ii (90% against I); others: Pr, Gd, Sa, Lud, Fl, Vo, M, N, D, P	P antigen. If the DL test is (+), specificity for the P Ag is indicated; reference lab help may be required	I or i have been observed or no specificity
Comments	*Rate of a (+) DAT without AIHA* (reported in normal blood donors): 1:13,000–1:14,000 *Rate of autoantibody in pregnancy:* 1:50,000 vs. 0.2:50,000 in an age-comparable control	*Pathogenic cold Ab AIHA:* High auto-Ab titer eg, >1:256 with high thermal range *1° CAS:* monoclonal IgM κ > λ ; *2° CAD:* Mono- or polyclonal IgM κ or λ *Nonpathogenic cold Abs* present in normal persons (<1:64)	*Donath-Landsteiner test:* Evaluates for the biphasic cold hemolysin (auto-Ab) that sensitizes RBCs at 0°–4°C (32°–39.2°F) by fixing C1 and hemolyzes RBCs at 37°C (98.6°F) A low titer, low thermal range DL antibody may persist for years	*Clinically significant cold antibodies:* High titer at 0°–4°C (32°–39.2°F) (eg, >1:1000) with a thermal amplitude ranging to >30°C (>86°F)

1°, primary; 2°, secondary

Serologic Features: Drug-Induced Immune Hemolytic Anemia*

Variable	Autoantibody	Drug-Dependent Antibodies (Abs)	
		Reacting with Drug-Treated RBCs	Reacting with RBCs in the Presence of Soluble Drug
DAT	(+) for poly-/IgG specific sera C3 usually (−)	(+) for poly-/IgG specific sera ± C3	(+) for poly-/IgG specific sera ± C3
Serum Ab testing†	(±) for routine IAT (±) for soluble drug (±) for drug-treated RBCs	(±) for routine IAT (−) for soluble drug (+) for drug-treated RBCs	(±) for routine IAT (+) for soluble drug (−) for drug-treated RBCs
RBC eluate Ab Testing†	(+) for routine IAT	Predominantly (−) or weakly (+) for routine IAT	Predominantly (−) or weakly (+) for routine IAT

*A diagnosis of DIIHA is made by clinical evidence of hemolysis associated with drug therapy and confirmed by serologic testing (Johnson ST et al. Transfusion 2007). Serologically indistinguishable (by DAT) from warm-Ab AIHA. May uncommonly present serologically similar to cold agglutinin disease (eg, ceftriaxone, levofloxacin)

†*Routine IAT:* Indirect antiglobulin test (incubated patient serum + reagent RBCs read before and after poly-/IgG specific sera added); *soluble drug:* incubated patient serum + putative drug solution + untreated RBCs tested by IAT; *drug-treated RBCs:* incubated e + RBCs + putative drug solution, then patient serum added and tested by IAT

Arndt PA, Garratty G. Semin Hematol 2005;42:137–144

Buetens OW , Ness PM. Curr Opin Hematol 2003;10:429–433

Engelfriet CP et al. Semin Hematol 1992;29:3–12

Gehrs BC, Friedberg RC. Am J Hematol 2002;69:258–271

Janvier D et al. Transfusion 2002;42:1547–1552

Johnson ST et al. Transfusion 2007;47:697–702

Packman CH. Blood Rev 2008;22:17–31

Petz LD. Blood Rev 2008;22:1–15

Petz LD, Garraty G. In: Petz LD, Garraty G, eds. Immune Hemolytic Anemias. Philadelphia, PA: Churchill Livingstone; 2004:61–131

Treatment Overview

Comment: The level of clinical evidence supporting the management of AIHA is derived from case reports, case series, and/or expert opinion. Randomized controlled trials of cytotoxic or immunosuppressive agents in AIHA have not been performed

Idiopathic and Secondary Warm Antibody AIHA

1. First-line
   a. Single-agent glucocorticoid therapy
   b. Disease-specific treatments for secondary etiologies* ± glucocorticoids
   c. Discontinue implicated drug if drug-induced
2. Second-line
   a. Splenectomy in surgical candidates who fail to benefit from glucocorticoid therapy
   b. Options in patients not surgical candidates for splenectomy: low-dose glucocorticoids ± danazol; rituximab as a splenectomy sparing procedure
3. Third-line
   a. Immunosuppressive agents (cyclophosphamide and azathioprine)
   b. Danazol
   c. Cyclosporine
   d. Rituximab
   e. Alemtuzumab
   f. High-dose cyclophosphamide
   g. Immune globulin (human) intravenous
   h. Plasmapheresis
   i. Splenic irradiation (reported in CLL)
   j. Mycophenolate mofetil

Comment: In patients with secondary warm antibody AIHA caused by underlying lymphoproliferative disorders or a solid tumor, therapy of the primary disorder may lead to AIHA remission

Cold Antibody AIHA (Cold-Agglutinin Syndrome [CAS])

Idiopathic (Primary) Cold-Agglutinin Syndrome (CAS)
1. First-line:
   a. Avoidance of cold; wearing warm clothing
2. Second-line or later (approaches that have produced responses in small groups of patients with CAS):
   a. Glucocorticoids (generally less effective than in warm Ab AIHA)
   b. Cytotoxic drugs (eg, chlorambucil)
   c. Plasma exchange
   d. Splenectomy in IgM (not IgG) CAS
   e. Rituximab
   f. High-dose cyclophosphamide
   g. Plasmapheresis

Secondary Cold-Agglutinin Syndrome (CAS)
1. First-line:
   a. Treat the underlying cause where identifiable
   b. Provide supportive care (spontaneous remissions of secondary AIHA have been observed in patients with infectious mononucleosis and *Mycoplasma pneumoniae* infections)
   c. Keep patient warm if the cold reactive antibodies demonstrate a high thermal amplitude
2. Second-line or later:
   a. Glucocorticoids
   b. Rituximab
   c. Plasmapheresis

Paroxysmal Cold Hemoglobinuria (PCH)
1. First-line
   a. Symptomatic therapy; transfusion support as indicated for brisk hemolysis; avoidance of cold; wearing warm clothing
   b. Corticosteroids are often added, but efficacy is difficult to evaluate because of transient nature of the hemolysis
   c. Plasmapheresis if PCH is life-threatening
   d. Treatment of syphilis if present

Mixed-Type Antibody AIHA
1. First-line
   a. Single-agent glucocorticoid therapy
   b. Disease-specific treatments for secondary etiologies ± glucocorticoids
2. Second-line
   a. Splenectomy in surgical candidates who fail to benefit from glucocorticoid therapy
   b. High-dose cyclophosphamide
   c. Rituximab

Drug-Induced Immune Hemolytic Anemia
1. First-line:
   a. Discontinuation of the suspected or causative agent is indicated
   b. Supportive care (also, see section on Purine Analog-Induced AIHA)
2. Second-line:
   a. Glucocorticoids if hemolysis is severe

Notes: Transfusion of RBCs in patients with symptomatic life-threatening AIHA is potentially indicated at any point along the disease or treatment continuum. The early collaboration of the treating physician with their blood bank or transfusion service is strongly recommended

REGIMEN

PREDNISONE

American College of Rheumatology Ad Hoc Committee on Glucocorticoid-Induced Osteoporosis. Arthritis Rheum 2001;44:1496–1503

Gehrs BC, Friedberg RC. Am J Hematol 2002;69:258–271

Hemolytic anemia resulting from warm-reacting antibodies. In: Lichtman MA et al. eds. Williams Manual of Hematology. 8th ed. New York, NY: McGraw Hill Medical; 2011:115–120

Murphy S, LoBuglio AF. Semin Hematol 1976;13:323–334

Petz LD. Curr Opin Hematol 2001;8:411–416

Petz LD, Garratty G. Blood transfusions in autoimmune hemolytic anemia. In: Petz LD, Garratty G, eds. Immune Hemolytic Anemias. 2nd ed. New York, NY: Churchill Livingstone; 2004:375–400

Petz LD, Garratty G. Management of autoimmune hemolytic anemias. In: Petz LD, Garratty G eds. Immune Hemolytic Anemias. 2nd ed. New York, NY: Churchill Livingstone; 2004:401–405

Rosse WF. Autoimmune hemolytic anemia. In: Handin RI, Lux SE, Stossel TP, eds. Blood: Principles and Practice in Hematology. Philadelphia, PA: JB Lippincott; 2005:1859–1885

Prednisone 1–1.5 mg/kg (≈40–60 mg) per day, *or* 0.5–0.75 mg/kg (≈20–30 mg) twice daily, orally, continually, for a minimum of 3–4 weeks before assessing efficacy

Supportive care:

Add a **proton pump inhibitor** during prednisone therapy

Calcium 400–600 mg elemental Ca per day; administer orally, continually, plus

Vitamin D$_3$ 800 units (calciferol or cholecalciferol 20 mcg) per day or an activated form of vitamin D; administer orally, continually. Supplementation is recommended for patients beginning or receiving prednisone (or prednisone equivalent ≥5 mg/day) for ≥3 months (American College of Rheumatology Ad Hoc Committee on Glucocorticoid-Induced Osteoporosis. Arthritis Rheum 2001). Monitor for hypercalcemia and hypercalciuria, especially if activated forms of vitamin D are used. Patients receiving prolonged glucocorticoid therapy should be assessed for hypogonadism, and if present, corrected if possible. Also see Chapter 44: Indications for Bisphosphonates in the Hematology Oncology Setting

Folic acid 1 mg/day; administer orally, continually, to prevent depletion of folate stores and megaloblastic anemia resulting from chronic hemolysis

Titration of prednisone in responding patients:

Murphy S, LoBuglio AF. Semin Hematol 1976;13:323–334

- Once Hgb is ≥10 g/dL, taper prednisone by 10–15 mg/week to a dose of 20–30 mg/day. This can usually be accomplished in 4–6 weeks
- If Hgb persists ≥10 g/dL, follow with a gradual reduction in 5-mg decrements to a dose of 10 mg/day over a period of 3 months
- If Hgb persists ≥10 g/dL, withdraw all therapy by slowly decreasing the dose over another 3-month period

or

Rosse WF. Autoimmune hemolytic anemia. In: Handin RI, Lux SE, Stossel TP, eds. Blood: Principles and Practice in Hematology. Philadelphia, PA: JB Lippincott; 2005:1859–1885

- Once Hgb is ≥10 g/dL, taper prednisone rapidly at first by 20 mg/day (0.3 mg/kg/day) each week to a dose of 20 mg/day. This can usually be accomplished in 2–3 weeks. The dose is then maintained for approximately 1 month to see if remission continues, *then*
- If Hgb persists ≥10 g/dL, switch to an alternating-day regimen over 2 months. In the first month, reduce the dose to 20 mg/dose every second day alternating with 10 mg/dose every second day. In the second month, reduce the dose to 20 mg/dose every second day, *then*
- If Hgb persists ≥10 g/dL, reduce the dose to 10 mg/dose every second day over the next month, *then*
- If Hgb persists ≥10 g/dL, reduce the dose to 5 mg/dose every second day over the next month, *then*
- If Hgb persists ≥10 g/dL, withdraw all therapy over another few months

Notes:

If the DAT is (+), a dose of 10 mg/every second day is maintained so long as remission continues
If at any point during dose reduction exacerbation of hemolysis occurs, increase the dose to the previous level and maintain that level. If the dose exceeds 20 mg (0.3 mg/kg) every second day, consider other therapeutic options

Indications

Initial therapy in:
- Patients with warm-antibody AIHA with clinically important signs and symptoms of anemia if there are no contraindications for its use
- Patients with mixed AIHA

Second-line therapy in others

Efficacy

Response within 1 Week	Most Patients
Hemolysis improved within 1–3 weeks	70–80%
Lasting remissions	20–30%
Unacceptable prednisone dose/no response	10–20%
Need low-dose prednisone maintenance	50%
Response rates in idiopathic types*	82%
Response rates in secondary forms*	60%

*Murphy S, Lobuglio AF. Semin Hematol 1976;13:323–334

Expert Opinion

Consider splenectomy, or if the patient is not a candidate for splenectomy, other immunosuppressive therapy if:

1. Response is not achieved after 3 weeks of prednisone treatment
2. Contraindications to prednisone therapy exist
3. Patient experiences intolerable side-effects
4. Prednisone doses of ≥15 mg/day are required to maintain a Hgb ≥10 g/dL

Toxicity

>10%: Insomnia, nervousness, increased appetite, indigestion

1–10%: Dizziness or lightheadedness, headache, hirsutism, hypopigmentation, glucose intolerance, diabetes mellitus, hyperglycemia, arthralgia, cataracts, glaucoma, epistaxis, diaphoresis

<1%* Cushing syndrome, edema, fractures, hallucinations, hypertension, muscle wasting, osteoporosis, pancreatitis, pituitary-adrenal axis suppression, seizures

*Limited to important or life-threatening

Dose Modifications

Note: Administer **prednisone** 0.6 mg/kg per day to patients who are older than age 70 years, immobilized or osteoporotic patients, and in a setting of active infection or other mitigating conditions

Prednisone tapering schedule for patients with AIHA who have achieved remission (based on the experience of the authors in the following reference):

Rosse WF, Schrier SL. Treatment of autoimmune hemolytic anemia: warm agglutinins. In: Mentzer WC, Landaw SA, eds. 2012 UpToDate, Version 19.3: January 2012:1–15 (accessed 1.30.12)

1. After a Hgb of >10 g/dL is achieved, maintain the prednisone dose at 60 mg/day for 1 week, *then*
2. Rapidly taper the prednisone dose to 20 mg/day over a period of 2 weeks. Maintain this dose for 1 month, *then*
3. If remission persists, gradually reduce the dose on alternate days to 10 mg/day. Maintain this regimen for 1 month
4. If remission persists, omit the dose on alternate days while maintaining the dose at 20 mg every other day
5. If remission persists, reduce the dose to 10 mg/day on alternate days. Tapering of glucocorticoids should be continued as long as the hemoglobin and haptoglobin levels remain improved and stable, LDH levels stay low, and the absolute reticulocyte count remains <100,000/mm³
6. Glucocorticoids can be stopped when there is normalization of the hemoglobin, haptoglobin, LDH, and absolute reticulocyte count, although the Coombs test may remain positive. The patient should be monitored for recurrence for a number of months following cessation of treatment

Notes:
If, at any time during the above prednisone tapering schedule, the remission is not maintained, other measures (eg, cytotoxic therapy or splenectomy), must be instituted. The authors state that this approach is also warranted in patients with AIHA who *do not respond* to prednisone after 2–3 weeks of therapy

SPLENECTOMY

ActHIB *Haemophilus* b conjugate vaccine (tetanus toxoid conjugate) for intramuscular injection; product label, November 2009. Sanofi Pasteur, Inc. Swiftwater, PA

Akpek G et al. Am J Hematol 1999;61:98–102

Bowdler AJ. Semin Hematol 1976;13:335–348

Coon WW. Arch Surg 1985;120:625–628

Hemolytic anemia resulting from warm-reacting antibodies. In: Lichtman MA et al., eds. Williams Manual of Hematology. 8th Ed. New York, NY: McGraw Hill Medical; 2011:115–120

Katkhouda N et al. Ann Surg 1998;228:568–578

Menactra (meningococcal [groups A, C, Y, and W-135]) polysaccharide diphtheria toxoid conjugate vaccine for intramuscular injection; product label, March 2011. Sanofi Pasteur, Inc., Swiftwater, PA

Menomune-A/C/Y/W-135 (meningococcal polysaccharide vaccine, groups A, C, Y and W-135 combined) Suspension for subcutaneous injection; product label, January 2009. Sanofi Pasteur, Inc. Swiftwater, PA

Menveo (meningococcal [groups A, C, Y, and W-1350] oligosaccharide diphtheria CRM$_{197}$ conjugate vaccine) solution for intramuscular injection; product label, March 2011. Novartis Vaccine and Diagnostics S.r.l., Bellaria-Rosia 53018, Sovicille (SI), Italy

Petz LD, Garratty G. Management of autoimmune hemolytic anemias. In: Petz LD, Garratty G, eds. Immune Hemolytic Anemias. 2nd ed. New York, NY: Churchill Livingstone; 2004:401–458

PNEUMOVAX 23 (pneumococcal vaccine polyvalent) sterile, liquid vaccine for intramuscular or subcutaneous injection; product label, Oct 2011. Merck & Co., Whitehouse Station, NJ,

Open or laparoscopic splenectomy depending on the surgeon's experience or patient requirements

Prior to splenectomy administer:

Pneumococcal vaccine: Pneumovax 0.5 mL; administer by intramuscular or subcutaneous injection in deltoid muscle or lateral mid-thigh

Haemophilus influenzae **type b vaccine (Hib)** 0.5 mL; administer by intramuscular injection only
Meningococcal vaccine:

    Menactra 0.5 mL; administer by intramuscular injection only in deltoid muscle, *or*

    Menomune 0.5 mL; administer by subcutaneous injection

Supportive care:
Folic acid 1 mg/day; administer orally, continually, to prevent depletion of folate stores and megaloblastic anemia resulting from chronic hemolysis

Efficacy

Bowdler AJ. Semin Hematol 1976;13:335-348

N = 9 Case Series; 308 AIHA Patients

All patients	57.5% remission

Bowdler AJ. Semin Hematol 1976;13:335-348

N = 2 Cases Series; 80 Patients

Idiopathic AIHA (N = 55)	52.7% remission
Secondary AIHA (N = 25)	32% remission

Coon WW. Arch Surg 1985;120:625–628

(N = 52)

Steroid terminated with a stable Hct ≥30%	64% (mean follow-up, 33 months)
Hct ≥30% on ≤15 mg/day of prednisone or equivalent	21% (mean follow-up, 73 months)

Akpek G et al. Am J Hematol 1999;61:98–102

(N = 27)

	Idiopathic (N = 11*)	Secondary (N = 16†)
Normal Hgb ≥6 months; no additional therapy (CR)	82%	19%
≥50% increase in Hgb; ± other therapy (PR)	18%	37%

*Median follow-up 18 months
†Median follow-up 11 months

Notes

1. Annual influenza vaccination is also recommended in asplenic patients
2. Patient education should include instruction as to early signs of potential OPSI and emphasis to seek early medical attention when present
3. For guidance on the prevention and treatment of OPSI and the use of vaccines in persons with altered immunocompetence see: BMJ 1996;312:430–434, Special Populations: patients with anatomical or functional asplenia. In: American College of Physicians Guide to Adult Immunization, 4th ed. American College of Physicians, 2011:87 (immunization.acponline.org accessed 2.12.12)

Indications

Recommended as second-line therapy in surgical candidates with AIHA who:
1. Do not benefit adequately from glucocorticoid therapy
2. Benefit initially from glucocorticoid therapy but suffer a relapse on taper
3. Require unacceptably high maintenance glucocorticoid doses (eg, >10–20 mg/day of prednisone) or have intractable side effects to glucocorticoid therapy

Note: Although considered ineffective in cold-agglutinin syndrome (CAS), a few cases of atypical CAS with hemolysins reactive at 37°C (98.6°F) and responsive to splenectomy have been reported (Petz LD, Garratty G. Management of autoimmune hemolytic anemias. 2004)

Toxicity (Complications)

1. Overwhelming postsplenectomy infection (OPSI):
   a. *Incidence:* Children <15 years (0.13–8.1%) vs. adults (0.28–1.9%), but may occur at any age
   b. *Risk factors:* Young age, history of hematologic disorders
   c. *Timing:* Most infections occur within 2 years after splenectomy; 42% reported within 5 years
   d. *Mortality:* 50–70% in older studies with >50% of deaths within the first 48 hours after hospitalization
2. Thrombocytosis
3. Deep venous thrombosis (reported to be increased in myeloproliferative disorders postsplenectomy)
4. Pseudohyperkalemia

REGIMEN

RITUXIMAB

Bussone G et al. Am J Hematol 2009;84:153–157
D'Arena G et al. Am J Hematol 2006;81:598–602
D'Arena G et al. Eur J Haematol 2007;79:53–58
Gupta N et al. Leukemia 2002;16:2092–2095
Narat S et al. Haematologica 2005;90:1273–1274
Petz LD, Garratty G. Blood transfusions in autoimmune hemolytic anemia. In: Petz LD, Garratty G, eds. Immune Hemolytic Anemias. 2nd ed. New York, NY: Churchill Livingstone; 2004:375–400
Rituxan (rituximab) injection for intravenous use; product label, April 2011. Genentech Inc., South San Francisco, CA
Wood AM. Am J Health Syst Pharm 2001;58:215–232

Premedication for rituximab:

Acetaminophen 650–1000 mg; administer orally, *plus*

Diphenhydramine 25–50 mg; administer orally or intravenously, 30–60 minutes before starting rituximab

Rituximab 375 mg/m^2; administer intravenously in 0.9% sodium chloride injection or 5% dextrose injection, diluted to a concentration within the range of 1–4 mg/mL, weekly for 4 consecutive weeks (total dosage/cycle = 1500 mg/m^2)

Notes on rituximab administration:

• Infuse initially at 50 mg/hour. If hypersensitivity or infusion reactions do not occur during the first 30 minutes, increase the rate by 50 mg/hour every 30 minutes as tolerated, to a maximum rate of 400 mg/hour. Subsequently, if previous administration was well tolerated, start administration at 100 mg/hour, and increase by 100 mg/hour every 30 minutes as tolerated, to a maximum rate of 400 mg/hour

• Interrupt rituximab administration for fever, chills, edema, congestion of the head and neck mucosa, hypotension, and other serious adverse events. Resume rituximab administration at a 50% reduction in rate after adverse events abate. Treat with IV diphenhydramine + acetaminophen, oxygen with bronchodilators, sodium chloride injection intravenously, and/or epinephrine subcutaneously as appropriate for managing hypersensitivity reactions

Supportive care:

Folic acid 1 mg/day; administer orally to prevent depletion of folate stores and megaloblastic anemia resulting from chronic hemolysis

Indications

Off-label use in the following adults with AIHA:

1. Patients with idiopathic or secondary AIHA with warm, cold, or mixed warm-cold hemolysins
2. Patients with persistent disease after immunosuppressive therapies

Alone (52%) or in combination (48%) with glucocorticoids, single or multiagent chemotherapy (lymphoproliferative disorders [LPD]), or IVIG

	Efficacy (N = 71) and Toxicity (Rituximab ± Other Therapy)				
	Author				
	Bussone, 2009	**D'Arena, 2007**	**D'Arena, 2006**	**Mehta, 2005**	**Gupta, 2002**
Patients, n (M/F)	27 (11/16)	11 (5/6)	14 (8/6)	11 (5/6)	8 (7/1)
Age (years)	49.7 (mean)	55 (mean)	64.0 (mean)	55 (median)	60 (median)
1°/2° AIHA (n)	17/10	10/1	0/11 (CLL)	3/8	0/8 (CLL)
Autoantibody	IgG (n = 7), IgG/C3 (n = 17), C3 (n = 2), IgA (1)	"All DAT (+)," warm antibody	"All DAT (+)," warm antibody	IgG/C3 (n = 2), IgG (n = 9)	"Positive Coombs pretreatment"
No. prior treatments for AIHA (median)	2	2	1	2	1; 2 prior chemo regimens for CLL
Regimen	R: 375 mg/m² IV weekly × 4 weeks	R: 375 mg/m² IV weekly × 4 weeks	R: 375 mg/m² IV weekly × 4 weeks	R: 375 mg/m² IV weekly × 4 weeks	R: 375 mg/m² IV Q 4 weeks + cyclophosphamide: 750 mg/m² IV D1 Q 4 weeks + Dex: 12 mg IV D1, 2; 12 mg PO D3–7 Q week
Response rate	93.0%	100%	71.4%	63.6%	100%
CR (%)	29.6 % DAT (−) in 3/8 CRs	54.6%	21.4%	27.2%	Not stated
PR (%)	36.4%	45.4%	50.0%	36.4%	Not stated
Median Hgb ↑	5.0 g/dL	3.3 g/dL	3.6 g/dL	6.2 g/dL	6.0 g/dL
Response duration	At 20.9 months follow-up: 75% in remission	At 604 days mean F/U: CR 73%, PR 27%	At 17 months median F/U: 57% alive	11 months (median); range: 2.5–20 months	13 months (median); range: 7–23 months. Time to maximum response (median): 5 weeks (range: 3–13)
Reported toxicity	2 mild infusion reactions; grade 4 neutropenia (n = 1), *Pneumocystis jirovecii* infection (n = 1)	1 each with infusion: fever, chills	First infusion side effects: fever (n=2), chills (n=1); ↑ transaminases (n = 1 patient with HCV); deaths: 2 with CHF + sepsis after third dose of rituximab	No significant acute side effects; 1 death caused by infection in CLL patient who was heavily pretreated	Most toxicities were grade 1/2; nausea (n = 2), mild headache (n = 2); 1 each: fever, rash, pruritus, ↓BP, grade 4 neutropenia

Key: 1°, primary; 2°, secondary; BP, blood pressure; CHF, congestive heart failure; CMP, comprehensive metabolic profile; CR, complete response; Dex, dexamethasone; F/U, follow-up; HCV, hepatitis C virus; Hgb, hemoglobin; IV, intravenously; PO, orally; PR, partial response; Q, every; R, rituximab

REGIMEN

ALEMTUZUMAB

Campath (alemtuzumab) injection for intravenous use; product label, August 2009. Genzyme Corporation, Cambridge, MA
Karlsson C et al. Leukemia 2007;21:511–514
Laurenti L et al. Leukemia 2007;21:1819–1821
Willis F et al. Br J Haematol 2001;114:891–898

Premedication for alemtuzumab:
Acetaminophen 500–1000 mg; administer orally 30 minutes before each dose and each dose escalation, *plus*
Diphenhydramine 50 mg; administer intravenously, 30–60 minutes before starting alemtuzumab and during escalation, then change to oral administration after escalation

Alemtuzumab dose escalation schedule:
Alemtuzumab 3 mg/day; administer intravenously diluted in 100 mL 0.9% sodium chloride injection (0.9% NS) or 5% dextrose injection (D5W) over 2 hours, daily until infusion-related adverse effects are grade ≤2, *then:*
Alemtuzumab 10 mg/day; administer intravenously diluted in 100 mL 0.9% NS or D5W over 2 hours, daily until tolerated (eg, infusion-related toxicities grade ≤2), *then:*
Alemtuzumab 30 mg/dose; administer intravenously diluted in 100 mL 0.9% NS or D5W over 2 hours as a maintenance dose (see below)

Alemtuzumab maintenance schedule:
Alemtuzumab 30 mg/dose; administer intravenously in 100 mL 0.9% NS or D5W over 2 hours as maintenance dose on alternate days for 3 doses per week (eg, Monday, Wednesday, Friday) not to exceed 90 mg/week

Notes on alemtuzumab administration:
If alemtuzumab is withheld for ≥7 days during treatment, restart with the dose-escalation schedule (this can usually be accomplished in 3–7 days)

Supportive Care
Antiemetic prophylaxis
Emetogenic potential is **MINIMAL**
See Chapter 39 for antiemetic recommendations

Hematopoietic growth factor (CSF) prophylaxis
Primary prophylaxis is NOT indicated
See Chapter 43 for more information

Antimicrobial prophylaxis
Risk of fever and neutropenia is HIGH
  Antimicrobial primary prophylaxis is recommended:
  • Antibacterial—*P. jirovecii* prophylaxis is recommended (eg, cotrimoxazole)
  • Antifungal—recommended
  • Antiviral—anti-herpes antivirals (eg, acyclovir or equivalent)
  • Continue antimicrobial prophylaxis for a minimum of 2 months after completing alemtuzumab or until the CD4+ count is ≥200 cells/mmn^3, whichever occurs later
See Chapter 47 for more information

Folic acid 1 mg/day orally, continually, to prevent depletion of folate stores and megaloblastic anemia resulting from chronic hemolysis

Indications

Off-label use has been reported in the following settings in adults with AIHA:
1. Patients with idiopathic or secondary AIHA with warm, cold, or mixed warm-cold hemolysins
2. Patients with persistent AIHA after immunosuppressive therapies
3. Alone or in combination with glucocorticoids (at lowest possible dose and tapered off when feasible)

Note: The FDA-approved indication for alemtuzumab is single-agent therapy for B-cell CLL

Efficacy (N = 12) and Toxicity

	Author		
	Karlsson (2007)	**Laurenti (2007)**	**Willis (2001)**
Patients, n (M/F)	5 (5/0)	3(3/0)	4 (1/3)
Age (median years)	66	53	52
1°/2° AIHA, n	0/5 (advanced B-CLL)	0/3 (advanced B-CLL)	4/0
Autoantibody	All DAT (+)	All DAT (+), IgG	IgG (n = 2), C′ (n = 2; 1 with weak IgG)
No. of prior treatments: AIHA (median)	3; 2 patients received prior rituximab	3 (median); no prior rituximab	3; no prior rituximab
Alemtuzumab regimen	3 or 10 mg SC injection in thigh or IV infusion escalated to 30 mg 3 times/week × 12 weeks	3 mg SC on day 1; then 10 mg SC TIW from day 3	*Pilot study of alemtuzumab:* 1 mg in 100 mL 0.9% NS IV over 1 hour, then 10 mg/day in 250 mL 0.9% NS IV over 4 hours daily for 10 days
Prophylaxis	Acetaminophen PO and antihistamine IV pretreatment day 1; Allopurinol 300 mg/day PO for the first 4 weeks; Valacyclovir 250 mg PO BID and cotrimoxazole 160 mg (TMP component) daily PO TIW for 8 weeks posttreatment	Acetaminophen 1000 mg PO and chlorpheniramine 10 PO pretreatment day 1; Acyclovir 800 mg PO BID up to 2 months posttreatment and cotrimoxazole 160 mg (TMP component) PO 2 doses on 2 days/week up to 1 year posttreatment	Oral ciprofloxacin, fluconazole, acyclovir, and chlorhexidine mouth washes (doses and schedules were not specified in the report)
Response criteria	Elimination of the need for RBC transfusions and a ≥2 g/dL rise in Hgb independent of transfusions	Independence of RBC transfusion and a concomitant ↑ of Hgb ≥2 g/dL	*Response:* Red cell transfusion independence and discontinuation of prednisolone; *PR:* either a >50% ↓ in red cell transfusion requirements or requirement for small doses (<10 mg) of prednisolone
Response	100%; *time to response:* SC regimen (n = 3): 4, 5, 7 weeks IV regimen (n = 2): 5, 5 weeks	100%; median time to response: 8 weeks	75% (1 response and 2 PRs; 1 PR had a partial relapse responding to low doses of prednisolone)
Response duration	SC regimen (n = 3): 2+, 12+, 13+ months IV regimen (n = 2): 10+, 13+ months	10 months (median duration)	3 of 4 patients alive at 5+, 11+, 10+ months follow-up
Median ↑ Hgb	4.7 g/dL	3.3 g/dL	Not specified numerically
Reported toxicity	First-day reactions were mainly grade 1: fever/rigors (n = 3); CMV reactivation responding to treatment (n = 1); *Escherichia coli* sepsis without neutropenia (n = 1); transient gastroenteritis (n = 1); grade 4 neutropenia (n = 2; 1 required filgrastim)	Therapy described as well tolerated, with mild hematologic and nonhematologic side effects such as fever, pruritus, rigor and headache (grade 1); no reported febrile neutropenia or bacterial/fungal infection	1 patient died 4 months after completion of treatment from intractable intravascular hemolysis and systemic venous thrombosis; specific toxicities referable to patients with AIHA were not specified in the report
Monitoring therapy	*Pretreatment:* Monitor CBC-diff, CMP, DAT During treatment: Weekly CBC-diff; if Hgb ≤8 g/dL transfuse	*Pre-treatment:* H&P; CBC-diff, CMP before each dose; retic count Q 2 weeks, CMV antigen (Ag) and CMV DNA Q 2 weeks, DAT/IAT Q 2 weeks Posttreatment: H&P, CMP, retic count, CMV Ag and DNA weekly × 8 wk, (DAT/) Q 2 wk), then monthly × 6 mo, then Q 3 mo	*Pretreatment:* CBC-diff, CMP, lymphocyte subsets, DAT, chest x-ray, ECG

1°, primary; 2°, secondary; BID, twice a day; CBC-diff, complete blood count and differential; CMP, comprehensive metabolic profile; CR, complete response; DAT, direct antiglobulin test; H&P, history and physical examination; IAT, indirect antiglobulin test; IV, intravenous; NS, 0.9% sodium chloride injection; PO, orally; PR, partial response; Q, every; R, response; retic count, reticulocyte count; SC, subcutaneous; TIW, three times per week; TMP, the trimethoprim component of cotrimoxazole (sulfamethoxazole + trimethoprim in a fixed 5:1 ratio)

Toxicity

Patient population: CLL (n = 296 from Campath product label, Aug. 2009): 147 previously untreated (mean alemtuzumab exposure: 11.7 weeks); 149 previously treated with ≥2 prior chemotherapy regimens (mean alemtuzumab exposure: 8 weeks)

Toxicity	% of Patients	
	Previously Untreated	Previously Treated
Neutropenia (grade 3/4)	42	64
Anemia (grade 3/4)	12	38
Thrombocytopenia (grade 3/4)	14	52
Infusion reactions (grade 3/4 pyrexia ± chills)	10	35
CMV infection	16 (≈ one-third serious or life-threatening); CMV testing weekly with PCR assay throughout treatment and Q 2 weeks × 2 months after treatment is completed	6 (nearly all life-threatening; data from studies where routine CMV surveillance was not required)

Patient population: Data reported across all studies (Campath product label, Aug. 2009)

Infections (other than CMV)\nSepsis (grade 3–5)\nInfection-related mortality	50%\n3–10%, higher in previously treated patients\nPreviously: untreated patients (2%); treated patients (16%)
Cardiac dysrhythmias	14% of previously untreated patients (grade 3/4 in 1%)\n• Most were tachycardias and were temporarily associated with infusion

The following serious, including fatal, infusion reactions have been identified in postmarketing reports: syncope, pulmonary infiltrates, acute respiratory distress syndrome (ARDS), respiratory arrest, cardiac arrhythmias, myocardial infarction, acute cardiac insufficiency, cardiac arrest, angioedema, and anaphylactoid shock

Notes

The treatment experience with alemtuzumab for AIHA is limited. Rare reports of treatment-related hemolysis have been reported with this agent: Galimberti S. J Immunother 2004;27:389–393; Wierda WG et al. Blood (Proc Am Soc Hematol) 2006;108:[abstract 2839a]

Therapy Monitoring

1. CBC with differential count weekly or more frequently if worsening neutropenia, anemia, and/or thrombocytopenia
2. Hold therapy for grade 3 or 4 infusion reactions (pyrexia, chills/rigors, nausea, hypotension, urticaria, dyspnea, rash, emesis, and bronchospasm
3. Discontinue alemtuzumab for any autoimmune thrombocytopenia or for worsening of baseline AIHA (if alemtuzumab is used for the treatment of AIHA)
4. Assess PCR for CMV at 6 weeks following initiation of alemtuzumab therapy
5. Irradiate blood products if they are required during therapy
6. Avoid live vaccine administration in patients who have recently received alemtuzumab

Hematologic Values	Dose Modification
Absolute Neutrophil Count (ANC) <250/mm³ and/or Platelet Count ≤25,000/mm³	
For first occurrence:	• Withhold alemtuzumab therapy\n• Resume alemtuzumab at 30 mg/dose when ANC ≥500/mm³ *and* platelet count ≥50,000/mm³
For second occurrence:	• Withhold alemtuzumab therapy\n• Resume alemtuzumab at 10 mg/dose when ANC ≥500/mm³ *and* platelet count ≥50,000/mm³
For third occurrence:	• Discontinue alemtuzumab therapy
≥50% Decrease from Baseline in Patients Initiating Therapy with a Baseline ANC ≤250/mm³ and/or a Baseline Platelet Count ≤25,000/mm³	
For first occurrence:	• Withhold alemtuzumab therapy\n• Resume alemtuzumab at 30 mg/dose upon return to baseline values
For second occurrence:	• Withhold alemtuzumab therapy\n• Resume alemtuzumab at 10 mg/dose upon return to baseline values
For third occurrence:	• Discontinue alemtuzumab therapy

REGIMEN FOR PURINE ANALOG-INDUCED AUTOIMMUNE HEMOLYTIC ANEMIA

Dearden C et al. Blood 2008;111:1820–1826
Johnson S et al. Lancet 1996;347:1432–1438
Leporrier M et al. Blood 2001;98:2319–2325
Robak T, Kasznicki M. Leukemia 2002;16:1015–1027
Steurer M et al. Cancer Treat Rev 2006;32:377–389

Epidemiology

The incidence of AIHA complicating purine analog therapy ranges from 1.8–5.6% among 3 prospective randomized controlled trials comparing single-agent purine analogs with alkylator-based regimens in the first-line treatment of patients with B-CLL (data from systematic review by Steurer M et al. Cochrane Database Syst Rev 2006;3:CD004270, shown below)

Study	Agent	AIHA by Treatment Cohort, Patient Number with AIHA/Total Patient Cohort (%)	
		Purine Analog	Alkylator-Based
Johnson et al., 1996	Fludarabine	2/53 (3.8)	0/52 (0.0)
Robak and Kasznicki, 2002	Cladribine	7/124 (5.6)	2/103 (1.9)
Leporrier et al., 2001	Fludarabine	6/336 (1.8)	3/588 (0.54)
Total:		15/513 (2.9)	5/743 (0.7)

The relative risk of AIHA with single-agent purine analog therapy compared with alkylator-based therapy for B-CLL: 3.36 (95% CI, 1.27–8.91)

Prognostic significance of a (+) DAT and AIHA in CLL: beneficial impact of fludarabine + cyclophosphamide (FC) vs. single-agent fludarabine (F) or chlorambucil (Dearden C et al. Blood 2008; LRF-CLL4 Trial: the largest prospective trial in CLL to examine these relationships)

Patient population: 783 Patients (2/99–10/04); DAT results available in 637 patients (82%) at study entry, 333 patients after first treatment, and 299 patients pre-/posttreatment. AIHA data available in 759 patients (DAT results available in 331)

Variable	Treatment Group		
	Chlorambucil	F	FC
(+) DAT at study entry in 637 patients	14%	13%	15%
(+) DAT after first treatment in 333 patients	13%	17%	10%

(continued)

(continued)

Variable	Treatment Group		
	Chlorambucil	F	FC
Results of 299 patients with DAT results available both pre-/posttreatment after 1 cycle, n (%)			
(+) At entry	11 (52)	9 (82)	5 (42)
(+) After treatment	10 (48)	2 (18)	7 (58)
(−) After treatment			
(−) At entry	4 (3)	6 (9)	3 (4)
(+) After treatment	112 (97)	62 (91)	68 (96)
(−) After treatment			
Development of AIHA			
Among 759 patients, n (%)	47 (12)	21 (11)	9 (5)
(+) Predictive value of a (+) DAT and development of AIHA, %	38	29	12
(−) Predictive value of a (−) DAT and the absence of AIHA, %	92	90	96

Additional outcome measures

Variable	AIHA		P Value
	Present	Absent	
Response to therapy for CLL	43/65 (66%)	530/654 (81%)	0.004
Progression-free survival, 5 years	9%	18%	0.003
Overall survival, 5 years	37%	58%	0.001

Notes

1. For patients treated with FC, the percent of DAT (+) patients decreased after treatment and increased with F monotherapy
2. Multivariate analysis showed that a pretreatment (+) DAT was associated with more advanced stage and ↑ β_2-microglobulin
3. The DAT result had an independent association with the development of AIHA: Risk of AIHA in a patient with a (+) DAT was 1:3; >90% of patients with a (−) DAT did not develop AIHA
4. Patients receiving chlorambucil or F alone were 3-fold more likely to develop AIHA than FC-treated patients
5. AIHA development was associated with older age, advanced stage, (+) DAT, and treatment modality

Purine Analog Rechallenge

In patients with purine analog-induced AIHA, there is published experience suggesting an increased risk of recurrent AIHA with purine analog rechallenge. A selection of this experience is outlined below:

1. Seven of 8 CLL patients with prior fludarabine-induced AIHA subsequently rechallenged with fludarabine developed recurrent AIHA of whom 3 died (Weiss RB et al. J Clin Oncol 1998;16:1885–1889)

2. Among 12 cases of fludarabine-induced AIHA observed among 52 patients with CLL, 6/8 patients rechallenged with fludarabine developed recurrent AIHA of whom 2 died (1 from hemolysis) (Myint H et al. Br J Haematol 1995;91:341–344)

3. Four (10%) relapsed CLL patients who were treated previously with cladribine developed a first-episode AIHA event after retreatment with cladribine (1 with cladribine alone, 2 with cladribine + prednisone, and 1 with cladribine + cyclophosphamide + mitoxantrone; "CMC" regimen) (Robak T et al. Eur J Haematol 2002;69:27–36)

Treatment

No prospective, randomized, controlled trials have been reported assessing the treatment of purine analog-induced AIHA in patients with CLL or other lymphoproliferative disorders. A recommended approach for the management and treatment of purine analog-induced AIHA, in lieu of more definitive evidenced-based guidance, is outlined below:

1. Discontinue purine analog treatment at the diagnosis of AIHA

2. Initiate corticosteroid therapy (see the section on prednisone for the treatment of AIHA)

3. If the AIHA is poorly responsive to initial corticosteroid therapy:

   a. Consider the use of an agent with a lower risk of associated myelosuppression (eg, cyclosporine or azathioprine; see pertinent sections in this chapter), *or*

   b. Consider alternative chemotherapy for the underlying lymphoproliferative disorder (eg, R-CVP or R-CHOP for CD20+ B-CLL based on Expert Opinion), *or*

   c. Consider the use of single-agent rituximab (see the section on rituximab for the treatment of AIHA and the "RCD" regimen for B-CLL)

   d. If the above measures fail to achieve remission of the AIHA or if the patient is intolerant to or declines the above measures, splenectomy should be considered

4. Among patients with a history of purine analog-induced AIHA, close monitoring is recommended with any subsequent treatment

Notes

Recurrent AIHA has been observed in a patient with CLL previously treated with fludarabine who, upon progression of disease, received chlorambucil 10 mg/day and developed rapid-onset hemolytic anemia (day 9). Despite the use of steroid therapy, the patient's Hgb fell further and the patient died (Orchard J et al. Br J Haematol 1998;102:1107–1113)

REGIMEN FOR REFRACTORY AUTOIMMUNE HEMOLYTIC ANEMIA

HIGH-DOSE CYCLOPHOSPHAMIDE

Brodsky RA et al. Ann Intern Med 2001;135:477–483
Moyo VM et al. Blood 2002;100:704–706

High-dose cyclophosphamide 50 mg/kg (ideal body weight) per day; administer intravenously in 100–1000 mL 0.9% sodium chloride injection (0.9% NS) or 5% dextrose injection (D5W) over 60 minutes, for 4 consecutive days, days 1–4 (total dosage/4-day course = 200 mg/kg ideal body weight)

Mesna 10 mg/kg per dose; administer intravenously, diluted within the range of 1–20 mg mesna/mL in 0.9% NS or D5W over 15 minutes starting at the same time as cyclophosphamide with repeated doses at 3, 6, and 8 hours after cyclophosphamide administration begun, for 4 doses/day on 4 consecutive days, days 1–4 (total dosage/day = 40 mg/kg; total dosage/4-day course = 160 mg/kg)

Supportive Care

Antiemetic prophylaxis
Emetogenic potential on days 1–4 is **HIGH**. *Potential for delayed symptoms*
See Chapter 39 for antiemetic recommendations

Hematopoietic growth factor (CSF) prophylaxis
Primary prophylaxis is indicated with one of the following:
   Filgrastim (G-CSF) 5 mcg/kg per day, by subcutaneous injection, *or*
   Pegfilgrastim (pegylated filgrastim) 6 mg/0.6 mL, by subcutaneous injection for 1 dose
   • Begin use on day 10 (6 days after completing cyclophosphamide)
   • Continue filgrastim beyond the ANC nadir until ANC recovers to ≥1000/mm[3]
See Chapter 43 for more information

Antimicrobial prophylaxis
Risk of fever and neutropenia is HIGH
   Antimicrobial primary prophylaxis is recommended:
   • Antibacterial—consider fluoroquinolone prophylaxis; *Pneumocystis jirovecii* prophylaxis is recommended (eg, cotrimoxazole)
   • Antifungal—recommended
   • Antiviral—antiherpes antivirals (eg, acyclovir)
See Chapter 47 for more information

Folic acid 1 mg/day, orally, continually, to prevent depletion of folate stores and megaloblastic anemia resulting from chronic hemolysis

Dose Modifications

No dose modification. Treatment criteria: (a) age ≤70 years, (b) cardiac ejection fraction >40%, (c) serum creatinine <2.5 mg/dL (<221 μmol/L), and (d) FVC/FEV/CO diffusion capacity at least 50% of predicted

Indications

High-dose cyclophosphamide with mesna and filgrastim support has been reported in a limited number of patients with severe refractory AIHA, defined as a need for transfusions and steroids >10 mg (prednisone)/day despite 2 therapies for idiopathic AIHA and at least 1 treatment for secondary AIHA

Clinical features of the enrolled patients included: Severe refractory AIHA (6, idiopathic; 3, secondary): warm Ab AIHA (N = 7), CAD (N = 1), mixed AIHA (N = 1). Median pretreatment Hgb: 6.7 g/dL (range: 5–10 g/dL). Median number of prior regimens = 3

Efficacy (N = 9)

Complete response*	67%[‡]
Partial response[†]	33%
15-month follow-up	
Continued response	100%
Maintained without steroids	77%

*Normal untransfused Hgb for age/sex while taking ≤10 mg/day of prednisone with the resolution of hemolysis
[†]Hgb of ≥10 g/dL and transfusion independence
[‡]Two CR patients became DAT-negative

Toxicity (N = 9)

Toxicity	Frequency
Nausea and vomiting	Common
Transient alopecia	Common
Neutropenia and fever	Common
Renal and LFT abnormalities	Infrequent
Hemorrhagic cystitis	Infrequent
SIADH	Infrequent

Parameter	Median Time
ANC ≥500/mm[3]	16 days
Platelet transfusion independence	15 days
RBC transfusion independence	19 days
Hospital stay	21 days

Notes

Benefits of therapy versus risks should be assessed

Use only by clinicians and medical centers with active experience in the use of "transplant doses" of cyclophosphamide and with the availability of appropriate ancillary clinical support and personnel

RED BLOOD CELL TRANSFUSION

Branch DR, Petz LD. Transfusion 1999;39:6–10
Buetens OW , Ness PM. Curr Opin Hematol 2003;10:429–433
Petz LD. Blood transfusion in acquired hemolytic anemia. In: Petz LD, Swisher SN, Kleinman S, Spence RK, Strauss RG, eds. Clinical Practice of Transfusion Medicine. 3rd ed. New York, NY: Churchill Livingstone;1996:469–499
Petz LD. Hematology 2002 (American Society of Hematology Educational Program) 449–454
Petz LD. Transfusion 2003;43:1503–1507
Petz LD, Garratty G. Blood transfusions in autoimmune hemolytic anemia. In: Petz LD, Garratty G, eds. Immune Hemolytic Anemias. 2nd ed. New York, NY: Churchill Livingstone; 2004:375–400
Rosenfield RE, Jagathambal. Semin Hematol 1976;13:311–321

RBC infusion: Volume and rate considerations:

Volume: The optimal volume of RBCs to be infused depends on the clinical setting. In general, the aim is to supply just enough RBCs to treat or prevent hypoxemia while avoiding overtransfusion

Rate: Administer RBCs slowly with a total volume not to exceed 1 mL/kg per hour

Monitoring considerations:

Hgb/Hct: In the setting of acute, life-threatening AIHA, the Hgb/Hct should be monitored at 2-hour intervals; at least every 12–24 hours in individuals less acutely ill

Volume status: During and following transfusion, assessments should be performed for the presence of congestive heart failure (CHF) or volume overload. Particular caution is advised for the development of fluid overload in the elderly and in patients with reduced cardiac reserve. Diuretic therapy should be used as clinically indicated

Other considerations:

Cold agglutinin syndrome: The patient should be dressed warmly and be in a warm environment

Efficacy

Not available. Goal of therapy is to stabilize red cell mass and reverse symptoms of acute anemia

Toxicity

Potential complications relevant to patients with AIHA may include:

1. Volume overload and congestive heart failure with attempts to raise the hematocrit too quickly
2. Acute hemolytic transfusion reactions
3. Development of alloimmunization
4. Posttransfusion hemoglobinemia or hemoglobinuria, particularly with large volumes of RBCs with ongoing auto-Ab production
5. Diffuse intravascular coagulation (DIC)
6. Thromboembolism
7. Death

Indications

Recommended in patients who are acutely ill with signs and symptoms compatible with acute hemolysis or in patients with progressive anemia where severe levels of hemolysis (eg, Hgb <5–6 g/dL) may probably be reached

General guidelines based on Hgb values and the probability of significant physiologic impairment:

Petz LD. Blood transfusion in acquired hemolytic anemia. In: Petz LD, Swisher SN, Kleinman S, Spence RK, Strauss RG, eds. Clinical Practice of Transfusion Medicine. 3rd ed. New York, NY: Churchill Livingstone; 1996:469–499

Note: The decision to transfuse should ultimately be guided by clinical assessments performed in individual patients

Hgb	Probability*	Recommendation
≥10 g/dL	Low	Avoid transfusion
8–10 g/dL	Low	Avoid transfusion, *or* Transfuse if improved after a transfusion trial
6–8 g/dL	Moderate	Transfuse if necessary, *or* Try to avoid transfusion
≤6 g/dL	High	Frequently requires transfusion
Stable	Low	Avoid transfusion

*Probability of significant physiologic impairment

Blood Product Selection

Note: Hemoglobin-based oxygen carriers (RBC Substitutes) have not received FDA approval for any indication

Warm Ab AIHA:

1. Most severe hemolytic transfusion reactions are caused by anti-A or anti-B antibodies. While a broadly reactive auto-Ab will make all units incompatible, with standard blood-banking techniques the ABO type can usually be identified permitting identical or compatible ABO type blood for transfusion

2. The blood bank should assess for alloantibodies (allo-Abs) that may be present from prior transfusion during the previous 3 months or pregnancy that may be masked by the presence of an auto-Ab. Allo-Abs have been reported to be present in 12–40% of patients with warm Ab AIHA. Allo-Abs have been reported in 209/647 (32%) of sera from patients with AIHA. Failure to identify the presence of allo-Abs may lead to worsening of the hemolysis, falsely increasing the perceived severity of AIHA following transfusion. The more common allo-Ab target antigens may include: *C, E, c, e, K, Fy*, Fy†, Jk*, Jk†, S,* and *s*

Cold agglutinin syndrome:

1. Compatibility testing should be done at 37°C (98.6°F). If testing cannot be performed strictly at this temperature, then it is recommended that 1 or 2 autoadsorptions be performed. Although high-titer cold agglutinins will not be completely removed with this maneuver, reactions that occur at 37°C (98.6°F) are likely to be eliminated

2. The specificity of cold agglutinins is often anti-*I*. Providing *I* antigen-negative blood may not be practical because of its rarity and may not be beneficial

3. There is controversy among experts as to the worth of blood warming in this setting. In patients with severe CAS or PCH, blood warming has been advocated. When an inline blood warmer is used, the temperature should be carefully regulated at body temperature to avoid RBC injury that can result in lethal in vivo hemolysis. Guidelines for the use of blood-warming devices have been published by the American Association of Blood Banks (AuBuchon, JP. Guidelines for the Use of Blood Warming Devices. Bethesda, MD: American Association of Blood Banks; 2001)

Paroxysmal cold hemoglobinuria:

1. The use of *p* or *pᵏ* RBCs (lacking the *P* antigen) is not practical because of its rarity and availability only from rare donor files. In this setting, transfusion of common *P* types should be provided

Notes

Initial communication between the clinician and the blood bank:

At the first indication that RBC transfusion may be required, the clinician should contact the blood bank or transfusion service. This communication should include:

1. An indication of the urgency for transfusion

2. An inquiry into the compatibility testing procedures used by the blood bank to assess the safety of the selected RBCs for transfusion, *and*

3. Clinical information that may help in assessing the risk of alloimmunization (eg, history of pregnancy, prior blood transfusion; particularly, during the past 3 months)

What the clinician should expect from the blood bank-transfusion service:

1. Notification of the diagnosis of AIHA made during compatibility testing for a requested transfusion

2. Information about the compatibility test procedures performed

3. RBCs selected for transfusion after excluding the presence of alloantibodies (eg, by adsorption techniques or by extended phenotype)

4. Assurances that the transfused cells are unlikely to cause an acute hemolytic transfusion reaction even though the RBCs cannot be expected to survive normally because of the autoantibody

PLASMAPHERESIS

Silva VA et al. J Clin Apher 1994;9:120–123
von Baeyer H. Ther Apher Dial 2003;7:127–140

Protocol for plasmapheresis alone:
Plasma exchange (PEX) and **albumin human** (HA) for IgM (IgA) Ab-mediated hemolysis and for IgG 1,2,4-mediated hemolysis
Daily PEX/HA at 1–1.5 times the plasma volume until hemolysis is controlled and transfusions are no longer required

Indications

von Baeyer H. Ther Apher Dial 2003;7:127–140

Therapeutic plasmapheresis in AIHA has been advocated under 2 conditions:

1. As an emergency bridging measure to eliminate auto-Abs until immunosuppressive therapy becomes effective
2. As therapy after failure of immunosuppressive therapy and splenectomy in an attempt to treat relapsing hemolysis

Efficacy (N = 20)

(15 Case Reports or Series of AIHA Treated with Plasmapheresis)

	% Responding
All patients (N = 20)	65%
Warm Ab (N = 10)	50%
Cold Ab (N = 6)	67%
Evans syndrome (N = 4)	100%
AIHA after BMT (N = 4)	25%

Notes

The American Association of Blood Banks and the American Society of Apheresis have assigned a Category III indication to plasmapheresis for AIHA, citing there is "insufficient data to determine the effectiveness of apheresis in which the results of clinical trials may be conflicting or in some circumstances where efficacy has been based on uncontrolled anecdotal reports." (Smith JW et al. Transfusion 2003;43:820–822)

Toxicity

Potential side effects to plasmapheresis include:
1. Complications associated with central venous catheter
2. Type I allergic hypersensitivity reactions

REGIMEN FOR REFRACTORY WARM ANTIBODY AUTOIMMUNE HEMOLYTIC ANEMIA

IMMUNOSUPPRESSIVE THERAPY
AZATHIOPRINE *or* CYCLOPHOSPHAMIDE

American College of Rheumatology Ad Hoc Committee on Glucocorticoid-Induced Osteoporosis. Arthritis Rheum 2001;44:1496–1503

Corley CC Jr et al. Am J Med 1966;41:404–412

Habibi B et al. Am J Med 1974;56:61–69

Hitzig WH, Massimo L. Blood 1966;28:840–850

Murphy S, LoBuglio AF. Semin Hematol 1976;13:323–334

Petz LD. Curr Opin Hematol 2001;8:411–416

Petz LD, Garratty G. Management of autoimmune hemolytic anemias. In: Petz LD, Garratty G, eds. Immune Hemolytic Anemias. 2nd ed. New York, NY: Churchill Livingstone; 2004:401–458

Rosse W et al. Challenges in managing autoimmune diseases. In: American Society of Hematology Educational Program 1997;92–94

Worrledge S. Immune hemolytic anemias. In: Hardesty RM, Weatherall DJ, eds. Blood and Its Disorders. Oxford, UK: Blackwell Scientific; 1982:479–513

Azathioprine 2 mg/kg per day; administer orally, continually (total dosage/week = 14 mg/kg), *or*

Azathioprine 75–200 mg/day; administer orally, continually (total dose/week = 525–1400 mg)

Note: Adjust therapy to maintain "slight thrombocytopenia or leukopenia." See Dose Modifications below

or

Azathioprine 80 mg/m² per day; administer orally, continually (total dosage/week = 560 mg/m²), *plus*

Prednisone 60 mg/day; administer orally, continually (total dose/week = 420 mg)

or

Cyclophosphamide 60 mg/m² per day; administer orally, continually (total dosage/week = 420 mg/m²), *plus*

Prednisone 60 mg/day; administer orally, continually (total dose/week = 420 mg)

Guidelines for tapering prednisone:

30 mg/day for 1 week; 20 mg/day for 1 week; 15 mg/day for 4 weeks; 10 mg/day for 4 weeks; 5 mg/day for 4 weeks; 5 mg every other day for 4 weeks; discontinue

Guidelines for tapering azathioprine, after 6 months of therapy:

60 mg/m² per day for 4 weeks; 35 mg/m² per day for 4 weeks; 15 mg/m² per day for 4 weeks; 25 mg every other day for 4 weeks; 25 mg twice weekly; discontinue

Guidelines for tapering cyclophosphamide after 6 months of therapy:

45 mg/m² per day for 4 weeks; 30 mg/m² per day for 4 weeks; 15 mg/m² per day for 4 weeks; 25 mg every other day for 4 weeks; 25 mg twice weekly; discontinue

Supportive Care

Antiemetic prophylaxis

Emetogenic potential with cyclophosphamide is **MODERATE**

Prednisone and azathioprine are not emetogenic

See Chapter 39 for antiemetic recommendations

Hematopoietic growth factor (CSF) prophylaxis

Primary prophylaxis is NOT indicated

See Chapter 43 for more information

Antimicrobial prophylaxis

Risk of fever and neutropenia is LOW

   Antimicrobial primary prophylaxis to be considered:

   • Antibacterial—not indicated

   • Antifungal—not indicated

   • Antiviral—not indicated unless patient previously had an episode of HSV

See Chapter 47 for more information

(continued)

Indications

Consider immunosuppressive therapy in patients with warm Ab AIHA who:

• Do not benefit from glucocorticoids

• Require unacceptable maintenance doses of glucocorticoids

• Are poor surgical candidates for splenectomy

• Experience a relapse following splenectomy

Efficacy

Percent responding	40–60%
Percent requiring low-dose glucocorticoids in addition to azathioprine or cyclophosphamide	≤50%

Toxicity

Potential side effects include:

1. Myelosuppression
2. Anemia
3. Thrombocytopenia
4. Infection
5. Renal and hepatic function abnormalities
6. Nausea and vomiting
7. Alopecia
8. Sterility
9. Secondary malignancies
10. Urinary tract hemorrhagic (cyclophosphamide)
11. SIADH (cyclophosphamide)

Therapy Monitoring

CBC with differential: Weekly during the first month, and weekly for a month after any dose increase. Otherwise, every 2 weeks until counts stabilize, and then, monthly

Notes

1. The rapid withdrawal of immunosuppressive agents may lead to a rebound phenomenon of hyperimmune responsiveness

2. If glucocorticoids have produced an incomplete remission before the initiation of immunosuppressive therapy, they should be continued until signs of clinical improvement

(continued)

Steroid-associated gastritis:
Add a **proton pump inhibitor** during prednisone use to prevent gastritis and duodenitis

Calcium and vitamin D supplementation in patients receiving long-term low- to medium-dose glucocorticoid therapy and who have normal levels of gonadal hormones (American College of Rheumatology Ad Hoc Committee on Glucocorticoid-Induced Osteoporosis. Arthritis Rheum 2001;44:1496–1503). See Chapter 44, Indications for Bisphosphonates in the Hematology-Oncology Setting

Folic acid 1 mg/day; administer orally, continually, to prevent depletion of folate stores and megaloblastic anemia resulting from chronic hemolysis

Treatment Modifications

Adjust azathioprine and cyclophosphamide therapy to maintain a "slight degree of marrow suppression" manifested as mild thrombocytopenia or leukopenia
Although "slight degree of marrow suppression" was not further defined in these studies, consider using National Cancer Institute Common Terminology Criteria for Adverse Events grade 1 toxicity as reasonable benchmarks; that is:
    WBC: 3000/mm^3 to the lower limit of normal
    ANC: ≥1500/mm^3 to <2000/mm^3
    Platelets: ≥75,000/mm^3 to the lower limit of normal
    Hemoglobin: 10 g/dL to the lower limit of normal

Adverse Event	Dose Modification
If WBC <3000/mm^3, ANC <1500/mm^3, *or* platelets <75,000/mm^3	Hold therapy for a minimum of 1 week. Restart only when WBC >3000/mm^3 *and* ANC >1500/mm^3 *and* platelets >75,000/mm^3. Then, start with a dosage adjustment for: Azathioprine decrease daily dosage by 0.5 mg/kg *or* decrease daily dose by 25–50 mg Cyclophosphamide, decrease daily dosage by 15 mg/m^2

REGIMEN FOR REFRACTORY WARM ANTIBODY AUTOIMMUNE HEMOLYTIC ANEMIA

DANAZOL

Ahn YS et al. Ann Intern Med 1985;102:298–301
DANAZOL capsules, USP, product label, revised April 2009, Barr Laboratories, Inc., Pomona, NY
Pignon J-M et al. Br J Haematol 1993;83:343–345

Danazol 200 mg/dose; administer orally 3–4 times/day, continually
(total daily dose = 600–800 mg)

Notes:
Danazol is usually added initially to medications previously employed for AIHA (eg, prednisone),
or is given concomitantly with prednisone 1 mg/kg per day

If a hematologic remission (HR) is attained, glucocorticoids are tapered to a minimal
requirement or discontinued. If a HR is maintained for >1 months without prednisone,
danazol is gradually tapered to 200–400 mg/day, and this dose is continued indefinitely as
long as there is no clinically important toxicity and Hgb remains >10 g/dL

Supportive Care
Antiemetic prophylaxis
Emetogenic potential with danazol is **MINIMAL**
See Chapter 39 for antiemetic recommendations
Note: Emetic symptoms may occur in association with benign intracranial hypertension,
a rare adverse event associated with danazol use

Hematopoietic growth factor (CSF) prophylaxis
Primary prophylaxis is NOT indicated
See Chapter 43 for more information

Antimicrobial prophylaxis
Risk of fever and neutropenia is LOW
   Antimicrobial primary prophylaxis to be considered:
- Antibacterial—not indicated
- Antifungal—not indicated
- Antiviral—not indicated unless patient previously had an episode of HSV
See Chapter 47 for more information

Steroid-associated gastritis:
Add a **proton pump inhibitor** during prednisone use to prevent gastritis and duodenitis

Calcium and vitamin D supplementation in patients receiving long-term low- to medium-dose
glucocorticoid therapy and who have normal levels of gonadal hormones (American College
of Rheumatology Ad Hoc Committee on Glucocorticoid-Induced Osteoporosis. Arthritis
Rheum 2001;44:1496–503). See Chapter 44, Indications for Bisphosphonates in the
Hematology-Oncology Setting

Folic acid 1 mg/day; administer orally, continually, to prevent depletion of folate stores and
megaloblastic anemia resulting from chronic hemolysis

Contraindications: Undiagnosed abnormal genital bleeding, pregnancy, breast feeding, porphyria,
"markedly impaired" hepatic, renal, or cardiac function

Indications

Patients with 1° (primary) or 2° (secondary) warm antibody AIHA:
1. In refractory disease despite prior therapy with glucocorticoids, splenectomy, and immunosuppressive therapy
2. Less frequently as initial therapy with prednisone

Efficacy

Pignon J-M et al. Br J Haematol 1993

Upfront Therapy with Prednisone (N = 10)

Hgb to ≥12.5 g/dL*	80%
Complete prednisone taper	75%
Low-dose every-other-day prednisone	25%
Mean response duration	18+ months (14+ to 37+ months)

Previously Treated with Prednisone, Splenectomy, and Immunosuppressive Therapy (N = 7)

Excellent response	43% (14–23+ months)
Partial response	14% (77+ months)
Treatment failure	43% (7–18 months)

*With prednisone decreased to ≤5 mg/day or discontinued
Ahn YS et al. Ann Intern Med 1985

1° (N = 7) or 2° (N = 5) Warm Ab AIHA

Hct increased to ≥40%	50%
Hct increased to ≥30%, but less than 40%	25%
Hct increased by 6% above baseline value with 50% reduction in steroids	25%
Time to response (weeks)	1–3
Remission sustained with steroids + danazol	58%
Remission sustained with danazol alone	42%

Malignant Warm Ab AIHA (N = 3)

Sustained remission	33%

1°, primary; 2°, secondary
Note: Nine of 15 patients without prior splenectomy achieved lasting remissions with addition of danazol, suggesting a splenectomy-sparing effect

Toxicity (Potential)

1. Virilization with facial hair growth, hair loss, and menstrual irregularities
2. Nervousness
3. Cushingoid features; glucose intolerance in patients with diabetes mellitus
4. Muscle cramps and myalgia
5. Elevations of LFTs
6. Fluid retention
7. Thromboembolism
8. Allergic skin reactions
9. Benign intracranial hypertension

Therapy Monitoring

1. Monitoring of LFTs at baseline and at least monthly or earlier as clinically indicated
2. Assessment for virilization since some signs may not be reversible

Treatment Modifications

Adverse Event	Dose Modification
G ≥2 LFTs*	Hold danazol until LFTs G ≤1

*National Cancer Institute Common Terminology Criteria for Adverse Events

REGIMEN FOR REFRACTORY WARM ANTIBODY AUTOIMMUNE HEMOLYTIC ANEMIA

CYCLOSPORINE

Emilia G et al. Br J Haematol 1996;93:341–344
Hershko C et al. Br J Haematol 1990;76:436–437

Starting dosage:
Cyclosporine 2.5 mg/kg per dose; administer orally twice daily for 6 days (total dosage/day = 5 mg/kg) *or*
Cyclosporine 2–3 mg/kg per dose; administer orally twice daily for 6 days (total dosage/day = 4–6 mg/kg)

Maintenance dosage:
Cyclosporine 1.5 mg/kg per dose adjusted to maintain a serum cyclosporine concentration between 200–400 ng/mL

Alternate Schedule

Starting dosage:
Cyclosporine 1.25 mg/kg per dose; administer orally twice daily, continually (total dosage/week = 17.5 mg/kg)

Maintenance dosage:
If no response, increase **cyclosporine** by 0.25 mg/kg per dose (0.5 mg/kg·day) increments every 2 weeks to a maximum of 2 mg/kg per dose (4 mg/kg·day; maximum total dosage/week = 28 mg/kg)

Note: Dosages vary with indication and AIHA is not an approved indication. Dosages and schedules for autoimmune diseases often fall within a broad range of 0.5–4 mg/kg per dose, administered orally every 12 hours. Generally, treatment is initiated at a low dosage and is titrated to the least dose that achieves a desired therapeutic effect
After that effect or a maximal response is achieved, an attempt should be made to gradually decrease the dose with the goal of discontinuing therapy

Supportive Care
Antiemetic prophylaxis
NOT indicated
See Chapter 39 for antiemetic recommendations

Hematopoietic growth factor (CSF) prophylaxis
Primary prophylaxis is NOT indicated
See Chapter 43 for more information

Antimicrobial prophylaxis
Risk of fever and neutropenia is LOW
  Antimicrobial primary prophylaxis to be considered:
  • Antibacterial—not indicated
  • Antifungal—not indicated
  • Antiviral—not indicated unless patient previously had an episode of HSV
See Chapter 47 for more information

Folic acid 1 mg/day, orally, continually, to prevent depletion of folate stores and megaloblastic anemia resulting from chronic hemolysis

AHFS Drug Information 2004:3625–3639
Emilia G et al. Br J Haematol 1996;93:341–344
Hershko C et al. Br J Haematol 1990;76:436–437

Indications

Cyclosporine has been administered in limited numbers of patients with refractory AIHA alone or in the setting of Evans syndrome

Efficacy

Emilia G et al. Br J Haematol 1996;93:341–344 (N = 5)

Coombs (+) AIHA (3 patients)	3 complete responses
ITP + AIHA (1 patient)	1 complete response
Evans' Syndrome (1 patient)	1 partial response

Note: Responses were dependent on continuation of cyclosporine. Two deaths (stroke and lung cancer). Median follow-up: 31 months (range: 13–62 months)

Hershko et al. Br J Haematol 1990;76:436–4367 (N = 3)

Coombs (+) AIHA + CLL (2 patients)	↑ Hgb/↓ steroids
Coombs (−) AIHA + CLL (1)	↑ Hgb/↓ steroids

Toxicity

Toxicity	Frequency
Mild-to-moderate hypertension	Common
Nephrotoxicity	Common/reversible
Hepatotoxicity	Common/reversible
Cyclosporine sensitivity	Infrequent
Cremophor EL sensitivity	Infrequent
Anaphylaxis	Infrequent (~1:1000)
Hypomagnesemia	Infrequent
Tremor	Infrequent
Hirsutism	Infrequent
Gum hypertrophy	Infrequent
Secondary malignancies	Infrequent
Hyperkalemia ± hyperchloremic metabolic acidosis	Infrequent
Thrombocytopenia and microangiopathic hemolytic anemia	Infrequent

Note: Contraindicated if patient has hypersensitivity to cyclosporine or Cremophor EL (polyoxyethylated castor oil)

Treatment Modifications

Adverse Event	Treatment Modification
First episode of serum creatinine >125% of baseline, confirmed within two weeks, or first episode of serum creatinine >150%	Reduce cyclosporine dosage by 25–50% for 6–10 days. If serum creatinine returns to baseline, resume original cyclosporine dosage. If serum creatinine does not return to normal, reduce cyclosporine dosage by an additional 25%
Second episode of serum creatinine >125% of baseline	Reduce cyclosporine dosage by 25–50%; do not attempt to reinstitute original dosage
Third episode of serum creatinine >125% of baseline	Discontinue cyclosporine
Increase in LFTs by 25–50% greater than baseline	Reduce cyclosporine dosage by 25–50% for 6–10 days. If LFTs return to baseline, resume original cyclosporine dosage. If LFTs do not return to normal, reduce cyclosporine dosage by an additional 25%
Second episode of LFTs 25–50% greater than baseline	Reduce cyclosporine dosage by 25–50%; do not attempt to reinstitute original dosage
Hypertension develops in a patient without a history of hypertension	Reduce cyclosporine dosage by 25–50% for 6–10 days. If blood pressure returns to baseline with or without treatment, resume original cyclosporine dosage. Consider calcium channel blockers or β-blockers as first-line therapy
Recurrent hypertension despite multiple cyclosporine dose reductions, or when adequate adjustment of antihypertensive therapy not possible	Discontinue cyclosporine
Tremor, headache, confusion, paresthesias, lethargy, or weakness, elevations of cholesterol and/or triglycerides of clinical concern	Reduce cyclosporine dosage by 25–50% for 6–10 days. If symptoms resolve, resume cyclosporine at the original dosage or a dosage 25% less than that in use when symptoms first appeared. If symptoms persist, reduce dosage by an additional 25%

Notes

Every 10 months (if ongoing use is required), discontinue cyclosporine for 2 weeks to evaluate for persistence of response

Cyclosporine levels correlating with AIHA response have not been systematically reported

Cyclosporine should only be used for therapeutic applications other than transplantation only by clinicians experienced in immunosuppressive therapy

Management of patients, during initiation or any change in, cyclosporine therapy should be performed in facilities equipped with adequate laboratory/supportive medical equipment and staffed with adequate medical personnel

Therapy Monitoring

1. *Baseline:* Serum creatinine (similar results on 2 occasions), BUN, CBC with differential, magnesium, potassium, uric acid, liver function tests, lipoproteins
Note: Serum lipoproteins are recommended because levels may increase modestly during therapy
2. *First 3 months:* Serum creatinine, BUN and other baseline lab measurements plus BP every 2 weeks; thereafter, stable patients monitored monthly
Note: Measure serum creatinine with initiation of new NSAID therapy or if a concomitantly used NSAID is increased in dose
3. *Cyclosporine levels:* Weekly for 2–3 months and then once per month. Increase monitoring frequency when potentially interacting drugs are introduced and withdrawn
Note: The type of cyclosporine assay used to monitor blood levels is important. Recommended trough levels for the cyclosporine parent compound depends on the type of assay used (HPLC vs. RIA vs. fluorescence polarization immunoassay) and vary by whole blood versus serum/plasma. Target levels are based on cyclosporine monitoring strategies in the transplant setting
Note: Monitor drug–drug interactions that may alter renal function and either increase or decrease cyclosporine concentrations

REGIMEN FOR REFRACTORY WARM ANTIBODY AUTOIMMUNE HEMOLYTIC ANEMIA

IMMUNE GLOBULIN INTRAVENOUS (HUMAN) (IVIG)

Anderson D et al. Transfus Med Rev 2007;21 (No. 2, Suppl 1): S9–S56
Centers for Disease Control and Prevention (CDC). MMWR Morb Mortal Wkly Rep 1999;48:518–521
Flores G et al. Am J Hematol 1993;44:237–242
Go RS, Call TG. Mayo Clin Proc 2000;75:83–85
Ratko TA et al. JAMA 1995;273:1865–1870

Hydration prior to immune globulin intravenous (human) (IVIG):
Ensure patients are not dehydrated before IVIG administration. Dehydration is a risk factor for renal failure. Patients who are well hydrated do not need additional hydration

Note: Patients at an increased risk for developing acute renal failure include those with any degree of preexisting renal dysfunction, diabetes, volume depletion, sepsis, paraproteinemia, age >65 years, and those receiving concomitant nephrotoxic drugs. The risk for renal impairment and thrombotic events associated with IVIG also correlate with administration rate, IgG product sucrose content, and product osmolality. The best recommendation is not to exceed the administration recommendations published in product labeling

Immune globulin intravenous (human) 0.4–0.5 g/kg per day; administer intravenously (consult product labeling for appropriate administration rates), daily for 2–5 days
Note: For sucrose-containing products, *do not exceed* a maximum infusion rate of 3 mg sucrose/kg (patient's body weight) per minute

Supportive Care
Folic acid 1 mg/day; administer orally, continually, to prevent depletion of folate stores and megaloblastic anemia resulting from chronic hemolysis

Indications

Ratko TA et al. JAMA 1995;273:1865–1870

A University Hospital Consortium Expert panel on IVIG and AIHA found that:
1. IVIG *may have a role* in patients with warm-type AIHA that does not respond to glucocorticoids
2. Evidence does not exist for the routine use of IVIG in AIHA

Efficacy

(Reports 1983–1987 and 3 case series, N = 62)

Response to therapy	54.5%
Hgb increased >2 g/dL	40%
Hgb increased >2 g/dL + peak Hgb ≥10 g/dL	14.5%
Days to achieve a response	10
Weeks Hgb elevated in responders	≥3

Treatment Modifications

Adverse Event or Condition	Dose Modification
Preexisting renal insufficiency	Decrease the rate of administration during subsequent immune globulin treatments. If permitted, dilute IVIG to decrease its osmolality
Diabetes mellitus	
Age >65 years	
Paraproteinemia	
Concomitant use of nephrotoxic drugs	
Sepsis	
Deteriorating renal function	Discontinue IVIG

Toxicity

Side effects with a frequency of 1–10%:
Infusion reactions*
Back or chest pain or tightness
Malaise and myalgia
Nausea and vomiting
Headache
Fever and chills
Renal damage†

Side effects with a frequency of <1%:
Thrombosis (myocardial infarct, stroke, spinal cord ischemia)
Aseptic meningitis syndrome, with doses ≥2 g/kg

*Fall in blood pressure and anaphylaxis even in patients without a prior history of sensitivity to Immunoglobulins
Note: Contraindications include a history of allergic response to thimerosal, systemic allergic response to gamma globulin or patients with anti-IgA Abs or isolated IgA deficiency
†Increased serum creatinine, oliguria, or renal failure. Ninety percent occurred with sucrose-containing IVIG; 61% with renal predisposing factors; 100% onset in 7 days; 40% required dialysis; 10 days mean recovery time; 15% died despite therapy

Therapy Monitoring

1. *Prior to IVIG:* BUN and serum creatinine
2. *Daily during IVIG administration:* BUN, serum creatinine, weight, and urine output monitoring

Notes

The National Advisory Committee on Blood and Blood Products of Canada and Canadian Blood Services convened a panel of experts on the use of intravenous immunoglobulin (IVIG) for the treatment of hematologic conditions as a basis for recommendations to Provincial Health Ministries (data reviewed from 1982–2004). The following recommendations were made relative to the use of IVIG for AIHA:
• IVIG is not recommended for routine use in either the acute or chronic treatment of AIHA
• IVIG may be considered among treatment options for severe life-threatening AIHA

(Anderson D et al. Transfus Med Rev 2007)

REGIMEN FOR REFRACTORY WARM ANTIBODY AUTOIMMUNE HEMOLYTIC ANEMIA

MYCOPHENOLATE MOFETIL (MMF)

CellCept (mycophenolate mofetil) product label, February 2010. Genentech USA, Inc., South San Francisco, CA
Howard J et al. Br J Haematol 2002;117:712–715
Zimmer-Molsberger B et al. Lancet 1997;350:1003–1004

Starting dose:
Mycophenolate mofetil 1000 mg/day; administer orally as a single dose, or 500 mg twice daily, continually, *or*

Mycophenolate mofetil 1000 mg/day; administer intravenously reconstituted and diluted with 5% dextrose injection (D5W) to a concentration of 6 mg/mL, over at least 2 hours daily, continually (total dose/week = 7000 mg)

Maintenance dose after 2 weeks:
Mycophenolate mofetil 1000 mg/dose; administer orally twice daily, continually

or

Mycophenolate mofetil 1000 mg/dose; administer intravenously reconstituted and diluted with D5W to a concentration of 6 mg/mL, over at least 2 hours twice daily, continually (total dose/week = 14,000 mg)

Supportive Care
Antiemetic prophylaxis
*Emetogenic potential is **MINIMAL** to **MODERATE***
See Chapter 39 for antiemetic recommendations

Hematopoietic growth factor (CSF) prophylaxis
Primary prophylaxis is NOT indicated
See Chapter 43 for more information

Antimicrobial prophylaxis
Risk of fever and neutropenia is LOW
   Antimicrobial primary prophylaxis to be considered:
   • Antibacterial—*Pneumocystis jirovecii* prophylaxis is recommended (eg, cotrimoxazole)
   • Antifungal—not indicated
   • Antiviral—not indicated unless patient previously had an episode of HSV
See Chapter 47 for more information

Folic acid 1 mg/day, orally, continually, to prevent depletion of folate stores and megaloblastic anemia resulting from chronic hemolysis

Toxicity

(Renal, Cardiac, and Hepatic Transplant)*

Toxicity	Incidence
Diarrhea	31–51%
Constipation	22–38%
Leukopenia (dose-related)	23–46%
Nausea	20–55%
Vomiting	33%
Hypertension	32–62 %
Infection	18–27 %
GI bleeding (with hospitalization)	1.7–5.4%
Severe neutropenia ($<500/mm^3$)	2–3.6%
Lymphoma and other malignancies	0.4–1%
Anemia; thrombocytopenia	26–43%; 23–46%
Headache	21–54%
Insomnia	41–52%
Death	2–5%

Risk of acquiring opportunistic infections (bacterial, fungal, viral) and PML increased with MMF

*Patients who received MMF 2000 mg/day or 3000 mg/day (PI); 41 cases of PRCA have been reported: alternative causes present (n = 10), unclear (n = 6), 16/25 cases reversed after dose reduction (n = 4) or discontinuation (n = 12)

Efficacy (N = 6)

	Author	
	Howard et al., 2002	**Zimmer-Molsberger et al., 1997**
Patients M/F	4/0	2/0
Ages, years	31, 52, 50, 74	84, 56
1°/2° AIHA, n	1/3	0/2
Auto-Ab	Present	Present, IgG
Prior Rx (median)	3 (2: prior splenectomy)	1
Regimen	MMF 500 mg PO BID, then 1000 mg PO BID after 2 weeks	MMF 1000 mg/day *then* 2000 mg/day
Hgb ↑ g/dL after MMF	2.1, 3.3, 1.4, 7.6	6, 1 (not stated)
Time to maximum response	4, 6, 9, 1 months	16 weeks, 4 weeks ↓ RBC needs
Treatment duration, months	15+, 6+, 9, 12; Prednisone ± cyclosporine tapered in 3 patients	8+, 1+

1°, primary; 2°, secondary

Treatment Modifications

Adverse Event or Condition	Treatment Modifications
ANC $<1300/mm^3$ estimated GFR <25 mL/min · 1.73 m²	Temporarily interrupt treatment or reduce dose and monitor as appropriate Avoid doses >1000 mg BID

Indications	Therapy Monitoring	Notes
MMF has been administered off-label to limited numbers of patients with 1° (primary) or 2° (secondary) AIHA treated with prior immunosuppressive regimens, including glucocorticoids ± splenectomy. Medications administered concomitantly with MMF have included prednisolone, cyclosporine, and IVIG	1. *CBC with differential:* Weekly during the first month, twice monthly during the second and third month, and then monthly, thereafter, for the first year 2. Periodic history and physical examination and performance of comprehensive metabolic profile as indicated	1. MMF use is recommended for clinicians who are experienced in renal, hepatic, or cardiac transplantation and in the management of immunosuppressive therapy 2. Patients receiving MMF should be instructed to report immediately any evidence of infection, gastrointestinal intolerance (nausea, vomiting, and/or diarrhea), change in neurological status, shortness of breath, unexpected bruising, bleeding, or any other manifestation of bone marrow suppression

REGIMEN FOR (IDIOPATHIC COLD-AGGLUTININ) AUTOIMMUNE HEMOLYTIC ANEMIA

CYTOTOXIC THERAPY
CHLORAMBUCIL

Hippe E et al. Blood 1970;35:68–72
Leukeran (chlorambucil) tablets, product label, November 2006. GlaxoSmithKline, Research Triangle Park, NC
Petz LD. Blood Rev 2008;22:1–15
Petz LD, Garratty G. Blood transfusion in autoimmune hemolytic anemias. In: Petz LD, Garratty G, eds. Immune Hemolytic Anemias. 2nd ed. New York, NY: Churchill Livingstone; 2004:375–400

Chlorambucil 2–4 mg/day, orally, continually, as a starting dose (total dose/week = 14–28 mg)

Notes:

- Increase dose in 2-mg increments every 2 months until a favorable response or dose-limiting toxicity occurs
- With achievement of a favorable response, additional options include intermittent treatment as required or maintenance therapy
- Although doses as high as 8–20 mg/day may be reached, with continued therapy these may have to be reduced to doses as low as 2 mg/day

Supportive Care
Antiemetic prophylaxis
Emetogenic potential is **MINIMAL**
See Chapter 39 for antiemetic recommendations

Hematopoietic growth factor (CSF) prophylaxis
Primary prophylaxis is NOT indicated
See Chapter 43 for more information

Antimicrobial prophylaxis
Risk of fever and neutropenia is LOW
Antimicrobial primary prophylaxis to be considered:
- Antibacterial—not indicated
- Antifungal—not indicated
- Antiviral—not indicated unless patient previously had an episode of HSV
See Chapter 47 for more information

Folic acid 1 mg/day, orally, continually, to prevent depletion of folate stores and megaloblastic anemia resulting from chronic hemolysis

Toxicity

Potential side effects include:
1. Leukopenia
2. Thrombocytopenia
3. Infection
4. Oral ulcers
5. Hypersensitivity and fever
6. Hepatotoxicity
7. Infertility
8. Seizures
9. Gastrointestinal toxicity
10. Interstitial pneumonitis
11. Secondary malignancy
12. Fetal harm (contraception recommended)

Therapy Monitoring

CBC with differential: Twice per week during the first 3–6 weeks of therapy or after a dose adjustment then weekly until counts stabilize and then every 2 weeks

Notes

The intermittent use of chlorambucil has been reported to be beneficial in limited numbers of patients with seasonal precipitation of symptomatic idiopathic CAS where the occupational environment required cold weather exposure. These reports predated clinical experience with agents such as rituximab

Indications

Patients with idiopathic cold agglutinin syndrome producing symptomatic anemia, Raynaud phenomena or cold-intolerance (off-label use)

Efficacy
(N = 15)

(Petz LD, Garratty G. Immune Hemolytic Anemias. 2nd ed. 2004)
Improvement with therapy: 67% (10/15)*

*Including 1 patient who had improvements in acrocyanosis, thermal amplitude, and cold agglutinin titer despite a falling Hgb on therapy

(Hippe E et al. Blood 1970)
Case series of 4 patients with idiopathic cold agglutinin syndrome:

Thermal amplitude:	Decreased a mean of 3.8°C
Hgb values:	Increased from 10.5–12.4 g/dL
IgM mean values:	Decreased from 8.8–2.2 g/dL
Raynaud's phenomena:	Resolved in all patients

Treatment Modifications

Adjust chlorambucil therapy to maintain a "slight degree of marrow suppression" manifested as mild thrombocytopenia or leukopenia
Although a "slight degree of marrow suppression" was not defined further in these studies, consider using NCI CTC* grade 1 toxicity as a reasonable benchmark:
WBC: 3000/mm³ to lower limits of normal
ANC: ≥1500/mm³ to <2000/mm³
Platelets: ≥75,000/mm³ to lower limits of normal
Hemoglobin: 10 g/dL to lower limit of normal

Adverse Event	Dose Modification
If WBC <3000/mm³ or ANC <1500/mm³ or platelets <75,000/mm³	Hold therapy for a minimum of 1 week. Restart only when WBC >3000/mm³ *and* ANC >1500/mm³ *and* platelets >75,000/mm³ *and* then starting with a dosage reduction of 25%

*National Cancer Institute Common Terminology Criteria for Adverse Events

Immune Hemolysis after Transplantation*

Variable	Minor ABO Blood Group iHSCT: Passenger Lymphocyte Syndrome†	Major ABO Blood Group iHSCT: Hemolysis of RBCs in Stem Cell Product	Major ABO Blood Group iHSCT: Hemolysis of RBCs Produced by Engrafted HSCs	Autoimmune Hemolysis after HSCT	RBC Alloantibodies‡ of non-ABO Blood Groups after HSCT Produced by: Engrafted Cells of Donor's Immune System	RBC Alloantibodies‡ of non-ABO Blood Groups after HSCT Produced by: Residual Cells of Recipient's Immune System	Immune Hemolysis with Solid-Organ Transplants
ABO Group or Rh: *-Donor* / *-Recipient*	O (any) / A (any)	O; O; A; B; O / A; B; AB; AB; AB	O; O; A; B; O / A; B; AB; AB; AB	Any / Any	Any (+) / Any (−)	Any (−) / Any (+)	O; O; non-AB / A; B; AB
Serology *-DAT* / *-Ab in serum* / *-Ab in eluate*	IgG ± C3 / anti-A, -B / anti-A, -B	IgM / anti-A, -B / anti-A, -B	IgG / anti-A, -B / anti-A, -B	IgG ± C3 > C3 / anti-Rh > anti-I, -Pr / anti-Rh > anti-I, -Pr	IgG / eg, anti-Rh, -K / eg, anti-Rh, -K	IgG / eg, anti-Rh, -K / eg, anti-Rh, -K	IgG ± C3; C3 / anti-A, -B, -Rh / anti-A, -B, -Rh
Source of Antibodies	Donor B-lymphocytes	Recipient	Recipient	Donor B-lymphocytes	Donor graft	Recipient	Donor B-lymphocytes
Target of Antibodies	Recipient RBCs	Donor RBCs	Donor RBCs	Donor RBCs	Recipient RBCs	Donor RBCs	Recipient RBCs
Pathogenesis of antibody formation	Proliferation and Ab production of "passenger" lymphocytes infused with the stem cell product	ABO incompatibility arising from persistent anti-A or anti-B in recipient plasma	ABO incompatibility arising from persistence of anti-A or anti-B of recipient origin after engraftment (mixed chimerism)	Caused by donor Abs produced against donor RBCs; warm and cold Abs have been reported, including Evan syndrome	Caused by engrafted marrow producing allo-Abs to recipient's original RBCs or transfused RBCs	Caused by residual recipient's immune system in setting of mixed chimerism (by Ig allotyping)	Proliferation and antibody production of "passenger" lymphocytes infused with organ transplanted
Clinical findings / Onset post-transplant / Severity	End of weeks 1–2 (Abs evident by days 5–17); May be severe with rapid onset; self-limiting; may be fatal	Potential of immediate onset; Severity depends on volume of transfused RBCs in iHSCT	With engraftment; transient; ABO Abs usually undetectable by second month	2–25 months (median: 8–10 months); Mild and transient to severe and chronic	May occur by days 45–330; No mild or transient hemolysis	Abs may persist for years; No mild or transient hemolysis	anti-ABO or -Rh Abs by days 3–24; Acute hemolysis, may be mild and self-limited
Treatment (see tables on the selection of blood products for ABO incompatible BMT and organ transplants)	Compatible blood products ± steroids, adequate renal perfusion, ± RBC or plasma exchange	Prevention: removal of RBCs from donor SC product or removal of allohemaglutinins from recipient. Transfuse compatible blood products. Delayed hemolysis is uncommon and is treated with supportive care and transfusion of group O RBCs.		Prednisone, compatible blood transfusion, adequate renal perfusion ± other immunosuppressant	High-titer allo-Abs may produce a (+) DAT and be detected in the recipients serum with the potential for hemolysis. Transfusion of compatible blood products if required; adequate renal perfusion		Compatible blood products often required; adequate renal perfusion; dialysis for renal failure

Ab, Antibody; iHSCT, incompatible hematopoietic stem cell transplant or infusion; SCs, stem cells; HSC, hematopoietic stem cell; Ig, immunoglobulin

*The differential diagnosis also includes other mechanisms for hemolysis: drug-induced IHA; microangiopathic hemolytic anemia; *Clostridium perfringens* septicemia; hemolysis associated with hemodialysis; infusion of: cryopreserved stem cell products, dimethylsulfoxide (DMSO); passive transfer of antibody from plasma products; other etiologies

†"Passenger lymphocyte syndrome after minor ABO blood group iHSCT is most likely to occur when the donor is group O and the patient group A; antibodies other than anti-A and anti-B have been reported (eg, anti-D, anti-E, anti-s, anti-Jk*)

‡One or more alloantibodies may be stimulated by disparities in various non-ABO blood groups: eg, Rh (various), Kell (K), Duffy (Fy), MNS, Lewis (Le), Lutheran (Lu)

Packman CH. Blood Rev 2008;22:17–31
Petz LD. Semin Hematol 2005;42:145–155
Sokol RJ et al. Transfusion 2002;42:198–204
Ting A. Transfusion 1987;27:145–147

Selection of Blood Products: Abo-Incompatible Bone Marrow Transplantation
(from preparative regimen until engraftment)

Recipient	Donor	RBCs	Platelets: First Choice	Platelets: Second Choice*	FFP*
Major incompatible					
O	A	O	A	AB, B, O	A, AB
O	B	O	B	AB, A, O	B, AB
A	AB	A	AB	A, B, O	AB
B	AB	B	AB	B, A, O	AB
O	AB	O	AB	A, B, O	AB
Minor incompatible					
A	O	O	A	AB, B, O	A, AB
B	O	O	B	AB, A, O	B, AB
AB	O	O	AB	A, B, O	AB
AB	A	A	AB	A, B, O	AB
AB	B	B	AB	B, A, O	AB
Major and minor incompatible					
A	B	O	AB	A, B, O	AB
B	A	O	AB	B, A, O	AB

FFP, fresh-frozen plasma; RBCs, red blood cells
Note: Engraftment occurs when forward and reverse types are of donor and the DAT is negative
*Avoid high-titer ABO antibodies
Adapted from Friedberg RC. Hematol Oncol Clin North Am 1994;8:1105–1116

Selection of Blood Products: Recipients of Abo-Mismatched Organs

Recipient ABO	Donor ABO	RBCs	Fresh-Frozen Plasma, Platelets: First Choice*	Platelets: Second Choice†
O	A	O	A, AB	B, O
	B	O	B, AB	A, O
	AB	O	AB	A, B, O
A	O	A, O	A, AB	B, O
	B	A, O	AB	B, A, O
	AB	A, O	AB	A, B, O
B	O	B, O	B, AB	A, O
	A	B, O	AB	A, B, O
	AB	B, O	AB	B, A, O
AB	O	AB, A, B, O	AB	A, B, O
	A	AB, A	AB	A, B, O
	B	AB, B	AB	B, A, O

RBCs, red blood cells
*Preferred ABO choice for platelets in order of preference
†Alternative ABO choice for platelets in order of preference, if the preferred ABO type is not available
Adapted from Petz L, Caljoun L. Preparation for blood and blood product replacement. In: Busuttil RW , Klintmaim GB, eds. Transplantation of the Liver. Philadelphia, PA: WB Saunders; 1998:442–448

61. Sickle Cell Disease: Acute Complications

James N. Frame, MD, FACP and Griffin P. Rodgers, MD, MACP

Individuals are diagnosed with sickle cell disease (SCD) if they have one of several genotypes that result in at least half of their hemoglobin (Hgb) being Hgb S. Sickle cell anemia (SCA) refers to the condition associated with homozygosity for the Hgb S mutation (Hgb SS). Other Hgb mutations may occur with Hgb S causing a similar but milder condition. In SCA, the presence of intracellular hemoglobin S polymerization leads to chronic hemolytic anemia, vasoocclusive crises of varying severity and frequency with cumulative organ damage and systemic manifestations that include impairment in growth and development, susceptibility to infection, and reduced quality and duration of life

Segal JB et al. Hydroxyurea for the Treatment of Sickle Cell Disease. Rockville, MD: Agency for Healthcare Research and Quality, 2008 Feb. Report No. 08-E007

Epidemiology

Incidence

Worldwide (SCD):	Millions
United States (SCD):	~1 in 500 African American births (~72,000)
	1 in 1000–1400 Hispanic babies each year
United States (Sickle cell trait):	1 in 12 African Americans (~2 million people)

Mortality*

U.S. median life expectancy for Hgb SS/SC males	42 years/60 years
U.S. median life expectancy for Hgb SS/SC females	48 years/68 years

*Mortality reductions have been attributed to several factors: development of sickle cell treatment programs, increased clinical research in sickle cell disease (SCD), and establishment of newborn screening programs coupled with penicillin prophylaxis

Platt OS et al. N Engl J Med 1994;330:1639–1644 (3764 patients. followed to determine life expectancy) Sickle Cell Research for Treatment and Cure. Bethesda, MD: NIH Publication No. 02-5214;2002:1–16 Dept. of Energy, Human Genome Project. www.nhlbi .nih.gov/resources/docs/scd30/scd30.pdf [accessed August 5, 2013]

Major Sickle Hemoglobinopathies: Laboratory Features

	Common Hematologic Findings in Adults					
				Percent of Hemoglobin		
Disorder	Percent*	MCV(fL)	Hgb (g/dL)	Hgb A/A$_2$	Hgb F	Hgb S
SCD-SS	65	80–100	6–10	0/2–3	2–15	>85
SCD-SC	25	75–90	10–12	0/0	1–7	50[†]
SCD-S β$^+$ thalassemia	8	65–75	8–12	5–30/3–6	2–10	70–90
SCD-S β-thalassemia	2	65–85	6–10	0/4–6	2–15	>85
SCD-S δβ thalassemia	<1	60–80	10–12	0/N-low[‡]	10–15	>80
S-HPFH pancellular	<1	80–90	12–13[§]	0/1–3	20–30	>70

*Approximate percent of U.S. patients determined by neonatal screening
[†]50% Hgb C
[‡]Hgb A$_2$ normal to low
[§]Hct 38–40%

Adams JG 3rd. Clinical laboratory diagnosis. In: Embury SH et al., eds. Sickle Cell Disease: Basic Principles and Clinical Practice. New York, NY: Raven Press; 1994:457–468
Bunn HF, Forget BG. Sickle cell disease—clinical and epidemiologic aspects. In: Hemoglobin: Molecular, Genetic and Clinical Aspects. Philadelphia, PA: WB Saunders; 1986:502–564
Glader BE. Anemia. In: Embury SH et al., eds. Sickle Cell Disease: Basic Principles and Clinical Practice. New York, NY: Raven Press; 1994:545–554
Kinney TR et al. Br J Haematol 1978;38:15–22
Murray N et al. Br J Haematol 1988;69:89–92

The Management of Sickle Cell Disease, 4th ed. NIH Publication No. 02-2117. Bethesda, MD: National Institutes of Health, National Heart, Lung, and Blood Institute, Division of Blood Diseases and Resources; 2002. www.nhlbi.nih.gov/health/prof/blood/sickle/sc_mngt.pdf [accessed August 5, 2013]

Acute Pain Syndrome

1. Most common type of pain
2. Unpredictably abrupt in onset
3. Sometimes migratory
4. Varies in intensity from a mild ache to a severe and debilitating pain
5. Acute pain may occur with chronic pain and frequent episodes of acute pain can resemble chronic pain
6. In adults, about one-third of episodes are associated with a preceding or concurrent infection
7. Factors that potentiate Hgb S polymerization may precipitate an acute painful episode. These factors include acidosis, hypoxia, and dehydration

Chronic pain
1. Caused by obvious pathophysiology (eg, leg ulcers, avascular necrosis, chronic osteomyelitis)
2. Intractable chronic pain with no obvious sign

Ballas SK. Current issues in sickle cell pain and its management. Hematology Am Soc Hematol Educ Program. 2007:97–105
Ballas SK. Semin Hematol 2001;38:307–314
Benjamin LJ et al. Guideline for the Management of Acute and Chronic Pain in Sickle-Cell Disease, APS Clinical Practice Guidelines Series, No. 1. Glenview, IL: American Pain Society; 1999:1–98
Castro O et al. Blood 1994;84:643–649
Rees DC et al. Br J Haematol 2003;120:744–752
The Management of Sickle Cell Disease, 4th ed. NIH Publication No. 02-2117. Bethesda, MD: National Institutes of Health, National Heart, Lung, and Blood Institute, Division of Blood Diseases and Resources; 2002. www.nhlbi.nih.gov/health/prof/blood/sickle/sc_mngt.pdf [accessed August 5, 2013]

Epidemiology

1. In SCD, pain is the most common complaint and reason for patients to consult doctors and to be admitted to the hospital
2. Among patients with SCD in the United States, an acute pain episode accounts for ~90% of visits to the ER and 70% of all hospitalizations
3. Mean rate per year of acute pain episodes
   Hgb SS (0.8)
   Hgb Sβ-thalassemia (1.0)
   Hgb SC (0.4)
4. The rate of painful crises increases over the first 3 decades of life and then declines as a consequence of the earlier mortality of adults with higher rates of pain

Treatment

Initial management of severe acute pain in the emergency department (ED)
1. **Arrival at ED to time +15–20 minutes after arrival**
   a. Assess for common SCD acute pain states
   b. Determine pain type (onset, duration, frequency)
      (1) *Pain is atypical for SCD:* Determine related symptoms (look for infections, complication, other comorbidities and precipitating factors). Next, assess pain, treat, and conduct work-up to determine etiology
      (2) *Pain is typical for SCD:* See next step
   c. Determine pain characteristics (intensity, location, and quality based on self-report)
      (1) Assess self-reported pain with an instrument such as a visual analog scale (VAS), Wong-Baker Faces Pain Rating Scale, or a simple verbal descriptor scale (0–10 scale; 0 = none, 10 = worst imaginable)
   d. Obtain treatment history (home meds, acute pain, hospital care, meds in past 24 hours, out-of-home meds)
   e. Examine pertinent physical factors
   f. Summarize assessment of profile and select treatment (based on characteristics of episode, prior treatment history, and physical findings)
      (1) *Not on chronic opioid therapy:* Start IV loading dose of short-acting opioid (eg, morphine or hydromorphone; see Table 61-1 for opioid dosages)
      (2) *On chronic opioid therapy:* Select medication and loading dose based on overall assessment and prior treatment history. Patient and family often know what medications and dosage have been effective in the past. Next, start IV loading dose of short-acting opioid. Administer SC if insufficient venous access
      (3) Begin IV hydration (see Acute Pain Syndrome, Notes Section)
2. **Time +15–30 minutes after ED arrival**
   a. Add combination therapy as indicated (eg, antiinflammatory and or antihistamine to improve response to therapy). See Acute Pain Syndrome Notes
   b. Assess degree of pain relief every 15–30 minutes; use a pain relief scale to assess response (eg, 0 = none, 1 = little; 2 = moderate; 3 = good; 4 = complete)
3. **Time +30 minutes to +2–8 hours after ED arrival**
   a. Assess pain relief every 15–30 minutes. If no pain relief achieved, administer one-quarter to one-half of initial loading dose of opioid to relief (see Table 61-1) with coanalgesic (see Acute Pain Syndrome, Notes Section, number 4)
   b. Admit to hospital if complications, treatment ineffective, or oral therapy cannot be maintained
   c. Discharge in absence of above admission criteria on oral analgesics to maintain adequate pain relief and refer to managing clinician

Notes

1. **Major barriers to effective pain management**

   (a) Clinicians' limited knowledge of SCD; (b) inadequate assessment of pain; (c) bias against opioid use; (d) inadequate understanding about opioid tolerance, physical dependence, and addiction; (e) unwarranted fear of addiction among patients and families

2. **Tolerance, physical dependence, addiction**

   (a) *Tolerance:* A physiologic response to opioid administration, the first sign of which is decreased duration of medication action. Larger doses or shorter intervals may be needed to achieve the same analgesic effect; (b) *physical dependence:* a physiologic response to opioid administration that requires no treatment unless withdrawal symptoms occur or are anticipated; (c) *addiction:* a psychological dependence with genetic, psychological, and social roots. Consultation with appropriate specialists in substance abuse is recommended. Estimates of the risk of addiction with opioid therapy in SCD appears to parallel that observed in the community at-large (Solomon LR. Blood 2008;111: 997–1003); (d) *pseudoaddiction:* is the seeking of additional medication because of undertreatment of pain

3. **Hydration.** (a) There is theoretical and empirical evidence that rehydration with a hypotonic solution (5% dextrose injection [D5W] or 5% dextrose/0.2% sodium chloride injection [D5W/¼NS]), unless contraindicated (eg, brain injury, severe hyponatremia, etc.), is preferable. Such therapy has been shown to swell red cells, reduce the MCHC and thereby reduce the rate and extent of intracellular Hgb S polymerization. (Rosa M et al. A study of induced hyponatremia in the prevention and treatment of sickle-cell crisis. N Engl J Med 1980;303:1138–1143.) (b) The Management of Sickle Cell Disease Guidelines (2002) recommends the use of 5% dextrose with 0.45% sodium chloride injection (D5W1/2NS) plus 20 mEq KCl/L adjusted for serum chemistry results given at a rate not exceeding 1.5 times maintenance (including volume for drug infusions)

4. **Hypovolemia should be corrected prior to the administration of ketorolac** and NSAIDs should be used with caution in patients with CHF, dehydration, hypovolemia, or any other condition that may compromise renal blood flow and increase the risk of developing renal toxicity. Ketorolac should be used with caution in patients with impaired hepatic function or a history of liver disease

   a. **Ketorolac is contraindicated in patients with:** (1) active peptic ulcer disease (PUD); (2) recent GI bleeding or perforation; (3) a history of PUD or GI bleeding; (4) advanced renal impairment or at risk for renal failure caused by volume depletion; (5) previously demonstrated hypersensitivity to ketorolac, other NSAIDs, or aspirin, or patients currently receiving aspirin or NSAIDs; and (6) suspected or confirmed cerebrovascular bleed, hemorrhagic diathesis, or incomplete hemostasis. Ketorolac should not be used in nursing mothers

   b. **Antiinflammatory medications, for example:**

      Ketorolac

      - *Multiple-dose treatment; adults <65 years old:* **Ketorolac** 30 mg; administer intravenously over at least 15 seconds or slowly by deep intramuscular injection every 6 hours (maximum daily dose = 120 mg)

      - *≥65 Years old, weight <50 kg, or renally impaired patients (see manufacturer's warnings):* **Ketorolac** 15 mg; administer intravenously over at least 15 seconds or by slow deep intramuscular injection every 6 hours (maximum daily parenteral dose = 60 mg)

   c. **Ketorolac (transition from IV/IM to oral)**

      - *<65 Years old:* **Ketorolac** 20 mg; administer orally initially, followed by 10 mg every 4–6 hours (maximum dose not to exceed 40 mg/24 hours)

      - *≥65 Years old, weight <50 kg, or renally impaired patients (see manufacturer's warnings):* **Ketorolac** 10 mg; administer orally every 4–6 hours (maximum dose not to exceed 40 mg/24 hours)

   Note: In adults, the maximum combined duration of ketorolac use (parenteral and oral) is limited to 5 days. The use of an H$_2$-blocker has been recommended to reduce GI side effects

   (See Perlin E et al. Am J Hematol 1994;46:43–47)

5. **Chronic hemolysis.** Routine supportive treatment should include folic acid 1 mg/day administered orally (Pearson HA, Cobb WT. J Lab Clin Med 1964;64:913–921)

Subacute management

1. *Moderate pain relief, acceptable toxicities:* Begin opioid analgesics on an around-the-clock (ATC) schedule (see Tables 61-1 and 61-2)

2. *Moderate pain relief, toxicities not acceptable:* Add **combination therapy** to include antiinflammatory medications; for example, **ibuprofen** 400–600 mg; administer orally every 6 hours (consider adding an H$_2$-blocker to reduce risk of GI side effects)

3. *Moderate pain relief not achieved:* Continue to adjust therapy by increasing the dose until pain is relieved. Increase dose in increments of 25–50% of the opioid analgesic loading dose

Table 61–1. Usual Starting Dosages for Moderate-to-Severe Pain in Sickle Cell Disease

	Opioid-Naïve Adults and Children*			
Medication	**Weight <50 kg**		**Weight ≥50 kg**	
Short-Acting Opioid Agonists†	Oral	Parenteral	Oral	Parenteral
Morphine immediate release‡	0.3 mg/kg q3–4h	0.1–0.15 mg/kg q2–4h	10–30 mg q3–4h	5–10 mg q2–4h
Hydromorphone‡ (Dilaudid)	0.06–0.08 mg/kg q3–4h	0.015–0.020 mg/kg q3–4h	7.5 mg q3–4h	1.5 mg q3–4h
Meperidine (Demerol)	NR; 1.1–1.75 mg/kg q3–4h only if deemed to be necessary after evaluation	NR; 0.75-1.0 mg/kg, 1.1–1.75 mg/kg q.3-4 h only if deemed necessary after evaluation	NR; 50–150 mg q3–4h only if deemed to be necessary after evaluation	NR; 50–150 mg every 3 hours only if deemed to be necessary after evaluation
Codeine^ϵ	—	—	15–60 mg q3–6h	N/A
Combination Opioid/ NSAID Preparations**	Oral	Parenteral	Oral	Parenteral
Codeine (with aspirin or acetaminophen)	0.5–1.0 mg/kg (codeine component) q3–4h	NR	60 mg (codeine component) q3–4h	N/A
Hydrocodone (in Lorcet, Vicodin, others)	0.15–0.20 mg/kg (hydrocodone component) q3–4h	N/A	10 mg (hydrocodone component) q3–4h	N/A
Oxycodone (in Roxicodone, Percocet, Percodan, Tylox, others)	0.15–0.20 mg/kg (oxycodone component) q3–4h	N/A	10 mg (oxycodone component) q4–6h	N/A
Long-Acting Opioid Agonists (controlled-release morphine or oxycodone, levorphanol, methadone)	• Because it is not possible to determine the appropriate starting dose of controlled-release opioids without knowing the patient's opioid requirements as determined by immediate-release preparation, usual starting doses are not listed for these medications • See chapter 52 on Cancer Pain for equianalgesic dose conversions between oral and parenteral opioid agonist preparations and for conversions between oral immediate-release and controlled-release opioid agonist preparations			

h, Hour; N/A, not available; NR, not recommended; q, every

Caution: Doses listed for body weight <50 kg cannot be used as initial starting doses in babies <6 months of age

†*Caution:* Recommended doses do not apply to patients with renal or hepatic insufficiency or other conditions that may affect pharmacokinetic behavior

‡*Caution:* For morphine and hydromorphone, rectal administration is an alternate route for patients unable to take oral medications, but equianalgesic doses differ from oral and parenteral routes primarily because of variable absorption after rectal administration both within and among patients

§There is general agreement that oral meperidine should not be used for acute or chronic pain and the parenteral use of meperidine for acute sickle pain is controversial. Chronic administration of meperidine may results in CNS stimulation: agitation, irritability, nervousness, tremors, myoclonic twitches, or seizures caused by accumulation of its neuroexcitatory metabolite, normeperidine. Meperidine should be reserved for brief use in patients who have benefited, or for patients with allergies or who are intolerant of other opioids, such as morphine and hydromorphone. Meperidine should not be used for more than 48 hours or at doses >600 mg/24 hours. **Meperidine is contraindicated for patients with impaired renal function and persons using monoamine oxidase inhibitor antidepressants**

ϵ*Caution:* Codeine doses >65 mg often are not appropriate because of diminishing incremental analgesia with increasing doses, but continually increasing nausea, constipation, and other side effects

***Caution:* Total doses of acetaminophen >4 g/day may be associated with hepatic toxicity. Aspirin is contraindicated in children in the presence of fever or viral disease because of its association with Reye syndrome

Note: Equianalgesic doses are approximations and recommendations for equivalent analgesia among opioid drugs vary among published tables. Pharmacodynamic responses are the criteria that must be applied for each patient; titration to clinical responses is necessary. Because cross-tolerance is not complete among opioid drugs, it is usually necessary to use less than an estimated equianalgesic dose when changing administration routes or replacing or combining opioid drugs and then retitrate to an optimal analgesic response

Benjamin LJ et al. Guideline for the Management of Acute and Chronic Pain in Sickle-Cell Disease. APS Clinical Practice Guidelines Series, No. 1. Glenview, IL: American Pain Society; 1999:31–32

The Management of Sickle Cell Disease, 4th ed. NIH Publication No. 02-2117. Bethesda, MD: National Institutes of Health, National Heart, Lung, and Blood Institute, Division of Blood Diseases and Resources; 2002. www.nhlbi.nih.gov/health/prof/blood/sickle/sc_mngt.pdf [accessed August 5, 2013]

Table 61–2. Opioid Side Effects and Their Treatment (Adults)

Side Effect	Frequency of Occurrence	Treatment
Sedation	Common	Decrease opioid dose if pain control can be achieved with less drug, or give lower doses of opioid more frequently to decrease peak concentration Consider changing opioid Consider addition of **caffeine** 100–200 mg orally q6h *or* **methylphenidate** 5–10 mg orally 1–3 times per day Assess for other causes of sedation (eg, hypoxia, dehydration, other sedating medications)
Nausea	Common	*Prevention:* Prescribe antiemetics with opioid prescription Consider **prochlorperazine** 10 mg orally q6h PRN **metoclopramide** 10–20 mg orally q6h PRN, or **thiethylperazine** 10 mg orally q6h PRN *Treatment:* Confirm whether and how PRN antiemetics are being used. If nausea persists despite appropriate use, consider **ondansetron** 8 mg orally TID for 1 week (use with caution as constipation is a side effect); consider oral disintegrating tablets or IV route if oral route is not tolerated
Pruritus	Common	**Hydroxyzine** 25–50 mg administer intramuscularly or orally q6h **Diphenhydramine** 25–50 mg IV or orally q6h **Promethazine** 12.5–25 mg IV (*must be* diluted for administration by IV infusion only via peripheral vascular access) or orally q6h **Naloxone** by continuous IV infusion at 0.25 mcg/kg per hour and titrate up to 1 mcg/kg per hour for relief of pruritus without decreasing analgesic effectiveness Consider change to another opioid if symptomatic management has failed
Constipation	Variable	*Prevention:* Provide a bowel prophylaxis regimen when initiating opioid use, based initially on stool softeners (eg, **docusate sodium** 100–300 mg/dose orally 1–3 times daily; **senna with docusate sodium** 2 tablets orally q am). Increase doses, frequency of use, or both when increasing opioid doses Encourage increased hydration and fiber intake Encourage patients to exercise, if feasible *Treatment:* For constipation, consider cause and severity; treat other causes if identified. Titrate medication doses with a goal of one unforced bowel movement every 1–2 days Consider: **Magnesium hydroxide** 30–60 mL/dose orally; **bisacodyl** 10–15 mg orally; **glycerin rectal suppository**, rectally; **lactulose** 30–60 mL/dose orally; **polyethylene glycol** 17 g (1 measuring capful)/dose in 8 oz. of water, orally; **magnesium citrate** 8 oz. orally; **Fleets or tap water enema**, rectally Consider promotility agent: **Metoclopramide** 10–20 mg orally QID
Dysphoria	Occasional	Adjust opioid doses or change opioid; consider nonopioid analgesics to supplement analgesia and decrease opioid doses
Respiratory depression (respiratory rate <10/min) or acute change in mental status	Uncommon in the setting of acute pain	Use reversal agents cautiously. Dilute 1 mL **naloxone** (0.4 mg/mL) in 9 mL 0.9% sodium chloride injection to produce a concentration = 0.04 mg/mL, administer 1–2 mL (0.04–0.08 mg) by intravenous injection every 30–60 seconds until improvement in symptoms. Be prepared to repeat the process. If patient is not responsive within 10 minutes after administering a total naloxone dose of 1 mg, consider other causes for changes in mental status *Additional monitoring interventions:* Pulse oximetry, apnea monitor, arterial blood gas (as needed)

Adapted in part from Adult cancer pain. Version 1. 2008. Management of opioid side effects. NCCN Clinical Practice Guidelines in Oncology (serial online) 2008. Available from: www.nccn.org (accessed March 1, 2009)

Benjamin LJ et al. Guideline for the Management of Acute and Chronic Pain in Sickle-Cell Disease. APS Clinical Practice Guidelines Series, No. 1. Glenview, IL: American Pain Society; 1999:29

Acute Chest Syndrome

Multicenter Acute Chest Syndrome Study (MACSS) definition: A pulmonary infiltrate consistent with consolidation, plus at least *1 of the following:*
- Chest pain
- Fever >38.5°C (>101.3°F)
- Tachypnea
- Wheezing
- Cough

Associated conditions:
- Pulmonary infarction (30%)
- Pulmonary fat embolization (16%)
- Infection (33%) including chlamydia (13%), mycoplasma (12%), viruses (12%), and bacterial isolates (8%) which included *Staphylococcus aureus*, *Streptococcus pneumoniae*, and *Haemophilus influenzae*

Ballas SK. Semin Hematol 2001;38:307–314
Bellet PS et al. N Engl J Med 1995;333:699–703
Charache A et al. N Engl J Med 1995;332:1317–1322
Emre U et al. J Pediatr 1993;123:272–275
Lacy CF et al., eds. Albuterol. In: Drug Information Handbook 2011. 20th ed. Hudson, OH: Lexi-Comp; 2011:49–51
Rosse WF et al. New views of sickle cell disease pathophysiology and treatment. Hematology Am Soc Hematol Educ Program 2000:2–17
The Management of Sickle Cell Disease, 4th ed. NIH Publication No. 02-2117. Bethesda, MD: National Institutes of Health, National Heart, Lung, and Blood Institute, Division of Blood Diseases and Resources; 2002. www.nhlbi.nih.gov/health/prof/blood/sickle/sc_mngt.pdf [accessed August 5, 2013]
Vichinsky EP et al. N Engl J Med 2000; 342:1855–1865

Epidemiology

1. Second most common cause of hospitalization in SCD
2. Most common complication of surgery and anesthesia
3. Incidence (per 100 patient-years):
   Hgb SS overall (12.8)
   Hgb SS ages 2–4 years (25.3)
   Hgb SS adults (8.8)
   Hgb Sβ-thalassemia (9.4)
   Hgb SC (5.2)
   Hgb Sβ$^+$ thalassemia (3.9)
4. In-hospital mortality:
   9% for adults
   <2% for children

Treatment

Carefully monitor oxygenation, hydration, and acid–base balance. Obtain daily weight, input/output, CBC, and appropriate serum chemistry panels. Measure baseline and pre-/posttransfusion Hgb S concentration. Follow CXR until stabilization is documented

Therapy:
1. **Oxygen**, by nasal cannula at a rate of 2 L/min or greater if needed to maintain a PaO_2 of 70–80 mm Hg (or oxygen saturation of ≥90%)
2. **Hydration** with 5% dextrose injection (D5W) or 5% dextrose/0.2% sodium chloride injection (D5W/¼NS) at a rate not to exceed 1.5 times maintenance (volume to include any drug infusions); also refer to Acute Pain Syndrome, Notes Section
3. Bronchodilator therapy for adults exacerbation of asthma (acute, severe):
   a. Albuterol nebulizer solution (5 mg/mL), administer 2.5–5 mg by nebulizer every 20 minutes up to 3 doses, followed by 2.5–10 mg every 1–4 hours as needed or 10–15 mg/hour by continuous nebulization. (For adults with bronchospasm, albuterol nebulizer solution [5 mg/mL], administer 2.5 mg 3–4 times daily as needed)
   b. Albuterol metered-dose inhaler (90 mcg/puff), administer 4–8 puffs every 20 minutes for up to 4 hours, then every 1–4 hours as needed. (For adults with bronchospasm, 2 puffs every 4–6 hours for quick relief)
4. **Institute opioids or other analgesic therapy** to prevent hypoventilation (see the Acute Pain Syndrome section)
5. **Incentive spirometry** protocol to prevent hypoventilation in patients able to perform it
6. **Transfuse packed RBCs** to achieve a Hgb S concentration <30–40%, or to a stable Hgb of 8–9 g/dL (see the section Red Blood Cell Transfusion)

Indications:
- Poor respiratory function
- PaO_2 <70 mm Hg on room air
- A decline in PaO_2 >10% from baseline in a patient with chronic hypoxia

Note: Exchange transfusion should be undertaken in patients with a high baseline Hgb in whom transfusion of RBCs is recommended (eg, goal to reduce the Hct to <30%), signs of increasing infiltrate on CXR, if the arterial PO_2 cannot be maintained above 70 Torr or if the patient is experiencing dyspnea or tachypnea (also see the section Red Blood Cell Transfusion)

Antibiotics should be given to febrile or severely ill patients. This should include:

A **third-generation cephalosporin:**
Ceftriaxone 1000 mg (maximum, 2000 mg); administer intravenously in 50–100 mL 5% dextrose injection (D5W) over 30 minutes every 24 hours, *and*

A **broad-spectrum macrolide or fluoroquinolone antibiotic:**
Azithromycin 500 mg; administer intravenously in 250–500 mL D5W over 60 minutes every 24 hours, *or*
Ciprofloxacin 400 mg; administer intravenously in 200 mL D5W over 60 minutes every 12 hours

Notes

1. Assess baseline oxygenation and continue to monitor ABGs as needed. The A-a gradient appears to be the best predictor of clinical severity

2. Limit hydration. Avoid fluid overload

3. Incentive spirometry is encouraged since it reduces the risk of ACS by 88% in patients hospitalized with thoracic bone ischemia/infarction

4. In 2010, a Cochrane Collaboration study was performed to assess the benefits and risks associated with the use of bronchodilators in sickle cell disease patients with acute chest syndrome. This study found no trials investigating the use of bronchodilators for acute chest syndrome in people with sickle cell disease. The authors' conclusions stated "if bronchial hyper-responsiveness is an important component of some episodes of acute chest syndrome in people with sickle cell disease, the use of inhaled bronchodilators may be indicated." Recommendations were proposed for well-designed, adequately powered randomized controlled trials to assess the risk and benefits of this treatment in patients with SSD acute chest syndrome. (Knight-Madden JM, Hambleton IR. Inhaled bronchodilators for acute chest syndrome in people with sickle cell disease (review). Cochrane Database Syst Rev 2010 Jul 11;CD003733. Available at: http://onlinelibrary.wiley.com/doi/10.1002/14651858.CD003733.pub2/abstract [accessed August 5, 2013])

5. Goal of transfusion therapy is to prevent progression of acute chest syndrome (ACS) to acute respiratory failure. Transfusions may not be required if the decline in A-a gradient is due to chest wall splinting that corrects with adequate analgesic therapy and incentive spirometry

6. Infection is a contributing factor as cause of death in 56% of ACS patients. Organisms include *Streptococcus pneumoniae*, *Escherichia coli*, *Haemophilus influenzae*, legionella, *Staphylococcus aureus*, cytomegalovirus, and chlamydia as well as atypical microorganisms (eg, *Chlamydia pneumoniae*, *Mycoplasma pneumoniae*)

7. In ACS patients it is often difficult to exclude a bacterial superinfection from a lung infarct

Acute Cholecystitis

Gilbert DN et al., eds. Gallbladder (cholecystitis). In: The Sanford Guide To Antimicrobial Therapy 2011, 41st ed. Speeryville, VA: Antimicrobial Therapy, Inc.; 2011:15
Nzeh DA et al. Pediatr Radiol 1989;19:290–292
The Management of Sickle Cell Disease, 4th ed. NIH Publication No. 02-2117. Bethesda, MD: National Institutes of Health, National Heart, Lung, and Blood Institute, Division of Blood Diseases and Resources; 2002. www.nhlbi.nih.gov/health/prof/blood/sickle/sc_mngt.pdf [accessed August 5, 2013]
Walker TM et al. J Pediatr 2000;135:80–85

Epidemiology

1. Cholelithiasis occurs as early as 2–4 years of age; incidence progressively increases with age; $\approx$30% of 18-year-old patients have cholelithiasis

2. Acute attacks of cholecystitis are difficult to differentiate from hepatic crisis. Biliary scintigraphy may be helpful in differentiating acute cholecystitis from sickle hepatic crisis but is not always diagnostic (D'Alonzo WA Jr, Heyman S. Pediatr Radiol 1985;15:395–398)

3. The natural history of asymptomatic cholelithiasis is unknown; however, up to 30% of patients may develop symptoms or complications within 3 years. The prevalence of cholelithiasis appears to be lower in patients co-inheriting α-or β-thalassemia

4. Patients with sickle cell trait have no increased risk of developing pigment stones

Treatment

The treatment of acute cholecystitis is similar to that of the general population

Therapy:

Hydration (as clinically indicated) with 5% dextrose injection (D5W) or 5% dextrose/0.2% sodium chloride injection (D5W/¼NS) at a rate not to exceed 1.5 times maintenance (volume to include any drug infusions). Also, refer to Acute Pain Syndrome, Notes Section

1. **Institute opioids or other analgesic therapy** as appropriate based on clinical symptoms with superimposed vasoocclusive crises (see the section Acute Pain Syndrome)

2. Antimicrobial therapy including

   Piperacillin sodium 3000 mg **+ tazobactam sodium** 375 mg; administer intravenously in 50–150 mL D5W or 0.9% sodium chloride injection (0.9% NS) over 20–30 minutes every 6 hours, *or*

   Imipenem 500 mg/**cilastatin** 500 mg; administer intravenously in 50–100 mL D5W or 0.9% NS over 20–60 minutes every 6 hours (if life-threatening)

3. **Elective cholecystectomy** is recommended several weeks after an acute episode subsides, given the greater operative risks during an episode of acute cholecystitis in SCD

Note:

• Although cholecystectomy in asymptomatic patients is controversial, an aggressive surgical approach has the benefit of reducing the risk of complications arising from cholecystitis and eliminating the gallbladder as a confounding diagnosis in RUQ pain (eg, sickle cell hepatic crises)

• Laparoscopic cholecystectomy on an elective basis in a well-prepared patient has been reported to be the standard surgical approach to symptomatic patients but does not reduce the risk of sickle cell-related complications as compared with open cholecystectomy

Acute Hepatic Sequestration (Right Upper Quadrant Syndrome)

Characterized by:

a. RUQ pain simulating acute cholecystitis

b. Fever

c. Jaundice

d. Elevations in hepatic transaminases

e. Marked elevations in serum bilirubin/ alkaline phosphatase

f. Progressive hepatomegaly

Note: The rapid decrease in transaminases with treatment differentiates hepatic crisis from the slower decline characteristic of acute viral hepatitis

Halton CS. Hepatic sequestration in sickle cell disease. BMJ 1985;290(6740):744

Rosse WF et al. New views of sickle cell disease: pathophysiology and treatment. Hematology Am Soc Hematol Educ Program. 2000:2–17

The Management of Sickle Cell Disease, 4th ed. NIH Publication No. 02-2117. Bethesda, MD: National Institutes of Health, National Heart, Lung, and Blood Institute, Division of Blood Diseases and Resources; 2002. www.nhlbi.nih.gov/health/prof/blood/sickle/ sc_mngt.pdf [accessed August 5, 2013]

Epidemiology

1. A rarely recognized complication of vaso-occlusive crisis in SCD

2. Prevalence in SCD is not well described

3. Approximately 10% of Hgb SS patients develop a transient and less-severe form of intrahepatic cholestasis that is usually self-limited

Treatment

Carefully monitor oxygenation, hydration, and acid–base balance. Obtain daily weight, input/output, CBC, and appropriate serum chemistry panels. Measure baseline and pre-/ posttransfusion Hgb S concentration

1. **Hydration** with 5% dextrose injection (D5W) or 5% dextrose/0.2% sodium chloride injection (D5W/¼NS) at a rate not to exceed 1.5 times maintenance (volume to include any drug infusions)

   Note: In the event of hypervolemia, the administration of diuretic therapy may be required. Also, refer to Acute Pain Syndrome, Notes Section

2. **Oxygen** by nasal cannula at a rate of 2 L/min or greater, if needed to maintain a PaO_2 of 70–80 mm Hg

3. **Institute opioids or other analgesic therapy** based on clinical symptoms (see the section Acute Pain Syndrome)

4. **Transfuse** packed RBCs to maintain Hgb close to baseline and Hgb S <30%

   Note:

   1. Exchange transfusion is the preferred method of transfusion although simple transfusion may be considered

   2. Fatal hyperviscosity syndrome may result from simple transfusion as an episode of hepatic sequestration resolves. A spontaneous and rapid increase in the serum hemoglobin from sequestered RBCs ("reverse sequestration") accounts for this clinical finding. Patients should be carefully monitored in the recovery phase of acute hepatic sequestration for an acutely rising Hgb that could place the patient at risk for hyperviscosity. If suspected, promptly institute exchange transfusion with a goal of reducing the Hct to <30% (also see the section Acute Splenic Sequestration: Hyperviscosity)

Notes

1. *Differential diagnosis of RUQ syndrome in a patient with a sickle cell disease who presents with RUQ pain and abnormal LFTs includes:* Acute cholecystitis, intrahepatic cholestasis, acute viral hepatitis, biloma, focal nodular hyperplasia in children, fungal ball, hepatic artery stenosis, hepatic infarct/abscess, hepatic vein thrombosis, mesenteric/colonic ischemia, pancreatitis, periappendiceal abscess, pericolonic abscess, pulmonary infarct/abscess, renal vein thrombosis

2. Patients should be taught to regularly monitor their liver size (and spleen size, especially in younger children and in adults coinheriting α-thalassemia who are at risk for acute splenic sequestration) in an effort to identify acute hepatic sequestration in its early stages

Acute Splenic Sequestration

1. Acutely enlarging spleen
2. Decrease in steady state Hgb concentration by at least 2 g/dL and evidence of increased erythropoiesis (eg, marked elevations in the reticulocyte count or nucleated RBCs)
3. In more severe episodes, hypovolemic shock may complicate precipitous drops in Hgb with marked splenic enlargement

Glader BE. Anemia. In: Embury SH et al., eds. Sickle Cell Disease: Basic Principles and Clinical Practice. New York, NY: Raven Press; 1994:545–554
Rosse WF et al. New views of sickle cell disease: pathophysiology and treatment. Hematology Am Soc Hematol Educ Program. 2000:2–17
Solanki DL et al. Am J Med 1986;80:985–990
The Management of Sickle Cell Disease, 4th ed. NIH Publication No. 02-2117. Bethesda, MD: National Institutes of Health, National Heart, Lung, and Blood Institute, Division of Blood Diseases and Resources; 2002. www.nhlbi.nih.gov/health/prof/blood/sickle/sc_mngt.pdf [accessed August 5, 2013]

Epidemiology

1. Majority of cases occur in children with Hgb SS before 2 years of age with almost all by age 6 years
2. Attacks may be associated with or preceded by bacterial or viral infections
3. Acute chest syndrome has been reported to complicate acute splenic syndrome in 20% of cases
4. Occurs less frequently in Hgb SC and Hgb S β$^+$-thalassemia disease, but may occur beyond childhood because of persistent splenomegaly
5. Occurrence in adults is rare, but may occur with persistent splenic function in patients with concurrent α-thalassemia
6. A mortality rate of 12% has been reported with first attacks in SCD-SS (Hgb SS)
7. Recurrent episodes may occur in 50% with a mortality rate of 20%

Treatment

Acute management:
Carefully monitor oxygenation, hydration, and acid–base balance. Obtain daily weight, input/output, CBC, and appropriate serum chemistry panels. Measure baseline and pre-/posttransfusion Hgb S concentration

Immediate treatment:
1. **Oxygen** by nasal cannula at a rate of 2 L/min or higher, if needed to maintain a PaO_2 of 70–80 mm Hg or oxygen saturation ≥90%
2. **Hydration** with 5% dextrose injection (D5W) or 5% dextrose/0.2% sodium chloride injection (D5W/1⁄4NS) at a rate not to exceed 1.5 times maintenance (volume to include any drug infusions). Also, refer to Acute Pain Syndrome, Notes Section
3. **Transfuse packed RBCs** by simple transfusion to maintain the baseline Hgb level

Following transfusion therapy and correction of hypovolemia, remobilization of sequestered RBCs may result in a Hgb increase greater than that predicted on the basis of the volume of administered RBCs. Because this can lead to hypervolemia, careful monitoring is indicated and use of diuretic therapy may be required

If hyperviscosity is contributing an important role in the pathogenesis of an acute complication of SCD, exchange transfusion using a mechanical device directed at reducing the hyperviscosity should be performed. The goal of this therapy would be to reduce the Hct to <30%

Chronic management:
Following an acute episode, subsequent management is influenced by the high recurrence rate of this syndrome
1. Chronic transfusions are recommended in children <2 years of age following a severe episode to keep Hgb SS levels <30% until splenectomy can be considered after 2 years of age
2. Splenectomy is recommended in patients who experience a life-threatening episode of acute splenic sequestration shortly after being placed on a chronic transfusion program. A splenectomy can also be considered in patients with chronic hypersplenism

Priapism

Sustained, painful, and unwanted erection resulting from vasoocclusive obstruction of penile venous drainage. Priapism has been classified as:
- Prolonged (>3 hours)
- Stuttering (>few minutes, <3 hours)

Mantadakis E et al. Blood 2000;95:78–82
Rackoff WR et al. J Pediatr 1992;120:882–885
The Management of Sickle Cell Disease, 4th ed. NIH Publication No. 02-2117. Bethesda, MD: National Institutes of Health, National Heart, Lung, and Blood Institute, Division of Blood Diseases and Resources; 2002. www.nhlbi.nih.gov/health/prof/blood/sickle/sc_mngt.pdf [accessed August 5, 2013]
Winter CC. J Urol 1978;119:227–228

Epidemiology

1. Mean age of onset: 12 years
2. By age 20 years, 89% of males will have experienced 1 or more episodes
3. Precipitating factors include:
   - Trauma
   - Infection
   - Drug use (eg, ethanol, cocaine, sildenafil, testosterone)
   - Prolonged sexual activity
   - Full bladder with infrequent urination
4. Complications include fibrosis of the penis and impotence

Treatment

Outpatient management:
1. Encourage oral fluid intake
2. Administer oral analgesics
3. Attempt to urinate as soon as priapism develops and encourage frequent urination

Instituting medication and conservative therapy within 4–6 hours of the onset of symptoms can usually lead to reduction of erection

In-patient management:
Carefully monitor oxygenation, hydration, and acid–base balance. Obtain daily weight, input/output, CBC, and appropriate serum chemistry panels, and baseline coagulation profile. Measure baseline and pre-/posttransfusion Hgb S concentration
1. **Hydration** with 5% dextrose injection (D5W) or 5% dextrose/0.2% sodium chloride injection (D5W/¼NS) at a rate not to exceed 1.5 times maintenance (volume to include any drug infusions). See Acute Pain Syndrome, Notes Section
2. **Oxygen** by nasal cannula at a rate of 2 L/min or greater if needed to maintain a PaO_2 of 70–80 mm Hg or oxygen saturation ≥90%
3. **Institute opioids or other analgesic therapy** as appropriate (see the section Acute Pain Syndrome)
4. **An urologist can perform penile aspiration** if more conservative measures fail to achieve detumescence within 1 hour. Use a **23-gauge needle** to aspirate blood from the corpus cavernosum followed by **irrigation with a 1:1,000,000 solution of epinephrine in 0.9% sodium chloride injection**
   Note: This is performed within 4–6 hours of onset and under conscious sedation and local analgesia. Successful in 15 young males on 37 of 39 occasions (Mantadakis E et al. Blood 2000;95:78–82)
5. **Transfusion of packed RBCs** is considered if penile aspiration with irrigation fails to achieve detumescence. Administer packed RBCs to reduce Hgb S to <30%
   Note: It is unclear if simple transfusion is equivalent to exchange transfusion

Management of recurrent priapism:
1. Chronic simple transfusion programs have been utilized to maintain the Hgb S <30%
   Note: Limit this approach to 6–12 months with frequent assessments
2. Penile shunting (*Winter procedure*) creates a shunt between the glans penis and the distal corpora with a Tru-Cut biopsy needle. This permits penile blood to drain from the distended corpora cavernosa into the uninvolved corpus spongiosa
   Note: Complications of priapism and its treatment:
   - Bleeding from the holes placed in the penis as part of the penile aspiration or shunting procedures
   - Infection, skin necrosis, damage, or strictures of the urethra, fistulas, and impotence

Transient Red Cell Aplasia (TRCA)

Characterized by a temporary suppression of erythropoiesis. Presenting manifestations may include:
- Preceding febrile illness
- Headache
- Fatigue
- Dyspnea
- More severe anemia than usual
- Reticulocytopenia* (eg, <1%)

*Reticulocytopenia begins 5 days post viral exposure and continues for 7–10 days. The hemoglobin nadir may reach values of 3–4 g/dL. Recovery is often associated with a massive increase in circulating nucleated RBCs (eg, >100 nRBC/100 WBC)

Anand A et al. N Engl J Med 1987;316:183–186
Bell LM et al. N Engl J Med 1989;321:485–491
Gilbert DN et al., eds. Parvo B19 virus (erythrovirus B19). In: The Sanford Guide to Antimicrobial Therapy 2011, 41st ed. Speeryville, VA: Antimicrobial Therapy; 2011:156
Kurtzman G et al. N Engl J Med 1989;321:519–523
Ohene-Frempong K, Steinberg MH. Clinical aspects of sickle cell anemia in adults and children. In: Steinberg MH et al., eds. Disorders of Hemoglobin: Genetics, Pathophysiology, and Clinical Management. New York, NY: Cambridge University Press; 2001:611–670
Serjeant GR et al. Lancet 1993;341:1237–1240
The Management of Sickle Cell Disease, 4th ed. NIH Publication No. 02-2117. Bethesda, MD: National Institutes of Health, National Heart, Lung, and Blood Institute, Division of Blood Diseases and Resources; 2002. www.nhlbi.nih.gov/health/prof/blood/sickle/sc_mngt.pdf [accessed August 5, 2013]
Young NS, Brown KE. N Engl J Med 2004;350:586–597

Epidemiology

In regions not endemic for malaria, 70–100% of episodes are caused by human parvovirus B19

Treatment

Transfuse packed RBCs to maintain Hgb close to baseline if ≥25% decrease in Hgb from baseline with declining or absent reticulocyte levels and symptomatic anemia

Transfuse small volumes cautiously to avoid hypervolemia and complications arising from an abrupt increase in serum viscosity

Notes:
1. Although TRCA is usually self-limited with resolution over a period of 2–3 weeks, transfusion support may be required to maintain the RBC mass and blood volume during this time period
2. If patients are beginning to show evidence of RBC production as determined by reticulocyte count, transfusion support may not be required
3. During the earliest phases of acute illness, obtain anti-B19 parvovirus IgM and IgG levels. If initial titers are negative, repeat in 1 week to assess for recent infection manifested by a rise in IgM levels

   Obtaining B19 parvovirus PCR (polymerase chain reaction) may be better for documenting acute infection
4. If there is failure to spontaneously resolve the B19 infection, discontinuing immunosuppressive therapy (if applicable) or instituting antiretroviral therapy in patients with HIV infection (if applicable) may terminate the underlying B19 viremia
5. In patients with persistent chronic B19 viremia and anemia requiring ongoing transfusion support, intravenous immunoglobulin containing viral neutralizing antibody may lead to a prompt decline in serum viral B19 viral DNA and accompanying reticulocytosis and increased Hgb production

Immune globulin intravenous (human) 400 mg/kg per day, intravenously, daily for 5 consecutive days, days 1–5 (total dosage/5-day course = 2000 mg/kg) or 1000 mg/kg IV for 3 consecutive days

Occasional responses to a single 400–mg/kg dose have been reported

Notes

1. Siblings and close contacts with SCD should be monitored for the development of aplastic crises
2. Complications reported to arise from TRCA in small series or single centers include bone marrow necrosis with pancytopenia, stroke, acute chest syndrome, splenic or hepatic sequestration, and glomerulonephritis
3. Most adults have acquired immunity to B19 parvovirus; however, susceptible individuals exposed to patients with active B19 parvovirus infection are at risk of contracting *erythema infectiosum*. Isolation precautions for pregnant staff are necessary

Stroke and CNS Disease

Cerebrovascular accidents (CVAs), transient ischemic attacks (TIAs), subarachnoid, intraparenchymal, and intraventricular hemorrhage

Broderick JP et al. Stroke 1999;30:905–915
Lansberg MG et al. Chest 2012;141(2_Suppl):
e601S–e636S. doi:10.1378/chest.11–2302
Malinow MR et al. Circulation 1999;99:178–182
Mayberg MR et al. Stroke 1994;25:231–232
Ohene-Frempong K et al. Blood 1998;91:288–294
The Management of Sickle Cell Disease, 4th ed. NIH
Publication No. 02-2117. Bethesda, MD: National Institutes
of Health, National Heart, Lung, and Blood Institute,
Division of Blood Diseases and Resources; 2002:83–94

Notes

- Without controlled trials in adults with SCD documenting the worth of transcranial Doppler (TCD) in reducing the risk of brain infarction, prevention should be based on standard recommendations applicable to adults without SCD

- In adults with SCD, the role of chronic transfusion in the prevention and treatment of stroke is unclear. However, chronic transfusion with the target of reducing Hgb S to less than 30% of total hemoglobin, as used in children, is an option. Moreover, the duration of time after which transfusion can be safely stopped has not been defined though some have suggested that transfusion may be safely withdrawn in older patients who have been extensively treated (Rana S et al. J Pediatr 1997;131:757–760). Management of iron overload must be managed with chelation

- In the event of intracranial hemorrhage complicating SCD in adults, consultation with a neurological specialty team is also indicated with stabilization in a neurological intensive care unit. A careful evaluation to rule out meningitis, sepsis, hypoxia, drug intoxication, or other metabolic arrangements is required (recommendations from children with SCD). A noncontrast cranial CT should be performed as soon as possible. The work-up and management should be approached based on the location of the blood on CT scan (eg, SAH, intraparenchymal hemorrhage, intraventricular hemorrhage). Initial management should include: IV normotonic fluids to avoid dehydration; a rapid search for coagulopathy (eg, PT, aPTT); complete blood count, comprehensive metabolic profile, Hgb S level; discontinuation of any medication with hemorrhagic risk and correction of any coagulopathy. A neurosurgical consultation should be obtained to advise for additional diagnostic studies and management as needed to identify aneurysms, arteriovenous malformations or hematoma that may require surgical intervention. The effect of transfusion on the course and outcome of intracranial hemorrhage complicating SCD is not know; however, reducing the Hgb S to <30% of total Hgb is recommended

Treatment

Compared with children, there is little information on the treatment and prevention of stroke in adults with SCD. Treatment and prevention recommendations for adults with SCD are therefore based primarily on current recommendations in adults without SCD. It is recommended that physicians with experience and skill in stroke management and interpretation of CT scans supervise treatment

General guidelines:
1. **Oxygen** by nasal cannula at a rate of 2 L/min or greater if needed to maintain a PaO_2 of 70–80 mm Hg for oxygen saturation of ≥90%
2. **Assess** the patient for cause of **pain and complications**. Conduct a rapid pain assessment with a simple self-reported pain scale. **Institute opioids or other analgesic therapy as appropriate** (see Acute Pain Syndrome)
3. **Hydration** (if required based on clinical evaluation to avoid dehydration) with normotonic fluids: eg, 5% dextrose solution (D5W)/normal saline (NS)

TIAS and CVAs:
Consult the Feburary 2012:141 (2 Suppl) *Antithrombotic Therapy and Prevention of Thrombosis, 9th ed: American College of Physicians Evidence-Based Clinical Guidelines* section on *Antithrombotic and Thrombolytic Therapy for Ischemic Stroke*. Specifics on inclusion/exclusion criteria for recombinant tissue plasminogen activator (r-TPA) as well as additional antithrombotic management recommendations for ischemic stroke/TIA and guidance in patients with a history of symptomatic primary intracerebral hemorrhage are expertly presented in this guideline

Subarachnoid Hemorrhage (SAH):
1. **Transfuse packed RBCs** to reduce Hgb S to <30%
Note: The effect of RBC transfusion on altering the course or outcome of SAH is unknown
2. Nimodipine (calcium channel antagonist) is indicated in adults with SAH from ruptured berry aneurysms to counteract delayed arterial vasospasm
Dosage: administer 60 mg orally every 4 hours for 21 days (one hour before or two hours after a meal; avoid grapefruit juice). Nimodipine may increase the blood pressure lowering effect of concomitantly administered antihypertensives and blood pressure should be carefully monitored; dose adjustment of the blood pressure lowering drug(s) may be necessary. Nursing mothers are advised not to breast feed their babies when taking nimodipine. Dosage should be reduced to one 30 mg capsule every 4 hours with close monitoring of blood pressure in patients with "severely disturbed liver function" (eg, liver cirrhosis). Strong inhibitors of CYP3A4 should not be administered concomitantly with nimodipine

The Management of Sickle Cell Disease, 4th ed. NIH Publication No. 02-2117. Bethesda, MD: National Institutes of Health, National Heart, Lung, and Blood Institute, Division of Blood Diseases and Resources; 2002. www.nhlbi .nih.gov/health/prof/blood/sickle/sc_mngt.pdf [accessed August 5, 2013]. (See chapter 13 on stroke and CNS disease in adults)

Work-up for Adults with TIA or Ischemic Stroke

CBC/diff; EKG; transthoracic echocardiogram with consideration given to TEE, especially in young patients; aPTT; PT; and a brain study to include MRI, DWI, and MRA, and/or TCD, and carotid duplex US or CT angiography to determine the status of the intracranial and extracranial vessels. Blood tests for protein C and S deficiency, homocysteine elevation, and anticardiolipin antibodies may be appropriate. Health care providers should consider etiologies seen in young patients with stroke without SCD: eg, CNS infection, illicit drug use and arterial dissection

Epidemiology

Cerebrovascular accidents (CVAs) are a leading cause of death in children and adults

Age-adjusted prevalence for CVAs:
Hgb SS (4.01%)
Hgb Sβ-thalassemia (2.43%)
Hgb Sβ+ thalassemia (1.29%)
Hgb SC (0.84%)

Among Hgb SS patients first CVAs were:
Infarctive (53.9%)
Hemorrhagic (34.2%)
TIA (10.5%)
Both infarctive/hemorrhagic (1.3%)

In all SCD patients recurrent CVAs occur in 16% of survivors of first-time CVAs Overall, the mortality rate for hemorrhagic CVA was 24–26% for Hgb SS patients

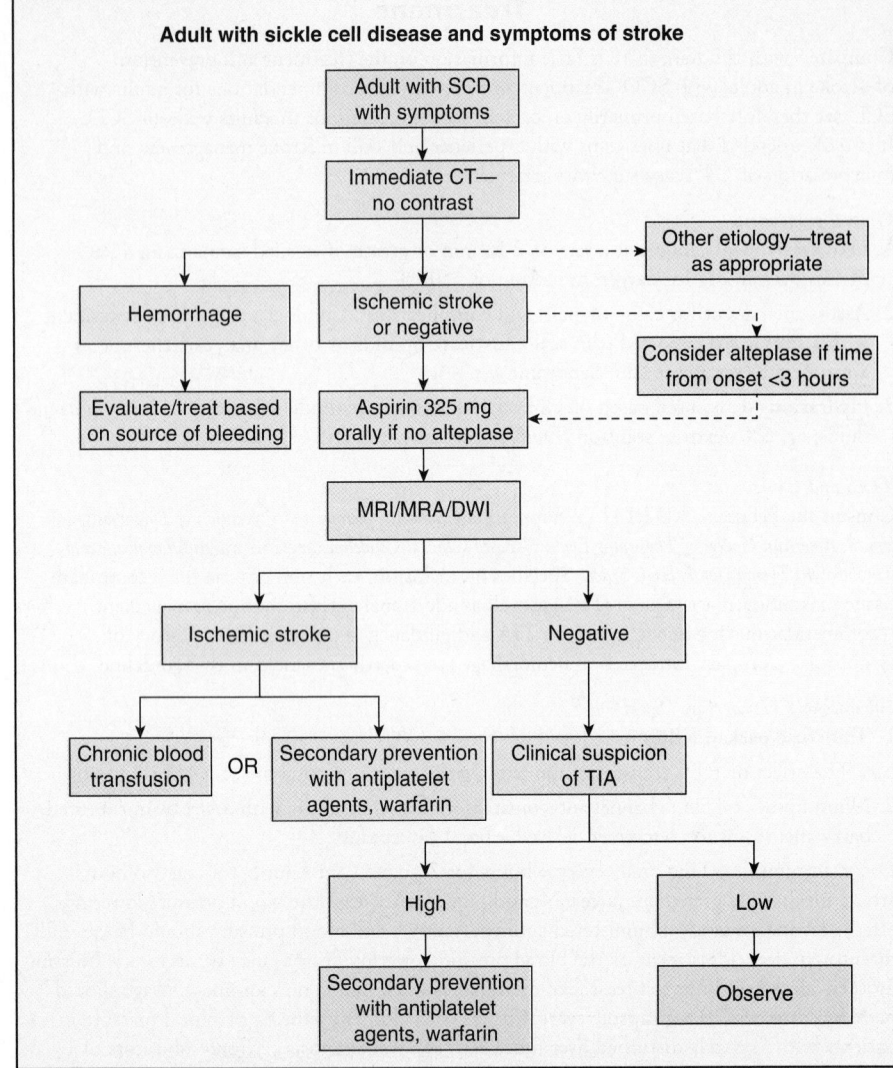

Adult with sickle cell disease and symptoms of stroke

Adult with SCD with symptoms → Immediate CT—no contrast

- Other etiology—treat as appropriate
- Hemorrhage → Evaluate/treat based on source of bleeding
- Ischemic stroke or negative → Consider alteplase if time from onset <3 hours → Aspirin 325 mg orally if no alteplase → MRI/MRA/DWI
  - Ischemic stroke → Chronic blood transfusion **OR** Secondary prevention with antiplatelet agents, warfarin
  - Negative → Clinical suspicion of TIA
    - High → Secondary prevention with antiplatelet agents, warfarin
    - Low → Observe

Adapted from The Management of Sickle Cell Disease, 4th ed. NIH Publication No. 02-2117. Bethesda, MD: National Institutes of Health, National Heart, Lung, and Blood Institute, Division of Blood Diseases and Resources; 2002. www.nhlbi.nih.gov/health/prof/blood/sickle/sc_mngt.pdf [accessed August 5, 2013]

Notes:
- r-tPA should not be given unless emergent care and appropriate treatment facilities available
- Antiplatelet agents are usually recommended for TIA in TIA's without SCD, but there are few data on the efficacy in SCD
- If antiplatelet therapy is administered in patients with acute ischemic stroke or TIA (after intracranial hemorrhage has been excluded), aspirin therapy at a dosage of 160–325 mg should be administered orally within 48 hours after symptom onset and reduced after 1–2 weeks to *secondary prevention* dosing (75–100 mg/day orally). Benefits: (1) fewer deaths: 9 per 1000; (2) good functional outcome at 30 days after ischemic stroke: 7 per 1000; (3) reduction in recurrent strokes: 7 per 1000. Risks: (1) nonfatal major extracranial bleeding events: 4 per 1000; (2) symptomatic intracranial hemorrhages: 2 per 1000
- Aspirin therapy for acute ischemic stroke or TIA should not be given for the first 24 hours after administration of r-tPA

According to established guidelines, alteplase (t-PA) is indicated when:
- The patient is at least 18 years old
- The patient's NIH Stroke Scale score is ≥4 (ischemic stroke in any circulation with a clinically significant deficit)
- Alteplase can begin within 3 hours after symptom onset
- Cranial CT shows no evidence of hemorrhage

It is not clear whether alteplase is appropriate for patients with SCD and hyperacute ischemic stroke; no experience with its use has been reported. However, there is no clear justification to exclude SCD patients. Caution is advised if severe stroke (<7% risk of symptomatic brain hemorrhage with an absolute risk of fatal ICH of 3.5% with IV r-tPA initiated within 3 hours in patients with acute ischemic stroke)

The 9th ed ACCP Guidelines on Antithrombotic and Thrombolytic Therapy for Ischemic Stroke (See reference by Lansberg MG et al. Chest 2012;141(2_Suppl): e601S–e636S. doi:10.1378/chest.11-2302) also recommends r-tPA use "in patients with acute ischemic stroke in whom treatment can be initiated within 4.5 hours but not within 3 hours of symptom onset"

Thrombolytic therapy cannot be recommended if:
- Evidence of intracranial hemorrhage (ICH) on pretreatment evaluation
- Suspicion of subarachnoid hemorrhage (SAH) on pretreatment evaluation
- Recent (within 3 months) intracranial or intraspinal surgery, serious head trauma or previous stroke
- History of ICH
- Minor neurological deficit
- Rapidly improving symptoms
- Uncontrolled hypertension at the time of treatment (eg, >185 mm Hg systolic or >110 mm Hg diastolic)
- Seizure at the onset of stroke
- Active internal bleeding
- Intracranial neoplasm, arteriovenous malformation, or aneurysm
- Known bleeding diathesis, including but not limited to: Current use of oral anticoagulants (eg, warfarin sodium) or an INR >1.7 or a PT >15 seconds

Administration of heparin within 48 hours preceding the onset of stroke and have an elevated aPTT at presentation
Platelet count <100,000/mm³
- Blood glucose of <50 mg/dL or >400 mg/dL

Chronic Pain Syndrome: Acute Osteomyelitis and Acute Septic Arthritis

Almeida A, Roberts I. Br J Haematol 2005;129:482–490
Gilbert DN et al., eds. Bone: osteomyelitis. In: The Sanford Guide to Antimicrobial Therapy 2011. 41st ed. Speeryville, VA: Antimicrobial Therapy; 2011:4
Glader BE. Anemia. In: Embury SH et al., eds. Sickle Cell Disease: Basic Principles and Clinical Practice. New York, NY: Raven Press; 1994:545–554
Keeley K, Buchanan GR. J Pediatr 1982;101:170–175
Rao S et al. J Pediatr 1985;107:685–688
Sickle cell disease: Clinical and epidemiologic aspects. In: Bunn HF, Forget BG, eds. Hemoglobin: Molecular, Genetic and Clinical Aspects. Philadelphia, PA: WB Saunders; 1986:502–564
Solanki DL et al. Am J Med 1986;80:985–990
The Management of Sickle Cell Disease, 4th ed. NIH Publication No. 02-2117. Bethesda, MD: National Institutes of Health, National Heart, Lung, and Blood Institute, Division of Blood Diseases and Resources; 2002. www.nhlbi.nih.gov/health/prof/blood/sickle/sc_mngt.pdf [accessed August 5, 2013]

Epidemiology

United States and most of the world:
Salmonella sp. are the most common causative organisms of osteomyelitis in Hgb SS patients (~60% or higher); *Staphylococcus aureus* is second most common, followed by Gram-negative enteric bacilli

Some regions of the world:
Gram-negative organisms, such as *Klebsiella* sp. may predominate

Treatment

1. **Assess** the patient for cause of **pain and complications.** Rapid pain assessment with simple self-reported pain scale
2. **Hydration** (as appropriate to the patient's clinical evaluation) with 5% dextrose injection or 0.9% sodium chloride injection at a rate not to exceed 1.5 times maintenance (volume to include any drug infusions); Also, refer to Acute Pain Syndrome, Notes Section
3. **Institute opioid therapy or other analgesics** as appropriate (see the section Acute Pain Syndrome)
4. **Institute appropriate antibiotics** (see below)

Adults with Acute Osteomyelitis

Empiric parenteral antibiotics that cover *Salmonella* sp., *Staphylococcus aureus*, and other Gram-negative organisms until culture results are available, for example:
Vancomycin 1000 mg; administer intravenously over 1 hour every 12 hours, *with*
Ciprofloxacin 400 mg; administer intravenously over 1 hour every 12 hours, *or*
Levofloxacin 750 mg; administer intravenously over 90 minutes every 24 hours

Note:
• Collect blood and bone cultures before empiric therapy
• If blood culture is negative, need culture of bone; culture of sinus tract not predictive of bone culture
• Definitive treatment is chosen according to in vitro susceptibility and continued for up to 6 weeks, depending on the nature and extent of the infection
• For the patient with suspected vertebral osteomyelitis ± epidural abscess, obtain MRI early to look for epidural abscess
• The doses identified are for adults with clinically severe (often life-threatening) infections and assume normal renal function and not severe hepatic dysfunction

Adults with Acute Monoarticular Septic Arthritis (Not at Risk for Sexually Transmitted Disease)

Empiric parenteral antibiotics (after collection of blood and joint fluid) that covers *Salmonella* sp., *Staphylococcus aureus*, and other Gram (−) organisms until culture results are available (see empiric antimicrobial coverage in section on Acute Osteomyelitis)

Note: Consider surgical drainage of the joint with the evacuation of exudates and breaking up joint loculations to reduce the risk of persistent infection and articular cartilage destruction

Notes

1. Osteomyelitis in SCD must be differentiated from acute bone infarction. Plain radiography and radionuclide bone imaging are of little or no use in differential diagnosis. However, radionuclide marrow imaging may be useful in depicting diminished uptake in infarction and normal uptake in infection
2. Despite progress made with various imaging techniques, a definitive diagnosis of osteomyelitis in SCD depends more upon clinical assessment and positive blood or bone cultures obtained by aspiration or biopsy
3. Consult institutional antimicrobial susceptibility profiles to guide selection of fluoroquinolone (in particular)

Systemic Fat Embolization

Characterized by embolization of necrotic marrow and fat in the setting of massive bone marrow infarction. Respiratory insuffi ciency and multiorgan failure from systemic emboli may occur with clinical signs dependent upon the organ involved and degree of involvement

Castro O. Hematol Oncol Clin North Am 1996;10:1289–1303
Milner PF, Brown M. Blood 1982;60:1411–1419
The Management of Sickle Cell Disease, 4th ed. NIH Publication No. 02-2117. Bethesda, MD: National Institutes of Health, National Heart, Lung, and Blood Institute, Division of Blood Diseases and Resources; 2002. www.nhlbi.nih.gov/health/prof/blood/sickle/sc_mngt.pdf [accessed August 5, 2013]
Vichinsky EP et al. N Engl J Med 2000;342:1855–1865

Epidemiology

1. A well-documented complication in the setting of acute chest syndrome
2. Responsible for symptoms in 8.8% of patients with acute chest syndrome
3. Systemic fat embolization can occur concurrently with an infectious agent
4. Risk factors:

   Hgb SC
   Pregnancy
   Prior corticosteroid treatment

Treatment

A high index of suspicion is required. All ACS patients are considered to be at risk. Treatment should not await proof of diagnosis

1. **Oxygen** by nasal cannula at a rate of 2 L/min, or greater if needed to maintain a PaO_2 of 70–80 mm Hg or oxygen saturation ≥90%. If needed, initiate critical care supportive measures to manage respiratory insufficiency
2. **Assess** the patient for cause of **pain and complications**. Conduct a rapid pain assessment with a simple self-reported pain scale. Institute **opioids** therapy or other analgesics based upon an individual patient's clinical evaluation (see the section Acute Pain Syndrome)
3. **Hydration** with 5% dextrose injection or 5% dextrose/0.2% sodium chloride injection at a rate not to exceed 1.5 times maintenance (volume to include any drug infusions). Also, refer to Acute Pain Syndrome, Notes Section
4. **Transfuse packed RBCs** to reduce Hgb S to <30%

Note: Case reports suggest that exchange transfusion may prevent some deterioration (see sections on Acute Chest Syndrome and Red Blood Cell Transfusion)

Notes

1. Clinical symptoms may include severe bone pain, fever, hypoxia, azotemia, liver damage, altered mental status or coma, progressive anemia and thrombocytopenia, and disseminated intravascular coagulation
2. Findings that prove systemic fat embolization: Fat droplets within retinal vessels or in biopsies of petechiae
3. Indirect evidence of systemic fat embolization: Positive fat stains in bronchial macrophages, lung microvesicle cells, or venous blood buffy coat
4. In the setting of acute chest syndrome patients with systemic fat embolization have a lower oxygen saturation at presentation, are more likely to have upper lobe infiltrates during hospitalization, and have a higher incidence of vasoocclusive events in comparison with patients with pulmonary infarction or infection
5. Systemic fat embolization may precipitate or coexist with acute chest pain syndrome (see treatment section for Acute Chest Syndrome)

Vichinsky EP et al. N Engl J Med 2000;342:1855–1865

Acute Multiorgan Failure Syndrome

Sudden onset of severe dysfunction of 2 or more major organ systems during an acute painful vasoocclusive episode. This syndrome may occur without an apparent predisposing event other than high baseline hemoglobin

Initial presentation:
Fever
Nonfocal encephalopathy
Evidence of rhabdomyolysis
Rapid decrease in Hgb and platelet count

Organ-specific manifestations:
Renal: hematuria or acute renal failure
Liver: acute hepatic necrosis or hepatic sequestration syndrome
Lung: pulmonary infiltrates, hypoxia
Bone marrow: generalized necrosis with fat emboli
Pancreas: pancreatitis

Notes:

1. For associated acute chest syndrome, see the section Acute Chest Syndrome
2. The use of granulocyte colony-stimulating factor has been associated with sickle cell crisis and multiorgan failure in 3 patients with sickle cell syndrome (2 patients after stem-cell mobilization with 1 death; 1 patient with stage II breast cancer treated with CMF chemotherapy + G-CSF)

Abboud M et al. Lancet 1998;351:959
Adler BK et al. Blood 2001;97:3313–3314
Bakanay SM et al. Blood 2005;105:545–547
Hassell KL et al. Am J Med 1994;96:155–162
Rosse WF et al. New views of sickle cell disease: pathophysiology and treatment. Hematology Am Soc Hematol Educ Program. 2000:2–17
The Management of Sickle Cell Disease, 4th ed. NIH Publication No. 02-2117. Bethesda, MD: National Institutes of Health, National Heart, Lung, and Blood Institute, Division of Blood Diseases and Resources; 2002. www.nhlbi.nih.gov/health/prof/blood/sickle/sc_mngt.pdf [accessed August 5, 2013]
Wei A, Grigg A. Blood 2001;97:3998–3999

Epidemiology

1. This syndrome is most commonly reported in Hgb S β-thalassemia but may occur in patients with classical Hgb SS disease with a high hematocrit
2. Second only to acute chest syndrome as the cause of sickle cell–related mortality

Treatment

Carefully monitor oxygenation, hydration, and acid–base balance. Obtain daily weight, input/output, CBC, and appropriate serum chemistry panels. Measure baseline and pre-/post-transfusion Hgb S concentration. Follow CXR until stabilization is documented

1. **Oxygen** by nasal cannula at a rate of 2 L/min, or greater if needed to maintain a PaO_2 of 70–80 mm Hg. Mechanical ventilation as appropriate to the clinical condition
2. **Hydration** with 5% dextrose injection or 5% dextrose/0.2% sodium chloride injection at a rate not to exceed 1.5 times maintenance (volume to include any drug infusions) with careful assessment of hydration status and fluid requirements in the setting of concomitant acute renal failure
3. **Assess** the patient for cause of **pain and complications**. Rapid pain assessment with simple self-reported pain scale if possible based on the underlying mental status. Institute **opioids** therapy **or other analgesics as appropriate** (see the section Acute Pain Syndrome)
4. **Perform aggressive transfusion** to reduce Hgb S to <30%:
   Simple transfusion (Packed RBCs) if Hgb <7 g/dL and no evidence of hyperviscosity, *or*
   Exchange transfusion using a mechanical device, if Hgb >7 g/dL or hyperviscosity is playing a role in the pathogenesis of the acute complication of SCD
   Note: Prompt initiation of transfusion therapy or exchange transfusion has the potential of reversing this syndrome
5. **Critical care** support is directed at the affected underlying organ systems
6. If narcosis is suspected:
   Try **Naloxone** 0.4 mg (1 mL) in 9 mL 0.9% sodium chloride injection to produce a concentration = 0.04 mg/mL, administer 0.5 mL (0.02 mg) by intravenous injection every 2 minutes, *or*
   Naloxone 0.4–2 mg/dose; administer intravenously, subcutaneously, or intramuscularly; may repeat every 2–3 minutes as needed to a maximum dose of 10 mg
7. Empiric antibiotics, pending culture results
   Antibiotics should be given to febrile or severely ill patients. These include (normal renal function):
   A **third-generation cephalosporin:**
   Ceftriaxone 1000 mg (maximum 2000 mg); administer intravenously in 50–100 mL D5W over 30 minutes every 24 hours, *and*
   A **broad-spectrum macrolide or fluoroquinolone antibiotic:**
   Azithromycin 500 mg; administer intravenously over 60 minutes every 24 hours, *or*
   Ciprofloxacin 400 mg; administer intravenously over 60 minutes every 12 hours

Notes

There are no reported prospective trials in the management of multiorgan failure syndrome complicating SCD. Treatment approaches are based upon clinical observations and expert opinion

FEVER

Epidemiology

1. Fever is a common presenting symptom in SCD and may represent the first indication of a serious infection and/or underlying SCD-associated clinical syndrome
2. Fever in SCD is presumed to be caused by infection and treated as such until proven otherwise

Clinical Features

1. Adult patients, parents, and children should be taught that a temperature ≥38.5°C (≥101.3°F) is an emergency and advised to seek immediate medical evaluation
2. Risk factors/etiologies for fever in SCD
   a. Functional asplenia
   b. *Clinical syndromes associated with SCD:* Acute chest syndrome (ACS), transient RBC aplasia, fat embolism, vasoocclusive crisis, sequestration syndromes (hepatic, splenic), acute cholecystitis, viral hepatitis, acute bone infarction, osteomyelitis, septic arthritis, skin ulceration, stroke, intracranial hemorrhage, multiorgan failure syndrome
   c. *Drug therapy:* Hydroxyurea (febrile neutropenia, drug-induced); allergic reactions to antimicrobial therapy, others; rare cases of ceftriaxone-induced AIHA
   d. Hemolytic transfusion reactions
   e. *Infections:* B19 parvovirus, HIV, meningitis, otitis media, PID, sinusitis, SBE, STDs, viral hepatitis

Management of Fever

1. Initial focused work-up

Assess for localized or systemic infection, pallor, liver/spleen size, neurologic status

Obtain vital signs, oxygen saturation, assess hemodynamic status of patient

Sign or Symptom	Clinical Finding in SCD
Pallor	Aplastic crisis, splenic or hepatic sequestration, other causes for reduced hemoglobin
Shortness of breath, chest pain, cough, splinting; new heart murmur	Vasoocclusive crisis, ACS, pneumonia, fat embolism; SBE
Abdominal pain, swelling (may be accompanied by jaundice)	Evaluate for change in size of liver and spleen from baseline that may suggest sequestration; RUQ pain syndrome; cholecystitis, hepatitis
Dysuria, flank or pelvic pain/fullness, vaginal discharge	UTI, pyelonephritis, PID, pregnancy, STD
Localized bone or joint pain, erythema, swelling	Marrow ischemia, osteomyelitis, septic arthritis
Skin redness, ulceration	Leg ulcer, cellulitis
Neck stiffness, altered MS, headache, focal neurologic signs	Meningitis, acute stroke, intracranial hemorrhage

2. Laboratory assessment
   a. CBC with differential, reticulocyte count (RPI), comprehensive metabolic profile (CMP), urinalysis, blood cultures; throat culture, nasopharyngeal swab as indicated; type and cross-match as indicated, request if available, minor antigen-matched, sickle-negative, leukodepleted RBCs), other cultures as indicated (eg, CSF, bone)

(continued)

Management of Fever (*continued*)

3. Empiric antibiotic use

    a. Administer antibiotics empirically before initial laboratory tests or imaging study results are available

    b. Empirically select antibiotics directed against common bacterial pathogens based on epidemiology and antimicrobial sensitivity (in the United States, most common include: *Streptococcus pneumoniae, Salmonella* sp., *Escherichia coli, Staphylococcus aureus*)

Pathogens to be Covered by Empiric Therapy

Clinical Situation	Pathogens to be Covered
Fever without source (rule-out sepsis)	*Streptococcus pneumoniae* *Haemophilus influenzae* type B Consider broadening to cover: Gram (−) enterics, *Salmonella*
Meningitis	*Streptococcus pneumoniae* *Haemophilus influenzae* type B Consider broadening to include: *Neisseria meningitidis*
Acute chest syndrome (ACS)	*Streptococcus pneumoniae* *Mycoplasma pneumoniae* *Chlamydia pneumoniae* Consider broadening to cover: *Legionella*, RSV
Osteomyelitis/septic arthritis	*Salmonella* *Staphylococcus aureus* *Streptococcus pneumoniae*
Urinary tract infection	*Escherichia coli* Other Gram (−) enterics

Empiric Antibiotics	Dose, Schedule (Normal Renal Function)
Ceftriaxone	Administer 1 g; administer intravenously over 30 minutes q24h; 2 g maximum dose *and* vancomycin
Vancomycin	Administer 15 mg/kg; administer intravenously over 1 hour q12h

- **Meningitis (bacterial, acute):** The goal is empiric therapy; then obtain CSF within 30 minutes. If a focal neurologic deficit is present, give empiric therapy, then head CT, then LP. *Primary regimen:* Administer **ampicillin** 2 g intravenously over 30 minutes q4h *and* **ceftriaxone** 2 g intravenously over 30 minutes q12h *and* **vancomycin** 500–750 mg intravenously over 60 minutes q6h **Dexamethasone** to block TNF production is administered at 0.15 mg/kg intravenously over 15 minutes q6h for 2–4 days with the first dose 15–20 minutes prior to or concomitant with the first dose of antibiotic (de Gans J, van de Beek D. N Engl J Med 2002;347:1549–1556; Tunkel AR, Scheld WM. N Engl J Med 2002;347:1613–1615)
- **ACS (if present):** Add a broad-spectrum macrolide or fluoroquinolone antibiotic (see the section Acute Chest Syndrome)

4. Further evaluation and management

    a. Goal-oriented management for associated SCD syndromes

    b. Review patient's most recent medical evaluation; assess for prior infections, surgical history, medications (current, OTC, recreational), allergies, communicable disease exposure; any changes in CBC/diff, reticulocyte count, CMP from baseline, and any change in size of liver and spleen from baseline

    c. LP for meningitis; joint fluid analysis for effusions; CXR for respiratory signs and symptoms (S×S); x-rays /scans for bone pain

    d. Consider abdominal ultrasound, liver function tests, amylase, and lipase for right upper quadrant pain, epigastric or severe abdominal pain (to rule out cholelithiasis, cholecystitis, pancreatitis)

    e. Orthopedic surgery consultation for aspiration and culture of bone or joint if osteomyelitis or septic arthritis are suspected

    f. Oxygen by nasal cannula or face mask if required to keep oxygen saturation ≥92% or ≥ patient's baseline value if ≥92%

(continued)

Management of Fever (*continued*)

  g. Type and crossmatch and consider RBC transfusion if Hgb is 1–2 g/dL or more below patient's usual baseline, if acute chest syndrome is suspected, or if the patient shows any signs of hemodynamic compromise from anemia

  h. Hydration with 5% dextrose injection (D5W) or 5% dextrose injection with 0.225% sodium chloride (D5W/¼NS) at a rate not to exceed 1.5 times maintenance (volume to include any drug infusions). *Note:* Increased fluids may be required if the patient is dehydrated or if insensible losses are increased with persistent fever; also refer to Acute Pain Syndrome, Notes Section

  i. Acetaminophen 15 mg/kg PO q4h (maximum daily dose: 75 mg/kg). Ibuprofen may be added at a dose of 10 mg/kg PO q6–8h if no contraindication (eg, coagulopathy, gastritis, ulcer or renal impairment). Limit more frequent dosing to the first 72 hours (maximum)

5. **Criteria for hospital admission**

   Any of the following:

   a. CXR infiltrate or abnormal oxygen saturation

   b. Hgb <5 g/dL (or ≥2 g/dL decline from baseline)

   c. WBC >30,000/mm³ or <5000/mm³

   d. Platelet count <100,000/mm³

   e. Hemodynamic instability

   f. Presence of identified SCD-associated syndromes

   g. History of sepsis

   h. Signs of meningitis

6. **Criteria for hospital discharge**

   a. Afebrile ≥24 hours with negative cultures ≥24–48 hours

   b. Able to take adequate fluids and PO medications, if applicable

   c. Resolution of pulmonary signs and symptoms or documentation of adequate room air oxygenation

   d. Stable hemoglobin and hematocrit without evidence of aplastic or sequestration crisis

   e. Appropriate follow-up arranged

CMP, Comprehensive metabolic profile; CT, computerized tomography; D/C, discharge; GU, genitourinary; LP, lumbar puncture; MS, mental status; PID, pelvic inflammatory disease; q, every; RSV, respiratory syncytial virus; SBE, subacute bacterial endocarditis; STD, sexually transmitted disease; S×S, signs and symptoms; TNF, tumor necrosis factor; UTI, urinary tract infection

Notes:

1. The majority of clinical evidence for the management of fever in SCD is derived from children instead of adults

2. Guidelines for empiric antibiotic treatment in adults are similar to guidelines for children unless altered by other identified problems

3. For a discussion on the management of specific SCD syndromes, refer to the sections on Acute Pain Syndrome, Acute Chest Syndrome, RUQ Syndrome, Hepatic Sequestration, Splenic Sequestration, Systemic Fat Embolization, Acute Cholecystitis, Transient RBC Aplasia, Acute Osteomyelitis and Acute Septic Arthritis, or Stroke and CNS Disease

Bernini JC et al. J Pediatr 1995;126(5 Pt 1):813–815

Gilbert DN et al., eds. Central nervous system: meningitis, bacterial, acute. In: The Sanford Guide to Antimicrobial Therapy 2011, 41st ed. Speeryville, VA: Antimicrobial Therapy; 2011:7–8

Hsu L, Adamkiewicz T. Care Path: inpatient management of fever. In: Sickle Cell Information Center Guidelines. Eckman J, Platt A, eds; April 1, 2001. http://scinfo.org/care-paths-and-protocols-children-adolescents/care-path-inpatient-management-of-fever. Accessed August 5, 2013. Sickle Cell Information Center, Georgia Comprehensive Sickle Cell Center at Grady Memorial Health System. The Sickle Cell Foundation of Georgia, Inc. Emory University School of Medicine, Department of Pediatrics, Atlanta, GA, Morehouse School of Medicine

Miller ST et al. J Pediatr 1991;118:30–33

Mountain States Regional Genetic Services Network. Sickle Cell Disease in Children and Adolescents: Diagnosis, Guidelines for Comprehensive Care, and Protocols for Management of acute and Chronic Complication. 2001

Poncz M et al. J Pediatr 1985;107:861–866

Section on Hematology/Oncology Committee on Genetics; American Academy of Pediatrics. Pediatrics 2002;109:526–535

The Management of Sickle Cell Disease, 4th ed. NIH Publication No. 02-2117. Bethesda, MD: National Institutes of Health, National Heart, Lung, and Blood Institute, Division of Blood Diseases and Resources; 2002. www.nhlbi.nih.gov/health/prof/blood/sickle/sc_mngt.pdf [accessed August 5, 2013]

Wright J et al. J Pediatr 1997;130:394–399

Zarkowsky HS et al. J Pediatr 1986;109:579–585

REGIMEN

HYDROXYUREA

Charache S et al. N Engl J Med 1995;332:1317–1322
Rodgers GP et al. N Engl J Med 1990;322:1037–1045
Steinberg MH. Hematology Am Soc Hematol Educ Program 2000:9–13
Steinberg MH et al. JAMA 2003;289:1645–1651
The Management of Sickle Cell Disease, 4th ed. NIH Publication No. 02-2117. Bethesda, MD: National
Institutes of Health, National Heart, Lung, and Blood Institute, Division of Blood Diseases and Resources; 2002
(chapters 26 and 29). www.nhlbi.nih.gov/health/prof/blood/sickle/sc_mngt.pdf [accessed August 5, 2013]

Initial dosing

Hydroxyurea 10–15 mg/kg per day (based on actual or ideal body weight, whichever is less); administer orally in a single daily dose for 6–8 weeks (total dosage/week = 70–105 mg/kg)

Initial Dose Adjustment Based on Renal Function

CrCl ≥60 mL/min (≥1 mL/s)	No dose adjustment
CrCl <60 mL/min	50% reduction
End-stage renal disease*	50% reduction

CrCl, Creatinine clearance

*Treatment should be given following hemodialysis

Maintenance Therapy

Adjust hydroxyurea dosage as outlined in the table of **Treatment Modifications**

Treatment Modifications

Note: If no major toxicity is observed, escalate hydroxyurea dosage by 5 mg/kg per day every 12 weeks until a maximum tolerated dose (the highest dose that does not produce toxic blood counts over a 24-week period) or 35 mg/kg per day is reached. In the study, 33% and 51% of patients received maximal doses of hydroxyurea (35 mg/kg per day) at 6 and 21 months, respectively

Notes:

1. A trial period of 6–12 months without transfusion support is adequate provided the patient does not suffer an intercurrent illness that suppresses erythropoiesis

2. Since hydroxyurea is a teratogen and its effects in pregnancy are unknown, contraception should be practiced and pregnancy should be avoided if the patient or their sexual partner is receiving hydroxyurea. Patients should be instructed to notify their physician if they plan to or become pregnant so treatment can be D/C'd

Supportive Care

Antiemetic prophylaxis
Emetogenic potential is **MINIMAL**
See Chapter 39 for antiemetic recommendations

Hematopoietic growth factor (CSF) prophylaxis
Primary prophylaxis is NOT indicated
See Chapter 43 for more information

Antimicrobial prophylaxis
Risk of fever and neutropenia is LOW
Antimicrobial primary prophylaxis to be considered:
- Antibacterial—not indicated
- Antifungal—not indicated
- Antiviral—not indicated unless patient previously had an episode of HSV

See Chapter 47 for more information

Patient Population Studied

The Multicenter Study of Hydroxyurea for Sickle Cell Anemia (MHS Study), a landmark prospective, double-blind, placebo-controlled, dose-escalation trial evaluated the effect of hydroxyurea on the frequency of painful vasoocclusive crises in adults with sickle cell disease and ≥3 painful crises/year. The MSH Study established hydroxyurea as the first clinically acceptable drug to prevent painful crises in adults with sickle cell anemia. Among 148 males and 151 females enrolled, 75% of patients took 80% of their capsules

Hydroxyurea has been recommended in the following settings (Management of SCD. In: The Management of Sickle Cell Disease, 4th ed. NIH Publication No. 02-2117. Bethesda, MD: National Institutes of Health, National Heart, Lung, and Blood Institute, Division of Blood Diseases and Resources; 2002. www.nhlbi.nih.gov/health/prof/blood/sickle/sc_mngt.pdf [accessed August 5, 2013])

1. Adults (FDA-approved indication), adolescents or children with Hgb SS after consultation with parents (children, adolescents) and physician

2. Hgb Sβ-thalassemia and frequent pain episodes

3. History of acute chest syndrome, other severe vaso occlusive events or severe symptomatic anemia

Efficacy

- Median rates of vasoocclusive crises were reduced by 44% with hydroxyurea
- There were no differences between the 2 arms in the rates of death, stroke, chronic transfusion, or hepatic sequestration

Event	HU (n = 152)	P (n = 147)	*P* Value
Median time to first crisis*	3	1.5	0.01
Median time to second crisis*	8.8	4.6	<0.001
Requirement for transfusion†	48	73	0.001
Units of blood transfused	336	586	0.004
Acute chest syndrome†	25	51	0.001
Median number of acute pain crises/year	2.5	4.5	<0.001
Discontinued treatment†	14	6	

HU, Hydroxyurea; P, placebo

*In months. Definition of painful crisis = visit to a medical facility that lasted >4 hours for sickling-related pain which was treated with a parenterally or orally administered opioid
†In number of patients

Treatment Modifications

Adverse Event	Treatment Modification
ANC ≥2500/mm^3, platelet count ≥95,000/mm^3, Hgb >5.3 g/dL, *and* reticulocytes ≥95,000/mm^3 if the Hgb is <9 g/dL	Escalate dosage by 5 mg/kg per day every 12 weeks until a maximum tolerated dose (the highest dose that does not produce toxic blood counts over a 24-week period) or 35 mg/kg per day is reached
ANC 2000–2500/mm^3, *or* platelet count 80,000–95,000/mm^3, *or* reticulocytes 80,000–95,000/mm^3 if the Hgb is <9 g/dL	Continue with same hydroxyurea dosage
ANC <2000/mm^3, *or* platelet count <80,000/mm^3, *or* reticulocytes <80,000/mm^3 if the Hgb is <9 g/dL	Stop hydroxyurea until ANC >2000/mm^3, *and* platelet count >80,000/mm^3, *and* reticulocytes >80,000/mm^3 if the Hgb is <9 g/dL. Then, restart hydroxyurea at a daily dosage decreased by 2.5 mg/kg*
Hematologic toxicity twice on 1 dosage	Do not administer or exceed this dosage again
Abnormal LFTs	There are no data that specifically guide dosage adjustment. Monitor hematologic parameters closely and adjust according to hematologic guidelines

*Subsequent doses may be titrated up or down every 12 weeks in 2.5-mg/kg per day increments, until the patient is at a stable dose for 24 weeks that does not result in toxicity

Side Effects of Hydroxyurea Treatment in People with Sickle Cell Disease

(Brawley O et al. Ann Intern Med 2008;148:932–938)

Side Effect	Comment
Leukopenia Thrombocytopenia Anemia	Frequent, expected, and dose-related; typically can be anticipated and prevented by temporary cessation of dose; usually resolves in 1–2 weeks

(continued)

Toxicity

Charache S et al. N Engl J Med 1995;332:1317–1322
Steinberg MH et al. JAMA 2003;289:1645–1651

1. Almost all patients had treatment temporarily stopped because of myelosuppression with counts usually recovering within 2 weeks
2. Leukemia has been reported in 4 adults with SCD treated with hydroxyurea from individual case reports and a single observational study (Lanzkron S et al. In: Hydroxyurea treatment for SCD. NIH Consensus Conference Feb 25–27, 2008:47–49a) http://consensus.nih .gov/2008/sicklecell.htm [Accessed August 8, 2013]

Treatment Modifications (*continued*)

Nausea (usually mild) Skin rash, Pneumonitis	Infrequent
Temporary decrease in sperm count or abnormalities	Not adequately evaluated
Increased risk for superficial skin cancer Hyperpigmentation	Infrequent
Permanently decreased sperm count	Not adequately evaluated

Notes

1. *Mechanism of action:* Hydroxyurea is a ribonucleotide reductase inhibitor that blocks ribonucleoside conversion to deoxyribonucleotides and interferes with DNA synthesis. Hydroxyurea induces Hgb F expression by a mechanism of erythroid regeneration that induces F-cell production. In adults, F-cells are rare erythrocytes that contain small amounts of Hgb F. Enhanced concentrations of Hgb F in F-cells can inhibit Hgb S polymerization and RBC sickling, and improve the course of SCD

2. *Duration of therapy:* A long-term observational follow-up study of mortality in patients with SCD in the original MSH trial (Multicenter Study of Hydroxyurea) was conducted from 1996–2001. Two-hundred thirty-three (77.9%) of the original 299 patients were enrolled in the MSH Patients' Follow-up: 52% and 16% received hydroxyurea for ≥1 year and <1 year, respectively. When analyzed according to original assignment (treatment vs. placebo) and regardless of a patient's postrandomization treatment choice, mortality rates were similar between groups (23.7% vs. 26.5%). Twenty-five percent of patients (N = 75) died during the original trial or during follow-up. Of these, 28% died from pulmonary disease and 12% died during SCD crisis

Notes:

- Continue treatment indefinitely in patients who benefit from therapy and have no toxicity
- If Hgb F (or MCV) does not increase, consider poor compliance or biological inability to respond. A trial period of 6–12 months without transfusion support is adequate provided the patient does not suffer an intercurrent illness that suppresses erythropoiesis

Cumulative mortality in the MSH trial analyzed according to clinical events and laboratory measurements at the conclusion of randomized treatment showed the following:

Clinical Variable at Conclusion of MSH Trial	Cumulative Mortality at 9 years (%)	*p* Value*
Hgb F[†]: <0.5 g/dL vs. >0.5 g/dL	28% vs. 15%	$p = 0.03$
Acute chest syndrome: presence vs. absence	32% vs. 18%	$p = 0.02$
Acute chest syndrome: ≥3 vs. <3 episodes/year	27% vs. 17%	$p = 0.06$
Reticulocytes: <250,000/mm³ vs. >250,000/mm³	37% vs. 18%	$p = 0.001$

*P values are reported as indicators of association, not tests of a priori hypotheses
[†]Hgb F expressed as absolute levels (g/dL) = Hgb F (%) × Hgb concentration (g/dL)

(*continued*)

Monitoring Therapy

Treatment monitoring end points include:
- Less pain
- Improved well-being
- Increase in Hgb F to 15–20%
- Increased Hgb level if severely anemic
- Acceptable myelotoxicity

Laboratory Monitoring:

Baseline:
1. CBC with differential, RBC indices, percent Hgb F, serum creatinine and BUN, liver function tests, renal panel, and pregnancy test in females

After initiation:
1. *Every 2 weeks:* CBC with differential
2. *Every 2–4 weeks:* Serum creatinine and BUN, LFTs, and renal panel
3. *Every 6–8 weeks:* Percent Hgb F

After a stable and nontoxic dose is reached:
1. *Every 4–8 weeks:* CBC with differential as long as ANC ≥2000/mm³ and platelets and reticulocytes are ≥80,000/mm³; periodic LFT monitoring is advised

Notes (continued)

Barriers to Hydroxyurea Treatment in Persons with Sickle Cell Disease

(Brawley OW et al. Ann Intern Med 2008;148:932–938)

Barriers	Patient	Parent/Family/ Caregiver	Provider
Fears or concerns about cancer, birth defects, infertility, and the uncertainty of long-term risks		X	X
Lack of knowledge about hydroxyurea as a therapeutic option	X	X	X
Lack of perception that hydroxyurea is currently the only therapy that directly modifies the disease process	X	X	X
Concern that the absence of FDA approval for hydroxyurea in children means that hydroxyurea is an experimental drug	X	X	
Difficulty in communication between patients and their caregivers regarding the use of hydroxyurea and other therapeutic options		X	
Need for frequent monitoring of response to hydroxyurea	X		
Lack of adherence to treatment program	X		
Provider bias and negative attitudes towards patients with sickle cell disease and their treatment			X
Lack of clarity of hydroxyurea treatment regimens and undertreatment in adults			X
Limited number of physicians who have expertise in the use of hydroxyurea for sickle cell disease			X
Failure to engage patients/caregivers in treatment decision making in a developmentally appropriate manner			X

Notes:

A systematic evidence review of the barriers to hydroxyurea found only 3 studies that specifically addressed this issue and none that tested interventions to overcome barriers to hydroxyurea treatment in SCD

System-level barriers included: (1) financing (lack of insurance, type of insurance, underinsurance, scope of coverage, copays, reimbursement, and payment structures); (2) lack of coordination between academic centers and community-based clinicians; (3) geographic isolation; (4) limited access to comprehensive care centers and care models; (5) problems in transitioning from pediatric to adult care; (6) limited access; (7) inadequate government, industry, and philanthropic support; (8) slow development and promotion of hydroxyurea because of lack of commercial interest; (9) lack of visibility/empowerment of SCD advocacy groups; (10) cultural and language barriers; and (11) inadequate information technology systems to support long-term care of SCD patients

RED BLOOD CELL TRANSFUSION

Hemolytic Transfusion Reactions. In: Petz L, Garratty G, eds. Immune Hemolytic Anemias. 2nd ed. Philadelphia, PA: Churchill Livingstone; 2004:541–572
Ohene-Frempong K. Semin Hematol 2001;38(1 Suppl 1):5–13
The Management of Sickle Cell Disease, 4th ed. NIH Publication No. 02-2117. Bethesda, MD: National Institutes of Health, National Heart, Lung, and Blood Institute, Division of Blood Diseases and Resources; 2002. www.nhlbi .nih.gov/health/prof/blood/sickle/sc_mngt.pdf [accessed August 5, 2013]
Vichinsky EP et al. N Engl J Med 1995;333:206–213

Most appropriate RBC product:

1. Phenotypically matched, sickle-negative, leukocyte-depleted packed RBCs
2. Administer washed RBCs if a patient had an allergic reaction to prior transfusions
3. Irradiation of RBCs is recommended in patients who are likely candidates for BMT

Methods of transfusion

1. Simple transfusion
   - Acute transfusion
     Note: Volume overload can occur when a large volume of blood is transfused too quickly. The administration of intravenous diuretics, slowing the rate of transfusion or partial removal of red cell supernatant fluid can help to prevent this complication
   - Chronic transfusion: Simple transfusion every 2–4 weeks to maintain a Hgb A level at 60–70%. The pretransfusion Hct should be between 25% and 30% and posttransfusion Hct ≤36% to prevent hyperviscosity
2. Exchange transfusion: The final Hgb should not exceed the range of 10–12 g/dL to avoid hyperviscosity and the percentage of Hgb A should meet the goals of therapy (60–70% normal Hgb A)
3. RBC apheresis

Review transfusion goals before starting

1. Assess for appropriate indication
2. Set goals for final posttransfusion hematocrit or Hgb and % Hgb S (avoid Hct >36%)
   - Major Surgery: Hgb 10 g/dL, Hgb S ~60% or less
   - Sudden severe illness: maintain Hgb S <30%

Patient Population Studied

Indications

1. Acute pain episodes complicated by sufficient physiologic derangement to result in heart failure, dyspnea, hypotension, or marked fatigue
2. Acute chest syndrome, systemic fat embolization, and stroke
3. Acute splenic sequestration
4. Multiorgan failure syndrome
5. Transient red blood cell aplasia or "aplastic crisis"
6. Severe anemia in patients with serious and potentially life-threatening infection
7. Hyperhemolysis where a Hgb level following transfusion is lower than that prior to transfusion; generally proposed to result from an increased rate of destruction of a patient's own RBCs. This may occur as a component of delayed hemolytic transfusion reactions or occasionally from an underlying G6PD deficiency, and may occur as a consequence of occult splenic sequestration or aplastic crises detected during a period of resolving reticulocytosis (Petz LD et al. Transfusion 1997;37:382–392)
8. Before major surgery
9. Consider administering in pregnant patients with complications such as preeclampsia, severe anemia, increasing frequency of pain episodes, women with previous pregnancy losses or who have multiple gestations

Controversial indications

1. Priapism
2. Leg ulcers

(continued)

Patient Population Studied (*continued*)

3. Preparation for infusion of hypertonic contrast media (gadolinium and nonionic contrast media lower the risk of RBC sickling)

4. Management of "silent" cerebral infarct and/or neurocognitive damage

Inappropriate indications and contraindications

1. Chronic steady-state anemia

2. Uncomplicated acute pain episodes

3. Uncomplicated infection

4. Minor surgery that does not require prolonged anesthesia (eg, myringotomy)

5. Aseptic necrosis of the shoulder or hip (except when surgery is required)

6. Uncomplicated pregnancies

Toxicity

1. *Alloimmunization.* The highest incidence is reported to be associated with SCD and AIHA. In a summary of 12 reports of 2818 transfused patients with SCD, alloimmunization occurred in 8–35% (mean and median, 25%)

   • Sickle cell hemolytic transfusion reaction: Manifestations of an acute or delayed hemolytic transfusion reaction where serologic studies may not provide an explanation for the hemolytic transfusion reaction

   • Development of symptoms suggestive of a sickle cell pain crisis that develop or are intensified by the hemolytic reaction

   • Development of a more severe anemia after transfusion than was previously present, with exacerbation of subsequent transfusions

   • Difficulty in finding compatible RBC units because of alloantibodies ± autoantibodies

2. *Delayed hemolytic transfusion reaction:* Four series in SCD reported an incidence of 4–22%; an incidence 10-times higher than for random transfused patients. Occurs 5–20 days after transfusion. Results from RBC antibodies are not present at the time of compatibility testing

3. Transfusion iron overload

4. Transmission of infection B19 parvovirus occurs in 1:40,000 RBC

5. Precipitation of pain episodes, strokes, acute pulmonary insufficiency

6. Hyperviscosity

7. Volume overload, when a large volume of blood is transfused too quickly

Notes

In a randomly assigned cohort of 551 patients with sickle cell disease undergoing 604 operations, a conservative transfusion regimen (designed to increase preoperative Hgb to 10 g/dL, regardless of Hgb S) was found to be as effective as an aggressive transfusion regimen (designed to maintain a preoperative Hgb at 10 g/dL; Hgb S ≤30%) in preventing serious complications (35% vs. 31%) and the development of acute chest (each regimen 10%), but was associated with half as many transfusion-associated complications (Vichinsky EP et al. N Engl J Med 1995;333:206–213)

62. Aplastic Anemia

Michael M. Boyiadzis, MD, MHSc and Neal S. Young, MD

Aplastic Anemia (AA)

Aplastic anemia is a distinct entity characterized by peripheral blood cytopenias and bone marrow hypocellularity. Aplastic anemia can be acquired or congenital. Acquired aplastic anemia is distinguished from iatrogenic marrow aplasia, the common occurrence of marrow hypocellularity after intensive cytotoxic chemotherapy

Epidemiology

Incidence: 2 per 1 million of population per year (West) and 2- to 3-fold higher in Asia

Male-to-female ratio: 1:1

Incidence of aplastic anemia. In: Kaufman DW et al., eds. The drug etiology of agranulocytosis and aplastic anemia. New York, NY: Oxford University Press; 1991:159–169
Young NS et al. Blood 2006;108:2509–2519

Disease Severity

Severe aplastic anemia
1. Bone marrow cellularity <25% of normal or 25–50% of normal with <30% residual hematopoietic cells, *and*
2. Two out of 3 criteria: (a) neutrophils <500/mm³; (b) platelets <20,000/mm³; (c) reticulocytes <1%

Very severe aplastic anemia
1. Bone marrow cellularity <25% of normal or 25–50% of normal with <30% residual hematopoietic cells, *and*
2. (a) Neutrophil count <200/mm³ and (b) platelets <20,000/mm³ or reticulocytes <1%

Moderate (nonsevere) aplastic anemia
Patients who do not fulfill the above criteria

Bacigalupo A et al. Br J Haematol 1988;70:177–182
Bacigalupo A et al. Semin Hematol 2000;37:69–80
Camitta BM et al. Blood 1976;48:63–70
Rosenfeld S et al. JAMA 2003;289:1130–1135
Young NS et al. Biol Blood Marrow Transplant 2010;16(1 Suppl):S119–S125

Etiology and Classification

I. Acquired aplastic anemia
A. Idiopathic (2/3 of all cases)
B. Secondary
  1. Drugs
    a. Predicted:
     (1) Cytotoxic chemotherapeutic agents
- Alkylating agents (busulfan, cyclophosphamide, melphalan)
- Antimitotics (vincristine, vinblastine)
- Antimetabolites (antifolate compounds, nucleotide analogs)

    b. Idiosyncratic:
     (1) Chloramphenicol
     (2) Antiprotozoal agents (quinacrine, chloroquine)
     (3) Nonsteroidal antiinflammatory drugs: ibuprofen, indomethacin, sulindac, diclofenac, naproxen, phenylbutazone
     (4) Anticonvulsants: hydantoins, carbamazepine, phenacemide, ethosuximide
     (5) Gold and arsenic
     (6) Sulfonamides
     (7) Antithyroid drugs (methimazole, methylthiouracil, propylthiouracil)
     (8) Oral hypoglycemic agents (tolbutamide, carbutamide, chlorpropamide)
     (9) Penicillamine
     (10) Mesalazine
  2. Chemicals: benzene, insecticides
  3. Radiation
  4. Viral infections:
    a. Parvovirus (rare, usually causes transient aplastic crisis, pure red cell aplasia)
    b. Hepatitis viruses (non-A, non-B, non-C hepatitis)
    c. Epstein-Barr virus
    d. Human immunodeficiency virus
  5. Immune disorders:
    a. Eosinophilic fasciitis
    b. Systemic lupus erythematosus
    c. Graft versus host disease, transfusion associated
    d. Hypoimmunoglobulinemia
    e. Thymoma and thymic carcinoma
  6. Paroxysmal nocturnal hemoglobinuria
  7. Pregnancy

II. Inherited aplastic anemia
  1. Fanconi anemia
  2. Dyskeratosis congenita
  3. Shwachman-Diamond syndrome
  4. Amegakaryocytic thrombocytopenia

Young NS. In: Young NS, ed. Bone Marrow Failure Syndromes. 1st ed. Philadelphia, PA: WB Saunders; 2000:1–46

Work-up

It is important to exclude other disorders that may present with pancytopenia and a hypoplastic bone marrow

CBC with differential	• All cell lineages may not be affected; bicytopenias or monocytopenias may occur • Decreased reticulocyte count • Red blood cells usually are normocytic but occasionally erythrocyte macrocytosis may be present • In the peripheral blood smear the remaining elements, while reduced, are morphologically normal
Bone marrow biopsy and aspiration	• The degree of bone marrow hypocellularity may not correlate with the peripheral blood count • Marrow morphology is usually normal or may have erythroid megaloblastoid changes • The marrow space is composed of fat cells and marrow stroma • Malignant infiltrates or fibrosis are absent
Cytogenetic analysis of marrow cells	• Usually normal in AA in contrast to MDS • However, presence of cytogenetic clones does not exclude AA Most common associated cytogenetics abnormalities with AA is monosomy 7 and trisomy 8. For myelodysplasia and leukemia, the cumulative long-term rate of clonal evolution is approximately 15%; evolution is not inevitable in aplastic anemia, and some cytogenetic abnormalities may be transient, or, as with trisomy 8, responsive to immunosuppressive treatments
Flow cytometry	To investigate for paroxysmal nocturnal hemoglobinuria (PNH); expression of the glycosylphosphatidylinositol-anchored proteins CD55 and CD5. Small PNH clones present at diagnosis usually remain stable over time but may expand sufficiently to produce symptomatic hemolysis
HLA typing	• For potential allogeneic hematopoietic cell transplantation candidates
Serology	• Hepatitis profile if liver function abnormalities and human immunodeficiency virus if clinically indicated

Young NS et al. Blood 2006;108:2509–2519

Differential Diagnosis of Pancytopenia

Pancytopenia with hypocellular bone marrow
1. Acquired aplastic anemia
2. Inherited aplastic anemia
3. Myelodysplasia syndromes (rare)
4. Aleukemic leukemia (rare)
5. Lymphomas of bone marrow (rare)

Pancytopenia with cellular bone marrow
Primary bone marrow diseases:
1. Myelodysplasia syndrome
2. Paroxysmal nocturnal hemoglobinuria
3. Myelofibrosis
4. Hairy cell leukemia
5. Myelophthisis
6. Bone marrow lymphoma

Secondary to systemic diseases:
1. Systemic lupus erythematosus
2. Sjögren syndrome
3. Hypersplenism
4. Vitamin B_{12} deficiency, folate deficiency
5. Alcoholism
6. Brucellosis
7. Ehrlichiosis
8. Sarcoidosis
9. Tuberculosis and atypical mycobacteria

Hypocellular bone marrow with or without cytopenia:
1. Q fever
2. Legionnaires' disease
3. Toxoplasmosis
4. Mycobacteria
5. Tuberculosis
6. Anorexia nervosa, starvation
7. Hypothyroidism

Treatment Options

Hematopoiesis can be restored in severe aplastic anemia with allogeneic hematopoietic cell transplantation (allo-HCT) or immunosupressive therapy. HCT is preferred when feasible as it is curative. However, most patients are not suitable candidates for optimal initial HCT because of lack of a matched sibling donor, lead time to identify a suitable unrelated donor, age, comorbidities, or access to transplantation. Patients <50 years old with severe aplastic anemia who have an HLA-compatible sibling should be offered allo-HCT as first-line treatment. The combination of ATG with cyclosporine is the standard for immunosuppressive therapy and should be considered for nonsevere transfusion-dependent AA patients or patients who lack an HLA-compatible sibling donor. Patients who do not respond at 6 months following ATG with cyclosporine should be considered for matched unrelated-donor HCT (children and young adults) or receive a second course of ATG + cyclosporine if no matched unrelated donor is available

Transplantation for AA from an HLA-identical sibling donor has improved over the years with a 70–80% chance of long-term cure. Graft failure rates following allo-HCT range from 4–14% and the development of chronic graft-versus-host disease range from 30–40% of patients. The correlation of increasing age with the risk of GVHD and the significant morbidity and mortality of this transplant complication continues to impact on the decision to pursue HCT versus immunosupressive therapy as initial therapy in adults with SAA. A report by the Center for International Blood and Marrow Transplant Research of more than 1300 severe aplastic anemia patients who were transplanted from 1991 to 2004, survival at 5 years for patients younger than 20 years of age was 82%, for those 20 to 40 years of age 72%, and for those older than 40 years, closer to 50%. Rates of GVHD increased with age, accounting for much of the decreased survival in older patients and the long-term morbidity. Thus, outcomes in the most favorable age group (children with matched sibling donor) resulted in long-term survival of approximate 80%

In severe aplastic anemia, peripheral blood stem cell results have been inferior to grafts of bone marrow origin. Higher rates of chronic GVHD were observed in patients of all ages undergoing HCT with peripheral blood compared with bone marrow derived stem cell grafts. It is recommended bone marrow stem cells be used rather than granulocyte-colony stimulating factor (G-CSF) mobilized peripheral blood stem cells

Gupta V et al. Haematologica 2010;95:2119–2125
Kojima S et al. Int J Hematol 2011;93:832–837
Scheinberg P, Young NS. Blood 2012;120:1185–1196
Young NS et al. Biol Blood Marrow Transplant 2010;16(1 Suppl):S119–S125

REGIMEN

APLASTIC ANEMIA THERAPY

LYMPHOCYTE IMMUNE GLOBULIN, ANTITHYMOCYTE GLOBULIN (EQUINE) (ATG) + CYCLOSPORINE

Rosenfeld S et al. Blood 1995; 85:3058–3065
Rosenfeld S et al. JAMA 2003;289:1130–1135
Scheinberg P et al. N Engl J Med 2011;365:430–438 + supplementary information available online at: www.nejm.org/doi/full/10.1056/NEJMoa1103975

Premedication:

Diphenhydramine 25–50 mg; administer orally 60 minutes before each antithymocyte globulin treatment

Lymphocyte immune globulin, antithymocyte globulin* (equine) (ATG) 40 mg/kg per day administered through a high-flow (central) vein, vascular shunt, or arteriovenous fistula in a volume of 0.9% sodium chloride injection (0.9% NS), 5% dextrose and 0.2% sodium chloride injection (D5W/0.2% NS), or 5% dextrose and 0.45% sodium chloride injection (D5W/0.45% NS) sufficient to produce a solution with antithymocyte globulin concentration ≤4 mg/mL, over at least 4 hours for 4 consecutive days, on days 1–4 (total dosage/course = 160 mg/kg)

Notes:

1. ATGAM (antithymocyte globulin [equine]) product labeling recommends intradermal skin testing prior to administration. Patients with a reactive skin test may still receive antithymocyte globulin after desensitization

2. Always administer antithymocyte globulin through a 0.2- to 1-μm pore size inline filter

3. After dilution, ATG should be allowed to come to room temperature before administration begins

4. The initial infusion rate should be 10% of the total volume per hour. For example, for a total volume of 500 mL, start at a rate of 50 mL/hour for the first 30 minutes. If there are no signs of an adverse reaction, the infusion rate can be advanced to complete the infusion over no less than 4 hours

Prednisone 1 mg/kg per day; administer orally starting prior to the first dose of ATG, and continuing for a total of 10 days; the daily dose is gradually decreased (tapered) over the following 7 days, and then discontinued

Adults:

Cyclosporine (initially) 6 mg/kg per dose; administer orally every 12 hours, continually for 6 months, commencing on day 1. Starting at 6 months, gradually decrease cyclosporine doses over the subsequent 18 months (taper to discontinuation)

Children:

Cyclosporine (initially) 7.5 mg/kg per dose; administer orally every 12 hours, continually for 6 months, commencing on day 1. Starting at 6 months, gradually decrease cyclosporine doses over the subsequent 18 months (taper to discontinuation)

Notes:

1. Cyclosporine doses are adjusted to maintain serum concentrations within the range of 200–400 mcg/L (166–333 nmol/L), and as a factor of renal and hepatic toxicity

2. *Prophylaxis for Pneumocystis jirovecii:* Pentamidine 300 mg by inhalation every 4 weeks beginning the first month of therapy, and continue for at least 6 months

3. Antibacterial, antiviral, and antifungal prophylaxes are not routinely administered with standard equine ATG and cyclosporine treatment

Patient Population Studied

A total of 120 consecutive patients, 2–77 years of age, were randomly assigned to horse ATG or rabbit ATG (60 patients in each group)

Efficacy

Scheinberg P et al. N Engl J Med 2011;365:430–438

Response	Horse (equine) ATG (n = 60)	95% CI	Rabbit (lepine) ATG (n = 60)	95% CI	P Value
At 3 months	37(62)	49–74	20(33)	21–46	0.002
At 6 months	41(68)	56–80	22(37)	24–39	<0.001

At 3 years, the survival rate was 96% (95% CI, 90–100) in the horse-ATG group as compared with 76% (95% CI, 61–95) in the rabbit-ATG group (P = 0.04) when data were censored at the time of stem-cell transplantation, and 94% (95% CI, 88–100) as compared with 70% (95% CI, 56–86; P = 0.008) in the respective groups when stem-cell–transplantation events were not censored

Disposition among nonresponders at 6 months to immunosuppression:
Among the 17 nonresponders to horse-ATG, 5 underwent stem-cell transplantation, 4 from a histocompatible sibling and 1 from a matched unrelated donor. Eight patients underwent second-line immunosuppression (rabbit-ATG plus cyclosporine or alemtuzumab). Of the 29 nonresponders in the rabbit-ATG group, 23 patients received second-line immunosuppression (horse-ATG plus cyclosporine or alemtuzumab). Four patients underwent stem-cell transplantation, 3 from a histocompatible sibling and 1 from an unrelated donor. Six patients who did not respond to second-line immunosuppression went on to receive a stem-cell transplantation, 1 from a histocompatible sibling, 4 from an unrelated donor, and 1 patient received a haploidentical/umbilical cord transplant

Toxicity

Adverse Events	Horse ATG	Rabbit ATG
Related to immunosuppression		
Serum sickness	2	5
Chest pain	1	0
Hemolysis*	0	1
SVT	0	1
Azotemia	1	0
PRES	0	1
Hemorrhage		
CNS	0	1
Vitreous	0	1
Hematemesis	0	1
Epistaxis	1	1
Menorrhagia	2	0
Hemoptysis	1	0

(continued)

Toxicity (continued)

Adverse Events	Horse ATG	Rabbit ATG
Infection		
Neutropenia and fever, negative cultures	23	16
Neutropenia and fever, positive cultures	17	14
Polymicrobial[†]	0	6
Pneumonia[‡]	1	3
Necrotizing fasciitis[§]	0	1
Clostridium difficile	2	2
Retropharyngeal abscess	0	1
Perirectal abscess	0	1
Periorbital cellulitis	1	0
Tonsillitis/pharyngitis	2	1
Appendicitis/typhlitis	0	4
Otitis media	1	0
Epididymitis	0	1
Upper respiratory infection	5[ᵉ]	1
Other	9	11

PRES, Posterior reversible encephalopathy syndrome; SVT, supraventricular tachycardia; CNS, central nervous system
Serious adverse events depicted are those that resulted in prolonged hospitalization, hospital admission, or death
Events shown are those that occurred after the first cycle of immunosuppression. Repeated hospitalizations in the same subject were counted as separate events
*Hemolysis occurred after ATG infusion in a patient with a large underlying paroxysmal nocturnal hemoglobinuria clone
[†]Patients with multiple microbial isolates and/or different sites of infection are categorized as having polymicrobial infection. The organisms recovered and sites for each of the patients were: (a) Escherichia coli, Staphylococcus epidermidis, Enterococcus faecium, Acinetobacter baumannii (all in blood); Enterococcus sp., Staphylococcus sp., and mold (left turbinate biopsy); (b) Pseudomonas sp., Klebsiella sp., Staphylococcus epidermidis, Streptococcus viridans, Staphylococcus hemolyticus, Enterococcus faecium, and Stenotrophomonas maltophilia (all in blood); (c) Enterobacter cloacae, Pseudomonas aeruginosa (respiratory cultures); Acinetobacter baumannii, Mycobacterium gordonae, Fusarium sp., Acinetobacter baumannii, Enterococcus faecalis (sinus culture), Corynebacterium sp. (blood), Proteus mirabilis (urine); (d) Propionibacterium acnes, Staphylococcus aureus, Candida albicans (throat); (e) Streptococcus sp. (blood), Trichosporon asahii (sinus), Candida albicans (skin); (f) Enterococcus faecium, Staphylococcus epidermidis (blood), Klebsiella pneumoniae (urine)
[‡]One case of fungal pneumonia in each group
[§]Caused by Clostridium sp
[ᵉ]In 3 subjects viral infection was confirmed by nasopharyngeal wash

Clonal evolution:

The cumulative incidence of clonal evolution at 3 years (in all patients, those with and those without a response) was 21% (95% CI, 7–33) in the horse-ATG group and 14% (95% CI, 1–25) in the rabbit-ATG group (P = 0.69). Among patients treated with horse-ATG, 1 each had deletion 3, deletion 5q, deletion 13q, deletion 20q, and leukemia, and 4 had monosomy 7. In 2 patients, monosomy 7 was preceded by t(12;13) and deletion 13q. In the rabbit-ATG group, 5 patients had monosomy 7, and 1 had deletion 13q

Therapy Monitoring

1. *During antithymocyte globulin infusion:* CBC with differential, LFTs, electrolytes
2. *After antithymocyte globulin therapy:* CBC monitoring is dependent on blood counts. If they are stable CBC with differential can be as infrequent as once every 2–3 weeks. Patients requiring platelets may need more frequent CBC
3. *Six months after the start of therapy:* Bone marrow biopsy and aspiration. If patients are stable based on blood counts, bone marrow biopsy may not need to be repeated

Therapeutic Drug Monitoring—Cyclosporine:

1. When initiating cyclosporine treatment and after any dose adjustments, monitor cyclosporine trough concentrations (sampled at the end of a dosing interval) every 4–7 days until stable concentrations are achieved
2. For patients on a stable cyclosporine regimen, monitor trough levels every 2 weeks
3. More frequent cyclosporine monitoring is recommended whenever cyclosporine dosage adjustments are made, serum creatinine increases, and when a patient's concomitantly administered medication regimen is changed (be wary of drugs that potentially perturb cytochrome P450 CYP3A subfamily enzymes expression, availability, or activity)
4. **Cyclosporine** doses are adjusted to maintain blood concentrations within the range of 200–400 mcg/L (166–333 nmol/L)

Notes

1. Avoid other nephrotoxic drugs concurrent with cyclosporine treatment

2. Granulocyte-colony stimulating factors (G-CSF) should be administered as clinically indicated, usually for evidence of infection such as fever or localized inflammation in the setting of severe inflammation. Emergence of monosomy 7 has been linked to exogenous use of G-CSF

   The role of G-CSF was evaluated in 192 patients with newly diagnosed severe AA not eligible for transplantation who were entered into a multicenter, randomized study to receive ATG/cyclosporine with or without G-CSF. Overall survival (OS) at 6 years was 76% ± 4%, and event-free survival (EFS) was 42% ± 4%. No difference in OS/EFS was seen between patients randomly assigned to receive or not to receive G-CSF, neither for the entire cohort nor in subgroups stratified by age and disease severity. Patients treated with G-CSF had fewer infectious episodes (24%) and hospitalization days (82%) compared with patients who did not receive G-CSF (36%; P = 0.006; 87%; P = 0.0003)

   Tichelli A et al. Blood 2011;117:4434–4441

3. Patients with AA usually receive irradiated blood products during and after ATG treatment. This policy should continue for at least as long as patients are receiving immune suppressive therapy

   Guidelines for administering antithymocyte globulin (ATG):

   - Severity and frequency of toxicities (rigors, fevers, oxygen desaturation, hypotension, nausea, vomiting, anaphylaxis) are greatest during the first day of infusion and diminish with each subsequent day. Toxicities generally subside after completing treatment
   - Adverse effects generally can be managed while continuing antithymocyte globulin infusion
   - Most patients receiving ATG will develop fever. Most fevers are not infectious in origin. Patients with fever and neutropenia should be treated with broad-spectrum antibiotics empirically

   Marsh J et al. Br J Haematol 2010;150:377–379

   Allergy skin testing prior to ATG administration:

   - Advise patients to avoid using H_1-receptor antagonists for 72 hours before skin testing
   - Antithymocyte globulin (equine) is freshly diluted (1:1000) with 0.9% sodium chloride injection (0.9% NS), to a concentration of 5 mcg/0.1 mL, and administered intradermally
   - Administer 0.1 mL 0.9% NS, intradermally in a contralateral extremity as a control
   - Observe every 15–20 minutes during the first hour after intradermal injection
   - A local reaction ≥10 mm with a wheal, erythema, or both, ± pseudopod formation and itching or a marked local swelling, is considered a positive test. For patients who exhibit a positive test result, consider desensitization prior to therapy
   - If antithymocyte globulin is administered after a locally positive skin test, administration should only be attempted in a setting where intensive life support facilities are immediately available and with the attendance of a physician familiar with the treatment of potentially life-threatening allergic reactions
   - Systemic reactions preclude antithymocyte globulin administration; for example, generalized rash, tachycardia, dyspnea, hypotension, or anaphylaxis

   Note: The predictive value of skin testing has not been proved clinically; that is, allergic reactions including anaphylaxis have occurred in patients whose skin test result is negative

   Monitoring during ATG administration:

   - Patients should remain under continual surveillance
   - Assess peripheral vascular access sites for thrombophlebitis every 8 hours
   - Monitor vital signs and assess for adverse reactions (flushing, hives, itching, SOB, difficulty breathing, chest tightness) before starting administration, then:
     - During initial dose: Continually during the first 15 minutes, then every 30 minutes × 2, then at least every hour until administration is completed
     - During subsequent doses: 30 minutes after initiating ATG infusion

Infusional Toxicities of Antithymocyte Globulin

Adverse Events	Interventions
Rigors	Antihistamines (eg, diphenhydramine 25–50 mg; administer intravenously or orally every 6 hours as needed) Meperidine 12.5–50 mg; administer intravenously every 3–4 hours as needed
Nausea, vomiting	Antiemetic rescue. Give antiemetic prophylaxis during subsequent antithymocyte globulin treatments (secondary prophylaxis)
Anaphylaxis*	Immediately STOP administration; administer steroids, assist respiration, and provide other resuscitative measures. DO NOT resume treatment
Thrombocytopenia, anemia	Blood product transfusions as needed[†]
Fever and neutropenia[‡]	Broad-spectrum antibiotics empirically, if ANC <500/mm^3. May give acetaminophen 650 mg orally every 4 hours
Hypotension	Fluid resuscitation
Refractory hypotension	May indicate anaphylaxis. Stop antithymocyte globulin infusion and stabilize blood pressure. Intensive Care Unit support
Oxygen desaturation	Oxygen therapy
Refractory oxygen desaturation	Discontinue antithymocyte globulin. Intensive Care Unit support
Respiratory distress	Discontinue antithymocyte globulin. If distress persists, administer an antihistamine, epinephrine, corticosteroids
Rash, pruritus, urticaria	Administer antihistamines and/or topical steroids for prophylaxis and treatment
Serum sickness-like symptoms[§]	Administer prophylactic glucocorticoids
Hepatotoxicity[ε]	Monitor LFTs

*Anaphylaxis (<3% of patients) most frequently occurs within the first hour after starting antithymocyte globulin infusion. After the first hour, adverse effects occur as result of a delayed immune response and generally can be managed while continuing the antithymocyte globulin infusion

[†]Concomitant administration of blood products should be avoided with antithymocyte globulin infusions to avoid confusing transfusion reactions with reactions to antithymocyte globulin

[‡]Most patients who receive antithymocyte globulin will develop fever as a result of the drug. Most fevers are not infectious in origin, but patients should receive broad spectrum antibiotics empirically until an infectious process is ruled out

[§]Type II hypersensitivity reactions/serum sickness consisting of fever, rash, and arthralgia develops in approximately 85% of patients between 7 and 14 days after ATG treatment. These symptoms can be managed with corticosteroids

[ε]An isolated increase in serum alanine aminotransferase (ALT) frequently has no clinical significance. Generally, liver function abnormalities are transient and return to normal within one month

Bevans MF, Shalabi RA. Clin J Oncol Nurs 2004;8:377–382

APLASTIC ANEMIA THERAPY
ANDROGENS

Bacigalupo A et al. Br J Haematol 1993;83:145–151
Besa EC. Semin Hematol 1994;31:134–145
Heimpel H. Acta Haematol 2000;103:11–15
Najean Y. Am J Med 1981;71:543–551
Passweg JR, Marsh JC. Hematology Am Soc Hematol Educ Program 2010:36–42 (review)

Oxymetholone 0.25–5 mg/kg per day; administer orally, continually
Danazol 600–800 mg per day; administer orally, continually

Indications

Androgens were used extensively in the treatment of AA for many decades before the availability of immunosuppressants

Patients with aplastic anemia who are not candidates for HSCT or who did not respond to immunosuppressive therapy

Efficacy

Response rate at 6 months	35–60%
5-year survival	25–50%

Therapy Monitoring

1. *Twice weekly to every 2–3 weeks:* CBC monitoring is dependent on blood counts. If they are stable, a CBC with differential can be obtained as infrequently as once every 2–3 weeks. Patients requiring platelets may need more frequent CBCs, but not more than twice weekly and usually only once weekly
2. *Monthly:* LFTs
3. *Periodic:* Serum HDL and LDL (anabolic steroids have been reported to lower the level of high-density lipoproteins and raise the level of low-density lipoproteins. These changes usually revert to normal on discontinuation of treatment)
   Serum iron and iron-binding capacity
   • Iron-deficiency anemia has been observed in some patients treated with steroids. If iron deficiency is detected, it should be appropriately treated with supplementary iron
4. *Every 6 months:* X-ray examinations of bone in prepubertal patients to determine the rate of bone maturation and drug effects on the epiphyseal centers

Notes

1. A trial of androgens for 3–6 months is recommended to evaluate a patient's response
2. Patients may respond to different androgen preparations. An alternative product may be used if the initially chosen androgen was not effective or no longer produces a therapeutic benefit
3. Hypoglycemic drug regimens may need to be adjusted in diabetic patients who receive anabolic steroids
4. Anabolic steroids may suppress clotting factors II, V, VII, and X, and increase prothrombin times
5. Danazol may produce symptoms of benign intracranial hypertension (papilledema, headache, nausea, vomiting, and visual disturbances). Advise patients who exhibit these symptoms to immediately discontinue danazol and refer them to a neurologist for further diagnosis and care
6. Contraindications to the use of androgens include undiagnosed abnormal genital bleeding, impaired hepatic function, impaired renal function, impaired cardiac function, pregnancy, porphyria, breast cancer in women with hypercalcemia, prostate cancer

Toxicity

Common: Acne, seborrhea, edema, emotional lability, nervousness, flushing, sweating, hair loss, hirsutism, menstrual disturbances, vaginal dryness and irritation, voice change, weight gain, changes in libido

Serious side effects: Cholestatic jaundice, peliosis (hemorrhagic liver cysts), hepatic tumors

Peliosis hepatis and hepatic adenomas may be silent until complicated by acute, potentially life-threatening intraabdominal hemorrhage

Hepatotoxicity occurs less frequently with parenteral preparations

Oxymetholone: Decreased serum HDL ± increased LDL. Cholestatic hepatitis and jaundice ± pruritus at low doses; may be associated with acute hepatic enlargement and RUQ pain. Continued therapy has been associated with hepatic coma and death

Danazol: Thromboembolism, thrombotic and thrombophlebitic events, including sagittal sinus thrombosis and life-threatening or fatal strokes; benign intracranial hypertension (pseudotumor cerebri)

63. Thrombotic Thrombocytopenic Purpura/ Hemolytic Uremic Syndrome

Arafat Tfayli, MD, Kiarash Kojouri, MD, MPH, and James N. George, MD

Thrombotic thrombocytopenic purpura (TTP) is defined clinically by the abnormalities caused by systemic thrombotic microangiopathy: thrombocytopenia and microangiopathic hemolytic anemia. Additional clinical features may include neurologic abnormalities, renal failure, and gastrointestinal symptoms

Hemolytic-uremic syndrome (HUS) is another clinical presentation of thrombotic microangiopathy. Like TTP, HUS is manifested by thrombocytopenia and microangiopathic hemolytic anemia with the additional abnormality of renal failure. Although it is commonly stated that HUS is manifested primarily by renal failure whereas TTP is manifested primarily by neurologic abnormalities, these 2 syndromes cannot be distinguished clinically, because many patients have both renal failure and severe neurologic abnormalities, or neither. The term HUS is often restricted to children. In adults, all syndromes are referred to as TTP, whether or not neurologic abnormalities or renal failure are present

Amorosi EL, Ultmann JE. Medicine (Baltimore) 1966;45:139–159
George JN. N Engl J Med 2006;354:1927–1935

Epidemiology

Incidence:

Inherited:	Very rare. Described in isolated case reports
Acquired:	11.3 cases/10^6 population/year for all patients diagnosed with TTP; 1.7 cases/10^6 population/year for patients with ADAMTS13 deficiency
Male-to-female ratio:	1:3
Age:	Rare in children, except for the typical diarrhea-associated HUS; TTP occurs in the complete age range of adults
Mortality:	Untreated, TTP is fatal in 90% of patients. With effective treatment, mortality is decreased to approximately 15%

Amorosi EL, Ultmann JE. Medicine (Baltimore) 1966;45:139–159
Terrell DR et al. J Thromb Haemost 2005;3:1432–1436
Vesely SK et al. Blood 2003;102:60–68

Classification

Congenital:
Patients with congenital TTP, presumably caused by inherited abnormalities of the *ADAMTS13* gene, may present in early childhood, as adults, or may remain asymptomatic. Also, congenital abnormalities of complement regulation can cause syndromes of HUS

Acquired:
1. *Idiopathic:* Most patients with TTP present without an associated condition or apparent etiology
2. *Allogeneic hematopoietic stem cell transplantation:* Although there are reports describing TTP as a specific complication of allogeneic hematopoietic stem cell transplantation, this may not exist as a specific entity. In most patients diagnosed with TTP following allogeneic hematopoietic stem cell transplantation, the clinical features suggesting thrombotic microangiopathy are caused by systemic infection (eg, aspergillus, cytomegalovirus), regimen-related toxicity, or acute graft-versus-host disease. These syndromes are now described as transplantation-associated thrombotic microangiopathy, not as TTP
3. *Pregnancy/postpartum:* Pregnancy is a risk factor for developing TTP, particularly in patients with congenital TTP. Congenital and acquired TTP typically occur near term or postpartum. Other pregnancy-related complications, such as severe preeclampsia and the HELLP (*H*emolysis, *E*levated *L*iver function tests, and *L*ow *P*latelets) syndrome may have clinical features identical to TTP
4. *Drug-associated, immune-mediated:* Hypersensitivity reactions to drugs can cause the complete syndrome of TTP. Most frequent is quinine hypersensitivity; also reported are ticlopidine, clopidogrel
5. *Drug-associated, dose-dependent toxicity:* The clinical and pathologic features of TTP can be caused by dose-dependent toxicity of chemotherapeutic agents, most commonly mitomycin, and immunosuppressive agents. Among the latter, most commonly cyclosporine
6. *Shiga toxin:* Enterohemorrhagic infections producing Shiga toxin, characteristically *Escherichia coli* 0157:H7, can cause all clinical features of TTP. Shiga toxin causes the characteristic HUS of young children, and may also cause TTP in adults, with or without renal abnormalities
7. *Association with established autoimmune disorders:* In some instances, the clinical syndrome of TTP occurs in a patient with an established diagnosis of an autoimmune disorder, such as systemic lupus erythematosus or the antiphospholipid antibody syndrome. Whether TTP is merely an additional manifestation of an established autoimmune disorder or should be considered a distinct entity, is never clinically clear

George JN et al. Semin Hematol 2004;41:60–67
Kojouri K et al. Ann Intern Med 2001;135:1047–1051
Kojouri K, George JN. Curr Opin Oncol 2007;19:148–154
Vesely SK et al. Blood 2003;102:60–68

Pathology

The clinical syndrome of TTP is caused by disseminated platelet thrombi obstructing arterioles and small vessels. The characteristic histologic pattern is described as thrombotic microangiopathy. TTP, like other thrombotic and vascular disorders, is the result of multiple etiologies and risk factors

1. ADAMTS13 deficiency. Best-described etiology is a congenital or acquired deficiency of the plasma von Willebrand factor-cleaving protease, ADAMTS13. Severe deficiency of ADAMTS13 results in an accumulation of unusually large von Willebrand factor multimers that can cause platelet agglutination in regions of high shear stress, resulting in platelet–von Willebrand factor thrombi
2. Shiga toxin damage of endothelial cells
3. Drug-dependent antibodies directed against platelets, granulocytes, and endothelial cells
4. Dose-dependent drug toxicity
5. Additional risk factors include factor V Leiden, female gender, African American ethnicity, and obesity

Moake JL. N Engl J Med 2002;347:589–600
Raife TJ et al. Blood 2002;99:437–442
Vesely SK et al. Blood 2003;102:60–68

Differential Diagnosis

The diagnosis of TTP is based on the observation of thrombocytopenia and microangiopathic hemolytic anemia without another clinically apparent cause. In rare instances, even these 2 cardinal features may not be present, as for example, patients with previously diagnosed episodes of TTP who subsequently have acute neurologic symptoms without thrombocytopenia or anemia, and are documented to have severe ADAMTS13 deficiency. Many years ago, TTP was diagnosed by a pentad of clinical features: thrombocytopenia, microangiopathic hemolytic anemia, neurologic abnormalities, renal insufficiency, and fever. In the current era, urgency of diagnosis is required to initiate effective treatment. Therefore only thrombocytopenia and microangiopathic hemolytic anemia are required to establish the diagnosis of TTP. Neurologic abnormalities, renal insufficiency, and fever are uncommon and not necessary for the diagnosis. Therefore the differential diagnosis includes all conditions associated with the clinical features of TTP

1. **Systemic infections**
   - Systemic fungal infections. Aspergillosis and other angioinvasive fungi can cause all clinical features of thrombotic microangiopathy
   - Viral infections. Disseminated CMV infection can cause all clinical features of thrombotic microangiopathy. HIV infection can also mimic TTP, typically related to additional opportunistic infections
   - Rickettsial infections. For example Rocky Mountain spotted fever
   - Bacterial sepsis, especially bacterial meningitis
2. **Systemic malignancy**

   Disseminated micrometastatic malignancies may mimic all clinical features of TTP, without apparent evidence by imaging studies. Although disseminated intravascular coagulation (DIC) can occur in patients with disseminated malignancy, systemic small-vessel metastases causing obstruction and thrombosis can occur without evidence of DIC. A syndrome mimicking TTP may occur with breast cancer, pancreatic cancer, gastric cancer, and non–small cell lung cancer
3. **Complications of pregnancy**

   Severe preeclampsia and the HELLP (*H*emolysis, *E*levated *L*iver function tests, and *L*ow *P*latelets) syndrome may mimic all clinical features of TTP
4. **Malignant hypertension**

   Severe hypertension may cause all clinical features of TTP, including thrombocytopenia, severe microangiopathic hemolysis, renal failure, and acute central nervous system abnormalities
5. **Autoimmune disorders**

   Patients with acute systemic symptoms related to systemic lupus erythematosus, antiphospholipid antibody syndrome, acute systemic sclerosis, polyarteritis nodosa, and other autoimmune disorders can have all clinical features of TTP

Downes KA et al. J Clin Apher 2004;19:86–89
Francis KK et al. Oncologist 2007;12:11–19
George JN et al. Semin Hematol 2004;41:60–67
McMinn JR, George JN. J Clin Apher 2001;16:202–209

Work-up

1. *CBC:* Thrombocytopenia and anemia should be present; the white blood cell count is typically normal

2. *Peripheral blood smear* should demonstrate polychromasia consistent with a high reticulocyte count and fragmented red blood cells (schistocytes)

3. *Serum chemistry profile:* Most remarkable should be the increased LDH level, a manifestation of severe systemic tissue ischemia as well as hemolysis. An elevated indirect bilirubin level indicates hemolysis. Elevated creatinine is commonly present

4. *Urinalysis:* Proteinuria and microscopic hematuria are nearly always present

5. *Imaging studies:* X-rays and scans are typically normal. Pulmonary manifestations are uncommon. The head CT scan is typically normal even in the presence of severe central nervous system abnormalities, because abnormalities are caused by diffuse small-vessel disease

6. *Microbiology:* Cultures and serologic tests for infectious etiologies should be negative in patients with TTP, though these studies are an essential part of the evaluation to exclude infections as an alternative etiology for the presenting signs and symptoms. Patients presenting with bloody diarrhea need a stool culture on special media to detect *E. coli* 0157:H7

7. *Plasma sample for assay of ADAMTS13 activity and ADAMTS13 inhibitor activity:* Normal values for ADAMTS13 activity do not exclude the diagnosis of TTP and do not suggest that plasma exchange treatment is not indicated. A severe deficiency of ADAMTS13 activity may be specific for TTP, but may also occur in asymptomatic individuals following recovery from an acute episode of TTP. ADAMTS13 activity may also be absent in patients with severe systemic infections or liver disease. The demonstration of severely decreased ADAMTS13 activity in association with a high-titer inhibitor is consistent with an autoimmune etiology and may predict a prolonged and severe course of illness and a 30–40% risk for relapse. ADAMTS13 circulates for several days in the plasma, therefore levels can be falsely elevated as a result of previous transfusions; patients with TTP are commonly transfused with red cells and platelets upon initial emergency room evaluation, and, therefore, plasma samples for ADAMTS13 activity are commonly inaccurate

Furlan M, Lämmle B. Best Pract Res Clin Haematol 2001;14:437–454
George JN. N Engl J Med 2006;354:1927–1935
Zheng XL et al. Blood 2004;103:4043–4049

Treatment Options

Congenital TTP

Plasma infusion:
Congenital TTP because of an abnormality of the *ADAMTS13* gene is caused by a deficiency of ADAMTS13 activity. These rare patients can be treated simply with plasma infusion to restore ADAMTS13 activity. Once the diagnosis of congenital TTP is established, regular infusions of 10 mL/kg of fresh-frozen plasma given at intervals of approximately 2–3 weeks are appropriate lifetime prophylactic treatment. Whole fresh-frozen plasma and cryoprecipitate-poor plasma are equivalent

Acquired TTP

Plasma exchange treatment is the key element for management of TTP. It is the one treatment with effectiveness documented by a randomized controlled clinical trial in which plasma exchange was compared with plasma infusion. Plasma exchange is urgently indicated in all patients with a clinical diagnosis of TTP. Although there are no data that clearly support the efficacy of glucocorticoids, they are commonly given in addition to plasma exchange as acquired TTP is commonly thought to have an autoimmune etiology. Many other immunosuppressive agents have been used in the treatment of TTP, such as rituximab and cyclosporine. These are used in patients with disease refractory to plasma exchange and glucocorticoids

Transfusion therapy:
Most patients with TTP will require red cell transfusions during their acute illness. Several well-publicized anecdotes of individual patients have suggested that platelet transfusions may be harmful in patients with TTP. However, many patients with TTP have received platelet transfusions appropriately given for overt bleeding or for invasive procedures without complications

Aspirin 81–325 mg/day may be used in patients with TIA or stroke symptoms, as in patients without TTP. However, it is prudent to avoid aspirin in patients with platelet counts <20,000/mm^3

Barbot J et al. Br J Haematol 2001;113:649–651
George JN. N Engl J Med 2006;354:1927–1935
Swisher KK et al. Transfusion 2009;49:873–887
Zheng X et al. Ann Intern Med 2003;138:105–108

REGIMEN

PLASMA EXCHANGE

(WHOLE FRESH-FROZEN PLASMA OR CRYOPRECIPITATE-POOR PLASMA)

Rock GA et al. N Engl J Med 1991;325:393–397

Prior to the start of therapy:
Insert a double-lumen dialysis catheter, placed in internal jugular, subclavian, or femoral vein, percutaneously at bedside when an elective procedure is not feasible, or when time and conditions allow, tunneled in the subclavian or internal jugular vein with sterile operating room conditions

Plasma exchange:
Use **whole fresh-frozen plasma or cryoprecipitate-poor plasma** to exchange 1 plasma volume per treatment each day. Continue daily exchanges until the platelet count reaches the normal range, indicating a hematologic response. Then discontinue exchanges either abruptly or gradually, depending on the patient's condition

Patients whose illness is responding slowly or who develop acute neurologic complications while on daily plasma exchange:
Use **whole fresh-frozen plasma or cryoprecipitate-poor plasma** to exchange 1.5 plasma volumes per treatment each day or 1 plasma volume twice daily

Indications

Plasma exchange is urgently indicated in all patients with a clinical diagnosis of TTP

Efficacy

1. Effectiveness documented in a randomized controlled clinical trial that compared plasma exchange with plasma infusion
2. Although some advocate cryoprecipitate-poor plasma because it is depleted of von Willebrand factor, 2 small, randomized clinical trials found equivalent clinical outcomes with whole fresh-frozen plasma and cryoprecipitate-poor plasma
3. Although the postulated mechanism for effectiveness of plasma exchange is removal of antibodies to ADAMTS13 by apheresis and replacement of ADAMTS13 by plasma infusion, plasma exchange probably has additional mechanisms for its effectiveness. Patients have been reported to achieve complete and durable remissions with plasma exchange treatment in spite of persistent severe ADAMTS13 deficiency and persistent inhibitor activity
4. Plasma exchange is not appropriate treatment for transplantation-associated thrombotic microangiopathy

George JN et al. N Engl J Med 2006;354:1927–1935
George JN et al. Transfusion 2004;44:294–304

Adverse Events

Insertion and maintenance of central venous catheters are associated with significant morbidity including bleeding, thrombosis and systemic infections

Plasma-related complications:
Hypotension
Anaphylaxis
Serum sickness
Hypoxia
Citrate toxicity

Rizvi MA et al. Transfusion 2000;40:896–901

Notes

Exacerbations of continuing disease requiring resumption of daily plasma exchange are common

REGIMEN

GLUCOCORTICOIDS

Bell WR et al. N Engl J Med 1991;325:398–403

Initial therapy:
Methylprednisolone 125 mg per dose twice daily, by intravenous injection or as an infusion in 10–50 mL 0.9% sodium chloride injection or 5% dextrose injection over 5–15 minutes, continually (total dose/day = 250 mg)

When a clinical response begins as evidenced by a sustained rise in the platelet count:
Prednisone 0.5–2 mg/kg per day orally, continually, until the platelet count reaches the normal or near-normal range, indicating a hematologic response, and then taper the dose gradually over 10 days to 2 weeks

Supportive Care
Steroid-associated gastritis:
Add a **proton pump inhibitor** during steroid use to prevent gastritis and duodenitis

Indications

As an adjunct to plasma exchange in the initial therapy of acquired TTP

Efficacy

Although there are no data that clearly support the efficacy of glucocorticoids, they are commonly given in addition to plasma exchange as acquired TTP is commonly thought to have an autoimmune etiology

Adverse Events*

Weight gain, facial swelling, hypertension, hyperglycemia, osteoporosis, cataracts, and mood and behavioral abnormalities

*Incidence and severity depend on the dose administered and the cumulative duration of administration

Notes

Glucocorticoids are important adjunctive therapy for patients with ADAMTS13 deficiency caused by autoantibody inhibitors

REGIMEN

RITUXIMAB

Scully M et al. Br J Haematol 2007;136:451–461

Premedication: Primary prophylaxis with **Acetaminophen** 650–1000 mg, *and* **diphenhydramine** 50–100 mg orally 30 minutes to 1 hour before rituximab administration to mitigate infusion reactions

Rituximab 375 mg/m^2 intravenously in 0.9% sodium chloride injection or 5% dextrose injection (D5W), diluted to a concentration within the range of 1–4 mg/mL, once weekly for 4 weeks (total dosage/4-week course = 1500 mg/m^2)

Infusion rate:
- Initially, at 50 mg/hour. If hypersensitivity or infusion reactions do not occur during the first 30 minutes, increase the rate by 50 mg/hour every 30 minutes, to a maximum rate of 400 mg/hour
- Subsequently, if previous administration was well tolerated, start at 100 mg/hour, and increase by 100 mg/hour increments every 30 minutes, to a maximum rate of 400 mg/hour

Supportive Care
Antiemetic prophylaxis
Emetogenic potential is **MINIMAL**
See Chapter 39 for antiemetic recommendations

Hematopoietic growth factor (CSF) prophylaxis
Primary prophylaxis is NOT indicated
See Chapter 43 for more information

Antimicrobial prophylaxis
Risk of fever and neutropenia is LOW
Antimicrobial primary prophylaxis to be considered:
- Antibacterial—not indicated
- Antifungal—not indicated
- Antiviral—not indicated unless patient previously had an episode of HSV

See Chapter 47 for more information

Indications

Adjunct to plasma exchange when disease does not respond to glucocorticoids or at a subsequent relapse

Efficacy

In patients who have high-titer inhibitors to ADAMTS13, rituximab has induced long-term remissions

All 25 patients with refractory/relapsing TTP attained complete clinical and laboratory remission after treatment with rituximab, in conjunction with plasma exchange therapy

Scully M et al. Br J Haematol 2007;136:451–461

Adverse Effects

Common Side Effects
(Generally are limited to time of infusion and may be of greatest severity during initial administration)

Fever	Diarrhea
Chills	Headache
Rigors	Asthenia
Nausea	Hypotension
Vomiting	Cardiac arrhythmias

"Black Box" Warnings
(For Severe Infusion Reactions)

Hypotension	Bronchospasm
Angioedema	

Hematologic Toxicities

Lymphopenia >> neutropenia	
Thrombocytopenia	Anemia

Rare, SEVERE Mucocutaneous Reactions

Stevens-Johnson syndrome

Vesiculobullous dermatitis

Lichenoid dermatitis

Toxic epidermal necrolysis

Hepatitis B reactivation with fulminant hepatic failure and death have been reported among chronic carriers of HBV

REGIMEN

OTHER IMMUNOSUPPRESSIVE AGENTS: CYCLOPHOSPHAMIDE AND VINCRISTINE

Zheng XL et al. Blood 2004;103:4043–4049

Cyclophosphamide 1–2 mg/kg per day (maximum daily dose of 150 mg), orally *in the morning*, continually until platelet count reaches normal or near-normal range

Ensure that patients consume plenty of liquids (64–80 ounces [1900–2400 mL] of nonalcoholic fluid) during the day to prevent hemorrhagic cystitis

or

Vincristine 1–2 mg per dose by intravenous injection over 1–3 minutes, once per week, continually until platelet count reaches normal or near-normal range (total dose/week = 1–2 mg)

Supportive Care
Antiemetic prophylaxis
Emetogenic potential for cyclophosphamide is **MINIMAL–LOW**
Emetogenic potential for vincristine is **MINIMAL**
See Chapter 39 for antiemetic recommendations

Hematopoietic growth factor (CSF) prophylaxis
Primary prophylaxis is NOT indicated
See Chapter 43 for more information

Antimicrobial prophylaxis
Risk of fever and neutropenia is LOW
  Antimicrobial primary prophylaxis to be considered:
  • Antibacterial—not indicated
  • Antifungal—not indicated
  • Antiviral—not indicated unless patient previously had an episode of HSV
See Chapter 47 for more information

Bowel prophylaxis:
Give **stool softeners** in a scheduled regimen, and saline, osmotic, and lubricant laxatives as needed for as long as vincristine use continues

Therapy Monitoring

Cyclophosphamide *or* vincristine
  CBC and differential initially weekly, then CBC and differential every other week
  Serum LFTs (with bilirubin) at baseline, then repeat serially at least every 3–4 weeks

Cyclophosphamide
  Serum creatinine at baseline, then repeat serially at least every 3–4 weeks
  Evaluate for hemoglobinuria at least monthly for as long as cyclophosphamide use continues

Vincristine
  Monitor deep tendon reflexes, neurological exam, and/or impaired bowel motility

Indications

Adjunct to plasma exchange when disease does not respond to glucocorticoids or at a subsequent relapse

Adverse Effects

Cyclophosphamide
Dose-related marrow suppression
Teratogenicity
Infertility
Alopecia
Hemorrhagic cystitis
Increased risk for developing AML associated with alkylating chemotherapy
Syndrome of inappropriate antidiuretic hormone (SIADH) secretion

Vincristine
Inflammation/thrombophlebitis at infusion site
Dose-related peripheral neuropathy
SIADH secretion
Constipation

Efficacy

Although there are no data that clearly support the efficacy of these agents, they are commonly given to patients whose disease does not improve with glucocorticoids in addition to plasma exchange since acquired TTP is commonly thought to have an autoimmune etiology. Use of rituximab has mostly replaced these drugs in current clinical practice

Notes

Immunosuppressive agents may be effective to suppress autoantibodies to ADAMTS13

REGIMEN

SPLENECTOMY

Kremer Hovinga JA et al. Haematologica 2004;89:320–324

Prior to splenectomy:

1. To enhance operative hemostasis, platelet transfusion can be considered if the platelet count is <20,000/mm^3

2. At least 2 weeks before surgery immunize with:
   - **Polyvalent pneumococcal conjugate vaccine** (13 serotypes conjugate vaccine, if available),
   - *Haemophilus influenzae* b (Hib polysaccharide) conjugate vaccine, *and*
   - **Quadrivalent meningococcal** (groups A, C, Y, and W-135) polysaccharide conjugate vaccine

3. Preoperative platelet transfusions are inappropriate if platelet count is >100,000/mm^3

Splenectomy can be performed by **open laparotomy** or **laparoscopy**, depending on surgeon's experience

Prognosis Following Recovery

1. **Risk for relapse:**
   Recurrent episodes of TTP occur almost exclusively in patients with severe ADAMTS13 deficiency without acute renal failure. In patients with severe ADAMTS13 deficiency, the rate of relapse may be 30–40% within 5 years. Most relapses occur within the first year following recovery. Most patients have only 1 relapse. The occurrence of repeated relapses is uncommon

2. **Chronic renal failure:**
   Patients who have acute renal failure as part of their initial acute episode commonly develop persistent renal failure. Even patients who initially recover may develop renal insufficiency and hypertension years later

3. **Cognitive deficits:**
   Preliminary data have documented long-term cognitive deficits, patients who appear to completely recover from an acute episode of TTP commonly describe problems with memory, concentration, and fatigue

4. **Risk of future pregnancies:**
   Because pregnancy appears to be a risk factor for the development of TTP, the safety of future pregnancies is a common issue. However, with the exception of a very rare female with congenital TTP, recurrence during subsequent pregnancy is uncommon. Women who have congenital TTP inevitably appear to have exacerbations of their recurrent episodes during pregnancy and require more frequent plasma infusion prophylaxis

Howard MA et al. J Clin Apher 2003;18:16–20
Vesely SK et al. Blood 2003;102:60–68
Vesely SK et al. Transfusion 2004;44:1149–1158

Indications

Recurrent episodes of TTP in a patient who has failed to respond to immunosuppressive treatment, including rituximab

Efficacy

Efficacy is documented only in case reports. However, the decreasing frequency of relapses over time may confound the interpretation of efficacy

Adverse Events

Laparoscopic splenectomy has less operative mortality and morbidity, as well as more rapid postoperative recovery

Notes

The mechanism for its effect is unknown, but may be related to removal of a major site of autoantibody production

64. Idiopathic Thrombocytopenic Purpura

Kiarash Kojouri, MD, MPH, Arafat Tfayli, MD, and James N. George, MD

Idiopathic Thrombocytopenic Purpura (ITP)

ITP is defined as isolated thrombocytopenia with no other clinically apparent associated conditions or causes of thrombocytopenia caused by accelerated destruction as well as impaired production of platelets by antiplatelet autoantibodies

Ballem PJ et al. J Clin Invest 1987;80:33–40
[British Committee for Standards in Haematology General Haematology Task Force] Br J Haematol 2003;120:574–596
George JN et al. Blood 1996;88:3–40
McMillan R. Semin Hematol 2007;44(4 Suppl 5):S3–S11

Epidemiology

Incidence:	1.6–$3.2/10^5$ per year, based on platelet count $<50,000/mm^3$. Incidence increases among elderly, reaching $4.6/10^5$ per year in persons >60 years old
Prevalence:	$10/10^5$
Median age:	56 years
Female-to-male ratio:	1.2–$1.7/1$; however, males and females are equally affected in the elderly
Mortality rate:	Most adults with ITP have no excess mortality when compared with that of the general population. However, those with persistent thrombocytopenia (platelet count $<30,000/mm^3$) at 2 years after initial presentation had higher mortality as compared to the general population (relative risk 4.2 [95% CI, 1.7–10.0]). The majority of deaths are a result of unrelated causes or complications of treatment, rather than hemorrhage

Frederiksen H, Schmidt K. Blood 1999;94:909–913
Neylon AJ et al. Br J Haematol 2003;122:966–974
Portielje JEA et al. Blood 2001;97:2549–2554
Segal JB, Powe NR. J Thromb Haemost 2006;4:2377–2383

Differential Diagnosis

1. Pseudothrombocytopenia (platelet clumping in the presence of EDTA by naturally occurring autoantibodies to normally concealed epitopes on glycoprotein IIb/IIIa)
2. Drug-induced thrombocytopenia (including nonprescription drugs and herbs)
3. Secondary autoimmune thrombocytopenia, for example, CLL, SLE, antiphospholipid antibody syndrome (isolated presence of antinuclear antibodies in a patient with immune thrombocytopenia, without other clinical features of SLE, does not imply a diagnosis of SLE, although some of these patients will eventually develop full-blown SLE)
4. Infectious disorders (HIV, HCV, EBV)
5. Bone marrow failure (myelodysplasia)
6. Congenital/hereditary nonimmune thrombocytopenia
7. Hypersplenism caused by occult liver disease
8. Incidental thrombocytopenia of pregnancy (also termed *gestational thrombocytopenia*)
9. Thrombotic thrombocytopenic purpura/hemolytic uremic syndrome
10. Chronic disseminated intravascular coagulation

[British Committee for Standards in Haematology General Haematology Task Force] Br J Haematol 2003;120:574–596
George JN et al. Ann Intern Med 1998;129:886–890
George JN et al. Blood 1996;88:3–40

Work-up

Objectives are to assess the type, severity, and duration of bleeding, and to exclude other etiologies

1. *CBC:* Pseudothrombocytopenia from EDTA-dependent platelet agglutination (occurs in $\approx 0.1\%$ of adults) or platelet adherence to neutrophils and monocytes (platelet rosetting) should be ruled out by examination of peripheral smear
2. *Peripheral blood smear:* Findings consistent with the diagnosis of ITP include thrombocytopenia with normal-sized or slightly larger than normal platelets, and normal red and white blood cell morphology
3. *Bone marrow examination:* The American Society of Hematology guidelines recommend bone marrow examination as appropriate to establish diagnosis in patients over age 60 years (because of the higher incidence of myelodysplasia), in those with atypical features in peripheral blood smear suggesting an alternative diagnosis, and if not previously performed, in patients considering splenectomy or second-line medical therapies that often cause prolonged immunosuppression or have other significant side effects. Bone marrow biopsy is inappropriate in patients <60 years old, with isolated thrombocytopenia, and no other atypical findings in medical history, clinical examination, and examination of CBC and peripheral blood smear. This view has been supported by several case series
4. *HIV and HCV serology:* Patients with relevant risk factors should be tested
5. *Autoimmune profile:* If suggested by history and physical findings (ANA, antiphospholipid antibodies)

If history, physical examination, and examination of CBC and peripheral blood smear are consistent with a diagnosis of ITP and no atypical features are present, no further tests are necessary for diagnosis

[British Committee for Standards in Haematology General Haematology Task Force] Br J Haematol 2003;120:574–596
George JN et al. Blood 1996;88:3–40
Jubelirer SJ, Harpold R. Clin Appl Thromb Hemost 2002;8:73–76
Mak YK et al. Clin Lab Haematol 2000;22:355–358
Westerman DA, Grigg AP. Med J Aust 1999;170:216–217

Classification

Childhood ITP: Usually an acute, self-limited disorder that characteristically resolves within 6 months with only supportive care. Males and females are equally affected, with a peak age at diagnosis of 2–4 years

Adult ITP: Usually a chronic disorder, with insidious onset of symptoms that rarely resolves spontaneously

Treatment Options

The goal of treatment is to achieve a safe platelet count while minimizing side effects of therapy. Achievement of a normal platelet count is not a goal of treatment. In general, observation is recommended for patients with platelet counts ≥30,000/mm³ unless they are undergoing a procedure likely to induce blood loss including surgery, dental extraction, or parturition. Glucocorticoids are considered the initial line of therapy in a patient with a platelet count <30,000/mm³, or a platelet count of 30,000–50,000/mm³ in the presence of clinically important bleeding (or significant risk for it). Splenectomy is recommended for patients with persistent thrombocytopenia despite steroids and for those who require steroids (>5 mg prednisone per day) for prolonged periods (>6 weeks) to maintain safe platelet count levels (≥30,000/mm³), but is considered inappropriate as initial therapy, or if the platelet count is >30,000/mm³. Treatment with rituximab may be considered when splenectomy is considered high risk or if a patient or physician wishes to defer splenectomy, but it should not routinely substitute for splenectomy because the frequency and durability of complete responses with splenectomy are greater than with rituximab. The majority of patients with persistent thrombocytopenia despite prior therapy with glucocorticoids and splenectomy can be managed with watchful observation. When treatment is needed however, it may be chosen from a list of available options, which include traditional immunosuppressive drugs, such as cyclophosphamide and azathioprine, or, more recently, and perhaps with a more favorable risk/benefit profile, rituximab and thrombopoietin receptor agonists, romiplostim and eltrombopag

Emergency Treatment

Hospitalization is required for severe, life-threatening bleeding regardless of the platelet count. Emergency treatment in addition to general supportive care measures, includes:
1. Platelet transfusions (can be given as bolus or continuous infusion)
2. High-dose parenteral glucocorticoids, for example, **methylprednisolone** 1000 mg/day intravenously in 50–1000 mL 0.9% sodium chloride injection or 5% dextrose injection over at least 30 minutes, daily for 1–3 consecutive days
3. **Immune globulin, intravenous (IVIG)** 1000 mg/kg (body weight) per dose intravenously. Refer to product-specific recommendations for administration rates (initial, escalation, and maximum rates). Repeat treatment on the following day if the platelet count remains <50,000/mm³
   (total dosage/1- to 2-day course = 1000–2000 mg/kg)
4. Other useful measures may include:

Aminocaproic acid oral rinse 5 mL (1.25 g) swish for 30 seconds 4 times per day for gingival bleeding
May be prepared extemporaneously from aminocaproic acid solution for intravenous use or compounded from aminocaproic acid tablets for oral administration
   Local application of **fibrin sealant** for intractable dental bleeding
   Medroxyprogesterone acetate to control excessive uterine bleeding

These modalities are given either alone or in combination

[British Committee for Standards in Haematology General Haematology Task Force] Br J Haematol 2003;120:574–596
George JN et al. Blood 1996;88:3–40

REGIMEN

OBSERVATION

[British Committee for Standards in Haematology General Haematology Task Force] Br J Haematol 2003;120:574–596
Cortelazzo S et al. Blood 1991;77:31–33
George JN et al. Blood 1996;88:3–40
Provan D, Newland A. Br J Haematol 2002;118:933–944
Vianelli N et al. Haematologica 2001;86:504–509

Indications

Patients with platelet counts exceeding 30,000/mm³ unless they are undergoing a procedure likely to induce blood loss including surgery, dental extraction, or parturition

Efficacy

1. In a consecutive series of 117 patients, no major hemorrhages occurred among 49 patients with platelet counts >30,000/mm³ who did not receive treatment and were followed for a median of 30 months
2. In another consecutive series of 310 patients followed for more than 10 years who generally were treated only if symptomatic or if platelet count <30,000/mm³, none of the patients who were only monitored without active therapy (N = 107) died of bleeding

Toxicity

None

Notes

Patients with low platelet counts (<30,000/mm³) may also be managed only with observation if they have no or minimal bleeding symptoms. This is especially appropriate in an individual patient with platelet count persistently <30,000/mm³ despite treatment, who proves over time that he/she does not bleed and is not at significant risk for major bleeding

REGIMEN

GLUCOCORTICOIDS

Ben-Yehuda D et al. Acta Haematol 1994;91:1–6
[British Committee for Standards in Haematology General Haematology Task Force] Br J Haematol 2003;120:574–596
Cheng Y et al. N Engl J Med 2003;349:831–836
George JN et al. Blood 1996;88:3–40
Mazzucconi MG et al. Blood 2007;109:1401–1407
Pizzuto J, Ambriz R. Blood 1984;64:1179–1183
Provan D, Newland A. Br J Haematol 2002;118:933–944
Stasi R et al. Am J Med 1995;98:436–442

Prednisone 1 mg/kg per day (dosage range, 0.5–2 mg/kg per day) orally for not more than 4–6 weeks (usually 2–4 weeks), after which, doses should be slowly tapered to the lowest effective dose, or tapered to discontinuation if an improvement in platelet count was not achieved
- The lowest effective dose may be continued for 4–6 weeks before attempting to slowly taper and discontinue steroids
- Splenectomy should be considered if steroids are required for prolonged periods to maintain safe levels of platelet count

or

Dexamethasone 40 mg per day orally as a single daily dose for 4 consecutive days. This treatment may be repeated 2 more times in 2-week intervals, or given once and repeated only upon relapse

In patients with severe, life-threatening bleeding, such as intracranial hemorrhage:
Methylprednisolone 1000 mg/day, intravenously in 100–250 mL 0.9% sodium chloride or 5% dextrose injection, over at least 30 minutes, daily for 3 consecutive days

Indications

Glucocorticoids are considered the initial line of therapy in a patient with
1. Platelet count <30,000/mm^3
2. Platelet count 30,000–50,000/mm^3 in the presence of clinically important bleeding

Notes

Glucocorticoids are the standard first-line and least-expensive treatment. A short course of dexamethasone may be less toxic and more effective than prolonged prednisone treatment

Adverse Events*

Weight gain, facial swelling, hypertension, hyperglycemia, osteoporosis, cataracts, and mood and behavioral abnormalities

*The incidence and severity of adverse effects generally correlates with the potency of the agents used, the dose administered, and duration of use

Efficacy

Prednisone:
1. Two randomized studies found equal efficacy between low versus high doses of glucocorticoids (prednisone: 0.5 vs. 1.5 mg/kg per day and 0.25 vs. 1 mg/kg per day)
2. In 1 large study, the incidence of prolonged complete remission was the same for patients treated for 4–6 weeks as for those treated for >3 months
3. About two-thirds to three-fourths of patients initially respond, but long-term remission without maintenance treatment occurs in only 10–30% following cessation of therapy

Dexamethasone:
1. In a consecutive cohort of 125 newly diagnosed adults with ITP, 85% of patients had an initial response; half of those had a sustained platelet count >50,000/mm^3 and required no further treatment during 2–5 years of follow-up
2. In another prospective study of 95 patients treated with four 4-day courses of dexamethasone 40 mg/day IV or PO given every 2 weeks, overall response rates after each consecutive cycle was 70%, 76%, 89%, and 86%, respectively

Methylprednisolone:
1. High-dose parenteral glucocorticoids, are reserved for severe, life-threatening bleeding, such as intracranial hemorrhage (see Emergency Treatment)

REGIMEN

SPLENECTOMY

[British Committee for Standards in Haematology General Haematology Task Force] Br J Haematol 2003;120:574–596
George JN et al. Blood 1996;88:3–40
Kojouri K et al. Blood 2004;104:2623–2634
PizzutoJ, Ambriz R. Blood 1984;64:1179–1183
Schwartz J et al. Am J Hematol 2003;72:94–98

Prior to splenectomy:

1. To enhance operative hemostasis, preoperative **immune globulin intravenous, (human)** (IVIG) if the platelet count is <20,000/mm³:

   IVIG 1000 mg/kg given as a single dose (total dosage/1-day course = 1000 mg/kg), *or*
   IVIG 1000 mg/kg per day for 2 consecutive days (total dosage/2-day course = 2000 mg/kg), *or*
   IVIG 400 mg/kg per day for 5 consecutive days (total dose/5-day course = 2000 mg/kg)
   • Administer intravenously
   • Refer to product-specific labeling for information about preparation (reconstitution and dilution when appropriate), administration rates (initial, escalation, maximum rates), and whether filtration during administration is needed or appropriate
   • If the platelet count remains <50,000/mm³ after a single treatment with IVIG 1000 mg/kg, repeat treatment on the following day

   or

   Prednisone 1 mg/kg per day orally as a single dose for 5–7 consecutive days if the platelet count is <20,000/mm³ (total dosage/5- to 7-day course = 5–7 mg/kg)

   or

   Dexamethasone 40 mg per day orally or intravenously as a single dose for 4 consecutive days if the platelet count is <20,000/mm³ (total dose/4-day course = 160 mg)

2. At least 2 weeks before surgery immunize with:
   • **Pneumococcal 13-valent conjugate vaccine,**
   • *Haemophilus influenzae* **b (Hib polysaccharide) conjugate vaccine,** *and*
   • **Quadrivalent meningococcal (A, C, Y, and W-135) polysaccharide conjugate vaccine**

3. Preoperative platelet transfusions are inappropriate if platelet count is >100,000/mm³

Splenectomy can be performed by **open laparotomy** or **laparoscopy**, depending on a surgeon's experience

Indications

Recommended in patients with:
1. Platelet counts <10,000/mm³, 6 weeks after initiation of medical therapy
2. Platelet counts <30,000/mm³, 3 months after initiation of medical therapy

Considered inappropriate:
1. As initial therapy
2. If the platelet count is >30,000/mm³

Adverse Events

Laparoscopic splenectomy has less operative mortality and morbidity, as well as more rapid postoperative recovery

Efficacy

66%	Long-term normalization of platelet count without maintenance medical therapy (complete remission)
10–15%	Safe platelet count level with or without further medical therapy (partial remission)

Fifteen to 25% of patients may relapse after an initial complete response to splenectomy and may require further treatment

Notes

1. The most effective treatment for achieving complete and durable remissions in adults with ITP
2. Consider in patients whose disease:
   • Does not respond to glucocorticoids
   • Recurs after an initial response
   • Requires continued steroid treatment to maintain safe platelet counts
3. Consider above immunizations at the time of initial diagnosis of ITP in an adult patient, because (a) immunizations may not be effective in the face of immunosuppressive therapy, and (b) splenectomy may occasionally need to be performed urgently

REGIMEN

ACCESSORY SPLENECTOMY

[British Committee for Standards in Haematology General Haematology Task Force] Br J Haematol 2003;120:574–596
Vesely SK et al. Ann Intern Med 2004;140:112–120

Prior to splenectomy:

1. To enhance operative hemostasis, preoperative **immune globulin intravenous (human)** **(IVIG)** if the platelet count is <20,000/mm³:

 IVIG 1000 mg/kg given as a single dose (total dosage/1-day course = 1000 mg/kg), *or*

 IVIG 1000 mg/kg per day for 2 consecutive days (total dosage/2-day course = 2000 mg/kg), *or*

 IVIG 400 mg/kg per day for 5 consecutive days (total dose/5-day course = 2000 mg/kg)

 • Administer intravenously

 • Refer to product-specific labeling for information about preparation (reconstitution and dilution when appropriate), administration rates (initial, escalation, maximum rates), and whether filtration during administration is needed or appropriate

 • If the platelet count remains <50,000/mm³ after a single treatment with IVIG 1000 mg/kg, repeat treatment on the following day

 or

 Prednisone 1 mg/kg per day orally as a single dose for 5–7 consecutive days if the platelet count is <20,000/mm³ (total dosage/5- to 7-day course = 5–7 mg/kg)

 or

 Dexamethasone 40 mg per day orally or intravenously as a single dose given on 4 consecutive days if the platelet count is <20,000/mm³ (total dose/4-day course = 160 mg)

2. Preoperative platelet transfusions are inappropriate if platelet count is >100,000/mm³

Indications

Many hematologists believe that accessory splenectomy is never indicated. However, in patients who fail to respond to splenectomy or relapse following an initial prolonged response, imaging studies to detect an accessory spleen have been suggested by some

Efficacy

Some case reports have described success with accessory splenectomy. However, these reports are difficult to evaluate and the experience of many hematologists is that accessory splenectomy is not effective

Adverse Events

Laparoscopy may not be appropriate to identify and remove small accessory spleens

Notes

Accessory spleens are present and removed in 15% of ITP patients undergoing splenectomy

REGIMEN

IMMUNE GLOBULIN INTRAVENOUS (HUMAN)
(POOLED NORMAL HUMAN IMMUNOGLOBULIN)

[British Committee for Standards in Haematology General Haematology Task Force] Br J Haematol 2003;120:574–596
George JN et al. Blood 1996;88:3–40
Godeau B et al. Blood 1993;82:1415–1421
Provan D, Newland A. Br J Haematol 2002;118:933–944

Immune globulin intravenous (human) (IVIG)*:
IVIG 400 mg/kg per day for 5 consecutive days (total dose/5-day course = 2000 mg/kg)

or

IVIG 1000 mg/kg per day for 2 consecutive days (total dosage/2-day course = 2000 mg/kg)

or

IVIG 1000 mg/kg given as a single dose (total dosage/1-day course = 1000 mg/kg)

*Refer to product-specific labeling for information about preparation (reconstitution and dilution when appropriate), administration rates (initial, escalation, maximum rates), and whether filtration during administration is needed or appropriate

Indications

1. As a temporary measure to increase platelet count
2. In a patient with a platelet count $<50,000/mm^3$ in the presence of severe bleeding
3. In a patient with a platelet count $<30,000/mm^3$ before splenectomy (or another major operation) to achieve hemostasis during surgery

Notes

The mechanism of action remains largely unknown but is reported to involve Fc receptor blockade on macrophages and monocytes, the presence of antiidiotype antibodies in IVIG that block autoantibody binding to circulating platelets, and immune suppression
IVIG products with high IgA content is contraindicated in persons with IgA deficiency

Efficacy

1. Seventy-five percent of patients respond to IVIG by increasing their platelet count
2. Approximately 50% achieve normal platelet counts
3. In almost all patients, the platelet count returns to pretreatment levels in 3–4 weeks
4. Five-day, 2-day, and single doses are equally efficacious

Adverse Events

Side effects are common, occurring in 15–75% of patients and may be severe. Hepatitis C infection has not been reported with viral inactivated products

Common	Rare
1. Headache	1. Aseptic meningitis
2. Backache	2. Alloimmune hemolysis
3. Nausea	3. Acute renal failure
4. Fever	4. Pulmonary insufficiency
	5. Thrombosis

REGIMEN

RH$_O$(D) IMMUNE GLOBULIN (HUMAN) FOR INJECTION (RH$_O$(D) IVIG)

[British Committee for Standards in Haematology General Haematology Task Force] Br J Haematol 2003;120:574–596
Gaines AR. Blood 2000;95:2523–2529
George JN et al. Am J Hematol 2003;74:161–169
Scaradavou A et al. Blood 1997;89:2689–2700

Rho(D) IVIG 50–75 mcg/kg*; administer ONLY by the intravenous route over 3–5 minutes (1 μg = 5 IU Rho(D) IVIG)

*Dosing Guidelines

Pretreatment Hemoglobin	Rho(D) IVIG Dose
<10 g/dL	50 mcg/kg
≥10 g/dL	75 mcg/kg

Notes:

- For patients with ITP it is recommended that before deciding to treat patients with Rho (D) IVIG the following be obtained: blood type, CBC, reticulocyte count, DAT, and dipstick urinalysis
- Administer Rho (D) IVIG only after confirming a patient is Rho (D)-positive
- An initial dose may be administered in two divided doses given on separate days
- Other treatments MUST be used in patients with evidence of hemolysis or patients at risk of hemolysis

  In patients with a hemoglobin level less than 8 g/dL, alternative treatments should be used due to the risk of increasing the severity of anemia

- The frequency and dose used should be administered based on a patient's clinical response by assessing platelet counts, red cell counts, hemoglobin, and reticulocyte levels
- Rho (D) IVIG is commercially available in a liquid formulation appropriate for intravenous administration without further dilution, or it may be diluted in 0.9% sodium chloride injection

Indications

Rho (D) IVIG is used to transiently elevate the platelet count in Rho (D)+ patients who have a spleen

Efficacy

In a single-institution experience, 70% of adult patients with ITP patients increased platelet count by ≥20,000/mm^3 within 2 days. In half of those patients, the response lasted 3 weeks or more

Adverse Events

1. The only clinically important adverse effect is alloimmune hemolysis. All Rho (D)+ patients develop a positive direct antiglobulin test after treatment, accompanied by a transient (1–2 weeks) decrease in hemoglobin concentration of approximately 0.5–2 g/dL
2. Severe intravascular hemolysis with DIC and acute renal failure has been reported as an adverse effect of Rho (D) IVIG

Notes

The mechanism of action is opsonization of Rho (D)+ red blood cells that are preferentially removed by the spleen, thus sparing autoantibody coated platelets through Fc receptor blockade

REGIMEN

CYCLOPHOSPHAMIDE, AZATHIOPRINE MYCOPHENOLATE MOFETIL

[British Committee for Standards in Haematology General Haematology Task Force] Br J Haematol 2003;120:574–596

George JN et al. Blood 1996;88:3–40

George JN et al. Semin Hematol 2000;37:290–298

Hou M et al. Eur J Haematol 2003;70:353–357

McMillan R. Ann Intern Med 1997;126:307–314

Provan D et al. Am J Hematol 2006;81:19–25

Quiquandon I et al. Br J Haematol 1990;74:223–228

Vesely SK et al. Ann Intern Med 2004;140:112–120

Cyclophosphamide 1–2 mg/kg per day (maximum dose = 150 mg/day), orally in the morning, continually if a response occurs (total dosage/week = 7–14 mg/kg; maximum dose/week = 1050 mg)

Encourage patients to increase their consumption of nonalcoholic fluid (64–80 ounces [1900–2400 mL]) to prevent developing hemorrhagic cystitis

or

Azathioprine 1–2 mg/kg per day (maximum dose = 150 mg/day), orally, continually if a response occurs (total dosage/week = 7–14 mg/kg; maximum dose/week = 1050 mg)

or

Mycophenolate mofetil 750–1000 mg/dose orally twice daily for a minimum of 12 weeks (total dose/day = 1500–2000 mg)

Supportive Care
Antiemetic prophylaxis
*Emetogenic potential with cyclophosphamide is **LOW***

*Emetogenic potential with azathioprine and mycophenolate mofetil is **MINIMAL–LOW***

See Chapter 39 for antiemetic recommendations

Hematopoietic growth factor (CSF) prophylaxis
Primary prophylaxis is NOT indicated

See Chapter 43 for more information

Antimicrobial prophylaxis
Risk of fever and neutropenia is LOW

Antimicrobial primary prophylaxis to be considered:

• Antibacterial—not indicated

• Antifungal—not indicated

• Antiviral—not indicated unless patient previously had an episode of HSV

See Chapter 47 for more information

Therapy Monitoring

Monitor CBC and leukocyte differential serially—initially at least weekly, then every other week

Notes

1. With cyclophosphamide, adjust dose to induce mild neutropenia
2. If no response occurs, discontinue after 3–4 months. If a response occurs, continue until maximum platelet count is achieved, then taper slowly and discontinue

Indications

Patients with persistent thrombocytopenia despite prior therapy with glucocorticoids and a prior splenectomy

Efficacy

1. Each can induce complete remission in approximately 15–20% and partial remission in another 30–50% of patients after glucocorticoids and splenectomy have failed
2. Responses may occur slowly over few months. Therefore, treatment should continue up to 4 months before being considered a failure

Advance Events

Cyclophosphamide
Dose-related marrow suppression
Teratogenicity
Infertility
Alopecia
Hemorrhagic cystitis
A risk for development of AML

Azathioprine
Reversible leukopenia
Small risk of developing malignancy
Teratogenicity

Mycophenolate mofetil
Headache
Diarrhea
Constipation
Nausea, vomiting
Myelosuppression
Hypertension
Peripheral edema

REGIMEN

CYCLOSPORINE

[British Committee for Standards in Haematology General Haematology Task Force] Br J Haematol 2003;120:574–596
Choudhary DR et al. Haematologica 2008;93(online):e61–e62
McMillan R. Ann Intern Med 1997;126:307–314
Vesely SK et al. Ann Intern Med 2004;140:112–120

Cyclosporine 1.25–2.5 mg/kg per dose, orally every 12 hours, continually if a response occurs (total dosage/day = 2.5–5 mg/kg)

Note: Cyclosporine is marketed as capsules for oral administration and in a microemulsion formulation. The formulations are not bioequivalent and cannot be interchanged

Cyclosporine may be given in combination with:
Prednisone 0.5–2 mg/kg per day, orally for not more than 4–6 weeks (usually 2–4 weeks), after which, doses should be slowly tapered to the lowest effective dose, or tapered to discontinuation if an improvement in platelet count was not achieved
• The lowest effective dose may be continued for 4–6 weeks before attempting to slowly taper and discontinue steroids

Supportive Care
Not emetogenic
See Chapter 39 for antiemetic recommendations

Hematopoietic growth factor (CSF) prophylaxis
Primary prophylaxis is NOT indicated
See Chapter 43 for more information

Antimicrobial prophylaxis
Risk of fever and neutropenia is LOW
   Antimicrobial primary prophylaxis to be considered:
   • Antibacterial—not indicated
   • Antifungal—not indicated
   • Antiviral—not indicated unless patient previously had an episode of HSV
See Chapter 47 for more information

Indications

Patients with persistent thrombocytopenia despite prior therapy with glucocorticoids and a prior splenectomy

Efficacy

Cyclosporine has been reported to induce rates of remissions comparable to azathioprine and cyclophosphamide with complete remission in 15–20% and partial remission in another 30–50% of patients

Responses occur slowly over few months. Treatment should continue up to 4 months before being considered a failure

Therapy Monitoring

Measure serum creatinine, LFTs and serum trough cyclosporine concentrations weekly for 1 month, then monthly or every 2 months*. Adjust cyclosporine dose as needed in increments or decrements of 0.5–0.75 mg/kg per day

*Measuring cyclosporine concentrations: for patients without hepatic impairment receiving cyclosporine every 12 hours:

   Obtain samples just before the fifth or seventh dose after starting treatment or after altering a dose or dosing interval, and periodically afterwards as above

   Generally, a target concentration range of 200–400 mcg/L (1.66–333 nmol/L [HPLC]) can be used as the reference

Note: Cyclosporine concentration monitoring is not a substitute for renal and liver function test monitoring

Adverse Events

Common	Frequent, Serious
Headache	Nephrotoxicity
Hirsutism	Hepatotoxicity
Nausea	Hypertension
Vomiting	
Diarrhea	
Gingival hyperplasia	
Tremor	

REGIMEN

VINCA ALKALOIDS

[British Committee for Standards in Haematology General Haematology Task Force] Br J Haematol 2003;120:574–596
George JN et al. Blood 1996;88:3–40
George JN et al. Semin Hematol 2000;37:290–298
Vesely SK et al. Ann Intern Med 2004;140:112–120

Vincristine 1–2 mg by intravenous injection over 1–3 minutes, once per week for 4–6 weeks (total dosage/week = 1–2 mg)

or

Vinblastine 5–10 mg by intravenous injection over 1–3 minutes, once per week for 4–6 weeks (total dosage/week = 5–10 mg)

Supportive Care
Antiemetic prophylaxis
Emetogenic potential is **MINIMAL**
See Chapter 39 for antiemetic recommendations

Hematopoietic growth factor (CSF) prophylaxis
Primary prophylaxis is NOT indicated
See Chapter 43 for more information

Antimicrobial prophylaxis
Risk of fever and neutropenia is LOW
  Antimicrobial primary prophylaxis to be considered:
  • Antibacterial—not indicated
  • Antifungal—not indicated
  • Antiviral—not indicated unless patient previously had an episode of HSV
See Chapter 47 for more information

Prophylaxis for decreased bowel motility
Give a bowel regimen to prevent constipation based initially on **stool softeners**
Note: Institute prophylaxis from the beginning of treatment, particularly when vincristine is used

Adverse Events

Vincristine	Vinblastine
For both drugs, tissue ulceration and necrosis are associated with soft-tissue extravasation	
Cumulative dose-related peripheral neuropathies (vincristine >> vinblastine) *Early:* ↓ DTRs and sensory neuropathies *Late*:* Motor and autonomic neuropathies *Occur > sensory neuropathies, but onset is variable	
Constipation → paralytic ileus (vincristine >> vinblastine)	
Syndrome of inappropriate antidiuretic hormone (SIADH) secretion	
Muscle weakness, myalgias (vincristine >> vinblastine)	
Leukopenia to a much greater extent than thrombocytopenia (vinblastine >> vincristine)	
Alopecia	

Indications

Patients with persistent thrombocytopenia despite prior therapy with glucocorticoids and a prior splenectomy

Efficacy

1. Either vincristine or vinblastine may produce a transient increase in platelet count, usually lasting 1–3 weeks, in approximately 50% of patients with persistent thrombocytopenia after splenectomy
2. Sustained responses are observed in less than 10% of patients
3. Results are comparable with both drugs

Therapy Monitoring

1. *Baseline and periodic neurologic examination:* monitor for the onset and development of neurologic adverse effects
2. *Weekly:* CBC and leukocyte differential counts
3. Baseline serum LFTs and bilirubin, repeated at least every other week

Note

Vincristine should be discontinued after 4–6 weeks or after dose-related peripheral neuropathy occurs, whichever is earlier

REGIMEN

RITUXIMAB

Arnold DM et al. Ann Intern Med 2007;146:25–33
[British Committee for Standards in Haematology
General Haematology Task Force] Br J Haematol 2003;
120:574–596
Godeau B et al. Blood 2008;112:999–1004

Premedication: Primary prophylaxis with
Acetaminophen 650–1000 mg, *and*
diphenhydramine 50–100 mg orally
30 minutes to 1 hour before rituximab
administration to mitigate infusion reactions

Rituximab 375 mg/m² intravenously in
0.9% sodium chloride injection or 5%
dextrose injection, diluted to a concentration
within the range of 1–4 mg/mL, once
weekly for 4 weeks (total dosage/4-week
course = 1500 mg/m²)

Infusion rate:
- Initially, at 50 mg/hour. If hypersensitivity
  or infusion reactions do not occur during
  the first 30 minutes, increase the rate by
  50 mg/hour every 30 minutes as tolerated,
  to a maximum rate of 400 mg/hour
- Subsequently, if previous administration
  was well tolerated, start at 100 mg/hour,
  and increase by 100 mg/hour every
  30 minutes as tolerated, to a maximum
  rate of 400 mg/hour

Supportive Care
Antiemetic prophylaxis
Emetogenic potential is **MINIMAL**
See Chapter 39 for antiemetic
recommendations

Hematopoietic growth factor (CSF) prophylaxis
Primary prophylaxis is NOT indicated
See Chapter 43 for more information

Antimicrobial prophylaxis
Risk of fever and neutropenia is LOW
Antimicrobial primary prophylaxis to be considered:
- Antibacterial—not indicated
- Antifungal—not indicated
- Antiviral—not indicated unless patient
  previously had an episode of HSV
See Chapter 47 for more information

Adverse Events
Black Box Warnings (excerpts)

1. Severe infusion reactions, including urticaria, hypotension, angioedema, hypoxia,
   bronchospasm, pulmonary infiltrates, acute respiratory distress syndrome, myocardial
   infarction, ventricular fibrillation, cardiogenic shock, and anaphylactoid events
2. Patients with preexisting cardiac or pulmonary conditions and those who experienced prior
   cardiopulmonary adverse reactions may be at increased risk for an adverse outcome from
   severe infusion reactions
3. Severe, including fatal, mucocutaneous reactions, including paraneoplastic pemphigus,
   Stevens-Johnson syndrome, lichenoid dermatitis, vesiculobullous dermatitis, and toxic
   epidermal necrolysis, with onset from 1–13 weeks after receiving rituximab
4. JC virus infection resulting in progressive multifocal leukoencephalopathy may occur in
   rituximab treated patients with autoimmune diseases and may result in death; most cases
   diagnosed within 12 months after a last treatment with rituximab

Common Side Effects
(Generally are limited to time of infusion and may
be of greatest severity during initial administration)

Fever	Diarrhea
Chills	Headache
Rigors	Asthenia
Nausea	Hypotension
Vomiting	Cardiac arrhythmias

Hematologic Toxicities

Lymphopenia >> neutropenia	
Thrombocytopenia	Anemia

Hepatitis B reactivation with fulminant hepatic failure and death have been reported among
chronic carriers of HBV

Therapy Monitoring

Weekly CBC and leukocyte differential
counts during treatment, and periodically
thereafter
Note: Avoid primary or booster vaccination
with live vaccines before and during
rituximab treatment

Indications

Patients with persistent thrombocytopenia
despite prior therapy with glucocorticoids
and a prior splenectomy

Notes

Optimal dose and schedule of rituximab in
treatment of ITP is not determined

Efficacy

1. A systematic review of 19 reports of
   rituximab in ITP, including 313 patients,
   nearly all of whom had previously
   received glucocorticoids, and half had
   also undergone splenectomy, reported
   62.5% overall response rate (platelet count
   >50,000/mm³). None of the included
   trials were controlled
2. In a recent prospective phase II trial
   of 60 patients with chronic ITP and
   platelet count <30,000/mm³, who were
   candidates of splenectomy, 4 weekly
   treatments of rituximab were able to
   safely defer splenectomy among 24 (40%)
   patients for 2 years

REGIMEN

THROMBOPOIETIN RECEPTOR AGONISTS
ROMIPLOSTIM AND ELTROMBOPAG OLAMINE

Bussel JB et al. N Engl J Med 2006;355:1672–1681
Bussel JB et al. N Engl J Med 2007;357:2237–2247
Kuter DJ et al. Lancet 2008;371:395–403
PROMACTA (eltrombopag) tablets, for oral use, product labeling dated 12/2011. GlaxoSmithKline, Research Triangle Park, NC
Nplate (romiplostim) for subcutaneous injection, product labeling dated 12/2011. Amgen Inc., Thousand Oaks, CA

Romiplostim dosing guidelines:
- Target a platelet count ≥50,000/mm^3 (a different platelet count target may be chosen for individual patients)
- Start 1 mcg/kg (actual body weight) once weekly as a subcutaneous injection, and check platelet count weekly
  - If platelet count <10,000/mm^3, give 2 mcg/kg every week
  - If platelet count 11,000–50,000/mm^3, give 2 mcg/kg every 2 weeks
- Once platelet count is in the desired target range (50,000–200,000/mm^3 in clinical trials)
  - Continue same dose weekly
  - Increase dosage by 1 mcg/kg every week to a maximum dosage of 10 mcg/kg per wk if platelet count drops to <10,000/mm^3
  - Increase by an additional 1 mcg/kg to a maximum dosage of 10 mcg/kg per wk after 2 consecutive weeks of platelet counts from 11,000–50,000/mm^3
  - Decrease by 1 mcg/kg after 2 consecutive weeks of platelet counts between 201,000–400,000/mm^3
  - Withhold if platelet count is >400,000/mm^3. Resume treatment after platelet count is <200,000/mm^3, and reduce subsequent doses by 1 mcg/kg
- DO NOT exceed the maximum weekly dose of 10 mcg/kg
  Discontinue romiplostim if the platelet count does not increase to a level sufficient to avoid clinically important bleeding after 4 weeks at the maximum dosage of 10 mcg/kg per day
Do not shake romiplostim vials during reconstitution

Eltrombopag olamine dosing guidelines:
- Use the lowest dose of eltrombopag needed to achieve and maintain a platelet count ≥50,000/mm^3 as necessary to reduce the risk for bleeding. Dose adjustments are based upon the platelet count response
- Do not use eltrombopag in an attempt to normalize platelet counts
- In clinical studies, platelet counts generally increased within 1–2 weeks after starting eltrombopag and decreased within 1–2 weeks after discontinuing eltrombopag

Initial Dose

Persons NOT of East Asian ancestry	Eltrombopag 50 mg once daily orally
Persons of East Asian ancestry (eg, Chinese, Japanese, Taiwanese, or Korean)	Eltrombopag 25 mg once daily orally
Persons who have mild-to-severe hepatic impairment (Child-Pugh Classes A, B, C)	
Persons of East Asian ancestry who have mild-to-severe hepatic impairment	Eltrombopag 12.5 mg once daily orally

Treatment Modifications

Platelet Count	Dose Adjustment or Response
<50,000/mm^3 after at least 2 weeks of eltrombopag	Increase daily dose by 25 mg to a maximum 75 mg/day. For patients taking 12.5 mg once daily, increase the dose to 25 mg daily before increasing the dose amount by 25 mg
≥200,000–≤400,000/mm^3 at any time	Decrease the daily dose by 25 mg. Wait 2 weeks to assess the effects of this and any subsequent dose adjustments
>400,000/mm^3	Stop eltrombopag. Increase the frequency of platelet monitoring to twice weekly

After the platelet count is <150,000/mm^3, reinitiate eltrombopag at a daily dose reduced by 25 mg

For patients taking 25 mg once daily, reinitiate eltrombopag at a daily dose of 12.5 mg |
| >400,000/mm^3 after 2 weeks of treatment at the lowest eltrombopag dose | Discontinue eltrombopag |

- Eltrombopag should be taken on an empty stomach, at least 1 hour before or 2 hours after a meal
- Patients should be advised not to take eltrombopag within 4 hours of other medications (eg, antacids), calcium-rich foods (eg, dairy products and calcium fortified juices), and mineral supplements containing polyvalent cations such as Fe, Ca, Al, Mg, Se, or Zn
- Do not administer more than one dose of eltrombopag within a 24-hour period
- Discontinue eltrombopag if the platelet count does not increase to a level sufficient to avoid clinically important bleeding after 4 weeks of therapy at the maximum daily dose of 75 mg
- Excessive platelet count responses or important liver test abnormalities also necessitate eltrombopag discontinuation

Adverse Events

Romiplostim

Commonly (mild to moderate): Headache, dizziness, fatigue, insomnia, arthralgia, myalgia, pain in extremity, back pain, abdominal pain, nausea, diarrhea

Progression from myelodysplastic syndromes (MDS) to acute myelogenous leukemia (AML) has been observed in clinical trials with romiplostim. Romiplostim is not indicated for the treatment of thrombocytopenia caused by myelodysplastic syndromes or any cause of thrombocytopenia other than chronic ITP

Romiplostim should be used with caution in patients with ITP and chronic liver disease

Eltrombopag olamine

Commonly (mild to moderate): Nausea, vomiting, myalgia, paresthesia
Eltrombopag has also been reported to cause hepatotoxicity and development or worsening of cataracts

Black Box Warnings for Eltrombopag Olamine

Eltrombopag may cause hepatotoxicity
1. Measure serum alanine aminotransferase (ALT), aspartate aminotransferase (AST), and bilirubin prior to initiating eltrombopag olamine, every 2 weeks during the dose adjustment phase, and monthly after a stable dose is established. If bilirubin is increased, perform fractionation
2. Evaluate abnormal serum LFTs with repeated testing within 3–5 days. If the abnormalities are confirmed, monitor serum LFTs weekly until abnormalities resolve, stabilize, or return to baseline levels
3. Discontinue eltrombopag olamine if serum ALT concentrations increase to ≥3× the upper limit of normal range and are:
   • Progressive, *or*
   • Persistent for ≥4 weeks, *or*
   • Accompanied by increased direct bilirubin, *or*
   • Accompanied by clinical symptoms of liver injury or evidence for hepatic decompensation
4. Reinitiating treatment with eltrombopag olamine is not recommended. If the potential benefit for reinitiating treatment is considered to outweigh the risk for hepatotoxicity, then cautiously reintroduce eltrombopag and measure serum liver tests weekly during the dose adjustment phase. If liver tests abnormalities persist, worsen, or recur, then permanently discontinue eltrombopag

Serious adverse events for both agents
1. *Bone marrow reticulin deposition:* Detection of peripheral smear abnormalities necessitates a bone marrow examination. If increased reticulin deposition is observed, discontinue treatment
2. Worsening thrombocytopenia after discontinuation of treatment (not caused by anti-TPO antibodies)

Although both romiplostim and eltrombopag olamine may increase the platelet count to levels greater than normal, no increased incidence of thromboembolic events has been reported in clinical trials

Both romiplostim and eltrombopag olamine have been subject to requirements of Risk Evaluation and Mitigations Strategy (REMS) programs. Prescribers are advised to consult the U.S. Food and Drug Administration Approved Risk Evaluation and Mitigation Strategies website at www.fda.gov/Drugs/DrugSafety/PostmarketDrugSafetyInformationforPatientsandProviders/ucm111350.htm or product manufacturers' websites for information about current REMS requirements

Efficacy

Both agents have been effective in randomized controlled clinical trials for increasing platelet counts in patients both before and after splenectomy. Both agents have been shown to increase platelet counts in patients in whom multiple previous therapies had failed

Therapy Monitoring

Romiplostim
• Obtain weekly CBCs and platelet counts during dose adjustment phases, monthly thereafter while patients are receiving romiplostim, and weekly for at least 2 weeks after discontinuing romiplostim. Consider alternative treatments for worsening thrombocytopenia

Note: Hyporesponsiveness or failure to maintain a platelet response with romiplostim should prompt a search for causative factors, including neutralizing antibodies to romiplostim

Product labeling provides information about submitting blood samples to Amgen, Inc., for analysis of antibody formation to romiplostim and thrombopoietin (TPO)

Eltrombopag olamine
• Baseline ocular examination, and periodically thereafter, particularly if visual change are noted during ongoing treatment
• Serum AST, ALT, and bilirubin prior to initiating eltrombopag olamine, every 2 weeks during the dose adjustment phase, and monthly after a stable dose is established (see Adverse Effects section for eltrombopag olamine [above])
• Weekly CBCs with differential leukocyte counts during dose adjustment phases until a stable platelet count has been achieved then monthly thereafter, and weekly for at least 4 weeks after discontinuing eltrombopag olamine

Notes

Both of these recently approved agents act by increasing production, mediated by stimulation of the thrombopoietin receptor Romiplostim is a novel thrombopoiesis-stimulating protein, with no sequence homology with endogenous thrombopoietin (TPO). It consists of 2 identical single-chain subunits, each consisting of human IgG_1-kappa Fc domain, covalently linked to a TPO receptor-binding peptide (a "peptibody") Eltrombopag is a nonpeptide, small molecule, thrombopoietin receptor agonist
In clinical trials, development of anti-TPO antibodies with neutralizing capability have not been reported with either agent

65. Hemochromatosis

James C. Barton, MD

Hemochromatosis is a heterogeneous group of heritable disorders that increase the risk of developing iron overload due to increased dietary absorption of iron. Most hemochromatosis is due to mutation(s) in genes that alter the expression, structure, or ferroportin binding of hepcidin, a liver polypeptide that is the central regulator of iron absorption. Deleterious mutations that cause hemochromatosis include those of the *HFE, HJV, TFR2, HAMP,* and *SLC40A1* genes. A rare mutation in the iron-responsive element of the *FTH1* gene caused hemochromatosis due to decreased ferritin heavy-chain ferroxidase activity. Because mechanisms to excrete iron are limited, some persons with hemochromatosis develop iron overload and consequent target organ injury

Epidemiology

Prevalence

HFE hemochromatosis:
- 4–10 per thousand (western European whites)
- 4–5 per thousand (non-Hispanic whites in United States)
- 1 in 200 (U.S. Vietnamese)

Non-HFE hemochromatosis:
Rare, based on pathogenic mutations and cases discovered in population samples

Race/ethnicity:

HFE hemochromatosis:
Predominantly European whites; some Native Americans, U.S. Vietnamese, Hispanics, African Americans
Non-HFE hemochromatosis:
Predominantly European whites; some Asians, Native Africans, African Americans, Japanese, Pacific Islanders

Male-to-female ratios in *HFE* hemochromatosis diagnosed in medical care:
- Hemochromatosis genotype: 1:1
- Elevated serum iron measures: 1.3:1
- Elevated hepatic transaminase levels: 2:1
- Diabetes mellitus: 4:1
- Cirrhosis: 5:1
- Primary liver cancer: 5:1

Age:

HFE hemochromatosis:
Severe iron overload typically occurs in subjects 40–60 years old but is rare before age 30 years
Non-HFE hemochromatosis:
Severe iron overload is common in children, adolescents, or young adults with *HJV, TFR2,* or "gain-of-function" *SLC40A1* hemochromatosis

Life expectancy:
Normal in treated patients without cardiomyopathy, cirrhosis, or diabetes mellitus, and in individuals who do not develop iron overload

Mortality rate in U.S. Adults:
- Men: 2.4/million
- Women: 1.2/million
- Whites: 1.9/million
- Nonwhites: 1/million

Barton JC et al. Genet Test 2007;11:269–275
Beutler E, Felitti VJ. Arch Intern Med 2002;162:1196–1197
Witte DL et al. Clin Chim Acta 1996;245:139–200
Yang Q et al. Ann Intern Med 1998;129:946–953

Etiology and Classification

Frequency	Transmission	Penetrance	Ethnicity	Presentation*	Clinical Presentations
Hereditary Hemochromatosis Type: Classic Hereditary (HFE) Hemochromatosis					
Common	AR (C282Y)	Low—Iron overload in <1% of heterozygotes	European whites (90% have *HFE* C282Y)	Second to fifth decades	Progressive iron overload *Advanced symptoms:* • Liver cirrhosis • Diabetes • Hypogonadism • Skin pigmentation *Early symptoms:* • Chronic fatigue • Joint and muscle pain • Decreased libido • Lethargy • Hepatomegaly
	AR (H63D, S65C, E168X)	—			• Iron overload, usually mild
	AR (IVS5+1 G/A)		Vietnamese		• Other liver disorders
Hereditary Hemochromatosis Type 2A: Hemojuvelin (HJV) Hemochromatosis (Juvenile Hemochromatosis)					
Uncommon	AR	High	European whites	First or second decades	• Arthropathy • Hypogonadism • Cardiomyopathy • Liver fibrosis or cirrhosis • Fatigue (*older patients*) • Diabetes mellitus (*older patients*) *With prolonged hypogonadism:* • Osteopenia • Osteoporosis
Hereditary Hemochromatosis Type 2B: Hepcidin (HAMP) Hemochromatosis					
Rare	AR or digenic HAMP/HFE		European whites	First or second decades	
Hereditary Hemochromatosis Type 3: Alternate Transferrin Receptor 2 (TFR2) Hemochromatosis					
Rare	AR	<100%	Italian and Japanese kinships	Second or third decades	• Cirrhosis • Hypogonadotrophic hypogonadism • Arthropathy • Diabetes mellitus (*uncommon*) • Cardiomyopathy (*uncommon*)
Hereditary Hemochromatosis Type 4: Ferroportin (SLC40A1) Hemochromatosis					
Uncommon	AD	Generally high	European whites		*"Gain-of-function" mutations:* • Similar to *HFE* or *HJV* *"Loss-of-function" mutations:* • Normal/low transferrin saturation • Anemia • Macrophage iron loading; serious liver disease is uncommon
Ferritin Heavy Chain (FTH1) Hemochromatosis					
Rare	AD	—	A Japanese kinship	—	Iron phenotypes similar to *HFE*
Familial Hemochromatosis Without Demonstrable Abnormality of Known Iron-Related Genes					
Rare	—	—	—	—	Iron phenotypes similar to *HFE*

AD, autosomal dominant; AR, autosomal recessive

*Classic hereditary (HFE-related) hemochromatosis usually becomes clinically apparent during the fourth or fifth decade of life. However, nowadays, thanks to the increased knowledge of this disease and to the higher frequency of screening laboratory tests, it is easier to recognize hereditary hemochromatosis at an earlier stage of its natural history

Camaschella C. Blood 2005;106:3710–3717
De Domenico I et al. Haematologica 2006;91:92–95
Kato J et al. Am J Hum Genet 2001;69:191–197
Papanikolaou G et al. Nat Genet 2004;36:77–82

Differential Diagnosis of Elevated Iron Measures

Non-hemochromatosis multiorgan iron overload:

1. Heritable anemias
   - Intermediate and severe β-thalassemia syndromes
   - X-linked sideroblastic anemia
   - Pyruvate kinase deficiency
   - Atransferrinemia
   - DMT-1 deficiency
   - Glutaredoxin deficiency
2. Hereditary aceruloplasminemia
3. Refractory anemia with ringed sideroblasts (myelodysplasia)
4. Transfusion iron overload
5. Chronic ingestion or injection of iron supplements
6. Excessive iron in total parenteral nutrition regimens
7. African iron overload
8. African American iron overload
9. Neonatal "hemochromatosis" (severe fetal liver injury because of maternal–fetal alloimmunity)

Liver disorders sometimes associated with iron overload:

1. Chronic viral hepatitis
2. Non-alcoholic fatty liver disease, including metabolic syndrome
3. Alcoholic liver disease
4. Porphyria cutanea tarda
5. Other advanced liver disease

Hyperferritinemia without iron overload:

1. Common liver disorders, especially non-alcoholic fatty liver, chronic viral hepatitis, and alcoholic liver disease
2. Other inflammation, tissue injury, or acute infection
3. Mean serum ferritin greater in healthy persons of Asian and Native sub-Saharan African descent than in European whites
4. *SLC40A1* Q248H polymorphism in Native Africans, African Americans
5. Hyporegenerative anemia
6. Autonomous ferritin production by malignancy
7. Hereditary hyperferritinemia-cataract syndrome

Work-Up

1. *CBC:* Hemoglobin, MCV often slightly increased; some patients with cirrhosis and portal hypertension have thrombocytopenia
2. *Serum chemistry profile:* Hepatic transaminase levels often mildly increased
3. *Serum iron measures:* Transferrin saturation often increased; unbound iron-binding capacity elevated; ferritin always elevated in iron overload
4. *Liver biopsy:* "Gold standard" for ascertaining occurrence, severity of iron overload. Recommended for patients with serum ferritin level >1,000 μ/L. Evaluate for morphology (hematoxylin and eosin stain), fibrosis (trichrome stain), and iron grade (Perls'/Prussian blue stain). Perform quantitative iron measurements, compute hepatic iron index
5. *Diabetes mellitus:* Use standard diagnostic criteria; type 2 diabetes is typical; evaluate for vascular, ophthalmic, and neurologic complications
6. *Anterior pituitary gland:* Evaluate gonadotroph function with testosterone, estradiol, luteinizing hormone, and follicle-stimulating hormone levels; evaluate pituitary iron content with MRI scanning
7. *Osteoporosis:* Evaluate patients with hypogonadism using DEXA scans
8. *Cardiac biopsy:* Endomyocardial biopsy indicated in young persons with cardiomyopathy attributed to iron overload; evaluate morphology as described for liver
9. *Imaging studies:* Use T2 or T2* MRI images of liver, heart, or pituitary to semiquantify iron content. Plain films of hands, hips, or knees detect arthropathy. In patients with cirrhosis, use CT scanning or liver ultrasonography to survey for primary liver cancer
10. *DNA-based testing:* HFE mutation analysis to detect alleles C282Y, H63D, and S65C is commercially available; testing for other *HFE* alleles or mutations in other hemochromatosis genes may be available from dedicated research or non-U.S. commercial laboratories
11. *Family screening:* Test first-degree family members of probands with transferrin saturation, serum ferritin. Perform DNA-based testing of family members with elevated iron measures
12. HLA-A and -B typing: For *HFE* hemochromatosis only. Persons HLA-identical to their sibling probands are assumed to have identical *HFE* genotypes and should be evaluated for iron overload

Treatment Options
Expert Opinion

Iron-depletion therapy:

1. Phlebotomy is the preferred treatment for patients with iron overload unassociated with severe anemia, especially *HFE* and other hemochromatosis syndromes, due to its efficacy, safety, and economy

2. Erythrocytapheresis, a phlebotomy variant, requires large intravenous catheters, is expensive, and is not widely available

3. The oral iron chelating agent deferasirox (DFX) or the parenteral iron chelator deferoxamine (DFO) can induce iron depletion in patients with hemochromatosis and in some patients with iron overload associated with anemia

4. DFX or DFO therapy alone reduces iron burdens slowly

5. Combined phlebotomy and iron chelation therapy is used to treat cardiomyopathy due to cardiac siderosis in some persons with early age-of-onset hemochromatosis, especially that due to *HJV* mutations

6. Combined chelation therapy is often used to decrease iron burdens in persons with beta-thalassemia major.

7. The oral iron chelating agent deferiprone is licensed in the U.S. for management of iron overload in persons with severe beta-thalassemia whose responses to other iron-chelating drugs have been inadequate

8. Manage compliant patients without iron-related organ injury whose serum ferritin levels are <300 μg/L (men) or <200 μg/L (women) with observation. Measure serum ferritin and hepatic transaminase levels yearly. Commence phlebotomy if serum ferritin levels increase above these limits, even in asymptomatic subjects

9. Patients with short life expectancy due to non-iron overload conditions are unlikely to benefit from iron depletion therapy

Dietary management:

1. No known dietary management removes absorbed iron

2. Avoiding consumption of iron-rich foods or use of iron cookware has no proven benefit

3. The daily ingestion of large amounts of tea reduces iron absorption in some patients with beta-thalassemia major and reduces maintenance phlebotomy requirements in some patients with hemochromatosis

4. Daily use of proton pump inhibitor drugs decreases iron absorption and thus reduces maintenance phlebotomy requirements in persons with hemochromatosis and *HFE* C282Y homozygosity

5. Permit iron-depleted patients without hepatic injury to consume alcohol in moderation; advise others to abstain from ingesting alcohol

6. Advise patients not to ingest supplemental iron, including that in "one-a-day" preparations; limit supplemental vitamin C to 500 mg daily

7. Advise patients to avoid supplements containing minerals absorbed in pathways shared with iron (Zn, Mn, Co). If a mineral deficiency is diagnosed, prescribe and monitor specific replacement therapy

8. Advise patients not to consume raw shellfish, to prevent contact of wounds with seawater, and to avoid direct handling of uncooked saltwater finfish or shellfish

Complications of iron overload:

General medical management of liver disorders, diabetes mellitus, hypogonadism, heart conditions, arthropathy, osteoporosis, and infections in hemochromatosis patients is the same as it is for other patients. Increasing evidence suggests that iron overload is not the predominant cause of diabetes mellitus in men and women and of hypogonadotrophic hypogonadism in men with *HFE* hemochromatosis

REGIMEN

THERAPEUTIC PHLEBOTOMY

Barton JC et al. Ann Intern Med 1998;129:932–939
Brissot P, de Bels F. Hematology Am Soc Hematol Educ Program 2006;36–41

Indications:

1. Iron overload due to hemochromatosis or other iron overload unassociated with severe anemia
2. Initiate treatment if ferritin level ≥300 ng/mL (men) and ≥200 ng/mL (women)

Treatment

Before therapy:

1. Verify that venous access is adequate. Use implanted ports for phlebotomy only if venous access is inadequate
2. If anemia is present, correct if possible
3. Routine erythropoietin therapy is unnecessary unless relative or absolute deficiency of erythropoietin is demonstrated

Achieving iron depletion:

1. Ensure adequate hydration before and after each session
2. Evaluate CBC each treatment day to ensure hemoglobin >11.0 g/dL
3. Use personnel skilled in therapeutic phlebotomy
4. Use butterfly needle (19 gauge) connected to an extension tubing set and collect blood in an evacuated bottle
5. Large needles (14 gauge, 16 gauge) are less well tolerated than smaller needles; use extension tubing and gravity to collect blood in bags
6. For port phlebotomy, use a 19-gauge Huber needle connected to an extension tubing set and collect blood in an evacuated bottle
7. Remove 300–450 mL/session from average women, older patients; 450–500 mL/session from men, larger women
8. Repeat every 5–14 days according to iron overload severity, patient tolerance

Toxicity

1. Local discomfort of venipuncture
2. Transient hypovolemia
3. Mild fatigue
4. Iron deficiency (if phlebotomy is excessive)

Efficacy

1. 95% of patients comply to achieve iron depletion
2. Each unit of blood (450–500 mL) contains 200–250 mg Fe (~1 mg Fe/ 1 mL erythrocytes)
3. Serum ferritin ~20 μg/L indicates that iron depletion has been achieved and that potentially harmful iron deposits have been removed
4. Aggressive iron depletion of patients with cardiac siderosis can be lifesaving
5. Hypogonadotrophic hypogonadism improves or resolves in some cases
6. Hepatic fibrosis or cirrhosis improves in some cases
7. Improved control of diabetes mellitus or joint symptoms, or in fatigue and weakness in some cases
8. Maintaining normal body iron levels (serum ferritin <300 μg/L in men, <200 μg/L in women) after achieving iron depletion would prevent future iron overload complications, but health benefits may not accrue to all asymptomatic patients
9. Compliance with phlebotomy to maintain iron depletion decreases ~7% yearly

Monitoring Therapy

1. *Initiation:* CBC, serum ferritin, liver profile
2. *Each phlebotomy session:* CBC
3. Serum ferritin every 4 phlebotomy sessions in patients undergoing therapy to achieve iron depletion
4. After serum ferritin <200 μg/L, measure serum ferritin after every 1–2 phlebotomy sessions
5. When serum ferritin 20–50 ng/mL: discontinue phlebotomy, compute quantity of iron removed
6. Once-twice yearly after iron depletion: serum ferritin, liver profile
7. Start maintenance therapy when serum ferritin >300 μg/L (men) and >200 μg/L (women)

Notes

1. Do not monitor therapy using serum iron or transferrin saturation
2. Patients with greater iron burdens at diagnosis usually need more frequent maintenance phlebotomy. Some patients, especially women and older men, require little maintenance phlebotomy, if any
3. Many patients with "loss-of-function" ferroportin mutations have anemia, slow recovery of hemoglobin level after phlebotomy, and intolerance of normal iron stores; permit higher levels of ferritin in these cases than recommended for other types of hemochromatosis
4. Healthy patients can be voluntary blood donors in some circumstances, especially during maintenance therapy
5. Phlebotomy diminishes severity of hepatic fibrosis or cirrhosis, but it is unknown if risk of primary liver cancer is also reduced
6. Consider repeating liver biopsy 6–12 months after iron depletion in patients with hepatic fibrosis or cirrhosis at diagnosis to re-evaluate liver morphology
7. Primary liver cancer is presently unreported in non-*HFE* hemochromatosis but occurs in some patients with severe non-hemochromatosis iron overload

REGIMEN

IRON CHELATION THERAPY WITH DEFEROXAMINE MESYLATE (DFO)

Barton JC. Curr Gastroenterol Rep 2007;9:74–82
De Gobbi M et al. Haematologica 2000;85:865–867
Fabio G et al. Blood 2007;109:362–364
Nielsen P et al. Br J Haematol 2003;123:952–953

Indications:
1. Adjunct management of cardiomyopathy due to cardiac siderosis in patients undergoing concurrent therapeutic phlebotomy
2. Treatment of severe iron overload due to hemochromatosis in patients unable to tolerate or unwilling to undergo therapeutic phlebotomy

Treatment

Before therapy:
1. Verify that renal function is normal
2. Educate patients about the importance of compliance with DFO infusion schedules and manifestations of toxicity

Achieving iron depletion:
1. *Subcutaneous DFO:* Infuse deferoxamine mesylate 40 mg/kg by continuous subcutaneous infusion for 8–12 hours nightly for 5–7 nights weekly using a portable (ambulatory) pump
2. *Intramuscular DFO:* Deferoxamine mesylate 500–1000 mg by intramuscular injection, daily
3. *Oral vitamin C:* Ascorbic acid 200 mg on each day of DFO administration enhances iron excretion. DO NOT exceed this dose

Efficacy

1. Deferoxamine mobilizes iron from parenchymal cells and macrophages; iron removal from heart is less rapid than from other sites
2. Urinary iron excretion, typically 5–40 mg/24 hours. Elimination often wanes after several consecutive days of therapy
3. Deferoxamine half-life is very short a stringent infusion routine is required for optimal efficacy
4. Hypogonadotrophic hypogonadism or cardiomyopathy due to *HJV* or *TFR2* hemochromatosis improves or resolves in some cases
5. Hepatic fibrosis or cirrhosis regresses in some cases
6. In 3 *HFE* hemochromatosis patients who were unable to tolerate phlebotomy, subcutaneous deferoxamine treatment removed hepatocyte iron at a rate similar to that of weekly 500-mL phlebotomy

Toxicity

1. Local reactions (eg, discomfort, pruritus, erythema)
2. Systemic allergic or hypersensitivity reactions (eg, urticaria, angioedema, musculoskeletal pain, anaphylaxis)
3. Diverse ocular and auditory adverse effects (eg, high-frequency hearing loss, deafness, retinal damage)
4. Neutropenia, agranulocytosis, thrombocytopenia
5. Increased susceptibility to *Yersinia* sp. infections and mucormycosis
6. Zinc deficiency

Monitoring Therapy

1. *Initiation:* CBC, serum ferritin, liver, and renal profiles
2. *Monthly:* Reevaluate patient; measure CBC, renal, liver profiles, serum ferritin; indicated cardiac assessment in patients with cardiomyopathy
3. *Every 6 months:* Serum luteinizing hormone, follicle-stimulating hormone, and testosterone or estradiol
4. *When ferritin <300 ng/mL (men) and <200 ng/mL (women):* Discontinue deferoxamine
5. *Once or twice yearly after iron depletion:* Reevaluate patient; serum ferritin, liver profile
6. *Once or twice yearly in patients treated for prolonged intervals or those with new symptoms:* Visual acuity tests, slit-lamp examinations, funduscopy, audiometry

Notes

1. Therapy must be individualized to maximize compliance and iron excretion
2. Red or rusty urine indicates a satisfactory level of iron excretion
3. Iron excretion after 8–12 hours of deferoxamine infusion is the same as with the same deferoxamine dose given over 24 hours in many patients
4. Improvement in survival or disease-related symptoms has not been established for persons with hemochromatosis
5. Possible role of DFO therapy for "maintenance" of normal serum ferritin levels in persons with *HFE* hemochromatosis is unknown
6. Safety and efficacy of DFO when administered with other iron chelation agents have not been established in patients with *HFE* hemochromatosis

REGIMEN

IRON CHELATION THERAPY DEFERASIROX (DFX)

Barton JC. Curr Gastroenterol Rep 2007;9:74–82
Phatak P et al. Hepatology 2010;52:1671–1679
Adams PC, Barton JC. Blood 2010;116:317–325
Exjade (deferasirox) tablets, for oral suspension; product label May 2013. Novartis Pharmaceuticals Corporation, East Hanover, NJ

Indications:

Treatment of iron overload with DFX should be considered in persons with *HFE* hemochromatosis who have anemia, severe heart disease, poor venous access, or poor compliance with phlebotomy

The U.S. Food and Drug Administration has licensed deferasirox for management of chronic iron overload:

1. Caused by transfusion in persons ≥2 years of age

2. In patients ≥10 years of age with non–transfusion-dependent thalassemia syndromes and with liver iron concentration ≥5 mg Fe/g of liver dry weight and serum ferritin >300 μg/L

Notes

1. Approximately 30% of patients with *HFE* hemochromatosis do not tolerate or continue DFX therapy because of adverse events

2. Improvement in survival or disease-related symptoms has not been established

3. Possible role of DFX therapy for "maintenance" of normal serum ferritin levels in persons with *HFE* hemochromatosis is unknown

4. Safety and efficacy of DFX when administered with other iron chelation agents have not been established

Treatment

Before therapy:

1. Select target serum ferritin level

2. Exclude:
   - Males with hemoglobin <13 g/dL
   - Females with hemoglobin <12 g/dL
   - Current treatment with deferoxamine (DFO) or deferiprone (DFP)
   - Serum creatinine levels above the upper reference limit of normal range
   - Alanine aminotransferase (ALT) levels ≥2 × the upper reference limit of normal range
   - Diagnosis of hepatic cirrhosis

Achieving iron depletion:

1. **Deferasirox** 10 mg/kg per day orally, continually, is suggested for starting treatment (Deferasirox 5 mg/kg per day was less effective than 10 or 15 mg/kg per day in decreasing serum ferritin. Daily doses of deferasirox 15 mg/kg did not increase the rate of iron loss but caused more adverse events than 10 mg/kg per day)

2. Doses of DFX for iron overload because of *HFE* hemochromatosis are typically less than those used for other indications

Toxicity

1. Increased serum levels of ALT/AST

2. Increased serum creatinine level

3. Diarrhea, abdominal pain, nausea

4. Headache, fatigue, back pain, arthralgia

5. Bone marrow suppression, gastrointestinal bleeding are rare but potentially fatal

Efficacy

1. DFX mobilizes iron from parenchymal cells and macrophages; iron removal from heart is less rapid than from other sites

2. DFX and metabolites are primarily excreted in the feces (~84% of dose)

3. Renal excretion of DFX and metabolites is minimal (~8% of administered dose)

4. Mean elimination half-life ranges from 8–16 hours after oral administration

5. After 48 weeks of treatment, median serum ferritin levels in patients with *HFE* hemochromatosis decreased by 64%, 75%, and 74% in cohorts of patients who received deferasirox 5, 10, or 15 mg/kg per day, respectively

6. In all cohorts, median serum ferritin decreased to <250 μg/L after 48 weeks of treatment

Monitoring Therapy

1. *Initiation:* CBC, serum ferritin, and liver and renal function profiles

2. *Monthly:* Reevaluate patient; measure CBC, renal and liver function profiles, serum ferritin

3. Discontinue or interrupt therapy if serum ALT/AST or serum creatinine levels increase, or if unfavorable changes in neutrophil or platelet counts or hemoglobin levels occur

4. Risk of hepatic or renal toxicity may be increased in patients with low serum ferritin levels

5. Discontinue DFX when target serum ferritin level is reached

6. *Once-twice yearly after iron depletion is completed:* Reevaluate patient; serum ferritin, liver function profile

66. Myeloproliferative Neoplasms

Naseema Gangat, MD and Ayalew Tefferi, MD

Myeloproliferative neoplasms (MPN) are clonal disorders of hematopoietic stem cells that manifest clinically as overproduction of cells that contribute to the myeloid lineage

Classification
WHO Myeloproliferative Neoplasm (MPN) Categories

1. Classic MPN
   - Chronic myelogenous leukemia (CML); see Chapter 21
   - **Polycythemia vera (PV)***
   - **Essential thrombocythemia (ET)***
   - **Primary myelofibrosis (PMF)***
2. "Nonclassic" MPNs
   - Chronic neutrophilic leukemia (CNL)
   - Mast cell disease (MCD)
   - Chronic eosinophilic leukemia not otherwise categorized (CEL-NOC)
   - "MPN unclassifiable"

*BCR-ABL–negative classic MPN (PV, ET, and PMF)

Epidemiology

BCR-ABL–negative classic MPN
Polycythemia vera (PV), essential thrombocythemia (ET), and primary myelofibrosis (PMF)

Polycythemia vera (PV)
1. *Incidence:* 0.8–2.6/100,000
2. *Median age at diagnosis:* ≈60 years
3. *Median survival:* >15 years
4. *10-year risk of myelofibrosis:* <4%
5. *10-year risk of AML:* <2%

Note: Longer disease duration and evolution into myelofibrosis significantly increase the risk of leukemic transformation

Ania BJ et al. Am J Hematol 1994;47:89–93
Gangat N et al. Br J Haematol 2007;138:354–358
Gangat N et al. Leukemia 2007;21:270–276
Mesa RA et al. Am J Hematol 1999;61:10–15

Essential thrombocythemia (ET)
1. *Incidence:* 0.2–2.5/100,000
2. *Median age at diagnosis:* ≈60 years
3. *Median survival:* >15 years
4. *10-year risk of myelofibrosis:* ≈10%
5. *10-year risk of AML:* ≈6%

Note: Longer disease duration and evolution into myelofibrosis significantly increase the risk of leukemic transformation

Primary myelofibrosis (PMF)
1. *Incidence:* 0.4–1.5/100,000
2. *Median age at diagnosis:* ≈60 years
3. *Median survival:* <3 years to >10 years
4. *10-year risk of myelofibrosis:* N/A
5. *10-year risk of AML:* ≈20% based on the presence or absence of well-defined prognostic determinants
6. Most important indicators of adverse prognosis:
   - Age >65 years
   - Hemoglobin <10 g/dL
   - Leukocyte count >25,000/mm³
   - Circulating blasts ≥1%
   - Constitutional symptoms
   - Unfavorable karyotype included complex karyotype or single or two abnormalities including +8, −7/7q-, i(17q), −5/5q-, 12p-, inv(3), or 11q23 rearrangement
   - Thrombocytopenia <100,000/mm³

Cervantes F et al. Br J Haematol 1997;97:635–640
Dupriez B et al. Blood 1996;88:1013–1018
Gangat N et al. J Clin Oncol 2011;29:392–397
Passamonti F et al. Blood 2010;115:1703–1708
Tefferi A et al. Cancer 2007;109:2083–2088

Mutations in MPN

Chronology:

- *1951:* CML, PV, ET, and PMF recognized to have significant overlap in both clinical and biological features and felt to be related diseases
- *1960:* CML recognized as distinct entity after discovery of Philadelphia chromosome
- *Early 1980s:* Analysis of X chromosome inactivation patterns in women with CML, PV, ET, or PMF carrying a polymorphic variant of the glucose-6-phosphate dehydrogenase gene establishes all 4 diseases as clonal stem-cell disorders
- *2005:* Somatic mutation involving Janus Kinase 2 (*JAK2*) identified in patients with PV, ET, and PMF. Mutation at codon 617, [*JAK2*V617F] is a G→T transversion at nucleotide 1849 in exon 14 of *JAK2* gene, with substitution of valine by phenylalanine at codon 617
- *2006–2007:* Additional *JAK2* and *MPL* (thrombopoietin receptor) mutations described in these diseases; some induce PV-like (*JAK2*) or PMF-like (*MPL*) phenotype in mice

Adamson JW et al. N Engl J Med 1976;295:913–916
Dameshek W. Blood 1951;6:372–375
Fialkow PJ et al. Blood 1981;58:916–919

Mutations

1. *JAK2*V617F mutations: 20–95%
   (Most frequent mutation in *BCR-ABL*-negative chronic myeloid malignancies)
   - 95% in PV
   - 50% in ET
   - 50% in PMF
   - 20% in RARS-T
   - 20% in other "MPN or MDS/MPN, unclassifiable"
   - <5% in AML
   - <5% in MDS
2. *JAK2* exon 12 mutations (eg, N542-E543del): 3%
   - 3% of all PV cases [relatively specific to PV]; occur in virtually all *JAK2*V617F-negative PV cases
3. *MPL* (thrombopoietin receptor) mutations (eg, *MPL*W515L/K): 1–10%
   - 5–10% in PMF
   - 1–5% in ET

Baxter EJ et al. Lancet 2005;365:1054–1061. Erratum in: Lancet 2005;366:122
James C et al. Nature 2005;434:1144–1148
Kralovics R et al. N Engl J Med 2005;352:1779–1790
Levine RL et al. Cancer Cell 2005;7:387–397
Pardanani AD et al. Blood 2006;108:3472–3476
Pikman Y et al. PLoS Med 2006;3:e270
Scott LM et al. N Engl J Med 2007;356:459–468

Thrombosis in MPN

Thrombosis in ET and PV

- Incidence of major thrombosis, mostly arterial: 11–25% at diagnosis and 11–22% during follow-up
- As regards the pathogenesis of thrombosis, an increased presence of neutrophil-platelet aggregates has been demonstrated in ET patients. Moreover, it has been shown that neutrophils are activated and endothelial dysfunction occurs, which is indicated by increased neutrophil activation parameters such as CD11b and leukocyte alkaline phosphatase, as well as markers of endothelial damage
- These observations have been confirmed in recent clinical studies, suggesting that leukocytosis is associated with an increased risk of thrombosis in both PV and ET

Carobbio A et al. Blood 2007;109:2310–2313
Falanga A et al. Blood 2000;96:4261–4266
Landolfi R et al. Blood 2007;109:2446–2452

Thrombohemorrhagic events in ET

- Incidence of major hemorrhage: 2–5% at diagnosis and 1–7% during follow-up
- Pathogenesis of thrombohemorrhagic events in ET remains unclear
- A frequently accepted mechanisms for hemorrhage in ET patients has been the association of extreme thrombocytosis (platelet count >1,000,000/mm^3) with acquired von Willebrand disease characterized by loss of the large von Willebrand factor multimers

Note: An elevated platelet count >1,000,000/mm^3 has been loosely associated with an increased risk of hemorrhage but has not been shown to correlate with thrombotic complications

Elliott MA et al. Br J Haematol 2005;128:275–290
Tefferi A et al. Blood 2006;108:2493–2494
van Genderen PJJ et al. Br J Haematol 1997;99:832–836

Table 66–1. 2008 World Health Organization Diagnostic Criteria

Polycythemia Vera (PV)	Essential Thrombocythemia (ET)	Primary Myelofibrosis (PMF)
Diagnosis of PV requires meeting both major criteria and 1 minor criterion *or* The first major criterion and 2 minor criteria	Diagnosis of ET requires meeting all 4 major criteria	Diagnosis of PMF requires meeting all 3 major criteria and 2 minor criteria

Major Criteria		
1. Hgb >18.5 g/dL (men) Hgb >16.5 g/dL (women) *or* Hgb >17 g/dL (men) Hgb >15 g/dL (women) (If associated with a sustained increase of ≥2 g/dL from baseline that cannot be attributed to correction of iron deficiency) *or* Hgb or Hct >99th percentile of reference range for age, sex, or altitude of residence *or* Red cell mass >25% above mean normal predicted	1. Platelet count ≥450,000/mm³	1. Megakaryocyte proliferation and atypia* accompanied by either reticulin and/or collagen fibrosis *or* In the absence of reticulin fibrosis, the megakaryocyte changes must be accompanied by increased marrow cellularity, granulocytic proliferation and often decreased erythropoiesis (ie, prefibrotic PMF)
	2. Megakaryocyte proliferation with large and mature morphology No or little granulocyte or erythroid proliferation	
	3. Not meeting WHO criteria for CML, PV, PMF, MDS, or other myeloid neoplasm	2. Not meeting WHO criteria for CML, PV, MDS, or other myeloid neoplasm
2. Presence of *JAK*2V617F or similar mutation	4. Demonstration of *JAK*2V617F or other clonal marker *or* No evidence of reactive thrombocytosis	3. Demonstration of JAK2V617F or other clonal marker *or* No evidence of reactive marrow fibrosis

Minor Criteria		
1. BM trilineage myeloproliferation		1. Leukoerythroblastosis
		2. Increased serum LDH
2. Subnormal serum Epo level		3. Anemia
3. EEC growth		4. Palpable splenomegaly

Hgb, Hemoglobin; Hct, hematocrit; Epo, erythropoietin; EEC, endogenous erythroid colony; WHO, World Health Organization; CML, chronic myelogenous leukemia; MDS, myelodysplastic syndrome; LDH, lactate dehydrogenase
*Small to large megakaryocytes with aberrant nuclear/cytoplasmic ratio and hyperchromatic and irregularly folded nuclei and dense clustering

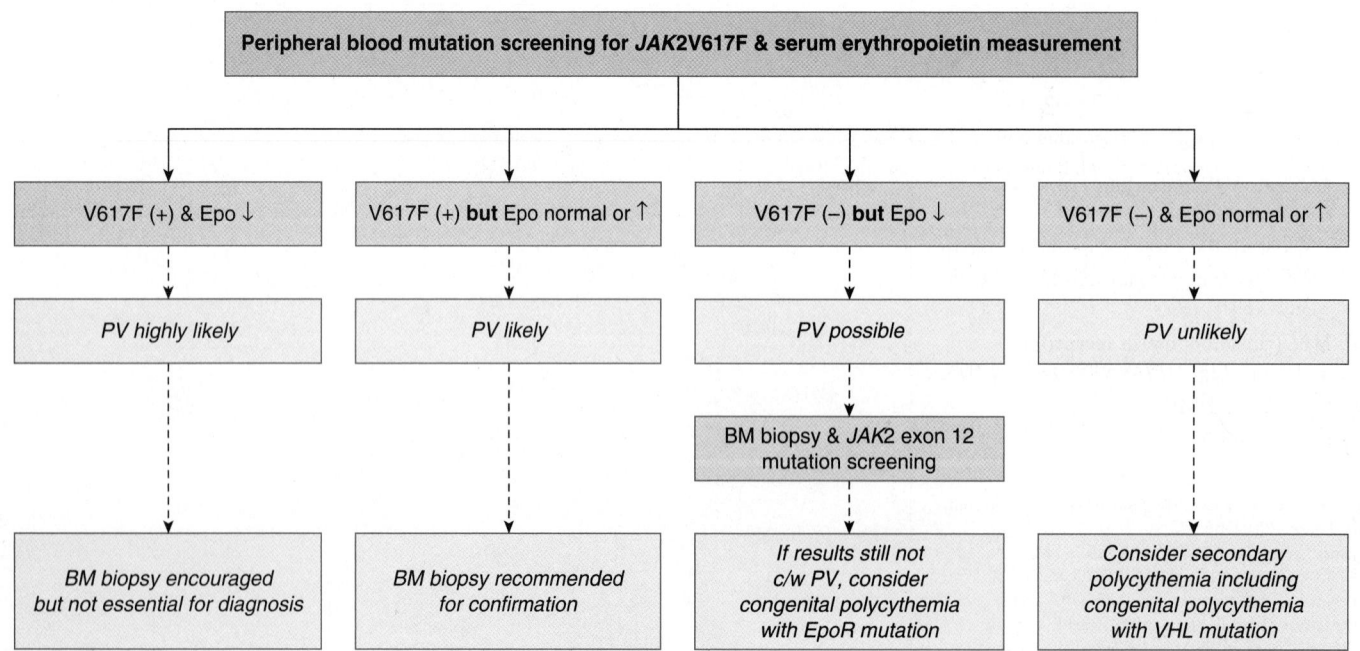

Figure 66–1. Diagnostic algorithm for suspected polycythemia vera. PV, polycythemia vera; SP, secondary polycythemia; CP, congenital polycythemia; BM, bone marrow; V617F, JAK2V617F; Epo, erythropoietin; EpoR, erythropoietin receptor; VHL, von Hippel-Lindau; c/w, consistent with

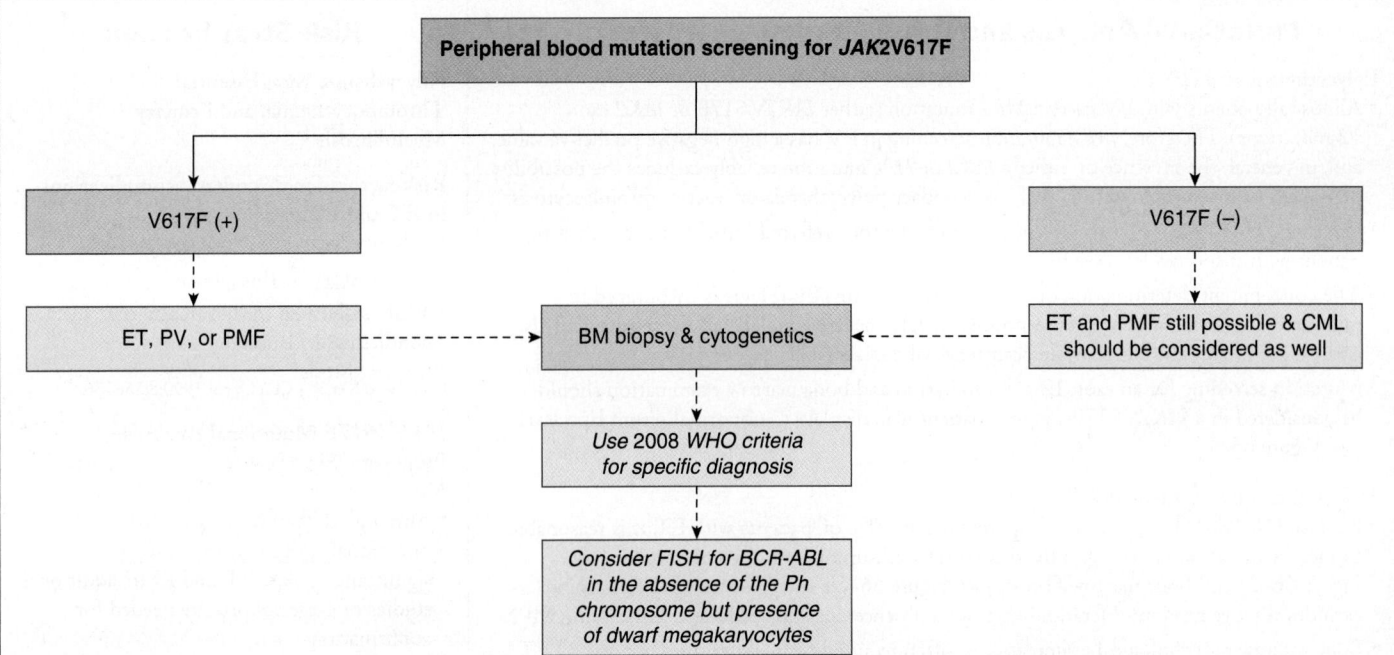

Figure 66–2. Diagnostic algorithm for suspected essential thrombocythemia. PV, polycythemia vera; ET, essential thrombocythemia; PMF, primary myelofibrosis; CML, chronic myeloid leukemia; MDS, myelodysplastic syndrome; MPN, myeloproliferative neoplasm; WHO, World Health Organization; RT, reactive thrombocytosis; FISH, fluorescent in situ hybridization; Ph, Philadelphia; BM, bone marrow; V617F, JAK2V617F

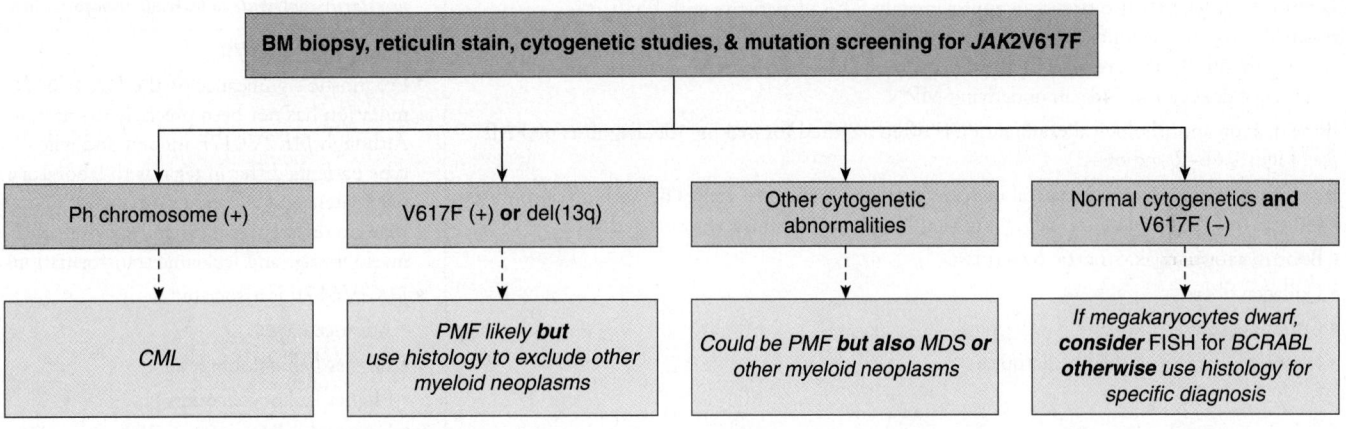

Figure 66–3. Diagnostic algorithm for suspected primary myelofibrosis. PMF, primary myelofibrosis; CML, chronic myeloid leukemia; MDS, myelodysplastic syndrome; FISH, fluorescent in situ hybridization; Ph, Philadelphia; BM, bone marrow; V617F, JAK2V617F

Mutational Analysis and Bone Marrow Examination

Polycythemia vera (PV)

- Almost all patients with PV carry a *JAK2* mutation (either *JAK2*V617F or *JAK2* exon 12 mutations). Therefore, *JAK2* mutation screening in PV has a high negative predictive value, and, in general, the presence of either a *JAK2* or *MPL* mutation reliably excludes the possibility of nonclonal myeloproliferation, such as secondary polycythemia or reactive thrombocytosis
- Peripheral blood *JAK2*V617F screening is currently the preferred initial test for evaluating a patient with suspected PV (see Figure 66–1)
- The concomitant determination of serum erythropoietin (Epo) level is encouraged to minimize the consequences of false-positive or false-negative molecular test results, and also address the infrequent but possible occurrence of *JAK2*V617F-negative PV
- Mutation screening for an exon 12 *JAK2* mutation and bone marrow examination should be considered in a *JAK2*V617F-negative patient who displays a subnormal serum Epo level (see Figure 66–1)

Essential thrombocythemia (ET)

- Because *JAK2*V617F also occurs in approximately 50% of patients with ET, it is reasonable to include mutation screening in the diagnostic work-up of both thrombocytosis (see Figure 66–2) and bone marrow fibrosis (see Figure 66–3); the presence of the mutation excludes reactive myeloproliferation whereas its absence does not exclude an underlying MPN
- Bone marrow morphological examination is often required for making the diagnosis of ET (see Figures 66–2 and 66–3)
- ET is the only MPN currently diagnosed by exclusion. ET may be diagnosed in patients with persistent thrombocytosis only in the absence of a known cause of reactive or clonal thrombocytosis

Primary myelofibrosis (PMF)

- Because *JAK2*V617F also occurs in approximately 50% of patients with PMF, it is reasonable to include mutation screening in the diagnostic work-up of bone marrow fibrosis (see Figure 66–3); the presence of the mutation excludes reactive myeloproliferation whereas its absence does not exclude an underlying MPN
- Bone marrow morphological examination is often required for making the diagnosis of PMF (see Figures 66–2 and 66–3)
- Bone marrow examination is critical in distinguishing between the causes of both myelophthisis and bone marrow fibrosis. In PMF, peripheral blood myelophthisis is associated with:
  - Bone marrow megakaryocytic hyperplasia
  - Collagen fibers
  - Osteosclerosis
  - Intramedullary sinusoidal hematopoiesis

Risk Stratification

Polycythemia Vera, Essential Thrombocythemia, and Primary Myelofibrosis

Risk factors for thrombotic complications in ET and PV patients

- Advanced age (age >60 years)
- Prior history of thrombosis
- Well-established cardiovascular risk; there is conflicting evidence

Cortelazzo S et al. J Clin Oncol 1990;8:556–562

*JAK2*V617F Mutational Analysis—Prognostic Significance

Notes:

- Although data suggest *JAK2*V617F mutational status may have prognostic significance in PV, ET, and PMF, additional studies of large cohorts are needed for confirmation
- *JAK2 (and myeloproliferative leukemia virus oncogene [MPL] mutations) are neither disease-specific nor contemporaneous with the ancestral clone of myeloproliferative neoplasms. Instead, they appear to constitute phenotype-modifying subclones that do not necessarily contribute to leukemic transformation*

ET and *JAK2*V617F

- Prognostic significance of the *JAK2*V617F mutation has not been precisely delineated. Although *JAK2*V617F mutant and wild-type patients differ in regards to laboratory parameters and clinical features there were no differences in overall survival, or myelofibrotic and leukemic transformations
- *JAK2*V617F is associated with:
  - Advanced age
  - Higher hemoglobin level
  - Higher leukocyte counts
  - Lower platelet counts
- In patients with *JAK2*V617F mutation, *allele burden* is directly correlated with:
  - Leukocyte count
  - Platelet count
  - Presence of palpable splenomegaly

Kittur J et al. Cancer 2007;109:2279–2284

PV and *JAK2*V617F

- *JAK2*V617F homozygous patients have:
  - Higher hemoglobin level
  - Higher leukocyte count
  - Lower platelet count
  - Increased incidence of pruritus
  - NO increased risk of thrombosis

(continued)

Treatment Options

Table 66–2. Current Management and Risk Stratification in Essential Thrombocythemia (ET), Polycythemia Vera (PV), and Primary Myelofibrosis (PMF)

Risk Categories	ET	PV	PMF Age <50 years	PMF Age ≥50 years
Low	Low-dose aspirin	Low-dose aspirin + Phlebotomy	Observation *or* Experimental drug therapy	
Low but with extreme thrombocytosis* for ET and PV Intermediate for PMF	Low-dose aspirin†	Low-dose aspirin† + Phlebotomy	Experimental drug therapy *or* RIC‡ transplant	Experimental drug therapy *or* Conventional drug therapy
High	Low-dose aspirin + Hydroxyurea	Low-dose aspirin + Phlebotomy + Hydroxyurea	Experimental drug therapy *or* Full transplant	Experimental drug therapy *or* RIC‡ transplant

Risk stratification for ET and PV:
High risk: Age ≥60 years *or* previous thrombosis
Low-risk: Neither of the above
Risk Stratification of Primary Myelofibrosis According to the Dynamic International Prognostic Scoring System Plus (DIPSS-plus):
age >65 years, hemoglobin <10 g/dL, leukocytes >25,000/mm³, circulating blasts ≥1%, constitutional symptoms, unfavorable karyotype, platelet count <100,000/mm³, transfusion status
Low risk: 0 adverse points (median survival, 180 months),
Intermediate-1 risk: 1 adverse point (median survival, 80 months)
Intermediate-2 risk: 2–3 adverse points (median survival, 35 months)
High risk: 4–6 adverse points (median survival, 16 months)

*Extreme thrombocytosis is defined as a platelet count ≥1,000,000/mm³
†Clinically significant acquired von Willebrand syndrome (ristocetin cofactor activity <30%) should be excluded before using aspirin in patients with a platelet count ≥1,000,000/mm³
‡RIC, reduced intensity conditioning

Treatment of Essential Thrombocythemia (ET)
Treatment recommendations:
1. Low-dose aspirin for all patients
2. Add hydroxyurea in high-risk patients

Barbui T et al. N Engl J Med 2005;353:85–86

Treatment options:
1. Antiplatelet therapy (eg, low-dose aspirin)
2. Cytoreductive therapy—hydroxyurea
3. Cytoreductive therapy—anagrelide
4. Cytoreductive therapy—interferon alfa (interferon-α, IFN-α)
5. Cytoreductive therapy—pipobroman
6. Cytoreductive therapy—busulfan

Note: There is no hard evidence to implicate any one of these agents, including hydroxyurea, as being leukemogenic in the treatment of ET
1. *Antiplatelet therapy (eg, low-dose aspirin)*
   - Has not been shown to influence survival or lower risk of disease transformation
   - Used to either alleviate microvascular symptoms or to prevent thrombohemorrhagic complications

(continued)

Risk Stratification (continued)

- In patients with *JAK2*V617F mutation, *allele burden* is directly correlated with:
  - Higher hemoglobin level
  - Higher leukocyte count
  - Lower platelet count
  - Increased incidence of pruritus
  - NO increased risk of thrombosis

Vannucchi AM et al. Blood 2007;110:840–846

PMF and *JAK2*V617F
- *JAK2*V617F mutation is associated with:
  - Poorer overall survival
  - Older age at diagnosis
  - Higher leukocyte count
  - Presence of pruritus
- *JAK2*V617F "homozygous" PMF patients have:
  - Even higher leukocyte count
  - Larger spleen size

Tefferi A et al. Leukemia 2008;22:756–761

Treatment Options (continued)

2. *Cytoreductive therapy—hydroxyurea*
- Treatment of choice in high-risk ET patients because of superior efficacy and less toxicity (see Table 66–1)
- Has not been shown to influence survival or lower risk of disease transformation
- Used to either alleviate microvascular symptoms or prevent thrombohemorrhagic complications
- *Two randomized controlled trials have evaluated hydroxyurea efficacy*
  Hydroxyurea vs. No Cytoreductive Therapy
  First study to demonstrate the benefit of cytoreductive therapy in ET patients
  - N = 114 patients
  - High-risk ET patients (age >60 years, or prior thrombosis)
  - Randomized to hydroxyurea (n = 56) or no cytoreductive therapy (n = 58)
  - Median follow-up = 27 months:
    - Two thromboses in hydroxyurea group (1.6% per patient-year)
    - Fourteen thromboses in control group (10.7% per patient-year; p = 0.003)

3. *Cytoreductive therapy—anagrelide*
- Anagrelide is inferior to hydroxyurea in every respect. The evidence does not support its role as first-line therapy. Can be considered for *use as a third-line agent in patients who have failed or are intolerant to hydroxyurea or interferon-α therapy*
  Hydroxyurea + Aspirin vs. Anagrelide + Aspirin (MRC PT-I trial)
  Superiority of hydroxyurea over anagrelide as first therapy for high-risk ET patients
  - N = >800 patients
  - High-risk ET patients (age >60 years, prior thrombosis or platelets >1,000,000/mm^3)
  - Randomized to hydroxyurea + aspirin or anagrelide + aspirin
  - Anagrelide plus aspirin
    - Decreased rate of venous thrombosis
    - Increased rate of arterial thrombosis,
    - Increased rate of major hemorrhage
    - Increased rate of transformation to MF
    - Increased rate of withdrawal from treatment

4. *Cytoreductive therapy—interferon alfa (IFN-α)*
- Single-agent activity
- Sometimes associated with modest reductions in *JAK2*V617F allele burden

5. *Cytoreductive therapy—pipobroman*
- Several single-arm studies have confirmed the efficacy of pipobroman in ET

6. *Cytoreductive therapy—busulfan*
- Several single-arm studies have confirmed the efficacy of busulfan in ET

Cortelazzo S et al. N Engl J Med 1995;332:1132–1136
Harrison CN et al. N Engl J Med 2005;353:33–45
Kiladjian J-J et al. Blood 2006;108:2037–2040

Treatment of Polycythemia Vera (PV)
Treatment options:
1. Phlebotomy
2. Antiplatelet therapy (eg, low-dose aspirin)
3. Cytoreductive therapy—hydroxyurea
4. Cytoreductive therapy—interferon alfa (interferon-α, IFN-α)
5. Cytoreductive therapy—pipobroman
6. Cytoreductive therapy—busulfan

Note: There is no hard evidence to implicate any one of these agents, including hydroxyurea, as being leukemogenic in the treatment of PV

(continued)

Treatment Options (*continued*)

Treatment recommendations:

1. Phlebotomy for all patients
2. Low-dose aspirin for all patients
3. Add hydroxyurea in high-risk patients

Barbui T et al. N Engl J Med 2005;353:85–86

1. *Phlebotomy*
   - Generally recommended to keep hematocrit levels at <45% in men and <42% in women
   - There is compelling evidence to support the use of phlebotomy in all patients
2. *Antiplatelet therapy (eg, low-dose aspirin)*
   - Has not been shown to influence survival or lower risk of disease transformation
   - Used to either alleviate microvascular symptoms or to prevent thrombohemorrhagic complications
3. *Cytoreductive therapy—hydroxyurea*
   - Treatment of choice in high-risk PV patients because of superior efficacy and less toxicity (see Table 66–1)
   - Has not been shown to influence survival or lower risk of disease transformation
   - Used to either alleviate microvascular symptoms or to prevent thrombohemorrhagic complications
   - *Studies have evaluated hydroxyurea efficacy*
     Hydroxyurea vs. pipobroman
     - Similar survival
     - Similar thrombosis risk
     - Similar leukemic transformation rate
     - Pipobroman associated with a lesser incidence of transformation into post-PV MF
     - Pipobroman is leukemogenic and is unsuitable for first-line therapy
4. *Interferon alfa (IFN-α)*
   - Single-agent activity
   - Sometimes associated with modest reductions in *JAK*2V617F allele burden
5. *Pipobroman*
   - Several studies have confirmed the efficacy of pipobroman in PV
   - Pipobroman is leukemogenic and is unsuitable for first-line therapy
6. *Busulfan*
   - Several single-arm studies have confirmed the efficacy of busulfan in PV

Finazzi G et al. Blood 2007;109:5104–5111
Kiladjian J-J et al. Blood 2006;108:2037–2040
Najean Y et al. Blood 1997;90:3370–3377

PHLEBOTOMY

POLYCYTHEMIA VERA (PV)

Marchioli R et al. N Engl J Med 2013;368:22–33
Streiff MB et al. Blood 2002;99:1144–1149

Indications:	• Prevent thrombosis by reducing the RBC mass. Indicated for all patients to normalize hematocrit • Treatment of choice for patients ages <50 years and all women during childbearing years
Goal:	• Achieve and maintain a hematocrit of 40–45% (Hct <45% in men and <42% in women)
Initial therapy:	• *Most patients:* 250–500 mL every other day to achieve a hematocrit of 40–45% • *Elderly and those with hemodynamic compromise:* 250–300 mL twice/per week
Maintenance therapy:	• CBC every 4–8 weeks • Phlebotomy if hematocrit >45% in men; >42% in women
Limitations:	• Phlebotomy unable to control leukocytosis, hyperuricemia, hypermetabolism, pruritus, and complications of splenomegaly seen in PV patients • Patients treated with phlebotomy alone have a higher incidence of serious thrombotic complications during the first 3 years of therapy when compared to patients treated with myelosuppression. True especially in those >60 years old • Elderly should be treated with cytoreduction in addition to phlebotomy

ANTIPLATELET (ANTITHROMBOTIC) THERAPY REGIMEN

ASPIRIN

Polycythemia Vera (PV)
Essential Thrombocythemia (ET)

Landolfi R et al. N Engl J Med 2004;350:114–124

Aspirin 50–100 mg/day; administer orally, continually
Notes:
- Dose used in clinical trial was 100 mg per day
- Although clinical trial enrolled patients with PV, the data is thought to support its use in ET as well

Patient Population Studied

Conducted by a network of 94 hematologic centers in 12 countries. Of the 1638 patients included in the ECLAP project, 1120 were entered into a prospective, observational cohort study, and the other 518 (32%) were enrolled in a double-blind, placebo-controlled, randomized trial to assess the efficacy and safety of low-dose aspirin (100 mg daily in an enteric-coated formulation [Bayer]). The main reasons for excluding patients in the ECLAP project from this aspirin trial were an indication for antithrombotic therapy (742 patients [66%]), a contraindication to aspirin therapy (271 patients [24%]), and a patient's unwillingness to participate (197 patients [18%]). Polycythemia vera was diagnosed on the basis of standard clinical and laboratory findings and criteria. Patients were eligible if they had no clear indication for aspirin treatment and no clear contraindication to it. There were no age limits. A total of 253 patients were randomly assigned to receive aspirin (100 mg daily), and 265 were randomly assigned to receive placebo. All patients received other recommended treatments: phlebotomy, cytoreductive drugs, and standard cardiovascular drugs as required. Data collection was recorded at follow-up visits at 12, 24, 36, 48, and 60 months. Compliance was monitored with the use of counts of aspirin or placebo pills and through attendance at follow-up visits

Efficacy

Rates and Relative Risks of Major Study End Points in the Two Groups*

	Aspirin (N = 253)	Placebo (N = 265)	Relative Risk (95% CI)	P Value
	Number (%)			
End Point				
Primary End Points				
Nonfatal myocardial infarction, nonfatal stroke, or death from cardiovascular causes	5 (2.0)	13 (4.9)	0.41 (0.15–1.15)	0.09
Nonfatal myocardial infarction, nonfatal stroke, pulmonary embolism, major venous thrombosis, or death from cardiovascular causes	8 (3.2)	21 (7.9)	0.40 (0.18–0.91)	0.03
Secondary End Points				
Nonfatal myocardial infarction, nonfatal stroke, or death from any cause	11 (4.3)	22 (8.3)	0.54 (0.26–1.11)	0.09
Nonfatal myocardial infarction, nonfatal stroke, pulmonary embolism, deep venous thrombosis, or death from any cause	13 (5.1)	29 (10.9)	0.47 (0.25–0.91)	0.02
Death from any cause	9 (3.6)	18 (6.8)	0.54 (0.24–1.20)	0.13
Death from cardiovascular causes	3 (1.2)	8 (3.0)	0.41 (0.11–1.53)	0.18
Cardiac	2 (0.8)	2 (0.8)	1.07 (0.15–7.58)	0.95
Acute myocardial infarction	1 (0.4)	1 (0.4)		
Other cardiac causes	1 (0.4)	1 (0.4)		
Vascular	1 (0.4)	6 (2.3)	0.18 (0.02–1.50)	0.11
Nonhemorrhagic stroke	0	4 (1.5)		
Intracranial hemorrhage	0	1 (0.4)		
Pulmonary embolism	0	1 (0.4)		
Other vascular causes	1 (0.4)	0		
Death from noncardiovascular causes	6 (2.4)	10 (3.8)	0.65 (0.24–1.79)	0.40
Major cerebrovascular events	3 (1.2)	10 (3.8)	0.32 (0.09–1.16)	0.08
Myocardial infarction	1 (0.4)	2 (0.8)	0.54 (0.09–23.57)	0.81
Major venous thrombosis	4 (1.6)	10 (3.8)	0.49 (0.13–1.78)	0.28
Deep venous thrombosis	2 (0.8)	6 (2.3)		
Pulmonary embolism	2 (0.8)	5 (1.9)		
Major or minor thrombosis	17 (6.7)	41 (15.5)	0.42 (0.24–0.74)	0.003
Minor thrombotic complications	10 (4.0)	22 (8.3)	0.47 (0.22–0.99)	0.049
Transient ischemic attack	4 (1.6)	9 (3.4)		
Peripheral arterial thrombosis	0	3 (1.1)		
Superficial venous thrombosis	2 (0.8)	6 (2.3)		
Erythromelalgia	4 (1.6)	5 (1.9)		

CI, Confidence interval
*Major cerebrovascular events include fatal and nonfatal stroke plus episodes of intracranial bleeding; minor thrombotic complications include transient ischemic attacks, superficial thrombophlebitis, peripheral arterial thrombosis, and erythromelalgia. Totals for categories may not equal the sum of the values for subcategories because some patients had more than 1 type of event

CYTOREDUCTIVE THERAPY REGIMEN

HYDROXYUREA

Polycythemia Vera (PV) and Essential Thrombocythemia (ET)

Cortelazzo S et al. N Engl J Med 1995;332:1132–1136 (ET)
[Editorial] Haematologica 1999;84:673–674 (PV)
Fruchtman SM et al. Semin Hematol 1997;34:17–23 (PV)

Note: Mechanism of action is believed to be inhibition of ribonucleotide reductase that is required for DNA repair by scavenging tyrosyl free radicals as they are involved in the reduction of nucleotide diphosphates

Initial dose:
Hydroxyurea 15–20 mg/kg; administer orally, every day after meals, as a single dose or divided into 2 doses (total dosage per week = 105–140 mg/kg)

Chronic therapy—optimal dose:
• Determined **empirically.** Adjust without causing leukopenia

• *Frequent monitoring of CBC:* Every 1–2 weeks for the first 2 months, every month thereafter, and after reaching a steady state, every 3 months

• Increase total daily dose by 25% to 50%, and assess effect after 7 days before further escalation. A dose of hydroxyurea 500–1000 mg/day is sufficient for the majority of patients; however, the total daily dose is extremely variable

Therapeutic goals:
PV
1. Control the hematocrit without causing leukopenia ($<3500/mm^3$) or thrombocytopenia ($<100,000/mm^3$). This may require significantly higher or lower doses than the initial dose
2. Patients requiring frequent phlebotomies or those with platelet counts $>600,000/mm^3$, increase the hydroxyurea dosage by 5 mg/kg per day at monthly intervals, with frequent monitoring until control is achieved
3. Supplemental phlebotomy is preferable to increased myelosuppression in controlling the hematocrit

ET
1. Achieve a target platelet count $<600,000/mm^3$ (greater protection from thrombosis if platelet count $<450,000/mm^3$) with care to avoid the development of significant leukopenia

Note: Very high doses carry a risk of prolonged aplasia

Emergency situations in polycythemia vera patients: **Decreased cerebral perfusion in setting of an elevated hematocrit or marked thrombocytosis:**
Phlebotomy: Daily to a hematocrit of 45% in men and 42% in women
Initial (loading) dose: **Hydroxyurea** 30 mg/kg per day; administer orally every day, after meals, as single dose or divided into 2 doses for 7 days (total dosage/week = 210 mg/kg), *followed by:*
Maintenance dose: **Hydroxyurea** 15 mg/kg per day; administer orally every day, after meals, as single dose or divided into 2 doses with close monitoring of CBC (total dosage/week = 105 mg/kg)
Note: Treatment of choice in high-risk PV and ET patients because of its superior efficacy and decreased toxicity

Supportive Care
Antiemetic prophylaxis
Emetogenic potential is **MINIMAL–LOW**
See Chapter 39 for antiemetic recommendations

Hematopoietic growth factor (CSF) prophylaxis
Primary prophylaxis is NOT indicated
See Chapter 43 for more information

Antimicrobial prophylaxis
Risk of fever and neutropenia is LOW
   Antimicrobial primary prophylaxis to be considered:
   • Antibacterial—*P. jirovecii* prophylaxis is recommended (eg, cotrimoxazole)
   • Antifungal—not indicated
   • Antiviral—not indicated unless patient previously had an episode of HSV
See Chapter 47 for more information

Treatment Modifications

Adverse Event	Treatment Modification
Hematologic Toxicity	
WBC $<3500/mm^3$ or platelet $<100,000/mm^3$	Hold hydroxyurea until WBC $>3500/mm^3$ and platelet $>100,000/mm^3$, then restart hydroxyurea at 50% of prior dose
Nonhematologic Toxicity	
G1	No dose modifications
G2/3	Hold hydroxyurea until toxicity G ≤1; restart at prior dose
Recurrent G2/3	Hold hydroxyurea until toxicity G ≤1; restart at 75% of prior dose
G4	Hold hydroxyurea until toxicity G ≤1; restart at 50% of prior dose
Recurrent G4	Discontinue hydroxyurea

Patient Population Studied

PV (Fruchtman SM et al. Semin Hematol 1997;34:17–23)
Patients with Philadelphia chromosome (Ph)-positive and Ph-negative myeloproliferative disorders

ET (Cortelazzo S et al. N Engl J Med 1995;332:1132–1136)
Fifty-six patients with essential thrombocythemia with median platelet count of 788,000/mm³

Toxicity

Hematologic side effects
1. Neutropenia is common
2. Thrombocytopenia is rare
3. Cytopenias often are rapidly reversible within 3–4 days but may take 7–21 days to recover after hydroxyurea is discontinued
4. High doses and/or failure to interrupt treatment despite cytopenia may result in prolonged aplasia

Nonhematologic Side Effects

Relatively Common	Rare
1. Gastrointestinal symptoms: • Stomatitis/mucositis • Anorexia • Mild nausea/vomiting • Diarrhea • Constipation 2. Acute skin reactions • Rash • Painful lower extremity ulcerations • Dermatomyositis-like changes • Erythema • Nail ridging or discoloration	1. Chronic skin reactions • Hyperpigmentation • Atrophy of skin and nails 2. Skin cancer 3. Alopecia 4. Headache 5. Drowsiness 6. Convulsions 7. Constitutional symptoms: • Fever • Chills • Asthenia 8. Renal impairment 9. Hepatic impairment

Boxed Warning (FDA approved product label):
Hydroxyurea is mutagenic and clastogenic, and causes cellular transformation to a tumorigenic phenotype. Hydroxyurea is thus unequivocally genotoxic and a presumed trans-species carcinogen that implies a carcinogenic risk to humans. Secondary leukemias have been reported in patients who received long-term hydroxyurea for myeloproliferative disorders, such as polycythemia vera and thrombocythemia. It is unknown whether this leukemogenic effect is secondary to hydroxyurea or is associated with a patients' underlying disease. Physicians and their patients must very carefully consider the potential benefits of hydroxyurea relative to the undefined risk of developing secondary malignancies

Efficacy

PV (Fruchtman SM et al. Semin Hematol 1997;34:17–23)
- Eighty percent of patients achieved control of blood counts with hydroxyurea and phlebotomy
- The other 20% of patients had refractory disease, could not tolerate therapy, or may develop leukopenia preventing further dose escalation

ET (Cortelazzo S et al. N Engl J Med 1995;332: 1132–1136)
- Patients treated with hydroxyurea had a lower incidence of thrombotic events compared to patients who received placebo
- Hydroxyurea is not universally successful in controlling thrombocytosis
- Resistance to hydroxyurea has been reported in 11–17% of cases

Therapy Monitoring

Frequent monitoring of CBC is necessary to prevent excessive marrow suppression. Obtain a CBC every 1–2 weeks for the first 2 months, every month thereafter, and, after reaching a steady state, every 3 months

CYTOREDUCTIVE THERAPY REGIMEN

ANAGRELIDE HCl

Polycythemia Vera (PV) and Essential Thrombocythemia (ET)

Anagrelide Study Group. Am J Med 1992;92:69–76 (ET)
Fruchtman SM et al. Annual Meeting of the American
Society of Hematology, Philadelphia, PA, 2002;
Abstract #256 (PV)
Storen EC, Tefferi A. Blood 2001;97:863–866 (PV, ET)
Tomer A. Blood 2002;99:1602–1609 (ET)

Note:
- Oral imidazoquinazoline compound for treatment of thrombocytosis associated with MPN

Initial dose:
Anagrelide HCl 0.5 mg/dose; administer orally every 12 hours for 7 consecutive days
Usual maintenance dose:
After 1 week at a dose of 0.5 mg orally every 12 hours, the dose should be increased by 0.5 mg/day at weekly intervals until response is achieved. The optimal dose is determined **empirically**, with frequent monitoring of platelet counts

Anagrelide HCl 0.5–1 mg/dose; administer orally, 2–4 doses/day to provide a total daily dose = 2–2.5 mg/day (doses need not be equal)

Note: Individual anagrelide doses should not exceed 2.5 mg; daily doses should not exceed 10 mg

Patient Population Studied

PV (Storen EC, Tefferi A. Blood 2001;97:863–866)
More than 2000 patients with both Philadelphia chromosome-positive and -negative MPDs have been studied

ET (Anagrelide Study Group. Am J Med 1992;92:69–76)
The Anagrelide Study Group included 335 patients with essential thrombocythemia

Treatment Modifications

Adverse Event	Treatment Modification
Hematologic Toxicity	
Platelet count <100,000/mm^3	Hold anagrelide until platelet count >100,000/mm^3; then restart at 50% of prior dose
Nonhematologic Toxicity > Initial 2 Weeks	
G1	No dose modifications
G2/3	Hold anagrelide until toxicity G ≤1; then restart at prior dose
Recurrent G2/3	Hold anagrelide until toxicity G ≤1; then restart at 75% of prior dose
G4	Hold anagrelide until toxicity G ≤1; then restart at 50% of prior dose
Recurrent G4	Discontinue anagrelide

Efficacy

PV
More than 75% of patients will achieve good platelet control. The remaining 25% will be either intolerant or have disease that is refractory to anagrelide

ET
- Anagrelide Study Group
- Purpose:
  - Evaluate the safety and efficacy of anagrelide when used to reduce platelet counts in patients with thrombocytosis and a diagnosis of a chronic myeloproliferative disease
  - **Anagrelide** 0.5–1 mg given orally 4 times per day

Patients and methods:
- 577 patients (504/577 previously but unsuccessfully treated with other modalities)
  - Essential thrombocythemia = 355
  - Chronic granulocytic leukemia = 114
  - Polycythemia vera = 68
  - Undifferentiated myeloproliferative diseases = 60

Results:
- 424/577 evaluable for response
- 396/424 (93%): Platelet count reduced by 50%, or to <600,000/mm^3, for ≥28 days
- Acquired resistance was not observed
- Major side effects: neurologic, gastrointestinal, and cardiac
- In >5 years, 16% of patients discontinued treatment because of side effects
- The MRC PT-1 trial (Medical Research Council clinical trial in patients with Primary Thrombocythemia) showed anagrelide is inferior to hydroxyurea in every respect, and does not support its role as first-line therapy; instead, *use as a third-line agent in patients who have failed or are intolerant to hydroxyurea or interferon-α therapy*

Notes:
- Initial studies suggested a specific effect on megakaryopoiesis and thrombocytosis. Anagrelide works by inhibiting the maturation of platelets from megakaryocytes. The exact mechanism of action is unclear, although it is known to be a potent inhibitor of phosphodiesterase-III (IC$_{50}$ = 36 nmol/L)

Toxicity*

Toxicity	Percent	Notes
Hematologic Toxicities		
↓ Hemoglobin[†]	36	
↓ WBC	—	
Leukemogenic	(2.6)[‡]	
Nonhematologic Toxicities		
Palpitations[§]	26	Administer carefully to elderly; avoid in patients with cardiac disease
Fluid retention[§]	20	
Headaches	43	Usually within 2 weeks after starting therapy; often diminishes in severity or resolves in 2 weeks with continued therapy
Diarrhea[ϲ]	25	
Nausea	17	
Abdominal pain	16	
Dizziness	15	

Less Common Nonhematologic Toxicities

Atrial fibrillation	Gastric/duodenal ulceration	Pulmonary hypertension
Cardiomegaly	Hair loss	Pulmonary infiltrates
Cardiomyopathy	Myocardial infarction	Renal impairment/failure
Cerebrovascular accident	Pancreatitis	Seizure
Complete heart block	Pericarditis	Weakness/fatigue
Congestive heart failure	Pulmonary fibrosis	

*Not to be used during pregnancy
[†]With long-term therapy, ↓ hemoglobin level up to 3 g/dL in 24% of patients
[‡]All patients who developed acute leukemia were previously exposed to other cytoreductive agents. There were no patients who transformed who were exposed only to anagrelide
[§]Related to drug's vasodilatory and inotropic properties. Minimize by starting with a low dose (0.5 mg twice daily), and gradually increase the dose until control of the platelet count is achieved
[ϲ]Occurs in patients with lactose intolerance because of the presence of lactose in commercially available products

Therapy Monitoring

Frequent platelet count monitoring is necessary to prevent excessive marrow suppression

1. *During period of initial dose adjustment:* Platelet count every 5–7 days
2. *When the peripheral blood count is maintained within acceptable range on a stable dose of anagrelide:* Lengthen interval to 2 weeks and then to 4 weeks

CYTOREDUCTIVE THERAPY REGIMEN

INTERFERON ALFA-2B

Polycythemia Vera (PV) and Essential Thrombocythemia (ET)

Elliott MA, Tefferi A. Semin Thromb Hemost 1997;23:463–472
Sacchi S et al. Ann Hematol 1991;63:206–209
Sacchi S. Leuk Lymphoma 1995;19:13–20
Silver RT. Cancer 2006;107:451–458
Silver RT. Semin Hematol 1997;34:40–50

Antipyretic primary prophylaxis:
Acetaminophen 650–1000 mg; administer orally, 1 hour before interferon administration, and then every 4 hours for a total of 3 doses, *or*
Ibuprofen 400–600 mg; administer orally, 1 hour before interferon administration, and then every 4 hours for a total of 3 doses

Secondary antiemetic prophylaxis:
If needed, use as primary prophylaxis with subsequent doses
Note: Have patients take interferon at bedtime, so they sleep through the period when symptoms are likely to be most severe

Initial dose:
Interferon alfa-(2a *or* 2b) 3 million IU per dose; administer subcutaneously on 3 nonconsecutive days per week; for example, Monday, Wednesday, and Friday (total dose/week = 9 million IU)

Maintenance doses:
• Increase interferon dose in increments of 1 million IU per dose to a dose of 5 million IU per dose; administer subcutaneously on 3 nonconsecutive days per. Dose adjustments should be performed no more frequently than once every 8 weeks, *thus:*
Interferon alfa-(2a *or* 2b) 5 million IU per dose; administer subcutaneously on 3 nonconsecutive days per (total dose/week = 15 million IU), *or*
Interferon alfa-(2a *or* 2b) 3 million IU per dose; administer subcutaneously on 5 days per week (total dose/week = 15 million IU)

Note: Interferon alfa is the agent of choice for PV and ET in high-risk women of childbearing age. It been safely used in pregnant women because it does not cross the placenta

Supportive Care
Antiemetic prophylaxis
Emetogenic potential is **MINIMAL**
See Chapter 39 for antiemetic recommendations

Hematopoietic growth factor (CSF) prophylaxis
Primary prophylaxis is NOT indicated
See Chapter 43 for more information

Antimicrobial prophylaxis
Risk of fever and neutropenia is LOW
  Antimicrobial primary prophylaxis to be considered:
  • Antibacterial—not indicated
  • Antifungal—not indicated
  • Antiviral—not indicated unless patient previously had an episode of HSV
See Chapter 47 for more information

Treatment Modifications

Adverse Event	Treatment Modification
Hematologic Toxicity	
ANC 1000–1500/mm^3	Reduce interferon dose by 50%; consider dose reescalation if ANC then increases to >1500/mm^3
ANC <500/mm^3 or platelet counts <25000/mm^3	Discontinue interferon therapy
Nonhematologic Toxicity > Initial 2 Weeks	
ALT/AST >5–10× upper limit of normal	Withhold therapy until ALT and AST return to pretreatment values, then resume interferon at 50% of the dose previously administered
G1	No dose modifications
G2/3	Withhold therapy until toxicity G ≤1, then resume interferon at 50% of the dose previously administered
Recurrent G2/3 at reduced interferon dosage	Discontinue therapy
G4	Withhold therapy until toxicity G ≤1, then resume interferon at 50% of the dose previously administered
Recurrent G4 at reduced interferon dosage	Discontinue therapy

Efficacy

Studied extensively in PV and ET with satisfactory responses in >80% of patients

PV

- Interferon alfa (IFN-α) has myelosuppressive activity and antagonizes the action of platelet-derived growth factor (PDGF), a product of megakaryopoiesis that initiates fibroblast proliferation

- In general, control of erythrocytosis occurs in approximately 76% of patients receiving subcutaneous IFN-α in doses ranging from 4.5–27 million units per week (usual dose: 3 million units subcutaneously 3 times per week)

- A similar degree of benefit was achieved in terms of reduction in spleen size and relief from intractable pruritus in other series

(Silver RT. Cancer 2006;107:451–458)

- Report of long-term use (median: 13 years) of IFN-α in 55 patients previously treated with phlebotomy alone or with phlebotomy + hydroxyurea

- Patients achieved partial response of their disease by 6 months, and complete response by 1–2 years (phlebotomy-free, Hct ≤45%, platelets ≤600,000/mm³); spleen size was reduced in 27 of 30 patients with prior splenomegaly

- *Initial dose:* 1 million IU 3 times/week for the majority of patients, with periodic dose increases as required and as tolerated

- *Maintenance dose:* Usually 3 million IU 3 times/week; decreased after the second year of treatment in half the patients. Toxicity was acceptable. Disease-free survival was marked by no thrombohemorrhagic complications reflecting both the effect of IFN-α and total patient care, effectively reduced phlebotomy requirements, thrombocythemia, splenomegaly, and thrombohemorrhagic events

ET

- Single-agent activity associated with modest reductions in JAK2V617F allele burden has been demonstrated in ET

- Results of several series indicate platelet counts can be reduced to <600,000/mm³ after approximately 3 months of therapy

(Sacchi S et al. Leuk Lymphoma 1995;19:13–20)

- In a total of 212 patients treated in 11 different clinical trials, a response rate of approximately 90% has been reported. At a dose of 3 million IU per dose, administered subcutaneously, 5 days/week, the median time to complete response with this dose is 3 months

Toxicity

General Comments

Drawback: IFN-α use is associated with many side effects and is not tolerated by a significant proportion of patients

Most frequent adverse effects are flu-like symptoms: increased body temperature, feeling ill, fatigue, headache, muscle pain, convulsion, dizziness, hair thinning, and depression. Erythema, pain and injection site induration are also frequently observed. Interferon therapy also causes immunosuppression and can result in infections manifesting in unusual ways. All known adverse effects are usually reversible and disappear a few days after the therapy has been discontinued

General Recommendations
Causes and Management of Acute Symptoms During Induction Therapy

Fever	
Bone and muscle pain	
Fatigue	Frequently controlled with acetaminophen
Lethargy	
Depression	

Symptoms Following Long-Term Administration

Mild weight loss	
Alopecia	
Thyroiditis and hypothyroidism	Autoimmune disorders
Hemolytic anemia	

Summary of Toxicities*

Application Site Disorders

Injection site inflammation	3% (1–5%)
All others	<5%

Blood Disorders

Anemia, leukopenia, neutropenia, thrombocytopenia	All ≤5%

Body as a Whole

Facial edema	<1% (<1–10%)
Weight decrease	3% (<1–13%)
All others	≤5%

Cardiovascular System Disorders

Angina, arrhythmia, cardiac failure, hypertension, hypotension	All <5%

Endocrine System Disorders

All toxicities	<5%

Flu-like Symptoms

Arthralgia	8% (3–19%)	Asthenia	11% (5–63%)	Back pain	6% (1–19%)
Chest pain	3% (1–28%)	Chills	46% (45–54%)	Dizziness	10% (7–24%)
Dry mouth	6% (1–28%)	Fatigue	65% (8–96%)	Fever	60% (34–94%)

(continued)

Therapy Monitoring

1. *Prior to initiation of therapy:* CBC and platelet counts, thyroid function tests including TSH
2. *Weeks 1 and 2 following initiation of therapy, and monthly thereafter:* CBC and platelet counts
3. LFTs at approximately 3-month intervals
4. Thyroid function tests at 3 and 6 months

Toxicity (continued)

Headache	52% (21–62%)	Influenza-like symptoms		65 (3–18%)	
Malaise	6% (3–14%)	Myalgia	40% (16–75%)	Rigors	23% (2–42%)
↑ Sweating	4% (1–21%)	Pain, unspecified	22% (<1–79%)	All others	<5%

Gastrointestinal System Disorders

Abdominal Pain	5% (1–21%)	Anorexia	40% (1–69%)	Constipation	3% (<1–14%)
Diarrhea	19% (2–45%)	Dyspepsia	4% (2–8%)	Gingivitis	5% (1–14%)
Loose stools	2% (<1–10%)	Nausea	23% (17–66%)	Taste altered	6% (<1–24%)
Vomiting	10% (2–32%)	All others	<5%		

Liver and Biliary Systems Disorders

Abnormal liver function tests		All <5%

Musculoskeletal Systems Disorders

Musculoskeletal pain	9% (1–21%)	All others	<5%

Nervous System and Psychiatric Disorders

Amnesia	<5% (1–14%)	Anxiety	3% (<1–9%)	Confusion	<5% (2–10%)
Decreased libido		1% (1–5%)		Depression	9% (3–40%)
Hypoesthesia	<5% (1–10%)	Impaired concentration		3% (<1–14%)	
Insomnia	5% (<1–12%)	Irritability	12% (1–13%)	Nervousness	2% (1–3%)
Paresthesia	6% (1–21%)	Somnolence	<5% (1–33%)	All others	<5%

Reproduction System

All toxicities		<5%

Resistance Mechanisms Disorders

Moniliasis	1% (<1–17%)	Herpes simplex	1% (1–5%)	

Respiratory System Disorders

Coughing	5% (<1–31%)	Dyspnea	5% (<1–34%)	Nasal congestion	3% (1–10%)
Nonproductive cough		2% (0–14%)		Pharyngitis	<5% (1–31%)
Sinusitis	3% (1–21%)	All other		<5%	

Skin and Appendages Disorders

Alopecia	26% (8–31%)	Dermatitis	2% (1–8%)	Dry skin	4% (<1–10%)
Pruritus	7% (1–11%)	Rash	9% (1–25%)	All others	<5%

Urinary Systems Disorders

↑ BUN	<5%	All other		<5%

Vision Disorders

All toxicities		<5%

*Excerpts from INTRON A, interferon alfa-2b, recombinant for injection; Aug. 2012 product labeling. Schering Corporation, a subsidiary of Merck & Co., Inc., Whitehouse Station, NJ. Percent toxicities are presented as median percent (range) reported for 3 to as many as 10 evaluations in a diverse group of disease states including malignant melanoma, follicular lymphoma, hairy cell leukemia, condylomata acuminata, AIDS-related Kaposi sarcoma, chronic hepatitis C, and chronic hepatitis B. The doses of interferon alfa-2b used ranged from 1 million IU/lesion to 30 million IU/m²

REGIMEN CYTOREDUCTIVE THERAPY

PIPOBROMAN

Polycythemia Vera (PV) and Essential Thrombocythemia (ET)

Kiladjian J-J et al. J Clin Oncol 2011;29:3907–3913
Passamonti F et al. Haematologica 2000;85:1011–1018

Pipobroman (NSC 25154) is a bromide derivative of piperazine and has structural resemblance to alkylating agents. It acts as a competitive inhibitor of pyrimidines

Kiladjian JJ et al.:
Initial regimen:
    Pipobroman 1.25 mg/kg per day; administer orally, daily, continually
Maintenance regimen:
    Pipobroman 0.4–0.7 mg/kg per day; administer orally, daily, continually

Passamonti et al.:
Initial regimen:
    Pipobroman 1 mg/kg per day; administer orally, daily, continually
Maintenance regimen:
    Pipobroman 0.3–0.6 mg/kg per day; administer orally, daily, continually

Notes:
- Give pipobroman at the starting dose until hematologic response (hematocrit <45% and platelets <400,000/mm³) then continue as maintenance therapy to keep the hematocrit/hemoglobin within normal ranges
- Pipobroman dosages up to 1.5–3 mg/kg per day may be required in patients refractory to other treatments, but *do not use* such doses until a dosage of 1–1.25 mg/kg per day has been given for at least 30 days with no improvement
- Pipobroman is no longer commercially available in the United States

Supportive Care
Antiemetic prophylaxis
Emetogenic potential is **LOW–MODERATE**
See Chapter 39 for antiemetic recommendations

Hematopoietic growth factor (CSF) prophylaxis
Primary prophylaxis is NOT indicated
See Chapter 43 for more information

Antimicrobial prophylaxis
Risk of fever and neutropenia is LOW
    Antimicrobial primary prophylaxis to be considered:
- Antibacterial—*P. jirovecii* prophylaxis is recommended (eg, cotrimoxazole)
- Antifungal—not indicated
- Antiviral—not indicated unless patient previously had an episode of HSV

See Chapter 47 for more information

Dose Adjustments

Adverse Event	Treatment Modification
Maintenance dose	Adjusted according to response to administer the lowest dose possible
WBC <3000/mm³ or platelet count <150,000/mm³	Temporarily discontinue pipobroman; resume cautiously and with monitoring of blood counts
G ≥2 anemia, leukopenia, thrombocytopenia	Permanently discontinue pipobroman
Rapid drop in hemoglobin, increased bilirubin levels, and reticulocytosis suggesting a hemolytic process	Permanently discontinue pipobroman

Patient Population Studied

Kiladjian J-J et al. J Clin Oncol 2011;29:3907–3913
French Polycythemia Study Group (FPSG) study that randomly assigned 285 patients younger than age 65 years with a diagnosis of polycythemia vera to hydroxyurea versus pipobroman as first-line therapy. Patients received either hydroxyurea 25 mg/kg per day followed by low-dose maintenance with hydroxyurea 10–15 mg/kg per day or pipobroman 1.25 mg/kg per day followed by low-dose maintenance with pipobroman 0.4–0.7 mg/kg per day. FPSG results were updated with a median follow-up of 16.3 years

Passamonti F et al. Haematologica 2000;85:1011–1018
A study of 163 untreated patients with polycythemia vera (median age: 57 years; range: 30–82 years) treated with pipobroman in a single institution for a median follow-up of 120 months. Diagnosis was made according to the Polycythemia Vera Study Group criteria. The study, conducted between June 1975 and December 1997, included patients with PV treated with pipobroman for more than 6 months. Patients lost to follow-up (4%) were censored at the date of their last visit

Efficacy

Kiladjian J-J et al. J Clin Oncol 2011;29:3907–3913

Median Survival in Intention-to-Treat Population (16.3 Years Follow-up)

Hydroxyurea	Pipobroman	P Value	Total Cohort
20.3 years 95% CI, 16.4–25.0	15.4 years 95% CI, 13.4–17.0	0.008	17 years 95% CI, 15.4–19.4

Passamonti F et al. Haematologica 2000;85:1011–1018

Efficacy (N = 163)

Complete response[*][†]	153/163 (94%)
Median time from the start of therapy to response	13 weeks (range: 6–48 months)
Resistance to pipobroman in responders	6/153 (4%)
Median time to resistance	80 months (range: 36–165 months)
Thrombocytosis (N = 53), complete response	100%
Time from the start of therapy to thrombocytosis response	2–4 months[†]

Median overall survival	215 months
Standardized mortality ratio	1.7
Cumulative risk of death at 7 years	11%
Cumulative risk of death at 10 years	22%
Cumulative risk of death at 12 years	26%
Cumulative risk of thrombotic events at 3 years	6%
Cumulative risk of thrombotic events at 7 years	11%
Cumulative risk of thrombotic events at 10 years	16%
Cumulative risk of thrombotic events at 12 years	20%
10-year cumulative risk of leukemia	5%
10-year cumulative risk of myelofibrosis	4%
10-year cumulative risk of solid tumors	8%

Logistic Regression Analyses

Correlations	P Values and Hazard Ratios
Age older than 65 years and higher risk of death	0.0001 (HR = 1.06; 95% CI, 1.03–1.09)
Thrombotic events at diagnosis and higher risk of death	0.001 (HR = 2.9; 95% CI, 1.6–5.2)
Female sex and thrombotic complications	0.02 (HR = 2.3; 95% CI, 1.08–7.91)
Age older than 65 years and thrombotic complications	0.01 (HR = 2.89; 95% CI, 1.30–6.42)
Age and leukemia[‡]	0.04 (HR = 1.09; 95% CI, 1.02–1.16)
Age and solid tumors[‡]	0.03 (HR = 1.06; 95% CI, 1.01–1.12)
Myelofibrosis	No significant risk factor

[*]Complete response defined as disappearance of all clinical sings and return to normal blood counts. After complete response, 142 patients (93%) received continuous maintenance therapy
[†]Maintained subsequently in the normal range by pipobroman therapy
[‡]Age was the only significant factor while the duration of pipobroman treatment did not influence these risks

Toxicity

Passamonti F et al. Haematologica 2000;85:1011–1018

G2 (WHO) leukopenia	2/163*
G4 thrombocytopenia	1/63*
Mild gastric pain or diarrhea	12/163 (7%)
Dry skin and acne	2/163

*Full hematologic recovery after pipobroman discontinued

Kiladjian J-J et al. J Clin Oncol 2011;29:3907–3913
Note: To account for treatment crossovers, statistical analyses were performed both for the intention-to-treat (ITT) population and according to the primary treatment (first treatment) received
Summary:
• Evolution to AML/MDS is the first cause of death
• Pipobroman is leukemogenic and is unsuitable for first-line therapy
• Incidence of evolution to AML/MDS with hydroxyurea was higher than previously reported

Outcome Hematologic Events in ITT and Main Treatment Received Analyses

Analysis	Follow-up (Years)	Hydroxyurea	Pipobroman	P Value	Total Cohort
Cumulative Incidence of AML/MDS					
ITT	10	6.6	13.1	0.004	9.8
	15	16.5	34.1		23.6
	20	24.2	52.1		33.9
Main Treatment	10	7.5	12.2	0.008	—
	15	14.3	37.5		
	20	21.9	55.9		
Cumulative Incidence of MF					
ITT	10	12.6	7.8	0.07	10.2
	15	19.4	15.7		17.7
	20	26.9	26.9		26.1
Main Treatment	10	15.4	5.1	0.02	—
	15	24.3	9.8		
	20	31.6	21.3		
Vascular Events (Thrombosis = 80; Hemorrhage = 5; Both = 5)					
ITT	10, 15, 20	Similar		0.61	
Main Treatment	10, 15, 20	Similar		0.32	

Note: Because 21% of patients received both drugs during follow-up, the data also was analyzed to assess the influence of switching with a time-dependent covariate introduced into a Cox model. In patients randomly allocated to treatment with hydroxyurea, switching to pipobroman during follow-up significantly increased the risk of death (hazard ratio, 2.06; 95% CI, 1.09–3.87; P = 0.026) following the switch, compared with patients who remained on hydroxyurea. In patients randomly assigned to pipobroman therapy, switching to hydroxyurea during follow-up did not modify the risk of death (hazard ratio, 1.37; 95% CI, 0.61–3.08; P = 0.45)

Therapy Monitoring

1. Bone marrow study prior to therapy and again at the time of maximal hematologic response
2. CBC with differential once or twice per week during the initial treatment phase (at the starting dose)
   • Continue testing until the desired response is obtained or until significant toxic effects intervene
3. CBC with differential while on maintenance therapy, every 4–8 weeks
4. Ancillary laboratory determinations, including liver and kidney function tests while on maintenance therapy, approximately every 6–12 months

CYTOREDUCTIVE THERAPY REGIMEN

BUSULFAN

Essential Thrombocythemia (ET)

Shvidel L et al. Leukemia 2007;21:2071–2072
Van de Pette JEW et al. Br J Haematol 1986;62:229–237

Notes:
- Busulfan is an alkylating agent with a specific action on megakaryocytic proliferation
- Because of concerns about leukemogenic potential busulfan use should be limited to older patients (>60 years of age) or patients intolerant of hydoxyurea

Busulfan 2–4 mg per day; administer orally, continually, until platelet count decreases to <400,000/mm³ (total dose/week = 14–28 mg)

Note: Once platelet count normalizes, long-term control of platelet count can be achieved with intermittent courses of busulfan given as follows:
Busulfan 2–4 mg per day; administer orally, continually, for 2 weeks after the platelet count increases to >400,000/mm³ (total dose/2-week cycle = 28–56 mg)

Supportive Care
Antiemetic prophylaxis
Emetogenic potential is **MINIMAL–LOW**
See Chapter 39 for antiemetic recommendations

Hematopoietic growth factor (CSF) prophylaxis
Primary prophylaxis is NOT indicated
See Chapter 43 for more information

Antimicrobial prophylaxis
Risk of fever and neutropenia is LOW
  Antimicrobial primary prophylaxis to be considered:
  - Antibacterial—*P. jirovecii* prophylaxis is recommended (eg, cotrimoxazole)
  - Antifungal—not indicated
  - Antiviral—not indicated unless patient previously had an episode of HSV

See Chapter 47 for more information

Treatment Modifications

Adverse Events	Treatment Modifications
WBC* <4000/mm³ but >3500/mm³	Reduce busulfan dose by 50%
WBC* <3500/mm³	Discontinue busulfan
LFTs 2–3 × UNL	Reduce busulfan dose by 50%
LFTs >3 × UNL	Hold busulfan until LFTs have returned to baseline values

*Regarding WBC monitoring and treatment modification. The product label for Myleran, a film-coated busulfan tablet (January 2004. GlaxoSmithKline, Research Triangle Park, NC), states: "A decrease in the leukocyte count is not usually seen during the first 10–15 days of treatment; the leukocyte count may actually increase during this period and it should not be interpreted as resistance to the drug, nor should the dose be increased. Since the leukocyte count may continue to fall for more than 1 month after discontinuing the drug, it is important that busulfan be discontinued prior to the total leukocyte count falling into the normal range. When the total leukocyte count has declined to approximately 15,000/μL, the drug should be withheld. With a constant dose of busulfan, the total leukocyte count declines exponentially . . . .
A decision to increase, decrease, continue, or discontinue a given dose of busulfan must be based not only on the absolute hematologic values, but also on the rapidity with which changes are occurring [in response to treatment]." Plotting weekly WBC counts on a semilogarithmic graph (WBC counts on the log axis; time on the linear axis) may aid in planning when to discontinue therapy

Patient Population Studied

Shvidel L et al. Leukemia 2007;21:2071–2072
Long-term outcome of 36 elderly patients with ET treated with busulfan and evaluated for thrombotic complications and blastic transformation. Thirteen men and 23 women; median age at treatment = 73 years (range: 60–91 years). Diagnosis of ET established according to Polycythemia Vera (PV) Study Group Criteria. Major risk factors for thrombosis: (a) old age (100%); (b) platelet count >1,500,000/mm³ or history of thrombosis (16/36, 44%); (c) at least 1 thrombotic event (12/36, 33%); (d) disturbances such as dizziness, headache, syncope, angina pectoris, erythromelalgia, or leg ulcers before busulfan therapy (21/36, 58%). The median platelet count at start of busulfan was 994,000/mm³ (range: 783,000–1,768,000/mm³)

Van de Pette JEW et al. Br J Haematol 1986;62:229–237

Thirty-seven patients with essential thrombocythemia treated with busulfan and followed for periods up to 25 years

Efficacy (N = 36)

Shvidel et al. Leukemia 2007;21:2071–2072*

Median follow-up time after therapy	72 months (range: 30–300 months)
Hematologic response (platelet count <400,000/mm³)	100%
Disappearance of thrombocytosis-related symptoms	100%
Cycles of busulfan administered	47[†]
Median duration of response in all the cycles given	38 months (range: 8+ to 207+ months)
Response duration following the first cycle	36 months[‡]
Response duration following subsequent cycles	38 months[‡]
Percent relapsed	47% (17/36)
Percent requiring additional treatment	33% (12/36)
Median time for next treatment	56 months (range: 22–116 months)
Actual survival at 7 years	78%
Percent dead during follow-up	36% (13/36)[§]
Leukemic transformation/other malignancies during follow-up	0

*To avoid the combination of multiple cytotoxic drugs, only 1 patient received hydroxyurea following busulfan. Two other patients in relapse were subsequently treated with anagrelide

[†]Twenty-six patients received 1 cycle, 9 patients received 2 cycles, and 1 patient received 3 cycles

[‡]No difference between response duration following the first and subsequent cycles

[§]One patient who was sequentially treated with busulfan and hydroxyurea, died of myelofibrosis with splenomegaly, thrombocytopenia, and bleeding 7 years after busulfan therapy. Among the other 12 patients, 9 >80 years of age died of cardiovascular disorders; all had normal platelet count at the time of death and causes of their death were thought to be related to old age/underlying diseases

Efficacy (N = 37)

Van de Pette JEW et al. Br J Haematol 1986;62:229–237

Cox regression analysis indicated only 2 prognostically important presenting features:
• Age → Strong inverse correlation with survival
• Vascular occlusive symptoms → Correlated with a better survival

Platelet count to <400,000/mm³	100%
Resolution of vascular occlusive symptoms	100%*
Median duration of survival on treatment	9.8 years
Deaths from thrombosis and malignant diseases, including leukemia	Not significantly different from the number expected
Progression of PT into myelofibrosis	24%
Development of polycythemia	9%

*Hemorrhagic symptoms often remained unaltered

Toxicity

Toxicity	Percent/Comment
Myelosuppression, all cell lines are equally affected*	Platelets can drop precipitously*
G1/2 nausea	>80%
G1/2 vomiting	>80%
G1/2 diarrhea	>80%
Skin hyperpigmentation	5–10%
Insomnia	Rare
Anxiety	Rare
Dizziness	Rare
Depression	Rare
Elevated LFTs	Rare
Pulmonary symptoms, cough, dyspnea, and fever	With long-term use in <5% of patients
Increased risk of secondary malignancy, especially AML	

*Failure to stop busulfan treatment may result in bone marrow failure with severe prolonged pancytopenia. Pancytopenia is potentially reversible, but recovery may take 1 month to 2 years

Therapy Monitoring

1. *Weekly:* CBC with differential and platelet count, and LFTs during period of busulfan therapy

   Note: Because sudden, unexpected marrow suppression may occur, frequent CBC monitoring is mandatory

2. *CXR as indicated:* For insidious onset of cough, dyspnea, and low-grade fever after months to years of therapy consider busulfan-related lung toxicity in differential diagnosis

CYTOREDUCTIVE THERAPY REGIMEN

RADIOACTIVE PHOSPHORUS (³²P)

Polycythemia Vera (PV) and Essential Thrombocythemia (ET)

Radioactive phosphorus (³²P) (sodium phosphate ³²P 18.5–185 MBq/mL injection) initial dose of 85.1 MBq (2.3 mCi)/m²; administer as an intravenous solution dosage form with a concentration of 24.8 MBq (0.67 mCi)/mL

Alternate dose (Najean Y, Rain J-D. Blood 1997;89:2319–2327):

Radioactive phosphorus (³²P) (sodium phosphate ³²P 18.5–185 MBq/mL injection) initial dose of 0.1 mCi/kg; administer intravenously with a concentration of 24.8 MBq (0.67 mCi)/mL

Notes:
- The dose administered depends upon the stage of disease and patient size
- Starting doses used: 2.5 mCi/m² or 0.1 mCi/kg
- Try not to exceed 185 MBq (5 mCi) although doses of 74–260 MBq (2–7 mCi) have been administered
- Reduce doses by 25% in patients >80 years of age
- Repeat doses must be adjusted to individual needs but should not be administered more often than every 12 weeks
- Subsequent doses are based on patient response. Doses of 111–185 MBq (3–5 mCi) ³²P sodium phosphate intravenously may be repeated in 12 weeks if needed
- Measure a patient's dose by a suitable radioactivity calibration system immediately prior to administration
- Parenteral drug products should be inspected visually for particulate matter and discoloration prior to administration, whenever solution and container permit
- Waterproof gloves should be used during the entire handling and administration procedure
- Maintain adequate shielding during the life of the product and use a sterile, shielded syringe for withdrawing and injecting the drug
- Oral administration of high specific activity in the fasting state may equal intravenous administration
- Phosphorus ³²P decays by beta emission with a physical half-life of 14.3 days
- Elimination is primarily renal; a very small percentage in the feces. In normal patients, 5–10% is eliminated in the urine within 24 hours and approximately 20% is eliminated within a week. Fecal excretion increases if ³²P sodium phosphate is administered orally

Indications:
- May have a role in elderly patients whose life expectancy is <10 years
- A rare, elderly patient who cannot tolerate oral agents or who does not have reliable access to laboratory monitoring may benefit from ³²P, which can be administered on a yearly basis by an expert

Contraindications:
- Discouraged in young patients because of its leukemogenicity
- ³²P sodium phosphate should not be used as a part of sequential treatment with a chemotherapeutic agent
- Patients who initially receive hydroxyurea and no longer respond or experience toxicity from hydroxyurea, and require another agent *should not* receive long-term ³²P therapy. Hydroxyurea and ³²P administered in this sequence is associated with an extremely high risk of leukemic transformation

Supportive Care

Antiemetic prophylaxis

Emetogenic potential is **MODERATE**

See Chapter 39 for antiemetic recommendations

Hematopoietic growth factor (CSF) prophylaxis

Primary prophylaxis is NOT indicated

See Chapter 43 for more information

Antimicrobial prophylaxis

Risk of fever and neutropenia is LOW

   Antimicrobial primary prophylaxis to be considered:
- Antibacterial—not indicated
- Antifungal—not indicated
- Antiviral—not indicated unless patient previously had an episode of HSV

See Chapter 47 for more information

Dose Modifications

Adverse Events	Dose Modification or Intervention
Patient with polycythemia vera and elevated hematocrit	Perform phlebotomy during the induction period before or after the administration of sodium phosphate ^{32}P to maintain hematocrit at normal levels
Patient with polycythemia vera with leukocyte count <5,000/mm³ or platelet count <150,000/mm³	Hold ^{32}P sodium phosphate until leukocyte count ≥5000/mm³ and platelet count ≥150,000/mm³

Efficacy

Treatment of polycythemia vera: Use of ^{32}P alone or in combination with maintenance therapy using hydroxyurea in 461 patients older than 65 years of age (N = 461)

Najean Y, Rain J-D. Blood 1997;89:2319–2327

- Patients older than 65 years of age
- ^{32}P dose = 0.1 mCi/kg (3.7 MBq with a maximum of 7 mCi)
- Phlebotomies used just before ^{32}P as emergency therapy if Hct level >55%, but not during follow-up
- Once complete remission (CR; normal Hb level and leukocyte and platelet counts) obtained >4 months, patients were randomized to either simple surveillance without treatment or maintenance treatment with low-dose hydroxyurea (10 mg/kg per day)
- Aspirin (100–250 mg/day) was only prescribed to patients with a history of thromboembolic events
- Patients observed every other month (blood examination) and twice/year (clinical examination)
- *Randomized to no hydroxyurea maintenance (N = 242):* ^{32}P resumed when the Hct level increased to 50% and the red blood cell volume was more than 125% of the normal value
- *Randomized to receive maintenance hydroxyurea >^{32}P-induced remission (N = 219):* Hydroxyurea treatment was delayed until the Hb level was >12 g/dL and the platelet count was >200,000/mm³

	^{32}P/No Hydroxyurea	^{32}P + Maintenance Hydroxyurea
CR by 3–4 months without additional ^{32}P doses	455/461 (98.7%)	
Median duration of CR	3 years*	60% at 14 years*
Median survival, intention-to-treat	11.2 years[†]	9.1 years[†]
Median survival, main therapy	10.9 years[‡]	9.3 years[‡]
Platelet count maintenance	No difference	
Risk of serious vascular accident	Not reduced by maintenance treatment	
Mean annual ^{32}P dose >2 years of observation	0.033 mCi/kg • years	0.009 mCi/kg • years
Leukemia risk, intention-to-treat		Increased[§]
Leukemia risk, main therapy		Increased[ᶜ]
Leukemia risk patients observed/surviving 5–10 years		Increased[**]
Leukemia risk patients observed/surviving >10 years		Increased[††]
Cancer risk, intention-to-treat		Increased[‡‡]
Cancer risk, main therapy		Increased[§§]

(continued)

Radiation Dosimetry

Absorbed Radiation Doses*

Tissue	Gray	RAD
Skeleton	9.45	945
Liver	0.93	93
Spleen	1.10	110
Brain	0.45	45
Testes	0.15	15
Ovaries	0.12	12
Total body	1.50	150

*Estimated absorbed radiation doses to an average patient (70 kg) following intravenous administration of 555 MBq (15 mCi) of sodium phosphate ^{32}P

Estimated Absorbed Radiation Dose*

Organ	mGy/MBq	RAD/mCi
Red marrow	11.00	40.74
Bone surfaces	11.00	40.74
Breast	0.92	3.41
Adrenals	0.74	2.74
Bladder wall	0.74	2.74
Kidneys	0.74	2.74
Large intestine wall (upper)	0.74	2.74
Large intestine wall (lower)	0.74	2.74
Liver	0.74	2.74
Lungs	0.74	2.74
Ovaries	0.74	2.74
Pancreas	0.74	2.74
Spleen	0.74	2.74
Small intestine	0.74	2.74
Stomach wall	0.74	2.74
Testes	0.74	2.74
Thyroid	0.74	2.74
Uterus	0.74	2.74
Other tissue	0.74	2.74

Note: Effective dose: 2.2 mSv/MBq (8.14 rem/mCi)
*For adults; intravenous injection. Data based on Task group of Committee 2 of the International Commission on Radiological Protection: ICRP Publication 53—Radiation Dose to Patients from Radiopharmaceuticals. New York, NY: Pergamon Press; 1988:83

Efficacy (continued)

	³²P/No Hydroxyurea	³²P + Maintenance Hydroxyurea
Cancer risk patients observed/surviving <5 years	No difference	
Cancer risk patients observed/surviving 5–10 years		Increased[ccc]
Cancer risk patients observed/surviving 5–10 years		Increased***

*$P < 0.01$
†$P = 0.1$
‡$P = 0.15$
§$P = 0.01$ (log-rank test)
¶$P = 0.03$ (log-rank test)
**$\chi 2$ test, $P = 0.03$
††$\chi 2$ test, $P = 0.05$
‡‡$P = 0.05$
§§$P = 0.08$
¶¶$P = 0.02$
***$P = 0.05$

Notes:
• The dose of ³²P received by patients who developed leukemia was moderately higher than that received by other patients (0.044 vs. 0.032 mCi/kg • years), but this difference was not statistically significant ($P > 0.05$, analysis of variance)
• In the group of patients who did not receive maintenance treatment and in the group who received maintenance treatment, no significant difference in the total ³²P dose was observed between patients who developed and those who did not develop a cancer (comparison of means and analysis of variance)
• The development of spent phase (hypersplenism in the absence of myelofibrosis) or overt splenic myeloid metaplasia did not occur before 5 years. The use of maintenance hydroxyurea after ³²P did not protect patients from this evolution, which was observed in approximately 30% of the cases at 15 years. A retrospective analysis of charts showed platelet count was generally >400,000/mm³ in 57% of the cases who developed myelofibrosis and myeloid metaplasia, against 31% of cases developing no such complication (difference of $P < 0.02$)
• Cases were considered to have severe polycythemia vera when, in the absence of complementary treatment, 2 injections of ³²P were required within 2 years or 3 injections were required in <4 years. Eighty-eight patients initially randomized in the nonmaintenance arm were included in this group, 38 of whom subsequently received maintenance treatment because of the need for repeated doses of ³²P. One-hundred seventeen less severe cases (no relapse during the first 2 years and still alive after 3 years) did not receive maintenance treatment. A significant survival difference (median: 8.2 years vs. 11.8 years, $P = 0.015$) was observed between severe and nonsevere cases treated using ³²P alone. The difference was because of an excess of leukemic transformation ($P = 0.05$) and vascular events ($P = 0.09$) in the group classified as having severe disease

Toxicity

Adverse Event	Frequency
Leukopenia*	Following administration of large therapeutic doses*
Thrombocytopenia*	
Anemia	
Acute leukemia	Long-term complications
Myelodysplasia	
Solid tumors	

*Moderate leukothrombocytopenia (approximately 3000/mm³ leukocytes and 100,000/mm³ platelets) generally observed at 4–6 weeks; usually resolve spontaneously by 4 months. More severe and prolonged pancytopenia (6–18 months) without any clinical consequence can be observed in patients >80 years of age

Therapy Monitoring

1. *Prior to therapy and at regular intervals during and after therapy:* Bone marrow studies
2. *Weekly, then monthly then at regular intervals:* Blood studies, including hemoglobin determinations and leukocyte, leukocyte differential, erythrocyte, and platelet counts

Note: Other tests may be warranted in some patients, depending on condition

Treatment-Related Risk Factors for Transformation to Acute Myeloid Leukemia and Myelodysplastic Syndromes in Myeloproliferative Neoplasms

Björkholm M et al. J Clin Oncol 2011;29:2410–2415

Conclusions: The risk of AML/MDS development after MPN diagnosis was **significantly associated with high exposures of ³²P and alkylators, but not with hydroxyurea treatment.** Twenty-five percent of patients with MPNs who developed AML/MDS were not exposed to cytotoxic therapy, supporting a major role for non–treatment-related factors

Risk of AML/MDS Transformation in Patients with MPNs in Relation to Cumulative Dose

| | Patient Cases | | Controls | | All Patient Cases and Controls | | | | | | Patient Cases and Controls With PV/ET | |
| | | | | | Risk of AML/MDS | | Risk of AML/MDS | | Risk of AML Only | | Risk of AML/MDS | |
Cumulative Dose	No.	%	No.	%	Crude OR	95% CI	Adjusted OR	95% CI	Adjusted OR	95% CI	Adjusted OR	95% CI
Total Number of Patients	162	100	242	100								
Hydroxyurea												
0 g	111	69	179	74	1.0	Ref	1.0	Ref	1.0	Ref	1.0	Ref
1–499 g	24	15	29	12	1.3	0.7–2.6	1.5	0.6–2.4	1.3	0.6–2.5	1.0	0.4–2.5
500–999 g	14	9	15	6	1.3	0.6–3.1	1.4	0.6–3.4	1.5	0.6–3.6	0.9	0.3–2.6
≥1000 g	13	8	19	8	1.0	0.4–2.3	1.3	0.5–3.3	1.1	0.4–3.0	1.2	0.5–3.2
Trend test P					0.510		0.320		0.370		0.600	
³²P Sodium Phosphate												
0 MBq	92	57	161	67	1.0	Ref	1.0	Ref	1.0	Ref	1.0	Ref
1–499 MBq	14	9	21	9	1.3	0.6–2.8	1.5	0.6–3.3	1.3	0.6–3.1	1.4	0.6–3.2
500–999 MBq	16	10	32	13	0.9	0.5–1.8	1.1	0.5–2.2	0.9	0.4–1.9	1.2	0.6–2.5
≥1000 MBq	40	25	28	12	4.0	1.9–8.3	4.6	2.1–9.8	4.8	2.0–9.9	4.4	2.0–9.6
Trend test P					0.006		0.002		0.006		0.003	
Alkylating Agents												
0 g	124	77	196	81	1.0	Ref	1.0	Ref	1.0	Ref	1.0	Ref
0.1–0.49 g	15	9	26	11	1.0	0.5–2.0	1.1	0.5–2.3	1.0	0.5–2.1	1.2	0.5–2.7
0.50–0.99 g	11	7	12	5	1.7	0.6–4.4	1.7	0.6–5.0	1.4	0.5–4.4	2.1	0.7–6.4
≥1.00	12	7	8	3	3.0	1.0–8.8	3.4	1.1–10.6	3.2	1.0–10.0	3.6	1.1–11.2
Trend test P					0.030		0.015		0.032		0.007	

AML, Acute myeloid leukemia; ET, essential thrombocythemia; MDS, myelodysplastic syndrome; Ref, reference.

Risk of AML/MDS Transformation According to Number of Cytoreductive Treatment Types

Treatment	OR	95% CI
None	1.0	Ref
P³² only	1.5	0.8–2.8
Alkylating agent only	0.9	0.4–2.1
Hydroxyurea only	1.2	0.6–2.4
Mixed treatment (2 or 3)	2.9	1.4–5.9

Ref, reference.

Treatment of (Primary) Myelofibrosis

- At present, only allogeneic hematopoietic stem cell transplantation (HSCT) is potentially curative in primary myelofibrosis (PMF). **However, the majority of patients are of advanced age, and, therefore, not good candidates for allogeneic HSCT, and such patients rely on palliative therapy to improve the quality of life,** although it may not prolong life
- Therapeutic options:
  - Autologous HSCT
  - Drug therapy
  - Splenectomy
  - Radiation therapy

Hematopoietic stem-cell transplantation
- In a retrospective, multicenter study of 66 consecutive patients, age was the major determinant of transplant outcome; 5-year survival was 62% in patients younger than 45 years of age and 14% in those who were older
- Other investigators have reported better survival in patients older than 44 years, and data suggest that transplant-related morbidity (TRM) in older patients may be positively influenced by the use of reduced-intensity conditioning regimens
- In the most recent communication of reduced-intensity, conditioning transplantation in myelofibrosis (n = 104; median age: 55 years [range, 32–68 years]; unrelated donors in 71 patients), 1-year mortality was 19% (27% if one excludes low-risk patients), and 32% of patients experienced chronic graft-versus-host disease. The 3-year overall survival, event-free survival, and relapse rate were 70%, 55%, and 29%, respectively

Conclusions: At present, it is reasonable to consider allogeneic HSCT (related or unrelated donor) *in high-risk patients who are younger than age 45 years.* In older patients with high-risk disease, it is reasonable to consider alternative transplantation options, including reduced-intensity allogeneic and autologous HSCT

Drug treatment
- Conventional drug therapy for anemia includes a combination of:
  - An **androgen** preparation (eg, fluoxymesterone 10 mg; administer orally twice daily, continually)
  - **Prednisone** 0.5 mg/kg per day; administer orally, continually
  - **Epoetin alfa** 40,000 units/week; administer subcutaneously in the presence of an endogenous blood erythropoietin concentration <100 mU/mL (<100 IU/L)
  - **Danazol** 200–800 mg/day; administer orally, continually
- **Low-dose thalidomide in combination with prednisone** has recently been identified as an effective combination for myelofibrosis-associated anemia, thrombocytopenia, and splenomegaly, with an approximate 50% overall response rate
- **Lenalidomide**, a thalidomide analog, has also been evaluated in myelofibrosis with 20–30% response rates in both anemia and splenomegaly. Lenalidomide response rates were increased in patients with myelofibrosis with the del(5q) abnormality. Therapy for symptomatic anemia in myelofibrosis should include lenalidomide in the presence of del(5q), and, in its absence, low-dose thalidomide and prednisone
- **Ruxolitinib**, a JAK1/JAK2 inhibitor, is approved for the treatment of patients with intermediate or high-risk myelofibrosis, including primary myelofibrosis, postpolycythemia vera myelofibrosis, and postessential thrombocythemia myelofibrosis. Two randomized studies confirmed the palliative value of ruxolitinib in terms of a partial response in splenomegaly and alleviation of constitutional symptoms. However, they did not show histopathologic, cytogenetic, or molecular remissions, and the drug was more likely to cause anemia and thrombocytopenia than to correct them. Notwithstanding the above, JAK–STAT remains an important drug target by virtue of its role in the production and activity of proinflammatory cytokines, which are overexpressed in myelofibrosis and probably contribute to disease symptoms. Ruxolitinib induces a rapid and marked suppression of these cytokines, in conjunction with its salutary effect on constitutional symptoms. Therefore, cytokine modulation might constitute its primary mode of action, although nonspecific myelosuppression probably contributes to the drug's effect on splenomegaly and blood counts

  In line with this assumption, cytokine rebound after drug withdrawal might explain the immediate and florid relapse of symptoms when ruxolitinib is discontinued; this relapse is sometimes accompanied by hemodynamic decompensation. Approximately 30% of patients with myelofibrosis present with ruxolitinib-sensitive symptoms, and the drug can be considered in these patients if they are not candidates for stem cell transplantation
- Hydroxyurea can also be used to control splenomegaly, leukocytosis, or thrombocytosis
- Other drugs that have been used in a similar setting include busulfan, melphalan, and cladribine
- In contrast, interferon alfa has limited therapeutic value in myelofibrosis with myeloid metaplasia (MMM)

Surgical treatment
- Splenectomy in myelofibrosis with myeloid metaplasia (MMM) is indicated in the presence of drug-refractory mechanical discomfort, portal hypertension, severe hypercatabolic symptoms, and heavy red blood cell transfusion requirements
- Operative mortality is approximately 9%, and 25% of patients may experience postsplenectomy thrombocytosis and progressive hepatomegaly

(continued)

Treatment of (Primary) Myelofibrosis (*continued*)

Radiation treatment
- Splenic irradiation (a total dose of 100–500 cGy in 5–10 fractions) may be considered an alternative treatment to splenectomy in poor surgical candidates
- Symptomatic pulmonary hypertension not secondary to a thromboembolic process has been associated with PMF and is believed to arise from diffuse pulmonary extramedullary hematopoiesis. Diagnosis is confirmed by a technetium-^{99m} sulfur colloid scintigraphy, which shows diffuse pulmonary uptake, and treatment with single-fraction (100 cGy) whole-lung irradiation has been shown to be effective

Björkholm M et al. J Clin Oncol 2011;29:2410–2415
Cervantes F et al. Br J Haematol 2006;134:184–186
Cervantes F et al. Haematologica 2000;85:595–599
Deeg HJ et al. Blood 2003;102:3912–3918
Guardiola P et al. Blood 1999;93:2831–2838
Kroeger N et al. Proc Am Soc Hematol 2007;110:683 [abstract]
Mesa RA et al. Blood 2003;101:2534–2541
Silver RT. Semin Hematol 1997;34:40–50
Tefferi A et al. Blood 2006;108:1158–1164

DRUG THERAPY REGIMEN

LOW-DOSE THALIDOMIDE IN COMBINATION WITH PREDNISONE (THAL-PRED)

Primary Myelofibrosis

Mesa RA et al. Blood 2003;101:2534–2541

Thalidomide 50 mg; administer orally, daily, by rigorously adhering to the Celgene *S.T.E.P.S.* **program** for thalidomide safety
Prednisone 0.5 mg/kg per day; administer orally for 1 month, *followed by:*
Prednisone 0.25 mg/kg per day; administer orally for 1 month, *followed by:*
Prednisone 0.125 mg/kg per day; administer orally for 1 month

Note: Patients showing any evidence of response after 3 months of combination therapy are treated for an additional 3 months with only 50 mg thalidomide daily

The System for Thalidomide Education and Prescribing Safety (*S.T.E.P.S.*) program is a Risk Evaluation and Mitigation Strategy program against the toxicity associated with fetal exposure to thalidomide, and to minimize the chance of fetal exposure to thalidomide
- To avoid fetal exposure, thalidomide is available only under a special restricted distribution program called *S.T.E.P.S. S.T.E.P.S.* requirements include, but are not limited to, the following:
  - Thalidomide must not be prescribed for female patients who are pregnant
  - Female patients taking thalidomide must not become pregnant, breastfeed a baby, or donate blood
  - Female patients able to become pregnant must use 2 methods of contraception 4 weeks before starting to use thalidomide and undergo pregnancy testing before receiving thalidomide and at prescribed intervals and during treatment
  - Male patients taking thalidomide must not impregnate a female, must not have unprotected sexual contact with a woman who is pregnant, and must use a latex condom every time they have sexual contact with women during thalidomide treatment and for 4 weeks after completing treatment
  - Only prescribers registered with *S.T.E.P.S.* can prescribe thalidomide
  - To receive thalidomide, patients must enroll in *S.T.E.P.S.* and agree to comply with the requirements of the *S.T.E.P.S.* program
- Information about thalidomide (THALOMID) and the *S.T.E.P.S.* program can be obtained by calling the Celgene Customer Care Center toll-free at 1-888-423-5436, or online from the U.S. Food and Drug Administration website for Postmarket Drug Safety Information for Patients and Providers, Approved Risk Evaluation and Mitigation Strategies (REMS) at: www.fda.gov/Drugs/DrugSafety/PostmarketDrugSafetyInformationforPatientsandProviders/ (last accessed August 30, 2013)

Supportive Care

Antiemetic prophylaxis
Emetogenic potential is **MINIMAL–LOW**
See Chapter 39 for antiemetic recommendations

Hematopoietic growth factor (CSF) prophylaxis
Primary prophylaxis is NOT indicated
See Chapter 43 for more information

Antimicrobial prophylaxis
Risk of fever and neutropenia is LOW
  Antimicrobial primary prophylaxis to be considered:
  - Antibacterial—not indicated
  - Antifungal—not indicated
  - Antiviral—not indicated unless patient previously had an episode of HSV
See Chapter 47 for more information

Thromboprophylaxis
Primary prophylaxis is not indicated
- Instruct patients to seek medical care if they develop shortness of breath, chest pain, or arm or leg swelling
- Consider thromboprophylaxis based on an assessment of an individual patient's underlying risk factors

Treatment Modifications

Adverse Event	Treatment Modification
Febrile neutropenia	Withhold therapy until fever abates, then resume therapy
G4 hematologic toxicity	Withhold therapy until ANC >750/mm^3 and platelets >500,00/mm^3, then resume therapy at a dose of thalidomide 25 mg/day
G3/4 nonhematologic toxicity	Interrupt therapy, follow clinically until toxicity remits to G ≤2, then resume therapy at a dose of thalidomide 25 mg/day
G ≥3 thalidomide neuropathy	Interrupt therapy, follow clinically until toxicity remits to G ≤2, then resume therapy at a dose of thalidomide 25 mg/day
If ANC nadir ≤1000/mm^3 or platelets nadir ≤50,000/mm^3	Continue treatment, but reduce thalidomide doses to 25 mg/day
G2 nonhematologic toxicity	Reduce thalidomide dose to 25 mg/day
G ≥3 nonhematologic toxicity	Discontinue thalidomide

Patient Population Studied

Patients met standard diagnostic criteria for myelofibrosis with myeloid metaplasia (MMM). All subtypes of MMM were eligible (agnogenic myeloid metaplasia [AMM], postpolycythemic myeloid metaplasia [PPMM], and postthrombocythemic myeloid metaplasia [PTMM]). All patients underwent bone marrow examination with cytogenetic and fluorescent in situ hybridization (FISH) studies to exclude occult chronic myeloid leukemia

Toxicity

Toxicity	Number of Patients Affected (Percent Affected)		
	Thalidomide + Prednisone	G2/G3 or Higher	Thalidomide 100–400 mg*
Leukocytosis[†]	8 (38)	6/2 (29/10)	2 (13)
Thrombocytosis[‡]	4 (19)	3/2 (14/10)	3 (20)
Constipation	8 (38)	3 (14)	9 (60)
Edema	5 (24)	2 (10)	3 (20)
Visual disturbance	4 (19)	2 (10)	2 (13)
Fatigue	2 (10)	2 (10)	10 (67)
Thrombosis	1 (5)	1/1 (5/5)	0
Paresthesias	6 (29)	1 (5)	4 (27)
Sedation	6 (29)	1 (5)	3 (20)
Neutropenia <1500/mm³	5 (24)	1 (5)	6 (40)
Neutropenia <1000/mm³	4 (19)	4 (19)	4 (27)
Anxiety	4 (19)	0	3 (20)
Rash	3 (14)	0	4 (27)
Orthostatic symptoms	0	0	5 (33)
Tremor	0	0	3 (20)
Myeloproliferative reaction	0	0	3 (20)
Dry mouth	0	0	2 (13)
Sinus bradycardia	0	0	2 (13)
Abdominal pain	0	0	2 (13)
Decreased hearing	0	0	2 (13)
Anorexia	0	0	1 (7)
Confusion	0	0	1 (7)
Dry eyes	0	0	1 (7)
Depression	0	0	1 (7)

*Elliott MA et al. Br J Haematol 2002;117:288–296
[†]One patient developed acute myeloid leukemia
[‡]A clinical consequence was observed in only 1 patient (deep venous thrombosis)

Therapy Monitoring

1. Monitor white blood cell count and differential on an ongoing basis, especially in patients who may be predisposed to develop neutropenia
2. Pregnancy testing
   • Females of childbearing potential
     ▪ Within 24 hours before commencing thalidomide treatment and at intervals explicitly prescribed by the *S.T.E.P.S.* program
3. Neurologic testing before starting thalidomide treatment (baseline), then every 3 months while receiving treatment

Efficacy (N = 21)

Objective and sustained clinical response in anemia	13 (62%; 95% CI, 38%–82%)*
Median increase in hemoglobin value	1.8 g/dL (range: 0.1–5.1 g/dL)
Response in RBC transfusion-dependent patients (n = 10)	7/10 (70%)[†]
Response in RBC transfusion-independent patients (n = 11; 7 patients [64%] with hemoglobin level <10 g/dL)	Hemoglobin increased by 2.1 g/dL (range: 0.1–5.1 g/dL)
Response in patients with clinically relevant thrombocytopenia (n = 8; platelet count <100,000/mm³)	8/8 (100%)[‡,§,€]
>50% decrease in palpable splenomegaly	4 (19%)[€]

*Improvements in anemia correlated with lower pretherapy CD34 cell counts in the peripheral blood (median: 81.2 CD34 cells/mm³ in responders vs. 554 CD34 cells/mm³ in nonresponders; P = 0.03) as well as lower numbers of circulating blasts (median: 0.8% in responders vs. 4.7% in nonresponders; P = 0.03)
[†]Four patients (40%) became transfusion independent and 3 (30%) had ≥50% decrease in transfusion requirements
[‡]Six patients (75%) had a more than 50% increase in their platelet count
[§]Improvements in clinically significant thrombocytopenia were associated with older ages (median: 71.4 years vs. 61.7 years; P = 0.04), smaller pretreatment spleens (median: 6.5 cm vs. 16.1 cm below the left costal margin; P <0.01), and hypocellular marrows (median cellularity: 18% vs. 58% for nonresponders; P <0.01)
[€]Responses in either splenomegaly or thrombocytopenia were strongly correlated with a concurrent response in anemia (P <0.01)

DRUG THERAPY REGIMEN

LENALIDOMIDE

Primary Myelofibrosis

Tefferi A et al. Blood 2006;108:1158–1164

Lenalidomide 10 mg/day; administer orally for 28 days, continually for 3–4 months (total dose/week = 70 mg)
- If initial platelet count is <100,000/mm^3, give **lenalidomide** 5 mg/day; administer orally for 28 days, continually for 3–4 months (total dose/week = 35 mg)

Note: Continue treat for 6–24 months if response is observed

Supportive Care
Antiemetic prophylaxis
*Emetogenic potential is **MINIMAL–LOW***
See Chapter 39 for antiemetic recommendations

Hematopoietic growth factor (CSF) prophylaxis
Primary prophylaxis is NOT indicated
See Chapter 43 for more information

Antimicrobial prophylaxis
Risk of fever and neutropenia is LOW
  Antimicrobial primary prophylaxis to be considered:
  - Antibacterial—not indicated
  - Antifungal—not indicated
  - Antiviral—not indicated unless patient previously had an episode of HSV
See Chapter 47 for more information

Thromboprophylaxis
  Primary prophylaxis is not indicated
  - Instruct patients to seek medical care if they develop shortness of breath, chest pain, or arm or leg swelling
  - Consider thromboprophylaxis based on an assessment of an individual patient's underlying risk factors

Efficacy

	Combined (n = 68)	Mayo Clinic* (n = 27)	MDACC† (n = 41)
	Number of Patients (% with Each Finding)		
Response‡ in anemia (patients with baseline hemoglobin <10 g/dL)	10/46 (22)	6/27 (22)	4/19 (21)
Major‡	8 (17)	4 (15)	4 (21)
Minor‡	2 (4)	2 (7)	0
Response‡ in palpable splenomegaly	14/42 (33)	6/22 (27)	8/20 (40)
Major‡	1 (2)	1 (5)	1 (5)
Minor‡	13 (31)	5 (23)	7 (35)
Response‡ in thrombocytopenia (patients with baseline platelet count <100,000/mm³)	6/12 (50)	Not available	6/12 (50)
Response‡ in hypercatabolic symptoms	4/10 (40)	4/10 (40)	Not available

(continued)

Dose Modifications

Adverse Event	Dose Modification
Platelet count <30,000/mm^3 on a lenalidomide dose of 10 mg/day	Interrupt lenalidomide treatment, follow CBC weekly, and when platelet count ≥30,000/mm^3, resume lenalidomide at 5 mg/day
Platelet count <30,000/mm^3 on a lenalidomide dose of 5 mg/day	Discontinue lenalidomide treatment
ANC <1000/mm^3 on a lenalidomide dose of 10 mg/day	Interrupt lenalidomide treatment, follow CBC weekly and resume lenalidomide when ANC ≥1000/mm^3 at 5 mg/day
ANC <1000/mm^3 on a lenalidomide dose of 5 mg/day	Discontinue lenalidomide treatment
Febrile neutropenia on a lenalidomide dose of 10 mg/day	Interrupt lenalidomide treatment, follow closely, and when fever is abated, resume lenalidomide at 5 mg/day
Febrile neutropenia on a lenalidomide dose of 5 mg/day	Discontinue lenalidomide treatment
G3/4 nonhematologic toxicity on a lenalidomide dose of 10 mg/day	Interrupt lenalidomide treatment, follow clinically, and when toxicity G ≤2, resume lenalidomide at 5 mg/day
G3/4 nonhematologic toxicity on a lenalidomide dose of 5 mg/day	Discontinue lenalidomide treatment

Starting Dose Adjustment for Renal Impairment in Multiple Myeloma (Days 1–21 of Each 28-Day Cycle)

Moderate renal impairment (30–60 mL/min [0.5–1 mL/s])	Lenalidomide 10 mg every 24 hours
Severe renal impairment (not requiring dialysis) (<30 mL/min [<0.5 mL/s])	Lenalidomide 15 mg every 48 hours
End-stage renal disease (requiring dialysis) (<30 mL/min [<0.5 mL/s])	Lenalidomide 5 mg/day. On dialysis days, administer a dose following dialysis

Efficacy *(continued)*

	Combined (n = 68)	Mayo Clinic* (n = 27)	MDACC† (n = 41)
More than 25% decrease in serum LDH	39/59 (66)	16/27 (67)	21/32 (66)
LDH normalized	20 (34)	8 (30)	12 (38)

*Treated at Mayo Clinic (lenalidomide dose = 10 mg/day)
†Treated at M.D. Anderson Cancer Center (MDACC lenalidomide dose = 10 mg or 5 mg/day)
‡Response criteria
• *Anemia:* Patients who entered the study as transfusion-dependent needed to maintain response for at least 3 months. Transfusion-independent patients needed to maintain response for at least 1 month to be considered responses. Major response indicates normalization of hemoglobin; minor response means either becoming transfusion-independent or having an increase in hemoglobin ≥2 g/dL
• *Spleen:* Patients needed to maintain response for ≥1 month to be considered responses. Major response indicates either becoming nonpalpable if baseline is palpable at >5 cm in maximum distance below left costal margin (LCM) or >50% decrease if baseline is ≥10 cm palpable below LCM. Minor response means either >50% decrease if baseline is <10 cm from LCM or >30% decrease if baseline is ≥10 cm from LCM
• *Thrombocytopenia:* Response indicates >50% increase from baseline and an absolute platelet count of 50,000/mm³
• *Hypercatabolic symptoms:* Patients needed to maintain response for ≥1 month to be considered responses. Response indicates complete resolution in patients with baseline fever, weight loss, or drenching night sweats

Toxicity*,†

	G1	G2	G3	G4	All Grades
Neutropenia					
Mayo Clinic‡	1 (4)	6 (22)	7 (23)	1 (4)	15 (56)
MDACC§	0	0	4 (10)	9 (22)	13 (32)
Fatigue					
Mayo Clinic	2 (7)	8 (30)	2 (7)	2 (7)	14 (52)
MDACC	0	0	3 (7)	0	3 (7)
Thrombocytopenia					
Mayo Clinic	5 (19)	3 (11)	2 (7)	0	10 (37)
MDACC	0	0	4 (10)	7 (17)	11 (27)
Pruritus					
Mayo Clinic	8 (30)	2 (7)	0	0	190 (37)
MDACC	8 (20)	0	1 (2)	0	9 (22)
Anemia					
Mayo Clinic	0	4 (15)	2 (7)	1 (4)	7 (26)
MDACC	0	0	0	0	0
Dyspnea/Hypoxia					
Mayo Clinic	0	1 (4)	4 (15)	0	5 (19)
MDACC	0	0	0	0	0
Rash					
Mayo Clinic	0	1 (4)	1 (4)	1 (4)	3 (11)
MDACC	8 (20)	6 (15)	2 (5)	0	16 (39)

*Adverse event episodes that occurred in more than 1 patient and were attributed as being possibly, probably, or definitely related to drug in patients with MMM
†Toxicity grades are according to the U.S. National Cancer Institute Common Terminology Criteria for Adverse Events, version 3.0
‡Treated at Mayo Clinic (lenalidomide 10 mg/day; n = 27)
§Treated at M.D. Anderson Cancer Center (MDACC; n = 41; lenalidomide 10 mg or 5 mg/day)

Patient Population Studied

Two separate phase II studies involving single-agent lenalidomide therapy in patients with myelofibrosis with myeloid metaplasia (MMM). Conventional criteria were used for the diagnosis of MMM including all subtypes of myeloid metaplasia: agnogenic (AMM), postpolycythemic (PPMM), and postthrombocythemic (PTMM). Patients with acute myelofibrosis or myelodysplastic syndrome with myelofibrosis were not eligible for participation

Therapy Monitoring

Monitor white blood cell count and differential on an ongoing basis, especially in patients who may be more prone to develop neutropenia

DRUG THERAPY REGIMEN

HYDROXYUREA

Primary Myelofibrosis

Löfvenberg E, Wahlin A. Eur J Haematol 1988;41:375–381
Martínez-Trillos A et al. Ann Hematol 2010;89:1233–1237

Hydroxyurea 500 mg/day; administer orally, continually (initial total dose/week = 3500 mg)

Notes:
- Modify dosage according to the efficacy and tolerability in each patient
- In the study by Martínez-Trillos et al., median maintenance daily hydroxyurea dose in responding patients was 700 mg (range: 500–2000 mg)
- Clinical end points for titrating the hydroxyurea dosage:
  - Disappearance of symptoms that motivated starting hydroxyurea
  - Improvement or normalization of clinical and hematologic parameters that led to using hydroxyurea (spleen size in case of symptomatic splenomegaly, and leukocyte and platelet counts in case of leukocytosis or thrombocytosis)

Cervantes F et al. Haematologica 2000;85:595–599

Supportive Care

Antiemetic prophylaxis
*Emetogenic potential is **MINIMAL–LOW***
See Chapter 39 for antiemetic recommendations

Hematopoietic growth factor (CSF) prophylaxis
Primary prophylaxis is NOT indicated
See Chapter 43 for more information

Antimicrobial prophylaxis
Risk of fever and neutropenia is LOW
Antimicrobial primary prophylaxis to be considered:
- Antibacterial—not indicated
- Antifungal—not indicated
- Antiviral—not indicated unless patient previously had an episode of HSV
See Chapter 47 for more information

Efficacy

Martínez-Trillos A et al. Ann Hematol 2010;89:1233–1237

	Number of Patients	Response Rate (%)*
Overall Clinical and Hematologic Responses According to EUMNET Criteria*		
Complete plus major response		30%
Moderate plus minor response		32%
Failure		38%[†]
Overall Clinical and Hematologic Responses According IWG-MRT Criteria*		
Clinical improvement	16/40	40%
Disappearance of palpable splenomegaly	4/40	10%
Reduction in spleen size ≥50%	12/40	30%
Hemoglobin value increase >2 g/dL	5/40	12.5%
Median duration of the response	13.2 months (range: 3–126.2 months)	
Alive[‡]	14 (35%)	
Dead[§]	26 (65%)	
Response by Specific Features in 40 Patients with Myelofibrosis Treated with Hydroxyurea*		
Constitutional symptoms	18	82
Symptomatic splenomegaly	8	45
Pruritus	2	50
Bone pain	2	100
Leukocytosis	9	81
Thrombocytosis	11	71

*The response was evaluated using the criteria of the European Myelofibrosis Network (EUMNET) and those of the International Working Group for Myelofibrosis Research and Treatment (IWG-MRT). The minimum time to assess the response was 3 months. Responses include complete plus partial responses according EUMNET criteria
[†]Among patients whose disease did not respond, 5 eventually developed acute transformation at a median of 18.8 months (range: 11.9–25.3 months) after the start of hydroxyurea, 2 received allo-HSCT and died from complications related to the procedure, and 2 required splenectomy or splenic radiation as salvage therapy for symptomatic splenomegaly
[‡]Thirteen patients were still receiving hydroxyurea maintenance
[§]Causes of death included disease progression (n = 8, including acute transformation in 5 patients), infection (n = 5), bleeding (n = 3), thrombosis (n = 3), complications of allo-HSCT (n = 2), liver failure and cardiac insufficiency (n = 1 each), and unknown causes (n = 3)

Patient Population Studied

Martínez-Trillos A et al. Ann Hematol 2010;89:1233–1237

Forty from among 157 subjects consecutively diagnosed with primary myelofibrosis (n = 127), or post-ET (n = 20), or post-PV (n = 10) myelofibrosis. Patients received hydroxyurea as treatment for hyperproliferative manifestations of myelofibrosis, including constitutional symptoms (weight loss, night sweats, low-grade fevers), symptomatic splenomegaly, pruritus, bone pain, leukocytosis, and thrombocytosis. The diagnosis of myelofibrosis was made according to the criteria accepted at the time patients were diagnosed, but in all cases, current WHO criteria were fulfilled

Toxicity

Hematologic Toxicity	**18/40 (45%)**
Appearance or worsening of a preexisting anemia*	14/40 (35%)
Required concomitant treatment for anemia*,†	26/40 (65%)
Concomitant epoetin alfa or darbepoetin alfa†	17/40 (42.5)
Concomitant danazol†	9/40 (22.5%)
Pancytopenia	4/40 (10%)
Nonhematologic Toxicity	**6/40 (15%)**
Oral or leg ulcers‡	5/40 (12.5%)
Gastrointestinal symptoms	1/40 (2.5%)

Toxicities Included in Product Labeling§

Hematologic Side Effects

1. Neutropenia common
2. Thrombocytopenia and anemia are less common than neutropenia, and seldom occur without preceding leukopenia
   a. Hydroxyurea causes macrocytosis which may mask incidental folic acid deficiency
      (1) Folic acid supplementation is recommended during treatment with hydroxyurea
3. Cytopenias often are rapidly reversible within 3–4 days, but may take 7–21 days to recover after drug discontinued
4. High doses and/or failure to interrupt treatment despite cytopenia may result in prolonged aplasia

Nonhematologic Side Effects

Relatively common	**Rare**
1. Gastrointestinal symptoms:	1. Chronic skin reactions
• Stomatitis/mucositis	• Hyperpigmentation
• Anorexia	• Atrophy of skin and nails
• Mild nausea/vomiting	2. Skin cancer
• Diarrhea	3. Alopecia
• Constipation	4. Headache
2. Acute skin reactions	5. Drowsiness
• Rash	6. Convulsions
• Painful lower extremity ulcerations	7. Constitutional symptoms:
• Dermatomyositis-like changes	• Fever
• Erythema	• Chills
• Nail ridging or discoloration	• Asthenia
	8. Renal impairment
	9. Hepatic impairment

*Median hydroxyurea dose received by patients who developed hydroxyurea-induced anemia was 643 mg/day (range: 143–1500 mg) versus 1000 mg/day (range: 143–1500 mg) for patients who did not require a specific treatment for anemia. The difference between groups was not significant (Mann-Whitney U test)
†Twelve patients responded to epoetin alfa or darbepoetin alfa, 7 patients responded to danazol, but in all cases, responses were short-lived
‡Median daily hydroxyurea dose in patients developing ulcers was 1340 mg (range: 500–2000 mg)
§Droxia—hydroxyurea capsule; product labeling, January 2012. Bristol-Myers Squibb Company, Princeton, NJ

Boxed warning (FDA approved product label):
Hydroxyurea is mutagenic and clastogenic, and causes cellular transformation to a tumorigenic phenotype. Hydroxyurea is thus unequivocally genotoxic and a presumed trans-species carcinogen that implies a carcinogenic risk to humans. Secondary leukemias have been reported in patients receiving hydroxyurea for long periods for myeloproliferative disorders, such as polycythemia vera and thrombocythemia. It is not known whether the leukemogenic effect is secondary to hydroxyurea or is associated with the underlying disease. Physicians and patients must very carefully consider the potential benefits of hydroxyurea relative to the undefined risk of developing secondary malignancies

Treatment Modifications

Adverse Event	Treatment Modification
Hematologic Toxicity	
WBC count <3500/mm³ or platelet count <100,000/mm³	Hold hydroxyurea until WBC >3500/mm³ and platelet >100,000/mm³, then restart hydroxyurea at 50% of prior dose
Nonhematologic Toxicity	
G1	No dose modifications
G2/3	Hold hydroxyurea until toxicity G ≤1, then restart at prior dose
Recurrent G2/3	Hold hydroxyurea until toxicity G ≤1, then restart at 75% of prior dose
G4	Hold hydroxyurea until toxicity G ≤1, then restart at 50% of prior dose
Recurrent G4	Discontinue hydroxyurea

Therapy Monitoring

Frequent monitoring of CBC is necessary to prevent excessive marrow suppression. Obtain CBC with leukocyte differential every 1–2 weeks for the first 2 months, every month thereafter, and every 3 months after reaching a steady state

DRUG THERAPY REGIMEN

RUXOLITINIB

Primary Myelofibrosis

Harrison C et al. N Engl J Med 2012;366:787–798
Verstovsek S et al. N Engl J Med 2012;366:799–807

- The recommended starting dose of **ruxolitinib** is based on platelet count (see table below). A complete blood count (CBC) and platelet count must be performed before initiating therapy
- Doses may be titrated based on safety and efficacy

Platelet Count	Ruxolitinib Starting Dose
>200,000/mm^3	20 mg; administer orally twice daily
100,000–200,000/mm^3	15 mg; administer orally twice daily

If efficacy is considered insufficient and platelet and neutrophil counts are adequate, doses may be increased in 5-mg twice-daily increments to a maximum of 25 mg twice daily:
1. Doses should not be increased during the first 4 weeks of therapy
2. Doses should not be increased more frequently than every 2 weeks

Consider dose increases in patients who meet all of the following conditions:
1. Failure to achieve either a reduction of 50% in palpable spleen length or a 35% reduction in spleen volume as measured by CT or MRI in comparison with pretreatment baseline
2. Platelet count >125,000/mm^3 at 4 weeks, and platelet count never <100,000/mm^3
3. ANC >750/mm^3

Consider dose adjustments as follows:
1. The recommended starting dose is **ruxolitinib** 10 mg; administer orally, twice daily for patients with a platelet count between 100,000 and 150,000/mm^3 and moderate (creatinine clearance
   [CrCl] = 30–59 mL/min; 0.5–0.98 mL/s) or severe renal impairment
   (CrCl = 15–29 mL/min; 0.25–0.48 mL/s)
2. Avoid ruxolitinib use in patients with end-stage renal disease (CrCl <15 mL/min; <0.25 mL/s) not requiring dialysis and in patients with moderate or severe renal impairment with platelet counts <100,000/mm^3
3. In patients with hepatic impairment, the recommended starting dose is **ruxolitinib** 10 mg; administer orally, twice daily for patients with a platelet count between 100,000–150,000/mm^3
4. Avoid ruxolitinib in patients with hepatic impairment with platelet counts <100,000/mm^3

Supportive Care
Antiemetic prophylaxis
*Emetogenic potential is **MINIMAL–LOW***
See Chapter 39 for antiemetic recommendations

Hematopoietic growth factor (CSF) prophylaxis
Primary prophylaxis is NOT indicated
See Chapter 43 for more information

Antimicrobial prophylaxis
Risk of fever and neutropenia is LOW
Antimicrobial primary prophylaxis to be considered:
- Antibacterial—not indicated
- Antifungal—not indicated
- Antiviral—not indicated unless patient previously had an episode of HSV

See Chapter 47 for more information

Dose Modifications

Adverse Event	Treatment Modification*
Platelet counts <50,000/mm^3	Interrupt treatment. If platelet counts recovers to >125,000/mm^3 resume treatment with ruxolitinib 20 mg twice daily
	Interrupt treatment. If platelet counts recovers to 100,000–125,000/mm^3, resume treatment with ruxolitinib 15 mg twice daily
	Interrupt treatment. If platelet counts recovers to 75,000–100,000/mm^3, resume treatment with ruxolitinib 10 mg twice daily for at least 2 weeks; if stable, dose may be increased to ruxolitinib 15 mg twice daily
	Interrupt treatment. If platelet counts recovers to >50,000–75,000/mm^3, resume treatment with ruxolitinib 5 mg twice daily for at least 2 weeks; if stable, dose may be increased to ruxolitinib 10 mg twice daily
	Interrupt treatment. If platelet counts remains <50,000/mm^3 continue to hold
No spleen size reduction or symptom improvement >6 months	Discontinue treatment
Concomitant use with strong CYP3A4 inhibitors	Reduce dose to ruxolitinib 10 mg twice daily

*When restarting ruxolitinib treatment, begin with a ruxolitinib dose at least 5 mg twice daily less than the dose given before treatment was interrupted

Efficacy

Verstovsek S et al. N Engl J Med 2012;366:799–807

	Ruxolitinib N = 129–139	Placebo N = 103–106	
Proportion of patients with ≥35% reduction in spleen volume at week 24	41.9%	0.7%	OR 134.4 P <0.001
Mean percent change in spleen volume	−31.6%	+8.1%	
Median percent change in spleen volume	−33.0%	+8.5%	
35% reduction in spleen volume maintained ≥48 weeks	67.0%		
Proportion of patients with ≥50% reduction in total symptom score from baseline to week 24	45.9%	5.3%	OR 15.3 P <0.001
Mean change symptom score from baseline to week 24	−46.1%*	+41.8%*	
Median change symptom score from baseline to week 24	−56.2%*	+14.6%*	P <0.001

Subgroups[†]

≥50% improvement in spleen-related symptoms[‡] with a reduction in spleen volume of ≥35%	62.7%		
≥50% improvement in spleen-related symptoms[‡] with a reduction in spleen volume of <35%	46.9%		
≥50% improvement in non-abdominal symptoms[§] with a reduction in spleen volume of ≥35%	58.6%		
≥50% improvement in non-abdominal symptoms[§] with a reduction in spleen volume of <35%	54.1%		
Mean percent change in spleen volume, patients with JAK2 V617F mutation	−34.6%	+8.1%	P = 0.07 For interaction
Mean percent change in spleen volume, patients without JAK2 V617F mutation	−23.8%	+8.4%	P = 0.07 For interaction
Mean change symptom score from baseline to week 24, patients with JAK2 V617F	−52.6%*	+42.8%*	P = 0.11 For interaction
Mean change symptom score from baseline to week 24, patients without JAK2 V617F	−28.1%*	+37.2%*	P = 0.11 For interaction

Biomarkers[ℰ]

Mean change in JAK2 V617F allele burden at week 24	−10.9%	+3.5%	
Mean change in JAK2 V617F allele burden at week 48	−21.5%	+6.3%	

*Note: −, means improvement in symptoms; +, means worsening of symptoms

[†]Across myelofibrosis subtypes (primary myelofibrosis, postpolycythemia vera myelofibrosis, and postessential thrombocythemia myelofibrosis), patients who received ruxolitinib had a decrease in spleen volume and improvement in the total symptom score; patients receiving placebo had increases in spleen volume (P = 0.52 for interaction) and worsening of the total symptom score (P = 0.46 for interaction)

[‡]As indicated by the sum of Myelofibrosis Symptom Assessment Form (version 2.0) scores for abdominal discomfort, pain under the ribs on the left side, and a feeling of fullness (early satiety)

[§]Night sweats, bone or muscle pain, and pruritus

[ℰ]Patients receiving ruxolitinib also had reductions in plasma levels of C-reactive protein and the proinflammatory cytokines, tumor necrosis factor-α, and interleukin-6, and increases in levels of plasma leptin and erythropoietin

Patient Population Studied

International Prognostic Scoring System—prognostic factors:
1. Age >65 years
2. Hemoglobin level <10 g/dL
3. Leukocyte count of >25,000/mm^3
4. ≥1% circulating myeloblasts
5. Presence of constitutional symptoms

Verstovsek S et al. N Engl J Med 2012;366:799–807

Patients with primary myelofibrosis, postpolycythemia vera myelofibrosis, or postessential thrombocythemia myelofibrosis according to 2008 World Health Organization criteria, with a life expectancy of ≥6 months, an International Prognostic Scoring System (IPSS) score of 2 (intermediate-2 risk) or 3 or more (high risk), an Eastern Cooperative Oncology Group (ECOG) performance status ≤3 (on a scale from 0 to 5, with higher scores indicating greater disability), <10% peripheral blood blasts, an absolute peripheral blood CD34+ cell count >20/mm^3, a platelet count >100,000/mm^3, and palpable splenomegaly (≥5 cm below the left costal margin). Patients had disease that was refractory to available therapies, had side effects requiring their discontinuation, or were not candidates for available therapies and had disease-requiring treatment

Harrison C et al. N Engl J Med 2012;366:787–798

Patients who had primary myelofibrosis, postpolycythemia vera myelofibrosis, or postessential thrombocythemia myelofibrosis and a palpable spleen ≥5 cm below the costal margin, irrespective of their JAK2 V617F mutation status. Eligible patients had 2 prognostic factors (intermediate-2 risk) or ≥3 prognostic factors (high risk) according to the International Prognostic Scoring System, a peripheral blood blast count <10%, a platelet count ≥100,000/mm^3, an ECOG performance status ≤3, and no prior treatment with a JAK inhibitor. In addition, eligible patients were not considered to be suitable candidates for allogeneic stem cell transplantation at the time of enrollment

(continued)

Efficacy (continued)

Harrison C et al. N Engl J Med 2012;366:787–798

	Ruxolitinib N = 149	Best Available N = 73
Proportion of patients with ≥35% reduction in spleen volume at week 24	32%*	0*
Proportion of patients with ≥35% reduction in spleen volume at week 48	28%*	0*
Mean percent change in spleen volume*,†	−29.2%*	+2.7%*
Mean percent change in spleen volume*,†	−30.1%*	+7.3%*
Median time to first observation on MRI or CT of a reduction ≥35% reduction in spleen volume from baseline	12 weeks	
The median duration of response	>12 months (80% at 12 months)	
Progression at 48 weeks	30%	26%
Mean Change from Baseline at 48 Weeks—EORTC QLQ-C30 Core Model Scores‡,§		
Global health status and quality of life§	+9.1	+3.4
Role functioning§	+3.4	−5.4
Mean Change from Baseline at 48 Weeks—EORTC QLQ-C30 Symptom Scores𝄆		
Fatigue𝄆	−12.8	+0.4
Pain𝄆	−1.9	+3.0
Dyspnea𝄆	−6.3	+4.8
Insomnia𝄆	−12.3	+6.0
Appetite loss𝄆	−8.2	+9.5
Mean Change from Baseline at 48 Weeks—FACT-Lym Scores§		
FACT-Lym Total Scores§ (6.5–11.2)**	+11.3	−0.9
FACT-TOI†† Score§ (5.5–11)**	+9.1	−0.9
FACT-G Total Scores§ (3–7)**	+8.9	+0.1
LymS Score§,‡‡ (2.9–5.4)**	+6.0	+0.7
Subgroups		
≥35% reduction in spleen volume at week 24 in patients with JAK2 V617F mutation	33%	0
≥35% reduction in spleen volume at week 24 in patients without JAK2 V617F mutation	14%	0

EORTC, European Organization for Research and Treatment of Cancer; FACT, Functional Assessment of Cancer Therapy; FACT-Lym, FACT–Lymphoma; FACT-TOI, FACT–Trial Outcome Index

*P <0.001
†Note: +, means reduction in size; −, means increase of size
‡For EORTC QLQ-C30 functioning and symptom subscales that are not shown, there were minimal between-group differences (ie, a difference of <10 points in the mean change in scores between the ruxolitinib group and the best-available-therapy (BAT) group at weeks 24 and 48)
§Note: +, means improvement in symptoms; −, means worsening of symptoms
𝄆Note: −, means improvement in symptoms; +, means worsening of symptoms
**The ranges in parentheses represent values for minimal clinically important differences
††FACT-TOI Scores: A summary of physical, functional, and disease-specific outcomes
‡‡FACT-LymS: Disease-specific subscale

Note: Levels of several proinflammatory cytokines, including interleukin-6, tumor necrosis factor-α, and C-reactive protein were reduced, whereas erythropoietin and leptin levels were increased

Therapy Monitoring

1. A complete blood count (CBC) with leukocyte differential and platelet count must be performed before initiating therapy, every 2–4 weeks until doses are stabilized, and then as clinically indicated

2. Renal and liver function tests before starting treatment with ruxolitinib (baseline), with serial reassessment as clinically indicated

Toxicity*

Verstovsek S et al. N Engl J Med 2012;366:799–807

	Ruxolitinib (N = 155)		Placebo (N = 151)	
	% All Grades	% G3/4	% All Grades	% G3/4
Nonhematologic fatigue	25.2	5.2	33.8	6.6
Diarrhea	23.2	1.9	21.2	0
Peripheral edema	18.7	0	22.5	1.3
Bruising†	23.2	0.6	14.6	0
Dyspnea	17.4	1.3	17.2	4.0
Dizziness‡	18.1	0.6	7.3	0
Nausea	14.8	0	19.2	0.7
Headache	14.8	0	5.3	0
Constipation	12.9	0	11.9	0
Vomiting	12.3	0.6	9.9	0.7
Pain in extremity	12.3	1.3	9.9	0
Insomnia	11.6	0	9.9	0
Arthralgia	11.0	1.9	8.6	0.7
Pyrexia	11.0	0.6	7.3	0.7
Abdominal pain	10.3	2.6	41.1	11.3
Weight Gain	7.1	0.6	1.3	0.7
Flatulence	5.2	0	0.7	0
Hematologic Abnormalities				
Anemia§	96.1	45.2	86.8	19.2
Thrombocytopenia§	69.7	12.9	30.5	1.3
Neutropenia§	18.7	7.1	4.0	2.0
↑Alanine transaminase (ALT)	25.2	1.3	7.3	—
↑Aspartate transaminase (AST)	17.4	0	6	—
↑Cholesterol	16.8	0	0.7	—

*National Cancer Institute Common Terminology Criteria for Adverse Events (CTCAE), version 3.0
†Includes contusion, ecchymosis, hematoma, injection site hematoma, periorbital hematoma, vessel puncture site hematoma, increased tendency to bruise, petechiae, purpura
‡Includes dizziness, postural dizziness, vertigo, balance disorder, Meniere disease, labyrinthitis
§Presented as worst-grade values regardless of baseline

Data from Verstovsek et al., and from JAKAFI (ruxolitinib) tablets, for oral use; product label, November 2011. Incyte Corporation, Wilmington, DE

(continued)

Toxicity (*continued*)

Harrison C et al. N Engl J Med 2012;366:787–798

Adverse Event	Ruxolitinib (N = 146)		Best Available Therapy (N = 73)	
	All Grades	G3/4	All Grades	G3/4
	Number of Patients (Percent)			
Nonhematologic				
Diarrhea	34 (23)	2 (1)	9 (12)	0
Peripheral edema	32 (22)	0	19 (26)	0
Asthenia	26 (18)	2 (1)	7 (10)	1 (1)
Dyspnea	23 (16)	1 (1)	13 (18)	3 (4)
Nasopharyngitis	23 (16)	0	10 (14)	0
Pyrexia	20 (14)	3 (2)	7 (10)	0
Cough	20 (14)	0	11 (15)	1 (1)
Nausea	19 (13)	1 (1)	5 (7)	0
Arthralgia	18 (12)	1 (1)	5 (7)	0
Fatigue	18 (12)	1 (1)	6 (8)	0
Pain in extremity	17 (12)	1 (1)	3 (4)	0
Abdominal pain	16 (11)	5 (3)	10 (14)	2 (3)
Headache	15 (10)	2 (1)	3 (4)	0
Back pain	14 (10)	3 (2)	8 (11)	0
Pruritus	7 (5)	0	9 (12)	0

Hematologic	G1	G2	G3	G4	G1	G2	G3	G4
Anemia	24 (16)	55 (38)	50 (34)	12 (8)	16 (23)	28 (40)	15 (21)	7 (10)
Thrombocytopenia	46 (32)	42 (28)	9 (6)	3 (2)	11 (16)	4 (6)	3 (4)	2 (3)

Serious		
Abdominal pain	3 (2)	1 (1)
Pyrexia	3 (2)	1 (1)
Esophageal varices	3 (2)	0
Dyspnea	2 (1)	3 (4)
Pneumonia	1 (1)	4 (5)
Actinic keratosis	0	2 (3)
Ascites	0	2 (3)
Peritoneal hemorrhage	0	2 (3)
Respiratory failure	0	2 (3)

67. Myelodysplastic Syndromes

Michael M. Boyiadzis, MD, MHSc and Neal S. Young, MD

Myelodysplastic syndromes (MDSs) are clonal disorders characterized initially by ineffective hematopoiesis and subsequently by the development of acute leukemias. Peripheral blood cytopenias in combination with a hypercellular bone marrow exhibiting dysplastic changes are the hallmark of MDS

Epidemiology

Incidence: Increases with Age

Mean age: 68 years	Male-to-female ratio: 1:1
Overall:	4.1 per 100,000
Ages 50–59 years:	0.3 per 100,000
Ages 60–69 years:	15 per 100,000
Ages 70–79 years:	49 per 100,000
Ages >80 years:	89 per 100,000

Dunbar CE, Saunthararajah Y. Myelodysplastic syndromes. In: Young NS, ed. Bone Marrow Failure Syndromes. Philadelphia, PA: WB Saunders; 2000:69–98 Greenberg P et al. Blood 1997;89:2079–2088. Erratum in: Blood 1998;91:1100. Comment in: Blood 1997;90:2843–2846, Blood 2001;98:1985

Work-up

CBC with differential
Serum liver function tests, electrolytes, serum creatinine
Bone marrow biopsy and aspiration with iron stains, flow cytometry, cytogenetics
HLA typing for patients who are candidates for allogeneic stem cell transplantation
RBC folate, serum B_{12}, serum iron/TIBC/ferritin, serum erythropoietin level (prior to RBC transfusion)
HIV testing if clinically indicated
Thyroid function tests to rule out hypothyroidism
HLA-DR15 typing to assist determination of response to immunosuppressive therapy
Evaluate patients with chronic myelomonocytic leukemia (CMML) for 5q31–33 translocations and/or PDGFRβ gene rearrangements
JAK2 mutation in patients with thrombocytosis

Frequent Chromosomal Aberrations in MDS

Numerical		Translocations		Deletions	
Cytogenetics	(%)	Cytogenetics	(%)	Cytogenetics	(%)
+ 8	19	inv 3	7	del 5q	27
−7	15	t (1;7)	2	del 11q	7
+21	7	t (1;3)	1	del 12q	5
−5	7	t (3;3)	1	del 20q	5
		t (6;9)	<1	del 7q	4
		t (5;12)	<1	del 13q	2

−, Loss of chromosome; +, additional chromosome; inv, inversion; t, translocation; del, deletion
• Clonal cytogenetic abnormalities: 30–79%
• Deletions are more frequent than translocations

Classification Systems for MDS

French-American-British Classification of MDS

FAB Subtype	% of Bone Marrow Blasts	% of Peripheral Blasts
Refractory anemia (RA)	<1	<5
Refractory anemia with ringed sideroblasts (RARS)	<1	<5
Refractory anemia with excess blasts (RAEB)	<5	5–20
Refractory anemia with excess blasts in transformation (REAB-t)	≥5	21–30
Chronic myelomonocytic leukemia (CMML) (>1000 monocytes/μL blood)	<5	5–20

Bennett JM et al. Proposals for the classification of the myelodysplastic syndromes. Br J Haematol 1982;51:189–199

2008 World Health Organization Classification of MDS

Subtype	Blood	Bone Marrow
Refractory cytopenia with unilineage dysplasia (RCUD)*	Single or bicytopenia	Dysplasia in ≥10% of 1 cell line, <5% blasts
Refractory anemia with ring sideroblasts (RARS)	Anemia, no blasts	≥15% of erythroid precursors w/ring sideroblasts, erythroid dysplasia only, <5% blasts
Refractory cytopenia with multilineage dysplasia (RCMD)	Cytopenias, monocytes <1000/μL	Dysplasia in ≥10% of cells in ≥2 hematopoietic lineages, ±15% ring sideroblasts, <5% blasts
Refractory anemia with excess blasts-1 (RAEB-1)	Cytopenias, ≤2–4% blasts, monocytes <1000/μL	Unilineage or multilineage dysplasia, no Auer rods, 5–9%
Refractory anemia with excess blasts-2 (RAEB-2)	Cytopenias, 5–19% blasts, monocytes <1000/μL	Unilineage or multilineage dysplasia, No Auer rods ±10–9% blasts
Myelodysplastic syndrome, unclassified (MDS-U)	Cytopenias	Unilineage dysplasia or no dysplasia but characteristic MDS cytogenetics, <5% blasts
MDS associated with isolated del (5q)	Anemia, platelets normal or increased	Unilineage erythroid dysplasia, isolated del (5q), <5% blasts

*This category encompasses refractory anemia (RA), refractory neutropenia (RN), and refractory thrombocytopenia (RT)

Swerdlow SH, Campo E, Harris NL et al. In: World Health Organization Classification of Tumours of Haematopoietic and Lymphoid tissue. 4th ed. Lyon, France: International Agency for Research on Cancer, 2008.

Classification Systems for De Novo MDS

International Prognostic Scoring System (IPSS)

Survival and AML Evolution

Prognostic Variable	Score Value				
	0	**0.5**	**1.0**	**1.5**	**2.0**
Marrow blasts (%)	<5	5–10	—	11–20	21–30
Karyotype*	Good	Intermediate	Poor		
Cytopenia†	0/1	2/3			

Risk Category (% IPSS Pop.)	Overall Score	Median Survival (Years) in the Absence of Therapy	25% AML Progression (Years) in the Absence of Therapy
LOW (33)	0	5.7	9.4
INT-1 (38)	0.5–1.0	3.5	3.3
INT-2 (22)	1.5–2.0	1.1	1.1
HIGH (7)	≥2.5	0.4	0.2

*Cytogenetics:
Good = normal, −Y alone, del (5q) alone, del (20q) alone
Poor = complex (≥3 abnormalities) or chromosome 7 anomalies
Intermediate = other abnormalities
Note: Categorization excludes karyotypes t(8;21), inv 16, and t(15;17), which are considered to be AML not MDS
†Cytopenias: neutrophil count <1800/μL, platelets <100,000/μL, Hb<10 g/dL

Greenberg P et al. Blood 1997;89:2079–2088. Erratum in: Blood 1998;91:1100. Comment in: Blood 1997;90: 2843–2846, Blood 2001;98:1985

IPSS-R, Revised International Prognostic Scoring System

Prognostic Variable	0	0.5	1	1.5	2	3	4
Cytogenetics*	Very good	—	Good	—	Intermediate	Poor	Very poor
BM blast, %	≤2	—	>2% to <5%	—	5%–10%	>10%	—
Hemoglobin	≥10	—	8 to <10	<8	—	—	—
Platelets	≥100	50 to <100	<50	—	—	—	—
ANC	≥0.8	<0.8	—	—	—	—	—

—, Indicates not applicable
*Cytogenetics:
Very good = −Y, del(11q)
Good = normal, del(5q), del(12p), del(20q), double including del(5q)
Intermediate = del(7q), +8, +19, i(17q), any other single or double independent clones
Poor = −7, inv(3)/t(3q)/del(3q), double including −7/del(7q), complex: 3 abnormalities
Very poor = complex >3 abnormalities

(*continued*)

Differential Diagnosis of Hypo-Productive Cytopenias

Hematologic Conditions	Nonhematologic Conditions
1. Congenital Hereditary sideroblastic anemia Congenital dyserythropoietic anemia Fanconi anemia Diamond-Blackfan syndrome Shwachman syndrome Kostmann syndrome 2. Nutritional Vitamin B₁₂ deficiency Folate deficiency Iron deficiency 3. Aplastic anemia 4. Paroxysmal nocturnal hemoglobinuria 5. Systemic mastocytosis 6. Hairy cell leukemia 7. Large granular lymphocyte disease 8. Myeloproliferative neoplasms Idiopathic myelofibrosis Polycythemia vera Chronic myelogenous leukemia Essential thrombocytosis	1. Toxins Alcohol Postchemotherapy or radiation Medications 2. Chronic diseases Renal failure Collagen-vascular diseases Chronic infections 3. Viral infections Parvovirus B19 Cytomegalovirus Human immunodeficiency virus 4. Malignancy Marrow infiltration Paraneoplastic syndrome

Classification Systems for De Novo MDS (continued)

Risk Category	Risk Score
Very low	≤1.5
Low	>1.5–3
Intermediate	>3–4.5
High	>4.5–6
Very high	>6

	Very Low	Low	Intermediate	High	Very High
Median survival, years	8.8	5.3	3.0	1.6	0.8
	(7.8–9.9)	(5.1–5.7)	(2.7–3.3)	(1.5–1.7)	(0.7–0.8)
25% AML progression, years	NR	10.8	3.2	1.4	0.73
	(14.5–NR)	(9.2–NR)	(2.8–4.4)	(1.1–1.7)	(0.7–0.9)

NR, not reached

Greenberg PL et al. Blood 2012;120:245–2465

WHO–based Prognostic Scoring System (WPSS)

	Variable Scores			
Variable	0	1	2	3
WHO category	RCUD, RARS, MDS, with isolated deletion (5q)	RCMD	RAEB-1	RAEB-2
Karyotype*	Good	Intermediate	Poor	—
Severe anemia (Hb <9 g/dL in males or <8 g/dL in females)	Absent	Present	—	—

WPSS Risk	Sum of Individual Variable Scores
Very low	0
Low	1
Intermediate	2
High	3–4
Very high	5–6

*Cytogenetics:
Good = normal, −Y alone, del (5q) alone, del (20q) alone
Poor = complex (≥3 abnormalities) or chromosome 7 anomalies
Intermediate = other abnormalities

Malcovati L et al. Hematologica 2011;95:1433–1440

International Working Group Treatment Response Criteria for MDS

Cheson BD et al. Blood 2000;96:3671–3674

Complete remission (CR)	• <5% myeloblasts with normal maturation of all cell lines • No evidence of dysplasia • Hemoglobin >11 g/dL (untranfused; patient not on cytokine support) • Neutrophils ≥1500/µL (patient not on cytokine support) • Platelets ≥100,000/µL (patient not on cytokine support)	
Partial remission (PR)	Same as CR except blast decreased by 50% or more over pretreatment	
Stable disease	Failure to achieve at least PR, but without evidence of progression for at least 2 months	

Hematologic Improvement

Erythroid Response

Major	Pretreatment hemoglobin <11 g/dL	>2 g/dL increase in hemoglobin
	RBC transfusion-dependent patients	Transfusion independence
Minor	Pretreatment hemoglobin <11 g/dL	1–2 g/dL increase in hemoglobin
	RBC transfusion-dependent patients	50% decrease in transfusion requirement

Platelet Response

Major	Pretreatment platelet count <100,000/µL	Absolute increase of ≥30,000/µL in platelet count
	Platelet transfusion-dependent patients	Stabilization of platelet counts and transfusion independence
Minor	Pretreatment platelet count <100,000/µL	≥50% increase in platelet count with a net increase of 10,000/µL–30,000/µL

Neutrophil Response (ANC = Absolute Neutrophil Count)

Major	Pretreatment ANC <1500/µL	≥100% increase in ANC, or an absolute increase of >500/µL whichever is greater
Minor	Pretreatment ANC <1500/µL	≥100% increase in ANC, but absolute increase <500/µL

Cytogenetic Response

Major	No detectable cytogenetic abnormality, if preexisting abnormality was present
Minor	50% or more reduction in abnormal metaphases

Treatment Options

IPSS: low/intermediate-1
WPSS: very low, low, intermediate

Patients with symptomatic anemia and del(5q) chromosomal abnormalities should receive lenalidomide. Other patients with anemia can be treated based on their levels of serum erythropoietin (sEPO). Those with levels of ≤500 mU/mL (≤500 IU/L) may be treated with recombinant human epoetin alfa or darbepoetin alfa either with or without granulocyte colony-stimulating factor. Patients with IPSS low or intermediate-1 risk, with moderate-to-severe anemia (hemoglobin below 10 g/dL), serum erythropoietin level <500 mU/mL and/or a red cell transfusion requirement <2 RBC unit per month should be considered for therapy with epoetin alfa or beta at an initial dose ranging from 30,000 to 60,000 IU/week. Patients who do not respond to epoetin alone after 8 weeks of treatment should be given granulocyte-colony stimulating factor (G-CSF 300 μg/week in 2–3 divided doses) in combination with epoetin alfa

Nonresponders should be considered for immunosuppressive therapy with equine thymocyte immune globulin (ATG; ATGAM) and cyclosporine (if there is a high likelihood of response: ≤60 years old, HLA-DR15–positive, PNH-positive clone, or hypoplastic MDS), or treatment with decitabine or azacitidine. Anemic patients with sEPO levels >500 mU/mL who have a low probability to respond to immunosuppressive therapy should be considered for treatment with lenalidomide, decitabine, or azacitidine

Patients with other serious cytopenias (thrombocytopenia, neutropenia) should be considered for treatment with decitabine or azacitidine. Nonresponders should be considered for immunosuppressive therapy with ATG and cyclosporine or allogeneic hematopoietic cell transplantation (allo-HCT)

IPSS: intermediate-2, high
WPSS: high, very high

Allogeneic HCT is the only treatment that can induce long-term remission in patients with MDS. Such therapy, however, is not applicable for many patients, because the median age at diagnosis exceeds 65 years and associated comorbidities. Allo-HCT for MDS is associated with a high rate of treatment-related death (approximately 30% at 1 year and 3 years) and suboptimal disease-free survival (approximately 40% at 1 year and 3 years). The decision to offer HCT as therapy for MDS remains an individual "personalized" decision. Age at transplantation is one of the most important prognostic factors: the older the age, the shorter the overall and disease-free survival. In addition, disease risk according to the IPSS and presence of comorbid disease are among the most relevant clinical variables to be considered in order to judge a patient's eligibility for allo-HCT

The optimal timing of myeloablative allo-HCT from HLA identical siblings was studied in patients <60 years of age. Low and intermediate-1 IPSS groups, delayed transplantation maximized overall survival. Transplantation prior to leukemic transformation was associated with a greater number of life years than transplantation at the time of leukemic progression. For intermediate-2 and high IPSS groups, transplantation at diagnosis maximized overall survival. Also, the use of reduced intensity conditioning allo-HCT regimens in de novo MDS was examined in patients aged 60-70 years. For patients with low/intermediate-1 IPSS MDS, reduced-intensity conditioning transplantation life expectancy was 38 months versus 77 months with non-transplantation approaches. For intermediate-2/high IPSS MDS, reduced-intensity conditioning transplantation life expectancy was 36 months versus 28 months for non-transplantation therapies. The study concluded that for low/intermediate-1 IPSS, non-transplantation approaches are preferred. For intermediate-2/high IPSS, reduced intensity conditioning transplantation offers overall and quality-adjusted survival benefit

For patients who are candidates for transplantation, the first choice of a donor is a HLA matched sibling, although results with HLA-matched unrelated donors have improved to levels comparable to those obtained with HLA-matched siblings. Consider intensive chemotherapy for patients who are eligible for intensive therapy but lack a stem cell donor, or those whose marrow blast count requires reduction. Patients who are not candidates for allo-HCT should receive supportive care and therapies similar to low-risk patients

Cutler CS et al. Blood 2004;104:579–585
Koreth J et al. J Clin Oncol 2013;31:2662–2670
Hellström-Lindberg E et al. Br J Haematol 1997;99:344–351
Hellström-Lindberg E et al. Br J Haematol 2003;120:1037–1046
Malcovati L et al. Blood 2013;122:2943–2964

Supportive Care

Hematopoietic cytokine support should be considered for patients with refractory symptomatic cytopenias

Aminocaproic acid and other antifibrinolytic agents may be used for bleeding episodes refractory to platelet transfusions or for profound thrombocytopenia

For patients with chronic RBC transfusion needs, serum ferritin levels and associated organ dysfunction should be monitored. Iron chelation therapy should also be considered in patients with MDS who have life expectancy of at least several years and have received at least 20 units of RBCs over 1 year or more, serum ferritin level persistently ≥1000 μg/L, clinically relevant iron overload or if allogeneic hematopoietic cell transplantation is planned

Symptomatic anemic patients should receive red blood cell transfusions (using leukocyte-poor products) and for potential allogeneic hematopoietic cell transplantation candidates CMV-negative (for patients who are serologically CMV-negative) and irradiated transfused blood products

Iron depletion needs to be verified before instituting epoetin alfa or darbepoetin alfa therapy. If no response occurs with these agents alone, the addition of a granulocyte colony-stimulating factor (G-CSF) should be considered. G-CSF, and, to a lesser extent, granulocyte-macrophage colony-stimulating factor (GM-CSF) have synergistic erythropoietic activity when used in combination with erythropoiesis stimulating agents and markedly enhance erythroid responses. A predictive model for response to epoetin alfa or beta and G-CSF in MDS patients was developed and validated in prospective studies. Three groups of patients were identified (high probability of response group, intermediate, and poor) based on serum erythropoietin levels (<500 mU/mL or ≥500 mU/mL) and transfusion needs (<2 RBC units/month or ≥2 RBC units/month) with response rates according to study response criteria to treatment of 74%, 23% and 7%

Greenberg P et al. Blood 1997;89:2079–2088.
Erratum in: Blood 1998;91:1100. Comment in: Blood 1997;90:2843–2846, Blood 2001;98:1985
Greenberg PL. Br J Haematol 2010;150:131–143
Hellström-Lindberg E et al. Br J Haematol 1997;99:344–351
Hellström-Lindberg E et al. Br J Haematol 2003;120:1037–1046
Malcovati L et al. Blood 2013;122:2943–2964
Steensma DP. J Natl Compr Canc Netw 2011;9:65–75
Tefferi A, Vardiman JW. N Engl J Med 2009;361:1872–1885

REGIMEN
DECITABINE

Kantarjian H et al. Blood 2007;109:52–57
Kantarjian H et al. Cancer 2006;106:1794–1803
Steensma DP et al. J Clin Oncol 2009;27:3842–3848

Decitabine 20 mg/m^2 per day; administer intravenously in a volume of cold* 0.9% sodium chloride injection (0.9% NS), 5% dextrose injection (D5W), or lactated Ringer's injection (LRI) sufficient to result in a solution concentration within the range of 0.1–1 mg/mL, over 60 minutes for 5 consecutive days, on days 1–5, every 4 weeks (total dosage per 5-day course = 100 mg/m^2)

or

Decitabine 15 mg/m^2 per dose; administer intravenously in a volume of cold* 0.9% NS, D5W, or LRI sufficient to result in a solution concentration within the range of 0.1–1 mg/mL, over 3 hours, every 8 hours for 3 consecutive days (total dosage/day = 45 mg/m^2; total dosage/3-day course = 135 mg/m^2)

• Patients should receive either regimen for a minimum of 4 cycles; however, it may take longer than 4 cycles to achieve a complete or partial response

*Cold vehicle solutions must be used if a decitabine product will not be used within 15 minutes after preparation is completed. See Chapter 40 for more information

Supportive Care
Antiemetic prophylaxis
Emetogenic potential is **MINIMAL**
See Chapter 39 for antiemetic recommendations

Hematopoietic growth factor (CSF) prophylaxis
Primary prophylaxis may be indicated for patients with refractory symptomatic cytopenias
See Chapter 43 for more information

Antimicrobial prophylaxis
Risk of fever and neutropenia is HIGH
Antimicrobial primary prophylaxis is recommended:
• Antibacterial—consider fluoroquinolone prophylaxis; *P. jirovecii* prophylaxis is recommended (eg, cotrimoxazole)
• Antifungal—recommended
• Antiviral—antiherpes antivirals (eg, acyclovir, famciclovir, valacyclovir)
See Chapter 47 for more information

Patient Population Studied

Ninety-nine patients with MDS (median age: 72 years; range: 34–87 years) including IPPS risk groups: high (24%), intermediate-2 (32%), intermediate-1 (28%), and low (4%). FAB classifications: RA plus RARS (37%), RAEB plus RAEB-T (52%), CMML (11%). At baseline, 67% of patients were RBC-transfusion dependent and 15% were platelet transfusion dependent

Efficacy

Response by 2006 IWG Criteria	ITT (N = 99) %
Overall complete response rate, CR + mCR	32
Overall response rate, CR + mCR + PR	32
Overall improvement rate, CR + mCR + PR + HI	51
Rate of stable disease or better, CR + mCR + PR + HI + SD	75
CR	17
mCR	15
PR	0
HI	18
SD	24
PD	10
	15

IWG, International Working Group; ITT, intention to treat; CR, complete response; mCR, marrow CR; PR, partial response; HI, hematologic improvement; SD, stable disease; PD, progressive disease

Activity was demonstrated across investigator-assessed IPSS risk groups, with an overall improvement rate of 50% for intermediate-1 patients, 61% for intermediate-2 patients, and 43% for high-risk patients
The 1-year survival rate for patients treated with decitabine was 66%. Median survival was 19.4 months. Patients who were classified as having CMML (n = 11) had a 73% improvement rate. Among 66 patients who were RBC transfusion-dependent at baseline, 22 patients (33%) became RBC transfusion-independent during the study. Of the 15 patients who were platelet transfusion-dependent at baseline, 6 patients (40%) became transfusion-independent during the course of the study

Adverse Effects

Event	% of Patients Grades 1–2	Grades ≥3
Hematologic		
Neutropenia	1	31
Thrombocytopenia	2	18
Febrile neutropenia	3	14
Anemia	5	12
Nonhematologic		
Fatigue	26	5
Nausea	26	1
Pyrexia	17	0
Diarrhea	12	0
Anorexia	12	0
Constipation	11	0
Pneumonia	1	11
Vomiting	10	1
Chills	10	0

Of the 619 cycles administered, 198 (32%) were delayed, primarily because of myelosuppression, with a median delay of 8 days, and there were 119 hospitalizations (19% of cycles were associated with a hospitalization)
Eleven patients (11%) died within 30 days after receiving decitabine

Treatment Modifications

REGIMEN 1: Decitabine 20 mg/m² per day; administer intravenously over 60 minutes, once daily for 5 consecutive, days 1–5, every 4 weeks (100 mg/m² per 5-day course)

Hematologic Adverse Effects

Cycles ≥ 2 (4-week cycles):

Day 1 ANC ≥1000/μL and platelets ≥50,000/μL	Begin a new treatment cycle at the same decitabine dosage and schedule previously given
Day 1 ANC <1000/μL or platelets <50,000/μL	Delay treatment and continually monitor ANC and platelet counts until recovery to ANC ≥1000/μL and platelets ≥50,000/μL, *then:* Begin a new treatment cycle at the same decitabine dosage and schedule previously given

Nonhematologic Adverse Effects

Cycles ≥ 2, for: • Serum creatinine ≥2 mg/dL (≥177 μmol/L) • Serum ALT (SGPT) or total bilirubin ≥2 times ULN • Active or uncontrolled infection	Withhold decitabine treatment until the toxicity is resolved, *then* Begin a new treatment cycle at the same decitabine dosage and schedule previously given

REGIMEN 2: Decitabine 15 mg/m² per dose; administer intravenously over 3 hours, every 8 hours for 3 consecutive days, days 1–3 (45 mg/m² per day; 135 mg/m² per 3-day course)

Hematologic Adverse Effects

Cycles ≥ 2, 4 weeks after a previous cycle:

If ANC ≥1000/μL and platelets ≥50,000/μL	Begin a new treatment cycle at the same decitabine dosage and schedule previously given
If ANC <1000/μL or platelets <50,000/μL	Delay treatment for up to 6 weeks after the last cycle began, and continually monitor ANC and platelet counts

Cycles ≥ 2, 6–8 weeks after a previous cycle:

Recovery to ANC ≥1000/μL and platelets ≥50,000/μL requiring >6 weeks, but <8 weeks	Delay treatment for up to 8 weeks after the last cycle began until ANC ≥1000/μL and platelets ≥50,000/μL, *then* Begin a new treatment cycle with decitabine dosage decreased to 11 mg/m² per dose every 8 hours for 3 consecutive days (33 mg/m² per day; 99 mg/m² per 3-day course)
If ANC <1000/μL or platelets <50,000/μL	Delay treatment for up to 10 weeks after the last cycle began, and continually monitor ANC and platelet counts

Cycles ≥ 2, 8–10 weeks after a previous cycle:

Recovery to ANC ≥1000/μL and platelets ≥50,000/μL requiring >8 weeks, but <10 weeks	1. Delay treatment for up to 8 weeks after the last cycle began until ANC ≥1000/μL and platelets ≥50,000/μL 2. Evaluate bone marrow (BM) aspirate for evidence of disease progression (PD). If BM aspirate is negative for PD, *then:* 3. Begin a new treatment cycle with decitabine dosage decreased to 11 mg/m² per dose every 8 hours for 3 consecutive days (33 mg/m² per day; 99 mg/m² per 3-day course) 4. Maintain or increase decitabine dosage during subsequent cycles as clinically indicated

Nonhematologic Adverse Effects

Cycles ≥ 2, for: • Serum creatinine ≥2 mg/dL (≥177 μmol/L) • Serum ALT (SGPT) or total bilirubin ≥2 times ULN • Active or uncontrolled infection	Withhold decitabine treatment until the toxicity is resolved, *then* Begin a new treatment cycle at the same decitabine dosage and schedule previously given

Therapy Monitoring

1. Complete blood counts, leukocyte differential, and platelet counts should be performed as needed to monitor response and toxicity; that is, at least once weekly
2. Consider bone marrow biopsy every 2 cycles until CR is confirmed
3. Liver chemistries and serum creatinine should be obtained prior to initiation of treatment

Notes

Decitabine is indicated for treatment of patients with myelodysplastic syndromes (MDS) including previously treated and untreated, de novo and secondary MDS of all French-American-British subtypes (refractory anemia, refractory anemia with ringed sideroblasts, refractory anemia with excess blasts, refractory anemia with excess blasts in transformation, and chronic myelomonocytic leukemia) and intermediate-1, intermediate-2, and high-risk International Prognostic Scoring System groups

REGIMEN

AZACITIDINE

Silverman LR et al. J Clin Oncol 2006;24:3895–3903
Silverman LR et al. J Clin Oncol 2002;20:2429–2440

Azacitidine 75 mg/m² per day; administer either by subcutaneous injection or intravenously for 7 consecutive days, days 1–7, every 4 weeks (total dosage/cycle = 525 mg/m²)

- If a beneficial effect is not seen after 2 cycles are completed and no adverse effects other than nausea and vomiting have occurred, dosage may be increased to **azacitidine** 100 mg/m² per day for 7 consecutive days, days 1–7, every 4 weeks (total dosage/cycle = 700 mg/m²)
- Patients should receive treatment for a minimum of 4–6 cycles; however, it may take longer than 4 cycles to achieve a complete or partial response
  - Treatment may be continued as long as a patient continues to benefit

Administration by subcutaneous injection
- Azacitidine is reconstituted to obtain a solution with concentration equal to 100 mg/mL
- Doses >100 mg (>4 mL) should be equally divided into 2 (or more) syringes and injected into 2 (or more) separate sites
- Rotate sites for each injection (thigh, abdomen, or upper arm)
- New injections should be given at least 1 inch from an old site and never into areas where the site is tender, bruised, red, or hard

Intravenous administration
- Azacitidine is diluted in 50–100 mL 0.9% sodium chloride injection or lactated Ringer's injection
- Administer a dose over 10–40 minutes. Dose administration must be completed within 60 minutes after product preparation

Supportive Care
Antiemetic prophylaxis
Emetogenic potential is MODERATE
See Chapter 39 for antiemetic recommendations

Hematopoietic growth factor (CSF) prophylaxis
Primary prophylaxis may be indicated for patients with refractory symptomatic cytopenias

Antimicrobial prophylaxis
Risk of fever and neutropenia is HIGH
  Antimicrobial primary prophylaxis is recommended:
  - Antibacterial—*P. jirovecii* prophylaxis is recommended (eg, cotrimoxazole)
  - Antifungal—recommended
  - Antiviral—antiherpes antivirals (eg, acyclovir, famciclovir, valacyclovir)
See Chapter 47 for more information

Patient Population Studied

In the Cancer and Leukemia Group B (CALGB) Protocols 8421, 8921, and 9221, 268 patients were treated with azacitidine, of whom 220 were treated with subcutaneous azacitidine and 48 were treated with intravenous azacitidine; 41 patients received best supportive care on the observation arm of Protocol 9221

Efficacy

Best Response for All Patients Using IWG Response Criteria for MDS in Protocols 8421, 8921, and 9221

| IWG Response | Protocol 8421: IV Azacitidine (n = 48) % | Protocol 8921: SC Azacitidine (n = 70) % | Protocol 9221 | | | Protocols 8921 and 9221: SC Azacitidine (n = 169) % |
			SC Azacitidine* (n = 99) %	Observation Only† (n = 41) %	SC Azacitidine After Observation (n = 51) %	
CR	15	17	10	0	6	13
PR	2	0	1	0	4	1
HI‡	27	23	36	17	25	31
Erythroid response, major	21	16	22	2	16	20
Erythroid response, minor	4	4	8	10	8	7
Platelet response, major	19	9	21	5	6	16
Platelet response, minor	0	3	3	0	2	3
Neutrophil response, major	4	0	8	2	4	5
Neutrophil response, minor	0	0	0	0	0	0
Overall: CR + PR + HI‡	44	40	47	17	35	44

IWG, International Working Group; MDS, myelodysplastic syndrome; IV, intravenous; SC, subcutaneous; CR, complete remission; PR, partial remission; HI, hematologic improvement
*Patients randomly assigned to azacitidine
†Patients randomly assigned to observation who did not cross over to azacitidine
‡Patients with HI (major or minor) were counted only once in the overall response

(continued)

Efficacy (continued)

Summary of Hematology Shifts by Maximum NCI CTC Grade Criteria (Hematology) in Protocol 9221

Maximum NCI CTC Grade Baseline Value	Post-baseline* Maximum NCI CTC Grade			
	All Azacitidine Patients[†] (n = 150)			
	No. of Patients	Grades 0–2 %	Grade 3 %	Grade 4 %
Hemoglobin				
Grades 0–2	105	26	59	15
Grade 3	29	7	59	35
Grade 4	9	0	33	67
WBCs				
Grades 0–2	117	42	40	18
Grade 3	27	0	33	67
Grade 4	5	0	0	100
Absolute neutrophil count				
Grades 0–2	66	18	17	65
Grade 3	22	9	0	91
Grade 4	23	9	4	87
Lymphocytes				
Grades 0–2	71	32	44	24
Grade 3	28	0	46	54
Grade 4	9	11	22	67
Platelets				
Grades 0–2	80	43	24	34
Grade 3	34	0	21	79
Grade 4	24	0	0	100

NCI CTC, National Cancer Institute Common Toxicity Criteria
*Post-baseline toxicity grade is the maximum grade after baseline and before the end of study
[†]Includes all patients exposed to azacitidine, including patients who crossed over to azacitidine from observation
Note: The number (n) for each treatment group is the number of patients with a baseline toxicity grade and at least 1 post-baseline toxicity grade

Treatment Modifications

For patients with baseline (start of treatment) WBC ≥3000/μL, ANC ≥1500/μL, and platelets ≥75,000/μL, adjust the dose as follows, based on nadir counts for any given cycle:

Nadir Counts		% Dose During the Next Course
ANC (/μL)	Platelets (/μL)	
<500	<25,000	50%
500–1500	25,000–50,000	67%
>1500	>50,000	100%

For patients whose baseline counts are WBC <3000/μL, ANC <1500/μL, or platelets <75,000/μL, dose adjustments should be based on nadir counts and bone marrow biopsy cellularity at the time of the nadir as noted below, unless there is clear improvement in differentiation (percentage of mature granulocytes is higher and ANC is higher than at the onset of that course) at the time of the next cycle, in which case the dose of the current treatment should be continued

WBC or Platelet Nadir % Decrease in Counts from Baseline	Bone Marrow Biopsy Cellularity at Time of Nadir (%)		
	30–60	15–30	<115
	% Dosage During the Next Course		
50–75	100	50	33
>75	75	50	33

- If a nadir has occurred as defined in the table above, the next course of treatment should be given 28 days after the start of the preceding course, provided that both the WBC and platelet counts are >25% above the nadir and rising
- If a >25% increase above the nadir is not seen by day 28, counts should be reassessed every 7 days
- If a 25% increase is not seen by day 42, then the patient should be treated with 50% of the scheduled dose

Toxicity

Most Frequently* Observed Adverse Events (NCI CTC Grades 1–4) by Patient-Years of Exposure in Protocol 9221

Adverse Event‡	All Azacitidine Patients† (n = 150)	
	Patients With Events Per Patient-Year of Exposure§	No. of Patients
Total exposure, patient-years	138.2	
At least 1 adverse event	1.09	150
Anemia NOS	0.77	107
Thrombocytopenia	0.74	102
Nausea	0.72	100
Pyrexia	0.56	77
Leukopenia NOS	0.55	76
Vomiting NOS	0.52	72
Fatigue	0.42	56
Constipation	0.42	58
Diarrhea NOS	0.39	54
Neutropenia	0.37	51
Injection site erythema	0.35	49
Cough	0.34	47
Dyspnea NOS	0.34	47
Ecchymosis	0.32	44
Weakness	0.32	44
Rigors	0.28	39
Injection site pain	0.26	36
Arthralgia	0.26	36
Headache NOS	0.25	34
Pain in limb	0.25	34
Anorexia	0.23	32
Pharyngitis	0.23	32
Contusion	0.22	31

NCI CTC, National Cancer Institute Common Toxicity Criteria; NOS, not otherwise specified
*More than or equal to 20.0% frequency
†Includes all patients exposed to azacitidine, including patients who crossed over to azacitidine from observation
‡Multiple reports of the same adverse event term for a patient are only counted once within each treatment group
§Total exposure for azacitidine is the cumulative time from the first dose to the end of study (30 days after last dose), and for observation, total exposure is the cumulative time from random assignment to withdrawal from study or day before cross over

Among the 150 patients treated, infections was the cause of death in 3 patients (2%)

Therapy Monitoring

1. Complete blood counts, leukocyte differential, and platelet count should be performed as needed to monitor response and toxicity; that is, at least once weekly
2. Consider bone marrow biopsy every 2 cycles until CR is confirmed
3. Serum liver chemistries and creatinine should be obtained prior to initiation of treatment

Notes

Azacitidine is a nucleoside metabolic inhibitor indicated for the treatment of patients with the following FAB myelodysplastic syndrome (MDS) subtypes: refractory anemia (RA) or refractory anemia with ringed sideroblasts (RARS; if accompanied by neutropenia or thrombocytopenia or requiring transfusions), refractory anemia with excess blasts (RAEB), refractory anemia with excess blasts in transformation (RAEB-T), and chronic myelomonocytic leukemia (CMMoL)

In a phase III, international, multicenter, controlled, parallel-group, open-label trial, patients with high-risk myelodysplastic syndromes were randomly assigned, one-to-one, to receive azacitidine (75 mg/m² per day by subcutaneous injection for 7 days every 28 days) or conventional care (best supportive care, low-dose cytarabine, or intensive chemotherapy as selected by investigators before randomization)

In the study, 358 patients were randomly assigned to receive azacitidine (n = 179) or conventional care regimens (n = 179). After a median follow-up of 21.1 months (IQR 15.1–26.9), median overall survival was 24.5 months (9.9; not reached) for the azacitidine group versus 15 months (5.6–24.1) for the conventional care group (hazard ratio 0.58; 95% CI, 0.43–0.77; stratified log-rank p = 0.0001). At last follow-up, 82 patients in the azacitidine group had died, compared with 113 patients in the conventional care group

At 2 years, on the basis of Kaplan-Meier estimates, 50.8% (95% CI, 42.1–58.8) of patients in the azacitidine group were alive compared with 26.2% (18.7–34.3) in the conventional care group (p <0.0001) Peripheral cytopenias were the most common grade 3–4 adverse events for all treatments

Fenaux P et al. Lancet Oncol 2009;10:223–232

REGIMEN

LENALIDOMIDE

List A et al. N Engl J Med 2006;355:1456–1465

Lenalidomide 10 mg per day; administer orally, continually (total dose/week = 70 mg)

Supportive Care
Antiemetic prophylaxis
*Emetogenic potential is **MINIMAL–LOW***
See Chapter 39 for antiemetic recommendations

Hematopoietic growth factor (CSF) prophylaxis
Primary prophylaxis may be indicated for patients with refractory symptomatic cytopenias
See Chapter 43 for more information

Antimicrobial prophylaxis
Risk of fever and neutropenia is HIGH
Antimicrobial primary prophylaxis is recommended:
- Antibacterial—*P. jirovecii* prophylaxis is recommended (eg, cotrimoxazole)
- Antifungal—recommended
- Antiviral—antiherpes antivirals (eg, acyclovir, famciclovir, valacyclovir)

See Chapter 47 for more information

Patient Population Studied

A study of 148 patients with MDS who were treated with lenalidomide, of whom 46 were treated on the 21-day schedule and 102 received continuous daily dosing. Of the patients, 64% had either refractory anemia or refractory anemia with ringed sideroblasts, and 81% were at low or intermediate-1 risk according to the IPSS scores

Treatment Modifications

Dose Adjustments for Hematologic Toxicities During MDS Treatment

Platelet Counts

If thrombocytopenia develops WITHIN 4 weeks of starting treatment at 10 mg daily in MDS

If baseline ≥100,000/μL

When Platelets	Recommended Course
Fall to <50,000/μL	Interrupt **lenalidomide** treatment
Return to ≥50,000/μL	Resume **lenalidomide** at 5 mg daily

If baseline <100,000/μL

When Platelets	Recommended Course
Fall to 50% of the baseline value	Interrupt **lenalidomide** treatment
If baseline ≥60,000/μL and returns to ≥50,000/μL	Resume **lenalidomide** at 5 mg daily
If baseline <60,000/μL and returns ≥30,000/μL	Resume **lenalidomide** at 5 mg daily

If thrombocytopenia develops AFTER 4 weeks of starting treatment at 10 mg daily in MDS

When Platelets	Recommended Course
<30,000/μL or <50,000/μL with platelet transfusions	Interrupt **lenalidomide** treatment
Return to ≥30,000/μL (without hemostatic failure)	Resume **lenalidomide** at 5 mg daily

Patients who experience thrombocytopenia at 5 mg daily should have their dosage adjusted as follows:

If thrombocytopenia develops during treatment at 5 mg daily in MDS

When Platelets	Recommended Course
<30,000/μL or <50,000/μL with platelet transfusions	Interrupt **lenalidomide** treatment
Return to ≥30,000/μL (without hemostatic failure)	Resume **lenalidomide** at 2.5 mg daily

Patients who are dosed initially at 10 mg and experience neutropenia should have their dosage adjusted as follows:

Absolute neutrophil counts (ANC)
If neutropenia develops WITHIN 4 weeks of starting treatment at 10 mg daily in MDS

If baseline ANC ≥1000/μL

When Neutrophils	Recommended Course
Fall to <750/μL	Interrupt **lenalidomide** treatment
Return to ≥1000/μL	Resume **lenalidomide** at 5 mg daily

If baseline ANC <1000/μL

When Neutrophils	Recommended Course
Fall to <500/μL	Interrupt **lenalidomide** treatment
Return to ≥500/μL	Resume **lenalidomide** at 5 mg daily

(continued)

Therapy Monitoring

1. Complete blood counts, leukocyte differential, and platelet count should be performed as needed to monitor response and toxicity; that is, at least once weekly
2. Consider bone marrow biopsy after 8 weeks of treatment
3. Serum liver chemistries and creatinine should be obtained prior to initiation of treatment

Treatment Modifications (*continued*)

If neutropenia develops 4 weeks AFTER starting treatment at 10 mg daily in MDS

When Neutrophils	Recommended Course
<500/μL for ≥7 days or <500/μL associated with fever (≥38.5C)	Interrupt **lenalidomide** treatment
Return to ≥500/μL	Resume **lenalidomide** at 5 mg daily

Patients who experience neutropenia at 5 mg daily should have their dosage adjusted as follows:

If neutropenia develops during treatment at 5 mg daily in MDS

When Neutrophils	Recommended Course
<500/μL for ≥ 7 days or < 500/μL associated with fever (≥38.5C)	Interrupt lenalidomide
Return to ≥500/μL	Resume lenalidomide at 2.5 mg daily

Other Grade 3/4 Toxicities in MDS

For other Grade 3/4 toxicities judged to be related to **lenalidomide**, hold treatment and restart at next lower dose level when toxicity has resolved to ≤ Grade 2

Starting Dose Adjustment for Renal Impairment in Myelodysplastic Syndromes (Days 1–28 of Each 28-Day Cycle)

Category	Renal Function (Cockcroft-Gault)	Dose
Moderate renal impairment	Clcr 30–60 mL/min (0.5–1 mL/s)	5 mg every 24 hours
Severe renal impairment	Clcr <30 mL/min (not requiring dialysis)	2.5 mg every 24 hours
End-stage renal disease	Clcr <30 mL/min (requiring dialysis)	2.5 mg once daily. On dialysis days, administer the dose following dialysis

Efficacy

Frequency of Cytogenetic Response According to Karyotype Complexity

Complexity	Patients Who Could be Evaluated*	Cytogenetic Response	Complete Cytogenetic Remission
Isolated 5q deletion–no. (%)	64	49 (77)	29 (45)
5q deletion + 1 additional abnormality–no. (%)	15	10 (67)	6 (40)
Complex (≥3 abnormalities)–no. (%)	6	3 (50)	3 (50)
P value		0.27	0.93

*Patients who could be evaluated were those with at least 20 analyzable cells in metaphase at baseline and at least 1 follow-up assessment. P values are for the association between karyotypic complexity and cytogenic response or complete cytogenetic remission

Among 148 patients, 99 (67%) no longer needed transfusions by week 24; the remaining 13 patients had a reduction of 50% or greater in the number of transfusions required. The median time to transfusion independence was 4.6 weeks (range: 1–49)

The rate of transfusion independence was significantly lower among patients with baseline thrombocytopenia than among patients with platelet counts >100,000/μL at baseline (39% vs. 73%, p = 0.001)

Toxicity

Grade 3 and 4 Treatment-Related Adverse Events

	Grade 3		Grade 4		Grades 3 and 4
	Continuous Daily Dosing*	21-Day Dosing*	Continuous Daily Dosing*	21-Day Dosing*	Both Schedules
	(N = 102)	(N = 46)	(N = 102)	(N = 46)	(N = 148)
Adverse Event	Number of Patients (%)				
Neutropenia	20 (20)	8 (17)	45 (44)	8 (17)	81 (55)
Thrombocytopenia	37 (36)	14 (30)	7 (7)	7 (15)	65 (44)
Anemia (not otherwise specified)	4 (4)	2 (4)	4 (4)	0	10 (7)
Leukopenia (not otherwise specified)	3 (3)	2 (4)	4 (4)	0	9 (6)
Rash	5 (5)	4 (9)	0	0	9 (6)
Febrile neutropenia	2 (2)	1 (2)	2 (2)	1 (2)	1 (1)
Pruritus	2 (2)	2 (4)	0	0	4 (3)
Fatigue	2 (2)	2 (4)	0	0	4 (3)
Muscle cramp	3 (3)	0	0	0	3 (2)
Pneumonia	1 (1)	2 (4)	1 (1)	0	4 (3)
Nausea	3 (3)	1 (2)	0	0	4 (3)
Diarrhea	4 (4)	0	0	0	4 (3)
Deep vein thrombosis	3 (3)	1 (2)	0	0	4 (3)
Hemorrhage	1 (1)	2 (4)	1 (1)	1 (2)	4 (3)
Hypokalemia	1 (1)	1 (2)	0	0	2 (1)
Pyrexia	1 (1)	0	0	0	1 (1)

*Lenalidomide 10 mg/day

Notes

Lenalidomide is indicated for patients with transfusion-dependent anemia because of low- or intermediate-1–risk myelodysplastic syndromes (MDS) associated with a deletion 5q abnormality with or without additional cytogenetic abnormalities

Lenalidomide may cause fetal harm when administered to a pregnant woman
In a phase III, randomized, double-blind study assessed the efficacy and safety of lenalidomide in 205 red-blood-cell-(RBC)-transfusion-dependent patients with International Prognostic Scoring System low-/intermediate-1–risk del5q31 MDS. Patients received lenalidomide 10 mg/day on days 1–21 (n = 69) or 5 mg/day on days 1–28 (n = 69) of 28-day cycles; or placebo (n = 67). Crossover to lenalidomide or higher dose was allowed after 16 weeks. More patients in the lenalidomide 10- and 5-mg groups achieved RBC-transfusion independence (TI) for ≥26 weeks (primary end point) versus placebo (56.1% and 42.6% vs. 5.9%; both P <0.001)

The median duration of RBC-TI was not reached (median follow-up: 1.55 years), with 60–67% of responses ongoing in patients without progression to acute myeloid leukemia (AML). Cytogenetic response rates were 50% (10 mg) versus 25% (5 mg; P = 0.066)

For the lenalidomide groups combined, 3-year overall survival and AML risk were 56.5% and 25.1%, respectively
RBC-TI for ≥8 weeks was associated with 47% and 42% reductions in the relative risks of death and AML progression or death, respectively (P = 0.021 and 0.048)

Fenaux P et al. Blood 2011;118:3765–3776

REGIMEN

LYMPHOCYTE IMMUNE GLOBULIN, ANTI-THYMOCYTE GLOBULIN [EQUINE] (ATG)

Atgam® (lymphocyte immune globulin, anti-thymocyte globulin, [equine] sterile solution) November 2005 product labeling. Distributed by Pharmacia & Upjohn Co., Division of Pfizer Inc., New York, NY

Molldrem JJ et al. Ann Intern Med 2002;137:156–163

Molldrem JJ et al. Br J Haematol 1997;99:699–705

Sloand EM et al. J Clin Oncol 2008;26:2505–2511

Saunthararajah Y et al. Blood 2003;102:3025–3027

U.S. National Heart, Lung, and Blood Institute intramural clinical trial, 09-H-0183

Premedication:

Acetaminophen 650 mg; administer orally 60 minutes before each antithymocyte globulin treatment, *plus*

Diphenhydramine 25–50 mg; administer orally 60 minutes before each antithymocyte globulin treatment

Prednisone 1 mg/kg per day or 40 mg/day (whichever dose is greater); administer orally starting prior to the first dose of ATG

• The daily prednisone dose is gradually decreased (tapered) starting on day 10 or when signs of serum sickness have resolved, whichever occurs later

• Prednisone dose is tapered with a dose decrement every 2 days over the following 8 days, and then is discontinued

• Patients with serum sickness may require greater prednisone doses to achieve clinical resolution and dose tapering over a longer duration

Lymphocyte immune globulin, anti-thymocyte globulin, [equine] (see Note 1 below) 40 mg/kg per day administered through a high-flow (central) vein, vascular shunt, or arteriovenous fistula in a volume of 0.9% sodium chloride injection (0.9% NS), 5% dextrose and 0.2% sodium chloride injection (D5W/0.2% NS), or 5% dextrose and 0.45% sodium chloride injection (D5W/0.45% NS) sufficient to produce a solution with antithymocyte globulin concentration ≤4 mg/mL, over at least 4 hours for 4 consecutive days, on days 1–4 (total dosage/ course = 160 mg/kg)

Notes:

1. Lymphocyte immune globulin, anti-thymocyte globulin [equine] (ATG) product labeling recommends intradermal skin testing prior to administration. Patients with a reactive skin test may still receive antithymocyte globulin after desensitization

2. Always administer anti-thymocyte globulin through a 0.2–1.0-μm pore size inline filter

3. After dilution, ATG should be allowed to come to room temperature before administration begins

4. The initial infusion rate should be 10% of the total volume per hour. For example, for a total volume of 500 mL, start at a rate of 50 mL/ hour for the first 30 minutes. If there are no signs of an adverse reaction, the infusion rate can be advanced to complete the infusion over no less than 4 hours

Cyclosporine orally every 12 hours, continually, starting on day 14

Patients ≥12 years of age: **Cyclosporine** 3 mg/kg per dose; administer orally every 12 hours (total daily dose = 6 mg/kg)

• Dosing is based on actual body weight (ABW) except in obese patients (defined as a body mass index >35 kg/m² in patients >20 years of age and >95th percentile for ages 12–20 years

• For obese patients, cyclosporine dosage is based on an *adjusted body weight* that is calculated as the midpoint between the ideal body weight (IBW) and ABW, thus:

$$\text{Adjusted Body Weight} = \text{IBW} + (\text{ABW} - \text{IBW})/2$$

• Cyclosporine is continued for 6 months, after which:

▪ In responding patients, the dose is gradually decreased by 5% per week, and then is discontinued

▪ In nonresponding patients, cyclosporine is discontinued

• Cyclosporine doses are adjusted for increases in serum creatinine and to maintain serum cyclosporine concentrations within the range of 200–400 mcg/L (166–333 nmol/L) by radioimmunoassay

Notes:

▪ Avoid other nephrotoxic drugs concurrent with cyclosporine treatment

▪ Granulocyte-colony stimulating factors (G-CSF) should be administered as clinically indicated, usually for evidence of infection such as fever or localized inflammation in the setting of severe inflammation. Emergence of monosomy 7 has been linked to exogenous use of G-CSF

Allergy skin testing prior to ATG administration:

1. Anti-thymocyte globulin (equine) is freshly diluted (1:1000) with 0.9% sodium chloride injection (0.9% NS), to a concentration of 5 mcg/0.1 mL, and administered intradermally

2. Administer 0.1 mL 0.9% NS, intradermally in a contralateral extremity as a control

3. Observe every 15–20 minutes during the first hour after intradermal injection

   a. A local reaction ≥10 mm with a wheal, erythema, or both, ± pseudopod formation and itching or a marked local swelling is considered a positive test. For patients who exhibit a positive test result, consider desensitization prior to therapy

Notes:

▪ Advise patients to avoid using H_1-receptor antagonists for 72 hours before skin testing

▪ The predictive value of skin testing has not been proved clinically; that is, allergic reactions including anaphylaxis have occurred in patients whose skin test result is negative

(continued)

(continued)

- If antithymocyte globulin is administered after a locally positive skin test, administration should only be attempted in a setting where intensive life-support facilities are immediately available and with the attendance of a physician familiar with the treatment of potentially life-threatening allergic reactions
- Systemic reactions preclude antithymocyte globulin administration; for example, generalized rash, tachycardia, dyspnea, hypotension, or anaphylaxis

Guidelines for administering antithymocyte globulin (ATG):
- Severity and frequency of toxicities (rigors, fevers, oxygen desaturation, hypotension, nausea, vomiting, anaphylaxis) are greatest during the first day of infusion and diminish with each subsequent day. Toxicities generally subside after completing treatment
- Adverse effects generally can be managed while continuing antithymocyte globulin infusion
- Most patients receiving ATG will develop fever. Most fevers are not infectious in origin

Monitoring during ATG administration:
- Patients should remain under continual surveillance
- Assess peripheral vascular access sites for thrombophlebitis every 8 hours
- Monitor vital signs and assess for adverse reactions (flushing, hives, itching, SOB, difficulty breathing, chest tightness) before starting administration, *then:*
  - *During initial dose:* Continually during the first 15 minutes, then every 30 minutes × 2, then at least every hour until administration is completed
  - *During subsequent doses:* 30 minutes after initiating ATG infusion

Supportive Care
Antimicrobial prophylaxis
Risk of fever and neutropenia is HIGH
  Antimicrobial primary prophylaxis is recommended:
  - Antibacterial—*P. jirovecii* prophylaxis is recommended (eg, cotrimoxazole or aerosolized pentamidine)
    - Begin during the first month of therapy, and continue throughout the duration of cyclosporine use
  - Antifungal—recommended
  - Antiviral—antiherpes antivirals (eg, acyclovir, famciclovir, valacyclovir)
See Chapter 47 for more information

Toxicity

Twelve patients required temporary admission to an intensive care unit during ATG treatment. Six patients did not complete 4 planned days of ATG treatment: 3 developed shaking chills, 2 experienced hypotension associated with shaking chills, and 1 died from alveolar hemorrhage associated with leukemic pulmonary infiltrates. One patient died shortly after receiving ATG from alveolar hemorrhage

Infusional toxicities of antithymocyte globulin:
- Severity and frequency of toxicities are greatest during the first day of ATG administration and diminish with each subsequent day. Toxicities generally subside after completing treatment

Adverse Events	Interventions
Rigors	Antihistamines (eg, diphenhydramine 25–50 mg, intravenously or orally every 6 hours as needed) Meperidine 12.5–50 mg, intravenously may be repeated every 10 minutes
Nausea, vomiting	Antiemetic rescue. Then give antiemetic prophylaxis during subsequent antithymocyte globulin treatments (secondary prophylaxis)
Anaphylaxis*	Immediately STOP administration; administer steroids; assist respiration; and provide other resuscitative measures. DO NOT resume treatment
Thrombocytopenia, anemia	Blood product transfusions as needed[†]
Fever and neutropenia[‡]	Broad-spectrum antibiotics empirically, if ANC <500/mm³. May give acetaminophen 650 mg orally every 4 hours
Hypotension	Fluid resuscitation
Refractory hypotension	May indicate anaphylaxis. Stop antithymocyte globulin administration and stabilize blood pressure. Intensive Care Unit support

Patient Population Studied

Sixteen patients had low IPSS risk, 94 patients intermediate-1 (int-1) IPSS, 13 patients int-2 IPSS, and 6 patients high risk IPSS. Seventy-four patients received equine ATG, 42 patients received a combination of ATG and cyclosporine (maintaining cyclosporine levels >100 mcg/L [>83 nmol/L] for up to 6 months), and 13 patients received cyclosporine alone on the same schedule

(continued)

Toxicity (*continued*)

Adverse Events	Interventions
Oxygen desaturation	Oxygen therapy
Refractory oxygen desaturation	Discontinue antithymocyte globulin. Intensive Care Unit support
Respiratory distress	Discontinue antithymocyte globulin. If distress persists, administer an antihistamine, epinephrine, steroids
Rash, pruritus, urticaria	Administer antihistamines and/or topical steroids for prophylaxis and treatment
Serum sickness-like symptoms§	Administer prophylactic glucocorticoids
Hepatotoxicity∈	Monitor LFTs

*Anaphylaxis (<3% of patients) more frequently occurs within the first hour after starting antithymocyte globulin infusion. After the first hour, adverse effects occur as result of a delayed immune response and generally can be managed while continuing the antithymocyte globulin infusion
†Concurrent administration of blood products should be avoided with antithymocyte globulin infusions to avoid confusing transfusion reactions with reactions to antithymocyte globulin
‡Most patients who receive antithymocyte globulin will develop fever as a result of the drug. Most fevers are not infectious in origin
§Type II hypersensitivity reactions/serum sickness consisting of fever, rash, and arthralgia develops in approximately 85% of patients between 7 and 14 days after ATG treatment. These symptoms can be managed with steroids
∈An isolated increase in serum alanine aminotransferase (ALT) frequently has no clinical significance. Generally, liver function abnormalities are transient and return to normal within 1 month

Bevans MF, Shalabi RA. Clin J Oncol Nurs 2004;8:377–382

Efficacy

Eighteen (24%) of 74 patients (95% CI, 14–34%) responded to ATG, 20 (45%) of 42 patients (95% CI, 32–63%) responded to ATG plus cyclosporine ($P = 0.01$), and 1 (8%) of 13 patients responded to cyclosporine. Thirty-one percent (12 of 39 patients; 95% CI, 16–46%) of the responses were complete, resulting in near-normal blood counts and transfusion independence; 32 (82%) of 39 (95% CI, 70–94%) of the responders achieved either bi-lineage or tri-lineage responses. Of the partial responders, all but 1 became transfusion independent

In multivariate analysis, young age was the most significant factor favoring response to therapy. Other favorable factors affecting response were HLA-DR15 positivity and combination ATG plus cyclosporine treatment ($P = 0.001$ and $P = 0.048$, respectively). Patients were seen at yearly follow-up from the start of IST. Seventy patients survive with a median follow-up of 3 years. Patients treated with ATG plus cyclosporine had superior response rates compared with patients treated with ATG alone, although there were no survival differences between these groups

Therapy Monitoring

1. *During antithymocyte globulin infusion:* CBC with differential, LFTs, electrolytes
2. *After antithymocyte globulin therapy:* CBC monitoring is dependent on blood counts. If WBC, ANC, and platelet counts are stable, a CBC with differential may be as infrequent as once every 2–3 weeks. Patients who require platelets may need more frequent CBCs, but not more than twice weekly and usually only once weekly
3. *Six months after the start of therapy:* Bone marrow biopsy and aspiration. If patients are stable based on blood counts, bone marrow biopsy may not need to be repeated

Therapeutic drug monitoring for cyclosporine:

- When initiating cyclosporine treatment and after any dose adjustments, monitor cyclosporine trough concentrations (sampled at the end of a dosing interval) every 4–7 days until stable concentrations are achieved
- For patients on a stable cyclosporine regimen, monitor trough levels every 2 weeks
- More frequent cyclosporine monitoring is recommended whenever cyclosporine dosage adjustments are made, serum creatinine increases, and when a patient's concomitantly administered medication regimen is changed (be wary of drugs that potentially perturb cytochrome P450 CYP3A subfamily enzymes expression, availability, or activity)
- Cyclosporine doses are adjusted to maintain blood concentrations with the range of 200–400 mcg/L (166–333 nmol/L) by radioimmunoassay

REGIMEN
ALEMTUZUMAB

Sloand EM et al. J Clin Oncol 2010;28:5166–5173

Premedication given before all alemtuzumab doses including test doses:
Diphenhydramine 25–50 mg orally or intravenously 30 minutes prior to alemtuzumab injection, *and*
Acetaminophen 650 mg; orally 30 minutes before alemtuzumab

Test dose: **Alemtuzumab** 1 mg intravenously in 100 mL 0.9% sodium chloride injection (0.9% NS) or 5% dextrose injection (D5W) over 1 hour on the day before the first full (10-mg) dose of alemtuzumab is administered

Treatment: If a test dose was tolerated, give **alemtuzumab** 10 mg/day intravenously in 100 mL 0.9% NS or D5W over 2 hours for 10 consecutive days, on days 1–10 (total dose/10-day course, including a test dose = 101 mg)

Supportive Care
Antiemetic prophylaxis
Emetogenic potential is **MINIMAL**
See Chapter 39 for antiemetic recommendations

Hematopoietic growth factor (CSF) prophylaxis
Primary prophylaxis may be indicated
- *Note:* In the study by Sloand et al, the use of erythropoietin-stimulating agents and/or granulocyte colony-stimulating factor (G-CSF) to treat severe anemia and/or neutropenia was permitted, but hematologic responses were ascertained after 4 weeks of withholding erythropoietin-stimulating agents and/or G-CSF

See Chapter 43 for more information

Antimicrobial prophylaxis
Risk of fever and neutropenia is HIGH
Antimicrobial primary prophylaxis is recommended:
- Antibacteria—**Pentamidine** 300 mg; administer aerosolized pentamidine by inhalation every 4 weeks beginning the first month of alemtuzumab therapy, and continue for at least 6 months. If at 6 months CD4+ cells are <200/μL, continue *Pneumocystis jirovecii* prophylaxis until CD4+ cells >200/μL
- **Ciprofloxacin** 500 mg orally twice daily until ANC >500/μL
- Antiviral—**Valacyclovir** 500 mg orally once daily for at least 2 months regardless of HSV serology status. If at 2 months CD4+ cells are <200/μL, continue antiviral prophylaxis until CD4+ cells ≥200/μL

See Chapter 47 for more information

Patient Population Studied

Study of 31 evaluable patients (median age: 57 years) with de novo MDS without known preceding aplastic anemia or prior chemotherapy. According to IPSS, 2 patients were classified as low risk, 22 patients were classified as intermediate-1 (Int-1) risk, and 7 patients were classified as intermediate-2 (Int-2) risk

For study entry, 1 or more of the following criteria were necessary: transfusion dependence (≥2 units RBCs or ≥5 units of platelets per month for 8 weeks before enrollment), thrombocytopenia (platelet count ≤50,000/μL), neutropenia (neutrophil count ≤500/μL), and anemia (hemoglobin <9 g/dL or absolute reticulocyte count of <60,000 cells/μL) based on the mean of 3 blood counts within 2 weeks before enrollment. HLA-DR1—negative patients in whom the sum of the age plus months of RBC transfusion dependence was <58 and HLA-DR15-positive patients in whom the sum of the age plus months of RBC transfusion dependence was <72 were eligible for the study

Treatment Modification

Withhold alemtuzumab during serious infection or other serious adverse reaction until resolution

Toxicity (N = 31)

SAE	No. of Patients	No. of Days to SAE
Infection		
Bacterial pneumonia	1	45
Cellulitis	1	428
Clostridium difficile diarrhea	2	78,123
Neutropenia and fever	3	7,31,329
Fever without neutropenia	2	35,162
Shingles	1	381
Sinusitis	1	173
URI symptoms	1	55
Infusion reaction		
Hypotension	1	1
Hematologic		
Autoimmune thrombocytopenia	1	84
Dermatologic		
Molluscum contagiosum skin lesion	1	217

SAE, severe adverse event; URI, upper respiratory tract infection

Nonhematologic AEs	No. of Patients		
	G2	G3	G4
Cardiovascular			
Hypertension		1	
Constitutional			
Asthenia	2		
Fatigue	1		
Stiffness	1		
Dermatology/skin			
Facial flushing	1		
Pruritus	1		
Rash	2		
Urticaria	3		

(continued)

Efficacy

Twenty-one patients (68%) achieved either hematologic improvement in 1 or more lineages or a CR

Seventeen (77%) of 22 evaluable patients with Int-1 MDS and 4 (57%) of 7 patients with Int-2 MDS responded to treatment
Median time to response was 3 months. Among the responders, 2 (11%) of 18 patients had a CR at 3 months, 3 (18%) of 17 evaluable responders had a CR at 6 months, and 5 (56%) of 9 evaluable responders had a CR at 12 months

Of the 25 patients who were RBC transfusion dependent before treatment, 10 (40%) achieved transfusion independence by 3 months. Seven (78%) of 9 of responders evaluable at 1 year were transfusion independent

Thirteen (65%) of 20 neutropenic patients had hematologic improvement or complete neutrophil response and 9 (38%) of 24 thrombocytopenic patients had a platelet response

Four of 7 responding patients with abnormal karyotype before treatment had cytogenetic CRs by 1 year

Therapy Monitoring

On treatment monitoring: CBC with differential (daily) and renal, hepatic function every other day

Post treatment monitoring: Complete blood counts with differential, renal, hepatic function should be evaluated as needed to monitor response and toxicity; ie, at least once weekly
Bone marrow biopsy and aspiration at 6 months post-treatment

EBV and CMV monitoring: EBV and CMV PCR in the blood prior to treatment, repeated weekly for the first month, then every other week in the second month, monthly for another 6 months, and at 12 months. In case of a positive PCR for CMV, treatment will be instituted when clinical symptoms are attributed to CMV. EBV positivity by PCR will also be placed in context of clinical signs and symptoms

Notes

Patients who experienced relapse 3 months after an initial response to alemtuzumab were eligible to receive cyclosporine, unless otherwise contraindicated: cyclosporine 5 mg/kg per dose orally every 12 hours, continually (total dosage/day = 10 mg/kg). No-responders were removed from study at 6 months

Toxicity (N = 31) *(continued)*

Nonhematologic AEs	No. of Patients		
	G2	G3	G4
GI			
Diarrhea		1	
Nausea	1		
Infusion reaction	23		
Infection/febrile neutropenia			
Orchitis	1		
Pilonidal cyst	1		
Upper respiratory tract	9		
Mycobacterium chelonae	1		
Lymphatic			
Hand swelling	1		
Metabolic			
Decreased phosphate		1	
Elevated AST, ALT		7	1
Elevated LDH		1	
Elevated creatinine		1	
Neurologic			
Dizziness	1		
Pain			
Headache	2		
Muscle cramps	3		
Neuropathic	1		
Renal/genitourinary			
Darkened urine	1		

AE, adverse even; LDH, lactate dehydrogenase; URI, upper respiratory tract infection

Twenty-four patients had infusion reactions of rigors, malaise, and elevated transaminases, and 1 patient developed hypotension after the first alemtuzumab dose. Infusion reactions were seen most frequently with the initial test dose, but became attenuated with successive infusions

Among 31 evaluable patients, all were seropositive for EBV, and 22 (71%) were seropositive for CMV. Of the EBV patients, 15 experienced reactivation of EBV. Of the CMV-seropositive patients, 5 (23%) experienced CMV reactivation. All reactivations were subclinical and self-limited; no patient developed EBV- or CMV-related disease or required pre-emptive antiviral therapy

Index

Toxicity

Rates and Relative Risks of Bleeding Episodes in the Two Groups*

Type of Bleeding Episode	Aspirin (N = 253)	Placebo (N = 265)	Relative Risk (95% CI)	P Value
	Number (%)			
Any bleeding	23 (9.1)	14 (5.3)	1.82 (0.94–3.53)	0.08
Major bleeding	3 (1.2)	2 (0.8)	1.62 (0.27–9.71)	0.60
Gastrointestinal	2 (0.8)	0		
Intracranial	1 (0.4)	2 (0.8)		
Minor bleeding	20 (7.9)	12 (4.5)	1.83 (0.90–3.75)	0.10
Hematoma	2 (0.8)	2 (0.8)		
Gastrointestinal	7 (2.8)	3 (1.1)		
Hematuria	1 (0.4)	3 (1.1)		
Epistaxis	9 (3.6)	1 (0.4)		
Other	2 (0.8)	4 (1.5)		

CI, confidence interval
*Major bleeding was defined as any bleeding episode that was fatal or necessitated transfusions or hospitalization. Totals for categories may not equal the sum of the values for subcategories because some patients had more than one type of bleeding episode

Study Conclusion

The authors noted the moderate increase in the risk of bleeding episodes associated with the long-term use of aspirin in polycythemia vera. The relative risk of major bleeding complications of 1.62 was felt to be consistent with estimates from 5 primary prevention trials involving subjects who did not have polycythemia, although the occurrence of a limited number of events precluded the precise estimation of the risk of bleeding. The authors concluded they believed that the risk of aspirin-induced bleeding in patients with PV has been overemphasized and recommended the use of aspirin to prevent thrombotic complications in patients with polycythemia vera who have no contraindication to this treatment

Notes:

- **Low-dose aspirin** 50–100 mg/day orally, continually, is beneficial in reducing arterial thrombosis in patients with PV and ET
- Microcirculatory disturbances, particularly erythromelalgia, are alleviated by aspirin. However, the use of aspirin in PV and ET requires the absence of clinically relevant acquired von Willebrand syndrome (AvWS), which might occur in patients with extreme thrombocytosis (platelet count >1,000,000/mm³). Use a ristocetin cofactor activity cutoff level of 30% to decide on aspirin therapy
- Aspirin significantly lowered the combined risk of cardiovascular death, nonfatal myocardial infarction, nonfatal stroke, pulmonary embolism, or major venous thrombosis (relative risk 0.40; 95% CI, 0.18–0.91)
- The study was insufficiently powered to detect significant differences between aspirin and placebo in the rates of any bleeding